# FIFTH EDITION
# Outdoor Emergency Care

Editor
**EDWARD C. MCNAMARA, BS, NREMT-P**

Medical Editor
**DAVID H. JOHE, MD**

Associate Editor
**DEBORAH A. ENDLY, BA, DH, NREMT-B**

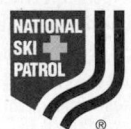

Brady
is an imprint of
Pearson

Boston  Columbus  Indianapolis  New York  San Francisco  Upper Saddle River  Amsterdam  Cape Town  Dubai  London  Madrid  Milan
Munich  Paris  Montréal  Toronto  Delhi  Mexico City  São Paulo  Sydney  Hong Kong  Seoul  Singapore  Taipei  Tokyo

Library of Congress Cataloging-in-Publication Data

Outdoor emergency care / National Ski Patrol ; edited by Edward C.
McNamara, David H. Johe, Deborah A. Endly.—5th edition.
   p. ; cm.
   Includes bibliographical references.
   ISBN-13: 978-0-13-507480-0
   ISBN-10: 0-13-507480-0
   1. Outdoor medical emergencies. I. McNamara, Edward C. II. Johe,
David H., 1952-  III. Endly, Deborah A. IV. Bowman, Warren D. Outdoor
emergency care. V. National Ski Patrol (U.S.), author.
   [DNLM: 1. Emergency Treatment—methods. 2. Critical Care—methods.
3. Emergencies. 4. Rural Health Services. WA 292]
   RC88.9.O95O93 2011
   616.02'52—dc22

                                               2010044467


Publisher: Julie Levin Alexander
Publisher's Assistant: Regina Bruno
Editor-in-Chief: Marlene McHugh Pratt
Medical Editor: Edward T. Dickinson, MD, FACEP
Senior Managing Editor for Development: Lois Berlowitz
Project Manager: Susan Simpfenderfer
Editorial Assistant: Jonathan Cheung
Director of Marketing: David Gesell
Executive Marketing Manager: Katrin Beacom
Marketing Manager: Brian Hoehl
Marketing Specialist: Michael Sirinides
Managing Editor for Production: Patrick Walsh
Production Liaison: Yagnesh Jani/Faye Gemmellaro
Production Editor: Heather Willison, S4Carlisle Publishing Services
Manufacturing Manager: Alan Fischer
Cover and Interior Design: Kathryn Foot
Front Cover Images: Man with goggles © Marco Matteucci/ Alamy; photo
   inside goggles: Edward McNamara, NSP
Back Cover Images: Hikers: © Blend Images/Alamy; Family canoeing: ©
   Image Source/Alamy; Cyclists: © imagebroker/Alamy; Equestrian:
   Edward McNamara, NSP
Historical Timeline Photos: Courtesy of NSP
Editorial Media Manager: Amy Peltier
Media Project Manager: Lorena Cerisano
Composition: S4Carlisle Publishing Services
Printer/Binder: LSC Communications
Cover Printer: Lehigh-Phoenix Color

---

Pearson® is a registered trademark of Pearson plc.

## DISCLAIMER

The National Ski Patrol is the premier provider of training and education
programs for emergency rescuers who serve the outdoor recreation community. The National Ski Patrol recognizes that rendering first aid in the
outdoors and on ski slopes creates a unique environment that presents
many factors for outdoor emergency care providers to consider. Therefore, nothing in *Outdoor Emergency Care* is intended to replace the good
judgment of outdoor emergency care providers in providing proper first-
aid care and managing an accident situation.

   This edition of *Outdoor Emergency Care* also sets forth accepted techniques that have been applied throughout the United States in providing
first aid in outdoor environments, although the techniques, suggestions,
and ideas contained in this manual are not intended to replace actual experience and training and cannot be considered absolute recommendations. Moreover, the National Ski Patrol recognizes that every state has
been evolving their own laws and regulations associated with rendering
first aid and providing emergency medical assistance. Consistent with the
National Ski Patrol's Joint Statement of Understanding with the National
Ski Areas Association, the National Ski Patrol is not responsible for the
day-to-day activities of its patrollers or for those who render outdoor
emergency care pursuant to those first-aid techniques set forth in this
manual. It is the responsibility of individual outdoor emergency care
providers, and the areas where they provide first-aid care (whether it be a
ski area or otherwise), to ensure that they comply with their individual
state's laws and regulations, as well as any other local or other applicable
regulations and guidelines, regarding first aid and outdoor emergency care
medical procedures. The reader should also note that the development of
new regulations, guidelines, and practices may require changes in some
techniques, suggestions, and ideas contained in this material.

   Although the information contained in this manual is believed to be reliable and correct at the time of original publication, neither the publisher
nor the authors make any warranty, expressed or implied, with respect to
the use of any techniques, suggestions, and ideas disclosed in this manual.
The publisher and authors disclaim any and all liability for any damages of
any kind or character, including without limitation any compensatory, in-
cidental, direct or indirect, special, punitive, or consequential damages,
loss of income or profit, loss of or damage to property or person, claims of
third parties, or other losses of any kind or character arising out of or in
connection with the use of this book or the accuracy of the information
contained herein, even if the publisher or authors have been advised of the
possibility of such damages or losses.

5  17

V011

                ISBN-10 0-13-507480-0
                ISBN-13 978-0-13-507480-0

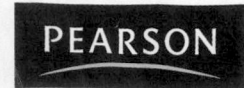

**Brady**
is an imprint of

**PEARSON**          www.bradybooks.com

# Dedication

This book is dedicated to members of the National Ski Patrol System, and specifically to patrollers past, present, and future. Patrollers spend countless hours in often-dismal weather conditions and on difficult terrain—performing rescue missions, checking trails, and conducting avalanche control to ensure the safety of those who relish the opportunity to recreate in outdoor environments. The keystone of our organization, the Patroller, provides outdoor enthusiasts a safety net so they can feel free to enjoy recreational activities during the winter and all other seasons of the year. Patrollers dedicate innumerable hours to training and becoming proficient in skills such as skiing, toboggan handling, outdoor emergency care, mountain travel and rescue, avalanche control, and lift evacuation, among others. But it's not all work. Patrollers also enjoy the early morning "fresh tracks" and the camaraderie that comes from being a member of a world-renowned rescue organization.

The 5th Edition OEC team would like to recognize and dedicate this edition of *Outdoor Emergency Care* to:

Patrollers: Past, Present, and Future.

We celebrate your enthusiasm and commitment.

Editor

Medical Editor

# CONTENTS

Letter to Students  xiii

Preface  xiv

Acknowledgments  xvi

About the Editors  xxiv


**Section 1**
**PREPARING TO BE AN OEC TECHNICIAN**  1

## Introduction to Outdoor Emergency Care  1

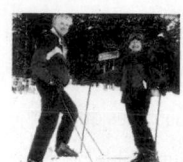

**National Ski Patrol's Early Years**  4
The National Ski Patrol Goes to War  4 • The Birth of OEC  6

**OEC Today**  7
Training: The Focus of the OEC Program  8 • Certification and Recertification Requirements  11 • Working in Outdoor Environments  12

**Ethical and Legal Issues**  13
Ethical Issues Facing OEC Technicians  15 • Good Samaritan Laws and Duty to Act  15 • Abandonment  17 • Negligence and Breach of Duty  18 • Assumption of Risk  18 • Preparing Documentation  19 • Scope of Training  20 • Standard of Training versus Standard of Care  20 • Joint Statement of Understanding  21 • Patient's Consent  21 • Refusal  23 • Assault and Battery  23 • Judgment  24 • Training  24 • EMS System Regulations  25 • Privacy Laws  25 • Teamwork  25

## Emergency Care Systems  31

**The History of Emergency Care**  33
EMS Agenda for the Future  35

**Levels of Emergency Personnel**  38
Emergency Medical Responder  39 • Emergency Medical Technician  39 • Advanced Emergency Medical Technician  39 • Paramedic  40 • Other EMS Personnel  40

**Emergency Facilities**  40

**Continuity of Care**  41

**The Importance of Commonality in Emergency Care Systems**  42

**The Relationship of Emergency Care Systems to Public Health**  43

**The Role of Research in Emergency Care Systems**  45

**Communication Systems in Emergency Care Systems**  46
Radio Etiquette  47 • Radio Terminology  48 • NATO Phonetic Alphabet  48 • Military Time  48

**Medical Oversight in Emergency Care Systems**  49

**Emergency Care Protocols**  50

**The Importance of Documentation in Emergency Care**  50

**Quality Improvement in Emergency Care Systems**  50

**Continuing Education in Emergency Care**  51

## Rescue Basics  56

**Anatomy and Physiology**  58
Temperature Regulation  58 • The "Fight or Flight" Response  61 • The Immune Response  62

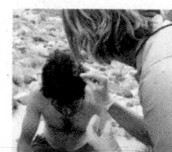

**Preparing to Work Outdoors**  63
Environmental Considerations  63 • Mental Preparedness  63 • Physical Fitness  64 • Proper Equipment  65 • Hydration  70 • Prolonged Rescue Response Preparation  71

**Protecting Yourself from Disease**  71
Contamination  73 • Common Infectious Diseases  74 • Personal Protective Equipment  77 • Decontamination  80

**Assessing Emergency Situations**  82
Scene Safety  82 • Mechanism of Injury  84 • Number of Patients and Need for Additional Resources  85

**Dealing with Hazardous Materials**  85

**Crime Scene Management**  87
Relations with the Media  88

**Dealing with Stress**  89

# Incident Command and Triage 98

### The National Incident Management System 99

### Incident Command System 101
Incident Command 104 • Operations Section 105 • Planning Section 106 • Logistics Section 107 • Finance/Administration Section 109

### ICS and the OEC Technician 110

### Triage 114
Triage Tags 118 • Triage Methods 119

# Moving, Lifting, and Transporting Patients 126

### The Body Mechanics of Lifting 128

### Devices and Equipment 131
Transfer Flat 131 • Long Spine Board 131 • Orthopedic Stretcher 132 • Portable Stretcher 133 • Basket Stretcher 134 • Short Spine Board and Vest-Type Lifting/Immobilization Devices 134 • Sitting Lifting Device 135

### Moving a Patient 135
Urgent Moves 136 • Nonurgent Moves 138 • Special Moving Situations 141

### Lifting the Patient 141
Power Grip 142 • Power Lift 142 • Other Types of Lifts 143

### Transporting Patients 146
Ground Transport 146 • Motorized Transport Vehicles 153 • Air Transportation 154 • Special Transport Tactics 157

### CPR during Transport 157
Sled CPR Method 158 • Leap Frog CPR Method 158

## Section 2
## THE BASICS OF PATIENT CARE 167

# Anatomy and Physiology 167

### Anatomy and Physiology 168
Terms for Planes and Directional Terms 168 • Terms for Movements 170 • Terms of Position 170

### Body Cavities 171

### Body Systems 174
The Respiratory System 174 • The Cardiovascular System 176 • The Nervous System 183 • The Gastrointestinal System 187 • The Urinary System 191 • The Endocrine System 191 • The Integumentary System 195 • The Skeletal System 195 • The Muscular System 199 • The Reproductive System 201 • The Lymphatic System 206

### Homeostasis 206

# Patient Assessment 213

### Scene Size-Up 215
General Impression 216 • Chief Complaint 216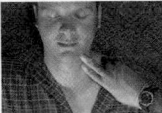

### Patient Assessment 217
The Primary Assessment 217 • The Secondary Assessment 226 • Special Assessment Considerations 244 • Reassessment 246

# Medical Communications and Documentation 264

### Communication Basics 267

### Forms of Communication 267

### Medical Communications 268
Oral Communication 268 • Written Communication 271 • Essential Content of Medical Communications 282

## Section 3
## CRITICAL INTERVENTIONS 291

# Airway Management 291

### Anatomy and Physiology 292

### Airway Management 294
Opening the Airway and Mouth 295 • Clearing the Airway 297 • Keeping the Airway Open and Clear 300

### Oxygen Therapy 306
Oxygen Containers 306 • Oxygen Cylinder Set-Up and Breakdown 307 • Oxygen Flow Duration Rates 308 • Oxygen Safety 309 • Indications for Oxygen Therapy 310 • Oxygen Delivery/Ventilation Adjuncts 311 • Pulse Oximetry 315 • Gastric Distention 315

## Shock  329

### Anatomy and Physiology  331
The Heart  332  •  Blood Vessels  332  •
Blood  332  •  Physiologic Compensation and the Stages
of Shock  335

### Types of Shock  336
Hypovolemic Shock  336  •  Cardiogenic Shock  339
•  Distributive Shock  339  •  Obstructive Shock  342

### Factors Affecting Shock  344

### Assessment  345

### Management  347

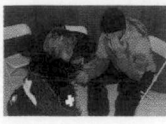

### Section 4
### MEDICAL EMERGENCIES  355

## Altered Mental Status  355

### Anatomy and Physiology  356

### Altered Mental Status  359
Causes of Altered Mental Status  359  •  Conditions
Associated with Altered Mental Status  363  •  Patient
Assessment  372  •  Patient Management  377

### Violent Behavior and Altered Mental Status  381

## Substance Abuse and Poisoning  386

### Anatomy and Physiology  387
Physiologic Actions  387  •  Body Systems Affected
by Substance Exposure  389

### Commonly Abused Substances and Poison-Related Emergencies  390
Commonly Encountered Substances  393

### Assessment  396

### Management  398
Reduce Further Exposure  398  •  Reduce
Absorption  399  •  Specific Interventions  400  •  Help
Is Only a Phone Call Away  401

## Respiratory Emergencies  406

### Anatomy and Physiology  408
Lower Airway  410  •  Normal Breathing  412

### Common Respiratory Emergencies  412
Obstruction/Choking  413  •  Chronic Obstructive
Pulmonary Disease  413  •  Asthma  414  •
Hyperventilation Syndrome  414  •  Pulmonary
Embolism  415  •  Spontaneous Pneumothorax  416  •
Other Respiratory System-Related Conditions  416

### Assessment  418

### Management  424

### The Use of Inhalers  424

## Allergies and Anaphylaxis  434

### Anatomy and Physiology  435

### Common Causes of Allergies and Anaphylaxis  438
Mild Allergic Reactions  439  •  Moderate Allergic
Reactions  440  •  Severe Allergic Reactions  440  •
Prevention  440

### Assessment  443
Mild Allergic Reaction  444  •  Moderate Allergic
Reaction  444  •  Severe Allergic Reaction  444  •
Anaphylactic Shock  445

### Management  446
Severe Allergic Reactions  446

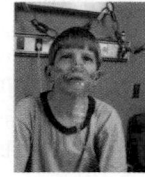

## Cardiovascular Emergencies  457

### Anatomy and Physiology  459
The Heart  459  •  Blood Vessels  460  •  Blood  462

### Cardiovascular Emergencies  464
Atherosclerosis  464  •  Hypertension  465  •
Congestive Heart Failure  465  •  Pulmonary
Edema  466  •  Angina Pectoris  466  •  Myocardial
Infarction  466  •  Cardiac Arrhythmias  467  •
Cardiogenic Shock  468  •  Sudden Cardiac
Arrest  468  •  Thromboembolism  468  •  Pericarditis
and Pericardial Tamponade  469  •  Aortic Aneurysm/
Aortic Dissection  469  •  Heart Valve Disorders  470  •
Concurrent Cardiovascular Diseases  470

### Assessment  472
Hypertension  474  •  Angina and Myocardial
Infarction  474  •  Cardiogenic Shock  474  •
Congestive Heart Failure  475  •  Pericardial
Tamponade  475  •  Aortic Aneurysm/Dissection  475  •
Thromboembolism  476

**Management** 476
Care for Patients in Cardiac Arrest  476  •  Hospital Care of MI Patients  484  •  Cardiovascular Patients Who Are Not in Cardiac Arrest  485

 **Gastrointestinal and Genitourinary Emergencies** 494

**GI/GU Anatomy & Physiology** 495

**The Acute Abdomen** 499
Causes of Acute Abdomen  500

**Common Gastrointestinal Ailments** 505
Gastroenteritis  505  •  Indigestion  505  •  Nausea and Vomiting  505  •  Colic  506  •  Diarrhea and Bloody Stool  506  •  Viruses, Protozoa, and Bacteria  506  •  Constipation  506

**Assessment** 508
ABCDs  508  •  Physical Exam  509

**Management** 510

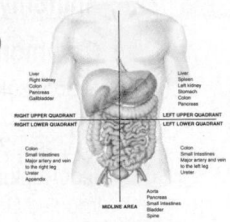

**Section 5
TRAUMA** 516

 **Principles of Trauma** 516

**Kinematics** 517

**Pathophysiology and Mechanisms of Injury** 521
Blunt Injury  522  •  Penetrating Injury  522  •  Rotational Injury  522  •  Crush Injury  523  •  Blast Injury  523

**The Three Phases of Injury** 525
Pre-Injury Phase  525  •  Injury Phase  525  •  Post-Injury Phase  526

**Trauma Systems** 526
Level I  527  •  Level II  527  •  Level III  527  •  Levels IV and V  528  •  Pediatric Trauma  528

**Assessment** 530

**Management** 532

 **Soft-Tissue Injuries** 537

**Anatomy and Physiology of Skin** 539
Skin Anatomy  539  •  Physiology of Bleeding and Clotting  540

**Types of Soft-Tissue Injuries** 542
Closed Injuries  542  •  Open Injuries  545  •  Burns  549

**Assessment** 551

**Management** 552
Direct Pressure  553  •  Dressings  553  •  Tourniquet  553  •  Treatment for Specific Soft-Tissue Injuries  555  •  Dressing and Bandaging  558

 **Burns** 579

**Anatomy and Physiology** 580

**Types of Burns** 581
Thermal Burns  581  •  Chemical Burns  582  •  Electrical Burns  583  •  Radiation Burns  584

**The Classification of Burns** 585
Superficial Burns  585  •  Partial-Thickness Burns  586  •  Full-Thickness Burns  586

**Assessment** 588

**Management** 591

**Thermal Burns** 593
Chemical Burns  593  •  Electrical Burns  594  •  Radiation Burns  595

**Further Care and Transport** 595

 **Musculoskeletal Injuries** 601

**Anatomy and Physiology** 602
The Skeleton  603  •  Joints  606  •  Ligaments  607  •  Muscle  608  •  Tendons  609

**The Physiology of Movement** 609
The Healing Process  610

**Common Musculoskeletal Injuries** 612
Sprains  612  •  Strains  612  •  Ruptured Tendons  613  •  Fractures  613  •  Dislocations  615  •  Multiple Simultaneous MS Injuries  616

**Assessment** 617
Signs and Symptoms of Common MS Injuries  620  •  Assessment of Upper Extremity Injuries  622

**Assessment of Lower Extremity Injuries** 630
Hip and Pelvis Injuries  630  •  Femur Fractures  631  •  Knee Injuries  632  •  Tibia and Fibula Injuries  634  •  Ankle Injuries  635  •  Foot and Toe Injuries  636

Axial Skeleton Injuries   638

**Management**   639

Splinting   640   •   Caring for Specific Extremity
Injuries   649   •   Lower Extremity Injuries   659

**Boot Removal**   670

Stabilized Extrication and Transfer: "Jams and Pretzels"   673

# 21  Head and Spine Injuries   697

**Anatomy and Physiology**   699

**Common Mechanisms of Injury**   702

**Increased Intracranial Pressure (ICP)**   703

**Coup-Contrecoup Injury**   703

**Common Injuries**   704

**Head and Brain Injuries**   704

Injuries of the Scalp   704   •   Skull Fractures   704   •
Traumatic Brain Injury   705   •   Concussion   705   •
Recurrent Traumatic Brain Injury   708   •   Cerebral
Contusion   708   •   Cerebral Hematoma   709   •
Diffuse Axonal Injury   710   •   Intracerebral
Hemorrhage   711

**Spinal Injuries**   711

Neurogenic Shock   712

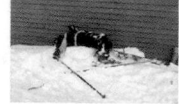

**Patient Assessment**   714

**Mini-Neurologic Exam**   715

**Management**   719

Sizing and Applying a Cervical Collar   720   •   Placing a
Patient on a Long Spine Board   720   •   Procedure for
Removing a Helmet (Lying Patient)   724

# 22  Face, Eye, and Neck Injuries   742

**Anatomy and Physiology**   743

Facial Structures   743   •   Auditory and Balance
System   744   •   Visual System   744   •   Neck
Anatomy   747

**Common Face, Eye, and Neck Injuries**   749

Face Injuries   749   •   Eye Injuries   751   •   Neck
Injuries   751

**Assessment**   754

Assessment of the Eye   754   •   Assessment of the
Mid-Face and Nose   755   •   Assessment of the
Mouth   755   •   Assessment of the Ear   755   •
Assessment of the Neck   756

**Management**   756

Management of Facial Injuries   757   •   Management
of Ear Injuries   758   •   Management of Eye
Injuries   759   •   Management of Neck Injuries   763

# 23  Thoracic Trauma   770

**Anatomy and Physiology of the Chest**   772

**Chest Injuries**   774

Mechanisms of Injury   774   •   Types of Chest
Injury   774   •   Environmental Factors   782

**Assessment**   783

**Management**   784

# 24  Abdominal and Pelvic Trauma   793

**Anatomy and Physiology**   794

**Common Abdominal and Pelvic Injuries**   798

Abdominal Wall Contusion   798   •   Liver
Injuries   798   •   Spleen Injuries   798   •   Pancreas
Injuries   798   •   Vascular Injuries   799   •   Diaphragm
Tear/Rupture   799   •   Intestinal Tear/Rupture   799   •
Impaled Objects   799   •   Evisceration   799   •   Pelvic
Fractures   800   •   Hip Injuries   800   •   Lower Urinary
Tract Injuries   801   •   Straddle Injuries   801   •   Genital
Injuries   801

**Assessment**   801

**Management**   805

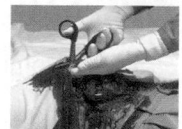

## Section 6
## ENVIRONMENTAL CONDITIONS   813

# 25  Cold-Related Emergencies   813

**Anatomy and Physiology**   815

**Common Cold-Related Emergencies**   818

Frostnip and Frostbite   818   •   Hypothermia   819   •
Afterdrop   820   •   Windburn   821

**Rescuer Preparation for Cold Weather
Rescue**   821

**Assessment of Cold Injuries**   824

Frostbite   824   •   Hypothermia   825

**Management**   827

Frostnip 827 • Frostbite 827 • Hypothermia: Prevent Heat Loss 828

**Evacuation and Transportation** 832

# Heat-Related Emergencies 838

**Anatomy and Physiology** 839

**Common Heat-Related Emergencies** 842
Heat Illness 842 • Heat-Related Illness Prevention 845 • Sunburn 845 • Lightning 848

**Assessment** 850
Heat-Induced Syncope 850 • Heat Cramps 851 • Heat Exhaustion 851 • Heat Stroke 852 • Sunburn 852 • Lightning Strikes 852

**Management** 852
Heat-Induced Syncope 852 • Heat Cramps 852 • Heat Exhaustion 852 • Heat Stroke 853 • Sunburn 854 • Lightning Strikes 855

# Plant and Animal Emergencies 861

**Anatomy and Physiology** 862

**Adverse Effects and Emergencies from Common Plants and Fungi** 863
Plants Toxic to the Skin 863 • Plants Toxic upon Ingestion 865 • Poisonous Mushrooms 870

**Adverse Effects from Various Animals** 871
Spiders 871 • Scorpions 874 • Ticks 874 • Bees, Wasps, and Hornets 875 • Mosquitoes, Fleas, and Biting Flies 876 • Ants 876 • Reptiles 878 • Marine Creatures 880 • Mammals 882

**Assessment** 885
Plants and Mushrooms 886 • Spiders and Scorpions 886 • Tick Bites 886 • Bee Stings 886 • Mosquito, Insect, and Ant Bites 886 • Reptile Bites 887 • Injuries Caused by Marine Animals 887 • Injuries Caused by Mammals 887

**Management** 887
Care of Cases Involving Plant Toxins 888 • Care of Cases Involving Ingested Plant and Mushroom Toxins 888 • Care for Cases Involving Biting and Stinging Creatures 888 • Care of Snake Bites 889 • Care of Injuries by Marine Creatures 889 • Care for Animal Bites 889 • Large Animal-Related Trauma 890

# Altitude-Related Emergencies 896

**Altitude Physiology** 898
Altitude Classifications 899 • Altitude Acclimatization 902

**Altitude-Related Problems** 903
Acute Mountain Sickness 903 • High-Altitude Pulmonary Edema 904 • High-Altitude Cerebral Edema 905 • Other Altitude-Related Problems 906

**Prevention of Altitude Illnesses** 909

**Patient Assessment** 911

**Patient Management** 912
General Management 912 • AMS Treatment 913 • HAPE Treatment 913 • HACE Treatment 913 • Khumbu Cough Treatment 913 • Treatment of Other Problems 914

# Water Emergencies 919

**Anatomy and Physiology** 921
Boyle's Law 923 • Henry's Law 923 • Dalton's Law 923

**Common Water Emergencies** 924
Submersion Injuries 924 • Barotrauma 927 • Nitrogen Narcosis 929 • Swimmer's Ear 929 • Breath Holding 929 • Trauma 930 • Injuries by Aquatic Animals 930 • Aggravation of Existing Conditions 931

**Preventing Water Emergencies** 931

**Patient Assessment** 933

**Patient Management** 934

**Section 7**
**SPECIAL POPULATIONS AND SITUATIONS** 942

# Pediatric Emergencies 942

**Anatomy and Physiology** 943
**Human Growth and Development** 946

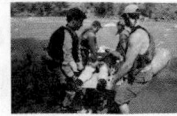

The Newborn Stage 947 • Infancy 947 • The Toddler Stage 947 • The Preschool Period 947 • The School-Age Period 948 • Adolescence 949

**Common Pediatric Illnesses and Injuries** 950
Airway Problems 950 • Respiratory Failure and Cardiac Arrest 952 • Abdominal Pain 953 • Nausea, Vomiting, and Diarrhea 953 • Seizures 953 • Meningitis 954 • Poisoning 954 • Sudden Infant Death Syndrome 957 • Trauma 957 • Burns and Electrocutions 959 • Child Abuse and Neglect 960 • Shock 961

**Assessment** 963
Scene Size-Up, MOI, and Consent 963 • Primary Assessment 965 • Secondary Assessment 966

**Management** 975

**31 Geriatric Emergencies** 985

**Physiologic Changes of Aging** 987
Neurological Changes 988 • Cardiovascular Changes 988 • Respiratory Changes 988 • Gastrointestinal Changes 988 • Changes in Renal Function and Electrolyte Balance 989 • Musculoskeletal Changes 989 • Integumentary and Endocrine Changes 989

**Common Geriatric Illnesses and Conditions** 991

Altered Mental Status 991 • Hypertension 991 • Myocardial Infarction 992 • Congestive Heart Failure 992 • Syncope 992 • Stroke 992 • Chronic Obstructive Pulmonary Disease 992 • Abdominal Emergencies 993

**Medication Use in the Elderly** 993

**Trauma Considerations in Elderly Patients** 996
Falls 996 • Hip and Pelvic Fractures 997 • Traumatic Brain Injury 997 • Cervical Spine Injury 998

**Elder Abuse** 998

**Additional Considerations** 999
Artificial Joints 999 • Implantable Devices 999 • External Openings, Ports, and Apparatus 1000 • Advanced Directives 1000 • Communicating with Elderly Patients 1000

**Assessment** 1001

**Management** 1003

**32 Outdoor Adaptive Athletes** 1009

**Common Disabilities** 1011
Intellectual Disabilities 1012 • Cognitive Disabilities 1013 • Intellectual Difficulties 1013 •

Physical Disabilities 1015 • Visually and Hearing Impaired Adaptive Athletes 1018 • Combined Physical and Intellectual Disability 1018

**Adaptive Equipment** 1019
General Equipment 1020 • Snow Sports Equipment 1022 • Warm Weather Sports Equipment 1025

**Assessment** 1028
Assessing Athletes with Intellectual Disabilities 1029 • Assessing Adaptive Athletes with Physical Disabilities 1030

**Management** 1031
Lift Evacuation Considerations 1033

**33 Behavioral Emergencies and Crisis Response** 1039

**Anatomy and Physiology** 1041

**Common Behavioral Emergencies** 1042
Medical Disorders 1042 • Chemical Exposures 1043 • Trauma 1043 • Behavioral Conditions 1043

**Death and Grief** 1047
Obvious Signs of Death 1047 • Grief 1048 • Post-Traumatic Stress Disorder 1049

**Assessment** 1051
Scene Safety 1051 • Patient Assessment 1051

**Management** 1056
Restraints 1058 • Critical Incident Stress 1060

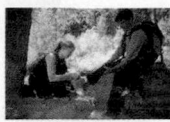

**34 Obstetric and Gynecologic Emergencies** 1068

**Anatomy & Physiology** 1069
Ovaries 1070 • Fallopian Tubes 1070 • Uterus 1071 • Vagina 1071 • Perineum 1071 • The Reproductive Cycle 1071

**Common Obstetrical and Gynecological Emergencies** 1073
Abdominal Pain 1073 • Vaginal Bleeding 1075 • Gynecological Trauma 1075 • Sexual Assault 1075

**Pregnancy: Normal Physiologic Changes** 1077

**Complications of Pregnancy** 1078
Hemorrhage 1078 • Pregnancy-Induced Hypertension (PIH) 1078 • Miscarriage 1078 • Supine Hypotensive Syndrome 1079

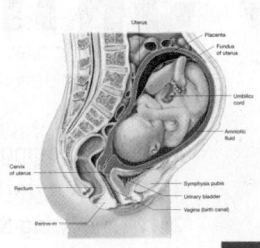

**Childbirth**  1079

**Basic Care of Newborns**  1085

**Trauma During Pregnancy**  1088

**Assessment**  1089

**Management**  1091


**Section 8**
**BEYOND OEC**  1100

**35** **Special Operations and Ambulance Operations**  1100

**Ambulance Operations**  1101
Preparing for a Call  1102  •  Responding to a Call  1103  •  Arriving at the Scene  1103  •  Transferring Patients  1105  •  Extricating a Patient from a Vehicle  1105

**Disaster Response**  1108
National Disaster Medical System (NDMS)  1110  •  Medical Reserve Corps (MRC)  1111  •  Community Emergency Response Team (CERT)  1111

**Hazardous Materials Response**  1111
Mechanism of Action of Nerve Agents  1116  •  Recommended Dosing Schedules for Exposure to a Nerve Agent  1116

**Search and Rescue**  1118
Avalanche Rescue  1120  •  Low-Angle Rescue  1123  •  Confined Space Rescue  1125  •  Water Rescue  1128

**Fire Ground Operations**  1128

**36** **ALS Interface**  1136

**Advanced Life Support**  1138
Transition of Care to ALS Providers  1138  •  Advanced Airway Management  1141  •  Mechanical Ventilators  1152  •  Metered-Dose Inhaler/ Nebulizer  1153  •  Intravenous (IV) Therapy  1156  •  Cardiac Monitoring and Electrical Therapy  1159  •  Electrical Therapy  1160  •  Medication Administration  1162

**Working and Moving as a Team**  1165

**Ambulance Stretcher Operation**  1165


**APP A    SURVIVAL: The Rule of Threes**  1171
**APP B    Student OEC Skill Guide**  1173
**APP C    Emergency Care Equipment**  1175
**Glossary**  1179
**Answer Key**  1198
**Index**  1219

# OEC Skills

**3-1**   Removing Contaminated Gloves, 91

**5-1**   Multiple Person Direct Ground Lift, 160

**5-2**   Bridge/BEAN Lift, 161

**7-1**   Patient Assessment, 248

**7-2**   Patient Assessment—Trauma Patient, 249

**7-3**   Patient Assessment—Medical Patient, 249

**7-4**   Assessing Pupils, 250

**7-5**   Assessing Pulse, 250

**7-6**   Assessing Respiration Rate, 251

**7-7**   Obtaining a Blood Pressure by Auscultation, 251

**9-1**   Suctioning a Patient's Airway, 317

**9-2**   Inserting a Nasopharyngeal Airway, 318

**9-3**   Inserting an Oropharyngeal Airway, 319

**9-4**   Oxygen Tank Set-Up and Breakdown, 320

**10-1**   Shock Management, 350

**13-1**   Auscultation of Breath Sounds, 426

**13-2**   Assisting with a Metered-Dose Inhaler, 427

**14-1**   Administration with an Auto-injector: EpiPen™, 450

**14-2**   Adiministration with an Auto-injector: Twinject™, 451

**14-3**   Adiministration with an Auto-injector: Twinject™ Additional Dose, 452

**15-1**   AED Use, 490

**18-1**   Controlling Bleeding, 566

**18-2**   Applying a Tourniquet, 567

**18-3**   Treating Closed Soft-Tissue Injuries, 568

**18-4**   Emergency Care for an Amputated Part, 569

**18-5**   Stablizing an Impaled Object, 570

**18-6**   Using a Self-Adhering Roller Bandage, 571

**18-7**   Using an Occlusive Dressing, 571

**18-8**   Using a Triangular Bandage Bandana Wrap, 572

**18-9**   Bandaging a Finger, 573

**19-1**   Caring for Burns, 597

**20-1**   Applying Sling and Swathe, 676

**20-2**   Creating and Applying a Figure Eight Splint, 677

**20-3**   Reducing a Posterior Sternoclavicular (S/C) Injury, 678

**20-4**   Applying a Blanket Roll Splint to a Shoulder, 678

**20-5**   Splinting a Humerus Fracture Using a Rigid Splint, 679

**20-6**   Rigid Splint Fixation of an Injured Elbow, 679

**20-7**   Splinting a Forearm Fracture, 680

**20-8**   Splinting to Immobilize the Hand, 680

**20-9**   Applying a Traction Splint to a Femur, 681

**20-10**   Applying an Airplane Splint, 682

**20-11**   Applying a Quick Splint, 682

**20-12**   Replacing a Quick Splint with a Cardboard Splint, 683

**20-13**   Immobilizing a Tib-Fib Fracture with Two Rigid Splints, 683

**20-14**   Removing a Boot, 684

**21-1**   Manual Spine Stabilization, 727

**21-2**   Sizing and Applying a Cervical Collar, 727

**21-3**   Supine Patient: Log Roll onto a Long Spine Board, 728

**21-4**   The Axial Drag, 728

**21-5**   Securing the Patient onto a Long Spine Board, 729

**21-6**   Immobilizing a Seated Patient, 729–730

**21-7**   Immobilizing a Standing Patient, 730

**21-8**   Removing a Helmet from a Lying Patient, 731

**22-1**   Treatment of an Impaled Object in the Eye, 765

**24-1**   Pelvic Stabilization, 808

**33-1**   Physical/Mechanical Restraint of a Patient, 1062

**34-1**   Assisting with Childbirth, 1092–1093

**36-1**   Preparing a Set-up for IV Therapy, 1167

# Letter to Students

Dear Student:

Welcome to the world of outdoor emergency care. No other program currently on the market offers the specific training needed to handle outdoor medical emergencies as comprehensively as this one. This text was developed primarily for the members of the National Ski Patrol. It is, however, relevant to all emergency first responders in outdoor environments.

The contributing authors and reviewers are highly respected experts in education in the outdoor emergency care community. The editors and reviewers, for the most part, have been active members, medical experts, and teachers in the National Ski Patrol for many years, serving the public at their local ski areas. The vast experience of these individuals, amounting to a total of over 90 years of EMS work and ski patrolling from the editors alone, has been incorporated into the chapters of this book, providing you with a learning environment that is rich in practical knowledge.

When you begin this course, we encourage you to scan through this text and learn how it is organized. Each chapter provides you with a Case Study; Stop, Think, Understand self quizzes; Chapter Review exercises; and a Scenario, all designed to provide you the best possible learning environment to practice what you have learned. You will also find information on the first page of each chapter related to the NSP's history providing insight on how and why our organization was founded.

Before the development of this book, many patrollers, OEC instructors, and representatives from other outdoor programs were interviewed to determine what information would be valuable in this program, and how best to present it to you. Our primary goal of this textbook was to make the OEC program both educational and enjoyable. We hope this is the case for you. This book is intended not only as your text during your training but also as a valuable reference manual you can keep on your bookshelf for future use. The information is current Emergency Medical System information and will be valuable to you during your future refresher training programs.

We hope you find this text valuable as you enjoy many years of service as an Outdoor Emergency Care Technician. Good luck to you all.

Editor

Medical Editor

# Preface

Welcome to the National Ski Patrol's (NSP) *Outdoor Emergency Care*, Fifth Edition. Medical education for ski patrollers has evolved over the years. In 1985, *Winter Emergency Care*, the precursor to *Outdoor Emergency Care (OEC)*, was written primarily by Warren Bowman, MD. Dr. Bowman was the principal author for the next two editions as well. He was responsible for changing the book's name to *Outdoor Emergency Care*, as content began to provide information pertaining to all four seasons. Other emergency medical providers who will benefit from this book can include river-rafting guides, park rangers, hunting and fishing guides, mountain biking organizations, or first responders who work in police or fire departments.

As *OEC* evolved, other prehospital medical authorities have increased their participation in the creation of the text. In *OEC4*, editors Dr. Bowman and Dr. David Johe called on multiple authors and reviewers. In this edition (*OEC5*), the NSP partnered with a new publisher—Brady—to develop and evolve *OEC* to new levels of publishing and performance excellence. Now over 40 authors, nearly 100 reviewers, and many other people affiliated with the NSP have spent many volunteer hours working on this project. One individual, Ed McNamara, was the glue and the driving force behind the book. His leadership was instrumental in keeping the team together and focused.

Completion of this project has been a pleasure and a rewarding pursuit that has taken well over four years. In 2006, Dr. Michael Millin and Ed McNamara proposed the development of *OEC5* to Larry Bost, National Education Chair, and to the NSP Board. After receiving approval, they began developing the Table of Contents, recruiting authors, and starting the manuscript-writing process. Many of these authors are leading authorities in their respective fields.

In the summer of 2007, Denis Meade was hired by the NSP to serve as its National Education Director, and he immediately joined the *OEC5* team. Realizing the need for additional assistance with the project, Ed McNamara appointed Deborah Endly, Assistant National OEC Program Director, as Chair of the *OEC5* Collaterals Committee, which brings to you the excellent teaching and student support package beyond this textbook.

Toward the end of the initial writing process, Dr. Millin stepped down as National Medical Advisor. However, he continued to participate in *OEC5*, reviewing and completing several chapters, and was a truly important part of the process. In January 2008, Dr. David Johe was appointed National Medical Advisor and joined the *OEC5* team.

In the fall of 2007, the National Ski Patrol decided to evaluate various noteworthy publishers throughout the country and to select one that is respected by the EMS profession and would provide our members the best program possible. After exhaustive research, our staff recommended that the *OEC5* team partner with Brady/Pearson Education.

Although *OEC4* was very successful, the team working on *OEC5* worked from the ground up to put the text into one voice and to make all the chapters consistent. This edition contains all-new material, and each chapter was written and completed using the most recent evidence-based medical information.

This text contains material that has never appeared in previous editions. It is also a combination textbook-workbook in which users write their answers to questions concerning core content.

+ The feature *Stop, Think, Understand* incorporates workbook-style exercises throughout each chapter to check the user's comprehension.
+ The first chapter includes some of the history of the NSP and OEC and has an important discussion of some of the legal aspects that we all face when caring for a patient.

- All OEC Technicians need to be familiar with current EMS language and need to be able to communicate among each other and with other EMS providers using the same vernacular. Chapters on both communication and documentation are included for this purpose.

- Patient assessment is now presented in the same way patients are assessed in the health care system. In addition, the A&P section has been expanded in each chapter, the format for case management has been modified for easier use, and skill guides have been included in many chapters to enable users to readily assess their abilities in the practical training sessions.

- Chapters also contain new information that is up to date with current prehospital patient care. Some examples include new assessment modules, the use of pulse oximeters, an expanded role for OEC Technicians in assisting patients with medications, use of Mark 1 kits, discussions of the enhanced role of tourniquets, some new ways to apply bandages and splints, and more in-depth discussions of anatomy.

- The material in this edition meets—and in many cases exceeds—the National EMS Education Standards for Emergency Medical Responders. However, this material is presented in a format that combines the disciplines of urban EMS and wilderness medical rescue.

- In addition, this edition was updated to incorporate relevant 2010 ECC recommendations for CPR. The editors, with the counsel of medical experts, modified some content to comply with their interpretation of the new guidelines.

- The last chapter of the text, Chapter 36, was authored by a physician who has written extensively for the wilderness medicine field, and it helps OEC Technicians understand what advanced EMS providers do. When asked to assist these providers, OEC Technicians—when legally allowed to do so—can provide this assistance. It is important to note that *this chapter is NOT part of the OEC curriculum and can be taught only by personnel with advanced training after receiving approval from mountain management, the Mountains patrol Medical Director, and in compliance with state and local regulations.*

- Beyond the textbook, students have access to an online resource called *myNSPkit*. This web-based tool includes additional exercises and multimedia examples to reinforce content and skills. Instructors have access to a PowerPoint presentation, a test bank, an Instructor Manual, and other materials needed to teach this course.

The National Ski Patrol is a unique organization that has provided training and care to countless individuals in outdoor environments. Originally, it was designed for ski patrollers. As ski patrollers joined other first-responder organizations such as Search and Rescue and Emergency Medical Services, they found that the training they received is widely accepted by those organizations. And in some states successful completion of an OEC course allows the individual the opportunity through reciprocity to obtain an EMS Emergency Medical Responder card. Because of the strength of the OEC program, many other agencies now look to the NSP for OEC courses as a primary education program for Emergency Medical Responders. We expect this audience to expand following the release of this new approach to training.

---

### Special Tribute

National Ski Patrol pays special tribute to Doug Howlett, who was actively involved in the National Ski Patrol from 1971 until he passed away in 2010. As a member of the Collateral Committee for *Outdoor Emergency Care*, Fifth Edition, Doug contributed to the development of the PowerPoint program.

# Acknowledgments

Thank you to every writer and participant who brought this teaching package together. We would like to especially thank NSP's Larry Bost, Terry Laliberte, Bela Musits, Bob Scarlett, and Tim White for providing their guidance and this opportunity.

Representatives from Brady were extremely helpful in providing guidance and direction in the development and production of this book. In particular, we would like to thank Marlene Pratt, Editor-in-Chief, and Lois Berlowitz, Senior Managing Editor, for their ongoing support and willingness to provide insight and guidance at any time during the development of the program. Finally, we want to thank Susan Simpfenderfer of Triple SSS Press Media Development, Inc., for her tremendous time and effort in the development, reviewing, editing, and production process. Susan made herself available to us days, nights, weekends, and holidays. She constantly provided support, direction, editorial assistance, and encouragement as we moved forward through development of this book. This project would not have been successfully accomplished without her dedication and professional involvement. Many thanks to Brady and Triple SSS.

## Contributors

We wish to acknowledge the remarkable talents and efforts of the following people who contributed to this edition of *Outdoor Emergency Care*. Individually, they worked with extraordinary commitment on this program. Together, they form a team of highly dedicated professionals who have upheld the highest standards of EMS instruction.

### CHAPTER 1 Introduction to Outdoor Emergency Care

**Warren Bowman, MD, FACP**
*Member, U.S. Ski Patrol*
*National #3537*

**David Johe, MD**
*Orthopedic Surgeon*
*Current NSP National Medical Advisor*
*Member, Holiday Valley Ski Patrol*
*Ellicottville, NY*
*National #8690*

**Robert Scarlett, Esq.**
*NSP National Legal Counsel*
*Member, Ski Liberty Ski Patrol*
*Carroll Valley, PA*
*National #8118*

### CHAPTER 2 Emergency Care Systems

**Denis Meade, MA, EMTP**
*Former NSP Education Director*
*Owner, Curriculum by Design*
*Littleton, CO*

**Michael G. Millin, MD, MPH, FACEP**
*Assistant Professor*
*Department of Emergency Medicine*
*Johns Hopkins University School of Medicine*
*Member, Ski Liberty Ski Patrol*
*Carroll Valley, PA*

### CHAPTER 3 Rescue Basics

**Eric P. Bowman, MD, FACEP, FAWM**
*Section of Wilderness Medicine Director*
*Department of Emergency Medicine*
*York Hospital*
*Member, Ski Liberty Ski Patrol*
*Carroll Valley, PA*

**Paul Murphy, MS, MA, EMT-P**
*Paul Murphy Consulting, Inc.*
*Member, Bear Mountain Ski Patrol*
*California*

### CHAPTER 4 Incident Command and Triage

**Denis Meade, MA, EMTP**
*Former NSP Education Director*
*Owner, Curriculum by Design*
*Littleton, CO*

**Edward McNamara, BS, NREMTP**
*Executive Director, Central MA EMS Corp*
*National OEC Program Director; Sterling Fire Dept. Dep. Fire Chief*
*Member, Wachusett Mountain Ski Patrol*
*Princeton, MA*
*National #7858*

### CHAPTER 5 Moving, Lifting, and Transporting Patients

**Jonathan Politis, EMT-P**
*Member, Willard Mountain Ski Patrol*
*Greenwich, NY*
*National #10996*

## CHAPTER 6 Anatomy and Physiology

**David Markenson, MD, FAAP, EMT-P**
*Chief Pediatric Emergency Medicine*
*Maria Fareri Children's Hospital*
*New York Medical College*
*Member, Sterling Forest Ski Patrol*
*Tuxedo, NY*

## CHAPTER 7 Patient Assessment

**Michael G. Millin, MD, MPH, FACEP**
*Assistant Professor*
*Department of Emergency Medicine*
*Johns Hopkins University School*
*of Medicine*
*Member, Ski Liberty Ski Patrol*
*Carroll Valley, PA*

**Denis Meade, MA, EMTP**
*Former NSP Education Director*
*Owner, Curriculum by Design*
*Littleton, CO*

## CHAPTER 8 Medical Communications and Documentation

**Jonathan Busko, MD, MPH, EMT-P**
*Medical Director, Maine Region, Eastern Division, NSP*
*Medical Director, Hermon Mountain Ski Patrol*
*Medical Director, Maine EMS Region 4*
*Emergency Physician, Eastern Maine Medical Center*
*Member, Hermon Mountain Ski Patrol*
*Stockton Springs, ME*

## CHAPTER 9 Airway Management

**Scott E. McIntosh, MD, MPH**
*Assistant Professor*
*Division of Emergency Medicine*
*University of Utah*

## CHAPTER 10 Shock

**Michael Levy, MD, FACP, FAAEM**
*Emergency Medicine*
*Alaska Regional Hospital*
*EMS Areawide Medical Director*
*Anchorage Fire Deparment*
*Member, Alaska Admin Patrol*
*Alaska*

## CHAPTER 11 Altered Mental Status

**John S. Nichols, MD, PhD, FACS**
*St. Anthony Hospital*
*Department of Neurosurgery*
*Medical Advisor*
*NSP Rocky Mountain Division*
*Member, Winter Park Pro Patrol*
*Colorado*

**Nici Singletary, MD, FACEP**
*Clinical–Associate Professor*
*Department of Emergency Medicine*
*University of Virginia*
*Charlottesville, VA*
*The Medical Clinic of Big Sky*
*Member, Northern Admin Patrol*
*National #7474*

## CHAPTER 12 Substance Abuse and Poisoning

**Maurus Sorg, MD, MPH, FAWM**
*Diplomate American Board of Family Practice*
*Diplomate of American Board of Emergency Medicine*
*Member Wilderness Medical Society*
*Fellow of Academy of Wilderness Medicine*
*Department of Emergency Medicine*
*Elk Regional Health Center*
*Saint Marys, PA*

## CHAPTER 13 Respiratiory Emergencies

**Fred A. Severyn, MD, FACEP**
*Associate Professor of Surgery*
*Division of Emergency Medicine*
*University of Colorado Denver School of Medicine*

## CHAPTER 14 Allergies and Anaphylaxis

**Denis Meade, MA, EMTP**
*Former NSP Education Director*
*Owner, Curriculum by Design*
*Littleton, CO*

## CHAPTER 15 Cardiovascular Emergencies

**John Latimer, MD**
*Department of Emergency Medicine*
*Wachusett Emergency Physicians*
*Medical Director Wachusett Mountain Ski Patrol*
*Princeton, MA*

**Roxanne Latimer, MD**
*Assistant Professor*
*Department of Family Medicine*
*University of Massachusetts Medical School*
*Member, Wachusett Mountain Ski Patrol*
*Princeton, MA*

**Michael G. Millin, MD, MPH, FACEP**
*Assistant Professor*
*Department of Emergency Medicine*
*Johns Hopkins University School of Medicine*
*Member, Ski Liberty Ski Patrol*
*Carroll Valley, PA*

**Edward McNamara, BS, NREMTP**
*Executive Director, Central MA EMS. Corp*
*National OEC Program Director; Sterling Fire Dept. Dep. Fire Chief*
*Member, Wachusett Mountain Ski Patrol*
*Princeton, MA*
*National #7858*

## CHAPTER 16 Gastrointestinal and Genitourinary Emergencies

**Denis Meade, MA, EMTP**
*Former NSP Education Director*
*Owner, Curriculum by Design*
*Littleton, CO*

**Michael G. Millin, MD, MPH, FACEP**
*Assistant Professor*
*Department of Emergency Medicine*
*Johns Hopkins University School of Medicine*
*Member, Ski Liberty Ski Patrol*
*Carroll Valley, PA*

## CHAPTER 17 Principles of Trauma

**Seth C. Hawkins, MD, FAWM**
*Assistant Professor, Wilderness Emergency Medical Care,*
*Western Carolina University*
*Executive Director, Appalachian Center for Wilderness Medicine*
*Sylva, NC*

## CHAPTER 18 Soft-Tissue Injuries

**David Johe, MD**
*Orthopedic Surgeon*
*Current NSP National Medical Advisor*
*Member, Holiday Valley Ski Patrol*
*Ellicottville, NY*
*National #8690*

## CHAPTER 19 Burns

**Jane Lee Fansler, MD**
*Resident*
*Department of Surgery, Division of*
*Emergency Medicine*
*Stanford Hospital and Clinics*

## CHAPTER 20 Musculoskeletal Injuries

**David Johe, MD**
*Orthopedic Surgeon*
*Current NSP National Medical Advisor*
*Member, Holiday Valley Ski Patrol*
*Ellicottville, NY*
*National # 8690*

## CHAPTER 21 Head and Spine Injuries

**John S. Nichols, MD, PhD, FACS**
*Neurological Surgeon*
*St. Anthony Hospital*
*NSP Rocky Mountain Division*
*Member, Winter Park Pro Patrol*
*Colorado*

**Michael Bateman, EMT-B, OEC Technician**
*Member, Winter Park Pro Patrol*
*Colorado*

## CHAPTER 22 Face, Eye and Neck Injuries

**Bruce Evans, MD**
*Assistant Professor*
*University of Colorado Denver, Division of*
*Emergency Medicine, Department of*
*Surgery, School of Medicine*
*Member, Alumni*
*Colorado*

## CHAPTER 23 Thoracic Trauma

**James Geiling, MD, FACP, FCCM**
*Chief, Medical Service: VA Medical Center*
*Associate Professor of Medicine*
*Dartmouth Medical School*
*Member, Dartmouth Skiway Ski Patrol*
*Hanover, NH*

**Matthew Fulton, BA, NREMTP**
*Patrol Director, Dartmouth Ski Patrol*
*Member, Dartmouth Skiway Ski Patrol*
*Hanover, NH*

## CHAPTER 24 Abdominal and Pelvic Trauma

**Eric M. Lamberts, MD, FAAFP, ASAM certified**
*Far West Medical Advisor*
*National Ski Patrol*
*Clinical Professor Psychiatry*
*University of Nevada School of Medicine*
*Member, Sky Tavern Pro Patrol*

## CHAPTER 25 Cold-Related Emergencies

**Marion C. McDevitt, DO**
*Emergency Medicine University of Utah*
*Wilderness Medicine and EMS Fellow,*
*Emergency Medicine University of Utah*
*Member, Park City Ski Patrol*
*Park City, UT*

**Gregory A. Bala, MS**
*Chair, Outdoor Emergency Care Refresher Committee*
*Member, Kelly Canyon Ski Patrol*
*Ririe, ID*
*National # 9128*

**Colin K. Grissom, MD**
*Professor Medicine, University of Utah*
*Critical Care Medicine, Shock Trauma*
*Intensive Care Unit*
*Intermountain Medical Center*
*Member, Park City Ski Patrol*
*Park City, UT*

## CHAPTER 26 Heat-Related Emergencies

**Gregory A. Bala, MS**
*Chair, Outdoor Emergency Care Refresher Committee*
*Member, Kelly Canyon Ski Patrol*
*Ririe, ID*
*National # 9128*

**Colin K. Grissom, MD**
*Professor Medicine, University of Utah*
*Critical Care Medicine, Shock Trauma*
*Intensive Care Unit*
*Intermountain Medical Center*
*Member, Park City Ski Patrol*
*Park City, UT*

**Marion C. McDevitt, DO**
*Emergency Medicine University of Utah*
*Wilderness Medicine and EMS Fellow,*
*Emergency Medicine University of Utah*
*Member, Park City Ski Patrol*
*Park City, UT*

## CHAPTER 27 Plant and Animal Emergencies

**Joshua Kucker, MD**
*Attending Physician*
*Santa Rosa Memorial Hospital Emergency*
*Department/Trauma Center*
*Clinical Instructor*
*Stanford University School of Medicine,*
*Division of Emergency Medicine*

## CHAPTER 28 Altitude-Related Emergencies

**Luanne Freer, MD, FACEP, FAWM**
*Medical Director, Yellowstone National Park*
*Founder/Director, Everest ER*
*Past President, Wilderness Medical Society*
*Member, Yellowstone Club Medical Ski Patrol*
*Bozeman, MT*

## CHAPTER 29 Water Emergencies

**Jeffrey Druck, MD, FACEP**
*Associate Professor, Emergency Medicine*
*University of Colorado Denver*
*School of Medicine*
*Associate Residency Director*
*Denver Health Residency Program in Emergency Medicine*

## CHAPTER 30 Pediatric Emergencies

**David C. Walker, MD, FAAP**
*Clinical Assistant Professor*
*Rainbow Babies and Children's Hospital*
*Case-Western Reserve Medical School*
*Member, Ohio Nordics*
*Concord Township, OH*
*National #10550*

**Brigitte Schran Brown, M.Ed, EMT**
*Clinical Case Manager, Academy Trainer,*
*Medical Assistant*
*Washington State Dept. of Social and*
*Health Services Child Protective Services*
*Member, Summit at Snoqualmie Ski Patrol*
*Snoqualmie, WA*
*LCA #8205*

## CHAPTER 31 Geriatric Emergencies

**Ricky Kue, MPH, MD, FACEP**
*Associate Medical Director*
*Boston EMS*
*Assistant Professor,*
*Boston University School of Medicine*

## CHAPTER 32 Outdoor Adaptive Athletes

**Bruce Evans, MD**
*Assistant Professor*
*Division of Emergency Medicine and*
*Emergency Services*
*University of Colorado Denver, Division of*
*Emergency Medicine, Department of*
*Surgery, School of Medicine*
*Member, Alumni*
*Colorado*

## CHAPTER 33 Behavioral Emergencies and Crisis Response

**Matthew J. Levy, DO, MS, NREMTP**
*Chief Resident*
*Department of Emergency Medicine*
*Johns Hopkins University School of*
*Medicine*
*Member, Donner Ski Ranch*
*Norden, CA*

## CHAPTER 34 Obstetric and Gynecologic Emergencies

**Nici Singletary, MD, FACEP**
*Cl. Associate Professor*
*Department of Emergency Medicine*
*University of Virginia*
*Charlottesville, VA*
*The Medical Clinic of Big Sky*
*Member, Northern Admin*
*National #7474*

## CHAPTER 35 Special Operations and Ambulance Operations

**Denis Meade, MA, EMTP**
*Former NSP Education Director*
*Owner, Curriculum by Design*
*Littleton, CO*

**Michael G. Millin, MD, MPH, FACEP**
*Assistant Professor*
*Department of Emergency Medicine*
*Johns Hopkins University School of*
*Medicine*
*Member, Ski Liberty Ski Patrol*
*Carroll Valley, PA*

**Rick King**
*Patroller–NSP MTR Program Director*
*Member, Perfect North Slopes Patrol*
*Lawrenceburg, IN*
*National #9998*

**Howard "Mike" Laney**
*Patroller–NSP Avalanche Program*
*Director*
*Member, Sugar Bowl Ski Patrol*
*Norden, CA*
*National #4411*

**Frank Rossi**
*Patroller–PACNW MTR Advisor*
*Member, Summit East Ski Patrol*
*Snoqualmie Pass, WA*
*National #3459*

## CHAPTER 36 ALS Interface

**Jamie A. Jenkins, MD**
*Attending Emergency Department*
*Physician*
*Washington Hospital Center/Union*
*Memorial Hospital*
*Ultrasound Fellow*

**Paul S. Auerbach, MD, MS, FACEP, FAWM**
*Redlich Family Professor of Surgery*
*Division of Emergency Medicine*
*Stanford University School of Medicine*
*Stanford, CA*
*Co-Founder and Past President,*
*Wilderness Medical Society*
*Medical Committee, National Ski Patrol*
*System*
*Consultant, Divers Alert Network*

# Reviewers

The following reviewers were commissioned by the National Ski Patrol. We wish to thank them for providing invaluable feedback and suggestions in preparation of *Outdoor Emergency Care*, Fifth Edition. Individuals with gold star by their name are recognized for reviewing and providing feedback on a significant number of chapters.

**Larry Bost** ★
*Chairman, National Education Committee*
*National #9538*
*U.S. Ski Patrol-Admin.*
*Denver, CO*

**Bill DeVarney, CSP, EMT**
*Eastern Division OEC Chief*
*Administrative Supervisor*
*National #9170*

**Carol Fountain, RN, MN, ONC**
*OEC Instructor, OEC IT*
*Instructor Development Instructor, ID IT*
*National #5980*
*Boise, ID*

**Paul D. Brooks, BS, MS, MICP**
*OEC Supervisor, Alaska Division*
*National Appointment #7751*
*OEC Instructor, IT*
*Pro Patrol, Alyeska Resort*

**Micaela Saeftel, MBA**
*European Division OEC Supervisor*
*OEC Instructor, OEC IT*
*Heidelberg Ski Patrol*

**Bill Cathey, JD**
*OEC IT; Northern Division Director*

**Keith Tatsukawa, MD**
*Far West Division (FWD) Medical*
*Advisor*
*FWD OEC Supervisor*
*Squaw Valley, CA, Ski Patrol*
*Squaw Valley, CA*

**Chris Fletcher**
*OEC Instructor/OEC IT*
*Instructor Development Advisor*
*Wachusett Mountain Ski Patrol*

**David Hemendinger**
*EMARI Regional OEC Administrator*
*OEC Instructor, OEC IT, EMT*
*Yawgoo Valley Ski Patrol, RI*

**Karen Anderson-Hadden, RN, BS**
*Bronson Methodist Hospital,*
*Kalamazoo, MI*
*Central Division OEC Supervisor,*
*OEC IT*
*National #8329*
*TimberRidge Ski Patrol Gobles, MI*

**Robert L. Andre, DVM** ★
*OEC IT*
*Sr OEC TE*
*Hunt Hollow Ski Patrol*
*Naples, NY*

**Paula Knight**
*Southington Public Schools*
*Southington, CT*
*Gifted and Talented Resource Teacher*
*OEC Assistant Supervisor Eastern*
*Division; OEC IT*
*National #7249*
*Mount Southington Ski Patrol*

**Scott R. Rockefeller, MA**
*EMT-B, EMT Instructor, EMT-*
*Examiner*
*Lee Volunteer Ambulance Squad*
*Eastern Division OEC Assistant*
*Supervisor*
*LCA #8345*
*Ski Butternut*
*Barrington, MA*

**Randy Harrison**
*Regional OEC Advisor*
*OEC and Nordic IT*
*Southern Idaho Region, PNWD*
*Boise, ID*

**Michael Parnell, DVM, PhD**
*Northern Division, OEC Supervisor*
*Miles City, MT*

**Dan Schaefer**
*Northern OEC Assistant Supervisor*
*Huff Hills Ski Patrol*
*Mandan, ND*

**Steven L. Thompson**
*OEC Instructor, OEC IT*
*National #4668*
*Montana Snow Bowl Ski Patrol*
*Missoula, MT*

**Bill Mills**
*OEC Instructor, OEC IT*
*National #6007*
*Lost Trail Powder Mountain*
*Darby, MT*

**William Lay**
*OEC Instructor, OEC IT*
*National #14924*
*Great Falls Ski Patrol*
*Great Falls, MT*

**Kim Lees**
*Central Division, SW Region ROA*
*Seven Oaks Ski Patrol*
*Boone, IA*

**Robert B. Scarlett, Esquire**
*Volunteer National Legal Counsel*
*Ski Liberty Ski Patrol, PA*
*Carroll Valley, PA*

**Teresa T. Stewart, BHS, MHS,**
**CEM(c), EMT-B**
*Administrative Officer—NDMS/SC-1*
*Senior Auxiliary, Division ID Supervisor,*
*OEC IT, Southern Cross*
*Hawksnest/Smoky Nordic Patrols*
*Charlotte, NC*

**Charles L. Lentz**
*OEC Instructor, Instructor Development*
*Instructor*
*National #8320*
*Appalachian Ski Patrol, Southern Division*
*Boone, NC*

**Cathy LaMarre**
*OEC Instructor, EMT-B*
*National #10464*
*Appalachian Ski Patrol*
*Boone, NC*

**Jennifer Laitala, AS, EMT**
*OEC Instructor, Sr OEC TE*
*National #10738*
*Wachusett Mountain Ski Patrol*
*Princeton, MA*

**E.M. "Nici" Singletary, MD, FACEP**
*Associate Professor of Emergency Medicine*
*University of Virginia*
*Charlottesville, VA*

**James R. Kopp, MD, FACS ★**
*Orthopedic Surgeon*
*Medical Advisor Pacific Northwest*
*Division*
*OEC Instructor, OEC IT,*
*National #8504*
*Anthony Lakes Ski Patrol*
*La Grande, OR*

**Kathy Mahoney, MD, FACOG ★**
*Assistant Clinical Professor of Medicine*
*Tufts University*
*Boston, MA*
*OEC Instructor*
*Okemo Mountain Resort Ski Patrol*
*Ludlow, VT*

**Eugene Eby, MD, FACEP**
*EMS Medical Director Littleton, Porter*
*and Parker Hospitals*
*Medical Director Littleton Fire*
*Department*
*Denver, CO*

**Pamela Bourg, RN, MS, ANP, CNS**
*Director Trauma Services Program*
*St. Anthony Central Hospital*
*Denver, CO*
*OEC Instructor*
*Copper Mountain Ski Patrol, Denver, CO*

**Ian Archibald, MD, FAAOS, FACS**
*Carolina Orthopedics and Sports Medicine*
*Clinic, Gastonia, NC*
*Medical Advisor, Southern Division NSP*
*Snowshoe Ski Patrol, WV*

**John B. Woodland, MD**
*Vail Valley Emergency Physicians*
*Vail Pro Patrol*
*Vail, CO*

**Milton (Skeet) Glatterer, Jr., MD,**
**FACS**
*Cardiothoracic and Vascular Surgery*
*Mountain Rescue Association: Chairman,*
*Medical Committee*
*Alpine Rescue Team, Evergreen, CO*
*OEC IT*
*Copper Mountain Ski Patrol, CO*

**Forest Harris, MD, FACP**
*Medical Advisor, Ski Liberty*
*Fairfield, PA*

**Thomas Pulling, MD**
*Sports Medicine*
*Maine Medical Center*
*Portland, ME*
*OEC Instructor*
*Alpine and Nordic Ski Patrols*
*Portland, ME*

**James A. Margolis, MD**
*OEC IT*
*Medical Advisor ESR*
*LCA #8387*
*Homewood Ski Patrol*
*Homewood, CA*

**James Brady, MD ★**
*MedExpress Urgent Care*
*Arkansas Valley Regional Medical Center, CO*
*Medical Associate, OEC Instructor*
*Seven Springs Ski Patrol*
*Champion, PA*

**Kristi A. Ball, MBA, RN, NREMT-B**
*Emergency Department Manager*
*IS7-Mayo Health System*
*OEC IT, Nat. #10112*
*Three Rivers Park District Ski Patrol*
*Bloomington, MN*

**Chuck Clements II, MD**
*Professor of Clinical Medicine*
*Director of Wilderness Medicine*
*Marshall University School of Medicine*
*Winterplace Ski Patrol*
*Huntington, WV*

**Mami Aiello Iwamoto, MD, FACS**
*Ophthalmic Consultants of Boston*
*Instructor of Ophthalmology*
*Harvard Department of Ophthalmology*
*Boston, MA*
*OEC TE, S&T TE*
*Sunday River Ski Patrol*
*Newey, ME*

**Cassandra H. Proctor, RN**
*Orthopedic Nurse*
*Sparrow Health Systems*
*OEC Instructor*
*Caberfae Peaks Ski Patrol*

**Edith McNamara, RN, EMT** ★
*Sterling, MA*
*OEC IT, Senior EMM TE, S&T TE*
*National #8068*
*Wachusett Mt. Ski Patrol*
*Princeton, MA*

**Jamie A. Jenkins, MD**
*Emergency Ultrasound Fellow*
*Department of Emergency Medicine*
*Washington Hospital Center/Union*
*Memorial Hospital*
*Washington, DC*

**Bryant F. Hall, MBA, BS (MT), NREMT-P** ★
*Monongalia Emergency Medical Services, Paramedic*
*Tucker County Emergency Medical Services, Paramedic*
*National #10076*
*OEC Instructor, OEC IT*
*Canaan Valley Ski Patrol*
*Davis, WV*

**Jim Derzon**
*OEC/S&T Instructor*
*Ski Liberty*
*Carroll Valley, PA*

**Steve Donelan**
*OEC Instructor, OEC IT*
*Pinecrest Nordic Ski Patrol*
*Pinecrest, CA*

**John T. Henderson, Jr., JD, EMT**
*New Cumberland Fire Department*
*New Cumberland, PA*
*Liberty Mountain Resort Ski Patrol*
*Carroll Valley, PA*

**Jack D. Bogdon, BS, EMT-B**
*OEC Instructor*
*Camelback Mountain Ski Patrol*
*Tannersville, PA*

**Timothy R. Thayer, BS, EMT-B**
*EMS Instructor*
*Anoka Technical College, Anoka, MN*
*OEC Instructor*
*Afton Alps Ski Patrol*
*Hastings, MN*

**Brigitte Schran Brown, MEd, MA, EMT**
*Foundation for Care Management*
*Vashon Island, WA*
*National #8205*
*Summit Central Ski Patrol*
*Snoqualmie Pass, WA*

**John J. Clair**
*National Chair, 1996–2000*
*EMT & OEC Instructor*
*National #4115*
*Brighton, UT Ski Patrol*

**Jay Reidy, MA, PhD**
*OEC, CPR Instructor*
*Pasadena, CA*

**Bernie Goddard**
*National #7535*
*OEC Instructor, OEC IT*
*Summit at Snoqualmie,*
*Snoqualmie, WA*

**Michelle R. Landry, MPH**
*Project Director, Center for Health Policy & Research,*
*UMASS*
*Worcester, MA*
*OEC Instructor, Senior EMM T/E*
*Wachusett Mountain Ski Patrol,*
*Princeton, MA*

**Karen Majors, RD**
*Wild Mountain Ski Patrol*
*Taylor Falls, MN*

**Susan Mullenix**
*OEC Instructor*
*Central Division Section 2,*
*Lutsen Mountain Ski Patrol*
*Lutsen, MN*

**Tom Olander, BA, NREMT-P**
*National #6198*
*OEC Instructor*
*Massanutten Ski Patrol*
*Harrisburg, VA*

**Cheryl Gall Tiernan**
*OEC IT*
*National #8622*
*Central Division, Section 1, Western Michigan Region*
*Bittersweet Ski Patrol*
*Ostego, MI*

**Elizabeth (Liz) Dodge**
*OEC Instructor, OEC IT*
*National #6464*
*Region Director, NW Region, PNWD*
*Summit At Snoqualmie–Central Ski Patrol*
*Snoqualmie, WA*

**Neil P. Blackington, EMT-T**
*Deputy Superintendent–Commander of Support Services*
*City of Boston Emergency Medical Services*
*OEC Instructor*
*Bradford Ski Patrol*
*Haverhill, MA*

**Carrie L. Vondrus**
*OEC Instructor, OEC IT*
*OEC Supervisor, 2006–2009*
*Intermountain Division—Alumni*
*Ogden, UT*

**Jeffrey P. Burko, EMA-II, EMT-I, ACLS-P**
*OEC Instructor*
*Peak Emergency Response Training*
*British Columbia, Canada*

**Stephen Francisco**
*OEC IT*
*National #8928*
*June Mountain Ski Patrol*
*June Lake, CA*

**Paul Rauschke**
*OEC Instructor*
*Colorado Mountain College*
*Leadville, CO*

**Erik Forsythe**
*EMT-P, OEC, WALS*
*Professional Division OEC Supervisor*
*Director, Crested Butte Professional Ski Patrol*
*Crested Butte, CO*

**John E. Mirus, MBA, EMT-I**
*OEC IT*
*Keystone Ski Patrol*
*Keystone, CO*

**Col. John J. Teevens (USAF Ret.) BS, MA, NREMT-P, OEC**
*Instructor NSP National #10800*
*Keystone Ski Patrol*
*Keystone, CO*

**Frederick Fowler, EMT-P**
*Executive Director*
*Southeastern Massachusetts EMS Council*
*Middleboro, MA*
*Past Member—Willard Mountain Ski Patrol*
*Middleboro, MA*

**Walt Alan Stoy, PhD, EMT-P**
*Professor and Director, Emergency Medicine Program*
*University of Pittsburgh*
*OEC Instructor*
*Hidden Valley Ski Patrol*
*Hidden Valley, PA*

**Diane M. Barletta, MEd, EMT-B**
*Assistant Director*
*Central MA EMS Corp.*
*Holden, MA*

**Bob Elling, EMT-P, MPA**
*Clinical Instructor, Albany Medical Center*
*Paramedic—Colonie EMS Department*
*Paramedic—Whiteface Medical Services*
*Area*
*Lake Placid, NY*

**David P. Fending, NREMT-P**
*Faculty, Pickens Technical College*
*Adjunct Faculty, Arapahoe and Red Rocks*
*Community College Aurora, Lakewood,*
*and Littleton, CO*

**John J. McAuliffe, LT/EMT**
*Sterling Fire Department Dive Rescue*
*Public Safety Diving Instructor and Ice*
*Rescue Instructor*
*Sterling, MA*

**Derrick Congdon, EMT-P**
*Assistant Regional Director*
*Mass Region 4 EMS*
*Burlington, MA*

**Janet L. Read, EMT I/C, NSP IT,**
**EMT-B**
*EMT Educator*
*Training Specialist*
*American Red Cross of Central Mass*
*Worcester, MA*

**Stephanie Dralle**
*Disaster Preparedness/EMS Coordinator*
*Advocate South Suburban Hospital*
*Hazel Crest, IL*

**Marc A. Minkler, NREMT-P,**
**CCEMT-P**
*Paramedic/Firefighter*
*Maine State EMS Instructor Coordinator*

**Adam Lee Taylor-Vaughan, MS,**
**RN, ACNP, BC, NREMT-P,**
**CCRN-CSC**
*Instructor of Surgery/Paramedic/Acute*
*Care Nurse Practitioner*

**Wesley R. Shifflett, EMT-P**
*EMT Instructor*
*Page County Fire–EMS*
*Luray, VA*

**Mark Podgwaite, NREMT-I,**
**NECEMS I/C**
*Training Coordinator*
*Vermont EMS District 6*

**Charles L. Parmley**
*Program Coordinator*
*North Tech High School Fire/EMS*
*Academy*

**David Jay Kleiman, NREMT-P,**
**CCEMT-P**
*Paramedic Instructor*

**Melissa K. F. Johnson, BA,**
**NREMT-P**
*AHA Instructor–BLS and ACLS*
*PHTLS Instructor*
*PEPP Instructor*
*VA EMT Instructor and ALS Coordinator,*
*EMS Captain*
*James City County Fire Department*

**Robert E. Sippel, MS, LP, NREMT-P**
*Assistant Professor*
*University of Texas Health Science Center*
*San Antonio, TX*

**Evelyn D. Barnum, CCEMTP/IC,**
**PhD**
*Lansing Community College*
*Health & Human Services*
*Lansing, MI*

**Richard Davis, JD**
*Rocky Mt. Division Legal Advisor*

**Robert Ferris, AAS, FF2/NREMT-P**
*EMS Specialist*
*Memorial Health System*
*Black Forest Fire Rescue*
*Colorado Springs, CO*

**Ann Gassman**
*Rocky Mt. Division OEC Supervisor*
*National #7602*

**Steven Hauser, EMT-P**
*Director*
*Strategic Emergency Response Training*
*and Consultation*
*Sheridan, CA*

**Bela Musits, EMT-B**
*Gore Mt. Patrol*
*National #7175*
*North Creek, NY*

**Stephen Simi**
*OEC IT*
*Far West Division*

## NSP Office Staff

**Timothy G. White**
*Executive Director*
*National Ski Patrol*
*Sol Vista Ski Patrol*
*Lakewood, CO*

**Carol Hudson, AA-Science**
*Education Assistant,*
*National Ski Patrol*
*OEC, Auxiliary Patroller*
*Sol Vista Ski Patrol*
*Granby, CO*

**Denise D. Cheney, BS**
*Outdoor Recreation, Cal Poly, Pomona*
*Executive Assistant, National Ski Patrol*
*OEC Instructor, Senior Auxiliary*
*Loveland Volunteer Ski Patrol*
*Loveland Basin, CO*

## Contributing Medical Editor

**Michael G. Millin, MD, MPH,**
**FACEP**
*Assistant Professor*
*Department of Emergency Medicine*
*Johns Hopkins University School of*
*Medicine*

# Collateral Committee

We wish to thank the following instructors and physicians who worked on development of the text's appendices, the art and photo program, and the student exercises, as well as on the preparation of instructor resources that accompany *Outdoor Emergency Care*, Fifth Edition.

## Associate Editor for Collateral Student and Instructor Materials

**Deborah A. Endly, BA, DH, NREMT-B**
*Senior Investigator, State of Minnesota*
*Minneapolis, MN*
*National Assistant OEC Program Director*
*Three Rivers Patrol-Hyland*
*Bloomington, MN*

## Appendices

**Chuck Clements, II, MD**
*Professor, Clinical Medicine*
*Director of Wilderness Medicine*
*Marshall University School of Medicine*
*Huntington, WV*
*Southern Division Medical Committee*
*Winterplace Ski Patrol*
*Ghent, WV*

**Kathleen A. Mahoney, MD, FACOG**
*Assistant Clinical Professor of Medicine*
*Tufts University*
*Boston, MA*
*OEC Instructor*
*Okemo Mountain Resort Ski Patrol*
*Ludlow, VT*

**Jeannine Mogan, EMT-B**
*Alpine Patrol Supervisor*
*Three Rivers Park District*
*Plymouth, MN*
*Patrol Representative, Central Division*
*Supervisor-Introduction to Patrolling*
*Three Rivers Patrol-Hyland*
*Bloomington, MN*

**Mary Ellen Walker, MD, MPH**
*Family Physician*
*Seattle, WA*

## Art and Photo Program

**Catharine V. Setzer, BS, MEd**
*Slippery Rock, PA*
*OEC IT, OEC Refresher Committee*
*Boyce Park Ski Patrol*
*Pittsburgh, PA*

**Edith S. McNamara, RN, EMT**
*Sterling, MA*
*OEC IT, Sr OEC & S&T Examiner*
*CPR Instructor*
*National #8068*
*Wachusett Mountain Ski Patrol*
*Princeton, MA*

**Deborah Foss, RT, EMT**
*West Boylston, MA*
*OEC IT, CPR Instructor*
*National #9824*
*Wachusett Mountain Ski Patrol*
*Princeton, MA*

## Student Exercises

**Brigitte Schran Brown, MEd, MA, EMT**
*Medical CME*
*Foundation for Care Management*
*Vashon Island, WA*
*OEC IT, OEC Refresher Committee*
*Summit at Snoqualmie Pass Central Ski Patrol*
*Snoqualmie Pass, WA*

**Timothy Thayer, BS, EMT-B**
*EMS Instructor*
*Anoka Technical College*
*Anoka, MN*
*OEC Instructor*
*Afton Alps Ski Patrol*
*Afton, MN*

## Instructor Manual

**Kathy Glynn, LPN, NREMT-B**
*Eagan, MN*
*OEC IT, Central Division OEC Supervisor*
*Three Rivers Patrol-Hyland*
*Bloomington, MN*

**Vicki R. Zierden**
*Bloomington, MN*
*OEC IT*
*Three Rivers Patrol-Hyland*
*Bloomington, MN*

## MyNSPkit and PowerPoint Program

**Geoffrey S. Ferguson, MD**
*Director, Vascular and Interventional Radiology*
*Evergreen Hospital Medical Center*
*Kirkland, WA*
*Medical Auxiliary Ski Patrol, Snoqualmie Pass EMT Supervisor*
*Alpental Ski Patrol*
*Snoqualmie Pass, WA*

**Steve Achelis, WEMT-I**
*Software/Book Author*
*Salt Lake City, UT*
*OEC Instructor*
*Brighton Ski Patrol*
*Brighton, UT*

**Traci Tenhulzen, BS**
*Exercise Physiology/Ergonomics*
*American Red Cross CPR/FA/AED Instructor*
*Woodinville, WA*
*Summit at Snoqualmie Central Ski Patrol*
*Snoqualmie Pass, WA*

**Janet Glaeser, BA, MEd**
*National Board Member, Education Committee*
*Boston Mills/Brandywine Ski Patrol*
*Parma, OH*

**Douglas W. Howlett, BA, MS, EdD**
*Former National Instructor Development Program Director*
*Former OEC IT*
*Somerdale, NJ*
*Spring Mountain Ski Patrol*
*Mount, PA*

**Alida Moonen**
*Boston Mills/Brandywine Ski Patrol*
*Sagamore Hills, OH*

**Matt Kurjanowicz**
*Summit at Snoqualmie Pass Central Ski Patrol*
*Snoqualmie Pass, WA*

**Nancy Pitsick, BA, MT (ASCP)**
*Vice President, Immunology*
*Division Manager ARUP Laboratories*
*Salt Lake City, UT*
*OEC Refresher Committee*
*Brighton Ski Patrol*
*Salt Lake City, UT*

## Test Program

**Shelia Daly, RN, MS, CPHQ**
*President and CEO Clinton Hospital*
*Clinton, MA*
*OEC IT, Assistant Patrol Director*
*Wachusett Mountain Ski Patrol*
*Princeton, MA*

**Scott R. Rockefeller, MA, EMT-B**
*EMT Instructor & Examiner*
*American Heart Association Faculty Member, Fairview Hospital*
*Lee, MA*
*Eastern Division Assistant OEC Supervisor*
*Ski Butternut*
*Lee, MA*

# About the Editors

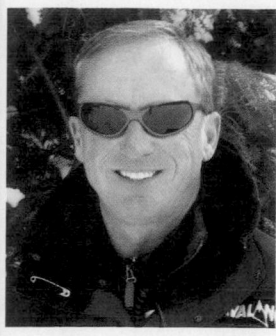

## EDWARD C. MCNAMARA, *BS, NREMT-P*

Edward C. McNamara is a Founding Incorporator and Executive Director of the Central Massachusetts Emergency Medical Systems Corporation, where he has served for the past 34 years. In addition, he is Deputy Chief of Sterling Massachusetts Fire Department and Safety Officer/Paramedic for Massachusetts 2 DMAT (Disaster Medical Assistance Team). He has also served as an EMT since 1974 and as a National Registry Paramedic for the past 12 years.

Before beginning his career in Health Administration, Mr. McNamara received his BS in Education from Norwich University and then spent three years in the Army. In 2001 he retired as a Colonel from the Massachusetts Army National Guard after 30 years of service. He currently serves as the Chair of the MA Central Region Homeland Security Council, a member of the state's Interoperability Executive Committee, and on other EMS-related committees. Mr. McNamara was also a paramedic instructor at the community college level and is an AHA Regional Faculty member.

For the past eight years, Mr. McNamara has served as the National OEC Program Director for the National Ski Patrol, and as a member of the NSP Medical Advisory Committee. Mr. McNamara, a 30-year patroller, is also a former Eastern Division OEC Supervisor, Patrol Director, Regional Director, Regional OEC Administrator, and Chief Senior OEC Trainer Evaluator. He is the recipient of 2 purple, one blue and several yellow merit stars and the Distinguished Service Award. He was the winner of the 2005 National Administrative Patroller of the Year, and he currently patrols at Wachusett Mt. Ski Area in Princeton, MA. He has been awarded National #7858.

**Personal Acknowledgement:** I would like to thank my wife, advisor, and best friend Edee for her tremendous support and extraordinary patience these past five years during the production of this book.

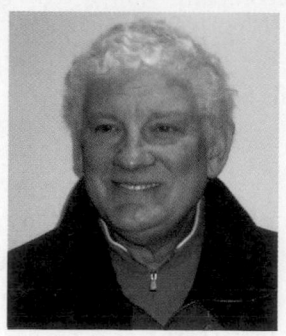

## DAVID H. JOHE, *MD*

David H. Johe, MD, is an orthopedic surgeon in private practice, Saint Mary's, Pennsylvania. He has practiced orthopedics in northwestern Pennsylvania and western New York since 1982. He attended medical school at West Virginia University, Morgantown, West Virginia; completed his internship at Hartford Hospital, Hartford, Connecticut; and completed his residency at University Hospitals of Cleveland, Cleveland, Ohio. David is currently affiliated with Elk Regional Health Center, Saint Mary's, PA; Allegheny Health Systems, Bradford Division, Bradford, PA; and Kane Hospital, Kane, PA.

David is a member of the American Medical Association and the Pennsylvania Orthopedic Society, and is a Founding Board Member, EMCO East, which provides prehospital care to northwestern Pennsylvania.

David has been a member of the Holiday Valley Ski Patrol, Ellicottville, NY, since 1990. In addition, he is an OEC Instructor, is the National Medical Advisor for the National Ski Patrol, and is Chairman of National Medical Advisory Committee National Appointment (NSP) #8690.

David's other interests include restoration of antique cars and raising Braque d'Auvergne bird dogs.

**Personal Acknowledgement:** For Roslyn, a very special thank you for your support.

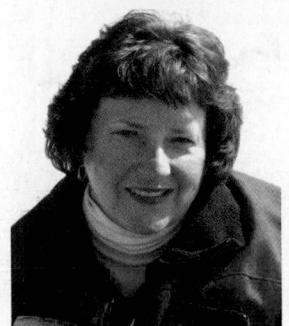

## DEBORAH A. ENDLY, *BA, DH, NREMT-B*

Deborah A. Endly has been a Senior Investigator for the State of Minnesota and Compliance Officer for the Minnesota Board of Dentistry since 1995. Ms. Endly received her A.S. degree in Dental Hygiene and a B.A. in Business Administration and Human Resource Management. She has also taught university-level dental hygiene courses at Argosy University, Eagan, MN.

In addition, Ms. Endly is a Minnesota-licensed Dental Hygienist as well as an NREMT-B and a Basic Life Support Instructor for the American Heart Association. Prior to earning her EMT licensure, Ms. Endly was registered in the State of Minnesota as a First Responder. She also has served on and has training in her local Citizen Emergency Response Team (CERT) and currently serves as one of the blood-borne pathogen trainers for Three Rivers Park District in Minnesota.

Ms. Endly has been a member of the National Ski Patrol since 1993. She has served as the Chair of the Collateral Committee for *Outdoor Emergency Care*, Fifth Edition, since August 2007 and was appointed National Assistant OEC Program Director in August 2008. Before accepting these national positions, Ms. Endly served as the Central Division OEC Supervisor for eight years and also served as the Region OEC Administrator before her Division appointment.

Additional National Ski Patrol positions include local patrol refresher Instructor of Record and OEC candidate class. Ms. Endly is also an Instructor Trainer in both OEC and Instructor Development and was one of the team members who developed the OEC Practical Final and continues to work with that team. She has been the recipient of multiple Yellow Merit Stars, the Central Division Outstanding Supervisor Award, the Region Director Award, Region Outstanding Administrative Patroller, as well as Outstanding Instructor and Patroller at the local level. She currently patrols and serves as a shift leader at the Three Rivers Patrol-Hyland, in Bloomington, MN, National #8305.

# Guide to Key Features

## Historical Timeline
Each chapter begins with a visual timeline that documents history and key events from the National Ski Patrol's archives.

### Introduction to Outdoor Emergency Care

David Johe, MD
Warren Bowman, MD
Robert Scarlett, Esquire

#### OBJECTIVES

Upon completion of this chapter, the OEC Technician will be able to:

1-1 Describe the evolution and purpose of the National Ski Patrol's OEC program.
1-2 Describe the history of the National Ski Patrol.
1-3 Identify the founder of the National Ski Patrol.
1-4 Describe the role of National Ski Patrol in the formation of the U.S. Army's 10th Mountain Division.
1-5 Compare and contrast the OEC textbook and OEC course/curriculum.
1-6 Describe the organization of the OEC worktext and its use during an OEC course or OEC refresher course.
1-7 Describe the OEC certification and recertification processes.
1-8 Contrast the standard of training and standard of care.

*continued*

#### Chapter Overview
Society today has many varied outdoor activities, especially sporting ones, during which injuries or illness may occur. Among the many winter sporting events, most people enjoy either skiing or snowboarding. The National Ski Patrol (NSP) has created a course called **Outdoor Emergency Care** to provide emergency medical care for individuals injured outdoors. The Outdoor Emergency Care program is the backbone of the National Ski Patrol's medical training program. It is also the standard of training for other organizations involved with outdoor recreation.

*continued*

#### HISTORICAL TIMELINE

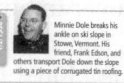 Minnie Dole breaks his ankle on ski slope in Stowe, Vermont. His friend, Frank Edson, and others transport Dole down the slope using a piece of corrugated tin roofing.

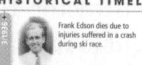 Frank Edson dies due to injuries suffered in a crash during ski race.

Minnie Dole publishes an article in an annual American ski publication summarizing ski accident causes and prevention.

---

## STOP, THINK, UNDERSTAND

### Multiple Choice
Choose the correct answer.

1. Which of the following is not a physical response to stress?_____
   a. nausea
   b. rapid breathing
   c. dilated pupils
   d. constricted pupils

2. When the core body temperature drops below 98.6°F, numerous events take place to conserve body heat and increase heat production. What of the following events does not help with heat production or heat conservation?_____
   a. shivering stops
   b. shivering increases
   c. metabolism increases
   d. blood vessels in the skin constrict

3. Which of the following are leukocytes?_____
   a. red blood cells
   b. white blood cells
   c. pathogens
   d. antibodies

4. When dressing for outdoor winter activities, what is the optimal number of layers to wear?_____
   a. 4
   b. 3
   c. 2
   d. 1

5. Which of the following is not a recommended way to purify surface water?_____
   a. boiling
   b. iodine tablets
   c. chlorine dioxide tablets
   d. solar radiation

### Fill in the Blank

1. During the "fight or flight" response, blood flow increases to the_____ and _____ muscles.

2. _____, _____, and _____ can weaken the immune system.

3. _____ clothing has no insulating value and takes a long time to dry, and thus it is a poor choice for outdoor winter activities.

4. Heat always transfers from the _____ object to the _____ object.

### Matching
Match each mechanism of heat transfer with the correct description at right.

_____ 1. conduction
_____ 2. convection
_____ 3. radiation
_____ 4. evaporation

a. the transfer of heat when a gas or liquid moves past your body
b. the transfer of heat when a liquid becomes a gas
c. the absorption or reflection of electromagnetic waves
d. the transfer of heat from a warmer object to a cooler one through direct contact

## Stop, Think, Understand
These exercises (including multiple-choice, matching, true/false, and short answer questions, and labeling activities) make this a true "work-text" where readers can test and internalize their knowledge.

---

## Chapter Objectives
Also placed in margins, these appear next to content that meets the objective.

**1-1** Describe the evolution and purpose of the National Ski Patrol's OEC program.

**1-2** Describe the history of the National Ski Patrol.

**1-3** Identify the founder of the National Ski Patrol.

---

5-11 Describe and demonstrate how to safely move when near a helicopter.
5-12 Describe the use of CPR during transport.

#### KEY TERMS

basket stretcher, p. 131
body mechanics, p. 128
carry, p. 131
drag, p. 136
high-Fowler position, p. 146
landing zone (LZ), p. 155

lift, p. 143
long spine board (LSB), p. 131
move, p. 135
orthopedic stretcher, p. 131
patient package, p. 127
Rothberg position, p. 146

semi-Fowler position, p. 146
stair chair, p. 152
Trendelenburg position, p. 146

Of all the tasks performed by OEC Technicians, moving, lifting, and transporting patients present some of the greatest challenges and risks. The reason is that OEC Technicians must perform these tasks under difficult conditions, often with limited resources. In addition to moving and lifting patients from awkward positions, OEC Technicians often must carry, lift, or transport a **patient package** weighing more than 300 pounds. Even when this weight is shared between two or more rescuers, carrying and/or sliding a heavy weight over snow, ice, and uneven terrain is tough, back-breaking work, even under the best of circumstances.

**patient package** the combination of the patient, any equipment needed to care for the patient, and the device used to transport the patient.

**Figure 5-1a** Sometimes injured patients can assist with their extrication.
Copyright Scott Smith

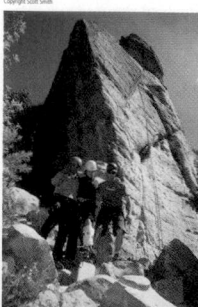

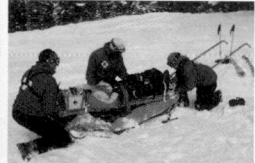

**Figure 5-1b** This injured alpine skier must be transported by toboggan.
Copyright Scott Smith

## Key Terms
These are listed with page references at the start of each chapter. Additionally, each key term is placed in the margin with its full definition, next to where it is first covered in the text.

---

### CASE PRESENTATION

You are ski patrolling alone for the first time after having completed all of your OEC training. You receive a call to respond to an accident in the parking lot of a condominium complex next to the resort. Although this condominium is not part of the ski resort, your management has an agreement to provide medical coverage to adjacent properties such as this because most guests staying there are also guests of the resort.

The call involves an eight-year-old girl who apparently was hit by a car that has left the scene. Upon your arrival, you find the child lying on the ground holding her leg. She is crying and asks repeatedly for her parents. An adult man says he was walking by and found the child. He states that he is not related to the child and has never met her.

**What should you do?**

niche of prehospital care. River rafters, cavers, park rangers, mountain bike race personnel, search-and-rescue personnel, rescuers at large sporting events, cruise-ship medical personnel, and medical rescuers at large outdoor concerns will find the information in this text invaluable when providing care for patients.

The prospective OEC Technician will learn how to function with minimal equipment in outdoor environments while assisting and caring for the sick and injured. As important as medical knowledge is the demeanor of the OEC Technician in dealing with patients, the public, and other emergency personnel. This text emphasizes the OEC Technician's ability to interact well with patients and their families, the public, peers, management, and other medical personnel (Figure 1-2■).

This chapter opens with a brief history of the National Ski Patrol and Charles Minor "Minnie" Dole, its founder. It also includes the history of OEC and of Dr. Warren Bowman, the man who is credited with its inception. The last portion of the chapter gives a brief overview of the medical-legal issues that OEC Technicians may encounter. We will review ethical considerations, reporting requirements, **confidentiality**, negligence, and abandonment.

prehospital care   any medical care rendered prior to arrival at a medical facility.

**1-1** Describe the evolution and purpose of the National Ski Patrol's OEC program.

**1-2** Describe the history of the National Ski Patrol.

**1-3** Identify the founder of the National Ski Patrol.

**confidentiality** the nondisclosure of personal information except to an authorized person with the need to know.

**Figure 1-2** An OEC Technician giving emergency care to a mountain biker.
Copyright Mike Fabisiak

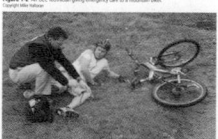

**CASE PRESENTATION**

It is a chilly afternoon with moderate cloud cover. You have just entered the mid-mountain lodge and are looking forward to a well-earned bowl of hot soup when you are summoned to respond to a skier who has fallen approximately 30 feet from a chairlift. The skier reportedly landed on a rock pile and is unconscious. You notify dispatch that you are responding.

Upon arrival, you see that the patient has fallen into a ravine, and that extrication will require specialized equipment and other rescuers. Two other OEC Technicians are already on scene and have initiated care of the patient. One of the technicians is Peter, the newest member of your patrol, who has been assigned to you for mentoring. He is at the patient's head while the other technician is assessing the patient for injuries. You note that Peter is wearing only a sweater and a lightweight outer shell.

As you approach, Peter looks up, smiles nervously, and then gives you a brief report on the patient's condition. As he speaks, you note that he is shivering slightly. It is then that you realize that Peter is not wearing a hat and that his gloves appear to be soaked. A light, freezing rain begins to fall.

***Do you have one patient to address, or two?***

## Case Study
Threaded through each chapter, these are introduced as the Case Presentation, followed up in the Case Update, and concluded in the Case Disposition.

 **CASE UPDATE**

Reaching into your pack, you hand Peter your spare wool hat and a dry set of waterproof gloves. You then assist the other technician in treating the injured patient. Still other rescuers arrive and begin setting up a rescue plan. As you continue to work, the weather becomes more severe as a mixture of snow and hail begins to fall. The temperature starts to drop and the wind increases. Peter's coat is not waterproof, and within minutes he is soaked. His fingertips are becoming numb and he repeatedly takes off his gloves to blow on his hands. You are about to say something to him when his stomach growls loudly. Embarrassed, he looks at you and says, "It was a late night last night, and I skipped breakfast." Glancing at your watch, you note that it is 1:30 p.m.

***What is the best way to help both the patient and Peter?***

 **CASE DISPOSITION**

Pulling Peter aside, you instruct him to remove his wet jacket, and you give him your backup waterproof jacket. You also hand him two of your energy bars. As the rescue efforts continue, Peter realizes that he was not prepared for the scene. You instruct another rescuer to take Peter back to the ski area first-aid station so that he can be checked and warmed up. A few minutes later, Peter is heading to the first-aid room on the back of a snowmobile, covered with a wool blanket. Although Peter survived this event without any major complications, he learned some valuable lessons about being appropriately prepared, both physically and mentally.

## OEC Skills
Many chapters end with a OEC skill, a visual guide to the skills covered. Some conclude with Skill Guides—checklists for skills performance.

**OEC SKILL 9-3** | Inserting an Oropharyngeal Airway

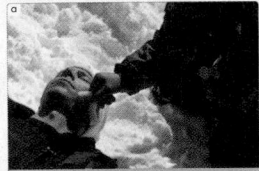
Size the airway by measuring from the corner of the mouth to the ear.
Copyright Scott Smith

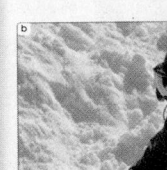
Insert the airway using the crossed-finger technique to open the mouth.
Copyright Scott Smith

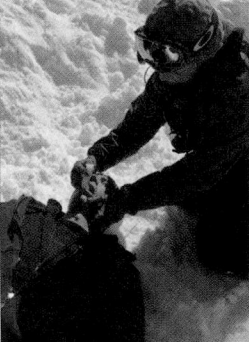

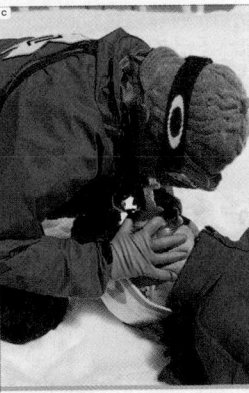
Check for airway patency by ventilating the patient.
Copyright Scott Smith

### Skill Guide

Date: _____

(CPI) = Critical Performance Indicator

Candidate: _____

Start Time: _____

End Time: _____

**Inserting an Oropharyngeal Airway (OPA)**

**Objective:** To measure and insert an oral airway into an adult.

| Skill | Max Points | Skill Demo | |
|---|---|---|---|
| Initiate Standard Precautions. | 1 | | (CPI) |
| Hold the adjunct against the side of the face with the flange adjacent to the corner of the patient's mouth. Size the airway by measuring from the patient's earlobe to the corner of the mouth or from the corner of the mouth to the angle of the jaw. | 1 | | (CPI) |
| Open the patient's mouth with the cross-finger technique. Hold the airway upside down with your other hand. Insert the airway with the tip facing the roof of the mouth and slide it in until it is half way into the mouth. | 1 | | (CPI) |
| Rotate the airway 180°. Insert the airway until the flange rests on the patient's lips. | 1 | | (CPI) |

| Must receive 4 out of 4 points. |
|---|

Comments: _____

Failure of any of the CPIs is an automatic failure.

Evaluator: _____ NSP ID: _____

PASS    FAIL

# 🛡️ Chapter Review

## Chapter Summary

The skills of lifting, moving, and transporting using good body mechanics must be mastered by every OEC Technician, because an understanding of the techniques involved is essential for the care of the patient, and for the patient's and the rescuers' safety. On occasion, a patient will be located in an area that poses an immediate threat to life and must be urgently moved to a safe location. These emergency moves are best accomplished by a "long-axis drag," which helps keep the patient's spine in proper alignment.

As part of their training, OEC Technicians must master the equipment and devices they will use in all conditions. Extreme care must be exercised with patients to avoid handling them roughly or dropping them, which is likely to aggravate their condition. OEC Technicians must learn how to properly package patients for transportation.

The helicopter is an amazing rescue tool that can save lives due to its ability to bring both rescuers and equipment to the scene rapidly, to extract patients from remote locations, and to speed the transport of patients to definitive care. It is essential that everyone on the scene have a basic understanding of landing zone selection and procedures for operating in and around a helicopter. Toboggan transport of a patient in full arrest is difficult. Decide the best method for your ski area, which will vary depending on terrain. Practice this skill often so that when it is needed, you are prepared.

## Remember...

1. Back injuries may be prevented through exercise, weight maintenance, and good body mechanics.
2. Plan each move carefully; get help when lifting.
3. Keep your back straight and lift with your legs.
4. Do not drop the patient.
5. Urgent moves require preserving the long axis of the spine.
6. Used properly, equipment can facilitate a move or a lift.
7. A landing zone should be at least 100 feet by 100 feet.
8. Do not approach a helicopter unless instructed to do so by the pilot or a crew member; keep your head low.
9. Never approach a helicopter from the rear.

## Chapter Questions

### Multiple Choice

Choose the correct answer.

1. In what position would a patient with a lower extremity injury be transported off the hill?_____
   a. sitting on a snowmobile
   b. injury facing downhill
   c. head uphill
   d. head downhill

2. In what position would a patient with an upper extremity injury be transported off the hill?_____
   a. sitting on a snowmobile
   b. injury downhill
   c. feet uphill
   d. feet downhill

3. Which of the following is *not* a basic LZ guideline?_____
   a. The site must be free of overhead obstructions and wires.
   b. The site should be well lit.
   c. The site must be a minimum of 100 feet by 100 feet.
   d. Point spotlights toward the aircraft.

---

4. Which of the following is *not* a backsmart tip?_____
   a. Turn with your feet, not your hips.
   b. Bend at your waist.
   c. Keep objects close to your body.
   d. Do not reach over your head.

5. All of the following are used by OEC Technicians to move, lift, or carry a patient *except*_____
   a. a long spine board.
   b. an orthopedic stretcher.
   c. rescue parallel bars.
   d. a short spine board.

6. What is the first principle of medicine?_____
   a. Use Standard Precautions.
   b. Do no harm.
   c. Help others who cannot help themselves.
   d. Maintain scene safety.

7. Which of the following is a long-axis drag?_____
   a. blanket drag
   b. human crutch
   c. chair carry
   d. two-person assist

## Matching

Match each of the following patient conditions with the most common position for transport.

_____ 1. semi-Fowler position
_____ 2. high-Fowler position
_____ 3. supine position
_____ 4. Rothenberg position
_____ 5. Trendelenburg position

a. a patient who is experiencing breathing problems
b. a patient with spinal injuries
c. a patient with chest pain and a suspected heart attack
d. a patient in shock
e. a patient who is awake and for whom no spinal injury is suspected

## Short Answer

List six basic principles of helicopter safety.

_____
_____
_____

## Scenario

You receive a call to the tubing park to aid an injured party. Once on scene, you find a 30-year-old male whose right lower leg is wedged between two trees. The patient is responsive and alert but has slurred speech. He complains of severe pain to his lower right leg. The patient states he was "horsing around" with two friends while tubing down the slope. He tells you he was "bumped," which forced him off the lane and into the trees. His friends state that he hit the trees "feet first." The patient denies striking his head, neck, or back and reports no pain in those areas. The friends admit to having been drinking.

Assessment of the patient's leg leads you to suspect a possible closed fracture of the right leg.

1. What type of move is needed for this extrication?_____
   a. a nonurgent move
   b. an urgent move
   c. a shoulder drag
   d. a fore and aft carry

After closing the outside lane and securing the scene, you request assistance and equipment. Another OEC Technician arrives and you formulate an extrication plan.

2. Most back injuries to rescuers are caused by_____
   a. not enough rescuers.
   b. adverse terrain.
   c. poor body mechanics.
   d. oversized patients.

---

Other rescuers arrive with the treatment and transport equipment. The patient is packaged and ready to load in the toboggan. Due to intense pain, the patient is not able to assist in moving himself to the toboggan. You decide to cravat his legs together and lift him. You have a total of four patrollers at the scene to help.

3. Which of the following types of lift is appropriate for placing the patient into the toboggan?_____
   a. Extremity lift
   b. BEAM lift
   c. Direct ground lift
   d. BEAN lift

## Suggested Reading

Lipke, Rick. 2009. *Technical Rescue Riggers Guide*, Second Edition, Conterra, Inc. Bellingham, WA.

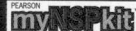

EXPLORE myNSPkit PEARSON

Please go to www.myNSPkit.com. Under Student Resources, you will find animations, videos, web links, and games related to this chapter—and much more. Look for additional information on the lifts covered in this chapter.

Register your access code from the front of your book by going to www.myNSPkit.com and selecting the appropriate links. If the in-cover access code has been redeemed, go to www.myNSPkit.com and follow links to **Buy Access**.

---

# Chapter Review

Included here are a Chapter Summary, Remember . . . , Chapter Questions, Scenario, Suggested Reading, and Explore myNSPkit, an online resource.

## Photography

A completely new, dynamic, and visually appealing photo program captures the spirit and skill of working in the outdoors.

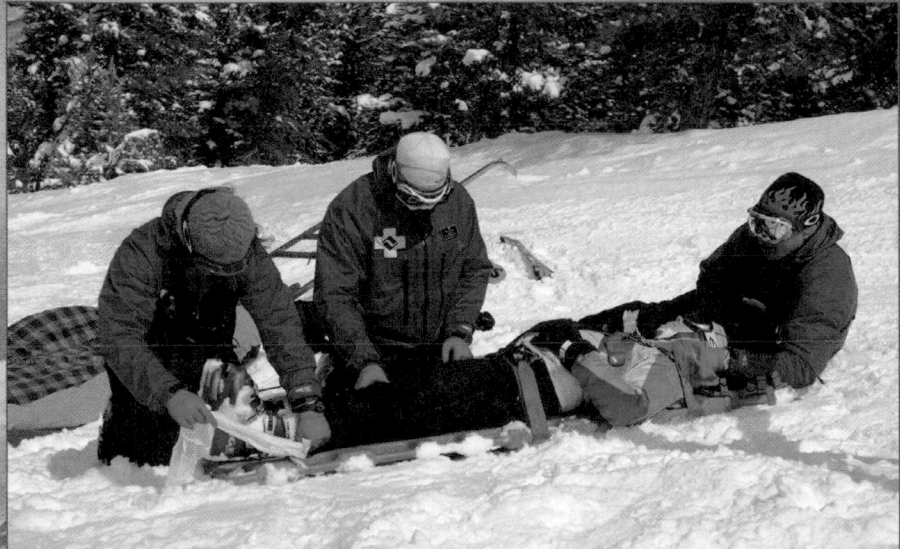

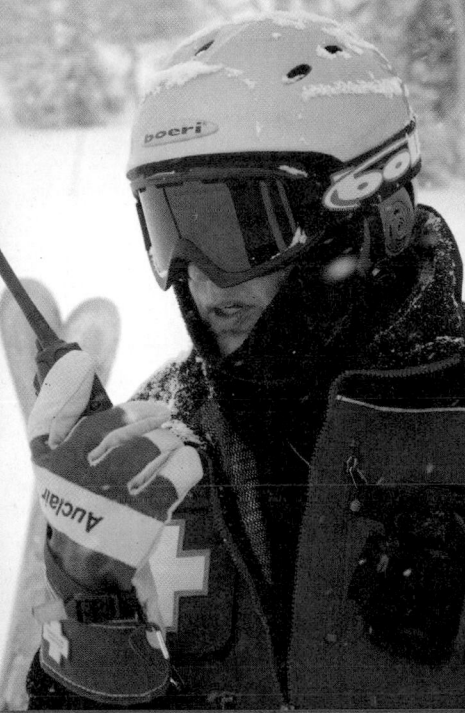

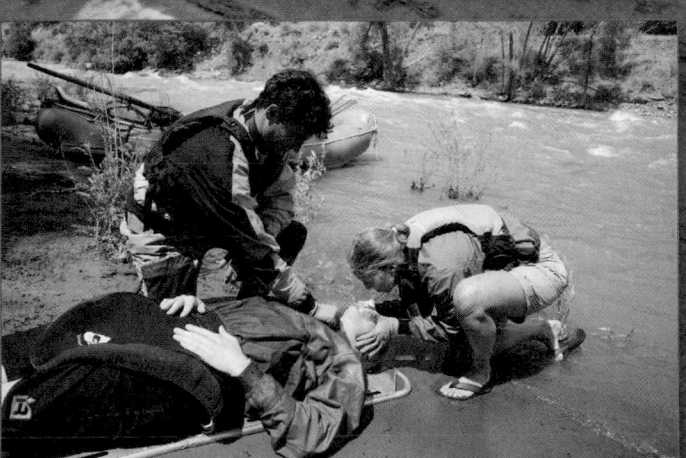

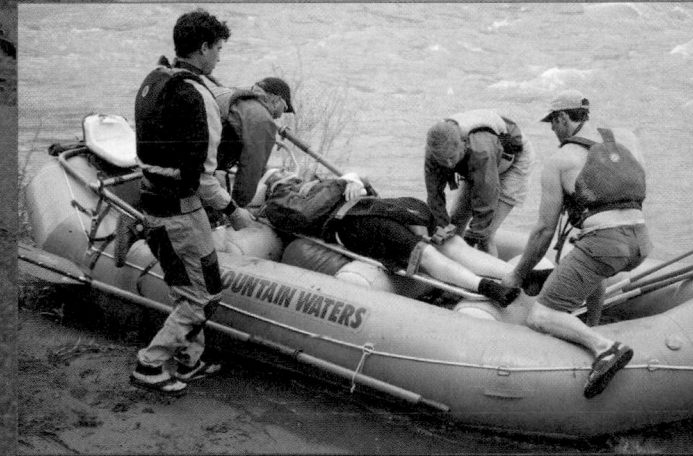

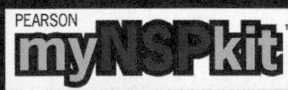

## myNSPkit

A one-stop shop for all online instructor and student resources, including lesson plans, testing program, and PowerPoints (for instructors), and quizzes, animations, audio glossary, games, and web links (for instructors and students).

EXPLORE **PEARSON myNSPkit™**

Please go to www.myNSPkit.com. Under Student Resources, you will find animations, videos, web links, and games related to this chapter—and much more. Look for information on disaster preparedness and triage simulation.

Register your access code from the front of your book by going to www.myNSPkit.com and selecting the appropriate links. If the in-cover access code has been redeemed, go to www.myNSPkit.com and follow links to **Buy Access.**

# Introduction to Outdoor Emergency Care

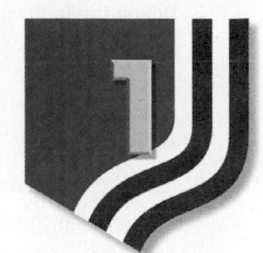

David Johe, MD
Warren Bowman, MD
Robert Scarlett, Esquire

## ✛ OBJECTIVES

**Upon completion of this chapter, the OEC Technician will be able to:**

**1-1** Describe the evolution and purpose of the National Ski Patrol's OEC program.

**1-2** Describe the history of the National Ski Patrol.

**1-3** Identify the founder of the National Ski Patrol.

**1-4** Describe the role of National Ski Patrol in the formation of the U.S. Army's 10th Mountain Division.

**1-5** Compare and contrast the OEC textbook and OEC course/curriculum.

**1-6** Describe the organization of the OEC worktext and its use during an OEC course or OEC refresher course.

**1-7** Describe the OEC certification and recertification processes.

**1-8** Contrast the standard of training and standard of care.

*continued*

## Chapter Overview

Society today has many varied outdoor activities, especially sporting ones, during which injuries or illness may occur. Among the many winter sporting events, most people enjoy either skiing or snowboarding. The National Ski Patrol (NSP) has created a course called **Outdoor Emergency Care** to provide emergency medical care for individuals injured outdoors. The Outdoor Emergency Care program is the backbone of the National Ski Patrol's medical training program. It is also the standard of training for other organizations involved with outdoor recreation.

*continued*

## HISTORICAL TIMELINE

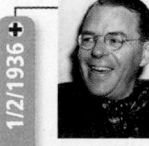

**1/2/1936** — Minnie Dole breaks his ankle on ski slope in Stowe, Vermont. His friend, Frank Edson, and others transport Dole down the slope using a piece of corrugated tin roofing.

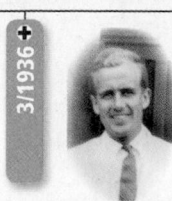

**3/1936** — Frank Edson dies due to injuries suffered in a crash during ski race.

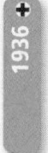

**1936** — Minnie Dole publishes an article in an annual American ski publication summarizing ski accident causes and prevention.

**1-9** Define the following legal terms:

- abandonment
- assault
- battery
- breach of duty

- consent
- duty to act
- negligence

**1-10** Describe the following forms of consent:

- expressed consent
- implied consent

- informed consent
- minor consent

**1-11** Describe the impact of Good Samaritan laws on volunteer rescuers.

## ⊕ KEY TERMS

abandonment, *p. 17*

assault, *p. 23*

battery, *p. 23*

breach of duty, *p. 18*

Charles Minot "Minnie" Dole, *p. 4*

confidentiality, *p. 3*

consent, *p. 21*

doctrine of public reliance, *p. 17*

duty to act, *p. 18*

Emergency Medical Responder (EMR), *p. 20*

ethics, *p. 15*

expressed content, *p. 21*

Good Samaritan laws, *p. 15*

Health Insurance Portability and Accountability Act (HIPAA), *p. 25*

informed consent, *p. 21*

implied consent, *p. 22*

minor consent, *p. 21*

National Medical Advisor, *p. 6*

National Medical Committee, *p. 11*

National OEC Program Committee, *p. 11*

National OEC Program Director, *p. 12*

National OEC Refresher Committee, *p. 12*

National Ski Patrol System, Inc. (NSP), *p. 4*

negligence, *p. 18*

Outdoor Emergency Care (OEC), *p. 1*

prehospital care, *p. 3*

refresher, *p. 12*

scenario, *p. 9*

standard of care, *p. 21*

standard of training, *p. 21*

**Outdoor Emergency Care (OEC)**   a course of medical instruction developed and taught by National Ski Patrol.

*Outdoor Emergency Care*, is the primary resource for a student who wants to become a ski patroller or an OEC Technician, but it also has value for other outdoor enthusiasts (Figure 1-1■). National Ski Patrol OEC Technicians, people who are enjoying the outdoors, or other rescuers can use this text as an educational tool. It bridges the gap between medical responders with access to an ambulance and advanced equipment, and wilderness search-and-rescue personnel who are several hours from advanced care. No other comprehensive medical textbook covers this

**Figure 1-1** These covers show the evolution of the *Outdoor Emergency Care* texts, which teach intermediate care to outdoor enthusiasts. The textbook has progressed from the American Red Cross First Aid to this Fifth Edition.
Copyright Caleb Hund

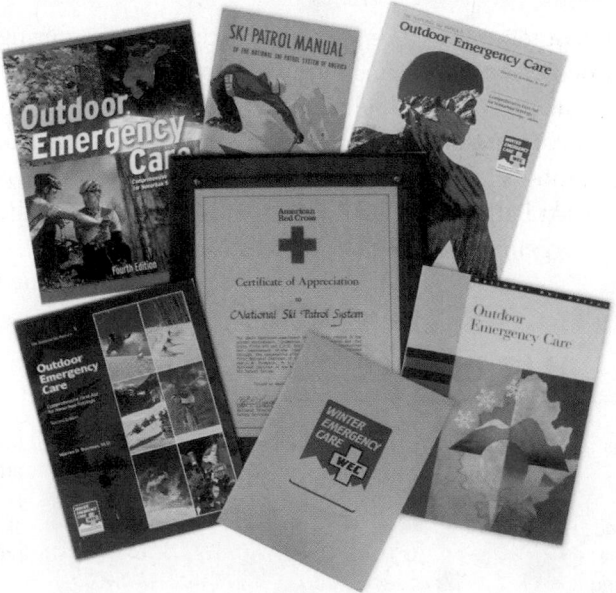

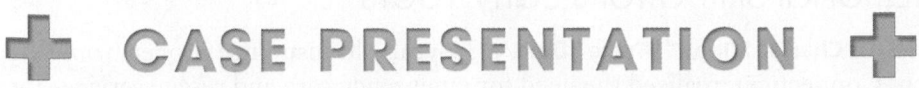

# CASE PRESENTATION

You are ski patrolling alone for the first time after having completed all of your OEC training. You receive a call to respond to an accident in the parking lot of a condominium complex next to the resort. Although this condominium is not part of the ski resort, your management has an agreement to provide medical coverage to adjacent properties such as this because most guests staying there are also guests of the resort.

The call involves an eight-year-old girl who apparently was hit by a car that has left the scene. Upon your arrival, you find the child lying on the ground holding her leg. She is crying and asks repeatedly for her parents. An adult man says he was walking by and found the child. He states that he is not related to the child and has never met her.

*What should you do?*

niche of **prehospital care**. River rafters, cavers, park rangers, mountain bike race personnel, search-and-rescue personnel, rescuers at large sporting events, cruise-ship medical personnel, and medical rescuers at large outdoor concerts will find the information in this text invaluable when providing care for patients.

The prospective OEC Technician will learn how to function with minimal equipment in outdoor environments while assessing and caring for the sick and injured. As important as medical knowledge is the demeanor of the OEC Technician in dealing with patients, the public, and other emergency personnel. This text emphasizes the OEC Technician's ability to interact well with patients and their families, the public, peers, management, and other medical personnel (Figure 1-2■).

This chapter opens with a brief history of the National Ski Patrol and Charles Minot "Minnie" Dole, its founder. It also includes the history of OEC and of Dr. Warren Bowman, the man who is credited with its inception. The last portion of the chapter gives a brief overview of the medical-legal issues that OEC Technicians may encounter. We will review ethical considerations, reporting requirements, **confidentiality**, negligence, and abandonment.

**prehospital care** any medical care rendered by trained personnel prior to arrival at a hospital.

**⊕ 1-1** Describe the evolution and purpose of the National Ski Patrol's OEC program.

**⊕ 1-2** Describe the history of the National Ski Patrol.

**⊕ 1-3** Identify the founder of the National Ski Patrol.

**confidentiality** the nondisclosure of personal information except to an authorized person with the need to know.

**Figure 1-2** An OEC Technician giving emergency care to a mountain biker.
Copyright Mike Halloran

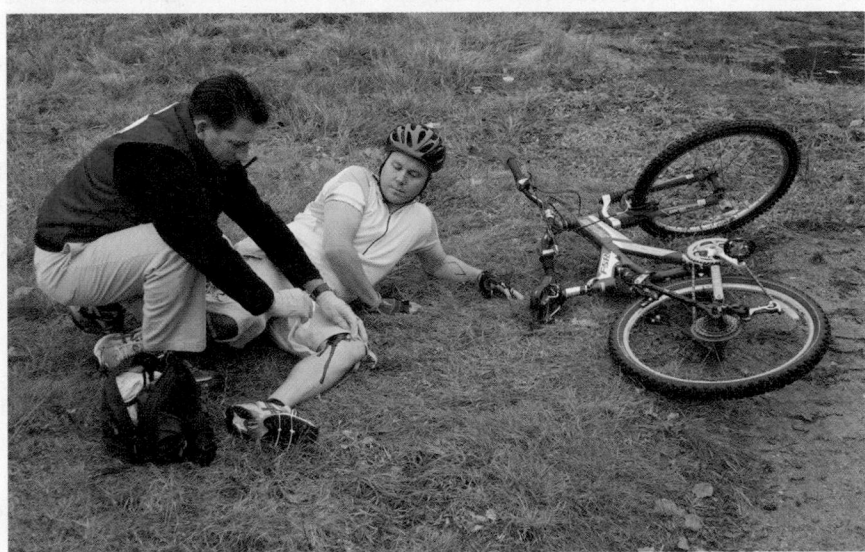

# National Ski Patrol's Early Years

**Charles Minot "Minnie" Dole**   the founder and creator of the National Ski Patrol.

In 1936, **Charles Minot "Minnie" Dole**, a 36-year-old insurance broker from Greenwich, Connecticut, realized the need for emergency care and rescue services for injured skiers following a personal mishap while skiing. Dole was skiing at Stowe, Vermont, with his wife, Jane, and their friends Frank and Jean Edson, when he heard a bone snap in his ankle, fell, and lay helpless in the snow. Frank stayed with Minnie while Jane and Jean skied down the mountain for help.

> **NOTE**
>
> ### The National Ski Patrol's Mission and Vision Statement (2009)
>
> The National Ski Patrol (NSP) is a member-driven professional organization of registered ski patrols striving to be recognized as the premier provider of training and educational programs for emergency rescuers serving the outdoor recreational community. To meet that goal and promote the safe enjoyment of snow sport enthusiasts, the NSP supports its members through accredited education and training in leadership, outdoor emergency care, safety programs, and transportation services.

The first person they met was a local farmer who told the women that people who were foolish enough to ski deserved whatever fate they met and then went on his way. Jane and Jean finally located two people who hauled Minnie off the hill two and half hours later on a makeshift toboggan improvised from a piece of corrugated tin roofing from an old shed. No splint was available to immobilize his ankle, and the resulting ride down the hill was quite painful. X-rays later showed the injury to be a severely displaced ankle fracture. During the 1930s, such injuries were difficult to treat, and Dole's doctor told him he might never walk again, let alone ski. He was determined to recover, and from this incident came the seed for the National Ski Patrol.

Two months later while still in a cast, Dole received word that his friend Frank Edson had been killed in a ski race. Dole was determined to develop a rescue program for skiers. Following a suggestion by the president of the Amateur Ski Club of New York, Roland Palmedo, Minnie was put in charge of a ski safety committee for the club. In March 1938, Dole organized a volunteer "ski patrol" for the National Downhill Races at Stowe, Vermont. Roger Langley, president of the National Ski Association (NSA)—now the United States Ski Association (USSA)—was so impressed with this patrol that he asked Dole to organize a national patrol. This marked the birth of the National Ski Patrol, which originated as a subcommittee of the NSA. Minnie Dole continued to chair the **National Ski Patrol System, Inc. (NSP)**, as it was then known, until 1950 (Figure 1-3a■ and Figure 1-3b■).

**National Ski Patrol System, Inc. (NSP)**   the largest winter rescue group in the world, as recognized by the United States Congress under Title 36 of the United States Code; is the premier snow sports rescue organization in the United States.

The NSP separated from the NSA in 1953, incorporating in Colorado and becoming an independent organization. Thanks to a distinguished legacy of altruistic service, the National Ski Patrol was recognized with a federal charter by the U. S. Congress in 1980. This is a coveted endorsement that only a few other U. S. institutions have earned, including the American Red Cross, the YMCA, and the Boy Scouts. Accordingly, the NSP annually reports directly to Congress.

As a leading authority of recreational outdoor safety and patient care, especially for ski areas, the NSP is dedicated to serving the public and the outdoor recreation industry by providing education and accreditation to emergency-care and safety-service providers. The organization is made up of more than 26,000 members, including alpine, nordic, and auxiliary OEC Technicians, who serve on over 600 ski patrols. NSP's members work on behalf of local ski and snowboard areas to improve the overall experience for outdoor recreation guests (Figure 1-4■).

## The National Ski Patrol Goes to War

By 1942, the United States was at war with both Germany and Japan. During this time, there were 180 registered patrols with more than 4,000 medically trained personnel, which included women for the first time. Also in 1942, the National Ski Patrol System (NSPS) initiated the first Air Force Search and Rescue units in collaboration with Second and Fourth Air Force Groups. The Ski Patrolmen completed 52 missions and saved at least eight lives. Still at the forefront of the NSP, Min-

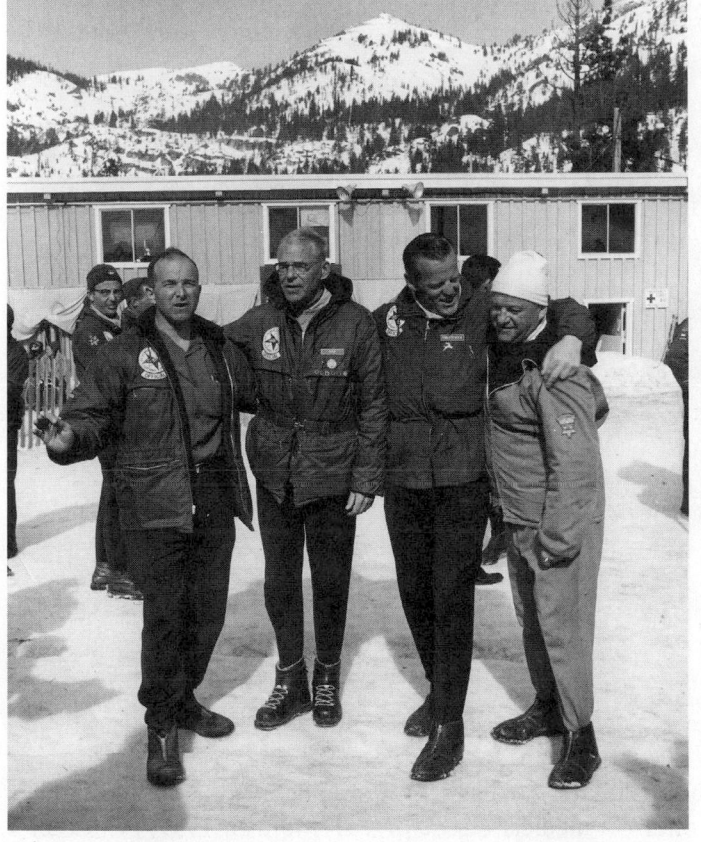

**Figure 1-3a** Minnie Dole (second from the left), the founder and creator of the National Ski Patrol, in 1938.
Copyright NSP

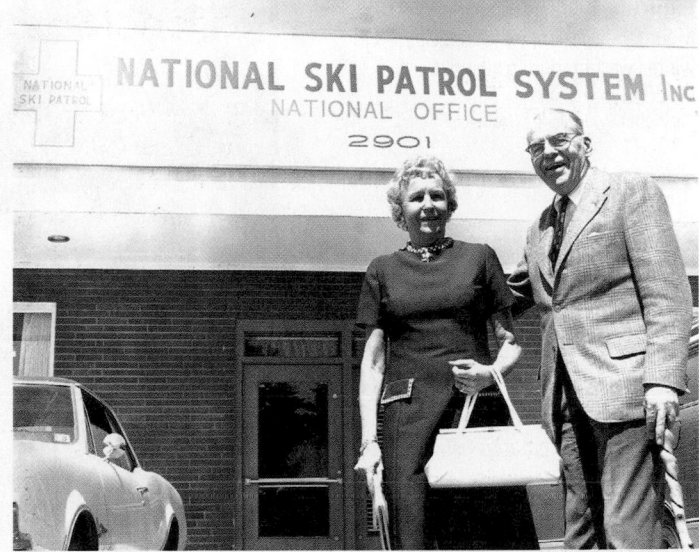

**Figure 1-3b** Minnie Dole and his wife outside the national office of the National Ski Patrol.
Copyright NSP

**1-4** Describe the role of National Ski Patrol in the formation of the U.S. Army's 10th Mountain Division.

**Figure 1-4** Memorabilia from the archives of the NSP, including the federal Charter by the US Congress of 1980.
Copyright Caleb Hund

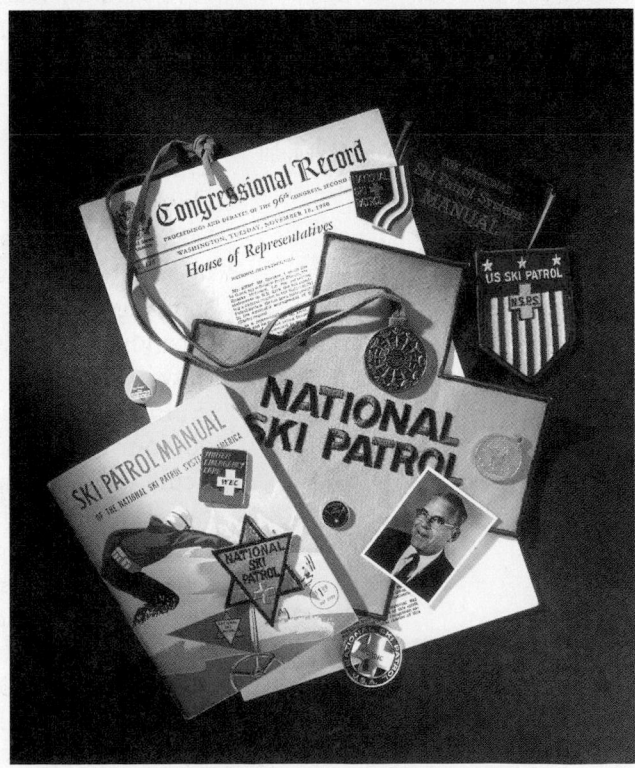

nie Dole convinced the U.S. Army's Chief of Staff, General George C. Marshall, of the value of a winter warfare unit. This concept originated with the Norwegian army when they created a cold weather unit to fight German troops.

Soon after, the 87th Mountain Infantry Regiment was activated at both Mt. Rainier and Fort Lewis, Washington. This regiment was transferred to Camp Hale, Colorado, in 1943 and was expanded to become the famous 10th Mountain Division. The NSP, the only civilian organization ever authorized to recruit for the armed forces, gathered 7,000 volunteers.

In 1944, the "Tenth" was transferred to Italy, where it performed with distinction in combat, capturing mountain strongholds that other units had been unable to take. One example is Riva Ridge, the impenetrable mountain that the Tenth took while spearheading a drive to the Po River. The ski run at Vail named Riva Ridge honors the men who participated in this assault. General Mark Clark called the Tenth the finest division he had ever seen. Following the war's end in 1945, many members of the Tenth Mountain Division who had been ski patrollers before the war returned home to become leaders—ski area owners and managers, and ski equipment manufacturers—in the growing U.S. skiing industry (Figure 1-5■).

**Figure 1-5** The members of the 10th Mountain Division, which specialized in winter warfare during World War II, included many ski patrollers.
Copyright New England Ski Museum

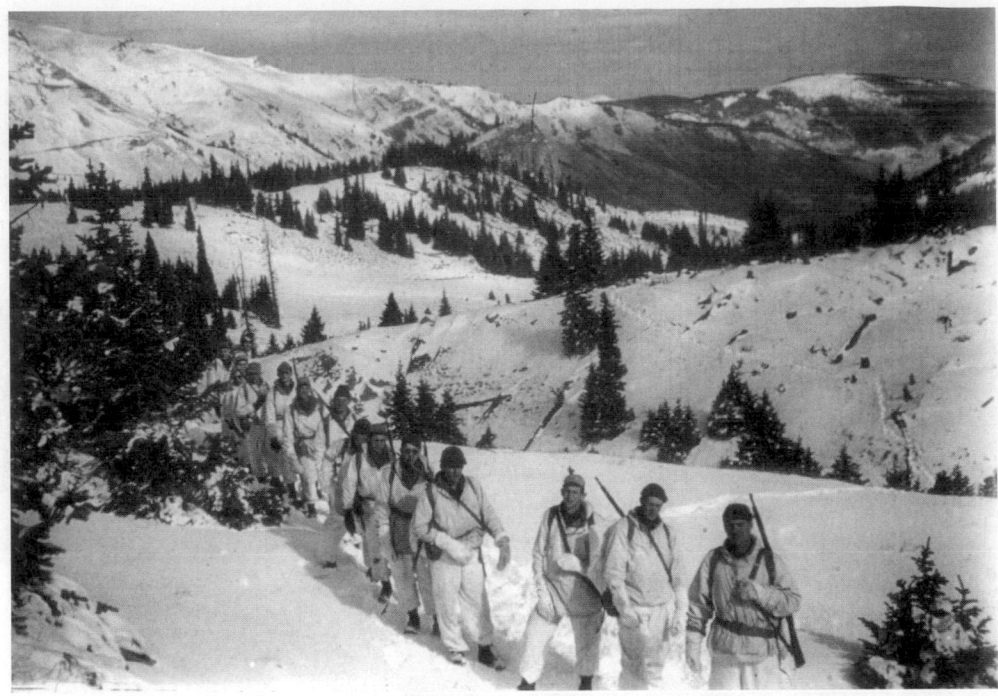

**National Medical Advisor**    a licensed physician, MD, or DO with an interest in outdoor/wilderness medicine and ski patrolling, who is appointed by the National Ski Patrol's chairman and approved by the National Ski Patrol's board of directors to serve the NSP in all matters of medical concern; chairs the National Medical Committee.

## The Birth of OEC

Since its founding, the National Ski Patrol has evolved from a handful of ski patrollers into the world's largest nonurban medical rescue organization. In 1939, NSP established an affiliation with the American Red Cross (ARC). Out of this relationship came the publication "Ski Safety and First Aid," which was written by an ARC officer, L. M. Thompson, who became the first Chairman of the NSP's Medical Advisory Committee. This position later became the **National Medical Advisor**.

For many years the American Red Cross First Aid Course proved very useful as a basic tool for ski patrollers. However, it became clear in the early 1980s that patrollers required additional training to care for patients during cold weather and at high altitude. As a result, in 1985 Dr. Warren Bowman, an internist from Billings, Montana, created an emergency responder textbook exclusively for ski patrollers, entitled *Winter Emergency Care (WEC)*. Three years later, this textbook was revised and renamed *Outdoor Emergency Care*. The new text was expanded to include information about a variety of illnesses and injuries in outdoor enthusiasts and for the first time included information about nonwinter emergencies and care for the sick and injured during sporting activities other than skiing. Those changes were made to better reflect the expanding role of OEC Technicians in providing year-round emergency care in a variety of settings.

In *Outdoor Emergency Care*, Dr. Bowman created the concept of "intermediate" outdoor medical care. OEC was positioned between the urban and wilderness curricula while emphasizing both. His idea—that OEC Technicians would begin the care of a patient in a wilderness situation, would continue care during transportation (usually using a toboggan in a ski area), and would further continue care in a first aid room or ski-area clinic—was unique to the prehospital emergency services community. The concept was widely successful, and the OEC text/curriculum was awarded the years "Best Educational Program Based on the Needs of Industry or Professional Associations" by the American Society of Association Executives (ASAE) in 1989. Truly, Warren Bowman, MD is the father of Outdoor Emergency Care (Figure 1-6■, Table 1-1■).

**⊕ 1-5**    Compare and contrast the OEC textbook and OEC course/curriculum.

# OEC Today

The field of emergency medicine is ever changing. As a result, the OEC curriculum has improved to meet the needs of ski patrollers and other outdoor emergency care professionals. Today, the OEC curriculum is the primary curriculum taught to ski patrollers at nearly every ski area in the United States, as well as to ski patrollers in Canada, Europe, Asia, and the Middle East. It also is used by others who may have need to provide emergency care in an outdoor setting, such as mountain guides and river guides, bike patrollers, law enforcement personnel, and various government agency personnel.

For over 70 years the National Ski Patrol has trained ski patrollers throughout the United States and in other parts of the world to provide emergency medical care for outdoor enthusiasts (Figure 1-7■). The National Ski Patrol's emergency care program began with the vision of its founder, Minnie Dole, and continues today in the training set forth in the OEC curriculum.

The OEC curriculum contains applicable baseline knowledge and skills identified in the U.S. Department of Transportation's (DOT) Emergency Medical Technician (EMT) National Standard Curriculum necessary for the nonurban environment. The training of OEC Technicians has been accepted and utilized by ski areas and in other outdoor environments throughout the country as the level of training of individuals who respond to accidents and deliver essential emergency care in the non-urban environment. In addition, the information and skills contained in the

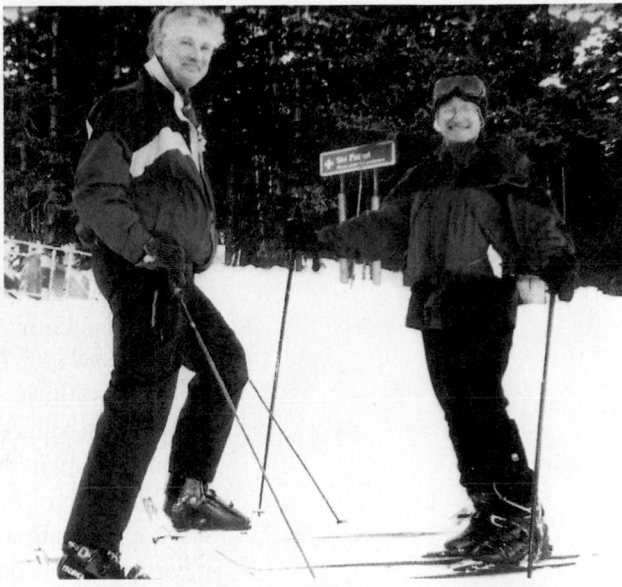

**Figure 1-6** Dr. Warren Bowman, right, the father of *Outdoor Emergency Care*, developed the concept of "intermediate" outdoor medical care. Dr. David Johe is on the left.
Copyright NSP Archives

| Table 1-1 | The National OEC Medical Advisors |
|---|---|

Warren Bowman, MD, 1970–2001
David H. Johe, MD, 2001–2007
Michael Millin, MD, 2007–2008
David H. Johe, MD, 2008–present

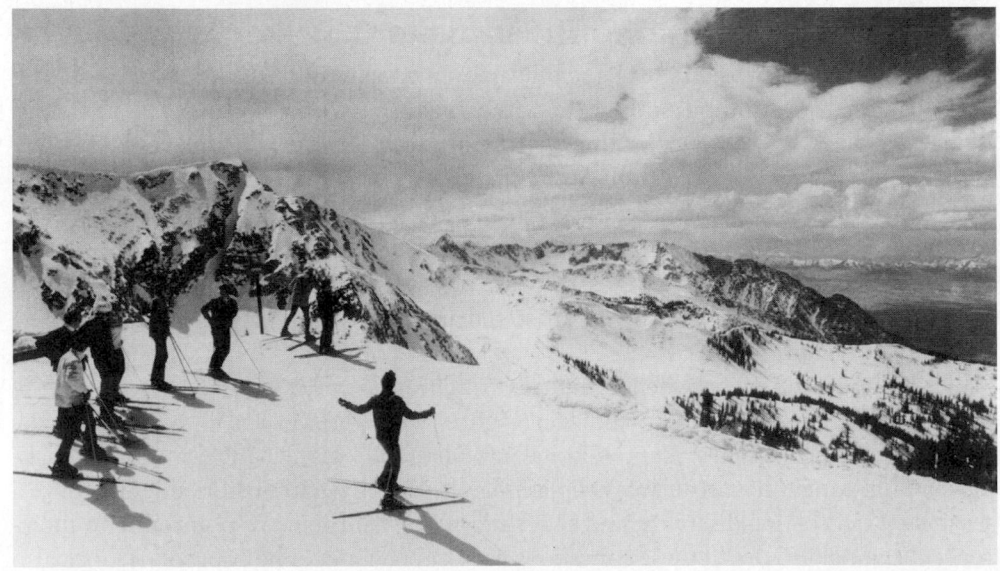

**Figure 1-7** For over 70 years the National Ski Patrol has trained people throughout the world to provide emergency care for outdoor enthusiasts.

OEC curriculum exceed the knowledge and skill level identified in the U.S. DOT's Education Standards for Emergency Medical Responder (EMR) training.

Now in this fifth edition, *Outdoor Emergency Care* is still considered the gold standard for anyone interested in becoming a ski patroller or in providing emergency care in nonurban environments. *OEC* Fifth Edition is written following the principle of "evidence-based medicine." Reviews of published, scientifically controlled studies plus retrospective evaluations of the outcomes of Emergency Medical Systems care enable us to formulate appropriate care for future patients.

Many older emergency medicine publications based training on personal observation, also known as anecdotal information. For instance, the ARC publication *First Aid Textbook* (1957, page 117) described "A Technique for Administering Manual Artificial Respiration" in which the emergency responder would place the patient on the stomach and push on the upper back with both hands (allowing inhalation), followed by pulling up on the elbows to let the air out of the lungs at a rate of 12 times a minute! This procedure was based purely on past observation and had no scientific basis. NSP has come a long way since that time, improving its course curriculum as new medical information becomes available.

Much of the current information in *OEC* on prehospital first-aid treatment comes from scientifically reviewing what works and what does not in warfare and urban trauma. What does work has been adapted throughout the OEC curriculum. Interestingly, many of the concepts of splinting, bandaging, and basic soft-tissue first aid presented in *OEC* First Edition (1988) are still appropriate today. Much of the equipment ski patrollers use today results from years of work by seasoned OEC Technicians who have made their tasks easier by creating different splints, toboggans, and other rescue equipment that work in outdoor environments. However, this edition of the text contains new information, discusses new equipment, and presents the terminology used by the prehospital community in 2010.

Throughout NSP's history, its members have devoted a significant part of their lives to providing the public emergency care, rescue services, and educational programs that promote safety and the enjoyment of outdoor recreation. As a result, hundreds of thousands of injured and ill persons have received prompt, skillful emergency care, and countless lives have been saved.

> ### The Creed of Service and Safety
>
> **NOTE**
>
> The National Ski Patrol adheres to the creed of "Service and Safety," which was established more than 70 years ago. As the ski industry has evolved, so too has the NSP. The emergence of new snow sports such as snowboarding, tubing, and snow-skating has introduced new equipment and has involved new terrain, which has required that new safety and rescue techniques and new emergency care methods be developed and taught. In addition, greater access to the backcountry has required new training and new regimens for NSP members as well.

## Training: The Focus of the OEC Program

⊕ 1-6  Describe the organization of the OEC worktext and its use during an OEC course or OEC refresher course.

To become proficient as an OEC Technician, you must first master the basic concepts of human anatomy and physiology. Without this background, you will be unable to "speak the language" of prehospital providers or understand the concepts of body functions that are so important to providing emergency care (Figure 1-8a■).

The next step is learning how to assess patients (Figure 1-8b■). This process requires much diligence and practice. Another important task to be mastered is documentation, using simple time-proven methods that are common to all prehospital and hospital providers. Only after these basics are mastered are you ready to begin learning specific medical interventions.

Learning to intervene when a patient's condition is critical is the next step in the process of becoming an OEC Technician (Figure 1-8c■). In every encounter with a critical patient, it is important that prehospital providers address the basic principles of making sure the patient has an airway, is breathing, has effective circulation, does not have a significant neurologic disability, and that they understand their responsibility to intervene when one or more of these conditions has not been met. The concept of shock also

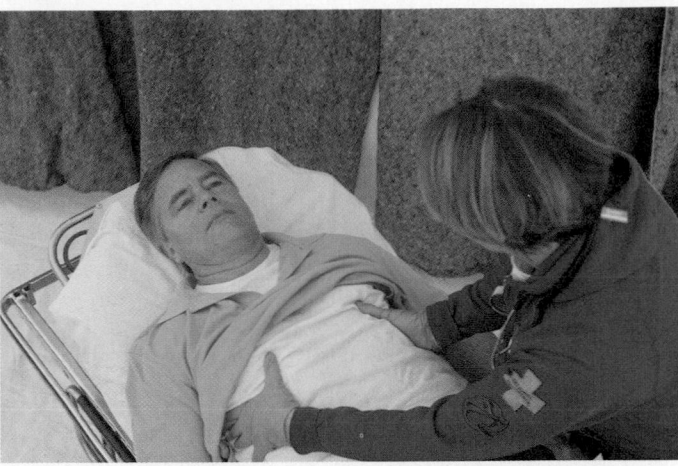
**Figure 1-8b** A student learning to perform an assessment.
Copyright Mike Halloran

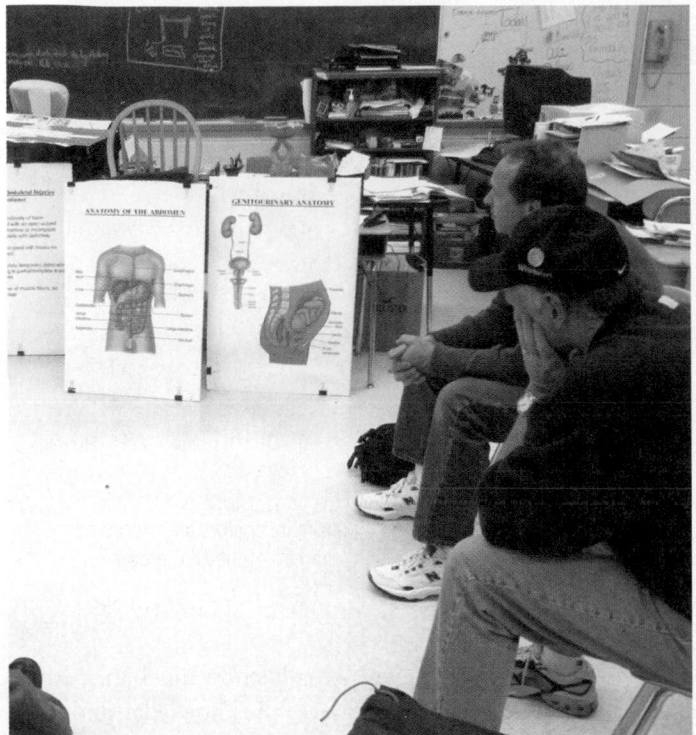
**Figure 1-8a** An OEC class learning abdominal and pelvic anatomy and physiology.
Copyright Edward McNamara

**Figure 1-8c** A student learning to intervene when the ABCDs are compromised in a critical patient.
Copyright Scott Smith

must be understood. Repeated training in evaluation, intervention, and continued care for critical patients is the best method to become proficient in helping very sick or severely traumatized patients.

By learning the functions of the body's various systems, you will be able to provide care in both medical and traumatic emergencies. Spend time to learn the body's systems, and then apply this knowledge when caring for a patient who has injured a specific body part or who has an illness affecting one or more body systems. From a broken arm to a cardiac event requiring cardiopulmonary resuscitation, OEC Technicians must be able to respond consistently to any emergency, even though the care provided will vary in different situations (Figure 1-8d■).

It is important that OEC Technicians learn the concepts and the procedures for patient care in special conditions related to high altitude, extremes of temperature, and bodies of water. Members of special populations—children, the elderly, the psychologically impaired, and individuals with special needs—have unique problems. As a certified OEC Technician, you will have the tools to care for all these people in all these special situations.

In most teaching systems, practice is an effective way to master technical skills. By learning concepts and then applying those concepts during training using the **"scenarios"** contained within both this text and the supplemental materials (e.g., Instructor Guide and the online resource MyNSPKit), OEC Technicians will be able to perform effectively in real-life situations outdoors.

As part of your OEC training, instructors will use performance-based objectives to evaluate your progress in becoming an OEC Technician. These objectives are learned through repeated practice in a variety of situations and settings (Figure 1-8e■). Once you

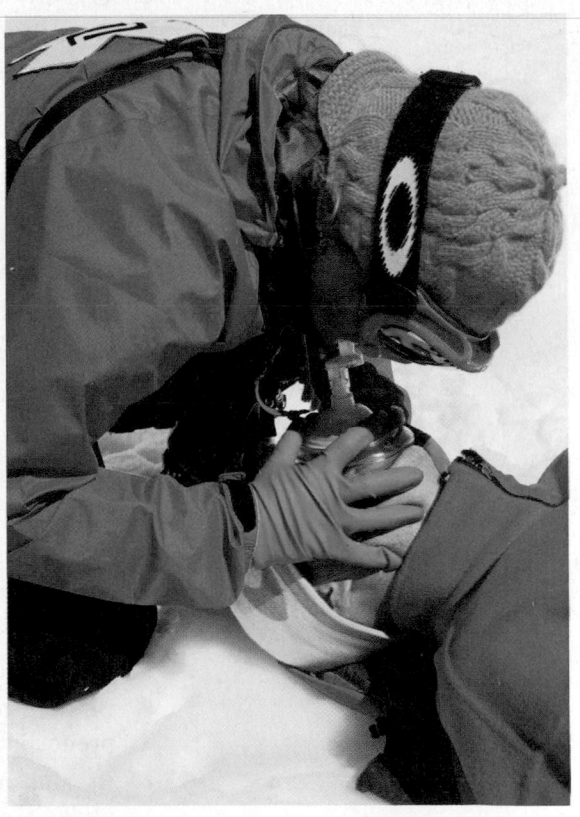

**scenario** a simulated problem that mimics a real-life medical situation.

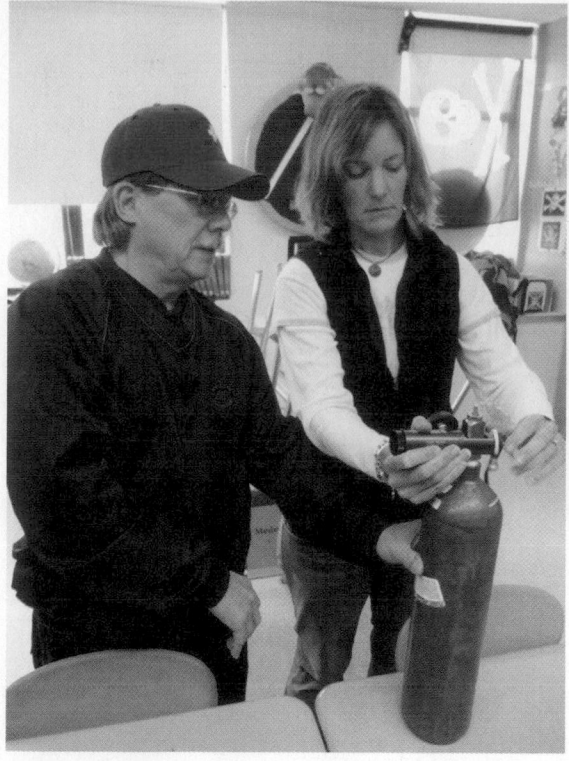

**Figure 1-8d** The OEC curriculum incorporates many opportunities for "hands on" practice of technical skills, which has been proven to be an effective learning method.
Copyright Edward McNamara

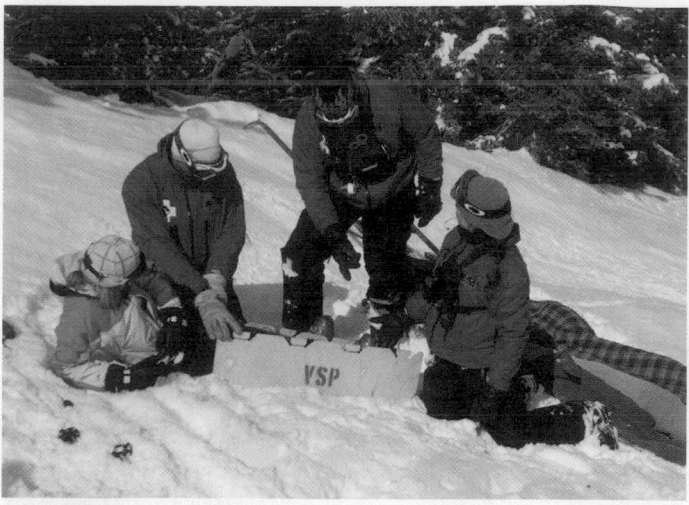

**Figure 1-8e** Evaluation and correction from instructors are important contributors to the quality and the high standard of the OEC program.
Copyright Scott Smith

have completed an OEC course, you will actually know much more than what is contained in the following list of some of the knowledge and skills goals an OEC Technician should master:

+ Assess safety, and maintain it at a rescue scene.
+ Use proper techniques to prevent unprotected contact with body fluids (Standard Precautions).
+ Assess a patient's level of responsiveness.
+ Establish and maintain an airway.
+ Assess respiration, and provide adequate ventilation.
+ Provide oxygen when necessary.
+ Assess perfusion of blood to body tissues.
+ Control bleeding.
+ Identify and address life-threatening problems, including shock.
+ Obtain a medical history of the patient.
+ Assess and provide specific care for various injuries.
+ Assess and provide care for medical illness.
+ Understand the nuances in the assessment and treatment of individuals in special populations.
+ Be able to splint or immobilize various body parts, including the spine.
+ Learn the concept of triage, and be able to help in a mass-causality situation.
+ Be able to use rescue equipment and to pack your rescue pack appropriately.
+ Understand your role as a team player in prehospital care.
+ Be able to communicate with patients, peers, and other medical providers in prehospital settings.
+ Be able to document care rendered in a form that all medical personnel can understand.
+ Understand your ski area's management needs, and interface with management.
+ Be able to identify the names of the more common medications and to describe their basic actions.

⊕ 1-7  Describe the OEC certification and recertification processes.

## Certification and Recertification Requirements

The OEC program is a prehospital emergency care course that has been developed and continuously improved by the National Ski Patrol, in conjunction with the OEC Program Director (Table 1-2■), the **National OEC Program Committee**, and the National Education Committee, with input and advice from the **National Medical Committee**. One may complete the course without having the ability to ski or snowboard. To become an "on the hill" OEC Technician, you will be required to demonstrate a level of skiing and toboggan handling proficiency to care for and transport an injured skier. You also will need to be able to perform other duties as required by the area where you patrol.

To receive an OEC certificate of completion, OEC candidates must successfully complete the OEC course. As part of this process, OEC Technicians must successfully complete a written examination developed under the direction of the OEC Program Director and distributed by the NSP's national office. In addition, prospective OEC Technicians must successfully complete a practical examination, which is also developed under the direction of the OEC Program Director and provided by the NSP National office, that may be conducted outdoors using scenarios that include simulated patients. The test is conducted by trained OEC instructors who function under the supervision and direction of a certified OEC Instructor/Trainer (Figure 1-9■).

Under current NSP guidelines, OEC certification is valid for three years (Figure 1-10■). To maintain your OEC certification, you must complete an annual

**National OEC Program Committee**   a committee composed of all Division OEC Supervisors and the National Medical Advisor, and chaired by the National OEC Program Director; provides insight and guidance to the Board of Directors annually on matters related to the functioning of the OEC program.

**National Medical Committee**   a group of physicians that includes one doctor from each division of the National Ski Patrol, the National OEC Program Director and other physicians selected at large, and the National Medical Advisor.

| Table 1-2   The Outdoor Emergency Care National Program Directors |
| --- |
| Mary Murrett, 1992–2002 |
| Larry Bost, 2002–2003 |
| Edward McNamara, 2003–present |

**Figure 1-9** Once you have successfully completed the OEC course, you'll have the important tools needed for treating people in outdoor environments.
Copyright Scott Smith

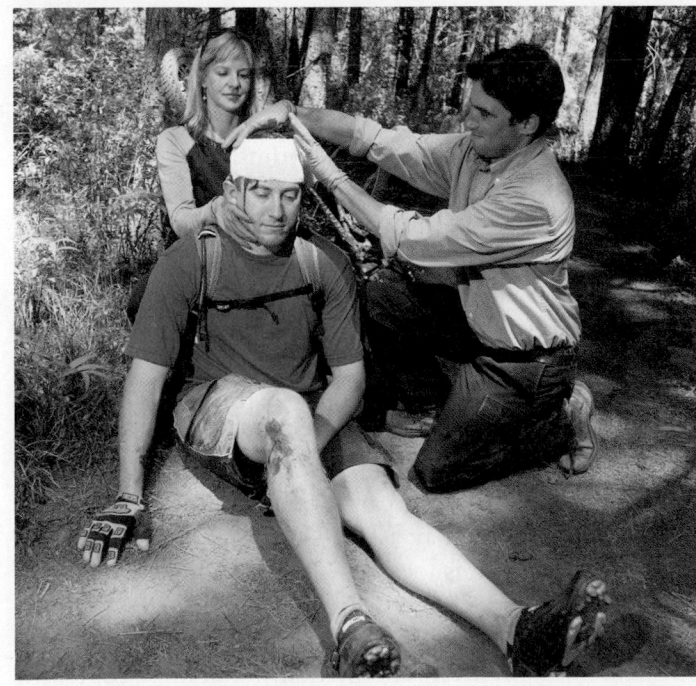

**Figure 1-10** The OEC Certificate of completion is awarded to individuals who have completed all course requirements, including successful completion of a final written exam and a practical evaluation.
Copyright NSP

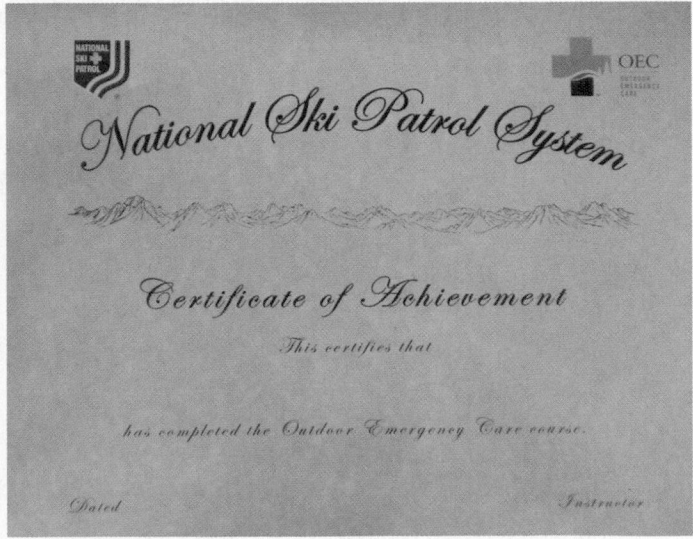

**refresher**   annual required continuing education training, usually given each year in the fall, that covers one-third of topics taught in the OEC curriculum.

**National OEC Refresher Committee**   committee appointed and supervised by the National OEC Program Director; is responsible for developing the annual OEC Refresher program.

**National OEC Program Director**   a National Ski Patrol member who is an active specialist in the field of outdoor medicine; is appointed by the NSP chairman and confirmed by the NSP board of directors; is responsible to the board for the effective management and operation of the national OEC program. This individual also chairs the national OEC Program Committee and serves as a member of the National Education Committee and the National Medical Committee.

⊕ **1-8**   Contrast the standard of training and standard of care.

**Figure 1-11** Members of the public see OEC Technicians in many different roles.
Copyright Studio 404

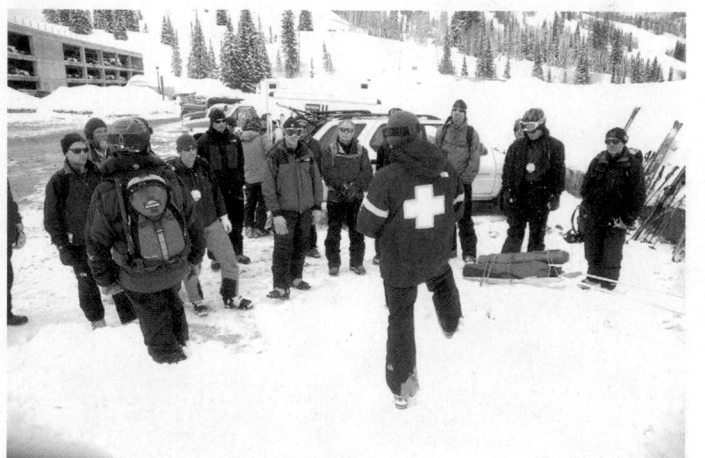

OEC **refresher** course, which may be provided by any currently certified OEC instructor. Each year, NSP develops a continuing education program that enables OEC Technicians to "refresh" their knowledge and skills. One-third of the total OEC curriculum is reviewed each year. Refreshers are primarily a "hands-on" learning experience, enabling OEC Technicians to demonstrate proficiency in the skills needed to care for a patient. Upon the completion of 3 consecutive refresher years (cycle a, b, and c) the OEC Technician will be issued a new OEC card. The refresher is developed annually by the **NSP National OEC Refresher Committee**, under the direction of the **National OEC Program Director**, and the curriculum is provided to NSP instructors.

According to NSP's policies and procedures, all NSP OEC Technicians must successfully complete the OEC course and annual refreshers to be eligible to patrol. Additionally the NSP has developed other programs that enable OEC Technicians to continue to develop leadership skills in the OEC arena.

Annually, or as required by the CPR certifying agency, each active member of the NSP must successfully complete a course given by one of the NSP-recognized organizations that teaches professional level CPR and the use of an automated external defibrillator (AED). OEC Technicians must also annually demonstrate the skill portion of this CPR curriculum to a recognized CPR instructor, regardless of how long the CPR certificate is good for.

Anyone may take an OEC course. However, because of the specific requirements for providing hands-on care, it may be difficult for all individuals to complete the course successfully. Because of the Americans with Disabilities Act (ADA) of 1990, state and government programs and services must be provided to all people. The NSP is not a state or government agency and is not regulated by laws regarding public accommodations. However, the NSP encourages its patrols to attempt to provide reasonable accommodations to students with disabilities, based on time and financial considerations. If an OEC instructor judges that students cannot complete the course with reasonable accommodations or could harm themselves or others while participating, that instructor has sole discretion in limiting those students to all or part of the course. These limitations may be necessary if others in the class are hindered in learning in a timely fashion.

## Working in Outdoor Environments

As an OEC Technician, you will have to master many roles. Your responsibilities will include that of scene manager, caregiver, patient advocate, and role model for the management who has trusted you to care for recreational enthusiasts. Your training will give you the tools to assess and help many people in outdoor environments.

Each time you respond to an incident, others will be assessing you: your appearance, presentation, demeanor, and interaction with members of the public. Their assessments will reflect on you, on your local ski area or responder agency, and on the National Ski Patrol (Figure 1-11■).

As an OEC Technician, you will provide guidance to others in nonmedical ways as well. The family of a patient, a scared child with a painful broken leg, or an autistic teen who is separated from his caregiver will all look to you for guidance. Someone may ask you a simple question about where the restroom is located. Act professionally in a kind and helpful way at all times (Figure 1-12■).

There will be times when OEC Technicians will be stressed, both physically and mentally. You must cope with

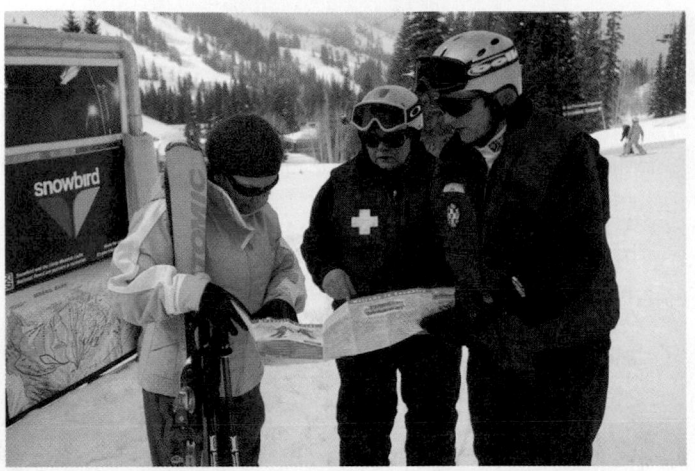

**Figure 1-12** At times OEC Technicians will interact with the public in nonmedical ways.
Copyright Studio 404

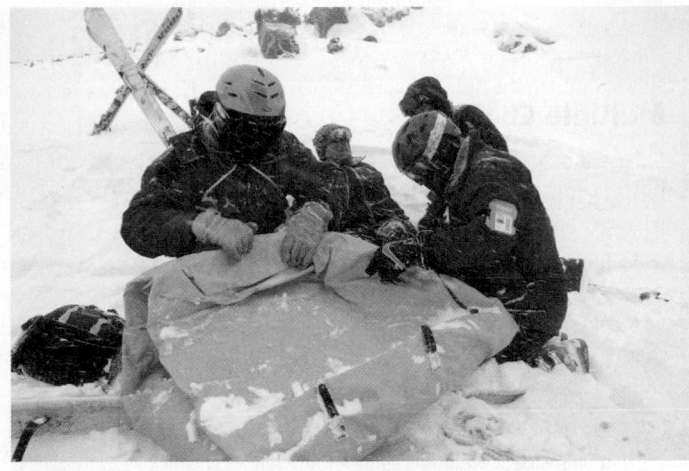

**Figure 1-13** At some accident scenes, OEC Technicians may be challenged both physically and mentally.
Copyright Studio 404

this stress during and after providing care to severely ill or injured patients. The well-being of each OEC Technician is the responsibility of everyone in your patrol or rescue agency. Working as a team, your group will provide help to each member during stressful situations (Figure 1-13■). When a rescue has been unsuccessful—as some will be, even though everything possible was done to help the patient—you may be needed to assist a peer cope with the aftermath. At other times you will need others to help you cope with an unfortunate situation.

Once you are a member of an emergency service team, you will have the unique opportunity to be the first person to help someone who could die, were it not for your initial care. Other members of the EMS community, such as ambulance crews, will interact with you (Figure 1-14■). You will be working with and delivering patients to EMTs, paramedics, nurses, and physicians who will take over the patient's care following your initial evaluation, stabilization, and transport. You will need to learn how to communicate with other members of the prehospital team to speed the patient's entry into the next phase of care. The more knowledge you have of the whole emergency care picture, the better you will be in providing your part of the patient's care.

This book includes information about the whole picture, not only to enable you to provide a higher level of medical care, but so that you also understand the complete package of prehospital care. After you give a higher level medical person a concise report about a critical patient during handoff—explaining what the patient's problem is, what you have done as an OEC Technician, and what your concerns are—and then seeing the patient seamlessly off to the hospital for definitive care, you will realize that all the effort and OEC training was worth it.

# Ethical and Legal Issues

Just as you must learn to manage an accident scene or the medical aspects of patient care, you also must learn to manage the legal aspects of rendering emergency care. Understanding how to reduce legal risk arising out of an accident situation is an important part of patrolling. The pertinent

**Figure 1-14** OEC Technicians interact with members of the local EMS system, such as ambulance services.
Copyright Mike Halloran

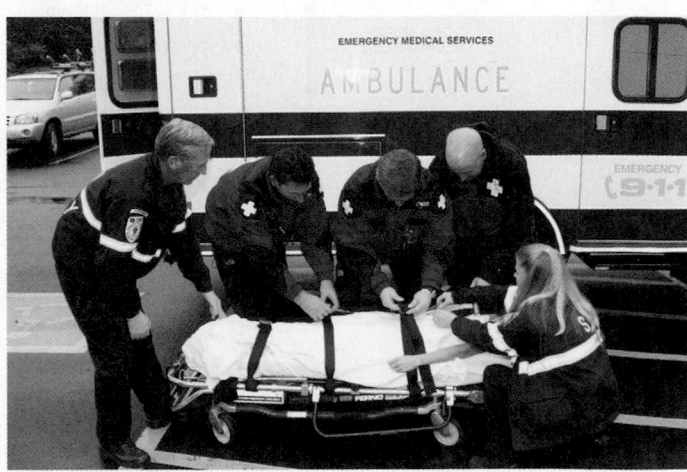

# STOP, THINK, UNDERSTAND

## Multiple Choice

Choose the correct answer.

1. What is the creed of the National Ski Patrol? _____
   a. Safety First
   b. Service and Safety
   c. Safety First, Then Service
   d. Outdoor Emergency Care Service

2. Who is responsible for forming the National Ski Patrol? _____
   a. Frank Edson
   b. President Franklin Delano Roosevelt
   c. The United States Congress, in 1938
   d. Charles "Minnie" Dole

3. Who is considered the father of Outdoor Emergency Care? _____
   a. Charles "Minnie" Dole
   b. Dr. Warren Bowman
   c. Edward McNamara
   d. Dr. David Johe

4. In what year was the National Ski Patrol recognized by the United States Congress with a federal charter? _____
   a. 1939
   b. 1948
   c. 1964
   d. 1980

## Short Answer

1. List three groups/organizations other than the National Ski Patrol that may train individuals to OEC standards.

   _____

   _____

   _____

2. Explain the significance of the Tenth Mountain Division to the National Ski Patrol.

   _____

   _____

   _____

# CASE UPDATE

You realize that the young girl's parent is not available, but because of her injury, she needs care. You must not leave the girl. The adult who found her says he saw the car that hit her and remembers the license plate number. You ask him to stay so that you can get his information once the child has received care. You put in a call for more help and EMS transport, and you ask management to come to the scene to assist you in the legal matters that will face you. Other OEC Technicians arrive, and you instruct some of them to help you with the splinting and transportation of the girl; other helpers get information from the adult who found the girl. While one helper summons the police, another begins the process of finding the child's parent.

***What should you do now?***

legal principles, when properly applied, will help you function as an OEC Technician as you render care to patients and will reduce the legal risk inherent in any accident.

Throughout the history of NSP—since Minnie Dole started ski patrolling over 70 years ago—ski patrollers have developed a good image with the skiing public. Minnie was the ultimate role model in his approach to patrolling. This "good image," which patrollers have earned over NSP's long history, is a significant protection for the patroller. Being considered the Good Samaritans of the slopes has historically meant that patrollers are rarely sued. Therefore, maintaining the good image and friendly attitude toward the skiing and snowboarding public remains an important goal of your education as an OEC Technician (Figure 1-15■).

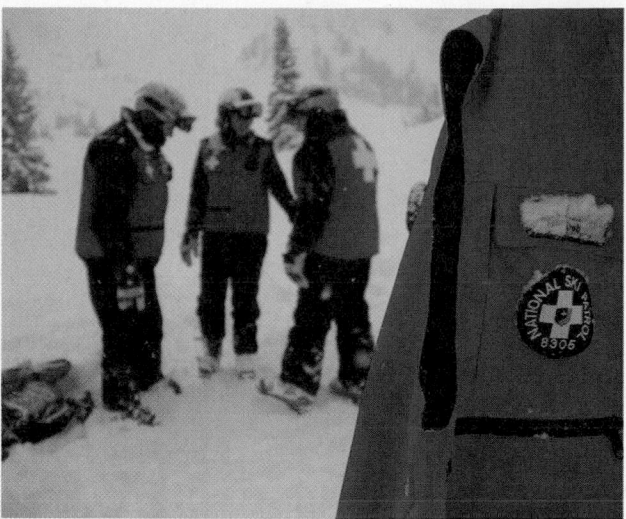

**Figure 1-15** The largest legal protection for OEC Technicians is our positive image and the respect we hold in our communities.
Copyright Studio 404

## Ethical Issues Facing OEC Technicians

As an OEC Technician, you should hold yourself to a high ethical standard. Historically, NSP patrollers and OEC Technicians have always maintained a high standard of ethical conduct with the public and with fellow OEC Technicians. Maintaining high **ethics** and the public's respect for OEC Technicians is one of the duties and privileges of the job.

The ethical principles used in resolving dilemmas in our daily lives also apply when helping a stranger who is a patient. Those principles are applied to all interpersonal relationships. OEC Technicians should follow the following five ethical principles (Beauchamp & Childress, 1979, 1994):

**ethics** the science (study) of morality or behavior that defines what is "good" or "right."

⊕ 1-11 Describe the impact of Good Samaritan laws on volunteer rescuers.

- Respect autonomy (independence). An individual has the right to act as a free agent. All are free to decide how they live their lives as long as their decisions do not harm the lives of others. Everyone has the right to exercise freedom of thought or choice. Under certain circumstances, people have the right to refuse care.

- Do no harm (nonmaleficence). OEC Technicians should not engage in any activities with the public that harm others. Any intervention provided should not cause further harm to the patient.

- Benefit others (beneficence). Our actions should actively promote the health and well-being of others. This principle is expressed in NSP's federal charter: ski OEC Technicians have a responsibility to promote skier safety.

- Be just (justice). Being just and fair balances the rights of one individual against those of others. This principle assumes three standards: impartiality, equality, and reciprocity. These standards are based on the Golden Rule, which states, "Treat others as you wish to be treated."

- Be faithful (fidelity). This principle involves loyalty, truthfulness, promise keeping, and respect of others.

## Good Samaritan Laws and Duty to Act

As previously discussed, the public has long viewed OEC Technicians as "Good Samaritans," people who help other people but expect nothing in return (Figure 1-16■). But what protects such "Good Samaritans" from legal harm when they help someone who could suffer irreversible physical harm or death, but a bad outcome ensues?

Over time, a group of laws—known as the **Good Samaritan laws**—have been enacted throughout the United States. These laws may protect voluntary OEC Technicians in providing first aid care. In general, they state that a volunteer rescuer is not civilly liable for any act or omission in giving any assistance or medical care, if (1) the act or omission is not one of gross negligence; (2) the assistance or medical care is

**Good Samaritan laws** laws that protect a person from legal liability when the person volunteers to perform an act to help someone else.

**Figure 1-16** OEC Technicians are seen as "Good Samaritans" by the public.
Copyright Edward McNamara

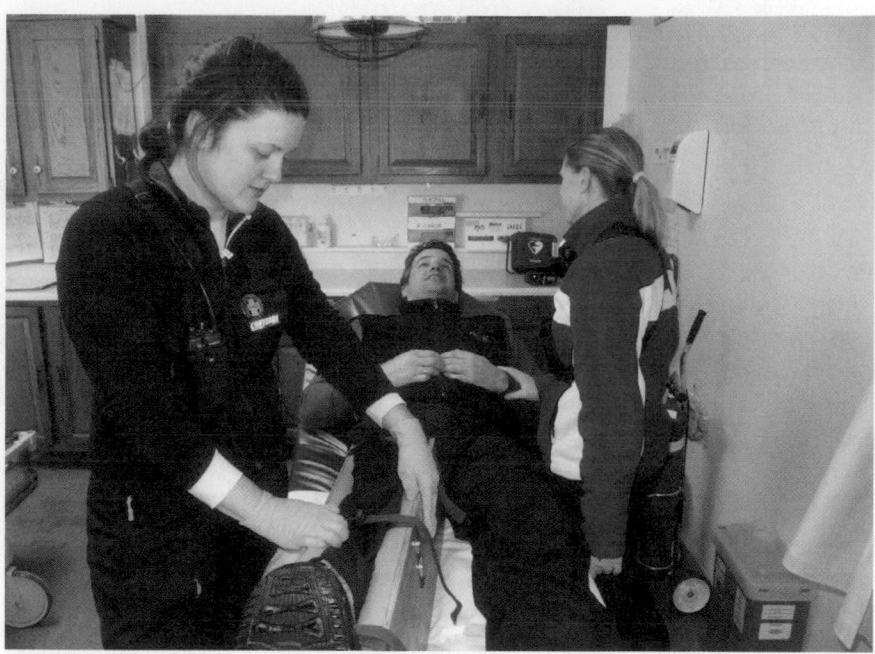

provided without fee or other compensation; and (3) the assistance or medical care is provided at the scene of an emergency, in transit to a medical facility, or through communications with personnel providing emergency assistance.

Good Samaritan laws may protect volunteer rescuers from negligent actions, but not from acts of gross negligence. *Gross negligence* has been defined as an intentional failure to perform a manifest duty in reckless disregard of the consequences as affecting the life or property of another, and it also implies a thoughtless disregard of the consequences without the exertion of any effort to avoid them. Gross negligence can also be considered a wanton or reckless disregard of the injured person by the rescuer. Consider, for example, the Colorado Good Samaritan law:

13-21-108. Persons rendering emergency assistance exempt from liability:

(1) Any person licensed as a physician and surgeon under the laws of the state of Colorado, or any other person, who in good faith renders emergency care or emergency assistance to a person not presently his patient without compensation at the place of an emergency or accident, including a health care institution as defined in section 13-64-202 (3), shall not be liable for any civil damages for acts or omissions made in good faith as a result of the rendering of such emergency care or emergency assistance during the emergency, unless the acts or omissions were grossly negligent or willful and wanton. This section shall not apply to any person who renders such emergency care or emergency assistance to a patient he is otherwise obligated to cover.

(2) Any person while acting as a volunteer member of a rescue unit, as defined in section 25-3.5-103 (II), C.R.S., notwithstanding the fact that such organization may recover actual costs incurred in the rendering of emergency care or assistance without compensation at the place of an emergency or accident shall not be liable for any civil damages for acts or omissions in good faith.

(3) Any person, including a licensed physician, surgeon, or other medical personnel while acting as a volunteer member of a ski patrol or ski area rescue unit, notwithstanding the fact that such person may receive free skiing privileges or other benefits as the result of his volunteer status, who in good faith renders emergency care or assistance without other compensation at the place

of an emergency or accident shall not be liable for any civil damages for acts or omissions in good faith.

Clearly, paragraph (3) of Colorado's law is intended to apply to ski patrollers specifically. Many other states have similar laws specifically worded to protect volunteer ski patrollers; however, OEC Technicians should be familiar with the laws of their own state because Good Samaritan laws vary from to state to state.

Good Samaritan laws are designed to encourage volunteers to provide first-aid care without the worry of being sued for negligence. These laws reflect the good work that voluntary rescuers provide the public. However, it is important that OEC Technicians make sure that the ski area or resort where they work has adequate insurance protection, and that they have adequate personal insurance.

A second important concept regarding an OEC Technician's legal obligation to provide care involves the "duty to rescue" (or "duty to act"). In general, an average citizen has no legal duty to rescue another individual who needs medical care. However, once OEC Technicians or other rescuers have put on a uniform, whether they are on duty or off, the public has a reasonable expectation that when injured a rescuer will come to them and provide care. The **doctrine of public reliance** is created whenever a rescuer may have a legal obligation to render first-aid care to an injured person in need of such care. The primary exception to this rule is when performing such care may place the safety of a rescuer or others at risk.

> **doctrine of public reliance** when the general public has been given a reasonable expectation that an OEC Technician has the ability and duty to provide first-aid services.

The legal issue as to whether an OEC Technician is required to provide first aid care when not on duty is primarily governed by individual state or provincial laws. Most states and provinces do not require OEC Technicians to provide such first-aid care. However, some states or provinces require individuals who are licensed by the state or province to render emergency care any time the person is present at an accident scene. Reviewing and understanding the relevant laws and codes concerning this legal point is important for an OEC Technician's own legal protection.

Anything that gives members of the public a reasonable expectation that an OEC Technician has the ability to provide first-aid services—for example, the wearing of a patrol jacket or other OEC insignia, even while off duty—may trigger the doctrine of public reliance. Therefore, even off-duty but identifiable OEC Technicians are representing to the general public that they have the ability to provide first-aid care, and thus those OEC Technicians should provide such first-aid care as is required.

OEC Technicians have both a moral duty and a legal duty to act. If you find someone who is injured or sick while you are off duty but are the only one around, you may have a *moral* duty to act, and you should be helped by the Good Samaritan laws. However, if you are on duty, you may have a *legal* duty to act, and you should follow the guidelines established by your management and state emergency medical system.

## Abandonment

An OEC Technician who does not provide first-aid care when legally required to do so could be liable under the legal doctrine of **abandonment**. Once you have started providing first-aid care in an emergency situation, you should continue providing such care until:

> **abandonment** to withdraw one's support or help from, especially in spite of duty, allegiance, or responsibility.

- all the care that is required has been given.
- the injured person has been transferred to another caregiver of equal or higher training and certification (Figure 1-17■).
- the injured person has specifically informed the rescuer that he or she no longer wants you to provide such emergency care.
- the patient is transported safely to a medical treatment facility.
- continuing such emergency medical care threatens the rescuer's safety.

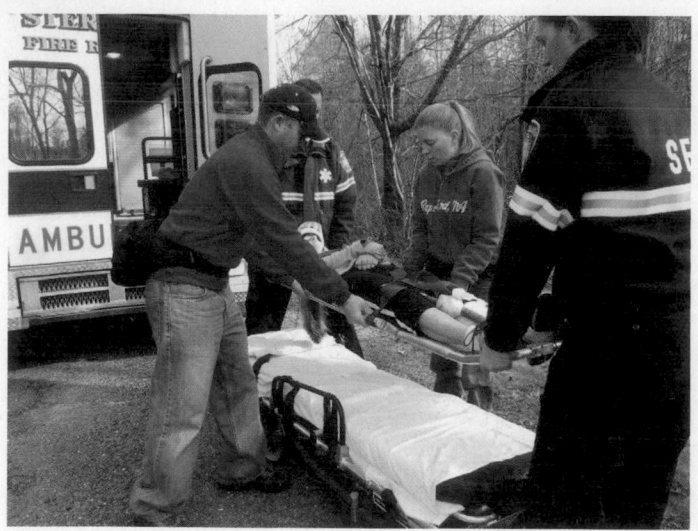

**Figure 1-17** An OEC Technician can hand off care of a patient only to personnel at an equal or higher level of care—in this case, an ambulance crew.
Copyright Edward McNamara

**breach of duty**   the failure to perform a promised act or obligation of due care.

**negligence**   the failure to exercise the care that a reasonably prudent person with similar training would exercise in a similar circumstance.

**duty to act**   a person's legal obligation to provide something to another individual.

Examples of abandonment include initiating care on an injured child and then leaving the child alone while you handle another accident, and leaving a patient awaiting ambulance transport alone in the aid room while the patient goes into shock. Once again, exceptions to the doctrine of abandonment are when providing such care could threaten a rescuer's own safety or when competent patients have informed a rescuer that they no longer want first aid care.

## Negligence and Breach of Duty

**Negligence** can occur when an OEC Technician harms an individual by not performing up to the technician's standard of training. Failure to provide care within the standard of training that a reasonable and prudent OEC Technician is expected to provide under the circumstances can also be negligence. For example, an improperly placed splint that results in further harm to the patient could be considered negligence. Therefore, it is important that a patroller exercise care and meet the standard of training when performing first aid activities in order to avoid legal negligence.

Once a **duty to act** is established, you are legally required to render appropriate care after you approach a patient. This duty of care is an obligation imposed on you as an OEC Technician that requires you to be reasonable in providing any care that could foreseeably harm the patient.

In many states, it is important to document evidence of any *contributory negligence* by the patient involved in an accident. In this situation, the patient actually contributes to his own harm. In such states, if the injured person was negligent in a manner that contributed to the cause of the accident, then the injured skier may not recover monetary damages as a result of the accident. A skier's statement that he or she was "going too fast" or "I was not looking ahead" could be considered an admission by the skier of contributory negligence and could prevent the skier from receiving a monetary recovery in court.

States that do not recognize the concept of contributory negligence might recognize the legal concept of *comparative negligence*. In such states, the legal system determines the degree or percentage of fault attributable to the patient and to other parties and then adjusts any monetary award for damages resulting from the accident based on those degrees of comparative fault.

In addressing either of these two legal principles, OEC Technicians should fully document the circumstances surrounding the accident and any care rendered, The OEC Technician should be familiar with the materials published by the National Ski Areas Association on documenting and investigating accidents.

## Assumption of Risk

A legal principle that protects patrollers is the doctrine of the *assumption of risk*. This doctrine means that when skiers or snowboarders choose to participate in these sports, they assume that the sport has inherent risks. Therefore, if a skier or snowboarder is injured while skiing or snowboarding, it is their fault. In many courts, a finding that the skier or snowboarder "assumed the risk" is all that is needed to end the legal proceeding. However, this principle is also the reason why accidents involving lifts or the transportation of these outdoor enthusiasts by the snowsports area are of greater legal concern. The skier or snowboarder might not be considered to assume the risk of being transported up the mountain, and thus injuries occurring while they are going up the mountain present a much greater potential for legal liability than injuries of those going down the mountain.

OEC Technicians should record the details of such accidents with great attention to "how" the accident was caused. They should complete the accident report in such a way that the forms indicate that the snowsports area made proper efforts to inform skiers how to go up the mountain safely. Many of the accidents that occur as skiers or snowboarders go up the mountain occur because skiers do not properly follow directions. If a skier or snowboarder does not follow the proper procedures, make sure that such information is recorded on the accident forms.

The same principle also applies to accidents that involve equipment such as snowmobiles. Collisions with such objects should be carefully documented because encountering this type of equipment might not be considered part of the "inherent risk" of skiing.

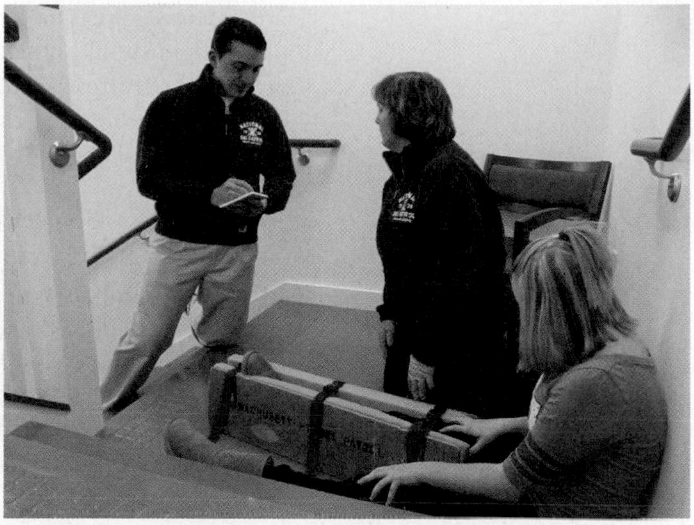

**Figure 1-18** Documentation is an important legal component of patient care. Copyright Edward McNamara

## Preparing Documentation

As part of your OEC training, you will learn to document what occurred at the accident scene. This documentation is extremely important because it might be the only reliable source of information for reconstructing in court what happened at the accident scene many years earlier. Doing a good job in preparing such documents and accident forms is a vital part of your training and a critical part of the risk management of an accident scene (Figure 1-18■).

Proper documentation includes a detailed description of the accident situation; pictures, when appropriate; names of all OEC Technicians involved in working at the accident scene; and names, addresses, and phone numbers of all witnesses. It is very important to document any statement the injured makes concerning the accident. Proper documentation and preservation of all evidence are the best legal protections for OEC Technicians and thus are skills that must be learned. However, to the extent permitted by the circumstances, OEC Technicians should always record completely and accurately all of the facts involved in the accident, as those facts are presented to them.

It is part of an OEC Technician's learned skills in the risk management of accidents to preserve statements by the injured person or any witnesses concerning either the good job performed by OEC Technicians or any admissions of fault made by the injured person. Writing down these types of statements is known as "preservation of evidence." Should an accident attended by an OEC Technician proceed to litigation, both you and the snow sports resort will appreciate the fact that the accident forms reflect the preservation of evidence.

OEC Technicians should understand that evidence that is vital to their protection can be destroyed by such events as changing snow conditions or replacement of signage; therefore, it is important that they preserve all of the evidence and accounts of the events involving an accident in a timely way. Preserving evidence is vital not only to winning legal cases, but also in preventing such cases from ever being filed (Figure 1-19■).

Preserving all evidence requires good sense, judgment, and lots of patience, so it is important to take the time to do a thorough job of completing the accident form documentation. Write everything down on the accident form neatly, completely, and with careful attention to preserving evidence that supports the fact that the patrollers did a good job. Remember that media such as photos or video are often helpful in documenting the condition of the accident scene, and that witness statements can be important in establishing what caused the accident.

**Figure 1-19** Vital evidence at an accident scene may be altered by changing weather conditions or due to a change in signage; important documentation needs to be continually updated in a log. Copyright Studio 404

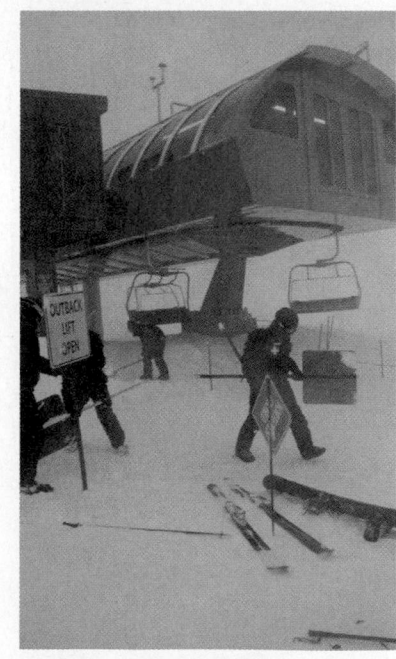

Most ski areas have a risk-management program to preserve this type of evidence. Patrollers should understand what is expected of them when a serious accident that requires the preservation of evidence and additional investigation occurs at their ski area. Understanding the area's risk-management system is a vital part of the teamwork a patrol and patrollers have with the area's management.

## Scope of Training

As previously indicated, OEC Technicians are trained in the NSP Outdoor Emergency Care curriculum, in the local protocols for emergency care required in their areas, and in the requirements of the state laws and regulations that govern first aid care. Some training, such as use of special equipment, may be unique to the local rescue unit or patrol. This scope of training will combine with what you have learned in the OEC curriculum class to become part of the level of training you are expected to perform in your local area.

The scope of training may be different for different members of a medical response team. **Emergency Medical Responders (EMRs)** and OEC Technicians usually assess the patient, provide emergency life-saving care, and perform noninvasive interventions. Other medical providers may perform invasive or advanced medical procedures. It is important for members of the medical response team to understand their roles and the limitations that are placed on them pursuant to their level of training (Figure 1-20■).

## Standard of Training versus Standard of Care

When providing first-aid services, OEC Technicians must remember that they are trained in the National Ski Patrol's Outdoor Emergency Care curriculum. OEC Technicians and EMRs are not physicians and are not trained to provide advanced life-support techniques, such as administering drugs. OEC Technicians are taught to use their judgment and, when the accident situation requires it, to request additional medical support from someone with a higher level of training. This is part of managing the legal aspects of an accident. However, acting within OEC Technicians' *standard of training* is fundamental to reducing their legal risk. It is when OEC Technicians perform procedures they are not trained to do that legal issues arise.

**Emergency Medical Responder (EMR)**   any trained individual who is first to respond on scene at a medical emergency; renders immediate care to the patient and continues care until care is assumed by a person with higher medical training.

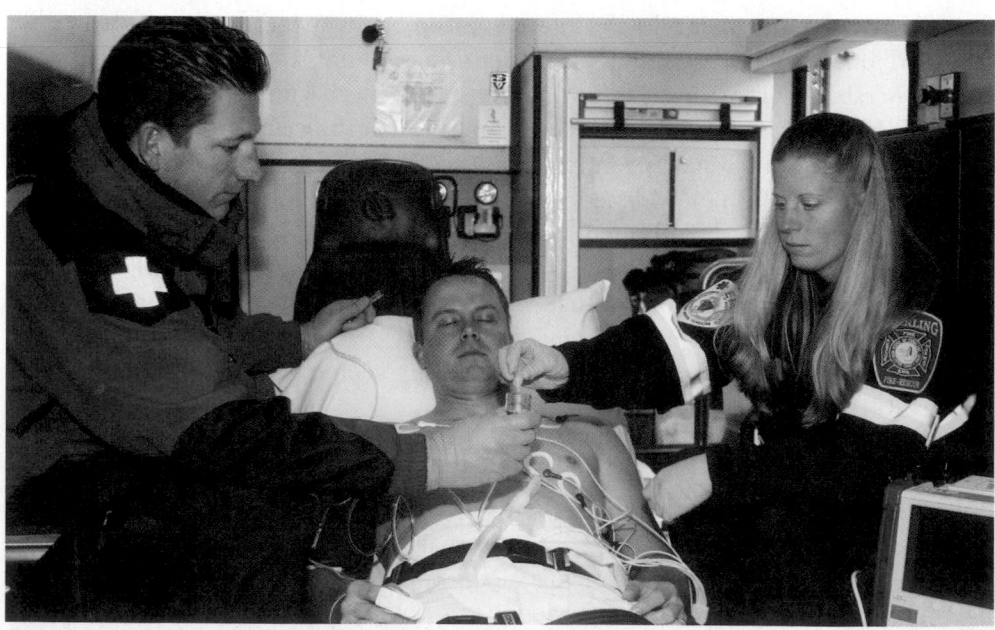

**Figure 1-20** Other "level of care" providers within EMS may be able to perform more advanced procedures.
Copyright Mike Halloran

Understanding the limits of the **standard of training** is important in reducing your legal risk as an OEC Technician. Simply put, you must know your limitations. It is important to understand that the information set forth in this textbook does *not* define the **standard of care** of an OEC Technician; the information only sets forth the standard of training that is taught by NSP's Outdoor Emergency Care program.

The standard of care an OEC Technician might be required to perform includes the training set forth in this textbook, but it also includes but may not be limited to the local area's protocols; the state's emergency medical services restrictions, laws, and procedures; and circumstances within the geographic area in which the rescuer works. It is each OEC Technician's responsibility to understand these additional elements, which, in conjunction with the training set forth in this textbook, define the standard of care that OEC Technicians should provide.

In addition to the training OEC Technicians receive in NSP's Outdoor Emergency Care, patrollers need to be familiar with the local first-aid protocols established by each OEC Technician's ski area. Those protocols, which become part of the standard of care the OEC Technician provides to the skiing public, vary from mountain to mountain. They are important because if patrollers do not perform under both the OEC standard of training and the local protocol standards, OEC Technicians might be placing themselves at legal risk.

There is an exception when working either professionally or voluntarily as an OEC Technician with OEC training. In most states when an OEC Technician is a physician, nurse, or an individual who is trained at a higher level of medical care than an OEC Technician, the OEC Technician must provide first aid at the higher standard of care, being the standard of care created by training.

## Joint Statement of Understanding

When you work as an OEC Technician at a ski area, you should be aware that you are patrolling as an "agent" of the ski area, and not on behalf of the National Ski Patrol. This distinction conforms to an agreement between the National Ski Patrol and the National Ski Areas Association in a document entitled "The Joint Statement of Understanding." This agreement states that it "is specifically agreed and understood that NSP does not control the patrol activities of OEC Technicians while they are patrolling at their respective ski areas." As such, it is understood, and may be asserted, that the ski area bears legal responsibility for patrolling activities that fall within the scope of duties of OEC Technicians. It is also understood and agreed that NSP provides educational training to individual OEC Technicians in the classroom and on the slopes, including (but not limited to) toboggan handling training, and OEC certification.

## Patient's Consent

Before providing first-aid care, OEC Technicians should obtain permission from the patient for that care. The same is true for any other medical provider. When you approach the patient, simply ask, "May I help you?" If the answer is yes, then you have permission to provide care.

OEC Technicians should be familiar with several forms of **consent**, including **expressed consent**, **informed consent**, implied consent, and **minor consent** involving minors. Expressed consent is given when a competent injured person specifically gives an OEC Technician permission to provide first aid treatment and transportation. To be competent, and to be informed consent, injured persons should sufficiently understand what first aid will be rendered in order for them to make an independent decision.

In order to provide expressed and informed consent, the injured person must be told what he or she is giving an OEC Technician consent to do. So, as a general rule it is important that OEC Technicians tell the injured person what they plan to do, so the

---

**standard of training** the training of National Ski Patrol OEC Technicians as set forth in the OEC course, using this text as a reference.

**standard of care** a level of care an OEC Technician must render based on OEC training, local medical protocols, and the requirements of a state's emergency medical system.

⊕ **1-9** Define the following legal terms:
- abandonment
- assault
- battery
- breach of duty
- consent
- duty to act
- negligence

⊕ **1-10** Describe the following forms of consent:
- expressed consent
- implied consent
- informed consent
- minor consent

**consent** to give permission or approval to something proposed or requested.

**expressed consent** consent given when a competent injured person gives permission to provide first aid treatment and transportation.

**informed consent** consent a person gives based upon an appreciation and understanding of the facts, implications, and possible future consequences of an action.

**minor consent** consent a parent or legal guardian gives for the treatment of a minor because legally the minor is not competent to give consent to medical treatment; the ability to provide such consent varies among states.

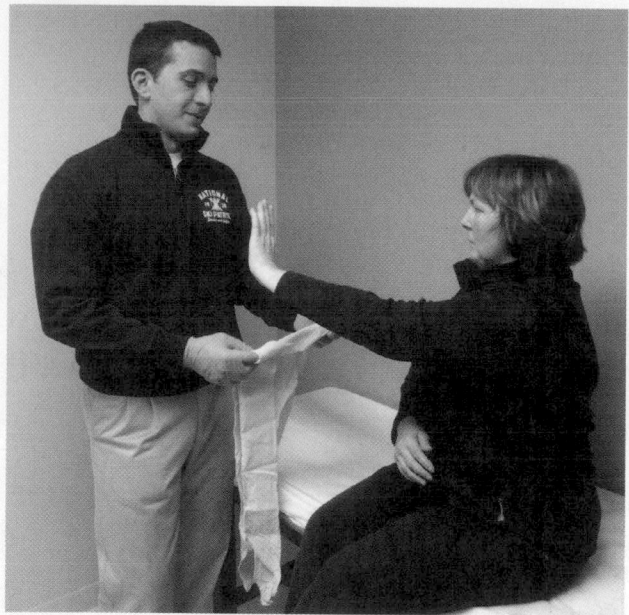

**Figure 1-21** Patients have the right to refuse treatment. However, OEC Technicians should have written documentation stating that refusal of treatment places the patient's health at risk.
Copyright Edward McNamara

**implied consent**   a form of consent that is not expressly granted by a person, but instead is inferred from a person's actions and the facts and circumstances of a particular situation.

**Figure 1-22** Implied consent gives health care providers permission to treat some patients, even if the patient's verbal authorization has not been given.
Copyright Edward McNamara

injured person can provide the necessary expressed consent. When you arrive on scene and approach the patient, simply say, "I'm David with the ski patrol, may I help you?" Once you have collected the history, ask, "May I examine you, care for you, and transport you?" If the patient says yes, then you have obtained express consent and you may treat the patient. Before rendering first aid, and if the circumstances permit, inform the injured person of the first-aid procedures you are going to perform, such as "I am going to put your leg in a quick splint," so the injured person can provide his or her expressed consent.

The concept of expressed consent can become complex at an accident scene. For example, an injured skier might provide a ski patroller with expressed consent to provide basic first aid; however, the injured skier might refuse to allow a patroller to transport him or her down the mountain. This situation involves both expressed consent and a refusal of care. If there is a refusal of care and the patroller, using a patroller's good judgment, believes that the refusal places the injured skier at risk, then the patroller should create an accident form, and the injured skier's refusal should be carefully documented (Figure 1-21■).

Another type of consent is **implied consent**. In general when an injured individual is not capable of providing expressed consent, implied consent may apply. Implied consent means that the patient would request first-aid care if he could provide the consent (Figure 1-22■). A classic example of such a situation is when an OEC Technician arrives at an accident scene and finds an unresponsive injured skier. In such situations, the general law allows the OEC Technician to assume that that skier has given the consent necessary for the OEC Technician to provide first aid to that skier. Other examples of situations in which implied consent applies are when the injured skier is delusional or unresponsive as a result of taking alcohol or drugs, and when the injured skier is otherwise physically unable to give expressed consent. In some situations, consent can be given by a spouse or a parent of an injured skier who is unable to provide such consent.

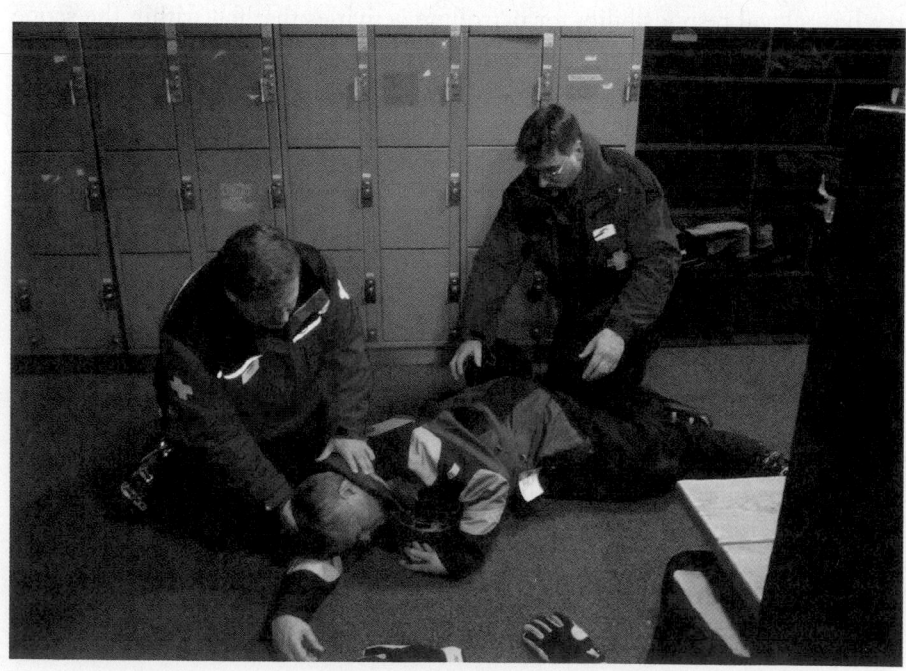

Consent Involving Minors

Some states have determined that minors do not to have the judgment necessary to provide expressed consent. In those instances OEC Technicians should attempt to obtain such consent from a parent or legal guardian. However, if a parent or legal guardian is not available, implied consent allows OEC Technicians to conduct first aid and provide transportation. In addition, in many ski areas groups of minors provide group leaders or chaperones written consent-to-treatment forms. Therefore, if a parent or guardian is not available, OEC Technicians should look to the group leader or chaperone to obtain expressed consent after ascertaining that the group leader or chaperone has the authority to provide such consent. Even though there may be no legal obligation to do so, OEC Technicians should use their good judgment and try to contact the parent or the legal guardian by telephone to keep that parent or legal guardian informed as to the minor's immediate first-aid needs.

## Refusal

Allowing an injured skier the opportunity to refuse first aid is important. If the injured skier denies an OEC Technician's offer to provide first-aid assistance, this denial should be carefully documented. It is important to document that you have explained the risks the patient is taking by refusing care. Without proper documentation, OEC Technicians may be exposing themselves to risk according to the doctrine of abandonment. Therefore, if a skier refuses first aid, OEC Technicians should document the refusal in writing, signed by the injured skier and, if possible, witnessed by another OEC Technician.

If a patient refuses first-aid treatment, attach a *written* refusal of first aid to an accident form in which all the required basic information has been entered. If the injured skier refuses to cooperate in preparing such a form, the OEC Technicians involved should carefully document that refusal and complete an accident form that includes the circumstances surrounding the injured skier's refusal of first aid. Having another OEC Technician as a witness on the completed form verifies that the injured skier refused first aid. In such circumstances, OEC Technicians should consider notifying the ski area's risk-management personnel.

When an injured skier is competent to provide consent or when a risk of serious injury or death exists if treatment is not provided, it is usually best to provide the treatment. The legal risk of not providing treatment outweighs the legal risk of not complying with the directions of the injured skier, who might later be found incompetent to have provided such directions.

## Assault and Battery

OEC Technicians who continue to provide first aid after receiving a competent refusal of such first aid are placing themselves at legal risk of being accused of **assault** and **battery**. This situation could lead to both civil and criminal offenses. Touching someone who does not desire to be touched is known as battery, whereas placing a person in a position in which he reasonably fears that battery will occur is known as assault.

The use of physical force is very rarely justified. An example in which some force is justified is restraining an injured skier who has a head injury and is thrashing around on the ground in order to protect the individual from further trauma.

If a skier threatens you with the use of force, back away and call for more patrollers and area security staff. If possible, isolate the individual from the rest of the skiing public and, if appropriate, request assistance from local authorities who are authorized to forcibly restrain the individual, if necessary.

OEC Technicians should be trained to avoid finding themselves in a position in which they could be accused of assault or battery. In such circumstances, OEC Technicians are trained to request assistance from management and from the local police. All

**assault**  placing somebody into a position where he or she reasonably fears that battery will occur.

**battery**  the act of touching someone without his or her consent.

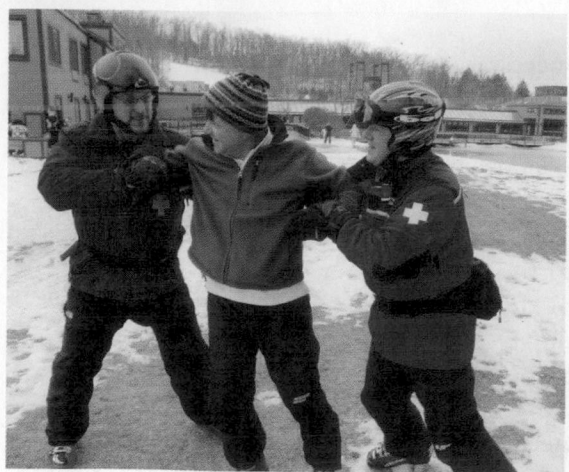

**Figure 1-23** Disorderly, unruly patients sometimes require special handling.
Copyright Edward McNamara

OEC Technicians should become familiar with their ski area's policies on the forcible restraint of individuals (Figure 1-23■).

## Judgment

One of the core skills of OEC Technicians is learning to use proper judgment. OEC Technicians are trained to rely on their "judgment" because each accident situation is different. If an OEC Technician sees that the people at an accident scene are escalating emotionally, or if an adversarial relationship is developing between the injured skier and witnesses concerning the accident, the OEC Technician should immediately request additional help. The assistance of additional OEC Technicians can help calm such situations, and it also provides excellent witnesses to assist the patroller at the accident scene. Obtaining additional help to control the skiing traffic near the accident scene is only good judgment.

Using good judgment to manage an accident scene both helps provide the proper emergency medical care required and reduces legal risk. As an OEC Technician, you should remember to (1) provide the first-aid care within your standard of training, (2) practice and maintain your skills so you can remain proficient in providing first-aid care, and (3) use good judgment and planning to manage the medical and legal aspects of the accident scene in a safe manner.

## Training

Training OEC Technicians poses its own legal risks. By the very nature of training, trainers must challenge the skills of their trainees so that each trainee's skills grow and improve. Since ski patrolling can be inherently dangerous, training OEC Technicians can be dangerous. Controlling that danger through risk management and proper supervision is part of what a trainer must do. But the legal obligations and responsibilities go both ways; trainees also must recognize that they have limited skills and should not place themselves during training in a situation that does not only stretch their skills but instead places themselves and other trainees in danger. Trainees must accept the responsibility for their own risks, and trainers must be skilled enough to train trainees properly, without exposing them and others to unnecessary risk (Figure 1-24■).

**Figure 1-24** During training events, instructors are responsible for minimizing some of the risks that may make the learning of skills dangerous.
Copyright Scott Smith

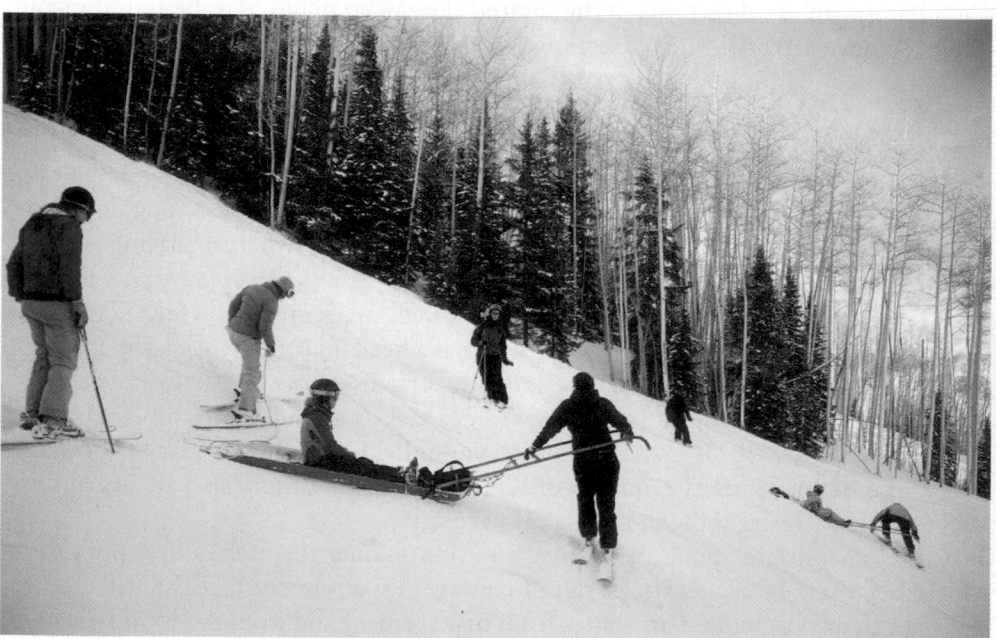

## EMS System Regulations

Each state has its own emergency medical system, known as EMS. Different states prohibit the use of different types of first-aid procedures unless proper training and certification has been obtained from the state or province. The National Ski Patrol has not designed the information in *Outdoor Emergency Care*, Fifth Edition, for any particular state or province but has, instead, designed the text to provide the best outdoor emergency care training for OEC Technicians everywhere. Therefore, it is important that OEC Technicians understand the level of care they can provide to patients based on their particular state's or province's EMS laws, rules, and regulations.

## Privacy Laws

The general trend of current laws is to keep medical information about injured persons private. To that end, the U.S. Congress passed the **Health Insurance Portability and Accountability Act** of 1996, also known as **HIPAA**. HIPAA was enacted to protect the privacy of an individual's medical information. The act specifically pertains to care providers who are compensated for the care they provide when the patient's information is transferred electronically.

HIPAA likely does not apply to volunteer patrolling activities because patrollers do not receive direct compensation for the medical services they render to injured skiers, and patrollers generally do not bill for medical services electronically or transfer medical information electronically.

However, the application of HIPAA could vary from ski area to ski area. For example, some ski areas operate a medical clinic as part of the ski area's medical facility. Because the clinic might be governed by HIPAA regulations, a patrol should ensure that its base of operations is physically separate from the clinic, so that the public can distinguish between patrol operations and clinic operations.

Additionally, some paid patrols might be subject to HIPAA requirements. Failure to comply with HIPAA laws may result in serious consequences, including fines and criminal prosecution. The determination of whether HIPAA applies to your patrolling activities must be made by your ski area. It is not a National Ski Patrol decision. Check with your area management to find out whether HIPAA laws apply to you.

Even though most volunteer patrols are exempt from HIPAA laws, that exemption does not mean there should be no attempt to keep private the medical information obtained from an injured skier. Simply put, OEC Technicians should always be conscious of the privacy of injured skiers and should not use their names or provide any information that could identify them, unless absolutely necessary.

**Health Insurance Portability and Accountability Act (HIPAA)** a law that addresses the confidentiality of the electronic transmission of medical records; applies to medical personnel who are compensated for service.

## Teamwork

One of the best ways to manage the legal aspects of an accident scene is for OEC Technicians to remember that they are part of a team of fellow OEC Technicians. Making the decision to call for additional help is one important way to manage an accident situation properly. Additional OEC Technicians assisting at an accident scene not only help OEC Technicians with the first-aid needs of the patient but also act as witnesses, preventing the situation in which it is a skier's word against a single OEC Technician's word. This team's ability to support an OEC Technician's account of events at the accident scene reduces that OEC Technician's legal risks.

# STOP, THINK, UNDERSTAND

## Multiple Choice

Choose the correct answer.

1. All of the following are ethical principles that should be followed, except _____
   - a. be just (justice).
   - b. do no harm (nonmaleficence).
   - c. be genuine (genuineness).
   - d. be faithful (fidelity).

2. Before leaving a patient who is refusing care, OEC Technicians should do all of the following except _____
   - a. explain the risk the patient is taking by refusing care.
   - b. document that you have explained the risks the patient is taking by refusing care.
   - c. have the patient sign a refusal of care document, if possible witnessed by another OEC Technician.
   - d. wish the patient well and leave the scene.

3. Which of the following situations represents the best example of expressed consent? _____
   - a. a frightened 6-year-old female who says nothing and allows you to provide care
   - b. a drunken 22-year-old male who agrees to let you provide care
   - c. a college roommate who provides consent for his diabetic, unresponsive friend
   - d. a 37-year-old snowboarder who requests your help

4. What type of consent would be in effect for an unresponsive 14-year-old male snowboarder? _____
   - a. expressed consent
   - b. implied consent
   - c. informed consent
   - d. assumed consent

## Short Answer

1. What is the purpose of Good Samaritan laws?

   _____

   _____

   _____

2. Explain the difference between *standard of training* and *standard of care*.

   _____

   _____

   _____

## Matching

Match each of the following numbered terms with the appropriate description.

_____ 1. abandonment
_____ 2. assault
_____ 3. battery
_____ 4. breach of duty
_____ 5. consent
_____ 6. duty to act
_____ 7. negligence

- a. to give permission or approval to something proposed or requested
- b. the act of touching someone without their consent
- c. to withdraw one's support or help from, especially in spite of duty, allegiance, or responsibility
- d. placing somebody into a position in which he or she reasonably fears battery will occur
- e. the failure to perform a promised act or obligation of due care
- f. a person's legal obligation to provide something to another individual
- g. the omission or neglect of reasonable care, precaution, or action

 CASE DISPOSITION

You care for the girl, rendering first aid until the ambulance arrives. Following your report to the EMT and paramedic, they take over transporting her to the hospital. Management arrives, as do the police, and you direct them to the witness, so that his statement may be obtained. The girl's parents are found in their condominium, and you explain to them what happened. While the mother accompanies her daughter to the hospital, you go back to the aid room and complete your paperwork. The next day, the mother calls the patrol room to tell you her daughter has a new cast on her leg and will be all right. Management informs you that the police found the driver who hit the girl.

# ✚ Chapter Review

## Chapter Summary

Becoming an OEC Technician requires commitment, diligence, understanding, perseverance, and good judgment. As one looks at the history of the NSP and specifically of OEC, you can see why the NSP'S OEC training is the most respected program for the snow sports industry, and now for many other EMS entities as well. Other outdoor emergency first-aid care providers are now turning to the OEC training to satisfy their needs.

Once completed, this course will give you the knowledge and tools you need to provide first aid to any patient in any outdoor (or indoor) environment, including cold and high-altitude conditions, wilderness and urban settings, and specifically at a ski resort. No other curriculum does this. No other curriculum is so extensive. By participating in annual OEC refreshers, you will keep your skills up to date and learn additional information to provide high-quality care to your patients.

OEC Technicians have a long history of successfully managing accident scenes, both medically and legally. This success is a testament not only to the quality of OEC Technicians, but to their good training. When OEC Technicians are managing the legal aspects of an accident scene, they should use their good judgment and render care within the standard of their training. When OEC Technicians are performing their many tasks, they should always remember to properly document the accident and the ensuing events. Once you have completed the OEC curriculum using this text, you will understand the role and practice of being an OEC Technician.

## Remember...

1. NSP was founded in 1938 by Minnie Dole.
2. OEC certification is a standard of training, not a standard of care.
3. The terminology used in this textbook is the same terminology used by all prehospital providers.
4. Your local management in conjunction with medical direction will establish the standard of care at your ski area.
5. Whenever possible, obtain consent before making physical contact with a patient.

## Chapter Questions

### Multiple Choice

Choose the correct answer.

1. All of the following are included in proper documentation, except _____
   a. the names of all OEC Technicians involved in the accident.
   b. the names, addresses, and phone numbers of the ambulance crew to whom you transferred the patient.
   c. a detailed description of the accident situation.
   d. the names, addresses, and phone number of all witnesses.

2. Upon successful completion of an OEC course, how long is OEC Technician certification valid? _____
   a. 1 year
   b. 2 years
   c. 3 years
   d. 4 years

3. The Outdoor Emergency Care curriculum is designed to exceed the U.S. DOT's standards for _____
   a. Emergency Medical Responder.
   b. Emergency Medical Technician.
   c. Advanced Emergency Medical Technician.
   d. Paramedic.

4. Leaving a patient without transferring them to another qualified individual is considered _____
   a. negligence.
   b. breach of duty.
   c. abandonment.
   d. assault.

5. A competent adult may do all of the following except _____
   a. grant you permission to provide care to a friend.
   b. refuse care at any time.
   c. accept care at any time.
   d. grant you permission to care for their child.

## Short Answer

1. List ten knowledge/skill sets that an OEC Technician should master.

_____
_____
_____
_____
_____
_____
_____
_____
_____
_____

2. Explain the process for maintaining one's OEC certification.

_____
_____
_____

# Scenario

*Today is the first day of the season at High Top Ski Area. You completed your OEC course last season and were promoted to full-status patroller. As you prepare to begin your first shift, your shift mentor approaches you. Together, you reflect on the many hours of training you received during your OEC course and recount some of the key points of being a patroller.*

*OEC Technicians must obtain permission to care for a patient.*

1. In which of the following cases is consent implied? _____
   a. The patient is fully responsive and has a laceration on his arm.
   b. The patient is a minor child.
   c. The patient is in cardiac arrest.
   d. The patient has crushing chest pain and requests your help.

*In the state where you patrol, there are laws that protect volunteer rescuers from liability while providing emergency care to a patient.*

2. The law(s) are collectively called the _____
   a. Minnie Dole Protection Act.
   b. Good Samaritan Law.
   c. Volunteer Rescuer Liability Law.
   d. First Responder Liability Act.

3. In order for OEC Technicians to maintain their certification, they must _____
   a. retake the OEC course every 4 years.
   b. apply for a new OEC card every 3 years.
   c. participate in an online EMS refresher course annually.
   d. attend a registered NSP refresher course annually.

*Although laws vary by state or province, an OEC Technician may have a duty to act and be required to render emergency care.*

4. The doctrine of public reliance is created when _____
   a. an OEC Technician is in uniform, whether on or off duty.
   b. the patient has a paid resort pass.
   c. the patient asks for help, even with untrained bystanders.
   d. the patient is responsive and in a public place.

5. While you are performing the duties of an OEC Technician, which of the following is NOT true? _____
   a. You must maintain a professional appearance and manner at all times.
   b. You should wear a clean and easily identifiable uniform.
   c. You should be nonjudgmental and not react negatively or aggressively.
   d. You should identify yourself as an EMT (if you are certified).

*Lawsuits can result from improper care, lack of care, or abandonment of care to the patient.*

6. Abandonment of care is best defined as _____
   a. the intentional stoppage of care without a legal excuse.
   b. treating a patient without first obtaining permission.
   c. failure to provide care equal to the standard of care.
   d. failure to respond to an injured party while on duty without just cause.

# Suggested Reading

Beauchamp, Tom L., and James F. Childress. 1994. *Prinicples of Biomedical Ethics*, Fourth Edition. New York, New York: Oxford University Press.

Besser, Gretchen R. 1983. *The National Ski Patrol: Samaritans of the Snow*. Woodstock, Vermont: Countryman Press.

EXPLORE **PEARSON myNSPkit**™

Please go to www.myNSPkit.com. Under Student Resources, you will find animations, videos, web links, and games related to this chapter—and much more. Look for information on EMS systems and organizations that are resources to the OEC Technician.

Register your access code from the front of your book by going to www.myNSPkit.com and selecting the appropriate links. If the in-cover access code has been redeemed, go to www.myNSPkit.com and follow links to **Buy Access.**

# Emergency Care Systems

Denis Meade, MA, EMT-P
Michael G. Millin, MD, MPH, FACEP

**2**

## ⊕ OBJECTIVES

**Upon completion of this chapter, the OEC Technician will be able to:**

**2-1** List six attributes of an emergency care system.

**2-2** List four nationally recognized prehospital emergency care provider levels.

**2-3** Compare and contrast direct medical oversight and indirect medical oversight.

**2-4** Describe the purpose of quality improvement.

## ⊕ KEY TERMS

**Advanced Emergency Medical Technician (AEMT),** *p. 39*

**emergency care system,** *p. 32*

**emergency medical dispatcher (EMD),** *p. 42*

**Emergency Medical Responder (EMR),** *p. 38*

**emergency medical services (EMS),** *p. 35*

**Emergency Medical Technician (EMT),** *p. 39*

**medical director,** *p. 42*

**medical oversight,** *p. 45*

**National Highway Traffic Safety Administration (NHTSA),** *p. 35*

**Outdoor Emergency Care (OEC) Technician,** *p. 32*

**Outdoor First Care (OFC) Provider,** *p. 32*

**paramedic,** *p. 39*

**prehospital provider,** *p. 38*

**protocols,** *p. 50*

**"Scope of Practice,"** *p. 39*

## Chapter Overview

Each day, tens of thousands of people around the world are involved in an emergency medical situation. Often these individuals require treatment before reaching a medical facility. In the past, people who became acutely ill or injured had to rely on friends, relatives, or strangers to come to their aid and transport them to a hospital. As a result, victims often suffered permanent, debilitating problems or died because they did not receive timely, effective medical care. Today, patient outcomes are significantly better,

*continued*

## HISTORICAL TIMELINE

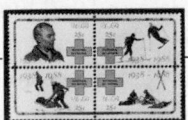

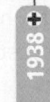 **1938** National Ski Patrol is founded.

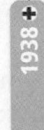 **1938** First Ski Patrol created in Estes Park, CO.

**1938** National Patrolmen, a higher rank than locals, wore this patch, designed by Livingston Longfellow.

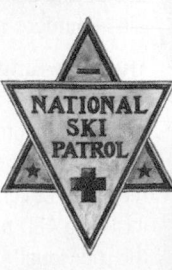

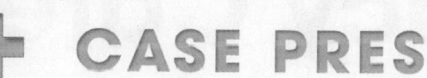 

# CASE PRESENTATION

While you are on vacation and skiing with a group of friends, one of your companions takes a hard fall. As you and the other members of your party ski up to him, you find him lying on his side, clutching his ankle. He is moaning loudly and appears to be in great distress. A quick examination reveals intense pain in the man's right lower leg/ankle, which is bent at an unnatural angle. He is awake and has no other apparent injuries but is unable to stand, let alone get down the mountain on his own.

**What is the first thing you should do?**

**emergency care system**
a network of specially trained personnel, equipment, facilities, and other resources that respond to medical emergencies. See EMS.

thanks to the advent of modern **emergency care systems**, which bring specifically trained personnel and resources to the scene of an emergency shortly after the situation occurs or symptoms become apparent. This coordinated response is part of an organized continuum of care that begins the moment the emergency care system is activated and continues long after the patient reaches the hospital.

Emergency care systems have been in use around the world since before the Pharaohs. Most early systems were conceived and implemented by the military, but they provided little more than the transportation of wounded soldiers from battlefields to nearby doctors. Today, modern emergency care systems are complex networks designed primarily for civilian use, and they bring a broad range of medical services and resources directly to the patient on scene and throughout transport to the hospital.

An emergency care system is a formal, organized network of specially trained personnel, equipment, and facilities that responds to medical emergencies, regardless of cause, location, or the patient's ability to pay. It is a portion of the overall public health system, and its purpose is to bring specialized resources to the scene of a medical emergency as soon as possible so that potential life-saving procedures can be implemented. Depending on the situation, treatment may begin at the scene and be continued until the patient arrives at a care facility. If the situation warrants it, treatment may be rendered only at the scene, thereby delaying or negating the need for additional treatment (Figure 2-1■).

In the United States, emergency care systems were born out of federal legislation enacted in the 1960s in response to the large number of highway fatalities. Later, these systems were expanded to decrease the growing number of out-of-hospital cardiac arrest-related deaths. Today's emergency care systems are designed to respond to and manage a wide variety of emergencies, both natural and human-caused. As with all aspects of health care, emergency care systems are constantly evolving to meet the ever-changing needs of the communities they serve and to reflect changes in medical knowledge, procedures, and technology. Regular monitoring helps to ensure that emergency care systems are in a constant state of readiness and will function as designed. An emergency care system requires considerable coordination and oversight to ensure that services are delivered to the highest level of quality possible and are provided in accordance with local, area, and state practices.

**Outdoor First Care (OFC) Provider** a person who has completed the NSP's Outdoor First Care course and is trained to render basic first aid in outdoor, nonurban environments.

**Outdoor Emergency Care (OEC) Technician** a provider who has successfully completed the NSP's OEC course and has kept his annual refresher requirement current. CPR training, including AED training, are required of this individual.

In many parts of the world, ski patrols, **Outdoor First Care Providers (OFC Providers)**, and **Outdoor Emergency Care Technicians (OEC Technicians)** interface with the local emergency system as they provide emergency assistance and transportation services to patients located in outdoor nonurban settings typically not served by traditional 9-1-1

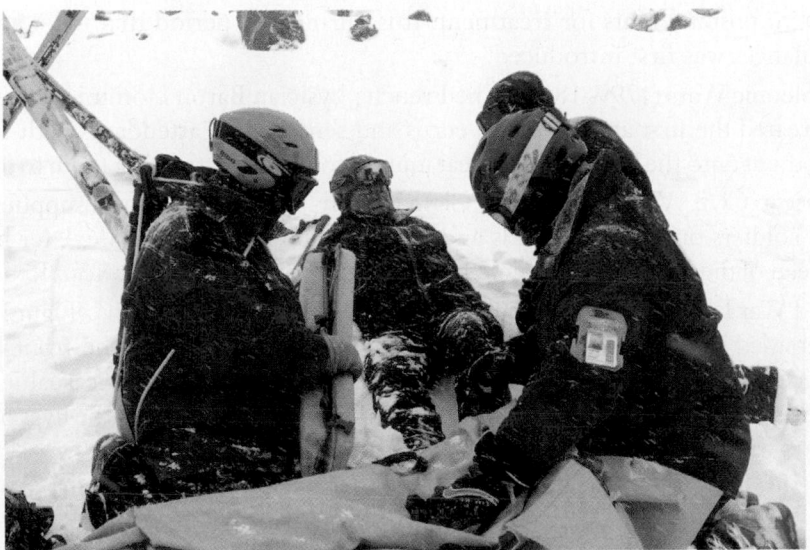

**Figure 2-1** An emergency care system is a formal, organized network of specifically trained personnel, equipment, and facilities. Two patrollers work together to provide aid to a patient.

providers. Having a basic understanding of what makes an emergency care system effective will help OEC Technicians operate more effectively and better serve their patients (Figure 2-2■).

# The History of Emergency Care

Rendering first aid to a critically ill or injured patient before the person reaches a hospital or transporting a patient from the field to a medical facility are not new concepts, as history yields numerous examples of such practices:

+ Crusades (the eleventh century): The Knights of St. John provided basic first aid to injured soldiers from both sides of the conflict and transported them on horse

**Figure 2-2** Ski patrols and OEC Technicians are an integral part of the local pre-hospital emergency care system. Ski patrollers hand off a patient to a local EMS squad.
Copyright Scott Smith

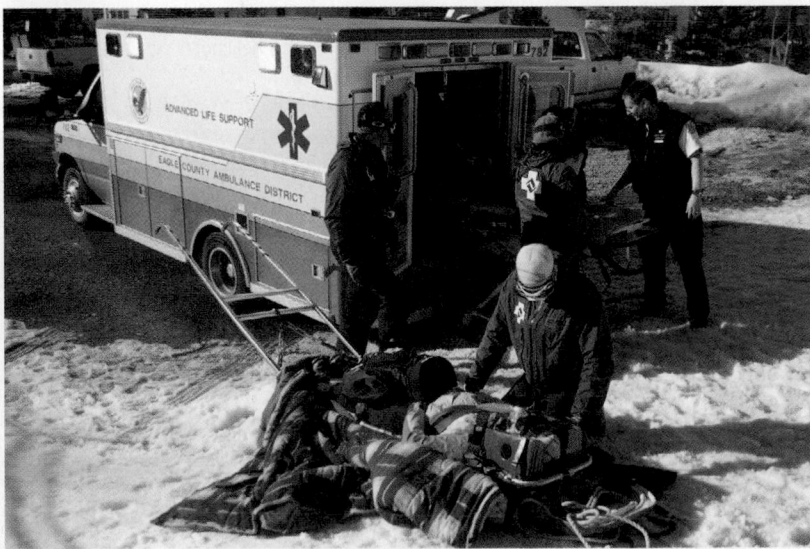

litters to hospital tents for treatment. It is during this period that the concept of ambulances was first introduced.

- Napoleonic Wars (1799–1815): The French physician Baron Dominique Jean Larrey created the first army medical corps and sent trained attendants with medical equipment onto the battlefield to treat injured soldiers and to bring them to doctors.
- American Civil War (1861–1865): Clara Barton distributed medical supplies to injured soldiers on the battlefields and nursed wounded soldiers. She later became the head of the Union Army's field hospitals and founded the American Red Cross.
- World War I (1914–1918): Ambulances used during the "Great War" (Figure 2-3a■) had trained attendants who transported wounded soldiers from the front lines, a practice that greatly reduced the mortality rate among wartime casualties. The Thomas half ring traction splint was first used in the field and saved the lives of many soldiers with broken femurs.
- Royal Flying Doctors of Australia (1928): Using fixed-wing aircraft, physicians were flown into remote locations in the Australian outback to treat patients with serious illnesses and injuries.
- World War II (1941–1945): In 1943, large fixed-wing multi-patient ambulance airplanes were developed to transport wounded soldiers back to the United States following initial care abroad.
- Korean War (1950–1953): Air evacuation using helicopters or "air ambulances" was introduced. This innovation significantly reduced the time a soldier spent between being wounded and receiving treatment at a mobile army surgical hospital, or M.A.S.H. unit (Figure 2-3b■). Air evacuation dramatically increased survival rates and was later perfected during the Vietnam War. It also served as the blueprint for modern civilian-based aero-medical transportation services.

Today's emergency care systems reflect the lessons learned from these and other historical milestones in medicine. Although civic-based ambulance services have existed in the United States since the early 1900s, it was not until 1966 when the National Academy of Science released its landmark report entitled "Accidental Death and Disability: The Neglected Disease of Modern Society" (The "White Paper") that

**Figure 2-3a** Modern-day ambulances evolved from primitive vehicles like this horse-drawn rig used during World War I.
Copyright Jerry Young/Dorling Kindersley Media Library

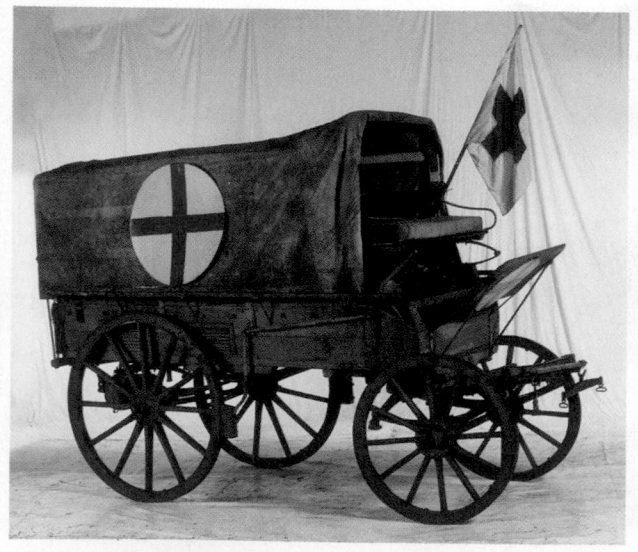

**Figure 2-3b** Air evacuation using helicopters or "air ambulances" was introduced during the Korean War. This helicopter was used in the evacuation of patients during Hurricane Katrina.
Copyright Edward McNamara

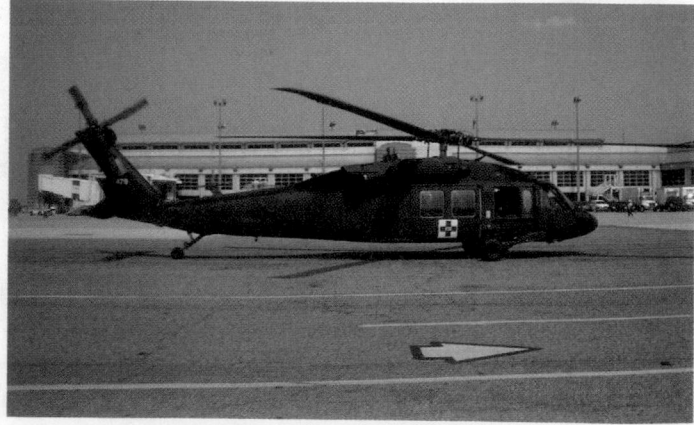

the groundwork for the modern emergency care system was laid. This paper exposed the causes, inherent problems, and high costs associated with highway crash–related deaths and pressed public officials to take action to mitigate the problem. Until that time, prehospital emergency transportation was provided primarily by funeral homes and volunteer rescue squads using lay persons with little or no formal medical training.

Later that same year, the newly enacted Highway Safety Act required states to adopt formal highway safety programs to decrease the number of traffic fatalities. This act provided funding for the development of state **emergency medical services (EMS)** offices and directed the creation of national education curricula for EMS providers. It also permitted the **National Highway Traffic Safety Administration (NHTSA)** to withhold highway funds from those states that did not comply. Modern ambulance and rescue services and prehospital practitioners emerged from the Highway Safety Act. Over the next decade, legislators passed additional federal and state laws, including the Emergency Medical Services Act of 1973, to address the need for the standardization of training, ambulance equipment, and emergency medical practices. The EMS Act identified 15 essential components for emergency medical services (Table 2-1■).

## EMS Agenda for the Future

In 1996, the National Highway Traffic Safety Administration (NHTSA), the federal agency tasked with overseeing the development of emergency care systems in the United States, released a report entitled *EMS Agenda for the Future*, which outlined key goals and 14 attributes of an effective emergency care system and provided strategies for fully integrating prehospital activities with the overall health care system. Agenda goals include the ability to "identify and modify illness and injury risks" and to "provide acute treatment and injury care and follow-up." The attributes are interrelated and are congruent with the National Ski Patrol's federal charter, mission, and vision. The 14 attributes and their relevance to ski patrollers and OEC Technicians are as follows:

1. **Integration of Health Services** Integration helps to ensure that ski patrols and OEC Technicians are included in the overall local health care system, and that the treatment they render is consistent with current evidence-based medical practices.

2. **Research** Research helps to identify patterns of injuries and illnesses to which skiers and outdoor recreation enthusiasts are most susceptible. Research can be used to assess the causes of various medical problems and the effectiveness of the treatment OEC Technicians provide. This information may be used to make outdoor activities safer, to identify future ski patroller training and equipment needs, and to identify new and more effective nonurban prehospital treatments.

3. **Legislation and Regulation** Legislation and regulation can help promote skiing and outdoor safety, and they may serve as sources of future funding of ski patrol–related activities and NSP-based outdoor safety initiatives.

**emergency medical services (EMS)**  a network of services, including rescue operations, prehospital emergency care, ambulance transportation, emergency department services, and public education, for treating victims of illness or injury. See emergency care system.

**National Highway Traffic Safety Administration (NHTSA)**  an agency of the Executive Branch of the U.S. Government, part of the Department of Transportation, whose mission is "Save lives, prevent injuries, reduce vehicle-related crashes."

⊕ **2-1**  List six attributes of an emergency care system.

---

| Table 2-1 | Fifteen Essential Components of an EMS System (1973) |
|---|---|
| 1. Manpower | 9. Access to Care |
| 2. Training | 10. Patient Transfer |
| 3. Communications | 11. Record Keeping |
| 4. Transportation | 12. Public Education |
| 5. Facilities | 13. System Evaluation |
| 6. Critical Care Units | 14. Disaster Response |
| 7. Public Safety Agencies | 15. Mutual Aid |
| 8. Consumer Participation | |

4. **System Finance** Proper finance helps to ensure that the overall health care system will have the resources it needs to manage emergencies within a given geographic response area. The National Ski Patrol must have a solid financial foundation if patrols are to continue providing high-quality educational services to the outdoor recreation public. Local ski patrols, who work under the direction of ski area operators, must have financial resources to execute their mission.

5. **Human Resources** To continue serving the outdoor recreation public, the National Ski Patrol must have a steady supply of qualified, competent, and dedicated personnel. Skilled OEC Technicians are the organization's greatest assets.

6. **Medical Direction** Ongoing medical oversight is the hallmark of quality health care and is the best method of ensuring that the treatment rendered by ski patrollers meets or exceeds both customers' expectations and the national education standards for emergency medical personnel.

7. **Education Systems** High-quality education is the wellspring from which high-quality patient care flows. The use of proven educational processes and systems that incorporate adult learning methods and learning technologies helps to ensure that patrollers receive the most up-to-date information and training in a timely and easily comprehensible manner.

8. **Public Education** Public education helps to safeguard outdoor recreation enthusiasts by promoting safety, which in turn helps reduce the incidence of injuries. Education also helps to ensure that lay persons know what to do should they encounter an emergency situation.

9. **Prevention** Prevention is the most effective method for reducing the incidence of injury or illness in skiing or other outdoor recreational activities. Participating in prevention initiatives is the responsibility of every OEC Technician and is an essential element of the NSP federal charter.

10. **Public Access** The public must be able to access appropriate emergency medical care promptly, regardless of setting or ability to pay. As specialists in providing emergency care in outdoor, nonurban settings, OEC Technicians render care in locations not serviced by traditional 9-1-1 systems, and they must be prepared to respond to an emergency at a moment's notice.

11. **Communication Systems** Communications help OEC Technicians interact with other components of the emergency care system and facilitate the coordination of rescue operations and related activities during emergencies.

12. **Clinical Care** Providing timely, effective aid is the goal of every OEC Technician. The clinical care and transportation services OEC Technicians provide has evolved since the NSP's founding and will continue as new equipment, practices, and procedures emerge. By incorporating the use of proven "best practices," patrollers provide their patients the highest quality of care possible, and help patients resume their preferred outdoor recreational activities as soon as possible (Figures 2-4a-g■).

13. **Information Systems** Data collection helps both NSP personnel and researchers better understand the nature, types, and sources of outdoor recreation–related injuries and illnesses. This information can help OEC Technicians better prepare for the emergencies they will most likely encounter. Additionally, access to information on a patient's history helps rescuers provide better emergency care.

14. **Evaluation** Assessing the effectiveness of every attribute of the emergency care system helps to ensure that the goals of the system are realized. Evaluation helps guide strategies that will make the emergency care system more effective.

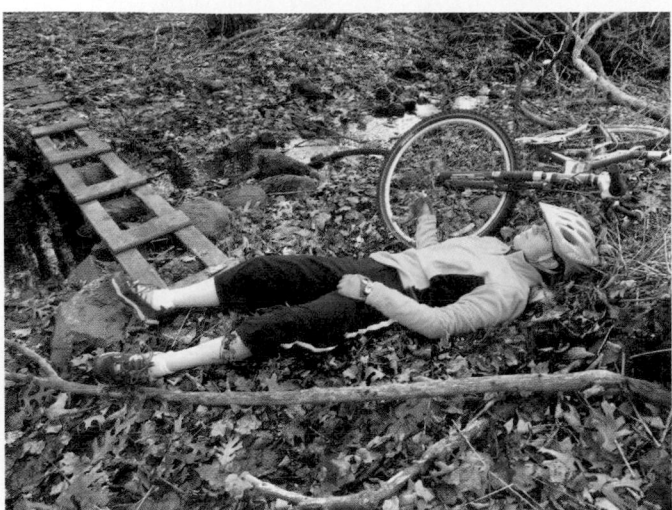

**Figure 2-4a** A mountain biker is injured on the trail.
Copyright Edward McNamara

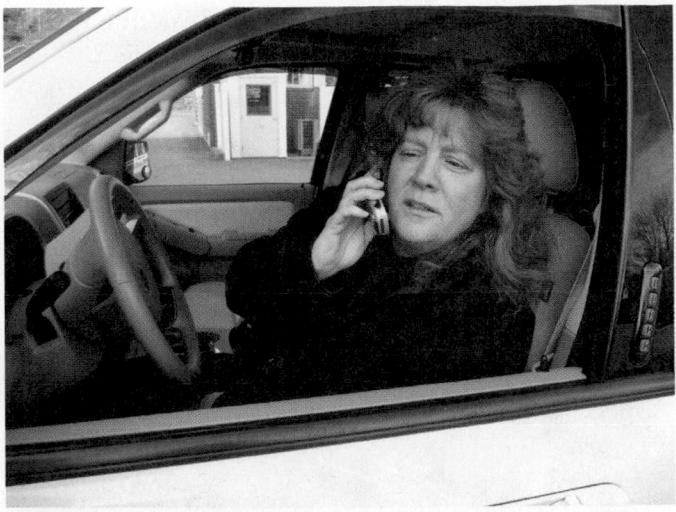

**Figure 2-4b** A passing motorist sees an accident and calls 911 on her cell phone.
Copyright Edward McNamara

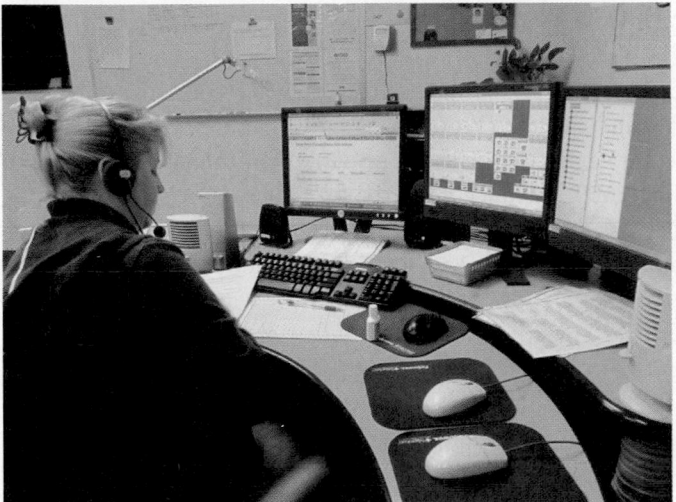

**Figure 2-4c** An emergency medical dispatcher receives a call and allocates resources.
Copyright Edward McNamara

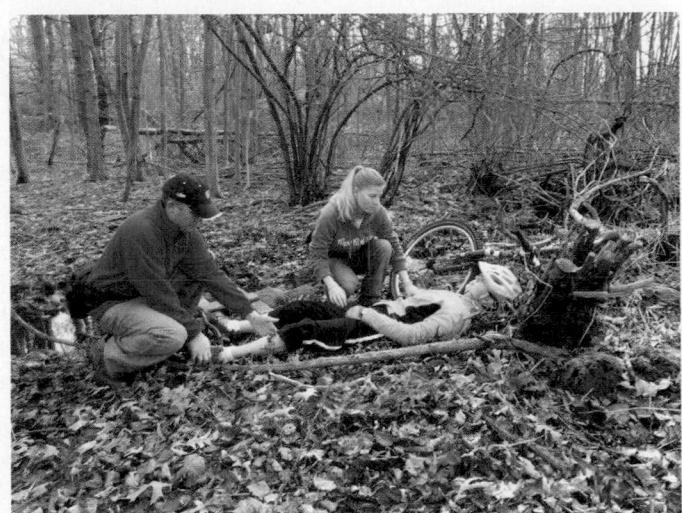

**Figure 2-4d** OEC Technicians provide medical care to the injured mountain biker.
Copyright Edward McNamara

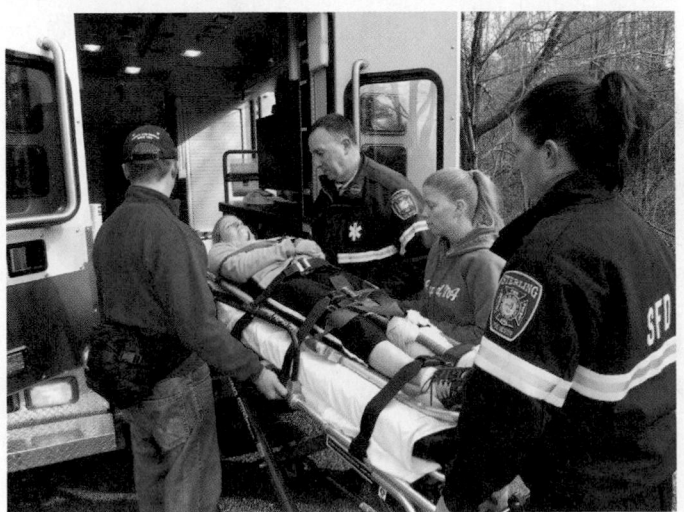

**Figure 2-4e** OEC Technicians handing a patient off to a local EMS provider.
Copyright Edward McNamara

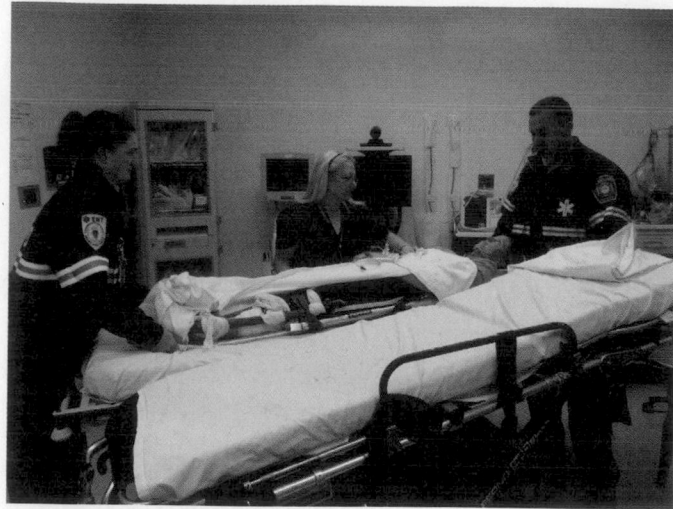

**Figure 2-4f** A local EMS provider hands off the patient for further treatment at a hospital.
Copyright Edward McNamara

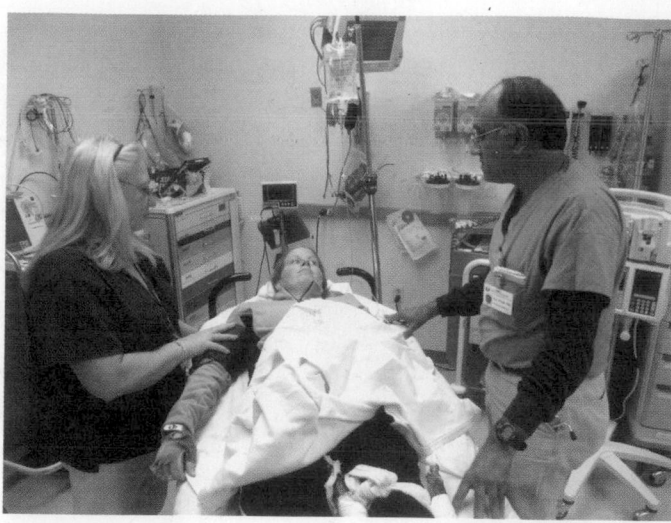

**Figure 2-4g** The chain of care continues at the hospital.
Copyright Edward McNamara

**prehospital provider** a person who is specially trained to render medical care to a patient outside of a hospital or medical care facility.

**Emergency Medical Responder (EMR)** a person who is specially trained to provide medical care to patients in prehospital settings. There are many types of EMRs, each with various training requirements and scopes of practice.

# Levels of Emergency Personnel

In the United States, emergency care systems utilize specially trained **prehospital providers** to deliver on-scene medical care (Figures 2-5a–d■). These providers are divided into four nationally recognized categories: **Emergency Medical Responder (EMR)**; **Emergency Medical Technician (EMT)**; **Advanced Emergency Medical Technician (AEMT)**; and **Paramedic**. Each category has different training requirements, scopes of practice, and recertification requirements. In 2006, a consensus document entitled the "National EMS Scope of Practice Model," or "**Scope of Practice**," was published as a set of rules, regulations, and ethical considerations that define the extent, boundaries, and limitations of a prehospital provider's duties (Figures 2-5a–d).

**Figure 2-5a** In many communities, fire departments not only provide fire suppression but are also Emergency Medical Responders.
Copyright Scott LaPrade

**Figure 2-5b** Ski patrollers are Emergency Medical Responders.
Copyright Studio 404

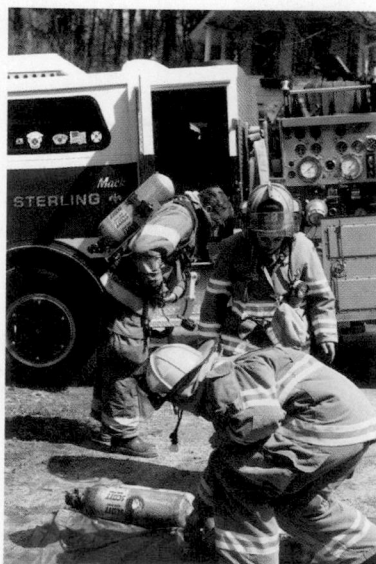

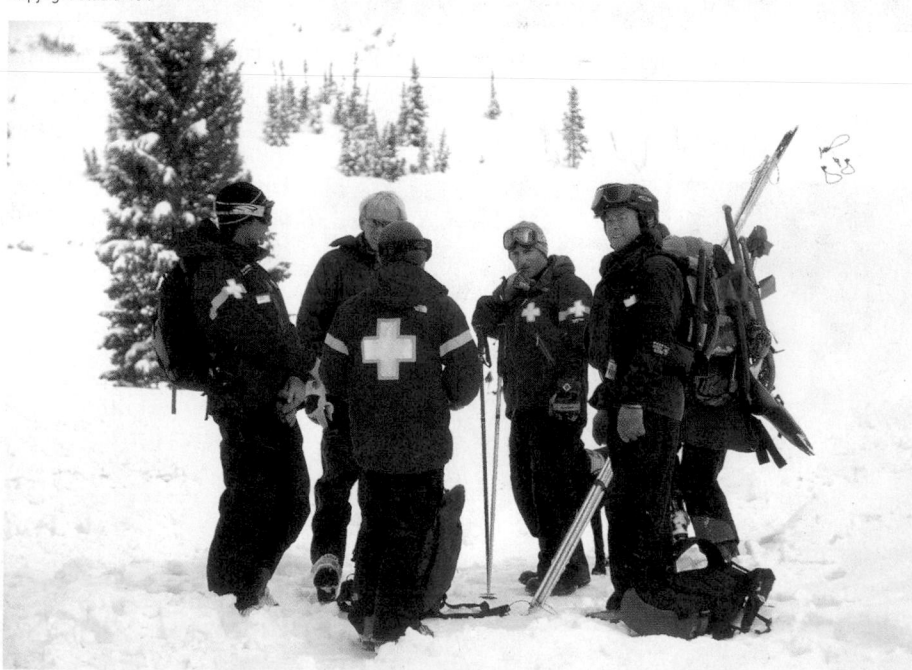

## Emergency Medical Responder

An EMR serves as the first responder of an emergency care system and is often the first formally trained health care provider to reach the patient. EMR-level personnel are trained to provide immediate life-saving treatment and stabilization to critically ill or injured patients while awaiting additional emergency response. Treatment is generally rendered using minimal equipment. EMR-level personnel also assist higher-level EMS providers, both at the scene and during transport.

The training requirements for EMR-level personnel vary depending on subsequent certification, and may or may not include minimum course or examination requirements. EMR-level training generally does not include hands-on training in a clinical environment. Whether EMR-level personnel may or may not function under medical oversight depends on the emergency care system design, although such oversight is recommended. OEC Technician training and qualifications meet or exceed the training requirements of an EMR.

## Emergency Medical Technician

An EMT is an individual who has completed an NHTSA-approved EMT National Standard training course or its equivalent. EMT courses must meet minimum national training standards, which consist of a minimum number of hours of didactic and practical instruction as well as clinical experience in an acute care setting (e.g., an emergency department, an ambulance, an intensive care unit). EMTs function with medical oversight to provide basic life support interventions, such as assessing clinical status, splinting fractures, administering certain medications, administering electrical therapy using an automatic external defibrillator, performing CPR, and transporting patients to a medical facility. With additional training in specific modules, EMTs may be authorized to use certain diagnostic devices or to perform more advanced therapeutic interventions, such as electrocardiography (EKG), intravenous therapy, or advanced airway management procedures. EMTs may also be involved in injury or illness prevention initiatives.

## Advanced Emergency Medical Technician

An AEMT is a person who has completed an NHTSA-approved AEMT National Standard training course or its equivalent, which includes didactic and practical instruction as well as clinical internships in one or more acute care settings. AEMTs

**Emergency Medical Technician (EMT)**  a basic-level technician who has successfully completed an NHTSA-approved EMT course or its equivalent and is authorized to provide basic life support.

**Advanced Emergency Medical Technician (AEMT)**  an intermediate-level technician who has successfully completed an NHTSA-approved Advanced EMT course or its equivalent and is authorized to provide both basic and intermediate life support.

**paramedic**  an allied health care professional who has successfully completed an NHTSA-approved paramedic course or its equivalent and is trained to deliver both basic and advanced life support.

**"Scope of Practice"**  a set of rules, regulations, and ethical considerations that define the extent, boundaries, and limitations of a prehospital provider's duties.

---

⊕ **2-2**  List four nationally recognized prehospital emergency care provider levels.

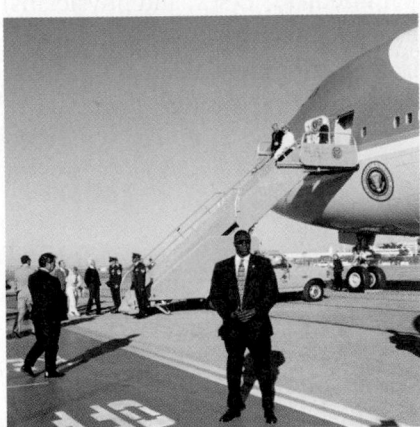

**Figure 2-5c** Executive protection personnel such as the Secret Service agent shown here are also Emergency Medical Responders, as are many park rangers, lifeguards, athletic trainers, and military combat lifesavers.
Copyright CORBIS-NY

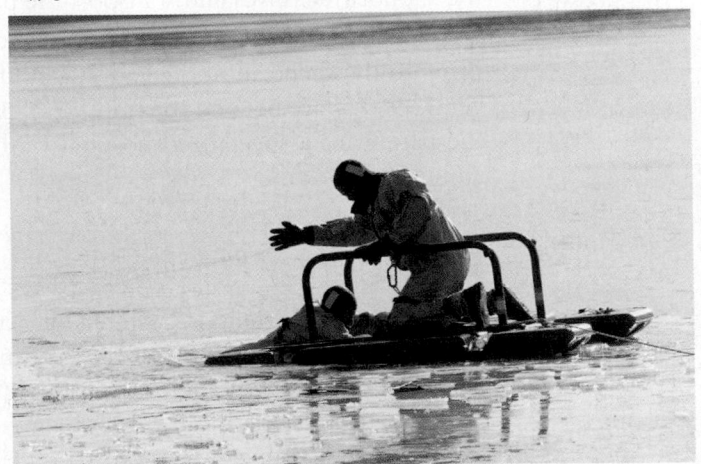

**Figure 2-5d** Within the EMR system are specialists in specific disciplines, such as hazardous materials rescues, high angle rescues, ice rescues, swift water rescues, and cave rescues. This is an example of an ice rescue.
Copyright Tina Gianos

function under medical oversight and may perform all of the skills performed by EMTs, as well as other intermediate therapeutic interventions using basic and advanced equipment and medications typically found on an ambulance. Equipment may vary by county, state, or province.

## Paramedic

A Paramedic is an allied health care professional who has successfully completed an NHTSA-approved Paramedic course, which includes extensive didactic, practical, and clinical training requirements. Paramedics operate under medical oversight and provide a higher level of prehospital care than all EMTs using a variety of basic and advanced equipment and medications, including narcotics.

EMTs, AEMTs, and Paramedics must complete an approved state EMS or other authorized agency training program and be certified or licensed by the state or province in which they work.

## Other EMS Personnel

Other members of the emergency care system include physicians (M.D. and D.O.), physicians assistants (PAs), nurse practitioners (NPs), registered nurses (RNs), licensed practical nurses (LPNs), and allied health care professionals (such as respiratory therapists, phlebotomists, laboratory technicians, radiology technicians, and EKG technicians) who provide definitive health care services within a hospital or medical facility. Under special circumstances (such as natural or human-caused disasters), these providers may assist prehospital personnel in the field. It is for this reason that the resources within a local emergency care system must be fully integrated and coordinated, so that they may be quickly mobilized when needed.

Most emergency care systems deploy personnel to emergencies using a stratified, or tiered, approach based on the patient's current condition or anticipated needs. This approach helps to ensure that adequate system resources are available should other emergencies arise.

**Tier 1:** EMRs arrive quickly at the scene and initiate basic emergency care while awaiting the arrival of higher-level emergency providers. In certain settings, EMRs (e.g., ski patrols, search and rescue teams, or wilderness first responders), may transport the patient to a location that is more accessible to rescue vehicles.

**Tier 2:** EMTs arrive shortly after EMRs and provide basic life support measures. If the situation warrants, EMTs may either await the arrival of advanced life support (ALS) providers or transport the patient to a definitive care facility.

**Tier 3:** AEMTs and paramedics arrive after EMRs/EMTs. They provide advanced life support measures and transport the patient to a definitive care facility.

**Tier 4:** Critical care providers (e.g., critical care paramedics, nurses, and physicians) bring to the scene additional advanced life support equipment, therapies, and interventions that are beyond the traditional paramedic scope of practice. They transport the patient to a specialized hospital via helicopter, fixed-wing aircraft, critical care ambulance, or other means.

# Emergency Facilities

Medical facilities such as hospitals or acute care clinics are important parts of the emergency care system and are the settings in which definitive patient treatment is delivered. Ideally, the facilities are part of a network that is integrated with the local public health system, but this is not always the case, most notably if the facility is located in a geographically remote area. Depending on the types of acute care services provided, facilities may be accredited or designated to provide either the full range of treatment to acutely ill and injured patients or the management of specific types of patients or medical conditions. Examples include designation as a trauma center (levels I–IV), an acute pediatric care facility, a burn center, a stroke center, or a toxicology center. Facility designations may be local or regional. A ski patrol's designated medical facility may be either the closest facility used to stabilize patients or (in the case of a critical patient) the closest trauma center equipped to handle patients transported by air.

# Continuity of Care

Continuity of care is the seamless delivery of high-quality emergency medical care while patients transition from their initial contact with an EMR through definitive treatment. It is a complex continuum involving each attribute of the emergency care system (Figures 2-6a–c■). Consider the following situation, which illustrates how continuity of care might occur in an outdoor, nonurban setting:

> A middle-aged man is snowmobiling with friends in the backcountry and gets stuck in a snowdrift. While attempting to get himself unstuck, he begins having severe chest pain. Sensing the seriousness of the sit-

**Figure 2-6a** OEC Technicians assess the patient and prepare for transport.
Copyright Studio 404

**Figure 2-6b** The team transfers the patient to the ambulance crew, where paramedics will continue to monitor and treat.
Copyright Studio 404

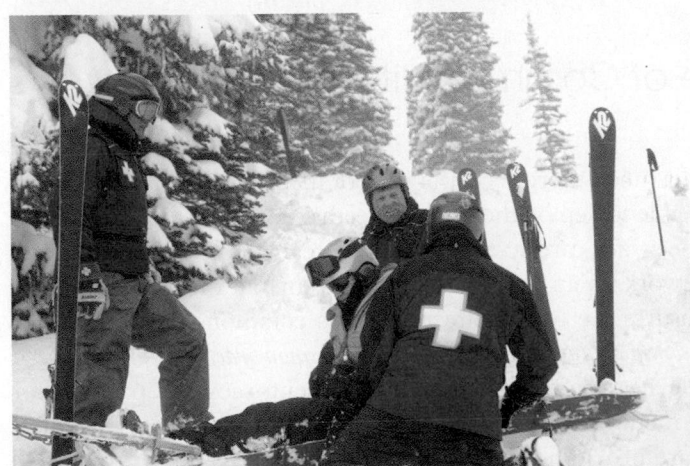

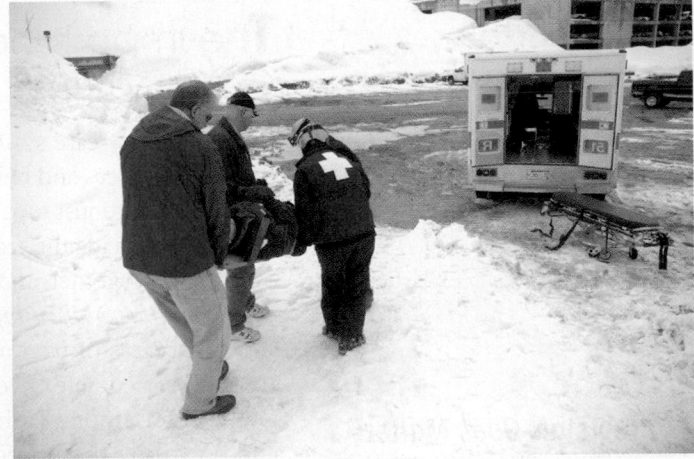

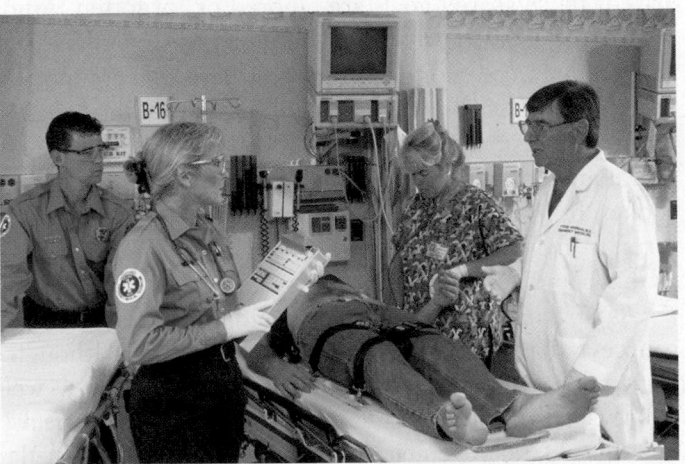

**Figure 2-6c** The physicians and nurses in the Emergency Department will continue to assess and further stabilize the patient as needed.

**emergency medical dispatcher (EMD)** a person who has been trained to provide emergency medical advice and instructions over the telephone.

**medical director** a physician who is responsible for ensuring and evaluating the appropriate level and quality of care throughout an emergency care system. Also referred to as a medical advisor or physician supervisor.

uation, one friend stays with the man while two others go to summon help. They encounter a Forest Service employee who calls 911 for assistance.

The **emergency medical dispatcher (EMD)** notifies nearby Nordic patrollers, who reach the man a short time later. OEC Technicians assess the man and place him on oxygen. Believing the man is having a heart attack, they request that a toboggan be brought to the scene and that an advanced life support ambulance meet them at the trailhead. Soon, snowmobiles arrive with two more ski patrollers and a paramedic. She establishes intravenous access. Next, she administers medication to lessen the damage to the heart. Together, the patrollers load the man into the toboggan, and the snowmobile team transports the man to an awaiting ambulance. The team transfers the patient to the ambulance crew, and paramedics monitor his heart while enroute to a regional cardiac center.

During the trip, the man's symptoms worsen. The paramedic notifies a doctor **medical director** at the hospital by radio, who orders other medicines to be administered. The man's symptoms stabilize. At the hospital, the man is taken to the emergency department, where his condition is further stabilized by physicians and nurses before he is transferred to the catheter lab. Following heart surgery to open a clogged blood vessel, the man spends three days in the critical care unit before being sent home to recuperate. He makes a complete recovery.

From the moment the man was initially contacted by ski patrollers to his discharge from the hospital, he received continuous care from trained medical professionals. At each transition, the level of medical care provided to the patient increased, which ultimately contributed to the man making a full recovery. Had there been a break in the continuity of care or had at any time the care provided not followed local practices, the outcome might not have been so favorable. This team approach is one of the hallmarks of an effective emergency care system.

## The Importance of Commonality in Emergency Care Systems

An emergency care system is much more than the sum of its parts. Simply having the proper resources and being able to deploy them when needed does not guarantee effectiveness. As we just saw, emergency care systems require a team approach. People and resources provide the framework for an emergency care system, but the glue that holds everything together and ensures the team's effectiveness is commonality: specifically, *having common goals, using a common language, and following common practices and procedures.*

Regardless of training level, type of working environment, scope of practice, or resources available, every member of an emergency care system shares common goals, chief among which are providing the best possible patient care (Figure 2-7■) and returning the emergency scene to normalcy. These shared goals serve as the banner around which all rescuers and medical providers must gather. Difficulties will arise if these shared goals are ignored or forgotten. Among the ways to ensure that these goals are achieved are the use of a common language and shared practices.

Having a common language is an essential component of any profession, as it is the foundation upon which mutual understanding is built. Using a shared vocabulary ensures precision, which in turn helps eliminate errors. This is why the OEC curriculum contains both medical and rescue terms and phrases; they reflect the language spoken by two different members of the emergency care system. In addition, these terms convey professionalism and enable OEC Technicians to communicate their findings and actions to other providers with greater precision.

As with any language, medical and rescue terminology is derived from numerous sources and is constantly growing and changing. Although heavily derived from Latin, it includes terms and phrases from other languages, as well as acronyms, mnemonics, abbreviations, and even military jargon. "Medical-speak" permeates every aspect of health care and the emergency care system, and it is used to describe human anatomy

**NOTE**

### Precision *Does* Matter!

Consider these examples involving commonality of language:

*"The patient has a broken leg."*
Do you know *which* leg is broken?

*"The patient has a broken left leg."*
Do you know *where* on the leg the break is located?

*"The patient has a mid-shaft fracture of the left femur."*
Can you now locate the exact site of the injury?
*Which description is most precise? Which one sounds most professional?*

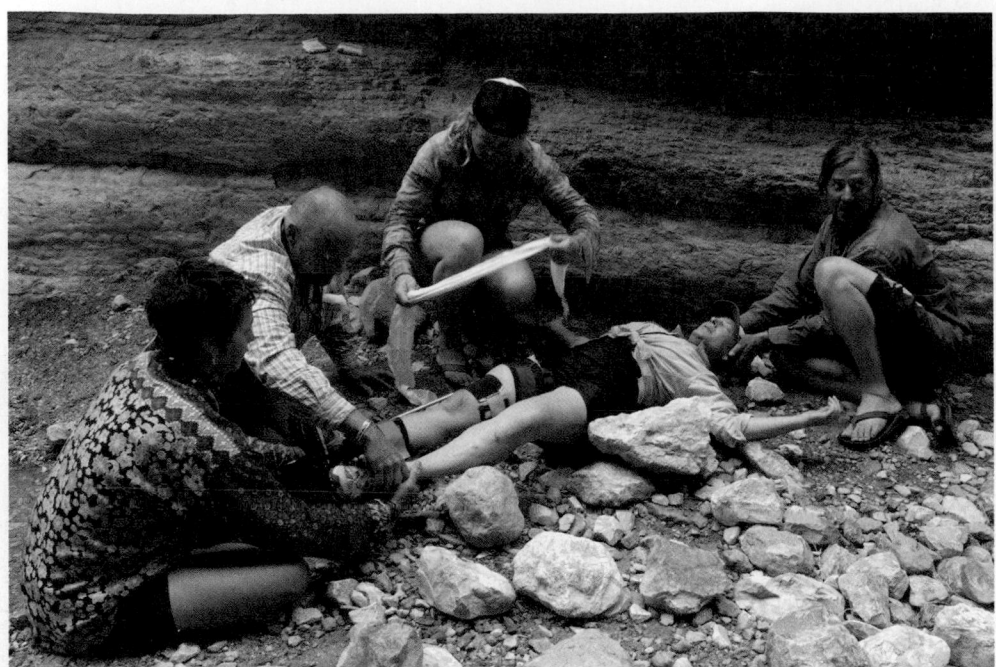

and physiology, assessment findings, treatments, equipment, and rescue operations. As new practices, procedures, equipment, and medications come into use, new terminology that more precisely describes rescue-related activities is put into use.

The use of common practices and procedures is as important as a common language, because they help to streamline processes, reduce redundancy and waste, and facilitate continuity of care. This is especially important when dealing with life-threatening emergencies. Imagine, for a moment, the ramifications if OEC Technicians began CPR on a cardiac arrest victim only to have other rescuers halt the life-saving procedure and instead transport the patient to the hospital. How might this difference in practice detract from the common goal of providing the patient the best possible care? Does this difference reflect effective continuity of care? Could it ultimately affect the patient's outcome?

Consider another situation involving multiple patients. Most emergency care systems employ a standardized approach that prioritizes patients according to the severity of their injuries. Using this approach, the most seriously injured victims receive treatment first and are transported to the hospital before those with less serious injuries. But what might happen if rescuers utilized different approaches or used different criteria to make these decisions? How might this affect the patients' outcomes?

Commonality enables rescuers within an emergency care system to focus on the same priorities, to speak the same language, and to perform rescue-related activities in a similar fashion, regardless of training level or clinical setting. This approach to teamwork enables rescuers to work together more effectively and to provide the best possible outcome for patients.

## The Relationship of Emergency Care Systems to Public Health

Public health is the umbrella under which every facet of health care, including emergency care systems, is sheltered, and it is concerned with issues that affect both society as a whole and its subgroups. Typical public health concerns center on epidemiology,

# STOP, THINK, UNDERSTAND

## Multiple Choice

Choose the correct answer.

1. Emergency care systems deploy personnel to emergencies using a tiered approach. How many tiers are there? _____
   a. 1
   b. 2
   c. 3
   d. 4

2. Which of the following is not an important aspect of commonality in the EMS system? _____
   a. having common goals
   b. having common uniforms
   c. using a common language
   d. following common practices/procedures

3. Which agency was tasked with developing an emergency care system? _____
   a. OSHA (Occupational Safety and Health Administration)
   b. EPA (Environmental Protection Agency)
   c. FEMA (Federal Emergency Management Agency)
   d. NHTSA (National Highway Traffic Safety Administration)

4. Which provider is *not* specially trained to deliver prehospital, on-scene medical care? _____
   a. a nurse
   b. an Emergency Medical Provider
   c. a paramedic
   d. an Advanced Emergency Medical Technician

## Short Answer

1. List 6 of the 14 attributes of the emergency care system.
   a. _____
   b. _____
   c. _____
   d. _____
   e. _____
   f. _____

2. Describe continuity of care.

   _____
   _____
   _____
   _____
   _____

 **CASE UPDATE**

You activate the emergency care system by sending someone to obtain ski patrol assistance, and you keep the patient calm and warm while awaiting assistance. You are careful not to move the person, however, you do stabilize the ankle and leg. Once ski patrollers arrive, you assist them by providing information about the incident and the patient. The patrollers assess the patient and initiate treatment. They splint the leg to prevent further injury and transport the patient to an awaiting ambulance crew, who administer pain medication and transport the patient to a definitive care facility.

***What is your next responsibility?***

injury prevention, and policy and program development, all of which are designed to promote healthier living. Epidemiology is the branch of medicine that monitors the incidence and prevalence of disease in large populations and detects the sources and causes of epidemics involving infectious diseases.

Public health activities are coordinated by state and county public health departments, which research emerging disease trends and monitor the effectiveness of health-related programs and initiatives. These departments also play pivotal roles in the development of emergency care systems by coordinating system activities and resources, offering specialized training, and providing **medical oversight** and a host of other services to rescue personnel. As members of an emergency care system, OEC Technicians have an obligation to assist public health officials in such department-sponsored activities as assisting with research projects, helping in disaster relief efforts, identifying outdoor safety issues, promoting safety in outdoor recreation, and conducting mass immunizations. The completion of accident and/or medical reports is another way in which OEC Technicians can assist public health endeavors, as this information is used to identify trends that can inform future public health reports, policies, or initiatives.

**medical oversight**   the process by which a physician monitors the quality of medical care rendered to patients and provides assistance and guidance to prehospital providers and emergency care systems.

## The Role of Research in Emergency Care Systems

Research plays an essential role in health care and serves many purposes. It is used to identify epidemiological and pathological trends, to report clinically relevant findings, and to introduce new technologies, practices, and techniques. According to *Taber's Cyclopedic Dictionary*, research is the "scientific and diligent study, investigation, or experimentation to establish facts and analyze their significance." It serves as the scientific basis for the universal understanding that enables medical professionals to manage injuries and diseases effectively.

In the past two decades, emergency care systems and the field of emergency medicine have evolved dramatically, largely because of the quality of prehospital research that has been conducted. In years past, new techniques, equipment, and medications were often introduced or adopted for field use without a clear understanding of the clinical benefits. As a result, so-called "technological advancements" were either no better than what they replaced or failed to achieve desired results. Some were even harmful. Today, *evidenced-based* research is the driving force behind the latest innovations in emergency medicine technology. Such research has helped reshape how prehospital care is delivered, the types of equipment and procedures used by field providers, and the training requirements of emergency care system personnel.

Medical research directly affects OEC Technicians and other prehospital providers, who increasingly will be called upon to help collect data, identify potential areas of study, and even manage research projects. The information gained from these activities will be used to develop safety policies and safer equipment, injury prevention programs, and clinical procedures that reduce snow sport–related injuries. It will also enable OEC personnel to provide high-quality care that has been scientifically proven to benefit patients.

By actively participating in research, patrollers and OEC Technicians help expand the growing body of medical knowledge and enable NSP to better fulfill its federal charter to improve skier safety (Figure 2-8■).

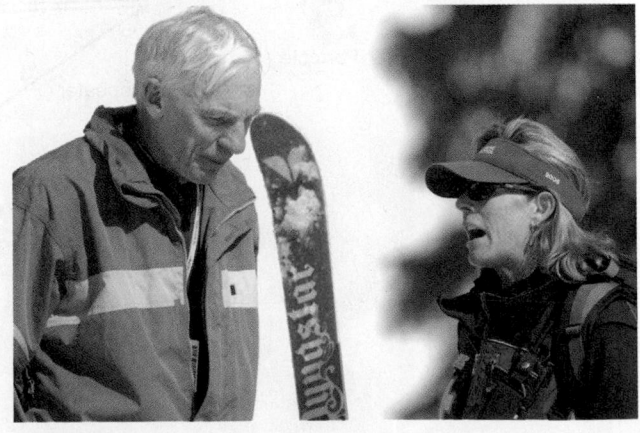

**Figure 2-8** A researcher (at left) is interviewing a ski patroller. Evidence-based research is the driving force behind innovations in medical technology. Copyright Snowbird

# Communication Systems in Emergency Care Systems

Communication systems are the vital links that connect all the components of the emergency care system and enables them to work together in a coordinated fashion (Figure 2-9■). A typical EMS communication system consists of hardware (e.g., telephones, cell phones, radio communications equipment, and computers), software, and specialized professionals who manage these resources. Effective communications improve patient outcomes and are essential for successful rescue operations. Although communication technology has vastly improved in the past decade, communicating in prehospital environments, especially in backcountry and nonurban areas, is extremely difficult. It is for this reason that OEC Technicians should have a fundamental understanding of both the common problems that can compromise radio communications and the various NSP resources available to help make your patrol's communication system more effective.

In the United States, radio communications systems are regulated by two agencies: the Interdepartment Radio Advisory Committee (IRAC) of the Department of Commerce, which regulates radio use by federal agencies, and the Federal Communications Commission (FCC), which regulates radio use by nonfederal entities. Radio frequencies used by ski patrols must be licensed by the FCC. Unauthorized communications or unlicensed operation can result in substantial fines. The National Ski Patrol has volunteer telecommunications advisors who will assist ski patrols in complying with FCC licensing requirements. If you are a rescuer for another nonfederal agency, contact the FCC (www.fcc.gov) for licensing information.

OEC Technicians communicate with each other and with other members of the emergency care system by various means, including two-way radios, landline telephones, and cell phones. Of these, portable radios are the daily workhorses for OEC Technicians (Figure 2-10■). However, because of topography, portable radios used in

**Figure 2-9** An overview of the transmission pathway of a radio communications call.

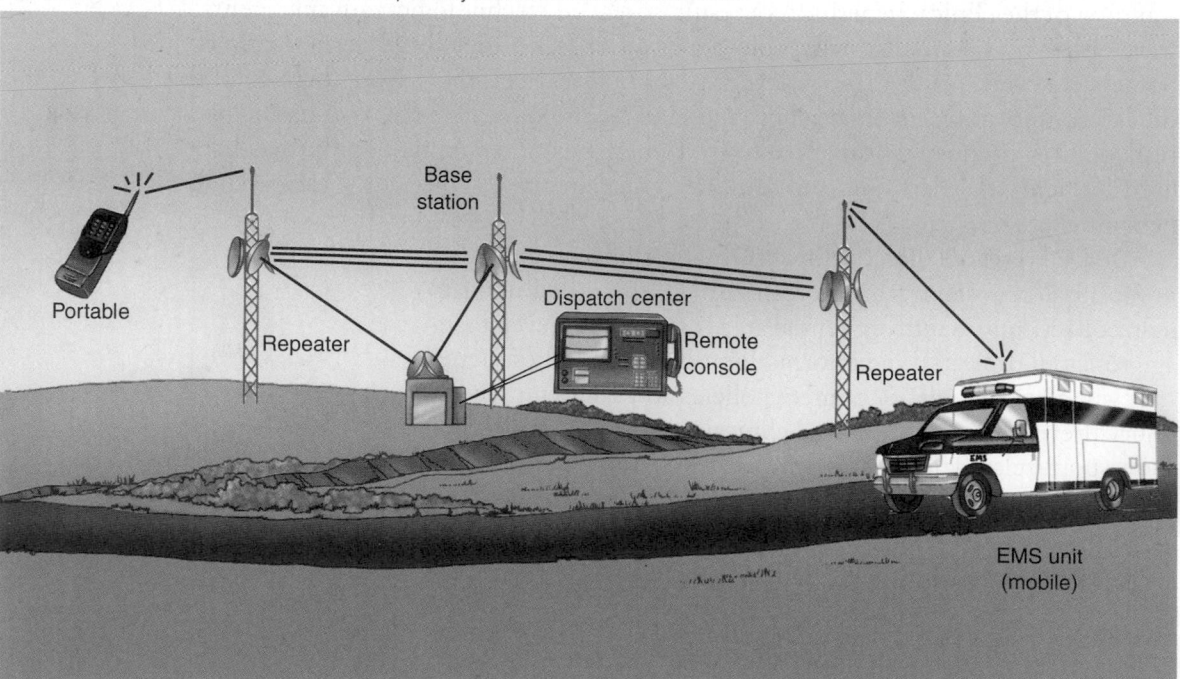

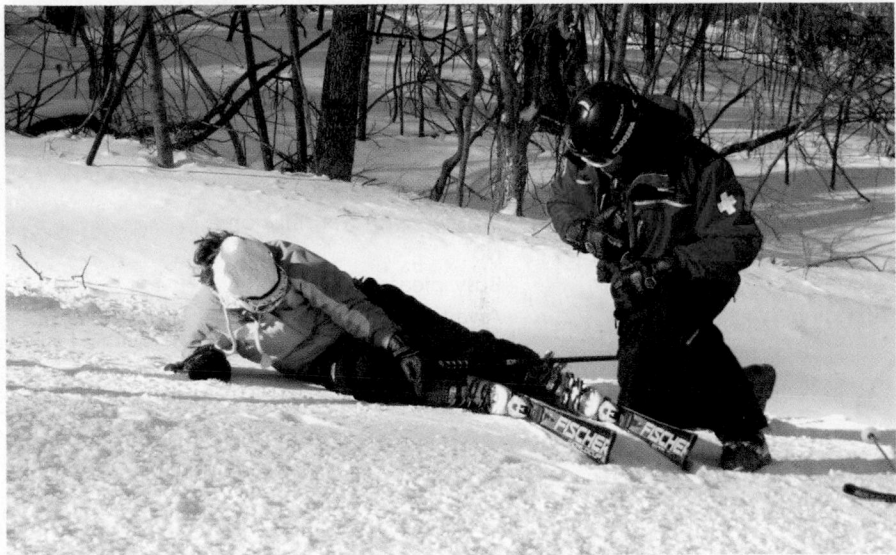

**Figure 2-10** When using a portable radio, patrollers must be clear, concise, and accurate in communicating with others; using a radio entails great responsibility.
Copyright Edward McNamara

direct, unit-to-unit communications have a limited range. This limitation can be overcome by using base stations, repeaters, or other infrastructure. NSP's volunteer telecommunications advisors can assist patrols by recommending ways to improve signal coverage.

## Radio Etiquette

Communicating with others by radio entails great responsibility and must be done clearly, concisely, and accurately. This is best accomplished by observing basic radio etiquette and universally accepted terms and practices. This is especially true when lives hang in the balance and time is of the essence. Additionally, emergency radio transmissions are often monitored and recorded by other rescuers, public safety organizations, and civilian organizations such as news media, and any recordings made may be subpoenaed during legal proceedings. It is essential that OEC Technicians maintain a professional demeanor at all times when communicating via radio. Common radio etiquette tips include the following:

- Listen before beginning to transmit a message (to prevent inadvertently cutting off another rescuer's transmission).
- Press the transmit key firmly and hold it for 1–2 seconds before speaking (to prevent inadvertently cutting off the beginning of your transmission).
- Speak directly into the microphone. (Shield the microphone from wind to improve communications.)
- Speak clearly and slowly, with a normal voice. Do not shout.
- Be concise; make each transmission less than 30 seconds long.
- When finished speaking, wait 1–2 seconds before releasing the transmit key (to prevent inadvertently cutting off the end of your transmission).
- Acknowledge receipt of all transmissions.
- Do not use profanity or offensive terms.
- Do not say the patient's name (this may violate privacy laws).
- Limit communications to official business only.

> **NOTE**
>
> ### Factors That Can Adversely Affect Radio Communications
>
> - Radio transmitter power
> - Antenna size
> - Antenna/repeater/cell tower location
> - Repeater power
> - Terrain (open versus mountainous)
> - Buildings
> - Weather
> - High-power lines
> - Nearby microwave signals or fluorescent lights
> - Competing electronic signals (e.g., GPS receivers, RADAR)
> - Overlapping signals (e.g., multiple users on the same frequency)
>   - Equipment damage (e.g., broken antenna)
>   - Incompatible equipment, radio frequencies

| Table 2-2 | Common Radio Terms |
|---|---|
| **Term** | **Meaning** |
| Affirmative | Yes |
| Acknowledge | Message received, understood |
| Confirm/Say Again | Please repeat |
| Go Ahead | Proceed with transmission |
| Negative | No |
| Stand By | Busy, please wait |
| Standing By | Awaiting further information or instructions |

## Radio Terminology

The use of common language and terms is especially critical when communicating via radio and is a key factor in improving mutual understanding among rescue personnel. Using universally accepted terms enables information to be conveyed quickly and precisely. Commonly used radio terms are presented in Table 2-2■.

When speaking to others over the airwaves, plain English is preferred over the use of radio codes such as the "10 codes" that were often used in the 1970s and 1980s. Radio codes have fallen into disfavor because they are not used in a uniform way and are often specific to a single organization. This lack of uniformity can cause significant problems, especially in situations involving multiple public safety agencies.

## NATO Phonetic Alphabet

Occasionally, unusual words, acronyms, or critical combinations of letters must be communicated to others via radio. This is easily accomplished by using the NATO phonetic alphabet, in which each letter is represented by a universally accepted word (Table 2-3■). To use the phonetic alphabet, simply state the corresponding phonetic word for each letter, pausing briefly between each word. For example, to communicate the vehicle license plate number OEC 2011, say "Oscar . . . Echo . . . Charlie . . . Two . . . Zero . . . One . . . One." Do not say "O as in Oscar, E as in Echo, C as in Charlie, Two thousand and eleven" because this introduces nonessential words that can be misinterpreted (especially if the transmitted signal breaks up) and is also an inefficient use of airtime.

| Table 2-3 | NATO Phonetic Alphabet |
|---|---|
| A | Alpha |
| B | Bravo |
| C | Charlie |
| D | Delta |
| E | Echo |
| F | Foxtrot |
| G | Golf |
| H | Hotel |
| I | India |
| J | Juliet |
| K | Kilo |
| L | Lima |
| M | Mike |
| N | November |
| O | Oscar |
| P | Papa |
| Q | Quebec |
| R | Romeo |
| S | Sierra |
| T | Tango |
| U | Uniform |
| V | Victor |
| W | Whiskey |
| X | X-Ray |
| Y | Yankee |
| Z | Zulu |

## Military Time

Ski patrols, like other rescue groups, express time using military or "universal" time, a precise method for stating the time that is based on a 24-hour clock (see Table 2-4■). This convention is different from civilian or "regular" time, which is based on a 12-hour clock. Under regular time, any given time occurs twice in a day and is followed by either a.m. or p.m. (e.g., 7:00 a.m. and 7:00 p.m.).

Under military time, each 24-hour time period begins at one minute past midnight and continues until the following midnight. Military time is expressed using four digits to signify the hours and minutes; the first two digits represent the hour, and the second two digits represent the minutes. Accordingly, a given time can only occur once each day: 7:00 a.m. is 0700, whereas 7:00 p.m. is 1900.

| Table **2-4** | Military Time | |
|---|---|---|
| **Military time** | **Regular time** | **Pronunciation** |
| 0001 | one minute past midnight | zero, zero, zero, one |
| 0015 | fifteen minutes past midnight | zero, zero, fifteen |
| 0030 | twelve-thirty a.m. | zero, zero, thirty |
| 0100 | one a.m. | zero, one hundred |
| 0200 | two a.m. | zero, two hundred |
| 1100 | eleven a.m. | eleven hundred |
| 1200 | twelve p.m. (noon) | twelve hundred |
| 1300 | one p.m. | thirteen hundred |
| 1400 | two p.m. | fourteen hundred |
| 2300 | eleven p.m. | twenty-three hundred |
| 2400 | twelve p.m. (midnight) | twenty-four hundred |

The hours from 1:00 a.m. to 12:00 p.m. are the same as they appear on the clock. Morning hours up to 9:59 a.m. are preceded by a zero: 0959. From 1:00 p.m. to midnight, add 12 to the hours displayed on the clock. Both systems calculate minutes and seconds in exactly the same manner. Thus, 6:00 a.m. is expressed as 0600 and is pronounced "zero six hundred," whereas 4:25 p.m. is expressed as 1625 (12 + 4 hours = 16 hours + 25 minutes = 1625) and is pronounced "sixteen twenty-five."

It is important to learn your local ski patrol's radio protocol, and it is recommended that your patrol uses universally accepted terms and military time. More detail on specific radio communications appears in Chapter 8.

# Medical Oversight in Emergency Care Systems

In the United States and many other countries, a licensed physician must assume legal responsibility for a patient's care throughout an emergency, from the time an EMR begins care through discharge from the emergency care system. Such medical oversight by a physician ensures continuity of care and that the patient receives proper treatment in accordance with local care guidelines (Figure 2-11■).

There are two types of medical oversight: direct oversight and indirect oversight. Direct oversight, or online medical control, involves real-time voice contact with a licensed physician who helps guide decisions concerning patient care. Direct oversight is usually conducted via telephone or radio, but it may also occur using video conferencing or other communication devices. The presence of a physician who oversees a patient's treatment at the scene is yet another form of direct medical oversight. Direct oversight is used primarily to oversee the provision of advanced care procedures or medications. It also serves as a means by which prehospital providers may consult with a physician to discuss complex cases or to obtain specific clinical, technical, or procedural information.

By contrast, in indirect oversight, or offline medical control, prehospital providers are not required to contact a physician before initiating specific treatments. This form of medical oversight is designed to expedite patient care and is commonly used for "preauthorizing" both routine procedures such as oxygen administration and advanced life-saving procedures or medications that must

 **2-3** Compare and contrast direct medical oversight and indirect medical oversight.

**Figure 2-11** This physician is on the radio, communicating with emergency medical personnel.
Copyright Edward McNamara

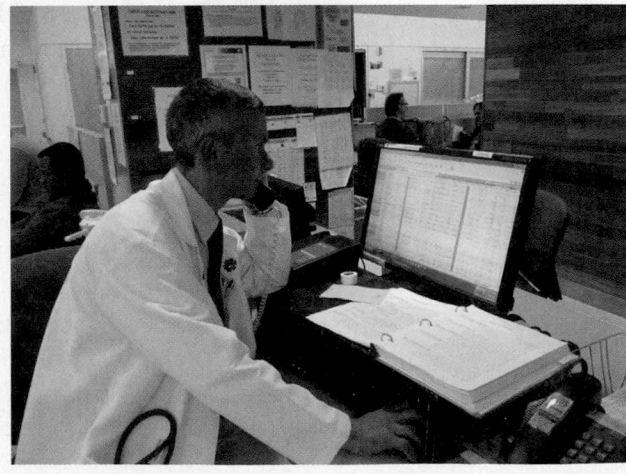

**protocols**  written procedures for assessing, treating, and transporting a patient. Protocols are generally written by a team of emergency care professionals and managed by a medical director.

be urgently administered. Both types of medical oversight are provided using preestablished medical orders, known as **protocols**, which have been approved by the local medical authority.

# Emergency Care Protocols

Protocols are written instructions that describe what should be done in a given situation. They serve as guidelines that identify the assessment and treatment considerations for commonly encountered emergencies. Protocols are developed on a local level by emergency care professionals who are familiar with the area's medical needs, available resources, system capabilities, and local standard of care. They should be reviewed annually and revised as needed to reflect changes in policies, procedures, equipment, medications, or other key system-related factors.

Given the complexities and variables associated with outdoor emergency medicine, protocols should be considered fluid instruments; they cannot be expected to address *every* situation that one might face. As such, OEC Technicians will likely confront situations for which no specific protocol exists. When these situations—known as "gray areas"—occur, use your good judgment to ensure that the patient receives the best possible medical care. Should there ever be doubt as to the proper course of action or treatment to follow, consultation with online medical control, if available, is recommended.

# The Importance of Documentation in Emergency Care

Good documentation is one of the hallmarks of a true medical professional, and it serves many purposes that go well beyond simply providing a record of events. Documentation provides pertinent clinical details that improve the continuity of care. It also can be used as a research tool; to provide legal protection for care providers, patrols, and ski areas; and to improve the quality of care. A full discussion of documentation is presented in Chapter 8.

# Quality Improvement in Emergency Care Systems

**2-4**  Describe the purpose of quality improvement.

Providing the best patient care possible is a common goal among emergency care personnel, a goal that is best achieved through the implementation of a quality improvement program. Quality improvement, or QI, is an ongoing process designed to ensure that the products and services provided meet or exceed customer expectations. In health care, QI involves careful examination of each step in the case, from initial entry into the emergency care system through definitive care, as well as the implementation of changes that ensure that the care the patient receives is delivered in accordance with local protocols and guidelines.

There are three types of quality improvement: prospective, concurrent, and retrospective. *Prospective quality improvement* centers on preventing problems from occurring. Two commons examples of prospective QI are providing training and developing protocols. Training ensures that a person has the necessary knowledge and skills to perform job-related tasks, whereas protocols ensure that each task will be completed in accordance with preestablished guidelines. *Concurrent quality improvement* centers on both preventing problems and taking corrective actions, as needed, while tasks are being performed. Examples of concurrent QI are online medical direction and following another on-scene rescuer's instructions in changing a treatment under consideration. *Retrospective quality improvement* addresses situations after they have occurred.

The purposes of retrospective QI are to identify acceptable or exceptional care and to identify ways to improve future care. Examples of retrospective QI are case reviews, after-action reports, and remedial training. Case reviews and after-action reports are used to compare what was supposed to happen and what actually occurred, whereas remedial training ensures that personnel know what, when, and how to perform specific procedures and tasks. An essential component of an effective case review or after-action report is accurate documentation.

## Continuing Education in Emergency Care

Continuing education, or CE, is an essential requirement of any professional license or certification (Figure 2-12■). It is the additional, on-going training that individuals receive following their initial schooling to increase their knowledge about a given topic or skill. CE enhances a person's ability to perform job-related tasks by providing them the most up-to-date information available. As part of their certification requirements, OEC Technicians must receive continuing education through required annual OEC refresher coursework.

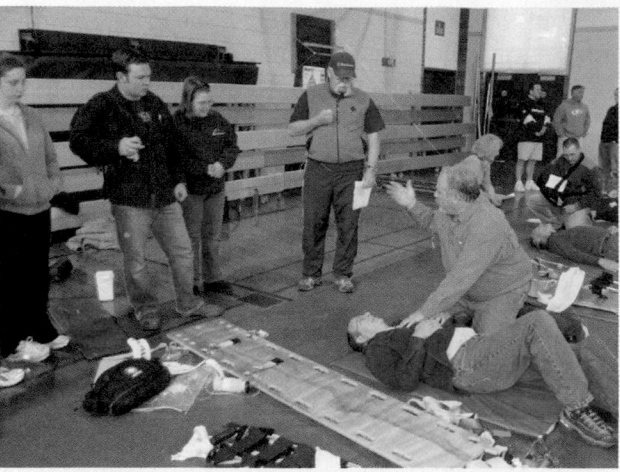

**Figure 2-12** Every patroller is required to complete an annual review of OEC skills.
Copyright Edward McNamara

---

 **CASE DISPOSITION**

Thanks to your quick thinking in activating the local emergency care system, the patient makes a full recovery, continues to enjoy skiing, and later becomes a member of your patrol.

---

# Chapter Review

## Chapter Summary

Today's emergency care systems have come a long way from their early beginnings, and they provide a broad range of services to acutely ill or injured patients. These systems are constantly evolving in response to the ever-changing needs of the communities they serve and will continue to grow as new treatments and technologies emerge. An effective emergency care system consists of many interrelated, interdependent components that work together to ensure that the system's common goals—chief of which is that patients receive the highest-quality medical care possible—are realized.

OEC Technicians are essential parts of the emergency care system and provide emergency assistance and transportation to patients not served by traditional 911 providers. As members of this system, OEC Technicians must be aware of the attributes of an effective emergency care system and must take an active role in the system's development and improvement. By taking an active role, OEC Technicians help the National Ski Patrol fulfill its federal charter and assist other rescue agencies in providing care. The result is the improved safety and health of everyone who works and plays in nonurban, outdoor environments.

## Remember...

1. An emergency care system is a network of specially trained personnel, equipment, facilities, and other resources that respond to emergencies.

2. Ski patrols and ski patrollers are part of the emergency care system.

3. An effective emergency care system has 14 distinct attributes.

4. In the United States, there are four types of prehospital emergency care providers: Emergency Medical Responders (EMRs), EMTs, Advanced EMTs, and Paramedics.

5. Emergency care system resources are deployed using a tiered approach based on specific needs.

6. Common goals, a common language, and common practices enable the components of an emergency care system to function as a team.

7. Effective communications permits emergency care systems to operate in a coordinated manner.

8. Time is expressed using military or universal time.

9. Medical oversight and quality improvement ensure that the care patients receive is in accordance with area medical guidelines.

10. By using prospective, concurrent, and retrospective quality improvement methods, OEC Technicians can improve the care they provide.

## Chapter Questions

### Multiple Choice

Choose the correct answer.

1. Common radio etiquette includes all of the following except _____
   a. speak rapidly, yet clearly.
   b. limit communication to official business only.
   c. be concise (less than 30 seconds).
   d. speak directly into the microphone.

2. Which of the following are protocols? _____
   a. Verbal guidelines that describe what should be done in a given situation.
   b. Written instructions that describe what should be done in a given situation.
   c. Written guidelines given by NHTSA (the National Highway Traffic Safety Administration).
   d. Verbal guidelines given by NHTSA (the National Highway Traffic Safety Administration).

3. What is the vital link that connects all the components of an EMS system and allows the system to work in a coordinated fashion? _____
   a. communication systems
   b. public health agencies
   c. medical oversight
   d. research

4. What is 5:28 p.m. in military time? _____
   a. 1428
   b. 1528
   c. 1628
   d. 1728

**5.** What is 10:43 p.m. in military time? _____ C
   **a.** 2043
   **b.** 2143
   **c.** 2243
   **d.** 2343

**6.** Using the NATO phonetic alphabet, how do you say the letters MLK? _____ C
   **a.** Mary, Lima, Kilo
   **b.** Mike, Lucky, Kilo
   **c.** Mike, Lima, Kilo
   **d.** Mary, Lucy, Kilo

**7.** Using the NATO phonetic alphabet, how do you say the letters WYZ? _____ a
   **a.** Whiskey, Yankee, Zulu
   **b.** Whiskey, Yankee, Zebra
   **c.** Whiskey, Yo-Yo, Zulu
   **d.** Whiskey, Yo-Yo, Zebra

**8.** The current EMS system was established in _____ b
   **a.** 1984, after the EMT curriculum was developed.
   **b.** the 1960s, in response to the large number of highway fatalities.
   **c.** 1980, to decrease the number of prehospital cardiac arrests.
   **d.** 1994, with the DOT National Registry program.

**9.** The four levels of EMS providers in the United States are _____ d
   **a.** EMR (Emergency Medical Responder), FR (First Responder), EMT (Emergency Medical Technician), and EMT-P (EMT Paramedic).
   **b.** FR (First Responder), EMT (Emergency Medical Technician), AEMT (Advanced Emergency Medical Technician (Intermediate), and EMT-P (EMT Paramedic).
   **c.** EMT (Emergency Medical Technician), AEMT (Advanced Emergency Medical Technician), Paramedic, and Medical Control.
   **d.** EMR (Emergency Medical Responder), EMT (Emergency Medical Technician), AEMT (Advanced Emergency Medical Technician), and Paramedic.

## Matching

**1.** Match each category of EMS provider with the correct description. Each answer may be used more than once, and each description may have more than one answer.

_cf_ **1.** Emergency Medical Responder (EMR)

_a g_ **2.** Emergency Medical Technician (EMT)

_a e g_ **3.** Advanced Emergency Medical Technician (AEMT)

_a b d e g_ **4.** Paramedic

   **a.** functions with medical oversight to provide basic life support interventions
   **b.** operates with medical oversight and provides the highest level of prehospital care
   **c.** is typically the first formally trained provider to reach the patient.
   **d.** uses a variety of basic and advanced equipment and medications, including narcotics
   **e.** may perform intermediate therapeutic interventions using basic and advanced equipment and medications typically found on an ambulance
   **f.** renders treatment using minimal equipment and often performs without medical oversight
   **g.** provides life support interventions such as making assessments, splinting fractures, and assisting patients in taking certain prescribed and over-the-counter medications

2. Match the type of quality improvement (QI) to each of the following characteristics. QI types may be used more than once.

___d d___ **1.** prospective QI

___c f___ **2.** concurrent QI

___b e___ **3.** retrospective QI

**a.** involves training

**b.** addresses situations after they occur

**c.** centers on taking corrective action as needed, while tasks are being preformed

**d.** involves protocols

**e.** includes case reviews and after-action reports

**f.** may involve online medical direction

## Labeling

Label the following descriptions with either DO (direct oversight) or IO (indirect oversight).

___IO___ **a.** Involves offline medical control.

___DO___ **b.** Is usually conducted by telephone or radio.

___DO___ **c.** Involves real-time voice contact with a licensed physician, who helps guide patient care decisions.

___IO___ **d.** Is designed to expedite patient care and is commonly used for "pre-authorizing."

___DO___ **e.** Is used primarily to oversee the provision of advanced care procedures or medications.

## Short Answer

Describe the prehospital role of Outdoor Emergency Care (OEC) Technicians.

their role is to assess, stabilize, and if necessary transport a patient to a higher level of provider while documenting the patient's conditions and circumstances surrounding the incident.

## Scenario

*As a new OEC Technician, you are working in your State Park system. A serious accident has occurred, and you have requested treatment equipment and an ALS (advanced life support) or paramedic ambulance.*

1. To what tier level is an ALS /paramedic assigned? ___4___

   **a.** 1

   **b.** 2

   **c.** 3

   **d.** 4

*Proper radio etiquette is an important factor in effective communications.*

2. When using a radio frequency to share patient information, which of the following should not be spoken over the radio? ___C___

   **a.** the patient's chief complaint

   **b.** the patient's vital signs

   **c.** the patient's name

   **d.** the patient's age

*Radio communication must be clear and precise. To be effective, radio communication should use a common set of terminology.*

3. It is suggested that OEC Technicians use which of the following to communicate letters and numbers? _____ a
   a. NATO phonetic alphabet
   b. Latin common alphabet
   c. Greek medical alphabet and abbreviations
   d. Medical abbreviation alphabet

*While treating the injured park visitor, the EMT contacts the physician of the receiving emergency department to obtain medical direction.*

4. This type of medical oversight is called _____ c
   a. indirect oversight or offline medical control.
   b. medical direction oversight.
   c. direct oversight or online medical control.
   d. prehospital medical direction.

# Suggested Reading

Brennan, John A., and Jon R. Krohmer. 2006. *Principles of EMS Systems*, Third Edition. [Sudbury, Massachusetts]: Jones & Bartlett Learning (ACEP).

National Highway Transportation Safety Administration. 1996. *EMS Agenda for the Future*. Washington, DC: NHTSA.

Page, James O. 1989. "A Brief History of EMS." *JEMS* 14(8): S11.

Public Law 93-154. 1973. Washington, DC.

Thomas, Clayton Lay. 1997. *Taber's Cyclopedic Dictionary*, Eighteenth Edition. Philadelphia: F.A. Davis.

Walz, Bruce J. 2002. *Introduction to EMS Systems*. Albany, NY: Delmar.

# Rescue Basics

Eric P. Bowman, MD, FACEP, FAWM
Paul Murphy, MS, MA, EMT-P

## ⊕ OBJECTIVES

**Upon completion of this chapter, the OEC Technician will be able to:**

**3-1** Describe how the body regulates temperature.

**3-2** Describe the four mechanisms of heat exchange.

**3-3** Describe the "fight or flight" response.

**3-4** Describe the steps an OEC Technician can take to be prepared when responding to a request for assistance.

**3-5** Describe how layering clothing can help preserve body heat.

**3-6** Describe the five modes of disease transmission.

**3-7** Define the following terms:
- pathogen
- Standard Precautions
- body substance isolation (BSI)
- hazardous material

**3-8** List common personal protective equipment used by OEC Technicians.

**3-9** Describe the four components of the scene size-up.

**3-10** Describe and demonstrate how to ensure scene safety.

**3-11** Describe chain of custody.

**3-12** Demonstrate how to safely put on and remove disposable medical gloves.

## Chapter Overview

OEC Technicians must be prepared to respond to a wide variety of situations (Figure 3-1■). Some situations will involve assessment and basic treatment of a single patient in mild weather. Others will be complicated by such factors as darkness, rain, snow, and steep terrain. Because of this potential, it is essential

*continued*

## HISTORICAL TIMELINE

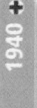
**1940**

Minnie Dole writes to President Franklin D. Roosevelt with the idea of creating an elite military unit composed of skiers.

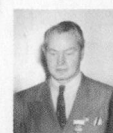
John E. P. Morgan (NSP National #11) becomes first NSP Treasurer.

**1940**

NSP adopts the American Red Cross First-Aid training program.

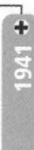
**1941**

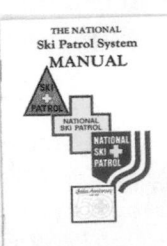

First NSP Ski Patroller's Manual published.

Women are allowed to join NSP.

## ⊕ KEY TERMS

**body substance isolation (BSI),** *p. 76*
**conduction,** *p. 59*
**contamination,** *p. 73*
**convection,** *p. 60*
**decontamination,** *p. 80*
**disease transmission,** *p. 80*
**evaporation,** *p. 60*
**hazardous materials (HazMat),** *p. 85*

**homeostasis,** *p. 58*
**immunity,** *p. 62*
**material safety data sheet (MSDS),** *p. 86*
**metabolism,** *p. 70*
**nutrition,** *p. 62*
**occupational exposure,** *p. 79*
**pathogen,** *p. 62*

**personal protective equipment (PPE),** *p. 77*
**radiation,** *p. 60*
**scene safety,** *p. 82*
**scene size-up,** *p. 82*
**Standard Precautions,** *p. 76*
**ultraviolet radiation,** *p. 69*

that you have an awareness of your overall well-being, are able to adapt to environmental changes, and are conscious of scene dynamics. You must also have a basic understanding of infectious diseases and hazardous materials.

One of the most important skills that you must master as an OEC Technician is taking care of yourself. Many responders have been injured or killed during rescue operations, further complicating rescue efforts and endangering others. Such tragedies often result from inadequate preparation and/or failure to ensure one's personal safety. As an OEC Technician, you will be exposed to many dangers. In order to perform your duties safely, you must learn how to adapt safely to your environment. Adjustments include functioning in temperature extremes and identifying and mitigating potential hazards. You also must learn how to manage stress during and after a rescue operation.

Contagious disease is another hazard you will face routinely. You must learn how communicable diseases are transmitted and how to protect yourself from becoming infected; how to adopt a standardized approach to all patients, don appropriate protective equipment, and properly decontaminate equipment after each patient encounter; and how to understand and manage strategies for reducing the risk of occupational exposures.

This chapter repeatedly emphasizes the importance of scene safety. It is your responsibility to look out for your own safety and the safety of others when approaching each and every patient. This is one of the most important lessons in this text.

The end of this chapter addresses hazardous materials (HazMats) and crime scenes. Although the details of these topics are beyond the scope of this text, it is important that you understand your role should you encounter them.

As an OEC Technician, your ability to put the contents of this chapter into practice will ensure your safety as well as that of your colleagues. The chapter also will discuss ways to provide optimal, safe care for patients. Being prepared and aware of your environment is essential and will likely contribute directly to your success as an OEC Technician.

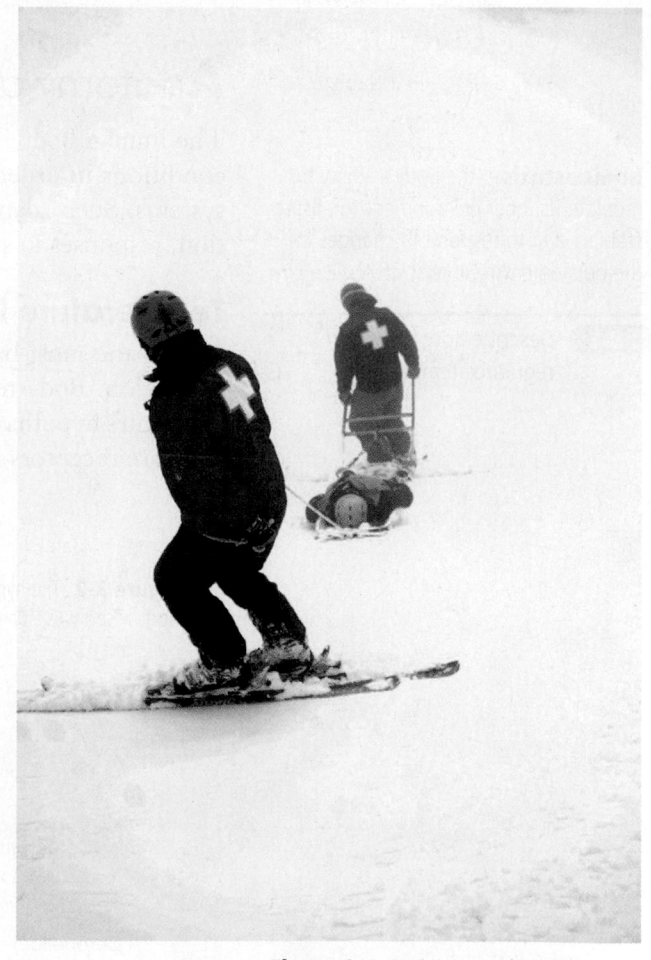

**Figure 3-1** Environmental conditions and hazards may expose OEC Technicians to dangerous situations.
Copyright Studio 404

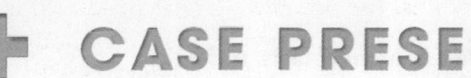 

## CASE PRESENTATION

It is a chilly afternoon with moderate cloud cover. You have just entered the mid-mountain lodge and are looking forward to a well-earned bowl of hot soup when you are summoned to respond to a skier who has fallen approximately 30 feet from a chairlift. The skier reportedly landed on a rock pile and is unconscious. You notify dispatch that you are responding.

Upon arrival, you see that the patient has fallen into a ravine, and that extrication will require specialized equipment and other rescuers. Two other OEC Technicians are already on scene and have initiated care of the patient. One of the technicians is Peter, the newest member of your patrol, who has been assigned to you for mentoring. He is at the patient's head while the other technician is assessing the patient for injuries. You note that Peter is wearing only a sweater and a lightweight outer shell.

As you approach, Peter looks up, smiles nervously, and then gives you a brief report on the patient's condition. As he speaks, you note that he is shivering slightly. It is then that you realize that Peter is not wearing a hat and that his gloves appear to be soaked. A light, freezing rain begins to fall.

**Do you have one patient to address, or two?**

# Anatomy and Physiology

**homeostasis** the body's ability to regulate its inner environment to ensure stability and to respond to changes in the outside environment.

The human body is an amazing organism that is capable of adapting to a variety of conditions in order to maintain **homeostasis**, the tendency toward stability of body systems. Such adaptation can be passive or active and includes temperature regulation, responses to stress, and defense against disease.

⊕ **3-1** Describe how the body regulates temperature.

## Temperature Regulation

One of the most basic adaptive features of the human body is internal temperature regulation. Body temperature regulation occurs automatically and is controlled by the brain's hypothalamus (Figure 3-2■), using neural feedback mechanisms from temperature receptors located throughout the body.

**Figure 3-2** The hypothalamus is in the region of the brain that is active in regulating the automatic body responses, such as "fight or flight."

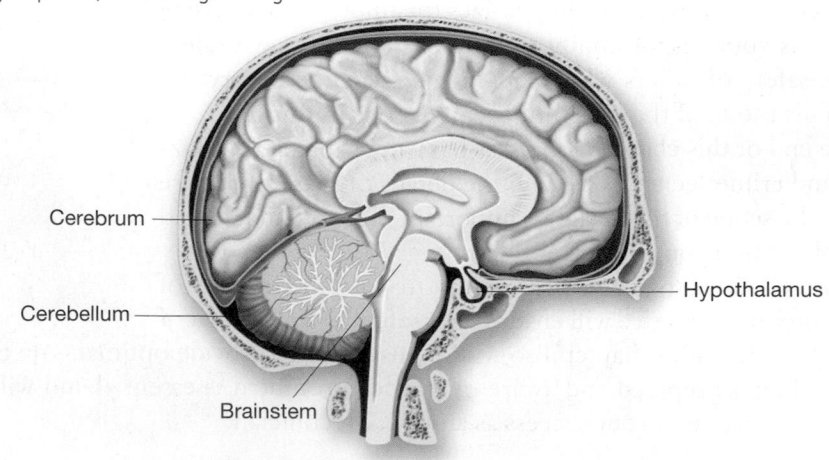

Cerebrum

Hypothalamus

Cerebellum

Brainstem

The process of metabolism by each cell in the body results in the production of heat. As the body's metabolic rate increases, the amount of heat produced also increases. This explains why body temperature rises during exercise. The body's internal thermostat is quite good at keeping body temperature near 98.6°F (37°C). Throughout a day body temperature can fluctuate about 1°F. Normal body temperature also varies slightly among individuals.

The body reacts to ambient temperature changes with the goal of maintaining body temperature at or near 98.6°F. If the core temperature drops below this temperature, several mechanisms act to conserve body heat and to increase heat production. For instance, blood vessels in the skin constrict, reducing blood flow to the body surface, reducing heat loss. In addition, the body may release chemicals such as epinephrine (adrenaline), which speeds up metabolism and helps to produce heat through increased muscular activity, or shivering. When the body becomes too hot, it cools itself through the combination of dilating peripheral blood vessels, which moves more warm blood to the skin's surface, and by sweating, which releases heat into the environment through evaporation.

Heat is lost or gained by the body in the form of thermal energy. Heat always transfers from a warmer object to a cooler object. The four mechanisms of heat transfer are conduction, convection, radiation, and evaporation (Figure 3-3■).

## Conduction

**Conduction** is the transfer of heat from a warmer object to a cooler object through direct contact. For instance, when you lie on the cold snow, heat is transferred directly from your body to the snow (Figure 3-4■). Conduction is the reason snow melts when it is in direct contact with your body. It is also why when you walk barefoot on hot pavement, your feet become hot.

**conduction**    a form of heat exchange in which heat transfers from a warmer object to a cooler object through direct contact.

**Figure 3-3** A poorly dressed climber is losing heat through the four mechanisms of heat transfer.

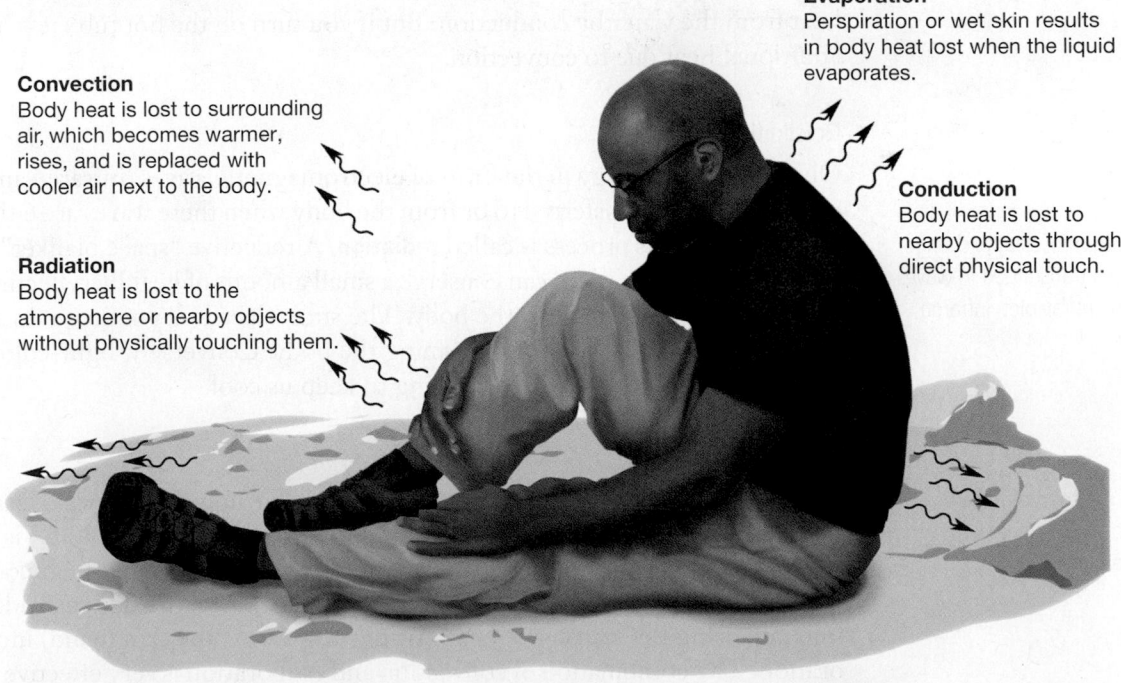

**MECHANISMS OF HEAT LOSS**

**Evaporation**
Perspiration or wet skin results in body heat lost when the liquid evaporates.

**Convection**
Body heat is lost to surrounding air, which becomes warmer, rises, and is replaced with cooler air next to the body.

**Conduction**
Body heat is lost to nearby objects through direct physical touch.

**Radiation**
Body heat is lost to the atmosphere or nearby objects without physically touching them.

**Figure 3-4** This person is experiencing heat loss. As patrollers, we must remain vigilant of our body temperature, the prevailing environmental conditions, and the mechanisms of heat transfer.
Copyright Edward McNamara

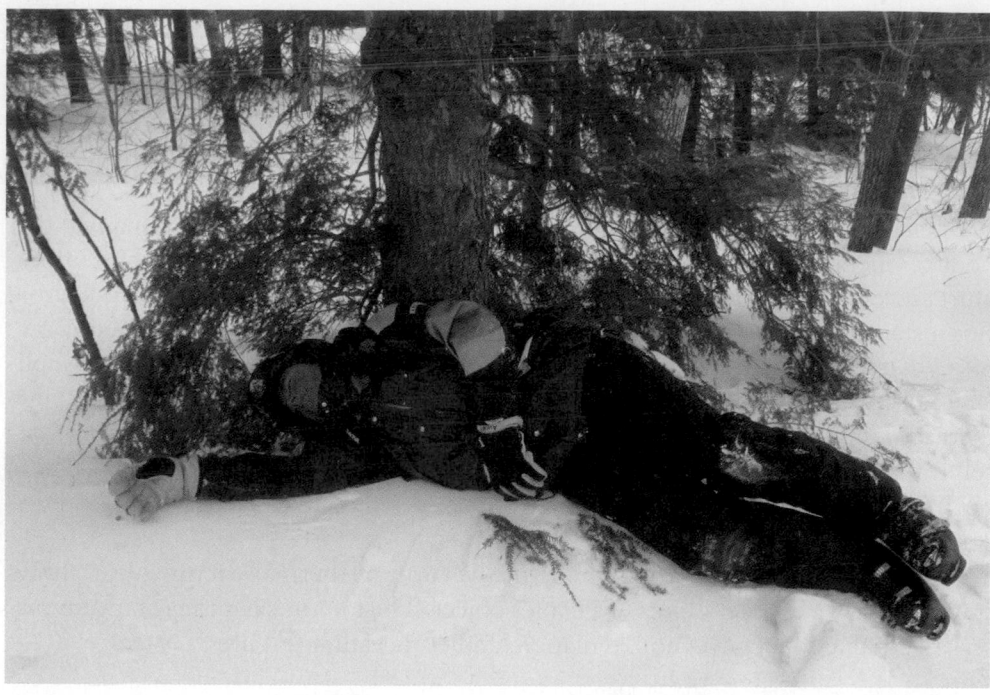

**⊕ 3-2** Describe the four mechanisms of heat exchange.

**⊕ 3-3** Describe the "fight or flight" response.

**convection** a form of heat exchange that occurs when a gas or a liquid moves past the surface of an object.

**radiation** a form of heat exchange in which energy is transmitted in waves (electromagnetic, ultraviolet, infrared) through space.

**evaporation** a form of heat exchange that occurs when a liquid converts to a gas.

## Convection

Convective heat exchange occurs when your body surface is exposed to the movement of a liquid or a gas. Imagine yourself in a body of cold, still water. As you just learned, you will lose heat to the water by conduction. If the water starts moving (or you start swimming), you will lose additional heat by **convection**, even though the water temperature remains constant.

Consider another example: when you are sitting outside on a cold day, you lose heat to the air via conduction. If it gets windy, you will lose additional heat by convection even though the air temperature remains constant. Conversely, imagine sitting in a hot tub of water that is warmer than your body temperature. You will gain heat from the water by conduction. But if you turn on the hot tub's jets, you will gain additional heat due to convection.

## Radiation

Objects radiate energy in the form of electromagnetic waves (infrared and ultraviolet energy). Heat is transferred to or from the body when these waves are either absorbed or reflected. This process is called **radiation**. A reflective "space blanket" is not effective as an insulator, but it can conserve a small amount of heat by reflecting the body's own radiant energy back to the body. The sun's electromagnetic waves are absorbed by bare skin or dark clothing, warming the body. Conversely, light-colored clothing reflects some of the sun's rays, helping to keep us cool.

## Evaporation

**Evaporation** involves the transfer of heat when a liquid becomes a gas. When we sweat, water forms on the skin. If the water vapor in the air (humidity) is low, the water on the skin evaporates, and heat is transferred to the air, which cools the body (Figure 3-5■). When humidity is high, sweat remains on the skin instead of evaporating, impairing the transfer of heat. Air moving across the skin (wind) increases evaporation. The combination of convection and evaporation is very effective in removing large amounts of heat quickly, so they are commonly used to cool a patient in the field.

## The "Fight or Flight" Response

It is important that OEC Technicians be aware of how the body responds to stressful situations. A stress response is stimulated by one or more of the body's five senses: sight, smell, hearing, taste, or touch. Seeing a grossly deformed body part, smelling the stench of a decaying animal, hearing someone retch, tasting foul water, or feeling broken bones move are all sensory cues that can make an OEC Technician feel physically ill.

Stress responses are controlled by the nervous system. When stressed, the body exhibits numerous physical signs and symptoms, such as nausea, diarrhea, dry mouth, sweaty palms, increased heart rate, rapid breathing, and dilated pupils. The stages of a stress response and related signs and symptoms are listed in Tables 3-1■ and 3-2■.

The "fight or flight" response is a function of the autonomic nervous system, the part of the central nervous system that we do not control voluntarily. Breathing, heart rate, and digestion are a few of the functions the autonomic nervous system controls. The release of chemicals such as epinephrine (adrenaline) during stress affects the autonomic nervous system, causing elevated heart rate and blood pressure, pupil dilation, increased respiratory rate and airway capacity, and

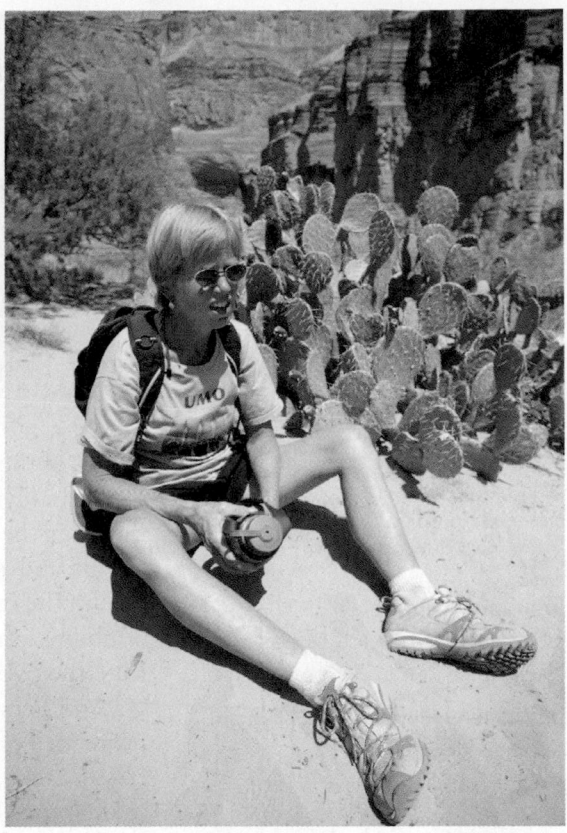

**Figure 3-5** The evaporation of sweat is helping to keep this hiker's body from overheating. Additionally, her peripheral blood vessels dilate, her respiration rate increases, and she becomes thirsty so that she will drink to replace water lost through perspiration.
Copyright Craig Brown

**Table 3-1** Body's Reaction to Stress

| Stage | When the stage begins | Typical signs and symptoms |
|---|---|---|
| Stage I: Alarm | At first exposure to the stressor | Increased heart rate, pupil dilation, increased breathing, sweating, nervousness |
| Stage II: Resistance | When individual begins to adapt to the stressor | Compensation occurs through the use of coping methods, pulse and blood pressure may return to normal |
| Stage III: Exhaustion | As prolonged exposure to same stressor exhausts the person's adaptation energy | Signs and symptoms of the alarm stage return and are more difficult to control |

Adapted from Bledsoe, B., R. Porter, and B. Shade. 1997. *Paramedic Emergency Care,* Third Edition. Upper Saddle River, NJ: Brady.

**Table 3-2** Possible Reactions to Stress

| | | |
|---|---|---|
| Chills | Nausea, vomiting | Confusion |
| Diarrhea | Tremors | Decreased attention span |
| Rapid heart rate | Lack of coordination | Difficulty making decisions |
| Muscle aches | Sweating | Memory lapses |
| Dry mouth | Visual problems | Inability to concentrate |
| Fatigue | Difficulty sleeping | Increased blood pressure |
| Chest tightness | Difficulty breathing | Dizziness |

Adapted from Bledsoe, B., R. Porter, and B. Shade. 1997. *Paramedic Emergency Care,* Third Edition. Upper Saddle River, NJ: Brady.

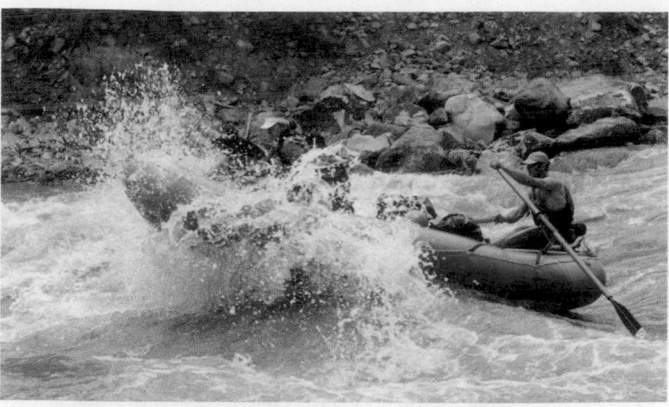

**Figure 3-6** These rafters are physiologically stressed, causing increased heart rate, increased respirations, and increased blood flow to the muscles.
Copyright Scott Smith

**immunity** the state of being protected from a disease, especially an infectious disease.

**pathogen** an infectious agent that can cause disease or illness.

**nutrition** the body's process of utilizing food substances needed for growth and the maintenance of life.

⊕ 3-4    Describe the steps an OEC Technician can take to be prepared when responding to a request for assistance.

increased blood flow to the muscles of the arms and legs (Figure 3-6■). The extra blood flow to muscles provides the additional oxygen and nutrients needed for rapid skeletal movement in the "fight or flight" response.

## The Immune Response

The immune system consists of a network of specialized cells and organs that defend the body from viruses, bacteria, parasites, and other foreign invaders by producing **immunity** or an **immune response**. Components of the immune system include the spleen, thymus, lymphatic system, bone marrow, antibodies, hormones, and leukocytes (white blood cells).

Produced in the bone marrow, leukocytes are the workhorses of the immune system. They are transported to where they are needed via the blood and lymphatic systems. For example, when **pathogens** such as viruses or bacteria enter the body and are detected, leukocytes converge at the site of invasion and engulf and destroy the invaders (Figure 3-7■). Occasionally the pathogens overwhelm the initial defense system. When this occurs, they can multiply quickly, often doubling in number every 20–30 seconds. If the leukocytes cannot completely eradicate the pathogens, an infection or illness will result.

Another way the immune system responds to some pathogens is by producing protective proteins called antibodies that may remain in the circulation indefinitely. If you contracted chicken pox as a child, your body created antibodies specifically against the chicken pox virus. Those antibodies remain in your body and protect you from future attacks by the chicken pox virus.

Many government health authorities have instituted aggressive vaccination programs to prevent the spread of such diseases as influenza, mumps, measles, polio, and tetanus. Smallpox has been essentially eradicated from the world by the most extensive and successful immunization campaign in history. Massive immunization programs have helped reduce the spread of influenza, including H1N1 ("swine flu").

On occasion, the immune system will target healthy cells in a self-destructive process known as an "autoimmune disorder," resulting in diseases such as rheumatoid arthritis and one type of diabetes. Although the immune system is robust, several factors, including inadequate sleep and poor **nutrition**, can affect the immune system's ability to protect you from disease and stressors (Table 3-3■). As an OEC Technician, you should consider lifestyle changes that might reduce your risk of exposure to illnesses and stressors. If you have a medical condition that could affect your immune system, consult your physician to discuss your role as an OEC Technician.

**Figure 3-7** When an invader (a bacterium or a virus) enters the body and is detected, leukocytes come to the site and engulf and destroy the invader.

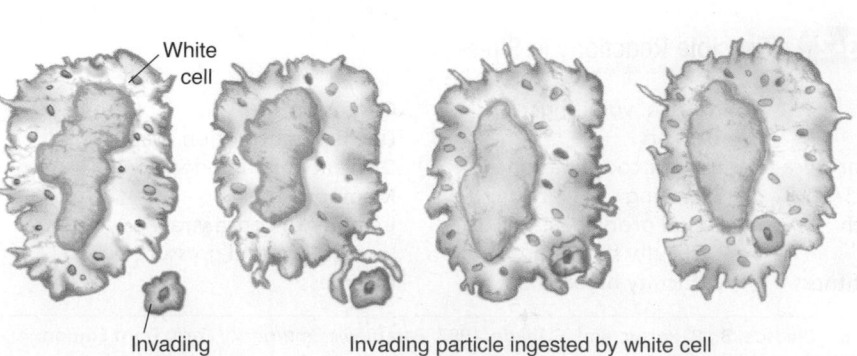

White cell

Invading particle

Invading particle ingested by white cell

| Table **3-3** Factors That Affect the Immune System | |
| --- | --- |
| **Factors that are within your control:** | **Medical conditions that affect your immune system:** |
| Smoking | Diabetes |
| Inadequate sleep | Chemotherapy |
| Poor nutrition | Corticosteroids prescribed for an illness |
| Alcohol abuse | Chronic infections |
| Illicit drug use | HIV, peripheral vascular disease, renal failure |

# Preparing to Work Outdoors

It has been said that proper preparation prevents poor performance. This section addresses several factors that can either enhance or impair your abilities to function as an effective rescuer in outdoor environments.

## Environmental Considerations

OEC Technicians frequently work outdoors, where they are exposed to all types of conditions (Figure 3-8a■). It is essential that you continually monitor the weather, for each change in environmental conditions poses a different set of challenges. There is a major difference between providing care on a warm summer day and providing the same care during a blizzard. Excessive exposure to heat can lead to heat cramps, heat exhaustion, and heatstroke. Exposure to cold can cause frostnip, frostbite, and hypothermia. By being prepared, taking proactive measures during changing weather, and using knowledge of the four mechanisms of heat exchange, an OEC Technician can maintain a normal body temperature and avoid becoming a patient (Figure 3-8b■).

## Mental Preparedness

Mental preparedness is an important step in maintaining well-being. It begins by having a positive attitude. OEC Technicians should always be prepared to encounter the worst-case scenario. Being mentally prepared helps you to overcome developing

**Figure 3-8a** Environmental conditions such as terrain, temperature, and weather conditions may affect the amount of effort involved in caring for and extricating patients.
Copyright Scott Smith

**Figure 3-8b** OEC Technicians give care to a patient in poor weather conditions and difficult terrain.
Copyright Studio 404

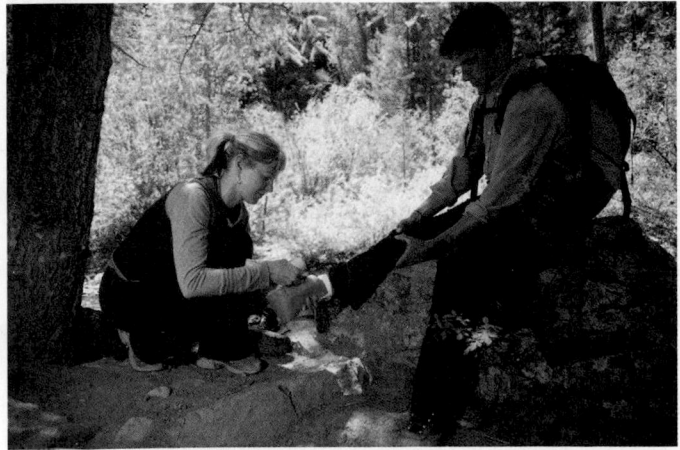

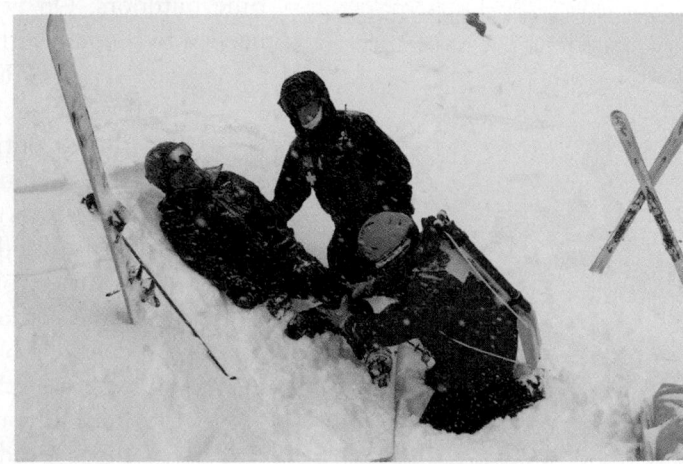

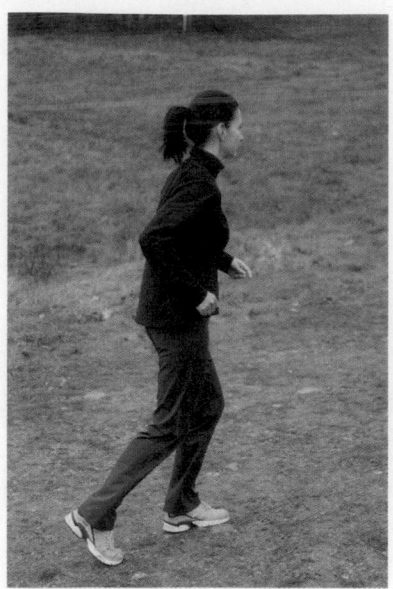

**Figure 3-9** This jogger is maintaining physical condition. OEC Technicians need to be in good physical and mental condition to meet the demands of the job. Preseason training is a must!
Copyright Mike Halloran

problems, including inclement weather, interference by bystanders, equipment failure, and emotionally disturbing situations. As you mentally adapt to changing conditions and stress, you will be better able to concentrate on making critical decisions and providing life-saving treatment.

## Physical Fitness

Physical fitness benefits overall well-being by reducing stress, improving cardiovascular and respiratory function, reducing blood pressure, enhancing physical endurance, strengthening muscles and bones, reducing cancer risks, and controlling weight (Figure 3-9■). To prepare yourself for the mental and physical rigors associated with rescue work, it is recommended that you develop an exercise routine. The routine need not be intense and can involve such activities as swimming, walking, hiking, or cycling. If you are starting a new exercise routine, begin slowly to avoid injury. Depending on your age and overall health, you may decide to consult a physician before embarking on a new workout routine. As progress is made, you can add new activities and include variations in your routine.

### Sleep and Fatigue

A lack of proper rest can cause a host of health-related problems. Sleep deprivation and fatigue may reduce both mental and physical awareness, as well as harm the immune system. Try to maintain a regular sleep schedule. Ideally, humans should receive 7–9 hours of uninterrupted sleep each night. Being well rested reduces fatigue and promotes recovery from physical exertion. Fatigue can affect mood, reduce the ability to adjust to new environments, and impair judgment, which can lead to errors in caring for patients.

### Food and Nutrition

The body must have energy in order to function. Energy is obtained from carbohydrates, fats, and proteins in the diet. The first fuels the body uses are carbohydrates: simple sugars and glycogen (a complex sugar stored in the muscles and liver). During periods of increased activity and reduced dietary carbohydrate intake, metabolic pathways that utilize stored fats sustain us, but peak performance during prolonged activity requires carbohydrate supplementation. In times of starvation, once fat is depleted, metabolic pathways use proteins from our tissues for energy. When our tissues' proteins are used, the body becomes weaker.

Being well nourished makes a significant difference in your ability to participate in strenuous outdoor activities such as rescue operations. You should anticipate the need for highly nutritious, lightweight, high-calorie foods if you are spending much time outdoors. On very strenuous rescues, eating something every hour may be needed to keep up with your body's caloric needs.

OEC Technicians should try to eat healthful, nutritious foods whenever possible (Figure 3-10■). Good nutrition is recommended for overall fitness, optimal body function, and recovery from stress. Table 3-4■ provides a summary of the USDA's daily recommendations for well-rounded meals. It is a good idea to have extra food available during a strenuous call. Nuts, dried fruit, and peanut butter and crackers are perennial favorites. A variety of "energy" bars are also available. Not all energy bars are the same. Packaging, taste, ingredients, carbohydrate content, and price vary considerably. Some products are intended to replace an entire meal, whereas others are intended to provide an energy boost until your next meal. If you decide to include energy bars as part of your routine, sample them ahead of time to ensure that the products you select are satisfactory.

**Figure 3-10** The Food Pyramid. Orange: grains; green: vegetables; red: fruits; yellow: oil; blue: milk (including cheese and yogurt); purple: protein (meat and beans).
Copyright USDA

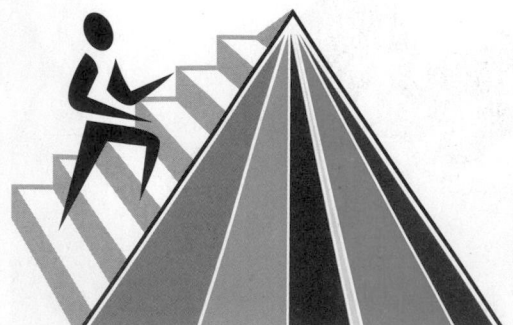

**Table 3-4**  Food Options & the USDA's Tips from the USDA

| Food | Tips |
|---|---|
| Bread, cereal, rice, pasta | 1/2 of grains should be whole |
| Vegetables | Variety is the key |
| Fruit | Primary focus as a food group |
| Milk, yogurt, cheese | Calcium assists in strong bones |
| Meat, poultry, fish, beans, eggs, nuts | Go lean with protein and vary with fish, beans, and nuts |
| Fats, oils, sweets | Use sparingly and use vegetable oil for lower cholesterol |

Adapted from: http://www.nal.usda.gov/fnic/Fpyr/pmap.htm

### Alcohol and Substance Abuse

You should avoid any substance that may compromise central nervous system function or lessen your sense of well-being. Alcohol, for example, can impair your thought processes, judgment, coordination, and decision-making abilities. Any resulting errors can place you, the patient, and others in immediate danger. Chronic substance abuse can injure organs such as the kidneys or liver and suppress your immune system. You should strive to be well rested, healthy, and substance-free before responding to any incident. Providing care while under the influence of any substance is unethical, dangerous, and fraught with medical and legal risks.

## Proper Equipment

Proper preparation includes having the appropriate equipment. This section discusses the importance of proper gear selection. In outdoor rescue work, you need to carry gear in a first-aid pack for providing patient care plus personal gear for maintaining your own well-being.

### First Aid and Survival Pack

As an OEC Technician, you should carry basic first-aid equipment to each incident. The selection of equipment and supplies will be influenced by various factors, including your personal preferences, availability of the equipment, and the type of incident. In some cases you may prefer to design your own custom pack. Your first-aid equipment will include, but not be limited to, the items listed in Appendix C.

**3-5** Describe how layering clothing can help preserve body heat.

### Clothing

Select proper clothing for the work you will be performing. Be sure to factor in possible weather changes when selecting clothing. In choosing safe and proper attire, consider the climate, elevation, time of year, and a multitude of site-specific factors. It is important to have additional layers of clothing available should the air temperature suddenly drop or if you are caught in a storm. It is surprising how cold you can become due to a soaking rain or cool breeze. Because environmental conditions can change rapidly, consider carrying extra clothing in case those you are wearing become wet or unusable, or in the event that you need to share clothing with patients or others.

Many synthetic fabrics have been engineered to protect the body from the elements. These materials can wick perspiration away from the body, provide lightweight insulation, repel water, block the wind, or do a combination of all four. Wool is probably the best natural material used in winter clothing because it is an excellent insulator even when wet, although it does take a long time to dry. Cotton is one of the worst materials for cold-weather use outdoors: it breathes well but is a poor insulator. In addition, wet cotton has almost no insulating value and takes a long time to dry. Cotton may be appropriate in hot, dry environments but is a poor choice for cold, windy, and wet conditions.

Having the right type of clothing is part of the safety equation (Figure 3-11■). Knowing which clothing to wear when, and how to wear it, are equally important. There are many ways to adjust your layers of clothing as the temperature changes. Keep an extra layer available in a backpack, and remove layers when not needed. Proper clothing includes items that protect your feet, hands, head, and face.

In sunny, warm weather, wear white lightweight clothes that cover the skin. This approach prevents sunburn and keeps you cool. Clothing is rated using the sun protection factor (SPF) scale. Most summer-weight clothing provides an SPF of 6.5. Sun-protective clothing can have an SPF as high as 30, which is the recommended SPF to prevent sunburn. Synthetic materials (polyester, nylon) and cotton are best for warm-weather clothing. A hat with a broad brim protects the face and back of the neck.

In cold weather, an OEC Technician's wardrobe should include warm, waterproof gloves and glove liners, synthetic or wool socks, a neck gator or balaclava, goggles, and a hat or helmet. In the winter, think in terms of three layers: base, middle, and outer layers.

+ Base layer. The base layer usually lies tight against the skin, helping to retain heat while allowing moisture to be transferred toward the exterior, a process known as wicking. Ideally, base layers should be made of silk or a synthetic material such as polyester.
+ Middle layer. The middle layer serves as the insulating layer by trapping warm air. Common insulating materials are fleece, wool, and down.
+ Outer layer. The outer layer is designed to be water repellant and wind repellant and should provide protection from sharp objects such as sticks or thorns.

Zippers should be waterproof and have an attached "pull" so that they can be manipulated easily with a gloved hand. A hood that can be folded into the jacket's collar

**Figure 3-11** An example of the many items of clothing you can wear to keep yourself safe. The choices of which items to wear are based on the ambient temperature and the activity being undertaken.
Copyright Mike Halloran

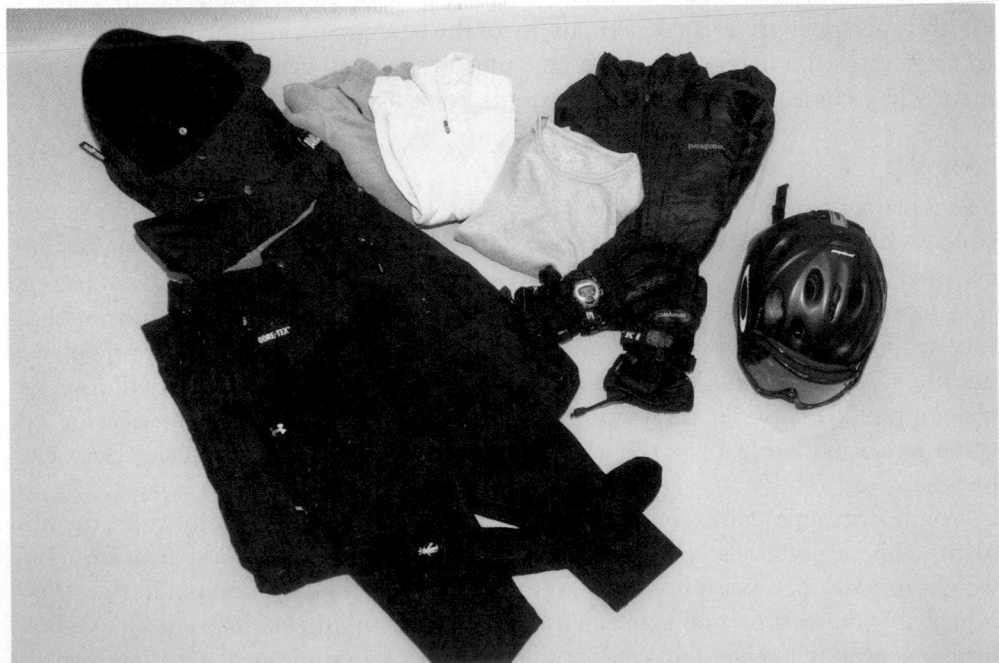

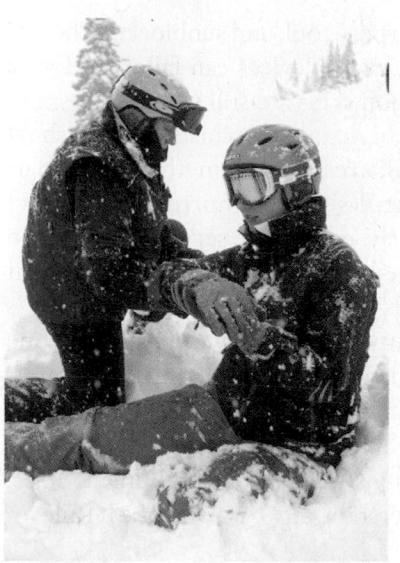

**Figure 3-12a** Helmets are strongly recommended during certain outdoor activities.
Copyright Studio 404

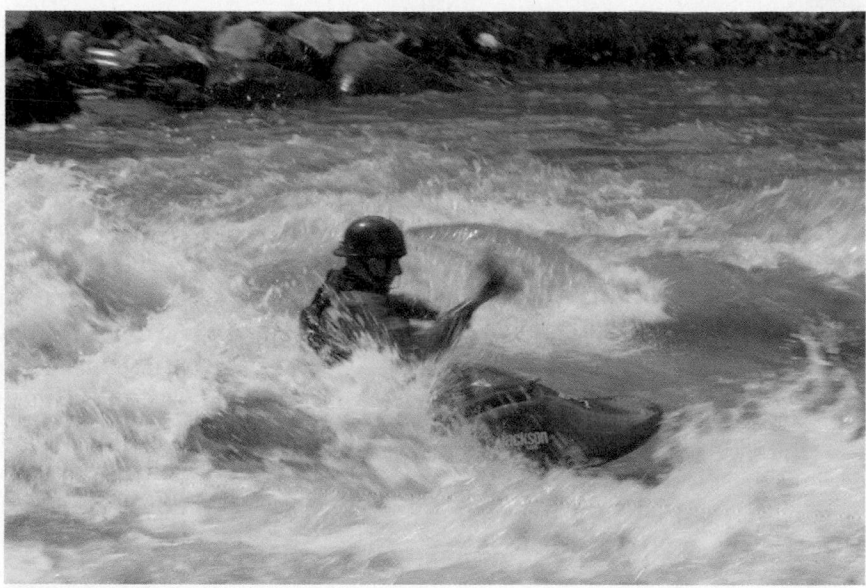

**Figure 3-12b** A kayaker wearing a helmet.
Copyright Studio 404

and opened as needed offers additional neck and head protection. Detachable sleeves may be useful in converting a coat into a vest. External and internal pockets and cargo pockets may be useful for carrying smaller rescue equipment.

The National Ski Patrol strongly recommends that OEC Technicians wear a helmet when engaging in such activities as skiing, snowboarding, snow machine riding, rafting, kayaking, biking, and technical climbing. In addition to protecting the head and keeping it warm, wearing a helmet sends a strong safety message to members of the public, who often adopt the equipment and philosophies they see professional rescuers using. Advances in technology have enabled helmets to offer the combination of protection, comfort, and ventilation (Figures 3-12a■ and 3-12b■).

As with clothing, it is wise to carry extra equipment. If you are going into the backcountry, pack a small survival kit that includes items to help with fire starting, navigation, and signaling (Figure 3-13■). Consider packing waterproof matches or a magnesium fire block, because they are more reliable than a lighter. Take a flashlight,

**Figure 3-13** A personal survival kit.
Copyright Andy Crawford/Dorling Kindersley Media Library

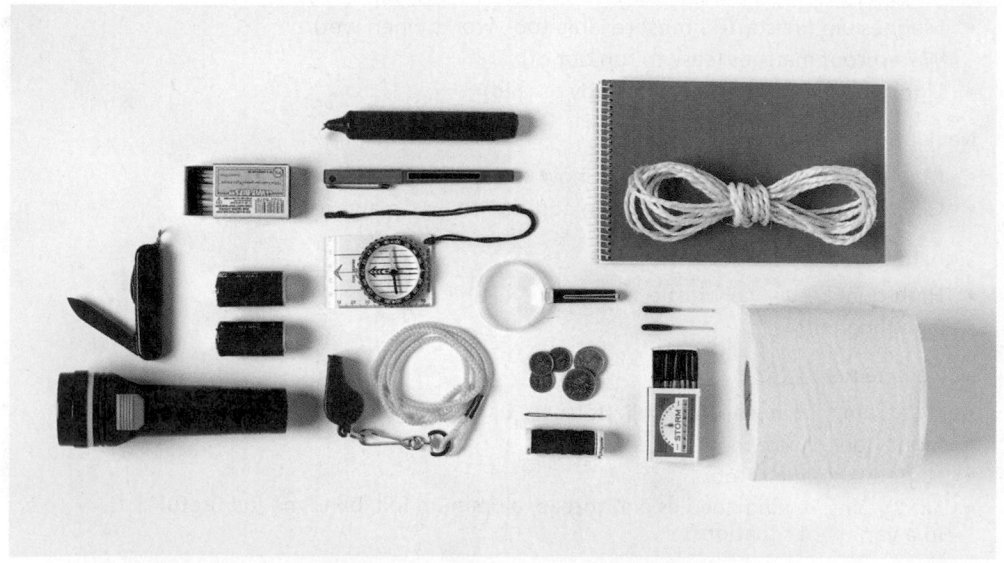

NOTE

## Survival—The "Rule of Threes"

- Three minutes: you can die if you are without oxygen for three minutes.
- Three hours: you may die from exposure within three hours without proper shelter.
- Three days: you may die within three days without a water supply.
- Three weeks: you can survive up to three weeks without food.
- Three months: This is variable, but it has been shown that the will to survive dwindles when one is without human contact for prolonged periods of time.

a carabiner, a high-quality multipurpose tool, and sunblock. Although GPS units are becoming popular, these devices can fail, therefore a map, a compass, and good navigation skills are still necessary.

Your kit should also include a high-quality whistle. Three short blasts is the international sign of distress. Other methods of signaling include radios, cell phones, and signaling mirrors (a compact disk works well as a mirror). Clearly, cell phone service is limited in many wilderness locations. However, there has been a significant increase in search-and-rescue calls using cell phones. Although it is unwise to completely rely on any mechanical device (especially one with batteries), you should consider the use of cell phones or satellite phones, if you are in areas with cell signals. For a complete list of items to include in your survival kit, see Table 3-5■.

Many survival classes, including some military training courses, mention a helpful tool for understanding survival: the "Rule of

### Table 3-5 Survival Kit Checklist

**Oxygen**

- Avalanche tools (beacon, probe, shovel)
- SCUBA divers: appropriate backup gear and rescue equipment

**Shelter**

- Large heavy-duty trash bag (50-gallon plastic drum liner works great)
- 50 feet of parachute cord (multiple purposes)
- Knowledge of how to build a debris hut or snow shelter

**Water**

- Container to hold and transport water
- Water purification methods (see Table 3-6■)
- Knowledge of how to procure water from the environment

**Food**

- Consider a few granola bars, dried fruit, bouillon cubes, honey packets
- Food is a low priority since we can survive without food for weeks
- Knowledge of how to procure food from the environment

**Fire**

- Magnesium fire starter (most reliable tool, works when wet)
- Waterproof matches (easy to run out of)
- Lighter (difficult to use when windy or cold)

**Navigation**

- Map, compass, and knowledge of how to use them
- GPS can be helpful, but use only in addition to a map and compass

**Signaling**

- High-quality survival whistle
- Signaling mirror

**Miscellaneous**

- Head lamp, or at least a flashlight (spare batteries and bulbs)
- Eight-hour candle
- High-quality multi-tool
- Safety pins, sewing needles and thread, aluminum foil, bandana (all useful in a variety of situations)

Threes." Even though it is an oversimplification, it can help you prioritize your goals if you find yourself in a life-threatening situation. Each situation is different, but the concept is valid.

## Skin and Eye Protection

Most rescues occur during daylight hours. A small amount (an hour) of daily direct sunlight on skin not covered by clothing is beneficial in promoting the production of vitamin D. Too much sun exposure puts your skin and eyes at risk from **ultraviolet radiation (UVR)**. Excessive exposure to UVR can cause sunburn, skin damage, cataracts, and skin cancer. You can take measures to protect your eyes and skin. See Chapter 26, for more information about the harmful effects of UVR.

A variety of products are available for protecting the skin from the sun's harmful rays. Sunscreen comes as a lotion, spray, gel, or paste that absorbs or reflects UVR. Most products include an SPF rating; higher numbers provide greater protection. Consider using a sunscreen with a minimum SPF of 30. Follow all manufacturer recommendations when using sunscreen, paying close to attention to reapplication recommendations. Adverse skin reactions, such as burning, itching, and rash, can occur from sunscreens. Before adopting a specific skin protection product for regular use, apply a small amount to the back of your hand and watch for signs of skin irritation. Reactions may be delayed for two to three days.

Proper eye protection is easily overlooked, but it is essential. Long-term exposure to sunlight can cause cataracts and damage your retinas and corneas, so reducing the amount of UVR that reaches the eyes helps prevent ocular damage. Sunglasses are an easy way to reduce UVR exposure (Figure 3-14a■). The "wraparound" style of sunglasses or those with side panels provide the greatest protection against solar UVR. It should be noted that UVR is present even on overcast days.

Unprotected eyes are at risk for a kind of damage to the cornea called ultraviolet (UV) keratitis (Figure 3-14b■). A common risk factor for this disorder is spending time on highly reflective surfaces such as water and snow, which is why this disorder is commonly called "snow blindness." Just as for sunburn of the skin, you remain unaware of this condition until you experience eye pain hours after exposure.

If you wear contact lenses, you should consider keeping an extra set of contacts or a pair of glasses available with you at all times in the event a contact lens is lost. You

**ultraviolet radiation** waves of solar energy that are beneficial in small amounts but harmful to the skin and eyes upon overexposure.

**Figure 3-14a**  This person is wearing sunglasses to protect his eyes from solar ultraviolet radiation.
Copyright Edward McNamara

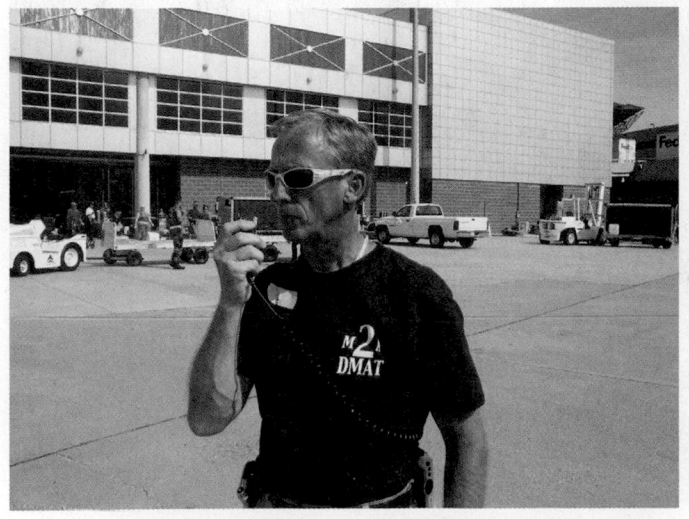

**Figure 3-14b**  Eye damage from the UV rays in sunlight.
Copyright Dorling Kindersley Media Library

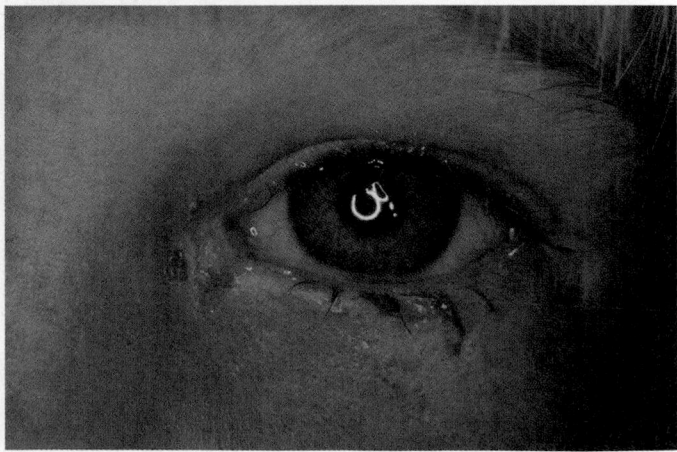

might also consider carrying small vials of saline solution to help keep your eyes and contacts moist.

## Hydration

Dehydration is a major concern not only in survival situations, but also in any outdoor activity. Given an ambient temperature of about 70°F and an average rate of **metabolism**, each day your body loses an average of 1 liter of water through respiration, 0.5 liter through perspiration, and about 1 liter through urination. During exercise or physical activity, especially when performed in a warm environment, you can lose up to 2 liters of fluid per hour. At high altitude, you can lose much more than a liter per day through the lungs just from an increased respiratory rate. To maintain homeostasis and peak performance, you must remain well hydrated.

The organs primarily responsible for maintaining normal fluid balance are the kidneys, which respond to dehydration by reducing urine production. Fluid excesses are handled by increasing urine output. Prolonged and severe dehydration can lead to kidney failure.

In order to remain properly hydrated, OEC Technicians should carry replacement fluids. Several commercial "sport" beverages contain electrolytes and other essential components that are specifically intended to support optimal hydration. Adding these fluids during prolonged physical activity may be beneficial. Some of these fluids contain large amounts of sugar and thus can cause diarrhea if consumed too rapidly. In most situations, water is sufficient. Carry more water than you think you will need.

In a survival situation, water in a lake, a pond, a stream or snow can be consumed. However, these surface water sources are usually contaminated by microorganisms or chemicals that can make you severely ill. If surface water is used, it should be disinfected, either by boiling or by using other means such as water filters, ultraviolet (UV) water purification lamps, iodine tablets, or chlorine dioxide tablets (Figure 3-15■). See Table 3-6 for a comparison of these various water purification methods.

**metabolism** the chemical processes occurring within a living cell or organism that are necessary for the maintenance of life.

**Figure 3-15** Surface water should be purified before consumption by boiling or the use of water filters, UV water purification lamps, iodine tablets, or chlorine dioxide tablets.

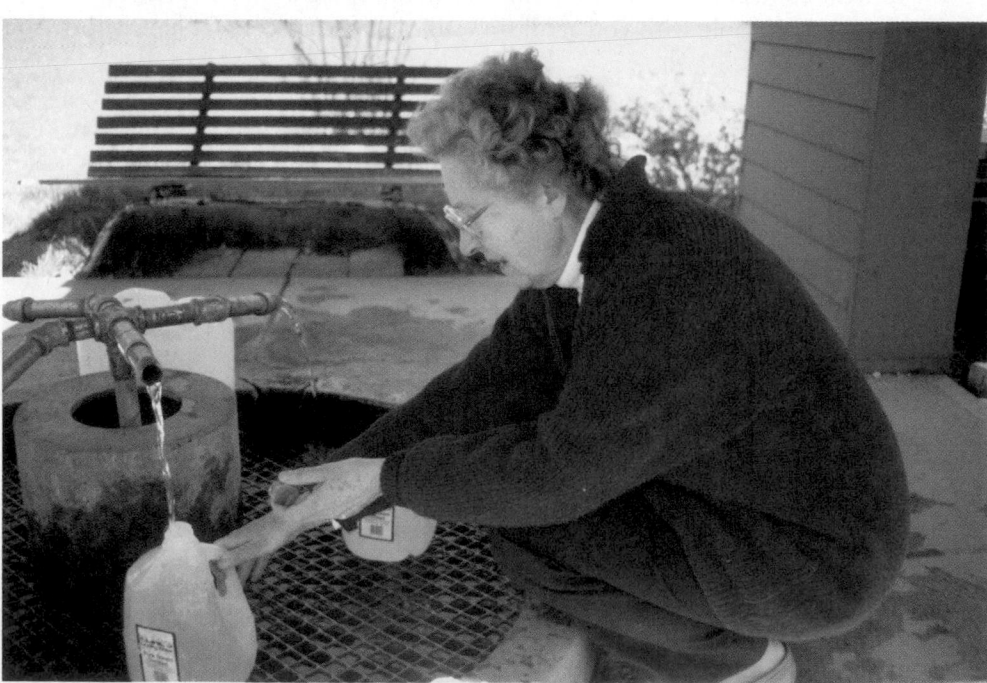

| Table 3-6 | Water Purification Methods | |
|---|---|---|
| **Method** | **Advantages** | **Disadvantages** |
| Heat (boiling water) | Reliable, simple | Limited by fuel source |
| Filtration (water filters) | Simple, no added taste, immediate | Heavy, somewhat expensive, bulky; will gradually clog |
| Chemicals | Inexpensive, lightweight | Unpleasant taste; must follow directions carefully; must wait defined period of time before drinking |
| Chlorine | Readily available | Requires knowledge and experience to use safely |
| Iodine | Very cheap for large number of tablets | Very short shelf life, especially once bottle is opened |
| Chlorine dioxide | Individually wrapped tablets | None |
| UV-light devices | Eliminates all pathogens, easy and quick to use | Expensive, somewhat heavy and bulky; can fail (use batteries and can be broken); are technique sensitive |

## Prolonged Rescue Response Preparation

Unlike a response in bounds at a ski area, a response to a request for assistance in the backcountry can be as brief as an hour or may span several hours or even days (Figure 3-16■). You should always be prepared for the possibility of a prolonged response. Preparation may include carrying a water purification device and a supply of nonperishable food. Always sample the foods before taking them on a response. Make sure ahead of time that your body tolerates the foods you choose, especially energy bars, which can cause gastrointestinal problems in some people.

Consider including an emergency shelter and bedding among your gear. A compact, single-person tent and ground tarp may be sufficient. In the event that the weather becomes extreme, you may seek shelter in an existing structure, such as a cave entrance or under rock formations, or you may need to construct a shelter using available materials found in the immediate area. Digging a snow cave or building a snow shelter can be life-saving.

## Protecting Yourself from Disease

When you are working as an OEC Technician, it is always possible that you will be exposed to an infectious, communicable disease. A *communicable disease* is an illness that can be transmitted from one individual to another. *Infectious diseases* are caused by microorganisms called pathogens, which invade the body. This section focuses on pathogens that cause the most common infectious diseases that OEC Technicians may encounter.

Infectious diseases are transmitted in five ways: by direct contact, by indirect contact, via airborne transmission, through ingestion, and via vector-borne transmission:

♦ Direct contact. Involves close person-to-person contact. Good examples of diseases spread by direct contact are hepatitis B, HIV, herpes simplex, gonorrhea, and mononucleosis.

**✛ 3-6** Describe the five modes of disease transmission.

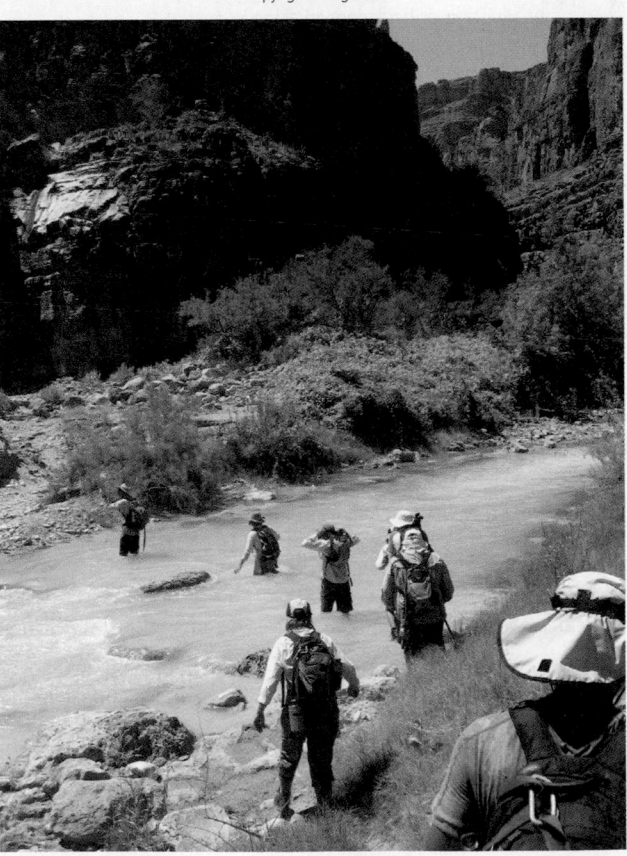

**Figure 3-16** OEC Technicians should be prepared with appropriate supplies when responding to a request for backcountry assistance; there is the potential of a prolonged response.
Copyright Craig Brown

+ Indirect contact. Involves physical contact with an object contaminated with pathogens, including clothing, dressings, towels, soil, and bedding. Examples of diseases that may be contracted through indirect contact are athlete's foot (from shower stalls) and lice (from bed linens).

+ Airborne transmission. Occurs from inhaling droplets containing infectious pathogens propelled into the air by coughing or sneezing, or by acts of bioterrorism. Examples of diseases that may be contracted through airborne transmission are the common cold, influenza, meningitis, chicken pox, and tuberculosis.

+ Ingestion (fecal-oral route). Involves ingestion of food or water that has been contaminated with feces. These diseases can be contracted by (1) eating food that was

# STOP, THINK, UNDERSTAND

## Multiple Choice

Choose the correct answer.

1. Which of the following is not a physical response to stress?_____
   a. nausea
   b. rapid breathing
   c. dilated pupils
   d. constricted pupils

2. When the core body temperature drops below 98.6°F, numerous events take place to conserve body heat and increase heat production. What of the following events does not help with heat production or heat conservation?_____
   a. shivering stops
   b. shivering increases
   c. metabolism increases
   d. blood vessels in the skin constrict

3. Which of the following are leukocytes?_____
   a. red blood cells
   b. white blood cells

   c. pathogens
   d. antibodies

4. When dressing for outdoor winter activities, what is the optimal number of layers to wear?_____
   a. 4
   b. 3
   c. 2
   d. 1

5. Which of the following is not a recommended way to purify surface water?_____
   a. boiling
   b. iodine tablets
   c. chlorine dioxide tablets
   d. solar radiation

## Fill in the Blank

1. During the "fight or flight" response, blood flow increases to the_____ and _____ muscles.

2. _____, _____, _____, and _____ can weaken the immune system.

3. _____ clothing has no insulating value and takes a long time to dry, and thus it is a poor choice for outdoor winter activities.

4. Heat always transfers from the _____ object to the _____ object.

## Matching

Match each mechanism of heat transfer with the correct description at right.

_____ 1. conduction

_____ 2. convection

_____ 3. radiation

_____ 4. evaporation

a. the transfer of heat when a gas or liquid moves past your body
b. the transfer of heat when a liquid becomes a gas
c. the absorption or reflection of electromagnetic waves
d. the transfer of heat from a warmer object to a cooler one through direct contact

# CASE UPDATE

Reaching into your pack, you hand Peter your spare wool hat and a dry set of waterproof gloves. You then assist the other technician in treating the injured patient. Still other rescuers arrive and begin setting up a rescue plan. As you continue to work, the weather becomes more severe as a mixture of snow and hail begins to fall. The temperature starts to drop and the wind increases. Peter's coat is not waterproof, and within minutes he is soaked. His fingertips are becoming numb and he repeatedly takes off his gloves to blow on his hands. You are about to say something to him when his stomach growls loudly. Embarrassed, he looks at you and says, "It was a late night last night, and I skipped breakfast." Glancing at your watch, you note that it is 1:30 p.m.

**What is the best way to help both the patient and Peter?**

either handled by an infected individual who did not wash his hands after defecating or grown in fecally contaminated soil, or (2) drinking from a water source contaminated with feces. One can also become ill from ingesting food or water contaminated by substances other than feces. Common diseases that are contracted through ingestion are gastroenteritis (caused by *Salmonella*, *Shigella*, or *Giardia*) and hepatitis A.

✦ Vector-borne transmission. Involves the transmission of pathogens to humans by other animals such as ticks and mosquitoes. Bites from infected ticks can cause many disorders, including Lyme disease and Rocky Mountain spotted fever. Mosquitoes transmit malaria, West Nile virus, encephalitis, and a host of other illnesses worldwide. Rabies is transmitted through the bite of a rabid animal.

## Contamination

**Contamination** occurs once an individual comes into contact with enough organisms to cause symptoms. After the individual becomes exposed and the disease has been acquired, there is a highly variable incubation period. During this time, the offending pathogens multiply until the individual may start to manifest symptoms. In many cases, the person can infect others during the incubation period. Consider the following situation:

> While you are taking care of a skier who has broken her arm but does not otherwise seem ill, she sneezes. Unknown to you, the patient is in the early phase of an upper respiratory infection. When she sneezed, thousands of viral particles filled the air, which you then inhaled with your next breath (Figure 3-17■). For the next several days you are in an incubation period during which the virus particles multiply. During this time, you are unwittingly contagious and expose others, including your family, friends, coworkers, and patients, to the virus. A few days later, you start to manifest symptoms. Once you start to feel better, your ability to contaminate others declines. However, because you infected others, illness spreads quickly. In a close work setting such as that of patrols and rescue teams, the disease can infect nearly everyone.

### Common Ways of Contracting Diseases

The two most common ways OEC Technicians contract a communicable disease are direct contact with a patient's bodily fluids and inhalation of pathogens during breathing.

**contamination** soiling of an object, water, or air by foreign material such as dirt, debris, bodily fluids, or radiation.

**Figure 3-17** This photograph reveals the thousands of germ-laden droplets expelled during a sneeze.

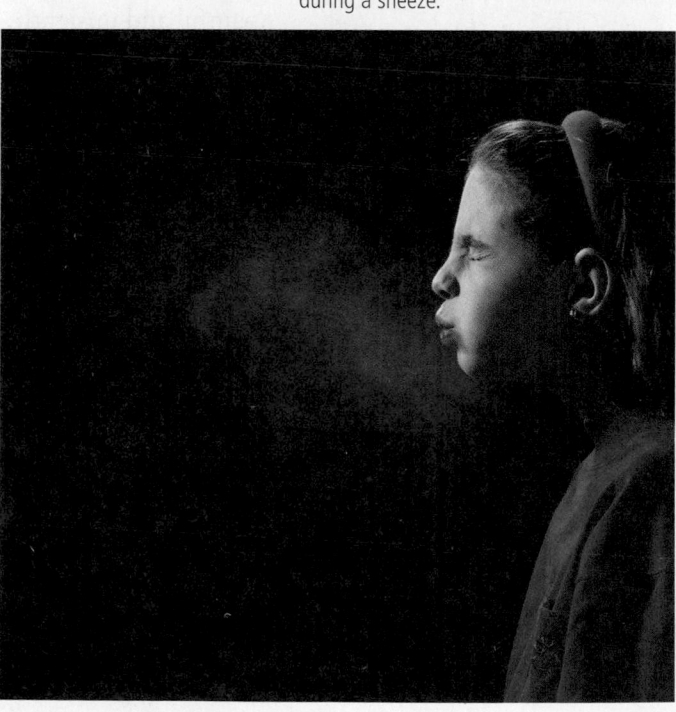

## Common Infectious Diseases

In this section we consider some of the more common and serious infectious diseases to which OEC Technicians might be exposed.

### Upper Respiratory Infections and Pneumonia

Common colds are caused by many different viruses. Simply inhaling enough viruses following someone's sneeze or cough is all it takes to become infected. Pneumonia involves infection of the lung by bacteria, viruses, or fungi. The individuals most at risk are those older than 65, those younger than 2, and those who already have health problems such as pulmonary disease or a weakened immune system.

Common colds are characterized by runny or stuffy nose, sore throat, cough, and transient fever. Pneumonia also presents with cough and fever but is more likely to produce chest pain, shortness of breath, prostration, and persistent fever.

### Influenza

Influenza, or the seasonal "flu," is caused by a virus that infects the respiratory tract. It is easily transmitted among humans and each year results in many deaths worldwide. Transmission most commonly occurs via the airborne route but also can occur indirectly following contact with a contaminated surface. The viruses can survive for up to two days on a hard, nonporous surface such as a doorknob. Recent outbreaks of the H1N1 virus, also known as "swine flu," increase the chances that you will be exposed to the flu virus outside of the normal flu season, which typically extends from November to April.

### Herpes Simplex Infections

Herpes simplex is a virus that causes the formation of small blisters, most often around the mouth. Also known as "fever blisters" or "cold-sores," this condition is transmitted through direct contact with the bodily fluids of an infected individual. The most common method of transmission among outdoor rescuers is the sharing of lip balm or water bottles. For this reason, such sharing is strongly discouraged. There is no known cure for herpes, and no vaccine to prevent its transmission. Once an individual becomes infected, blisters may break out several times a year and can be both painful and unsightly.

### Hepatitis

Infectious hepatitis is an acute viral illness that causes inflammation of the liver. There are several common forms of hepatitis. Hepatitis A is acquired by the fecal-oral route, usually by the ingestion of contaminated food or water. Hepatitis B and C are transmitted by exposure to blood, semen, or other bodily fluids; contaminated needles; or sexual contact. Conditions that can develop following hepatitis include liver failure, a chronic form of liver disease called cirrhosis, and liver cancer.

Hepatitis can cause fever, weakness, loss of appetite, nausea, vomiting, jaundice, dark-colored urine, and light-colored stools. Administration of a hepatitis B vaccine is recommended for all health care workers, including OEC Technicians. No vaccine is available for hepatitis C. Review your local protocols regarding receiving your hepatitis B vaccine series. For more information about hepatitis, review the appropriate section of Chapter 16.

### Chicken Pox

Chicken pox is a highly contagious viral disease that is spread through both airborne transmission and direct contact with an infected individual. The disease is caused by the varicella-zoster virus and results in red and itchy blisters that burst, dry out, and crust over within a few days. The condition lasts approximately 5–10 days, during which new crops of blisters continue to form. Patients with chicken pox remain contagious until all lesions have developed crusts.

## Tetanus

Tetanus is a serious disease caused by a toxin produced by bacteria that enter the body through a laceration or puncture wound. The disease results in painful tightening of muscles, including jaw spasms. The lay term for this condition is "lockjaw." Due to an effective vaccine program, tetanus is very uncommon except in underdeveloped countries. Once an individual has been vaccinated as a child, a booster is recommended every 10 years. In certain types of high-risk wounds, your doctor may update your vaccination if you received your last tetanus vaccine over five years ago. If you sustain a wound and have not had a tetanus vaccine within the past five years, consult your physician.

## Human Immunodeficiency Virus / Acquired Immunodeficiency Syndrome

Human immunodeficiency virus (HIV) is a pathogen that is transmitted either through direct contact with bodily fluids containing the virus or through the transfusion of blood containing the virus. It may take up to six months following exposure until HIV infection can be detected by blood tests. HIV frequently impairs the immune system, resulting in acquired immune deficiency syndrome (AIDS).

AIDS patients are susceptible to opportunistic infections such as pneumonia, meningitis, and encephalitis, and to some cancers. Although some antiviral therapies can dramatically help individuals infected with this virus, there is still no effective vaccine to prevent HIV infection or effective cure for AIDS. Prevention of infection is of paramount importance.

## Tuberculosis

Tuberculosis (TB) is a bacterial infection most commonly spread by the airborne route. The disease usually involves the lungs but can affect many other body systems as well. Signs and symptoms include cough, fever, night sweats, weight loss, fatigue, and coughing up blood. TB is detectable and treatable, but the active phase of the infection can be difficult to treat and often requires lengthy antibiotic therapy. A resurgence of TB in recent years has coincided with the emergence of strains that are resistant to commonly used antibiotics. Many health care facilities provide annual skin testing to detect exposure or early illness. Refer to your local protocols regarding recommendations for TB testing.

## Meningitis

Meningitis, an inflammation of the membranes that surround the spinal cord and brain, can be caused by bacteria or viruses. Signs and symptoms can include headache, nausea and vomiting, stiff neck, chills, fever, confusion, rash, altered mental status, and irritability. Seizure and coma also may occur.

Viral meningitis is usually self-limited, but bacterial meningitis can be a devastating illness that requires early recognition and aggressive treatment. Certain types of bacterial meningitis are highly contagious, and individuals who have had close contact with patients, including exposed but unprotected health care workers, may need to take prophylactic antibiotics.

## Rabies

Rabies is a serious viral disease transmitted through the bite of a diseased animal. Bats, raccoons, skunks, foxes, dogs, cats, groundhogs, wolves, weasels, and other animals can be infected with the rabies virus. Once symptoms of rabies develop, usually 30–50 days after infection, the disease is uniformly fatal. Fortunately, a highly effective vaccine is available and should be given immediately to anyone bitten by a rabid animal. It is essential that you contact a physician immediately after any animal bite in order to manage the wound and to determine if rabies vaccination is indicated.

### Measles

Measles is a disease caused by an infrequently encountered virus that infects the respiratory system and produces a characteristic rash. It is highly contagious and is spread through airborne transmission. Due to effective immunization programs, measles is rare in the United States.

### Vaccination Recommendations

Because of the potential exposure to communicable diseases, it is recommended that OEC Technicians be properly vaccinated against the diseases in Table 3-7■. In the United States, Canada, and Europe, most children are vaccinated for common communicable diseases as part of a childhood immunization program. OEC Technicians should undergo hepatitis B vaccination and should consider receiving an annual seasonal influenza vaccine. They also should consider being tested annually for TB. A valuable resource on vaccinations can be found at the Centers for Disease Control and Prevention website: http://www.cdc.gov.

### Standard Precautions and Body Substance Isolation

In order to reduce the number of health care workers acquiring illness from patients, the Centers for Disease Control and Prevention (CDC) has developed guidelines called **Standard Precautions**. Following these guidelines, health care workers treat every patient as potentially infectious. Central to this approach is the concept of **body substance isolation (BSI)**, in which measures are taken to prevent the patient's bodily

---

⊕ **3-7** Define the following terms:
- pathogen
- Standard Precautions
- body substance isolation (BSI)
- hazardous material

**Standard Precautions** the practice of protecting health care workers from exposure to bodily fluids based on the assumption that all patients are potentially infectious.

**body substance isolation (BSI)** the practice of isolating all bodily substances (blood, urine, tears, feces, and so on) of patients from rescuers in order to decrease disease transmission.

---

**Table 3-7** Vaccine Recommendations

| Vaccine | Schedule | Indication |
|---|---|---|
| HepB (hepatitis B) | Three doses | Advisable due to risk of exposure to blood and other bodily fluids |
| Seasonal influenza ("the flu") | Annual | All health care workers (HCW), especially those with high-risk medical conditions or who are older than 65 years |
| MMR (measles, mumps, rubella) | Usually given in childhood | Vaccination should be considered for all health care personnel who lack proof of immunization |
| Varicella zoster (chicken pox) | Two doses | Indicated for health care personnel who lack a history of varicella infection or evidence of immunization |
| Meningococcal (meningitis) | —— | Not routinely indicated for health care personnel, but prophylaxis after exposure may be recommended |
| Tetanus and diphtheria (Td) | Three doses initially (usually given in childhood); booster given every 10 years | All adults |
| Tdap (tetanus, diphtheria, and pertussis) | One-time dose for adults | Considered in lieu of the Td vaccine due to a resurgence of pertussis in some areas |
| Pneumococcal (pneumonia) | One dose; revaccination considered more than 5 years after first dose | Certain adults at risk due to underlying medical conditions or age greater than 65 years |

Resources: CDC, MMWR Recommendations and Reports, December 26, 1997/46(RR-18); 1–42.

Immunization of Health-Care Workers: Recommendations of the Advisory Committee on Immunization Practices (ACIP) and the Hospital Infection Control Practices Advisory Committee (HICPAC).

http://www.cdc.gov/mmwr/preview/mmwrhtml/00050577.htm
http://www.cdc.gov/ncidod/dhqp/wrkr_immune.html#2

fluids from contacting any unprotected portions of the rescuer's person. Standard Precautions and BSI are designed to prevent the transmission of pathogens. It is essential that OEC Technicians be protected from patients' bodily fluids (Figure 3-18▪). Bodily fluids include:

+ Blood
+ Saliva and sputum
+ Vomit
+ Tears
+ Nasal secretions
+ Urine
+ Cerebrospinal fluid
+ Fcccs
+ Menstrual blood or vaginal secretions
+ Placental fluid
+ Synovial (joint) fluid
+ Pericardial fluid (from within the heart sac)
+ Peritoneal (abdominal) fluid
+ Pleural (lung) fluid
+ Semen

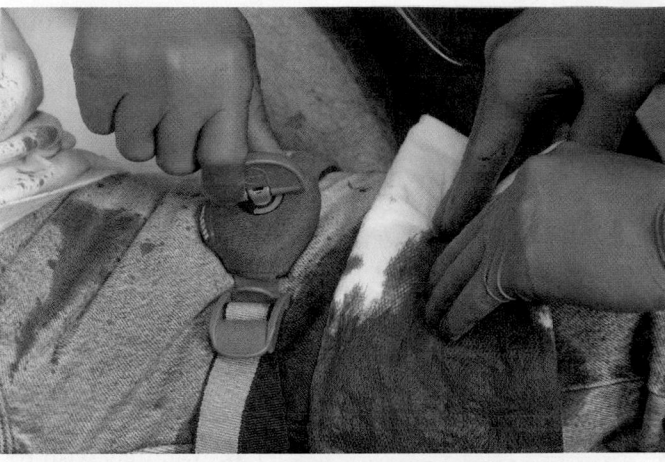

**Figure 3-18** Unprotected contact with bodily fluids may put OEC Technicians at risk.

Also, be wary of any objects that may be contaminated with bodily fluids, including bandages, equipment, towels, blankets, clothing, paper products, and a patient's other belongings. It is your responsibility to practice Standard Precautions on every patient that you encounter, regardless of the patient's clinical signs, condition, age, or background. Do not succumb to the temptation of assuming that the patient is "safe."

Using the concept of Standard Precautions ensures that all patients are treated as though they harbor potentially contagious pathogens. Because many patients with a communicable disease have no obvious signs of illness, it is important that a protective barrier is placed between you and each patient. This protective barrier prevents the transmission of disease through the use of specialized protective medical equipment known as personal protective equipment.

## Personal Protective Equipment

**Personal protective equipment (PPE)** is designed to safeguard rescuers from exposure to infectious agents in the patient's bodily fluids. Although intact skin acts as a good barrier to infection, skin is vulnerable to damage and to dermatologic conditions that can weaken this barrier. Additionally, your mucous membranes (eyes, nose, and mouth) are particularly susceptible to the entry of pathogens. As an OEC Technician, you will need to determine what level of personal protection is appropriate for each specific circumstance.

### Disposable Medical Gloves

Before touching any patient, you should first put on a pair of disposable gloves. You should carry several pairs of gloves with you at all times when you are away from the first-aid area. Because many people are allergic to natural latex rubber, use gloves made from latex-free materials such as polyvinyl chloride (PVC), nitrile, or other synthetic materials. Remember that any item you touch is then potentially contaminated

⊕ 3-8   List common personal protective equipment used by OEC Technicians.

**personal protective equipment (PPE)**   items worn by medical providers, including gloves, mask, safety eyeglasses (or mask with shield), and gown, to protect them from bodily fluids.

⊕ 3-12   Demonstrate how to safely put on and remove disposable medical gloves.

and must be thoroughly cleaned at the end of an incident. Additionally, anyone who touches potentially contaminated equipment with an ungloved hand is also potentially contaminated and might become infected or spread the disease.

Use the following procedure to put on a pair of disposable medical gloves:

1. Whenever possible, wash your hands before donning gloves. Use antimicrobial gel if soap and water are not available.
2. Grasp one glove using your nondominant hand.
3. Slide your dominant hand into the glove, with fingers slightly spread apart. Wiggle your fingers to ensure a snug fit with no air pockets.
4. With the gloved hand, pick up a second glove.
5. Place the remaining hand into the glove as described in step 3.
6. You may wish to interlock the fingers of both gloved hands to ensure a snug fit and to remove any remaining air pockets.

It is imperative to change gloves after every encounter with a patient, and before touching another patient, in order to prevent the transmission of pathogens from one patient to another, a condition known as cross-contamination. Make sure all contaminated items, including medical gloves, do not come into contact with anything else. Any item touched, such as a cell phone, should be considered contaminated.

To prevent self-contamination, you must remove your gloves properly and dispose of them with other contaminated waste. Do not place contaminated gloves into your pocket or medical kit! The time-tested key to removing gloves is "dirty to dirty and clean to clean." That is, a contaminated surface (gloved hand) should only touch another contaminated surface (the external surface of the glove), whereas a clean surface (ungloved hand) should only touch another clean surface (the interior surface of the glove).

Use the following procedure to remove disposable gloves after use (OEC Skill 3-1■):

1. Using your dominant hand, grasp the exterior of the opposite glove at the wrist.
2. Carefully fold the glove over and peel it back, turning it inside out. Once removed, hold the glove in your gloved dominant hand.
3. Place your ungloved fingers inside the cuff of the glove on your dominant hand, being careful not to touch the exterior. Carefully peel the glove off the hand, turning the glove inside out as you remove it. When finished, both gloves should be turned inside out, with the second glove serving as a container for the first glove.

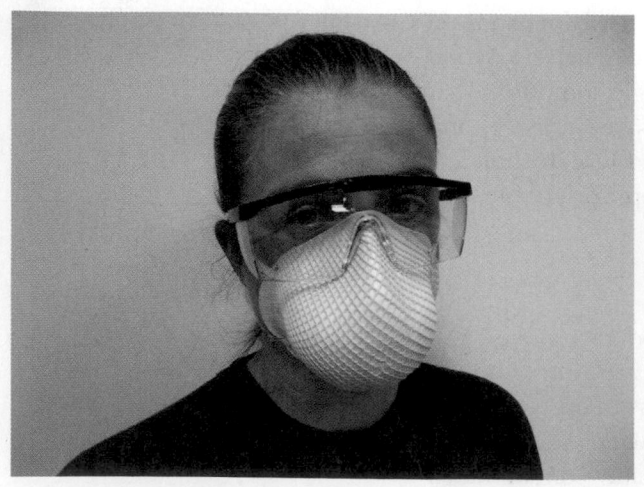

**Figure 3-19** An OEC Technician wearing eye protection, and a mask as well.
Copyright Edward McNamara

### Eye Protection

Eye protection should be worn during every encounter with a patient (Figure 3-19■). Wearing eye protection is especially important when there is a risk of bodily fluids getting splashed or splattered into your eyes. For skiers, ski goggles may serve as an emergency substitute for safety glasses, but they may be difficult to clean if they become contaminated. Sunglasses and prescription glasses also offer some protection, they but provide a less-effective barrier than safety glasses. In order to provide better protection, sunglasses and prescription glasses should have attached side shields.

### Surgical Mask / N95 Mask

Surgical masks provide an effective barrier to airborne droplets and protect your nose and mouth from exposure to bodily fluids

(Figure 3-19). Some masks have attached shields that protect the eyes. Masks also protect the patient from any pathogens that you may have. Use of a mask is especially important if you are suffering from a cold, influenza, or other airborne-transmitted disease. Additionally, you should place a mask on any patient who has, or is suspected of having, an airborne-transmitted disease, especially influenza or TB.

The use of a properly fitted NIOSH-approved N95 mask is recommended when taking care of a patient with TB. Follow your local protocols for dealing with patients with known or suspected TB.

## Medical Gown

To complete your PPE, you should consider wearing a medical gown. Although not all situations warrant the use of a gown, you should wear one if there is a risk of bodily fluids being splashed or sprayed (such as a nose bleed or arterial bleed). For ski patrollers, most ski parkas and pants are waterproof and should suffice in protecting you while on patrol. However, if your clothing becomes exposed, you should thoroughly decontaminate it immediately after the incident.

## Hand Washing

According to the CDC, hand washing is one of the most effective methods for preventing the spread of disease. You should wash your hands *before and after* every contact with a patient. You may use soap and water or a waterless alcohol-based antimicrobial product. Many diseases are transmitted via contaminated hands, so diligent hand washing is mandatory for all OEC Technicians (Figure 3-20■).

## Occupational Exposure

Despite your best efforts to follow Standard Precautions using proper body substance isolation and PPE, you may still sustain an **occupational exposure**. Your risk of becoming infected depends on many factors, including the type of pathogen, type of bodily fluid involved, and route of exposure. Injection of blood confers the highest risk, followed by a contaminated needle stick (Figure 3-21■). Exposure of mucous membranes and broken skin is still a concern but entails less risk, and exposure to intact skin is a low risk. You must report all exposure incidents to your supervisor.

Local protocols should be in place to assist any rescuer who has sustained an occupational exposure. In the meantime, you should immediately decontaminate the

**occupational exposure** an event in which a worker comes into contact with a bodily fluid or hazardous material while on the job.

**Figure 3-20** Hand washing is one of the most effective methods for preventing the spread of disease.
Copyright Edward McNamara

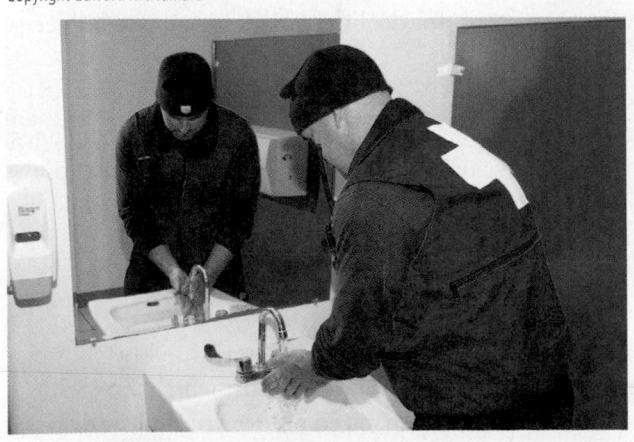

**Figure 3-21** An accidental needle stick.
Copyright Edward McNamara

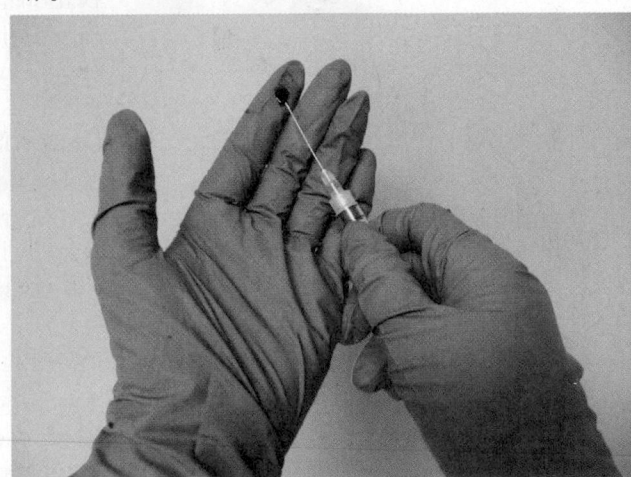

site of exposure. Immediately rinse the affected area with water. If the exposure site is your eyes, flush them copiously with water. If the exposure site is your skin, use soap and rinse thoroughly with water.

Postexposure prophylaxis (PEP) is any preventive treatment that is started immediately after exposure to a pathogen in order to prevent infection and the development of disease. Decisions surrounding postexposure prophylaxis are complex and involve the nature of the exposure as well as the medical history of the source patient. The source patient may be asked to provide blood for testing for HIV infection and hepatitis, and you also may be asked to be tested in order to provide a baseline. Your medical provider will determine appropriate treatment. Effective prevention is time sensitive and thus should be initiated promptly, if indicated.

## Decontamination

Medical equipment used during patient care will have come into contact with dirt and microorganisms—that is, it has become contaminated. Before this equipment can be used again, it must be exposed to one or more of the following processes:

+ Cleaning. The removal of foreign material such as dust or soil from equipment. In most cases, this can be accomplished using hot water and soap.
+ **Decontamination**. The removal of disease-producing organisms. Once an item is decontaminated, it is safe to handle.
+ Disinfection. The actual destruction of disease-producing organisms using special chemicals.

Decisions to clean and/or to disinfect vary and are based on a review of the activities that occurred during the call. Before cleaning or decontaminating equipment, consult with your local protocols and guidelines regarding the recommended procedure.

When cleaning or disinfecting equipment, use appropriate PPE. This is especially important if you have any open wounds on your hands. The use of heavier and more durable utility gloves, such as household rubber gloves, may be considered as well. In addition, to avoid accidental exposure through the mouth or nose, as well as splashes to the eyes, use a mask with an eye shield. The amount of PPE to be worn when cleaning equipment should be guided by the amount of cleaning that will be needed and the potential for splashing. Durable goods should be cleaned and disinfected following manufacturer recommendations.

In the following sections we consider the procedures recommended by the National Institute for Occupational Safety and Health (NIOSH), in collaboration with the Center for Infectious Diseases (CID) and the Centers for Disease Control and Prevention (CDC), for dealing with contaminated objects.

### Disposable Items

Many items that rescuers use are disposable, including gloves, bandages, cardboard splints, cervical collars, and paper sheets. Dispose of them appropriately in biohazard (red) containers or in bags (Figure 3-22■). Double bag if there is any possibility of leakage.

### Infectious Waste

The procedures for disposal of infective waste are determined by the relative risk of **disease transmission** and by local regulations, which vary widely. In all cases, local regulations should be consulted before you follow disposal

**decontamination** the process of rendering an object, person, or area free of harmful substances such as bacteria, poison, gas, and radiation.

**disease transmission** transfer of illness from an infected individual to a healthy individual.

**Figure 3-22** The use of a biohazard bag to dispose of infectious or contaminated material.

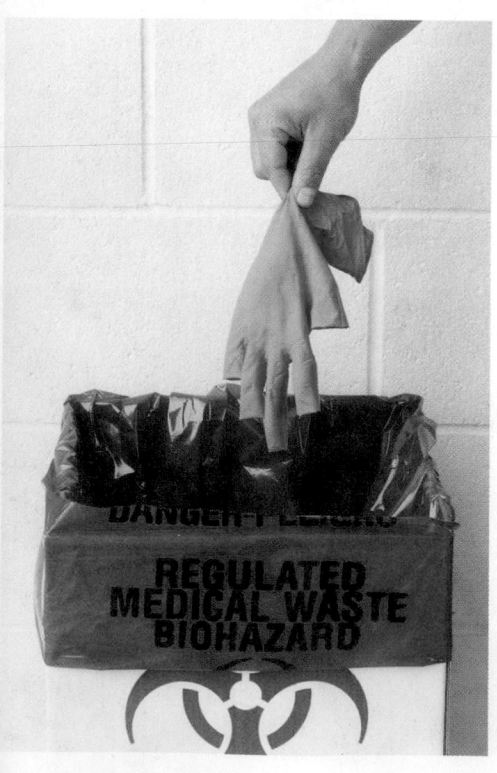

procedures. In general, infective waste should either be in-cinerated or decontaminated before disposal in a sanitary landfill. Where it is permitted, bulk blood, suctioned fluids, excretions, secretions, and infectious wastes that can be ground up may be carefully poured down a drain connected to a sanitary sewer.

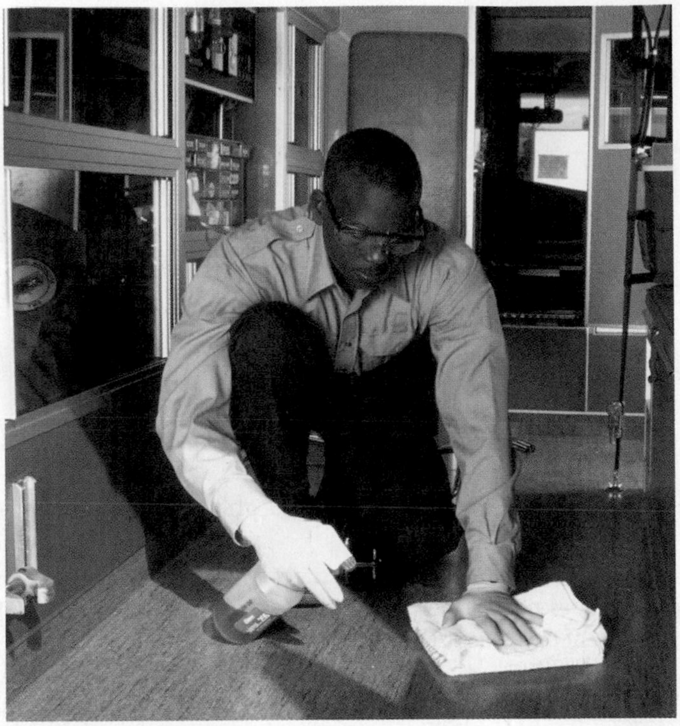

### Bed Linens, Blankets, and Contaminated Clothing

Any nondisposable linen or clothing that is contaminated with blood or other body fluids should be placed into and trans-ported in red hazard bags or containers that prevent leakage. Personnel involved in the bagging, transport, and laundering of contaminated clothing should wear gloves. The clothing should be washed and dried according to manufacturer in-structions. Boots and leather goods may be brush-scrubbed with soap and hot water using Standard Precautions. Most items can simply be laundered, but use caution with certain specialty items, such as ski jackets. Follow the clothing label instructions to avoid damage to these items.

### Spills

While observing Standard Precautions, first remove visible spilled material using dis-posable towels or other appropriate means (Figure 3-23a■). If splashing is anticipated, wear protective eyewear and an impervious gown or apron that provides an effective barrier to splashes. Then decontaminate the spill area using an EPA-approved germi-cide or a 1:10 solution of household bleach, and decontaminate your equipment and supplies as well (Figure 3-23b■). Wash your hands following the removal of gloves. Where snow is contaminated with blood or other bodily fluids, remove the contami-nated snow by shovel to an area away from the public and treat it with one of the pre-viously mentioned solutions; then treat the shovel with the same solution. As an alternative, you may use one of the commercially available "spill kits" to assist with the

**Figure 3-23a** A bodily fluid spill requires a special cleaning and disinfection process.

**Figure 3-23b** Safe workplace procedures include the use of facilities for cleaning contaminated equipment and supplies.

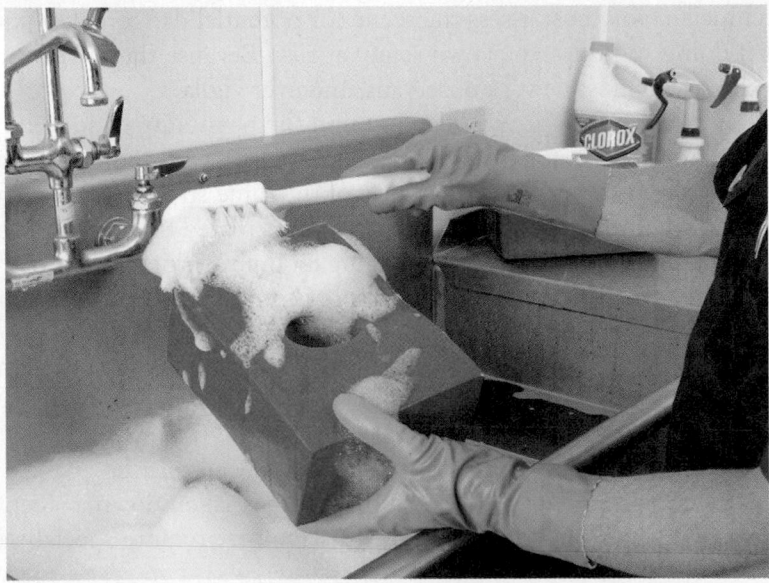

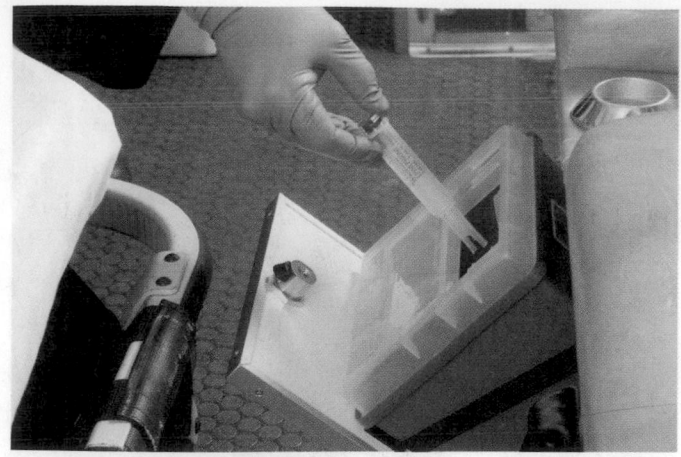

**Figure 3-24** The disposal of a syringe and needle into a sharps container.

**3-9** Describe the four components of the scene size-up.

**scene size-up** the first step of the assessment process, consisting of four components: scene safety, mechanism of injury, total number of patients involved, and the need for additional resources.

**3-10** Describe and demonstrate how to ensure scene safety.

**scene safety** the process of assessing the site of an accident or disaster and making it safe for rescuers to enter.

cleanup process. Most kits convert the spilled liquid into a solid for easy pickup and have been shown to be effective even on some porous surfaces such as snow.

### Sharps

Handle all sharp objects, or "sharps," with extreme caution. Being stuck or cut by a sharp object that is contaminated by bodily fluid carries a significant risk for HIV infection and hepatitis. Commonly encountered "sharps" include needles and broken glass. Place the sharp objects into an approved "sharps container," which should include a lid and rigid walls to prevent accidental punctures and spills.

Needles usually have a safety cap. Because many needle sticks occur when attempting to replace the caps, it is preferable to place used needles directly into a "sharps container" without recapping them. Safer needle caps, which recover the needle without risk, are now in use and have significantly reduced exposures by needle stick. Never touch the needle itself. Instead, handle the syringe only (Figure 3-24■).

## Assessing Emergency Situations

The assessment process starts the moment you arrive on the scene of an emergency. It begins with a **scene size-up,** in which you assess the nature and scope of the overall problem before turning your attention to the patient(s). The scene size-up usually takes only a few moments, but it may take longer depending on the situation. A scene size-up has four components: scene safety, the mechanism of injury (MOI) involved or nature of illness (NOI), the total number of patients involved, and need for additional resources.

### Scene Safety

For OEC Technicians, safety measures extend well beyond simply ensuring that you are healthy, are properly clothed, have proper equipment, and observe Standard Precautions. It also includes ensuring that the environment is free of hazards. This concept is known as **scene safety**. The "scene" is the location in which a potentially ill or injured patient is located. As a component of ensuring your own well-being as an OEC Technician, you must assess the scene for potential dangers. Do not approach a patient if doing so places your own safety at risk. Because the list of possible dangers is endless, you must be very observant, and ever vigilant.

Scene safety requires that you keep in mind the possibility of succumbing to the same fate as your patient, for the same danger may still exist. You could fall into the same crevasse, or you could drown because of the same strong water current. However, some hazards are not related to the event that created the victim's problem. For example, you might find yourself approaching an injured skier, and if you are observant you may recognize that this particular spot is not easily seen by oncoming skiers, putting you and your patient at risk for a collision. Or the scene might feature an overhanging cornice that could suddenly break free. Weather may be a safety issue, too, including blowing debris in high winds, lightning, and flooding. Do not approach a scene in which fire or electrical hazards exist. If someone has a weapon at the scene, do not risk your life until the weapon has been secured.

It may be tempting to approach a victim who has fallen down a steep slope, but you could become a victim yourself. This situation may require special rescue experience. In some situations, you may be able to remove the potential hazard by yourself; in other instances the problem can be rectified only with assistance from others, such as law enforcement personnel or specialized rescue teams.

Move the patient away from danger whenever possible. In order to recognize dangers, you must carefully assess your surroundings. Before making contact with a patient, mark the scene as well as you can to keep others from entering. If you are caring for a patient on a ski slope, prevent others from skiing directly into your patient care area by marking the scene with skis, ski poles, packs, brightly colored clothing, or snow fencing, preferably well upslope of your location (Figure 3-25■).

## STOP, THINK, UNDERSTAND

### Multiple Choice
Choose the correct answer.

1. How long can influenza survive on hard, nonporous surfaces?_____
   a. two minutes
   b. two hours
   c. two days
   d. two weeks

2. Which of the following procedures is most effective for preventing the spread of disease? _____
   a. wearing disposable gloves
   b. washing your hands
   c. wearing a surgical mask / N95 mask
   d. wearing all the personal protective equipment (PPE) while in contact with a patient

3. Which of the following is *not* a symptom of hepatitis? _____
   a. constipation
   b. jaundice (yellow skin)
   c. vomiting
   d. dark-colored urine

4. How often is a booster shot recommended for tetanus?_____
   a. every 2 years
   b. every 5 years
   c. every 10 years
   d. every 15 years

5. What are the most common methods by which OEC Technicians may contact a communicable disease? _____
   a. direct contact and indirect contact
   b. airborne and vector-borne routes
   c. airborne route and indirect contact
   d. direct contact and airborne route

### Fill in the Blank

_____, _____, _____, _____, and _____ are the five modes by which infectious diseases can be transmitted.

### Matching
Match each of the following diseases with the correct mode of transmission.

_____ 1. salmonellosis
_____ 2. Rocky Mountain spotted fever
_____ 3. mononucleosis
_____ 4. malaria
_____ 5. tuberculosis
_____ 6. hepatitis "A"
_____ 7. hepatitis "B"
_____ 8. athlete's foot
_____ 9. lice infestation
_____ 10. common cold

a. direct contact
b. indirect contact
c. airborne transmission
d. ingestion
e. vector-borne transmission

## NOTE

### Common Life-Threatening Conditions

Here are some life-threatening conditions commonly encountered by OEC Technicians:

- A snowboarder with an open head injury sustained from a collision with a tree
- An unconscious climber who fell 45 feet to the ground
- A skier with a penetrating chest wound from a broken ski pole
- An elderly guest at the lodge who is sweaty and complaining of chest pain
- A biker who was stung by a bee and is complaining of shortness of breath, itching, and a swollen tongue
- A confused diabetic whose friends state that she has not eaten anything all day

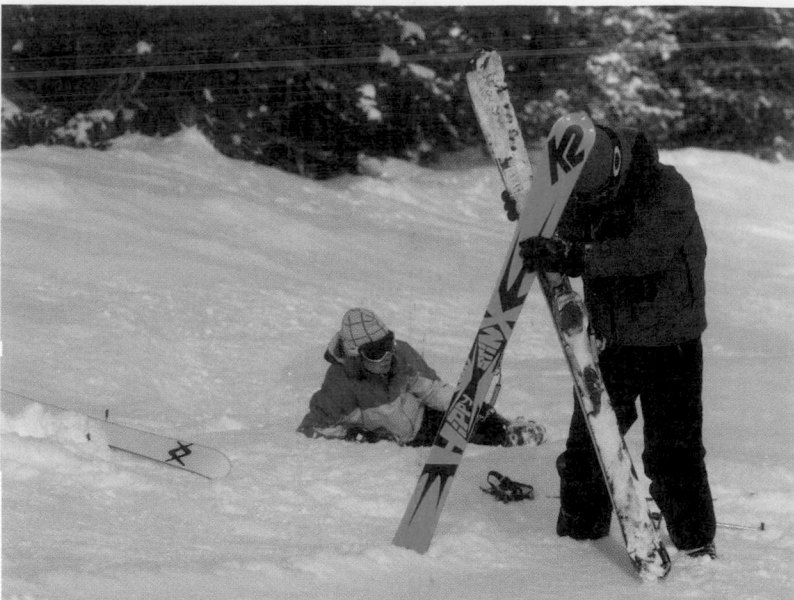

**Figure 3-25** Scene safety includes making the scene more visible. Some of the ways to do this include the use of skis, snowboard, ski poles packs, bright clothing, or snow fencing.
Copyright Scott Smith

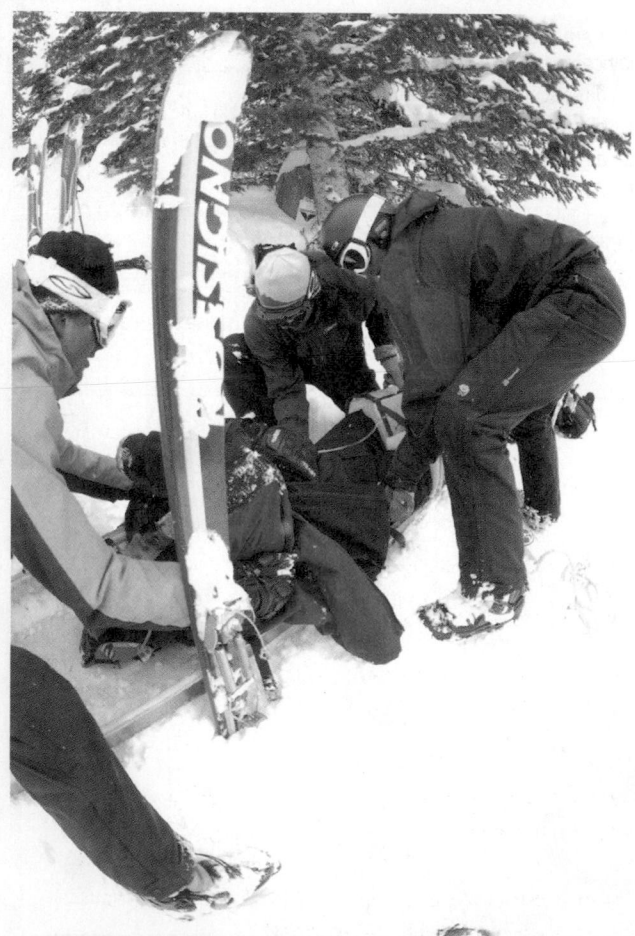

**Figure 3-26** The patient has been moved from a hazardous area to a safer location prior to being treated.
Copyright Studio 404

Similarly, if you are located on a busy mountain biking trail, you may need to strategically position one or more bikes or people to effectively cordon off a safe working zone. Use whatever resources you have on hand to form a protective barrier around the accident scene. If personnel are available, position someone away from the immediate scene in order to warn others to keep away (Figure 3-26■).

Surveying the scene for hazards and controlling them is an ongoing process that must be repeated continually because new hazards may arise while you are caring for the patient.

## Mechanism of Injury

In assessing a trauma situation, an important step is to determine the mechanism of injury (MOI). This will help you determine the mechanical forces involved in producing the patient's injuries (Figure 3-27■). In the event of a medical disorder, you will need to determine the nature of the illness (NOI).

Determining the MOI or NOI helps to identify critically injured or ill patients, who require rapid assessment, rapid treatment, and rapid transport. Life-threatening problems encountered may include any condition that (1) affects the airway and cannot be immediately corrected, (2) affects the exchange of oxygen in the lungs, or (3) has compromised the heart's ability to pump blood. A patient who is not responsive, has uncontrolled bleeding, or might go into shock also needs rapid care.

Mechanism of injury (MOI) and nature of illness (NOI) will be discussed in further detail in Chapter 17.

## Number of Patients and Need for Additional Resources

As part of your assessment, determine the total number of patients involved in the incident (Figure 3-28■). This information will directly affect what resources you will need and is especially important whenever on-scene resources are distant or likely to be limited. In many instances you will be able to manage the patient with the equipment you have on hand. But in some cases you will need special equipment that is not immediately available. When a patient must be placed on a backboard or in a specialized splint, additional providers are required. In nonurban, outdoor environments, it is essential that the need for additional resources be identified early, so that they can be requested and mobilized quickly.

Your initial radio call will include, among other information, the number of patients involved and the resources that are needed.

Consider the following examples of situations in which additional equipment or manpower is needed:

+ It is late in the afternoon, and while searching for a lost child in mountainous terrain you hear a faint cry for help. Peering over the edge of a ravine, you see the child, trapped on a narrow ledge 20 feet below you. You have no climbing equipment with you.
+ You respond to a report that a person has fallen from the chairlift. You arrive on scene to discover three people lying in the snow. Two are unconscious and one is screaming in pain from a broken leg.
+ While patrolling a backcountry trail, you are informed of a nearby avalanche involving victims. As you near the scene, you see a person frantically digging in the snow. He yells to you that he cannot find his friend.

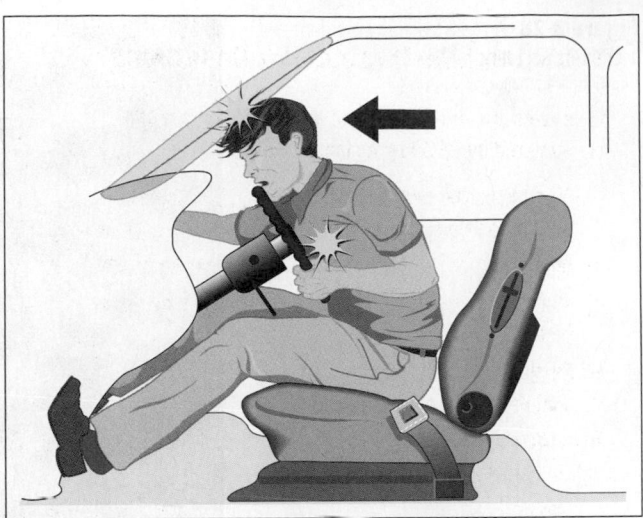

**Figure 3-27** Determining the MOI (in this case, in an automobile collision) is helpful in understanding the forces that cause the injuries observed.

### Common MOIs

- Blunt force (fall from a bike, car crash, punch in face by a fist)
- Penetrating force (gunshot wound, knife wound, puncture from a broken tree branch or ski pole)
- Twisting or rotational force (knee injury from catching an edge while skiing, hurt back from bending at an awkward angle to pick up something)
- Explosive force (injury sustained from the shock waves of an explosion)

## Dealing with Hazardous Materials

As part of the scene size-up and assessment for dangers, you may encounter **hazardous materials (HazMat)**. A hazardous material is any solid, liquid, or gas that has the potential to cause harm to humans, animals, or the environment, either by itself or through interaction with other factors. Hazardous materials include materials that are radioactive, flammable, explosive, or corrosive, as well as pathogens, allergens, and other biohazardous substances. Examples of HazMat are avalanche explosives, chlorine, cleaning chemicals, gasoline, and propane. Some hazardous materials can cause health problems if ingested or inhaled; others can be dangerous upon contact with intact skin or the eyes. Many chemicals cause immediate health problems, such as respiratory distress and loss of vision; others are more insidious and may take years to manifest, as is the case with asbestos, which poses a long-term risk of lung cancer.

It is your job to recognize any material that may be hazardous. If you identify a potential HazMat situation, call 9-1-1 and report the incident. Most locales have HazMat

### Common NOIs

- Altered mental status
- Respiratory problems
- Cardiac problems
- Gastrointestinal problems
- Substance-related problems
- Environment-related problems

**hazardous materials (HazMat)** substances that have the potential to harm people, animals, or the environment.

**Figure 3-28** A mass casualty incident—
a chairlift accident.
Copyright Mike Halloran

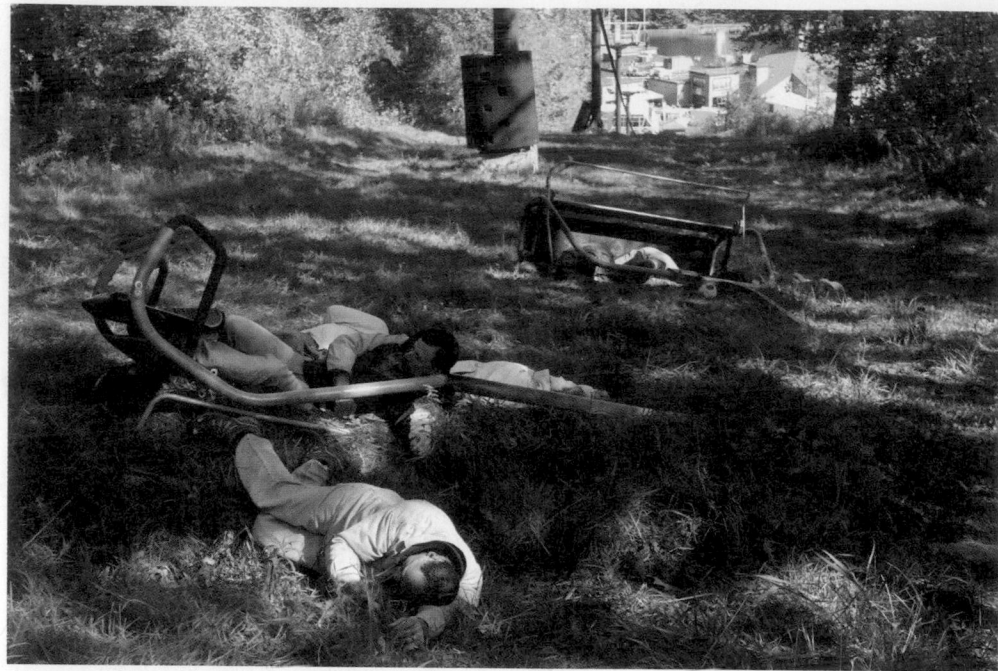

teams that are trained to manage these scenes safely. Your job is to prevent yourself and others from becoming contaminated by the substance. As a general rule, you should stay uphill and upwind from any potentially hazardous material.

Most resort facilities utilize and store hazardous substances, including cleaning solvents, fertilizers, petroleum-based products, and explosives. Hazardous materials stored at your facility may be identified by safety placards (Figure 3-29■). Your facility also should have readily available information concerning any hazardous materials that are on site. In the United States, this information is available on the manufacturer's **material safety data sheet (MSDS)**. The MSDS for a given substance

**Figure 3-29** The Department of Transportation (DOT) requires the use of placards to identify materials as flammable, radioactive, explosive, and/or poisonous.
U.S. Department of Transportation, Pipeline and Hazardous Materials Safety Administration

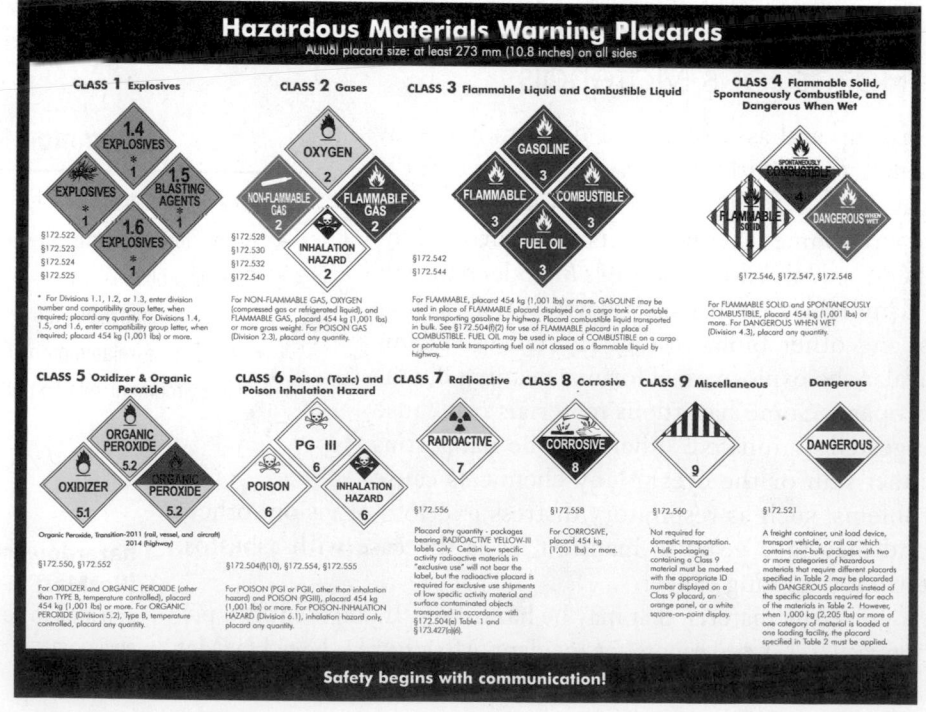

describes known health risks and provides information on the safe handling of the substance. When you respond to a scene involving hazardous materials, first ensure your own personal safety. In major HazMat situations, it is recommended that you stay at least 250 feet from the scene. If you are downwind, it is recommended you stay 500 feet away. You may need to delay care of patients until the scene is secured by trained HazMat personnel. Delaying the care of patients is difficult to do and against our instincts, but it is the best option in a HazMat incident.

MSDSs provide an overview of the materials, including instructions for handling, storing, decontamination, and emergency care. If you work in an area that has a high potential for a HazMat situation, consider taking additional specialized training. For more information about hazardous materials, refer to Chapter 35, Special Operations and Ambulance Operations.

## Crime Scene Management

OEC Technicians may occasionally encounter crime scenes. If you discover a potential crime scene, notify law enforcement immediately. The responding law enforcement officer is in charge of the crime scene. If no law enforcement personnel are present, do not assume that the scene is safe to enter. If a law enforcement officer is present, do not approach the scene until the officer notifies you that it is safe to do so.

Take care to follow instructions so that you do not disturb the scene. Make sure the area is cordoned off (Figure 3-30■), and that members of the public do not enter the scene. Take precautions not to remove, move, or otherwise disturb anything in the environment, except as is absolutely necessary to provide critical care to patients. Any mishandling of evidence can make it inadmissible in court. To avoid this problem, it is important to create an accurate "paper trail," or "chain of custody," accounting for the location of the evidence at each step, from the time of its discovery to its presentation in court. Let law enforcement personnel handle any materials that could be used as evidence.

Examples of crime scenes include sites at which homicides, hostage situations, domestic violence, and assaults occurred. If you have any doubt about how to proceed, consult with the law enforcement officer in charge of the scene. For more information about crime scenes, refer to Chapter 35, Special Operations and Ambulance Operations. See Table 3-8■ for additional tips concerning crime scene preservation.

**material safety data sheet (MSDS)** a form that contains relevant information pertaining to a specific substance, with a focus on the hazards it poses to workers.

⊕ **3-11** Describe chain of custody.

**Figure 3-30** A crime scene.

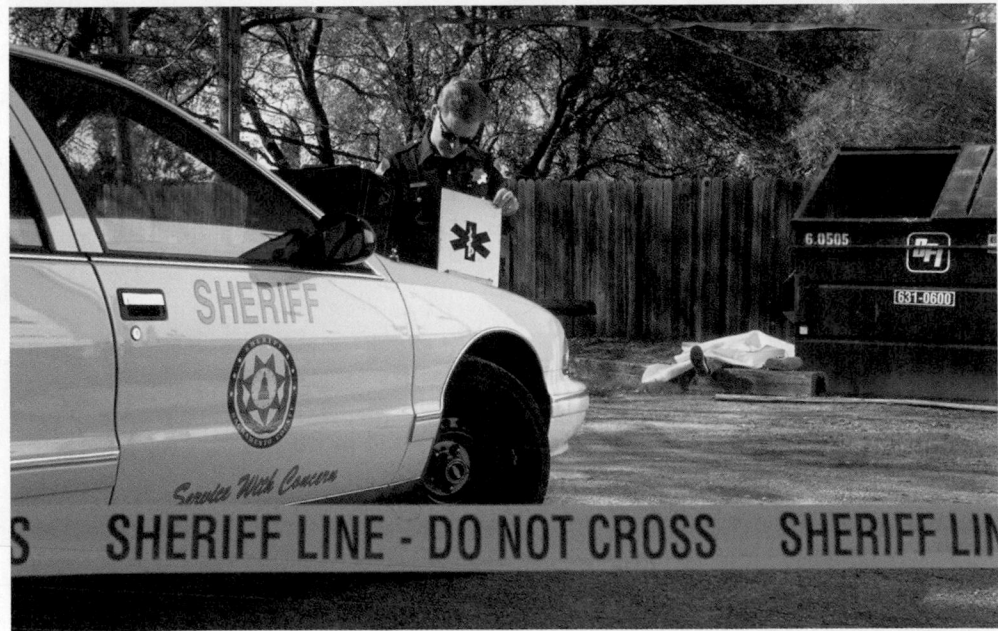

| Table **3-8** | Crime Scene Preservation Tips |
| --- | --- |

Approaching the Scene:

- Identify the minimum number of rescuers needed. (Consider if one rescuer is sufficient.)
- Send in the most trained rescuer.
- Take the minimum amount of needed equipment to the scene.
- Minimize contact to only what is needed to take care of the patient.

Entering the Scene:

- Minimize disturbance of the scene.
- While coming into the scene, pay attention to where you put your feet. (Do not kick or step in anything.)
- Do not wander around the scene.
- Unless necessary in caring for a patient, do not change the lighting, position of the drapes, TV or radio, furniture position, and so on.
- While in the scene, do not smoke, eat, drink, or use the bathroom.

Weapons and Ropes:

- Assume that all guns are loaded.
- If a weapon must be moved in order to care for a patient, only one *gloved* person (preferably a law enforcement officer) should handle the grip of the weapon.
- Before moving a weapon, mark or outline its location.
- If a rope needs to be removed to care for a patient, make sure that in doing so no knots are either cut or untied.

Clothing:

- Do not shake or turn clothing inside out.
- Minimize destruction of clothing.
- Cut around (not through) any bullet hole, puncture, or other damaged areas.
- Leave all removed clothing with law enforcement personnel.

Providing Care:

- Use gloves.
- Keep medical equipment close to the patient.
- Stay close to the victim.
- Keep your hands out of pooled blood.
- Collect and remove all packaging, wrappers, and used bandages.

Treating the Patient:

- If deceased do not disturb any belongings, and do not clean or cover the body.
- Do not allow victims of sexual assault to wash, clean, change clothes, or use the bathroom until after medical/forensic examination.
- If resuscitation is required, transfer the victim from the scene to an ambulance as soon as possible.
- Remind EMS that any sheets used under the victim for transport should be "bagged" because they may contain evidence.

Remember: Although crime scene preservation and patient care occur in tandem, patient care takes priority.

## Relations with the Media

Any incident to which you respond may involve the media. Reports can be generated and subsequently appear on media outlets even if no "official" media personnel are at the scene: given today's technology, *anyone* can become an "on-scene reporter" and begin transmitting reports on events, including text, pictures, audio, and streaming video.

While working at the scene, always be careful what you say and how you say it. Statements or comments spoken while on scene, your actions while caring for patients, your interactions with bystanders, and the overall scene dynamics all can be broadcast to a wide audience within minutes (Figure 3-31■). As a health care provider, you must respect the privacy of patients, treating all information regarding their care as confidential. You may need to insist that bystanders and media personnel relocate. Mountain hosts, safety patrollers, and law enforcement officials may be able to assist with keeping media away from the scene. Take every possible measure to ensure that scene safety and patient care remain the top priority. Media relations are a secondary concern.

Always consult management before speaking to the media. Many organizations have a designated, formally trained public information officer who is authorized to speak to the media.

## Dealing with Stress

Providing medical care under emergent conditions is very stressful and can lead to a variety of health problems. Stress is not intrinsically harmful, but when it begins to affect a person's cognitive, emotional, or behavioral well-being, that person may need help. Abnormal stress responses may be immediate (acute), delayed, or result from cumulative stress.

During an abnormal acute stress response, a person may experience chest pain, breathe rapidly, cry, scream, or lose the ability to think rationally. Rescuers who have become overwhelmed by difficult circumstances and cannot adapt to the situation should be removed from the scene and receive care from appropriate personnel.

Even when stress is managed appropriately, OEC Technicians may experience stress-related symptoms (Figure 3-32■) that may occur days, weeks, or even months

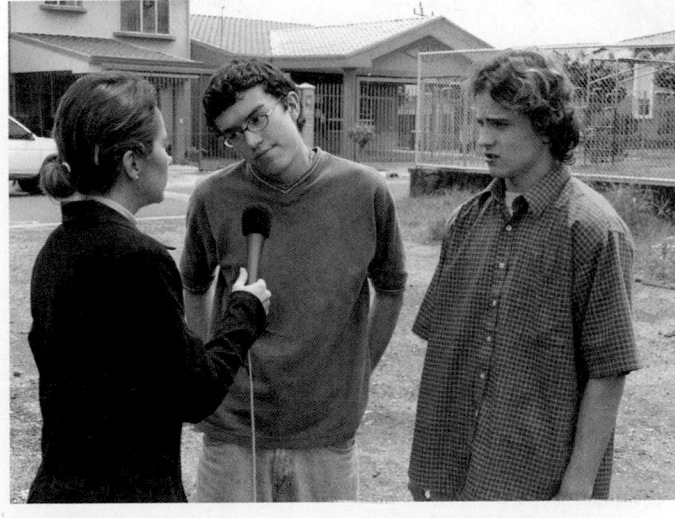

**Figure 3-31** Media interactions: a reporter interviewing two individuals.

**Figure 3-32** The warning signs of stress.

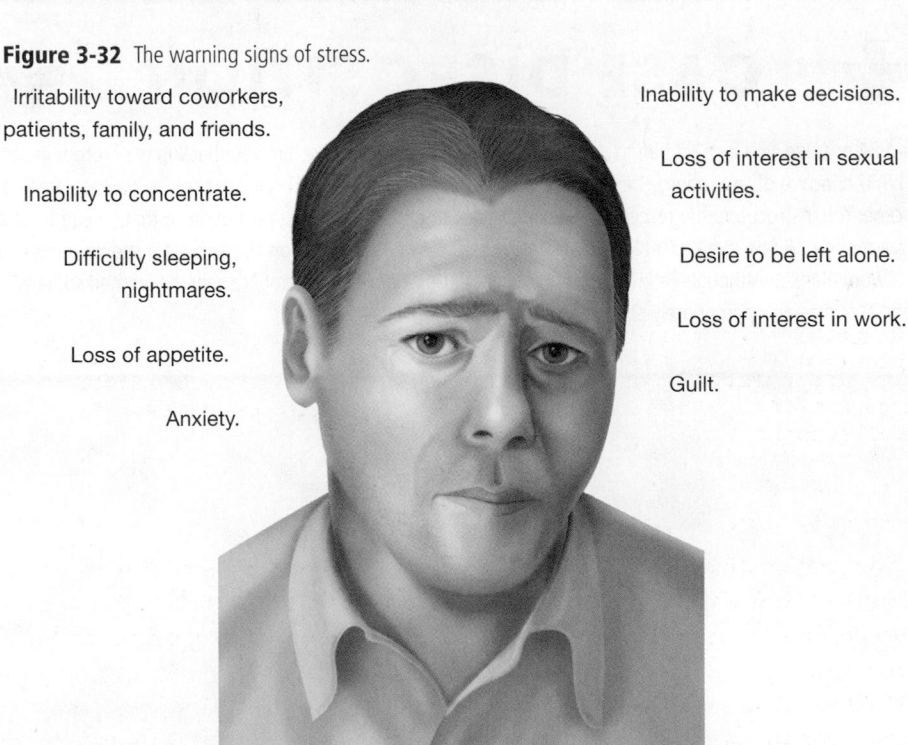

Irritability toward coworkers, patients, family, and friends.

Inability to concentrate.

Difficulty sleeping, nightmares.

Loss of appetite.

Anxiety.

Inability to make decisions.

Loss of interest in sexual activities.

Desire to be left alone.

Loss of interest in work.

Guilt.

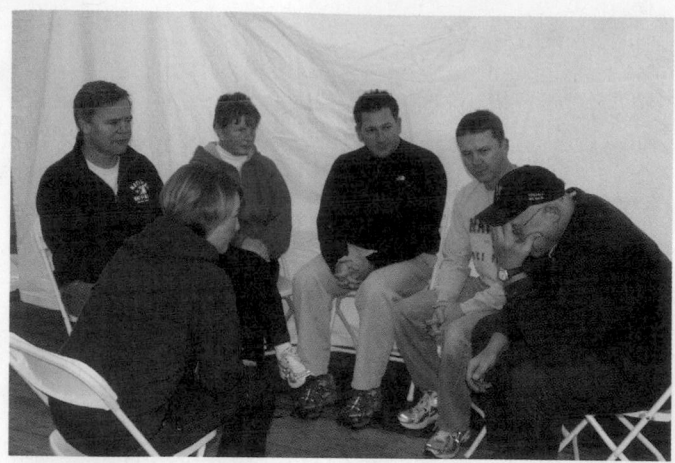

**Figure 3-33** A critical incident debriefing: a group session.
Copyright Mike Halloran

following the incident. Symptoms can include irritability, flashbacks to the incident, bad dreams, sleep problems, detachment, lack of concentration, and interpersonal relationship difficulties. Such a delayed stress response (DSR) is a form of post-traumatic stress disorder (PTSD).

One of the more common causes of DSR for OEC Technicians is the death of a patient despite their best efforts. Fortunately, DSR and PTSD are treatable, and many resorts and organizations have developed formal "stress debriefing" programs to help OEC Technicians manage their stress (Figure 3-33■). These programs are typically conducted by a health professional trained in critical incident stress management (CISM). OEC Technicians should refer to local protocols regarding available CISM resources.

The effects of stress also may be cumulative and affect OEC Technicians who have experienced numerous stressors. This is a cumulative stress reaction, more commonly known as "burnout." This condition usually starts with anxiety, apathy, and a feeling of exhaustion. People who experience burnout may complain of abdominal pain, headache, or muscle aches. Sleep disturbances, irrational anger, withdrawn behavior, and depression also are common. Those suffering from burnout may abuse alcohol, nicotine, or other substances. Loss of sexual drive, poor work performance, and inappropriate outbursts may also occur.

OEC Technicians must be able to recognize abnormal reactions to stress in themselves and in coworkers, so that medical help can be obtained. These issues are presented in more detail in Chapter 33, Behavioral Emergencies and Crisis Response.

 # CASE DISPOSITION

Pulling Peter aside, you instruct him to remove his wet jacket, and you give him your backup waterproof jacket. You also hand him two of your energy bars. As the rescue efforts continue, Peter realizes that he was not prepared for the scene. You instruct another rescuer to take Peter back to the ski area first-aid station so that he can be checked and warmed up. A few minutes later, Peter is heading to the first-aid room on the back of a snowmobile, covered with a wool blanket. Although Peter survived this event without any major complications, he learned some valuable lessons about being appropriately prepared, both physically and mentally.

**OEC SKILL 3-1** | Removing Contaminated Gloves

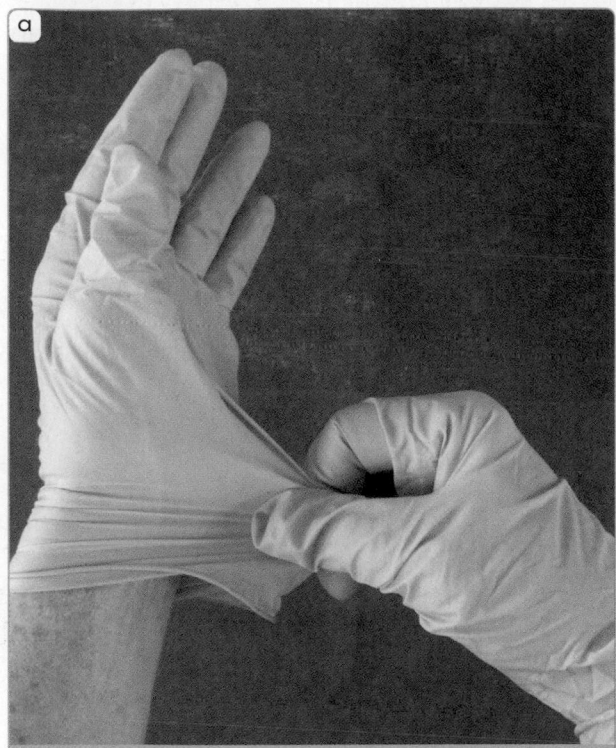

Glove Removal— Using your dominant hand, grasp the exterior of the opposite glove at the wrist.
Copyright Edward McNamara

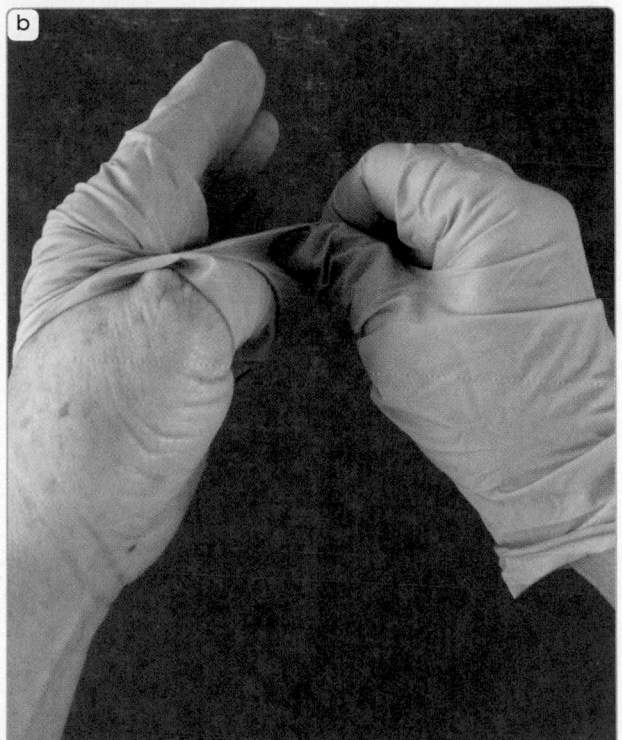

Carefully fold the glove over and peel it back, turning it inside out.
Copyright Edward McNamara

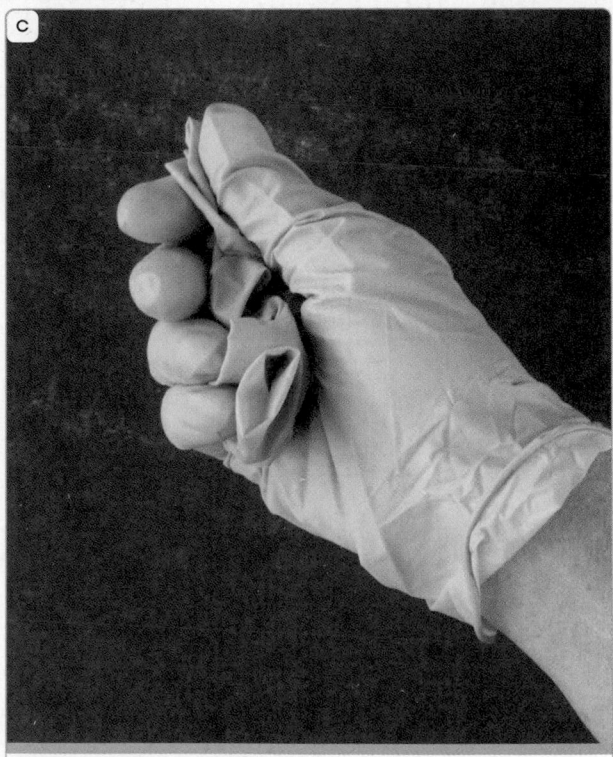

Once removed, hold the glove in your gloved dominant hand.
Copyright Edward McNamara

*continued*

# OEC SKILL 3-1 | Removing Contaminated Gloves *continued*

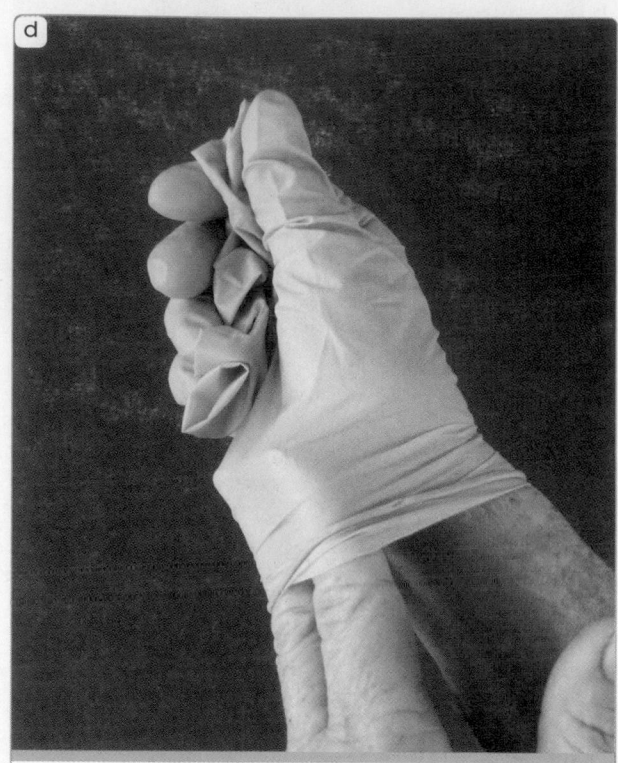

Place your ungloved fingers inside the opposite cuff, being careful not to touch the exterior of the glove.
Copyright Edward McNamara

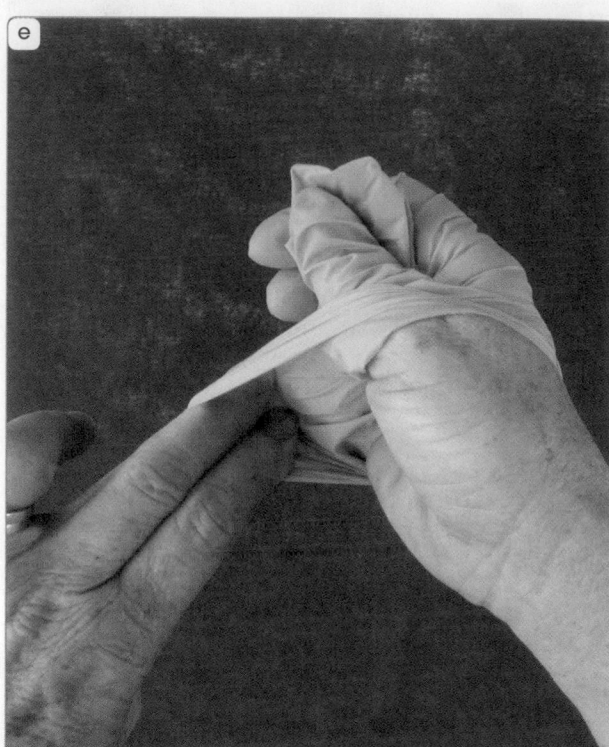

Carefully peel the glove off the hand, turning the glove inside out as you remove it.
Copyright Edward McNamara

## Skill Guide

Date: _____

(CPI) = Critical Performance Indicator

Candidate: _____

Start Time: _____

End Time: _____

## Removing Contaminated Gloves

**Objective:** To remove contaminated gloves.

| Skill | Max Points | Skill Demo | |
|---|---|---|---|
| Using dominant hand, grasp exterior of the opposite glove at the wrist, ensuring that you do not contaminate your skin. | 1 | | (CPI) |
| Starting at wrist, fold glove over and peel it back, turning it inside out as you remove the glove. | 1 | | |
| Place the removed glove in the palm of your gloved dominant hand. | 1 | | |
| Place ungloved fingers inside the cuff of the gloved hand, making sure you do not touch exterior of gloved hand. | 1 | | (CPI) |
| Peel the glove off of your hand, turning it inside out as you remove it. | 1 | | |
| Gloves should be turned inside out, with the second glove serving as a container for the first glove. | 1 | | |

Must receive 4 out of 6 points.

Comments: _____

Failure of any of the CPIs is an automatic failure.

Evaluator: _____ NSP ID: _____

PASS      FAIL

# ⛨ Chapter Review

## Chapter Summary

This chapter has presented a tremendous amount of information that will serve you well in your future as an OEC Technician. Although there is much anatomy and physiology yet to learn, you have learned about the "fight or flight" response and the basics of the immune system. You also learned about how the body regulates temperature and the various mechanisms of heat exchange (conduction, convection, radiation, and evaporation), and how those topics apply to rescue situations.

Proper preparation is an essential part of being an effective rescuer and aids your performance at a rescue scene. Preparation occurs before you respond to a call for help and includes not only proper mental and physical preparedness, but also knowledge of and experience with different environments and weather extremes. To maximize performance, it is critical that you obtain sufficient sleep and avoid poor nutrition and substance abuse.

You also have learned about the importance of proper equipment selection. When responding to a rescue situation, you need to arrive with the correct equipment. Although Appendix C will guide you in preparing a well-stocked first-aid kit, this chapter provided a solid basis for being prepared for the unexpected. What you carry on each of your trips into the backcountry should include enough gear to enable you to survive for at least 24 hours without assistance.

You also learned that your primary shield and front line of defense against the elements is your clothing. In addition to shelter and clothing, a key priority is remaining hydrated. Always plan on carrying more water than you expect to need. It is important to know how to purify water if you procure water from the environment. Proper skin and eye care is also essential.

As a rescuer you are likely to be exposed to a variety of infections. This chapter listed and briefly discussed many of those diseases, as well as the five modes of disease transmission. Strategies to mitigate your risk from infectious diseases include implementing Standard Precautions, body substance isolation (BSI), and the proper use of personal protective equipment (PPE). This section concluded with a discussion of occupational exposures and decontamination.

As an OEC Technician, you will need to perform a proper scene size-up on every scene that you encounter. Each scene size-up consists of four components: scene safety, mechanism of injury (MOI) or nature of illness (NOI), the number of patients involved, and an anticipation of needed resources. Some special circumstances may be encountered, such as HazMats, crime scenes, and the presence of media. The primary message of this section is scene safety.

The chapter concluded with an overview of the effects of stress on OEC Technicians, including a review of the symptoms of stress, effective stress management techniques, and professional resources that may be useful. OEC Technicians will find that supporting others following a stressful situation is a valuable component of being a team player.

The contents of this chapter have been presented in a manner that is intended to support each OEC Technician's overall well-being and success. While not every scenario can be anticipated or predicted, OEC Technicians that have done their due-diligence in being as prepared as possible are more likely to be successful than are those who are less-well prepared. The more prepared OEC Technicians are, the more likely they are to achieve positive patient outcomes.

## Remember...

1. Rescuer safety is always the #1 priority.
2. Manage the four mechanisms of heat exchange to your advantage.
3. Adequately prepare yourself for rescue operations.
4. Physical fitness, adequate sleep, and proper nutrition are important.
5. Your personal pack should include appropriate first-aid gear and personal gear.
6. Learning the Rule of Threes may save your life.
7. Standard Precautions, BSI, and PPE are essential for preventing the transmission of disease.
8. "Dirty to dirty and clean to clean" is helpful in removing disposable medical gloves.
9. The scene size-up includes an assessment of scene safety, the mechanism of injury, the total number of patients involved, and the need for additional resources.
10. Look for dangers at a rescue scene and be aware of changing scene dynamics.
11. Request assistance in HazMat and crime-scene situations.
12. Do not be afraid to ask for help if you are having difficulty coping with stress.

# Chapter Questions

## Multiple Choice

Choose the correct answer.

1. For which of the following diseases is a vaccination available? _____
   a. HIV
   b. Tuberculosis (TB)
   c. Meningitis
   d. Hepatitis "B"

2. What method does the body use to cool itself? _____
   a. It stops sweating.
   b. It increases shivering.
   c. It dilates peripheral blood vessels.
   d. It stops shivering.

3. Which of the following is not a component of the immune system? _____
   a. red blood cells
   b. the spleen
   c. the lymphatic system
   d. antibodies

4. The concept of scene safety is designed for whose protection? _____
   a. rescuers
   b. the victim(s)
   c. bystanders
   d. bystanders, rescuers, and the victim(s)

5. Help sessions for OEC Technicians suffering from PTSD are usually conducted by health professionals trained in _____
   a. delayed stress response.
   b. critical incident stress management (CISM).
   c. cumulative stress reaction.
   d. depression.

6. Which one of the following is not an aspect of the scene size-up? _____
   a. number of victims
   b. scene safety
   c. mechanism of injury
   d. description of injuries

7. As a general rule, during outdoor activities, how much water should you carry to remain properly hydrated? _____
   a. less than 2 liters
   b. more than 2 liters
   c. more than you think you need
   d. as much as you can comfortably carry

8. Which of the following diseases is not contracted through direct contact? _____
   a. Mononucleosis
   b. Tuberculosis
   c. Hepatitis "B"
   d. Chlamydia

**9.** Which of the following is not considered personal protective equipment? _____
   **a.** shoe coverings
   **b.** surgical mask / N95 mask
   **c.** disposable medical gloves
   **d.** eye protection

**10.** In which position should you be during a HazMat situation? _____
   **a.** downwind and downhill
   **b.** downwind and uphill
   **c.** upwind and downhill
   **d.** upwind and uphill

**11.** Which combination of heat transfer mechanisms is commonly used for cooling patients in the field? _____
   **a.** conduction and evaporation
   **b.** conduction and convection
   **c.** evaporation and radiation
   **d.** convection and evaporation

**12.** Put a check next to each of the following items that is a common mechanism of injuries (MOIs).
   _____ **a.** indirect force
   _____ **b.** gastrointestinal problems
   _____ **c.** blunt force
   _____ **d.** altered mental status
   _____ **e.** direct force
   _____ **f.** twisting or rotational force
   _____ **g.** cardiac problems
   _____ **h.** penetrating force
   _____ **i.** environmental-related problems

## Fill in the Blank

**1.** A(n) _____, _____, _____, and a(n) _____ are four essential items you should bring in your backcountry survival kit.

**2.** State the purpose of a winter base layer.

_____

_____

_____

**3.** State the purpose of the middle layer in winter.

_____

_____

_____

## Scenario

○○○○○○○○○○○○○○○○○○○○○○○○○○○○○○○○○○○○○○○○○○○○○○○○○○○○

*You have been recruited as a new member of the local community Search and Rescue team because of your OEC skills and training in mountaineering, search, and rescue. As a part of this team, you have been advised to prepare a "Load-n-go" pack that will enable you to function for two days in any environment. You start researching the equipment you will need, and then you make a trip to a local store specializing in outdoor gear. Knowing that changeable weather is one of the major factors you must consider in outfitting yourself, you start with eyewear. Available models have spring loaded bows, anti-fogging coating, and UVR protection.*

*Your base layer of clothing should allow for wicking.*

1. The type of cold-weather clothing material that allows wicking is_____
   a. a nylon and cotton blend.
   b. polypropylene.
   c. a cotton and rayon blend.
   d. silk or polyester.

*Search and Rescue can take the OEC Technician into many areas with unstable footing, which could result in a fall.*

2. Equipment that provides important warmth and body protection is/are_____
   a. heated boots.
   b. a helmet.
   c. a water-bouyancy vest.
   d. ear muffs.

## Suggested Reading

○○○○○○○○○○○○○○○○○○○○○○○○○○○○○○○○○○○○○○○○○○○○○○○○○○○○

Centers for Disease Control and Prevention website: www.cdc.gov , Emergency Preparedness and Response section.

Mitchell, Jeffrey, and H. Resnick. 1986. *Emergency Response to Crisis.* Upper Saddle River, NJ: Brady.

*Rosen's Emergency Medicine: Concepts and Clinical Practice*, Fifth Edition. 2002. St. Louis: Mosby.

West, Katherine. Basic Principles of Cleaning, Decontamination and Disinfection for EMS. Accessed March 4, 2009, http://www.emsresponder.com/print/Emergency-Medical-Services/Bug-PATROL/1$6546

EXPLORE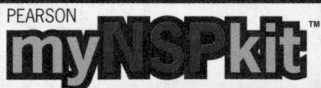

# Incident Command and Triage

Denis Meade, MA, EMTP
Edward McNamara, BS, EMTP

## ⊕ OBJECTIVES

**Upon completion of this chapter, the OEC Technician will be able to:**

**4-1** Define incident command system.

**4-2** Describe the primary responsibilities of each of the five functional areas of the incident command system.

**4-3** Describe and demonstrate how to use the "ID-ME" triage system.

**4-4** Describe and demonstrate how to use the START system of triage.

## ⊕ KEY TERMS

facility, *p. 107*
incident, *p. 99*
Incident Command System (ICS), *p. 101*
Incident Commander (IC), *p. 104*
multi-agency coordination system (MACS), *p. 100*

multiple casualty incident (MCI), *p. 114*
National Incident Management System (NIMS), *p. 98*
resource, *p. 100*
Section Chief, *p. 104*

span of control, *p. 100*
START, *p. 119*
strike team, *p. 105*
task force, *p. 105*
triage, *p. 114*

## Chapter Overview

Emergencies can happen at any time, in any place, and under a variety of circumstances. Each emergency is unique and presents rescue personnel with countless challenges, so OEC Technicians must be prepared to respond to and manage a wide variety of situations, whether they are natural or man-made, small or large, or simple or complex (Figure 4-1 ■). Fortunately, in managing any type of emergency, patrollers will use the federally mandated **National Incident Management System (NIMS)**.

## HISTORICAL TIMELINE

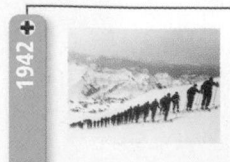

**1942**

Soldiers of the 87th training on Mt. Ranier in the winter of 1942.

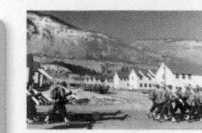

**1942**

Construction begun at Camp Hale near Pando, Colorado.

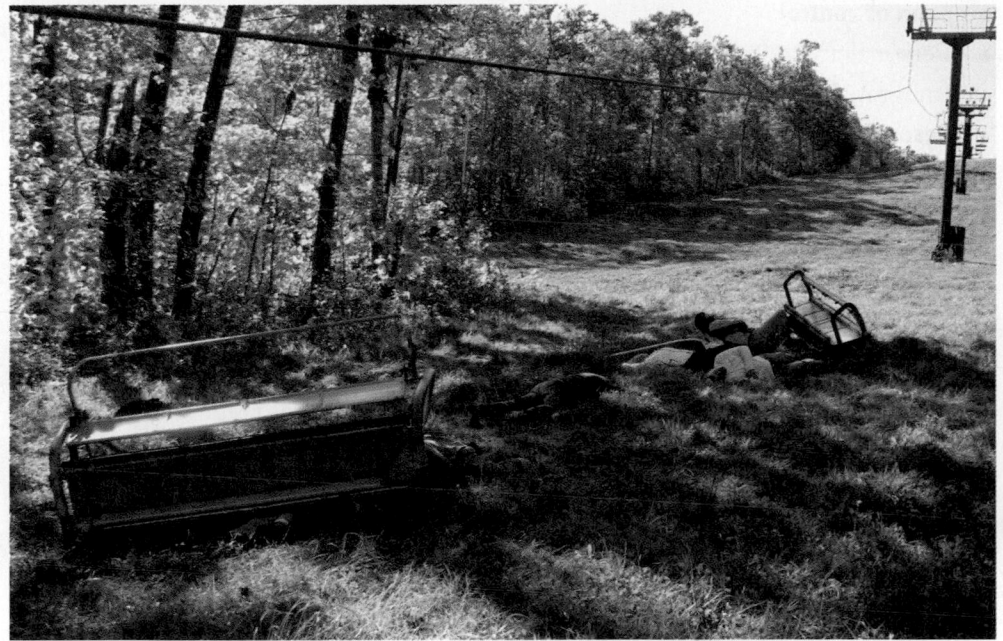 CASE PRESENTATION

You and three other patrollers are eating lunch in the mid-mountain cafeteria when you are dispatched to respond to "a skier that has fallen from a lift and may be hurt." As you walk out of the lodge, you see a large group of people standing at the top of the slope. You observe that many individuals are hastily removing their skis and then running over to the edge. As you ski over to their location, you quickly see the source of their concern. Looking downhill, the scene before you is pure chaos. All the way down the lift line, people are frantically clinging to lift chairs. Several appear to have fallen from the lift, some as much as 40 feet. Small groups of bystanders have gathered around some the patients and appear to be rendering aid. People are frantically waving both upslope and downslope, trying to get attention. You hear muffled yells for help and screaming in the distance.

**What is the first thing you and the other patrollers should do?**

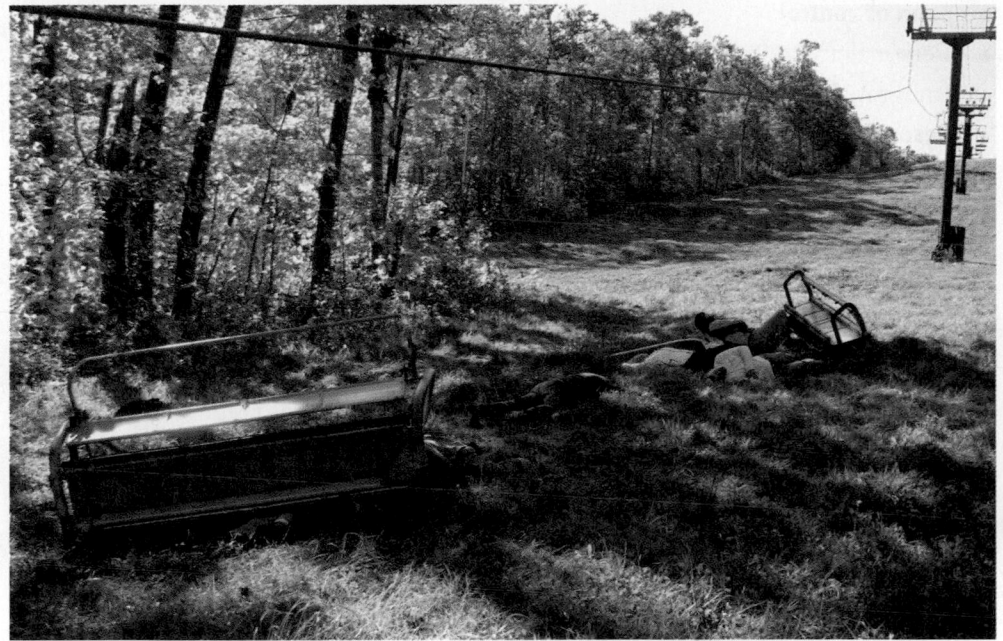

**Figure 4-1** In this chairlift accident, lift chairs have fallen to the ground. How many injuries are there? How will this event be handled?
Copyright Mike Halloran

# The National Incident Management System

NIMS is a standardized framework for responding to, and managing, emergencies or situations involving multiple jurisdictions. NIMS was established in 2003 by President George W. Bush, who signed Homeland Security Presidential Directive-5 in response to the terrorist attacks of September 11, 2001. NIMS is a national "all-hazard" model for incident management that provides "*a consistent nationwide approach for federal, state, tribal and local governments to work effectively and efficiently together to prepare for, prevent, respond to, and recover from domestic incidents, regardless of cause, size, or complexity*" (HSPD-5). An **incident** is defined as "*anything out of ordinary day-to-day activities that necessitates a response*" and includes medical emergencies, search and rescue

**National Incident Management System (NIMS)** a federally mandated "all hazards" method for responding to and managing an incident; was created as a result of Homeland Security Presidential Directive-5.

**incident** anything out of ordinary day-to-day activities that necessitates a response (e.g., emergencies, disasters, outbreaks, vaccination programs, important meetings or conferences).

missions, natural disasters, fires, terrorist/weapons of mass destruction (WMD) events, disease outbreaks, public vaccination programs, and such planned events as important meetings, conferences, or large public events.

NIMS is designed to improve overall incident management interoperability, integration, and coordination. It is federally mandated for use by all government and civilian organizations and personnel whose duties include responding to and managing emergency situations. This mandate extends to ski patrols and OEC Technicians, who may be called upon to take the lead in managing an incident involving external public safety organizations or to assist other public safety agencies during an incident.

NIMS provides numerous benefits that enable rescuers from different agencies to work together effectively at an incident. Among these benefits are the standardization of roles, functions, processes, terms, and forms; modularization, which allows rescuers to use only those components they need; and, flexibility, which permits rescue leaders to create special solutions to resolve unique incident-related challenges. Additionally, NIMS provides the following managerial benefits:

**span of control**   the total number of individuals or resources supervised by a single person; usually 3–7 individuals or resources.

**resource**   an individual, a single piece of equipment and its personnel complement, or a crew or team of individuals with an identified work supervisor, that can be used at an incident.

**multi-agency coordination system (MACS)**   a process for managing an incident in which multiple agencies that have different command structures and communication capabilities are participating.

+ A formal chain of command
+ Management by objectives
+ **Span of control**
+ Personal accountability
+ Integrated communications
+ **Resource** management

NIMS activities consist of four major components:

+ Command and management: focuses on managing incidents using standardized processes, the **multi-agency coordination system (MACS)**, and public information systems (Figure 4-2■).
+ Preparedness: emphasizes planning, training, practical exercises, standards and certification, mutual aid, and information and publications (Figure 4-3■).

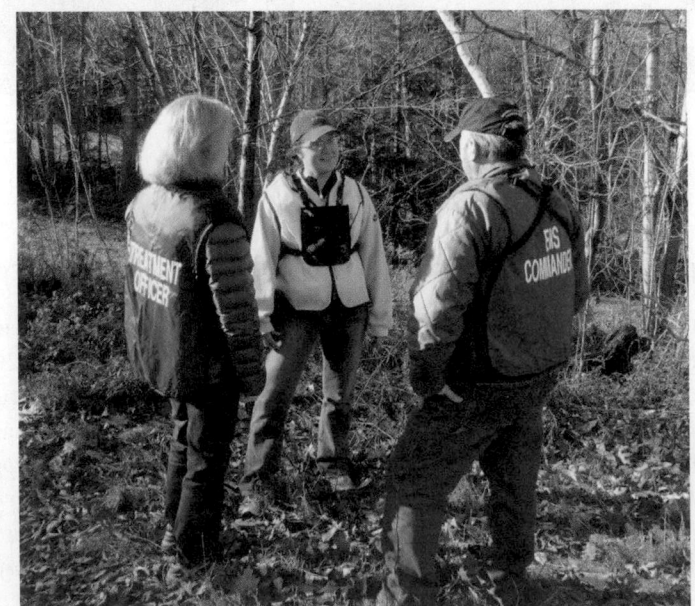

**Figure 4-3** A command and management "on hill" meeting to discuss the team's preparedness for the incident.
Copyright Edward McNamara

**Figure 4-2** The Incident Commander directs the response and coordinates the resources at a mass-casualty incident.

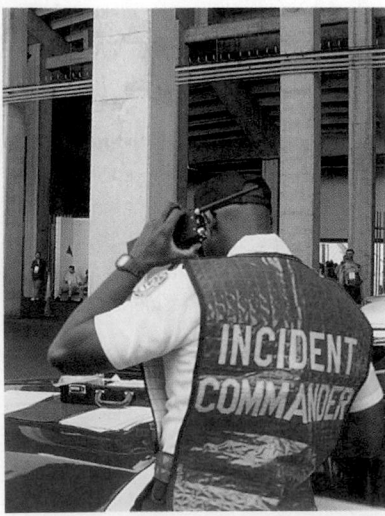

- Resource management: used to identify and categorize incident resources; to certify and credential personnel; and to acquire, inventory, mobilize, track, recover, and rehabilitate incident resources (Figure 4-4■).
- Communications and information management: deals with interoperability and the flow and use of NIMS and incident-related information.

As part of NIMS's federal mandate, all rescue organizations within the United States must adopt the **Incident Command System (ICS)**.

# Incident Command System

The Incident Command System provides a method for managing any incident, regardless of its cause, size, scope, or complexity. Developed in the 1970s as a method for managing California wildfires, ICS has evolved into an all-hazard management plan that provides a core set of doctrines, concepts, principles, terminology, and organizational processes that help responding organizations operate in a standardized fashion. The system improves efficiency, reduces confusion, and provides a safer work environment for rescue personnel. ICS provides considerable flexibility in that it can grow or shrink to accommodate the needs of each incident.

The ICS structure consists of five functional areas, each of which has specific responsibilities. The areas are interdependent and, depending on the size of the incident, may either be combined and managed by a single person or expanded and individually managed. The functional areas are (Figure 4-5■):

- Incident Command
- Operations Section
- Planning Section
- Logistics Section
- Finance/Administration Section

**Incident Command System (ICS)** a formal, organized method for managing an incident, regardless of its cause, size, scope, or complexity.

**4-1** Define incident command system.

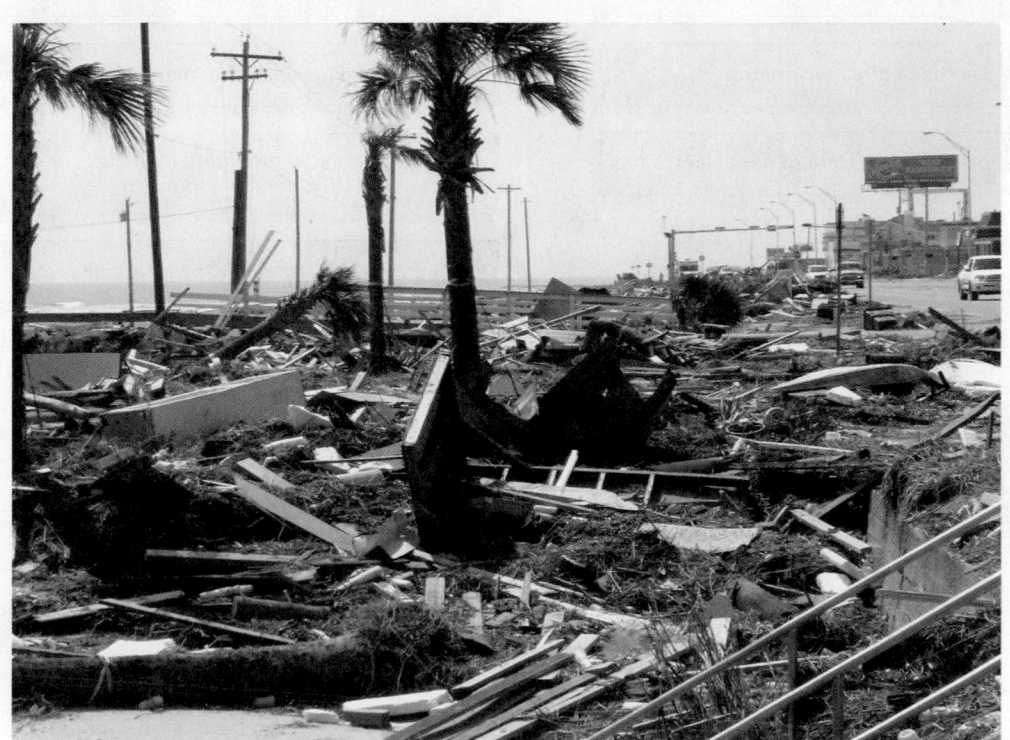

**Figure 4-4** The damage from Hurricane Katrina highlighted the need for disaster preparedness.
Copyright Edward McNamara

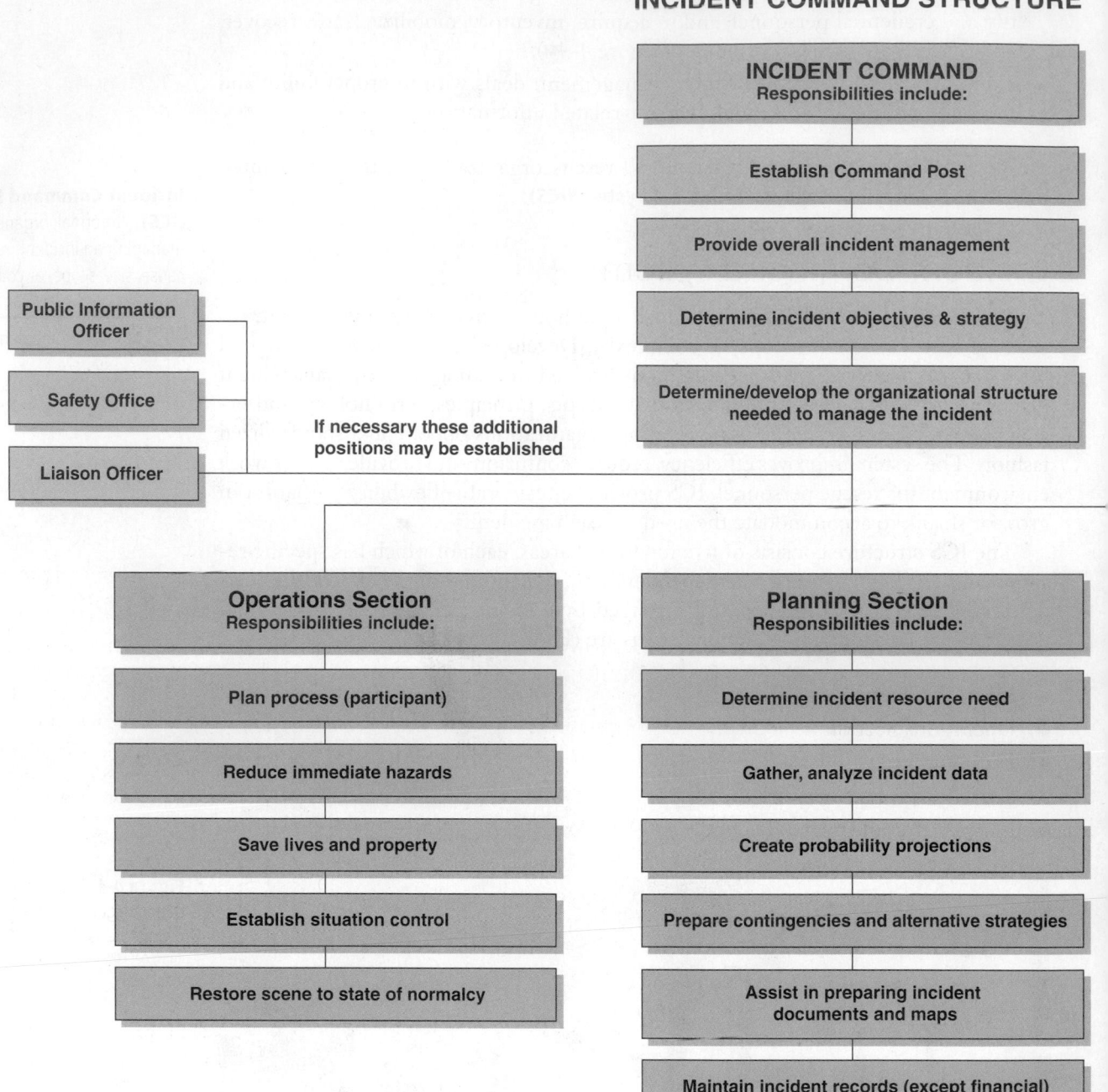

**Figure 4-5** ICS Organizational Chart.

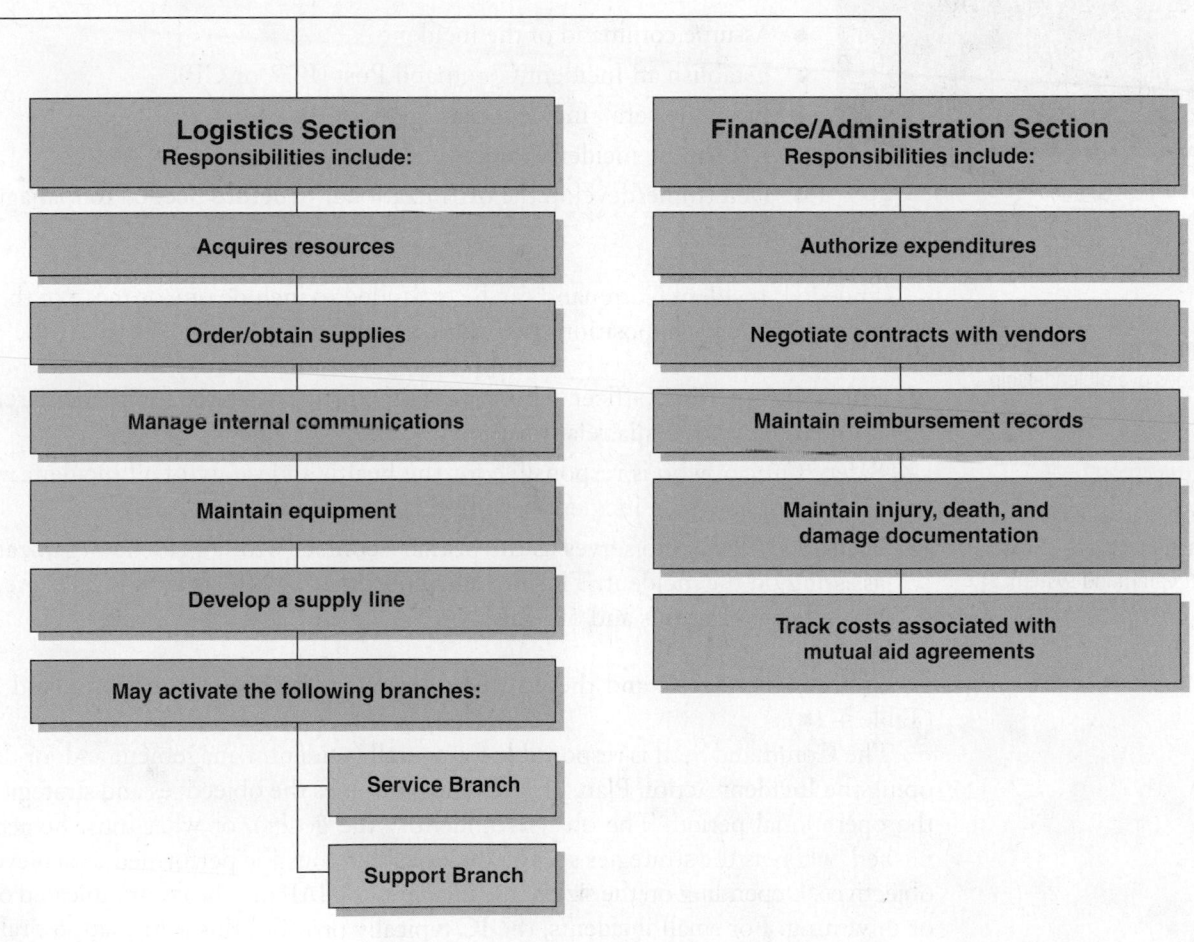

**Logistics Section**
Responsibilities include:

Acquires resources

Order/obtain supplies

Manage internal communications

Maintain equipment

Develop a supply line

May activate the following branches:

Service Branch

Support Branch

**Finance/Administration Section**
Responsibilities include:

Authorize expenditures

Negotiate contracts with vendors

Maintain reimbursement records

Maintain injury, death, and damage documentation

Track costs associated with mutual aid agreements

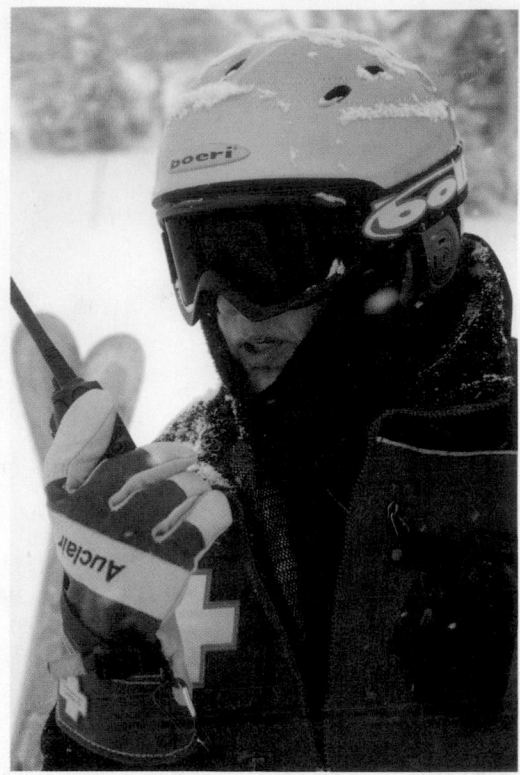

**Figure 4-6** A patroller acting as an IC of an incident uses the radio to communicate pertinent information.
Copyright Studio 404

**Incident Commander (IC)**   the person who provides overall leadership at an incident.

⊕ 4-2   Describe the primary responsibilities of each of the five functional areas of the incident command system.

**Section Chief**   the head of a functional area within the Incident Command System.

## Incident Command

Of the five functional areas, Incident Command is the first to be established at any incident and is managed by an **Incident Commander (IC)**. Identification of the IC is essential, as this person provides overall leadership and direction for managing the incident. The role of IC is typically assumed by the most senior person among the initial responders arriving at the scene.

After conducting an initial assessment of the scene, the IC establishes a Command Post, or CP, which serves as the IC's base of operations while managing the incident. The CP must be established in a safe, secure location that is near the incident but is away from any hazards (Figure 4-6■). The IC serves in this capacity until one of the following occurs: the incident is over, the IC is relieved by another qualified IC, or, the IC's operational period (specified amount of work time) is complete. Ideally, an operational period should not exceed 12 hours, and it can be much shorter depending on the nature of the incident and the task to be performed. To avoid confusion, there is only one IC at a time per incident. The IC's several key responsibilities include the following tasks:

+ Assume command of the incident.
+ Establish an Incident Command Post (ICP, or CP).
+ Provide overall incident management.
+ Determine incident objectives and strategies.
+ Determine/develop the organizational structure needed to manage the incident.

If needed, Incident Command can be expanded to include one or more of the following three additional positions that can assist the IC:

1. Public Information Officer, who serves as the primary source for incident-related information and media relations.
2. Safety Officer, who is responsible for the health and safety of all incident workers and for assessing incident hazards.
3. Liaison Officer, who serves as the primary contact with all rescue organizations assisting on the incident. This includes coordinating efforts with local, state, and federal organizations and officials.

Collectively, the IC and these three officers are known as the Command Staff (Table 4-1■).

The Command Staff is responsible for overall incident management and for developing the Incident Action Plan, or IAP, which outlines the objectives and strategies for the operational period. The objectives identify the goal(s), or what must be accomplished, whereas the strategies specify the tasks that must be performed to achieve the objectives. Depending on the size of the incident, the IAP may be communicated orally or in writing. For small incidents, the IC typically provides this information orally to his subordinates, whereas for large incidents this information is given to the chief of each of the four sections orally and in writing to execute their specific section-related tasks. **Section Chiefs** constitute the General Staff and report directly to the IC.

Large incidents involving multiple jurisdictions or multiple agencies may need to be organized under a "Unified Command" structure in which the commanders from each on-scene agency work together to achieve the overall incident goals and objectives while simultaneously carrying out their respective jurisdictional activities.

## Table 4-1  Titles and Organization of ICS Personnel

| Organizational Level | Supervisory Title | Reports To | Support Position (if needed) |
|---|---|---|---|
| Command Staff | Incident Commander (IC) | — | Deputy IC |
| | Staff Officers | | |
| | –Information Officer | IC | Asst. Information Officer |
| | –Safety Officer | IC | Asst. Safety Officer |
| | –Liaison Officer | IC | Asst. Liaison Officer |
| General Staff | Section Chiefs | | |
| | –Operations Chief | IC | Deputy Operations Chief |
| | –Planning Chief | IC | Deputy Planning Chief |
| | –Logistics Chief | IC | Deputy Logistics Chief |
| | –Finance Chief | IC | Deputy Finance Chief |
| Branches | Branch Directors | Section Chief | Deputy Branch Director |
| Groups/Divisions | Group Officers | Branch Director | NA |
| | Division Supervisors | Branch Director | NA |
| Units | Unit Leaders | Section Chief | Unit Manager/coordinator |

## Operations Section

Operations is the next section to be established at an incident and is the functional area responsible for executing the strategies of the IAP. This functional area is managed by an Operations Chief who oversees the following responsibilities:

+ Participating in the planning process (to create the IAP)
+ Reducing immediate hazard(s)
+ Saving lives and property
+ Establishing situational control
+ Restoring the scene to normalcy

The Operations Chief achieves these goals by constantly assessing the nature and scope of the incident, as well as the hazards present, and by determining the resources needed to achieve the IAP. A resource is defined as "*an individual, a piece of equipment and its complement, or a crew or team of individuals with an identified work supervisor that can be used at an incident.*" Resources are the assets, both physical and human, that are used to execute incident-related tasks. Depending on incident size, the Operations Chief may create one or more branches to perform specific tasks (see Table 4-1). Branches can be named using specific predesignated ICS names (e.g., Medical Branch, Police Branch, Fire Branch, Air Operations Branch) or can be named for a specific operational need (e.g., Search Branch, Avalanche Branch). Branches are managed by a Director who reports directly to the Operations Chief.

If needed, branches can be expanded to include one or more groups or divisions. For instance, under the Medical Branch, groups are often created for triage, treatment, and transportation of patients. Given their medical expertise, OEC Technicians are commonly assigned to these groups. Groups are managed by an Officer, whereas Divisions are managed by a Supervisor. Both roles report directly to the Branch Director (see Table 4-1). If needed, resources may be formed into strike teams or task forces to perform specific operational tasks. A **strike team** consists of resources of the same type (e.g., a group of Nordic Patrollers or river guides) and is managed by a strike team leader, whereas a **task force** includes a combination of different resources (e.g., a sheriff's deputy, an NSP alpine patrol, and a search-and-rescue team) with common communications

**strike team** a group of resources of the same size or type that is managed by a strike team leader (e.g., a group of Nordic Patrollers).

**task force** a combination of different resources with common communications that is managed by a task force leader (e.g., a sheriff's deputy, an NSP alpine patrol, and a search-and-rescue team).

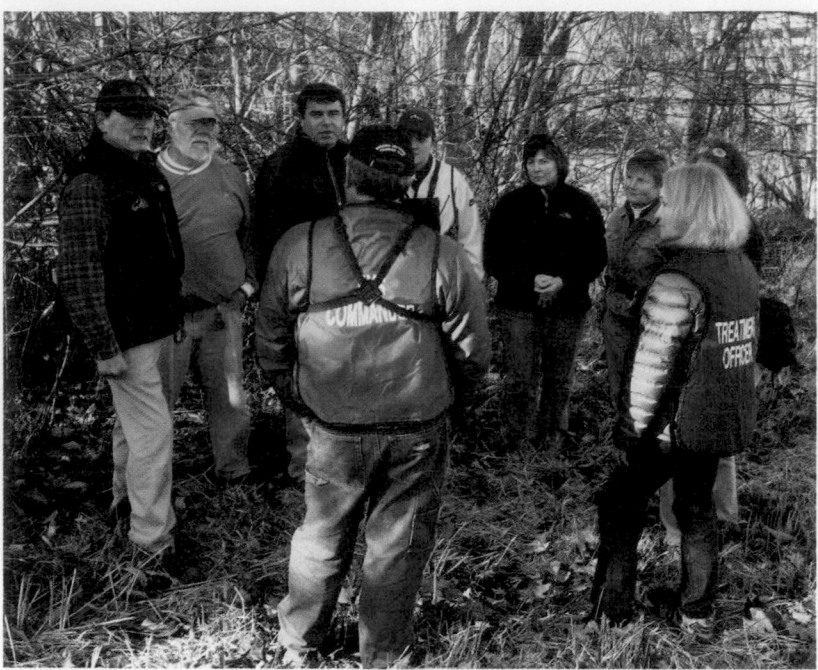

**Figure 4-7** Ski patrollers confer with the Branch Director at an MCI.
Copyright Mike Halloran

and is managed by a task force leader. The leaders from both groups report directly to the Branch Director under which they are operating (Figure 4-7■).

Command and operations sections are established on every incident, although they may be managed by a single individual on small, isolated incidents. The next three functional areas—Planning, Logistics, and Finance/Administration sections—are usually established only on large incidents that last days, weeks, or even months (e.g., natural disasters or human-caused incidents).

## Planning Section

The Planning Section collects, assesses, distributes, and uses incident-related data (Figure 4-8■). It also coordinates the preparation of the IAP and other incident documents. This section achieves its goals by performing the following activities (see Figure 4-5):

- Determine incident resource needs.
- Gather and analyze incident-related data.
- Create probability projections (e.g., incident needs, outcomes).
- Prepare contingencies and alternative strategies.
- Assist in the preparation of incident documents and maps.
- Maintain incident records (except financial records).

The section is managed by the Planning Chief, who chairs all planning meetings. If needed, the Planning Chief may activate one or more of the following units:

- Resources unit: responsible for maintaining the status of every resource at the incident.
- Situation unit: responsible for obtaining up-to-date information about the incident and providing that information to the Information Officer.

- Documentation unit: responsible for providing ICS paperwork, clerical support, and incident documentation (except financial documentation) to incident personnel.
- Demobilization unit: responsible for rehabilitating equipment, personnel, and the environment, and for overall incident clean-up efforts.

Each unit is managed by a Unit Leader who reports directly to the Planning Chief. If needed, the Planning Chief may also request assistance from technical specialists to help gather information, evaluate the situation, or prepare projections and forecasts.

## Logistics Section

The Logistics Section provides support for all the functional areas and has the following responsibilities (see Figure 4-5):

- Acquire resources (e.g., personnel, equipment, services).
- Order/obtain supplies (e.g., food, water).
- Manage internal communications equipment.
- Maintain equipment.
- Develop a transportation system/supply line (to support operational needs).

The Logistics Section is managed by the Logistics Chief who, in addition to these duties, is also responsible for ensuring that all incident facilities meet specified needs. A **facility** is any primary work area in or around the incident in which incident-related activities are planned, organized, directed, or conducted (Figure 4-9■). Depending on the nature of the incident, one or more of the following facilities may be established:

- Incident Command Post (ICP): site where all command functions are undertaken. Every incident must have an ICP. The command post is the first incident facility created and is named after the incident (e.g., Bridger Command).

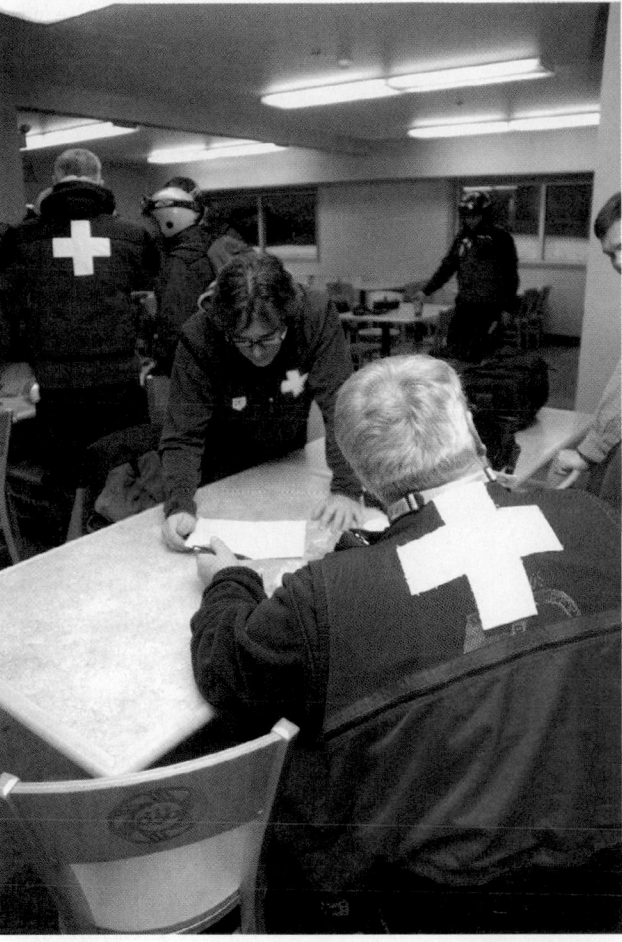

**Figure 4-8** A ski patroller reviews planning documents with others.
Copyright Studio 404

**facility** any primary work area in or around an incident in which incident-related activities are planned, organized, directed, or conducted.

**Figure 4-9** A ski patrol base facility.
Copyright Studio 404

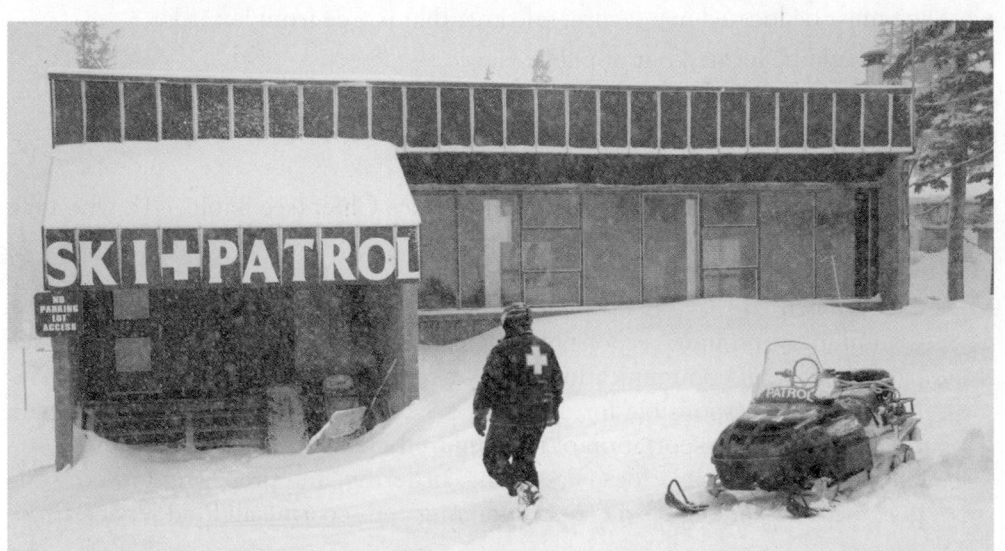

- Base: site where logistics functions are coordinated/administered. There is only one base per incident, and it is often adjacent to the command post. The base is named after the incident (e.g., Hayman Base) and is managed by a Base Manager, who reports to either the Facilities Unit Leader or the Logistics Chief.
- Staging areas: one or more sites where resources are kept until assigned. Staging areas may be near to or remote from the incident and are numbered (e.g., Staging Area 1). They are managed by a Staging Area Manager, who reports to the Operations Chief. Resources in a staging area are considered out of service until assigned.
- Camps: sites where incident personnel may eat, sleep, and rehabilitate. Camps are numbered (e.g., Camp 1) and are run by Camp Managers, who report to either the Facilities Unit Leader or the Logistics Chief. Personnel located in camps are considered assigned.
- Helibase: site from which helicopter operations are conducted. Helibases are named for the incident (e.g., Buffalo Creek Helibase) and are managed by the Helibase Manager, who reports to either the Air Operations Branch Director or the Operations Chief.
- Helispot/landing zones (LZ): temporary or permanent sites where helicopters can safely land and take off. Helispots and landing zones are numbered (e.g., H1 or LZ1) and are managed by a Helispot Manager, who reports to the Helibase Manager.

Note that not every facility must be established at every incident. Some incidents may require only a command post, whereas others may require each type of facility. Other facilities that may be found at an incident include the following:

- A communications center: the primary site at which all incident-related communications are coordinated.
- A rehabilitation center: the site where the physical condition of incident personnel is monitored.
- A demobilization center: the site where incident resources are discharged from the incident.

Regardless of the type of facility established, all incident facilities share several key characteristics:

- They must be located in a secure, safe area that is free from hazards.
- They should be located out of public view.
- They must be able to grow in size as needed.
- They must be accessible to incident personnel.

The Logistics Section is managed by a Logistics Chief (see Table 4-1), who may activate any of the following branches and units:

- Service Branch
  - Communication unit: responsible for installing, testing, maintaining, and repairing incident communications equipment (Figure 4-10■).
  - Medical unit: responsible for developing a medical plan that provides for the treatment and transportation of ill or injured incident personnel.
  - Food unit: responsible for (1) assessing, ordering, and preparing food to support incident personnel and (2) maintaining and securing all food service areas.

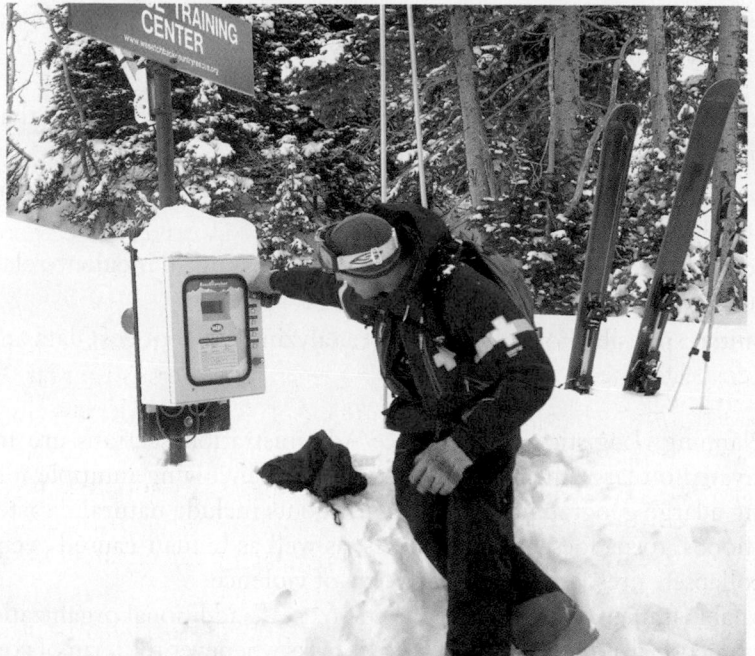

**Figure 4-10** A ski patroller testing an emergency communications box.
Copyright Snowbird

- Security unit: responsible for assessing and mitigating security risks to incident personnel and facilities and for establishing a secure perimeter around the incident.
+ Support Branch
  - Supply unit: responsible for ordering, receiving, storing, and processing all incident resources (personnel and supplies).
  - Facilities unit: responsible for setting-up, maintaining, and demobilizing all incident support facilities.
  - Ground support unit: responsible for monitoring, fueling, maintaining, and repairing incident equipment and for providing support transportation for incident operations.

## Finance/Administration Section

The Finance/Administration Section is responsible for providing financial management, accountability, and administrative services to support incident management activities. This section is responsible for the following activities:

+ Authorize expenditures.
+ Negotiate contracts with vendors.
+ Maintain reimbursement records.
+ Maintain injury, death, and damage documentation.
+ Tracks costs associated with mutual aid agreements.

The information gathered and documented is required to ensure that all incident-related expenses are tracked and paid, and it is especially crucial for incidents related to a President-declared disaster because these expenses are reimbursed under the federal Robert T. Stafford Disaster Relief and Emergency Assistance Act, also known as the Stafford Act (Public Law 100-707).

The Finance/Administration Section is managed by the Finance Chief, who may activate any of the following units:

+ Time unit: responsible for recording the amount of time resources that are used at the incident.
+ Procurement unit: responsible for administering all financial and vendor contracts and leases.
+ Compensation/Claims unit: responsible for processing all incident-related claims and injury compensation.
+ Cost unit: responsible for collecting and analyzing incident cost data and for providing cost estimates.

The Planning, Logistics, and Finance/Administration sections are most commonly activated on large incidents, especially those involving multiple jurisdictions or spanning a large geographic area. Such incidents include natural disasters such as wildfires, floods, tornadoes, and hurricanes, as well as human-caused events such as building collapses, fires, civil unrest, and acts of violence.

As a scalable framework, ICS allows users to create additional organizational levels within the functional areas to perform specific tasks whenever the span of control—the total number of individuals or resources supervised by a single person—becomes greater than one person can manage effectively. Under ICS, span of control is limited to 3–7 resources, with 5 being the average. Span of control ensures that each individual at the incident reports to only one supervisor. This greatly improves communications and the overall effectiveness of managing incident resources.

## ICS and the OEC Technician

When an incident occurs at a ski slope or other outdoor venue, OEC Technicians are generally the first rescuers to arrive on scene (Figure 4-11■). As a result, they will likely serve in a variety of key ICS roles. Among the roles that an OEC Technician may assume or be assigned are:

+ Incident Commander
+ Operations Chief
+ Medical Branch Director
+ Triage, Treatment, and/or Transportation Group Officers

Depending on the nature and scope of the incident, these roles may be combined as necessary. As Incident Commander or Operations Chief, an OEC Technician is responsible for performing all section-related tasks, as previously described. The first task of the IC is to assume command of the incident by notifying dispatch. The second task is to establish a command post. For ski patrollers, the CP is often located at the bottom of a ski lift, especially if the incident involves a lift. Once the CP is established, the IC identifies key tasks to be performed, assigns resources to complete the tasks, and manages the overall incident. When serving as the Operations Chief, OEC Technicians perform and/or oversee all rescue and patient treatment activities. On large or complex incidents, the Operations Chief may wish to establish a Medical Branch, which is managed by a Medical Branch Director who, if desired, can expand this branch into three groups: the Triage, Treatment, and Transportation groups.

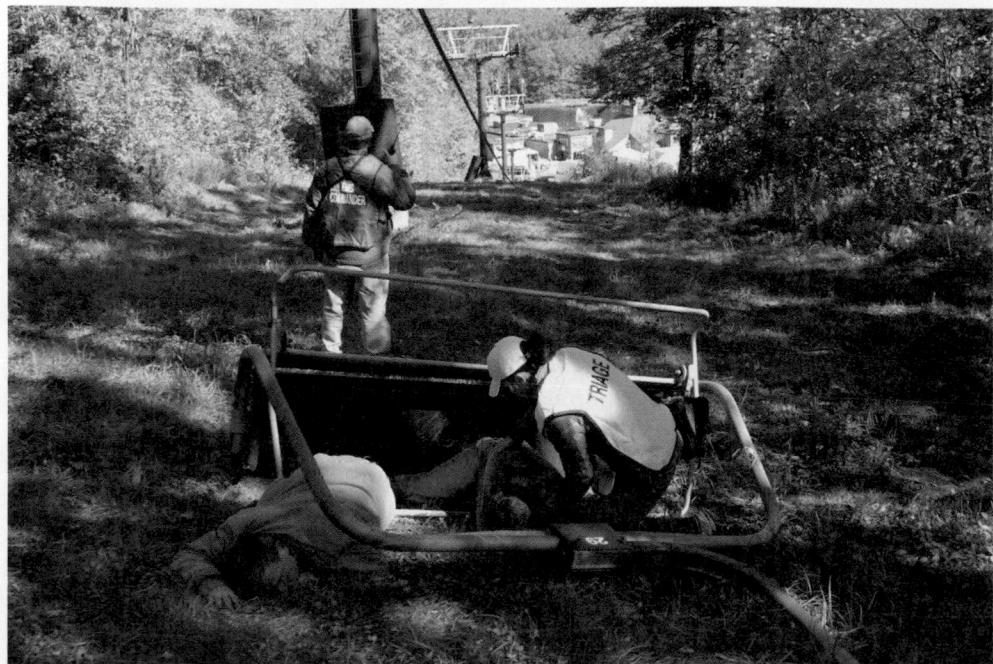

**Figure 4-11** Ski patrollers are the first to respond to the chairlift MCI scene.
Copyright Mike Halloran

**1.** Triage Group

The Triage Group is responsible for identifying, collecting, and sorting patients (Figure 4-12■). It is managed by a Triage Officer, who may perform the group's tasks himself or delegate them to others. Depending on the nature of the incident and available resources, the Triage Officer may establish near the greatest concentration of patients a "triage funnel," which serves as the entry point to the EMS Branch and is designed to speed the identification and removal of patients

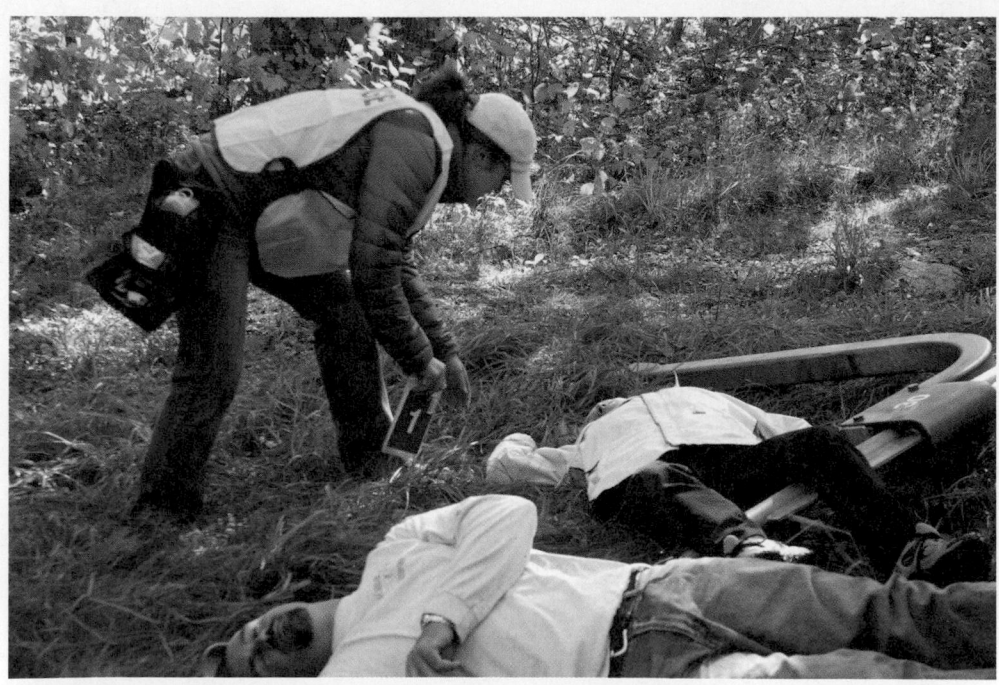

**Figure 4-12** Triage tagging at the chairlift MCI scene.
Copyright Mike Halloran

from the incident. OEC Technicians who are assigned to the Triage Group are tasked with the following duties:

- Prioritize patients for treatment according to injury severity and likelihood of survival (primary triage).
- Provide minimal care (open the airway, control life-threatening bleeding).
- Move patients to the treatment area.

Triage is covered in more detail in the next section of this text.

2. **Treatment Group**

The Treatment Group is responsible for providing on-scene care to patients that have been triaged by the Triage Group. The group is managed by a Treatment Officer, who oversees the group's activities. OEC Technicians who are assigned to the Treatment Group perform one or more of the following tasks:

- Establish an easily identifiable treatment area that has been approved by the IC (may include individual color-coded areas for each triage category).
- Reassess each patient's triage status (secondary triage).
- Provide emergency care to patients in accordance with state and local protocols.
- Provide an updated casualty report to the EMS Branch Officer.
- Prepare patients for transport.
- Move patients to the transport area.
- Maintain a written record of activities.

3. **Transportation Group**

The Transportation Group oversees the movement of patients from the incident to one or more medical facilities. Depending on the size of the incident, the total number of patients, the severity of patients' injuries, and the resources available, these facilities may include the patrol's mountain aid station. The Transportation Group is managed by a Transportation Officer who, like other group officers, may perform the group's tasks himself or delegate them to others. The Transportation Group is responsible for determining the number of patients in each triage category that each facility within the emergency care system can receive. This report, known as a hospital capacity status report, helps to ensure that patients are properly distributed, and it lessens the chance that any one facility will become overwhelmed by too many patients. Among the group's other responsibilities are:

- Identifying transport needs (i.e., determining how many toboggans, ATVs, ambulances, helicopters, and so on are needed).
- Coordinating the transport and distribution of patients to medical facilities (i.e., determining the mode of transport for each patient, and sending patients according to the hospital capacity report and/or in accordance with state, regional, or local protocols).
- Tracking patients (i.e., obtaining key patient data and recording which facility each patient was sent to).
- Providing updates to the EMS Branch Director (informing the director of current transport needs, how many patients remain on scene, and so on).

On a large incident, the Transportation Officer may wish to have an individual serve as a Transport Coordinator, who helps ensure the smooth departure of patients from the scene.

In addition to their primary duties, each group is responsible for maintaining a written record of its activities and for submitting individual group reports to the Medical Branch Director, as requested. Once a group has completed all of its assigned tasks, group personnel and resources may be reassigned to perform other incident-related tasks.

# STOP, THINK, UNDERSTAND

## Multiple Choice

Choose the correct answer.

1. Which of the following is one of the four major activity components of NIMS? _____
   a. span of control
   b. standardization of roles
   c. preparedness
   d. personal accountability

2. Which of the following describes the responsibilities of the Operations Section of NIMS? _____

   a. collects, assesses, distributes, and uses incident related data
   b. provides support for all the functional areas
   c. provides financial management
   d. executes the strategies of the Incident Action Plan (IAP)

3. What does NIMS stand for?_____
   a. National Initial Management Structure
   b. National Incident Management System
   c. National Initial Management System
   d. National Incident Management Structure

## Fill in the Blank

Fill in the blank boxes in the following ICS organizational chart.

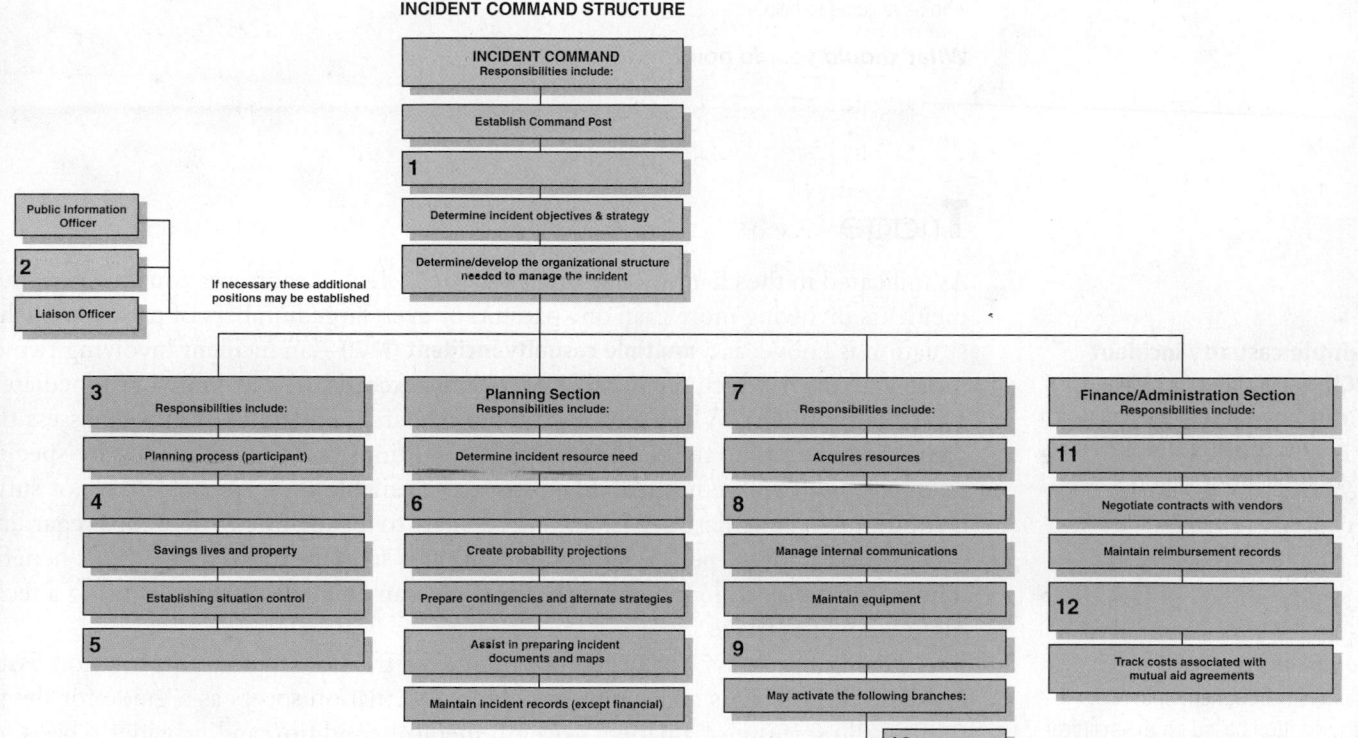

**INCIDENT COMMAND STRUCTURE**

INCIDENT COMMAND
Responsibilities include:

Establish Command Post

**1**

Determine incident objectives & strategy

Determine/develop the organizational structure needed to manage the incident

Public Information Officer

**2**

Liaison Officer

If necessary these additional positions may be established

**3** Responsibilities include:

Planning process (participant)

**4**

Savings lives and property

Establishing situation control

**5**

Planning Section
Responsibilities include:

Determine incident resource need

**6**

Create probability projections

Prepare contingencies and alternate strategies

Assist in preparing incident documents and maps

Maintain incident records (except financial)

**7** Responsibilities include:

Acquires resources

**8**

Manage internal communications

Maintain equipment

**9**

May activate the following branches:

**10**

Support Branch

Finance/Administration Section
Responsibilities include:

**11**

Negotiate contracts with vendors

Maintain reimbursement records

**12**

Track costs associated with mutual aid agreements

# CASE UPDATE

You contact patrol dispatch to declare a major mass casualty incident, give a brief situation report, and call for additional resources. You also identify yourself as the Incident Commander. As IC, you then start to determine the nature and extent of the incident by sending your fellow patrollers downhill to assess the situation. At the same time, you establish a Command Post in the lift operator's booth, which gives you a sweeping view of the scene. Given the number of patients you can see, you decide that an Operations Section should be created, and you inform dispatch that you need additional resources, both from the ski area and from the local emergency care system.

A patroller calls you on the radio and tells you that there are "at least 30 patients on the ground and least 120 trapped on the lifts." With this information you begin to formulate your Incident Action Plan.

A few minutes later, the patrol director enters the CP and assumes the role of IC. You give her a quick verbal report of the situation and what you have done so far. The transfer of incident command to the patrol director is announced over the radio so that everyone is aware of the change. She then designates you as the Operations Chief and directs you to go to the scene to lead the rescue efforts. Upon your arrival, a patroller informs you that the lift has collapsed and that *"there are patients all the way down to the bottom!"* Before you can catch your breath, a person approaches you and identifies himself as a doctor. He tells you that he is one of several emergency physicians who have come to help.

**What should you do now?**

# Triage

As indicated in the chapter's opening case, OEC Technicians occasionally encounter incidents involving more than one patient, or even large numbers of patients. Such a situation is known as a **multiple casualty incident (MCI)**—an incident involving two or more patients in which the number of patients exceeds the capability of immediately available resources. When such an incident occurs, rescuers must quickly assess the victims to determine the severity of their conditions and to rapidly identify specific resources that will be needed. The resources available on scene are often not sufficient to meet immediate needs, forcing rescuers to make difficult decisions regarding how to best allocate personnel, equipment, and supplies to maximize their benefit. These decisions, while fraught with emotions, can be made objectively using a technique known as triage.

**Triage** is a process of prioritizing patients for treatment and transportation based on their clinical signs and symptoms. This information serves as a guide for determining the severity of a patient's overall medical condition and provides a basis for predicting their outcome in a setting of limited resources. Using this systematic approach, rescuers can assess large numbers of patients in a relatively short period of time. This approach facilitates decision making so that precious resources can be allocated to *"do the most good for the most people."*

The word *triage* originates from the French verb *trier,* which means "to sort." The concept was first introduced by Baron Dominique Jean Larrey, chief surgeon of Napoleon's Grande Armée, who developed the practice during the Peninsular Wars of the early nineteenth century as a means of prioritizing the medical needs of battlefield casualties. The practice enabled French physicians to rapidly identify soldiers whose injuries were survivable and who could be made fit to return to active duty in a relatively short period of time. Today, triage is the preferred method for evaluating large numbers of casualties and is a fundamental rescue skill that all OEC Technicians must master.

**multiple casualty incident (MCI)**   an incident involving two or more patients or an incident in which the number of patients exceeds the capability of local resources.

**triage**   a process of prioritizing patients for treatment and transportation based on their clinical signs and symptoms.

Triage is typically implemented only when the sheer volume of patients, the severity of injuries, or on-scene problems overwhelm emergency care personnel or outstrip available resources. On small incidents (fewer than 5–10 patients), the IC may elect to perform triage himself. The process provides a means of organizing patients into categories based on their medical needs. The most widely used triage categorization system in the world is "ID-ME" (pronounced "I.D. Me"), an acronym that represents the four specific triage categories used by NATO forces, National Disaster Life Support, public safety agencies, and search-and-rescue groups. The ID-ME triage categories are:

**4-3** Describe and demonstrate how to use the "ID-ME" triage system.

I    Immediate
D    Delayed
M    Minimal
E    Expectant (Table 4-2■)

The ID-ME triage system is often simplified for civilian use during natural disasters by adding color-coding, Roman numerals, or universally understood graphics.

The "Immediate" (Red)(rabbit) category is used to identify patients with detectable vital signs and injuries so severe that the person will die unless they receive immediate (within 2 hours) medical treatment (Figure 4-13■). Most patients who fall

**Table 4-2** Triage Categories

| Triage Category | Color | Prioritization Number | Universal Graphic |
|---|---|---|---|
| Immediate | Red | I | Rabbit |
| Delayed | Yellow | II | Turtle |
| Minimal | Green | III | Crossed-out ambulance |
| Expectant | Black | 0 | Cross |

**Figure 4-13** Triage tag #1, RED indicates immediate (I) transport needed.
Copyright Edward McNamara

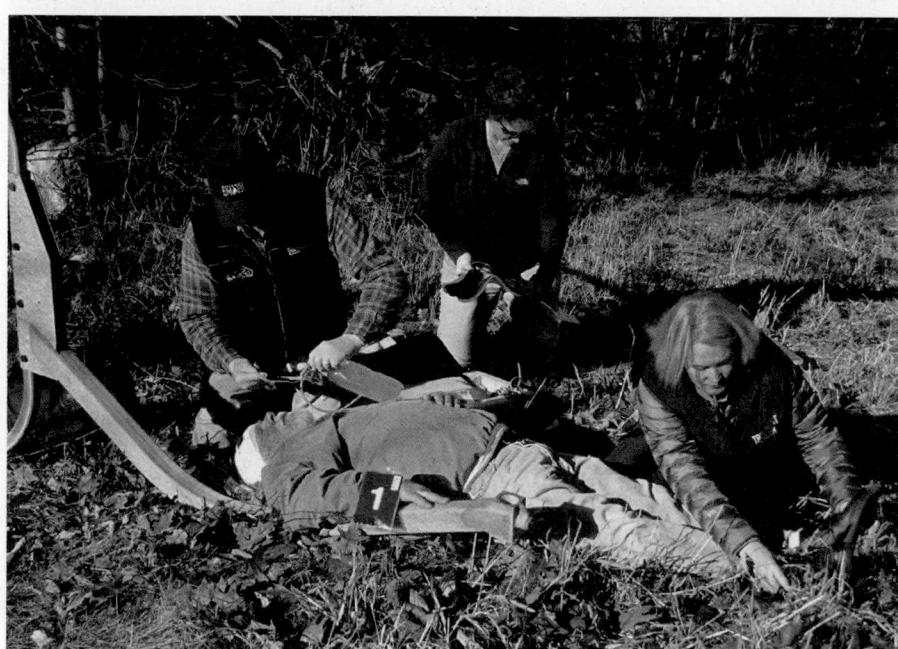

into this category have a complication involving their airway, breathing, or circulation. Conditions commonly classified as "Immediate" include:

+ A head injury with altered mental status
+ Severe respiratory distress
+ Tension pneumothorax
+ Extensive second- or third-degree burns of the face
+ Uncontrolled bleeding
+ Decompensated shock
+ Extensive thoracic, abdominal, or pelvic injuries
+ Amputation above the elbow or knee
+ Complicated obstetrics delivery

Patients categorized as "Delayed" (Yellow)(turtle) include anyone with a serious injury or medical condition who obviously needs medical attention but will not rapidly deteriorate if treatment is delayed for up to 4 hours (Figure 4-14■). Conditions commonly categorized as "Delayed" are:

+ Moderate shortness of breath
+ Compensated shock
+ Moderate-to-severe bleeding that is controlled
+ Penetrating injury without airway compromise
+ Open fractures
+ Compartment syndrome
+ Uncomplicated cervical spine injury
+ Severe abdominal pain with stable vital signs

**Figure 4-14** Triage tag #2, YELLOW indicates delayed (D) transport needed.
Copyright Edward McNamara

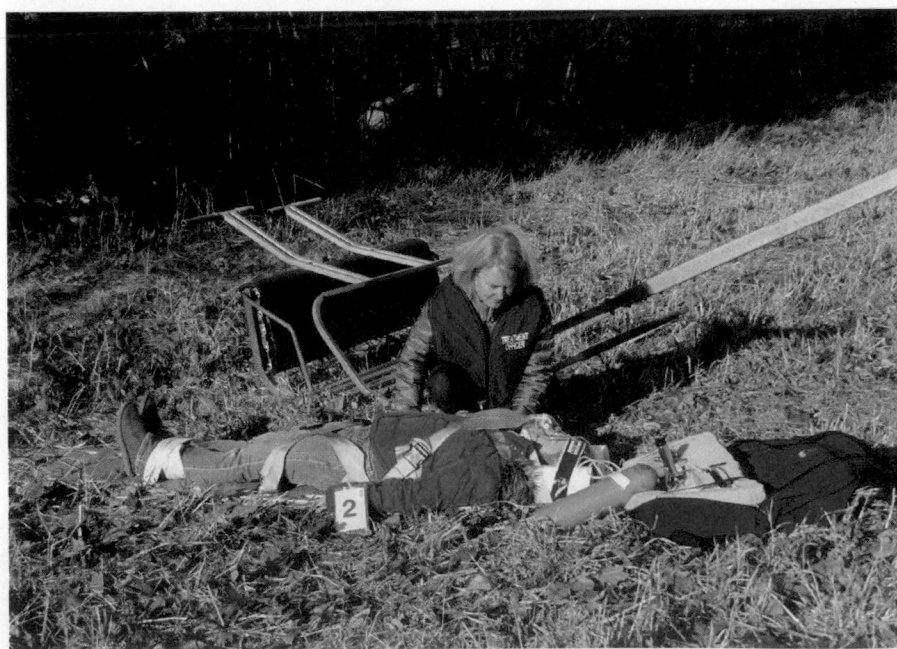

Patients categorized as "Minimal" (Green) (crossed-out ambulance) are individuals that have minor injuries that can go untreated for more than 4 hours or even days without serious complications. These patients are commonly referred to as the "walking wounded," meaning that they may be injured or ill but are fully conscious, able to understand commands, able to move under their own power, and, if conditions require it, able to take care of themselves for an extended period of time (Figure 4-15■). Conditions commonly categorized as "Minimal" include:

+ Mild respiratory distress
+ Closed fractures or dislocations without accompanying shock
+ Minor-to-moderate bleeding that is controlled
+ Burns involving less than 20% of body surface area (BSA) and not involving the head, face, or joints
+ Isolated penetrating injury to an extremity without accompanying shock
+ Frostbite
+ Strains and sprains
+ Minor head injury

Patients categorized as "Expectant" (Black cross) have little, if any, chance to survive their injuries or illness. This category is reserved for those unfortunate patients who are already dead or will likely (are "expected" to) die even if they receive immediate medical treatment (Figure 4-16■). Examples of patients who are categorized as "Expectant" include:

+ Cardiac arrest (from any cause)
+ Severe head or brain injury
+ Second- or third-degree burns involving more than 70% BSA (see Chapter 19)

**Figure 4-15** Triage tag #3, GREEN indicates minimal (M) transport needed.
Copyright Edward McNamara

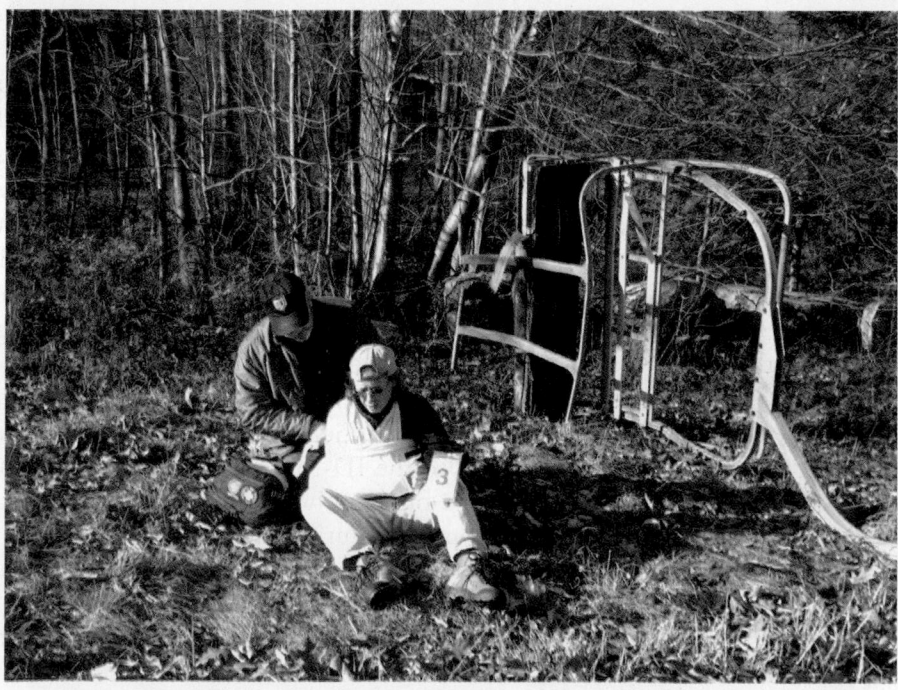

**Figure 4-16** Triage tag #0, BLACK indicates (E) expectant/dead.
Copyright Mike Halloran

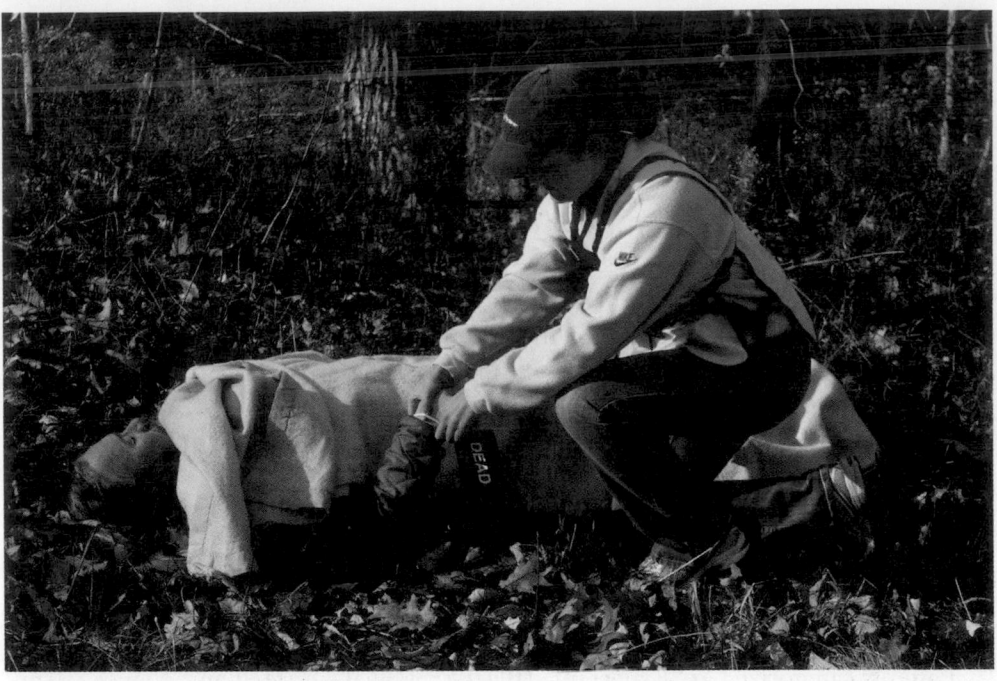

+ Irreversible shock
+ Gunshot wounds to the head with a GCS (Glasgow Coma Scale) of 5 or less

Once a victim has been categorized into an ID-ME category, this information must be conveyed to other rescuers, both those on scene and at the hospital, because it serves as the basis for both the patient's entry into the emergency care system and the order in which the patient is treated and transported. In most emergency care systems, this information is conveyed by the use of triage tags.

## Triage Tags

Triage tags are all-weather cards that are physically attached to the patient or their clothing to indicate the ID-ME category to which the person has been assigned. They enable rescuers to see this information "at a glance," without the need to reassess the patient.

Several types of triage tags are commonly used in the United States, including the Medical Emergency Triage tag or METTAG (Figure 4-17a■), the All-Risk Triage tag, and the SMART triage tag (Figure 4-17b■). Of these, the METTAG and the SMART tag are the two types that OEC Technicians will most likely encounter—unless the incident results in a federal response that includes mobilization of National Guard units, which utilize a military triage tag known as the Field Medical Card, or FMC. Although all three civilian tags correspond to the ID-ME triage categories, both the METTAG and START tags incorporate other universal features (previously described) that allow them to be used by lay persons during large disasters. All three tags include a unique identifier number, which helps rescuers track patients as they move through the emergency care system. The METTAG and SMART tags also have barcoding numbers that enable new computerized systems to track patients as they move through the medical system.

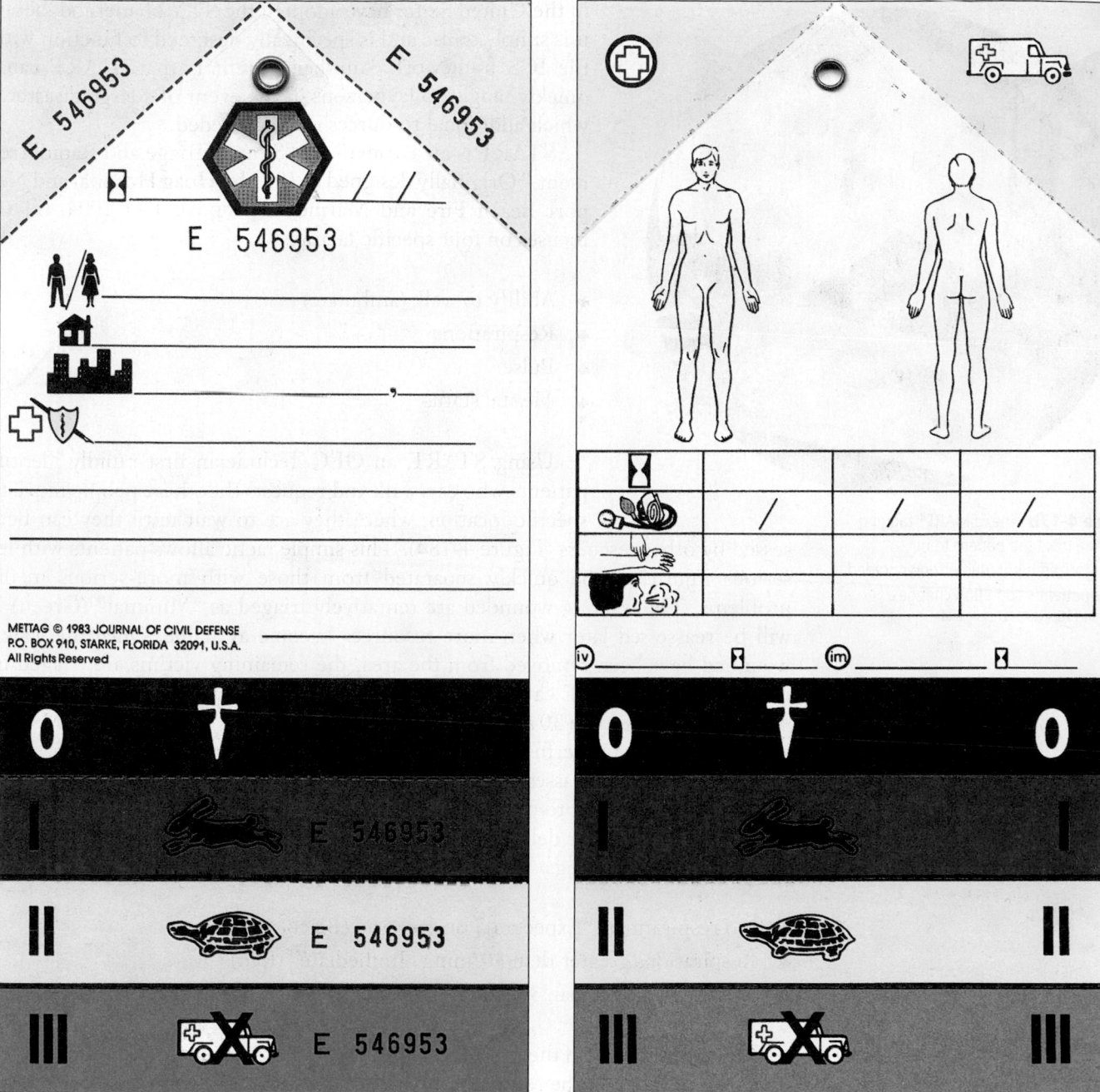

**Figure 4-17a** The "METTAG" system is used to identify Priority 1, 2, 3, and 0 patients.

## Triage Methods

Among the many methods for triaging patients used by emergency services and military personnel around the world are **START**, SALT (Sort, Assess, Life Saving Triage), MASS (Move, Assess, Sort, Send), and CIT (Continuous Integrated Triage). Additionally, comprehensive triage systems such as SMART are available. The SMART system offers a full range of ICS/triage resources, including triage tags, triage personnel vests, and the START triage protocol, in one comprehensive package.

Check with your state to determine which triage system you should use. Some states require all emergency care systems to utilize a single system, whereas others are less stringent. Of the systems identified, most public safety and rescue organizations

**START** a triage system commonly used by public safety personnel; an acronym for Simple Triage and Rapid Treatment.

⊕ **4-4** Describe and demonstrate how to use the START system of triage.

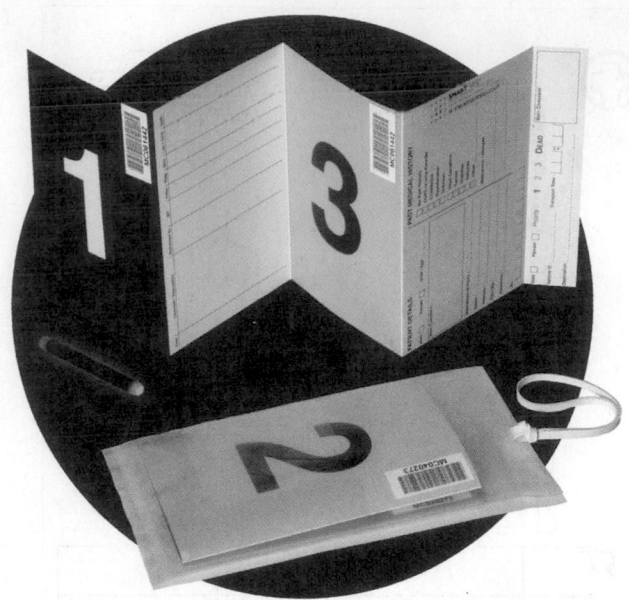

**Figure 4-17b** The "SMART" tagging system allows the patient to be recatagorized, upgraded or downgraded, as the patient's condition changes. Copyright ISG Assoc. LLP, England

in the United States have adopted the START method, because it is simple to use and is specifically designed to function within the ICS framework. Another benefit is that START can be quickly taught to laypersons in the event of a large disaster for which additional resources may be needed.

START is an acronym for "Simple Triage and Rapid Treatment." Originally designed in 1983 by Hoag Hospital and Newport Beach Fire and Marine, and updated in 1994, START focuses on four specific factors:

+ Ability to walk (ambulate)
+ Respirations
+ Pulse
+ Mental status

Using START, an OEC Technician first rapidly identifies patients who can walk and requests that these people move to a specific location, where they are to wait until they can be assessed by other rescuers (Figure 4-18■). This simple tactic allows patients with less-serious injuries to be quickly separated from those with more-serious medical problems. The walking wounded are tentatively triaged as "Minimal" (Green) but will be reassessed later when more resources become available. Once the walking wounded have been removed from the area, the remaining victims are triaged into one of the four ID-ME categories. Using START, this process can generally be accomplished in less than 30 seconds and centers on assessing the patient's RPMs—that is, their respirations, perfusion, and mental status.

The first step is to assess whether or not the patient is breathing. If the person is not breathing, attempt to open the airway, using no equipment or medical aids. Obvious foreign bodies or debris should be removed. The patient is then triaged based on the following findings:

+ No respirations: "Expectant" or deceased (Black)
+ Respirations greater than 30/min.: "Immediate" (Red)
+ Respirations less than 30/min.: Go to the next assessment criterion: perfusion

Next, check to see if the victim has a heartbeat by assessing the radial pulse or capillary refill. Based on the results of this assessment, the patient is triaged as follows:

+ No radial pulse or capillary refill takes longer than 2 seconds: "Immediate" (Red)
+ Radial pulse present and skin is pink and warm, or capillary refill occurs in less than 2 seconds: Go to the next assessment criterion: mental status

Determine whether or not the person can follow simple commands. Based on the result, the patient is triaged as follows:

+ Unable to follow simple commands or unresponsive: "Immediate" (Red)
+ Able to follow simple commands: "Delayed" (Yellow)

An easy way to remember the assessment findings of START is "**30–2-Can Do**"—*30* respirations, capillary refill of *2* seconds, and whether or not the patient *Can Do* (can

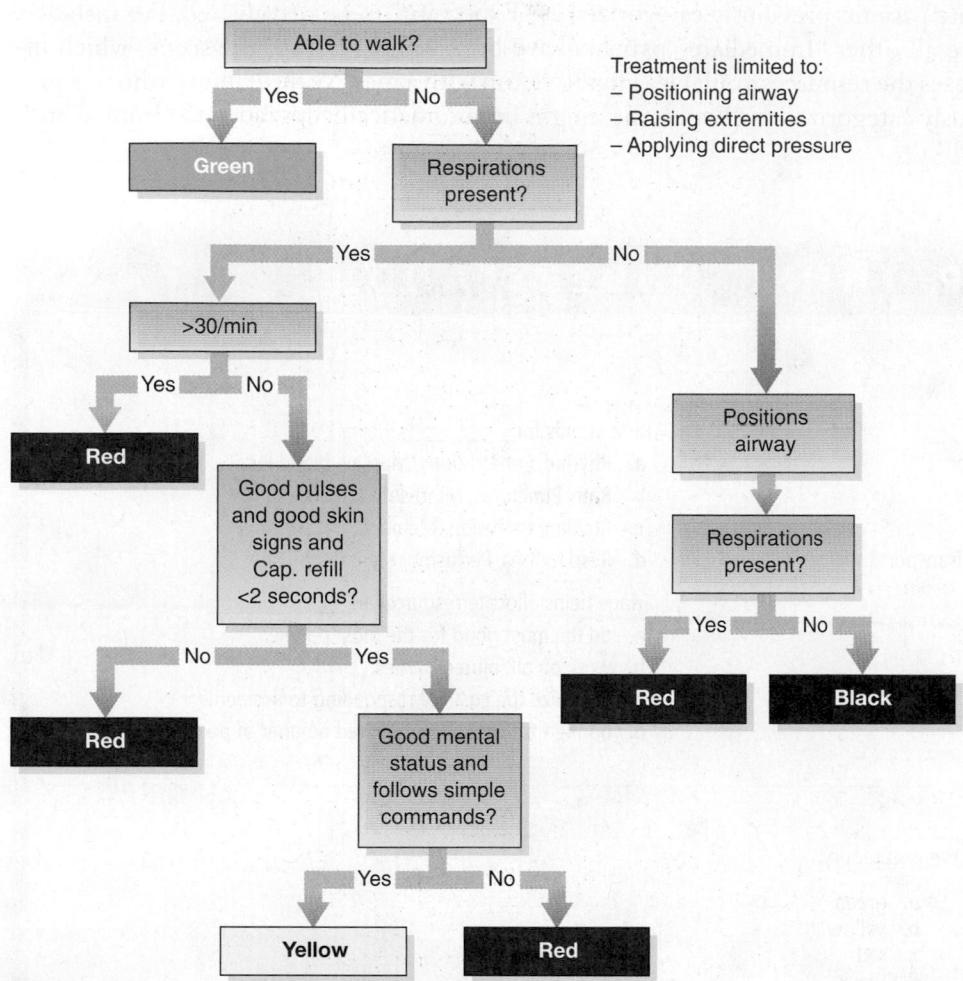

**Figure 4-18** The START triage flowchart.

follow) simple commands. This approach may not be suitable in all environments, however, as capillary refill is often delayed in a cold climate. In these situations, the presence (or lack) of a radial pulse is a better guide for determining the patient's perfusion status.

Triage should be considered a dynamic process that may need to be performed more than once. This is especially true for incidents involving large numbers of patients, because a person's condition can improve or deteriorate over time (Figure 4-19■). For instance, a patient who is found unconscious with a bleeding head wound may initially be triaged as "Immediate," but if the person wakes up and the head wound is found to be a minor laceration that has stopped bleeding, the patient may then be categorized as "Delayed" or even as "Minimal." Conversely, a person with apparent anxiety might initially be triaged as "Minimal" and subsequently be triaged as "Immediate" if the signs and symptoms begin to suggest that the patient is experiencing a heart attack.

Triage may also need to be performed again as additional resources or more-highly trained personnel arrive,

**Figure 4-19** Triage should be an ongoing process: reassessment may require changing a patient's tag number and transport needs.
Copyright Edward McNamara

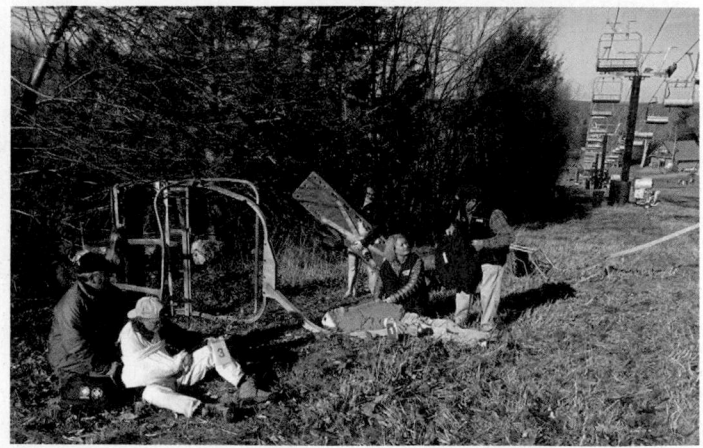

or as patients are transported to definitive care facilities, thereby allowing on-scene personnel to assume additional duties. An increase in available resources may allow living patients previously categorized as "Expectant" to be reevaluated. For instance, once all other "Immediate" patients have been removed from the scene, which increases the resources available, a living victim with a massive head injury who was previously categorized as "Expectant" might be automatically upgraded to "Immediate."

## STOP, THINK, UNDERSTAND

### Multiple Choice
Choose the correct answer.

1. START stands for_____
   a. Selective Triage and Recovery Transport.
   b. Safe Triage and Responsive Transport.
   c. Simple Triage and Rapid Treatment.
   d. Sophisticated Triage and Responsive Transport.

2. MCI stands for_____
   a. Multiple Casualty Incident.
   b. Many Casualty Incident.
   c. Multiple Casualty Injuries.
   d. Multiple Crises Incident.

3. RPM stands for_____
   a. Rhythm, Penetrations, Massive blood loss.
   b. Rate, Punctures, Mind-set.
   c. Rhythm, Perfusion, Memory.
   d. Respirations, Perfusion, Mental status.

4. Triage helps allocate resources to_____
   a. do the most good for the most people.
   b. work on all injured parties.
   c. minimize the costs of responding to accidents.
   d. do the most good for a limited number of people.

### Matching
Match each of the colors with the appropriate triage category.

_____ 1. immediate
_____ 2. delayed
_____ 3. minimal
_____ 4. expectant

a. green
b. yellow
c. red
d. black

##  CASE DISPOSITION

You soon have several patrollers and ski resort staff members on scene. To maintain a proper span of control, you inform the IC that you are creating two operations branches: a Rescue and Evacuation Branch and a Medical Branch. You assign a director to each. The Rescue Branch is tasked with evacuating stranded skiers from the lift while the Medical Branch is tasked with assessing, treating, and transporting the patients. The Medical Branch is expanded into three divisions: Triage, Treatment, and Transportation. A supervisor is assigned to manage each division. Physicians are assigned to the Triage and Treatment divisions to help care for the patients. Primary triage reveals the following distribution of patients: 11 "Immediate" (Red), 18 "Delayed" (Yellow), 21 "Minimal" (Green), 0 "Expectant" (Black). As more resources arrive, they are assigned to one of the two branches.

This incident took more than 4 hours to manage, during which time the Operations Section evacuated 220 people from the lift and treated or transported more than 100 patients, including 50 who had fallen from the lift.

# ⛉ Chapter Review

## Chapter Summary ○○○○○○○○○○○○○○○○○○○○○○○○○○○○○○○○○○○○○○○○○○○○○○○○○○

Incidents, both small and large, can present enormous challenges to OEC Technicians when sufficient resources to manage the situation are not readily available. These challenges are further compounded when an incident includes mass casualties, because the immediate medical needs of patients can quickly overwhelm local emergency care system resources. When such incidents occur, it is essential that they be managed in accordance with nationally accepted practices.

NIMS and ICS are powerful tools that can be used to manage any type of incident, regardless of cause, size, or scope. These tools provide a formal, standardized organizational structure, common terminology, and standardized procedures that enable rescue personnel from different organizations to work together

to return the scene to normalcy. The use of this all-hazard approach to incident management is federally mandated for all rescue organizations and personnel in the United States that respond to and manage emergency situations. This includes ski patrols, ski patrollers, and OEC Technicians who provide emergency care and transportation services in nonurban settings.

By using the principles and techniques inherent to NIMS, ICS, and triage, OEC Technicians will be better able to manage any type of emergency they encounter and will help ensure that resources are used to provide the greatest benefit to the most people. In accomplishing this, ski patrols and patrollers are an effective component of the national incident management team.

## Remember... ○○○○○○○○○○○○○○○○○○○○○○○○○○○○○○○○○○○○○○○○○○○○○○○○○○○○○○○

1. All rescue organizations and personnel are federally mandated to use the Incident Command System.
2. Every incident must have an Incident Commander.
3. There are five ICS functional areas: Incident Command, Operations Section, Planning Section, Logistics Section, and Finance/Administration Section.

4. The four triage categories can be remembered using the acronym ID-ME: Immediate, Delayed, Minimal, Expectant.
5. Triage is a dynamic process that may need to be performed more than once.
6. Use the START triage system.

## Chapter Questions ○○○○○○○○○○○○○○○○○○○○○○○○○○○○○○○○○○○○○○○○○○○○○○○○

### Multiple Choice

Choose the correct answer.

1. START assessments can generally be accomplished in less than _____
   a. 15 seconds.
   b. 30 seconds.
   c. 60 seconds.
   d. 90 seconds.

2. Which of the following are the responsibilities and logistics in NIMS? _____
   a. collects, assesses, distributes, and uses incident-related data
   b. provides support for all the functional areas
   c. executes the strategies of the Incident Action Plan (IAP)
   d. acquires resources

3. Which of the following is *not* a benefit of NIMS? _____
   a. early warning system for incidents
   b. standardization of roles
   c. standardization of processes
   d. modularization

4. Which of the following is *not* a key responsibility of the Incident Commander? _____
   a. Determine incident objectives and strategies.
   b. Provide overall incident management.
   c. Establish the Incident Command Post (ICP).
   d. Evaluate the injured.

5. Which of the following is *not* one of the five functional areas of the Incident Command Structure (ICS)? _____
   a. Operations Section
   b. Terminology Section
   c. Planning Section
   d. Finance/Administration Section

6. The role of the Incident Commander is typically assumed by whom? _____
   a. The most senior person among the initial arriving responders.
   b. The most qualified responder on duty.
   c. The most senior responder on duty.
   d. The most senior and qualified responder on duty.

7. What does "ID-ME" stand for? _____
   a. Immediate, Delayed, Maximum, Exceptional
   b. Immediate, Delayed, Minimal, Exceptional
   c. Immediate, Detain, Minimal, Expectant
   d. Immediate, Delayed, Minimal, Expectant

## Matching

A bullwheel on a chairlift collapsed, causing numerous people to be thrown off the lift. The chair has stopped moving, and there is no danger of another collapse, or any other dangers. For each of the following patients (A–J), write the number of the correct START system color code in the blank.

1. red
2. yellow
3. green
4. black

_____ a. A 48-year-old male patient is lying in the snow. Respirations are 31/minute, and he is able to follow simple commands.

_____ b. A 12-year-old female states that her ankle "hurts a little" and she wants to go find her parents in the chalet.

_____ c. A 36-year-old female complains of neck pain. She is ambulatory and able to follow instructions.

_____ d. A 16-year-old female snowboarder is unresponsive and has no pulse or respirations.

_____ e. A 55-year-old male is sitting on the side of the run, his respirations are 27/min, and his skin is pale and cool; capillary refill takes 4 seconds.

_____ f. A 61-year-old male complains of right shoulder pain. He is oriented and ambulatory.

_____ g. A 34-year-old Ski Patroller, a good friend of yours, has a massive head injury and no respirations.

_____ h. A 24-year-old male has a ski pole impaled in his left forearm. There is a small amount of bleeding from the wound.

_____ i. A 29-year-old female has severe abdominal pain; vital signs are stable.

_____ j. A 31-year-old conscious male has uncontrollable bleeding from an open head wound.

## Scenario

*Your ski area is sponsoring a large rock concert on a hot and humid July evening. From the base you notice clouds off in the distance. All of a sudden, a microburst storm quickly passes over the concert position, and a bolt of lightning strikes in the middle of the concert crowd. You realize that some of the concert goers have been struck. You wait for this quick-moving storm to pass and for the scene to become safe. Grabbing a battery-operated bullhorn, you head into "ground zero" and take charge.*

1. Your role in this situation is called_____
   a. Operations Chief.
   b. Logistics Chief.
   c. Planning Chief.
   d. Incident Commander.

*Using the bullhorn, you request that the uninjured head for the indoor lodges. The number of injured appears to be about 20 people. If the number had exceeded 100 and resulted from a criminal act, assistance would be provided by multiple agencies.*

2. This type of command is called _____
   a. multi-response.
   b. multi-organizational.
   c. simplified.
   d. unified.

*From your position and using your portable radio, you organize the MCI team and call EMS and the local dispatcher, declaring the MCI and requesting help.*

*Primary and secondary triage officers are assigned. They grab the MCI kit and head to the incident site. Using the START Triage method, the breathing of the more-seriously injured patients is checked.*

**3.** If the respiratory rate is greater than 30 per minute, the triage classification is _____

    **a.** "Immediate."                           **c.** "Minimal."

    **b.** "Expectant."                             **d.** "Delayed."

*The "walking wounded" are asked to move to a safer area under cover, leaving the more seriously injured patients out in the open. You assign a patroller to the "walking wounded" until a triage tag can be assigned to each.*

*What would the classification of the following patients be?*

**4.** A patient with second- and third-degree burns from the lightning and altered mental status _____

    **a.** "Expectant."                           **c.** "Minimal."

    **b.** "Delayed."                              **d.** "Immediate."

**5.** A patient with uncontrolled bleeding _____

    **a.** Green.                                   **c.** Yellow.

    **b.** Black.                                   **d.** Red.

**6.** A patient with a deformity on the forearm who is not in shock and is capable of following commands _____

    **a.** Green.                                   **c.** Yellow.

    **b.** Black.                                   **d.** Red.

**7.** A patient with an open fracture of the radius and neck pain _____

    **a.** Green.                                   **c.** Yellow.

    **b.** Black.                                   **d.** Red.

## Suggested Reading

Born, C. T., S. M. Briggs, D. L. Ciraulo, E. R. Frykberg, J. S. Hammond, A. Hirshberg, D. W. Lhowe, and P. A. O'Neill. 2007. "Disasters and Mass Casualties: I. General Principles of Response and Management." *J. Am. Acad. Orthop. Surg.* 15(7):388–396.

Department of Homeland Security. 2004. *National Incident Management System.* Washington D.C.

FEMA Emergency Management Institute. Introduction to Incident Command System, ICS-100. http://training.fema.gov/EMIWeb/Is/is100.asp

FEMA Emergency Management Institute. FEMA ICS Resource Center. www.training.fema.gov/EMIWeb/IS/ICSResource/index.htm

Maniscalco P. M., and H. T. Christen. 1999. "EMS Incident Management: Emergency Medical Logistics. *Emerg. Med. Serv.* 28(1):49–52.

Sasser S. 2006. "Field Triage in Disasters." *Prehosp. Emerg. Care* 10(3):322–323.

Thomas, T. L., E. B. Hsu, H. K. Kim, S. Colli, G. Arana, and G. B. Green. 2005. "The Incident Command System in Disasters: Evaluation Methods for a Hospital-based Exercise." *Prehosp. Disaster Med.* 20(1):14–23.

 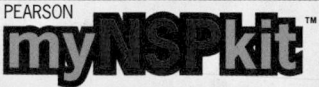

# Moving, Lifting, and Transporting Patients

Jonathan Politis, MPA, NREMT-P

## ⊕ OBJECTIVES

**Upon completion of this chapter, the OEC Technician will be able to:**

**5-1** Define body mechanics.

**5-2** Describe and demonstrate a power grip.

**5-3** Describe and demonstrate a power lift.

**5-4** Describe the basic guidelines for safely moving a patient.

**5-5** Explain the difference between an urgent move and a nonurgent move.

**5-6** List and describe various devices used to move and transport patients.

**5-7** Describe and demonstrate the following drags, lifts, and carries:

- Shoulder drag
- Extremity lift
- Bridge/BEAN lift
- Human crutch
- Fore and aft carry
- Chair carry
- BEAM lift
- Draw sheet carry

**5-8** List and demonstrate the proper use of equipment to move, lift, and carry a patient.

**5-9** Compare and contrast common transportation devices.

**5-10** List the components of a safe landing zone (LZ).

*continued*

## Chapter Overview

Patients who become sick or injured in an outdoor setting often require additional treatment or follow-up care in a definitive care facility. As a result of their condition, backcountry and ski slope patients often are unable to evacuate under their own power. In these instances, OEC Technicians are required to assist patients who are partially mobile and then arrange transportation (Figure 5-1a■), or to physically carry those who are immobile (Figure 5-1b■).

*continued*

## HISTORICAL TIMELINE

**7/15/1943** 10th Mountain Division activated.

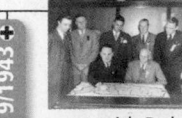

**9/1943** Minnie Dole recruits 3,500 to join the 10th Mountain Division. Two staff officers meet with Dole, upper right, and John E. P. Morgan, next to Dole.

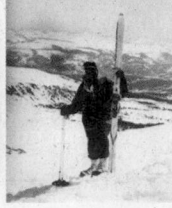

**1943** George Wesson joined the 10th Light Division and trained at Camp Hale. He is seen here on Homestake Peak.

**5-11**  Describe and demonstrate how to safely move when near a helicopter.

**5-12**  Describe the use of CPR during transport.

## ⊕ KEY TERMS

| | | |
|---|---|---|
| **basket stretcher,** *p. 131* | **lift,** *p. 143* | **semi-Fowler position,** *p. 146* |
| **body mechanics,** *p. 128* | **long spine board (LSB),** *p. 131* | **stair chair,** *p. 152* |
| **carry,** *p. 131* | **move,** *p. 135* | **Trendelenburg position,** *p. 146* |
| **drag,** *p. 136* | **orthopedic stretcher,** *p. 131* | |
| **high-Fowler position,** *p. 146* | **patient package,** *p. 127* | |
| **landing zone (LZ),** *p. 155* | **Rothberg position,** *p. 146* | |

Of all the tasks performed by OEC Technicians, moving, lifting, and transporting patients present some of the greatest challenges and risks. The reason is that OEC Technicians must perform these tasks under difficult conditions, often with limited resources. In addition to moving and lifting patients from awkward positions, OEC Technicians often must carry, lift, or transport a **patient package** weighing more than 300 pounds. Even when this weight is shared between two or more rescuers, carrying and/or sliding a heavy weight over snow, ice, and uneven terrain is tough, back-breaking work, even under the best of circumstances.

**patient package**   the combination of the patient, any equipment needed to care for the patient, and the device used to transport the patient.

**Figure 5-1a** Sometimes injured patients can assist with their extrication.
Copyright Scott Smith

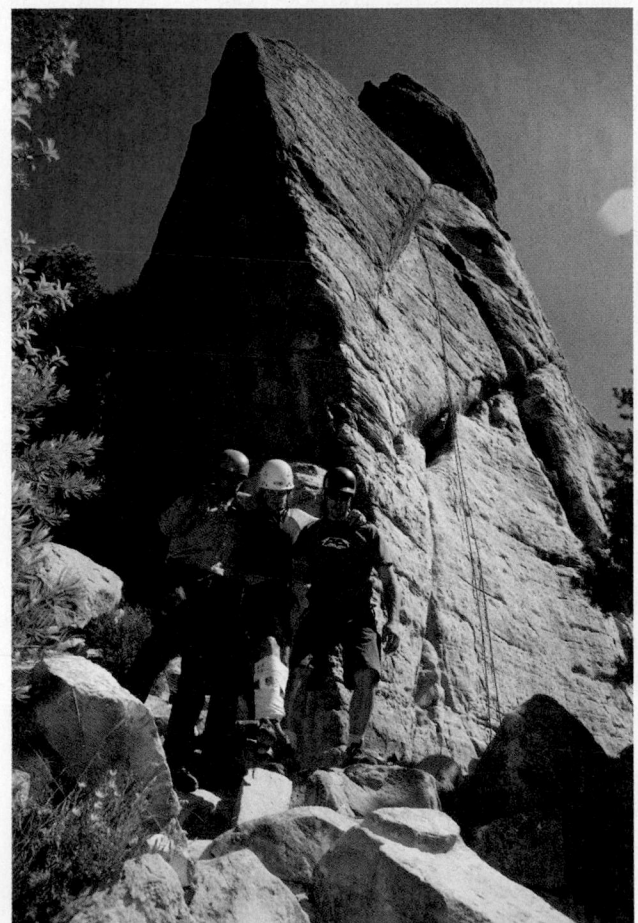

**Figure 5-1b** This injured alpine skier must be transported by toboggan.
Copyright Scott Smith

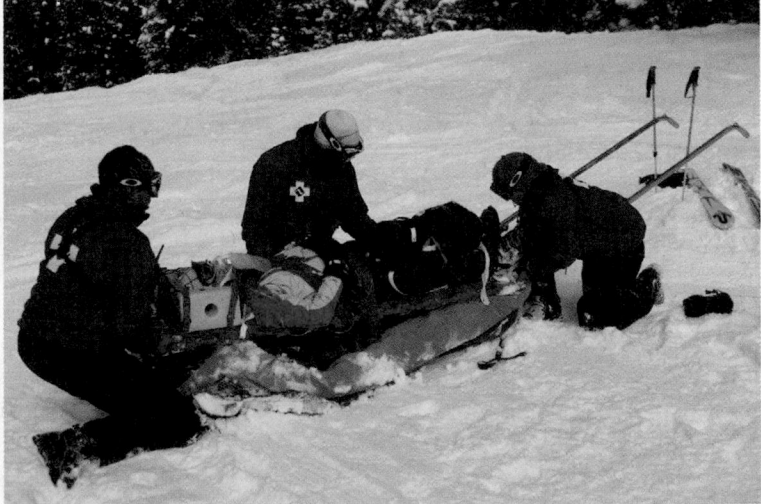

## ➕ CASE PRESENTATION ➕

You receive a report of a fire in the lower maintenance building. You arrive to find flames and smoke coming out of the back of the building. One of the workers stumbles out the front garage door, shouting for help. The man states that his coworker is unresponsive and is lying just outside the door in front of the groomer. Apparently, the two men were fixing a hydraulic leak when a fire broke out in the back of the building. The man states that during their attempt to leave the building, his coworker struck his head on a low hanging pipe and collapsed just outside the front door. The man speaking to you is obviously frightened but appears unhurt. He refuses any assistance, instead yelling at you to "Save my buddy!" He points to the nearby garage door, where you can see a man lying unresponsive on the ground, near the entrance. Smoke is slowly billowing out the door.

*What are the first steps you should take?*

Transporting patients is one of the essential roles of OEC Technicians and is a task that is performed on a regular basis. In some situations, the most important intervention that OEC Technicians can provide is rapid transportation to definitive care. Transport can be performed on foot while the patient walks with assistance, by skiing down a slope with the patient in a toboggan, by carrying the patient in an improvised litter, or by using motorized ground or air vehicles. Transport decisions are based on various factors, including available manpower, safety, weather, available equipment, and specific patient needs that require advanced care. Transport can be a complex task that requires careful planning, because poor packaging/transportation can cause a patient to be dropped, aggravating existing injuries and/or injuring the rescuers.

This chapter will help OEC Technicians learn how to lift, move, and transport a patient in a safe and efficient manner. It also describes body mechanics and proper lifting techniques. Urgent and nonurgent moves are also covered, as are commercial and improvised moving and transporting devices. The chapter concludes with a discussion about basic helicopter operations and safety during backcountry rescue operations.

## The Body Mechanics of Lifting

In the world of emergency rescue work, it is not difficult to find someone who has sustained a back injury. The National Institute of Occupational Safety and Health (NIOSH) estimates that 20% of all workplace injuries are back related. National EMS organizations also report that as many as 50% of EMS workers have sustained a back injury that resulted in the loss of time from work. Sadly, many dedicated patrollers and rescuers have had to stop patrolling or leave emergency rescue work because of chronic back injuries. Fortunately, many work-related injuries can be prevented by understanding the **body mechanics** of lifting and by practicing good lifting techniques. The key to reducing back injuries is to understand the mechanics of lifting and moving and to perform these tasks using proper technique.

The human spine is a collection of vertebrae (Figure 5-2■). Between each pair of adjacent vertebrae is a cartilaginous pad, known as a "disc," that cushions the vertebrae, preventing direct "bone-on-bone" contact. Spinal nerves arise from the spinal cord and leave it through holes between

**➕ 5-1** Define body mechanics.

**body mechanics** the proper use of body movement in daily activities to prevent problems associated with posture.

**Figure 5-2** The human spine is a collection of vertebrae arranged in alignment.

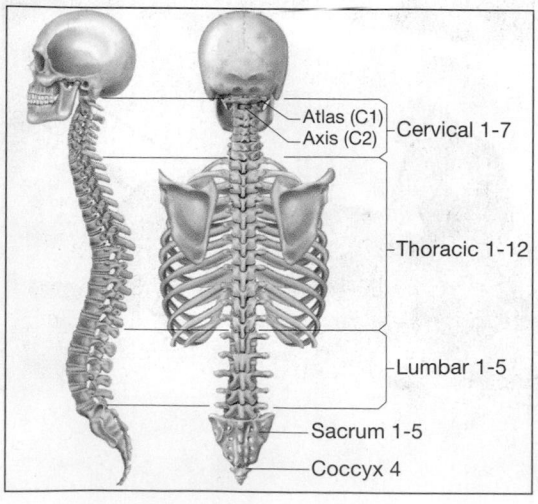

Atlas (C1)
Axis (C2)
Cervical 1-7

Thoracic 1-12

Lumbar 1-5

Sacrum 1-5

Coccyx 4

the vertebrae, and these nerves provide nervous system control to various parts of the body. Muscles attach directly to each vertebra, helping to keep the spine in proper alignment.

To stand upright and to maintain proper anatomical alignment of the spine, humans must have strong abdominal and back muscles. To maintain this alignment when moving or lifting heavy objects, the weight being lifted must be evenly transferred throughout the lifter's body (Figure 5-3■). The leg muscles, especially the upper thigh muscles, are especially well suited for lifting because they are among the strongest muscles in the body.

Most back injuries are caused by using poor body mechanics. Our bodies are capable of moving and lifting heavy weights, but only if we use good body mechanics. Good body mechanics, when combined with good lifting and moving techniques, lessen one's chance of injury.

When a person exhibits good body mechanics and lifts properly, the spine is in a straight line, with the weight evenly distributed to the vertebrae and the discs. The use of good mechanics—called axial loading—distributes the weight evenly, down the entire spinal column, through the pelvis, and to the bones of the legs. The shoulders need to be aligned over the spine, not in front or behind the upright spine (Figure 5-4a■).

When a person exhibits poor body mechanics and lifts improperly (Figure 5-4b■), the vertebrae are misaligned. This misalignment causes the load to be unevenly distributed across the discs. The resulting shearing force can damage the discs, spinal nerves, and/or adjacent spinal muscles and ligaments.

To stack the odds in your favor, OEC Technicians are encouraged to practice good body mechanics. In addition, you should engage in a program of regular exercise that is designed to strengthen your back and abdominal muscles. Also, lose excess weight, because every extra pound you carry in your abdomen pulls on the spine, increasing the pressure on the discs.

Making lifting safe requires some planning. Begin by asking yourself the following questions before you move or lift a heavy object: How heavy is the object? What type of terrain is involved? Which carrying device will work best for the situation?

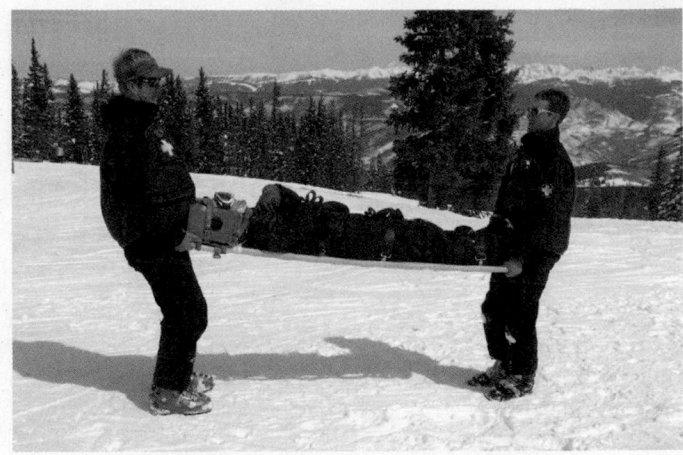

**Figure 5-3** Proper anatomical position is needed to distribute the weight of a patient evenly throughout the rescuer's entire body.
Copyright Scott Smith

**Figure 5-4a** The proper position when preparing to lift.
Copyright Scott Smith

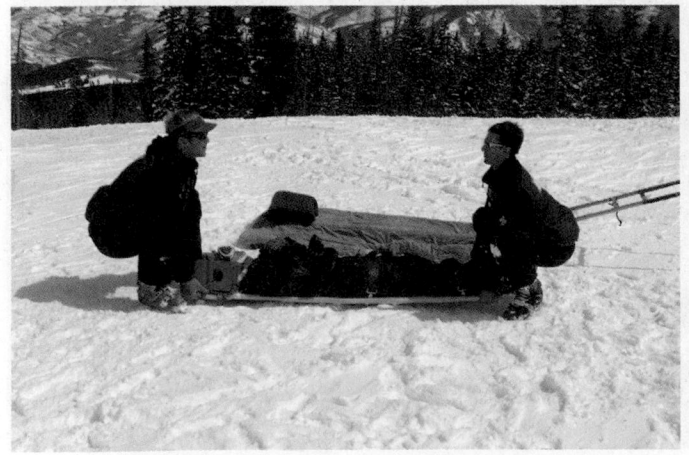

**Figure 5-4b** Using these improper lifting positions could very well injure your back.
Copyright Scott Smith

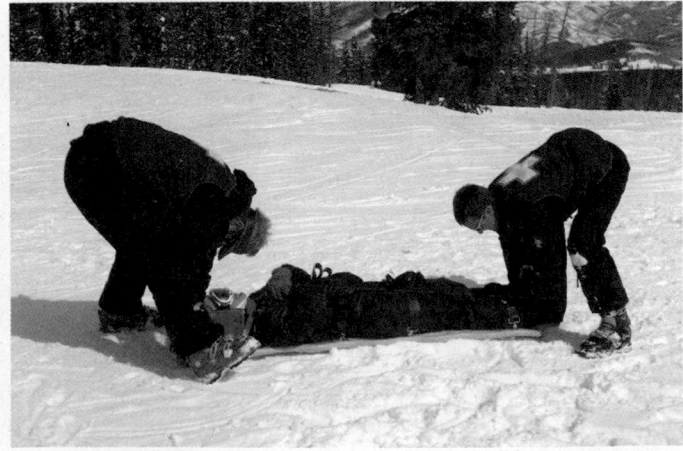

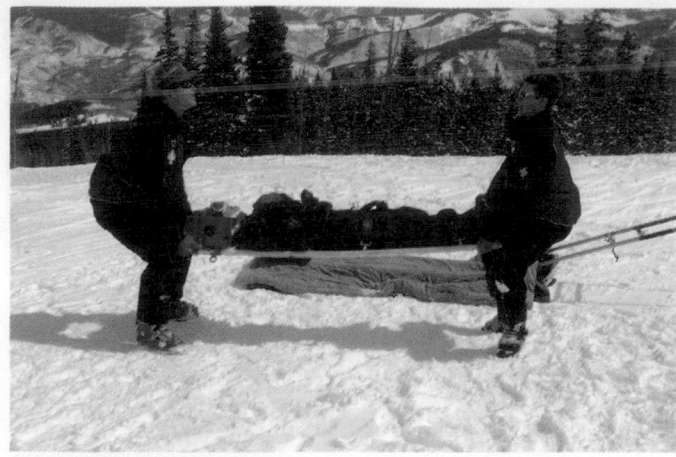

**Figure 5-5** Proper lifting uses the strong and large thigh and buttock muscles.
Copyright Edward McNamara

Then, always follow these back-smart tips, which help reduce your chances of sustaining a lift-related back injury:

+ Know your physical limitations.
+ Plan the move and/or lift.
+ Get help! Do not try to move or lift an object that is too heavy to handle by yourself.
+ Keep your feet a shoulder's width apart.
+ Keep your back straight. (Do not bend at the waist.)
+ Do not overreach over your head.
+ Get a good grip on the object being lifted.
+ Bend your knees.
+ Lift with your legs, not with your back (Figure 5-5■).
+ Keep your shoulders centered over the upright, aligned spine.
+ Keep the object close to your body.
+ Keep your head up as you lift.
+ Turn with your feet, not your hips. (Avoid twisting and turning your back at the same time.)

It has been said that many hands make light work. In addition to other rescuers, most emergency scenes have bystanders who can lend a hand. Develop the leadership skills needed to use assistants safely and effectively. It is much easier for four people to lift 300 lbs than it is for two. Look at the terrain and plan accordingly. Lifting and carrying a patient up and down hills or over uneven or slippery terrain requires planning and extreme care to prevent falling or dropping the patient (Figure 5-6■). The winter environment and snow can be used to your advantage by using the surface to

**Figure 5-6** Transporting a patient over uneven or slippery terrain may require more assistance; plan the details of the move *before* you get started to avoid getting into trouble.
Copyright Edward McNamara

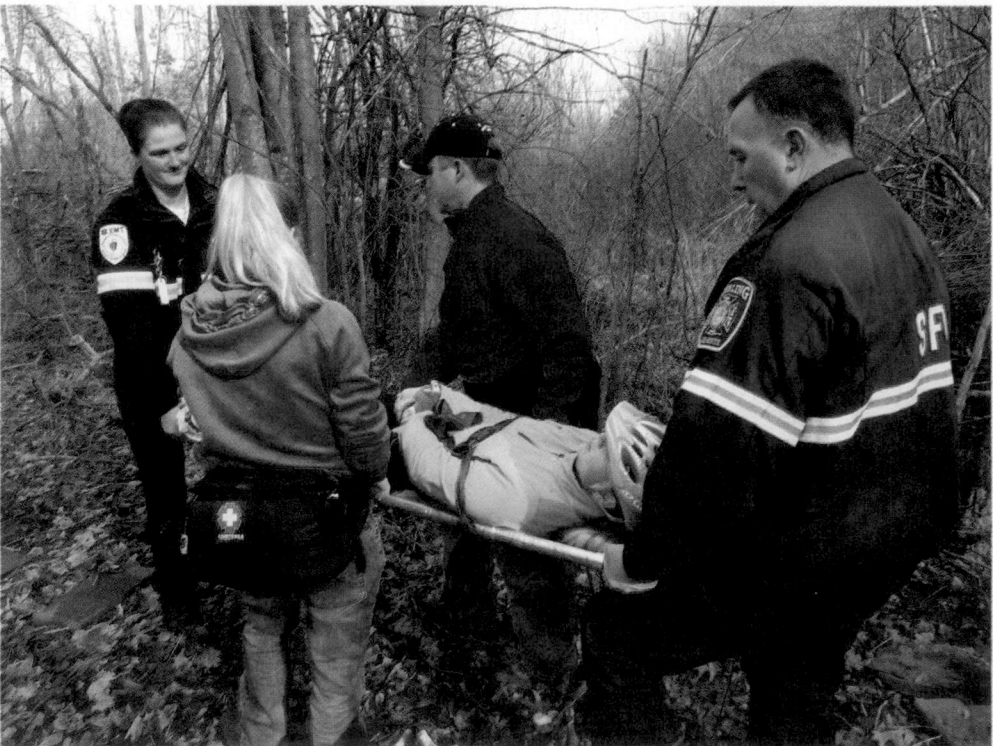

slide the patient in a rescue sled rather than attempt a **carry**. A backboard can be used for carrying the patient short distances. Longer distances require special litters or carrying methods. Using the right method and the right equipment for the situation are additional keys for reducing the risk of injury.

# Devices and Equipment

Many commercial devices are available to aid in moving, lifting, or carrying a patient. Used properly, this equipment facilitates good body mechanics and lessens one's risk of injury. Additionally, the transport equipment listed in Table 5-1■ is very useful in handling patients.

The more common equipment used by OEC Technicians to move, lift, or carry a patient include the following devices:

+ Transfer flat
+ **Long spine board (LSB)**
+ **Orthopedic stretcher**
+ Portable stretcher
+ **Basket stretcher**/stokes
+ Short spine board and vest-type lifting/immobilization devices
+ Sitting lifting device

## Transfer Flat

When it comes to lifting an overly large, heavy, or obese patient, there often is no easy solution besides obtaining as much help as possible. More hands mean the weight can be more evenly distributed among more people. However, it can be difficult to find a secure place to hold on to. Draw sheets are usually not practical because they are not strong enough to bear the load. To solve this problem, many rescue organizations and hospitals use a so-called "transfer flat" to lift large and heavy patients.

A transfer flat is constructed of thick, reinforced material and has both load-bearing straps and handles sewn into the device. The device may be laid next to the patient. The patient can either move onto the transfer flat or, if he is unable, rescuers may roll the patient onto the device using a special technique known as a log roll (described in detail in a later chapter).

## Long Spine Board

A long spine board (LSB) is one of the most commonly used pieces of medical equipment in emergency care today (Figure 5-7■). It is a rectangular board, 16 inches wide by 72 inches long, onto which a patient with a spinal injury is placed and then secured

**carry**    the act of taking or supporting the movement of a person from one location to another.

**long spine board (LSB)**    a long rectangular board, 16 inches wide by 72 inches long, on which a patient with a spinal injury is placed.

**orthopedic stretcher**    a two-piece device that is slightly concave and has an open center section; is used to transport a patient; also called a "scoop" stretcher.

**basket stretcher**    a lightweight device used to transport a patient during a backcountry rescue; sometimes called a "Stokes" stretcher.

| Table 5-1 | Transport Equipment |
|---|---|

- LSB with straps
- Head blocks
- Cervical collars
- Two or three blankets
- Pillow
- Rope
- Splints
- Waterproof covering

**Figure 5-7** A long spine or back board being readied for use.
Copyright Scott Smith

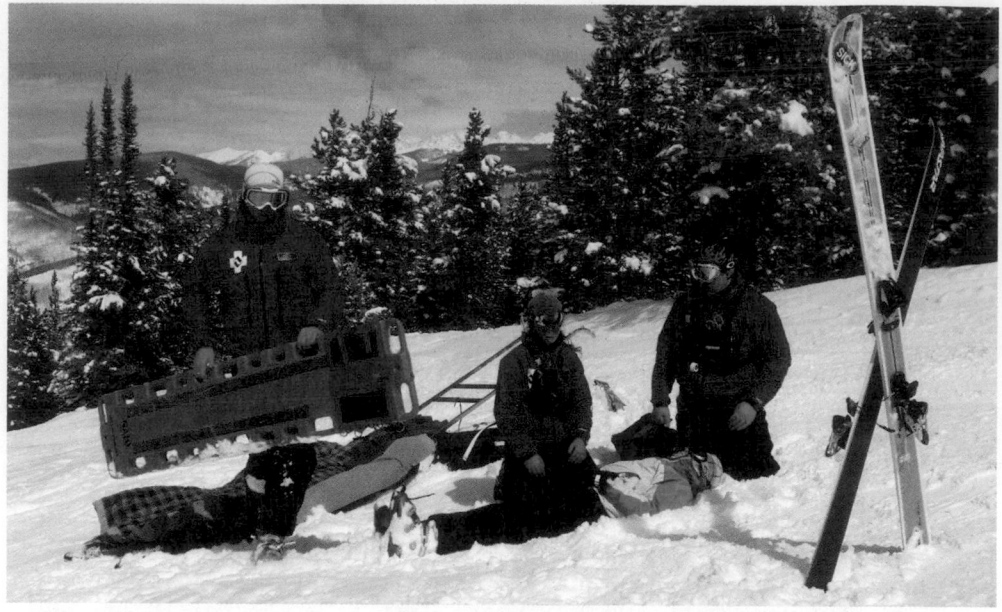

for transport. Longer, wider, and extra-strength LSBs are available for patients who are very tall, very broad, or especially heavy.

Some LSBs are tapered on both ends. Tapered boards are sometimes used in combination with a basket stretcher because many square boards will not otherwise fit. Most LSBs are manufactured from specially coated marine-grade plywood or lightweight plastic that is impervious to blood, body fluids, water, and snow.

Long spine boards are used for a variety of purposes including to immobilize suspected fractures of the spine, hip, pelvis, or femur; to carry a patient over short distances; and to facilitate transferring a patient between beds and transportation devices. It also is an excellent tool for extrication because of the ease of sliding patients onto it. It is not intended to be carried long distances. The patient should be placed onto a long spine board using one of the proper lifting methods previously described or, in cases involving suspected spine injury, using a log roll.

When deciding to immobilize a patient on a long spine board, remember how much time the patient will be committed to lying on its hard surface. Studies show that lying on a backboard, even for short periods of time, may cause profound back pain. It is for this reason that all gaps in the board should be padded. Padding can be accomplished with anything from closed-cell foam pads to towels and jackets. Once the patient has been placed on an LSB, use straps, cravats, or a commercially available product to secure the patient before lifting and carrying (Figure 5-8■).

## Orthopedic Stretcher

An orthopedic stretcher, or "scoop" stretcher, is a two-piece aluminum or high-density thermoplastic device that is slightly concave and has an open center section, allowing it to conform to the patient's body (Figure 5-9■). The wide end of the device is used to support the head and torso, whereas the narrow end is used to support the lower legs and feet; it can also be adjusted to match the patient's height. "Scoop"

### LSBs and Patient Care

**NOTE**

Prolonged contact with a hard surface can cause back pain and increase the chances that skin ulcers/pressure sores will develop in just a few hours. This is especially important in any backcountry rescue operation in which a patient will be placed on an LSB for over two hours. Thus OEC Technicians are encouraged to pad the LSB with a closed cell foam pad, if available. Additionally, all gaps in the board should be filled with towels, shirts, or other padding to reduce the incidence of pressure sores.

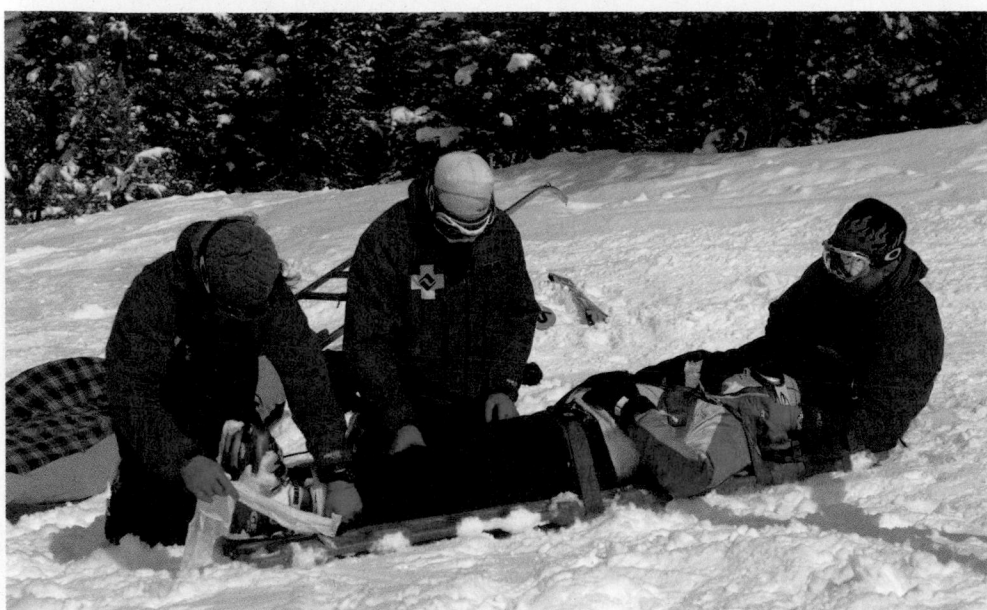

**Figure 5-8** The patient must be secured to the board; various strapping techniques are available to achieve this goal.
Copyright Scott Smith

stretchers have limited application in rugged or cold settings because they are heavier than most long spine boards, do not function well in cold environments, and are difficult to use by rescuers wearing gloves.

To use an orthopedic stretcher (Figures 5-10a–c ■):

1. Disconnect the two sides of the stretcher by pressing the button in the center of the mechanical fitting at either end.
2. Release the adjusting lever located on each side where the device narrows.
3. Place the two parts of the stretcher beside the patient, one on either side of the patient (Figure 5-10a).
4. Extend each side of the stretcher so that it is 1–3 inches longer than the patient. Ensure that both sides are the same length by checking that the number of exposed holes in the tubing is the same on both sides.
5. Slide both parts of the stretcher beneath the patient until the mechanical fittings at each end touch. Do not lift the patient.
6. Reconnect the two sides of the stretcher by firmly pressing the two ends back together until you hear a loud "click" at each end (Figure 5-10b).
7. Secure the patient to the device using straps, tape, or commercial device (Figure 5-10c).
8. To remove the stretcher, reverse the procedure.

⊕ **5-6** List and describe the various devices used to move and transport patients.

**Figure 5-9** An orthopedic stretcher or "scoop" stretcher, which can be placed under patients without moving them much, is also useful in tight spaces.

## Portable Stretcher

A portable stretcher consists of an aluminum frame and a vinyl-coated platform (Figure 5-11 ■). Slightly wider than a standard LSB, the device has cut-outs for the rescuer's hands at each corner and along each side to facilitate carrying by multiple rescuers. This device is available as either a one-piece stretcher or as a folding stretcher. Both devices are lightweight and are impervious to blood, body fluids, and water. A patient is moved onto the device using one of the techniques described in the section on lifting in this chapter.

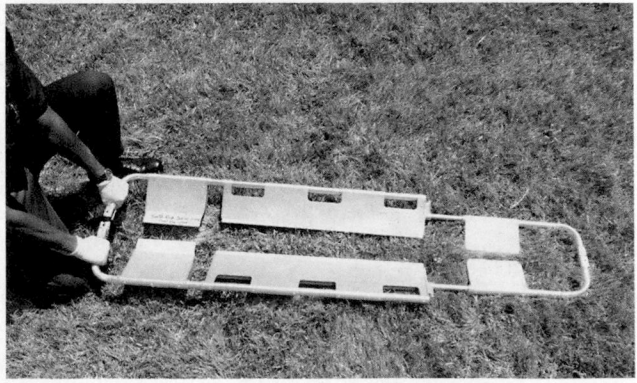

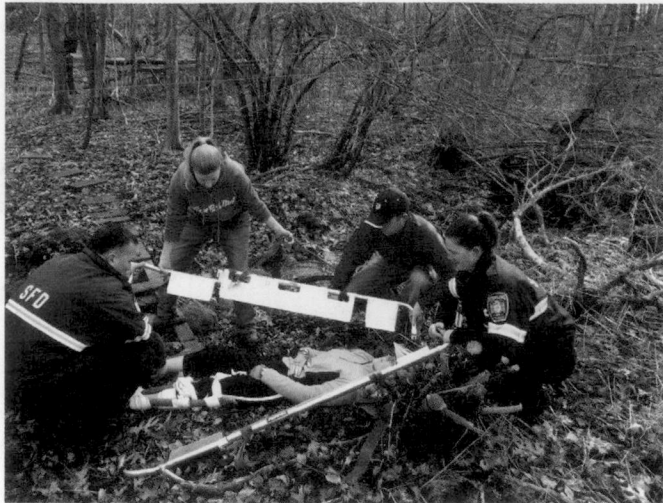

**Figure 5-10a** Place the two sections of the "scoop" stretcher beside the patient, one on either side.
Copyright Edward McNamara

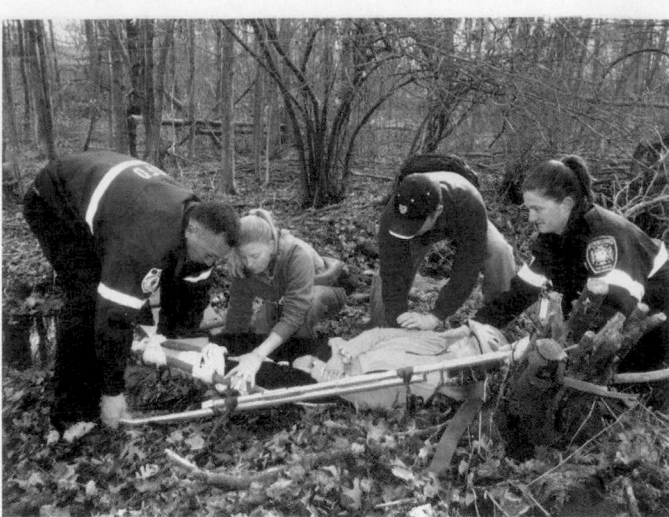

**Figure 5-10b** Slide the two sections under the patient until they clip together top and bottom.
Copyright Edward McNamara

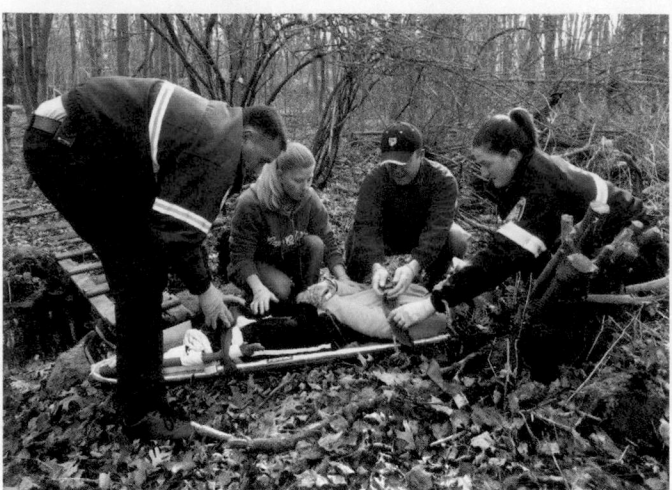

**Figure 5-10c** Secure the patient to the device carefully.
Copyright Edward McNamara

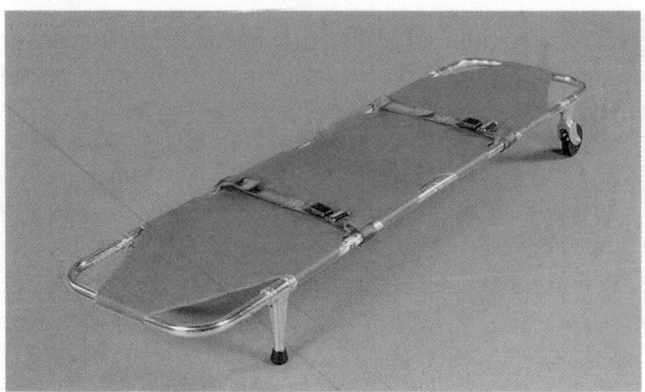

**Figure 5-11** A portable ambulance stretcher.

## Basket Stretcher

The basket stretcher or "Stokes" stretcher has evolved considerably from its initial use by the military for transferring patients between ships to its current use in back-country rescue operations (Figure 5-12■). Originally constructed of metal and wire mesh, today's basket stretchers are constructed from high-impact plastics and ultra-light materials such as Kevlar and titanium. Some can even be disassembled into two parts, making them easy to carry and reassemble at the point of use. This is especially convenient for backcountry operations that require the rescue team to carry their equipment over great distances to reach the patient.

**Figure 5-12** A basket stretcher or "Stokes" stretcher is used in backcountry rescue; current models are constructed of ultra-lightweight materials.

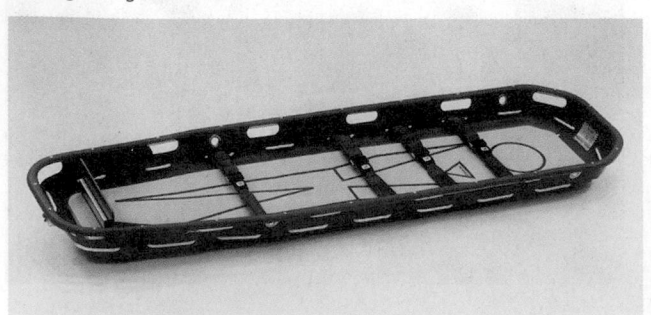

## Short Spine Board and Vest-Type Lifting/Immobilization Devices

These devices are typically used to move a sitting patient into supine position on a long spine board (Figure 5-13■). Although these devices are commonly used by ambulance personnel, who frequently must extricate injured patients from vehicles, they are infrequently used in outdoor emergency care. Seated patients in need of extrication who cannot be easily moved to a long spine board are rare.

## Sitting Lifting Device

Made from 3/4-inch or 1-inch plywood, this device allows a patient to sit on a board with one leg extended (Figure 5-14a■). Handholds cut into the wood enable two rescuers (or three rescuers, when one stabilizes the injured leg) to carry the patient for a short distance. It often is used to carry a nonambulatory patient from an aid room to a car for transport to a hospital when an ambulance is not needed (Figure 5-14b■). This device is especially useful for lower extremity injuries that have been immobilized in a cardboard splint. It is not used for spinal immobilization.

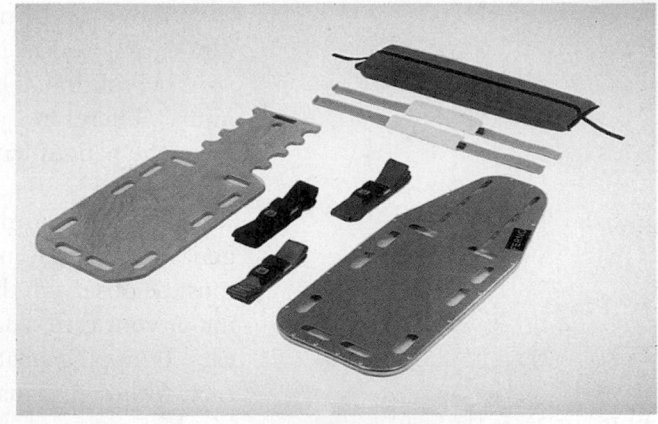

**Figure 5-13** A short spine board with accompanying straps and head immobilizer.

# Moving a Patient

A **move** is defined as the passage of a patient from one location to another. Depending on the nature and severity of the patient's condition and other factors, a move may be just a few inches, or it can be several feet. A move may be performed in a hurried fashion using one or two rescuers, or in a more controlled manner using multiple rescuers. Some patients require minimal assistance in moving, whereas others cannot move on their own and must be physically moved by others. During a rescue, OEC Technicians move a patient a minimum of three times:

+ From the ground to a toboggan or basket stretcher
+ From a toboggan or basket stretcher to an examination table
+ From an examination table to an ambulance stretcher or vehicle

**move** the passage of a patient from one location to another.

⊕ 5-4  Describe the basic guidelines for safely moving a patient.

**Figure 5-14a** A sitting lifting device.
Copyright Edward McNamara

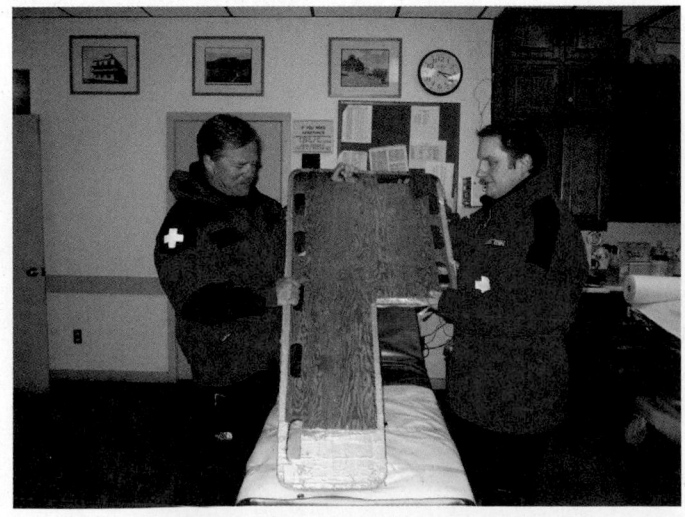

**Figure 5-14b** A patient using a sitting lifting device, which is especially useful in transferring a nonambulatory patient between an aid room and a car.
Copyright Edward McNamara

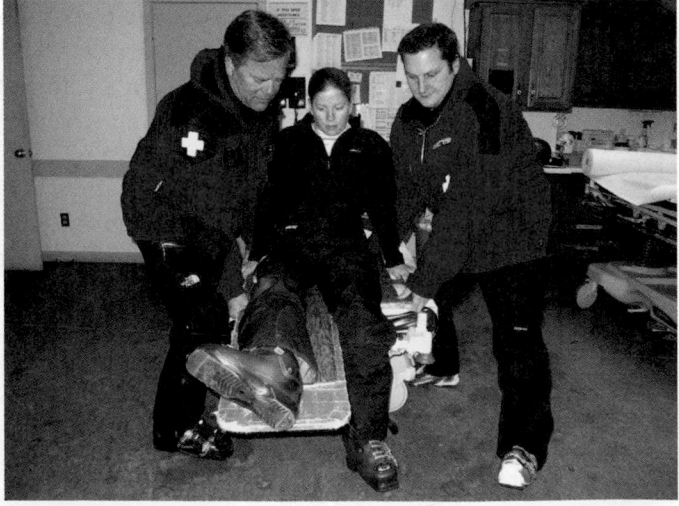

A move can be traumatic for a patient, especially one who is in great pain due to illness or physical injury. Each move entails a risk of further aggravating the patient's condition. The greatest concern when moving a patient is causing spinal cord injury. Therefore, you must ask yourself two questions before moving a patient: Does the patient have a suspected spinal injury? Does the patient need to be moved immediately?

Depending on the situation, OEC Technicians perform two types of moves: urgent moves and nonurgent moves. Regardless of the type of move, one cardinal rule must be observed: the patient cannot be dropped or allowed to fall. Once a patient is under your care, you are responsible for his safety, unless the patient refuses further care. Dropping a patient is one of the greatest areas of liability in outdoor emergency care. Although it may be appropriate to allow a patient to assist in a move, do not allow him to move unassisted. Remember, the first principle of medicine is, "Do no harm," so protect your patients from harm at all times.

If a spinal injury is suspected, protect the patient's spine. Specific techniques and equipment to protect the spine are addressed in Chapter 21, Head and Spine Injuries. If no spinal injuries are suspected, the patient may be asked to assist in the move, provided the request neither exposes the patient to a risk of aggravating his condition nor places him at risk of falling.

## Urgent Moves

As the name implies, an urgent move is reserved exclusively for situations in which the patient and/or rescuer must move quickly to safety or the patient's medical condition is life threatening and requires immediate transport. The primary indication for an urgent move is the presence of a hazard that could prove life threatening to the patient, the rescuer, or both. In outdoor settings, this could include situations in which the risk of avalanche, rock fall, or rising waters is high, or situations involving wild animals, fire, inclement weather, or other hazards, whether natural or human-caused.

An urgent move also may be needed if care cannot be adequately rendered where the patient is located. For instance, a patient may need to be moved from an uneven or cramped location to a flat or more open area so that a rescuer can administer CPR. In most instances, an urgent move is performed before the patient is assessed. However, because the dynamics of a scene can change quickly, an urgent move may be performed at any time, especially when the patient must be moved quickly and there is insufficient time or resources to perform the move in a more controlled or leisurely fashion. Among the many factors that determine the difficulty of an urgent move are the terrain, the patient's size and weight, and the number of rescuers available to assist. The greatest risks posed by an urgent move are delaying life-saving interventions (e.g., opening the airway or controlling external bleeding), aggravating an existing injury, and injuring a rescuer. Therefore, most urgent moves are usually less than 100 feet (30.5 m).

**drag**   a method of moving a patient on the ground to another location.

Because the patient may be unresponsive or incapacitated, urgent moves generally involve some type of **drag**, a method of pulling a patient on the ground to another location. Most drags protect the head, but they may allow the spine to flex or move, which can aggravate any spinal injury that is present.

To minimize this potential, observe two basic principles: keep the patient's spine in the best anatomical alignment possible, and minimize movement. A simple way to remember this is to keep the patient's "nose, navel, and toes" in a straight line, which keeps the long axis of the spine in proper alignment. If the patient is unresponsive, it will be necessary to move him using a long-axis drag.

There are four types of long-axis drags:

1. Shoulder drag (Figure 5-15■)
   - Bend down on one knee and grab the patient's clothing at the shoulders.
   - Support the patient's head with both of your forearms.
   - Raise your head while moving from kneeling to standing.
   - Drag the patient to the desired location.
2. Underarm-wrist drag (Figure 5-16■)
   - Place the patient in seated position.
   - Bend down on one knee and reach under the patient's arm pits and grasp the wrists.
   - Raise your head while moving from kneeling to standing.
   - Drag the patient to the desired location.
3. Blanket drag (Figure 5-17■)
   - It is often easier to hold on to a blanket than the patient, Hazards or time constraints may not permit the extra move to a device, however a blanket is often readily available.
   - Using any of the three previous techniques, drag the patient onto a blanket.
   - Bend down on one knee and firmly grasp the blanket either with one or both hands.
   - Raise your head while moving from kneeling to standing.
   - Drag the patient to the desired location.
4. Feet drag
   - Of the four drag techniques, this is the least desirable because it exposes the patient's head to considerable movement. The head also may be injured as it contacts the ground.

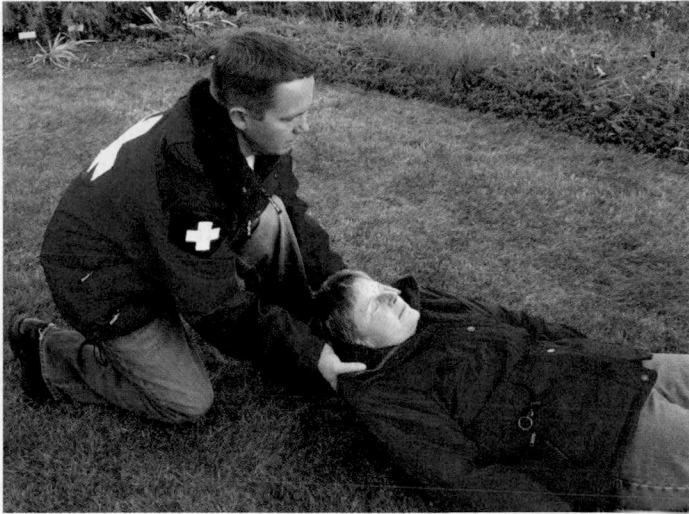

**Figure 5-15** A one-rescuer shoulder drag.
Copyright Edward McNamara

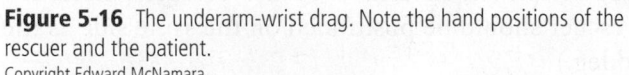

**Figure 5-16** The underarm-wrist drag. Note the hand positions of the rescuer and the patient.
Copyright Edward McNamara

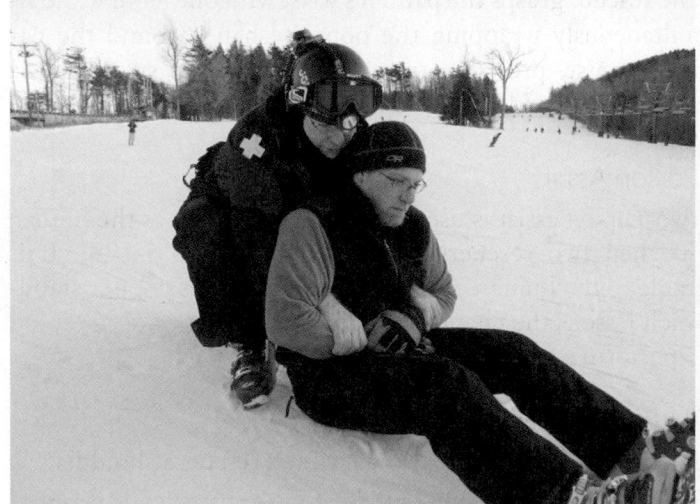

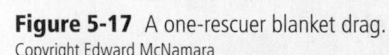

**Figure 5-17** A one-rescuer blanket drag.
Copyright Edward McNamara

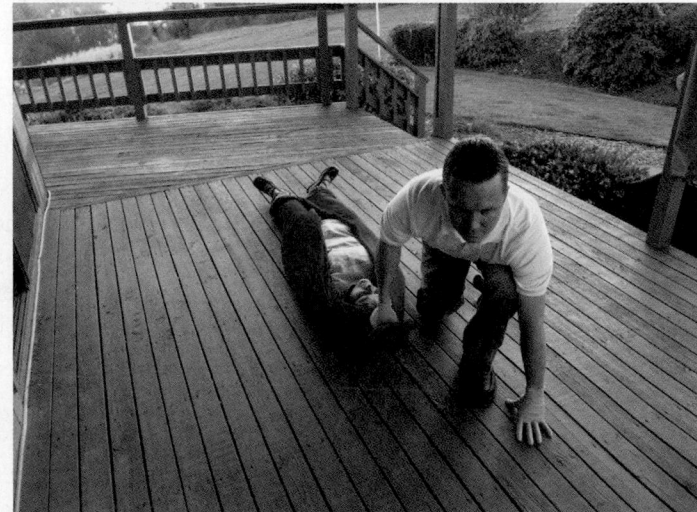

- Bend down on one knee and grasp the patient's feet/ankles.
- Raise your head while moving from kneeling to standing.
- Drag the patient to the desired location.
- An alternative method for this drag is to pull on a rope or sheet that is placed between the legs and tied around the ankles.

## Nonurgent Moves

A nonurgent move is used whenever a patient may be moved in a controlled fashion. Nonurgent moves often require a rescuer to either *assist* the patient (move the patient with the help of other rescuers) or *carry* the patient (move the patient to another location by physically lifting and moving them). Depending on available resources, a nonurgent move may be performed with little or no equipment, or using highly specialized equipment designed specifically for this purpose.

The nonurgent moves most commonly used by OEC Technicians are:

- Human crutch
- Two-person assist
- Chair carry
- Fore and aft carry

### Human Crutch

The human crutch, also known as a one-person assist, is one of the most common methods used to help a patient in a backcountry setting travel down a slope or trail (Figure 5-18■). It also can be used to help a patient move from the patrol room to a vehicle or from a vehicle to a stretcher. When performing this technique, the rescuer acts as a crutch by taking the weight off an injured lower extremity, thereby helping the patient walk with assistance. To perform the human crutch:

1. Place the patient in a standing position.
2. The patient places an arm over the rescuer's shoulder. (The rescuer should be positioned on the same side as the injured leg.)
3. The rescuer grasps the patient's wrist with one hand while simultaneously wrapping the opposite hand around the patient's waist, providing support. (For added support, the rescuer may hold onto the patient's belt or pants.)

### Two-Person Assist

The two-person assist is used in the same manner as the human crutch when two rescuers are available (Figure 5-19■). It is preferable to the human crutch in that it provides greater stability, which lessens the chance of falling.

To perform a two-person assist:

1. Place the patient in a standing position.
2. The patient places one arm over each rescuer's shoulder.
3. Each rescuer grasps one of the patient's wrists while simultaneously wrapping the opposite hand around the patient's

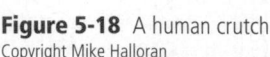

**⊕ 5-5** Explain the difference between an urgent move and a nonurgent move.

**⊕ 5-7** Describe and demonstrate the following drags, lifts, and carries:

  **a.** Shoulder drag
  **b.** Extremity lift
  **c.** Bridge/BEAN lift
  **d.** Human crutch
  **e.** Fore and aft carry
  **f.** Chair carry
  **g.** BEAM lift
  **h.** Draw sheet carry

**Figure 5-18** A human crutch.
Copyright Mike Halloran

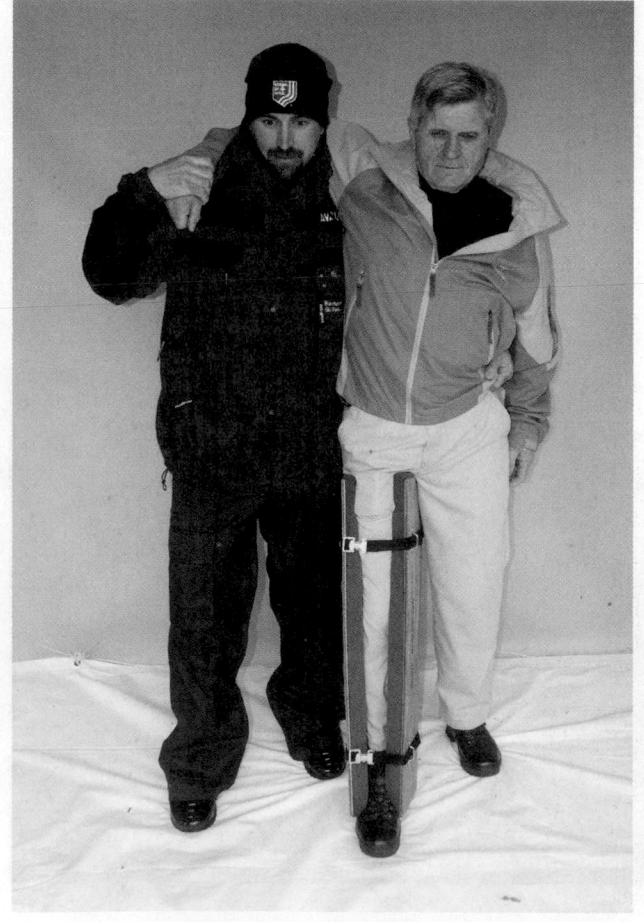

waist, providing support. (For added support, the two rescuers may hold onto the patient's belt or pants on opposite sides.)

## Chair Carry

A chair carry may be used to move a patient who is able to sit up unassisted. This technique requires two rescuers. Depending on the strength of the rescuers and the size of the patient, this technique is effective for carrying a person over short-to-moderate distances. To perform a chair carry:

1. You and another rescuer stand on either side of the patient.
2. Both rescuers squat down next to the patient using good body mechanics and allow the patient to place her arms around the shoulders and necks of the rescuers.
3. Extend your dominant arm out in front of your body.
4. Grasp your extended arm just below the elbow with your other hand.
5. Each rescuer reaches across and grasps the other rescuer's forearm (just below the elbow), creating a seat for the patient Figure 5-20a■).
6. Slowly bring the seat under the patient (Figure 5-20b■), and then lift the patient off the ground (Figure 5-20c■).

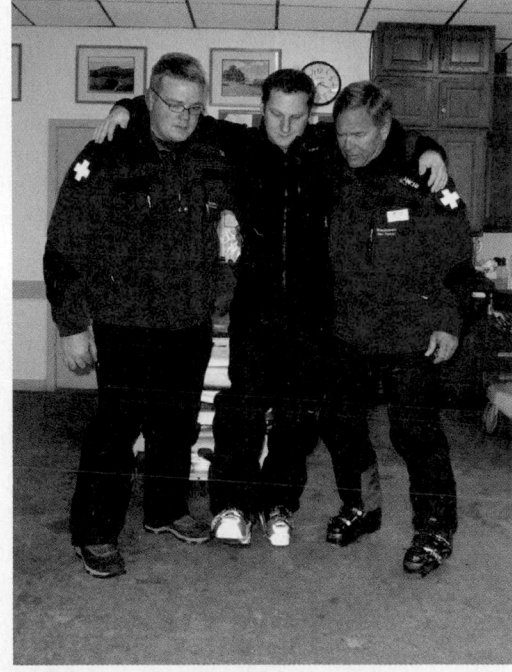

**Figure 5-19** A two-person assist.
Copyright Edward McNamara

**Figure 5-20a** Hand placements for the chair carry showing the cross-arm grip.
Copyright Mike Halloran

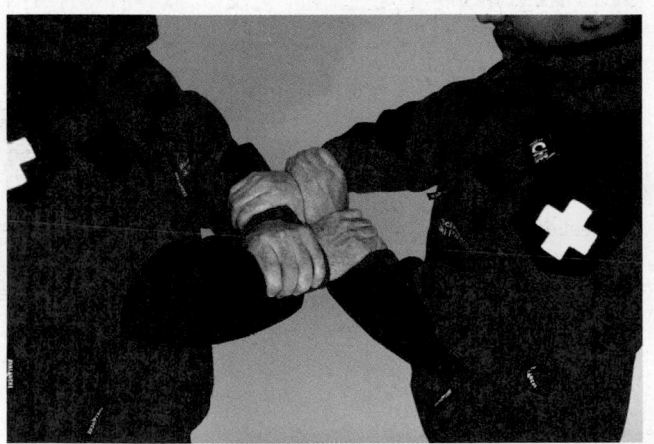

**Figure 5-20b** These rescuers are using good body mechanics to raise this patient.
Copyright Mike Halloran

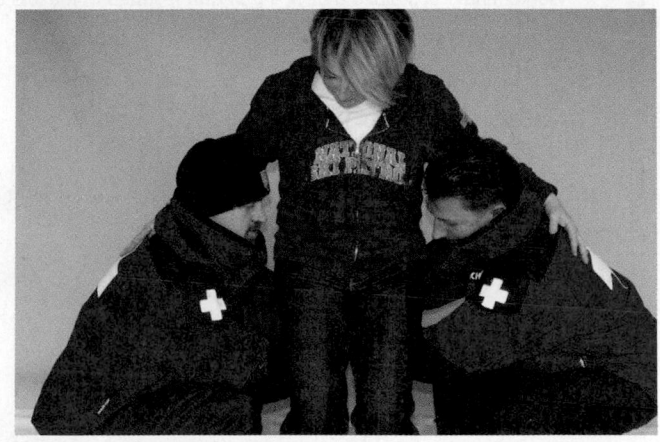

**Figure 5-20c** A completed chair carry lift, which is used for short-to-moderate distances.
Copyright Mike Halloran

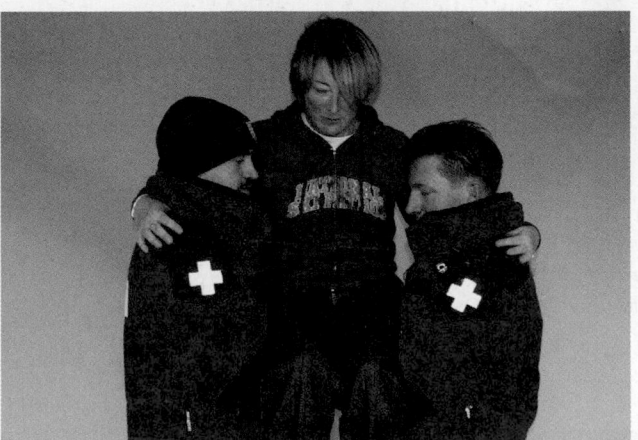

Fore and Aft Carry

This technique, used in conjunction with the extremity lift (described later in the chapter), is performed by two rescuers to carry a patient over short-to-moderate distances. To perform a fore and aft carry:

1. Place the patient into a sitting position, with legs extended along the ground. If the patient is supine, Rescuer #1 (located at the patient's feet) grasps the patient's wrists and leans back to pull the patient into a sitting position.
2. Rescuer #2 (the taller of two rescuers, located at the patient's head) folds the patient's arms across the patient's chest, reaches under the arm pits, and grabs the wrists.
3. Facing away from the patient, Rescuer #1 kneels between the patient's legs and either places his hands behind the patient's knees or grasps the patient's lower legs.
4. On the count of three, both rescuers move to a crouching position, and then lift the patient in unison (Figure 5-21■).
5. Once both rescuers are standing, they may carry the patient.

# STOP, THINK, UNDERSTAND

## Multiple Choice
Choose the correct answer.

1. According to national EMS organizations, what percentage of EMS workers have sustained a back injury that resulted in the loss of work time?_____
   a. 10%
   b. 20%
   c. 25%
   d. 50%

2. Which of the following would *not* be considered a situation for an urgent move?_____
   a. risk of an avalanche
   b. risk of a rock fall
   c. risk of fire
   d. risk of slipping on ice

3. Which of the following is *not* taken into consideration when making a transportation decision?_____
   a. nature of last oral intake
   b. weather
   c. safety
   d. available manpower

4. While performing a long-axis drag, the three parts of the body that should line up are the_____
   a. nose, sternum, and pubis.
   b. nose, navel, and toes.
   c. nose, navel, and pubis.
   d. nose, pubis, and toes.

5. Which long-axis drag would you not use if you suspect a spinal injury?_____
   a. feet drag
   b. underarm-wrist drag
   c. blanket drag
   d. shoulder drag

6. How many times will an OEC Technician most likely move a patient?_____
   a. 1
   b. 2
   c. 3
   d. 4

## Short Answer

1. What three questions should you ask yourself before moving or lifting a heavy object?

2. What two questions must OEC Technicians ask themselves before moving a patient?

3. Describe axial loading.

4. Define urgent move.

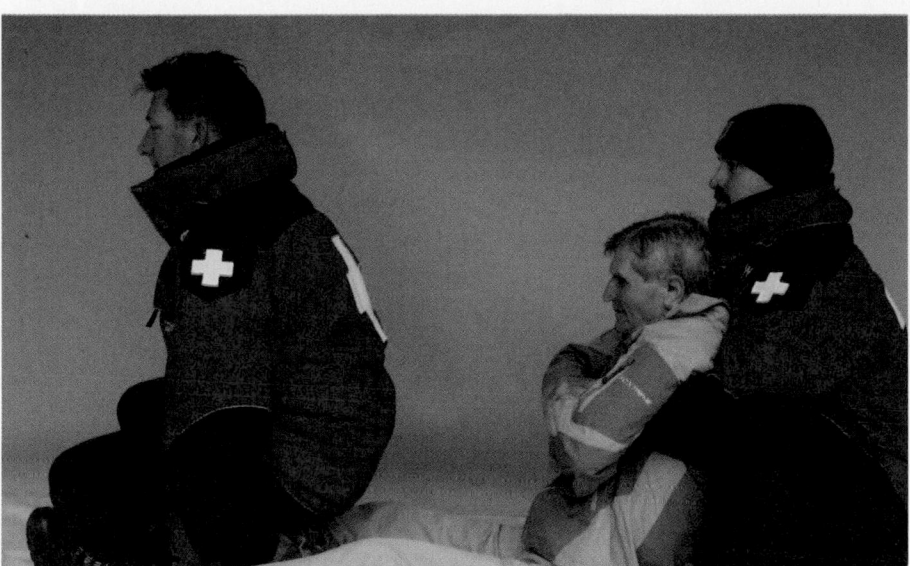

**Figure 5-21** A fore and aft carry.
Copyright Mike Halloran

 **CASE UPDATE**

You confirm that no one is in the building. You then notify dispatch to call the fire department and to request more help and equipment, including oxygen. You run to the patient near the entrance of the building. The intensity of the fire is growing, and it is obvious that the unresponsive man needs to be moved away from the fire. Grabbing him by both feet, you perform a long-axis drag, pulling him away from the building. After pulling him about 10 feet, a partner comes to assist you. Together, you perform an underarm-wrist drag to support the patient's head while moving approximately 50 feet from the building and from any other potential hazards. Fire and ambulance personnel arrive.

**What should you do now?**

## Special Moving Situations

OEC Technicians often will encounter situations in which a patient who must be moved has a spine, pelvis, hip, or extremity injury. Unless faced with an urgent move, these injuries are typically managed before moving the patient. These situations and specific management techniques are addressed in other chapters.

## Lifting the Patient

When providing outdoor emergency care, lifting a patient is a frequent occurrence. Some of the reasons to lift a patient include ensuring the safety of patient and/or rescuer, facilitating patient movement, transferring the patient to a lifting device, and preparing the patient for transport. Most lifts are nonurgent in nature, but in certain circumstances they may need to be performed urgently. As with moving a patient, the potential for injury when lifting a patient is great if it is not performed correctly. To reduce the chance of injury, OEC Technicians should use two techniques that make lifting safer and easier: the power grip and the power lift.

⊕ 5-8 List and demonstrate the proper use of equipment to move, lift, and carry a patient.

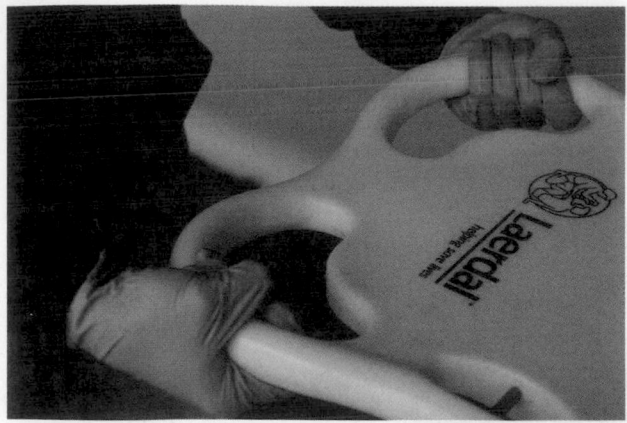

**Figure 5-22** The power grip is the tightest grip and maximizes the strength of the entire arm.
Copyright Mike Halloran

---

**5-2** Describe and demonstrate a power grip.

---

**5-3** Describe and demonstrate a power lift.

## Power Grip

The power grip maximizes the force of the hands and enables you to firmly grip and hold on to an object. This technique is used in conjunction with the power lift (described shortly) when lifting or moving a patient. The power grip provides the tightest grip possible by ensuring that the palms and fingers are in constant contact with the object. It also allows you to hang the weight from the bones of your upper extremity. To perform a power grip (Figure 5-22■):

1. Place your hands, palms up, approximately 10 inches apart.
2. Reach underneath and firmly grasp the object.
3. If possible, loop your thumb over your index and middle fingers.

## Power Lift

Weight lifters have long known the importance of proper form and have developed a technique that enables them to lift heavy objects without becoming injured. This technique, known as the "power lift," combines optimal anatomical position with good body mechanics and the power of leg muscles, which serve as the primary lifting muscles. The power lift is the best method of lifting because it properly aligns the spine and evenly distributes the weight to be lifted. To perform a power lift (Figure 5-23a–c■):

1. Maintain a wide stance by placing your feet shoulder-width apart (approximately 15 inches).
2. Bend your knees and squat down, keeping your back as straight as possible and your shoulders over the spine.
3. Firmly grasp the item to be lifted with your palms up.

**Figure 5-23a** A power lift: bend your knees and squat down while keeping your back as straight as possible.
Copyright Mike Halloran

**Figure 5-23b** A power lift: keep your back muscles and abdominal muscles tight and your head in a neutral position.
Copyright Mike Halloran

**Figure 5-23c** A power lift: straighten your legs by engaging the large leg and buttock muscles to lift the object.
Copyright Mike Halloran

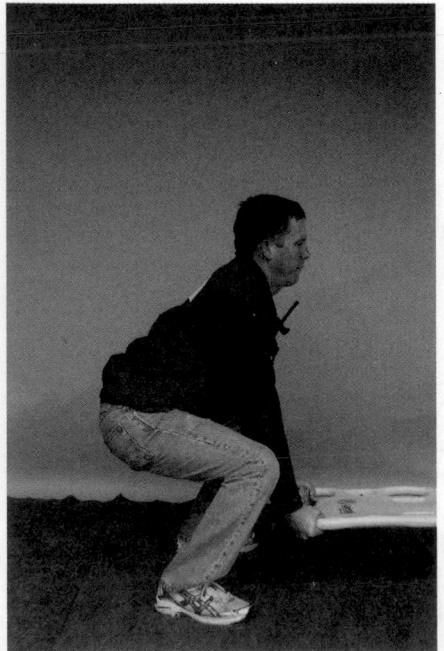

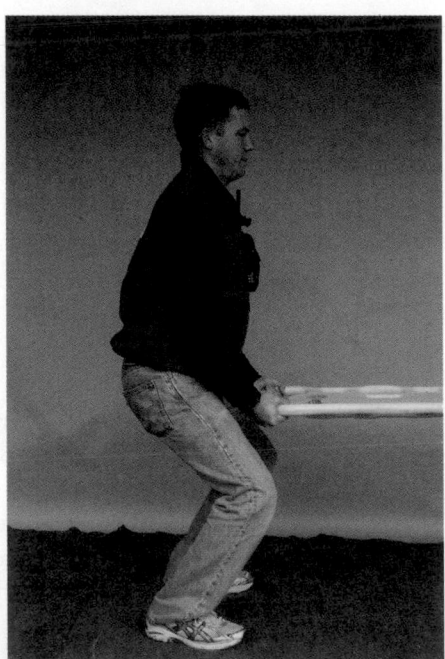

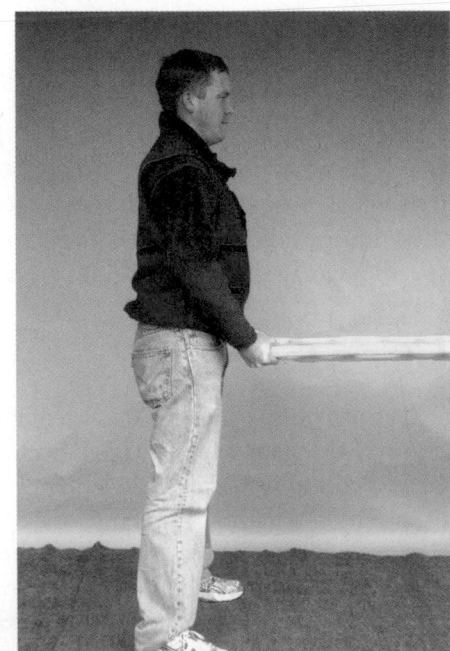

**4.** Keeping your back muscles tight, keep your head up.

**5.** Straighten your legs to lift the object.

## Other Types of Lifts

A **lift** is defined as a means to raise a person from a lower position to a higher position. In outdoor emergency care, this can mean lifting a patient from the ground to a stretcher, lifting the patient out of a vehicle, or simply lifting the patient from one surface to another. OEC Technicians commonly use five types of lifts:

+ Extremity lift
+ Direct-ground lift
+ BEAN lift
+ BEAM lift
+ Draw-sheet lift (transfer flat)

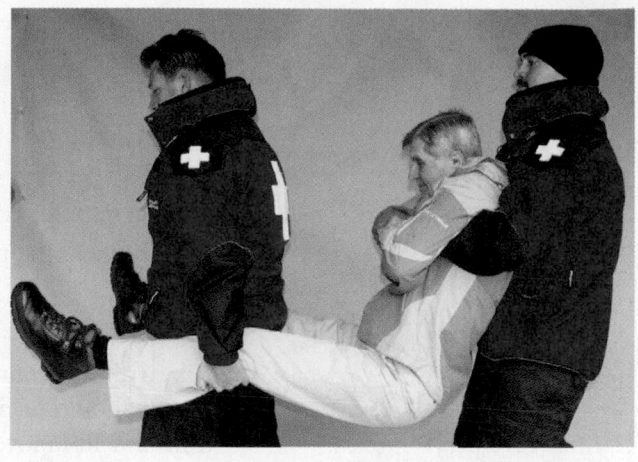

**Figure 5-24** An extremity lift.
Copyright Mike Halloran

**lift** the act of raising a person from a lower position to a higher position.

### The Extremity Lift

One of the most commonly used lifts in rescue operations is the extremity lift (Figure 5-24■). When properly performed by two rescuers, both rescuers keep their backs straight throughout the lift. This method is most often used to lift a patient onto a transportation device or onto an examination table in the patrol room. It is indicated for any patient who does not have a suspected spine injury or who must be quickly moved from one location to another. The patient may be responsive or unresponsive, lying on the ground, or sitting. A word of caution: this lifting method places pressure on the patient's chest and thus may not be tolerated by all patients, especially elderly patients and patients with breathing disorders. It is not recommended for patients who are very heavy or obese.

To perform an extremity lift:

**1.** Place the patient into a sitting position. If the patient is supine, Rescuer #1 grasps the patient's wrists and leans back to pull the patient into a sitting position.

**2.** Rescuer #2 folds the patient's arms across the patient's chest, reaches under the arm pits, and grabs the wrists.

**3.** Rescuer #1 holds and supports the patient's legs at the knees.

**4.** On the count of three, both rescuers move to a crouching position, and then lift the patient at the same time.

**5.** Once both rescuers are standing, they may carry the patient.

### Direct Ground Lift

A direct ground lift is used to raise a patient who is lying on his back and place him onto a flat surface such as a backboard, stretcher, bed, or table (OEC Skill 5-1■). This lift is only used for patients that do not have a suspected spinal injury. This technique may be performed with as few as two rescuers, but ideally it is performed using three or four rescuers. The patient is first placed in the supine anatomical position and then is lifted while all rescuers maintain a safe back position.

To perform a direct ground lift (OEC Skill 5-1):

**1.** All the rescuers kneel along the same side of the patient.
   • If there are two rescuers, they should be at the patient's chest and knees.
   • If there are three rescuers, they should be at the patient's head, waist, and knees.

- If there are four rescuers, they should be at the patient's head, chest, waist, and knees.

2. The rescuers place their arms under the patient.

3. The rescuer closest to the patient's head directs the lift.

4. On the count of three, the rescuers roll the patient toward their chests.

5. On another count of three, the rescuers all stand in unison.

6. To lower the patient, the steps are reversed.

## BEAN Lift

Like a direct ground lift, a BEAN lift is used to raise a patient who is lying on his back. There should be no suspicion of spinal injury. BEAN is an acronym for "body elevation and nonmovement." Previously, this lift was referred to as a bridge lift. The BEAN technique uses four to six rescuers and involves keeping the patient in proper anatomical alignment and raising the patient from the ground while a long spine board is slid under her (OEC Skill 5-2■).

To perform a BEAN lift:

1. Two or three rescuers kneel on either side of the patient, staggering their positions. An additional rescuer or bystander will be required to move the backboard into position at the appropriate time.
   - If there are four rescuers, they should be at the patient's head, chest, waist, and knees. An additional rescuer or bystander will be required to move the backboard into position at the appropriate time.
   - If there are five rescuers, they should be at the patient's head, chest, waist, thighs, and knees. An additional rescuer or bystander will be required to move the backboard into position at the appropriate time.
   - It is recommended that rescuers rehearse the lift by placing their hands on top of the patient to determine where their hands will be placed under the patient. The hands are alternately sequenced to ensure sufficient coverage.

2. Rescuers then place their arms under the patient, following the same pattern as rehearsed. Ideally, the rescuers' arms should be nearly touching.

3. One rescuer prepares the long spine board or other device.

4. The rescuer closest to the patient's head directs the lift.

5. On the count of three, the rescuers move to a crouching position while simultaneously raising the patient off the ground.

6. On another count of three, rescuers raise the patient about 5–6 inches.

7. The long spine board is positioned under the patient, sliding it up from the patient's feet.

8. To lower the patient, the steps are reversed.

## BEAM Lift

The BEAM lift is performed in the same manner as the BEAN lift, except that the patient without suspected spinal injury is lifted and carried a short distance. BEAM is an acronym for "body elevation and movement." From the patient's perspective, the BEAN lift and the BEAM lift are the most comfortable ways to be lifted and moved to a long spine board. While these techniques involve more people than other techniques, such as a log roll (described in a later chapter), both techniques can be safely performed by one OEC Technician and several assistants. If needed, bystanders can be trained quickly to perform this lifting technique.

## Draw-Sheet Lift

This technique is used to lift a patient without a suspected spinal injury a few inches or to transfer a person over a very short distance. It may be used when transferring a patient from a ski toboggan on a cart to an examination table, or to an ambulance stretcher from an examination table. A draw-sheet lift, or flat transfer, is accomplished with a sheet of plastic or fabric that is placed under a patient and then used to raise the patient or slide him from one surface to another. A draw sheet may be improvised using a standard bed sheet or blanket, or it may be commercially produced. Commercial products are favored because they generally have handles, which facilitate the lift.

Of the four lifting techniques described, this method has the lowest risk of back injury to rescuers because it does not involve raising the patient very high. Instead, it involves pushing and pulling the patient. However, great caution must be used when lifting/transferring a large or heavy patient because the fabric can rip.

To perform a draw-sheet lift or flat transfer:

1. Gently place a sheet or blanket beneath the patient (Figure 5-25a■), using a log roll if necessary.
2. One to three rescuers should position themselves on either side of the patient.
3. Roll the edges of the sheet up to the patient's sides (Figure 5-25b■).
4. On the count of three, gently lift while sliding the patient to the destination bed, table, or other flat surface (Figure 5-25c■).

**Figure 5-25a** A draw-sheet lift: place a sheet or blanket beneath the patient.
Copyright Edward McNamara

**Figure 5-25b** A draw-sheet lift: roll the sheet or blanket up close to the patient for a better grip on a firmer lifting device.
Copyright Edward McNamara

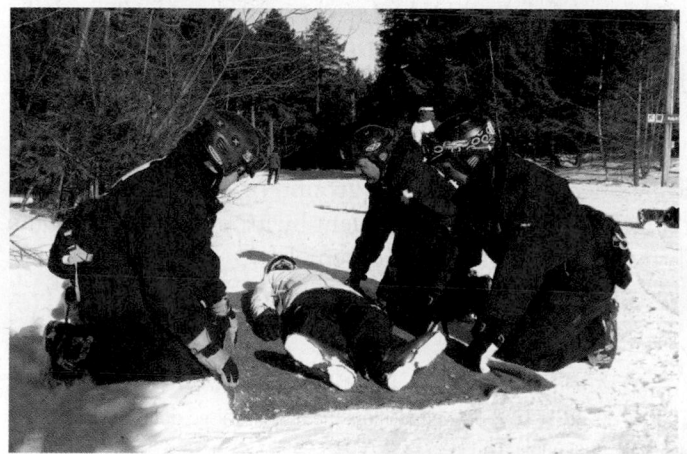

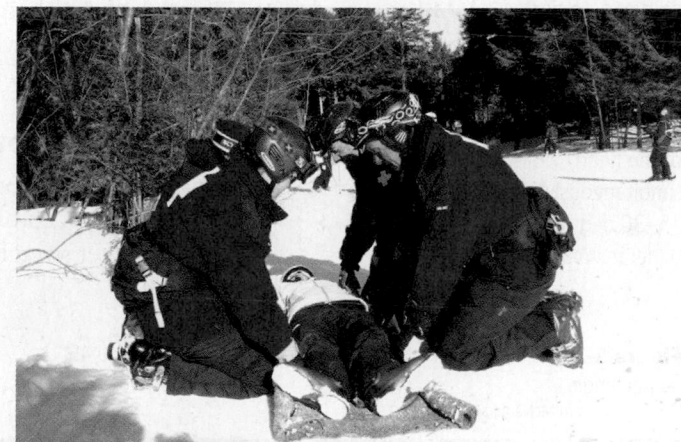

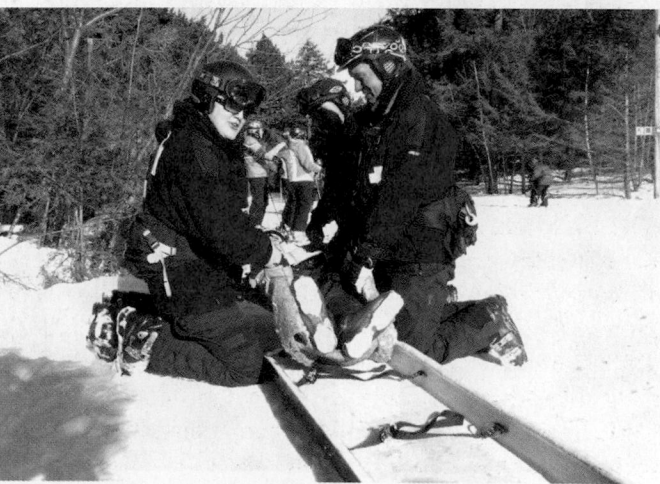

**Figure 5-25c** A draw-sheet lift: on this transfer, the patient is lifted up and a sled is pushed into position under the patient.
Copyright Edward McNamara

A commercial flat transfer also may be used to perform this lift and is advisable when lifting large, heavy, or obese patients.

# Transporting Patients

Patients who require further care beyond what is provided at the scene must be transported to a setting where care can be rendered. This may be to a patrol hut, medical tent, or definitive care facility. When transporting patients, it is important that they are properly positioned to make them more comfortable and to lessen the chance of aggravating their injuries or illness. OEC Technicians most commonly transport patients using the following positions:

+ **Semi-Fowler position.** This is a sitting position in which the patient's upper body is raised to 45 degrees (Figure 5-26a■). This position is commonly used for patients who are awake and are not suspected to have a serious injury or illness.
+ **High-Fowler position.** This is a sitting position in which the patient's head is raised until the body is at a 90 degree angle (Figure 5-26b■). It is typically used for patients who are experiencing severe breathing problems.
+ Supine position. The patient is lying flat on her back, face up (Figure 5-26c■). This position is used for patients who have a suspected spinal injury.
+ **Rothberg position.** The patient's upper body is raised at a 45-degree angle, the abdomen is flat, and the legs are elevated by flexing the hips 15 degrees or bending the knees (Figure 5-26d■). This position is most often used for patients who are experiencing chest pain due to a suspected heart attack.
+ **Trendelenburg position.** The patient's head is lowered 15–30 degrees (below the level of the heart) while the feet are simultaneously raised approximately 15–30 degrees (Figure 5-26e■). This position is generally used for patients who are in shock.

## Ground Transport

Patients can be transported by one of two means: by ground or by air. In the backcountry, the most common methods to transport a patient by ground are a toboggan or sled, a basket stretcher/litter, and various transport vehicles.

---

⊕ 5-9    Compare and contrast common transportation devices.

**semi-Fowler position**    a sitting position in which the patient's upper body is raised to 45 degrees; is commonly used for patients who are awake and are not suspected of having a serious injury or illness.

**high-Fowler position**    a sitting position with the patient's body bent at the waist to 90 degrees; is typically used for patients who are experiencing severe breathing problems.

**Rothberg position**    a sitting position in which the patient's upper body is raised 45 degrees and the knees are slightly bent; is used often for patients who are experiencing chest pain or a suspected heart attack.

**Trendelenburg position**    a position in which the patient's head is lowered 15–30 degrees (below the level of the heart) while the feet are simultaneously raised approximately 15–30 degrees; is generally used for patients who are in shock.

---

**Figure 5-26a** Semi-Fowler position: the upper body is raised to a 45-degree angle.
Copyright Edward McNamara

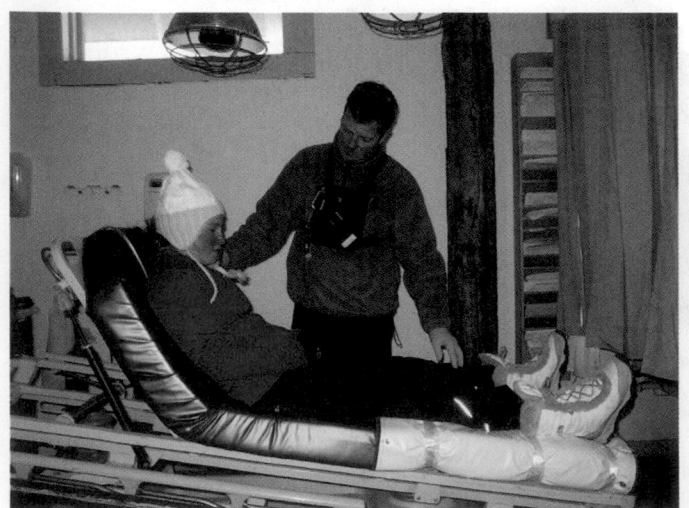

**Figure 5-26b** High-Fowler position: the head is raised until the body is at a 90-degree angle.
Copyright Edward McNamara

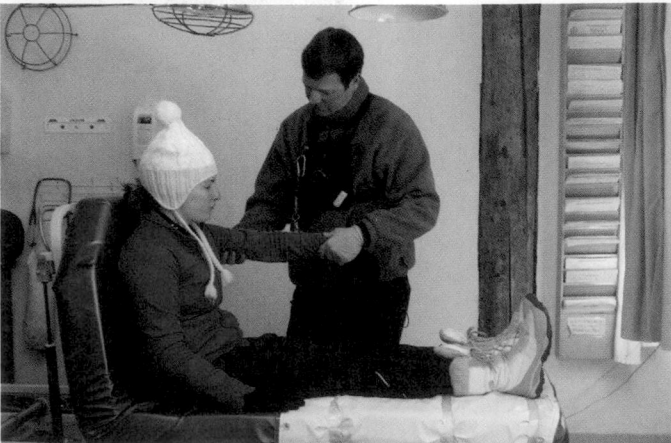

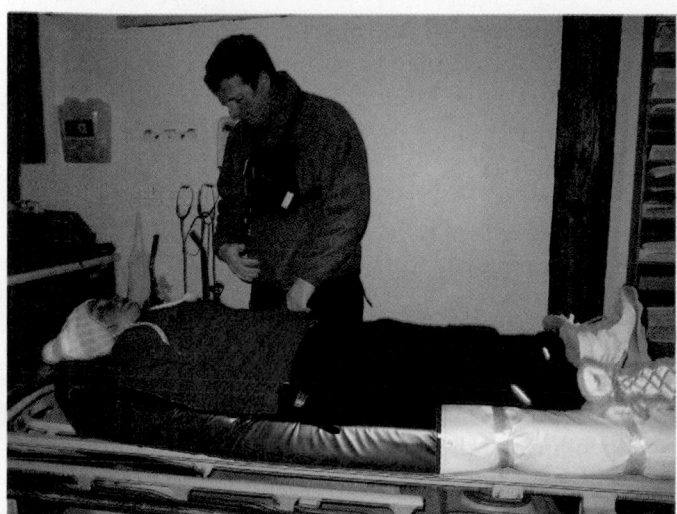

**Figure 5-26c** Supine position: lying flat on the back, face up. Remember "supine is on the spine."
Copyright Edward McNamara

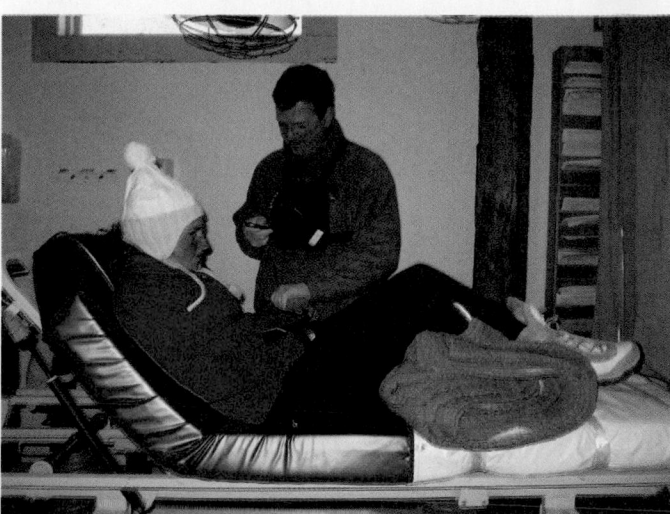

**Figure 5-26d** Rothberg position: the upper body is at a 45-degree angle, the abdomen is flat, and the legs are elevated.
Copyright Edward McNamara

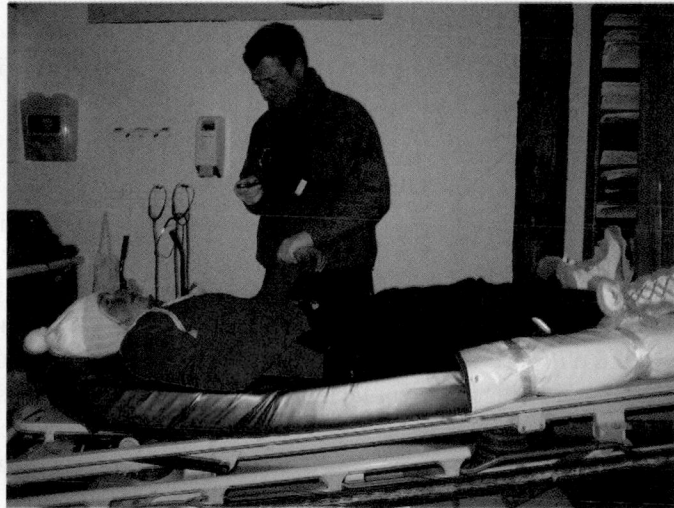

**Figure 5-26e** Trendelenburg position: this is the shock treatment position.
Copyright Edward McNamara

## Toboggan or Sled

The toboggan or sled is the primary method for transporting patients by ski patrollers (Figure 5-27■). At the dawn of patrolling, the toboggan was a simple wooden sled that was outfitted with handles and skied off the mountain. Today's sleds are made of reinforced fiberglass, aluminum, and steel and are highly specialized to perform the function of sliding down the mountain carrying a patient. When the handles are locked into place, the sled is easy to use, even in difficult snow conditions.

Most ski patrol rescue toboggans are equipped with a basic "sled pack," which contains blankets, splinting materials, and other items necessary for routine operations. In addition, many patrols have a toboggan with a specialized sled pack to handle major emergencies on the mountain. Additional equipment such as oxygen or an AED should be requested, if needed.

The toboggan must be prepared before the patient is loaded into it. The patient is lifted into the toboggan or sled using a lifting or moving technique that best suits the injury or illness involved. If the patient does not have a suspected head or spine injury, a thicker pad may be placed under the patient to improve overall comfort. If

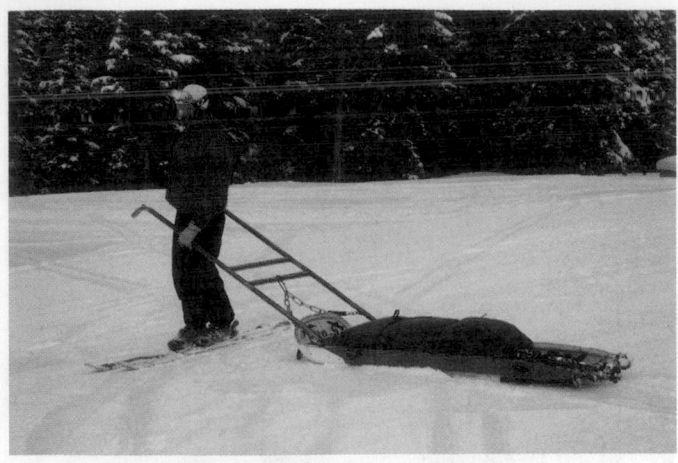

**Figure 5-27** One of the types of toboggan used to transport patients.
Copyright Scott Smith

the patient is on an LSB, the board is loaded into the toboggan or sled. The LSB may have thin padding attached to it, but the padding should not allow the patient to slide on the board. When on a slope, it is best to lift the patient uphill into the toboggan.

## Packaging a Patient

To reduce the chances that further injury or a worsening of symptoms occurs during transport, the patient must be properly "packaged." Packaging is a process by which the patient is adequately prepared for transport, and it occurs after you have completed all on-scene care. Packaging needs vary depending on the patient's injuries or illness and environmental conditions. For instance, when packaging a patient during a winter rescue, it is important that the patient remain warm during transport. Likewise, if the patient has a broken leg, it is important that the leg is properly secured to prevent unnecessary movement during transport. If any special equipment is used, it must be packaged with the patient.

In general, proper patient packaging consists of four steps:

1. The patient is properly positioned on the transportation device (Figure 5-28a■), typically with the injury uphill.
2. The patient is made as comfortable as possible (Figure 5-28b■).
3. The patient is securely fastened within the transportation device (Figure 5-28c■).
4. All necessary medical equipment is transported with the patient (Figure 5-28d■).

The first step in packaging the patient is deciding whether the patient's head should be positioned uphill or downhill. This decision is based on the patient's injuries or illness and the care that has been rendered. The most comfortable way to transport the patient is to place the injury uphill. The reason for this is that on steep terrain, gravity will cause increased weight on the injured part, which could cause problems. For instance, consider a patient whose broken upper leg has been placed in a traction splint. If the patient is placed in a head-uphill position, is it harder to maintain traction on the injured leg's boot or foot because gravity is working against

**Figure 5-28a** When packaging a patient, most of the time, place the injury uphill in the toboggan.
Copyright Scott Smith

**Figure 5-28b** Make the patient as warm and comfortable as possible.
Copyright Scott Smith

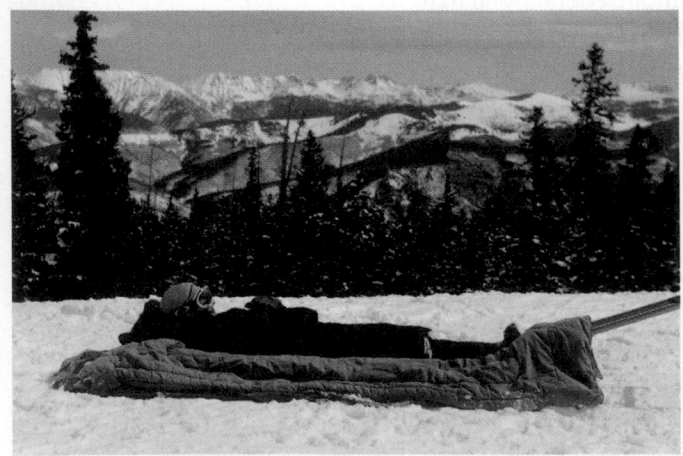

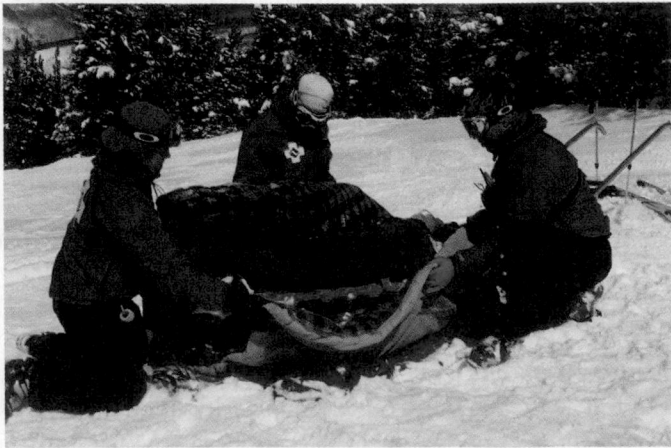

maintaining traction. Additionally, the patient will tend to slide downhill, toward the front of the toboggan or transportation device, making traction less effective. For this reason, patients with lower extremity injuries are placed in a (head-downhill) position.

The three major exceptions to the "injury uphill" principle are:

✦ Patients who are having breathing difficulty. Most patients who experience breathing problems want to sit up. Unfortunately, this creates a high center of gravity for the load (the patient) and increases the risk of the transportation device tipping over. These patients should be placed in a head-uphill position that allows them to breathe more easily because there is less pressure from the abdominal contents pushing upward. Propping the chest up with a pack or blanket behind the patient's back may be needed. Putting a second person in the sled to hold the patient up is difficult.

✦ Patients who are in shock. These patients should be placed in a head-downhill position so that more blood is available to perfuse vital organs. Unfortunately, this position pushes the abdominal contents upward, which can make breathing more difficult. If both shock and respiratory distress are present, the patient should be placed in a head-uphill position because breathing takes precedence over circulation in the ABCDs.

✦ Patients with a serious head injury. It is recommended that patients who are unresponsive or who have significant head injury should be transported in a head-uphill position. If the patient has head trauma and is in shock, the head-uphill position is still used.

Patients with multiple injuries present unique challenges. In these cases, you must prioritize and place the more-significant injury uphill. For example, if a patient has a possible broken arm and a broken leg, the leg injury is placed uphill.

In nearly all instances, it is best to place patients on their backs. Rarely, as with a patient with an anterior dislocated hip whose leg is positioned posteriorly, the patient may be placed in the toboggan on his stomach. This should be avoided whenever possible, however, because lying prone is a difficult position for the patient to maintain, can create breathing problems, and is typically uncomfortable, especially over long transports. Another option is to place the patient on his good side in the toboggan.

**Figure 5-28d** Securely fasten all medical equipment that needs to be transported with the patient, such as an AED and/or oxygen.
Copyright Edward McNamara

**Figure 5-28c** Securely fasten the patient for transportation, because uneven terrain may give the patient a rough ride.
Copyright Scott Smith

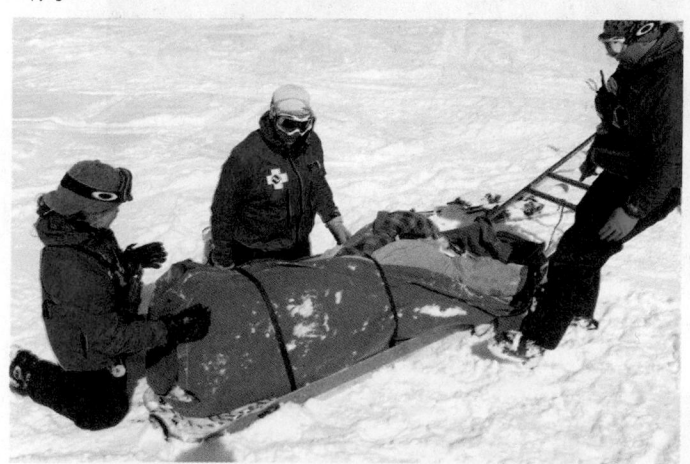

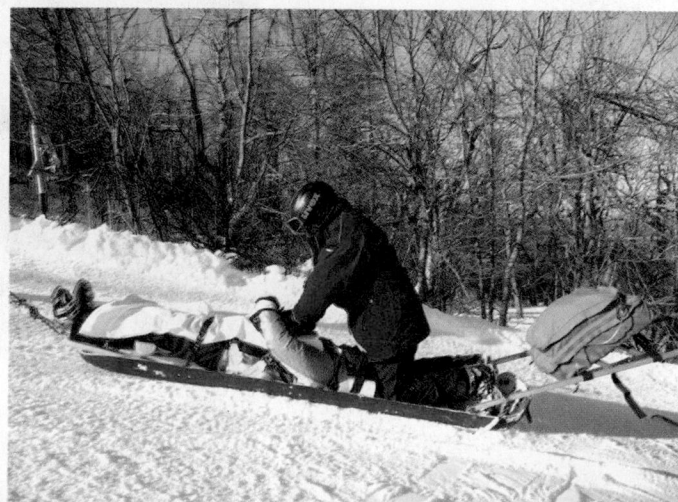

There may be instances for which patients may need to be placed on their sides. For instance, a pregnant woman should be placed on her left side. When positioned in this way, the vena cava is not compressed by the gravid uterus, and blood can return to the heart. Being on the side is especially useful if the patient cannot stop vomiting.

Being transported during an emergency can be a nerve-wracking, uncomfortable experience for patients. Therefore, the next step in packaging the patient is to make the patient as comfortable as possible. In cold conditions, it is important to insulate the patient from the elements. Cover the patient first with blankets and then (if used in your area) with a large "wrapper" (e.g., a large plastic sheet) that is impervious to snow and rain. Cover the patient completely, except for the face. Conversely, in warm or hot climates it may be necessary to provide some shade for the patient. Use padding to lessen the effects of the inevitable bumps that occur during transport. If neck, back, or spine injuries are not suspected, a pillow may be placed under the patient's head or knees to provide additional comfort for the ride down the mountain.

Use the attached straps to secure the patient to the toboggan or transport device to keep the patient from falling out. Extremities that are splinted must remain securely in place and must not be allowed to move around. Be careful not to make the straps too tight because this can hinder the patient's breathing. Whenever possible, avoid placing straps directly over known injuries.

When packaging the patient, it is important that essential medical equipment remain with the patient. For instance, if the patient is receiving oxygen, the oxygen tank should accompany the patient. Oxygen tanks, suction equipment, and AEDs are commonly placed in the toboggan or transport device with the patient. These are best placed between the patient's legs or to the outside of an uninjured leg. Equipment must be secured within the toboggan with appropriate straps, without putting pressure on an injured body part. Some oxygen delivery systems can be attached to the handle bars of the toboggan. Avoid placing any equipment near the patient's head. It is best not to place unused rescue or personal equipment in the toboggan with the patient. Instead, have other patroller(s) perform "clean up" and carry these items to the aid room. Refer again to Table 5-1 for supplies to carry in a rescue bag to accompany a toboggan.

Ski patrollers learn how to drive a ski toboggan in the transport portion of their training. The patroller at the front handles "drives" the sled and determines the route down the hill while the patroller on the tail rope acts as a backup and ensures that the tail of the sled stays in the fall line (Figure 5-29■). A critical part of becoming an

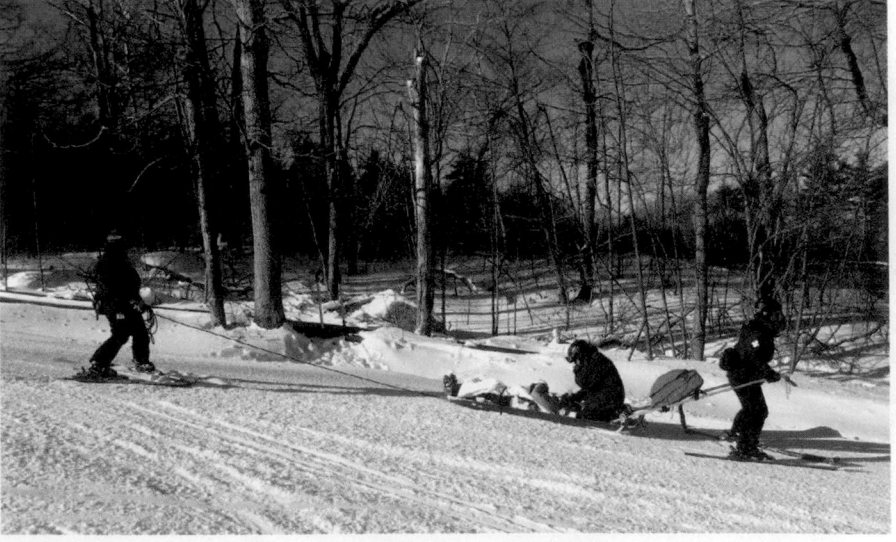

**Figure 5-29** Competent toboggan handling skills—the ability to drive it and to use a tail rope—are critical attributes of alpine ski patrollers.
Copyright Edward McNamara

alpine patroller is qualification on "driving" and "tail roping" a rescue toboggan. Many practice hours are required to develop competence in handling a toboggan on all terrain in all conditions.

Sleds also are used for transport, and some of them use the patient's skis as part of the transport system. One example is the Brooks-Range Sled, which is available as a small, rolled package. The system has spacer bars that hold the patient's skis together and a plastic sheet to hold the patient. Another device is the SKED, which is a large sheet of thick plastic that is wrapped around the patient. Lightweight and easy to store, this device is best used for sliding a patient over snow or ice (Figure 5-30■).

## Basket Stretchers/Litters

Basket stretchers (previously described) and other types of litters are commonly used in transporting a patient out of the backcountry. The basket stretcher, considered to be the "backcountry ambulance," is commonly used to transport patients by hand or by technical rescue systems. The device may be carried by a litter team, typically composed of four to six people. It can be used alone or in combination with other devices such as an LSB, scoop stretcher, or portable stretcher.

Depending on the manufacturer, some basket stretchers may be outfitted with a litter or "trail" wheel to make transportation over uneven or rough terrain easier by reducing the number of litter bearers required.

Ideally, litter bearers should be of similar height; this helps to distribute the load evenly among the bearers. Six rescuers are best, with one rescuer at each corner and one along either of the two long sides of the basket or litter. In this manner, the average carrying speed will be about 1 mile per hour over moderate trail terrain. Off-trail movement can take much longer. Four rescuers can be used, but this requires more effort by each individual.

Transporting a patient by basket stretcher or litter is back-breaking work (Figure 5-31■). To avoid fatigue, a fresh group of litter bearers should be rotated onto the team at regular intervals, usually every few minutes.

## Wheeled Ambulance Stretcher

Due to their interactions with other emergency care system providers, OEC Technicians likely will encounter ambulance stretchers on a regular basis (Figure 5-32■). This device is standard equipment for ambulances and is rugged in its design and durability. The standard ambulance stretcher, or cot, is slightly longer and wider than

**Figure 5-30** A SKED device for transport in use on the mountain.
Copyright Jon Politis

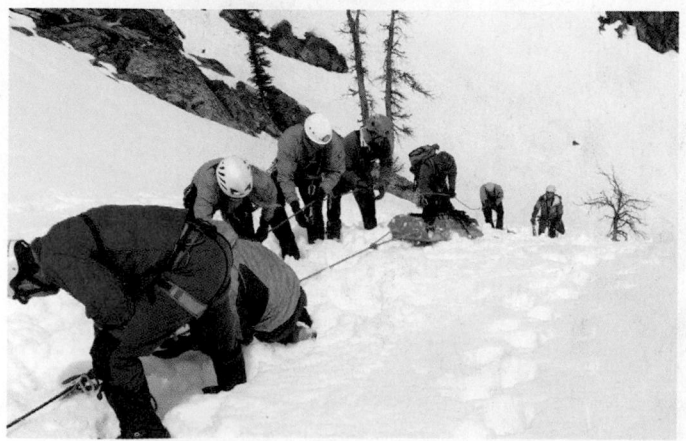

**Figure 5-31** A basket stretcher is excellent for transport over rough terrain but is very hard work.

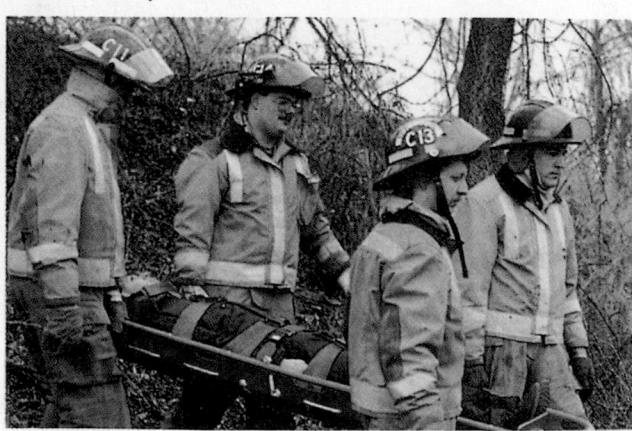

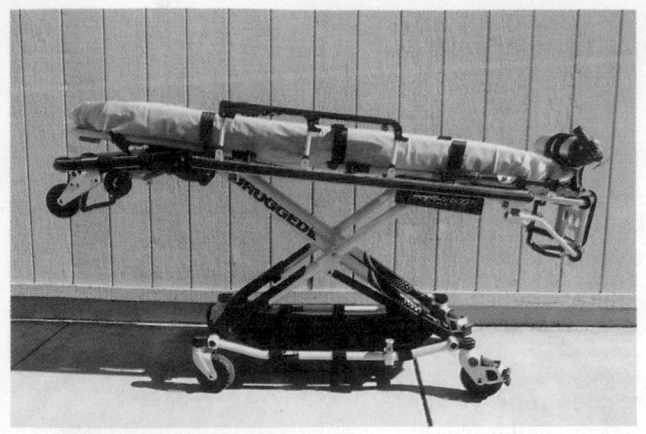

**Figure 5-32** A wheeled ambulance stretcher.

a standard LSB. It can be adjusted to various heights and positions. Due to its weight (average is 75 lbs/34 kg) and low ground clearance, the use of an ambulance stretcher in the backcountry is simply not practical.

A wheeled ambulance stretcher is best used for carrying a patient over smooth surfaces for short or medium distances. Some ski patrols use it to transport patients inside the patrol base first-aid facility.

Wheeled ambulance stretchers are made by numerous manufacturers; most models have the same basic features:

+ Adjustability for placing the patient in various positions, ranging from Trendelenburg position to high-Fowler position

+ Adjustability in raising and lowering the stretcher to several heights, from ground level to waist height

When an ambulance stretcher is used to transport a patient over smooth ground, one person is positioned at the head of the stretcher and a second one is placed at the foot of the stretcher. The wheels are set on casters, making it easy to roll in different directions. Some also have wheel locks that can be set to prevent the stretcher from rolling. Just like the rescue toboggan, handling an ambulance stretcher requires "hands on" training to develop proficiency, and it is not without some inherent hazards. For instance, when the stretcher is loaded and in the full "up" position, it can be unstable, especially when used on rough or uneven terrain, making it prone to tipping over.

When a stretcher is used in rough terrain or on snow-packed ground, it is suggested that one rescuer be placed at each of the four corners of the stretcher (Figure 5-33■). This maximizes stretcher stability and reduces the risk of tipping.

### Evacuation Chair

**stair chair**  a portable evacuation chair that enables a patient to be transported in a seated position.

An evacuation chair or **stair chair** is a portable stretcher that allows a patient to be transported in a seated position (Figure 5-34■). This lightweight device has both wheels and handles that enable it to be maneuvered in tight spaces, including up and down stairs. Newer evacuation chairs include such features as built-in sliding bars,

**Figure 5-33** A demonstration of the technique used for carrying a wheeled stretcher over rough terrain.

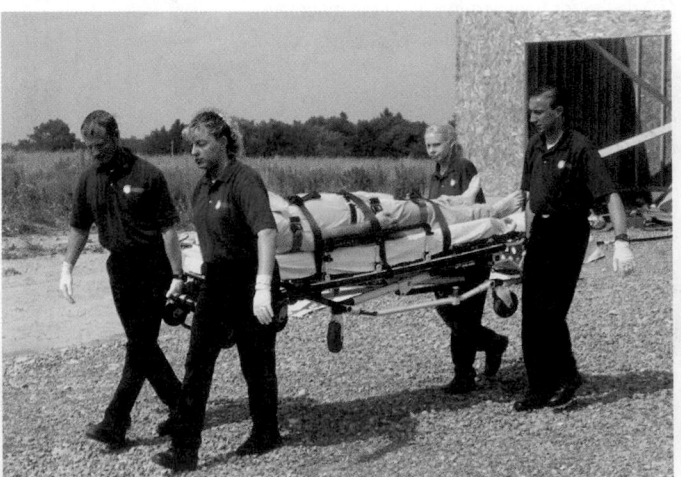

oxygen cylinder holders, and the ability to lay a patient flat, adding yet more versatility to this popular transport device.

## Improvised Litters

Occasionally, the evacuation of a supine patient must be conducted using only the equipment at hand. On most overnight backcountry trips the party has some of the following items that can be used to make an improvised litter:

+ Climbing rope (Figure 5-35■)
+ Closed cell foam pad
+ Trekking poles
+ Skis
+ Pack frames
+ Raft oars or paddles
+ Sleeping bag

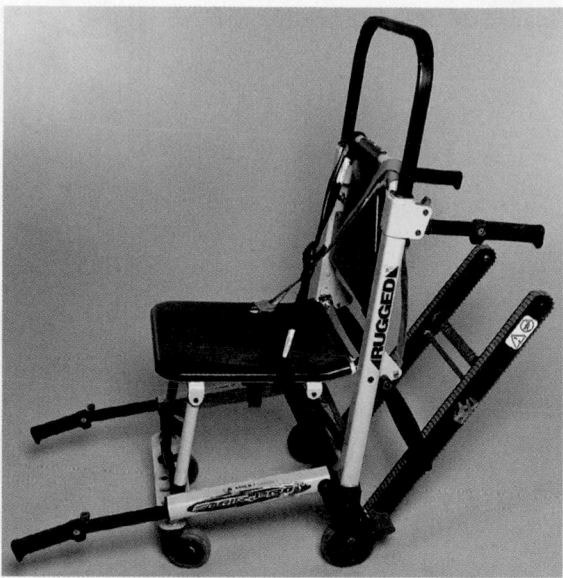

**Figure 5-34** An evacuation chair or stair chair is much easier than a stretcher to maneuver in tight places such as stairs.

All of these items can be used to help construct a crude litter for improvised transportation. The first step is construction of a rigid frame for dragging/carrying. Skis, paddles, or available wood is lashed together to make a rigid frame for carrying (Figure 5-36■). Next the patient is placed in a sleeping bag, and the closed cell foam pad is placed between the patient and frame.

## Motorized Transport Vehicles

OEC Technicians may have access to various engine-powered transport vehicles such as all-terrain vehicles (ATVs), snow machines, and golf carts (Figure 5-37■). Transport vehicles enable patients to be transported over relatively long distances in a short period of time, depending on terrain. Some ATVs and golf carts have special racks or decks to which a backboard or basket litter can be attached. The use of transport vehicles requires additional training that goes beyond the scope of this text. Once a patient arrives at a trailhead, access road, or patrol hut, additional ground transportation options, such as ambulances or private vehicles, may be available.

**Figure 5-35** An improvised litter made from a rope.
Copyright NSP

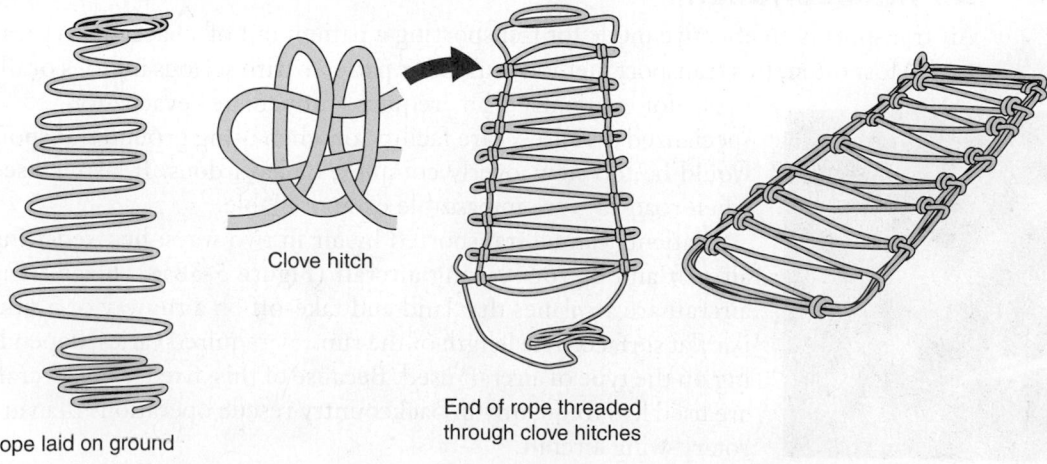

Rope laid on ground

Clove hitch

End of rope threaded
through clove hitches

**Figure 5-36** The use of two poles and two jackets to make an improvised litter. Copyright Edward McNamara

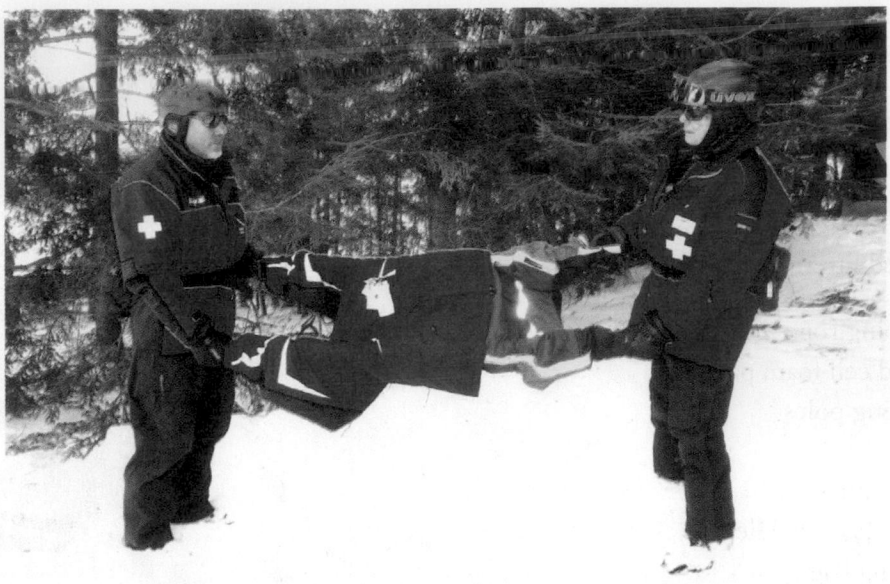

**Figure 5-37** Among the motorized transport vehicles available to OEC Technicians are snow machines and ATVs. Copyright Edward McNamara

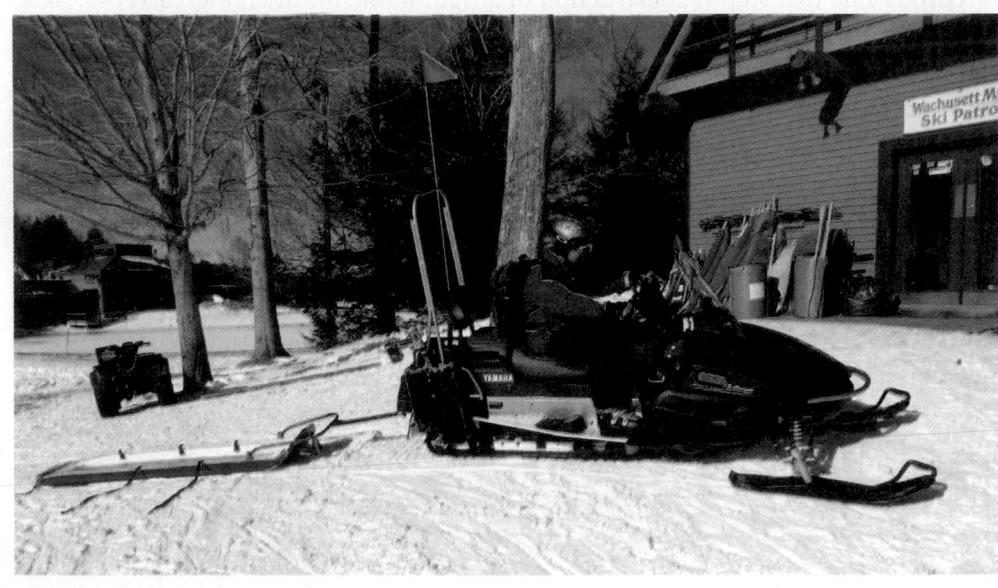

⊕ **5-10** List the components of a safe landing zone (LZ).

**Figure 5-38a** Both helicopters and fixed-wing airplanes are used in EMS. Copyright REACH, Inc.

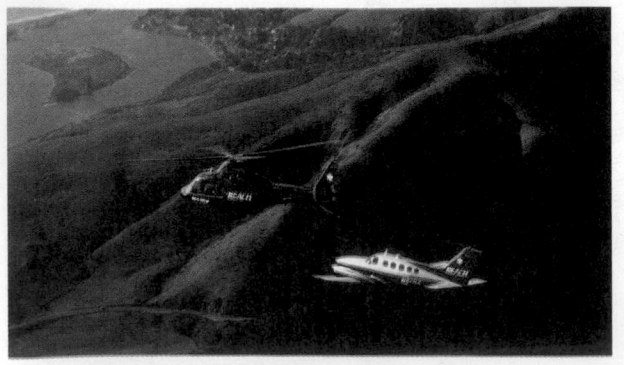

## Air Transportation

Air transport is an effective mode for transporting a patient out of a backcountry setting. Most often, this transport method is used for patients with serious injuries or illness, for patients who require immediate evacuation to a specialized definitive care facility, or when using ground transport would be too slow, overly complex, or hazardous. It also is used when roadways are impassable or unavailable.

Patients can be transported by air in two ways: by fixed-wing aircraft and by rotary-wing aircraft (Figure 5-38a■). Fixed-wing aircraft are airplanes that land and take-off on a runway or a similar flat surface. The length of the runway required varies, depending on the type of aircraft used. Because of this, fixed-wing aircraft are used less frequently in backcountry rescue operations than are rotary-wing aircraft.

Rotary wing aircraft (helicopters) are marvelous modes of transport that have revolutionized mountain rescue operations. Their ability to carry people and equipment, hover, and land in tight spaces make them logical rescue and transport vehicles. While standard aircraft must usually take-off and land at designated landing sites in controlled air space, rescue helicopters can land near where they are needed (Figure 5-38b■). However, helicopters have limitations regarding their use, including factors relating to weather, altitude, ambient temperature, weight, time of day, and area needed to land.

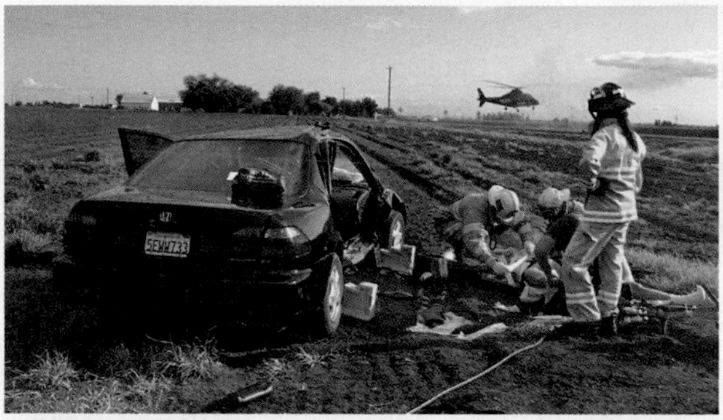

**Figure 5-38b** A helicopter may be able to land right at the emergency scene.
Copyright REACH, Inc.

## Weather Limitations

Aircraft operate under rules established by the U.S. Federal Aviation Administration (FAA). For take-offs and landings, aircraft operate under one of two strict, weather-based guidelines: visual flight rules (VFR) or instrument flight rules (IFR). Visual flight rules require the pilot to be able to see outside the cockpit and to generally see where the aircraft is going in order to avoid hazards such as other aircraft. Most rescue operations, with the exception of the U.S. Coast Guard and military services, operate under VFR. Because visibility is needed both for safety and to accomplish a rescue mission, a helicopter may not be launched if the weather is below established minimum standards. While weather standards vary, a good rule of thumb for visual flight rules is:

Day: 500-foot cloud ceiling and 1 mile of visibility
Night: 1,000-foot cloud ceiling and 3 miles of visibility

> ### Night Flight Operations
>
> Night flight operations are much more dangerous than day operations due to decreased visibility. Visibility is crucial in rescue operations because of the need to maintain visual contact with the ground team to receive flight instructions and information regarding any obstructions near the landing zone.
>
> **NOTE**

## Altitude and Temperature Limitations

Altitude plays an important role in aircraft performance in rescue operations. The ability of a helicopter to sustain a hovering pattern is crucial to its utility as a rescue and transport aircraft. As altitude increases, air density decreases. Thus, at higher altitudes, a helicopter requires more power to continue hovering. In addition to altitude, ambient air temperature plays a role in a helicopter's overall performance. In general, the warmer the temperature, the less dense the air is, and the more power is needed to remain hovering.

## Space and Load

Helicopters are very weight and space sensitive. The size of the aircraft and number of engines are also factors that must be considered. Some helicopters are large enough to carry many people and have the ability to hoist large loads. Others are small and cannot accommodate much more than a pilot, one patient, one crew member, and basic medical supplies. Every aircraft is different, and pilots are responsible for ensuring that their aircraft are not overloaded. If an aircraft is heavily loaded, it may be able to land but then be unable to take off without first off-loading nonessential gear or (in some cases) nonessential personnel.

## Helicopter Safety

Most helicopter evacuations require the aircraft to land on the ground. The patient is then loaded on board and the aircraft lifts off, taking the patient and crew to a medical facility. Though this process seems simple, it requires coordination to ensure that it is performed safely. When ordering a helicopter to respond to the scene of a backcountry emergency, numerous factors must be considered, including **landing zone** selection, ground-to-air communications, and ground operations (Figure 5-39■).

**landing zone (LZ)** an area used to land a helicopter; for fixed wing aircraft, the LZ is a temporary runway.

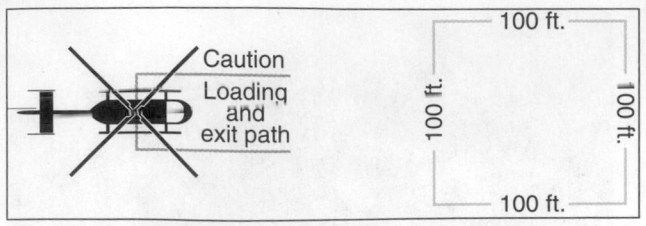

**Figure 5-39** Some characteristics of a helicopter landing zone (LZ).

**Landing Zone Selection** Most aeromedical crashes occur during take-off or landing. For this reason, the landing zone (LZ) should be an area at least 100 feet by 100 feet (Figure 5-39). The LZ also should be flat or have no more than an 8° slope. Ideally, the area should be free of overhead obstructions such as wires and power lines, which are nearly invisible to the pilot (even if visibility is excellent) and thus present serious hazards. If overhead obstructions are present, notify the pilot of their locations over the radio well before the helicopter's arrival.

Likewise, loose objects in the LZ can create a dangerous situation, both for the helicopter crew and for rescuers on the ground. A helicopter's rotors can generate winds in excess of 100 miles per hour. Small stones, loose clothing, and lightweight gear should be removed from the LZ or secured to prevent them from being blown away or into the rotors.

The LZ should be well lit. Headlights from cars can light the ground up to 100 feet outside the zone, so that the pilot can see the ground. Place chemical light sticks or small strobe lights on all four corners of the LZ, securing them in place with tent stakes or by other means. Do not shine spotlights toward the helicopter because they can temporally blind the pilot (and cause a potentially fatal accident).

The LZ must be secured. No pedestrians, animals, or traffic should be within 100 feet of the aircraft. No one other than the landing coordinator is allowed within the LZ area during take-off or landing. Table 5-2■ summarizes the guidelines for establishing landing zones.

**Ground-to-Air Communications** Good communication between the pilot and the ground crew is an essential component of safe rescue operations involving aircraft. As a rule, participation in helicopter landings and take-offs should involve only those personnel, including OEC Technicians, who have been formally trained in the procedures.

Before the helicopter arrives, the landing coordinator should contact the pilot to obtain both an estimated time of arrival (ETA) and the direction of arrival. This information should be conveyed to other rescuers on the ground to ensure that the LZ remains clear of personnel, gear, and any potential obstructions. In return, the landing coordinator should provide the pilot with the LZ coordinates and current weather conditions, including wind direction, if known. As the helicopter makes its final approach to the LZ, the landing coordinator should use universal ground-to-air signals.

**Ground Operations** Once the helicopter is safely on the ground, do not approach the aircraft until signaled to do so by the pilot or crew chief. Often, a crew member will exit the aircraft to escort you to it. If signaled to approach the helicopter unescorted, maintain eye contact with the pilot or crew chief, and only approach from the front of the craft so that you remain in the pilot's field of vision (Figure 5-40■).

⊕ 5-11 Describe and demonstrate how to safely move when near a helicopter.

| Table 5-2 | Landing Zone Guidelines |
|---|---|

- The LZ must be a minimum of 100 feet by 100 feet.
- The site must be free from overhead obstructions and wires.
- The site should be on firm ground (avoid areas with loose debris).
- The site should be well lit.
- Keep emergency lights on, but do not point spotlights toward the aircraft.
- Keep pedestrians and vehicles at least 100 feet from the LZ.

Never approach a helicopter from the rear. The tail rotor spins so fast that it is nearly invisible and is lethal if inadvertently walked into. Stay low and avoid holding anything above your head because the main rotor may be lower than you think. Depending on the grade of the LZ, the overhead rotor blades may be no more than a few feet above the ground. Avoid wearing anything loose or long (like a scarf) that can be blown away or pulled into the blades by the rotor wash. Take off your hat.

## Special Transport Tactics

Special tactics are high-risk operations and include activities such as hoisting, flying with an external load, or rappelling from an aircraft. Under FAA regulations, these activities may be performed only during emergency situations, "life and death" situations, and humanitarian relief efforts. Special training beyond the scope of this text is required to become proficient in these skills.

Some aircraft are equipped with mechanical hoists to lower people to the ground (insert them) and raise people from the ground (extract them). These devices are most commonly found on military and some public safety aircraft. A variety of devices are used to attach the patient to the hoist cable for lifting into the helicopter. Hoisting operations require the helicopter to hover in a fixed position. The time needed to hoist an object depends on the speed of the hoist and the amount of cable to be let out. A special insertion and extraction (SPIE) line is a special cable or rope used to carry rescuers, equipment, or the patient beneath the helicopter for short distances. Also called a "short haul" technique, this method of transport was developed by mountain rescue teams in Europe and by Parks Canada. It is commonly used with light-duty aircraft that lack hoisting capabilities to both insert and extract rescuers and victims.

Generally, a weighted and backed up rope system is attached to a cargo hook or belly band of a helicopter. Specially trained rescuers who are in direct communication with the pilot are clipped into the other end of the line. As the helicopter ascends, the rescuers dangle beneath the aircraft as they are flown to the target area. There, they are gently lowered into the desired insertion point. Once safely on the ground, the rescuers disconnect from the line, allowing the helicopter to ascend to a safe altitude. When the patient and rescuers are ready to be extracted, the helicopter flies into position and hovers over the extraction point. The ground team clips the litter or themselves to the SPIE line. The helicopter then ascends and flies the patient and rescuers to a designated area, where they are off-loaded. The use of a SPIE is a high-risk operation and is usually undertaken only by specialized rescue teams during emergency situations.

## CPR during Transport

Caring for a patient in full cardiac arrest in outdoor environments is difficult. Techniques for performing CPR are discussed in Chapter 15, Cardiovascular Emergencies, whereas methods for transporting a patient in full arrest are described here.

If an AED is available, transport the device to the patient as rapidly and safely as possible. Defibrillation using an AED is most effective when done within 5 to 10 minutes after the onset of sudden cardiac arrest. If the patient is not close to an AED, it

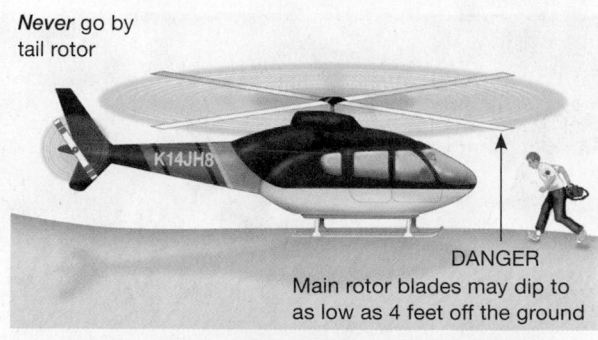

*Never* go by tail rotor

DANGER
Main rotor blades may dip to as low as 4 feet off the ground

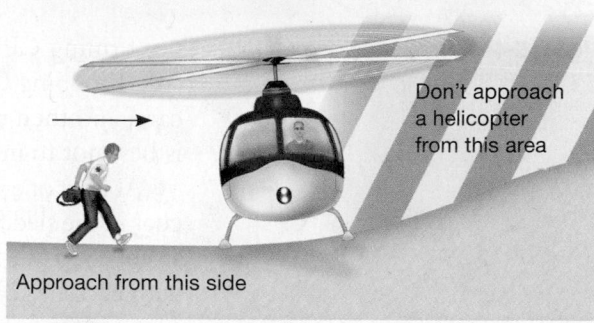

Don't approach a helicopter from this area

Approach from this side

**Figure 5-40** Be alert to the dangers of being near a helicopter on the ground!

### Basic Helicopter Safety

- Do not approach a helicopter unless signaled to do so or escorted by a crew member.
- Always approach a helicopter from the front. (Never approach the helicopter from the rear, where tail rotor is located.)
- Remain in sight of the pilot at all times.
- Stay low.
- Do not hold anything above your head.
- Take off your hat.
- Remove any loose clothing (e.g., hats, scarves, lightweight items) when in or near the LZ.

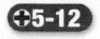

NOTE

⊕5-12 Describe the use of CPR during transport.

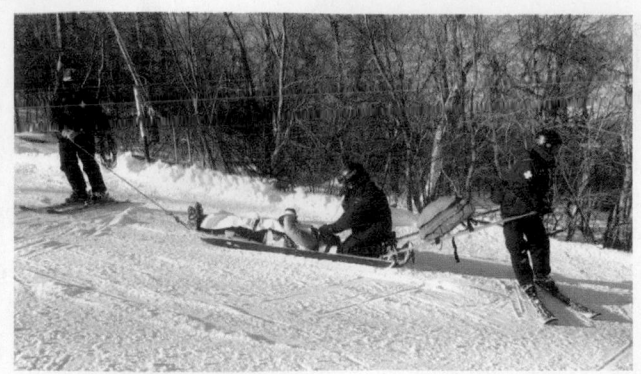

**Figure 5-41** CPR continues as a patient is being transported.
Copyright Edward McNamara

may be necessary to move the patient and the AED toward each other. When the patient and the AED meet, the AED should be used immediately. This practice can significantly reduce the time that elapses before the first defibrillating "shock" is administered in outdoor settings.

It is important for OEC Technicians to become familiar with the best way to transport a patient receiving ongoing CPR (Figure 5-41■). At a ski area, on-hill procedures like this are typically developed in conjunction with your medical adviser and management to suit your area's individual needs. Moving a patient in cardiac arrest off a ski slope is not an easy task. Likewise, performing CPR in a moving toboggan going down a steep slope is extremely difficult. Stopping CPR long enough to move a patient a short distance toward definitive care, and then resuming CPR, is not ideal, but at times it may be the only choice. It is best not to interrupt CPR once started unless you have no other choice.

At least one manufacturer makes a double sled specifically designed to position a rescuer in the sled for performing CPR. Some patrols use mechanical CPR devices that are strapped to the patient's chest and provide chest compressions and oxygen in accordance with current CPR guidelines. Both pieces of equipment are expensive. In relatively flat areas, a "tow toboggan" carrying a rescuer performing CPR on the patient can be pulled behind a snowmobile. If a double sled or mechanical CPR device is not available for use on steep slopes, other methods may need to be used. Any method used should be tailored to your area's needs. There are two alternatives to continuing CPR while moving a patient down the mountain: the sled CPR method and the leap frog CPR method.

## Sled CPR Method

Three rescuers are needed to perform the sled CPR method of managing a patient in cardiac arrest. Begin by assessing the ABCDs. Perform CPR after calling for ALS and arranging for a pack containing an AED and oxygen to meet you. Stop CPR briefly to log roll the patient onto a backboard. Continue CPR while securing the patient to the backboard with cravats or quick clips. Use head blocks to stabilize the head with the airway open after using the head-tilt/chin-lift maneuver.

Place a blanket in the head end of the toboggan for the rescuer who will be in the sled with the patient. The lightest patroller should move into position, kneeling on the blanket in the front of the toboggan. Strap the legs of that patroller into the toboggan, using the toboggan strap at the head end.

Stop CPR briefly and load the backboard bearing the patient into the sled. The backboard will extend approximately 12–18 inches out the back end of the toboggan. Once the patroller has knelt in the toboggan close to the head of the patient, the patroller should immediately take over one-person CPR while performing chest compressions from the patient's head. If this is not possible, just give chest compressions. It is best to administer oxygen using a bag-valve mask attached to the patient's head. The oxygen tank is secured between the patient's knees.

Secure the backboard into the toboggan with the toboggan straps, and secure the back end of the backboard by tying it with cravats to the back toboggan straps. The strongest skier then transports the toboggan down the mountain at a slow, steady speed while the person in the toboggan performs one-person CPR and the third person runs the tail rope for safety reasons. If the AED arrives, use it immediately.

## Leap Frog CPR Method

Another approach to transporting a patient in cardiac arrest is the leap frog CPR method. Five people are needed to perform this technique, which includes two-person

CPR. This method is less effective in maintaining CPR without interruption, as the American Heart Association recommends. It is used on steep terrain or moguls, where it is impossible for an OEC Technician to kneel in the toboggan with the patient.

To begin, determine that the person is in cardiac arrest, begin CPR and have someone call for ALS personnel. Instruct someone to bring an AED and portable oxygen in an emergency pack to meet you, explaining the route you will take down the slope. After the toboggan has arrived, briefly stop CPR and move the patient onto a spine board that has been placed next to the patient. Resume CPR once the patient is secured on a backboard and head blocks are used to secure the head in a way that keeps the airway open. CPR is stopped only long enough to load the patient into the toboggan.

Two OEC Technicians perform CPR for five cycles (approximately two minutes). Then, as rapidly and safely as possible, a strong skier transports the patient downhill for 20 to 30 seconds to two other OEC Technicians, who then perform CPR for five cycles. The first two OEC Technicians continue down the slope to await the arrival of the patient for the next cycle of CPR. The two teams of CPR-performing OEC Technicians continue "leap frogging" each other until the patient is at the bottom of the slope. If only three people are available, one-man CPR is used.

As soon as the AED arrives, stop CPR and use it. These actions take considerable coordination and practice to be effective. Using the two methods just described effectively while transporting a patient in cardiac arrest requires frequent practice. Remember, the sooner an AED is used on the patient, the more likely is the person's survival.

Neither of these methods is perfect, so some improvisation may be needed to perform CPR while trying to get a patient in full cardiac arrest off a ski slope. Tailor one of these methods to meet your patrol's needs, and then practice it often.

## STOP, THINK, UNDERSTAND

### Multiple Choice
Choose the correct answer.

1. Back injuries may be prevented by_____
   a. exercise, planning your move, and lifting with your arms.
   b. exercise, weight maintenance, and good body mechanics.
   c. exercise, weight maintenance, and bending at the waist.
   d. exercise, numerous lifters, and lifting with your arms.

2. When you have no suspicions of a spinal injury, which lift is used to raise a patient so that a long board may be slid under them?_____
   a. BEAN lift
   b. BEAM lift
   c. extremity lift
   d. direct ground lift

3. This lift is performed in the same manner as BEAN lift, but the patient is lifted and carried only a short distance._____
   a. draw-sheet lift
   b. BEAM lift
   c. extremity lift
   d. direct ground lift

4. Which lift has the lowest risk of back injury for the rescuer?_____
   a. BEAN lift
   b. draw-sheet lift
   c. extremity lift
   d. direct ground lift

5. Which of the following techniques combines optimal anatomical position with good body mechanics and the power of leg muscles?_____
   a. power squat
   b. power drag
   c. power grip
   d. power lift

6. Which of the following is one of the most commonly used lifts in rescue operations?_____
   a. direct ground lift
   b. extremity lift
   c. BEAN lift
   d. BEAM lift

7. This type of lift is used on patients who are not suspected of having a back injury and need to be raised onto a flat surface._____
   a. BEAN lift
   b. BEAM lift
   c. draw-sheet lift
   d. direct ground lift

*continued*

## STOP, THINK, UNDERSTAND *continued*

## Matching

Write the letter of the following descriptions in the blank beside the correct position.

_____ 1. high-Fowler position

_____ 2. semi-Fowler position

_____ 3. Trendelenburg position

_____ 4. Rothberg position

_____ 5. supine position

a. head is 15–30 degrees lower than the heart while the feet are raised 15–30 degrees

b. patient is lying on the back, face up

c. patient is in a sitting position, with the upper body raised 45 degrees

d. most often used for patients experiencing chest pain due to a suspected heart attack

e. patient is in a sitting position, with the body bent at 90 degrees

## Short Answer

1. What is the role of the patroller located at the front handles of the toboggan?

_____

2. What is the role of the patroller on the tail rope?

_____

3. List seven objects that may be used to make an improvised litter while on an overnight camping trip.

_____

_____

4. List five limitations regarding rotary-wing aircraft (helicopters) in rescue operations.

_____

_____

 # CASE DISPOSITION

The patient quickly becomes responsive. You decide that he should be transported quickly. Together with the ambulance personnel, you and your partner perform a four-person direct ground lift onto the ambulance stretcher. The ambulance crew transports the patient to a nearby care facility. The next day, you get word that the patient did well and was discharged having recovered from a mild concussion.

## OEC SKILL 5-1  Multiple Person Direct Ground Lift

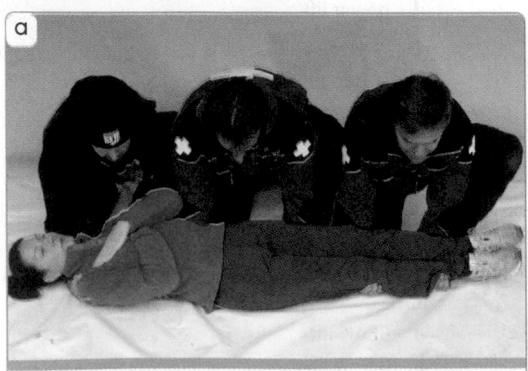

a

A direct ground lift involving three rescuers; the rescuer at the head directs the lift.
Copyright Mike Halloran

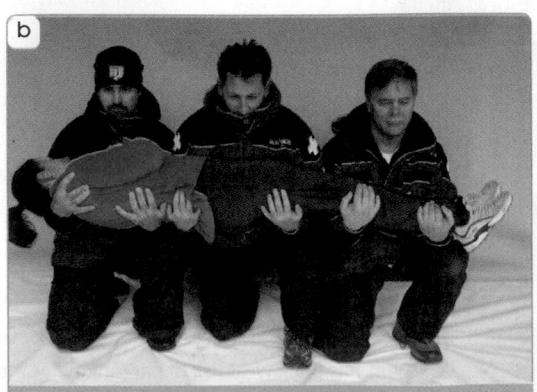

b

The rescuers' arms are almost touching, enabling a lifting action that keeps the entire length of the body stable.
Copyright Mike Halloran

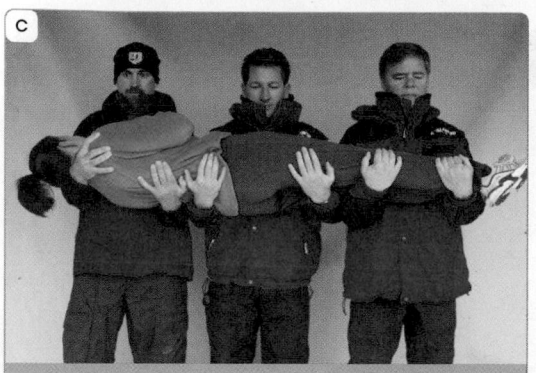

**c**

On the count of three, the rescuers roll the patient toward the rescuers' chests; then, on the next count of three, the rescuers stand in unison.
Copyright Mike Halloran

## OEC SKILL 5-2 | Bridge/BEAN Lift

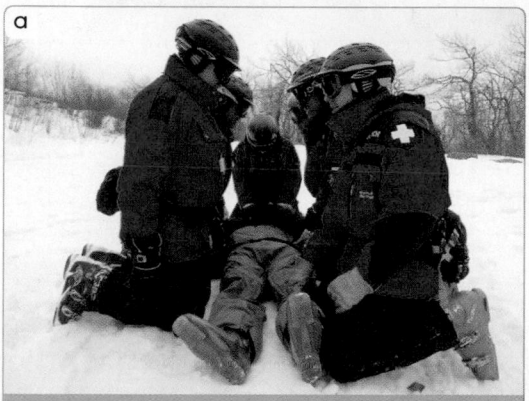

**a**

Two to five rescuers kneel on either side of the patient, staggering their positions.
Copyright Edward McNamara

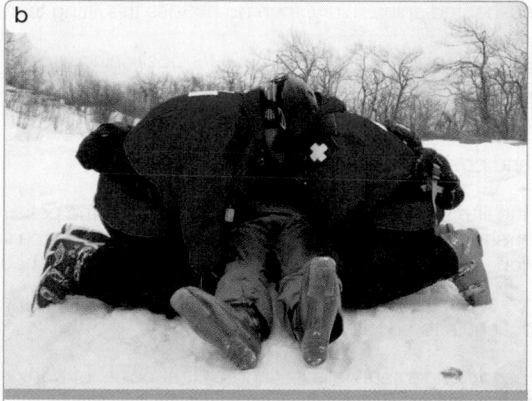

**b**

The rescuers then place their arms, nearly touching, under the patient, following the same pattern as rehearsed.
Copyright Edward McNamara

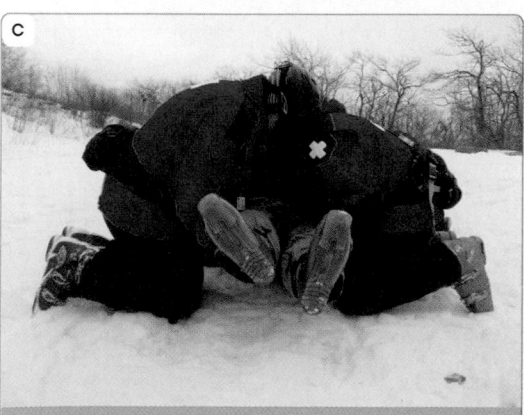

**c**

On the count of three, rescuers move to a crouching position while simultaneously raising the patient off the ground.
Copyright Edward McNamara

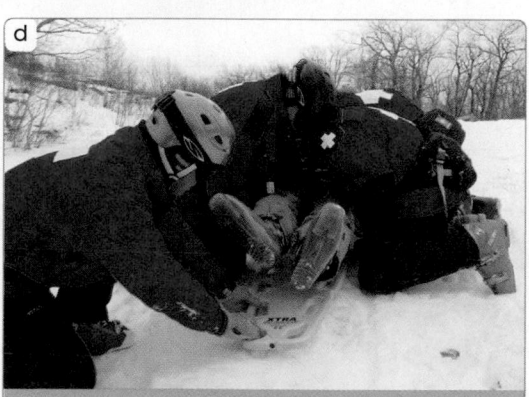

**d**

On another count of three, rescuers raise the patient 5–6 inches and a long spine board is positioned under the patient.
Copyright Edward McNamara

## Skill Guide

Date:_____

(CPI) = Critical Performance Indicator

Candidate: _____

Start time: _____

End time: _____ Time allowed: 10 min.

## Lifting Techniques: Bridge/BEAN Lift

| **Objective:** To demonstrate manual lifting techniques to move patients onto other devices. |
| --- |

| Skill | Max Points | Skill Demo | |
| --- | --- | --- | --- |
| Initiates Standard Precautions. | 1 | | (CPI) |
| If pt. has suspected spinal injury, then do not use this lifting technique. | 1 | | |
| Determines the number of lifters available for positioning:<br>• 4 people—position at head, chest, waist, and knees<br>• 5 people—position at head, chest, waist, thighs, and knees | 1 | | |
| Prepares and position all of the equipment needed. | 1 | | |
| Positions the lifters and have them form a bridge over the patient, head-to-shoulder or shoulder-to-shoulder. (Note: all lifters must use the same configuration whether it is head-to-shoulder or shoulder-to-shoulder.) | 1 | | |
| Explains the commands, procedures, and hand positions for the lift, including distance patient is to be lifted. | 1 | | |
| Positions hands underneath the patient to lift at points of body mass (shoulders, hips). Rescuer at head directs lift. | 1 | | |
| Executes the lift. Another rescuer slides the device into place starting at the pt.'s feet. Lower the patient as a unit. | 1 | | (CPI) |

| Must receive 6 out of 8 points. |
| --- |

Comments: _____

Failure of any of the CPIs is an automatic failure.

Evaluator: _____ NSP ID:_____

PASS     FAIL

## Skill Guide

Date: _____

(CPI) = Critical Performance Indicator

Candidate: _____

Start time: _____

End time: _____ Time allowed: 10 min.

## Lifting Techniques: Multiple Person Direct Ground Lift

**Objective:** To demonstrate manual lifting techniques to move patients onto other devices.

| Skill | Max Points | Skill Demo | |
|---|---|---|---|
| Initiates Standard Precautions. | 1 | | (CPI) |
| If patient has suspected spinal injury, does not use this lifting technique. | 1 | | (CPI-if pt. has spinal injury) |
| Determines the number of lifters available for positioning:<br>• 3 people—position at head, waist, and knees—on same side of pt.<br>• 4 people—position at head, chest, waist, and knees—on same side of pt. | 1 | | |
| Prepares and position all of the equipment needed. | 1 | | |
| Explains the commands, procedures, and hand positions for the lift, including distance patient is to be lifted. | 1 | | |
| Positions arms under pt. Rescuer closest to pt. head directs lift. | 1 | | |
| Executes the lift, rescuers rolling pt. toward their chest. Position into place, lifting and lowering the patient as a unit. | 1 | | (CPI) |

Must receive 5 out of 7 points.

Comments: _____

Failure of any of the CPIs is an automatic failure.

Evaluator: _____ NSP ID: _____

PASS     FAIL

# ♛ Chapter Review

## Chapter Summary

The skills of lifting, moving, and transporting using good body mechanics must be mastered by every OEC Technician, because an understanding of the techniques involved is essential for the care of the patient, and for the patient's and the rescuers' safety. On occasion, a patient will be located in an area that poses an immediate threat to life and must be urgently moved to a safe location. These emergency moves are best accomplished by a "long-axis drag," which helps keep the patient's spine in proper alignment.

As part of their training, OEC Technicians must master the equipment and devices they will use in all conditions. Extreme care must be exercised with patients to avoid handling them roughly or dropping them, which is likely to aggravate their con-

dition. OEC Technicians must learn how to properly package patients for transportation.

The helicopter is an amazing rescue tool that can save lives due to its ability to bring both rescuers and equipment to the scene rapidly, to extract patients from remote locations, and to speed the transport of patients to definitive care. It is essential that everyone on the scene have a basic understanding of landing zone selection and procedures for operating in and around a helicopter. Toboggan transport of a patient in full arrest is difficult. Decide the best method for your ski area, which will vary depending on terrain. Practice this skill often so that when it is needed, you are prepared.

## Remember...

1. Back injuries may be prevented through exercise, weight maintenance, and good body mechanics.
2. Plan each move carefully; get help when lifting.
3. Keep your back straight and lift with your legs.
4. Do not drop the patient.
5. Urgent moves require preserving the long axis of the spine.
6. Used properly, equipment can facilitate a move or a lift.
7. A landing zone should be at least 100 feet by 100 feet.
8. Do not approach a helicopter unless instructed to do so by the pilot or a crew member; keep your head low.
9. Never approach a helicopter from the rear.

## Chapter Questions

### Multiple Choice

Choose the correct answer.

1. In what position would a patient with a lower extremity injury be transported off the hill?_____
   a. sitting on a snowmobile
   b. injury facing downhill
   c. head uphill
   d. head downhill

2. In what position would a patient with an upper extremity injury be transported off the hill?_____
   a. sitting on a snowmobile
   b. injury downhill
   c. feet uphill
   d. feet downhill

3. Which of the following is *not* a basic LZ guideline?_____
   a. The site must be free of overhead obstructions and wires.
   b. The site should be well lit.
   c. The site must be a minimum of 100 feet by 100 feet.
   d. Point spotlights toward the aircraft.

**4.** Which of the following is *not* a backsmart tip?_____
   **a.** Turn with your feet, not your hips.
   **b.** Bend at your waist.
   **c.** Keep objects close to your body.
   **d.** Do not reach over your head.

**5.** All of the following are used by OEC Technicians to move, lift, or carry a patient *except*_____
   **a.** a long spine board.
   **b.** an orthopedic stretcher.
   **c.** rescue parallel bars.
   **d.** a short spine board.

**6.** What is the first principle of medicine?_____
   **a.** Use Standard Precautions.
   **b.** Do no harm.
   **c.** Help others who cannot help themselves.
   **d.** Maintain scene safety.

**7.** Which of the following is a long-axis drag?_____
   **a.** blanket drag
   **b.** human crutch
   **c.** chair carry
   **d.** two-person assist

## Matching

Match each of the following patient conditions with the most common position for transport.

_____ **1.** semi-Fowler position
_____ **2.** high-Fowler position
_____ **3.** supine position
_____ **4.** Rothberg position
_____ **5.** Trendelenburg position

**a.** a patient who is experiencing breathing problems
**b.** a patient with spinal injuries
**c.** a patient with chest pain and a suspected heart attack
**d.** a patient in shock
**e.** a patient who is awake and for whom no spinal injury is suspected

## Short Answer

List six basic principles of helicopter safety.

_____

_____

# Scenario  ○○○○○○○○○○○○○○○○○○○○○○○○○○○○○○○○○○○○○○○○○○○○○○○○○○○○○○

*You receive a call to the tubing park to aid an injured party. Once on scene, you find a 30-year-old male whose right lower leg is wedged between two trees. The patient is responsive and alert but has slurred speech. He complains of severe pain to his lower right leg. The patient states he was "horsing around" with two friends while tubing down the slope. He tells you he was "bumped," which forced him off the lane and into the trees. His friends state that he hit the trees "feet first." The patient denies striking his head, neck, or back and reports no pain in those areas. The friends admit to having been drinking.*

*Assessment of the patient's leg leads you to suspect a possible closed fracture of the right leg.*

**1.** What type of move is needed for this extrication?_____
   **a.** a nonurgent move
   **b.** an urgent move
   **c.** a shoulder drag
   **d.** a fore and aft carry

*After closing the outside lane and securing the scene, you request assistance and equipment. Another OEC Technician arrives and you formulate an extrication plan.*

**2.** Most back injuries to rescuers are caused by_____
   **a.** not enough rescuers.
   **b.** adverse terrain.
   **c.** poor body mechanics.
   **d.** oversized patients.

*Other rescuers arrive with the treatment and transport equipment. The patient is packaged and ready to load in the toboggan. Due to intense pain, the patient is not able to assist in moving himself to the toboggan. You decide to cravat his legs together and lift him. You have a total of four patrollers at the scene to help.*

**3.** Which of the following types of lift is appropriate for placing the patient into the toboggan?_____

    **a.** Extremity lift                     **c.** Direct ground lift

    **b.** BEAM lift                           **d.** BEAN lift

## Suggested Reading

Lipke, Rick. 2009. *Technical Rescue Riggers Guide*, Second Edition, Conterra, Inc. Bellingham, WA.

# Anatomy and Physiology

David Markenson, MD, FAAP, EMT-P

## ⊕ OBJECTIVES

**Upon completion of this chapter, the OEC Technician will be able to:**

**6-1** Define the following terms:

- anatomy
- body system
- cell
- homeostasis

- organ
- physiology
- tissue

**6-2** Identify various anatomical terms commonly used to refer to the body.

**6-3** Identify at least four body positions.

**6-4** List the five body cavities.

**6-5** Identify and describe the fundamental anatomy and physiology of the 11 body systems.

**6-6** Describe homeostasis and its importance for good health.

**6-7** Identify and properly use various anatomical terms to describe body direction, location, and movement.

## ⊕ KEY TERMS

**anatomy,** *p. 168*
**body system,** *p. 174*
**cell,** *p. 174*

**circulatory system,** *p. 174*
**endocrine system,** *p. 191*
**gastrointestinal system,** *p. 187*

**integumentary system,** *p. 195*
**lymphatic system,** *p. 206*
**muscular system,** *p. 199*

*continued*

## Chapter Overview

The human body is complex, containing 11 body systems that work together to keep it functioning properly. These systems control movement, provide structure, maintain nutritional status, circulate nutrients and oxygen to body tissues for continuous use, and perform other functions to maintain life.

As an OEC Technician, it is important that you have a basic understanding of normal human structure (anatomy) and function (physiology). Each of the 11 body systems

*continued*

## HISTORICAL TIMELINE

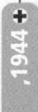
**1944** On Thanksgiving Day, Major General George P. Hays assumes command of the 10th Mountain Division.

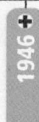
**1946**
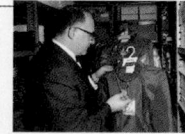
NSP adopts "Rainier Red" colored jackets from White Stag company as the official NSP patroller jacket.

**1946**
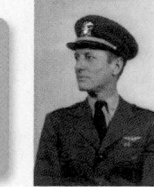
Roland Palmedo, one of the creators of the National Ski Patrol.

**nervous system,** *p. 183*        **reproductive system,** *p. 201*        **tissue,** *p. 174*
**organ,** *p. 171*                    **respiratory system,** *p. 174*        **urinary system,** *p. 191*
**physiology,** *p. 168*               **skeletal system,** *p. 195*

⊕ **6-1**   Define the following terms:

- anatomy
- body system
- cell
- homeostasis
- organ
- physiology
- tissue

**anatomy**  the study of human and animal structures, including gross anatomy (structures that can be seen with the unaided eye) and microscopic anatomy (structures visible only through a microscope).

**physiology**  the study of how living organisms function (e.g., movement or reproduction).

depends on other systems to function properly. Injury or illness to one system may cause problems in others. Therefore, understanding the anatomy and physiology of the body systems, and how they interact with each other, will help you more easily recognize and understand injuries and illnesses (Figure 6-1■).

In this chapter you will study the basic anatomy and physiology of the 11 body systems. You also will study key terms that will help you understand the relationship of each system to the others. This information will be used each time you assess and manage a patient and will help you communicate more effectively with other health care providers.

# Anatomy and Physiology

Human **anatomy** is the study of the structure of the body. It includes gross anatomy (i.e., structures that can be seen with the unaided eye) and microscopic anatomy (i.e., structures that can be seen only under a microscope). Human **physiology** is the study of the mechanical, physical, and biochemical functions of humans.

## Terms for Planes and Directional Terms

Among the terms universally used to communicate with other emergency medical personnel are terms that refer to planes (Figure 6-2■) and the following directional terms (Figure 6-3■):

**Figure 6-2** The anatomical planes of the body.

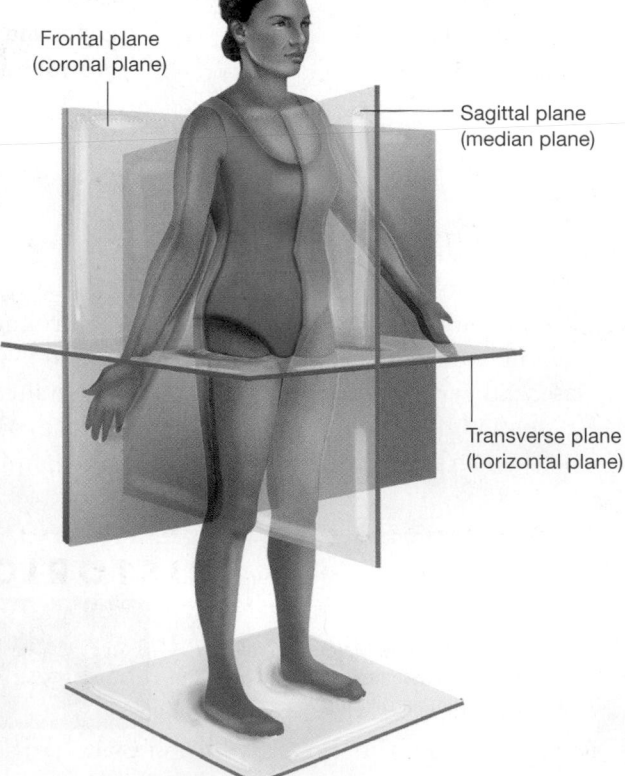

Frontal plane
(coronal plane)

Sagittal plane
(median plane)

Transverse plane
(horizontal plane)

**Figure 6-1** OEC Technicians must have a good understanding of basic anatomy and physiology.
Copyright Edward McNamara

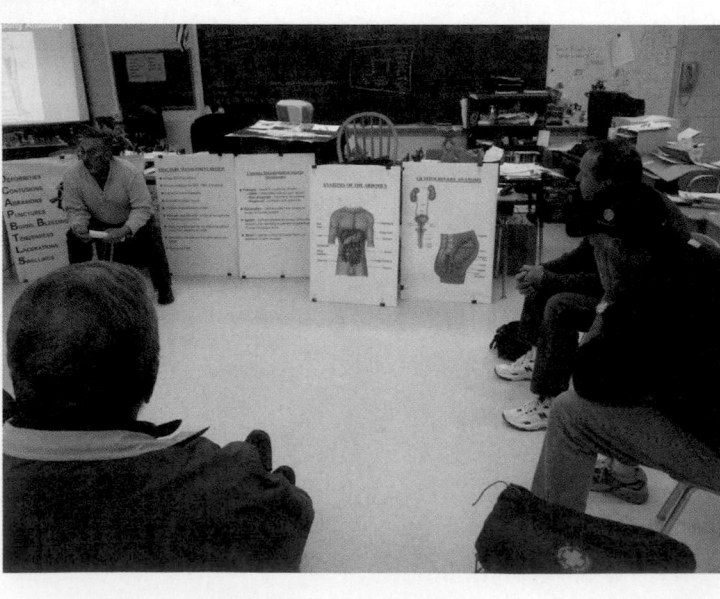

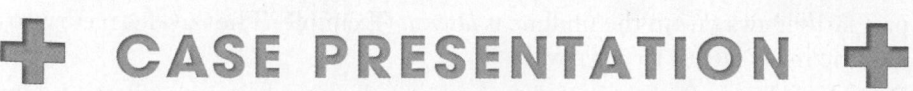

**CASE PRESENTATION**

You respond to an emergency involving two skiers who have collided. As you size up the scene, both people appear to be injured. The first person, a woman, is sitting on the ground with her knees drawn up toward her chest. She is clutching her left side and is groaning in pain. The second person, a man, is lying on the ground. His left leg is bent at an awkward angle and he repeatedly asks, "What happened?"

**What should you do? What body systems and structures might be involved?**

**Figure 6-3** Directional terms used to describe locations on the body and the relationships between parts of the body.

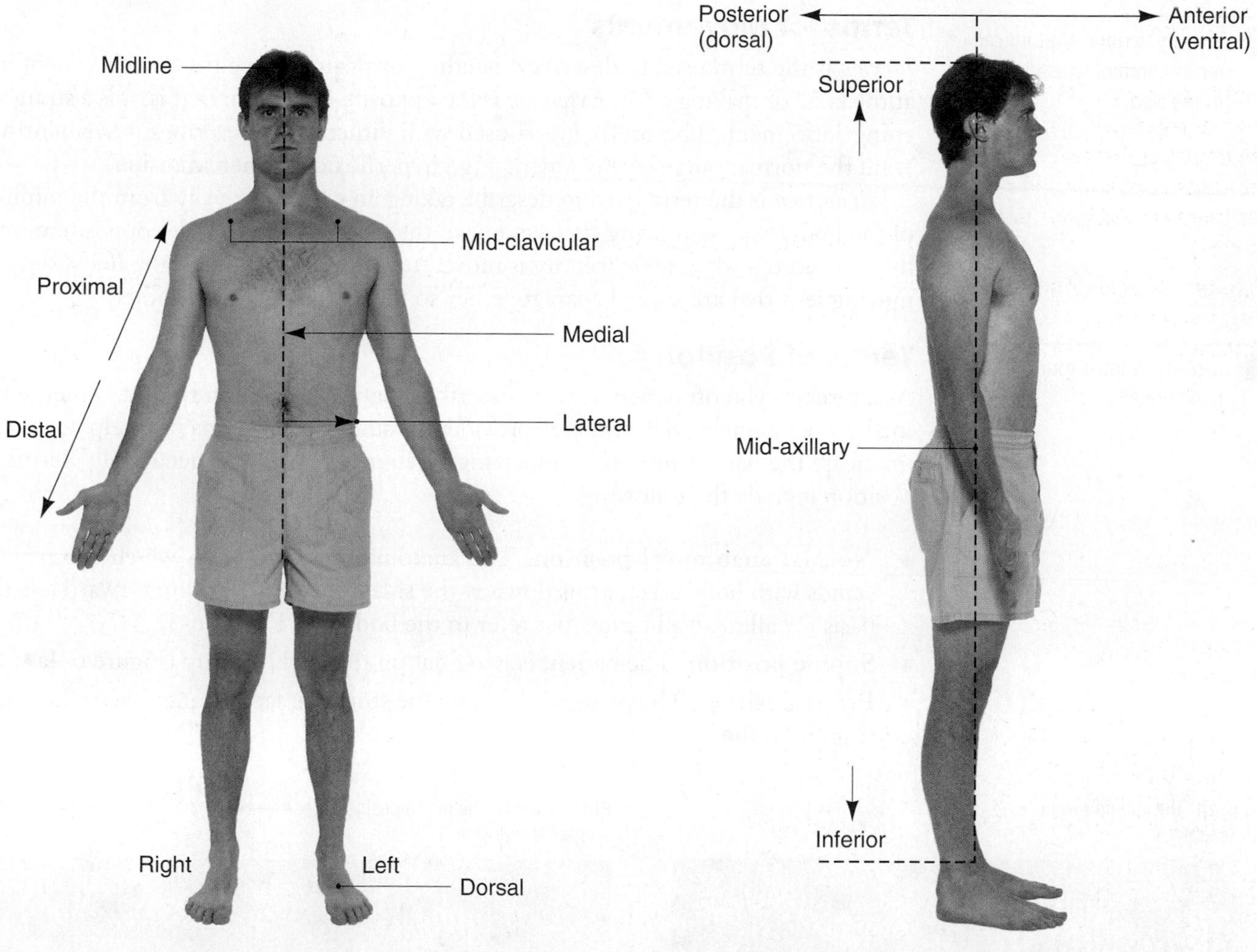

Posterior (dorsal) — Anterior (ventral)
Superior
Midline
Mid-clavicular
Proximal
Medial
Distal
Lateral
Mid-axillary
Right    Left
Dorsal
Inferior

- **Anterior/posterior.** The term *anterior* refers to the front of the body, whereas *posterior* refers to the back of the body. (Example: The jaw is anterior to the ears; the ears are posterior to the jaw.)
- **Superior/inferior.** *Superior* describes any part nearer the patient's head, whereas *inferior* describes any part nearer the patient's feet. (Example: The jaw is superior to the neck; the neck is inferior to the jaw.)
- **Medial/lateral:** The terms *medial* and *lateral* are based on the midline, an imaginary line that runs down the middle of the body from the head to the ground and

**6-7** Identify and properly use various anatomical terms to describe body direction, location, and movement.

creates right and left halves. Any part closer to the midline is *medial*, whereas any part farther away from the midline is *lateral*. (Example: The navel is medial to the hip; the hip is lateral to the navel.)

+ **Proximal/distal.** *Proximal* refers to any part close to the trunk (chest, abdomen, and pelvis), and *distal* refers to any part away from the trunk and nearer to the extremities (arms and legs). (Example: The shoulder is proximal to the elbow; the elbow is distal to the shoulder.)

+ **Superficial/deep.** *Superficial* refers to any part near the surface of the body, whereas *deep* refers to any part far from the surface. (Example: The skin is superficial to the bones; the bones are deep to the skin.)

+ **Internal/external.** *Internal* refers to the inside, whereas *external* refers to the outside. (Example: The liver is an internal organ; the skin is an external organ.)

+ **Right/left.** *Right* and *left* always refer to the patient's right and left, not yours.

## Terms for Movements

**⊕ 6-2** Identify various anatomical terms commonly used to refer to the body.

*Flexion* is the term used to describe a bending or flexing movement, such as bending at the knee or making a fist. *Extension* is the opposite of flexion; that is, it is a straightening movement. The prefix *hyper-* used with either term describes movement beyond the normal range of movement (e.g., hyperflexion, hyperextension).

*Abduction* is the term used to describe taking an extremity away from the midline of the body, such as moving the arm out to the side. *Adduction* is the opposite movement; it occurs when an extremity is moved toward the midline of the body, such as moving legs that are spread apart together so that they touch each other.

## Terms of Position

**⊕ 6-3** Identify at least four body positions.

As a rescuer, you often will need to describe a patient's position to other emergency medical personnel and health care providers. Using correct terms will help you communicate the nature and extent of a patient's injury quickly and accurately. Terms of position include the following:

+ **Normal anatomical position.** The anatomical position—in which the patient stands with body erect, arms down at the sides, and palms facing forward—is the basis for all medical terms that refer to the body (see Figure 6-3).

+ **Supine position.** The patient is lying flat on the back, face up (Figure 6-4a■).

+ **Prone position.** The patient is lying on the stomach, face to one side or the other (Figure 6-4b■).

**Figure 6-4a** The supine position.
Copyright Mike Halloran

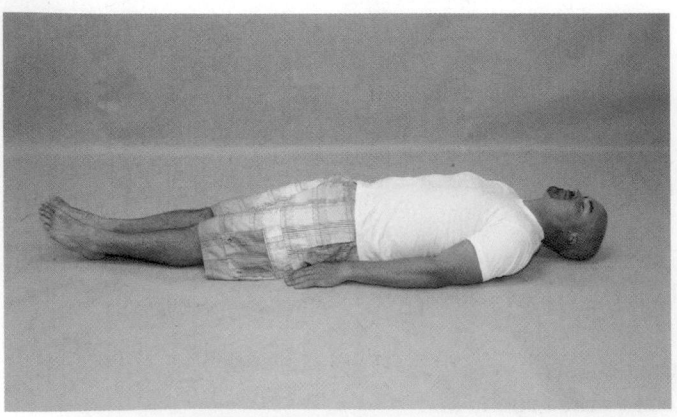

**Figure 6-4b** The prone position.
Copyright Mike Halloran

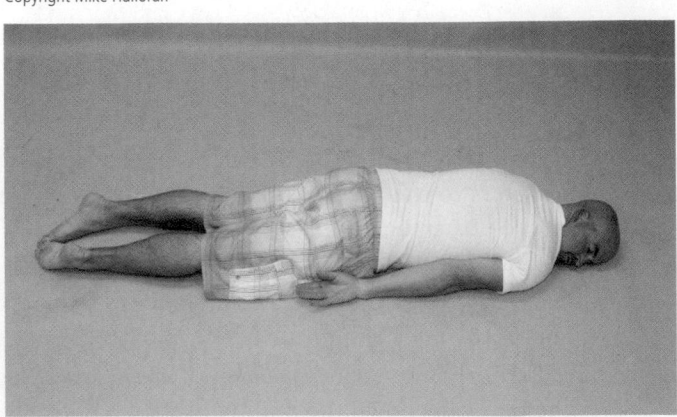

- **Right or left lateral recumbent position (recovery position).** The patient is lying on the right side or the left side (Figure 6-4c■).
- **Semi-Fowler position.** The patient is lying on his back with the upper body elevated at a 45° to 60° angle (Figure 6-5■).
- **High-Fowler position.** The patient is on his back with the upper body elevated at a 90° angle at the waist.
- **Trendelenburg position.** The patient is lying on his back, forming an inclined plane in which the legs are elevated above the head (Figure 6-6■).

# Body Cavities

The **organs** of the body, with the exception of the skin, are located within hollow spaces in the body referred to as body cavities. The five major body cavities are (Figure 6-7■):

- **Cranial cavity.** Located inside the skull, the cranial cavity contains the brain and the membranes that surround it.
- **Spinal cavity.** This cavity extends from the bottom of the skull (where the brain ends) to the tailbone and is a canal formed by the vertebrae of the spinal column. The spinal cavity contains the spinal cord and the membranes that surround it.
- **Thoracic (chest) cavity.** Located in the central part of the body, or trunk, between the diaphragm and the neck, the thoracic cavity contains the lungs, heart, and great vessels. The rib cage, sternum, and the upper portion of the spine protect it. The diaphragm separates it from the abdominal cavity.
- **Abdominal cavity.** Located in the trunk below the ribs, between the diaphragm and the pelvis, the abdominal cavity is described as having four quadrants: the right and left upper quadrants, and the right and left lower quadrants (Figure 6-8■). The abdominal cavity contains the organs of digestion, including the liver, gallbladder, pancreas, stomach, and intestines. The abdominal cavity also includes the spleen, which is an organ of the lymphatic system. The kidneys are located just outside and posterior to the abdominal cavity.
- **Pelvic cavity.** The pelvic cavity is located just inferior to the abdomen and is encased by the pelvic bones and the lower portion of the spine. It contains the bladder, the rectum, and the internal reproductive organs.

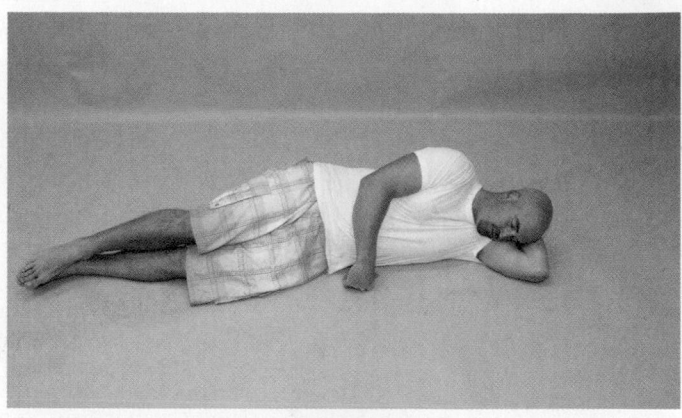

**Figure 6-4c** The lateral recumbent position.
Copyright Mike Halloran

**⊕ 6-4**  List the five body cavities.

**organ**  a structure containing similar tissues that act together to perform specific body functions.

**Figure 6-5** Semi-Fowler position.

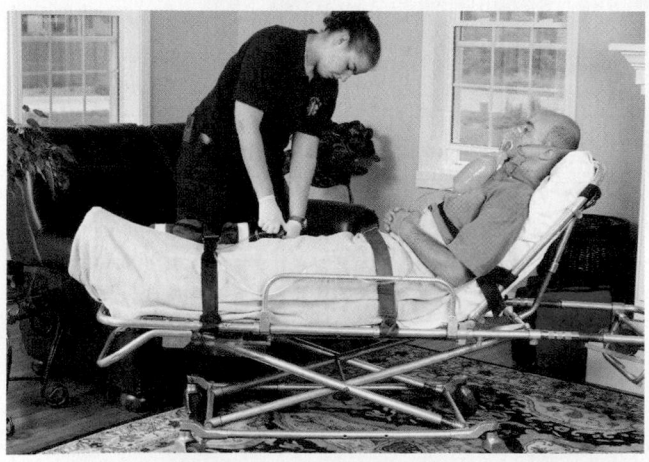

**Figure 6-6** Trendelenburg position.

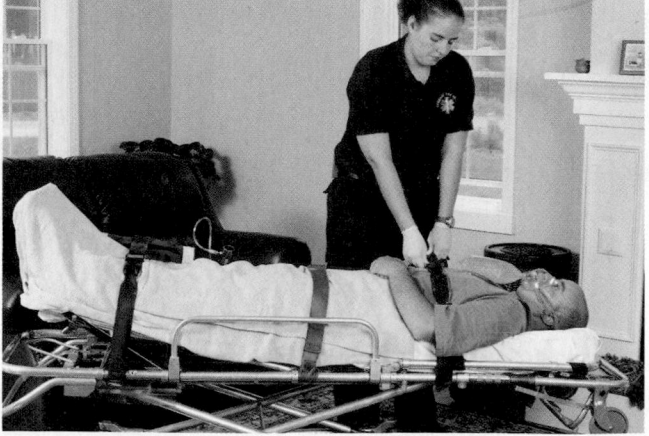

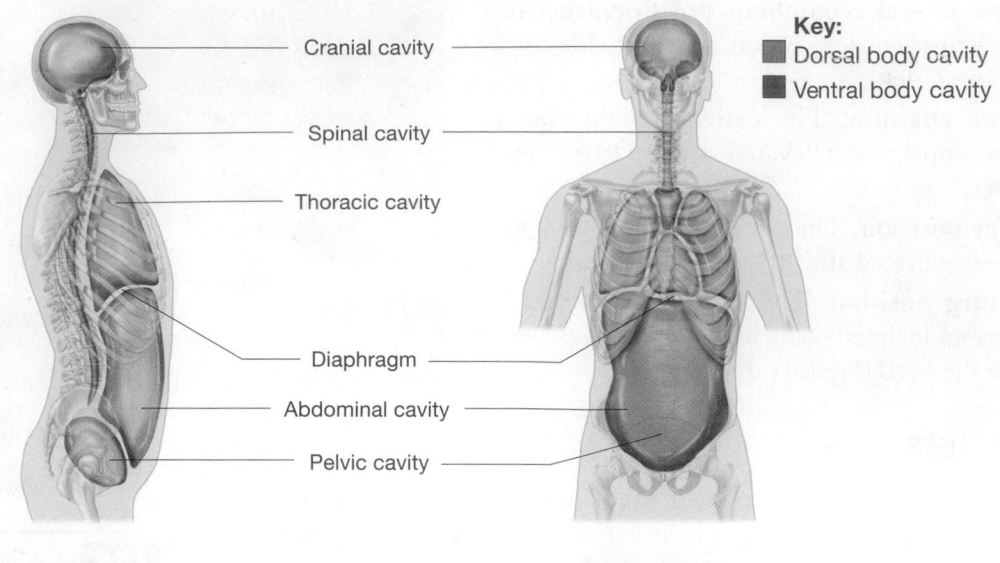

Cranial cavity
Spinal cavity
Thoracic cavity
Diaphragm
Abdominal cavity
Pelvic cavity
Key:
Dorsal body cavity
Ventral body cavity
Lateral view
Anterior view

**Figure 6-7** The five major body cavities: the cranial, spinal, thoracic, abdominal, and pelvic cavities.

**Figure 6-8** The four quadrants of the abdomen.

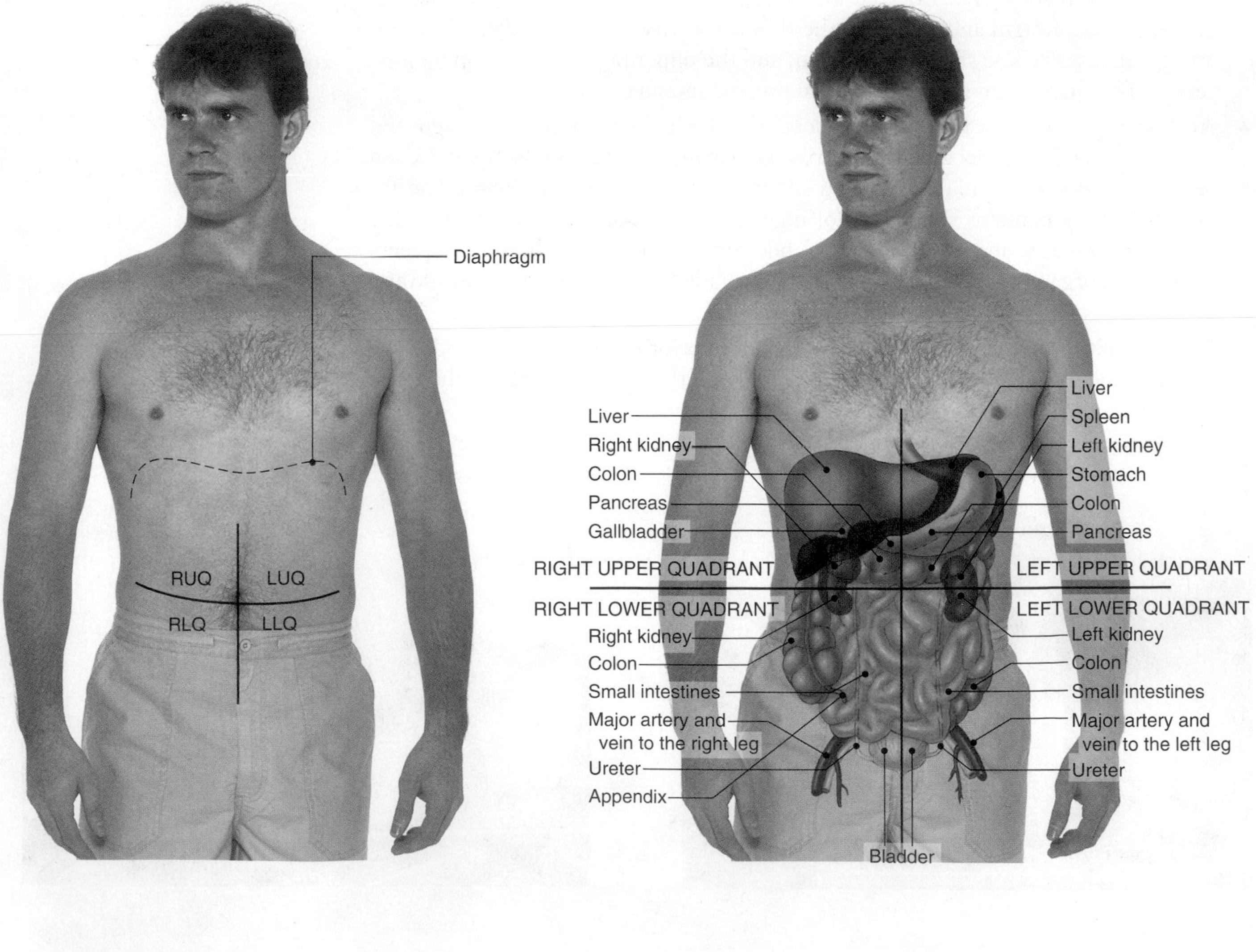

Diaphragm
RUQ
LUQ
RLQ
LLQ
Liver
Right kidney
Colon
Pancreas
Gallbladder
RIGHT UPPER QUADRANT
RIGHT LOWER QUADRANT
Right kidney
Colon
Small intestines
Major artery and vein to the right leg
Ureter
Appendix
Liver
Spleen
Left kidney
Stomach
Colon
Pancreas
LEFT UPPER QUADRANT
LEFT LOWER QUADRANT
Left kidney
Colon
Small intestines
Major artery and vein to the left leg
Ureter
Bladder

In addition to the cavities just described, health care providers often refer to body cavities in combination (e.g., the thoracoabdominal cavity or the abdominopelvic cavity). This is commonly used in describing suspected injuries involving more than one body cavity. For example, an OEC Technician might report that "The patient struck a tree and has potential thoracoabdominal injuries."

## STOP, THINK, UNDERSTAND

### Multiple Choice

Choose the correct answer.

1. How many organ systems does the human body have?_____
   a. 3
   b. 8
   c. 11
   d. 15

2. Which of the following statements best describes the functioning of the organ systems?_____
   a. They are independent entities that do not overlap at all.
   b. They are independent entities that overlap somewhat.
   c. They are dependent systems that rely on each other to function properly.
   d. They are actually one large, singular system.

3. A patient has hyperextended his knee. What does this mean?_____
   a. He has straightened his knee beyond the normal range of movement.
   b. He has bent his knee beyond the normal range of movement.
   c. He has pushed his knee cap too far to the right or left.
   d. He has straightened his knee into a normal position.

4. During an evaluation, a patient is unable to raise her arm over her head while trying to move it straight out from the side of her body. In your short report you describe the patient as being unable to _____
   a. adduct her arm.
   b. abduct her arm.
   c. hyperflex her arm.
   d. hyperextend her arm.

5. A patient complains of shortness of breath, and you decide to place him in the semi-Fowler position. This means that you will place this patient on his _____
   a. left side.
   b. right side.
   c. back with his legs elevated higher than his head.
   d. back with his upper body elevated at a 45–60° angle.

6. A snowmobiler comes to a sudden, abrupt stop and strikes his abdomen and chest against his handlebars. The location of possible internal injuries is best described as _____
   a. cranioabdominal.
   b. thoracoabdominal.
   c. abdominopelvic.
   d. supraspinal.

7. This large muscle separates the thoracic and abdominal cavities._____
   a. Vastus
   b. Deltoid
   c. Diaphragm
   d. Scapula

### Matching

Match each of the following directional terms with the best description at right.

_____ 1. anterior
_____ 2. deep
_____ 3. distal
_____ 4. external
_____ 5. inferior
_____ 6. internal
_____ 7. lateral
_____ 8. medial
_____ 9. posterior
_____ 10. proximal
_____ 11. superficial
_____ 12. superior

a. closer to the trunk
b. in the back of the body
c. near the patient's head
d. close to the midline
e. near the surface of the body
f. refers to the inside
g. refers to the outside
h. far from the surface
i. near the patient's feet
j. in the front of the body
k. away from the trunk and nearer to the extremities
l. away from the midline

### Fill in the Blank

The lungs, heart, and great vessels are located in the _____ cavity.

**6-5** Identify and describe the fundamental anatomy and physiology of the 11 body systems.

**cell**   the basic unit of all living tissue.

**tissue**   a collection of cells acting together to perform a specific body function.

**body system**   a group of organs and other structures that work together to perform specific functions.

**circulatory system**   a group of organs and other structures that transport blood and other nutrients throughout the body.

**respiratory system**   a group of organs and other structures that bring oxygen in the air into the body and eliminate carbon dioxide into the air through a process called breathing or respiration.

# Body Systems

The human body is a miraculous machine. It performs many complex functions, each of which helps us live. The human body is made up of billions of **cells** of different types that contribute in special ways to keep the body functioning normally. Cells form **tissues**, which in turn form organs. Organs that perform similar or related functions work together and form a **body system**. A body system, also referred to as an organ system, consists of a group of organs and other structures that are specially adapted to performing specific body functions needed for life. For example, the **circulatory system** consists of the heart, blood, and blood vessels, and its main function is to transport many substances needed for life, including oxygen-rich blood.

The 11 organ systems in the human body are:

+ Respiratory system
+ Cardiovascular system
+ Nervous system
+ Gastrointestinal system
+ Urinary system
+ Endocrine system

+ Integumentary system
+ Skeletal system
+ Muscular system
+ Reproductive system
+ Lymphatic system

## The Respiratory System

The **respiratory system** consists of organs that move air into and out of the body and exchange gases between the air and the blood. The system delivers oxygen to body cells and removes carbon dioxide from those cells in a process called respiration. In a healthy person, the act of respiration is sufficient to meet the body's normal oxygen needs, and it also removes carbon dioxide, thereby helping to balance the body's internal pH (the degree of acidity or alkalinity of the blood).

### Anatomy of the Respiratory System

The respiratory system is divided into the upper and lower airways at roughly the level of the vocal cords within the larynx (Figures 6-9■ and 6-10■).

**Upper Airway**   The upper airway includes the nose, mouth and teeth, tongue and jaw, pharynx, larynx, and epiglottis. During inspiration, air enters the body through the nose and mouth, where it is warmed and moistened. Large particles are filtered by hairs within the nostrils.

Air entering through the nose passes through the nasopharynx (the part of the throat posterior to the nose), and air entering through the mouth travels through the oropharynx. The air then continues down through the larynx, which houses the vocal cords. To prevent foreign objects from entering the trachea during swallowing, the epiglottis, a leaf-shaped structure, folds down over the top of the trachea, the first structure of the lower airway.

**Lower Airway**   The lower airway consists of the trachea, bronchi, and the lungs, which contain the bronchioles and alveoli. Air passes through the larynx and travels down the trachea to the passageways within the lungs. The trachea contains rings of cartilage and can be felt in the anterior neck. Air moving down the trachea passes into the right and left bronchi to enter each lung. These bronchi continue to divide into smaller and smaller passages, called bronchioles, like the branches of a tree. The bronchioles have muscular walls that can constrict.

At the ends of each bronchiole are air collection areas called alveoli. Each alveolus is surrounded by tiny blood vessels, known as capillaries. The alveoli are the

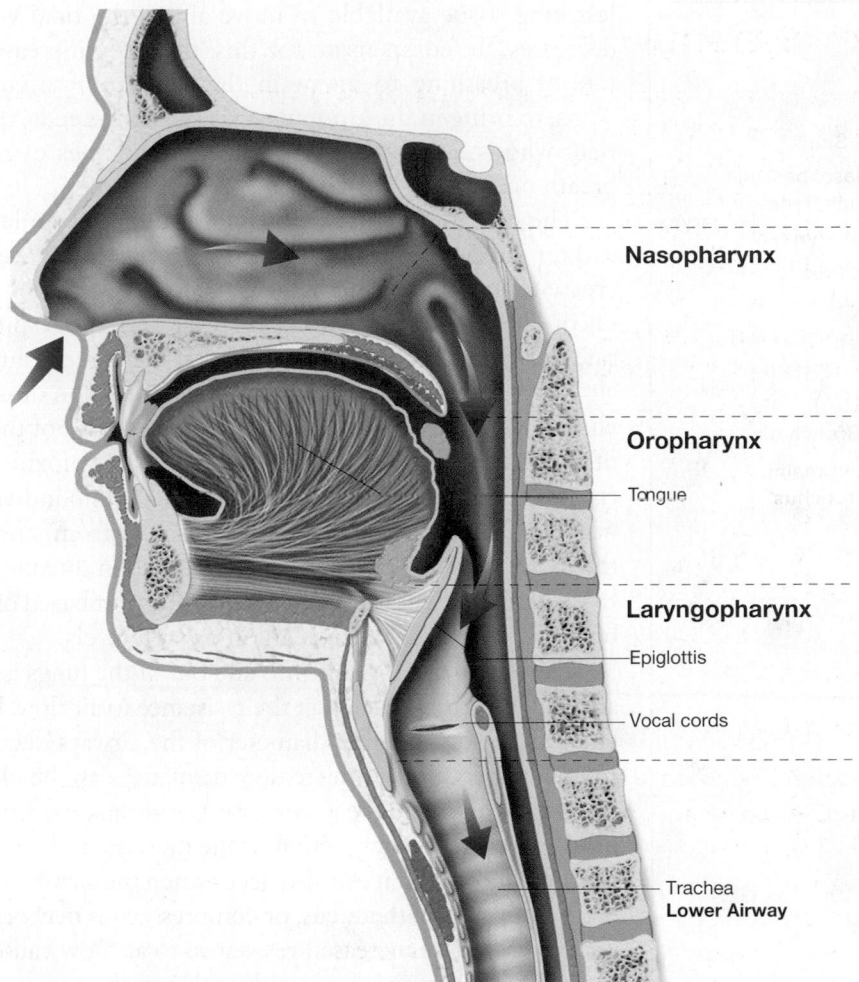

**Figure 6-9** The structures of the upper airway.

sites of carbon dioxide and oxygen exchange between the air and the blood. The lungs are thus the organs responsible for gas exchange, and they house thousands of alveoli.

## Physiology of the Respiratory System

Breathing, or ventilation, is the mechanical process of moving air into and out of the lungs to exchange oxygen and carbon dioxide between body tissues and the environment (Figure 6-11■). The flow of air into the lungs is caused primarily by contraction of the diaphragm, the large muscle that separates the thoracic and abdominal cavities. Contraction of the diaphragm results in the expansion of the lungs by creating negative pressure within the thoracic cavity, drawing air into the lungs. Air then flows out of the lungs in a passive process resulting from the combination of relaxation of the diaphragm and recoil of the chest wall, which together decrease the lung size. Accessory muscles between the ribs and in the neck are able to expand the chest directly, aiding inspiration, especially during labored or rapid breathing.

Each breath entails the movement of a volume of air into and out of the body. This volume is known as the minute ventilation and is the product of the respiratory rate (breaths per minute) and the tidal volume (volume of air moved per breath). Understanding minute ventilation will help you to understand how the body adapts to respiratory problems. For example, a person with a lung infection or a collapsed lung has

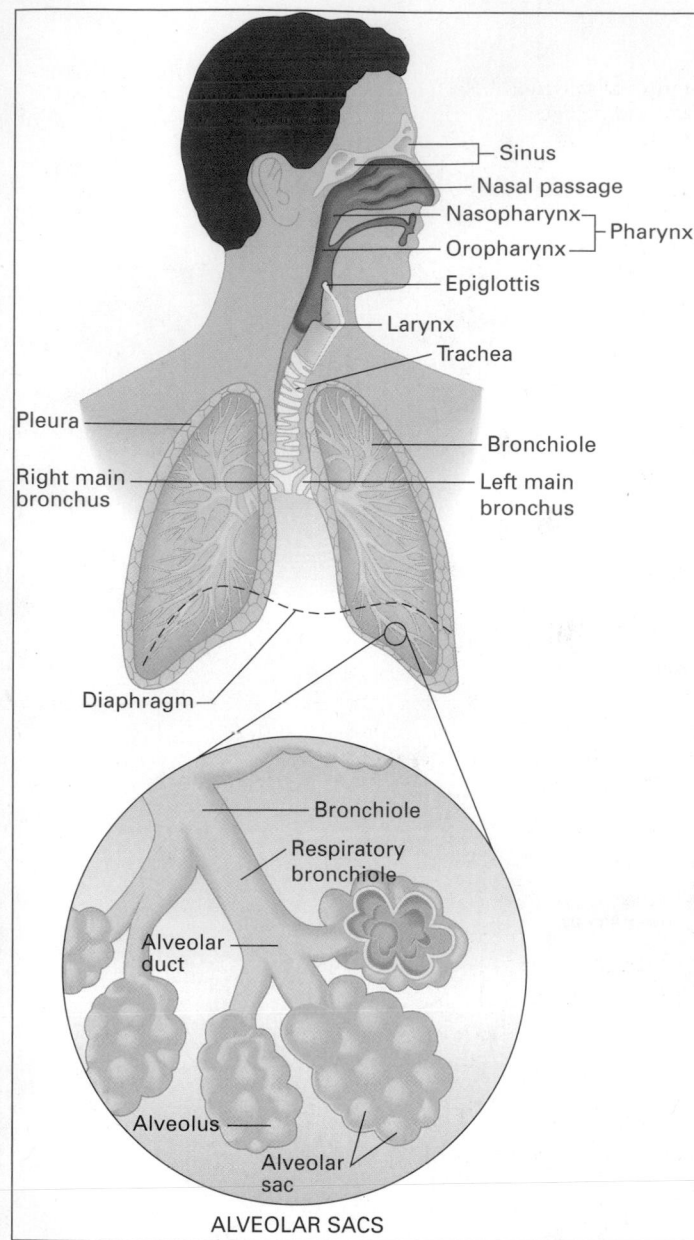

Sinus
Nasal passage
Nasopharynx
Oropharynx — Pharynx
Epiglottis
Larynx
Trachea
Pleura
Right main bronchus
Bronchiole
Left main bronchus
Diaphragm

Bronchiole
Respiratory bronchiole
Alveolar duct
Alveolus
Alveolar sac
ALVEOLAR SACS

**Figure 6-10** The anatomy of the respiratory system.

less lung tissue available to move air, so the tidal volume decreases. To compensate for this, the body increases the rate of breathing to maintain the same minute volume. Thus, to bring in the amount of air the body needs, the patient who is now breathing in smaller volumes of air per breath must breathe more times each minute.

The control of breathing is dependent on the level of carbon dioxide in the blood. If carbon dioxide levels increase (either due to increased production of carbon dioxide or due to decreased minute ventilation), the respiration rate increases automatically so that an increased volume of air is moved each minute until the excess carbon dioxide is eliminated. Therefore, in most individuals it is not the lack of oxygen, but instead the excess of carbon dioxide, that causes an increase in respiratory rate. In certain individuals who have significant lung disease, usually from smoking, the blood contains a chronically high carbon dioxide level. In these individuals the drive to breathe is not based on carbon dioxide levels, but instead on oxygen levels.

The ability to move air into and out of the lungs is often affected by factors that affect the resistance to air flow. Resistance increases when the diameter of the airways decreases. In the upper airway, decreased diameter can be due to swelling or injury. In the lower airway, resistance to airflow is most often due to constriction of the muscles in the walls of the bronchioles, but it can also occur when the airways are inflamed, plugged with mucus, or compressed (as may occur in pneumonia). The increased resistance to air flow causes the body to either move less air with each breath or to do more work to move the same volume of air. In most cases the body increases the work to maintain movement of the same volume of air. This increased effort to overcome the increased resistance is accomplished by use of the accessory muscles (previously identified). The use of accessory muscles is a sign that the body is compensating for a problem in the lungs or airways, or needs more oxygen due to ongoing exercise.

In addition to ventilation, the process of cellular respiration refers to respiration at the cellular level in all tissues. This metabolic process occurs within cells and across the cell's membrane, so the cells can obtain energy for the body to function and to remove the waste products of cellular activity. Cellular respiration involves the reaction of oxygen and glucose, both brought to the cells by the circulation of blood, to produce ATP, a chemical that cells use for energy, water, and carbon dioxide (a waste product).

## The Cardiovascular System

The cardiovascular (CV) system consists of the heart, blood vessels, and blood (Figure 6-12■). Also known as the circulatory system, the CV system is responsible for delivering oxygen, nutrients, and fluids to the body's cells, and for taking carbon dioxide and other waste products to the lungs and kidneys for excretion.

### Anatomy of the Cardiovascular System

**The Heart**  The heart is a highly efficient muscular organ that pumps blood throughout the body. It is about the size of a closed fist and is located in the thoracic

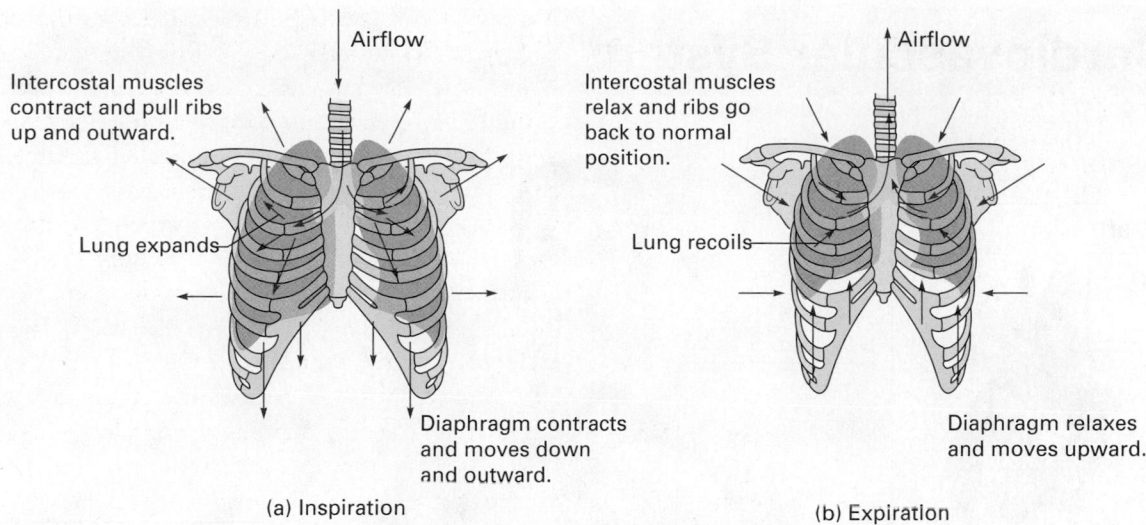

**Figure 6-11** (a) Breathing or ventilation is the mechanical process of moving air into and out of the lungs. (b) Ventilation includes inspiration and expiration.

cavity between the two lungs, posterior to the sternum and slightly to the left of the midline.

The heart is divided into four chambers: right and left upper chambers called atria, and right and left lower chambers called ventricles. The two chambers on the right side of the heart are separated from the two chambers on the left side by muscular walls called the interatrial septum and the interventricular septum. The right side of the heart pumps blood to the lungs; the left side pumps blood to the rest of the body (Figure 6-13a■).

Blood makes a complete circuit throughout the body (Figure 6-13b■). The body's veins take oxygen-depleted blood from the tissues and deliver it into the superior and inferior venae cavae, the largest veins in the body. The right atrium receives blood from the venae cavae and pumps it through a one-way valve into the right ventricle, which in turn pumps the blood through another one-way valve into the pulmonary arteries and on to the lungs for oxygenation (see Figure 6-13a). The left atrium receives this oxygen-rich blood from the lungs and delivers it through a valve to the left ventricle. The oxygen-rich blood is then pumped through another one-way valve into the aorta and then on to the arteries. The arteries travel throughout the body, carrying oxygenated blood to the tissues. The blood goes through the smallest blood vessels (capillaries) and then into veins of increasing sizes during its return to the heart. Nutrients and oxygen diffuse through the capillary walls to the cells while waste from the cells diffuse into the capillaries. Arteries that supply the heart itself, called the coronary arteries arise from the first part of the aorta (Figure 6-14a■).

The heart's coordination of pumping is regulated through an intricate electrical network of cells that "pace" the heart. These "pacemaker" cells create an electric current that is conducted through the heart and causes the heart's muscle cells to contract in a coordinated way. In actuality, all muscle cells in the heart can generate their own electric current, but under normal conditions the more dominant pacemaker cells provide the electric impulse for coordinated contractions. The electric impulse begins in the wall of the right atrium and spreads through both atria, causing contraction of both atria. The impulse then spreads to cells in the right and left ventricles, leading to a coordinated contraction of both ventricles. This electrical system causes the heart muscle to contract in such a way that blood is "pumped" out of the heart.

Pacemaker cells fire at a basic rate that can be modified by input from the autonomic nervous system (described later in this chapter). If one group of pacemaker

# Cardiovascular System

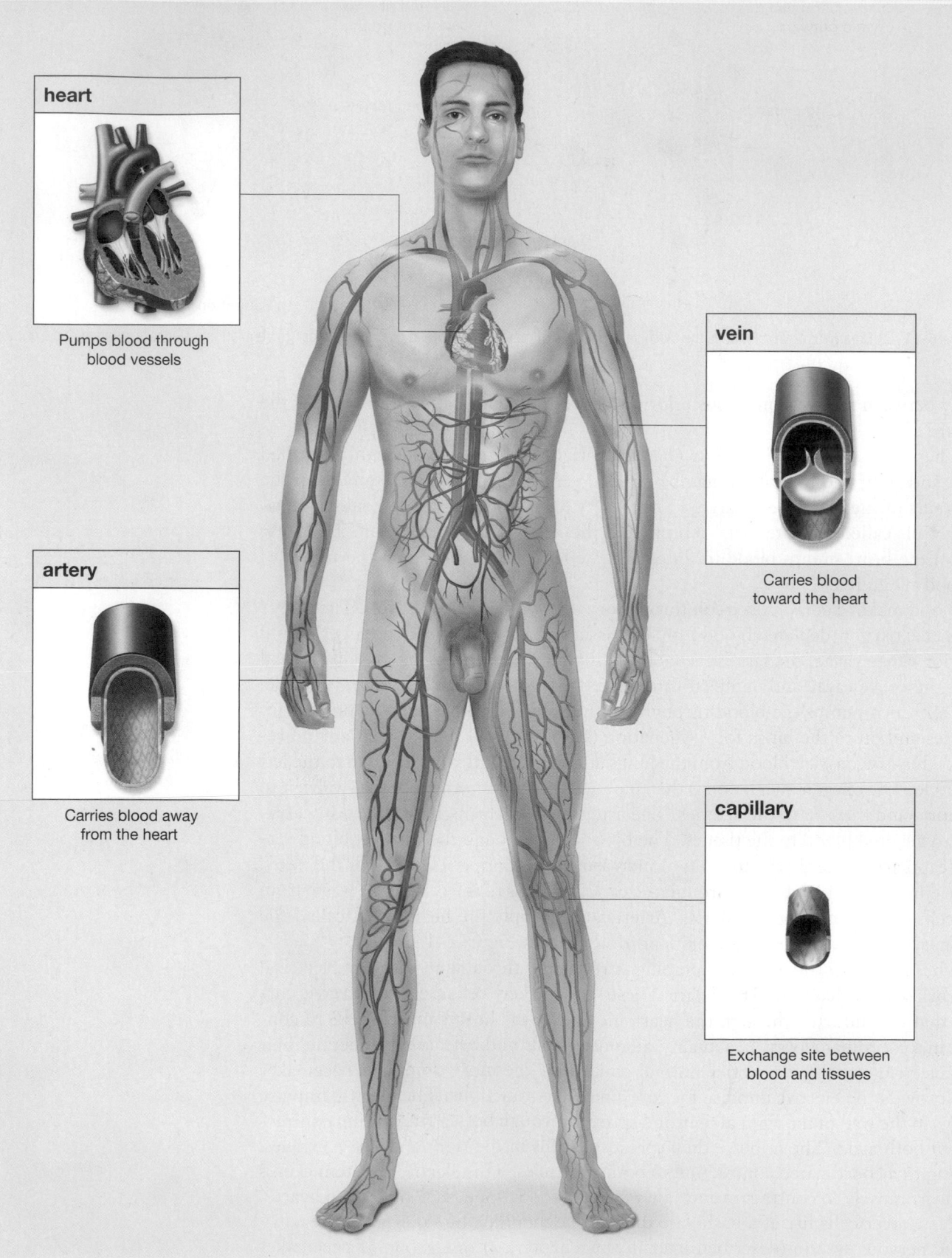

**heart**

Pumps blood through
blood vessels

**artery**

Carries blood away
from the heart

**vein**

Carries blood
toward the heart

**capillary**

Exchange site between
blood and tissues

**Figure 6-12** The cardiovascular system, also known as the circulatory system, consists of the heart, blood vessels, and blood.

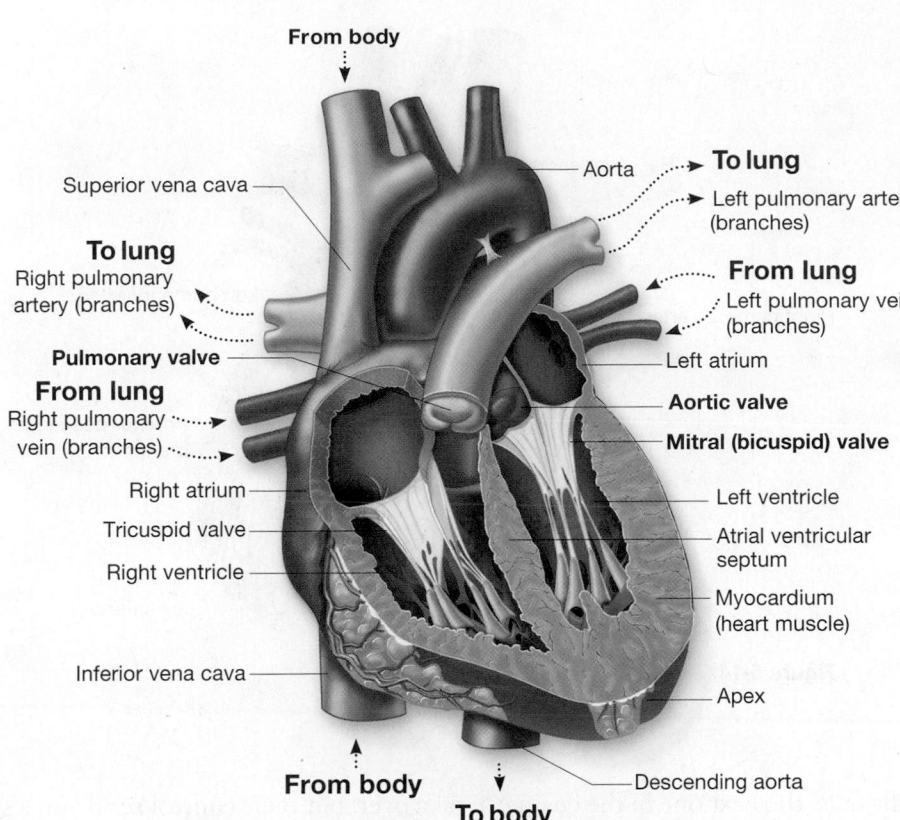

From body

Superior vena cava

Aorta

**To lung**
Left pulmonary artery (branches)

**To lung**
Right pulmonary artery (branches)

**From lung**
Left pulmonary vein (branches)

**Pulmonary valve**

Left atrium

**From lung**
Right pulmonary vein (branches)

**Aortic valve**

**Mitral (bicuspid) valve**

Right atrium

Left ventricle

Tricuspid valve

Atrial ventricular septum

Right ventricle

Myocardium (heart muscle)

Inferior vena cava

Apex

**From body**

Descending aorta

**To body**

**Figure 6-13a** Blood flow through the chambers of the heart. The heart's four valves ensure that blood flows in one direction only.

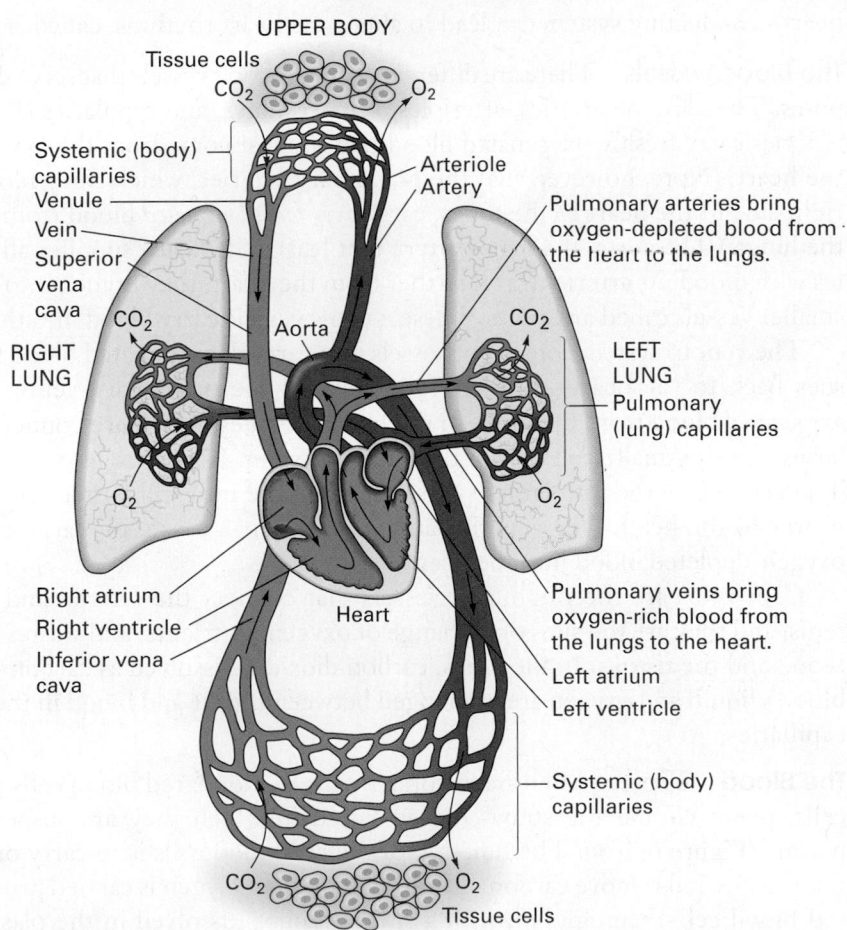

UPPER BODY

Tissue cells

$CO_2$     $O_2$

Systemic (body) capillaries

Arteriole
Artery

Venule

Vein

Superior vena cava

Pulmonary arteries bring oxygen-depleted blood from the heart to the lungs.

$CO_2$

Aorta

$CO_2$

RIGHT LUNG

LEFT LUNG

Pulmonary (lung) capillaries

$O_2$

$O_2$

Right atrium

Right ventricle

Heart

Inferior vena cava

Pulmonary veins bring oxygen-rich blood from the lungs to the heart.

Left atrium

Left ventricle

Systemic (body) capillaries

$CO_2$     $O_2$

Tissue cells

LOWER BODY

**Figure 6-13b** Blood flow throughout the entire cardiovascular system.

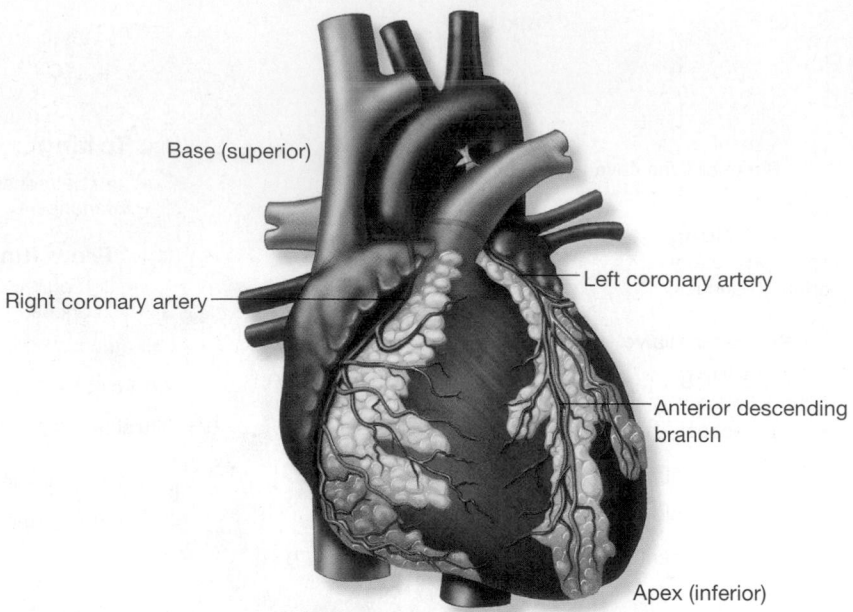

Base (superior)

Right coronary artery

Left coronary artery

Anterior descending branch

Apex (inferior)

**Figure 6-14** The coronary arteries.

cells fails, the next one in the chain can take over, but their control results in a slower heart rate, and often less-coordinated contractions. In addition, abnormalities in the heart's conducting system can lead to abnormal heart rhythms, called arrhythmias.

**The Blood Vessels** There are different types of blood vessels that serve different purposes. They are the arteries, arterioles, veins, venules, and capillaries (Figure 6-15■). Arteries carry freshly oxygenated blood that has just come from the lungs away from the heart. (Note, however, that the pulmonary arteries, which carry blood from the right side of the heart to the lungs, carry *oxygenated-depleted* blood from the heart to the lungs.) The aorta, the major artery that leaves the heart, supplies all other arteries with blood. As arteries travel farther from the heart, they branch into increasingly smaller vessels called arterioles. These narrow vessels carry blood into the capillaries.

The venous system consists of vessels that carry deoxygenated blood from the tissues back to the heart—with the exception of the pulmonary veins, which carry *oxygenated* blood from the lungs to the heart. Venules, which are connected to capillaries, are the smallest vessels in the venous system. Like arteries, veins vary in size. The venules merge into larger veins, which merge into still larger veins as they get nearer to the heart. The superior and inferior venae cavae, the largest veins, drain oxygen-depleted blood into the heart.

Capillaries are the tiny blood vessels that connect the arterial and venous systems, and they are the sites of exchange of oxygen, nutrients, and wastes between the blood and the tissues. In the lungs, carbon dioxide, dissolved as carbonic acid in the blood's liquid and oxygen are exchanged between the air and blood in the pulmonary capillaries.

**The Blood** There are four main components of blood: red blood cells, white blood cells, platelets, and the straw-colored liquid in which they are suspended, called plasma (Figure 6-16■). The function of the red blood cells is to carry oxygen to the body's cells and remove carbon dioxide from them. Oxygen is carried primarily by the red blood cell's hemoglobin, with a small amount dissolved in the plasma. Carbon dioxide is dissolved primarily in the plasma, with a small amount carried by the red

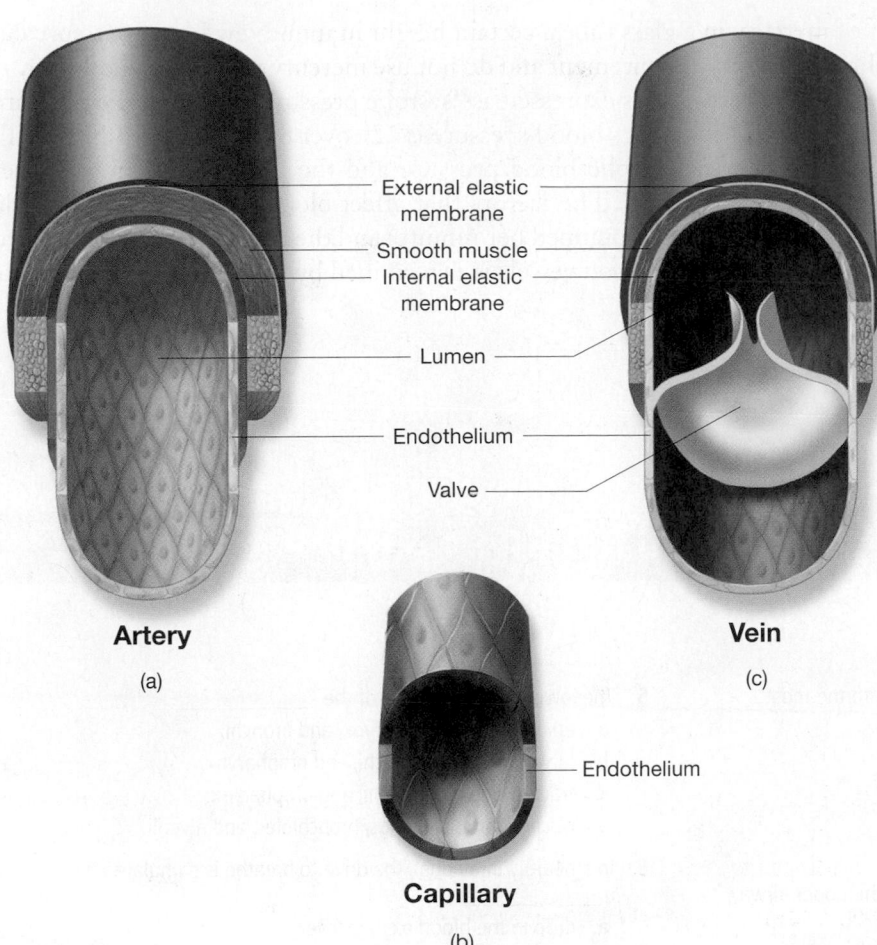

**Figure 6-15** The three major types of blood vessels: arteries, capillaries, and veins.

**Figure 6-16** The main components of blood: red blood cells, white blood cells, and platelets, which are suspended in the plasma.

blood cells. The iron in the hemoglobin of red blood cells gives blood its red color and is necessary for oxygen transport.

White blood cells are part of the body's immune system helping the body defend itself against infection. There are several types of white blood cells, each providing defense against different microorganisms. Platelets are the component of blood that (along with specialized proteins in the plasma) forms blood clots to stop the loss of blood during hemorrhaging. Plasma is the straw colored or clear liquid component of blood that carries the blood cells and nutrients to the tissues, as well as waste products away to the organs involved in excretion.

## Physiology of the Circulatory System

As the heart pumps blood from the left ventricle to the body, a wave of pressure referred to as blood pressure can be felt by palpating arterial pulse points. Blood pressure consists of two measures: the systolic pressure (when the left ventricle maximally contracts) and the diastolic pressure (when the left ventricle is at rest). The blood pressure is measured in millimeters (mm) of mercury, or the amount of pressure needed to raise a

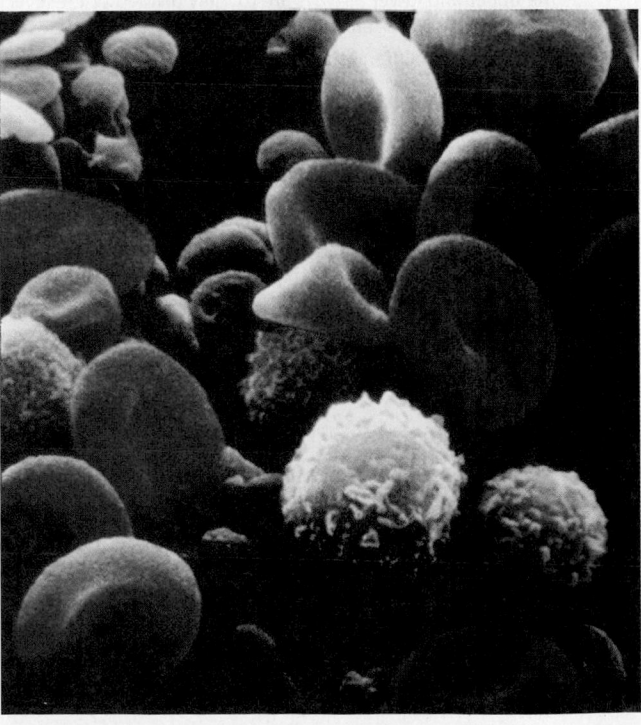

column of mercury in a glass tube a certain height in mm. New blood pressure cuffs are calibrated for this measurement and do not use mercury in a glass tube as they did in the past. Blood pressure is expressed as "systolic pressure over diastolic pressure," which means that the patient's blood pressure is 120 over 80 (written as 120/80). The difference between the systolic blood pressure and the diastolic blood pressure is known as the pulse pressure. The factors that affect blood pressure are the cardiac output (the volume of blood pumped per minute) and the resistance in the blood vessels. The resistance in the blood vessels is determined by the amount of constriction or dilation in the arterioles.

## STOP, THINK, UNDERSTAND

### Multiple Choice
Choose the correct answer.

1. The correct sequence from the simplest system to the most complex system is_____
   a. body system, organs, tissues, cells.
   b. organs, tissues, body system, cells.
   c. cells, tissues, organs, body system.
   d. cells, organs, tissues, body system.

2. What is the correct sequence for structures in the upper airway, from superior to inferior?_____
   a. Epiglottis, larynx, pharynx, jaw, tongue, teeth, mouth, nose
   b. Nose, mouth, teeth, tongue, jaw, pharynx, larynx, epiglottis
   c. Nose, mouth, pharynx, bronchi, alveoli, epiglottis
   d. Pharynx, epiglottis, larynx, alveoli, bronchioles

3. The upper and lower airways are roughly divided at the level of the _____ and _____.
   a. diaphragm; intercostal muscles
   b. nose; throat
   c. vocal cords; larynx
   d. epiglottis; bronchi

4. Nasopharynx refers to _____, whereas oropharynx refers to_____.
   a. the part of the throat posterior to the nose; the posterior portion of the mouth to the throat
   b. the tip of the nose; the teeth and tongue
   c. the epiglottis; the vocal cords
   d. the bronchi; the lungs

5. The lower airway consists of the_____
   a. epiglottis, pharynx, larynx, and bronchi.
   b. larynx, pharynx, bronchi, and oropharynx.
   c. trachea, larynx, bronchi, and oropharynx.
   d. trachea, bronchi, lungs, bronchioles, and alveoli.

6. In a healthy individual, the drive to breathe is stimulated by a_____
   a. drop in the blood oxygen level.
   b. rise in the blood oxygen level.
   c. drop in the blood carbon dioxide level.
   d. rise in the blood carbon dioxide level.

7. Which of the following is the correct sequence for the blood circulating through the heart, beginning with the superior and inferior venae cavae?_____
   a. Right atrium, right ventricle, pulmonary arteries, lungs, left atrium, left ventricle, aorta, arteries, capillaries, veins
   b. Left atrium, left ventricle, pulmonary arteries, lungs, right atrium, right ventricle, capillaries, veins
   c. Right ventricle, right atrium, pulmonary veins, lungs, pulmonary arteries, right ventricle, left ventricle, aorta, capillaries, veins
   d. Left ventricle, left atrium, pulmonary veins, lungs, pulmonary arteries, right atrium, left atrium, aorta, capillaries, veins

### Fill in the Blank

1. The mechanical process of breathing occurs when: _____.
2. The cardiovascular system consists of the _____, _____, and _____.
3. The four primary components of the blood are _____, _____, _____, and _____.
4. Basically, arteries carry _____ blood_____the heart, whereas veins carry_____blood_____the heart.

# The Nervous System

The **nervous system** is the most complex of all the body systems. The center of the nervous system, the brain, is responsible for the control of all the other body systems. The brain coordinates the function of sensation, regulates the motor system, and integrates consciousness, memory, emotions, and the use of language.

**nervous system** a group of organs and other structures that regulate all body functions.

## Anatomy of the Nervous System

The nervous system can be divided into two main anatomical parts: the central nervous system and the peripheral nervous system (Figure 6-17■). The central nervous system consists of the brain and spinal cord. Both are encased in bone (the brain within the skull, and the spinal cord within the vertebrae).

The brain can be divided into three major portions: the cerebrum, the cerebellum, and the brainstem (Figure 6-18■). The cerebrum, the largest and outermost structure of the brain, is responsible for higher functions such as thought, memory, and the voluntary use of muscles. The cerebellum is beneath the cerebrum and is responsible for certain constant and involuntary functions such as coordinating movement. Lastly, the brainstem is the most primitive part of the brain and is the brain's connection with the spinal cord. The brainstem is the control center for vital functions, including respiration, cardiac function, and vasomotor status (dilation and constriction of the blood vessels). The pons and the medulla oblongata are parts of the brainstem.

The brain and spinal cord are covered by three protective layers, collectively known as the meninges (Figure 6-19■), which are in turn protected by the bones of the skull, the vertebrae and soft tissues. Circulating within these layers, bathing the brain and spinal cord and providing further protection, is cerebrospinal fluid (CSF).

The outer meningeal layer, known as the dura mater, is a tough, fibrous membrane that lies just inside the skull and within the vertebral canal and covers the brain and spinal cord like a sheet. In several places, the dura mater folds inward to separate the larger portions of the brain from each other, providing support for the brain and dispersing forces generated in a traumatic injury. The middle meningeal layer, the arachnoid mater, is transparent and gets its name from the web-like pattern its cells exhibit when viewed under a microscope. The pia mater is the finest of the meninges and lies in intimate contact with the convoluted surface of the brain.

Cerebrospinal fluid (CSF) is a clear, colorless fluid that is produced inside the brain and circulates throughout the central nervous system in a network of canals within the meninges. The CSF provides three beneficial properties:

+ **Buoyancy.** The brain and CSF are of similar density, so the brain neither sinks nor floats in CSF but exists in suspension.
+ **Cushioning/protection.** CSF protects the brain from striking the inside of the skull.
+ **Chemical stability.** The flow of CSF carries metabolic wastes away from the nervous system tissues and helps regulate chemical concentrations and pH.

The cerebrum constitutes the majority (approximately 75%) of the brain's mass and is responsible for higher functions such as sense perception, voluntary movement, speech, thought, and memory. It is divided along the longitudinal fissure into left and right cerebral hemispheres. Much of the cerebrum's mass is white matter: nerve fibers (tracts) that connect "pools" of nerves. The rest of the cerebrum's mass is gray matter, composed mainly of neuron bodies. The cerebellum lies inferior to the posterior aspect of the cerebrum and superior to the brainstem. Like the cerebrum, it is divided into left and right hemispheres, and has an outer cortex composed of gray

# Nervous System

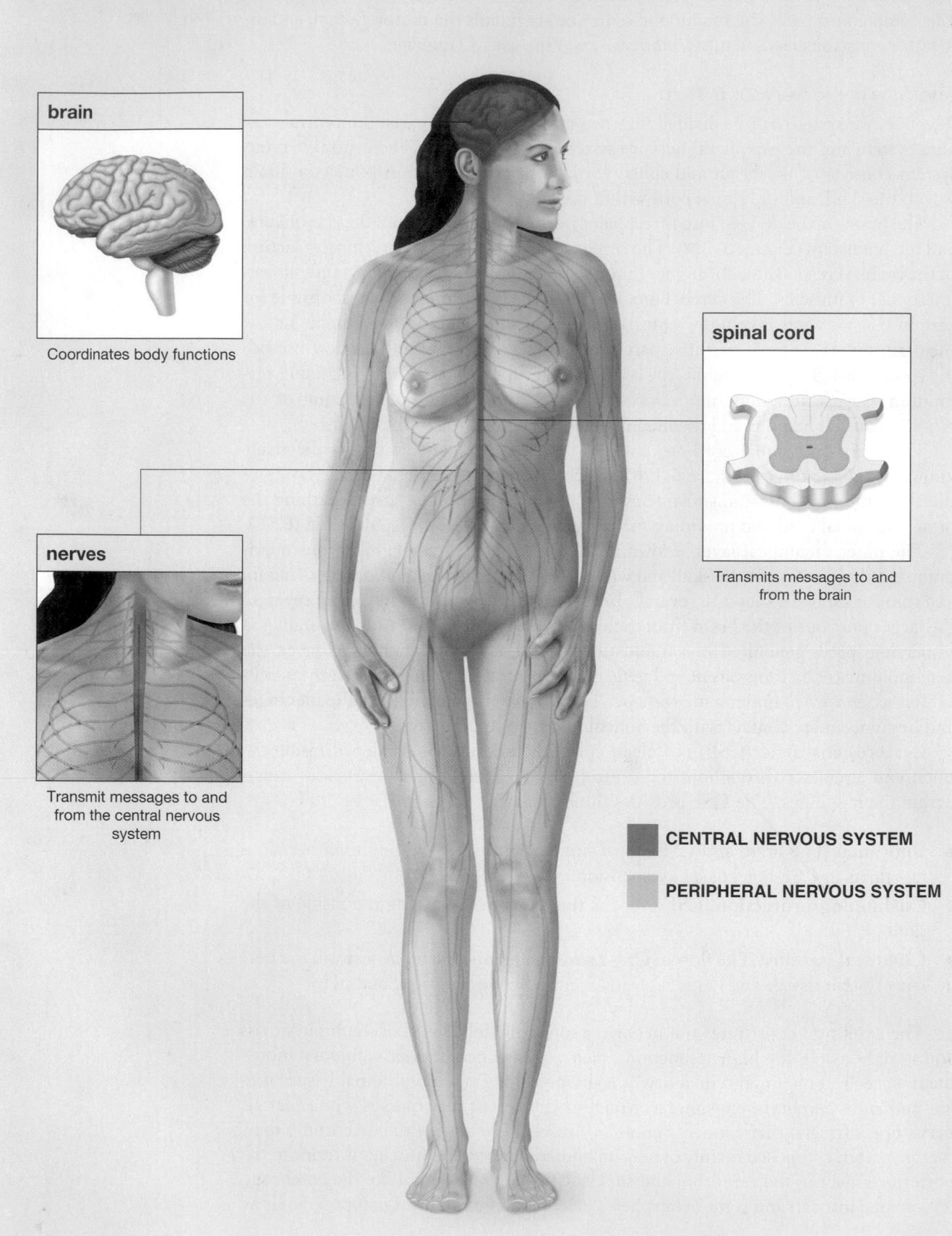

**brain**

Coordinates body functions

**spinal cord**

Transmits messages to and from the brain

**nerves**

Transmit messages to and from the central nervous system

■ CENTRAL NERVOUS SYSTEM

□ PERIPHERAL NERVOUS SYSTEM

**Figure 6-17** The nervous system, which is composed of the central nervous system and the peripheral nervous system.

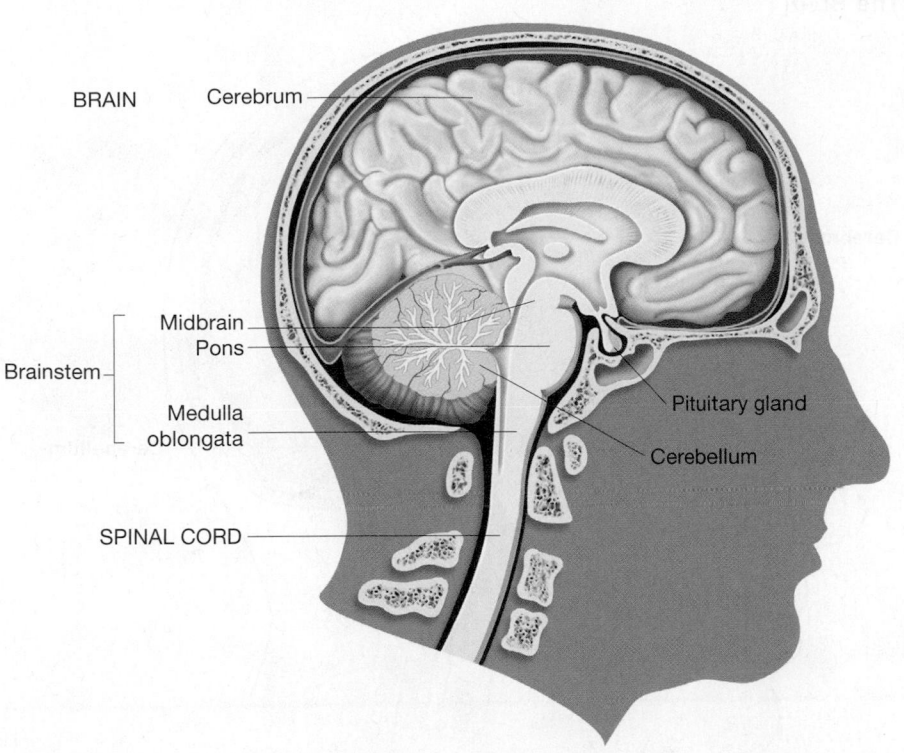

BRAIN
Cerebrum

Midbrain
Pons
Brainstem
Medulla
oblongata

Pituitary gland

Cerebellum

SPINAL CORD

matter surrounding an inner layer of white matter. Deep to the cerebellum is the brainstem. The brainstem gives rise to 12 cranial nerves that support important functions such as smell, sight, facial movement, and hearing, as well as the nerve fibers that become the spinal cord. In addition, the brainstem controls the most fundamental life-support functions of the body (Figure 6-20■).

The nerve fibers of the brain exit the base of the skull through the foramen magnum as the spinal cord, a ropelike bundle of nervous tissue that travels in the vertebral canal to about the level of the first lumbar vertebra (L1). Like the brain, the spinal cord is protected by CSF and the three layers of the meninges, and it is also protected

**Figure 6-19** The meninges, the layers of protective membranes covering the brain and spinal cord.

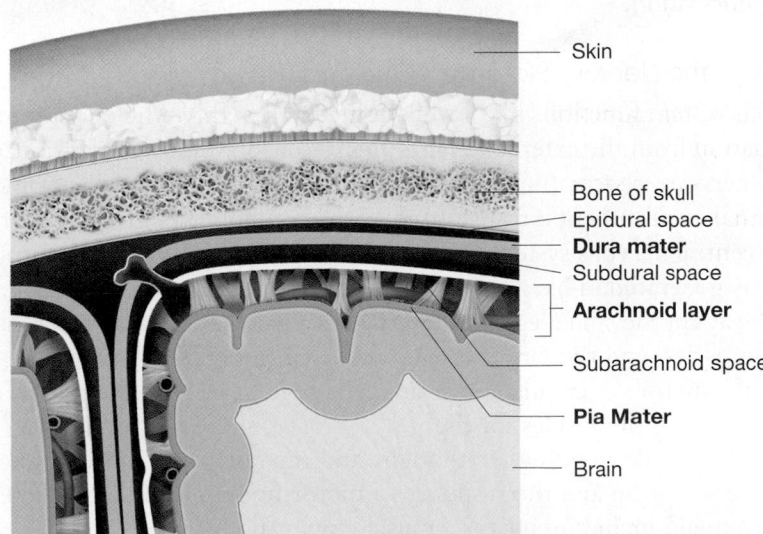

Skin

Bone of skull
Epidural space
**Dura mater**
Subdural space

**Arachnoid layer**

Subarachnoid space

**Pia Mater**

Brain

**Figure 6-20** A section showing some of the anatomical features of the brain.

**The Brain**

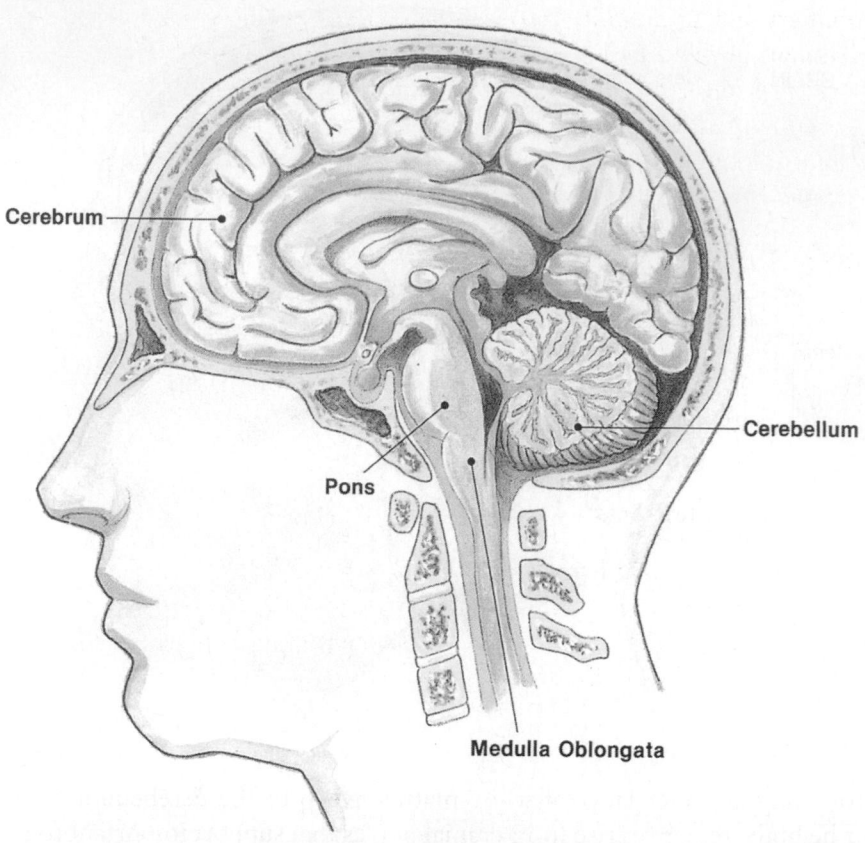

Cerebrum

Cerebellum

Pons

Medulla Oblongata

by the vertebral bodies. Below the level of L1, the nerve fibers of the spinal cord fan out in a structure known as the cauda equina, or "horse's tail," which represents the distal portion of the spinal cord.

The peripheral nervous system is the portion of the nervous system located outside the brain and spinal cord. It includes the nerves that attach to the spinal cord. These nerves carry sensory information from the body to the spinal cord and then the brain, and motor instructions from the brain through the spinal cord to the muscles. The neuron, the fundamental functional unit of the nervous system, is the cell that conducts information.

## Physiology of the Nervous System

The nervous system functions like a well-trained and highly efficient command center. Information from the external environment (sensory input) is transmitted by the peripheral nervous system (nerves and their branches), and information from the body's internal environment is transmitted by the autonomic (automatic) nervous system to the central nervous system (brain and spinal cord), where it is interpreted and a response is generated. This response is then transmitted from the brain, through motor pathways in the spinal cord, to target organs such as the heart, adrenal glands, or skeletal muscles, and the target organs act accordingly. For example, in response to a threat, the motor system may cause an increase in heart rate, the release of adrenaline, or the tensing of muscles for flight.

The cerebrum controls higher thought and memory and coordinates both the perception of sensation and the response of motor functions. The cerebellum coordinates movement, including posture, muscle tone, and balance.

The nervous system also can be divided into two functional systems: the voluntary and autonomic systems. The voluntary system controls movement of the muscles and transmits sensations from the sensory organs to the brain and spinal cord. The autonomic (or automatic) system is involuntary and controls the involuntary muscles of the organs and glands.

The autonomic system can be divided into two subsystems: the sympathetic and parasympathetic divisions. The sympathetic division controls the body's response to stressors such as pain, fear, or a sudden loss of blood. These actions are sometimes referred to as the "fight-or-flight" response. The effects of the parasympathetic division are the opposite of those of the sympathetic division (Figure 6-21■).

## The Gastrointestinal System

The **gastrointestinal (GI) system** consists of the organs that work together to process food and absorb water. Also known as the digestive system, the GI system is composed of the alimentary tract (food passageway) and several accessory organs that contribute to the digestive process. Together, the organs of the GI system break down food, absorb nutrients, and eliminate indigestible food components and some wastes (Figure 6-22■).

### Anatomy of the Gastrointestinal System

Food enters the digestive system through the mouth, is chewed, and then passes down the esophagus, the passageway to the stomach. The stomach and other major organs involved in this system are located in the abdominal cavity. Food travels from the stomach into the small intestine, where further digestion takes place and nutrients are absorbed through the intestinal wall into a group of venous blood vessels that collect blood from the small intestine called the hepatic portal system. The nutrients then go to the liver (for absorption and processing) before continuing on to the heart via the inferior vena cava. Waste products and substances that either cannot be digested or are undigested pass into the large intestine, or colon, where water is absorbed and the remaining waste is passed through the rectum and anus as feces. The large intestine also functions with other body systems in maintaining water balance. This is why patients with significant diarrhea can have such profound dehydration.

The liver, the largest organ in the abdomen, aids in the digestion of fats by producing bile. The gallbladder stores the bile. The liver also is responsible for breaking down many toxic substances absorbed through the intestines and for producing many of the major proteins needed in the body. The pancreas secretes pancreatic juices that aid in the digestion of fats, starches, and proteins. It is also where the sugar-regulating hormones insulin and glucagon (products of the endocrine system, to be discussed later) are produced.

Digestion occurs both mechanically and chemically. Mechanical digestion refers to the physical breaking down of food that begins with chewing, swallowing, and moving the food through the digestive tract. Chemical digestion refers to the process whereby chemicals break foods down into components the body can absorb, such as fatty acids and amino acids.

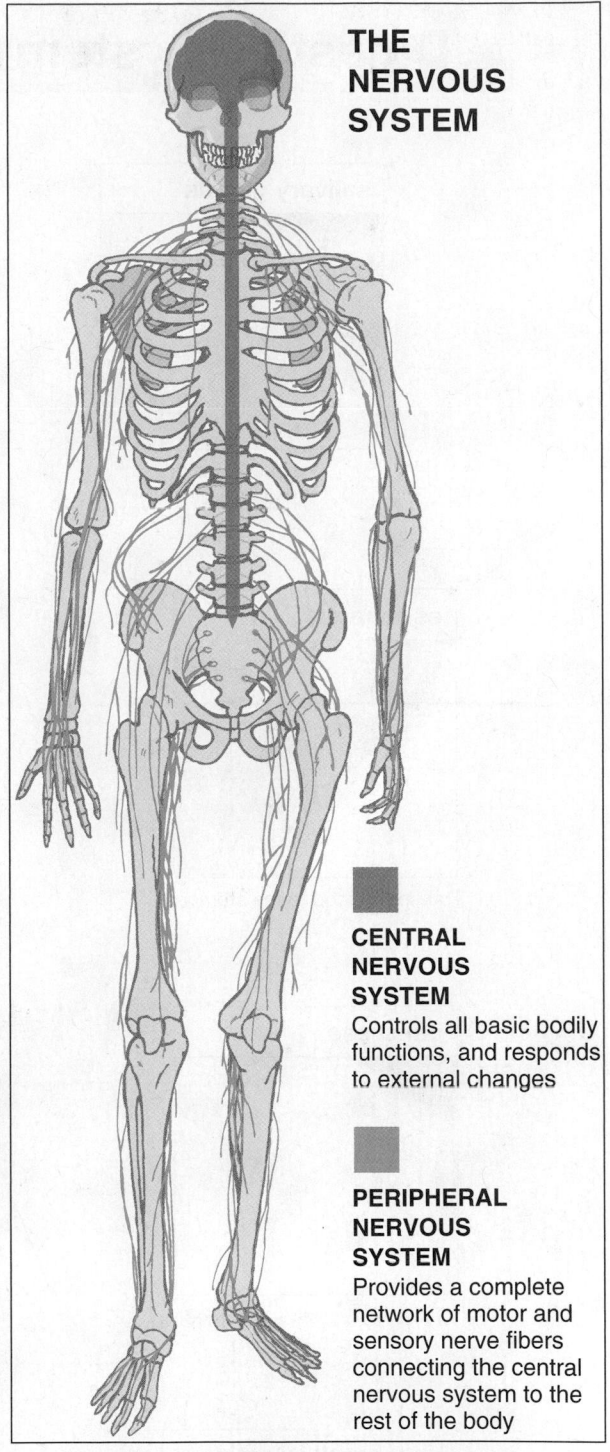

THE NERVOUS SYSTEM

**CENTRAL NERVOUS SYSTEM**
Controls all basic bodily functions, and responds to external changes

**PERIPHERAL NERVOUS SYSTEM**
Provides a complete network of motor and sensory nerve fibers connecting the central nervous system to the rest of the body

**Figure 6-21** The systems of the autonomic nervous system: the sympathetic and parasympathetic divisions and their effects on organs and the central and peripheral nervous system.

**gastrointestinal system** a group of organs and other structures that break down food and absorb nutrients into the body.

# Digestive System

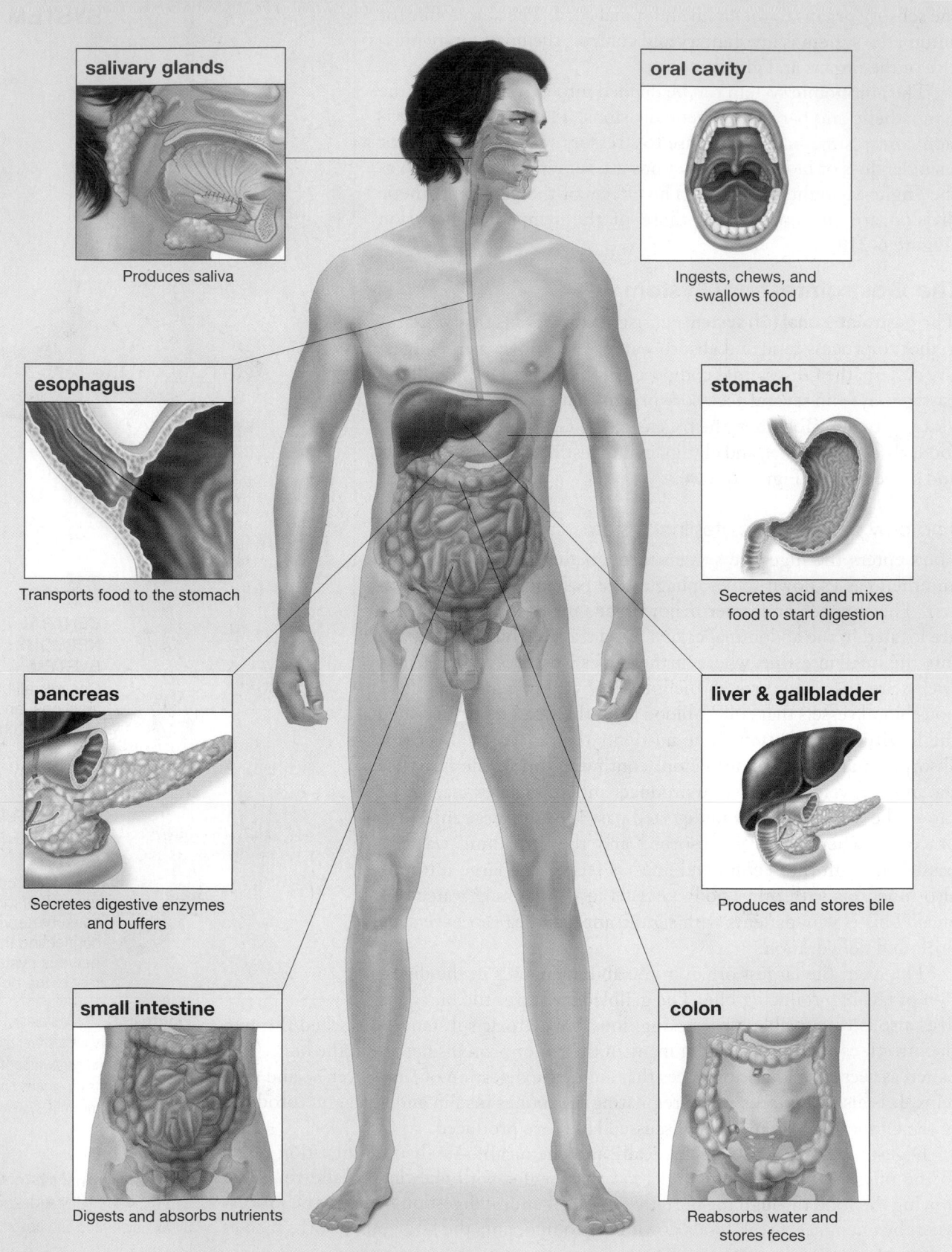

**salivary glands**

Produces saliva

**oral cavity**

Ingests, chews, and swallows food

**esophagus**

Transports food to the stomach

**stomach**

Secretes acid and mixes food to start digestion

**pancreas**

Secretes digestive enzymes and buffers

**liver & gallbladder**

Produces and stores bile

**small intestine**

Digests and absorbs nutrients

**colon**

Reabsorbs water and stores feces

**Figure 6-22** The organs of the digestive system break down food, absorb water and nutrients, and eliminate wastes.

## Physiology of Digestion

The process of chemical digestion begins in the mouth, where enzymes in saliva, produced by the salivary glands (Figure 6-23■), break starches down into sugars. Next, hydrochloric acid produced by cells that line the stomach digests the food into smaller elements. Pancreatic enzymes further break proteins and starches into amino acids and sugars, respectively. Bile, which is secreted by the liver and stored in the gall bladder, then breaks down fats into small absorbable units. Next, the small intestines absorb sugars, amino acids, and small fat units through the wall of the intestine into the bloodstream, using the rich vasculature present in the intestinal wall. Toxins also can be absorbed in this process. This nutrient-rich blood then passes through the liver, where some nutrients are processed, while other nutrients in the blood travel directly to the organs of the body. Toxins can harm the liver or may be neutralized by it.

Unused food and some wastes from the liver (including old red blood cells) end up in the large intestine. Stool, also known as feces, gets its characteristic brown color from the breakdown of old red blood cells. The material passing through the small intestines is liquid, so the large intestine absorbs water out of this material, making it solid, formed stool. Gas-forming bacteria that that are normal residents in the intestines aid in the digestion of the food, and they also create noxious gases, primarily methane. Both the stool and the gas are expelled from the anus.

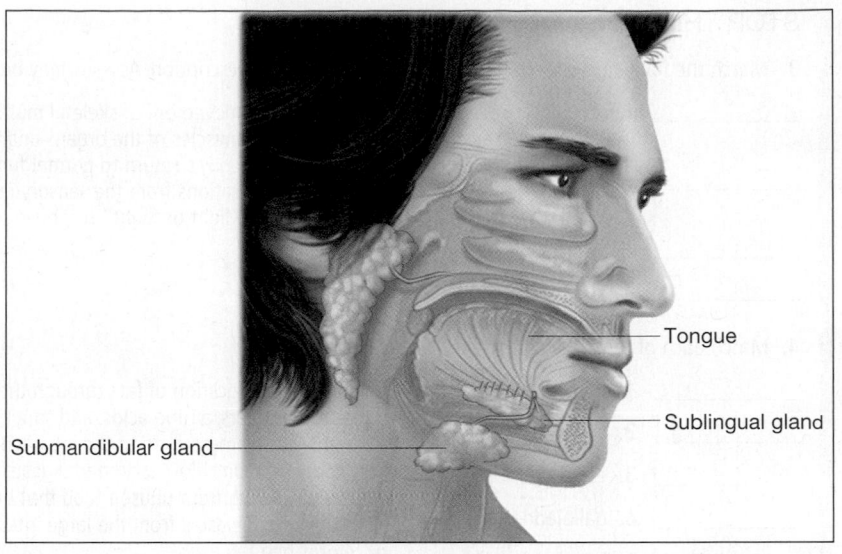

**Figure 6-23** The parotid, sublingual, and submandibular salivary glands, whose ducts empty into the oral cavity.

Tongue

Sublingual gland

Submandibular gland

# STOP, THINK, UNDERSTAND

## Multiple Choice

Choose the correct answer.

1. The central nervous system is protected by_____
   a. the cerebrum, pons, and medulla.
   b. the vertebrae, skull, meninges, and cerebrospinal fluid.
   c. the skull, cerebellum, cranium, and pons.
   d. the dura mater, glia mater, vertebra, and pia mater.

2. The cauda equina is best defined as:_____
   a. the site where the spinal cord leaves the brain through the foramen magnum.

   b. the center-most portion of the brain.
   c. the bony covering of the vertebrae that protects the spinal cord.
   d. the area below the first lumbar vertebra (L1) where the spinal cord fans out into a "horse's tail" structure.

3. Gas passed out of the anus is primarily_____
   a. ethanol.
   b. methane.
   c. glucagon.
   d. sulfur monoxide.

## Matching

1. Match each of the following portions of the brain with its description.

   _____ **1.** brainstem
   _____ **2.** cerebellum
   _____ **3.** cerebrum

   a. control center for vital functions, including respiration and cardiac function
   b. site of higher functions such as thought, memory, and voluntary use of muscles
   c. coordinates movement and balance

2. Match each of the following parts of the meninges with its description.

   _____ **1.** arachnoid mater
   _____ **2.** dura mater
   _____ **3.** pia mater

   a. tough, fibrous membrane that lies immediately deep to the skull and inside the vertebral canal; covers the brain and spinal cord like a sheet; provides support for the brain and disperses forces generated in traumatic injury
   b. transparent middle meningeal layer
   c. finest of the meninges; lies in direct contact with the convoluted surfaces of the brain

*continued*

STOP, THINK, UNDERSTAND *continued*

3. Match the following aspects of the nervous system to its description. Aspects may be used more than once.

_____ 1. involuntary (autonomic) system

_____ 2. parasympathetic division

_____ 3. sympathetic division

_____ 4. voluntary system

    a. controls the movement of skeletal muscles
    b. controls the muscles of the organs and glands
    c. controls the body's return to normal functions after such responses as "fight or flight"
    d. controls sensations from the sensory organs back to the brain and spinal cord
    e. controls the "fight or flight" response

4. Match each of the following structures to its description.

_____ 1. anus

_____ 2. colon

_____ 3. esophagus

_____ 4. gallbladder

_____ 5. large intestine

_____ 6. liver

_____ 7. pancreas

_____ 8. rectum

_____ 9. small intestine

_____ 10. stomach

    a. aids in the digestion of fats through the production of bile
    b. absorbs sugars, amino acids, and small fat units into the bloodstream
    c. transports chewed food to the stomach
    d. produces hydrochloric acid and digests food
    e. absorbs water from unused food that becomes feces
    f. moves solid wastes from the large intestine to the anus
    g. stores bile
    h. another word for large intestine
    i. creates juices that aid in the digestion of fats, starches, and proteins and produces insulin and glucagon
    j. moves solid and gaseous wastes out of the body

## Fill in the Blank

1. The central nervous system (CNS) consists of the _____ and _____.

2. The three beneficial properties of CSF are_____, _____, and _____.

3. Which of the following are true of the peripheral nervous system? (check all that apply)

_____ a. The PNS originates in the brain and spinal cord.

_____ b. The PNS is located outside of the brain and spinal cord.

_____ c. The PNS carries sensory information in the body to and from the spinal cord and brain.

_____ d. The PNS carries sensory information between the spinal cord and the brain.

_____ e. Neurons are the fundamental functional units of the nervous system.

_____ f. Capillaries are the fundamental functional units of the nervous system.

 # CASE UPDATE

You contact dispatch to request immediate assistance. You also request that equipment and two toboggans be brought to the scene. As you approach the woman, you see that she is sitting down, holding the left side of her abdomen just below the rib cage at the junction of the thoracic and abdominal cavities. She states that her "stomach and ribs hurt." The other patient is lying nearby on the ground and is grabbing at his left upper leg. He appears to be confused and complains of pain in his posterior neck. You perform a complete assessment on both patients. Based on your findings and your knowledge of anatomy, you suspect that the female patient may have injuries involving the skeletal, gastrointestinal, and circulatory systems. You are concerned that she may have internal bleeding within the thoracic cavity, the abdominal cavity, or both. You suspect the male patient has serious musculoskeletal, cardiovascular, and nervous system-related injuries.

***How would you more accurately describe these injuries to the arriving OEC Technicians?***

# The Urinary System

The **urinary system** consists of organs and other structures involved in the elimination of waste products that are filtered from the blood by the kidneys and excreted in urine. These waste products include the normal by-products of the body's metabolism and some toxins that may have been introduced into the blood.

## Anatomy of the Urinary System

The urinary system consists of the kidneys, ureters, urinary bladder, and urethra (Figure 6-24■). The kidneys are located in the lower back outside the abdominal cavity at the lower margin of the rib cage, one on each side. The ureters carry the urine from the kidneys to the bladder. The bladder is a small, muscular sac that stores the urine until it is excreted. The urethra carries the urine from the bladder and out of the body.

## Physiology of the Urinary System

The kidneys produce urine by filtering metabolic wastes from the circulating blood. The kidneys are under the control of several endocrine organs and regulate water balance in the body by either increasing or decreasing the amount of sodium chloride (a salt) that is excreted. If salt is retained, water is retained. If salt is excreted in the urine, water also is excreted. This system also functions in maintaining the balance of other electrolytes and in controlling the pH of the blood.

# The Endocrine System

The **endocrine system** is made up of ductless glands that secrete hormones, which are chemical substances that enter the bloodstream and influence a variety of functions in different parts of the body (e.g., strength, stature, hair growth, and behavior).

## Anatomy of the Endocrine System

The body contains several important endocrine glands (Figure 6-25■). The hypothalamus and pituitary glands are located in the brain and control many of the other endocrine glands. The pituitary gland, also known as the "master gland," secretes chemicals into the bloodstream that regulate growth and the activities of many other glands. The hypothalamus secretes hormones that act on the pituitary gland. The hypothalamus also helps control the regulation of water excretion by the kidneys.

The thyroid gland, located in the anterior neck, regulates metabolism, growth, and development. It also partially regulates nervous system activity.

The adrenal glands are located on top of the kidneys and secrete several hormones, including epinephrine (adrenalin) and norepinephrine (noradrenaline), which function in the "fight-or-flight" response and affect heart rate, digestive system function, and the contraction of smooth muscles, including those in the lungs and blood vessels. The pancreas, located in the middle of the abdomen, has both an endocrine function (the secretion of hormones that regulate blood glucose) and non-endocrine functions. The gonads (ovaries and testes) produce hormones that control reproduction and sex characteristics. The pineal gland is a tiny gland in the brain that helps regulate daily wake/sleep patterns.

## Physiology of the Endocrine System

One of the critical functions of the endocrine system is the control of blood glucose levels. The pancreas produces and secretes insulin, which lowers the level of glucose in the blood and permits cells to use glucose. The pancreas also releases glucagon, which raises the level of glucose in the blood by facilitating the conversion of stored carbohydrates into glucose.

# Urinary System

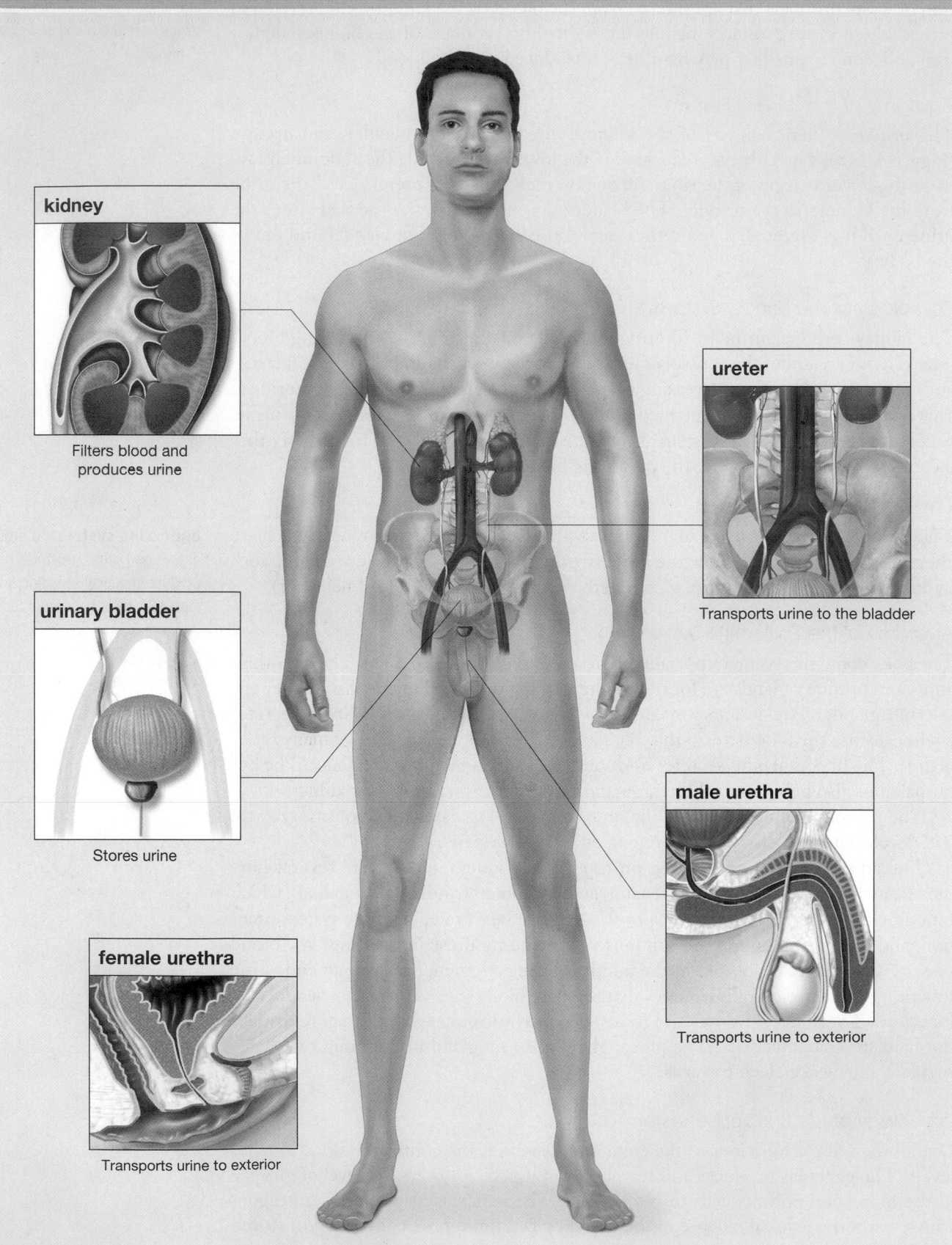

**kidney**

Filters blood and produces urine

**ureter**

Transports urine to the bladder

**urinary bladder**

Stores urine

**male urethra**

Transports urine to exterior

**female urethra**

Transports urine to exterior

**Figure 6-24** The kidneys, ureters, bladder, and urethra make up the urinary system.

# Endocrine System

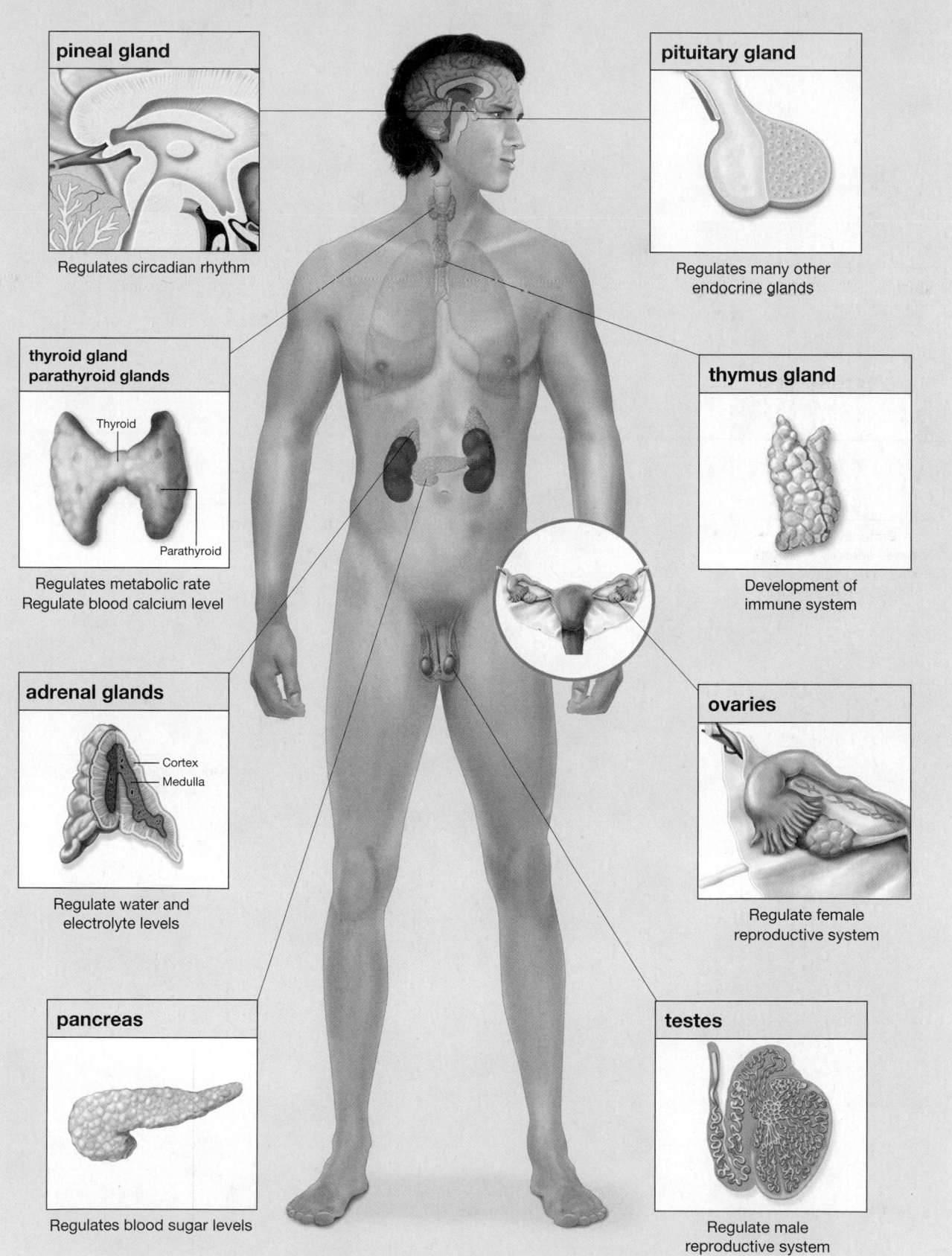

**pineal gland**

Regulates circadian rhythm

**pituitary gland**

Regulates many other
endocrine glands

**thyroid gland
parathyroid glands**

Thyroid

Parathyroid

Regulates metabolic rate
Regulate blood calcium level

**thymus gland**

Development of
immune system

**adrenal glands**

Cortex
Medulla

Regulate water and
electrolyte levels

**ovaries**

Regulate female
reproductive system

**pancreas**

Regulates blood sugar levels

**testes**

Regulate male
reproductive system

**Figure 6-25** The structures of the endocrine system secrete hormones that influence activity in different parts of the body.

# Integumentary System

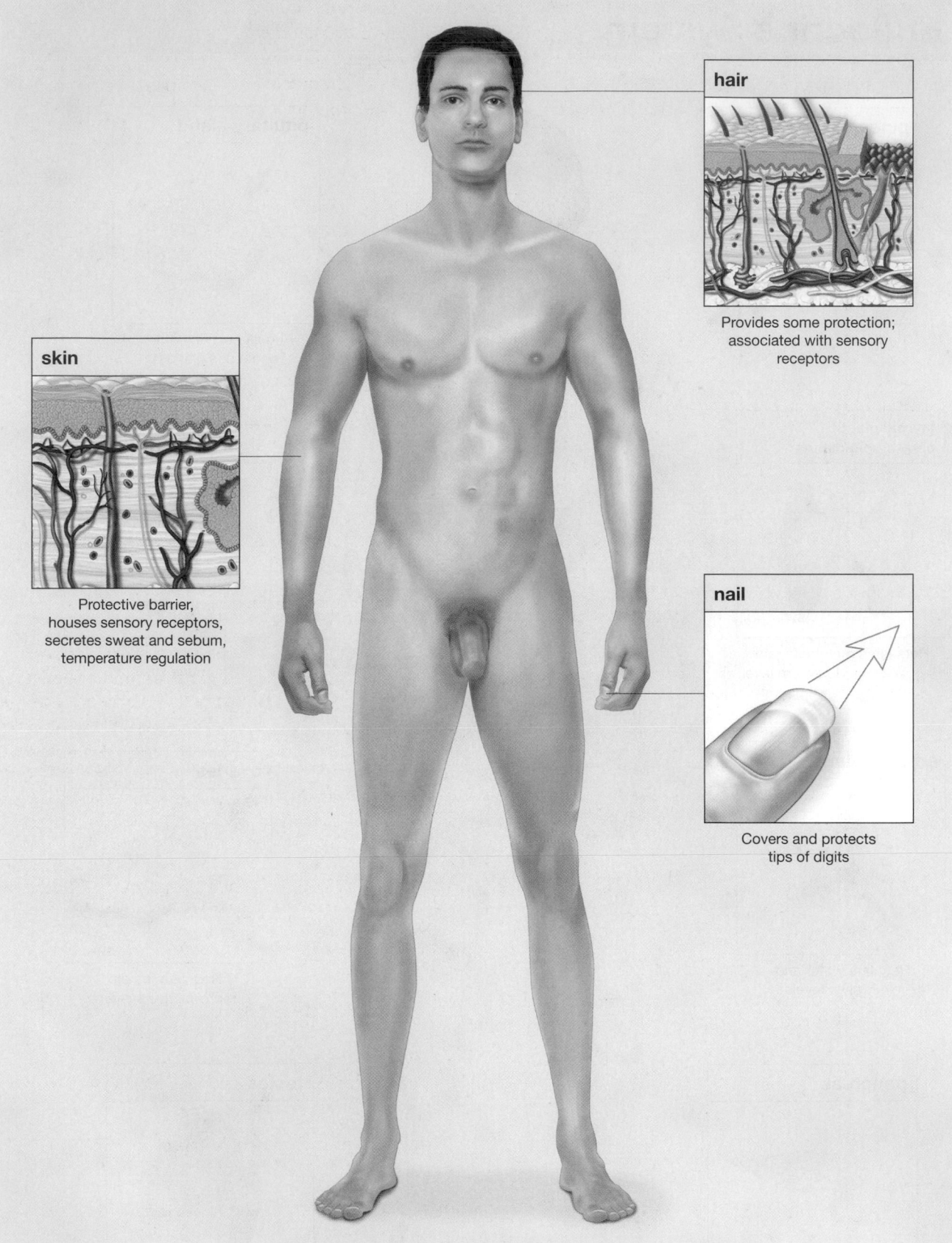

**hair**

Provides some protection; associated with sensory receptors

**skin**

Protective barrier, houses sensory receptors, secretes sweat and sebum, temperature regulation

**nail**

Covers and protects tips of digits

**Figure 6-26** The integumentary system consists of skin, hair, nails, sweat glands, and oil glands.

The sympathetic nervous system is regulated through the endocrine system. Adrenaline and noradrenaline, produced by the adrenal glands, cause multiple effects on the sympathetic system, including constricting of vessels, increased heart rate, and dilation of smooth muscles, including those that control respirations and the size of the bronchi.

The adrenal glands and pituitary gland affect kidney function by regulating water and salt balance.

## The Integumentary System

The **integumentary system** consists of the skin, hair, nails, sweat glands, and oil glands (Figure 6-26■). The skin provides a protective barrier that separates our tissues, organs, and other systems from the outside world.

### Anatomy of the Integumentary System

The skin is the body's largest organ. It has two major layers: the superficial epidermis contains the skin's pigmentation and the dermis contains blood vessels, nerves, glands, and hair and is the primary source of the skin's elasticity and strength. Under these layers is the deep subcutaneous layer, which is made up of fatty tissue (Figure 6-27■).

### Physiology of the Integumentary System

The skin not only is the largest organ system in the body, it also serves several major functions, which include protection of the body from injury and invasion from bacteria and other disease-producing pathogens. The skin serves as one of the major organs in the regulation of fluid balance and body temperature. When blood vessels in the dermis dilate, the blood circulates close to the skin's surface, allowing for the release of heat. When those blood vessels constrict, less blood flows to the skin's surface, causing the skin to appear pale or ashen and feel cool. This helps to conserve heat in the body by keeping the blood closer to the body's core. The evaporation of sweat produced by sweat glands in the skin also helps control body temperature.

## The Skeletal System

The **skeletal system** includes bones and ligaments that support the body's structure (Figure 6-28■). In addition, the skeletal system stores minerals such as calcium and is where the majority of blood cells are produced.

**integumentary system**    a group of specialized tissues that protect the body, retain fluids, and help prevent infection; the skin.

**skeletal system**    a group of specialized tissues that provide support to the body, provide attachment points for muscles, protect internal organs, allow movement, store minerals, and constitute one of the sites where blood cells are made; the bones.

**Figure 6-27** The two layers of the skin: the epidermis, dermis, and under these is the subcutaneous layer.

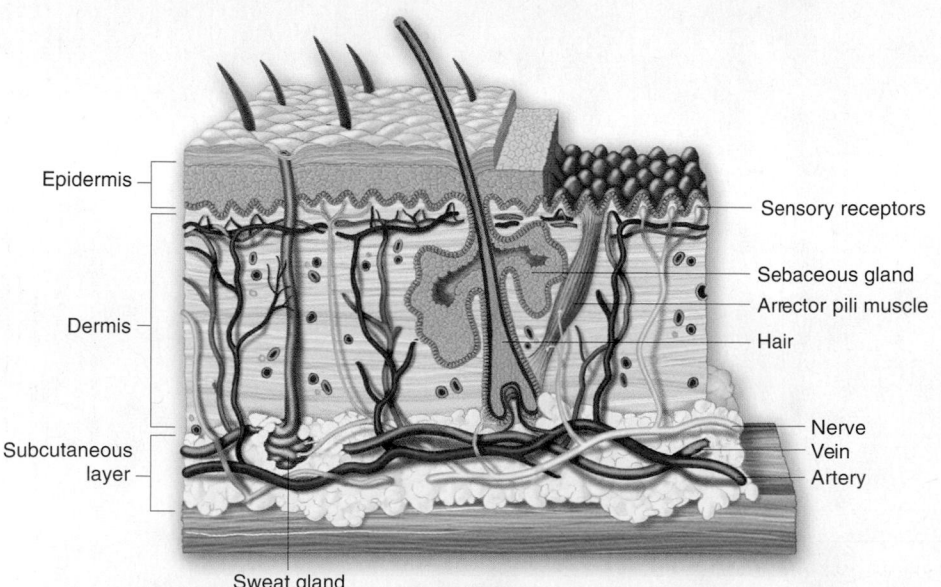

Epidermis

Dermis

Subcutaneous layer

Sweat gland

Sensory receptors

Sebaceous gland

Arrector pili muscle

Hair

Nerve
Vein
Artery

## Skeletal System

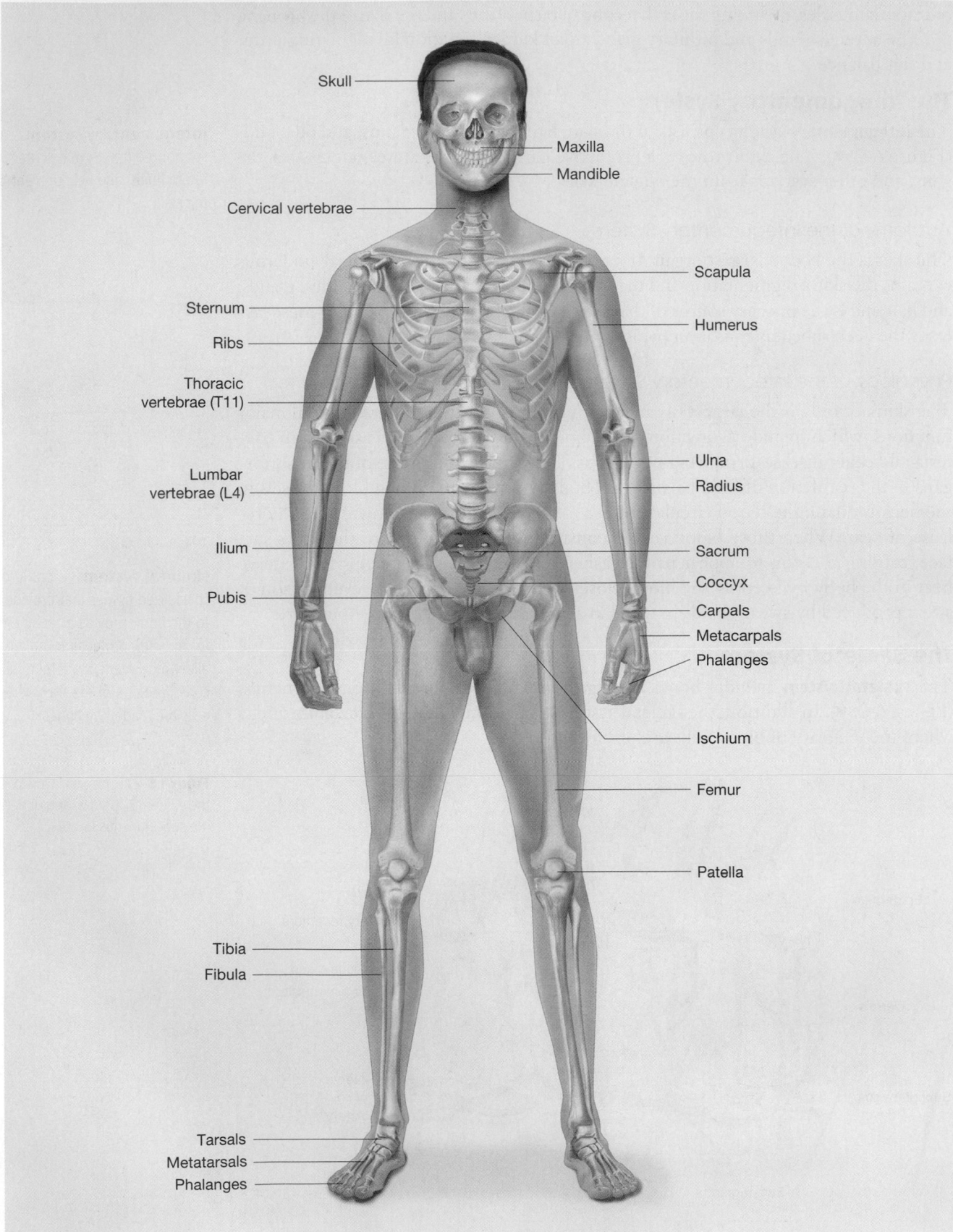

Skull

Maxilla

Mandible

Cervical vertebrae

Scapula

Sternum

Humerus

Ribs

Thoracic
vertebrae (T11)

Lumbar
vertebrae (L4)

Ulna

Radius

Ilium

Sacrum

Coccyx

Pubis

Carpals

Metacarpals

Phalanges

Ischium

Femur

Patella

Tibia

Fibula

Tarsals

Metatarsals

Phalanges

**Figure 6-28** An important function of the skeletal system is providing shape and form to the body.

## Anatomy of the Skeletal System

The adult skeleton has 206 bones. Bone is a hard, dense tissue that forms the skeleton. The outer region of a bone is called the cortex, and the inner region of the bone is the site of the marrow. Different bones have different sizes and shapes, enabling them to perform specific functions.

The skeleton forms the framework that supports the body. Where two or more bones join, they form a joint (Figure 6-29■). Strong, tough, fibrous bands called ligaments hold the bones at a joint together. Ligaments restrict joint movement based on their location. Most joints allow movement, but some (those in the skull) are immovable, and others (those in the pelvis) allow only slight movement. Movable joints have a normal range of motion—a distance they can move freely without causing injury.

The most common types of movable joints are the ball-and-socket joints such as the hip and shoulder, and hinged joints such as the elbow, knee, and finger joints. Different types of joints have different amounts of stability and allow different degrees of flexibility and types of movement.

Long bones generally form the arms and legs, whereas flat bones form the skull and pelvis. Spinal bones have a unique shape of their own.

The skeleton consists of six sections: the skull, spinal column, thorax, pelvis, and upper and lower extremities:

✦ **Skull.** The various bones that make up the skull can be divided into two main parts: the cranium and the face (Figure 6-30■). The cranium houses the brain. It

**Figure 6-29** Examples of types of freely movable joints.

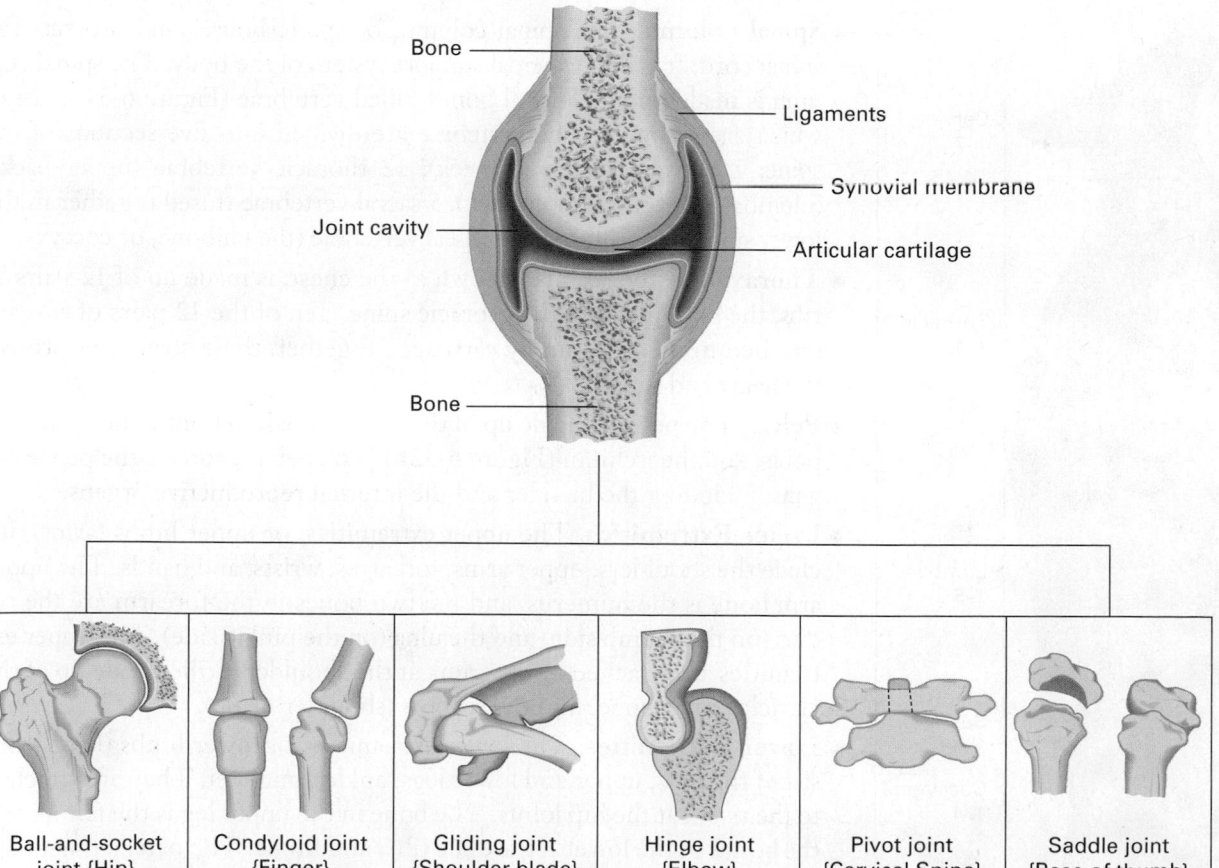

| Ball-and-socket joint {Hip} | Condyloid joint {Finger} | Gliding joint {Shoulder blade} | Hinge joint {Elbow} | Pivot joint {Cervical Spine} | Saddle joint {Base of thumb} |

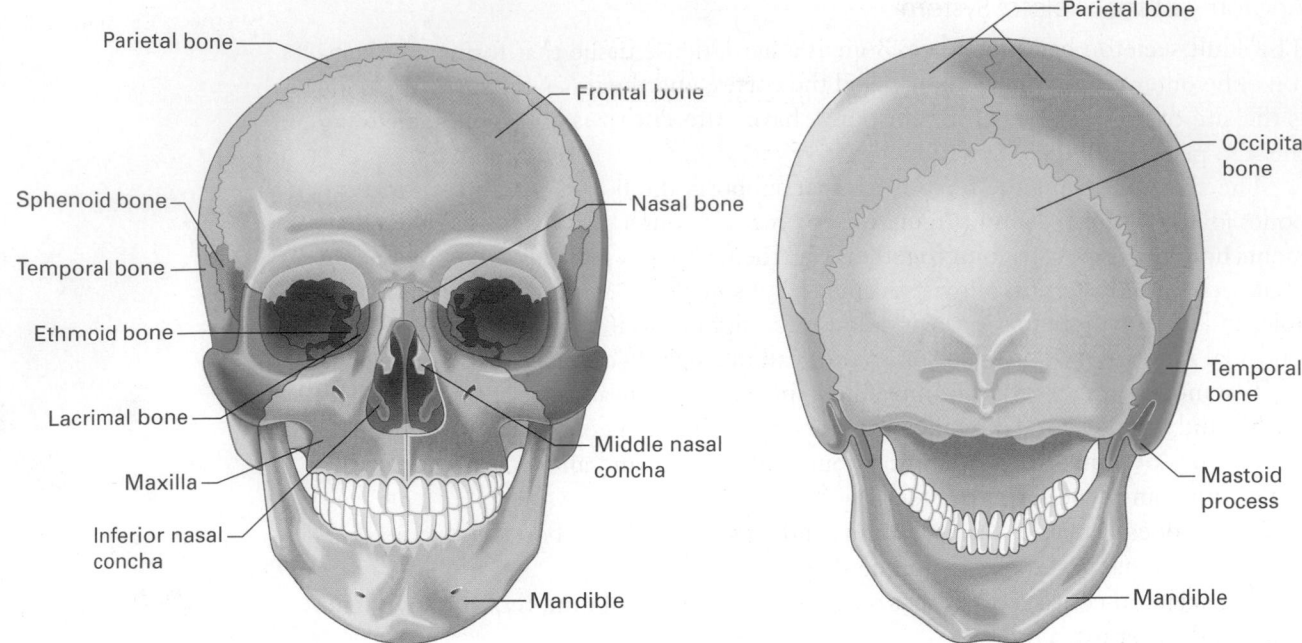

**Figure 6-30** The bones of the skull.

**Figure 6-31** The spinal column houses and protects the spinal cord and is divided into five sections.

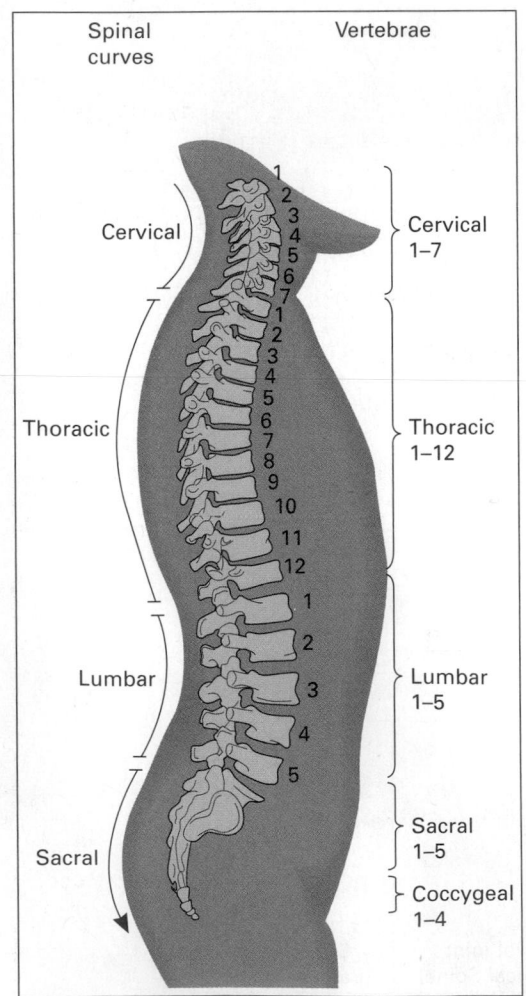

is made up of broad, flat bones that form the top, back, sides, front of the skull. Thirteen smaller bones plus the freely movable lower jaw (the mandible) make up the face.

+ **Spinal column.** The spinal column, or spine, houses and protects the spinal cord. It is the principal support system of the body. The spinal column is made up of 33 small bones called vertebrae (Figure 6-31■), 24 of which are movable. The vertebrae are divided into five sections of the spine: 7 cervical vertebrae (neck), 12 thoracic vertebrae (upper back), 5 lumbar vertebrae (lower back), 5 sacral vertebrae (fused together in the lower spine), and 4 fused coccygeal vertebrae (the tailbone, or coccyx).

+ **Thorax.** The thorax, also known as the chest, is made up of 12 pairs of ribs, the sternum, and the thoracic spine. Ten of the 12 pairs of ribs are attached to the sternum by cartilage. Together, these structures protect the heart and lungs.

+ **Pelvis.** The pelvis is made up of three sets of paired bones: the ilium, the pubis, and the ischium (Figure 6-32■). The pelvis protects the pelvic organs, including the bladder and the internal reproductive organs.

+ **Upper Extremities.** The upper extremities, or upper limbs (arms), include the shoulders, upper arms, forearms, wrists, and hands. The upper arm bone is the humerus, and the two bones in the forearm are the radius (on the thumb side) and the ulna (on the pinkie side). The upper extremities are attached to the trunk at the shoulder girdle, made up of the clavicle (collarbone) and the scapula (shoulder blade).

+ **Lower Extremities.** The lower extremities, or lower limbs (legs), consist of the hips, upper and lower legs, ankles, and feet. They are attached to the trunk at the hip joints. The bone in the upper leg is the femur, and the bones in the lower leg are the tibia and fibula. The patella (knee cap) is a small circular-shaped bone that protects the knee joint.

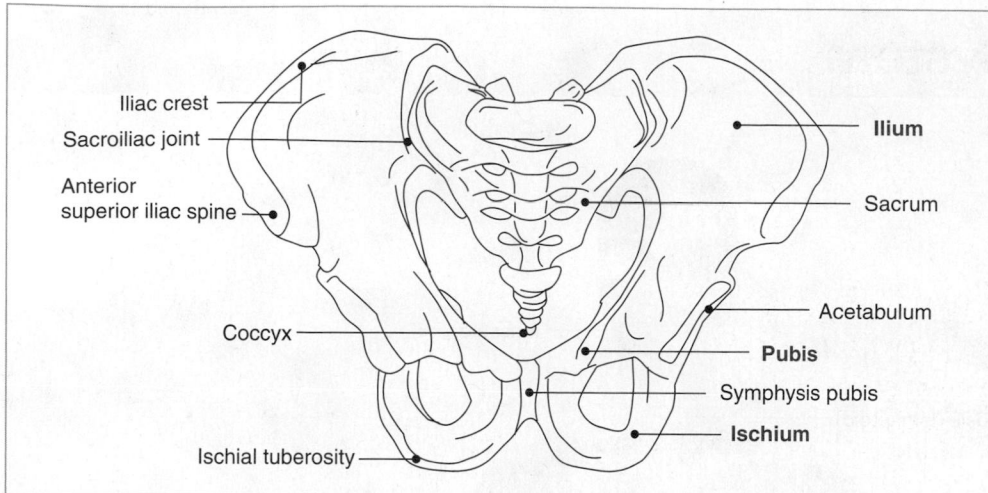

**Figure 6-32** The bones of the pelvis.

Iliac crest
Sacroiliac joint
Anterior superior iliac spine
Coccyx
Ischial tuberosity
**Ilium**
Sacrum
Acetabulum
**Pubis**
Symphysis pubis
**Ischium**

## Physiology of the Skeletal System

The primary function of the skeleton is to provide structure to the body. In addition, the bones are a large storage site for important minerals, especially calcium, needed for many of the body's functions. The bone marrow is the place where blood cells are made (Figure 6-33■). Red blood cells, white blood cells, and platelets are produced in the bone marrow and are released into the bloodstream. The bones of the skull, thorax, and pelvis protect internal structures from trauma.

## The Muscular System

Muscles are soft tissues. Contractions of **muscular system**, allow the body to move (Figure 6-34■). The body has over 600 muscles, most of which are attached to bones by strong tissues called tendons. A tendon is the extension of a muscle that connects the muscle to a bone. A tendon increases the mechanical advantage of a muscle by lengthening the lever arm across a joint. Muscle tissue attached to the skeleton has the ability to contract (become shorter and thicker) when stimulated by a nerve. Muscle cells, called fibers, are usually long and threadlike and are packed closely together in bundles, which are bound together by connective tissue.

### Anatomy of the Muscular System

There are three basic types of muscles (Figure 6-35■):

+ **Skeletal muscle.** Skeletal, or voluntary, muscles are under the control of the voluntary nervous system. These muscles help give the body its shape and make it possible to move when we walk, smile, talk, or move our eyes.
+ **Smooth muscle.** Smooth muscles, also called involuntary muscles, are found in the walls of tubelike organs, ducts, and blood vessels. They also form much of the intestinal wall.
+ **Cardiac muscle.** Cardiac muscle is found only in the walls of the heart and shares some of the properties of skeletal and smooth muscle. Cardiac muscle has the unique property of being able to generate its own electrical impulses independent of the nervous system. The primary purpose of cardiac muscle is to produce the pumping action of the heart.

**muscular system** a group of specialized tissues that allow movement of the body, movement within the organs of the digestive system, and the beating of the heart.

**Figure 6-33** The location of the bone marrow in a long bone.

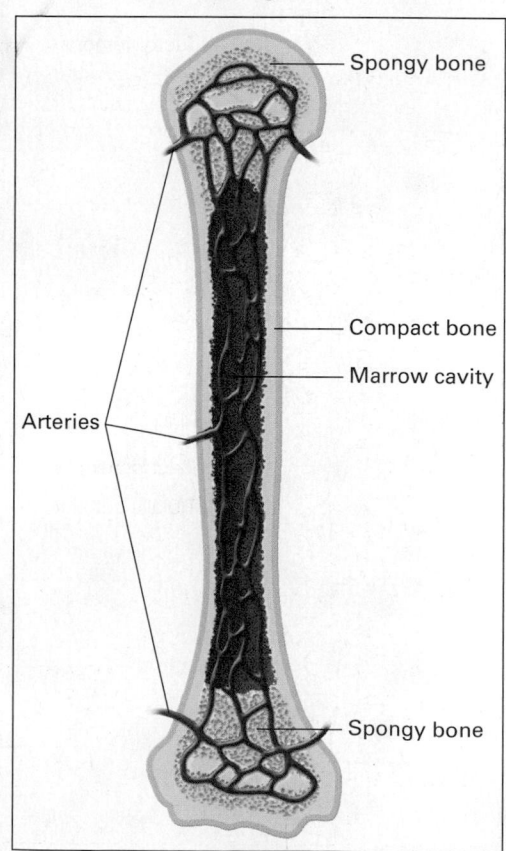

Spongy bone
Compact bone
Marrow cavity
Arteries
Spongy bone

# Muscular System

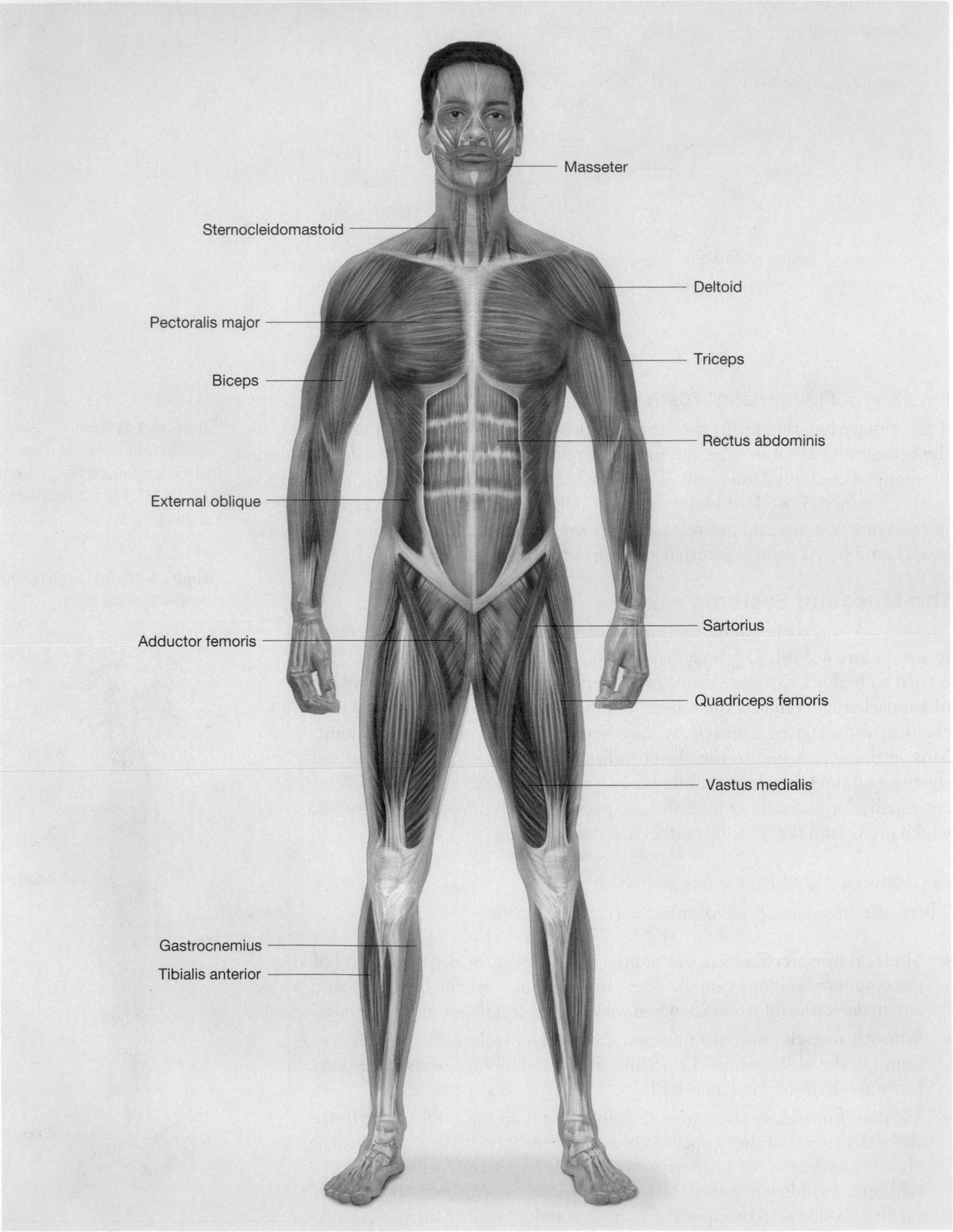

Masseter

Sternocleidomastoid

Deltoid

Pectoralis major

Triceps

Biceps

Rectus abdominis

External oblique

Adductor femoris

Sartorius

Quadriceps femoris

Vastus medialis

Gastrocnemius

Tibialis anterior

**Figure 6-34** Some major muscles of the muscular system.

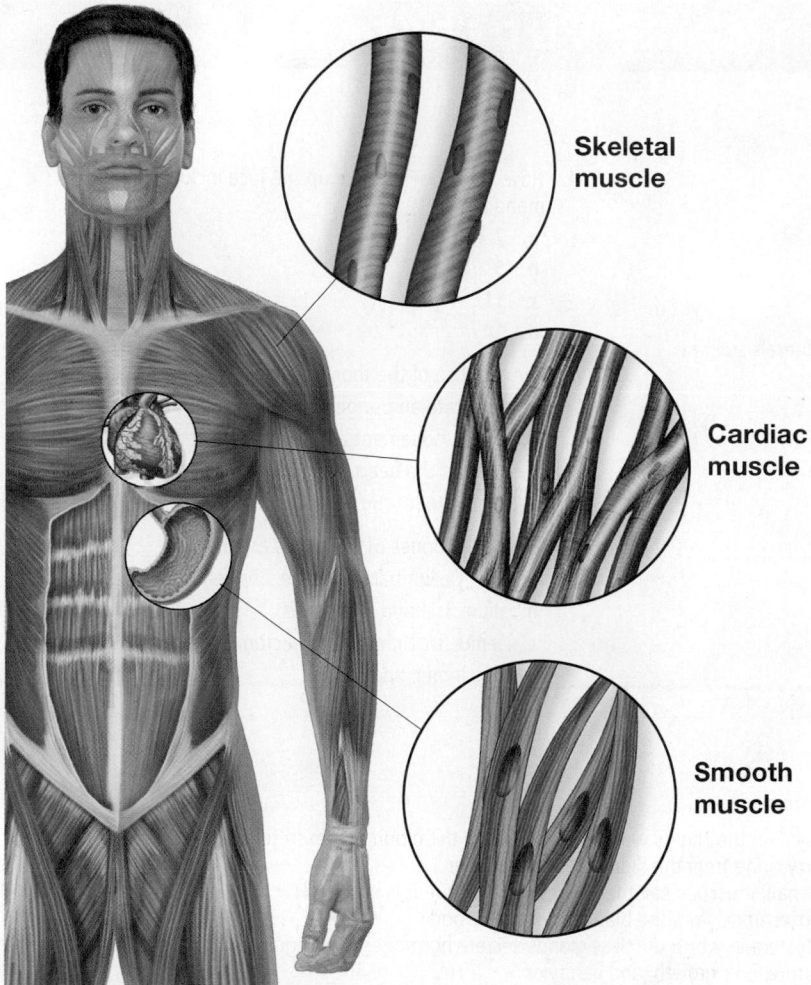

**Figure 6-35** The three basic types of muscle: skeletal, cardiac, and smooth.

## Physiology of the Muscular System

Contraction of a muscle results in movement. Skeletal muscle contraction will move the bones such that a person is able to walk or pick up a glass. Skeletal muscles are typically paired such that one set of muscles produces flexion of a joint, and a different set of muscles produces extension of a joint. For example, contraction of one set of muscles of the hand will produce flexion and allow for grasping a glass of water, whereas contraction of another set of muscles of the hand will produce extension and release the glass.

Contraction of skeletal muscle results in movement of the bones. Contraction of smooth muscle leads to movement within the organs of the body. Smooth muscle inside the wall of the intestines moves the food being digested along the gastrointestinal tract toward the anus. Contraction of cardiac muscle causes the pumping action of the heart that moves blood through the cardiovascular system.

## The Reproductive System

The **reproductive system** of both men and women include the organs for sexual reproduction. Puberty usually begins between the ages of 10 and 14 and is controlled by hormones secreted by the pituitary gland in the brain. Hormones secreted by the "master gland" influence the secretion of male or female sex hormones, which leads to the maturation of reproductive organs. These hormones also control what are

**reproductive system** a group of organs and other structures responsible for human reproduction.

# STOP, THINK, UNDERSTAND

## Multiple Choice

Choose the correct answer.

1. The two layers of the skin are_____
   a. integumentary and alimentary.
   b. pigmentary and dermis.
   c. epidermis and dermis.
   d. inguinal and sublingual.

2. Which of the following body systems stores minerals such as calcium?_____
   a. Skeletal
   b. Integumentary
   c. Endocrine
   d. Gastrointestinal

3. The hip and shoulder are what type of joint?_____
   a. Hinge
   b. Ball and socket
   c. Flat
   d. Static

4. How many bones make up the face including the mandible?_____
   a. 2
   b. 5
   c. 11
   d. 14

5. The purpose of the thorax is to _____
   a. facilitate an upright position.
   b. allow movement and expansion of the lungs.
   c. protect the heart and lungs.
   d. facilitate rotation and flexion of the spine.

6. The paired bones of the pelvis are the_____
   a. coccyx, lumbar vertebrae, and femoral head.
   b. ilium, ischium, and pubis.
   c. femur, trochanter, and sacrum.
   d. hip, femur, and coccyx.

## Matching

1. Match each of the following terms with its description.

   _____ 1. adrenal
   _____ 2. bladder
   _____ 3. endocrine
   _____ 4. gonads
   _____ 5. hypothalamus
   _____ 6. pancreas
   _____ 7. pineal
   _____ 8. pituitary
   _____ 9. thyroid
   _____ 10. ureters
   _____ 11. urethra
   _____ 12. urinary

   a. a system that filters waste products from the blood and excretes them from the body
   b. carry urine from the kidneys to the bladder
   c. a small, muscular sac that stores urine before it is excreted
   d. carries urine from the bladder out of the body
   e. a system in which ductless glands secrete hormones that regulate body functions such as strength, stature, hair growth, and behavior
   f. the "master gland" located in the brain that secretes chemicals that regulate growth and the function of other glands
   g. secretes hormones that act on the "master gland" and helps control regulation of water in the kidneys
   h. a gland located in the anterior neck that regulates metabolism, growth, and development; partially regulates nervous system activity
   i. a gland located on top of a kidney that secretes epinephrine and norepinephrine and affects heart rate, digestive system function, and lung/blood vessel function
   j. a gland in the posterior of the abdomen that secretes hormones that regulate blood glucose
   k. ovaries in females, testes in males; produce hormones that control reproduction and sex characteristics
   l. a gland that regulates daily sleep/wake patterns

2. Match each of the following types of vertebrae with its description.

   _____ 1. cervical
   _____ 2. coccygeal (coccyx)
   _____ 3. lumbar
   _____ 4. sacral
   _____ 5. thoracic

   a. contains fused vertebrae
   b. also known as the tailbone
   c. contains the first 7 vertebrae; begins at the foramen magnum
   d. the lower part of the back; contains 5 vertebrae
   e. the largest portion of the spinal column; contains 12 vertebrae

*continued*

## Fill in the Blank

1. The hair, skin, nails, sweat glands, and oil glands are part of the_____ system.

2. The body's largest organ is the _____.

3. The _____layer of the skin contains the blood vessels, nerves, glands, and hair.

4. The _____, the outermost layer of skin, contains the skin's pigmentation.

5. The _____layer below the skin contains fatty tissue.

6. The three primary functions of the skin are_____, _____, and _____.

7. The human skeleton consists of _____ and _____ and contains _____ (number) of bones.

8. The two main parts of the skull are the _____ and _____.

9. Another name for the thorax is the _____ (chest), and it is composed of the_____, _____, and the _____.

10. The six sections of the skeleton are the _____, _____, _____, _____, _____, and _____.

11. The five sections of the spinal column and the number of vertebrae in each are the _____, _____, _____, _____, and_____.

called secondary sex characteristics, such as facial hair in males, pubic hair, and breast development in females.

### Anatomy of the Male Reproductive System

Many of the male reproductive structures are located outside of the pelvic cavity and thus are more vulnerable to injury than are those of the females (Figure 6-36■). The two testicles hang from the underside of the penis in a sac-like structure called the scrotum. Inside the pelvic cavity are the prostate gland and the seminal vesicles. The urethra extends from the bladder to the tip of the penis. The penis, the prominent external phallus, is the terminal part of both the urinary and reproductive systems in males.

### Physiology of the Male Reproductive System

The testes produce sperm and testosterone, the primary male sex hormone. The prostate and seminal vesicles make and store the seminal fluid, the liquid part of the man's ejaculate. Sperm are small structures with a whiplike tail and a head that contains the genetic material needed to fertilize a woman's egg. Sperm made in the testicles combine with the seminal fluid to form semen, which is ejaculated during intercourse. Most of the urethra is part of the urinary system and transports urine from the bladder. The last part of the urethra also is part of the reproductive system through which semen is ejaculated. The sperm contributes half the genetic material to offspring.

### Anatomy of the Female Reproductive System

The female reproductive system consists of the ovaries, fallopian tubes, uterus, and vagina, and it is protected by the pelvic bones (Figure 6-37■). The external structures consist of two vertical lips called the labia, as well as the vulva and the clitoris. The breasts of a woman are sometimes included in this system because they produce milk for the newborn.

# Male Reproductive System

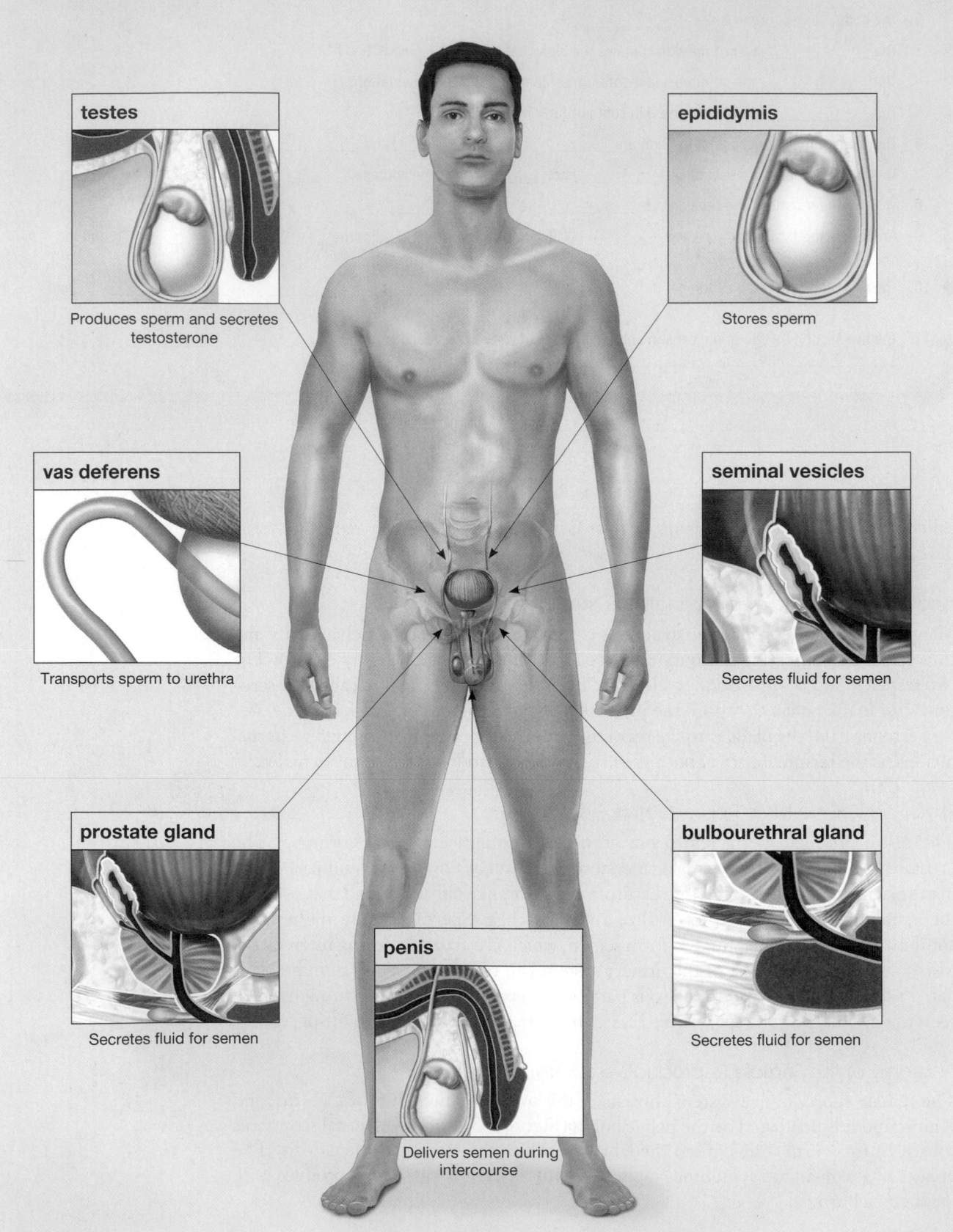

**testes**

Produces sperm and secretes testosterone

**epididymis**

Stores sperm

**vas deferens**

Transports sperm to urethra

**seminal vesicles**

Secretes fluid for semen

**prostate gland**

Secretes fluid for semen

**penis**

Delivers semen during intercourse

**bulbourethral gland**

Secretes fluid for semen

**Figure 6-36** The male reproductive organs are more susceptible to injury because of their external location.

# Female Reproductive System

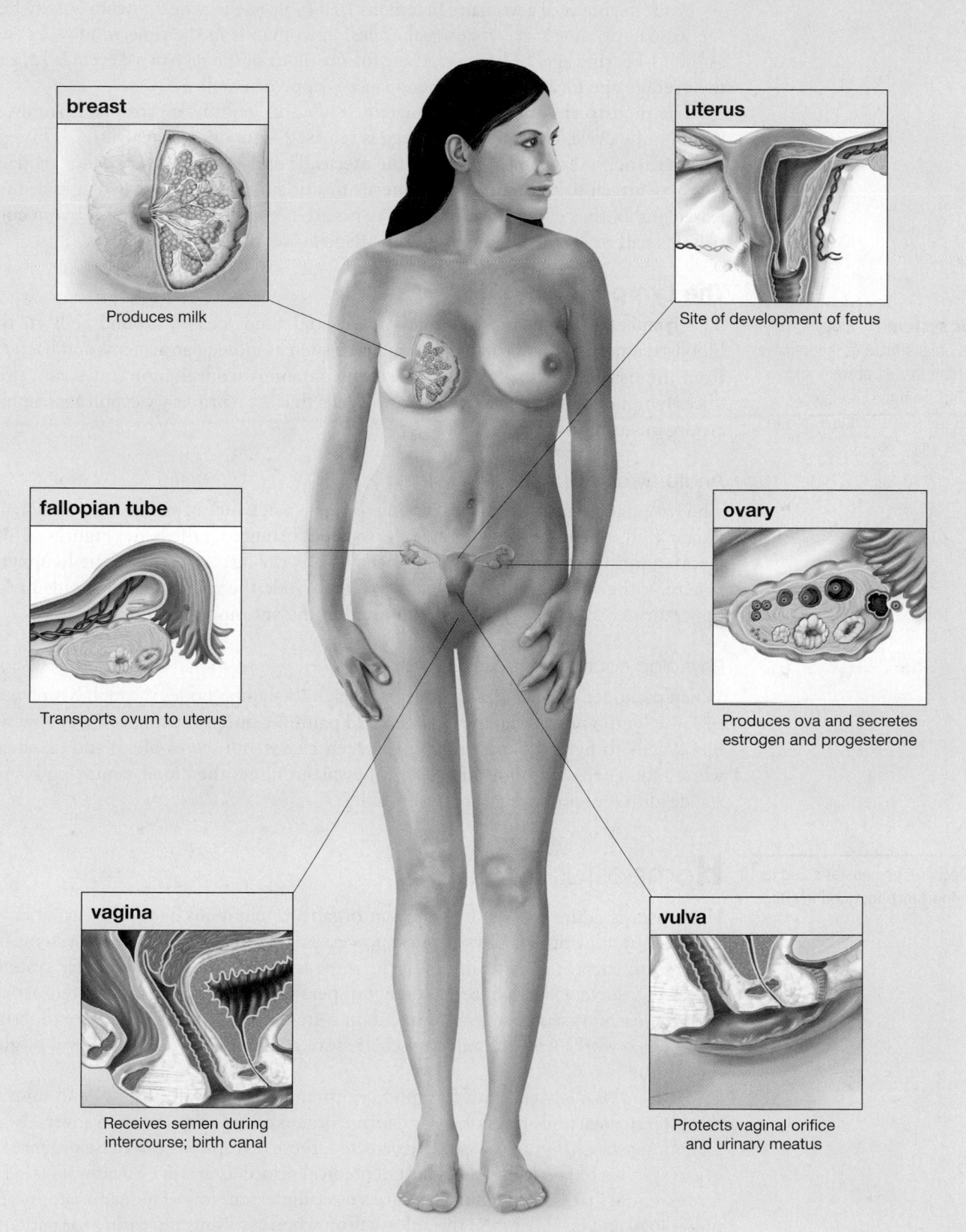

**breast**

Produces milk

**uterus**

Site of development of fetus

**fallopian tube**

Transports ovum to uterus

**ovary**

Produces ova and secretes estrogen and progesterone

**vagina**

Receives semen during intercourse; birth canal

**vulva**

Protects vaginal orifice and urinary meatus

**Figure 6-37** The female reproductive system.

### Physiology of the Female Reproductive System

Endocrine glands in the body, including the hypothalamus and pituitary glands, interact with the reproductive system by releasing hormones that control and coordinate the development and functioning of the female reproductive system.

From the onset of a woman's first menstrual cycle to the time of menopause (when the woman no longer has menstrual cycles), a woman is in the time window known as "child-bearing age." The average age for the onset of the menstrual cycle is 12, and the average age for the onset of menopause is approximately 52.

The menstrual cycle is approximately 28 days in length. Approximately midway through the cycle, typically a single egg is released from one of the ovaries. This egg travels through the fallopian tube to the uterus. If united with a sperm, the fertilized egg may attach to the lining of the uterus to initiate pregnancy. If two eggs are released and both are fertilized, fraternal twins are conceived. The female's ovum contributes half the genetic material to the offspring.

## The Lymphatic System

**lymphatic system**    a group of organs and other structures that remove extra fluid from tissues, absorbs and transports fats from the circulatory system, and transports immune cells to and from the lymph nodes.

The **lymphatic system** returns excess interstitial fluid located around cells to the bloodstream, transports particulate materials such as molecular proteins and bacteria from the tissues, absorbs fats and fat-soluble vitamins from the intestines, and produces lymphocytes, which are white blood cells that are a primary weapon against microorganisms invading the body.

### Anatomy of the Lymphatic System

The lymphatic system consists of various organs, a network of vessels that carry lymphatic fluid, and numerous lymph nodes located throughout the body (Figure 6-38■). Located in the left upper abdomen, the spleen is the largest organ of the lymphatic system. Other parts of the lymphatic system include the tonsils and adenoids in the upper airway, and the thymus gland located in the anterior neck.

### Physiology of the Lymphatic System

When pathogens from a nearby infection reach the lymph nodes through lymph vessels, the lymph nodes become enlarged and painful from producing additional white blood cells to fight the infection. The spleen cleans and stores blood and produces white blood cells that fight infection. The spleen filters the blood, removing bacteria, dead tissue, and foreign matter from it.

**6-6**  Describe homeostasis and its importance for good health.

# Homeostasis

Homeostasis is the process by which an organism maintains a stable internal environment by adjusting its physiological processes. In humans, the 11 body systems interact with each other. For instance, the integumentary and cardiovascular systems help to preserve a steady internal body temperature, and the nervous system works with the cardiovascular system to maintain a steady blood pressure. The endocrine system also works with the cardiovascular system to maintain a normal level of glucose in the blood.

Homeostasis is vital, both for good health and for survival. Illnesses and injuries that alter normal body physiology or damage organs or organ systems can adversely affect homeostasis (Figure 6-39■). Uncorrected, these disruptions can cause organs and organ systems to fail, leading to a host of medical disorders and even death. It is therefore essential that OEC Technicians have a basic understanding of human anatomy and physiology and be able to use this information when assessing and caring for patients.

# Lymphatic System

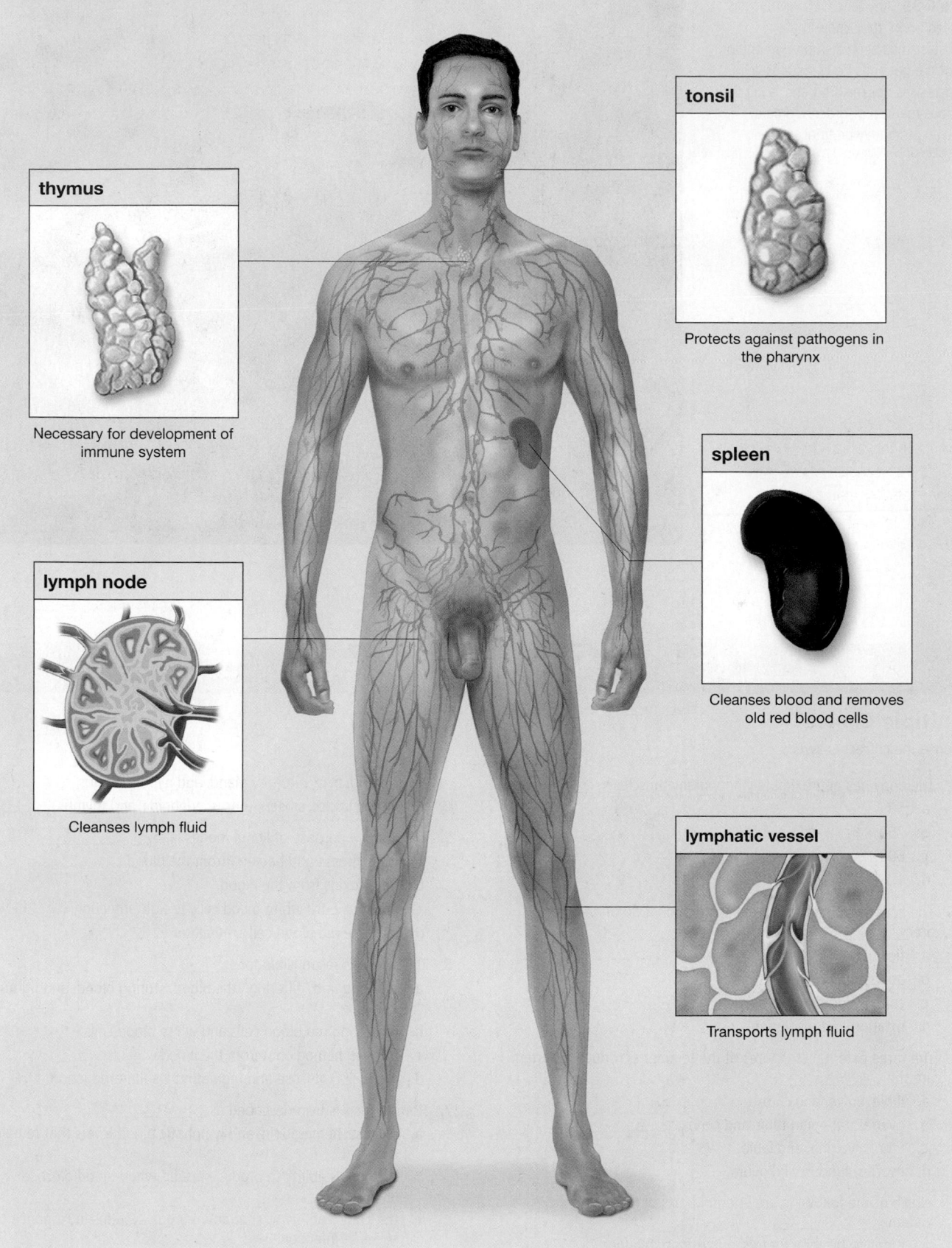

**thymus**

Necessary for development of immune system

**tonsil**

Protects against pathogens in the pharynx

**lymph node**

Cleanses lymph fluid

**spleen**

Cleanses blood and removes old red blood cells

**lymphatic vessel**

Transports lymph fluid

**Figure 6-38** The lymphatic system conducts lymphatic fluid through lymph vessels that connect the numerous lymph nodes.

**Figure 6-39** Any time OEC Technicians are called upon, they know that homeostasis has been disrupted in one or more of the patient's body systems. If homeostasis is not restored, the result will be various medical disorders, some of which can ultimately be fatal.
Copyright Edward McNamara

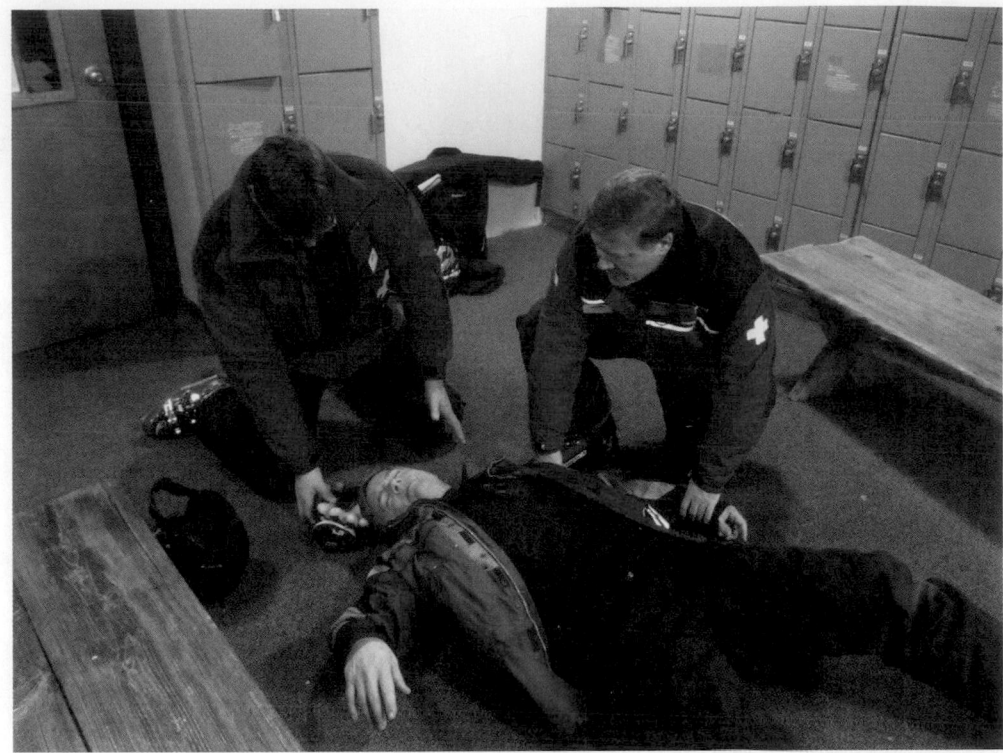

# STOP, THINK, UNDERSTAND

## Multiple Choice

Choose the correct answer.

1. The body has approximately how many muscles?_____
   a. 50
   b. 250
   c. 600
   d. 1,100

2. The actions that allow us to pick up and let go of an object are _____
   a. flexion and extension.
   b. abduction and adduction.
   c. contraction and release.
   d. rotation and resolution.

3. The three external structures of the female reproductive system are the _____
   a. labia, vulva, and clitoris.
   b. ovaries, fallopian tube, and cervix.
   c. uterus, vagina, and labia.
   d. ovaries, fundus, and ovum.

4. Which of the following are integral parts of the lymphatic system?_____
   a. Kidneys, urethra, ureters, and urinary bladder
   b. Lymph ducts, pancreas, adrenal glands, and pineal gland
   c. Thyroid, liver, pituitary gland, and hypothalamus
   d. Lymph nodes, spleen, tonsils, adenoids, and thymus

5. The primary purpose of lymph nodes is to _____
   a. filter viruses and bacteria from the blood.
   b. filter toxins from the blood.
   c. produce extra white blood cells to fight infection.
   d. increase red blood cell production.

6. The spleen is responsible for _____
   a. cleaning and "filtering" the blood, storing blood, and fighting infection.
   b. producing red blood cells and white blood cells.
   c. filtering hemoglobin from the blood.
   d. producing glucose and regulating insulin production.

7. Homeostasis is best described as _____
   a. glucose, hemoglobin, and lymphatic blood levels that remain constant.
   b. the body's ability to produce insulin when blood glucose levels fall.
   c. the body's ability to shut down organ systems in response to stress or infection.
   d. the ability of the body to maintain a stable internal environment by adjusting physiologic processes.

*continued*

## Matching

Match each of the following types of muscle with its description.

_____ **1.** smooth

_____ **2.** skeletal

_____ **3.** cardiac

**a.** a voluntary type of muscle that helps give us shape and makes it possible for us to move, walk, smile, talk, or move our eyes

**b.** this type of muscle can generate its own electrical impulses independent of the nervous system

**c.** also known as "involuntary" muscle; is found in the tubelike organs, ducts, blood vessels, and intestinal walls

## Fill in the Blank

Which of the following are functions of the lymphatic system? (check all that apply)

_____ **a.** Returns excess interstitial fluid to the bloodstream

_____ **b.** Removes proteins and bacteria from tissues

_____ **c.** Absorbs and distributes glucose

_____ **d.** Absorbs fats and fat-soluble vitamins from the intestines

_____ **e.** Produces glucagon, which helps control blood sugar levels

_____ **f.** Produces adrenaline, which aids in the "fight-or-flight" response and fights infection

 **CASE DISPOSITION**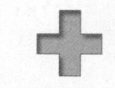

Other OEC Technicians soon arrive, bringing with them trauma packs, an oxygen kit, and two toboggans. You inform them that the female patient has pain in the left lower anterior thorax and the left upper abdominal quadrant, and that you suspect both rib fractures and a splenic injury. You describe the male patient as having a suspected head injury and a probable fracture of the left proximal femur. Working together, you and the other OEC Technicians correctly assess, treat, and package the two patients, load them into the toboggans, and transport them down the hill to waiting ambulances. You later learn that the woman was admitted with rib fractures and a ruptured spleen, and that the man did have a proximal femur fracture. He also was diagnosed with a mild concussion. Both patients were expected to make full recoveries.

# Chapter Review

## Chapter Summary

The 11 organ systems in the human body work together to maintain homeostasis, a relatively stable internal environment. All organ systems must work together and stay healthy in order to maintain homeostasis. An injury or illness in one system can and often will affect other systems, causing the human body to quickly lose its ability to function normally. Among the problems that could affect homeostasis are an injury to the brain or spinal cord, an injury to the chest resulting in difficulty breathing, an infection in the gastrointestinal system such as appendicitis, injury to the heart muscle from a heart attack, and extreme environmental conditions.

Each organ system has a specific function that is essential for life. Understanding the anatomy and physiology of the 11 organ systems will assist you in assessing your patients as you identify the systems that may not be functioning properly due to illness or trauma.

# Remember...

1. Human anatomy is the study of the structure of the human body.
2. Human physiology is the study of the function of the human body.
3. The 11 organ systems and their primary functions are:
   - **Respiratory system.** Brings oxygen into the body and removes carbon dioxide from the body.
   - **Cardiovascular system.** Moves blood and nutrients throughout the body; also called the circulatory system.
   - **Nervous system.** Controls other organ systems and thought processes.
   - **Gastrointestinal system.** Breaks down food and absorbs nutrients.

- **Urinary system.** Excretes wastes and toxins in urine.
- **Endocrine system.** Controls organ systems by producing hormones.
- **Integumentary system.** Protects the body; also called skin.
- **Skeletal system.** Provides structure to the body.
- **Muscular system.** Enables body movements.
- **Reproductive system.** Is responsible for human reproduction.
- **Lymphatic system.** Protects the body from harmful microorganisms.

# Chapter Questions

## Multiple Choice

Choose the correct answer.

1. A patient is using accessory muscles to breathe. This is _____
   a. normal.
   b. indicative that the body is compensating for a problem with the lungs or airway.
   c. indicative that this person has recently smoked a cigarette.
   d. a sign of less resistance to air flow and of an increase in the diameter of the airway.

2. The purpose of ligaments is to _____
   a. hold bones together at a joint and restrict movement.
   b. permit unlimited movement of a joint.
   c. allow the hyperflexion of a joint.
   d. attach bones to muscles.

## Matching

1. Match each of the following positions to its description.

| | |
|---|---|
| _____ **1.** high-Fowler | **a.** the basis for all medical terms that refer to the body |
| _____ **2.** left lateral recumbent | **b.** patient sitting with knees bent |
| _____ **3.** anatomical | **c.** patient lying on abdomen |
| _____ **4.** prone | **d.** patient lying on back with legs higher than the head and the body on an inclined plane (head down, legs raised) |
| _____ **5.** right lateral recumbent | **e.** patient lying on back with upper body elevated to a 90° angle |
| _____ **6.** Rothberg | **f.** patient lying on back with upper body elevated 45–60° |
| _____ **7.** semi-Fowler | **g.** patient lying face up on back |
| _____ **8.** supine | **h.** patient lying on left side |
| _____ **9.** Trendelenburg | **i.** patient lying on right side |

**2.** Place each of the following organs into its correct body cavity.

_____ **1.** abdominal

_____ **2.** cranial

_____ **3.** pelvic

_____ **4.** spinal

_____ **5.** thoracic

**a.** rectum, bladder, internal reproductive organs

**b.** brain

**c.** liver, gallbladder, pancreas, kidneys, stomach, intestines, spleen

**d.** lungs, heart, great vessels

**e.** spinal cord

**3.** Match each of the following body systems to its primary function.

_____ **1.** cardiovascular

_____ **2.** endocrine

_____ **3.** gastrointestinal

_____ **4.** integumentary

_____ **5.** lymphatic

_____ **6.** muscular

_____ **7.** nervous

_____ **8.** reproductive

_____ **9.** respiratory

_____ **10.** skeletal

_____ **11.** urinary

**a.** returns excess interstitial fluid around cells to the bloodstream, removes bacteria from tissues, absorbs fats, fights infections

**b.** eliminates waste products that are filtered from the blood by the kidneys

**c.** processes food and water; eliminates waste

**d.** moves air and into and out of the body; exchanges gases, removes $CO_2$, and helps manage the body's internal pH balance

**e.** regulates all body functions

**f.** secretes hormones that trigger puberty, and contains those organs that facilitate continuation of the species

**g.** is responsible for delivering oxygen, nutrients, and fluids to the body's cells and for removing carbon dioxide and other waste products

**h.** consists of ductless glands that secrete hormones that regulate strength, stature, hair growth, and behavior

**i.** contains specialized cells that protect the body, retains fluids, and helps prevent infection; skin

**j.** allows movement of the body, of the organs of the digestive system, and of the heart

**k.** provides support and protection for the body and is an attachment point for organs; stores minerals; contains one of the sites where blood cells are made

**4.** Match each of the following components of blood to its primary function.

_____ **1.** red blood cell

_____ **2.** white blood cell

_____ **3.** platelets

_____ **4.** plasma

**a.** clear liquid that carries blood cells, delivers nutrients to body cells, and dissolves and transports carbon dioxide ($CO_2$)

**b.** part of the body's immune system; fights infection

**c.** form blood clots to stop bleeding

**d.** contains iron; carries oxygen to the cells

**5.** For each of the descriptions of the circumstances of injury (a–e), indicate which of the lists of body structures (1–5) are *most likely* to be directly affected.

_____ **1.** reproductive, bladder, skeletal, muscular

_____ **2.** brain, spinal column (nervous system)

_____ **3.** gastrointestinal, circulatory (spleen, liver, intestines, stomach)

_____ **4.** skeletal, GI, nervous (hips, pelvis, coccyx, internal GI injuries, spinal)

_____ **5.** skeletal, circulatory, respiratory, muscular, nervous (ribs, heart, lungs, diaphragm, spinal)

**a.** a swimmer who dives into a creek and hits his head on a rock

**b.** a skier who misses a terrain park feature and lands straddling a rail

**c.** a female climber who falls approximately six feet and lands sitting on a rock

**d.** a bicyclist who flips over his handlebars and lands chest-first against a tree

**e.** an equestrienne who is kicked in the "gut" by a horse

## Fill in the Blank

1. The purpose of the bony pelvis is to protect the _____organs.
2. The functions of the skeletal system include which of the following? (check all that apply)

   _____ **a.** provides structure for the body   _____ **e.** produces WBCs

   _____ **b.** stores glucose   _____ **f.** produces platelets

   _____ **c.** stores calcium and minerals   _____ **g.** produces growth hormone

   _____ **d.** produces RBCs

## Scenario

*You respond to an injured skier. Upon arrival, you find an adult female down on the side of the trail. After marking and securing the scene, you start your primary assessment. The patient reports that she caught an edge and fell, striking her left knee on a rock and jamming her ski pole into her body just below the ribs on her right side.*

1. Which of the following pairs of terms does *not* refer to a direction or a location?_____

   **a.** Anterior/posterior   **c.** Superior/inferior

   **b.** Pedal/malleolus   **d.** Medial/lateral

*The patient is responsive, alert, and oriented to person, place, and time. In the secondary assessment you palpate the liver area and the patient reports pain.*

2. The liver is located in the_____

   **a.** pelvic cavity.   **c.** thoracic cavity.

   **b.** abdominal cavity.   **d.** endocrine cavity.

*You call for a toboggan, $O_2$, and an ALS ambulance. The patient denies any head, neck, or back pain. When help arrives, you ask for a splint to apply to the left knee and then load and go.*

3. The patient is sitting up with her knees bent. This position is called the_____

   **a.** Trendelenburg position.   **c.** High-Fowler position.

   **b.** Rothberg position.   **d.** Semi-Fowler position.

4. Trauma to the liver is a concern because the liver_____

   **a.** processes nutrient-rich blood.   **c.** produces hydrochloric acid.

   **b.** produces insulin.   **d.** produces amino acids.

## Suggested Reading

Bledsoe, B. E., et al. 2007. *Anatomy and Physiology for Emergency Care*, Second Edition. Englewood Cliffs, NJ: Prentice Hall.

Gray, H. 1985. *Gray's Anatomy*. 30th Ed., Philadelphia: Running Press.

 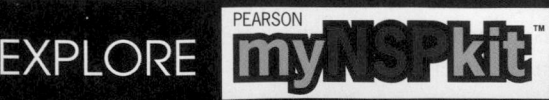

# Patient Assessment

Michael G. Millin, MD, MPH, FACEP
Denis Meade, MA, EMT-P

## ⊕ OBJECTIVES

**Upon completion of this chapter, the OEC Technician will be able to:**

**7-1** Describe the two parts of the overall assessment process.

**7-2** Describe the importance of scene safety.

**7-3** List the two parts of a patient assessment.

**7-4** Describe and demonstrate how to perform a primary assessment and manage the ABCDs.

**7-5** Describe and demonstrate how to perform a secondary assessment.

**7-6** Define the following terms:
- assessment
- chief complaint
- DCAP-BTLS
- sign
- symptom

**7-7** List and describe the key components of a patient history.

**7-8** Describe how environmental conditions can affect patient assessment.

**7-9** Describe and demonstrate how to obtain a SAMPLE history.

**7-10** Describe and demonstrate how to assess pain using the OPQRST mnemonic.

*continued*

## Chapter Overview

As you learned in Chapter 6, Anatomy and Physiology, the human body is composed of 11 interrelated body systems, each of which is responsible for various functions. Given the complex nature of these functions, it is inevitable that the organs and structures of those systems can malfunction due to disease or physical damage. When this occurs, body functions may cease to operate normally, resulting in clinical evidence that can be observed or measured by another person, or described by patients. Identifying those findings, which may be obvious or subtle, requires that you assess the

*continued*

## HISTORICAL TIMELINE

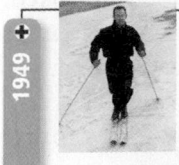

**1949** Edward Taylor accepts appointment as the first National Director of the NSP.

**1949** National office moved from New York City to Denver, CO.

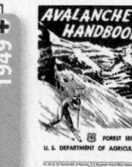

**1949** Monty Atwater publishes *Avalanche Handbook*.

**7-11**  Describe and demonstrate how to assess the eyes (pupils and movement).

**7-12**  Describe and demonstrate how to assess a patient's level of responsiveness using the following:

    a.  AVPU

    b.  Glasgow Coma Score

**7-13**  Describe and demonstrate the procedure for obtaining the following vital signs:

    a.  Respiratory rate

    b.  Blood pressure

    c.  Heart rate

**7-14**  Describe and demonstrate how to reassess a patient.

## ⊕ KEY TERMS

| | | |
|---|---|---|
| **abrasion**, *p. 230* | **distracting injury**, *p. 230* | **paresthesia**, *p. 224* |
| **assessment**, *p. 214* | **Glasgow Coma Scale**, *p. 222* | **PERRL**, *p. 232* |
| **AVPU**, *p. 222* | **hypoxia**, *p. 222* | **pulse**, *p. 220* |
| **avulsion**, *p. 230* | **laceration**, *p. 230* | **respiration**, *p. 239* |
| **blood pressure (BP)**, *p. 239* | **level of responsiveness (LOR)**, *p. 238* | **SAMPLE**, *p. 227* |
| **chief complaint**, *p. 216* | **mechanism of injury (MOI)**, *p. 216* | **sign**, *p. 227* |
| **contusion**, *p. 230* | **nature of illness (NOI)**, *p. 216* | **swelling**, *p. 230* |
| **DCAP-BTLS**, *p. 230* | **OPQRST**, *p. 228* | **symptom**, *p. 227* |
| **decerebrate posturing**, *p. 224* | **oxygenation**, *p. 246* | **vital signs**, *p. 238* |
| **decorticate posturing**, *p. 224* | **paralysis**, *p. 224* | |

patient and compare the results to normal values and known disorders to determine the underlying source of the problem. You can then use this information to formulate an appropriate treatment plan.

You will use an assessment process to gather information about the scene, the patient, the events leading up to the current situation, and pertinent historical facts, all of which can help you determine what may be going on with the patient. This information will be collected from a variety of sources, which can include the patient, the patient's family and friends, bystanders, and even other rescuers.

**assessment**   the act of determining the nature of a patient's injuries and illnesses.

As part of patient **assessment**, you will perform a primary assessment, the purpose of which is to identify life-threatening problems. You also will perform a secondary assessment, which includes recording the patient's vital signs and conducting a head-to-toe physical examination. While performing a patient assessment, you may identify significant medical problems that you will need to manage immediately. Thus, it is important to understand that patient assessment and patient management often occur simultaneously.

⊕ **7-1**   Describe the two parts of the overall assessment process.

Although performing a patient assessment may seem overwhelming at first, as you work through this chapter and begin performing assessments on your classmates and others, you will find that assessing the scene and the patient is actually quite straightforward and can be completed very rapidly. The key is to use a systematic, standardized approach for every emergency situation to ensure that potential medical problems do not go unrecognized and that key clinical information is not overlooked.

⊕ **7-6**   Define the following terms:

- assessment
- chief complaint
- DCAP-BTLS
- sign
- symptom

Patient assessment is the most important skill that you will use in your career as an OEC Technician. Because you will perform an assessment on every patient you will encounter, patient assessment is an essential and fundamental skill that every OEC Technician must master. The overall assessment process consists of two parts: the scene size-up and the patient assessment.

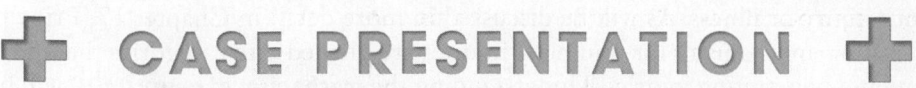

# CASE PRESENTATION

It is a sunny day and you are responding to a call to assist a patient who has fallen while rock climbing. When you arrive on scene, you find a male in his mid-50s sitting beside a trail next to a rock face. His wife reports that her husband was "bouldering," traversing along the rock face when he slipped, falling approximately 6 feet to the ground. She states that he was wearing a helmet and that he did not lose responsiveness. As you assess the man, he appears to be having difficulty breathing and is complaining of left upper-chest pain, saying that he "feels like I was hit with a baseball bat."

**What should you do?**

## Scene Size-Up

As was discussed in Chapter 3, Rescue Basics, your assessment of any incident begins with an assessment of scene safety before you make contact with the patient (Figure 7-1■). You will need to use your senses— of vision, hearing, and smell to evaluate potential dangers in the area. Hazards may be made by humans, such as downed electrical wires, or they may be natural, such as a wild animal. Even the terrain and the environment can present hazards. Taking care of a patient on a steep slope could put the rescuer at risk of a fall on ice or rocks and could expose the rescuer to a possible avalanche or rock fall. A rescue in bitter cold weather can present a risk of hypothermia to an OEC Technician. Whatever the hazard may be, you should do your best to mitigate all actual or potential hazards before initiating patient contact and care. Injury to yourself or to other rescuers while attempting to help someone else delays care to the patient and further complicates the situation.

**⊕ 7-2** Describe the importance of scene safety.

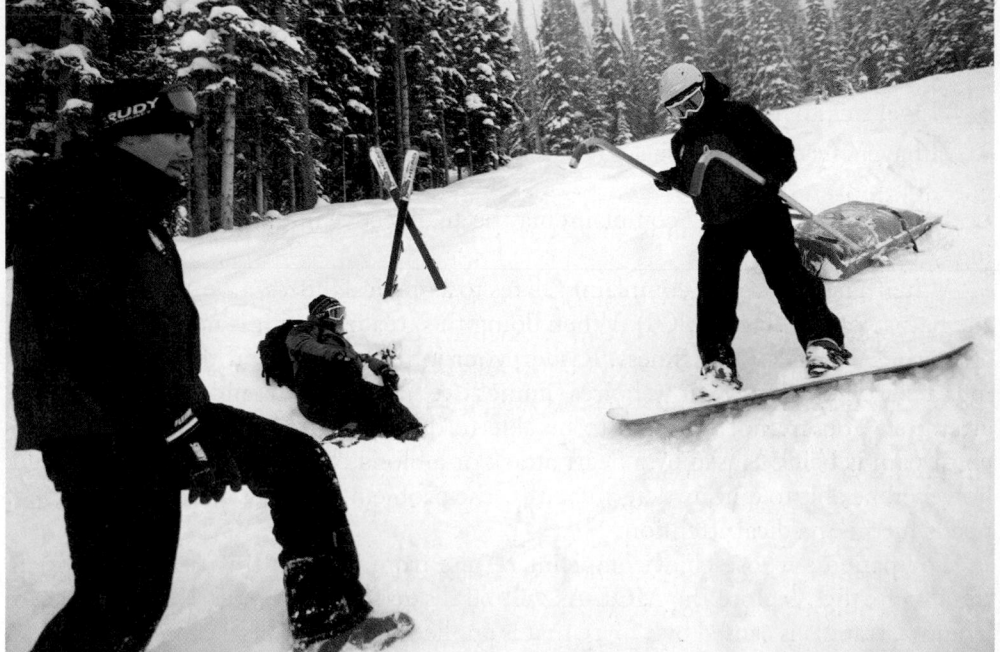

**Figure 7-1** As you approach an accident scene and evaluate scene safety, you may see clues about what may have happened or what injuries to expect.
Copyright J. Selkowitz

**mechanisim of injury (MOI)** the kind of force that acts on the body to cause injury; the method of trauma causing an injury.

**nature of illness (NOI)** evaluation to determine the type of medical illness present.

**chief complaint** the symptom or group of symptoms about which the patient is concerned.

As part of the scene size-up, you will begin to assess the events that led to the patient's injury or illness. As will be discussed in more detail in Chapter 17, Principles of Trauma, mechanisms for traumatic injuries are divided into categories that include blunt and penetrating injuries. Understanding the **mechanism of injury (MOI)** will help you determine what may be going on with the patient. In most cases, you will begin to assess the MOI as you enter the scene. Once you know the scene is safe, you should not delay the primary assessment (to be discussed later) in order to collect information on the mechanism of injury. For sick patients, coming to understanding the **nature of illness (NOI)** follows a process similar to that for understanding MOI.

## General Impression

OEC Technicians should be able to form a general impression rapidly based on the patient's chief complaint, the scene size-up, the mechanism of injury or nature of illness, and the patient's initial appearance. You should then establish priorities for care and transport based on this information. If the patient has a life-threatening problem or is unresponsive, immediately care for the life threat, seek help and rapidly transport. If the patient is responsive, ask what is wrong so that you can determine the patient's **chief complaint**.

It is important to introduce yourself to the patient and to ask for permission to provide care. This is done by simply saying, "Hello, I'm David with the ski patrol, may I help you?" If the answer is yes, then proceed. When the patient is unresponsive or is a child without a parent, you may proceed following the principle of implied consent explained in Chapter 1. If a parent is present, ask the parent for permission to treat.

## Chief Complaint

The most important piece of information that must be quickly identified is the chief complaint, which is defined as the primary reason the person is seeking medical care. The cause of the chief complaint may be traumatic or medical or both. If the patient has more than one problem, there may be more than one chief complaint. Examples of chief complaints that OEC Technicians routinely encounter are:

+ "My chest hurts."
+ "I can't breathe."
+ "My knee is killing me."
+ "My back hurts and my right arm hurts."
+ "I feel sick to my stomach."
+ "I have a terrible headache."

In some cases, the chief complaint may be an objective finding, such as "I'm bleeding" or "My arm is crooked."

When a patient's chief complaint relates to a medical illness, attempt to determine the nature of the illness (NOI). When doing this, realize that it is not your job to diagnose the exact cause of illness. Rather, your job is to identify if the patient is having a serious illness that requires immediate intervention and further medical attention. You are not expected to be able to determine, for example, if a patient's chest pain is being caused by a heart attack or a blood clot in the lungs. You should, however, be able to quickly determine that the problem is serious and that the patient needs further medical attention.

For patients whose chief complaint results from trauma, this is an appropriate time to further explore the MOI. As will be discussed in Chapter 17, Principles of Trauma, trauma is caused by a force that is applied to the body and causes injury. The

| Table 7-1 | Examples of Significant Mechanisms of Injury |
|---|---|
| **Mechanisms of Injury** | **Examples** |
| Falls | Adults: more than 20 feet |
| | Children: more than 10 feet |
| High-velocity crashes | Person hitting an object or another person at high speed |
| | Person being thrown a great distance |
| Other high-risk events | Death of another person in the crash |
| | Pedestrian hit by car or other motorized vehicle such as a snow cat going greater than 20 mph |

nature and extent of the injury are directly related to the forces applied. Penetration of the body by a tree branch will cause a different kind of injury than blunt force from hitting a tree at a high rate of speed. Therefore, understanding the mechanism of injury will help you determine the nature of a patient's injury. Table 7-1■ lists some significant mechanisms of injury.

Any patient who appears to be uninjured after some kind of significant mishap should still be a reason for concern. Do not assume that a patient in such circumstances is not injured simply because you have not yet identified the MOI; it is possible to have a major, even potentially lethal injury even if the mechanism by which it occurred is yet to be determined. An example would be a man falling down the stairs, immediately getting up, says he is fine, but in fact it turns out that he had ruptured his spleen. Therefore, the lack of a demonstrable MOI should never be used to rule out the possibility of major injury, even in a patient with no evidence of physical injury.

# Patient Assessment

Patient assessment is the formal process in which important clinical findings associated with various injuries and illnesses are identified. It consists of two parts: a primary assessment and a secondary assessment. Together, the information gathered from these assessments will help you identify the nature and origin of various medical disorders so that you can initiate proper treatment.

As stated previously, patient assessment is the most important skill that OEC Technicians perform, and it is one that you must master. Fortunately, the process need not be daunting. In fact, patient assessment is relatively simple when it is performed in a systematic, organized manner each and every time. The two parts of a patient assessment are equally important, and both are needed to obtain a complete and accurate understanding of the patient's current medical condition and needs.

**7-3** List the two parts of a patient assessment.

## The Primary Assessment

The purpose of a primary assessment is to quickly identify and correct any potential life-threatening problems that may be present. It is conducted on every patient, regardless of whether the problem is traumatic or medical in origin, and it should take only 30–60 seconds to complete. Refer to OEC Skill 7-1■, OEC Skill 7-2■ and OEC Skill 7-3■.

The assessment of an unresponsive adult patient follows a slightly different track. In the event you find a patient that appears unresponsive, you should do the following.

**7-4** Describe and demonstrate how to perform a primary assessment and manage the ABCDs.

1. Check for response by tapping the victims shoulder and shouting at the victim.
2. Simultaneously open the airway, check for breathing or absent breathing; which includes agonal breathing (which is occasional gasping), and check for carotid pulse, for no more than 10 seconds.

3. If breathing normally, continue primary assessment.

4. If there is no pulse, start chest compressions (CPR).

5. If there is a pulse but no breathing, start rescue breathing.

6. For additional CPR information see Chapter 15, Cardiovascular Emergencies.

A primary assessment consists of evaluating four parameters and immediately treating any abnormalities as they are found. These four parameters are collectively referred to as the ABCDs, each of which corresponds to a critical life function:

**A—Airway:** having an open and patent airway which will remain open

**B—Breathing:** being able to breathe, so that oxygen gets to the body's tissues effectively and carbon dioxide is removed

**C—Circulation:** having blood moving through the vessels to perfuse the tissues

**D—Disability:** having normal mental status and central and peripheral neurologic function, which includes having no spinal injury (Figure 7-2■)

> ### Assessing the ABCDs
>
> **NOTE**
>
> As a general rule, if a patient can talk to you and move their arms and legs in a normal fashion, the **A**irway is usually open and clear, the person is **B**reathing, blood is **C**irculating to the brain, and the patient does not have a neurologic or spinal **D**isability.

It is essential that you assess each life function, in order, and correct any problems that you discover before moving to the next life function. It cannot be overstated that failure to quickly identify and correct an ABCD-related problem can significantly affect the patient's outcome and can result in death.

### Airway

The first step of the primary assessment is to examine the patient's airway to ensure that it is open and clear of any obstructions that could restrict the free movement of air into and out of the lungs. The most common cause of airway obstruction is the tongue falling back and either partially or completely blocking the oral pharynx. Other common causes of airway compromise or blockage include vomit, bleeding, broken teeth, food or candy particles, other foreign bodies, and structural damage or swelling involving the face, nose, mouth, or neck.

**Figure 7-2** An OEC Technician assessing a patient's ABCDs.
Copyright J. Selkowitz

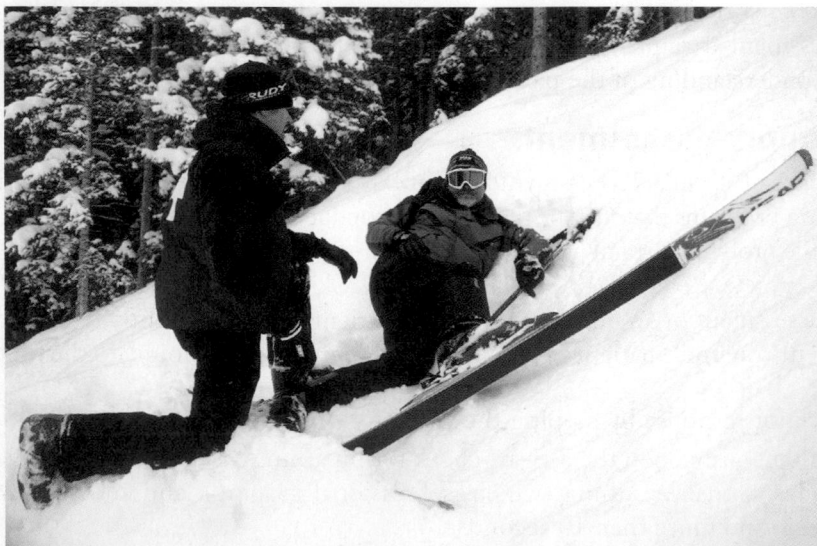

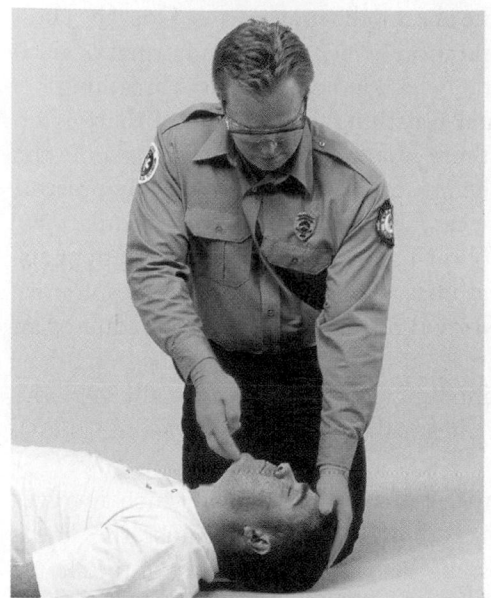 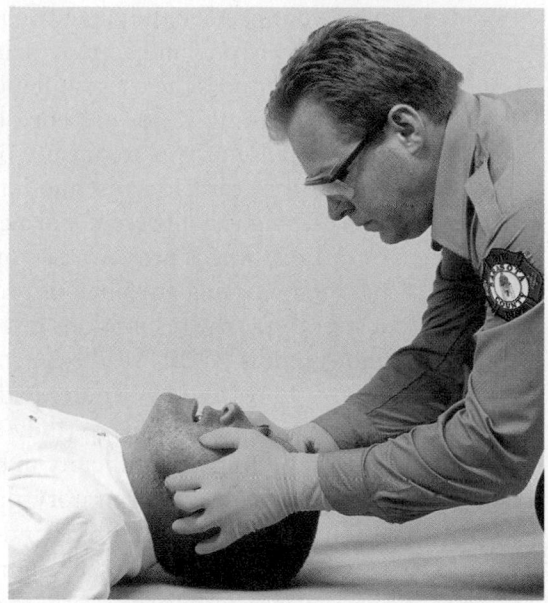

**Figure 7-3** An Emergency Medical Responder assessing a patient's airway. Left: the head-tilt, chin-lift maneuver; right: the jaw-thrust maneuver.

If an airway problem is discovered, it must be immediately corrected before proceeding. If no airway problems exist, the airway is said to be open, patent, or "intact." The easiest method to determine if the airway is intact is to talk to the patient as soon as you make contact. If the person is able to speak normally when replying to your simple questions, then the airway is generally considered open.

If the patient's airway appears to be compromised but there is no concern for cervical spinal trauma, open the airway using the head-tilt, chin-lift maneuver (Figure 7-3■). To perform this maneuver, use the hand that is nearer the patient's head to press gently downward on the patient's forehead while placing two or three fingers of the other hand under the patient's chin and lifting upward to stabilize the jaw.

If there is concern for cervical injury, open the airway with the jaw-thrust maneuver, in which you place your thumbs behind the patient's mandible and thrust the jaw forward (Figure 7-3). Always use the jaw-thrust maneuver to make sure that an unresponsive patient with a traumatic injury has an open airway, as unresponsiveness could be the result of cervical spinal trauma. If you are unable to open the airway with the jaw-thrust maneuver even in the setting of a potential spinal injury, use the head-tilt chin-lift maneuver. Both these techniques lift the tongue off the back of the throat to open the patient's airway (Figure 7-4■), and both techniques are described more fully in Chapter 9, Airway Management.

**Figure 7-4** How the head-tilt, chin-lift maneuver moves the tongue to open a patient's airway.

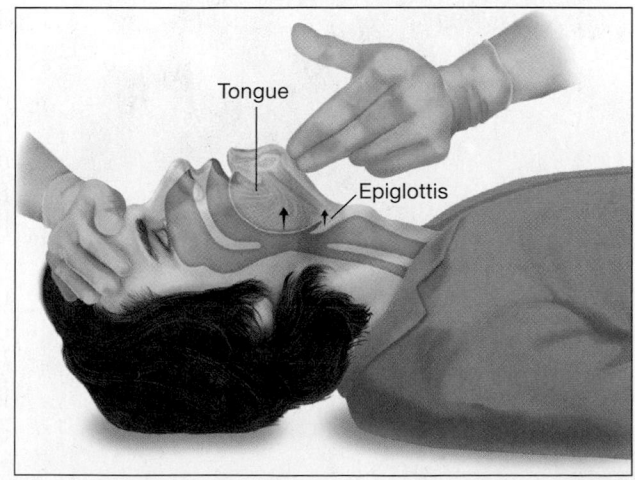

## Breathing

Once you make sure the patient's airway is intact, assess the patient's breathing using a process known as "Look, Listen, and Feel." In the unresponsive patient, simultaneously feel for the carotid pulse.

*Look* for evidence of breathing by watching to see if the chest rises and falls with each inhalation and exhalation. Place your ear near the patient's open mouth to *Listen* for the sound of breath moving in and out. Do you hear any unusual sounds when the patient breathes? *Feel* for air on your cheek during exhalation and place your hand on the patient's chest to *Feel* the chest wall's movements. Does the chest wall fully expand and contract with each respiration (which indicates normal or deep breaths), or does the chest wall move very little (which indicates shallow breathing)?

If breathing is not present or only agonal breathing is present and there is no carotid pulse or you are unsure of whether there is a pulse, you should presume the patient is in cardiac arrest and immediately begin compressions followed by breaths. If breathing is not present and a carotid pulse can be felt, begin assisting ventilations.

If breathing is present, ask yourself the following questions: Does the patient appear to be having any obvious problems breathing, a condition known as respiratory distress? Are the respirations fast or slow? Normal respiration rate for an adult or an adolescent is 12–20 breaths per minute, whereas normal respiration rate for an infant is 20–30 breaths per minute. Is the patient inhaling and exhaling normally? Are the patient's respirations deep (fully expand the chest), shallow (barely move the chest), or labored (indicate difficulty in breathing)?

Other signs of respiratory distress include a "tripod" position, which involves leaning forward with the hands or forearms braced near or against the knees (Figure 7-5■); breathing through pursed lips; marked rising and falling of the shoulder muscles with each breath; and flaring of the nostrils on inspiration. Another abnormal finding would be the unequal movement of the chest where, during inspiration, one side appears to expand while the other appears to contract. All of these findings indicate that the patient is experiencing a breathing problem.

Does the patient speak in complete sentences, or instead break sentences into small groups of words? As indicated previously, the ability to converse in full sentences is a good sign. Rarely will a person with a life-threatening respiratory problem be able to speak in complete sentences.

Even when the patient is unresponsive during the primary assessment, you can still effectively assess breathing using the "Look, Listen, and Feel" method. Simply look to see if the patient's chest rises and falls symmetrically with each breath, listen for breathing, and feel the chest move with each respiration by placing your hand on the person's chest.

**pulse**  rhythmic expansion of an artery caused by the movement of blood.

**Figure 7-5**  A sitting patient in the "tripod" position, which is indicative of respiratory distress.
Copyright Edward McNamara

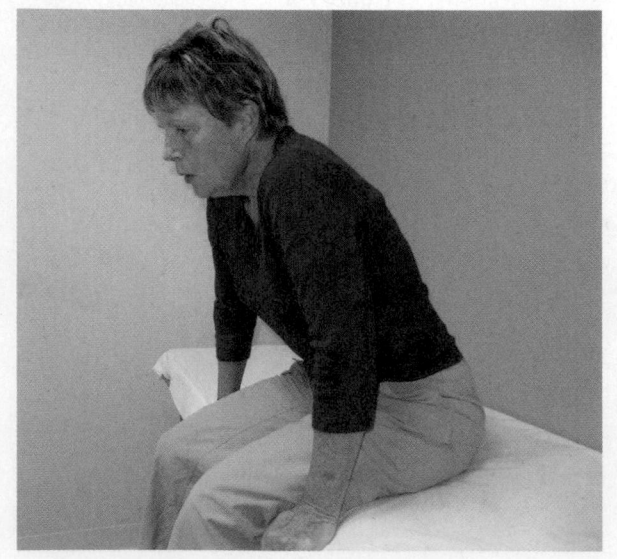

## Circulation

The circulatory system transports blood containing the nutrients and oxygen to the body's cells. Any condition that reduces blood flow can disrupt homeostasis. Assessment of the circulatory system, therefore, is performed to determine whether the vital organs (e.g., the heart, brain, lungs, kidneys) are receiving adequate blood flow.

To assess circulation, check for the presence of an arterial **pulse**. The pulse is most often checked first at the wrist over the radial artery (Figure 7-6■). If a pulse is present, you can easily determine the pulse rate by counting the number of pulses for 15 seconds and then multiplying that number by 4, obtaining a heart rate in beats per minute. You should also check the quality of the "beats." Are they fast or slow? Are they strong or weak? Is the pulse regular in time between each beat? Any patient who does not have a strong, steady radial pulse is a matter of concern because a weak or irregular pulse may indicate the presence of underlying medical or traumatic disorders. If no radial pulse is detected, check for a carotid pulse (Figure 7-7■). In children younger than 8 years of age, assess circulation by checking the brachial pulse (Figure 7-8■). If no pulse is detected at any of the sites assessed, the patient is considered "pulseless," and cardiopulmonary resuscitation (compressions fol-

## Table **7-2** Normal Vital Signs

|  | Adult | Child (1–8 years) | Infant (Birth–1 year) |
|---|---|---|---|
| Pulse | 60–100 beats per minute | 80–100 | 100–120 |
| Respirations | 12–20 respirations per minute | 15–30 | 25–50 |
| Blood Pressure |  |  |  |
|   Systolic | 90–140 mmHg | 80–100 | 75–95 |
|   Diastolic | 60–90 mmHg |  |  |
| Temperature | 36.1–38.0°C (97.0–100.4°F) | 36.1–38.0°C | 36.1–38.0°C |

lowed by breaths) must be initiated immediately. Table 7-2■ lists the normal values for several vital signs, including those for pulse rate.

Circulation is also dependent on having an adequate amount of blood. Check for any life-threatening external bleeding. If present, it will need to be controlled immediately using one of the methods described in a later chapter.

Once a pulse is detected, assess the patient's skin color and temperature (Figure 7-9■). Under normal conditions, the skin should have a pink or dark tone,

**Figure 7-6** Assessing the radial pulse.

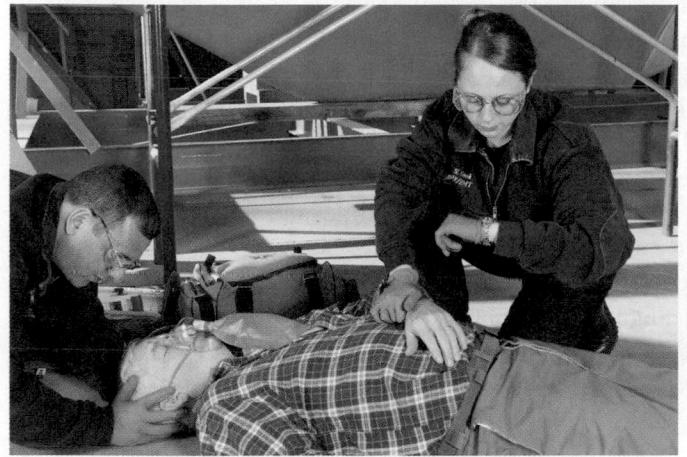

**Figure 7-7** Assessing the carotid pulse, found on either side of the trachea.

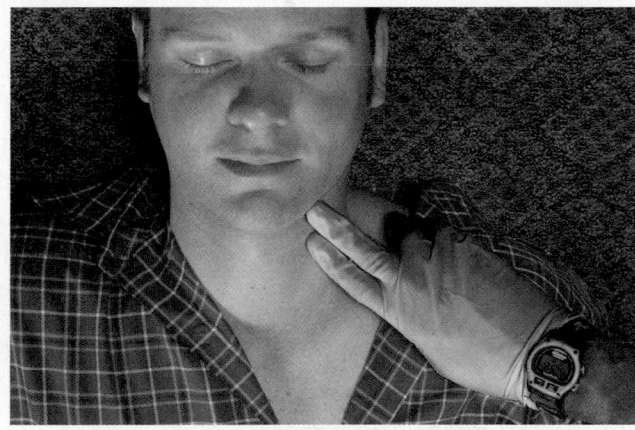

**Figure 7-8** Assessing the brachial pulse of an infant.

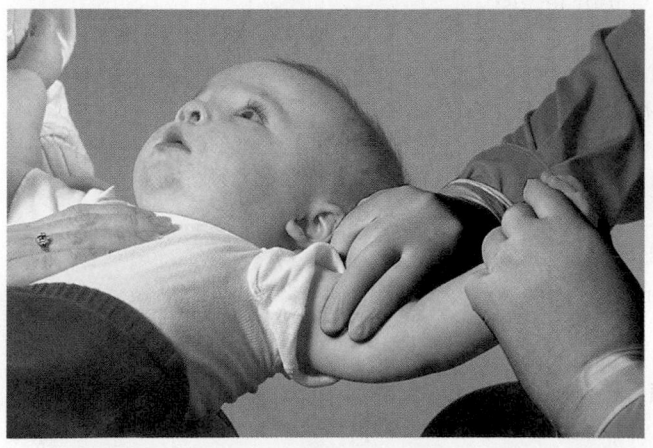

**Figure 7-9** Circulation perfusion is assessed by observing the color, temperature, and condition of the skin.

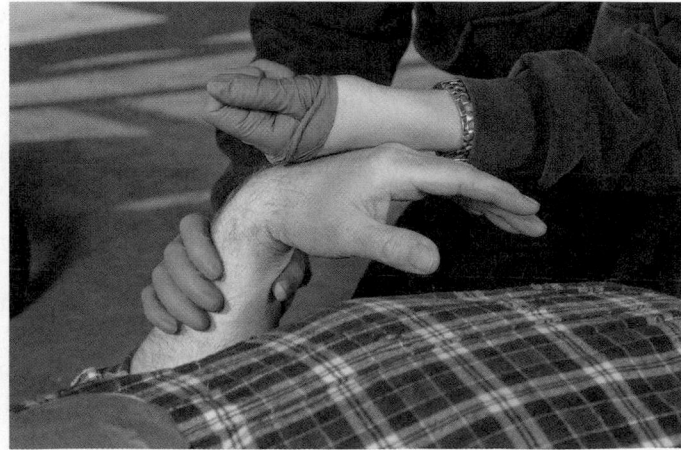

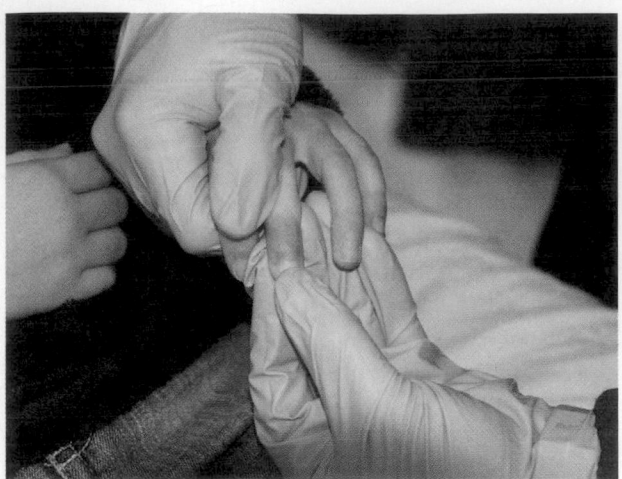

**Figure 7-10** Assessing capillary refill in a nail bed, an indication of circulation.
Copyright Mike Halloran

depending on pigmentation. Skin that is pale, gray, or blue (cyanosis) indicates that circulation is compromised. The skin is normally warm to the touch. In outdoor environments, skin color and temperature can be affected by such factors such as sunburn, exposure to wind or moisture (snow or rain), and cold or hot ambient temperatures.

Assess capillary refill by pressing on the nail bed of one of the patient's fingers and then quickly releasing the pressure (Figure 7-10■). Under normal conditions, the nail bed will blanch (turn white) when pressed and then return to its normal color in less than 2 seconds once the pressure is released. A nail bed that is cyanotic or does not return to its normal color within 2 seconds indicates that circulation is not normal. Cold environmental conditions cause the capillaries in the nail bed to be pale, blue, or slow to refill, because peripheral blood vessels are narrowed in response to the cold. An abnormal capillary refill exam (one in which refill takes longer than 2 seconds) should prompt you to investigate the underlying causes more thoroughly. Cyanosis also may be detected in the lips and earlobes.

### Disability

Next the patient is assessed for any life-threatening neurological disorders, including any problems affecting the brain or cervical spine. Begin by assessing the patient's level of responsiveness (LOR), a measure of the patient's awareness and responsiveness to the surrounding environment. Level of responsiveness is a continuum that ranges from the patient being fully alert to various levels of unresponsiveness. Under normal conditions, a patient is awake and oriented. A person who is oriented should know his name, where he is physically located, the approximate time of day, and the situation (e.g., what happened). When the patient can answer all these questions correctly, he is said to be awake, alert, and oriented to person, place, time, and situation (AAO × 4).

The inability to correctly answer even one question suggests a potential neurologic problem and is considered abnormal. An abnormal LOR can result from brain injury, **hypoxia**, and a wide range of medical conditions. Regardless of which method is used to assess the patient, it is important to initially assess the patient's LOR in the event that other care providers subsequently decide to assess the patient for any changes in LOR.

**hypoxia** a reduction in oxygen supply to a tissue.

**⊕ 7-12** Describe and demonstrate how to assess a patient's level of responsiveness using the following:

 a. AVPU

 b. Glasgow Coma Score

**AVPU** a mnemonic for assessing neurologic function; represents Awake or alert, responds to Verbal stimuli or Pain, Unresponsive.

**Glasgow Coma Scale** a method for assessing neurologic function (i.e., level of responsiveness, movement).

**AVPU and the Glasgow Coma Scale** Neurologic function also may be assessed using either the **AVPU** scale or **Glasgow Coma Scale.** Of the two, the AVPU scale is easier to use.

The AVPU scale consists of four levels:

**A—Alert:** the patient is fully awake, opens his eyes without prompting, and can speak to you; the patient is aware and responsive to the surroundings

**V—Verbal:** the patient does not open his eyes spontaneously, but responds to your voice by opening his eyes, making some type of vocal sound, or moving an extremity slightly

**P—Pain:** the patient responds to painful stimuli

**U—Unresponsive:** the patient does not respond to any type of stimulus

To assess the patient using the AVPU scale, first look at the patient to see if he appears to be awake and alert. If the patient is awake and alert, he is scored as "A" on the AVPU scale (Table 7-3■). If the patient does not appear to be alert or has his eyes

**Table 7-3** Methods for Assessing Mental Status

| | Glasgow Coma Scale | | AVPU | |
|---|---|---|---|---|
| Eyes | 4 | Opens eyes spontaneously | A | Alert |
| | 3 | Opens eyes to verbal stimuli | V | Unresponsive, but responds to verbal stimuli |
| | 2 | Opens eyes to pain | | |
| | 1 | Does not open eyes | P | Unresponsive, but responds to painful stimuli |
| Verbal | 5 | Speaks coherently | | |
| | 4 | Speaks confusedly | U | Unresponsive to pain |
| | 3 | Mutters words in response to pain | | |
| | 2 | Moans in response to pain | | |
| | 1 | No verbal response to pain | | |
| Motor | 6 | Follows commands | | |
| | 5 | Localizes pain | | |
| | 4 | Withdraws from pain | | |
| | 3 | Has a flexor response to pain | | |
| | 2 | Has an extensor response to pain | | |
| | 1 | Has no motor response to pain | | |

closed, talk to him. If the patient looks at you or merely opens his eyes, he is scored a "V" on the AVPU scale. If the patient does not respond to verbal stimuli, attempt to illicit a pain response in the patient using one of the techniques described in the next section. A patient that responds to pain is noted as "P" on the AVPU scale. If the patient does not respond to pain, then the patient is marked as "U" for unresponsive. Any score less than "A" is considered abnormal.

Another method to assess neurologic function is the Glasgow Coma Scale (GCS). Although more precise than the AVPU scale and more likely to uncover a neurologic abnormality, the GCS is more difficult to use than the AVPU scale and takes longer to perform. Use the AVPU scale for the initial assessment, and, if time permits complete a more detailed assessment using the GCS.

An OEC Technician should ideally calculate the GCS once the patient is in a more controlled environment such as a first aid room or transport vehicle. Alternatively, calculate the GCS in the field while waiting for transport to arrive. Even though the GCS provides valuable information, definitive care and transportation of the patient should never be delayed for the sole purpose of calculating the GCS. The GCS, which provides an objective measure of the patient's overall neurologic condition, has three components (Table 7-3):

+ The patient's best eye response
+ The patient's best verbal response
+ The patient's best motor response

Each component consists of a range of physical responses; each response is assigned a numerical value. The patient is assessed for the best response for each component, and then the sum of the assigned values represents the GCS score.

To calculate the GCS, begin by assessing the patient's eye response: select the description that best matches the patient's response. If, for example, the patient's eyes are initially closed but open as you first begin speaking to him, the score would be 3. If the patient's eyes remain closed regardless of what you do, the score would be 1. Next, assess the patient's best verbal response. As before, select the description that best matches the patient's response. For instance, if the patient speaks coherently and is able to carry on a normal conversation, the score is 5. If the patient only moans in response to pain, the score is 2.

Finally, assess the patient's best motor response. You might, for instance, ask the patient to hold up two fingers. If the patient can accurately follow your command, the score is 6. If the patient is unable to follow your command, you will need to assess whether or not the patient responds to painful stimuli using one of the techniques described in the next section. If the patient pushes away from the source of the pain, known as "localizing pain," the score is 5. If the patient moves his hands toward his chest in response (a flexor response), the score is 3. This response, known as **decorticate posturing**, is an ominous finding and indicates serious brain injury. If the patient moves his hands away from his body in response to the pain (an extensor response), the score is 2. This, too, is a grave finding known as **decerebrate posturing**. If there is no response at all to painful stimulus, the score is 1.

The GCS score may range from 3 to 15, and any score of 14 or less is considered abnormal. A total score of 13 or less, or any motor score less than 6, is associated with a high risk for major neurological injury. A score of 8 or less is associated with a high risk for long-term disability or death.

**Administering Painful Stimuli**    There are many different ways to illicit a pain response from a patient. The most common method used by OEC Technicians is a "trapezius pinch." To perform this technique, pinch and twist the patient's skin above the shoulder, over the trapezius muscle (Figure 7-11■). Another method is to pinch the patient's fingernail or ear lobe. The objective in using any of these techniques is to observe and document the patient's response. Do not be afraid to use these techniques, but be careful not to inflict significant tissue damage. Used appropriately, applying a painful stimulus provides valuable information about the patient's LOR. When attempting to illicit a pain response in an unresponsive patient with a known or suspected spinal cord injury, be careful not to move the patient's neck because neck movement in this setting may cause permanent neurologic damage.

Because any trauma patient with an abnormal LOR or a significant head injury is assumed to have a cervical spine injury, assessment of the cervical spine is included in the disability portion of a primary assessment. In addition, all alert trauma patients should be assessed for possible cervical spine injury at this point in the overall assessment process. Assess for cervical spine injury by determining whether the patient complains of any neck pain or shows a response to neck pain upon palpation. The person may complain of tingling or numbness in the arms or legs, a condition known as **paresthesia**, or may complain of weakness of one or more of the extremities. Unrecognized cervical spine injury can result in permanent **paralysis** or death.

**decorticate posturing**    abnormal flexing of the arms, clenching fists, and extending legs; due to an injury along the nerve pathway between the brain and spinal cord.

**decerebrate posturing**    abnormal extension of arms and legs, downward pointing of toes, and arching of the head; due to an injury to the brain at the level of the brainstem.

**paresthesia**    sensation of tingling, pricking, or numbness of a person's skin, or the feeling of "pins and needles" or a limb being "asleep."

**paralysis**    loss or impairment of motor function in a part of the body.

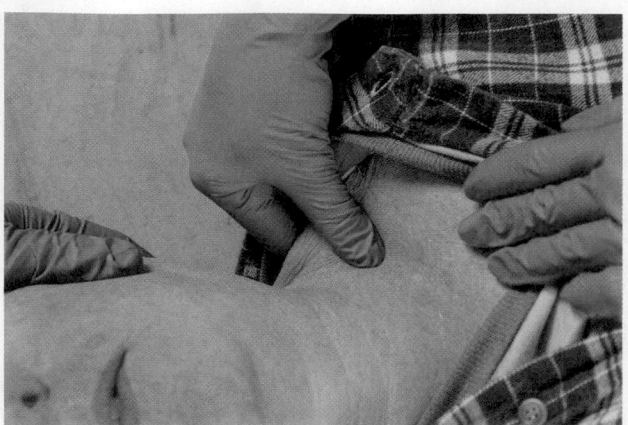

**Figure 7-11** A trapezius pinch, one method of assessing the response to pain stimuli.

### Managing Life-threatening Conditions

If at any time during the primary assessment you identify a significant life-threatening injury or illness, initiate interventions immediately and arrange for immediate transport to an appropriate higher level of care. Do not proceed with the rest of the assessment until you have managed the problem. In managing the problem, take corrective actions starting with the airway, then breathing, then circulation, and finally disability (ABCD). For instance, if the patient is not breathing, you must correct this problem before assessing the patient's circulation. Likewise, you must manage life-threatening bleeding before assessing disability.

If during the primary assessment you identify an abnormality in the ABCDs that in your judgment places the patient at imminent life-threatening risk, you should immediately expedite the rest of the assessment process and care. Focus on immediate life threats, and rapidly transport the patient to definitive care. Manage the ABCDs, protect the cervical spine, and initiate rapid transport.

## STOP, THINK, UNDERSTAND

### Multiple Choice

Choose the correct answer.

1. A scene size-up includes all of the following components *except*_____
   a. using your senses to evaluate potential dangers.
   b. determining the mechanism of injury (MOI).
   c. obtaining a patient's vital signs.
   d. determining how many victims there are.

2. Which of the following statements regarding the primary assessment is *not* true?_____
   a. Its purpose is to quickly identify and correct any potential life-threatening problems that may be present.
   b. It is conducted only on trauma patients.
   c. It should take 30–60 seconds to complete.
   d. Patient assessment and patient management often occur simultaneously.

3. The ABCDs of primary assessment stand for_____
   a. airway, breathing, circulation, disability.
   b. airway, bleeding, circulation, disability.
   c. airway, breathing, circulation, deformity.
   d. auscultation, blood pressure, correction, discovery.

4. The most consistent of the earliest observations that warns an OEC Technician of possible problems with ABCD is a patient_____
   a. with uneven pupils.
   b. who cannot stand up without assistance.
   c. who cannot grip your hands with equal grip strength.
   d. who is confused.

5. The normal respiratory rate for an adult is_____
   a. 6–10 breaths per minute.
   b. 12–20 breaths per minute.
   c. 20–30 breaths per minute.
   d. 32–38 breaths per minute.

6. The normal respiratory rate for an infant is_____
   a. 6–10 breaths per minute.
   b. 12–20 breaths per minute.
   c. 25–50 breaths per minute.
   d. 30–38 breaths per minute.

7. The pulse of a child younger than 8 years of age should be checked at which pulse point?_____
   a. brachial
   c. radial
   b. carotid
   d. femoral

8. Normal capillary refill time is_____
   a. less than 2 seconds.
   b. more than 2 seconds.
   c. less 5 seconds.
   d. immediate.

9. "AAO × 4" means_____
   a. awake, alert and oriented, checked four times at 5-minute intervals.
   b. awake, alert, and oriented to person, place, time, and situation.
   c. awake, alert, and oriented to person, place, and time.
   d. awake, alert, and oral answers are correct.

10. The three components of the Glasgow Coma Scale are_____
    a. best eye, verbal, and motor responses.
    b. assessment of pulse, respiration, and motor skills.
    c. assessment of pulse, respiration, and mentation.
    d. best response to grimace, circulation, and sensation.

11. If during your primary assessment you identify a serious abnormality in the ABCD, you should_____
    a. stop and correct the problem, and then continue with your assessment as usual.
    b. document the problem, expedite and continue with your assessment, and then correct the problem upon completion of the assessment.
    c. stop and correct any threats to life, expedite the rest of the assessment process, manage the ABCDs, protect the cervical spine (if indicated), and transport the patient to definitive care.
    d. stop the assessment, immediately treat threats to life, and transport the patient to definitive care.

### Fill in the Blank

1. List the signs of respiratory distress: _____, _____, _____, _____, _____, and_____.

2. AVPU stands for _____ _____, _____, _____.

Remember that every patient's condition is dynamic and can change over time. Therefore, do not assume that because no threats to life were identified among the ABCDs, the patient will remain stable. Instead, continually monitor the patient's ABCDs throughout the entire time you are with the patient.

Only after the patient's ABCDs have been assessed and any problems have been corrected can you move on to the next part of the patient assessment: the secondary assessment.

## The Secondary Assessment

**7-5** Describe and demonstrate how to perform a secondary assessment.

The purpose of a secondary assessment is to obtain additional information about the patient to ensure that no medical or traumatic problem is overlooked. This information will help you identify something as simple as a sprained knee to problems that could be life threatening. You may also discover other potential problems such as diabetes, which could result in long-term disability if they are not identified and appropriately managed.

A secondary assessment consists of three steps: taking a medical history, performing a physical exam, and assessing vital signs. Although these steps may be performed in this order, they can be performed concurrently, especially when other OEC Technicians are available to assist. For instance, you may obtain a medical history at the same time that a second rescuer is assessing vital signs. The key is that only one person at a time should ask the patient questions or perform the physical exam. Depending on the conditions and your findings, a secondary assessment may take 2–5 minutes to complete. In a hazardous setting, a secondary assessment may be performed very quickly or may be delayed until the patient can be moved to a safer location.

Many EMS programs differentiate the way to assess trauma patients from patients with a medical problem. It is important to remember that a patient could have sustained trauma and *simultaneously* have a serious medical problem. Even though two patients could be unresponsive, have life-threatening problems, and need immediate care, you will seek to identify the nature of injury (NOI) for a medical patient, and the mechanism of injury (MOI) for a trauma patient. In taking a medical history different questions may be used for medical versus trauma patients although the physical exam used for both types of patients is the same.

### Taking a Medical History

**7-7** List and describe the key components of a patient history.

A medical history is used to collect important historical information about the patient and the events surrounding his current condition. It consists of subjective data, known as symptoms, or evidence of disease that is qualitative in nature. Symptoms are typically provided by the patient, the patient's family or friends, or bystanders and are feeling- or emotion-based descriptions. Examples of symptoms include descriptions of pain, weakness, fatigue, nausea, blurred vision, impending doom, and the like (Figure 7-12■).

**Chief Complaint** In addition to identifying the patient's chief complaint and assessing potential causes, ask the patient about the possible presence of other associated symptoms—any other complaints the patient has that may be related to the chief complaint. Associated symptoms often indicate that something serious is causing the symptoms. For instance, a patient may complain of chest pain, but upon further questioning you discover that the patient is also short of breath. In this case, the shortness of breath is likely caused by the same mechanism(s) that is causing the patient's chest pain. Other examples of associated symptoms are nausea and vomiting associated with abdominal pain, and headache, dizziness, or visual disturbances associated with a head injury.

**7-9** Describe and demonstrate how to obtain a SAMPLE history.

**SAMPLE History** As part of the history, ask about other medical information, such as what medical problems the patient may have, what medications the patient is tak-

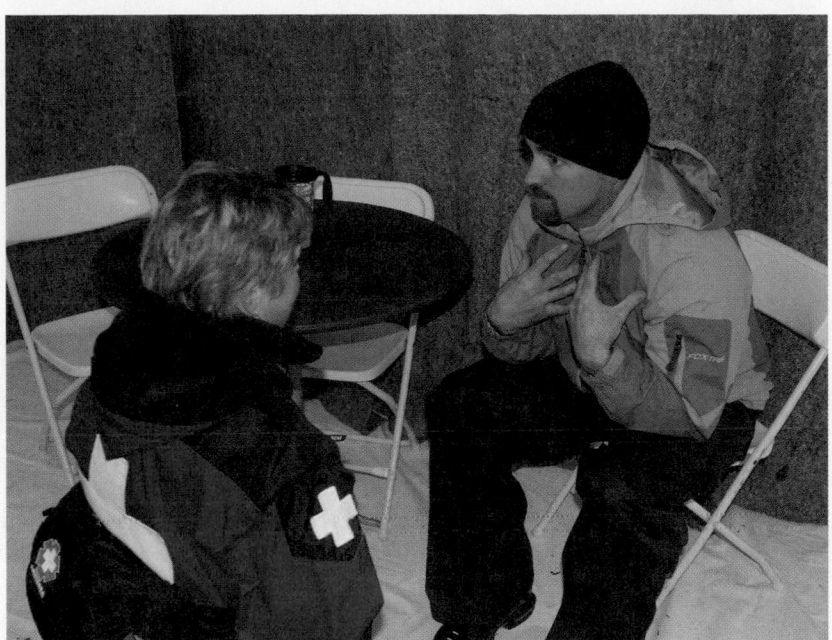

**Figure 7-12** Only one person at a time should interview a patient to obtain a medical history. This OEC Technician is obtaining a medical history from a patient.
Copyright Edward McNamara

ing, or if the patient has any known allergies. To facilitate the organized collection of this data, many rescuers use the acronym **SAMPLE**, which represents Signs and symptoms, Allergies and adverse reactions, Medications, Pertinent past medical history, Last time patient ate or drank, and Events leading up to the incident (Table 7-4■).

**S—Signs and symptoms:** Begin the SAMPLE history by assessing for any clinical signs that may be present. A **sign** is any objective finding or evidence of disease that you can detect using your senses (e.g., see, feel, hear, smell) or that you can quantify. Examples of signs are dilated pupils, a deformity, audible respiratory wheezing, a foul odor, and blood pressure. Next, ask the patient to identify each **symptom** he is having, preferably in the order in which they cause the most concern to the patient. Ask if the patient has ever experienced the symptoms before. If he has, ask what happened the last time the symptoms occurred. For instance, the patient may reply, "The last time I felt like this, I had a heart attack!"

**SAMPLE** an acronym used to obtain medical history information during the assessment process; refers to Signs/symptoms, Allergies, Medications, Past medical history, Last oral intake, Events leading up to present incident.

**sign** any objective finding that can be seen, heard, smelled, or measured; typically discovered during a physical exam (e.g., a bruise, the patient's blood pressure).

**symptom** a subjective finding that a patient experiences and can be identified only by the patient (e.g., pain, blurred vision).

**Table 7-4** Acronyms and Mnemonics for Taking Medical Histories

| SAMPLE History | |
| --- | --- |
| S | Signs and symptoms |
| A | Allergies |
| M | Medications |
| P | Pertinent past medical history |
| L | Last oral intake |
| E | Events leading to incident |
| | |
| **OPQRST (Pain Assessment)** | |
| O | Onset |
| P | Provocation and palliation |
| Q | Quality |
| R | Radiation |
| S | Severity |
| T | Time |

**A—Allergies:** Ask the patient if he has any known allergies or has had an allergic reaction in the past. This includes allergies to medications, foods, materials, insects, or animals. Knowing a patient's allergies, especially medication allergies, will be helpful for health care providers who continue the patient's care after you. Giving a patient a medication that causes an allergic reaction can be deadly.

**M—Medications:** Ask the patient if he is taking any medications or is supposed to be taking any medications, including prescription medications, over-the-counter medications, herbs, vitamin supplements, homeopathic remedies, and illicit drugs or alcohol. This information is very important because many of these substances can mask symptoms or react with one another. If the patient is taking a prescription medication, ask if he has been taking the medication as prescribed.

**P—Past medical history:** Ask the patient about his past medical history, including any previously diagnosed medical problems such as heart disease, a respiratory condition, diabetes, or high blood pressure, and any previous surgeries. Although these problems may have been resolved or are seemingly under control, this information may help you anticipate problems. For instance, knowing that a patient has a history of a previous heart attack is important if the person is complaining of chest pain or shortness of breath. Similarly, if you encounter a patient experiencing ankle pain after a fall, it is helpful to know that, for instance, the person has had ankle surgery and now has a metal plate in the ankle. Be direct. Ask the patient, "Do you have any significant medical problems?" or "Do you have any medical conditions for which you are seeing a physician or are supposed to be seeing a physician?" In some instances, you may need to be specific by asking, "Have you ever hurt your ankle before?"

**L—Last time patient ate or drank something:** Ask the patient when he last ate a meal or had any fluids, including any alcoholic beverages. This information may be helpful as you attempt to figure out if the patient's weakness is due to not eating or to drinking. It also will be helpful should the patient require surgery in the immediate future.

**E—Events leading up to the incident:** Ask the patient about the events leading up to the incident, especially what the patient was doing when the symptoms were first noticed. This information helps bring the pieces of the assessment puzzle together and helps you to treat the patient's injuries and/or illness more effectively. If appropriate, ask if the patient has or is feeling nauseated, and if the patient has vomited. If the answer is yes, ask how many times the patient vomited, over how long a period has the vomiting occurred, whether the vomit was clear or blood-tinged, and when the patient vomited last. This information helps you determine if the vomiting is a life threat. For example, blood in the vomit could be life threatening and repeated vomiting within a short period of time is also a serious situation.

**⊕ 7-10** Describe and demonstrate how to assess pain using the OPQRST mnemonic.

**OPQRST** In addition to the SAMPLE history, the **OPQRST** mnemonic can be helpful in gathering additional information about the patient's chief complaint and associated symptoms (Table 7-4). Although originally designed for assessing pain, the OPQRST mnemonic works equally well for assessing other complaints and symptoms. It can be used to assess both traumatic and medical complaints. OPQRST represents Onset, Provocation and palliation, Quality, Radiation, Severity, and Time.

**OPQRST** a mnemonic that is used in the assessment of a patient's chief complaint: represents Onset, Provocation and palliation, Quality, Radiation, Severity, and Time.

**O—Onset:** Query the patient about when the symptoms began. What was the patient doing when the complaint was first noticed? Depending on the circumstances, this may be obvious or not so clear. Attempt to find out if the pain came on suddenly or gradually. Determine whether the patient was at rest or engaged in a physical activity when the symptoms began. If the patient has a history of medical problems, ask if the onset feels like any previously experienced condition. Also, ask whether the current symptoms have been constant or come and go (are intermittent). Although questions of this nature may have been asked as part of the SAMPLE, they provide an opportunity to gather additional relevant information.

**P—Provocation and palliation:** Ask if the patient has any idea what might have caused the problem. If, for instance, the patient has been on a strenuous hike and has experienced progressive difficulties in breathing, the patient's condition may be connected to the hike. Additionally, ask if anything makes the problem either worse (is a provocation) or better (is a palliation). Attempt to determine if rest provides any relief from the problem, even if only slightly or momentarily. Using the previous situation, the patient may indicate that when he stopped hiking, his breathing became much easier.

**Q—Quality:** Ask the patient to describe the nature of his symptoms. For instance, if the patient presents with pain, ask him to describe the pain. Is it sharp, dull, or throbbing? Attempt to determine whether the symptoms have changed in any way since they were first noticed. For instance, the patient may initially have experienced only abdominal pain that has now resolved, only to be replaced by severe nausea.

**R—Radiation:** Ask the patient to locate the source of the problem by pointing to where the symptoms are most intense. If the problem involves a large area, ask the patient to draw a circle around the site using his fingers. Attempt to determine whether the symptoms move from this area to another location or remain in one spot. If the problem is pain, ask if pressing on the site of the discomfort causes pain in another part of the body.

**S—Severity:** Ask the patient to describe the severity of the symptoms. You may find it helpful to ask the patient to rate the severity using a 1–10 scale, with 1 being problem free and 10 being the worst pain they have ever felt. Repeat the question to monitor changes in the patient's perception of the severity over time.

**T—Time:** Ask how long the patient has had the problem. Also ask if the same problem has occurred previously.

The SAMPLE and OPQRST techniques are tools that may help you collect the patient's history. It is very important that you collect all the information on the patient's history that is outlined by the SAMPLE and OPQRST procedures.

## Physical Exam

A physical exam is a head-to-toe, hands-on assessment of the patient (Figure 7-13 ■). It is performed to identify specific clinical findings that will aid in determining the source of the patient's current medical problem or traumatic injury. As part of the

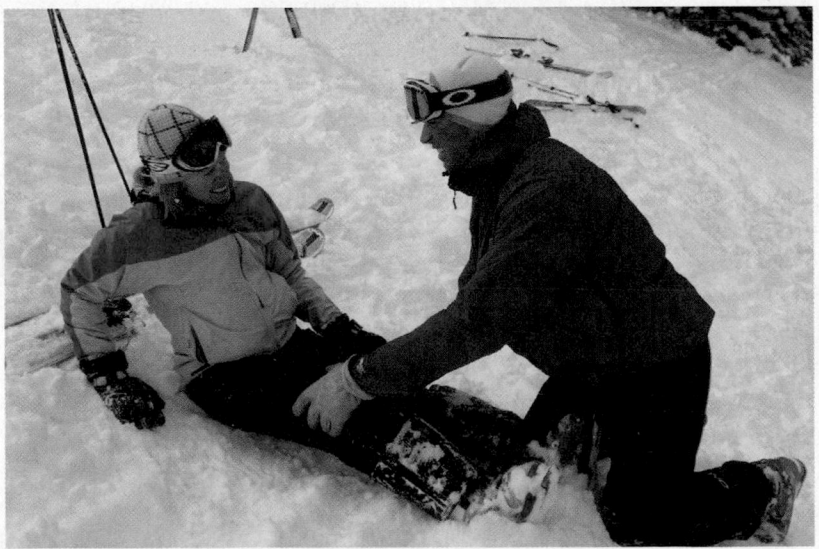

**Figure 7-13** A full-body examination is an important part of a secondary assessment.
Copyright Scott Smith

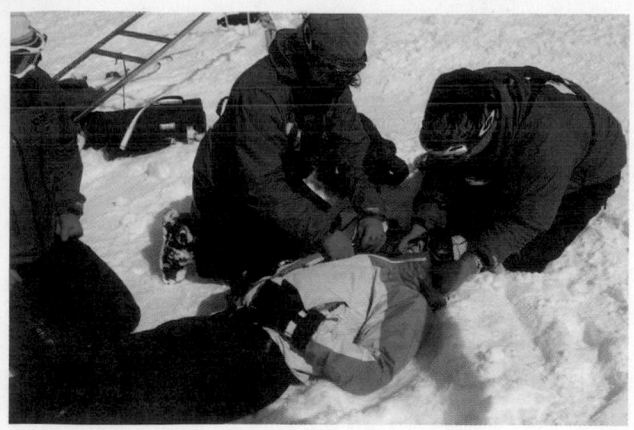

**Figure 7-14** During inclement weather, open bulky clothes to perform the examination and then close them again to keep the patient warm.
Copyright Scott Smith

**distracting injury**   any injury that directs the patient's attention away from the exam that is being performed by the rescuer.

**DCAP-BTLS**   a mnemonic for assessing trauma-related injuries; represents Deformity; Contusions; Abrasions and avulsions; Punctures and penetrations; Burns, bleeding, and bruises; Tenderness; Lacerations; and Swelling.

**contusion**   a bruise or soft tissue injury to a body part without a break in the skin.

**abrasion**   a rubbed or scraped area of skin.

**avulsion**   the tearing away of soft tissue, or a piece of soft tissue hanging as a flap.

**laceration**   an open soft tissue injury with smooth or jagged edges.

**swelling**   an enlargement of body tissue caused by an accumulation of excess fluid.

physical exam, you will note the patient's *signs*—any objective findings or evidence of a disease that you can detect using your senses (e.g., that you can see, feel, hear, smell) or that you can quantify. First look at the body part, then palpate it. You should open or remove clothes to examine each area of the body and then redress the patient, especially during inclement weather (Figure 7-14■).

Patients who have experienced spinal injury or head trauma should remain in spinal alignment during the exam. If help is available and it is practical to do so, maintain spinal alignment, including the neck, and log roll the person to the supine position to make the exam easier. Other trauma patients may be examined in the position found, or if it is practical and safe to do so based on the injury, may be placed in a supine or sitting position.

Patients with medical conditions will typically assume a position of comfort. When short of breath they will sit upright; when abdominal pain is present, they will want to bend their knees. The exam can be done in any position, but it goes more easily when the patient is made comfortable.

A physical exam is performed in a systematic manner and should take only a few minutes to complete, unless a serious problem is encountered. Do not be afraid to touch the patient; touching is an essential part of the exam process. Be aware of **distracting injuries**, and be aware that touching, also known as palpating, may cause the patient some physical discomfort, especially if you must palpate areas that are tender or swollen. Despite this possibility, you must perform a thorough physical exam, or potential problems might go undetected. If you encounter any body fluids, take appropriate precautions to avoid coming in contact with those fluids.

To facilitate the exam process, you may find it helpful to use the **DCAP-BTLS** mnemonic to help identify abnormalities (Table 7-5■). DCAP-BTLS was created by Dr. John Campbell, author of the acclaimed trauma textbook *Basic Trauma Life Support*. DCAP-BTLS refers to the following abnormalities:

**D**—Deformity                    **B**—Burns/bleeding/bruises
**C—Contusions**                  **T**—Tenderness
**A—Abrasions/avulsions**    **L—Lacerations**
**P**—Punctures /penetrations    **S—Swelling**

**Examining the Head**   Using the DCAP-BTLS method, begin the physical exam by palpating the patient's entire head, scalp, and face, moving from back to front (posterior to anterior) (Figure 7-15■). Look and feel for any irregularities or evidence of trauma. Look for blood or clear fluid draining from the ears or nose. Check the area

| Table **7-5**  Trauma Physical Exam Mnemonic |
|---|
| **DCAP-BTLS (Physical Exam)** |

| | |
|---|---|
| D | Deformity |
| C | Contusions |
| A | Abrasions/avulsions |
| P | Punctures/penetrations |
| B | Burns/bleeding/bruises |
| T | Tenderness |
| L | Lacerations |
| S | Swelling |

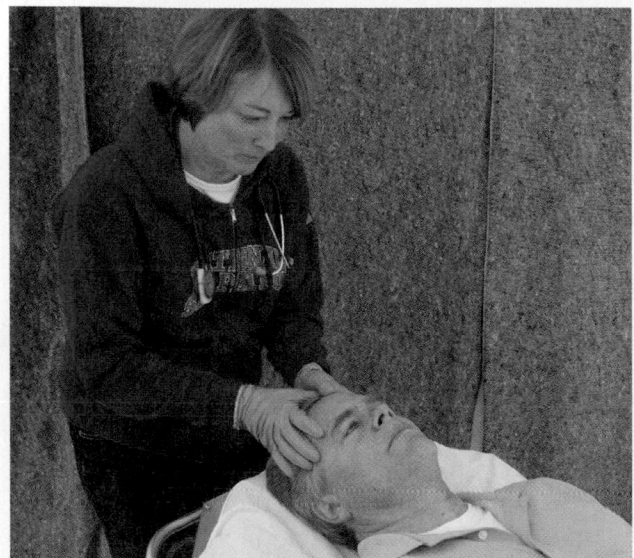

**Figure 7-15** Head assessment begins by feeling the entire head, including the scalp and face, for irregularities or trauma.
Copyright Mike Halloran

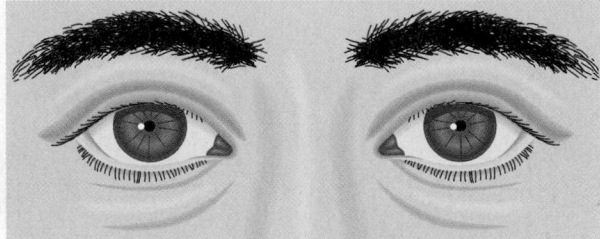

Constricted pupils

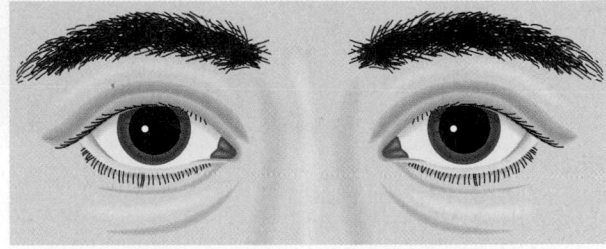

Dilated pupils

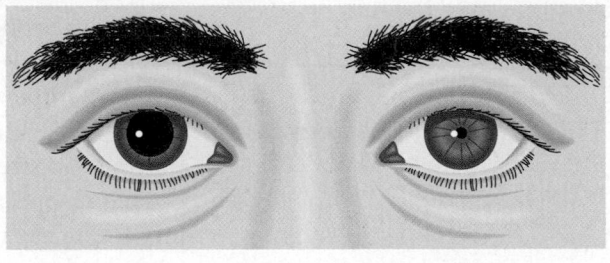

Unequal pupils

**Figure 7-16** Pupil assessment: constricted, dilated, or unequal?

behind the ears for discoloration. Is the white part of the eye yellow, indicating possible hepatitis or liver disease?

Next, examine the eyes for symmetry and to see if the pupils are constricted, dilated, or unequal (Figure 7-16■). To assess the pupils' reactions to light, conduct the following procedure, which requires the use of a penlight or a small flashlight (OEC Skill 7-4■):

1. Instruct the patient to stare at your nose or the center of your forehead.

2. Observe the pupils. Do they appear to be the same size? If not, the pupils are said to be asymmetrical. Asymmetry may be caused by an underlying medical or traumatic condition, or it may be normal.

3. Turn the penlight on.

4. Moving from the lateral side of the patient's face, briefly shine the light into the patient's left pupil (Figure 7-17■). Note the reaction of the pupil to the light. It should get smaller, or constrict, when the light is shined into it. In some cases, you may need to perform this step more than once. Move the light away from the left eye.

5. Shine the light into the left pupil a second time. Note the reaction of the right pupil, which also should constrict when the light is shined into the left pupil.

6. Repeat step #4, this time shining the light into the patient's right pupil. Again, note the pupillary reaction to the light. As before, the pupil should constrict when the light is shined into it.

7. Shine the light into the right pupil a second time, this time noting the pupillary reaction of the left pupil. The pupil should constrict.

You also may wish to assess eye movement. Unless the patient has an eye injury or a preexisting condition, the eyes should move together in unison. Medically, such eye movement is called

⊕ 7-11 Describe and demonstrate how to assess the eyes (pupils and movement).

**Figure 7-17** Checking the patient's left pupil for response to light.
Copyright Mike Halloran

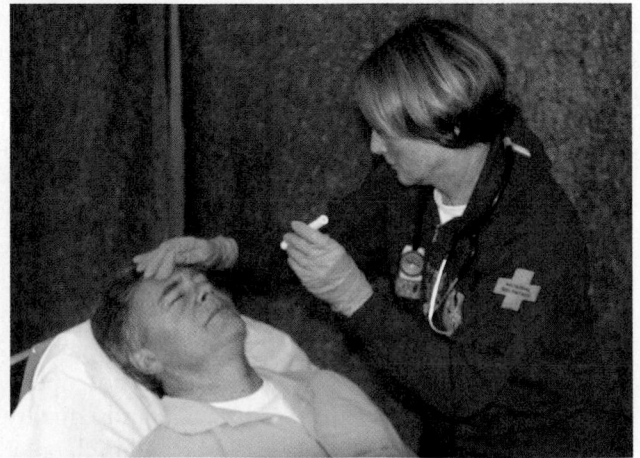

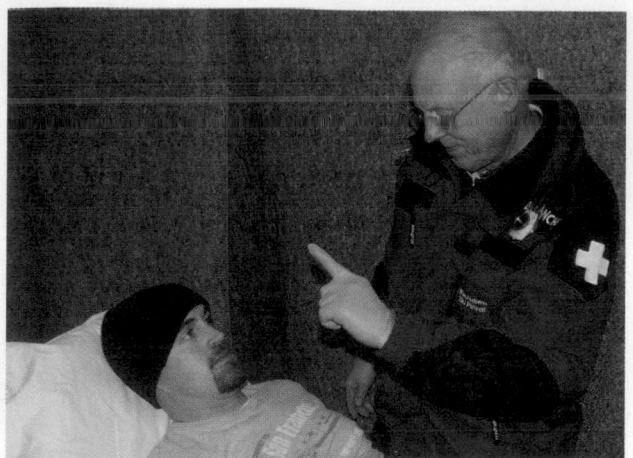

**Figure 7-18** Assessment of eye movement: the patient is instructed to follow the finger with his eyes without moving his head.
Copyright Mike Halloran

**PERRL** a mnemonic for assessing the eyes (i.e., Pupils Equal, Round, Reactive to Light).

extra-ocular movement. If the eyes move correctly, then extra-ocular movement is intact, or EOMI. To assess eye movement, follow these steps:

1. Ask the patient to stare at the center of your forehead (as previously described).
2. Hold up your index finger approximately 6–8 inches away from the patient's face (Figure 7-18■). Instruct the patient to follow the tip of your finger with his eyes without moving his head.
3. Slowly move your index finger from the center to the right, then back to center, then over to the left, and then back to center again. Then, slowly move your finger from the center upward, then downward past center, and then back up to the center. Next, slowly move your finger toward you a few inches, and then toward the patient's nose. Throughout this step, the patient's eyes should follow your finger and move in sync with one another.

If the light conditions are too bright to use a penlight, you can still assess the pupils by either shading the patient's eyes during the exam or by simply instructing the patient to close, then open, his eyes. Repeat this several times until you have assessed both pupils.

If the pupils are the same size, are both round, and both get smaller when a light is shined into each eye, they are noted as "**P**upils are **E**qual, **R**ound, and **R**eactive to **L**ight," or **PERRL**. As you are examining the eyes, note whether the light causes the patient any apparent discomfort. Look for any bleeding or fluid leaking from the eye. If the pupil appears elongated, the pupils are not symmetrical; this may indicate an injury to the eye itself or to the brain.

Next, look at the patient's face. Does it appear symmetrical, or does one side look different from the other? Are the muscles on one side of the face not working, making that side droop? Does the patient's overall color appear normal, or is it pale, yellow, or slightly blue? Check the stability of the facial bones by applying equal but gentle pressure, first on the cheekbones, then on the bone beneath the nose. Check the mouth for evidence of broken or loose teeth, cuts on the inside of the cheeks, swelling, or bleeding. Instruct the patient to clench his teeth and ask whether the teeth feel like they align normally.

**Examining the Neck** If you suspect a neck injury, begin by manually stabilizing the neck and spine. Examine the back of the neck. Can you see any bleeding or deformity? Palpate for tenderness at the base of the skull and down the back of the neck. Then, moving from the middle, palpate toward the sides (Figure 7-19■). Look at the front of the neck for symmetry, any deformity, swelling, or other signs of trauma. Palpate the front of the neck, noting any tenderness or crackling (Figure 7-20■). Listen for any abnormal sounds.

**Examining the Chest** Expose and look at the chest wall. Note the general color of the skin. Are there any signs of trauma, such as bruising or bleeding? Watch the patient breathe in and out. Does the chest movement appear equal? Ask the patient to breathe deeply. Does this cause the patient any discomfort? If not, place your hands on each side of the patient's chest, beneath the armpits, and squeeze firmly as the patient breathes in deeply. Does this cause any pain? If not, place one hand on the patient's sternum and the other on the patient's spine between the shoulder blades, squeezing gently. Ask the patient to breathe deeply. Again, does this cause any pain? If a stethoscope is available, listen to the breath sounds (Figure 7-21■). Note the presence and equality of breath sounds on both sides of the chest. This process is described in detail in Chapter 13, Respiratory Emergencies.

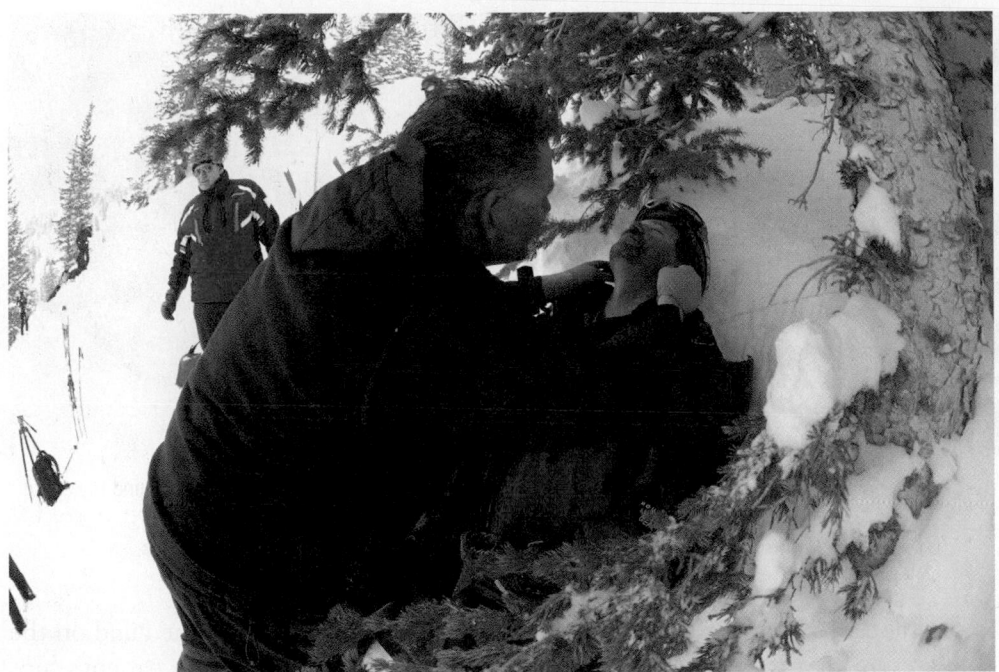

**Examining the Abdomen**   Expose and look at the abdomen. Does it appear flat or distended? Does it appear pale or otherwise discolored? Ask the patient where it hurts, and then palpate each of four quadrants in turn, always palpating the quadrant that hurts last (Figure 7-22■). Palpate firmly, but not too hard. Note any tenderness, rigidity, or masses.

**Examining the Back**   Look at the patient's back, noting the general color of the skin and any abnormalities that may be present. Using a flat, open hand, examine the entire back. Palpate the entire length of the spine from the neck to the tailbone (Figure 7-23■). Palpate either side of the spine. Feel for areas of tenderness or deformity. If a spinal injury is suspected, assess the back and spine gently, being careful not to move the spine.

**Figure 7-21** Chest assessment includes listening to see if breath sounds are present on the chest and back.
Copyright Mike Halloran

**Figure 7-20** Neck assessment should include gentle palpation of the front of the neck.
Copyright Mike Halloran

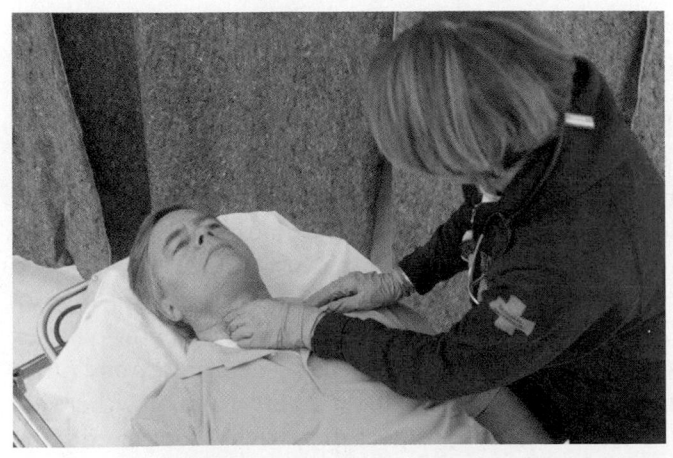

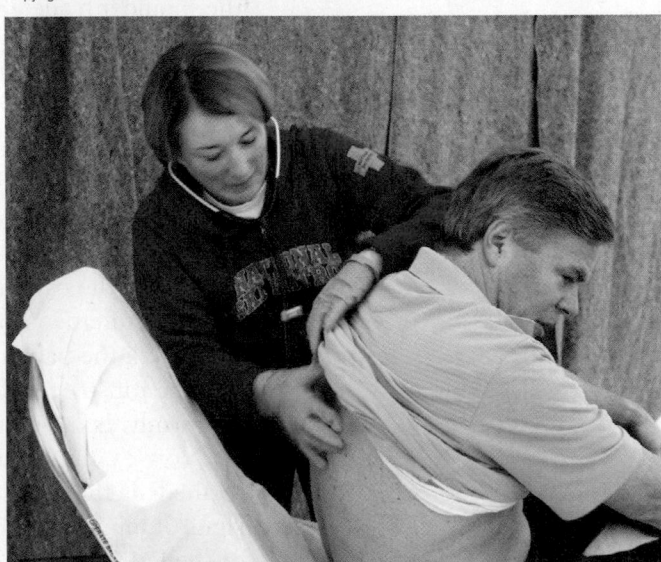

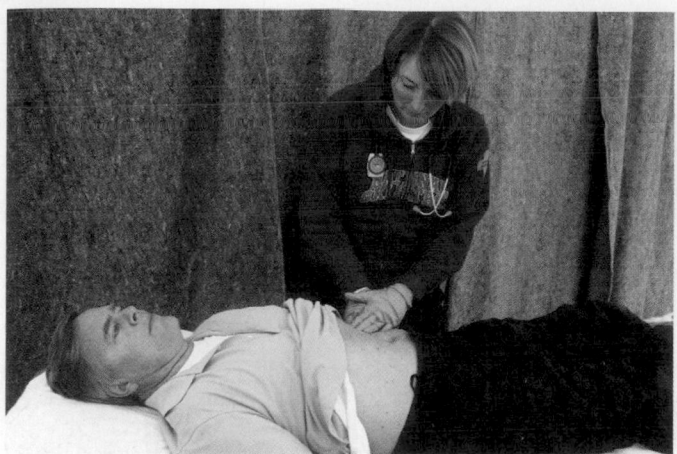

**Figure 7-22** This OEC Technician is palpating the left lower quadrant during an assessment of the abdomen.
Copyright Mike Halloran

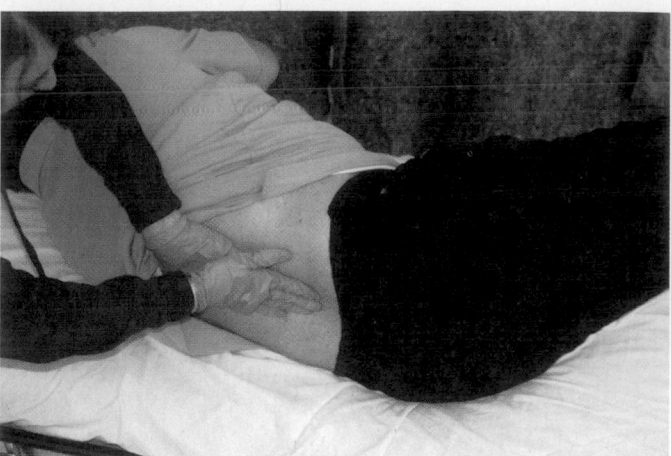

**Figure 7-23** An assessment of the back must include palpating the entire spine.
Copyright Mike Halloran

**Examining the Pelvis**    Palpate the bones of the pelvis by placing one hand on the iliac crests—that is, on each of the large pelvic bones just above the patient's hips (Figure 7-24■). Firmly but gently squeeze the bones inward (medially). This test should be performed only once because excessive manipulation of an unstable pelvis injury could cause potentially life-threatening bleeding. Note any instability or movement. If external bleeding is apparent, visually inspect the source of bleeding. Preserve the patient's modesty by covering the person with a blanket or jacket. The pelvis, groin, and genital area should be visually examined only if bleeding or other major injury to the area is suspected.

**Examining the Extremities**    Look at the arms and legs. Do they appear normal, or is one bent at an unnatural angle? Is visible bleeding apparent? Ask the patient if he has a wet and warm feeling under the clothes, indicating bleeding.

If the patient complains of arm or leg pain, ask the patient to point to where it hurts. Palpate the *non-injured* part of the extremity first, and then examine the painful part. Otherwise, the patient may pull away and not let you examine the rest of that extremity. This is especially true in children.

In assessing the arm, begin at the shoulder and move distally. Palpate lightly first on the shoulder blade, then wrap your hands around the upper arm and firmly palpate the entire arm down to the hand (Figure 7-25■). Note any palpable deformities or complaints of pain. Feel the bones of the hand. Do they feel intact? Note the color of the skin. Press on one of the nail beds; does the color immediately return? Ask the patient to make a fist, and then to straighten out his fingers and spread them apart. Check sensation on the palm side of the thumb and pinkie finger as well as the back of the thumb.

Repeat this entire exam for the other arm. When complete, feel for equality of pulses in both arms by checking the radial pulses at the same time. Do they feel the same? Ask the patient to grip and squeeze the middle and index fingers of both your hands simultaneously (Figure 7-26■). Is the patient's grip equal and strong on both sides? Ask the patient to hold his elbows up, straight out from each side of the body and then instruct the patient not to let you push his arms down. Push down slowly but firmly. Is the patient's strength equal on both sides?

Now examine the legs. Do they appear normal, or does one or both look deformed? Is there any evidence of bleeding or trauma? Feel for deformities and other signs of injury by palpating the entire length of one leg with one hand on either side of the leg (Figure 7-27■). If conditions permit, inspect the patient's foot, noting the

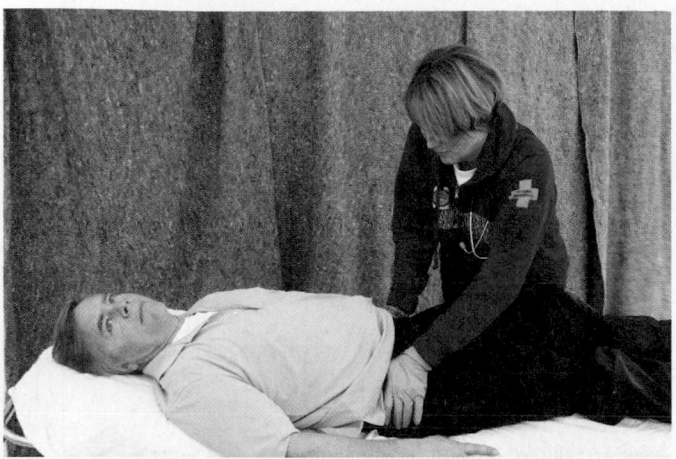

**Figure 7-24** An assessment of the pelvis includes an examination of the iliac crests on each side.
Copyright Mike Halloran

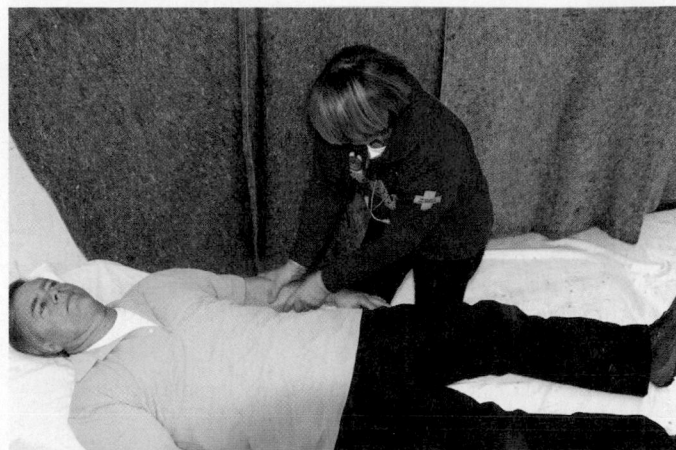

**Figure 7-25** Use both hands to palpate each arm from the shoulder blade to the fingers.
Copyright Mike Halloran

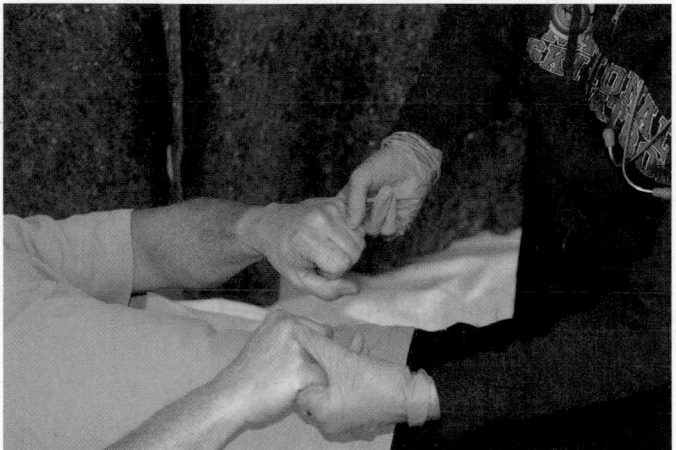

**Figure 7-26** Assessing hand grip strength to determine whether it is the same on each side.
Copyright Mike Halloran

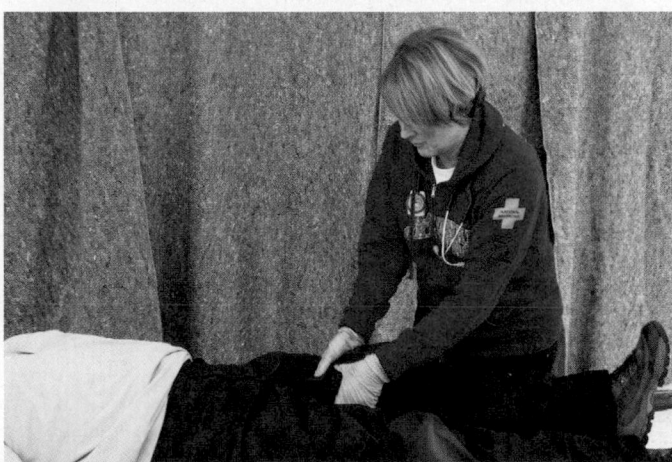

**Figure 7-27** During leg palpation, examine each leg by placing one hand on either side of the leg.
Copyright Mike Halloran

color, overall skin temperature, and presence or absence of a pedal pulse. Repeat the exam on the other leg. Next, place one hand against the bottom of each of the patient's feet and ask the patient to push against your hands with both feet. Strength should be equal on both sides of the patient's body. Touch the patient on both legs at the lateral and medial side of the ankle. The sensation felt by the patient should be described as being equal. If conditions do not permit a visual exam of the foot, have the patient wiggle his toes inside the boot; note whether the patient can feel the toes wiggle. Although not ideal, this method of assessment may have to suffice until later, when the boot may be taken off in a more controlled environment.

If there are no concerns for spinal injury and no findings of any leg injury, and you do not judge the patient to be at risk for falling, examine the patient's ability to walk (also known as testing for gait). Slowly bring the patient from a lying position to a sitting position, and then with assistance to a standing position. Then, while standing next to the patient, ask him to walk with one foot directly in front of the other (this is known as tandem gait). Abnormalities in tandem gait should make you concerned for a subtle injury or neurological deficit. Testing for gait is typically done in a controlled setting such as inside a first-aid room.

# STOP, THINK, UNDERSTAND

## Multiple Choice

Choose the correct answer.

1. What is the purpose of a secondary assessment?_____
   a. To obtain additional information about the patient.
   b. To ensure that no medical or traumatic problems that may need treatment are overlooked.
   c. To obtain medical history, vital signs, and a physical exam.
   d. All of the above

2. The medical history exam includes all of the following data *except*_____
   a. diagnosis.
   b. subjective complaints such as symptoms.
   c. the chief complaint.
   d. the nature of the illness.

3. In which of the following situations is the resulting MOI likely to be considered significant?_____ (more than one may apply)
   a. An adult climber who falls 22 feet off a ledge.
   b. A 10-year-old climber who falls 12 feet.
   c. A cross country skier struck by a snowmobile going 25 mph.
   d. A cross country skier struck by a snowmobile going 15 mph.
   e. A lift-operator struck by an out-of-control skier traveling at a high rate of speed.

4. What is an associated symptom?_____
   a. An additional complaint that may be related to the chief complaint.
   b. A symptom you observe but that the patient may not be unaware of.
   c. A cause and effect.
   d. A symptom inadvertently caused by the rescuer's intervention.

5. A patient fell out of a chair in the lodge cafeteria and your first judgment is that the patient suffered no significant injuries. However, the patient is complaining that his neck hurts and his fingers tingle. What is your *next* appropriate response?_____
   a. Continue your assessment without being overly concerned about the complaint because no significant injuries are apparent.
   b. Give the patient an ice pack and instruct him to see his physician if his neck still hurts in the morning.
   c. Stop the assessment and initiate full spinal precautions, including putting this patient on a back board.
   d. Have your partner stabilize the patient's head and neck, then rapidly continue your assessment.

6. Which of the following about MOI is true?_____
   a. If the patient has no complaints following a significant MOI, then an OEC Technician can safely assume that the patient is probably all right.
   b. Even if the patient has no complaints following a significant MOI, an OEC Technician should assume that a significant injury may still have occurred.
   c. An OEC Technician should never assume anything.
   d. None of the above are true.

7. Any trauma patient with an abnormal LOR or a significant head injury is automatically assumed to have what?_____
   a. a compromised airway
   b. a skull fracture
   c. a cervical spine injury
   d. an OEC Technician should never assume anything about a patient

8. Decerebrate posturing is defined as_____
   a. a slumped-forward position.
   b. a response in which a patient moves the hands toward the chest in response to painful stimuli.
   c. a response in which a patient moves the hands away from the body in response to painful stimuli.
   d. a situation in which a patient can hold the arms straight out in front of the body for 30 seconds.

9. SAMPLE stands for which of the following?_____
   a. Signs/symptoms, Allergies, Medications, Past medical history, Last oral intake, Events prior
   b. Signs/symptoms, Allergies, MOI, Plan/pulse, Limitations, Environment
   c. Subjective, Assessment, Medical history, Pain, LOR, Events
   d. Symptoms, Associated signs, MOI, Plan/pulse, Limitations, Emesis

10. What does the Q stand for in OPQRST?
    a. Quality
    b. Quiet
    c. Quick
    d. Quixotic

11. Which of the following questions are appropriate to ask a patient regarding their medication(s)?_____
    a. "Are you taking any herbs, supplements, or homeopathic remedies?"
    b. "Which prescription medications are you taking?"
    c. "Why are you taking this medication?"
    d. Privacy laws prohibit OEC Technicians from asking any of these questions.
    e. A, B, and C

12. Why is it important to ask a patient what caused them to fall?_____
    a. Dizziness or chest pains preceding or causing a fall could be indicative of a serious medical problem.
    b. Knowing what caused a fall might prevent a law suit.
    c. The cause of a fall is an indicator of a significant MOI.
    d. The cause of a fall is not important for an OEC Technician to determine.

*continued*

13. Which of the following statements regarding assessment is *not* true?_____
    a. An assessment must be performed in the same sequence every time.
    b. Whenever possible, an OEC Technician should establish and follow the same sequence of assessment every time.
    c. An assessment should be stopped to correct any serious problems encountered.
    d. An assessment may be modified depending on existing circumstances, including environmental considerations and rescuer safety and well-being.

## Sequence

Number the following components of a physical exam in the correct sequence for performing it:

_____ a. Assess the back of the neck.
_____ b. Palpate the head/scalp.
_____ c. Palpate the abdominal quadrants.
_____ d. Look at the chest; assess for symmetry of breathing.
_____ e. Look in the eyes and ears.
_____ f. Assess papillary reaction and eye symmetry.
_____ g. Palpate hips/pelvis.
_____ h. Assess the face.
_____ i. Examine the upper extremities.
_____ j. Examine the lower extremities.
_____ k. Examine the back/spine.

## Matching

Indicate whether each of the following items is a sign or a symptom by writing the correct letter in the blank.

_____ 1. sign
_____ 2. symptom

a. pain
b. dilated pupils
c. nausea
d. deformity
e. audible wheezing
f. low blood pressure
g. shortness of breath (SOB)
h. tripoding
i. elevated pulse
j. tightness in chest

# CASE UPDATE

You introduce yourself and ask permission to assess and treat the patient. The patient says, "Yes," so you perform a primary assessment while using spinal precautions because of the MOI. The patient is awake and speaks to you in two- or three-word sentences. You determine that his airway is open, but you are concerned that he appears to be having trouble breathing. You check his radial pulse, which is rapid (100/bpm) and strong. The patient is alert and oriented to person, place, and time. He opens his eyes spontaneously, speaks coherently, and is able to follow your commands.

In assessing his AVPU score, you assign him an "A" for "alert." The patient complains of a persistent pain on the left side of his chest. The history you take reveals that the patient was climbing approximately 6 feet off the ground when he began to feel weak and dizzy. He started having some pain in his chest and "lost my grip." He remembers hitting his lower back against a rock but does not believe that he lost consciousness. He describes the pain in his chest as "heavy." The pain does not radiate and is localized to the chest. He also reports being short of breath. He denies any other complaints. He reports no allergies to any medications but states that he takes aspirin on a daily basis because he had a heart attack ten years ago but has been doing quite well since then. He had been bouldering for about an hour and had taken several breaks during which he drank two bottles of a popular sports drink. His last rest break was about 15 minutes before he fell. He also ate a protein bar during that break. You obtain additional information using the OPQRST mnemonic.

***What should you do now?***

**vital signs**   the key objective findings used to evaluate a patient's overall condition; includes pulse rate, respiratory rate, blood pressure, temperature, and level of responsiveness.

## Assessing Vital Signs

**Vital signs** are an essential step of the overall assessment process and should be obtained on every patient. Also known as "vitals," vital signs are the key objective findings used to evaluate a patient's overall condition. They are used in conjunction with the information gathered from the medical history and during the physical exam both to identify medical problems and to evaluate the effectiveness of your treatment efforts. Whether they are normal or abnormal, vital signs provide valuable information about your patient. It is essential that you are able to distinguish between normal and abnormal vital signs for all age groups.

In most instances, a complete set of vital signs—consisting of level of responsiveness, pulse rate, respiration rate, blood pressure, and body temperature—is obtained both at the beginning and at the end of the secondary assessment. The first set of vital signs, known as "baseline vitals," establishes a reference point against which all other sets of vital signs are compared. Temperature and blood pressure may be difficult to obtain outdoors if equipment to measure these parameters is not available. However, obtain data on level of responsiveness, pulse rate, and respiration rate. Most EMS personnel assess vital signs in the following order: level of responsiveness, then pulse rate, then respiration rate (unless there is obvious respiratory difficulty), then blood pressure, and finally temperature.

**level of responsiveness (LOR)**   the degree of cognitive function and arousal of the brain; ranges from fully alert to unresponsive.

**Level of Responsiveness**   The first vital sign, **level of responsiveness (LOR)**, is immediately apparent when you begin your assessment. It is easiest to use the AVPU scale for this vital sign. OEC Technicians should reevaluate this vital sign frequently, especially for a patient with a head injury.

**Pulse**   Assess both the rate and quality of the pulse—that is, the number of times the heart beats in a minute and the strength of the heartbeat (OEC Skill 7-5■). The normal range of pulse rate for an adult is 60–100 beats per minute. A rate of less than 60 or greater than 100 is abnormal but does not necessarily mean there is a significant problem. In fact, trained athletes frequently have a normal resting pulse rate less than 60, whereas high pulse rates can result from exercise, pain, or fear. Nevertheless, the presence of an abnormal pulse rate should raise your suspicion concerning a potentially dangerous problem.

Following are the different pulse locations that can be found on the body:

**Figure 7-28** Assessing the carotid pulse.

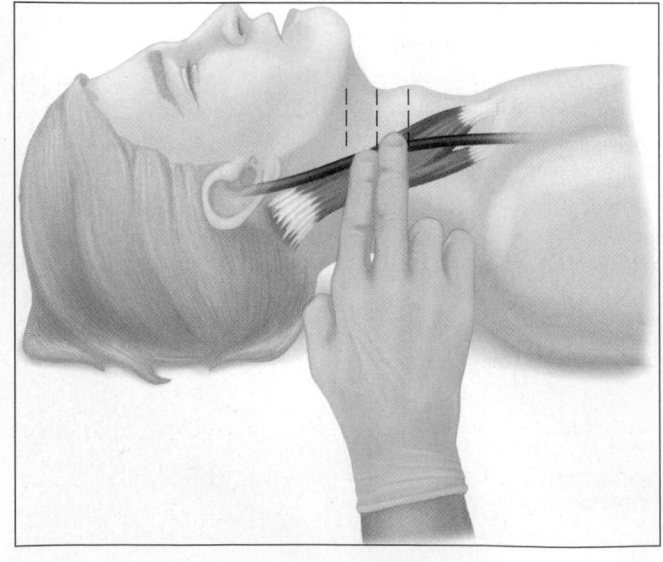

+ **Radial pulse.** The radial artery is the most common site used to assess pulse rate in a responsive patient. To feel for the radial pulse, place your index and middle fingers on the bony prominence of the thumb or radial side of the wrist, and slide them toward the palm side of the wrist until they fall into a groove.

+ **Carotid pulse.** To locate the carotid pulse, place your index and middle fingers on the thyroid cartilage (also known as the Adam's apple) and then slide them laterally into the first groove (Figure 7-28■). Due to the proximity of this site to the heart, the carotid pulse is usually the strongest arterial pulse and is frequently used first when assessing the pulse of an unresponsive patient.

+ **Brachial pulse.** To locate the brachial pulse, place your hand at the bony prominence at the ulnar side (medial side) of the elbow and then slide your fingers into the groove at the base of the biceps muscle in the medial aspect of the elbow (Figure 7-29■).

✦ **Femoral pulse.** To locate the femoral pulse, draw an imaginary line on the patient from the middle of the groin to the hip bone, or iliac crest, and then slide your fingers along this line about one-third of the way. The pulse can be detected along the crease between the leg and the lower abdomen (Figure 7-30■).

**Respiration Rate**    Assessment of **respiration** primarily consists of evaluating the respiration rate, but it also involves evaluating the quality of respirations. Begin by calculating the patient's respiratory rate, an objective measure of the number of times the patient takes a breath in a minute. One breath, or respiration, consists of one inhalation and one exhalation. The normal respiratory rate of an adult is 12–20 breaths per minute. A respiratory rate less than 12 or greater than 20 is abnormal and may indicate either a problem directly related to the respiratory system or some other serious medical disorder.

To count respirations, watch the patient breathe for 30 seconds, counting each time the patient inhales. Multiplying this number by 2 provides the respiratory rate. For instance, if the patient breathes eight times in 30 seconds, the respiratory rate is 16 times per minute.

If the patient is unresponsive or is wearing heavy clothing, you may have to be more creative to count respirations. In these instances, count respirations by watching or palpating the rise and fall of the patient's chest, or count breath sounds using your stethoscope. You may even need to put a hand up to the patient's mouth to count the number of exhalations. Patients sometimes purposely change their respiratory rate, so if the patient is alert, it may be best to count respirations without the person's knowledge. To do this, place your fingers on the patient's wrist as if you were checking the pulse; at the same time, tip your head slightly downward while moving your eyes upward to subtly watch the respirations. Calculate the respiratory rate in the manner previously described (OEC Skill 7-6■).

**Blood Pressure**    Adequate **blood pressure** (BP) is needed to perfuse vital organs and tissue with the blood they need to function. BP, which is measured in mmHg (millimeters of mercury), is a measure of the pressure of blood on the interior walls of the arteries. A blood pressure reading consists of two values: the systolic pressure, which is the pressure within the arteries when the ventricles are contracting, and the diastolic pressure, which is a measure of the pressure within the arteries

---

### Taking A Pulse

When checking for a pulse, make sure that you press gently. If you press too hard, you will close off the flow of blood through the artery and will not be able to feel the pulse. Assess pulse quality by determining whether it is regular or irregular and whether it is strong, bounding, (very strong or forceful) or weak.

**NOTE**

⊕ **7-13** Describe and demonstrate the procedure for obtaining the following vital signs:

a. Respiratory rate
b. Blood pressure
c. Heart rate

**respiration**    the act of breathing in and out; also, the act of taking in of oxygen and nutrients and giving off of carbon dioxide and waste products by a cell.

**blood pressure (BP)**    the pressure of the blood on the interior walls of the arteries.

---

**Figure 7-29** The brachial pulse is assessed just proximal to the elbow.
Copyright Edward McNamara

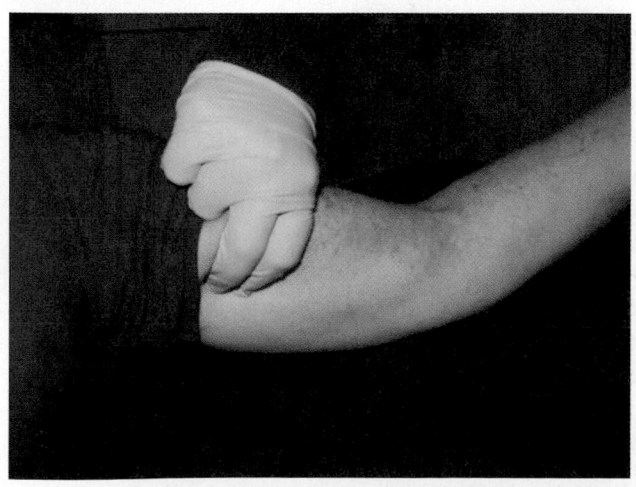

**Figure 7-30** The location of the femoral pulse. It is best to palpate this area with the patient's clothes removed while respecting the patient's privacy.
Copyright Edward McNamara

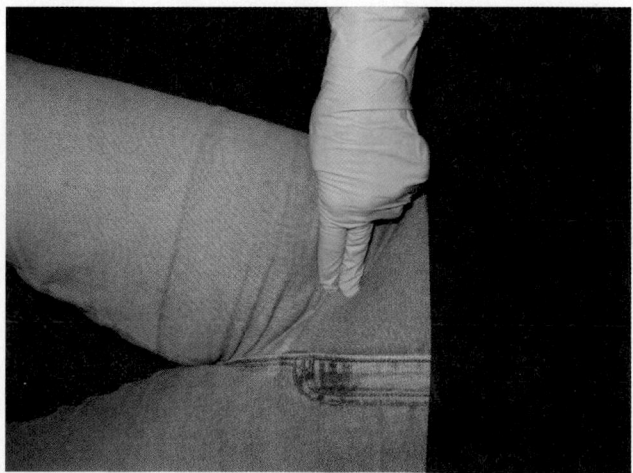

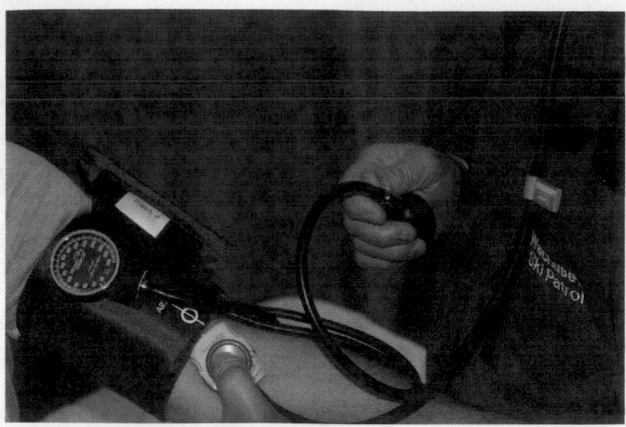

**Figure 7-31** Taking a blood pressure reading over the brachial artery using a stethoscope and a blood pressure cuff. Copyright Mike Halloran

while the heart is at rest. A blood pressure that is too high or too low may indicate serious illness. A normal blood pressure for an adult is 120/80, which is read as "one hundred twenty over eighty." In this case, the systolic pressure is 120 mmHg, and the diastolic pressure is 80 mmHg.

The most common place to check a blood pressure is over the brachial artery (Figure 7-31■). To auscultate (listen to) the blood pressure, you will need a blood pressure cuff and a stethoscope. A blood pressure cuff consists of four parts: a flexible rubber bulb with an attached thumb screw valve, a rubber bladder (cuff) and hoses, a sphygmomanometer, and a nylon or cloth bladder covering.

To obtain a blood pressure reading, perform the following procedure (OEC Skill 7-7■):

1. Unscrew the thumb screw valve on the flexible bulb and deflate the bladder of the cuff.
2. Place the cuff on the patient's upper arm with the hoses over the brachial artery. The cuff should be placed directly on the patient's skin because you will get a false reading if the cuff is placed over bulky clothing. The cuff should be snug, but not too tight.
3. Place the sphygmomanometer in a location that is easy for you to read without having to hold it. (Some cuffs have a clip on the sphygmomanometer that enables you to attach it to the patient's clothing or to a loop on the cuff while you are taking the pressure reading.)
4. Place the ear tips of the stethoscope in your ears. The tips should point forward.
5. Palpate the pulse of the brachial artery below the cuff at the crease of the elbow and then place the diaphragm of the stethoscope over the pulse point. (You will not hear a pulse at this time.)
6. Hold the stethoscope in place as you measure the pressure.
7. Using your other hand, tighten the thumb screw valve on the sphygmomanometer and inflate the cuff by repeatedly pumping the flexible bulb. Inflate the cuff to a pressure of 160 mmHg. If you can hear the pulse sound immediately, inflate the cuff to 200 mmHg. If you still can hear the heartbeat, inflate the cuff in 20 mmHg increments until you can no longer hear the pulse sound.
8. Gently open the thumb screw valve and slowly release the air from the cuff.
9. Listen for the first pulse sound (first "thump") as you slowly release air. The reading on the dial at this time is the systolic blood pressure.
10. Continue to slowly release the air from the cuff. The sound will become very soft and will eventually disappear. The reading on the dial when the sound disappears is the diastolic blood pressure.

In rare instances, you may continue to hear the pulse sound as you deflate the cuff down to a reading of 0 mmHg. Should this occur, wait a few seconds, reinflate the cuff, and slowly release the pressure again. This time, after noting the systolic blood pressure, continue to deflate the cuff, and listen *carefully*. At some point, you

> **NOTE**
>
> ### Quality of Respirations
>
> Assess the quality of respirations by determining if a patient's respirations are normal, deep, or shallow.

> **NOTE**
>
> ### Accurate Measurement of Blood Pressure
>
> If you inadvertently deflate the blood pressure cuff too quickly, fail to detect the systolic or diastolic pressure, or simply forget one of the two numbers, do not reinflate the cuff immediately. Instead, deflate the cuff completely and wait a few seconds before reinflating it. These steps will help ensure accurate readings when you repeat the procedure.

should detect a subtle change in the sound of the pulse sound. The number at which this change occurs is the diastolic blood pressure.

Once you are finished measuring the blood pressure you may remove the cuff, or you may leave it on the arm if you anticipate taking additional readings in a potentially unstable patient. If the BP cuff will be left in place, be sure it is completely deflated. Do not leave an inflated BP cuff on the arm for more than a few minutes because doing so can cut off blood flow to the distal arm and hand, which is painful.

If you do not have a stethoscope, or if it is too noisy to hear the pulse sound using the stethoscope, you can obtain an approximate measure of the systolic pressure with just the BP cuff and your fingers. Although not as accurate as an auscultated blood pressure, this method—known as a palpated blood pressure—provides a useful estimate of the patient's blood pressure.

To obtain a palpated blood pressure (Figure 7-32■):

1. Apply the blood pressure cuff in the fashion previously described (Figure 7-32a).
2. Find the patient's radial pulse.
3. Inflate the BP cuff until you can no longer feel the radial pulse.
4. Open the thumb screw and slowly release air from the cuff (Figure 7-32b).
5. The pressure at which you can again feel the radial pulse is the systolic blood pressure.

An example of how a palpated blood pressure reading would be verbally stated is: "The patient's blood pressure is ninety over palpation," or "The patient's blood pressure is ninety over palp." The pressure would be documented on the PCR as "90/Palp" or "90/P."

Even if you do not have a blood pressure cuff or are outside, you can still estimate the blood pressure by feeling the presence of an arterial pulse at various locations. A radial pulse correlates to a minimum systolic pressure of approximately 80 mmHg. A femoral pulse is equivalent to a systolic pressure of about 70 mmHg. A carotid pulse is equivalent to a systolic pressure of approximately 60 mmHg. Although these estimates correlate fairly well, you should not necessarily be reassured by a strong radial pulse. In the setting of trauma or suspected acute internal blood loss, a systolic blood pressure less than 90 mmHg can be life threatening.

> ### Estimates of Systolic BP for Various Pulse Points
>
> Radial pulse: 80 mmHg; femoral pulse: 70 mmHg; carotid pulse: 60 mmHg.
>
> **NOTE**

**Figure 7-32a** Taking a palpated blood pressure: apply the blood pressure cuff.

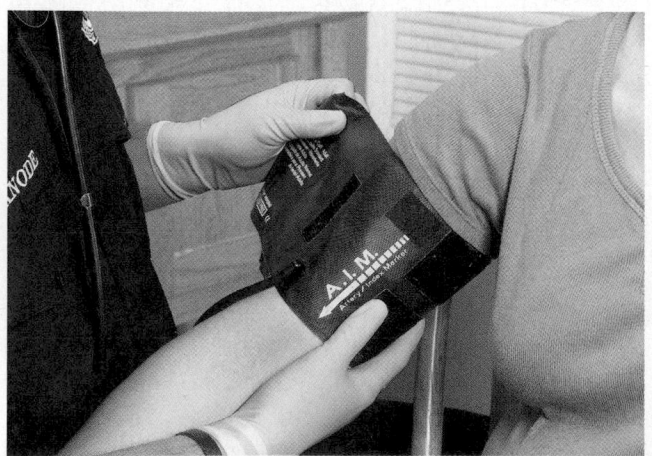

**Figure 7-32b** Taking a palpated blood pressure: slowly deflate the cuff until the radial pulse returns.

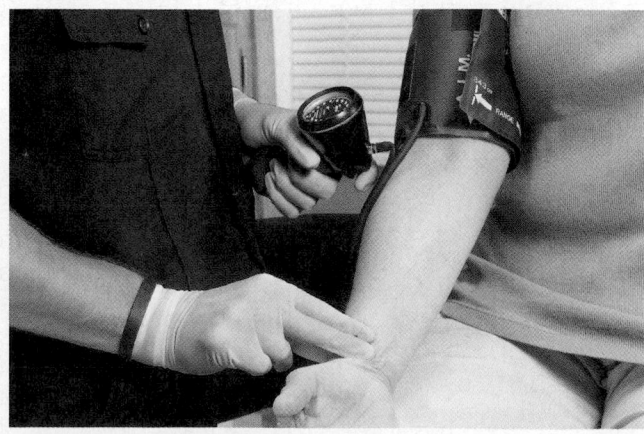

**Body Temperature**   Because of the potentially harsh conditions of outdoor environments, obtaining an accurate reading of a patient's body temperature in the field is extremely difficult. Getting an accurate core body temperature requires the use of a rectal thermometer; other methods of assessing temperature, such as placing a thermometer in the patient's arm pit or on the forehead, are not accurate. An oral thermometer can give reasonably accurate core temperature, and this is what will be most often used by OEC Technicians. Accordingly, assessing body temperature in the field beyond classifying the skin as hot, warm, cool, or cold has limited usefulness for OEC Technicians.

Normal body temperature ranges from 36° to 38° Celsius (96.8° to 100.4° Fahrenheit). Body temperatures below 35°C (95.0°F) are considered hypothermic, whereas temperatures above 39°C (102.2°F) are considered hyperthermic. Significantly abnormal temperatures in either direction are harmful to the patient (Table 7-6■).

**Oxygen Saturation Level**   In addition to the previously mentioned vital signs, your patrol may elect to measure another vital sign: the patient's oxygen saturation level. Oxygen saturation levels are measured using a device known as a pulse oximeter (Figure 7-33■). This device measures the percentage of oxygen in the blood using a probe that is attached to a patient's finger or earlobe. A pulse oximetry reading of less than 95 percent is abnormal and may indicate serious illness or injury. A more detailed description of pulse oximeters and their use is presented in Chapter 13, Respiratory Emergencies, and Chapter 36, ALS Interface.

**Orthostatic Blood Pressure Test**   When you are in an aid room or in another controlled environment assessing a patient in which trauma is not suspected, it may be helpful to check orthostatic, or postural, vital signs. The purpose of this evaluation is to assess for orthostatic hypotension (also known as postural hypotension), which is a sudden drop in blood pressure upon standing that could indicate dehydration or internal bleeding.

When a person stands, approximately 500–1,000 mL of blood move from the upper body to the lower body in response to gravity. To compensate, blood vessels in the lower extremities constrict so that more blood remains in the thorax to maintain

**Table  7-6**   Equivalent Fahrenheit and Celsius Body Temperatures

| Fahrenheit | Celsius | |
|---|---|---|
| 90° | 32.2° | |
| 91° | 32.7° | |
| 92° | 33.3° | |
| 93° | 33.8° | |
| 94° | 34.4° | |
| 95° | 35° | Abnormally low body temperature (hypothermia) |
| 96° | 35.5° | |
| 97° | 36.1° | |
| 98.6° | 37° | Normal body temperature (normothermia) |
| 100.4° | 38° | |
| 101° | 38.3° | |
| 102° | 38.8° | |
| 103° | 39.4° | Abnormally high body temperature (hyperthermia) |
| 104° | 40° | |
| 105° | 40.5° | |
| 106° | 41.1° | |

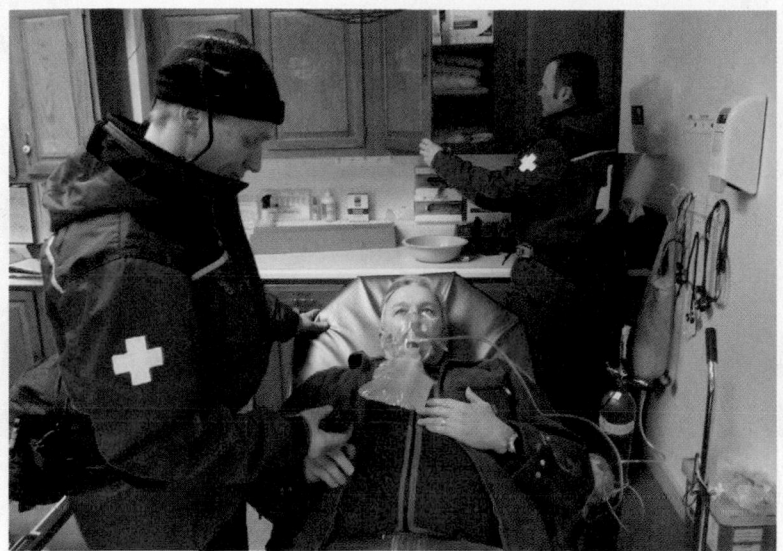

**Figure 7-33** Oxygen saturation levels are measured using a device known as a pulse oximeter.
Copyright Edward McNamara

cardiac output and homeostasis. This compensatory mechanism should occur within 3 minutes. However, if the patient's cardiac output is compromised due to injury or illness, the compensatory mechanisms may be overtaxed and unable to maintain sufficient cardiac output upon the sudden change in position. The result is a sudden drop in blood pressure. The pulse rate also may change, although current studies indicate that this is neither as reliable nor as predictive as a sudden change in blood pressure. Hypotension with a smaller compensatory increase in heart rate (10 beats per minute) suggests neurologic impairment; marked increase (>100 beats per minute or it has increased by >30 beats per minute) suggests hypovolemia.

Among the most common causes of orthostatic hypotension are the following:

- Hypovolemia from dehydration or hemorrhage (the number 1 cause)
- Medications: diuretics such as Lasix® and hydrochlorothiazide (for treating high blood pressure), nitroglycerine (for treating cardiac chest pain), and Flomax® (for treating an enlarged prostate)
- Neurological disease (e.g., spinal cord injury, brainstem stroke)

Clinically, orthostatic hypotension results in a drop of at least 20 mmHg in the systolic blood pressure or a drop of at least 10 mmHg in the diastolic blood pressure or both within 3 minutes of standing. A patient with orthostatic hypotension will generally experience dizziness and a rapid heart rate. Such patients also may be diaphoretic or pale. Although most patients experience these symptoms, some do not, which is a condition known as asymptomatic orthostatic hypotension. You may wish to check for orthostatic hypotension in any patient who complains of dizziness, a rapid heart rate, or dehydration, or in patients whose history suggests dehydration or hemorrhage. However, you should consider the possible risks before checking orthostatic vital signs.

In the setting of trauma, it is more important for you to protect the patient's spine than it is to check orthostatic vital signs. Accordingly, do not check orthostatic hypotension in a trauma patient. Additionally, during the procedure assist the patient to a standing position and protect the patient from falling. If the patient immediately becomes dizzy upon standing, assist the patient to a supine position and discontinue the test.

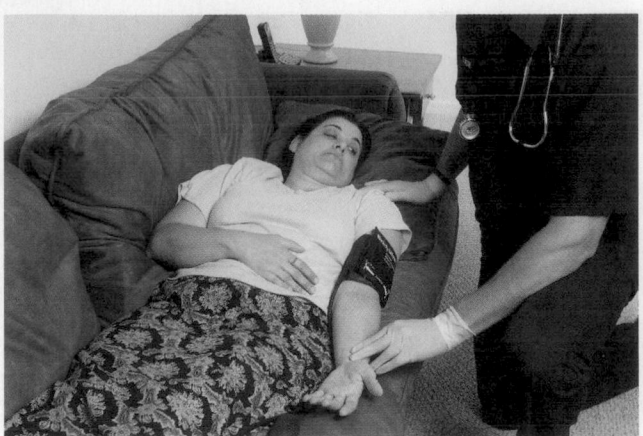

**Figure 7-34a** Assessing for orthostatic hypotension: obtain the patient's blood pressure and pulse rate while the patient is lying down.

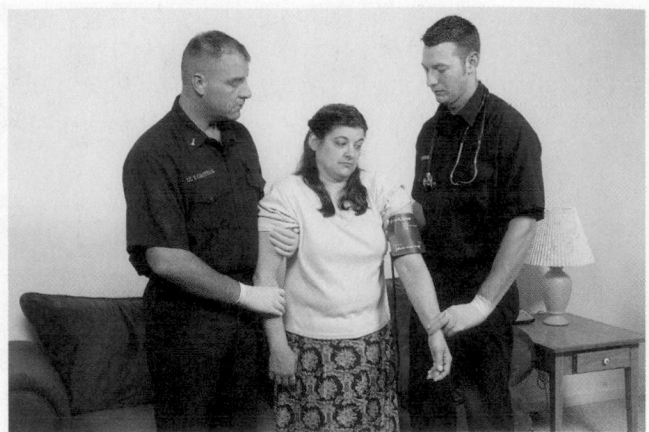

**Figure 7-34b** Assessing for orthostatic hypotension: assist the patient to a standing position, wait about 3 minutes, and then obtain the patient's blood pressure and pulse rate a second time.

To check for orthostatic hypotension, perform the following procedure:

1. Obtain the patient's blood pressure and pulse rate while the patient is lying down (Figure 7-34a■).
2. Assist the patient to a standing position. (If the patient feels dizzy, immediately help the patient to a supine position.) Wait approximately 3 minutes.
3. After 3 minutes, recheck the patient's blood pressure and pulse rate (Figure 7-34b■).

If the systolic blood pressure decreases by 20 mmHg or the diastolic blood pressure falls by 10 mmHg or more, the patient is said to be "positive" for orthostatic hypotension. If the systolic blood pressure remains the same, increases, increases or decreases less than 20 mmHg, the patient is said to be "negative" for orthostatic hypotension. Additionally if the heart rate increases by 10 or more beats per minute, the patient is "positive" for hypovolemic orthostatic hypotension. If the results for orthostatic hypotension are positive, assist the patient in lying back down and consider the possible causes previously mentioned.

## Special Assessment Considerations

### Assessment of Unresponsive Patients

Unresponsive patients present unique challenges. In many cases unresponsiveness requires that you begin CPR. As required for any unresponsive patient, the opening of the airway and simultaneous check for breathing and pulse should take no longer than 10 seconds. If the patient is in cardiac arrest, start compressions as soon as possible.

In a patient who has a pulse and is breathing, you will be unable to obtain a medical history or valuable feedback. If a relative or friend is present, some history may become available. Unless a witness says the patient became unresponsive without any trauma, you must assume that the patient has a cervical spine injury until proven otherwise.

Following the initial ABCD evaluation and treatment of life-threatening problems, it is essential that the ABCDs be continually monitored because if not quickly identified, even minor ABCD-related problems can become life threatening in an unresponsive patient. The most important thing an OEC Technician can do for an unresponsive patient with a pulse is maintain an open airway.

Time permitting, conduct a secondary assessment in the usual fashion. Note an exception, however: assessment of sensation and movement in the extremities is usually omitted. Ensure that as you are conducting your secondary assessment, you are not preventing the timely management of any problems involving the ABCDs. Do not delay transport of an unresponsive patient when a life-threatening problem exists.

## Other Assessment Situations

Sometimes the assessment process is complicated by one or more of a variety of factors, such as a communication barrier (deafness, differences in language), cultural differences, aggressive behavior by the patient, or a problem resulting from trauma (the patient's brain may not be getting enough oxygen or glucose because of a brain injury). Assessment of a patient with whom you are having a difficult time communicating can be especially difficult.

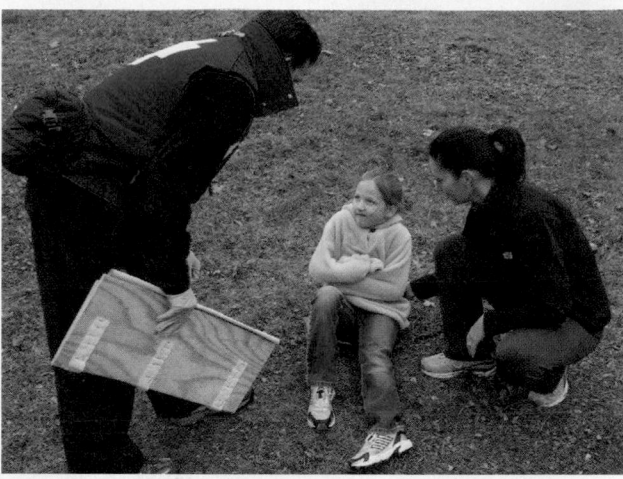

**Figure 7-35** Children may be afraid of strangers. Talk slowly and calmly as you walk up to begin your assessment.
Copyright Mike Halloran

Begin by staying calm. Getting frustrated and agitated will not help the situation. Always assume communication difficulties are the result of an illness or injury until proven otherwise. Look for companions of the patient who may be able to assist you in communicating with the patient. Smile at the patient to demonstrate that you are there to assist them; a smile is universally understood. Despite your best efforts, there will be times in which the patient will not able to understand you. In these cases, assess the patient to the best of your ability, and always act with the patient's best interests in mind. If the patient appears to be critically ill or injured but resists your assessment efforts, you may need to aid the patient under implied consent.

Children can be especially difficult to assess and are often scared by the presence of a stranger (Figure 7-35■). Depending on age, the child may not understand who you are. The problem may be compounded if the child is not with his parents. The child may be in pain. Be patient. Explain what is happening, using age-appropriate words the child can understand. Speak slowly and calmly. Fully explain what you are doing, and why, before you begin your assessment. Encourage the child to participate in the assessment process. Never stand over a child; instead, get down to the child's level during the assessment. Allow the child to examine your penlight or stethoscope before you use it. Other techniques for interacting with children are described in Chapter 30, Pediatric Emergencies.

You may encounter a patient who is combative or aggressive. As discussed in Chapter 3, Rescue Basics, never place yourself or others at risk of harm. Be aware, however, that combative or aggressive behavior can be a sign of significant illness or injury resulting from a lack of oxygen, decreased blood sugar, an intoxicating substance, or a brain injury. If you think the patient may harm himself or others, request assistance from other rescuers, area security, or law enforcement. Continue to talk to the person and maintain a calm demeanor until additional help arrives. Follow your area, state, or provincial protocols for managing this type of situation.

**Cultural Diversity**    As you are performing your assessment, be sensitive to differences in cultural norms among your patients. Whereas some patients will feel quite comfortable with your examining them, others may not feel so comfortable. Be respectful. Ask permission to perform your exam. Be prepared to fully explain what you want to do and the need for each step the physical exam. Depending on the patient's culture, you may need to seek permission, support, or advice from the patient's family or friends before making physical contact with the patient. Women of certain religions, such as Islam, may request privacy from men. In this case, a female OEC Technician, if available, should perform the exam.

**Environmental Considerations**    Performing a patient assessment in outdoor environments can be quite challenging and complex. Environmental conditions may

**7-8** Describe how environmental conditions can affect patient assessment.

prevent you from performing a physical examination of your patient. In addition, harsh environmental conditions may have contributed to your patient's injury and/or illness.

Take ambient temperature into account during the assessment process. If the weather is cold, the patient will likely be reluctant to let you remove any clothing. As a result, you may need to perform a secondary assessment over bulky clothes, or perhaps you can unzip them, quickly perform your assessment, and then zip them back up. If you suspect an injury that is associated with bleeding, expose the skin to the elements only as much as is needed to adequately assess and manage the injury. Cover the area with clothes or a blanket as soon as possible.

If you do not suspect bleeding, it may be more beneficial to expose the injury only after the patient has been moved to a more controlled environment. However, always expose the area if there is any possibility of bleeding. In a hot, sunny environment, it may be impossible to perform certain portions of the assessment properly; for instance, it may be impossible to assess the pupils in bright sun. Under such conditions, put your hand over one eye and then the other, allowing the covered pupil to dilate slightly and then watching it constrict as you remove your hand and allow sunlight into the pupil. In a windy, dusty, rainy, or dark environment, it may be very difficult to even see your patient clearly, let alone perform a thorough assessment. Regardless of the environmental conditions, at a minimum you should assess the patient's ABCDs before attempting to move him to a location that is better suited for a secondary assessment.

When faced with difficult conditions, you can do several things to make the assessment process easier. You can protect your patient from the elements: shade the patient's face with your hand while examining his face, cover the patient with a blanket when it is cold, or create a temporary cover or shelter to block the sun when it is hot. If the patient is located on a slope or steep incline, you may be able to cut a flat step into the slope or slide the patient down a bit to a more level spot. On the ski slope, kick your boots into the snow, or anchor yourself, your patient, and your equipment with ropes or skis.

No one thing works in every situation. Decide what to do by balancing how urgently you need information to assess the situation adequately and prepare for safe transport, against the length of time you must keep the patient exposed to a harsh environment.

## Reassessment

⊕ **7-14** Describe and demonstrate how to reassess a patient.

A patient's condition is dynamic and can change over time. For instance, if a patient is bleeding, his condition will worsen if the bleeding is not controlled. Similarly, a patient who is having a heart attack can become sicker if the process causing the problem is not reversed. Of course, a change in a patient's condition can be good; it can be an improvement. If you stabilize a fractured bone, the patient will likely be in less pain, and a patient with a breathing problem often feels much better after **oxygenation** has been achieved. Assessment is not a one-time activity, but instead an ongoing process that is used to evaluate both the progression of the patient's illness or injury and the effectiveness of your treatment.

**oxygenation** a process in which oxygen is added to the body's tissues.

Because your patient's condition may change over time, you must continually reassess the patient. As a general guide, patients who are considered stable (those without ABCD problems and with normal vital signs) should be reassessed every 10–15 minutes, whereas patients who are considered unstable (those with abnormal vital signs or ABCD-related problems) should be reassessed every 3–5 minutes. Continually monitor the ABCDs, and repeat the vital signs regularly. Changes in vital signs toward normal values generally indicate an improvement in the patient's condition, whereas changes in vital signs farther away from normal values generally indicate deterioration in the patient's condition.

# STOP, THINK, UNDERSTAND

## Multiple Choice

1. The mnemonic DCAP-BTLS is used to help with what process?_____
   a. the head-to-toe physical exam
   b. the correct sequencing of vital signs
   c. a classification for burns and wounds
   d. assessing and monitoring the patient's LOR

2. DCAP-BTLS stands for _____
   a. Distal, Circulation, Airway, Pulse, Breathing, Tenderness, LOR, Signs/symptoms.
   b. Dorsalis, Circulation, Assessment, Pulse, Bleeding, Tenderness, LOR, Signs/symptoms.
   c. Deformity, Contusions, Abrasions/avulsions, Punctures/penetrations, Burns/bleeding, Tenderness, Lacerations, Swelling.
   d. Deformity, Circulation, Airway, Pulse, Breathing, Touch, Location, Signs/symptoms.

3. "Baseline vitals" are _____
   a. the lowest level of vital signs (respiration rate, pulse rate, blood pressure, temperature) obtained on your patient.
   b. the first and last set of vital signs recorded by the first responder in the system.
   c. the first set of vital signs, which establishes a reference point against which all other sets of vital signs are compared.
   d. the average range of vital signs, which is calculated by adding up the individual values of each set (respiration rate, pulse, BP, and temperature) and dividing this number by the number of sets taken.

4. A complete set of vitals includes _____
   a. respiration rate, pulse rate, blood pressure, and touch.
   b. respiration rate, PEERL/pulse rate, blood pressure, temperature, and LOR.
   c. responsiveness, pulse rate, blood pressure, and temperature/touch.
   d. respiration rate, responsiveness, pulse rate, blood pressure, and temperature.

5. Which of the following can affect a person's pulse rate?_____
   a. pain
   b. fear
   c. trauma
   d. all of the above

6. Which of the following do you assess when checking a pulse? (check all that apply)
   a. regularity of rhythm
   b. rate
   c. strength
   d. palpability

7. BP measures _____
   a. sphygomanometric variations in pulse rate.
   b. tissue oxygen saturation levels.
   c. the pressure on the inside wall of an artery.
   d. the heart's ability to deliver blood to the body's tissues.

8. The two values of BP are _____
   a. sphygomanometric and dorsalis.
   b. symphysis and diastis.
   c. supine and distal.
   d. systolic and diastolic.

9. Blood pressure is defined as _____
   a. a measure of the pressure of blood on the interior walls of arteries.
   b. a measure of the pressure of blood on the interior walls of veins.
   c. the difference between the pulse rates measured at the carotid and femoral pulse points.
   d. the pressure the heart needs to keep the mitral and bicuspid valves open.

10. You have auscultated a patient's BP and heard the initial sound at 118, then lost the sound again at 64. This person's BP would be recorded as _____
    a. 118/64.
    b. 64/118.
    c. not recordable, because the pulse pressure value is missing.
    d. inaccurate, because you lost the second sound.

11. The most accurate method of determining BP is by _____
    a. palpation.
    b. auscultation.
    c. determining arterial pulses.
    d. none of the above.

12. BP by palpation measures which value(s)?_____
    a. pulse pressure
    b. systolic pressure over diastolic pressure
    c. systolic pressure only
    d. diastolic pressure only

13. The abbreviation mmHg stands for _____
    a. millimeters of hemoglobin.
    b. millimeters in histograms.
    c. millimeters of mercury.
    d. millimeters per sphygmomanometer.

14. A device used to measure body oxygen saturation levels is _____
    a. a pulse oximeter.
    b. an oxynamoter.
    c. a sphygmomanometer.
    d. a stethoscope.

## Fill in the Blank

The difference between the systolic pressure and diastolic pressure is known as the _____.

*continued*

STOP, THINK, UNDERSTAND *continued*

## Matching

1. Indicate the phase that applies to the events described in A–D:

_____ 1. diastolic phase

_____ 2. systolic phase

   **a.** the pressure within arteries when ventricles are contracting
   **b.** the pressure within arteries while the heart is at rest
   **c.** the first (upper) number in a blood pressure reading
   **d.** the second (lower) number in a blood pressure reading

2. Match each of the following pulse points to its approximate blood pressure value:

_____ 1. carotid pulse point

_____ 2. femoral pulse point

_____ 3. radial pulse point

   **a.** 80 mmHg
   **b.** 70 mmHg
   **c.** 60 mmHg

# CASE DISPOSITION

Suspecting that something concerning the patient's condition might be serious, you call for backup from your fellow OEC Technicians. You then perform a physical exam on the patient. During the exam, you notice some discoloration on the left upper portion of the patient's chest. You also discover that the patient has some tenderness in his lower back, near his spine, although there is no obvious damage to the skin. He has equal sensation and movement in all his extremities. Pulses in both the upper and lower extremities are equal and strong. The vital signs are normal. Other OEC Technicians arrive to assist you. Working together, you package the patient using spinal precautions and send him by ambulance to a nearby hospital. You later learn that the patient had a mild heart attack, which the doctors think may have caused him to become dizzy and fall. He also had a bruise to his chest. His spine was not injured.

## OEC SKILL 7-1 | Patient Assessment

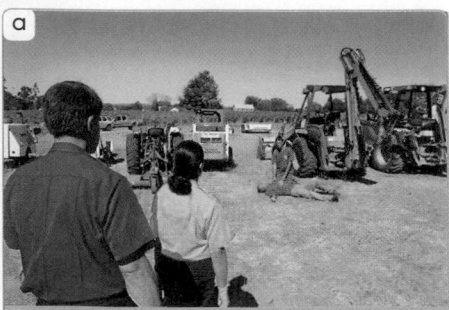

Perform scene size-up. Initiate Standard Precautions.

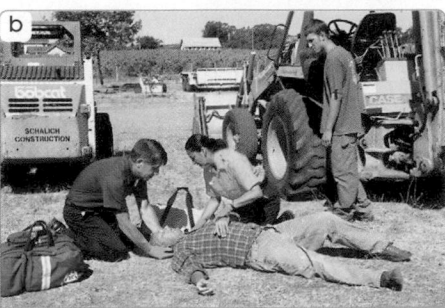

Perform a primary assessment and manage ABCDs.

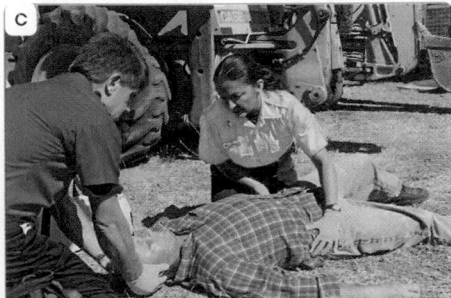

Perform a secondary assessment and provide intervention per your local protocols. Reassess the patient based on the patient's condition.

## OEC SKILL 7-2 | Patient Assessment—Trauma Patient

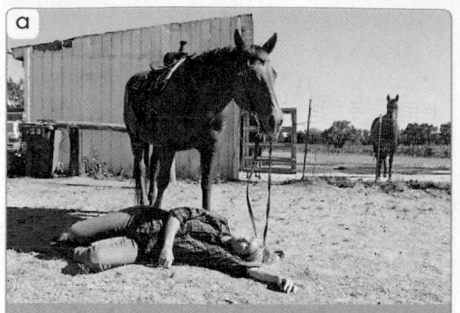

Perform scene size-up. Initiate Standard Precautions.

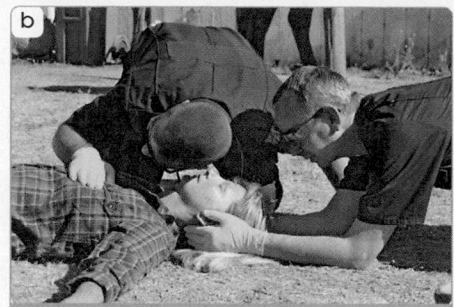

Perform a primary assessment and provide stabilization to the patient.

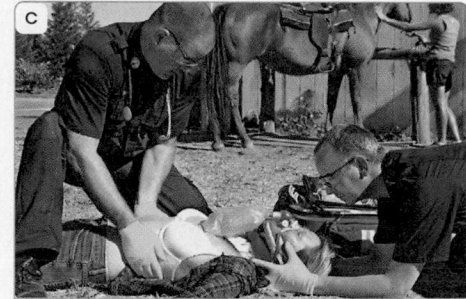

Perform a secondary assessment to detect any serious injuries. Take baseline vital signs. Then reassess as necessary.

## OEC SKILL 7-3 | Patient Assessment—Medical Patient

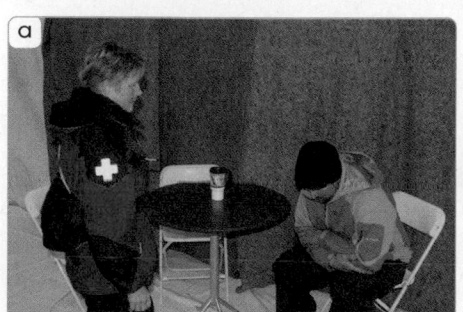

Patroller is conducting a scene size-up in this incident involving skier in the lodge.
Copyright Mike Halloran

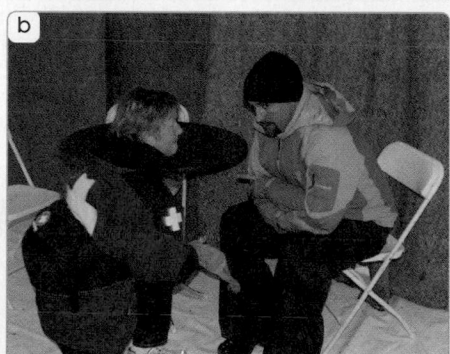

Patroller performs a primary assessment.
Copyright Mike Halloran

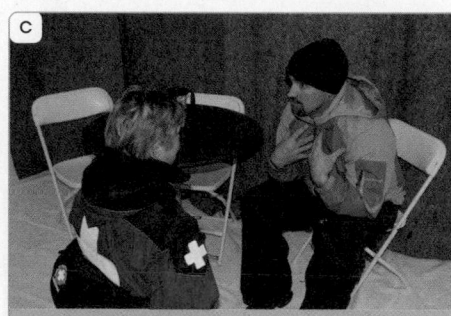

Listening to patient and examining him based on his chief complaint.
Copyright Mike Halloran

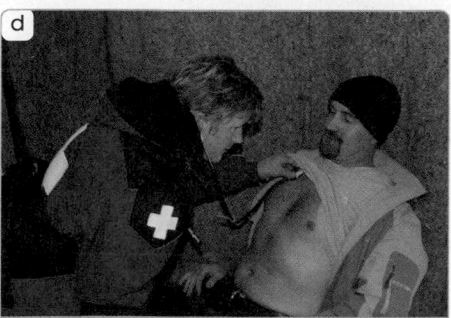

Performing a secondary assessment with a detailed examination.
Copyright Mike Halloran

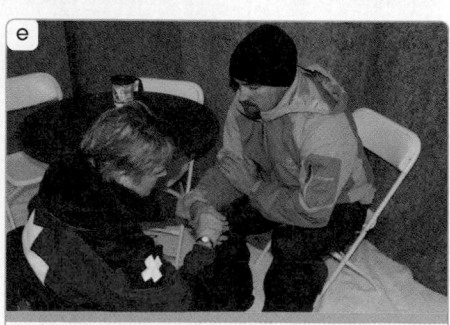

Obtaining a complete SAMPLE history.
Copyright Mike Halloran

## OEC SKILL 7-4 | Assessing Pupils

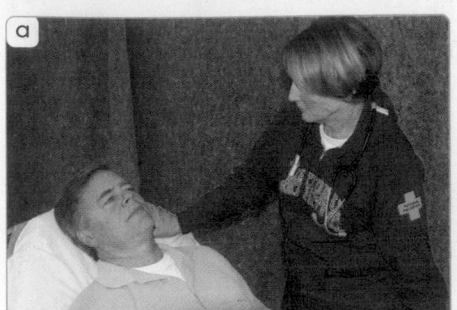

a

Instruct the patient to stare at your nose or the center of your forehead. Check that the pupils are equally sized and are round.
Copyright Mike Halloran

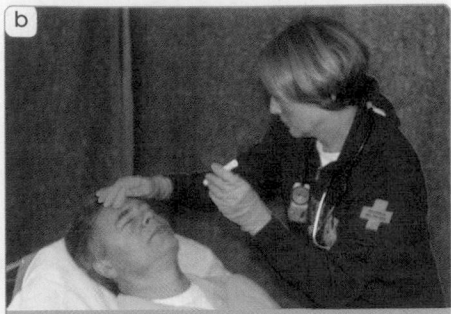

b

Moving laterally to medially, briefly shine the penlight into the patient's left eye and then do so a second time.
Copyright Mike Halloran

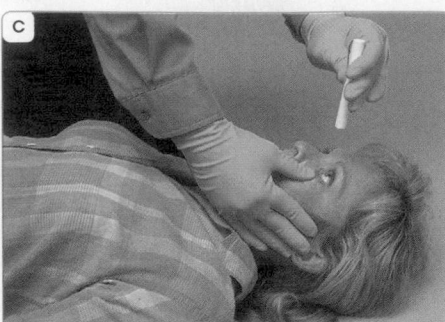

c

Next shine the light in the patient's right eye, and then do so a second time.

## OEC SKILL 7-5 | Assessing Pulse

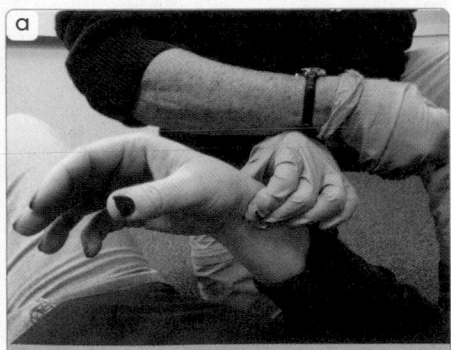

a

Locate the radial pulse on an adult.
Copyright Edward McNamara

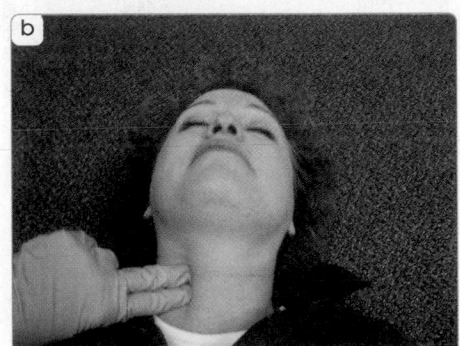

b

Locate the carotid pulse on an unresponsive adult. In each case, note the quality of the pulse.
Copyright Edward McNamara

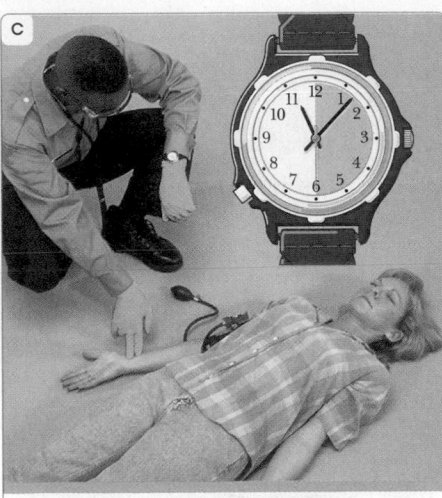

c

Assess pulse rate and quality.

## OEC SKILL 7-6  Assessing Respiration Rate

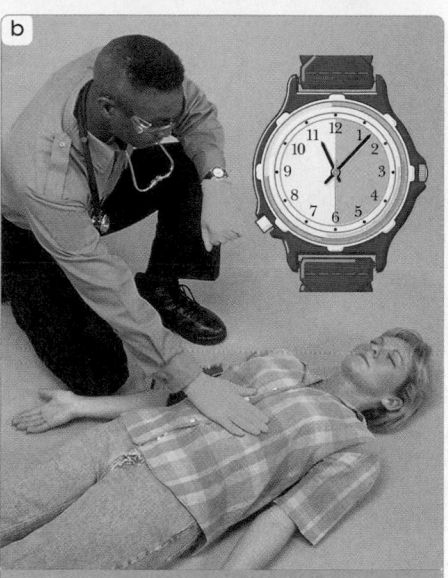

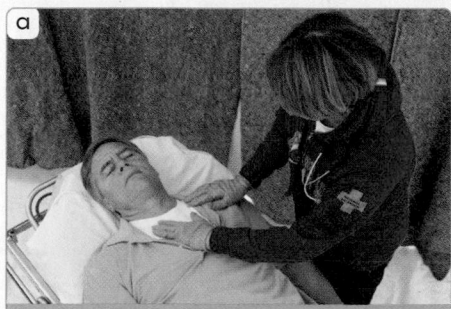

Look and feel for the patient's chest to rise and fall.
Copyright Mike Halloran

Assess the patient's respirations for rhythm, depth, effort, and noise to determine if the patient is breathing within normal limits.

## OEC SKILL 7-7  Obtaining a Blood Pressure by Auscultation

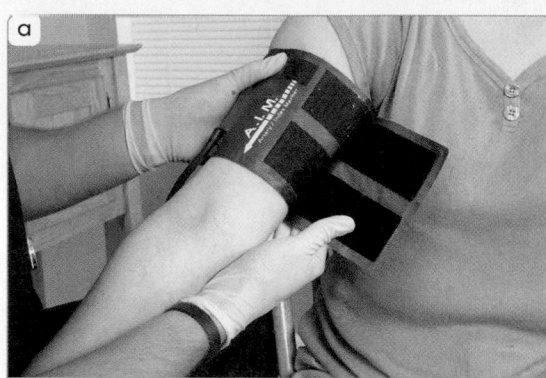

Place the cuff on the upper arm with the arrow pointing over the brachial artery. Place the stethoscope tips to your ears.

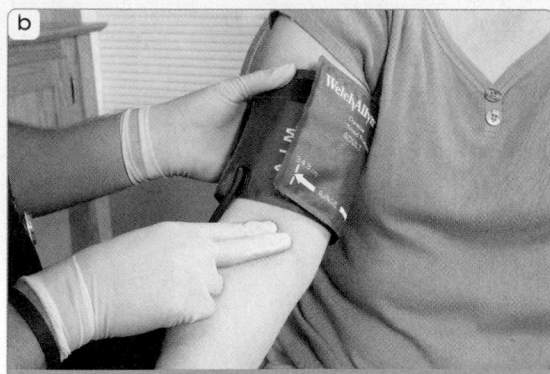

Palpate the brachial artery pulse and place the diaphragm of the stethoscope on the pulse. Hold the stethoscope in place as you measure the pressure.

## OEC SKILL 7-7 | Obtaining a Blood Pressure by Auscultation *continued*

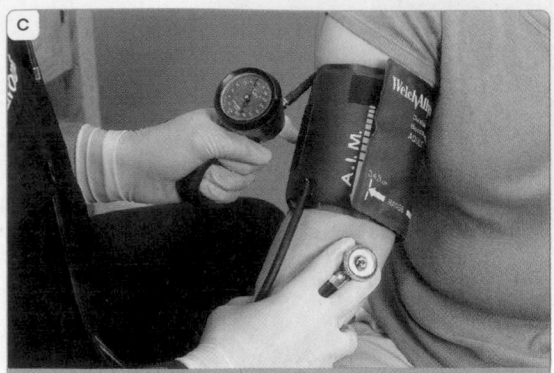

Using your other hand, tighten the thumb screw on the cuff, and inflate by repeatedly pumping the flexible bulb. Inflate the cuff to a pressure of 160 millimeters of mercury (mmHg).

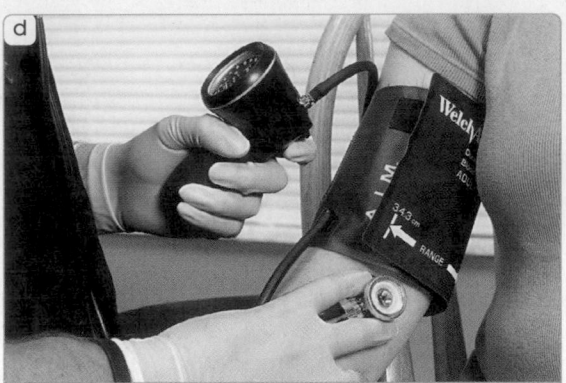

Pulse sound (first "thump") as you slowly release air from the cuff. This is the systolic blood pressure. Continue to slowly release the air from the cuff. The point at which the sound disappears is the diastolic blood pressure.

## Skill Guide

Date: _____

(CPI) = Critical Performance Indicator

Candidate: _____

Start Time: _____

End Time: _____

## Patient Assessment

**Objective:** To demonstrate the proper assessment of a patient, to determine a baseline, and to select the appropriate transport method.

| Skill | Max Points | Skill Demo | |
|---|---|---|---|
| Scene Size-Up | | | |
| Determines scene is safe. | 1 | | (CPI) |
| Introduces self, obtains permission to examine/treat. | 1 | | |
| Initiates Standard Precautions. | 1 | | (CPI) |
| Determines the MOI (mechanism of injury) and/or NOI (nature of illness)—patient's chief complaint. | 1 | | (CPI) |
| Identifies the number of patient(s) and the LOR of each. | 1 | | |
| Forms general impression—evaluates any extrication issues for each patient(s); considers c-spine stabilization/immobilization. | 1 | | |

*continued*

| Primary Assessment | | | |
|---|---|---|---|
| Assesses airway, breathing, circulation, disability (ABCDs). | 1 | | (CPI) |
| Provides any necessary interventions related to airway/breathing. | 1 | | (CPI) |
| Checks for and controls any major bleeding. | 1 | | (CPI) |
| Confirms and monitors LOR (AVPU or GCS). | 1 | | |
| Calls for transport, equipment, and/or additional assistance. | 1 | | |
| Secondary Assessment | | | |
| Performs detailed head-to-toe body assessment physical exam DCAP-BTLS. | 1 | | (CPI) |
| Obtains SAMPLE history from patient and/or witness (if available). | 1 | | (CPI) |
| Obtains baseline set of vitals. | 1 | | (CPI) |
| Provides interventions per protocols. | 1 | | |
| Treats for shock. | 1 | | |
| Maintains spinal immobilization if applicable. | 1 | | (CPI) |
| Prepares patient for transport. | 1 | | |
| Reassesses vital signs and primary assessment. | 1 | | |

| Must receive 17 out of 19 points. |
|---|

Comments: _____

Failure of any of the CPIs is an automatic failure.

Evaluator: _____ NSP ID:_____

PASS     FAIL

## Skill Guide

Date: _____

(CPI) = Critical Performance Indicator

Candidate: _____

Start Time: _____

End Time: _____

## Patient Assessment—Trauma Patient

**Objective:** To demonstrate the proper assessment of a trauma patient, to determine a baseline, and to select the appropriate transport method.

*continued*

SKILL GUIDE *continued*

| Skill | Max Points | Skill Demo | |
|---|:---:|:---:|:---:|
| Scene Size-Up | | | |
| Determines that scene is safe. | 1 | | (CPI) |
| Introduces self, obtains permission to assist/treat. | 1 | | |
| Initiates Standard Precautions. | 1 | | (CPI) |
| Determines the MOI (mechanism of injury)—patient's chief complaint. | 1 | | (CPI) |
| Identifies the number of patient(s) and the LOR of each. | 1 | | |
| Forms general impression—evaluates any extrication issues for each patient(s); considers c-spine stabilization/immobilization. | 1 | | |
| Primary Assessment | | | |
| Assesses airway, breathing, circulation, disability ( ABCDs). | 1 | | (CPI) |
| Manages/treats life threats. | 1 | | |
| Checks for and controls any major bleeding. | 1 | | (CPI) |
| Confirms and monitors LOR (AVPU or GCS). | 1 | | |
| Calls for transport, equipment, and/or additional assistance, EMS if needed. | 1 | | |
| Secondary Assessment | | | |
| Performs head-to-toe detailed body assessment. DCAP-BTLS. | 1 | | (CPI) |
| Exposes and inspects injury to identify level of emergency and formulate treatment plan. | 1 | | (CPI) |
| Obtains SAMPLE history from patient and/or witness (if available). | 1 | | (CPI) |
| Obtains baseline set of vitals. | 1 | | (CPI) |
| Provides interventions per local protocols. | 1 | | |
| Treats for shock. | 1 | | |
| Maintains spinal immobilization if applicable. | 1 | | (CPI) |
| Prepares patient for transport. | 1 | | |
| Reassesses vital signs and primary assessment. | 1 | | |

| Must receive 16 out of 20 points. |
|---|

Comments: _____

Failure to perform any of the CPIs is an automatic failure.

Evaluator: _____ NSP ID: _____

PASS     FAIL

## Skill Guide

Date: _____

(CPI) = Critical Performance Indicator

Candidate: _____

Start Time: _____

End Time: _____

## Patient Assessment—Medical Patient

Objective: To demonstrate the proper assessment of a medical patient, to determine a baseline with a specific complaint.

| Skill | Max Points | Skill Demo | |
|---|---|---|---|
| Scene Size-Up | | | |
| Determines that the scene is safe. | 1 | | (CPI) |
| Introduces self and obtains permission to examine/treat. | 1 | | |
| Initiates Standard Precautions. | 1 | | (CPI) |
| Determines NOI (nature of illness)—patient's chief complaint. | 1 | | (CPI) |
| Identifies the number of patient(s) and the LOR of each. | 1 | | |
| Forms general impression—evaluates any extrication issues and considers spinal precautions. | 1 | | |
| Primary Assessment | | | |
| Assesses airway, breathing, circulation, disability (ABCDs). | 1 | | (CPI) |
| Assists breathing, manages/treats life threats. | 1 | | (CPI) |
| Confirms and monitors LOR (AVPU or GCS). | 1 | | |
| Calls for transport, equipment, personnel, and EMS if needed. | 1 | | |
| Secondary Assessment | | | |
| Performs detailed head-to-toe body assessment/physical exam. | 1 | | |
| Obtains SAMPLE history. | 1 | | (CPI) |
| Based on the chief complaint, gathers information by asking OPQRST questions. | 1 | | (CPI) |
| Obtains baseline vital signs. | 1 | | (CPI) |
| Provides interventions per local protocols. | 1 | | (CPI) |
| Treats for shock. | 1 | | |
| Maintains spinal immobilization if applicable. | 1 | | (CPI) |
| Prepares patient for transport. | 1 | | |
| Reassesses vital signs and primary assessment. | 1 | | |

*continued*

SKILL GUIDE *continued*

Must receive 17 out of 19 points.

Comments: _____

Failure of any of the CPIs is an automatic failure.

Evaluator: _____ NSP ID: _____

PASS    FAIL

---

## Skill Guide

Date: _____

(CPI) = Critical Performance Indicator

Candidate: _____

Start Time: _____

End Time: _____

## Patient Assessment: Assessing Pupils

**Objective:** To demonstrate the ability to assess pupils.

| Skill | Max Points | Skill Demo | |
|---|---|---|---|
| Initiates Standard Precautions. | 1 | | (CPI) |
| Obtains permission from patient. | 1 | | |
| Notes initial size/shape as patient stares at examiners forehead. | 1 | | (CPI) |
| Shines a light into one eye, noting reaction of pupil. | 1 | | (CPI) |
| Shines light again into first eye noting if the reaction/size of other pupil gets smaller. | 1 | | |
| Shines light into other (2nd) eye, noting if pupil gets smaller. Shines light again into the second eye noting if the other eye reacts by getting smaller. | 1 | | (CPI) |
| Acknowledges if reactions are WNL. | 1 | | |

Must receive 5 out of 7 points.

Comments: _____

Failure of any of the CPIs is an automatic failure.

Evaluator: _____ NSP ID: _____

PASS    FAIL

## Skill Guide

Date: _____

(CPI) = Critical Performance Indicator

Candidate: _____

Start Time: _____

End Time: _____

## Patient Assessment: Assessing Pulse

Objective: To demonstrate the ability to locate, assess pulse, and obtain rate.

| Skill | Max Points | Skill Demo | |
|---|---|---|---|
| Initiates Standard Precautions. | 1 | | (CPI) |
| Obtains permission from patient. | 1 | | |
| Locates radial pulse (for child < 8 YOA, locate brachial pulse). Locates carotid pulse for unresponsive patient. | 1 | | (CPI) |
| Notes quality of pulse (strength/regularity). | 1 | | |
| Notes and verbalizes rate. | 1 | | (CPI) |
| Acknowledges if rate obtained is WNL. | 1 | | |

Must receive 4 out of 6 points.

Comments: _____

Failure of any of the CPIs is an automatic failure.

Evaluator: _____   NSP ID:_____

PASS     FAIL

## Skill Guide

Date: _____

(CPI) = Critical Performance Indicator

Candidate: _____

Start Time: _____

End Time: _____

## Assessing Respiration Rate

Objective: To evaluate patient's respiration rate.

| Skill | Max Points | Skill Demo | |
|---|---|---|---|
| Initiates Standard Precautions. | 1 | | (CPI) |
| Obtains permission to treat patient. | 1 | | |
| Determines if patient can speak in complete sentences. | 1 | | |
| Looks for chest rise and fall (On unresponsive patient, places hand on patient's chest or listen at mouth for respirations). | 1 | | |
| Determines if patient has breathing problems. | 1 | | |
| Assesses respirations for the following:<br>• Rhythm<br>• Depth<br>• Effort<br>• Noise | 1 | | |
| Counts number of breaths for 30 seconds and multiplies by two for respirations per minute; determines if patient is breathing within normal limits (12–20 adult) (15–30 child) (25-50 infant). | 1 | | (CPI) |

Must receive 5 out of 7 points.

Comments: _____

Failure of any of the CPIs is an automatic failure.

Evaluator: _____    NSP ID: _____

PASS    FAIL

## Skill Guide

Date: _____

(CPI) = Critical Performance Indicator

Candidate: _____

Start Time: _____

End Time: _____

## Obtaining a Blood Pressure by Auscultation

**Objective:** To measure a blood pressure by auscultation.

| Skill | Max Points | Skill Demo | |
|---|:---:|:---:|:---:|
| Initiates Standard Precautions. | 1 | | (CPI) |
| Obtains permission to treat patient. | 1 | | |
| Applies the cuff snugly to the humerus above the elbow, ensuring that arrow on cuff points to brachial artery. Places the sphygmomanometer in position that is easy for you to read. | 1 | | (CPI) |
| Palpates the brachial artery. | 1 | | |
| Places the stethescope diaphragm over the brachial artery and grasp the ball-pump. Turn the valve clockwise to close. | 1 | | |
| Pumps a pressure of 160mmHg, if you can hear the pulse sound immediately inflate to 200mmHg. If you can still hear the heartbeat inflate in 20mm increments until no sound is heard. Open the valve counterclockwise and let the air escape slowly. | 1 | | |
| Notes the number on the gauge where the first beat is heard (systolic pressure) as the needle descends. | 1 | | (CPI) |
| Notes the number on the gauge where the last beat is heard (diastolic pressure). | 1 | | (CPI) |
| Opens the valve, and quickly release remaining air. | 1 | | |

Must receive 7 out of 9 points.

Comments: _____

Failure of any of the CPIs is an automatic failure.

Evaluator: _____ NSP ID: _____

PASS      FAIL

# ⛨ Chapter Review

## Chapter Summary

Assessment is the most important skill you will learn as an OEC Technician because it is used during every patient encounter. Your overall assessment should begin with making sure the scene is safe for you and other rescuers to enter. Then look for life-threatening abnormalities of airway, breathing, circulation, and disability. Any of these abnormalities must be managed immediately. Continue the assessment by collecting information: the patient's medical history, findings of the physical exam, and the patient's vital signs. All of this information will help you figure out what is wrong with the patient.

Sometimes it will be appropriate to perform a complete assessment in an outdoor environment, and sometimes it will be more appropriate to do an abbreviated assessment and then complete the exam in a more stable environment. This decision should be made by taking into account abnormalities in the ABCDs, the patient's vital signs, and the prevailing environmental conditions. The key thing to remember is that the patient's condition is dynamic, and that you must continually reassess the patient's condition for changes.

## Remember...

1. Your first priority is scene safety.
2. Assess the ABCDs first.
3. The chief complaint is the patient's primary concern.
4. Stabilize all potential threats to life before performing a secondary assessment.
5. A significant MOI for a patient who has no signs of physical injury should raise your suspicions.
6. A minor MOI does not mean that the patient has no serious injury.
7. Use SAMPLE, OPQRST, and DCAP-BTLS when performing a secondary assessment.
8. Know the normal values of vital signs. Any abnormalities should raise your level of concern.
9. Reassess the patient frequently.

## Chapter Questions

### Multiple Choice

Choose the correct answer.

1. The assessment process can be complicated by which of the following factors? (check all that apply).
   a. communication or language barriers
   b. age differences
   c. cultural differences
   d. aggressive or combative behavior by the patient
   e. congenital disorders
   f. traumatic injuries
   g. medical problems
   h. environmental conditions

2. Which of the following statements regarding assessment is true?_____
   a. It is a one-time process.
   b. It is an ongoing process.
   c. It should not be interrupted.
   d. Changes in vital signs are always indicative of a deterioration of the patient's condition.

3. The most important component of assessment is_____
   a. ensuring scene safety.
   b. the ABCDs.
   c. recording accurate vital sign values.
   d. pulse oximetry.

4. Which of the following regarding scene safety is true?_____

a. Heroes go where angels fear to tread.

b. It is acceptable to rush into an unsafe scene and quickly pull a patient to safety if it is a matter of life or death.

c. You do not owe a patient your life.

d. None of the above are true.

5. The assessment referred to as tandem gait checks for_____

a. a subtle injury or neurological deficit.

b. whether or not the patient's arms move equally.

c. whether or not the patient's pupils react equally.

d. whether grip strength is equal in both hands.

6. A complete set of vitals consists of _____

a. respiration rate, pulse rate, level of responsiveness, blood pressure, and temperature.

b. respiration rate, pulse rate, pulse oximetry (PSAT), blood pressure, and temperature.

c. MOI, NOI, pulse rate, and blood pressure.

d. PSAT, Glasgow Coma Scale, AVPU, and SAMPLE.

7. You are taking a patient's blood pressure by auscultation. As you release the cuff, you continue to hear the patient's pulse all the way to the "zero" reading on gauge. What should you do?

a. Note that the patient has a diastolic reading of "0" and arrange for immediate transport to the closest medical facility.

b. Wait a few moments, reinflate the cuff, and listen again carefully to determine when the sound changes rather than disappears.

c. Wait a few moments and then reassess blood pressure because you obviously made a mistake.

d. Simply document the finding, because in some patients a diastolic reading of 0 is a normal condition known as hypophoresis.

8. Which of the following statements about taking a blood pressure reading is correct?_____

a. If you release the cuff too quickly and miss the diastolic reading, go ahead and reinflate the cuff immediately, then reassess the BP.

b. Releasing the cuff very slowly will give you a more accurate reading.

c. It does not matter how quickly or slowly you deflate the cuff.

d. None of the above are correct.

9. Orthostatic hypotension is defined as_____

a. a condition in which a patient has an abnormally low blood pressure.

b. a condition in which a patient's blood pressure increases when the patient stands up.

c. a condition in which a patient's blood pressure decreases suddenly when the patient stands up.

d. a condition in which blood pressure is controlled by taking antihypertension medication.

10. A drop in blood pressure during a postural BP check could indicate that_____

a. the patient's blood pressure is too high.

b. the patient is hypotensive.

c. the patient is dehydrated or bleeding internally.

d. the patient has a normal reaction for when a person goes from sitting to standing.

11. Which of the following regarding orthostatic hypotension is true?_____

a. It should only be performed on a patient who is not at risk for spinal cord injury.

b. The test should be discontinued if the patient begins to faint.

c. Some patients with orthostatic hypotension do not show a drop in pulse.

d. All of the above are true.

12. The most important thing an OEC Technician can do for an unresponsive patient with a pulse is_____

a. monitor and maintain the airway.

b. transport the patient immediately to the nearest medical facility.

c. record the GCS value.

d. perform CPR.

**13.** Which of the following statements regarding vital signs is true?

    **a.** A stable patient's vitals should be taken and recorded every 10–15 minutes, whereas a seriously injured or unstable patient's vitals should be recorded every 3-5 minutes.

    **b.** A patient's vitals should be taken every 5 minutes whether they are stable or not.

    **c.** Vital signs should not be taken in the field and are best performed in an aid station or in the back of an ambulance.

    **d.** A patient's temperature should be checked at the axilla (armpit) or using a forehead strip thermometer because these methods are the least invasive forms of recording temperature.

**14.** The normal respiratory rate for an adult is_____

    **a.** 8–24 breaths per minute.              **c.** 12–20 breaths per minute.

    **b.** 12–22 breaths per minute.            **d.** highly variable from person to person.

**15.** The normal pulse rate for an adult is_____

    **a.** 60–100 beats per minute.            **c.** 20–40 beats per minute.

    **b.** 50–90 beats per minute.             **d.** highly variable from person to person.

**16.** BP by auscultation is measured at which pulse point?_____

    **a.** Carotid                       **c.** Radial

    **b.** Brachial                     **d.** Femoral

**17.** Which is the best answer regarding patient assessment?_____

    **a.** It is a dynamic, ongoing process.

    **b.** It should be done systematically and by one rescuer only.

    **c.** A typical complete exam (primary and secondary assessments) should take only a few minutes to complete.

    **d.** All of the above are true.

## Matching

Match each of the following acronyms or mnemonics to its use.

_____ **1.** AVPU

_____ **2.** OPQRST

_____ **3.** PERRL

_____ **4.** SAMPLE

_____ **5.** DCAP-BTLS

_____ **6.** ABCD

    **a.** used to assess a patient's chief complaint

    **b.** used to assess a patient's pupils

    **c.** used for conducting a trauma assessment

    **d.** used to obtain a medical history during the assessment process

    **e.** used to assess a patient's level of responsiveness

    **f.** used to obtain critical information during a primary patient assessment

# Scenario

You receive a call that a visitor to the ski area is "down" in the cafeteria of the upper lodge. Upon arrival you find a 72-year-old man sitting on the floor holding his right wrist and arm. He appears to be slightly confused. The answers to your questions reveal that the patient had become dizzy and tripped and had landed on his right arm, that earlier today he drove 3 hours by car, and that he has left-sided dull chest pain (rated at 5 out of a possible 10, or "5/10") and mild difficulty breathing. The patient does not have a history of cardiac problems. He does take warfarin (blood thinner) for a clotting problem in his legs. Breakfast was at 7 a.m. The scene is secure. The patient's pulse rate is 90 per minute, and respiration rate is 28 per minute.

  **1.** In the SAMPLE interview, what information under "M" did the patient share?_____

    **a.** Breakfast was at 7 a.m.            **c.** He has no known allergies.

    **b.** He became dizzy and tripped.        **d.** He takes warfarin.

**2.** What information did you learn for the "E" in SAMPLE?_____
a. He became dizzy and tripped.
b. He has blood clots in his legs.
c. He ate breakfast at 7 a.m.
d. He has arm pain.

*There is minor swelling of the wrist. Upon palpation of the wrist and arm the patient indicates that the pain starts at the wrist and radiates up to the elbow. The patient denies any head, neck, or back pain. He is not wearing any medical alert tag. His skin is warm and dry.*

*The OPQRST mnemonic is used for evaluating pain in an illness. The patient informs you that he was having left-sided chest pain, rated as 5/10, and that it does not radiate.*

**3.** What information did the patient provide for the "R"?_____
a. The pain is 5/10.
b. The pain in his chest started just before he tripped.
c. He does not know why the pain started.
d. The pain is in the left side of the chest only.

**4.** What did the information provided by the patient for "S" concerning the chest pain reveal?_____
a. His pain was rated 5/10.
b. His pain is in the left side of his chest.
c. The pain started just before he tripped.
d. His pain is dull.

*You have called for O₂, an AED with a trauma bag, and an ALS ambulance to come directly to the lodge. Vitals are pulse rate: 90; BP: 130/70; and respirations: 28 and short. The right arm is properly immobilized.*

*O₂ is applied via a nonrebreather at 12 LPM (liters per minute) without any relief.*

*The patient is loaded into an ambulance and transported for treatment for a possible pulmonary embolism.*

## Suggested Reading

Bates, B. 2002. *A Guide to Physical Examination and History Taking,* Eighth Edition. Philadelphia: J. B. Lippincott Company.

Krost, W. S., J. J. Mistovich, and D. D. Limmer. 2006. "Beyond the Basics: Trauma Assessment." *Emergency Medical Services* 35(8): 71–75.

Stoy, W. A. 2001. "Patient Puzzle." *JEMS* 26(1): 24–33, 36–37.

## EXPLORE PEARSON myNSPkit™

Please go to www.myNSPkit.com. Under Student Resources, you will find animations, videos, web links, and games related to this chapter—and much more. Look for information on taking blood pressure and other vital signs, respiration rates, palpating peripheral pulses, developing rapport with your patients, and many other topics.

Register your access code from the front of your book by going to www.myNSPkit.com and selecting the appropriate links if the in-cover access code has been redeemed, go to www.myNSPkit.com and follow links to **Buy Access**.

# Medical Communications and Documentation

Jonathan Busko, MD, MPH, EMT-P

## ⊕ OBJECTIVES

**Upon completion of this chapter, the OEC Technician will be able to:**

**8-1** List the two types of medical communications.

**8-2** List the essential content that should be included in all verbal communications, using the acronym SAILER.

**8-3** List the components for the following methods used to complete a PCR:
  a. SOAP
  b. CHEATED

**8-4** List the characteristics of good report writing using the acronym FACTUAL-OEC.

**8-5** Describe and demonstrate how to correct an error on a written report.

**8-6** List two criteria that must be documented on a patient refusal.

**8-7** List four injuries or crimes that a mandated reporter must report to authorities.

**8-8** Demonstrate how to complete a sample patient care report with 100-percent accuracy.

**8-9** Demonstrate how to provide an oral report.

## Chapter Overview

As an OEC Technician, you evaluate and care for a variety of patients whose injuries or illnesses range from relatively minor to immediately life threatening. As part of this process, you collect valuable information about the patient and the case, including what happened, important clinical findings, the care the person received, and his response to treatment (Figure 8-1■). This information is critical in that it is used not only to formulate on-scene treatment plans but in many instances is also factored into the long-term care of the patient. It may even be used to determine both the patient's

*continued*

## HISTORICAL TIMELINE

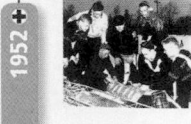

**1952** NSP European Division formed; Junior Ski Patrol program introduced.

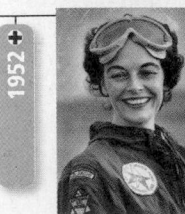

**1952** Edward Taylor, who valued women patrollers, clearly stated the position on equality of women in his 1952 edition of the *Ski Patrol Manual*.

**1/2/1953** Minnie Dole breaks leg while skiing (states, "I'll never ski on January second again.")

## ⊕ KEY TERMS

**capacity,** *p. 284*

**communication,** *p. 265*

**field care notes,** *p. 272*

**hand-off report,** *p. 269*

**history of present illness,** *p. 282*

**incident report forms,** *p. 271*

**mandated reporter,** *p. 286*

**patient care report,** *p. 273*

diagnosis and his prognosis. This information also may be critical to reducing legal risk in the event that a legal case is filed, because it may be the only source of information for reconstructing the incident scene years later. In fact, proper documentation can prevent legal cases from ever being filed.

For these reasons, OEC Technicians must be able to effectively obtain and properly document crucial medical information, and to accurately communicate that information to other members of the emergency care system and to the definitive care facility staff. OEC Technicians also must collect and document information from the incident scene to "preserve evidence" that could be used to reduce legal risk inherent to any patient care provided.

**Communication** is a process that enables information to be transmitted from one person to another and includes several components. In a health care setting, *mis*communication can adversely affect the patient's outcome. In a legal context, a breakdown of communications and the absence of the proper recording of facts involving an incident could result in the loss of vital evidence that could assist the OEC Technician in any ensuing legal proceeding.

Medical written communications are used by many people for many reasons. OEC Technicians, resort managers, insurers, patrol educators, medical advisors, and patrol representatives routinely use these data for activities that are both directly and indirectly related to patient care. The information is used in many ways, including efforts to improve the quality of care provided, insurance claims, and risk management evaluations. By doing your part to ensure the effective flow of medical communications, you will be helping to reduce morbidity and mortality and improve the safety of outdoor recreational activities.

**communication**  a process by which a message is transmitted from one person to another.

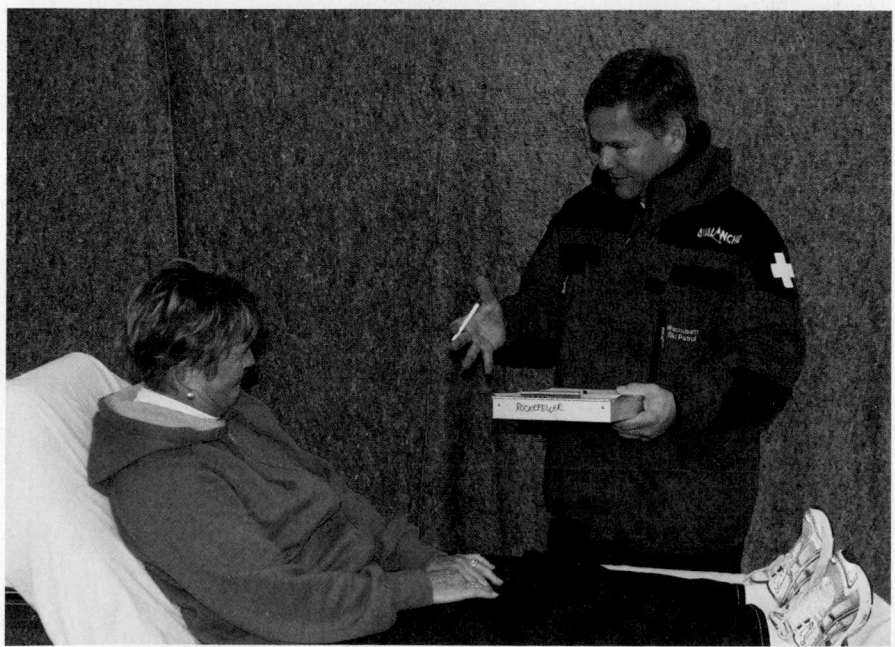

**Figure 8-1** Obtaining detailed information is very important in the interview process.
Copyright Mike Halloran

# ✚ CASE PRESENTATION ✚

You and your partner respond to the scene of a skier injured at the base of a large rock. Upon arrival, you find an adult male who is complaining of neck and back pain. Following your introduction, and after obtaining his permission to care for him, you perform a SAMPLE medical history, obtain vital signs, and begin to care for him. During your physical exam, you find that the patient does not have movement or sensation below the waist. Soon after, other patrollers arrive to assist you. On a small preprinted field-incident form you record the patient's information. Another patroller quickly interviews the patient's friend and witnesses to the incident and records their names, brief statements, and phone numbers. These bystanders are asked to come to the patrol hut to continue the interview. Following care and packaging, which includes spinal immobilization, you help load the patient into a toboggan, take his vital signs again, and accompany him to the aid room. Once there, you help move the patient to a stretcher.

*What should you do now?*

This chapter discusses the principles and practices OEC Technicians use to collect, record, and communicate essential medical and legal data, both during and after rescue operations. Because complete, accurate, and timely communication and documentation support excellent patient care, this chapter emphasizes the most common reports and forms that OEC Technicians are expected to complete and the essential information required for each. In addition, the chapter describes strategies that facilitate the medical communications process.

The ability to communicate effectively with others and properly record and document interactions with patients is one of the essential skills that every OEC Technician must possess (Figure 8-2■). It is a skill that, when mastered, is one of the hallmarks of a highly trained rescuer.

**Figure 8-2** This OEC instructor is teaching students the good communication skills they need to do their jobs effectively.
Copyright Mike Halloran

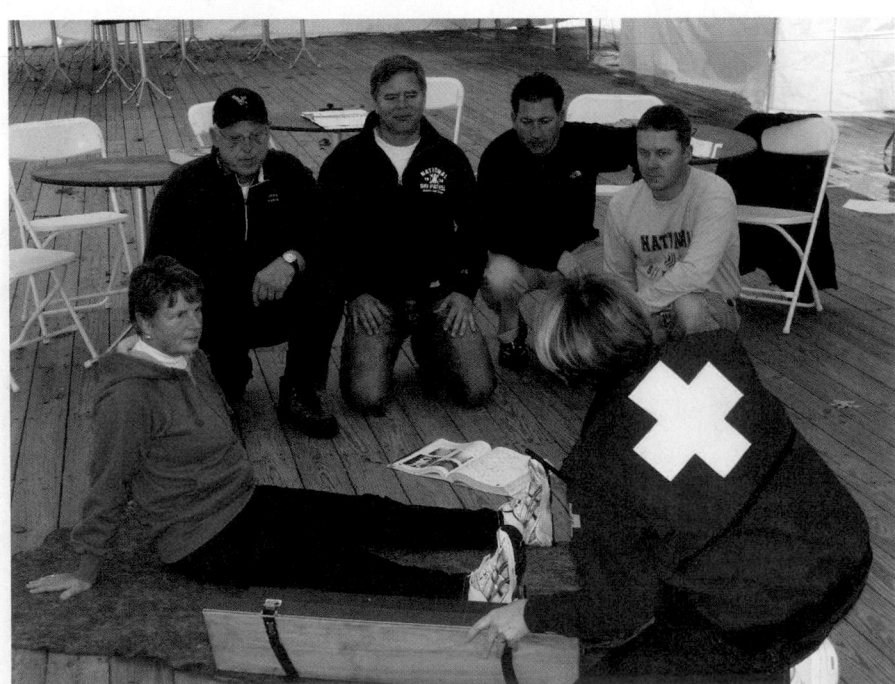

# Communication Basics

Communication is a process in which a message is transmitted from a sender to a receiver. The goal of communication is to deliver that message in a manner that is understood by the recipient. The communication process consists of the following six components:

+ Message: the information that you wish to convey
+ Sender: the person who is delivering the message
+ Encoding: the translation of the message into words or signals
+ Channel: the medium through which the encoded message is transmitted (e.g., a face-to-face discussion, a radio, a telephone, in writing)
+ Decoding: the translation of the message into meaning by the receiver(s)
+ Receiver: the person or group for whom the message is intended

Miscommunication occurs when the receiver does not interpret the message as originally intended by the sender. This can be due to any number of factors, known as noise, which can affect any or all of the components of communication. If, for instance, the original message was properly encoded, transmitted, and decoded by the receiver but was unclear to begin with, the message will likely be unclear. Similarly, factors affecting the channel used to transmit the message, such as a dead spot resulting in gaps in radio or cell phone transmission, can cause miscommunication. Even face-to-face conversations are not immune to communication problems; stress, information overload, and a host of other factors can adversely affect how a message is transmitted, received, or interpreted.

Because errors can arise anywhere along the communication process, it is important that senders obtain ongoing feedback from receivers to ensure that the intended message was both received and accurately interpreted. Such feedback will greatly improve the quality of communication and reduce errors.

**8-1** List the two types of medical communications.

# Forms of Communication

Humans communicate with one another through various forms, including verbally (including orally and in writing) and nonverbally. Verbal communication involves the use of words and is the primary means by which humans communicate with one another—especially face to face, or orally (Figure 8-3■). Studies show that most humans have a vocabulary of approximately 10,000 words and speak at a rate of 125–150 words per minute. However, they are capable of listening at a rate of 275–300 words per minute and can think at rates of up to 500 words per minute. This listening-to-speaking gap may help explain why people sometimes "tune-out" parts of conversations, which can result in miscommunication.

Written communication involves the use of words or symbols.

Nonverbal communication is defined as communicating without words and includes behaviors such as facial expressions, eye movements, hand gestures, touch, vocal tone, body posture, positioning, and movement (Figure 8-4■). Studies indicate that as much as 93 percent of communication between humans is nonverbal.

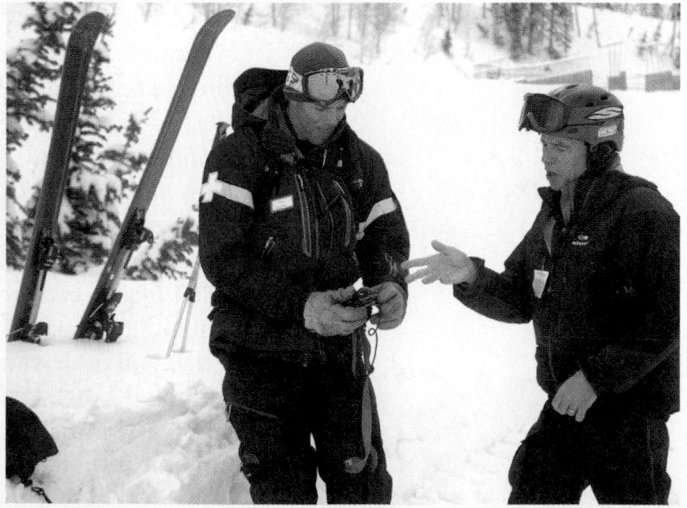

**Figure 8-3** Good oral communication skills are essential when in contact with the public.
Copyright Studio 404

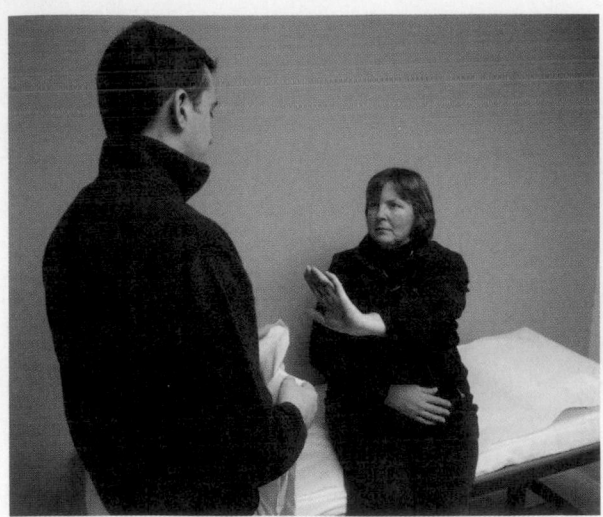

**Figure 8-4** This patient is communicating her denial of treatment nonverbally.
Copyright Edward McNamara

# Medical Communications

Medical communication is a specialized form of communication used to transmit health care–related data. Such data are communicated for many reasons, in many ways, and by many people. OEC Technicians use medical communication primarily to transmit information about an incident and a patient from one person to another. The sender of this data is typically the patient's primary care provider, and the receiver is typically the person who is either assisting in the patient's treatment or assuming primary care responsibilities. Because health care data typically contain personal information, medical communications are generally considered "privileged communications."

Patient information should be shared only with authorized personnel who have a direct need for the information. OEC Technicians that are members of a state or provincial emergency care system must safeguard medical communications and prevent unauthorized access to these sensitive data. Basic rules of patient privacy are applicable to OEC Technicians.

As a general rule, volunteer patrol members are not held to the higher HIPAA (Health Insurance Portability and Accountability Act of 1996) privacy requirements. Some of the requirements of this statute involve compensation via electronic communications. Given that volunteer OEC Technicians usually are not involved with electronic communications of medical billing, this law generally does not apply to OEC Technicians. However, this does not mean that maintaining medical information about an injured person should not be kept confidential. Questions regarding an area's medical information privacy policy should be directed to your area management.

Medical communication is an ongoing process that occurs throughout the patient care process. To ensure continuity and efficiency in the care of patients and to avoid misunderstanding, medical communications must be clear, concise, and accurate.

OEC Technicians must be familiar with and demonstrate proficiency in two types of medical communication: oral communication and written documentation. Depending on your role at the scene of an emergency, you will likely use one or both types of medical communication at every incident to which you respond.

⊕ 8-9  Demonstrate how to provide an oral report.

## Oral Communication

Oral communication is the transmission of information through spoken words. Most often, oral communication occurs in the form of face-to-face conversation, but it also can be accomplished using various communication devices such as a two-way radio or a telephone. The language used in oral communications must be commonly understood by other rescuers and medical providers, including advanced medical personnel. As indicated in Chapter 2, Emergency Care Systems, the use of plain English is preferred over radio codes, which are neither universally used nor accepted. OEC Technicians use oral communication as the primary means to convey information to dispatchers, to other rescuers, or when transferring the care of a patient to another health care provider. When communicating medical information orally, it is essential that you present the information in a clear, concise, and organized manner, and that you understand the level of training of the people with whom you are speaking (Table 8-1■).

After the initial evaluation of a patient, you should identify yourself in your radio communication to base. One method that OEC Technicians can use to communicate

**Table 8-1** Who Uses Medical Communications?

- Dispatchers (e.g., patrol, 9-1-1, law enforcement)
- Rescuers (OEC Technicians, EMS, firefighters, law enforcement personnel)
- Hospital personnel (physicians, nurses, physician assistants)
- Medical Advisor/Director
- Area management (patrol directors, managers)
- Legal professionals (attorneys, paralegals, judges)
- Insurance company personnel

with others concerning an incident is the acronym "SAILER," which represents the following pieces of information:

**S**—Sex of the patient

**A**—Age of the patient

**I**—Incident/chief complaint

**L**—Location of incident/patient

**E**—Equipment needed (e.g., splints, backboards, toboggans)

**R**—Resources needed (e.g., extra help, security personnel, management personnel, activation of EMS (BLS or ALS)

⊕ **8-2** List the essential content that should be included in all verbal communications, using the acronym SAILER.

Depending on your local protocols, this information may or may not be presented in that exact order. All the information, however, should be conveyed in your oral communications. With few exceptions, you should be able to convey the information in 30 seconds or less. Here is how information from the opening scenario (see "Case Presentation") might be presented to your area dispatcher:

> "This is patroller David. I have one patient, a 45-year-old male, who has hit a large rock near the top of The Wall on the skier's right. He is an urgent patient who requires immediate care and transport. Vital signs are stable. Send a toboggan with backboard, oxygen, and extra help. I need an ALS ambulance. Notify management of the incident."

Notice that this oral communication conveyed essential information only and was presented in a clear, concise manner. Always make sure that dispatch acknowledges your message. Ideally, the dispatcher should repeat the key portion of your message back to you so that miscommunication is much less likely, although local protocols will dictate the actual process to be followed (Figure 8-5■). The dispatcher might reply as follows:

> "Confirming, you are on scene with a 45-year-old male near the top of The Wall. Patient is urgent. Requesting toboggan, backboard, oxygen pack, assistance, ALS ambulance, and management."

Most radio protocols do not include the patient's name, unless there is a specific reason for that information, such as a need to find a lost child. Remember, anyone can listen to your transmissions using a scanner, and each patient's privacy should be protected.

As other rescuers arrive on scene, you should give each of them a concise oral report—known as a **hand-off report**—that includes a brief description of the patient's chief complaint and detailed directions regarding how that rescuer can help you (Figure 8-6■).

**hand-off report** an oral report given at the transfer of a patient from one provider to another.

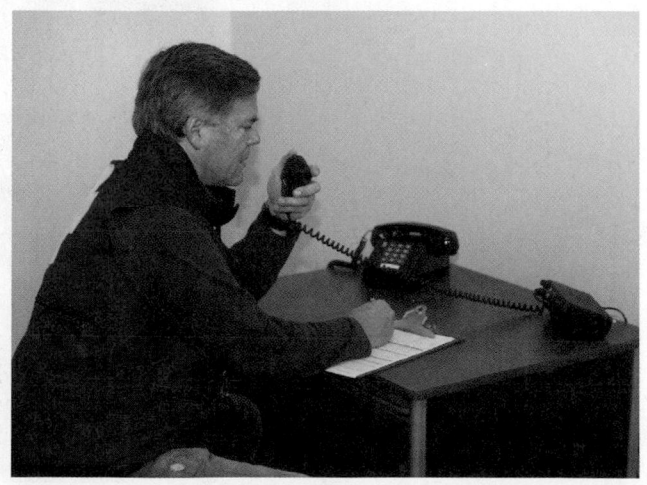

**Figure 8-5** A dispatcher must have excellent oral skills.
Copyright Mike Halloran

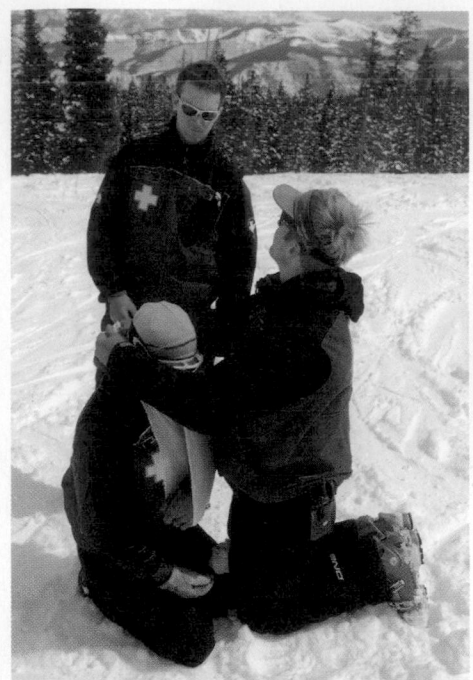

**Figure 8-6** An oral report should be given when handing off a patient.
Copyright Scott Smith

Direct your assistants in a clear, calm, and professional manner. Make sure they understand you. Continue to provide directions and communicate with all on-scene assistants as you render aid to the patient and prepare the person for transport. Listen to other rescuers' suggestions and, when appropriate, use their ideas while maintaining overall management of the incident. Effective communication increases the efficiency of rescue operations and decreases on-scene problems, especially during incidents involving multiple patients.

When the patient arrives at the first-aid station or medical facility, provide a concise oral hand-off report to the person who will be assuming the patient's care. This oral report should also be clear and concise, but it may include the following information, some of which was not communicated previously:

- The patient's name, if known
- The patient's age (approximate if the exact age is unknown)
- The nature of the injury or illness
- The patient's chief complaint
- All treatment that has been rendered
- The patient's response to that treatment
- Serial sets of vital signs, including the most current set
- Immediate patient care needs

The hand-off report usually to other medical personnel contains more detailed information about the patient than that provided to dispatch, and it should emphasize the patient's current condition and treatment needs (Figure 8-7■). After delivering your hand-off report, ask the personnel who are assuming the patient's care if they have any questions. Under normal circumstances, a hand-off report should take

**Figure 8-7** Transferring the hand-off report to ambulance personnel is an important step in protecting the patient's privacy.

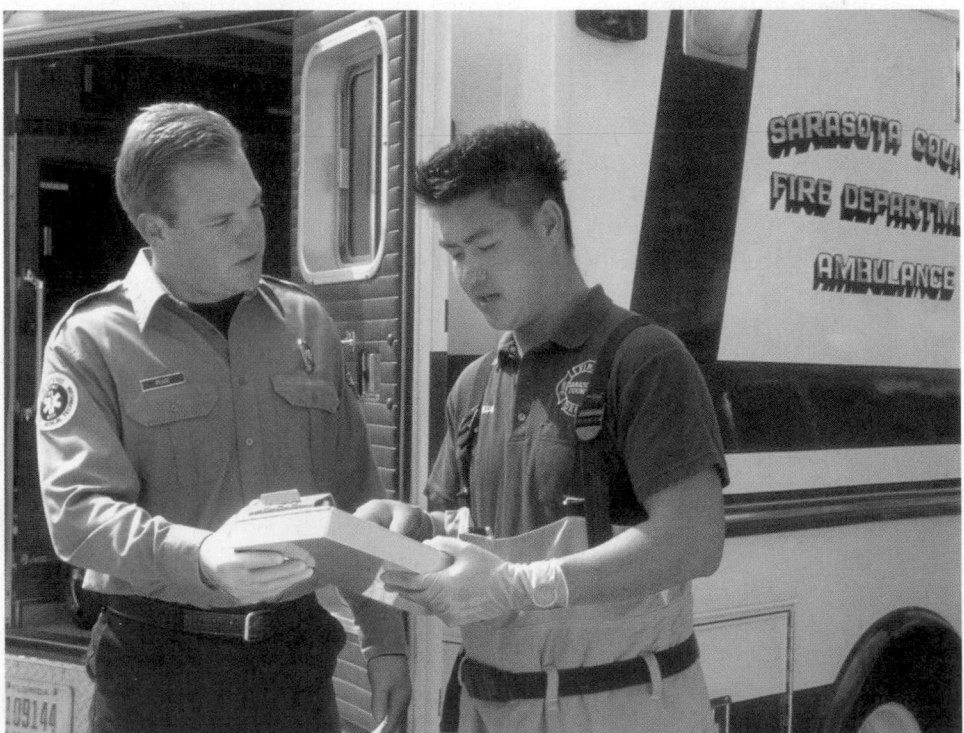

30–60 seconds to complete. To illustrate how a hand-off report might be presented, consider the following example:

> "This is John. He's a 45-year-old male who hit a large rock on the trail, The Wall, at moderate speed. He was wearing a helmet, and there was no loss of responsiveness. He is complaining of mid-thoracic back pain and has no movement or sensation below the waist. My secondary assessment showed no other injuries. His serial vital signs have been stable. He has no allergies, takes no medications, and we have placed him on oxygen."

## Written Communication

Written communication is used to document patient encounters and may become part of the patient's permanent medical record. Depending on local protocol, this information may be given to the care provider who assumes care of the patient. It also may be used for research purposes, to identify or document trends, for continuous quality-improvement endeavors, and to assist in risk management. Written reports also are used as medical-legal records. In most ski areas, these written incident reports become the cornerstone of incident risk management. Therefore, learning to properly document and preserve evidence from a patient encounter is vital for OEC Technicians and the ski area alike.

You may encounter the following three types of written communication:

1. field care notes
2. **incident report forms**
3. patient care reports

All these documents eventually become part of the completed incident report form. Unlike oral communication, in which only limited information is provided, written communication should be more detailed. From a legal perspective, written incident reports carefully document two types of facts: those concerning the parties involved, and those associated with the incident from when the OEC Technician's first heard of the incident until the OEC Technician's involvement was completed. These incident report forms not only include the medical information previously described but also should include the following:

+ A detailed, factual description of the incident.
+ The names of all of the patrollers involved in responding to the incident, including a description of what each patroller did at the incident.
+ The names, addresses, and phone numbers of all witnesses to the incident. Ski patrollers also may need to obtain a witness statement, if the incident is serious, which should include how the incident occurred and what the witnesses observed.
+ Take special care to document and preserve any statements that reveal that the patient knew or believes that he was at fault, such as, "I knew I was going too fast" or "I should not have been skiing that slope."

In addition to the previously mentioned documentation skills, OEC Technicians must know when to ask for help. Almost all areas have a designated risk manager. Recognizing a high-risk situation and notifying others—other patrollers if help is needed, or the area risk manager—is important for caring for injured patients and managing the legal risks associated with the incident. This skill, in combination with properly documenting and managing an incident scene, can reduce both the medical risk to the injured patient and the legal risk for OEC Technicians and their employers.

⊕ **8-8** Demonstrate how to complete a sample patient care report with 100-percent accuracy.

**incident report forms** forms provided by the National Ski Area Association, a ski resort, or an insurance carrier and used by OEC Technicians to document an incident; the forms include the circumstances leading to injury.

## Field Care Notes

It is common for OEC Technicians and other rescue personnel to take notes while they are involved with rescue operations. These notes, known as **field care notes**, generally include essential information about the incident, including the location, witnesses' names, and contact information (Figure 8-8■). If the incident involves one or more patients, the field care notes also include patient-specific information such as the person's name, level of consciousness, vital signs, medications, and other relevant data. Often the information is documented along a chronological time line and is later transferred to, or becomes a part of, a patient care report, an incident report form, or both. Field care notes may need to be attached to other reports, depending on your area's local protocol.

## NSAA Incident Report Form

Most OEC Technicians use incident reporting forms such as those published by the National Ski Areas Association (NSAA) or a ski area's insurance company. NSAA is one of NSP's most important ski-industry partners. NSP and NSAA have historically worked together to improve skiing safety and have developed incident reporting forms adopted throughout the ski industry. NSAA's incident report form (Figure 8-9■) contains all of the fundamental information needed to properly document an incident, including (but not limited to) sections that document the following information:

+ Patient identification information
+ Cause of the injury (mechanism of injury)
+ Names of individuals at the incident, including OEC Technicians and witnesses
+ Patient's statement concerning what caused the incident
+ Emergency care given at the incident scene
+ Emergency care given in the aid room
+ Further comments about the incident

Properly completing this form or one like it is a skill most OEC Technicians will learn if they patrol at ski areas. Understanding the limitations of the form, and the cir-

**Figure 8-8** This patroller is making careful field care notes at an incident scene.
Copyright Edward McNamara

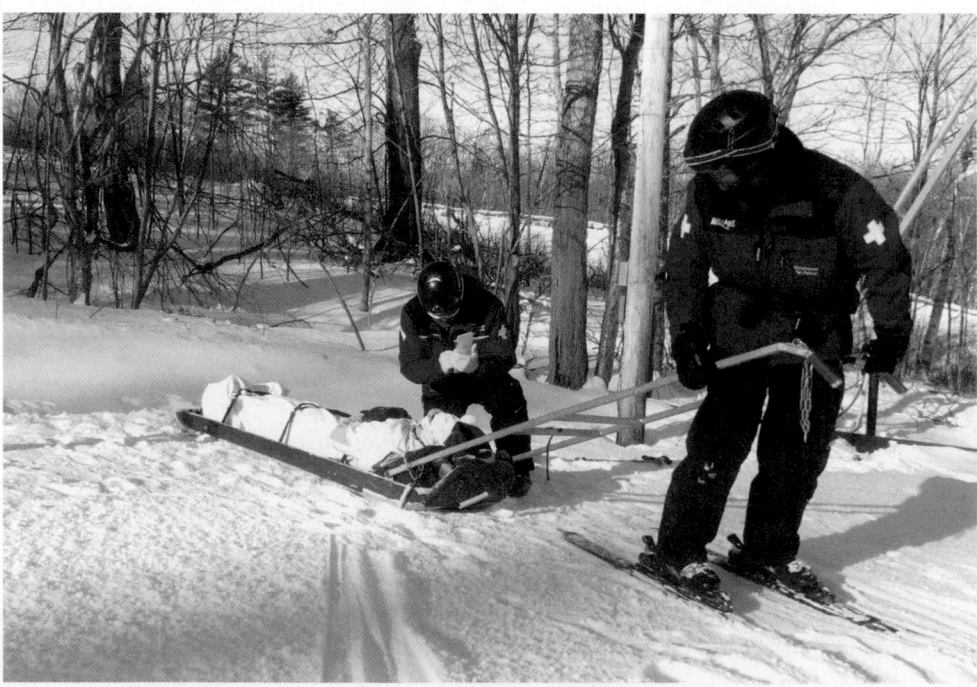

cumstances in which an OEC Technician must supplement it with additional forms and information, are things you should learn in becoming an OEC Technician.

## Patient Care Reports

In addition to becoming familiar with the NSAA incident form, OEC Technicians should be familiar with a **patient care report** (PCR). A PCR is used to record specific information about the medical care provided to the patient (Figure 8-10■). It is a document that may become part of the patient's permanent medical record. A copy of the PCR might accompany the patient to a definitive care facility, or be sent to the facility as soon as it is completed. PCRs have several formats, including closed, open, and mixed.

A closed-format PCR has a series of check boxes or limited fill-in-the-blank sections, allowing the PCR to be completed quickly. This form often is favored by

**patient care report** a report that documents a patient's complaints and past medical history, plus a chronological account of the examination and treatment of the patient; is a legal document.

NSAA

**INCIDENT REPORT FORM**

RESORT____

DATE____ DAY OF WK.____ TIME OF INCIDENT____ ☐ AM ☐ PM INCIDENT #____

| | | |
|---|---|---|
| LOCATION | ☐ ON-HILL ☐ LIFT ☐ PREMISE ☐ TUBING HILL | DESCRIBE SPECIFIC LOCATION: ☐ EASIER ○ ☐ MORE DIFFICULT ☐ ☐ MOST DIFFICULT ◆ ☐ EXPERTS ONLY◆◆ ☐ FREESTYLE TERRAIN▢ ☐ NOT APPLICABLE |
| INJURED PERSON | NAME____ ☐ MALE ☐ FEMALE DOB____ ADDRESS____ AGE____ CITY____ STATE____ ZIP____ HT____ HOME PH____ CELL PH____ OCCUPATION____ WT____ | |
| SKIING HISTORY | **ABILITY** ☐BEG ☐N/APP ☐INTERMEDIATE ☐ADV/EXPERT; **LESSONS** ☐ IN LESSON INSTR____ ☐ N/APPLICABLE; **NUMBER OF TIMES ON:** ☐TRAIL ☐TODAY____ ☐LIFT ☐PRIOR____ OTHER____ | **EQUIPMENT REMOVED BY:** ☐ FALL ☐ PATROL ☐ INJURED ☐ OTHER |
| PATIENT HISTORY | PRIOR INJURY/ILLNESS- DESCRIBE____ YEAR INJURED____ CORRECTIVE LENSES NEEDED? ☐YES ☐NO WORN? ☐YES ☐NO MEDICAL INSURANCE? ☐YES ☐NO LIST ANY MEDS TAKEN:____ TICKET TYPE____ ALLERGIES/MEDICAL ALERT DESCRIBE____ GROUP NAME____ | |
| EQUIPMENT | ☐ ALPINE ☐ NORDIC ☐ SNOWBOARD ☐ OTHER EQUIP:____ ☐ OWNED ☐ AREA RENTAL ☐ OTHER RENTAL ☐ BORROWED ☐ DEMO BINDING MAKE____ MODEL____ SKI/BOARD #____ BOOT #____ SHOP NAME____ ADDRESS____ HELMET WORN? ☐ YES ☐ NO HELMET AREA RENTAL? ☐ YES ☐ NO HELMET RENTAL #____ | LEFT DIN: TOE / HEEL; RIGHT DIN: TOE / HEEL |
| DESCRIPTION OF INCIDENT (Patient's words) | ____ **THE ABOVE STATEMENT IS TRUE AND CORRECT** INJURED'S SIGNATURE____ **PARENT/GUARDIAN SIGNATURE**____ I REFUSE FIRST AID: INJURED'S SIGNATURE (PARENT/GUARDIAN IF MINOR)____ | |
| PROBABLE INJURY | ☐ FRACTURE ☐SPRAIN/STRAIN ☐ PUNCTURE/LACERATION ☐ BRUISE/CONTUSION ☐ ABRASION ☐ CONCUSSION ☐DISLOCATION ☐ FROSTBITE ☐ MULTIPLE ☐ OTHER____ | |
| INJURY ZONE | ☐ LEFT ☐ RIGHT ☐ BOTH ☐ MULTIPLE | ☐ HEAD ☐ FACE ☐ EYE ☐ NOSE ☐ MOUTH ☐ TEETH ☐ NECK ☐ SHOULDER ☐ ARM ☐ WRIST ☐ HAND ☐ THUMB ☐ CHEST ☐ BACK ☐ ABDOMEN ☐ HIP ☐ UPPER LEG ☐ KNEE ☐ LOWER LEG ☐ ANKLE ☐ FOOT ☐ OTHER____ |
| FIRST AID RENDERED | ON HILL:____ AT FIRST AID STATION:____ | |
| PATROLLERS INVOLVED | AT SCENE:____ TRANSPORTING:____ AT FIRST AID STATION:____ | |
| TRANSPORT & DESTINATION | ARRIVED AT FIRST AID STATION BY: ☐ PATROL/TOBOGGAN ☐ WALK-IN ☐ OTHER | LEFT FIRST AID STATION BY: ☐ WALKED OUT ☐ ASSISTED TO CAR/BUS ☐ AMBULANCE **DESTINATION:** ☐ HOME ☐ LODGE ☐ RETURN SKIING ☐ MEDICAL FACILITY:____ |
| SITE CONDITIONS | **SURFACE AT SCENE:** ☐POWDER ☐CORN ☐VARIABLE ☐PACKED POWDER ☐LOOSE GRANULAR ☐FROZ GRAN/HARD PACKED ☐WET ☐OTHER____ | **VISIBILITY:** ☐ CLEAR ☐ OVERCAST ☐ FOG ☐ SNOWING ☐ RAINING ☐ SNOW BEING MADE NEAR SCENE **TEMPERATURE:** ☐ BELOW 0 ☐ 0-32 ☐ ABOVE 32 **WIND:** ☐ CALM ☐ MODERATE ☐ HIGH |
| WITNESSES | NAME____ PHONE____ ADDRESS____ CITY____ STATE____ ZIP____ NAME____ PHONE____ ADDRESS____ CITY____ STATE____ ZIP____ | |

SIGNATURE OF INDIVIDUAL COMPLETING REPORT:____ DATE REPORT COMPLETED:____
PRINT NAME:____ Rev. 9/06

**Figure 8-9** A sample of the National Ski Area Association's Incident Report Form.

members of multi-tiered emergency care systems in which the field care of the patient is routinely transferred to other providers.

In contrast, in an open-format PCR, information is organized under broad headings such as Patient Information, SOAP or CHEATED information, AMPLE, Vital Signs, Patient Condition, Treatment, and Transport. Beneath each heading is a blank

**Figure 8-10** A sample of closed-format ambulance patient care report.

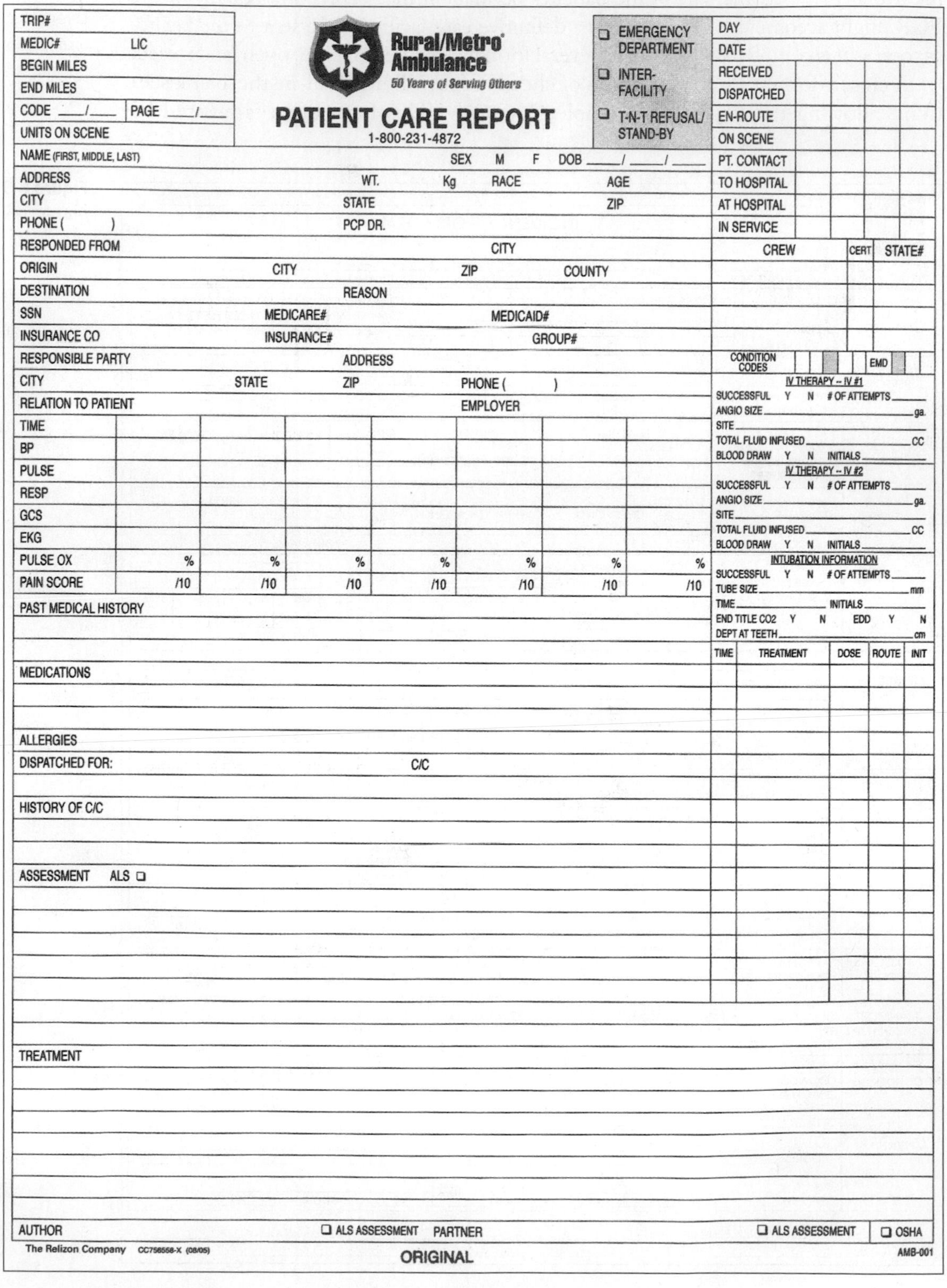

TRIP#
MEDIC# LIC
BEGIN MILES
END MILES
CODE ___/___ PAGE ___/___
UNITS ON SCENE

Rural/Metro Ambulance
50 Years of Serving Others
PATIENT CARE REPORT
1-800-231-4872

❑ EMERGENCY DEPARTMENT
❑ INTER-FACILITY
❑ T-N-T REFUSAL/ STAND-BY

DAY
DATE
RECEIVED
DISPATCHED
EN-ROUTE
ON SCENE
PT. CONTACT
TO HOSPITAL
AT HOSPITAL
IN SERVICE

NAME (FIRST, MIDDLE, LAST) SEX M F DOB ___/___/___
ADDRESS WT. Kg RACE AGE
CITY STATE ZIP
PHONE ( ) PCP DR.
RESPONDED FROM CITY
ORIGIN CITY ZIP COUNTY
DESTINATION REASON
SSN MEDICARE# MEDICAID#
INSURANCE CO INSURANCE# GROUP#
RESPONSIBLE PARTY ADDRESS
CITY STATE ZIP PHONE ( )
RELATION TO PATIENT EMPLOYER

CREW CERT STATE#

CONDITION CODES EMD

IV THERAPY -- IV #1
SUCCESSFUL Y N # OF ATTEMPTS
ANGIO SIZE ga.
SITE
TOTAL FLUID INFUSED CC
BLOOD DRAW Y N INITIALS

IV THERAPY -- IV #2
SUCCESSFUL Y N # OF ATTEMPTS
ANGIO SIZE ga.
SITE
TOTAL FLUID INFUSED CC
BLOOD DRAW Y N INITIALS

INTUBATION INFORMATION
SUCCESSFUL Y N # OF ATTEMPTS
TUBE SIZE mm
TIME INITIALS
END TITLE CO2 Y N EDD Y N
DEPT AT TEETH cm

| | | | | | | | |
|---|---|---|---|---|---|---|---|
| TIME | | | | | | | |
| BP | | | | | | | |
| PULSE | | | | | | | |
| RESP | | | | | | | |
| GCS | | | | | | | |
| EKG | | | | | | | |
| PULSE OX | % | % | % | % | % | % | % |
| PAIN SCORE | /10 | /10 | /10 | /10 | /10 | /10 | /10 |

| TIME | TREATMENT | DOSE | ROUTE | INIT |
|---|---|---|---|---|

PAST MEDICAL HISTORY
MEDICATIONS
ALLERGIES
DISPATCHED FOR: C/C
HISTORY OF C/C
ASSESSMENT ALS ❑
TREATMENT
AUTHOR ❑ ALS ASSESSMENT PARTNER ❑ ALS ASSESSMENT ❑ OSHA
The Relizon Company CC756558-X (08/05) ORIGINAL AMB-001

section in which the OEC Technician writes in all pertinent findings and incident-related content. Because they are more loosely structured, these forms generally take more time to complete than either closed- or mixed-format PCRs (Figure 8-11■).

A mixed-format PCR combines the two previous styles and includes both check boxes for common types of data and blanks into which specific comments or information are written (Figure 8-12■).

Nearly all PCRs include a section for recording serial sets of vital signs. A simple PCR that OEC Technicians might use for seriously ill or injured patients may contain places to record serial sets of vital signs, skin color, temperature, and level of consciousness. The SAMPLE acronym can also be found on many of these forms (Figure 8-13■). Most ski areas require OEC Technicians to fill out the NSAA form (or an equivalent), and when a patient needs further medical documentation because of significant injury or illness, a form like the one shown in Figure 8-13 may be used.

**Figure 8-11** A sample of a ski area open-format patient care report.
Courtesy of Dr. David Johe

**BLUE RIDGE SKI RESORT**
**PATIENT CARE REPORT**

Name: _____ Sex: _____ Age: _____

| S: | A: |
|----|----|
| O: | M: |
| A: | P: |
| P: | L: |
|    | E: |

**VITAL SIGNS**

| | Time | Pulse | Blood Pressure | Respirations | LOC |
|---|------|-------|----------------|--------------|-----|
| 1 | | | | | |
| 2 | | | | | |
| 3 | | | | | |
| 4 | | | | | |

**TREATMENT:**

| **PATIENT CONDITION:** | **TRANSPORT:** |
|------------------------|----------------|
| | |

**Figure 8-12** A sample of a mixed-format ambulance patient care form.

MAINE EMS

PRESS DOWN, YOU ARE MAKING THREE COPIES.

| RUN REPORT # | Mo. | Day | Year | M T W Th F S Sun | SERVICE NAME | SERVICE NO. | VEHICLE NO. | ALS ☐ Performed ☐ Back-up called | SERVICE RUN NO. |
|---|---|---|---|---|---|---|---|---|---|
| 746118 | | | | | | | | | |

NAME | BILLING INFORMATION

STREET OR R.F.D.

CITY/TOWN | STATE | ZIP

AGE/DATE OF BIRTH | ☐ Male ☐ Female | PHONE

INCIDENT LOCATION: | ADDRESS | CITY/TOWN

TRANSPORTED TO: | TREATING/FAMILY PHYSICIAN | CREW LICENSE NUMBERS

TRANSPORTATION/COMMUNICATIONS PROBLEMS

☐ Medical
☐ Cardiac
☐ Poisoning/OD
☐ Respiratory
☐ Behavioral
☐ Diabetic
☐ Seizure
☐ CVA
☐ OB/Gyn
☐ Other ________

☐ Trauma
☐ Multi-Systems Trauma
☐ Head
☐ Spinal
☐ Burn
☐ Soft Tissue Injury
☐ Fractures
☐ Other ________

☐ Code 99

| R | L | LUNG SOUNDS |
|---|---|---|
| ☐ | ☐ | CLEAR |
| ☐ | ☐ | ABSENT |
| ☐ | ☐ | DECREASED |
| ☐ | ☐ | RALES |
| ☐ | ☐ | WHEEZE |
| ☐ | ☐ | STRIDOR |

TYPE OF RUN
☐ Emergency Transport
☐ Routine Transfer
☐ Emergency Transfer
☐ No Transport
☐ Refused Transport

| TIME | CODE | | ODOMETER |
|---|---|---|---|
| | | Call Received | |
| | | Enroute | |
| | | At Scene | |
| | | From Scene | |
| | | At Destination | |
| | | In Service | |

☐ MEDICATIONS ☐ ALLERGIES

CHIEF COMPLAINT:

| TIME | PULSE | RESP | BP | PUPILLARY RESPONSE | SKIN | VERBAL RESPONSE | MOTOR RESPONSE | EYE-OPENING RESPONSE | CAPILLARY REFILL |
|---|---|---|---|---|---|---|---|---|---|
| | | | / | | | 5 4 3 2 1 | 6 5 4 3 2 1 | 4 3 2 1 | ☐ Normal ☐ Delayed ☐ None |
| | | | / | | | 5 4 3 2 1 | 6 5 4 3 2 1 | 4 3 2 1 | ☐ Normal ☐ Delayed ☐ None |
| | | | / | | | 5 4 3 2 1 | 6 5 4 3 2 1 | 4 3 2 1 | ☐ Normal ☐ Delayed ☐ None |

☐ MVA ☐ Concern AOB/ETOH SEAT BELTS: ☐ Used ☐ Not Used ☐ N/A ☐ Helmet Used

MUTUAL AID: Assisted/Assisted by Service # ________ Time Called: ________

PATIENT'S SUSPECTED PROBLEM: 746118

| | |
|---|---|
| Cleared Airway | Extrication |
| Artificial Respiration/BVM | Cervical Immobilization |
| Oropharyngeal Airway | KED/Short Board |
| Nasopharyngeal Airway | Long Board |
| CPR–Time: | Restraints |
| Bystander CPR | Traction Splinting |
| AED | General Splinting |
| Suction | Cold Application |
| Oxygen–LPMin ___ ☐ Nasal ☐ Mask | MAST Inflated |
| Pulse Oximetry | |
| Autovent | |

☐ Medication Administered | ☐ Defib Lic.# ________ | MEDICAL CONTROL ☐ Written Order/Protocol ☐ Verbal Order/Protocol

☐ Monitor | ☐ Chest Decomp | IV Total Attempts ☐ SUC LIC.# ________ ☐ UNSUC LIC.# ________

☐ Pacing | ☐ Cricothyrotomy

EOA Total Attempts ☐ SUC LIC.# ________ ☐ UNSUC LIC.# ________

ET Total Attempts ☐ SUC LIC.# ________ ☐ UNSUC LIC.# ________

| LIC # | EKG RHYTHM | TIME | MEDS/DEFIB/C-VERT | DOSE W/S | ROUTE |
|---|---|---|---|---|---|
| | | | | | |

NAME OF E.D. TREATING PHYSICIAN ________ SIGNATURE OF CREW MEMBER IN CHARGE ________ COPY 1 HOSPITAL

**PATIENT CARE RECORD**

**VITAL SIGNS FLOW SHEET**
(record every five minutes if possible)

Patient Name_____ Age_____

| Time | Pulse | Respiration | Blood Pressure* | Skin (& oral temp. if avail.) | Level of Consciousness (circle one) |
|---|---|---|---|---|---|
| | ____rate/min reg./irreg. strong/weak | ____rate/min normal/labored | | pale/normal/red moist/dry cool/warm/hot Temp____°F | **Alert** (knows name, day, & place) **Verbal** (responds to commands) **Pain** (responds to pain) **Unresponsive** |
| | ____rate/min reg./irreg. strong/weak | ____rate/min normal/labored | | pale/normal/red moist/dry cool/warm/hot Temp____°F | **Alert** (knows name, day, & place) **Verbal** (responds to commands) **Pain** (responds to pain) **Unresponsive** |
| | ____rate/min reg./irreg. strong/weak | ____rate/min normal/labored | | pale/normal/red moist/dry cool/warm/hot Temp____°F | **Alert** (knows name, day, & place) **Verbal** (responds to commands) **Pain** (responds to pain) **Unresponsive** |
| | ____rate/min reg./irreg. strong/weak | ____rate/min normal/labored | | pale/normal/red moist/dry cool/warm/hot Temp____°F | **Alert** (knows name, day, & place) **Verbal** (responds to commands) **Pain** (responds to pain) **Unresponsive** |
| | ____rate/min reg./irreg. strong/weak | ____rate/min normal/labored | | pale/normal/red moist/dry cool/warm/hot Temp____°F | **Alert** (knows name, day, & place) **Verbal** (responds to commands) **Pain** (responds to pain) **Unresponsive** |

* if unavailable, record whether radial pulse present (presence indicates systolic is 80 or greater)

<u>**AMPLE:**</u>

Allergies:

Medications:

Prior medical problems:

Last meal:

Events leading to situation:

**Figure 8-13** Additional forms such as this example that provide room for more patient information may need to be filled out in addition to the incident report form. Courtesy of Dr. David Johe

Among the many different open-format PCRs or medical charts, those that use the SOAP and CHEATED methods are generally preferred by OEC Technicians due to their structured formats. SOAP is an acronym that represents four report components:

**S**—Subjective: Contains all nonobjective, qualitative information that the patient describes, including the chief complaint, the history of the present illness, and the past medical history

**O**—Objective: Contains all observable, quantitative findings that you discover during the scene size-up and physical exam

**A**—Assessment: Your general impression of what the medical problem is

**P**—Plan: Includes all aspects of treatment that has been rendered to the patient

⊕ 8-3  List the components for the following methods used to complete a PCR:
a. SOAP
b. CHEATED

The CHEATED acronym for medical documentation represents the primary components of the assessment and management process:

**C**—Chief complaint: The patient's primary problem

**H**—History: SAMPLE history of the present illness and past medical history

**E**—Examination: Physical exam

**A**—Assessment: General impression of patient

**T**—Treatment: All aspects of treatment rendered, including that provided by bystanders

**E**—Evaluation: Changes in the patient's condition over time; the patient's response to treatment

**D**—Disposition: Information indicating whether the patient refused treatment, was treated and released or was taken to a higher level of care such as a hospital.

Used properly, both methods are effective and enable OEC Technicians to document the patient encounter quickly and accurately. All pertinent patient medical information should be documented on the PCR form. Because PCRs may be subpoenaed into court, they must accurately reflect all aspects of the patient encounter. Being able to accomplish these tasks is an important part of an OEC Technician's duties and is a vital part of medically and legally managing an incident scene.

Remember: "If it isn't documented, it didn't happen." Therefore, make sure you take the time needed to fully document (including taking photographs or making diagrams if appropriate) all the medical facts associated with the incident, all the scene facts (day, time, and conditions) of the incident, the names of all the patrollers and witnesses involved in the incident, the statements of the patient, the mechanism of injury, vital signs, and anything else that will enable you to review the documents even years later and accurately reconstruct what happened at the incident.

It is also important to document the incident scene and take pictures of a serious incident scene *as soon as possible* to preserve an accurate record of events. Any delay in documenting important information can result in the loss of that information, because, for example, the wind might blow away skier's tracks. If accomplishing this task promptly requires more help, remember that one of the skills of OEC Technicians is to ask for and manage such help. Your area's risk manager is usually willing to provide help and support for this task.

**NOTE**

## Emergency Documentation

In most cases, if emergency care is not carefully documented in writing, then it is presumed that the emergency care was not given. An incomplete or sloppy report can suggest that the emergency care given was also sloppy.

### Characteristics of Good Report Writing

Well-written communication does not simply happen. It is the result of determined professionalism and attention to detail. Because both the patient care report and incident report form are considered medical and legal documents, you must exercise care when filling out these forms.

OEC Technicians should adhere to the characteristics of good report writing, which can be remembered using the mnemonic FACTUAL-OEC:

**8-4** List the characteristics of good report writing using the acronym FACTUAL-OEC.

**F**—Facts: Include only information that is true and can be documented.

**A**—Accurate: Describe what you saw, heard, and did accurately.

**C**—Complete: Include all relevant information regarding the incident and the patient.

**T**—Terms: Use only accepted medical terms and abbreviations.

**U**—Unbiased: Information should be objective; avoid personal opinions.

**A**—Avoid slang: Do not use informal words or words that have multiple meanings.

**L**—Legible/legal: All written reports should be written in clear, easy-to-read language, with black or blue ink.

**O**—Organized: The report should present information in a logical manner; this is especially important when using an open-format PCR.
**E**—Error free: Ensure that all words are spelled correctly and that proper grammar is used.
**C**—Checked: Proofread the document before submitting it.

### Correcting Errors and Creating Addendums

During the course of filling out reports and forms, it is only natural that OEC Technicians will occasionally make a written error that needs to be corrected. To correct a written mistake, draw a single line through the error. Never scratch out, erase, or otherwise obliterate the error because doing so can suggest that the OEC Technician is attempting to hide something. Next, write in the correct information, either above or next to the error. Finally, place your initials—and ideally, the current date and time—next to the error (Figure 8-14■). Corrected forms should be reviewed by your area's risk manager.

Given the complexities of emergency medicine, it is understandable that occasionally some important information may be overlooked or require correction. When you want or need to correct or add information to a previously submitted report or form, follow your local area's protocol in providing an addendum—a form that supplements information provided in the primary incident report form. A standard procedure is to complete and sign the addendum and then attach it to the original form. The addendum should be completed as soon as the need for additional information is identified because any delay in its submission reduces its credibility and potential usefulness. If an addendum is created at any time other than that of the incident, the date and time should be noted on the document. Ensure that you sign the addendum, and that your area's risk manager reviews it.

*Computer-Generated Forms* Many agencies and some ski areas now fill out and submit incident-related forms electronically (Figures 8-15a■ and 8-15b■). The use of electronic

**⊕ 8-5** Describe and demonstrate how to correct an error on a written report.

---

> ### Wilderness Tips
>
> In a wilderness environment in which radio communication is not available, you may need to use hand-written field notes and runners (individuals who will carry the notes between the senders and receivers) to transmit information. These notes will generally include information concerning both patient care, equipment necessary and your needs for evacuating the patient. Although they are often retained as part of the rescue documentation, they are not usually considered part of the patient's medical record.

**Figure 8-14** An example of how to correct a written mistake.

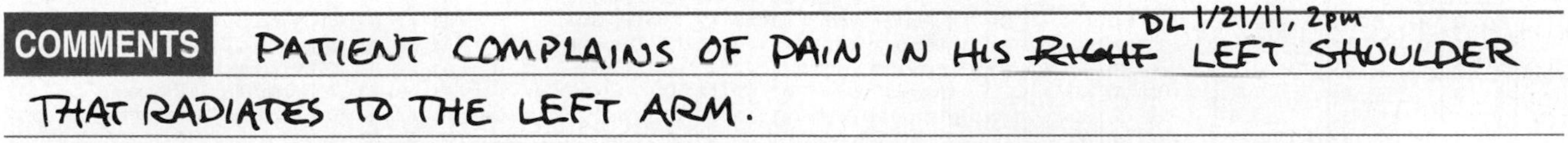

| COMMENTS | PATIENT COMPLAINS OF PAIN IN HIS ~~RIGHT~~ LEFT SHOULDER ^(DL 1/21/11, 2pm) THAT RADIATES TO THE LEFT ARM. |

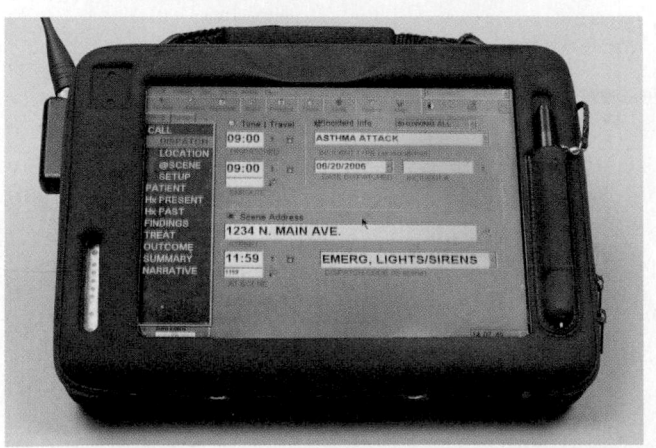

**Figure 8-15a** Some ski patrols use computers to input information concerning an incident such as this one at a ski area lodge.

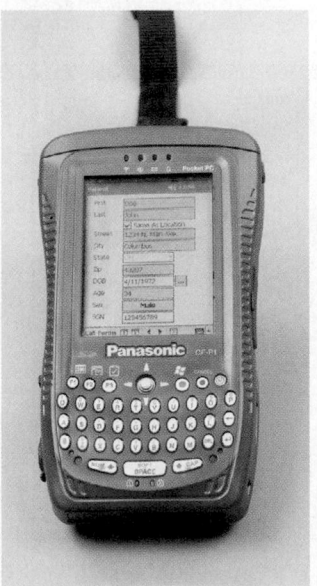

**Figure 8-15b** PDAs are also used by patrollers in some ski areas.

**Figure 8-16** An example of a computer-generated (scannable) incident report form.

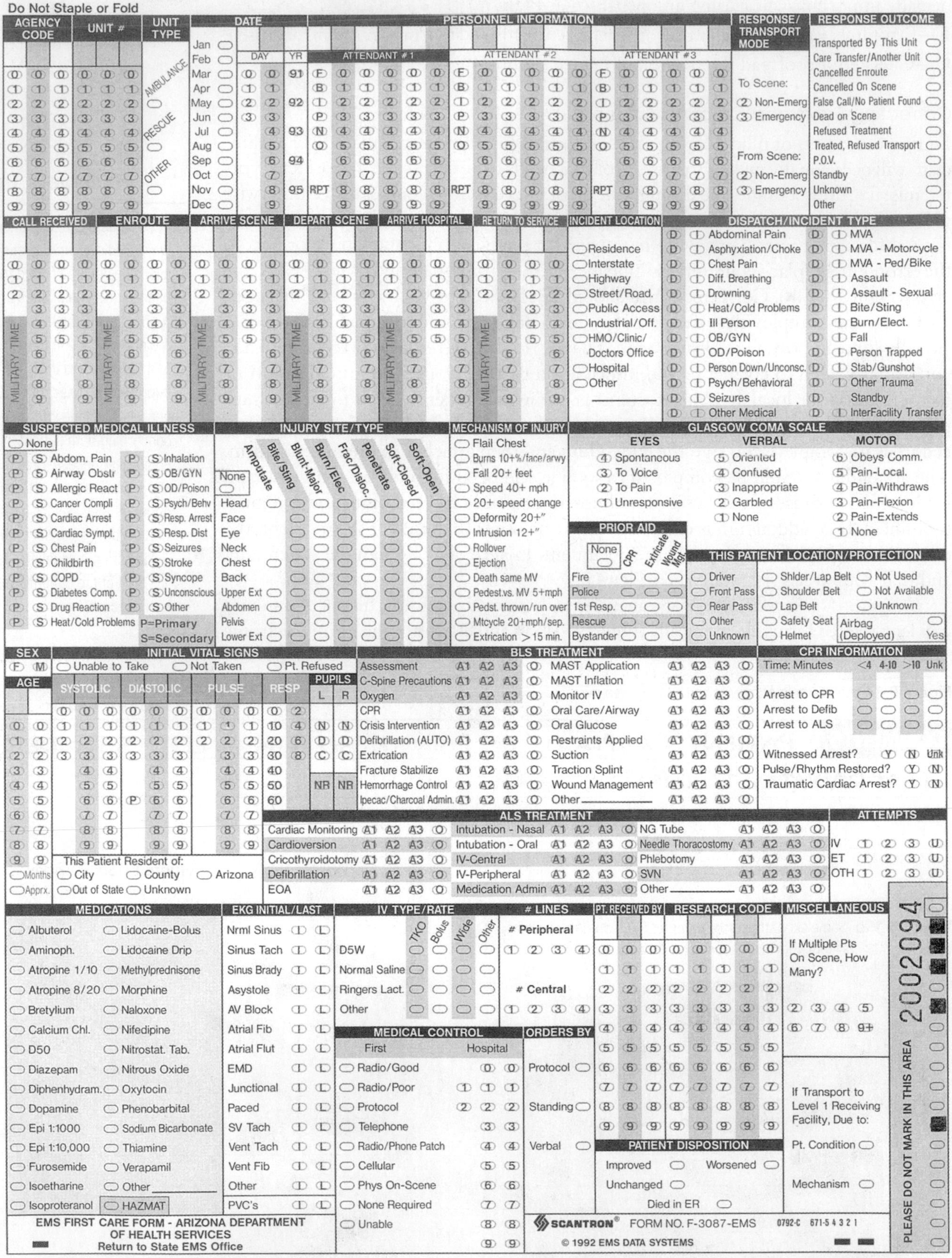

devices to prepare forms has the advantage of recording specific information needed to document any patient encounter in an easy-to-read format. However, these electronic devices often provide limited space to enter data, with the result that some critical data may not be included. Accordingly, OEC Technicians may need to supplement electronically prepared forms with additional written documentation. If the computer-generated form only allows you to list two patrollers but four patrollers were involved in the incident, or the form does not provide enough space to properly describe the events, treatment, or handling of the incident, then you will need to supplement the electronic form with a written list of the additional information needed.

There are advantages and disadvantages to using computer-scannable forms. These forms allow statistical information to be gathered (Figure 8-16■). OEC Technicians should appreciate the advantages while remaining mindful of the disadvantages in order to properly supplement such forms as the circumstances require.

# STOP, THINK, UNDERSTAND

## Multiple Choice
Choose the correct answer.

1. What are the two types of medical communication?_____
   a. verbal and nonverbal
   b. nonverbal and written
   c. verbal and written
   d. oral and nonoral

2. When a patient arrives at the first-aid station, you should provide a brief oral report called the_____
   a. pass-off report.
   b. hand-off report.
   c. tag-off report.
   d. trade-off report.

3. Which of the following is documentation that may be used as a medical-legal record? _____
   a. field care notes
   b. patient care reports (PCR)
   c. incident report forms
   d. all of the above

4. On what form would you most likely use the SOAP acronym?_____
   a. a patient care report (PCR)
   b. field care notes (FCR)

c. a hand-off report
d. a hand-off report and field care notes

5. An incident report form (IRF) is provided by the area's insurance carrier. What purpose does this form serve?_____
   a. It collects data concerning the patient and the circumstances surrounding the incident.
   b. It is designed to communicate medical information to other parties.
   c. It collects data regarding the circumstances surrounding the incident only.
   d. It collects data surrounding the incident, gathers patient data, and is used to communicate medical information to other parties.

## Short Answer

1. When you evaluate a patient, you collect information that includes what happened, clinical findings, the care the patient received, and the patient's response. How is this information used?
   _____
   _____.

2. What is the goal of communication?
   _____
   _____

3. List three forms of communication.
   a. _____
   b. _____
   c. _____

4. Define medical communication.
   _____
   _____

5. Use the SAILER acronym to communicate with the members of your patrol concerning the details of an incident involving a made-up patient.
   _____
   _____
   _____

# CASE UPDATE

Using your field care notes, you give an OEC Technician or the senior medical person on duty in the aid room or clinic an oral report about the patient. This report includes a complete description of your initial impressions of the patient, the nature of the patient's injury, the patient's level of responsiveness, results from the primary and secondary assessments, and the basic care you provided.

**What should you do now?**

## Essential Content of Medical Communications

When you communicate medical information to others, it is important that you provide an accurate "clinical picture," because the recipient of this communication rarely has prior knowledge of the circumstances surrounding the incident. Medical information should be presented clearly and succinctly in an organized manner, whether presented orally or in writing. Although medical communications and documents vary, the kinds of data contained within these communications are fairly standard (Table 8-2■). Understanding what data are required will enable you to document and communicate vital patient data more clearly and completely.

### Age and Gender

Human anatomy and physiology changes with age and differs slightly by gender. Because of this, it is important to report the patient's gender and actual or approximate age. These data allow health care providers to begin developing a "mental picture" of the patient.

### Chief Complaint

The chief complaint is what the patient tells you is wrong and should, whenever possible, be recorded in the patient's own words. The patient may give you a specific complaint ("my chest hurts"), may tell you what happened ("I ran into a tree"), or may tell you what he thinks is wrong ("I broke my ribs"). Unless the patient provides a specific complaint, ask questions to identify which body system(s) may be affected. For example, if the patient tells you "I ran into a tree," you might ask "Are you hurt?" to elicit a response such as, "My chest hurts, and I'm having trouble breathing," which indicates possible involvement of the musculoskeletal, cardiovascular, and respiratory systems.

### History of Present Illness

**history of present
illness** a description of the
circumstances surrounding the events of
an incident; includes all subjective
descriptions presented by the patient
(or a bystander, if the patient cannot
tell you).

The **history of present illness** (HPI) should provide a description of the circumstances surrounding the events of the incident and include all subjective descriptions presented by the patient. For an illness, this may be a description of the symptoms the

| Table 8-2 | Essential Medical Communications |
| --- | --- |
| Age and gender | Physical exam |
| Chief complaint | Impression |
| History of present illness | Treatment |
| Past medical history | Response to treatment |

patient experienced just before requesting help. For trauma, it may be a description of the incident that led to the injury. The HPI should include the "S," "L," and "E" portions of the SAMPLE history as well as an "OPQRST" assessment of the complaint, as discussed in Chapter 7, Patient Assessment. Include a review of any medical history that is relevant to the chief complaint. For example, for a patient with a chief complaint of "trouble breathing," the HPI should include "the patient has a history of asthma." The HPI should not include any physical findings; thus, it should not include a statement such as "the patient has a history of asthma and is wheezing" because "wheezing" is a physical finding.

### Past Medical History

The past medical history includes the "A," "M," and "P" portions of the SAMPLE history. Of these, only medical history and medications relevant to the chief complaint should be reported in an oral report given over the radio, whereas the entire past medical history should be presented during an oral hand-off or a written report.

### Physical Exam

The physical exam includes all the objective findings obtained during the primary and secondary assessments. These findings include both the level of responsiveness and all vital signs, although these data are usually recorded in separate sections of the PCR.

### Impression

An impression is what you think the medical problem is based on the subjective and objective information that you gathered during the scene size-up and patient assessment. Even though an impression is not a "diagnosis," you should formulate a medical impression because this information may be used to make treatment decisions. An example of a medical impression is "possible thoracic spine injury."

### Treatment

The treatment is a description of everything you've done in caring for the patient. It may include nothing more than "transported in the position of comfort," or it may include the various treatments provided during a full resuscitation. If you administered oxygen, applied a splint, or immobilized the spine, report those actions in the treatment section. Be sure to document what happened to the patient—also known as the disposition—after the patient was released from your care. Examples of the disposition include transferred to EMS, transported by family members, released on his own recognizance, or refused medical treatment.

### Response to Treatment

One of the most frequently overlooked aspects of medical communications is describing how the patient responded to the treatment rendered. High-quality treatment dictates that after you've done something for a patient, you monitor the patient's response. Make sure you report whether the patient got better, got worse, or stayed the same, and, if necessary, indicate whether any further interventions were needed and the subsequent response to them. For example, if you took care of a patient in respiratory distress who improved with treatment, you might state on your report that "the airway was opened using a head-tilt, chin-lift, and the patient developed spontaneous respirations at 12 breaths per minute with some snoring. A nasal airway was placed and the snoring stopped. Oxygen was applied at 15 liters per minute via non-rebreather mask, and distal cyanosis diminished."

Other important information that should be included, especially on the PCR, are the date and time of the incident and the location where the incident occurred, the latter of which might include GPS coordinates.

To illustrate how the essential components might be presented in a hand-off report, consider the following:

> "This is John. He is 45 years old and ran into a large rock at moderate speed. His friends state that John never lost consciousness and was responsive. Upon my arrival, the patient was A on the AVPU scale and complaining of mid-thoracic back pain. He has tenderness along his upper thoracic spine. There is no other obvious trauma, and he denies drinking any alcohol today. He has a history of high blood pressure and is compliant with his antihypertensive medication. Vitals are stable. He has no movement or sensation below the waist. I believe John may have a spinal injury, so we fully immobilized his neck and spine and provided oxygen at 15 liters per minute by nonrebreather mask. Do you have any questions?"

### Special Circumstances

As part of your duties as an OEC Technician, you will likely encounter special circumstances that require you to provide additional information. Among the most common incidents that require additional documentation or communications are the following:

+ A person who refuses medical care
+ Incidents that must be reported to authorities
+ Incident investigations

As described in Chapter 1, any patient who is 18 years of age or older has the legal right to refuse medical care so long as three criteria are met:

1. The person has the capacity to understand the nature of the medical problem.
2. The person understands the ramifications of refusing medical care.
3. The person is allowed by law to make their own decisions regarding their medical care.

**capacity** indicates the patient has normal decision-making abilities and whose judgment is not impaired.

The medical term **capacity**—is distinct from "competence"—indicates that a patient has normal decision-making abilities and judgment that is not impaired. Factors that can impair judgment include alcohol, certain prescription medications, illicit drugs, low blood sugar, head injury, hypoxia, and shock. A patient with demonstrated capacity may refuse any or all medical care. Likewise, a parent may refuse to allow care for his or her child, as can a legal guardian refuse care for a ward.

If the patient or guardian is refusing what you believe is necessary medical care, complete documentation of the refusal for care is critical. It is best to have a standardized form on which to document the refusal of medical assistance (Figure 8-17■). Your area or agency might provide you with such a form, also known as an A.M.A. or "against medical advice" form. Even if you do not have a standardized form, you must still completely document the refusal and obtain all appropriate signatures. The most important item to document is that the patient either understood the risks of refusal and accepted those risks, or refused to listen while you identified the risks.

⊕ **8-6** List two criteria that must be documented on a patient refusal.

Remember, in circumstances in which emergency care is being refused, ask another OEC Technician to witness the refusal, and then clearly indicate on the form the circumstances surrounding the refusal of care, including the name of your fellow patroller who also witnessed the refusal of care. Such refusals are serious events that may need to be reported to your area's risk manager pursuant to local area protocols.

If the patient refuses to sign the refuse treatment form, document this refusal as well and obtain the signature of a witness, preferably another OEC Technician who

GUIDELINES

## REFUSAL INFORMATION SHEET

**PLEASE READ AND KEEP THIS FORM!**

This form has been given to you because you have refused treatment and/or transport by the XYZ Mt. Ski Patrol. Your health and safety are our primary concern, so even though you have decided not to accept our advice, please remember the following:

1) The evaluation and/or treatment provided to you by the OEC Technician is not a substitute for medical evaluation and treatment by a doctor. We advise you to get medical evaluation and treatment.

2) Your condition may not seem as bad to you as it actually is. Without treatment, your condition or problem could become worse. If you are planning to get medical treatment, a decision to refuse treatment or transport by our OEC Technicians may result in a delay which could make your condition or problem worse.

3) Medical evaluation and/or treatment may be obtained by calling your doctor, if you have one, or by going to any hospital Emergency Department in this area, all of which are staffed 24 hours a day by Emergency Physicians. You may be seen at these Emergency Departments without an appointment.

4) If you change your mind or your condition becomes worse and you decide to accept treatment and transport by our OEC Technicians, please do not hesitate to contact us. We will do our best to help you.

5) DON'T WAIT! When medical treatment is needed, it is usually better to get it right away.

I have received a copy of this information sheet.

PATIENT SIGNATURE: _____ DATE: _____

WITNESS SIGNATURE: _____ DATE: _____

AGENCY INCIDENT #: _____ AGENCY CODE: _____

NAME OF PERSON FILLING OUT FORM: _____

G 11A

**Figure 8-17** Whenever a patient refuses treatment, it is crucial that a refusal form be filled out and signed.

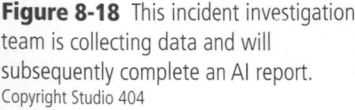

**8-7** List four injuries or crimes that a mandated reporter must report to authorities.

**mandated reporter** an individual (such as a social worker, physician, teacher, police, EMT, or counselor) who is required to report to the appropriate authorities certain types of injuries or the suspicion of specific crimes.

directly observed the patient's refusal. For more information about patient refusals, OEC Technicians should review the medical-legal material presented in Chapter 1.

In some states or provinces, patrollers and other OEC Technicians may be required to report certain types of injuries or the suspicion of specific crimes. To determine if you are such a **mandated reporter**, check with your area management and your state/provincial EMS laws and regulations. Among the conditions that may require reporting are the following:

+ Abuse (physical, sexual, of children, of the elderly)
+ Assault (physical, sexual)
+ Domestic violence
+ Gunshot wounds
+ Stab wounds
+ Animal bites
+ Communicable diseases (e.g., tuberculosis)
+ Any incident resulting in death (check with management)

Finally, your ski or recreational area may have an accident investigation (AI) team (Figure 8-18■). If it does, local protocols will dictate when and how this team is activated. The assistance of such a team is recommended for any serious incident. At many resorts, an AI team must be summoned to any incident involving a life-threatening condition, a death, or an accident in which liability is suspected. An AI team also may be required to respond to a lift-related accident or to an injury involving a motorized vehicle or other manmade object.

You may be requested to furnish AI team members with such things as maps, photos, witness statements, accident reports, PCRs, and other information, or you may be asked to assist the team in gathering these data. You may be asked to help the team complete other forms. Cooperate and assist the team as directed by your area management.

If you have questions regarding your role during an accident investigation, contact your area management or local patrol representative. Remember, in the event of a serious accident that utilizes many OEC Technicians, you have a duty to manage the OEC Technician coverage for the area while you are involved in handling the serious accident. It may be wise to call other OEC Technicians and patrollers into the area to provide additional support and coverage. Once again, this is part of the skill and judgment required of OEC Technicians when managing an accident scene.

**Figure 8-18** This incident investigation team is collecting data and will subsequently complete an AI report. Copyright Studio 404

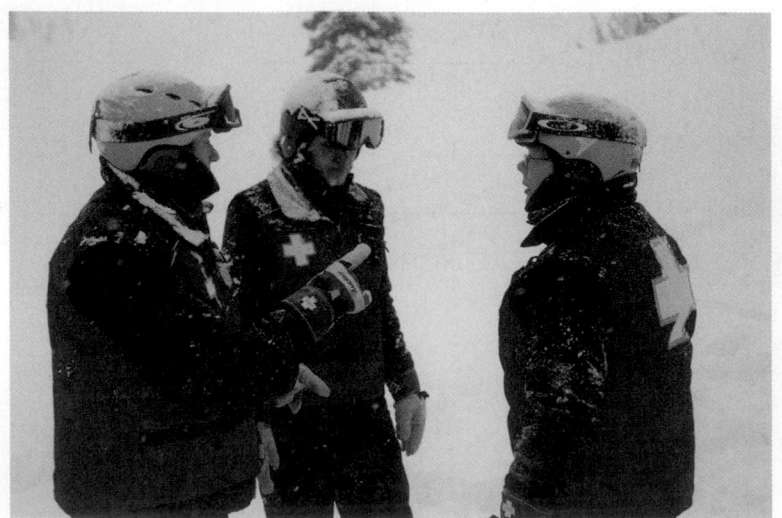

# CASE DISPOSITION

You begin writing a patient care report to document the case using the SOAP format. EMS arrives just after you have completed the report. You give the ambulance crew an oral hand-off report and a copy of your patient care report. You also complete an incident report form and place both documents into the patrol record box. You later discover that the patient was admitted to the hospital with a spinal fracture. The medical director identified the case as an excellent example of good documentation and asked the educational team to include the material anonymously in the next refresher cycle.

# Chapter Review

## Chapter Summary

The role of OEC Technicians is complex and goes well beyond simply providing high-quality emergency care to sick or injured patients in outdoor settings. It includes the ability to obtain and record essential medical information quickly and accurately and to effectively transmit these data to others. In addition, OEC Technicians should work with their risk manager to properly document the patient encounter.

Given their importance and daily use, medical communication and proper documentation are among the most important skills that OEC Technicians must master. To be effective, oral communication must be clear, concise, and accurate. Likewise, all written documentation must follow this basic tenet while documenting the patient encounter completely and objectively. As part of this process, OEC Technicians must be proficient in doc-

umenting special circumstances such as patient care refusals, and in knowing which injuries or suspected crimes must be reported to area management. OEC Technicians also must know how to correct written errors and how to properly submit additional information gathered after the fact.

Management will determine what information needs to be documented and what form should be used. Additionally, extra documentation using a PCR may be needed for certain patients.

By learning all these tasks and by applying strategies that facilitate effective medical communications, OEC Technicians will help to ensure the continuity of care that is a crucial aspect of an effective emergency care system while also reducing the legal risks to themselves and to the area.

## Remember...

1. Effective medical communications is one of the hallmarks of a highly skilled OEC Technician.
2. Careful documentation is important both for medical and legal reasons.
3. Medical communications include oral communication and written documentation.
4. Breakdowns in the communication process can create misunderstandings and errors.
5. An oral hand-off report should take less than 60 seconds to complete.
6. Patients who refuse medical assistance must have the capacity to do so.
7. Thoroughly document all patient refusals.
8. If it isn't documented, it didn't happen; document reports completely and accurately.
9. Write good reports by being a FACTUAL OEC Technician.

# Chapter Questions

## Multiple Choice

Choose the correct answer.

1. Rather than rewriting the whole report when an error is made, what is the best method for correcting errors on the report?_____
   a. Erase the error; then write the correct information and initial the change.
   b. Scratch the error out; then write the correct information and initial the change.
   c. Use Wite-Out to correct the mistake; then write the correct information and initial the change.
   d. Draw a single line through the error; then write the correct information, initial and date the change.

2. What is the best possible way to add information to a form that has already been submitted?_____
   a. Submit the additional information as an addendum to the report.
   b. Ask for the report back so you can add to it.
   c. It is impossible to add information; once a report is submitted you cannot gain access to it.
   d. Write the additional information on the copy of the form you kept for your records and resubmit form.

3. What is the prevailing maxim for medical-legal documentation?_____
   a. "If I wrote it, it will never be questioned."
   b. "All things were considered, even if they weren't written down."
   c. "If it isn't documented, it didn't happen."
   d. "If it isn't documented, it wasn't considered."

4. Which of the following situations is *not* a special case that would require you to complete extra documentation or provide additional communications?_____
   a. a person who refuses medical care
   b. accident investigations
   c. a diabetic whose blood sugars were abnormal
   d. incidents that must be reported to authorities

5. What is a patient care report (PCR) used for?_____
   a. To collect information regarding the circumstances surrounding an incident.
   b. To serve as an insurance report and risk-management tool.
   c. To record specific information regarding medical care for the patient.
   d. For taking notes during a rescue operation.

6. Written communications may be used for all of the following purposes except?_____
   a. to convey information to dispatchers.
   b. for research.
   c. for documenting trends.
   d. for validating insurance claims.

7. What purpose does the incident report form (IRF) serve?_____
   a. To record specific information regarding medical care given to a patient.
   b. To communicate medical information to other parties.
   c. To collect data regarding the circumstances surrounding the incident.
   d. To collect data concerning the incident, to gather patient data, and to communicate medical information to other parties.

## Short Answer

**1.** Most radio protocols do not include mentioning the patient's name. Why?

_____

_____

_____

**2.** List four groups of individuals (not including OEC Technicians) that may use medical communications.

**a.** _____

**b.** _____

**c.** _____

**d.** _____

## Fill in the Blank

In the following columns of blanks, write the listed words that complete the FACTUAL-OEC, SAILER, CHEATED, and SOAP acronyms. (words may be used more than once)

Sex of patient, Plan, History, Accurate, Error free, Subjective, Disposition, Age of patient, Unbiased, Facts, Resources needed, Objective, Avoid slang, Location of incident, Organized, Chief Complaint, Assessment, Incident chief complaint, Treatment, Legible/legal, Equipment needed, Terms, Examination, Evaluation, Complete, Checked.

| FACTUAL_OEC | SAILER | CHEATED | SOAP |
|---|---|---|---|
| _____ | _____ | _____ | _____ |
| _____ | _____ | _____ | _____ |
| _____ | _____ | _____ | _____ |
| _____ | _____ | _____ | _____ |

## Scenario

*You are dispatched to a black diamond trail to aid a skier who struck a tree. Upon arriving on the scene you do a quick scene size-up, secure the scene by placing the injured skier's skis in an "X" position, and take Standard Precautions.*

*You make a radio call to dispatch to acknowledge that you are "on scene" and that only one patient appears to be involved. You request base to stand by for additional information. Base acknowledges your message and repeats that base is standing by for additional information.*

**1.** Which of the following pieces of information will the dispatcher *not* need?_____

    **a.** your exact location

    **b.** the weight of the patient

    **c.** the age and sex of the patient

    **d.** the resources you need to attend to the situation

*After performing a primary assessment, you find that the 30-year-old patient has a patent airway, is alert, and is oriented according to person, place, date, and time (AAO x 4). The patient's chief complaint is pain in the right femur, which is deformed. You observe no external bleeding.*

*You make a radio request to dispatch for a toboggan, a backboard, oxygen, and an ALS or paramedic ambulance.*

*Additional patrollers arrive with the toboggan. The patient is packaged with a traction splint and transferred to a long board and then into the toboggan. Using a field note pad, you write down the patient's information, patient findings, vitals and time measured, the treatment begun, SAMPLE answers, and so on. You will pass a copy of this information to the paramedic team for use as baseline data.*

**2.** After the patient is packaged and securely placed in the toboggan, injury uphill, the OEC Technician should_____

    **a.** call dispatch and notify them of the transport and approximate time until arrival at base.

    **b.** try to reach the paramedic unit to give them updated information.

    **c.** call medical control via a cell phone and advise them of the injury.

    **d.** notify the hospital that the patient is coming.

*The patient arrives at the treatment room, and the ambulance is 10 minutes out. You pass the incident information from your field care notes to the base technicians. You complete the patient care report before you return to the top shack.*

**3.** Using the CHEATED format of report writing, what would be listed for "T"?_____

    **a.** patient has a metered-dose inhaler

    **b.** traction splint applied, $O_2$ applied, and full c-spine protection provided

    **c.** deformity noted on the right femur area with no external bleeding

    **d.** asthma and allergy to peanuts

*The next day you realize that the patient care report had incorrect information concerning the side of the injury. You had written "left femur" instead of "right femur."*

**4.** What action should you take?_____

    **a.** Correct the report by putting Wite-Out on "left" and inserting "right."

    **b.** Cross out the mistake with one straight line, initial and date the change, and write "right" above the crossed-out mistake.

    **c.** Rewrite the entire report correcting the error.

    **d.** Create an addendum stating what the error was and the correction needed.

*Treatment provided to this patient with a femur injury should be detailed in the narrative.*

**5.** In addition to outlining the treatment, you should not_____

    **a.** list the marital status of the patient.

    **c.** list all the treatments in chronological order.

    **b.** list the patient's response to the treatment.

    **d.** list the name(s) of the individuals providing the treatment.

## Suggested Reading

Joyce, S. M., K. L. Dutkowski, and T. Haynes. 1997. "Efficacy of an EMS quality improvement program in improving documentation and performance." *Prehospital Emergency Care* 1: 140–144.

Teich, J. M., and W. H. Cordell. 2006. "Chapter 202: Information Technology in Emergency Medicine." In *Rosen's Emergency Medicine: Concepts and Clinical Practice*, Sixth Edition, edited by J. Marx. Philadelphia: Mosby.

Weaver, J., K. H. Binsfield, and D. Dalphond. 2009X. "Prehospital refusal-of-transport policies: Adequate legal protection?" *Prehospital Emergency Care* 4: 53–56.

 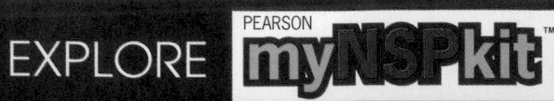

# Airway Management

Scott McIntosh, MD, MPH

## ⊕ OBJECTIVES

**Upon completion of this chapter, the OEC Technician will be able to:**

**9-1** List the major anatomical structures of the upper airway.

**9-2** Describe and demonstrate how to manually open the airway or mouth using the following techniques:

a. Head-tilt, chin-lift
b. Jaw thrust
c. Crossed finger

**9-3** Describe how to clear a patient's airway using the following methods:

a. Gravity
b. Finger sweep
c. Suction

**9-4** Describe how to place a patient into the recovery position.

**9-5** Compare, contrast, and demonstrate the usage of a rigid suction catheter and a flexible suction catheter.

**9-6** List the indications of and uses for the following airway adjuncts, and demonstrate the proper methods for choosing the correct size and inserting them:

a. Oropharyngeal airway
b. Nasopharyngeal airway

**9-7** Describe how to calculate the oxygen flow duration rate.

**9-8** Describe and demonstrate how to properly set up an oxygen tank for use.

**9-9** List four tips for the safe use of oxygen.

*continued*

## Chapter Overview

Having an open **airway** and adequate respiration is the most important factor for preserving homeostasis because every cell in the body depends on a constant supply of oxygen. This is why assessment of the airway and breathing is first in a primary assessment. Under normal conditions, the airway is open and clear, which permits the free and constant exchange of gas between the environment and the lungs.

*continued*

## HISTORICAL TIMELINE

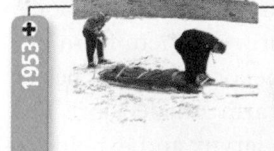

**1953** NSP incorporated in Colorado.

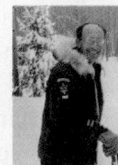

**1956** William R. Judd becomes first elected National Director of NSP.

**9-10** Describe and demonstrate how to use the following oxygen delivery, ventilation, and barrier devices:

a. Nasal cannula
b. Nonrebreather mask
c. Pocket mask

d. Bag-valve mask
e. Face shield

## ⊕ KEY TERMS

adjunct, *p. 300*
airway, *p. 291*
bag-valve mask (BVM), *p. 313*
epiglottis, *p. 292*
exhalation, *p. 294*
gastric distention, *p. 315*

head-tilt, chin-lift maneuver, *p. 295*
inhalation, *p. 294*
jaw-thrust maneuver, *p. 295*
nasal cannula (NC), *p. 311*
nasopharyngeal airway (NPA), *p. 300*
nonrebreather mask (NRB), *p. 312*

oropharyngeal airway (OPA), *p. 302*
pharynx, *p. 292*
pocket mask, *p. 305*
pulse oximeter, *p. 315*
suctioning, *p. 298*

---

**airway**   a natural passageway that allows air to enter and exit the lungs.

---

⊕ **9-1**   List the major anatomical structures of the upper airway.

**pharynx**   the passageway that extends from the nose and mouth to the larynx; consists of three parts: nasopharynx, oropharynx, and laryngopharynx.

**epiglottis**   a thin, leaf-shaped structure posterior to the tongue; covers the larynx when swallowing, preventing food or liquid from entering the airway.

**Figure 9-1** OEC Technicians are trained to provide medical care to patients in remote outdoor settings.
Copyright Scott Smith

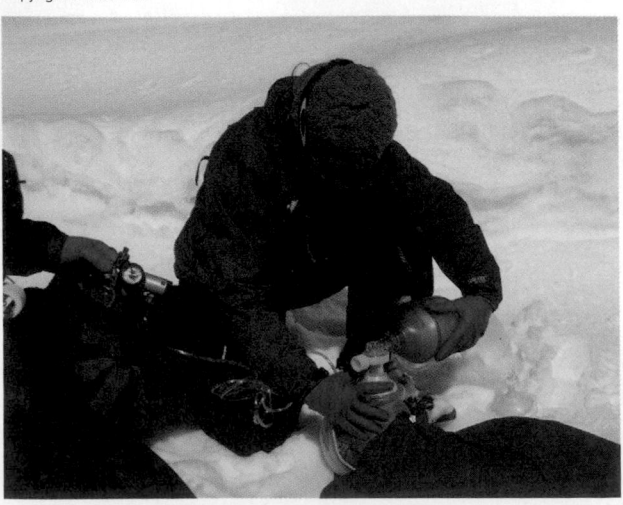

The human body is susceptible to a variety of physical, medical, and traumatic conditions that can adversely affect the breathing process. When problems occur, they must be managed quickly and effectively in order to restore respiration, because without a continuous source of oxygen, death occurs rapidly.

As members of the emergency care system, OEC Technicians are specifically trained to provide medical care to patients under austere conditions in remote outdoor settings (Figure 9-1■). Because OEC Technicians typically arrive at a patient's side well before other care providers, they must be able to assess a patient's airway quickly and immediately correct any problems that are discovered. As part of this process, technicians must be prepared to open, clear, and maintain the airway using a variety of methods. Technicians also must be able to deliver supplemental oxygen whenever it is indicated and stand ready to provide artificial ventilations if either spontaneous respirations are not observed or the patient's breathing efforts are ineffective. Each of these skills, fundamental to the OEC curriculum, can be life saving, and therefore we must become proficient in them.

An understanding of the principles and practices of airway management is crucial to an OEC Technician's ability to apply this information effectively in an emergency situation. Oxygen administration, airway maintenance, and ventilation assistance are essential skills that every OEC Technician must master.

## Anatomy and Physiology

The airway is divided into upper and lower components. The upper airway begins at the mouth and nose and ends at the larynx (Figure 9-2■). In between are the **pharynx** and **epiglottis**. The pharynx is subdivided into three parts: the nasopharynx, oropharynx, and the laryngopharynx. The nasopharynx, better known as the nasal cavity, warms and humidifies air as it enters the body. The hairs in it remove small particles to prevent them from entering the trachea and lower airway. The oropharynx, better known as the oral cavity, also helps to warm inhaled air. The laryngopharynx lies below and behind the larynx and extends to the esophagus.

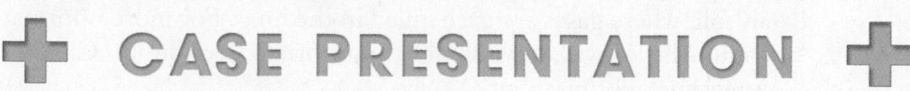

# ✚ CASE PRESENTATION ✚

You are called to the scene of an accident, where you find a middle-aged ice climber who is unresponsive to painful stimuli and has shallow respirations. He reportedly fell approximately 20 feet, striking his head and neck on a rocky outcrop. You note minor bleeding coming from the patient's mouth as well as a deep cut on his chin. His pulse is rapid at 108/minute. The climber's head and neck appear "crooked," and his left arm appears bent at an unnatural angle.

*What should you do?*

The epiglottis is a leaflike structure that directs air into the trachea and lungs and prevents food or liquids from entering the lower airway. Below the epiglottis is the larynx, or voice box, where sound originates when we speak.

The lower airway includes the trachea, bronchi, and alveoli (Figure 9-3■). The trachea is a tube, made in part of cartilage that ends at the two main stem bronchi, each of which extends into one lung. These bronchi continue as smaller bronchi,

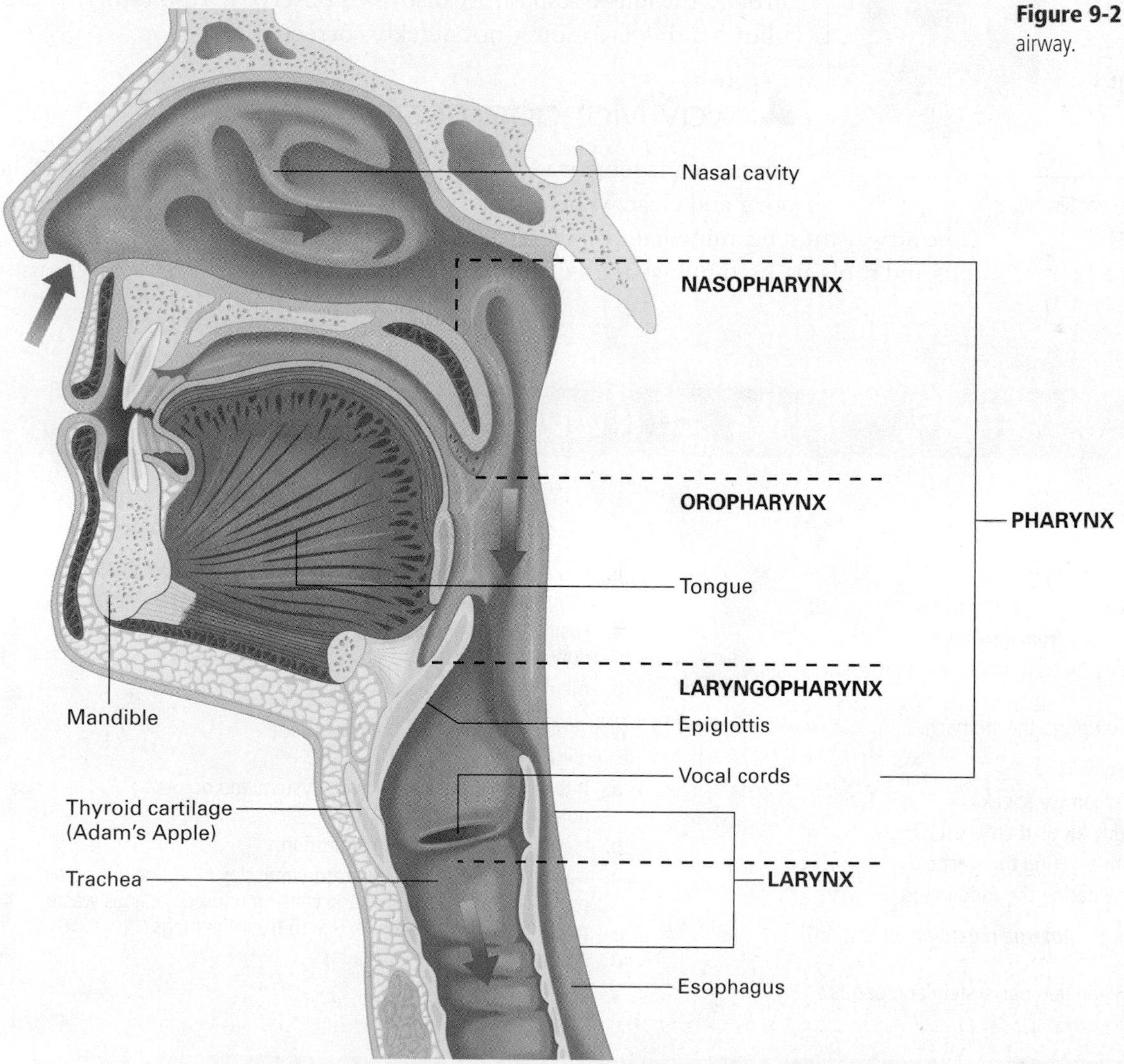

**Figure 9-2** Anatomy of the upper airway.

Nasal cavity

**NASOPHARYNX**

**OROPHARYNX**

**PHARYNX**

Tongue

**LARYNGOPHARYNX**

Mandible

Epiglottis

Vocal cords

Thyroid cartilage
(Adam's Apple)

**LARYNX**

Trachea

Esophagus

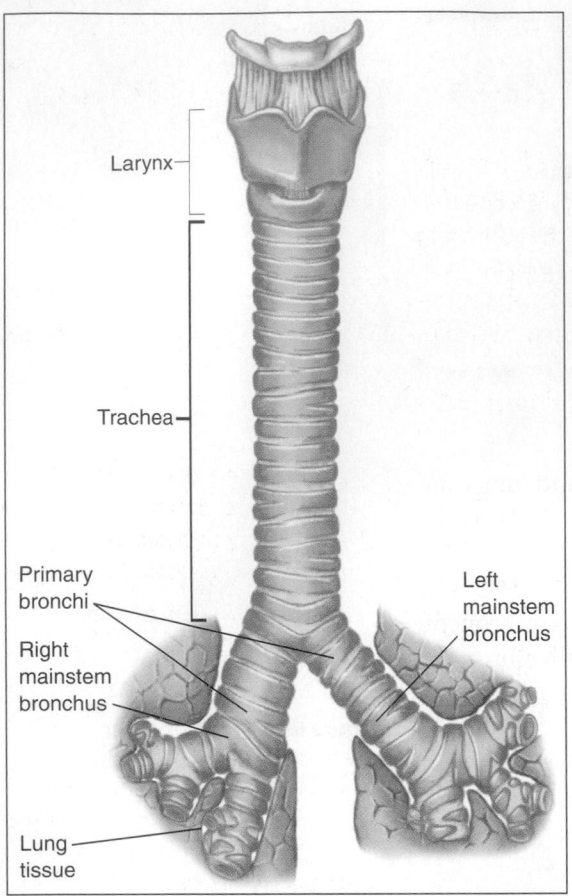

**Figure 9-3** Anatomy of the lower airway.

Labels: Larynx, Trachea, Primary bronchi, Right mainstem bronchus, Left mainstem bronchus, Lung tissue

eventually branching into many smaller bronchioles and end in the alveoli, where gases are exchanged in the lung. For more information about the airway, review the appropriate section in Chapter 6, Anatomy and Physiology.

Respiration, or breathing, is a biological process in which air enters the body and then is expelled back into the environment. Oxygen in the air enters the lungs, and carbon dioxide, a waste product, leaves the lungs. The conduit through which gas enters and exits the lungs is the airway. Breathing is a mechanical process, both active and passive in nature, consisting of two phases: **inhalation** and **exhalation**. Both phases are controlled by the nervous system and occur automatically.

Inhalation, also known as inspiration, is an active process during which the respiratory muscles contract, creating negative internal pressure in the chest cavity thereby causing air to flow inward. Exhalation, or expiration, is the passive phase of respiration. During this phase, the respiratory muscles relax, increasing pressure within the chest, thereby expelling any unused air and gaseous waste products from the lungs and out of the body. For more detailed information about the mechanics of breathing, refer again to Chapter 6.

If breathing is compromised and oxygen cannot get into the blood through the lungs, respiratory distress is observed. Respiratory failure follows if this situation is not quickly corrected.

## Airway Management

Airway management is the physical process that ensures the airway is open and clear. When the airway is closed, respiration cannot occur. The airway must be immediately opened to prevent injury or death. Numerous methods and tools are used to manage a partially or completely occluded airway. By learn-

# STOP, THINK, UNDERSTAND

## Multiple Choice

Choose the correct answer.

1. The purpose of the nasopharynx is to _____
   a. prevent food from entering the trachea.
   b. remove noxious gases from inhaled air.
   c. warm and humidify air as it enters the body and to remove small particles.
   d. prevent air from entering the stomach.

2. The purpose of the larynx is to _____
   a. generate sound when we speak.
   b. warm and humidify air as it enters the body.
   c. prevent food from entering the trachea.
   d. prevent air from entering the esophagus.

3. Which of the following is *not* true regarding inhalation? _____
   a. It is controlled by the nervous system and occurs automatically.
   b. It is an active process during which respiratory muscles contract.
   c. Positive internal pressure in the chest cavity permits air to flow inward.
   d. All of the above are correct.

4. Which of the following is *not* true about expiration? _____
   a. It is controlled by the nervous system and occurs automatically.
   b. It is the active phase of respiration.
   c. During this phase the respiratory muscles relax, increasing air pressure within the chest and causing unused gaseous waste products to be removed (exhaled) from the lungs.
   d. All of the above are true.

ing the principles of airway management and becoming proficient in each skill, OEC Technicians will greatly improve their patients' chances for survival.

## Opening the Airway and Mouth

Normal breathing requires that the airway be intact, open and clear. In addition, the structures that constitute the upper airway must be properly aligned to allow the free flow of air into and out of the lungs. In an unresponsive patient, the airway muscles may relax, and in certain body positions this may cause the tongue to fall back and occlude the airway (Figure 9-4■). When a patient's head is unnaturally flexed, hyperextended, or tilted acutely to one side, the airway may become compressed or blocked. The first step in effective airway management is to ensure that the airway is open and aligned. The two primary methods used by OEC Technicians to align and open a patient's airway are the head-tilt, chin-lift and the jaw-thrust maneuvers.

### Head-Tilt, Chin-Lift

The **head-tilt, chin-lift** method is the primary technique OEC Technicians use to open a patient's airway. Because this procedure manipulates the neck, it should be used only on patients who have no possibility of head, neck, or spine trauma. To perform the head-tilt, chin-lift procedure, take the following steps (Figures 9-5a–d■):

1. Kneel beside the patient's head.
2. Place one hand on the patient's forehead.
3. Place two or three fingers of your other hand under the patient's chin.
4. Gently pull the chin up while simultaneously pushing down on the forehead. Do not compress the soft tissue under the chin.
5. Maintain the position to ensure that the airway remains open.

### Jaw-Thrust

If the patient has sustained head, neck, or spine trauma or there is even a *concern* about a potential cervical spine injury, open the airway using the **jaw-thrust maneuver** (Figure 9-6■). This method opens the airway while allowing only minimal movement of the cervical spine. When performing a jaw thrust, it is essential that the neck

**inhalation**   act of drawing breath or air into the lungs.

**exhalation**   the act of expelling breath or air out of the lungs.

⊕ **9-2**   Describe and demonstrate how to manually open the airway or mouth using the following techniques:

   **a.** Head-tilt, chin-lift

   **b.** Jaw thrust

   **c.** Crossed finger

**head-tilt, chin-lift maneuver** a method to open a patient's airway; a process that involves tilting the patient's head backward while simultaneously lifting the patient's chin.

**jaw-thrust maneuver**   a method used to open a patient's airway by displacing the jaw forward; commonly used whenever spine injury is suspected because it helps to maintain cervical spine alignment.

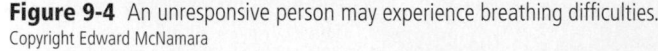

**Figure 9-4** An unresponsive person may experience breathing difficulties.
Copyright Edward McNamara

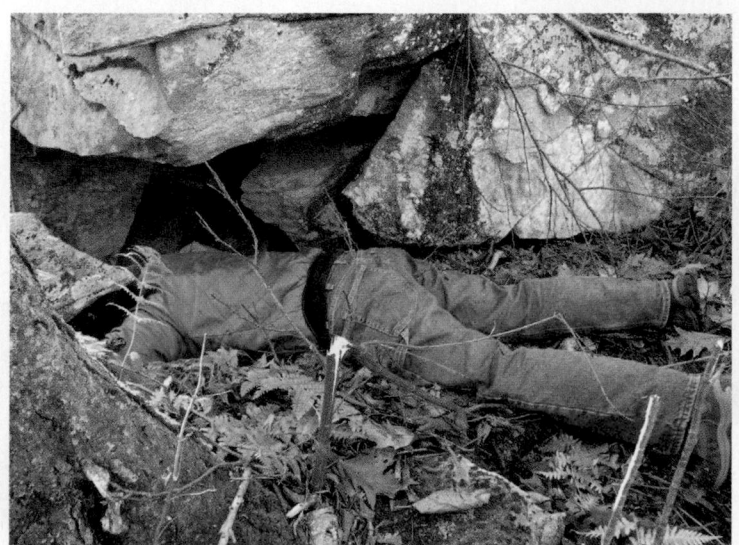

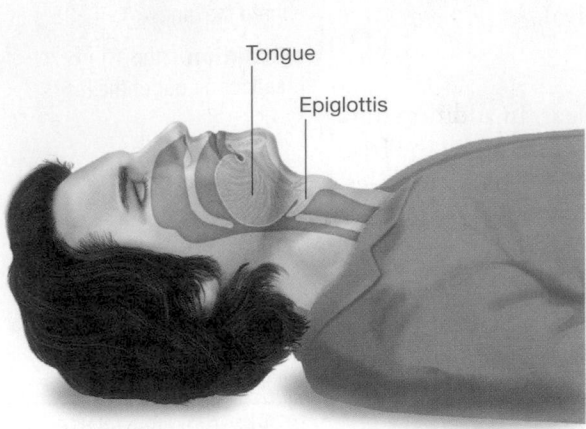

Tongue

Epiglottis

**Figure 9-5a** Anatomy of the adult in a neutral position.

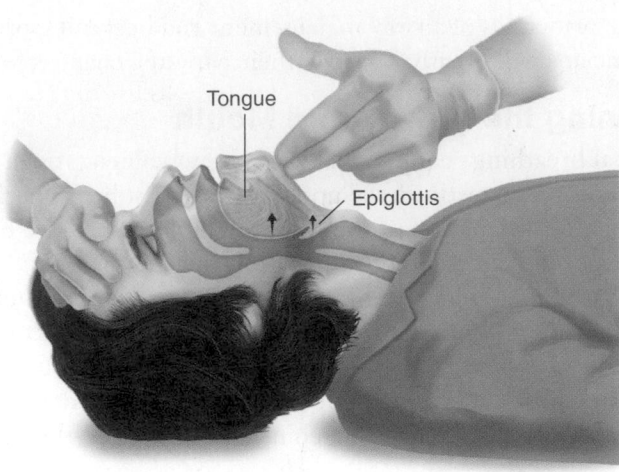

Tongue

Epiglottis

**Figure 9-5b** The head-tilt, chin-lift position; note the open airway.

**Figure 9-5c** The neutral starting position for the head-tilt, chin-lift maneuver in an adult.

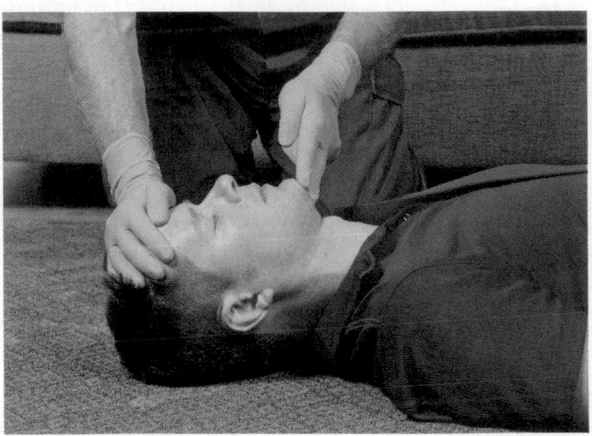

**Figure 9-5d** The final tilted position of the head-tilt, chin-lift in an adult.

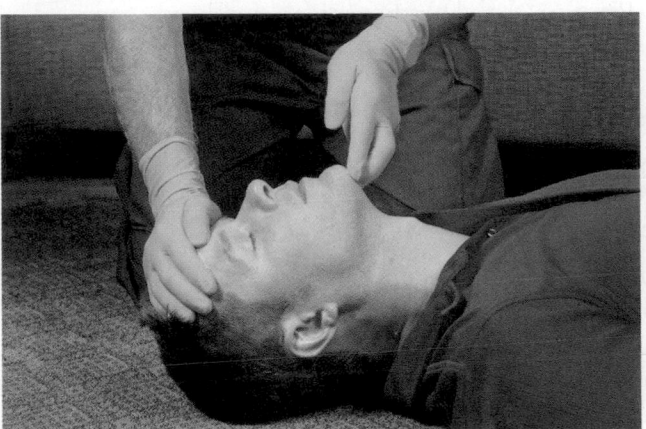

**Figure 9-6** The jaw-thrust maneuver is used to open the airway in patients with a suspected spinal injury.

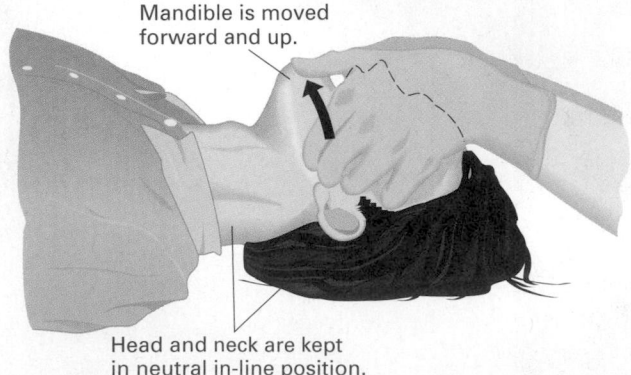

Mandible is moved forward and up.

Head and neck are kept in neutral in-line position.

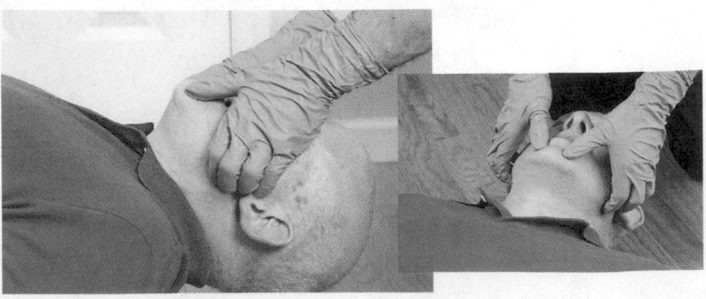

is not moved and remains in an anatomically neutral position, because any neck movement could result in spinal injury. To perform the jaw-thrust maneuver, take the following steps:

1. Kneel down above the patient's head, with your knees straddling the head. (You can use your knees to gently stabilize the head and cervical spine.)
2. Using the fingers of both hands, grasp the angle of the mandible on each side of the jaw.
3. Place your thumbs on the mandible.
4. Lift the mandible upward.

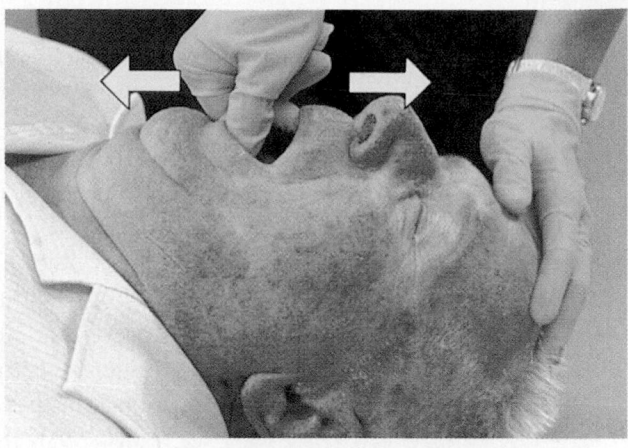

**Figure 9-7** Opening a patient's mouth using the crossed-finger technique.

### Opening the Mouth Using the Crossed-Finger Method

If you need to open a patient's mouth—to suction the oropharynx, to perform a finger sweep, or to insert an oral airway—the method most commonly used is the crossed-finger technique (Figure 9-7■). Always use Standard Precautions. To open the patient's mouth using this technique:

1. Using your dominant hand, cross your index finger under your thumb.
2. Place your thumb and index finger against the patient's upper and lower teeth. (Be careful not to insert either finger between the patient's teeth.)
3. Spread your thumb and finger apart to open the patient's mouth.

## Clearing the Airway

Effective breathing is difficult when any foreign material obstructs the airway. The airway-opening techniques just described keep the tongue from blocking the airway, but they are not effective in clearing other obstructions such as blood, mucus, fluids, broken teeth, foreign bodies, dirt, and food. Debris must be cleared quickly to ensure adequate oxygen flow and prevent aspiration of fluid or solids into the lungs. OEC Technicians can remove mechanical obstructions from the airway by three means: using gravity, a finger sweep, or suction.

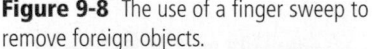

**⊕ 9-3** Describe how to clear a patient's airway using the following methods:
  **a.** Gravity
  **b.** Finger sweep
  **c.** Suction

### Gravity

Gravity is a time-honored method for quickly removing fluid and solids from the airway, and it requires no special equipment. This technique can be effective regardless of whether the patient is responsive or unresponsive. If the patient is responsive and is able to follow simple commands, instruct the person to lean forward with the head down (in a dependent position) to allow vomit, blood, and any solids to flow or fall out of the mouth or nose. If the patient is unresponsive, roll the person into the recovery position (discussed shortly). In the presence of a suspected spinal injury, the patient may be rolled onto his side while another rescuer maintains the patient's head and neck in a neutral position.

**Figure 9-8** The use of a finger sweep to remove foreign objects.

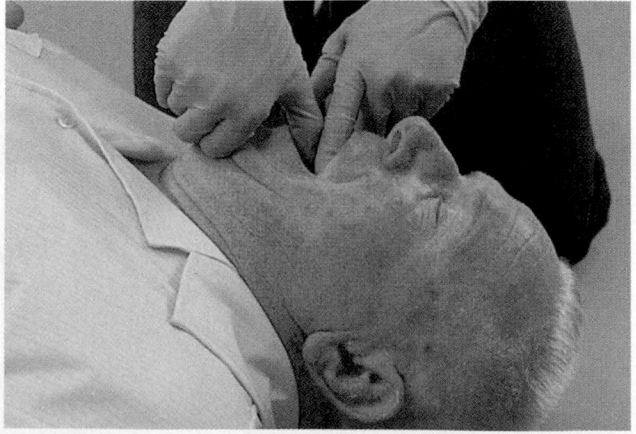

### Finger Sweep

Occasionally, vomit, unchewed food, or other objects can become trapped in the airway; if not removed, the airway can become obstructed. If gravity is not effective in removing these objects, it may be necessary to clear the airway using the finger sweep technique (Figure 9-8■). This technique is indicated only for patients who are unresponsive, because placing a finger into the airway of a person who is responsive could stimulate the gag reflex and induce even more vomiting, or it could cause the person to bite down, which could result in serious injury to the rescuer's finger. Do not do a "blind finger sweep" by inserting your finger further than you can see, as this might further compromise the patient's airway by pushing the object in farther. To perform a finger sweep on an unresponsive patient, use the following steps:

1. Observing all Standard Precautions, open the patient's mouth using the crossed-finger technique.
2. Insert your gloved index finger into the patient's mouth such that the tip of your finger is behind or beneath the foreign object. (Be careful not to push the foreign object farther into the airway.)
3. Curve your finger into a hook and remove the object. (You may need to repeat this technique more than once to completely clear the airway.)

### Suction

Another common method for clearing the airway is **suctioning**, which involves the use of negative air pressure to create a vacuum that is used to remove a liquid or solid. This procedure is very effective and is indicated any time the airway is compromised by fluid or particulate matter. Suctioning can be life saving and is especially crucial whenever repeated vomiting or active oral bleeding occurs.

OEC Technicians should be familiar with two basic types of suction devices: manually operated devices and powered devices. Portable devices are used primarily in the field, whereas fixed devices are generally used in an aid station, an ambulance, or a hospital. Become familiar with all the types of suction devices available to you, because suctioning is a life-saving skill that must be performed quickly and appropriately whenever the need arises.

Manually operated suction devices are lightweight, compact, and can provide adequate suction for short periods of time (Figure 9-9■). They require a continuous pumping action by the rescuer, who serves as the power source. These devices usually have a small container for collecting fluids and debris. The container fills quickly, so these devices may not be adequate during prolonged rescue operations.

Powered suction devices provide excellent suctioning capabilities (Figure 9-10■). Some are powered by an electric motor using AC current while others operate off a vacuum source from a vehicle engine (ambulance). Portable motorized units use rechargeable batteries. These devices are usually very reliable and provide consider-

**9-5** Compare, contrast, and demonstrate the usage of a rigid suction catheter and a flexible suction catheter.

**suctioning** a procedure that uses negative pressure to remove an object or a fluid.

**Figure 9-9** A manual suction device.

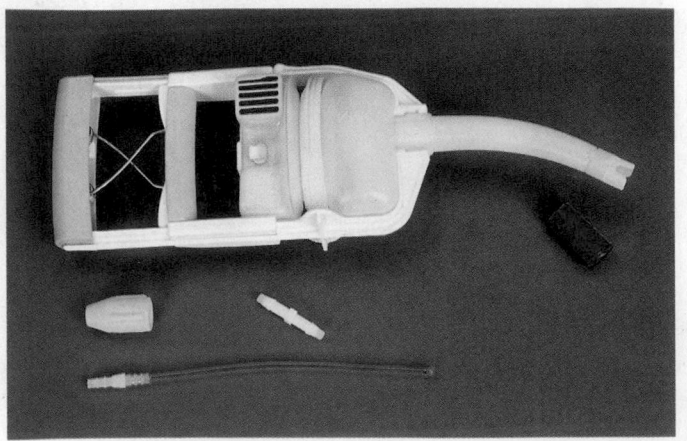

**Figure 9-10** A portable, battery-operated suction device.

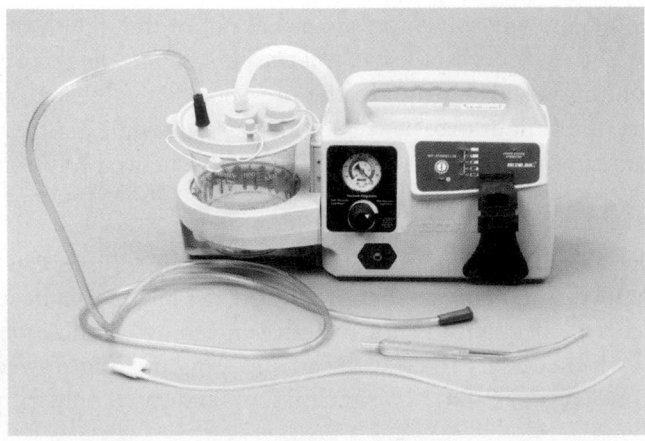

able suction for extended periods of time. However, because they can be heavy, they may not be ideal for all circumstances (e.g., a ski patrol backpack). Regardless of whether it is hand operated or powered, all suction devices must be capable of generating a strong vacuum.

Suctioning is performed using either a rigid or a flexible catheter. A rigid suction catheter, also known as a "tonsil tip" or "Yankauer" catheter, is made from clear plastic and is curved or angled. Ideally, it should have a port (hole) in the handle that enables the OEC Technician to control the flow of suction. When the hole is covered with the thumb, suction is applied. Conversely, little or no suction occurs when the hole is left uncovered. On one end the catheter has a connector to which suction tubing is attached. The other end of the catheter has one or more holes through which fluid and solid matter are removed. Rigid suction catheters are primarily used to suction the oropharynx but also can be used to suction around the external nares.

A flexible suction catheter is a soft tube constructed of clear silicone or plastic. Its pliable design allows it to enter narrow passageways. For this reason, it is used to suction the nasopharynx, but it also may be used for oropharyngeal suctioning. As with a rigid catheter, a flexible suction catheter has an adapter on one end that connects to a suction tube; the other end is open.

Of the two types, rigid suction catheters are used more often by OEC Technicians because they are less affected by temperature and other environmental conditions and can remove large volumes of debris rapidly. ALS personnel use sterile soft catheters for deep suctioning of the lower airways. Both types of suction catheters are connected to a collection container through a clear, flexible suction tube. Manually powered suction devices usually have an integrated suction catheter that is directly connected to a disposable collection container, which is replaced following use.

## Principles of Suctioning

If possible, "pre-oxygenate" the patient before suctioning by giving high-flow oxygen by mask to saturate the blood. Once you have prepared the suctioning device for use, open the patient's mouth and then look into the oral pharynx to locate the fluid or object you need to remove. Insert the tip of the suction catheter into the pharynx *before applying suction* (Figure 9-11■). Be careful not to insert the catheter farther than you can see because this may result in trauma to the soft oral tissues, initiate the gag reflex in a responsive or semi-responsive patient, or force a foreign body farther into the airway. To initiate suction, turn the machine on or cover the suction hole on the catheter. Suction only as deep as you can see to prevent pushing foreign matter farther into the airway. Using either a side-to-side or circular motion, suction the airway as you slowly withdraw the catheter from the airway. Remember to always protect the c-spine if you suspect any spinal trauma.

Apply suction for no more than 10–15 seconds at a time because the procedure does not remove fluid and debris only; it also removes oxygen, which could cause the patient's condition to worsen. In a child, suction the airway for only 5–10 seconds. Repeat the procedure as needed until the airway is clear. When active oral bleeding or repeated vomiting is involved, it may be necessary to use gravity and suction concurrently to clear the airway. Report to ambulance personnel what material you suctioned out, especially if it included blood.

After each incident, the suction unit must be thoroughly cleaned and disinfected before being placed back into service. Additionally, all disposable equipment, such as the suction catheter, suction tubing, and collection bag, must be replaced. If the device is battery

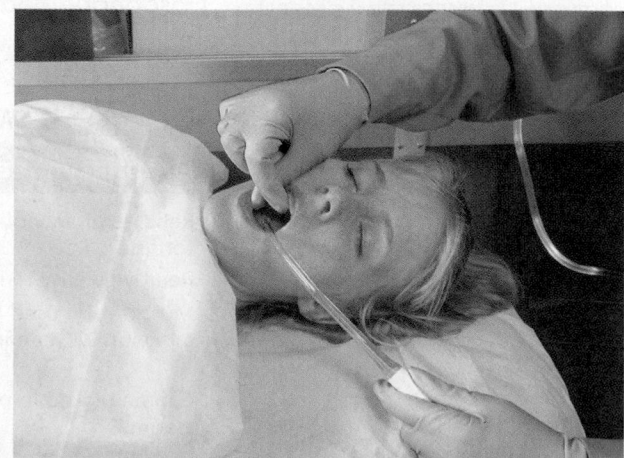

**Figure 9-11** Apply suction only after the catheter is in place.

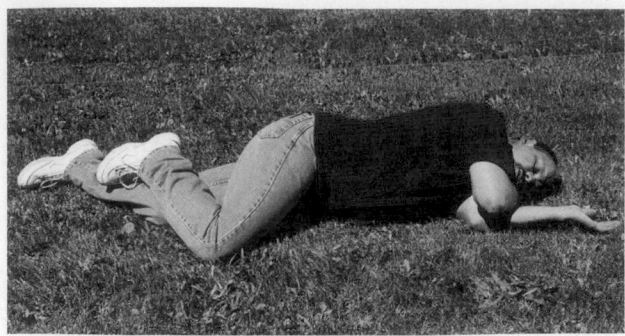

**Figure 9-12** The modified recovery position (or left lateral recumbent position) may be used to prevent aspiration in patients not suspected to have spinal injuries.

**⊕ 9-4** Describe how to place a patient into the recovery position.

**⊕ 9-6** List the indications of and uses for the following airway adjuncts, and demonstrate the proper methods of choosing the correct size and inserting them:

a. Oropharyngeal airway

b. Nasopharyngeal airway

**adjunct** a medical device that is used to assist the OEC Technician in providing patient care.

**nasopharyngeal airway (NPA)** a trumpet-shaped airway adjunct made from soft rubber or silicone that is inserted into the nostril to maintain a patent airway.

operated, replace or recharge the batteries as necessary to ensure satisfactory performance when the device is next used. If the suction unit is manually powered, replace the catheter-collection assembly. Always put disposable medical equipment in a biohazard container to dispose of it properly. See OEC Skill 9-1■.

## Keeping the Airway Open and Clear

### Recovery Position

Once the airway is opened and cleared, it must remain in this state to ensure adequate breathing. The easiest method to achieve this, until other airway equipment or rescue personnel are available, is to place the patient into the HAINES (High Arm In Endangered Spine) recovery position (Figure 9-12■). This position, also known as the coma or left lateral recumbent position, is indicated for any unresponsive patient in whom spine injury is *not* suspected. It also may be used for responsive patients and any patients with an altered level of responsiveness who cannot manage their airway. When alone, rescuers should use this technique to allow them to do other care-related tasks. To place a patient into the recovery position, perform the following procedure:

1. Kneel by the left side of the patient, preferably with your knees near the patient's hips or chest.
2. Extend the patient's left arm so that it extends over the person's head.
3. Gently roll the patient toward you onto his left side so that his head rests on his straightened arm.
4. The head should be tilted at a *slight* downward angle, with the mouth open, to allow secretions to flow out of the mouth.
5. Flex the patient's right knee at a right angle to anchor the patient into this position.
6. Position the patient's right arm so that it is in front of the patient and does not block the rescuer's access to the patient's airway.
7. Always make sure the airway remains open.

### Airway Adjuncts

Sometimes it is necessary to insert an airway **adjunct** in order to keep the airway open. The OEC Technician has two options—a nasopharyngeal airway or an oropharyngeal airway (Table 9-1■). One of these devices may be used depending on the patient's level of responsiveness.

**Nasopharyngeal Airway** A **nasopharyngeal airway (NPA)** is a flexible tube that is inserted into the nasopharynx (Figure 9-13■). It is made of soft, latex-free plastic. Also

| Table 9-1 | A Comparison of Oropharyngeal and Nasopharyngeal Airway Adjuncts |
|---|---|
| **Oropharyngeal Airway (OPA)** | **Nasopharyngeal Airway (NPA)** |
| Relieves airway obstruction caused by tongue | Relieves airway obstruction caused by the tongue or by mucus and nasal swelling |
| Relatively easy to insert | Easy to insert |
| Must not be used in a responsive patient or a person with an intact gag reflex | Can be safely used in responsive and semi-responsive patients or in a person with an intact gag reflex |
| Can be placed in patients who have nasal trauma | Caution required if used in patients who have oral trauma |

# STOP, THINK, UNDERSTAND

## Multiple Choice

Choose the correct answer.

1. Which of the following is *not* true about airway management?
   _____
   a. It is a physical process that ensures that the airway is open and clear.
   b. Respiration cannot occur through a closed or blocked (occluded) airway.
   c. It is a fundamental and crucial life-saving skill that OEC Technicians must learn.
   d. True airway maintenance is beyond the scope of OEC Technicians.

2. Which of the following is a method for opening the airway?_____
   a. head-tilt, chin-lift maneuver
   b. crossed-finger maneuver
   c. jaw-thrust maneuver
   d. both A and C

3. Which of the following is not correct regarding suctioning of an airway?_____ (check all that apply)
   a. Insert the catheter into the airway with the suction *on* (thumb hole covered).
   b. Insert the catheter only as deeply as you can see.
   c. Suction side to side for 10–15 seconds maximum in an adult, for 5–10 seconds maximum in a child.
   d. Insert the catheter tip into the airway with the suction *off* (thumb hole open).
   e. Suction only the outer nares and lips, allowing gravity to clear the remainder of the oropharynx and nasopharynx.
   f. Suctioning is not a skill that OEC Technicians may perform.

4. What can cause an airway to occlude and prevent adequate breathing? (check all that apply)
   _____ a. the tongue falling back into the pharynx
   _____ b. unnatural flexion, extension, or tilting of the patient's head
   _____ c. an inhaled foreign object such as food or a small toy
   _____ d. blood or vomitus
   _____ e. broken teeth

5. Which of the following methods may be used to remove fluid and solids (such as vomitus or broken teeth) from a *responsive* patient's mouth? (check all that apply)
   _____ a. placing the patient sitting forward with the head in a dependent position
   _____ b. placing the patient in the recovery position with or without spinal precautions, as indicated
   _____ c. using suction with a rigid or flexible catheter

6. Which of the following methods may be used to remove fluids or solids from an *unresponsive* patient's mouth? (check all that apply)
   _____ a. using a finger sweep
   _____ b. placing the patient in the recovery position with or without spinal precautions, as indicated
   _____ c. using suction with a rigid or flexible catheter

known as a nasal trumpet, this mechanical airway provides an unobstructed pathway from an external nares to the posterior nasopharynx, keeping the passageway open for air exchange. When properly sized, the adjunct is well tolerated, even in responsive patients, as it does not stimulate the gag reflex. NPAs come in a variety of sizes and can be used in all patients, from small children to large adults.

The indications for an NPA are fairly broad and include any patient in whom a mechanical airway is needed to keep the airway open. Indications include patients who

+ are unresponsive or semi-responsive,
+ have altered mental status and an intact gag reflex,
+ exhibit signs of partial airway obstruction (as when snoring),
+ have oral injuries and airway compromise, or
+ have had, or are having, a seizure and whose teeth are tightly clenched.

The adjunct is relatively contraindicated in patients with massive head injuries due to possible aggravation of the injury and/or damage to the nose.

Proper insertion of an NPA consists of the following four steps, which can be remembered using the acronym "SLIC" (OEC Skill 9-2■).

**Figure 9-13** Two nasopharyngeal (nasal) airways (NPAs).

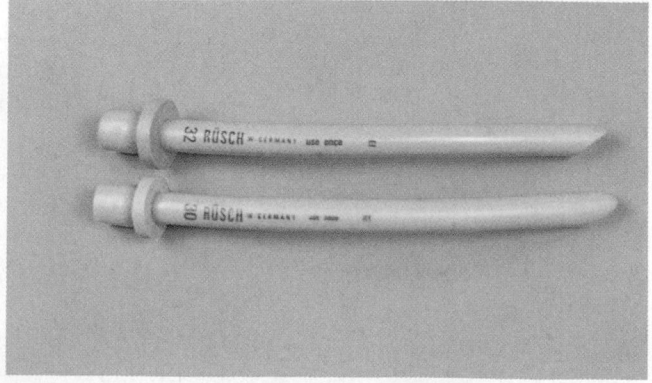

**S—Size the adjunct.** NPAs come in a variety of sizes. To be effective, the device must be sized appropriately. A tube that is too small may become blocked by the tongue, whereas a tube that is too large may enter the esophagus or stimulate the patient's gag reflex. To properly size an NPA, hold the tube against the side of the patient's face. For a tube that is the correct size, the flange should rest against the nostril, the end should just touch the patient's lower earlobe on the same side of the face, and the outside of the tube should be slightly smaller than the nostril into which it will be placed.

**L—Lubricate the adjunct.** Apply a small amount of water-based lubricant along the entire length of the NPA tube. Be careful not to apply too much lubricant, which could aggravate an existing airway problem. The goal is to provide a slippery surface so that the tube can slide gently into position.

**I—Insert the adjunct.** To insert an NPA:

- Hold the tube between your thumb and first two fingers.
- Place the bevel side of the tube toward the nasal septum.
- Gently insert the tube into the nostril while rotating the tube between your fingers until the flange is flush with the nostril. Do not force the tube into position because that can cause a nosebleed, an obstruction, or other injuries. If you meet an obstruction, pull the tube back slightly and reinsert, again while rotating the tube between your fingers. Properly placed, the curvature of the tube will follow the natural curve of the nasal passage and lie in the distal portion of the nasopharynx directly above the larynx.

**C—Check the adjunct.** Confirm proper placement of the tube by listening to the patient breathe. You should be able to hear or feel air movement through the tube. If no air is detected, check to see if the patient is still breathing. If the patient is not, assist the patient's ventilations. If the patient is breathing, the tube may be obstructed, may need to be repositioned, or may need to be removed and resized. Rarely, foreign material inside the nose can obstruct the opening of the NPA.

If the patient's level of responsiveness improves, you may need to remove the NPA. To accomplish this, simply grasp the NPA by the flange and withdraw the adjunct using a steady downward motion that follows the device's curvature.

**Oropharyngeal Airway**    An **oropharyngeal airway (OPA)** is a hard plastic device that is inserted into the oropharynx to help keep the airway open (Figure 9-14■). The device displaces the relaxed tongue and prevents it from lying across the epiglottis and occluding the airway. When the OPA is in place, the tongue rests within the curvature of the device. An OPA is indicated only for patients who do not have a gag reflex and are unable to protect the airway. The device is frequently used when assisting ventilations with a bag valve mask.

If you attempt to place an oropharyngeal airway into a patient who is either fully or partially responsive, it will stimulate the gag reflex, which may result in vomiting and possible aspiration of gastric contents. If when the soft palate is touched by the OPA and the person gags, remove the OPA and do not reinsert it.

Proper insertion of an OPA consists of the following three steps, which may be remembered using the mnemonic "SIC" (OEC Skill 9-3■).

**S—Size the adjunct.** OPAs come in several sizes ranging from #0 for infants to #6 for large adults. As with an NPA, an OPA must be properly sized to be effective. An OPA that is too small will force

**oropharyngeal airway (OPA)**
a rigid plastic airway adjunct that is inserted into the oropharynx to maintain a patent airway.

> **NOTE**
>
> **Oropharyngeal Airway**
>
> ALS providers may use an OPA as a bite block to protect the teeth. It may also be used as a spacer between the teeth that will prevent damage to an advanced airway device such as a breathing tube that is placed in the oral airway.

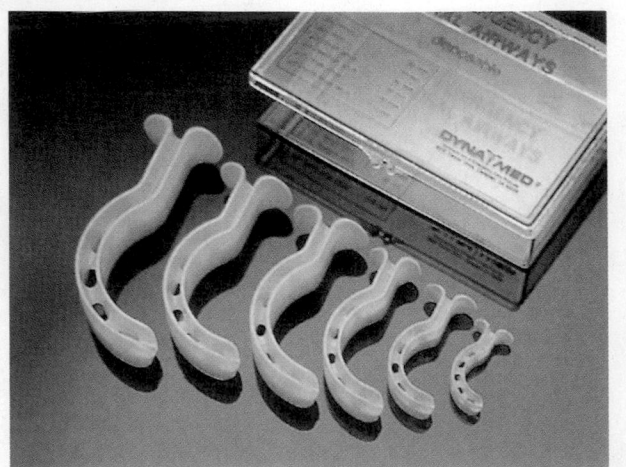

**Figure 9-14** A set of oropharyngeal (oral) airways (OPAs).

the tongue downward and block the oropharynx, whereas an OPA that is too large can enter the esophagus or damage the epiglottis or vocal cords.

To properly size an OPA, hold the adjunct against the side of the patient's face with the flange adjacent to the corner of the patient's mouth. The tip of the adjunct should touch the angle of the jaw on the same side of the face; alternatively, measure from the corner of the mouth to the earlobe on the same side of the face.

**I—Insert the adjunct.** To insert an OPA, open the patient's mouth using the crossed-finger technique. Insert the OPA, with the tip pointed up toward the roof of the mouth, until it is halfway into the mouth. Then rotate the adjunct 180 degrees such that the tip faces toward the patient's tongue. The tongue should now lie along the curve of the OPA, and the external flange should rest against the patient's lips.

An alternative method for placing an OPA involves the use of a tongue blade, bite block (device used to hold mouth open and prevent the patient from biting his tongue or the oral airway), or other smooth object. Using a tongue blade, depress the tongue toward the floor of the mouth. Then, insert the adjunct along the side of the mouth, with the tip pointing toward the inside cheek, until the OPA is halfway into the mouth. Rotate the OPA 90 degrees until the flange rests on the patient's lips.

**C—Check the adjunct.** Confirm proper placement by listening for breaths, watching the chest rise and fall, and feeling air moving in and out of the OPA. If the adjunct is properly placed, air should be able to move freely in and out of the airway (either spontaneously, or when using a ventilation assistance device such as a pocket mask or bag-valve mask). If air does not move freely, the tongue may have been pushed farther back into the posterior pharynx and may be blocking the airway. As before, remove the OPA, confirm that it is properly sized, and then reinsert it.

## STOP, THINK, UNDERSTAND

### Multiple Choice

Choose the correct answer.

1. The mnemonic SLIC stands for _____
   a. size, length, intubate, compress.
   b. suction, lubrication, insertion, compression.
   c. suction, lubrication, insertion, control.
   d. size, lubricate, insert, check.

2. Write either "NPA" or "OPA" in the blanks to correctly categorize the following descriptions.
   _____ a. indicated for use only in patients without a gag reflex
   _____ b. for use in unresponsive patients only
   _____ c. can be used on a seizing patient with clenched teeth
   _____ d. a soft, flexible device
   _____ e. contraindicated in patients with massive head trauma
   _____ f. a rigid, hard, plastic device
   _____ g. works by displacing the tongue
   _____ h. is tolerated by responsive patients
   _____ i. can be used on a patient with signs/symptoms of partial airway obstruction such as snoring
   _____ j. also known as a "nasal trumpet"
   _____ k. provides an unobstructed path from the external nare to the posterior pharynx

### Short Answer

You have inserted an OPA into an unresponsive patient. Under what two conditions could it be removed?

_____

_____

# CASE UPDATE

An assistant immediately performs a jaw-thrust maneuver to open the unresponsive patient's airway. As the assistant protects the patient's spine, you carefully roll the patient onto his side to allow blood to flow out of the airway. Noting several broken teeth in the patient's airway, you perform a finger sweep to remove the debris. Upon arrival of a suction device, you suction out the airway. Although the patient's pulse is strong, his respirations are becoming increasingly shallow and erratic. His lips are cyanotic.

*What should you do now?*

An OPA should be left in place until one of two conditions arises: either the patient begins to gag, or a more-advanced airway adjunct (Chapter 36) is inserted by an ALS provider. However, in the event that you need to remove an OPA, grasp the adjunct by the flanges and pull it both outward and slightly downward, following the natural contour of the tongue. Removal should be performed in one swift motion to reduce the incidence of vomiting and other complications. Have a suction device ready in case the patient vomits.

**⊕ 9-10** Describe and demonstrate how to use the following oxygen delivery, ventilation, and barrier devices:

a. Nasal cannula

b. Nonrebreather mask

c. Pocket mask

d. Bag-valve mask

e. Face shield

## Barrier Devices

OEC Technicians are sometimes the first rescuers to arrive at an incident, but they may not always have immediate access to certain medical equipment. Accordingly, be prepared for such contingencies by always carrying a few key items—including disposable medical gloves and a barrier device in the event you need to provide rescue breaths (Appendix C: Survival Kit).

Barrier devices are a form of personal protective equipment that provides a non-porous layer between you and the patient to prevent the transmission of communicable diseases (Figure 9-15■). Used properly, a barrier device is an effective way to ventilate a patient until more sophisticated airway equipment and oxygen become available.

Barrier devices permit OEC Technicians to provide rescue breaths using the residual oxygen in the rescuer's lungs. The mixture of gases in exhaled air contains approximately 15–16 percent oxygen, which is enough to provide effective oxygenation to a patient who is not breathing. Room air is 21 percent oxygen. The use of a barrier device will help to ensure Standard Precautions are maintained. The most common barrier devices used for this purpose are a face shield and a pocket mask.

**Face Shield**   A face shield is a clear plastic sheet, usually rectangular in shape, with a mouthpiece through which to administer rescue breaths. Some face shields also have an integrated one-way valve/bite block that directs air flow into the patient's airway while preventing the rescuer from becoming contaminated. To use a face shield, perform the following procedure:

1. Kneel at either side of the patient's head.
2. Remove the face shield from its protective package and place the shield over the patient's mouth and nose. If the device contains an integrated one-way valve/bite-block, place the valve into the patient's mouth, between the teeth.

**Figure 9-15** Examples of barrier devices.

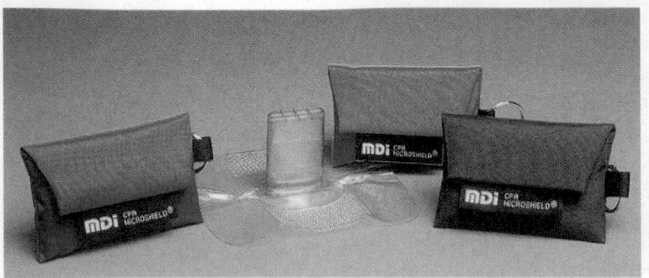

3. Pinch the patient's nose and seal your lips on the shield around the valve (as if you were performing normal mouth-to-mouth resuscitation) and provide rescue breaths. You should see the chest rise and fall with each breath.

**Pocket Mask** A **pocket mask** is a triangular or pear-shaped barrier device made from clear, soft plastic or silicone (Figure 9-16■). Some older styles are circular or donut shaped. The apex of the mask fits over the bridge of the patient's nose. Some pocket masks include a built-in oxygen port that allows the device to be connected to supplemental oxygen. Used correctly, a pocket mask provides an excellent seal on the patient's face and offers better protection from blood and secretions than a face shield.

A pocket mask generally consists of three parts: a mask, a one-way valve, and a breathing tube. To assemble a pocket mask, follow this procedure:

1. Remove the device from its protective package or case.
2. Open the mask (by pulling on the connector, if necessary).
3. Connect the one-way valve to the mask. (Follow the manufacturer's instructions to ensure that the valve is pointed toward the patient.)
4. Connect the breathing tube to the one-way valve.

To deliver rescue breaths using a pocket mask, follow these steps (Figures 9-17a■ and 9-17b■):

1. Assemble the pocket mask as previously described.
2. Kneel at the top of the patient's head, and open the airway using either the head-tilt, chin-lift or the jaw-thrust maneuver.
3. Fit the mask onto the patient, placing the apex of the triangle on the bridge of the patient's nose. The mask should be rocked down so that the base of the triangle fits in the groove between the patient's lower lip and chin. If the mask does not fit in the groove, the mask may not be the correct size, or it may need to be repositioned on the face.

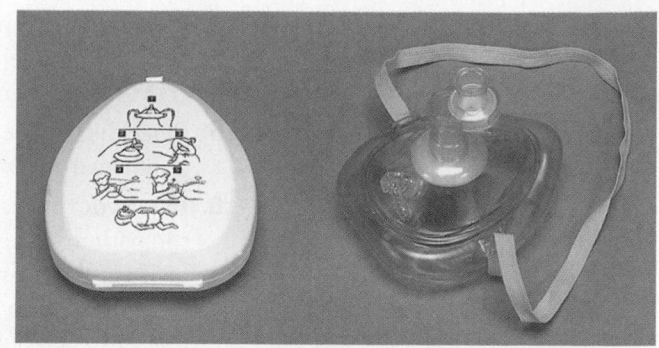

**Figure 9-16** A pocket mask with a one-way valve.

**pocket mask** a barrier device; a folding mask with an oxygen inlet valve that is used for artificial ventilation; may be used with or without supplemental oxygen.

**Figure 9-17a** Place the face mask on the patient; note the positions of the fingers.
Copyright Edward McNamara

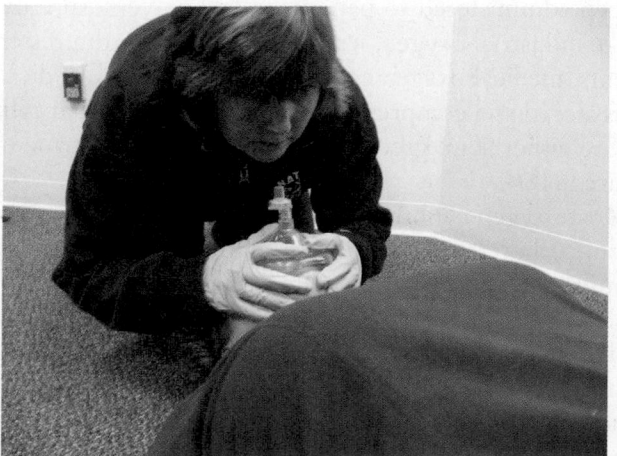

**Figure 9-17b** Deliver rescue breaths into the mask.
Copyright Edward McNamara

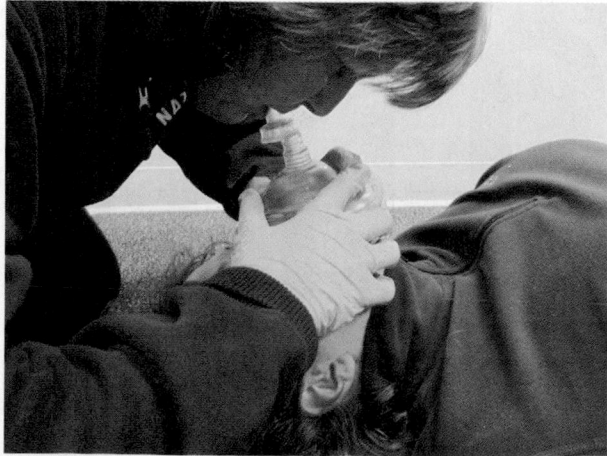

4. Place your thumbs on the top of the mask, near the bridge of the patient's nose, while simultaneously placing your index fingers on the bottom of the mask, which is over the section between the lower lip and chin.

5. Place the middle, ring, and little fingers of both your hands under the mandible and pull upward, toward the mask (as opposed to pushing the mask down onto the face).

6. Place your lips around the open port and deliver a rescue breath. You should see the patient's chest rise and fall with each breath. If the patient's chest does not rise or if you hear air escaping between the mask and the patient's face, reposition the device and then deliver another rescue breath. If the chest still does not rise, follow obstructed airway procedures.

Creating an adequate seal and delivering appropriate rescue breaths with a pocket mask is one of the most important skills in emergency airway and respiration care. Practice this skill until you are very comfortable with it.

# Oxygen Therapy

Oxygen, also known by its chemical symbol $O_2$, is an odorless, colorless, and tasteless gas that is essential to human survival. Ambient air consists of 78 percent nitrogen, 21 percent oxygen, and 1 percent other gases. The human body requires a constant supply of oxygen in order to function properly. If the body does not receive enough oxygen, cellular or tissue damage, organ failure, shock, or death can occur. Ensuring that a patient's blood is sufficiently oxygenated may require you to administer supplemental oxygen.

Administering oxygen—or providing oxygen therapy—is an essential part of an OEC Technician's training and treatment regimen. In some jurisdictions, OEC Technicians may administer oxygen as part of their regular care, whereas in others the administration of oxygen requires a physician order. Such an order may be provided by a patrol's medical advisor as either an indirect or direct order, or it may be obtained through the local emergency care system's medical command. It is best to develop a local protocol concerning oxygen delivery by incorporating input from a local doctor, management, and the patrol's leadership. In some areas, OEC Technicians are not legally permitted to administer oxygen. To determine if you are permitted to provide oxygen therapy in your state, province, or area, check with your patrol director, area management, or state EMS office.

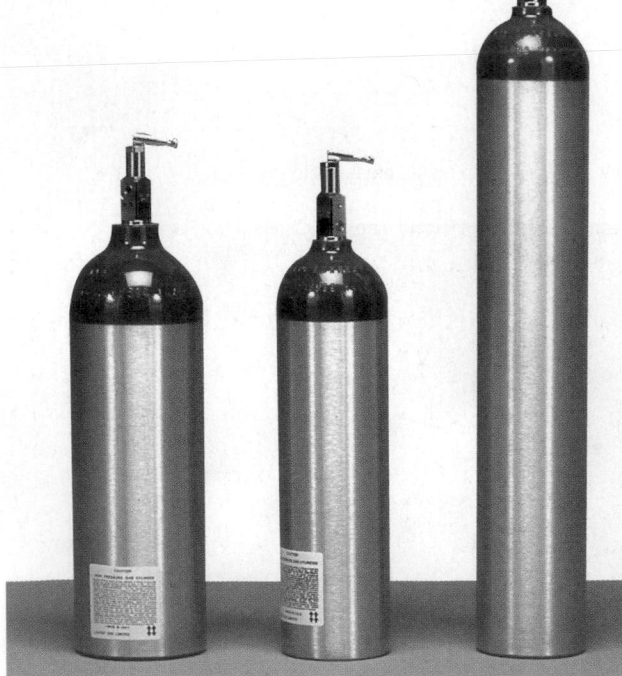

**Figure 9-18** Three oxygen cylinders. Left to right: jumbo D cylinder, D cylinder, and E cylinder.

## Oxygen Containers

Oxygen administered to patients is 100 percent pure oxygen. Unlike industrial oxygen, which should not be administered to patients, medical oxygen contains no impurities. Medical oxygen is stored as a compressed gas in specially marked cylinders that are either solid green or have a large green stripe on top (Figure 9-18■).

Most oxygen cylinders are constructed of lightweight aluminum, although older cylinders made from steel may still be encountered. Oxygen cylinders come in a variety of sizes (Table 9-2■). Smaller cylinders, such as C, D, and E cylinders, are lightweight, making them easy to carry and store. When full, these cylinders contain 350 to 625 liters of oxygen. Small cylinders are designed for short-term use. Large oxygen cylinders, such as M, H, and K cylinders, are more cumber-

## Table 9-2    Oxygen Cylinder Sizes and Volumes

| Size | Volume (Liters) |
| --- | --- |
| D | 350 |
| Super D | 500 |
| E | 625 |
| M | 3,000 |
| G | 5,300 |
| H, A, K | 6,900 |

some but contain several thousand liters of oxygen. Because of their size and weight, large oxygen cylinders are usually found on ambulances, in hospitals, and in ski patrol first-aid rooms or base camps.

An oxygen cylinder consists of three components: a cylinder, a neck, and a valve stem:

+ **Cylinder.** The cylinder serves as a reservoir in which highly compressed oxygen gas is stored. Depending on size, a full oxygen cylinder can hold between 350 and 6,900 liters of oxygen at a pressure of 2,000–2,200 pounds per square inch (psi).
+ **Neck.** The neck of an oxygen cylinder extends outward from the cylinder and contains three holes—a large hole toward the top and two smaller holes located directly beneath (Figure 9-19■). The location of these holes is universal to all medical oxygen cylinders and is part of the internal pin index system.
+ **Valve stem.** The valve stem is a small protrusion that extends approximately 0.5–1 inch beyond the neck and is used to turn the cylinder on and off.

In order to safely administer oxygen to a patient, the gas must first be routed through a pressure regulator, which significantly reduces its pressure to approximately 40–70 psi. Each type of gas has a unique pressure regulator that conforms to the universal pin index system. This safety precaution ensures that the regulator will fit only the type of gas cylinder for which it is intended. As a result, only oxygen gas can be administered through an oxygen regulator.

Several different types of commercial oxygen regulators are available. Most small oxygen cylinders (e.g., D, E cylinders) utilize a yoke regulator assembly, whereas large cylinders typically have a screw-on regulator assembly (Figure 9-20■). Yoke-type regulator assemblies usually have a large thumb screw for securing the regulator to the tank neck. The large hole inside the yoke assembly is surrounded by a dime-size plastic or silicone gasket, which prevents gas leaks. Oxygen regulators also have at least two gauges: a pressure gauge, which indicates the pressure in the tank, and a flow gauge, which indicates the number of liters of oxygen being administered per minute (LPM). A large knob enables you to control the rate of oxygen flow, which for most clinical applications is 2–15 LPM. A part of the regulator—a small graduated adapter known as a "Christmas tree"—connects to a tube that in turn connects to an oxygen delivery device.

## Oxygen Cylinder Set-Up and Breakdown

To set up an oxygen cylinder, you must first inspect the entire cylinder, including the gasket—an O-shaped plastic, silicone, or rubber disk that seals the regulator to the cylinder and helps prevent leaks. If the gasket is dry or cracked, replace it before continuing. Then, before attaching a regulator to a cylinder, "crack" the cylinder by opening the cylinder valve slightly for one second, and then close the valve. This clears the cylinder of any dirt or debris that has accumulated since the cylinder was used last.

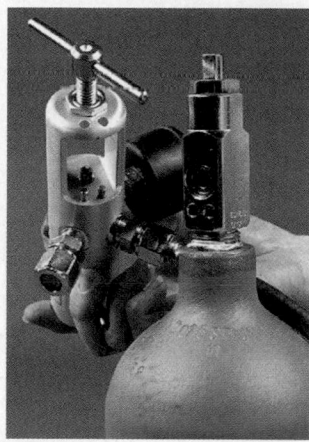

**Figure 9-19** The neck of the cylinder, which contains three holes with a yoke regulator.

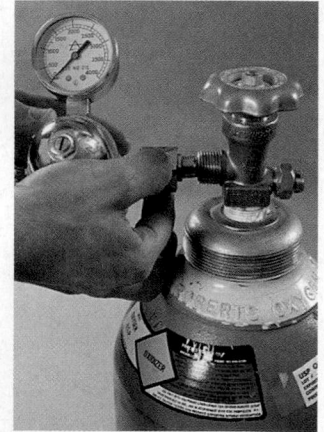

**Figure 9-20** A high-pressure regulator being placed on an E tank.

⊕ 9-8    Describe and demonstrate how to properly set up an oxygen tank for use.

To prepare the oxygen cylinder and oxygen regulator, align the large circular fitting and the two smaller pins on the regulator with the corresponding circular hole and two smaller holes on the neck of the oxygen cylinder. The pins and holes should match perfectly. Finger-tighten the screw bolt or knob until the fittings and pins fit snugly together. Do not over-tighten the screw or knob, as this could damage the assembly or cylinder and can make removal of the regulator very difficult, especially in extreme temperatures (OEC Skill 9-4■).

To open the oxygen system, turn the valve stem on the top of the cylinder counterclockwise, using a special oxygen wrench or key that should be stored with the cylinder. If you hear a hissing sound, the regulator is not seated correctly onto the cylinder. Turn off the oxygen flow, remove the regulator from the cylinder, check the gasket (replace if old, cracked, or dry), and reconnect the regulator. Check the pressure gauge indicator to determine the pressure in the cylinder. Check to make sure that the cylinder contains enough oxygen for its intended use—and make sure that it is not empty! If you will be performing an extended rescue or a medical operation, the cylinder should be full (approximately 2,000 psi). Oxygen cylinders should be refilled once they reach 500 psi or less.

To begin the flow of oxygen, turn the oxygen control knob counterclockwise. Use the oxygen flow gauge to set the amount of oxygen that you wish to administer.

To stop the flow of oxygen, simply reverse the process by turning the oxygen flow knob clockwise until it stops. To turn the cylinder off, turn the valve stem clockwise until it stops, being careful to not over-tighten it. At this point, the cylinder is closed, and oxygen is no longer flowing into the regulator. However, there is still a small amount of oxygen trapped within the regulator that must be released; otherwise, it can damage the regulator. The process of relieving this residual pressure is known as "bleeding the cylinder" and is performed as follows:

1. With the cylinder turned off, turn the oxygen flow knob counterclockwise (open) until you no longer hear gas escaping. Check the pressure gauge to ensure that the pressure is at 0 psi. (Again, be careful not to over-tighten the knob.)
2. Turn the oxygen flow knob clockwise (close) to close the system completely.

The oxygen delivery system is now completely turned off and drained and is ready to be used again or to be placed into storage until the next time it is needed. Oxygen equipment that will not be used again soon should be disassembled for storage. To remove the regulator from the cylinder, ensure that the cylinder is turned off, and that any remaining oxygen in the regulator has been bled. Turn the yoke screw counterclockwise, and remove the regulator from the cylinder.

⊕ **9-7**  Describe how to calculate the oxygen flow duration rate.

## Oxygen Flow Duration Rates

As you will learn in future chapters, oxygen therapy is an essential part of the care regimen for numerous medical and trauma conditions. In many cases, oxygen is the primary care rendered and is delivered in a specific amount known as a "flow rate." If you operate in an environment in which transport or extrication may be prolonged, you must carefully balance the flow rate you administer with the amount of oxygen available and the patient's anticipated oxygen needs; in fact, it may become necessary to ration the amount of oxygen that is administered to extend the time it is available.

To calculate the duration of oxygen flow from a single cylinder, use the following equation:

$$\text{Duration of flow} = \frac{(\text{Gauge pressure in psi} \; - \; \text{safe residual pressure}) \times \text{cylinder size constant}}{\text{Flow rate in LPM}}$$

| Table 9-3 | Oxygen Cylinder Size Constants |
| Cylinder Size | Cylinder Size Constant |
| --- | --- |
| D or Super D | 0.16 |
| E | 0.28 |
| M | 1.56 |
| G | 2.41 |
| H or K | 3.14 |

For most cylinders, the "safe residual pressure" is 200 psi; below this level, the oxygen pressure is dangerously low. For cylinder size constants, see Table 9-3■.

Knowing how to calculate how long your oxygen supply will last at a given flow rate enables you to make good patient care decisions. For example, suppose you respond to an incident carrying a full D cylinder containing 2,000 psi. (This is the most common oxygen cylinder size available to OEC Technicians and other rescuers.) If the oxygen flow rate is set at 4 LPM, for how long can you expect oxygen to continue flowing?

$$\text{Duration of flow} = \frac{(2{,}000 - 200) \times 0.16}{4 \text{ LPM}} = 72 \text{ minutes}$$

Thus, at 4 LPM, you can expect a maximum of 72 minutes of continuous oxygen flow.

Likewise, if the patient requires oxygen at 15 LPM, the same full cylinder will only last 19 minutes:

$$\frac{(2{,}000 - 200) \times 0.16}{15 \text{ LPM}} = 19.2 \text{ minutes}$$

As you can see from the latter example, when continuous oxygen therapy must be delivered in remote settings or during incidents when extrication or transport is prolonged, multiple oxygen cylinders may be needed.

## Oxygen Safety

Oxygen cylinders are vessels containing highly compressed gas and should be treated very carefully to prevent inadvertent damage and injury. As a rule, they should be laid on their side, kept in a protective carrier, or firmly secured to a wall to prevent them from falling. Before each use, inspect the cylinder for damage, including dents or cracks in the valve-gauge assembly or the cylinder. Other safety tips include the following:

♣ Never use oxygen near a spark or flame such as candles, a camp fire, a stove, or a heater.

♣ Do not allow a patient or others to smoke when oxygen is being used.

♣ Keep oil, grease, or other petroleum-based or combustible materials away from oxygen cylinders and oxygen regulators.

♣ Turn the oxygen cylinder off when it is not in use.

♣ Protect the valve stem from damage.

♣ Leave protective caps in place until the cylinder is ready for use.

♣ Clear valve stems of dust and debris before attaching the regulator.

♣ Do not over-tighten the valve stem, saddle screw, or regulator knobs.

9-9 List four tips for the safe use of oxygen.

## Indications for Oxygen Therapy

Oxygen should be administered to anyone who is short of breath. Patients with suspected cardiac or respiratory arrest, cardiac-related chest pain, stroke, significant blood loss, shock, decreased level of responsiveness, head injury, or a broken long bone should receive oxygen. By administering supplemental $O_2$, an OEC Technician increases the oxygen saturation of hemoglobin in the blood, providing more oxygen to the body's tissues. If not enough $O_2$ is supplied to the body's tissues, hypoxia results. Patients who have chronic lung disease (usually from smoking), those whose respiration rate has been decreased by an overdose of depressant drugs, or those who have a

# STOP, THINK, UNDERSTAND

## Multiple Choice

Choose the correct answer.

1. What is the chemical symbol for oxygen? _____
   a. $O_2$
   b. $CO_2$
   c. $O_3$
   d. Ox

2. Ambient air consists of _____
   a. 21% nitrogen, 78% oxygen, and 1% carbon dioxide.
   b. 50% oxygen, 50% nitrogen, and a trace of other gases.
   c. 78% nitrogen, 21% oxygen, and 1% other gases.
   d. 100% oxygen.

3. Which of the following statements about oxygen administration best describes an OEC Technician's role in its use? _____
   a. All OEC Technicians may administer oxygen.
   b. Oxygen administration is a skill in which OEC Technicians may *assist* a higher-level caregiver, but OEC Technicians may not administer oxygen themselves.
   c. Only paramedics and physicians may administer oxygen.
   d. The legality of oxygen administration by OEC Technicians varies from state to state and county to county; it is the responsibility of each OEC Technician to determine what local protocol is.

4. Which of the following statements is true? _____
   a. Medical oxygen cylinders contain 78% oxygen, 21% nitrogen, and 1% inert gases.
   b. Medical oxygen and industrial oxygen may be used interchangeably as long as a filter is applied to the regulator.
   c. Medical oxygen cylinders are green and contain 100 percent oxygen.
   d. On a low-flow setting, a small (C, D, or E) cylinder contains enough oxygen for use during a lengthy transport, because these cylinders are compact, lightweight, and efficient.

5. The abbreviations psi and LPM stand for _____
   a. pin securing index and last pressure measurement.
   b. portable site indicator and load per millimeter.
   c. pound at site inertia and liter pint metric.
   d. pounds per square inch and liters per minute.

6. The usual flow rate for the clinical administration of oxygen is _____
   a. 2–15 LPM.
   b. 1–10 LPM.
   c. 5–30 LPM.
   d. measured in psi.

7. The purpose of "cracking" a cylinder before use is _____
   a. to ensure that the cylinder is full.
   b. to bleed off enough pressure to lessen the chance of damaging the regulator.
   c. to clear the cylinder of dirt or debris before attaching the regulator.
   d. One should never "crack" an oxygen cylinder.

8. Upon attaching a regulator set at 0 LPM and opening the valve stem, you hear a loud hissing sound. This is indicative of what? _____
   a. The regulator is not sealed correctly onto the cylinder.
   b. The regulator is properly attached and $O_2$ is flowing properly.
   c. The cylinder is almost empty.
   d. The cylinder has been overfilled and should be bled before use.

9. At what level should an oxygen cylinder be refilled? _____
   a. 1,000 psi
   b. 500 psi
   c. 200 psi
   d. Only when it is completely empty

10. What is the purpose of bleeding residual air out of the regulator after use? _____
    a. It completely empties the cylinder of the final 200 psi so it can be safely refilled.
    b. It removes debris in the regulator neck.
    c. It fills the regulator with 25 psi so that it is ready for use on the next patient.
    d. It removes air trapped within the regulator and prevents regulator damage.

11. It is appropriate to give oxygen to which of the following patients? (check all that apply)
    _____ a. a patient who is in respiratory or cardiac arrest
    _____ b. any patient who is short of breath (SOB)
    _____ c. a patient with a decreased or deteriorating level of responsiveness
    _____ d. a patient who has suffered a severe blood loss
    _____ e. a patient with multiple fractures
    _____ f. a patient who is sweating, anxious, and complaining of chest pain

failing heart may be hypoxic and need oxygen. These signs and symptoms, and the conditions with which they are associated, are covered in other chapters.

## Oxygen Delivery/Ventilation Adjuncts

A number of different adjuncts are available for delivering oxygen to a patient or for assisting ventilations. The method of delivery you choose must be tailored to meet the patient's needs, and OEC Technicians must be very familiar with the indications, set-up, and use of each airway delivery adjunct. OEC Technicians may use the following oxygen-delivery devices:

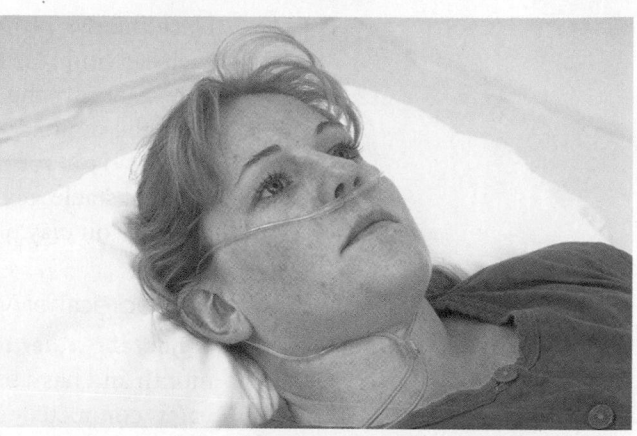

**Figure 9-21** A nasal cannula.

+ Nasal cannula
+ Nonrebreather mask
+ Bag-valve mask

### Nasal Cannula

A **nasal cannula (NC)** is a flexible, circular tube that is attached to a long clear hose (Figure 9-21■). It has two short, pliable hollow prongs for passively delivering small amounts of oxygen, or "low-flow" oxygen, into the patient's nostrils. When the two short prongs are inserted (concave down) into the patient's nostrils, the nasopharynx is filled with oxygen-enriched air that is then inhaled into the lungs. The range of flow rates of a nasal cannula is 1–6 LPM, with 2–4 LPM being the typical initial rate of administration (Table 9-4■). This delivers an oxygen concentration of 24–44 percent. The actual percentage of oxygen varies according to whether the patient breathes exclusively through the nose or also through the mouth. A nasal cannula is quite comfortable and is usually well tolerated.

Patients often prefer a nasal cannula over oxygen-delivery masks because it is less restrictive and because not covering the nose and mouth provokes less anxiety.

Nasal cannulas do have several drawbacks. Prolonged use is associated with drying of the nasal passages. In addition, at low rates (1–3 LPM) the delivery of oxygen is minimal. Thus this adjunct is not recommended for use on patients who require high concentrations of oxygen, such as those who exhibit signs of respiratory distress or shock or have severe chest pain. However, for patients who refuse to wear a mask that delivers a higher concentration of $O_2$, the use of a nasal cannula at 2–4 LPM is better than providing no supplemental oxygen at all.

To apply a nasal cannula, attach the connector at the end of the connecting tubing to the Christmas tree on the regulator. Set the oxygen regulator to the desired flow rate in LPM. Slide the lariat lock (a slide lock found on the nasal cannula tubing that is adjustable and holds the cannula in place on the patients face) to its full open position, and

**nasal cannula (NC)**  an airway adjunct that consists of plastic tubing with two open prongs that are inserted into the patient's nostrils; provides low-flow oxygen when connected to an oxygen source.

| Table 9-4 | Data on Oxygen Delivery Through a Nasal Cannula |
|---|---|
| **Flow Rate** | **Percentage of Oxygen Delivered** |
| 1 LPM | 24% |
| 2 LPM | 28% |
| 3 LPM | 32% |
| 4 LPM | 36% |
| 5 LPM | 40% |
| 6 LPM | 44% |

place the two prongs into the patient's nostrils while looping the cannula tubing over each ear. Slide the lariat lock up so that it holds the cannula in place. Check with the patient to ensure the lariat lock is not too tight and that the device is comfortable. Do not place the cannula completely over the patient's head because this is both uncomfortable and could put the patient in danger should a portion of the loose hose become snagged on an obstacle such as a tree branch or rock. If the patient tends to breathe through the mouth, you may place the two prongs at the entrance to the patient's mouth.

### Nonrebreather Mask

**nonrebreather mask (NRB)** an oxygen delivery device that has a mask, a one-way flow valve, and a reservoir bag; when connected to an oxygen tank, provides a high concentration of supplemental oxygen.

A **nonrebreather mask (NRB)** is a clear plastic mask that covers both the nose and mouth and has a bag (the reservoir) that hangs beneath the mask (Figure 9-22■). This bag is connected to connecting tubing that continually fills the reservoir with oxygen. Each time the patient takes a breath, oxygen within the reservoir is drawn into the mask and inhaled into the lungs. During exhalations, the flap valve on top of the reservoir closes while the flap valve(s) on each side of the mask open while the reservoir refills with oxygen. Thus, the patient cannot "rebreathe" expired gases and breathes only oxygen during inhalation.

As a result of this design, a nonrebreather mask can deliver 80–90 percent oxygen to the patient and has a flow rate of 10–15 LPM. The actual amount of oxygen delivered depends on the flow rate and the face seal (Table 9-5■).

A nonrebreather mask is the most common oxygen delivery device used by OEC Technicians and is appropriate for patients who have serious respiratory, cardiac, or trauma-related problems.

The main disadvantage of a nonrebreather mask is that the mask covers both the nose and the mouth, which can cause the patient anxiety. Communication with the patient can also be difficult due to the mask's position over the mouth and the noise of oxygen flow, especially at higher flow rates. Reassurance and calming techniques frequently relieve the patient's anxiety greatly.

To prepare an NRB for use, remove the mask from its protective wrapper and connect the attached connecting tubing to the regulator. Set the regulator at the desired flow rate, usually 12–15 LPM while simultaneously holding down the flap valve lo-

**Figure 9-22** A nonrebreather mask.

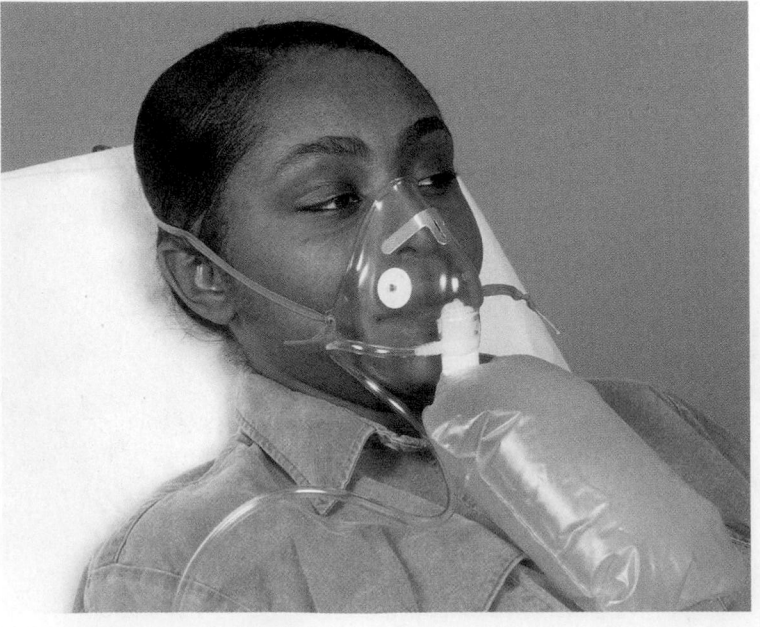
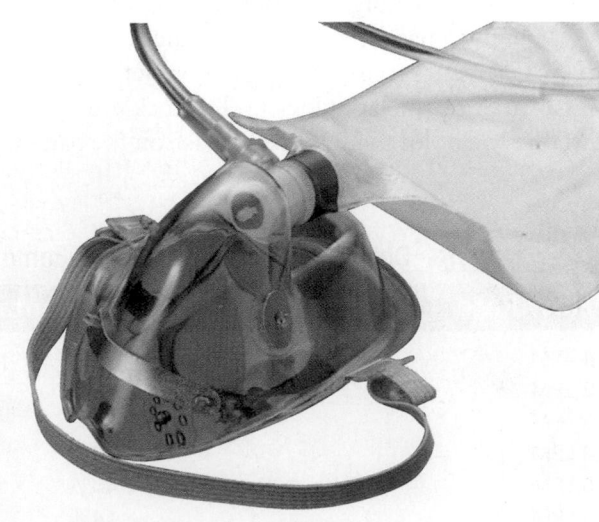

| Table 9-5 | Data on Oxygen Delivery Through a Nonrebreather Mask |
| --- | --- |
| **Flow Rate** | **Percentage of Oxygen Delivered** |
| 10 LPM | 80% |
| 11 LPM | 82% |
| 12 LPM | 84% |
| 13 LPM | 86% |
| 14 LPM | 88% |
| 15 LPM | 90% |

cated inside the nose piece of the mask until the reservoir completely inflates. Next, place the mask on the patient's face, placing the elastic strap behind the patient's head to help hold the mask in place. Once the mask is properly positioned on the patient's face, gently squeeze the aluminum nose piece to help ensure a good seal. Then, observe while the patient breathes. Upon each inspiration, the reservoir bag should deflate by about two-thirds of its total volume.

To conserve oxygen, such as might be required during a prolonged rescue operation, decrease the flow rate. However, do not lower the oxygen flow rate to the point at which the reservoir becomes completely empty between breaths. Adjust the oxygen flow to a level that nearly, but not completely, allows the bag to fully collapse when the patient inhales.

## Bag-Valve Mask

**Bag-valve mask (BVM)** is the device that OEC Technicians use most widely for ventilating patients who are not breathing, need assisted ventilation, or are critically ill or injured. The system typically consists of an oxygen reservoir, a football–size self-expanding bag, a one-way valve, a universal adaptor, and a clear flexible mask (Figure 9-23a■). The BVM is typically constructed from silicone, whereas the reservoir and universal adapter are generally fashioned from plastic. The unit should be latex free.

The system can deliver ambient air, or it may be connected to a supplemental oxygen supply. The flow rate for this device is 12–15 LPM, which delivers 80–100 percent oxygen, depending on the quality of the seal of the face mask. The volume delivered also can vary, depending on bag size and depth of ventilation (Table 9-6■).

BVMs come in three basic sizes: adult, child, and infant (Figure 9-23b■). When the appropriate size bag is used, the device should automatically deliver the correct

**bag-valve mask (BVM)** a manually operated resuscitator consisting of three components: a bag reservoir, a one-way flow valve, and a face mask; used to assist patient ventilations.

**Figure 9-23a** A bag-valve mask unit with an oxygen reservoir.

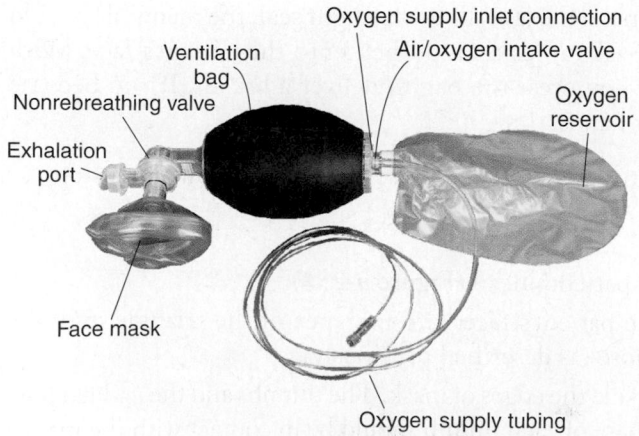

Oxygen supply inlet connection
Ventilation bag
Air/oxygen intake valve
Nonrebreathing valve
Oxygen reservoir
Exhalation port
Face mask
Oxygen supply tubing

| Table 9-6 | Bag-Valve Mask Ventilation Volumes |
| --- | --- |
| **Size** | **Volume** |
| Adult | 1,200–1,600 mL |
| Pediatric | 500–700 mL |
| Infant | 150–240 mL |

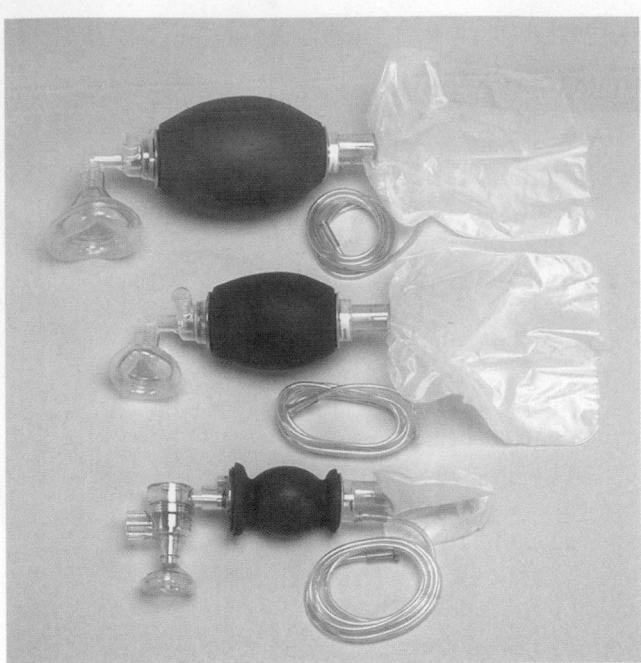

**Figure 9-23b** Bag-valve mask units for adults, children, and infants.

volume of oxygen per breath. As noted previously, a BVM can be used with or without supplemental oxygen. When available, oxygen should be used. A BVM is ergonomically designed to enable a rescuer to ventilate and deliver large quantities of oxygen to a patient for an extended period of time.

In addition, the system is hand operated, resulting in greater safety for the patient and less fatigue for the operator compared to either a face shield or pocket mask. However, the BVM setup is larger than some of the other oxygen-delivery devices and is usually included as part of a large medical backpack, not in a small medical belt or pack.

A BVM can be used effectively by one or two rescuers. Two people are recommended because this provides the most effective method for obtaining a good seal and more effective ventilations.

To use a BVM, it must first be assembled. Most rescuers store the self-expanding bag in its collapsed form, as this saves space in the rescue pack. Begin by pulling both ends of the bag outward to fully expand the bag. Connect the reservoir. Attach the oxygen tubing from the BVM to the oxygen regulator, and set the flow rate to 15 LPM. The reservoir should begin to fill immediately. Attach the universal, L-shaped adapter to the other end of the bag. Then, connect the face mask to the universal adapter. The system is now ready to use.

A properly sized oral or nasal airway should be inserted into the patient before using a BVM to help keep the airway open when assisting with ventilation.

**One-Rescuer BVM**    The one-rescuer BVM technique should be used only when other rescuers are not available to assist (Figure 9-24■). To perform one-rescuer BVM ventilations, follow these steps:

1. Kneel next to the top of the patient's head.
2. Place the mask on the patient's face with the apex (top) of the mask over the bridge of the patient's nose. The mask should be rocked down so that the base of the triangle fits in the groove between the patient's lower lip and chin. If it does not fit in this way, the mask may be an inappropriate size or may need to be repositioned.
3. With your nondominant hand, place your thumb on the mask over the bridge of the patient's nose, and your index finger on the mask over the patient's lower lip, forming a "C" shape around the mask-valve opening.
4. With your little, ring and middle fingers, grasp the underside of the patient's mandible.
5. Pull upward with the fingers on the jaw. To form a tight seal, the mandible should be pulled up toward the mask rather than pushed onto the patient's face. With your dominant hand, fully compress the bag to deliver a breath. If you become tired, you can reverse your hands.

**Figure 9-24** A one-rescuer breathing assist using a bag-valve mask.
Copyright Scott Smith

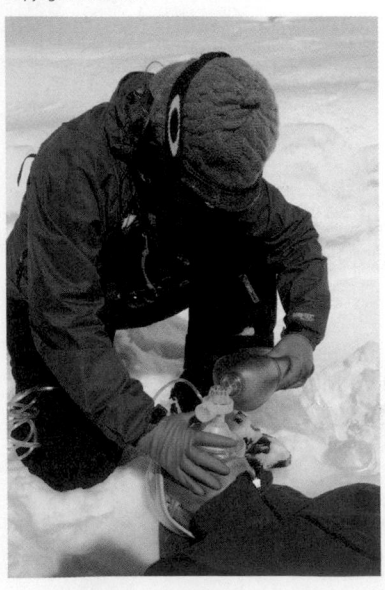

**Two-Person BVM**    To perform two-person BVM ventilations, follow these steps:

✦   Rescuer #1:
   1. Kneel to the side of the patient's head (Figure 9-25■).
   2. Place the mask onto the patient's face with the apex of the triangle over the bridge of the patient's nose (as described previously).
   3. Place your thumbs alongside the edges of mask. The thumbs and the padded portions of the palm at the base of each thumb should be in contact with the mask.

**4.** Using the middle, ring, and little fingers of each hand, grasp the underside of the mandible and pull upward. As before, the mandible should be pulled up toward the mask rather than pushing the mask onto the face.

+ Rescuer #2:

**1.** Kneel beside Rescuer #1, near the top of the patient's head.

**2.** Fully squeeze the bag with both hands to deliver the full volume of air in the bag.

## Pulse Oximetry

A pulse oximeter is a noninvasive device that evaluates oxygenation at the tissue level by measuring oxygen saturation of hemoglobin in red blood cells (Figure 9-26a■). The device has a photoelectric sensing probe that, when clipped onto a finger or an earlobe, measures the oxygenation of the blood in the capillaries (Figures 9-26b■ and 9-26c■). Under normal conditions, oxygen saturation should be above 95 percent when the patient is breathing ambient air at sea level.

Pulse oximetry is a useful tool because it provides quantitative data on the effectiveness of a patient's ventilation efforts. As a rule, patients with an oxygen saturation of less than 95 percent should be placed on oxygen. Patients with an $O_2$ saturation of greater than 95 percent but are experiencing difficulty breathing should likewise be placed on oxygen. When administering oxygen to a patient, adjust the flow rate such that an oxygen saturation level greater than 95 percent is achieved.

Pulse oximetry, like other diagnostic instruments, is not foolproof and should not be used as the sole method of assessing oxygenation because false readings can occur. Factors that can cause false readings include nail polish, cold weather, shock, carbon monoxide poisoning, a low red blood cell count, and device malfunction. Clinical assessment of the patient generally is more reliable than a **pulse oximeter**. Thus even if pulse oximetry indicates that a patient's oxygen saturation is 100 percent, if they are visibly in respiratory distress, administer supplemental oxygen as allowed by local protocol.

## Gastric Distention

Whenever artificial ventilations are provided, it is common for the patient's stomach to fill with air, which can lead to abdominal bloating, a condition more properly known as **gastric distention**. This condition occurs when the amount of ventilatory pressure exceeds the pressure keeping the opening of the esophagus closed, causing

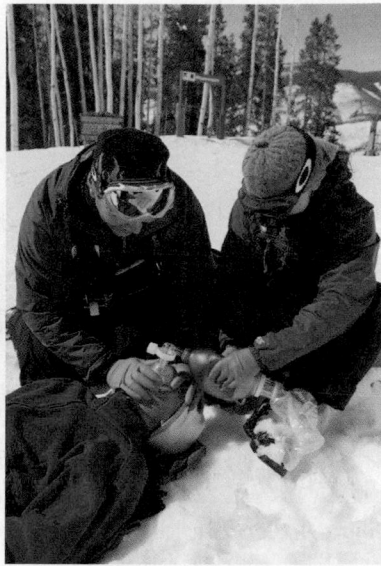

**Figure 9-25** A two-rescuer breathing assist using a bag-valve mask.
Copyright Scott Smith

**pulse oximeter** a device that attaches to a patient's finger, toe, or earlobe and photoelectrically measures blood oxygen content as percent of oxygen saturation.

**gastric distention** inflation of the stomach with air; can lead to vomiting.

**Figure 9-26a** A pulse oximeter, which evaluates oxygenation at the tissue level.

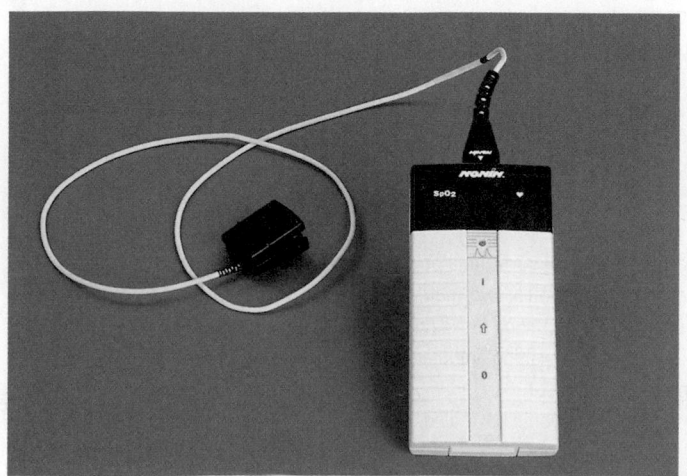

**Figure 9-26b** A pulse oximeter, as normally placed on the finger of an adult.

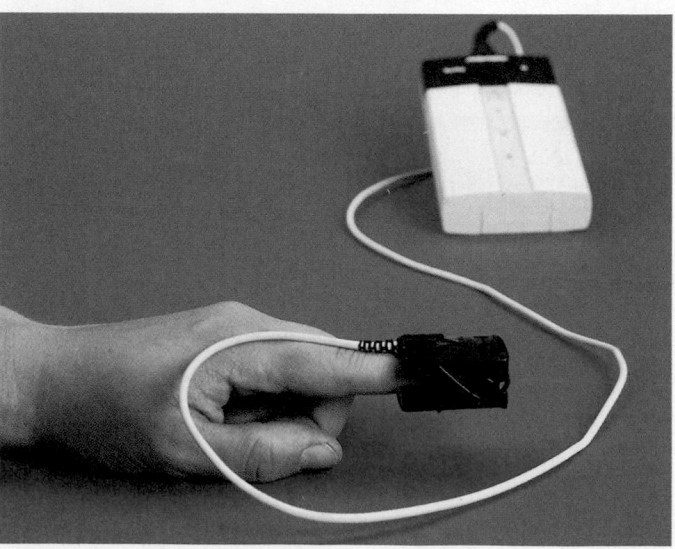

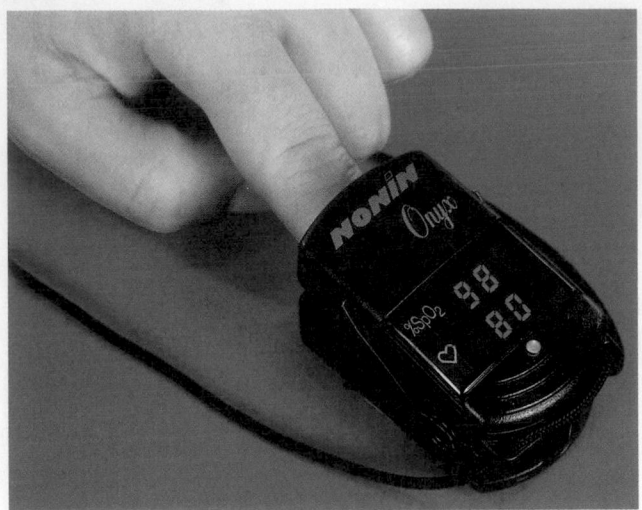

**Figure 9-26c** A mini "finger-sized" pulse oximeter.

air or oxygen to be directed down the esophagus and into the stomach. Partial or total obstruction of the upper airway also can cause gastric distention to occur. The condition is more common in children than in adults but can be prevented by administering slow, gentle breaths or by squeezing the bag over two full seconds.

Gastric distention is not without complications. It can cause vomiting or more-injurious aspiration of gastric contents into the lungs. In addition, gastric distention can restrict movement of the diaphragm, which can decrease the effectiveness of ventilations.

If the stomach becomes distended, make sure the airway is open. Do not push on a distended stomach because the result is nearly always vomiting, which can lead to aspiration of the vomit. If the patient does vomit, place the patient on his side, suction the airway, and then resume rescue breathing.

## STOP, THINK, UNDERSTAND

### Multiple Choice
Choose the correct answer.

1. Pulse oximetry provides rescuers with what data? _____
   a. hematocrit level
   b. patient's respiratory rate
   c. absolute data to determine whether or not oxygen administration is needed
   d. quantitative data regarding the effectiveness of a patient's ventilatory efforts

2. Under normal conditions and when breathing ambient air, in what range should a healthy individual's pulse oximetry level fall?
   _____
   a. 72–80 percent
   b. 82–90 percent

   c. 95–100 percent
   d. OEC Technicians cannot rely on pulse oximetry levels due to the adverse environment in which these parameters are usually measured.

3. Which of the following statements about gastric distension is true? _____
   a. It can be caused by artificial ventilations.
   b. It is caused when ventilatory pressure exceeds the pressure holding the opening of the esophagus closed.
   c. It is more common in children than adults.
   d. All of the above are true.

### Fill in the Blank

1. The three oxygen delivery adjuncts are _____, _____, and _____.

2. Some of the factors that can cause false pulse oximetry readings are _____.

 **CASE DISPOSITION**

You insert an OPA and begin providing artificial respirations using a pocket mask. As other providers and equipment arrive, you request that another OEC Technician assist you in two-man ventilation using a BVM, and you suction the patient as needed. You assist the team in immobilizing the patient's head and spine and placing him onto a toboggan. His arm was splinted. He is then transported to a waiting ambulance. You later learn that the patient had a severe head injury. The neurosurgeon who treated the patient credits you and your team for your effective airway management, without which, she states, the patient would have died.

# OEC SKILL 9-1 | Suctioning a Patient's Airway

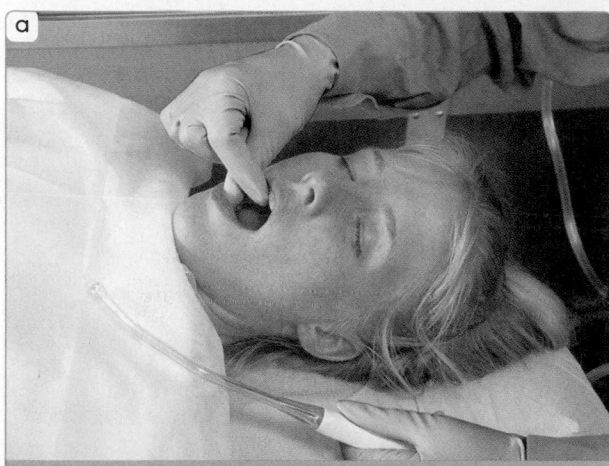

Open and clear the patient's mouth.

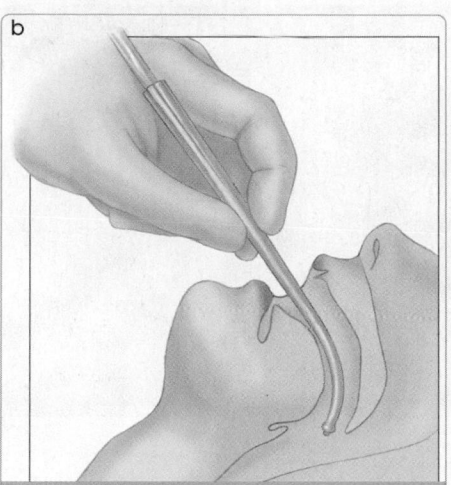

Insert the tip of the catheter no farther than the base of the tongue, making sure you can still see the tip of the catheter.

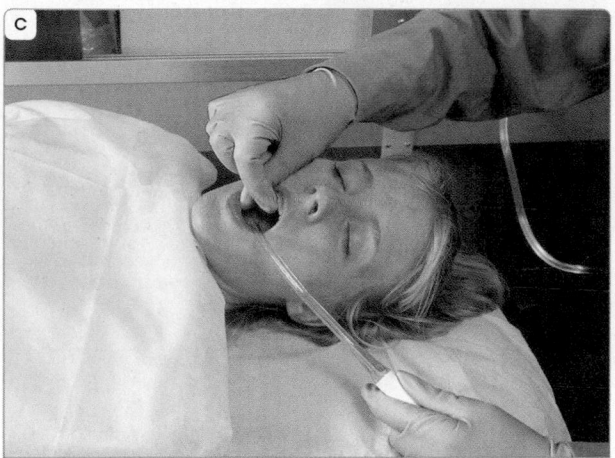

Suction while withdrawing the tip; suction for 10–15 seconds at a time in an adult.

# OEC SKILL 9-2 | Inserting a Nasopharyngeal Airway

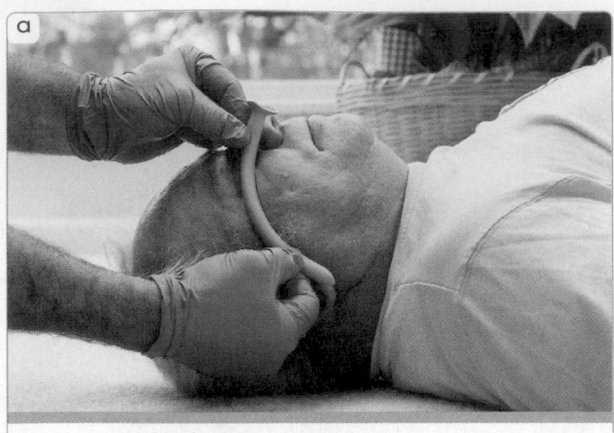

a

Measure the nasopharyngeal airway.

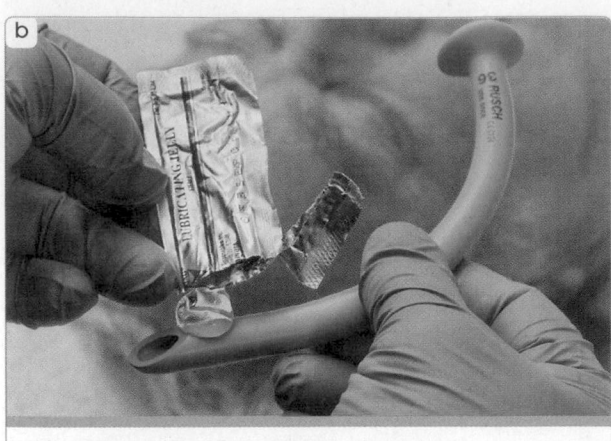

b

Moisten the airway with a water-soluble lubricant.

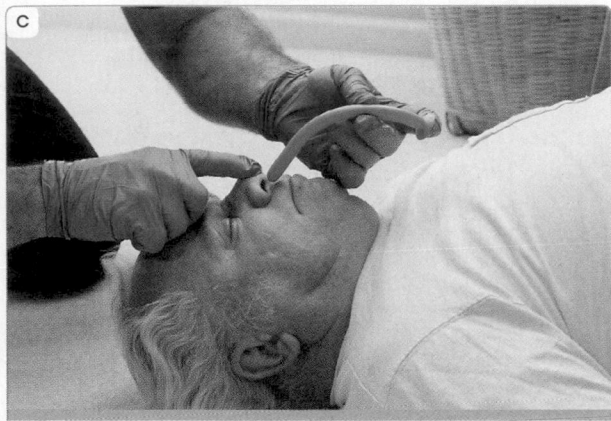

c

Insert the airway with the bevel toward the base of the tonsil.

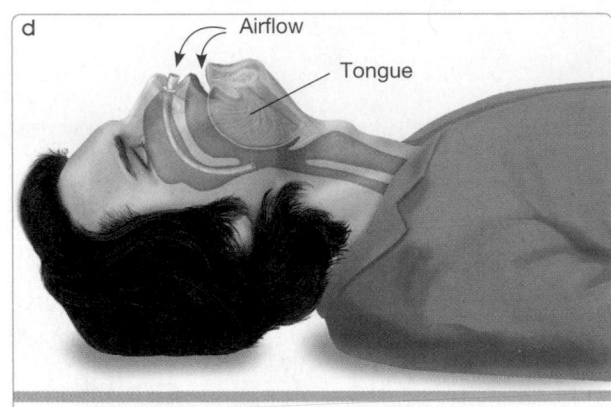

d

Airflow

Tongue

A nasopharyngeal airway that is properly placed.

# OEC SKILL 9-3 | Inserting an Oropharyngeal Airway

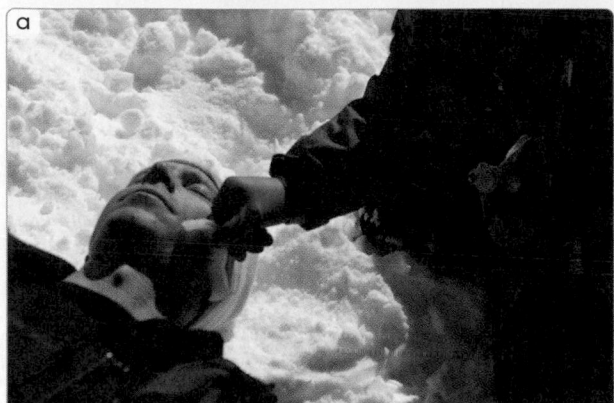

a

Size the airway by measuring from the corner of the mouth to the ear.
Copyright Scott Smith

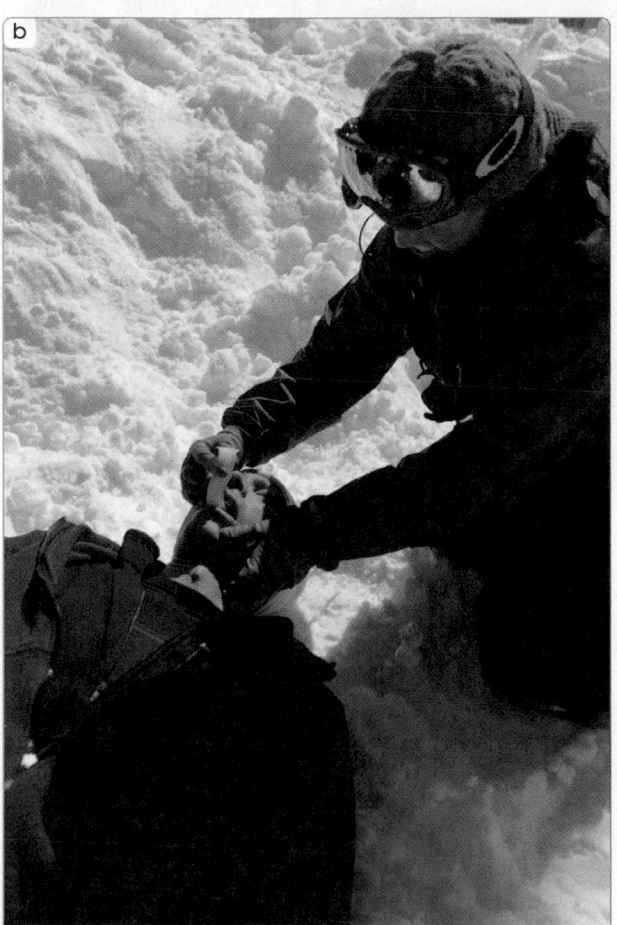

b

Insert the airway using the crossed-finger technique to open the mouth.
Copyright Scott Smith

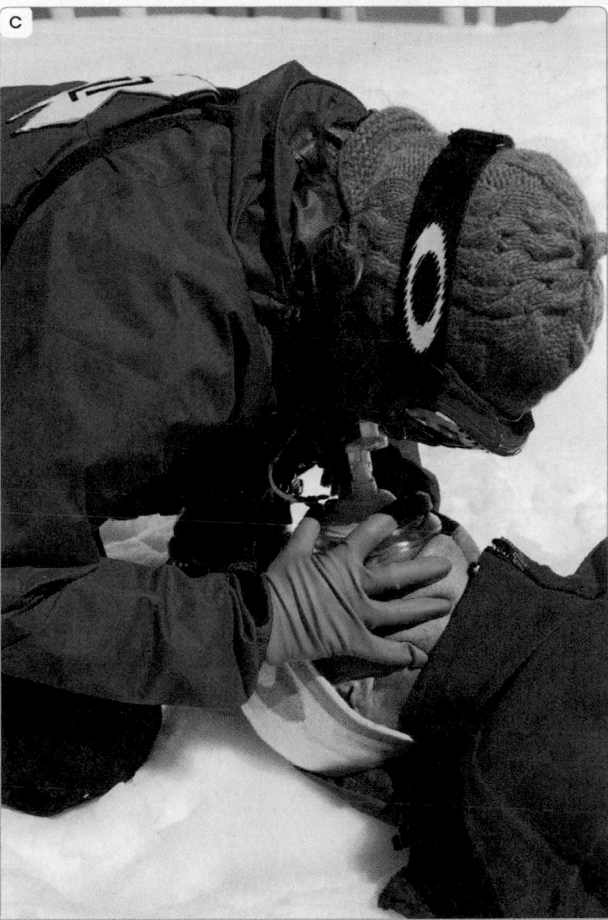

c

Check for airway patency by ventilating the patient.
Copyright Scott Smith

# OEC SKILL 9-4 | Oxygen Tank Set-Up and Breakdown

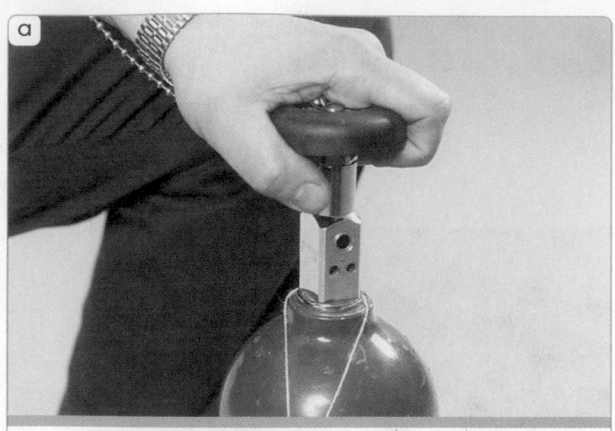

a

"Crack" the main valve for 1 second.

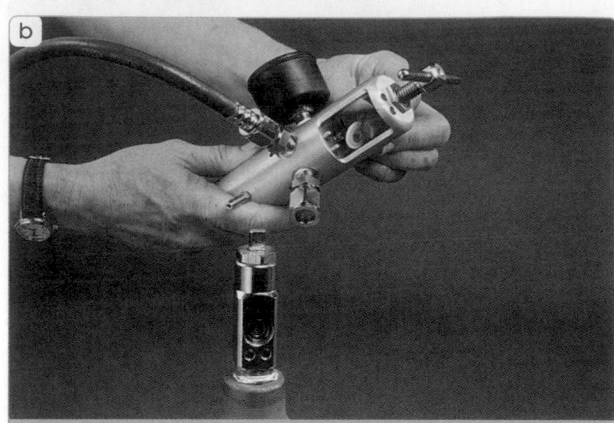

b

Select the correct pressure regulator and then place the cylinder valve gasket on the regulator oxygen port.

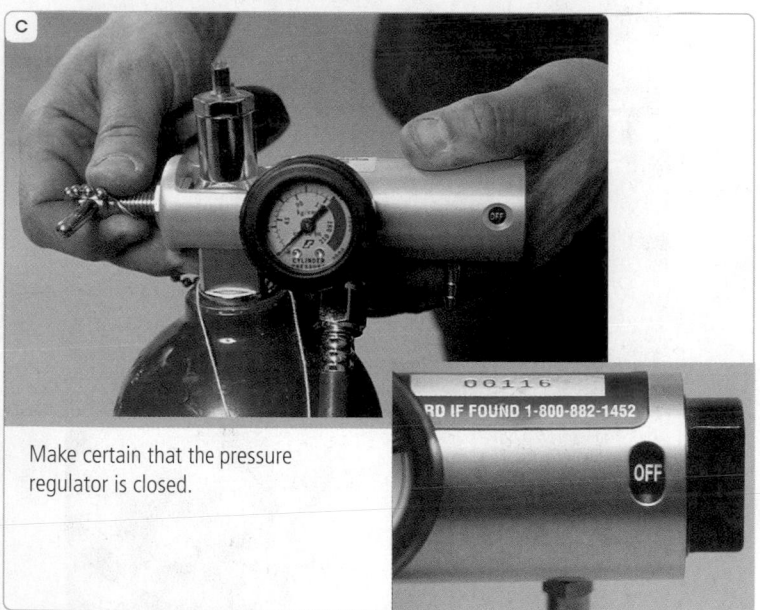

c

Make certain that the pressure regulator is closed.

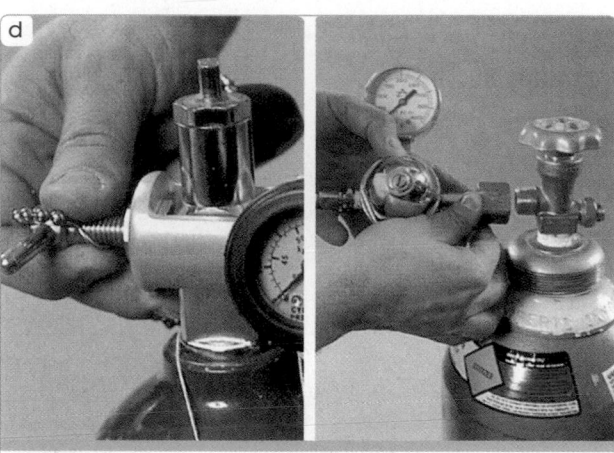

d

Align pins (left) or thread by hand (right).

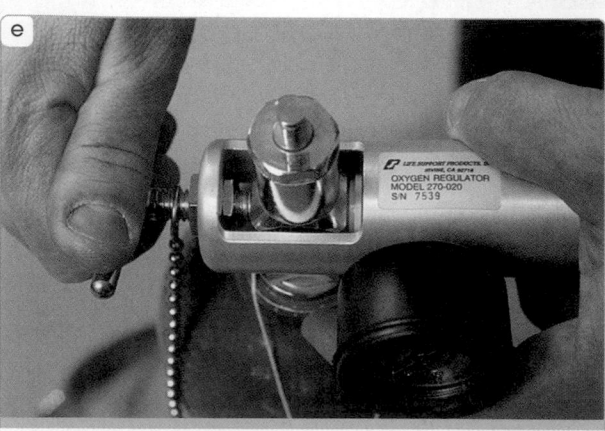

e

Tighten the T-screw for a pin yoke . . .

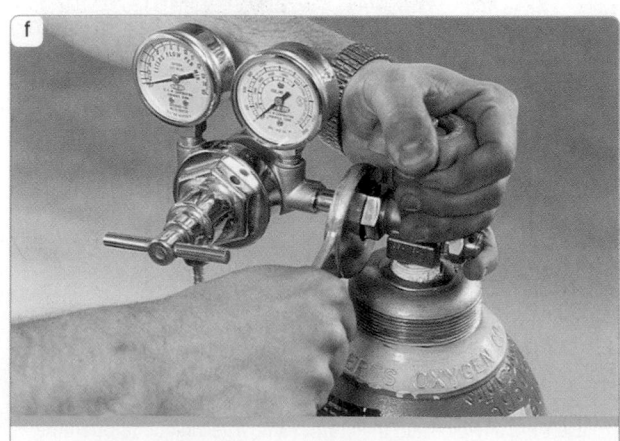

f

. . . or tighten a threaded outlet with a wrench or key.

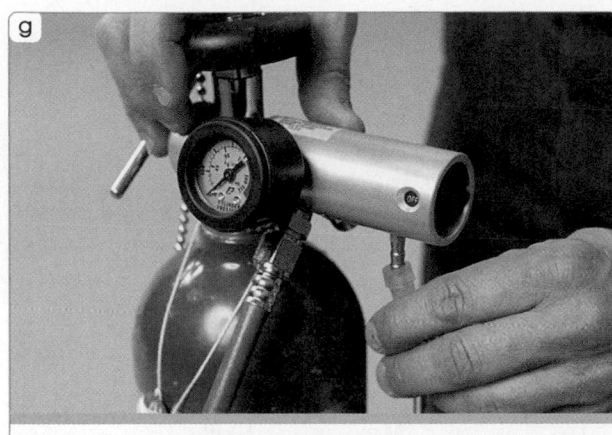

Attach tubing and delivery device.

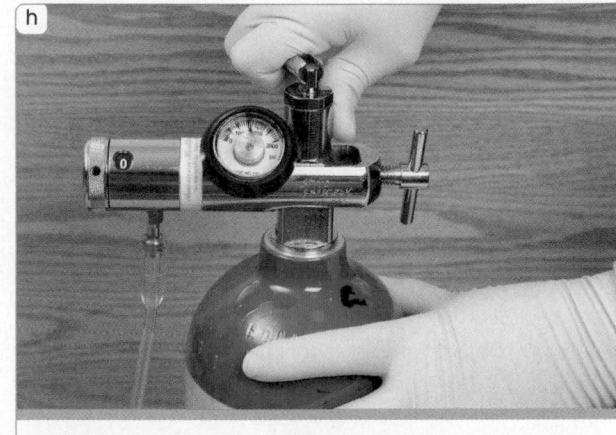

Turn the cylinder on by opening the main valve.

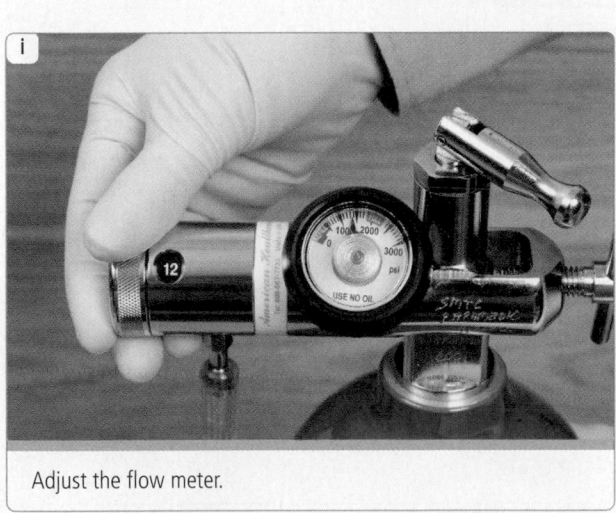

Adjust the flow meter.

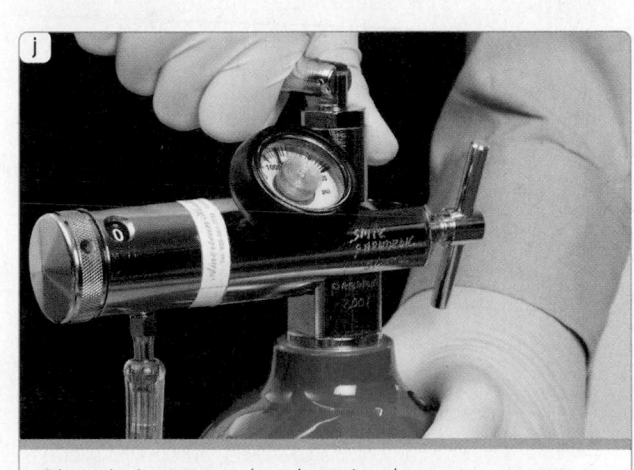

Discontinuing oxygen: close the main valve.

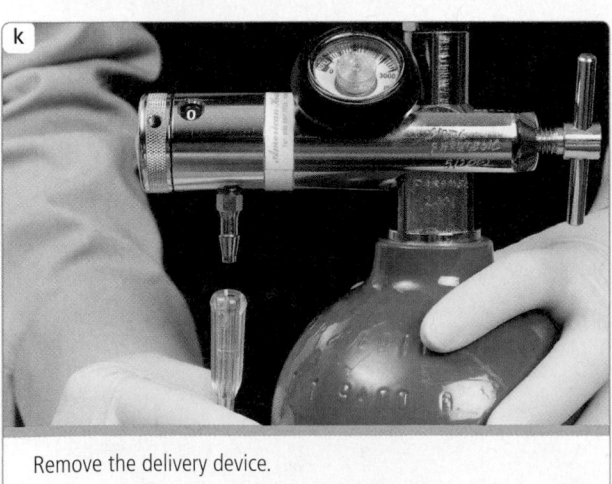

Remove the delivery device.

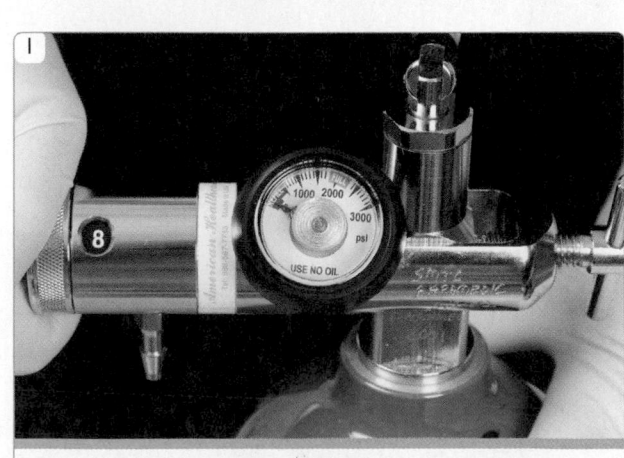

Bleed the flow meter: turn the oxygen flow knob counterclockwise (open) until you no longer hear air escape. Check the pressure gauge to ensure that the pressure is at "0" psi.

## Skill Guide

Date: _____

(CPI) = Critical Performance Indicator

Candidate: _____

Start Time: _____

End Time: _____

## Suctioning a Patient's Airway

**Objective:** To demonstrate proper suctioning of a patient's airway.

| Skill | Max Points | Skill Demo | |
|---|---|---|---|
| Initiate Standard Precautions. | 1 | | (CPI) |
| Make sure the suctioning unit is properly assembled and turn on the unit if using a power system. | 1 | | |
| Pre-oxygenate patient prior to suctioning. | 1 | | |
| Open the patient's mouth and insert the catheter only as far as you can see. | 1 | | (CPI) |
| Apply suction in a side to side or circular motion as you withdraw the catheter. | 1 | | |
| Do not suction an adult for more than 15 seconds. | 1 | | (CPI) |

Must receive 4 out of 6 points.

Comments: _____

Failure of any of the CPIs is an automatic failure.

Evaluator: _____  NSP ID: _____

PASS     FAIL

## Skill Guide

Date: _____

(CPI) = Critical Performance Indicator

Candidate: _____

Start Time: _____

End Time: _____

## Inserting Nasopharyngeal Airway (NPA)

**Objective:** To properly insert a nasopharyngeal airway into a patient.

| Skill | Max Points | Skill Demo | |
|---|:---:|:---:|:---:|
| Initiate Standard Precautions. | 1 | | (CPI) |
| Size the airway. Place the flange against the nostril, and the end should touch the patient's lower earlobe. Coat the tip and the entire length with a water-based lubricant. | 1 | | |
| Insert the lubricated airway into the larger nostril with the curvature following the floor of the nose. If you are using the right nare, the bevel should face the septum. If using the left nare, insert the airway with the tip of the airway pointing upward, which will allow the bevel to face the septum. | 1 | | (CPI) |
| Gently advance the airway. If using the left nare, insert the nasopharyngeal airway until resistance is met. Then rotate the nasopharyngeal airway 180 into position. This rotation is not required if using the right nostril. | 1 | | (CPI) |
| Continue until the flange rests against the skin. If you feel any resistance or obstruction, remove the airway and insert it into the other nostril. | 1 | | |

| Must receive 4 out of 5 points. |
|---|

Comments: _____

Failure of any of the CPIs is an automatic failure.

Evaluator: _____  NSP ID:_____

PASS      FAIL

## Skill Guide

Date: _____

(CPI) = Critical Performance Indicator

Candidate: _____

Start Time: _____

End Time: _____

## Inserting an Oropharyngeal Airway (OPA)

**Objective:** To measure and insert an oral airway into an adult.

| Skill | Max Points | Skill Demo | |
|---|---|---|---|
| Initiate Standard Precautions. | 1 | | (CPI) |
| Hold the adjunct against the side of the face with the flange adjacent to the corner of the patient's mouth. Size the airway by measuring from the patient's earlobe to the corner of the mouth or from the corner of the mouth to the angle of the jaw. | 1 | | (CPI) |
| Open the patient's mouth with the cross-finger technique. Hold the airway upside down with your other hand. Insert the airway with the tip facing the roof of the mouth and slide it in until it is half way into the mouth. | 1 | | (CPI) |
| Rotate the airway 180°. Insert the airway until the flange rests on the patient's lips. | 1 | | (CPI) |

| Must receive 4 out of 4 points. |
|---|

Comments: _____

Failure of any of the CPIs is an automatic failure.

Evaluator: _____ NSP ID: _____

PASS     FAIL

## Skill Guide

Date: _____

(CPI) = Critical Performance Indicator

Candidate: _____

Start Time: _____

End Time: _____

## Oxygen Tank Set-up and Breakdown

**Objective:** To prepare a new $O_2$ tank and apply the regulator for use.

| Skill | Max Points | Skill Demo | |
|---|---|---|---|
| Inspect the tank, regulator, and O ring or washer for any visible damage. | 1 | | |
| Using an oxygen wrench or the valve stem on the top of the cylinder turn the valve counterclockwise to slowly "crack" the cylinder for 1 second. | 1 | | (CPI) |
| Attach the regulator/flow meter to the valve stem using the two pin-indexing holes and make sure that the washer is in place over the larger hole. Do not overtighten. | 1 | | |
| Open the $O_2$ system by turning the valve stem on top of the cylinder or using the wrench, counterclockwise. | 1 | | |
| Check for/correct any leaks. Check for adequate pressure in tank. | 1 | | |
| Attach the oxygen connective tubing to the flow meter. | 1 | | |
| Set the regulator to the proper flow based on the delivery device. | 1 | | (CPI) |
| Secure the bottle from falling. | 1 | | (CPI) |
| Close regulator and release pressure from tank. | 1 | | (CPI) |
| Remove regulator from tank. | 1 | | |

| Must receive 8 out of 10 points. |
|---|

Comments:_____

Failure of any of the CPIs is an automatic failure.

Evaluator: _____ NSP ID: _____

PASS     FAIL

# ⛨ Chapter Review

## Chapter Summary

The ability to manage a patient's airway is among the most important and fundamental skills every OEC Technician must master. Without an intact, open, and clear airway, a patient will quickly die. As a result of their training, OEC Technicians have several options to open, clear, and maintain a patient's airway. In addition, they are able to provide a patient with supplemental oxygen using a variety of different delivery devices. The combination of these skills and adjuncts are all critical for ensuring that a patient's airway and breathing are preserved. By mastering airway procedures and initiating them quickly when indicated, patient survival can dramatically increase.

## Remember...

1. Airway management is a skill that every OEC Technician must master. PRACTICE OFTEN! The head-tilt, chin-lift maneuver is the preferred technique for medical patients; the jaw thrust must be used for trauma patients with a head or neck injury and may be used on medical patients. The recovery position can help keep a patient's airway clear.
2. NPA insertion is easy when you use "SLIC."
3. An OPA should be inserted only in a patient who does not have a gag reflex.
4. A barrier device should be used to provide rescue breaths until the arrival of a bag-valve mask and oxygen.
5. A nasal cannula can deliver 24–44 percent oxygen at 1–6 LPM.
6. A nonrebreather mask can deliver 80–90 percent oxygen at 10–15 LPM.
7. A BVM can deliver 80–100 percent oxygen at 12–15 LPM.
8. Continually monitor the airway to ensure that it remains open and clear.

## Chapter Questions

### Multiple Choice

Choose the correct answer.

1. What is the purpose of the three-hole system on medical oxygen cylinders? _____
   a. It has no purpose beyond correctly and securely attaching the regulator to the cylinder.
   b. It ensures that no other type of gas can inadvertently be administered to a patient requiring oxygen.
   c. It limits the maximum flow rate on a cylinder to between 2,000 and 2,200 psi.
   d. It fixes the flow rate on a cylinder to 15–25 LPM at 40–70 psi.

2. How long will an oxygen supply last (what is the duration of flow) on a D cylinder that contains 1,500 psi and is set at a flow rate of 15 LPM? _____
   a. less than 10 minutes
   b. just under 15 minutes
   c. between 20 and 30 minutes

## Fill in the Blank

1. Indicate whether you would use jaw thrust or head-tilt, chin-lift as the preferred method in each of the following situations:

   _____ **a.** An unresponsive 20-year-old snowboarder who overshot a terrain park feature and landed on his head

   _____ **b.** An 8-year-old who choked on a pretzel

   _____ **c.** A 14-year-old drowning victim

   _____ **d.** A 17-year-old mountain biker whose mouth is full of blood and broken teeth after he flipped over his handlebars and landed on a boulder

   _____ **e.** A 52-year-old female who has suffered a major heart attack

   _____ **f.** A 27-year-old female who landed head first after falling off her horse

2. Indicate which of the following airway adjuncts should be used for each of the following tasks:

   _____ **1.** suction

   _____ **2.** nasal cannula

   _____ **3.** nonrebreather

   _____ **4.** bag-valve mask

   _____ **5.** pocket mask

   _____ **6.** barrier device

   **a.** clearing an airway of vomitus

   **b.** administering low-flow, passive oxygen to a patient

   **c.** administering oxygen at 1–6 LPM, with 2–4 LPM being typical

   **d.** can deliver 80–90 percent oxygen

   **e.** can deliver 80–100 percent oxygen

   **f.** best device for use on a patient feeling claustrophobic or panicked

   **g.** best used for trauma patients who can breathe well on their own

   **h.** requires filling of a reservoir bag before use

   **i.** a form of personal protective equipment that provides a nonporous layer between you and the patient to prevent the transmission of communicable diseases

   **j.** used at a flow rate of 10–15 LPM

   **k.** used to clean vomit out of the mouth

   **l.** used to ventilate a patient manually when supplemental oxygen, a BVM, a mask, or a nasal cannula are not available

3. A patient who has suffered a major loss of blood and requires high-flow oxygen through a nonrebreather mask is refusing to allow you to place the mask on his face. What should you do?

   _____

   _____

## Scenario

○○○○○○○○○○○○○○○○○○○○○○○○○○○○○○○○○○○○○○○○○○○○○○○○○○○○○○○○○○○

*You are dispatched to aid a skier who has fallen and struck a snow-making machine. Because you are the first to arrive, you secure the scene. A 16-year-old unresponsive female is draped over the machine. Her head is bloodied. You assess her airway, and she is not breathing.*

1. What should you do? _____

   **a.** Make sure she isn't moved until help arrives and proper c-spine procedures can be applied.

   **b.** Apply direct, firm pressure to the wound on her head to control the bleeding.

   **c.** Carefully put her in a position that will enable you to secure an airway using the jaw-thrust technique.

   **d.** Open the airway with a tongue blade.

*You call for a toboggan, a backboard, the trauma pack, and an ALS unit. The requested help arrives. The patient's airway is patent, and she is breathing at 8 breaths per minute and shallow. You decide to insert an OPA to secure the airway.*

2. How should you measure for the correct size of the oropharyngeal airway? _____
   a. from the bottom of the ear to the middle of the mouth
   b. from the bottom of the ear to the tip of the nose
   c. from the bottom of the ear to the corner of the mouth
   d. from the center of the ear to the center of the mouth

*The toboggan and trauma pack now arrive. When attempting to insert the OPA, you are prepared for vomiting and have the manual suction pump assembled and at the patient's side. As the OPA is inserted, the patient presents with a gag reflex.*

3. Your response to the gag reflex is to _____
   a. remove the OPA and suction any vomitus material.
   b. remove the OPA and attempt to reinsert a smaller size.
   c. place the patient in the left lateral recumbent position.
   d. place the patient in a prone position.

*You remove the OPA, and the team uses a bag-valve mask with high-flow oxygen to assist the patient's breathing at a rate of one breath every five seconds.*

*You decide an NPA is the adjunct of choice, and using a water-soluble lubricant you insert the device with the bevel toward the septum in the larger nostril.*

4. Before insertion, the NPA is measured _____
   a. from the earlobe to the edge of the mouth.
   b. from the top of the ear to the middle of the nostril.
   c. from middle of the ear to the middle of the nostril.
   d. from the tip of the nose to the patient's earlobe.

# Shock

Michael Levy, MD, FACP, FAAEM
Jennifer Dow, MD, FACEP, FAWM

## ⊕ OBJECTIVES

**Upon completion of this chapter, the OEC Technician will be able to:**

**10-1** Define shock.

**10-2** Describe the basic components of the cardiovascular system:

    a. blood
    b. heart
    c. blood vessels

**10-3** Describe the key components of blood.

**10-4** Define cardiac output.

**10-5** Compare and contrast the three stages of shock.

**10-6** List the four types of shock.

**10-7** Describe how the body compensates for shock.

**10-8** List the classic signs and symptoms of shock.

**10-9** Describe and demonstrate the management of shock.

## ⊕ KEY TERMS

**anticoagulant,** *p. 345*
**cardiac output,** *p. 332*
**diaphoresis,** *p. 345*
**erythrocyte,** *p. 332*
**hemoglobin,** *p. 333*

**occult,** *p. 337*
**oxygen saturation,** *p. 333*
**platelets,** *p. 333*
**resistance blood vessel,** *p. 332*
**sepsis,** *p. 340*

**shock,** *p. 329*
**stroke volume,** *p. 332*
**tachycardia,** *p. 335*
**tachypnea,** *p. 335*

## Chapter Overview

The human body is a remarkable machine composed of a marvelous and complex web of interacting systems that produce a relatively constant internal environment known as homeostasis. When one or more of these systems becomes seriously impaired through injury or illness, the results can be life threatening. One of the most serious threats to life is the condition known as **shock**, or hypoperfusion. Shock is defined as failure of the circulatory system to maintain adequate blood flow to tissues, resulting

*continued*

## HISTORICAL TIMELINE

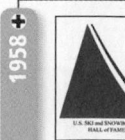

**1958**

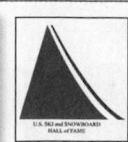

Minnie Dole inducted into the National Ski Hall of Fame.

**1959**

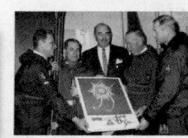

NSP established a national advisory committee related to ski safety.

## CASE PRESENTATION

While patrolling on a snowy ski day with some friends, you notice a gray-haired man leaning on his ski poles near the edge of a groomed run. He appears somewhat shaken, as if he may be taking stock of himself after a fall. You note that the area in which he is currently standing empties onto a slope that has numerous high-speed enthusiasts, despite the day's poor visibility. Skiing over to him, you discover that he was just "run over" by a hit-and-run snowboard rider. He says that the impact definitely "knocked the air out of me" but states that he is feeling better and "just wants to rest awhile." Smiling, the man tells you that even though he is 70, he is not ready to give up the sport he loves. You identify yourself and ask if you can examine him. As you begin your assessment, the man says that he's fine and really doesn't think any examination is necessary. Although he appears a little pale, his radial pulse seems normal, perhaps a little slow. As you gently touch his left upper abdomen and chest, he winces slightly. By now, your friends are calling for you to join them. The man repeats that he is fine and says, "Go on, I'm just going to stand here a little longer."

*What should you do?*

---

⊕ **10-1** Define shock.

**shock**  failure of the circulatory system to maintain adequate blood flow to tissues.

in a state of inadequate tissue perfusion in which cells do not receive sufficient amounts of oxygen and nutrients to meet their immediate metabolic needs. Although the potential causes of shock are numerous, shock occurs when one or more components of the cardiovascular system fail. This failure sets into motion a series of events that, unless corrected, may cause other body systems to fail and death to ensue.

Shock is one of the serious problems that OEC Technicians will encounter. Rarely observed alone, shock is frequently associated with various medical and traumatic conditions (Figure 10-1■). Unfortunately, shock is a condition in which the signs and symptoms may not initially be apparent because it may result from several factors. Poor underlying health, overtaxed physiologic compensating mechanisms, or the patient's age and medication use may be present, making shock more difficult to discern at first. For this reason, OEC Technicians must be keenly aware of the causes of shock and the body's responses to it. Using this information, OEC Technicians will

**Figure 10-1** Shock is often associated with many different medical and traumatic conditions.
Copyright Scott Smith

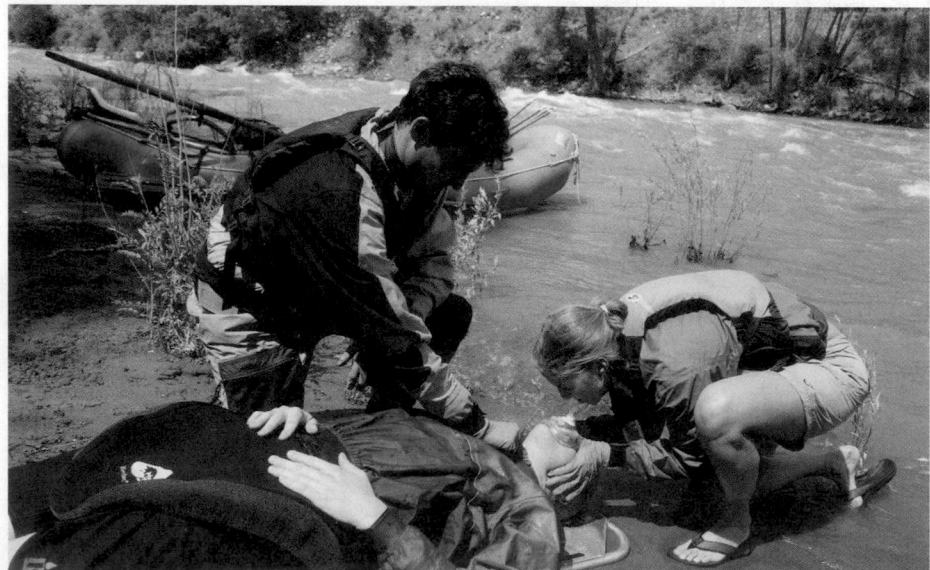

be better able to recognize shock and initiate appropriate treatment. Although the assessment and treatment of the specific causes of shock will be covered in later chapters, this chapter provides ski patrollers and other outdoor-based health care providers a firm understanding of shock, including its causes, its assessment, and treatment priorities.

## Anatomy and Physiology

The cardiovascular system (CVS), which was described in detail in Chapter 6, Anatomy and Physiology, includes the heart, blood vessels, and blood. When functioning properly, the heart pumps oxygenated blood through arterial vessels to the capillaries, where oxygen and carbon dioxide are exchanged at a cellular level. Deoxygenated blood travels through venous blood vessels to the heart, which pumps the blood on to the lungs. There, carbon dioxide is excreted into the atmosphere and the blood is oxygenated and returned to the heart, which begins the cycle anew (Figure 10-2■). Problems affecting any part of the cardiovascular system can disrupt this process, resulting in decreased blood flow, cellular hypoxia, and shock.

**⊕ 10-2** Describe the basic components of the cardiovascular system:

   a. blood

   b. heart

   c. blood vessels

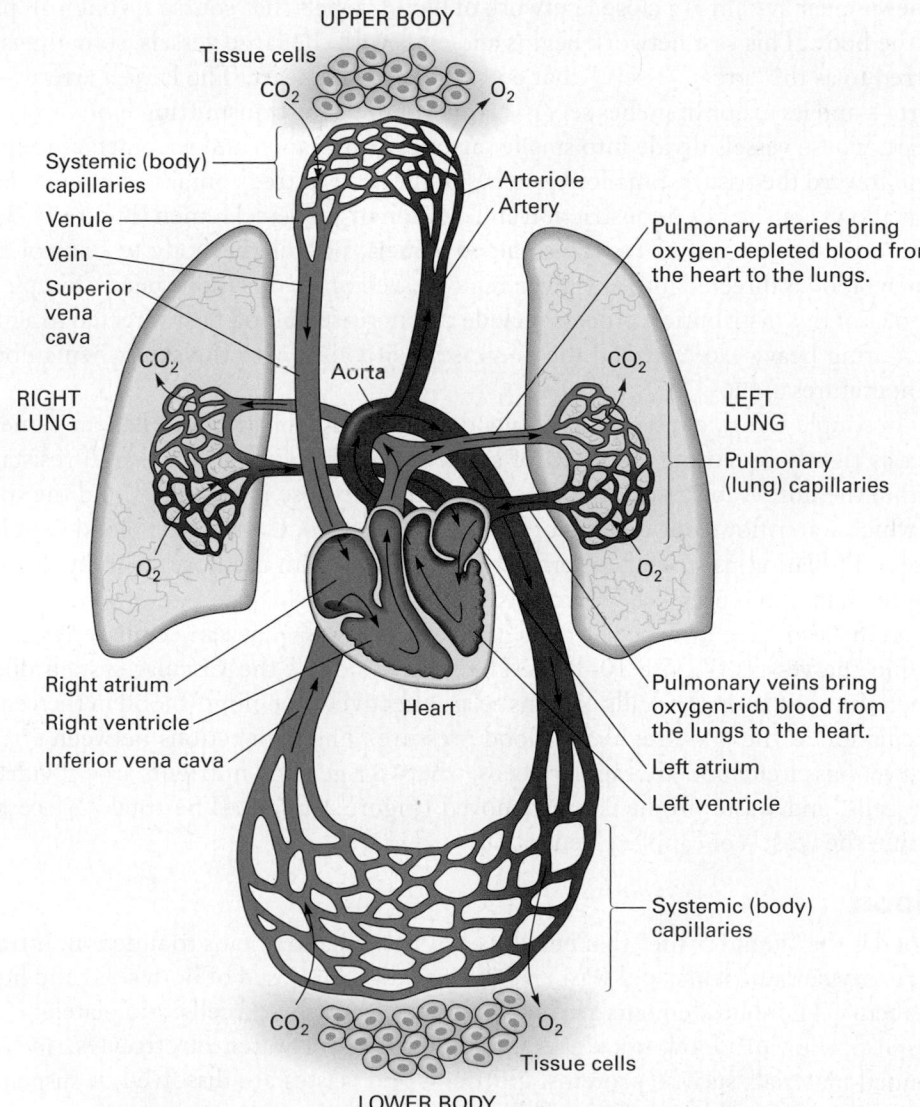

**Figure 10-2** The cardiovascular system circuit; tissue perfusion occurs adjacent to capillary beds throughout the body.

UPPER BODY

Tissue cells

$CO_2$          $O_2$

Systemic (body) capillaries

Arteriole
Artery

Venule

Vein

Superior vena cava

Pulmonary arteries bring oxygen-depleted blood from the heart to the lungs.

$CO_2$          Aorta          $CO_2$

RIGHT LUNG          LEFT LUNG

Pulmonary (lung) capillaries

$O_2$          $O_2$

Right atrium

Right ventricle          Heart

Inferior vena cava

Pulmonary veins bring oxygen-rich blood from the lungs to the heart.

Left atrium

Left ventricle

Systemic (body) capillaries

$CO_2$          $O_2$

Tissue cells

LOWER BODY

⊕ **10-4** Define cardiac output.

**cardiac output**   the volume of blood pumped out of the heart each minute.

**stroke volume**   the volume of blood pumped out of the heart's left ventricle per contraction.

**resistance blood vessel**   a small artery whose wall contains muscle cells capable of contraction; as a result, such vessels can constrict and dilate to redistribute blood flow.

⊕ **10-3** Describe the key components of blood.

**erythrocyte**   a red blood cell.

## The Heart

The heart is a four-chambered, double-sided pump about the size of a clenched fist. It is located near the center of the chest directly deep to the sternum. Specialized cells within the heart generate an electrical impulse that spreads through the walls of this muscular organ in a wavelike fashion, resulting in rhythmic contractions of the heart muscle. The heart's function is to pump blood through arteries to the tissues of the body.

With each contraction, the heart pumps 60–100 mL of blood. The volume of blood that is pumped in one minute is known as **cardiac output** and consists of two components: **stroke volume**, the amount of blood pumped by the heart's left ventricle with each contraction (heartbeat), and heart rate, the number of heartbeats per minute. The product of these two variables equals the cardiac output. For example, if the stroke volume is 80 mL and the heart rate is 70 beats per minute (bpm), then cardiac output is 80 mL x 70 bpm, or 5,600 mL (5.6 liters) per minute. If the heart begins to beat extremely fast, cardiac output is affected, and this formula does not work, because the heart's left ventricle does not have enough time to fully refill with blood. Factors that adversely affect either the heart rate or the stroke volume can reduce the cardiac output, which can lead to shock.

## Blood Vessels

The vascular system is a closed network of blood vessels that course through all parts of the body. This vast network begins and ends with the large vessels, sometimes referred to as the "great vessels," that enter and exit the heart. The largest artery—the aorta—and its major branches serve as large conduits for transmitting blood from the heart. These vessels divide into smaller arteries that branch and rebranch as they extend toward the tissues. Smaller branches of the arterial tree contain a muscular layer that allows considerable constriction and dilation of the vessel lumen (Figure 10-3a■). These vessels, known as **resistance blood vessels**, permit the body to control how much blood is directed into any given region based on its metabolic needs. Simple examples of this distribution process include the increased blood flow directed to a muscle during heavy exercise, and the decrease in blood flow to the skin when ambient temperatures are low.

In simple terms, constriction of blood vessels (vasoconstriction) has the same effect as tightly squeezing a section of a soft garden hose with your hand: resistance within the hose is increased, the pressure within the hose is increased, and the speed at which water flows out the end of the hose is reduced. Conversely, blood vessel relaxation (dilation) is similar to removing your hand from the hose, thereby decreasing resistance and pressure within the hose, and increasing the rate of water flow.

Veins also have a muscular layer in the vessel wall that can regulate resistance within the vessels (Figure 10-3b■). The venous side of the vascular system dilates when the muscles in the walls of veins relax, effectively "pooling" blood in the venous circulation as the body regulates blood pressure. The connections between arterial and venous circulation are capillary beds, where oxygen and nutrients are provided to the cells, and waste products are removed (Figure 10-3c■). The total surface area within the vessels of capillary beds is vast.

## Blood

Blood is the "liquid of life" that enables cells, tissues, and organs to function. It transports oxygen, nutrients, and waste products and is composed of both solid and liquid elements. The solid elements are red blood cells, white blood cells, and platelets. The liquid portion of blood, known as plasma, consists of water, electrolytes, and suspended materials such as proteins. Nutrients and wastes are dissolved or suspended in the plasma. Red blood cells or **erythrocytes** are particularly important because they

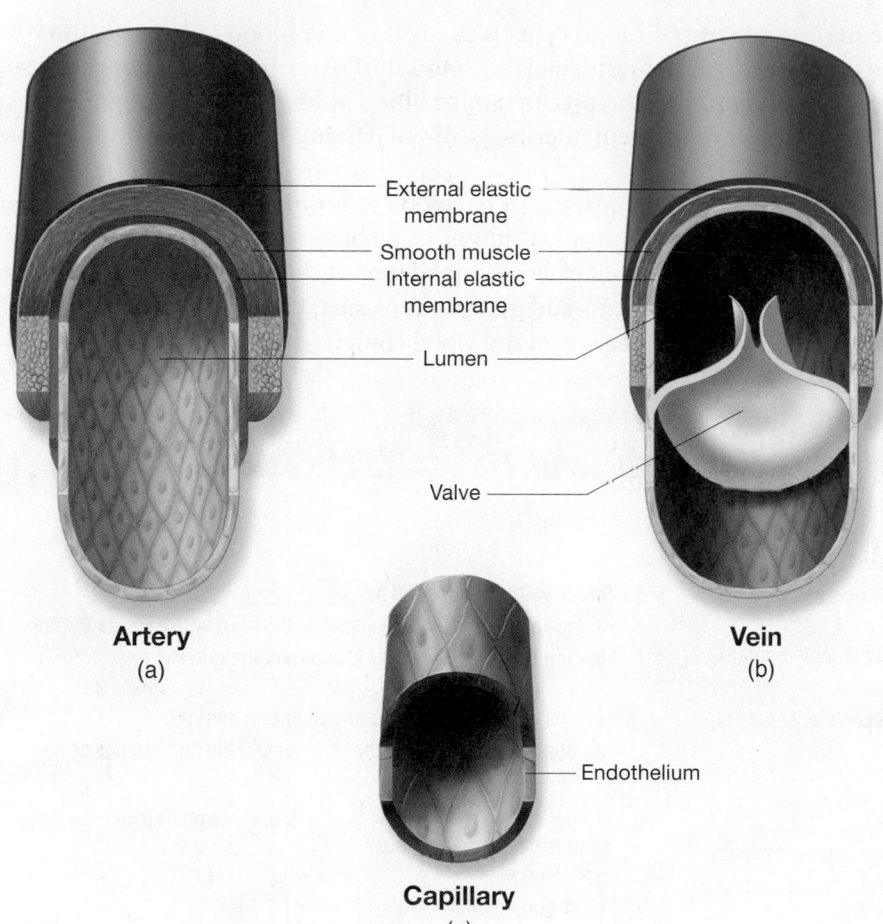

**Figure 10-3** (a) The structure of an artery. (b) The structure of a vein. (c) The structure of a capillary.

External elastic membrane

Smooth muscle

Internal elastic membrane

Lumen

Valve

**Artery**
(a)

**Vein**
(b)

Endothelium

**Capillary**
(c)

carry oxygen using a protein called **hemoglobin** (Figure 10-4a■). White blood cells fight infection (Figure 10-4b■). **Platelets** aid in clotting (Figure 10-4c■).

Hemoglobin in red blood cells has the remarkable property of rapidly and tightly binding oxygen where oxygen is plentiful (e.g., in the lungs) and releasing it in areas of low oxygen concentration (e.g., in the tissues). Almost all of the oxygen in the body is transported via hemoglobin; only a very small amount is transported in the blood dissolved in the plasma. The degree to which hemoglobin has bound to oxygen is referred to as **oxygen saturation**, which is often measured using a specialized device known as a pulse oximeter.

**hemoglobin** oxygen-carrying protein in red blood cells.

**platelets** solid elements in the blood that aid in clotting.

**oxygen saturation** the degree to which oxygen has bound to hemoglobin.

**Figure 10-4b** White blood cells or leukocytes help the body fight infections.

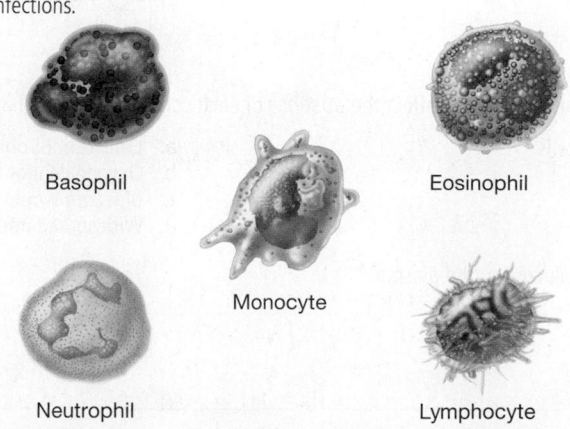

Basophil

Eosinophil

Monocyte

**Figure 10-4a** Red blood cells contain hemoglobin, which enables them to transport oxygen.

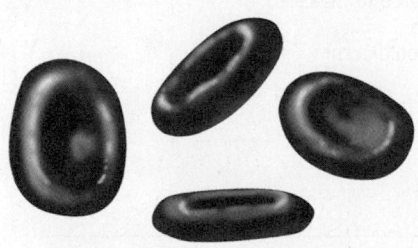

Neutrophil

Lymphocyte

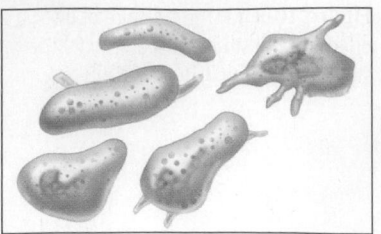

**Figure 10-4c** Platelets are smaller than red blood cells or white blood cells and help the blood to clot.

The percentage of red blood cells to the rest of the blood volume is important because it can dramatically influence the amount of oxygen that reaches the tissues. Under normal conditions, the proportion of blood volume that is composed of red blood cells—known as the hematocrit—is 38–46 percent in women, and 42–54 percent in men.

Thus, without a sufficient quantity of red blood cells or hemoglobin, oxygen cannot be effectively delivered to body cells. Without white blood cells, the body is susceptible to widespread infection. Without platelets, blood cannot clot and bleeding will continue unchecked. Without the proteins and glucose in plasma, cells cannot receive nourishment. Thus, problems affecting any of the blood components can result in shock.

# STOP, THINK, UNDERSTAND

## Multiple Choice

Choose the correct answer.

1. Which of the following is a definition or description of homeostasis?_____
   a. The body's ability to maintain a stable internal environment.
   b. A body that is well perfused.
   c. A condition in which tissues and organs receive adequate $O_2$, and dispose of waste products.
   d. All of the above.

2. Which of the following is *not* true about shock?_____
   a. The signs and symptoms of shock may not be apparent initially.
   b. Shock is rarely observed by itself; it is frequently associated with various medical and traumatic conditions.
   c. Patients can lose up to 30 percent of their blood volume before they exhibit signs or symptoms of shock.
   d. Shock is always preceded by some traumatic event.

3. With each contraction (heartbeat), how much blood does the heart pump?_____
   a. 40–60 mL          c. 100–140 mL
   b. 60–100 mL         d. 140–200 mL

4. Cardiac output, which is the volume of blood pumped by the heart in one minute, is calculated by multiplying _____
   a. tidal volume and heart rate.
   b. stroke volume and heart rate.
   c. systolic pressure and diastolic pressure.
   d. pulse pressure and heart rate.

5. Stroke volume is defined as_____
   a. the amount of blood pumped by the heart with each contraction.
   b. the amount of residual blood remaining in the heart after a contraction.
   c. the amount of blood pumped in one minute.
   d. the amount of blood that completely fills the arteries at any given time.

6. If a patient's stroke volume is 90 mL and her heart rate is 80 bpm, what is her cardiac output?_____
   a. 90 mL/min
   b. 1,700 mL/min
   c. 7,200 mL/min
   d. Cardiac output cannot be determined from the values provided.

7. Which of the following is an example of the redistribution process of blood flow?_____
   a. Increased blood flow to a muscle during heavy exercise.
   b. Increased blood flow to the GI tract after a heavy meal.
   c. Increased blood flow to the heart, lungs, and brain, and decreased blood flow to the extremities following trauma.
   d. All of the above.

8. The degree to which oxygen has been bound by hemoglobin is known as_____
   a. blood oximetrization.          c. hematocrit.
   b. platelet/hemoglobin saturation.   d. oxygen saturation.

## Matching

Match the following components of blood to the effect the *absence* of each component would have on the body:

_____ 1. white blood cells

_____ 2. red blood cells

_____ 3. platelets

_____ 4. proteins and glucose in the plasma

a. Cells cannot obtain adequate nourishment
b. Oxygen cannot be delivered to the cells
c. Bleeding would not stop
d. Widespread infection would occur

## Fill in the Blank

Shock is defined as _____.

# Physiologic Compensation and the Stages of Shock

Shock is a progressive disorder that can be divided into three stages: compensated shock, decompensated shock, and irreversible shock.

⊕ 10-5 Compare and contrast the three stages of shock.

## Compensated Shock

The body is instilled with an innate capacity to compensate for suboptimal conditions to maintain homeostasis. The body's systems have built-in redundancy and flexibility that correct adverse conditions without incurring a total shutdown of body systems or long-term organ damage. In times of stress or increased metabolic demand, the body activates various compensatory mechanisms that help restore homeostasis, but those mechanisms can function only for a while unless the problem is corrected. For example, if sensors in the body detect a decrease in the amount of blood being circulated or a sudden decrease in the amount of oxygen reaching the cells, the brain sends signals that stimulate the release of epinephrine, which causes the heart to contract more quickly and the ventricles to contract more forcefully with each contraction. Both changes increase the stroke volume, which enables more blood, oxygen, and nutrients to reach the tissues. In addition, blood vessels in the skin and extremities constrict, which redistributes blood flow away from those structures and to vital areas. At the same time, sensors within the respiratory center of the brain cause an increase in both the rate and depth of respirations to bring more oxygen into the body and expel more carbon dioxide. This combination of **tachycardia**, increased stroke volume, increased peripheral vascular resistance, and increased oxygen intake helps to stabilize the internal environment, at least temporarily.

**tachycardia**   a heart rate greater than 100 beats per minute in adults.

Compensated shock, therefore, is the body's ability to maintain blood perfusion to vital tissues under conditions that, if left uncorrected, would inevitably lead to death. It is important to keep in mind that the body's ability to compensate for shock can mask gravely serious circumstances and give an unsuspecting OEC Technician the false impression that the patient is less sick or less injured than is in fact the case.

The first pieces of evidence that the body may be in shock are tachycardia (heart rate greater than 100 bpm), **tachypnea** (respiratory rate greater than 20 rpm), delayed capillary refill (greater than 2 seconds), cool skin, altered mental status (GCS less than 15 or less than A in AVPU), and a *normal* blood pressure. Treated early, this form of shock is correctable and generally has no long-term adverse effects. Untreated, however, shock will progress until the body is no longer able to compensate. The cyclical series of events that occur in shock are depicted in Figure 10-5■.

**tachypnea**   respirations greater than 20 breaths per minute in adults.

## Decompensated Shock

If the body's compensatory mechanisms are unable to restore blood perfusion to the tissues, cellular hypoxia will worsen, and the body's systems will begin to fail. Heart rate will continue to rise, systolic blood pressure will begin to fall (to below 90 mmHg), and respirations may become shallow. The skin will become grossly pale or cyanotic and will be cool and moist to the touch. Capillary refill will be significantly delayed and may become undetectable due to the shunting of blood away from the extremities. The patient's level of responsiveness will decrease due to decreased oxygen levels in the brain. Treated early, decompensated shock may be corrected, but serious complications can result.

## Irreversible Shock

Once the body's compensating mechanisms fail, cells begin to die. This sets into motion a cascading effect that cannot be reversed. As more cells die, the tissues of various

CONTINUOUS CYCLE OF SHOCK

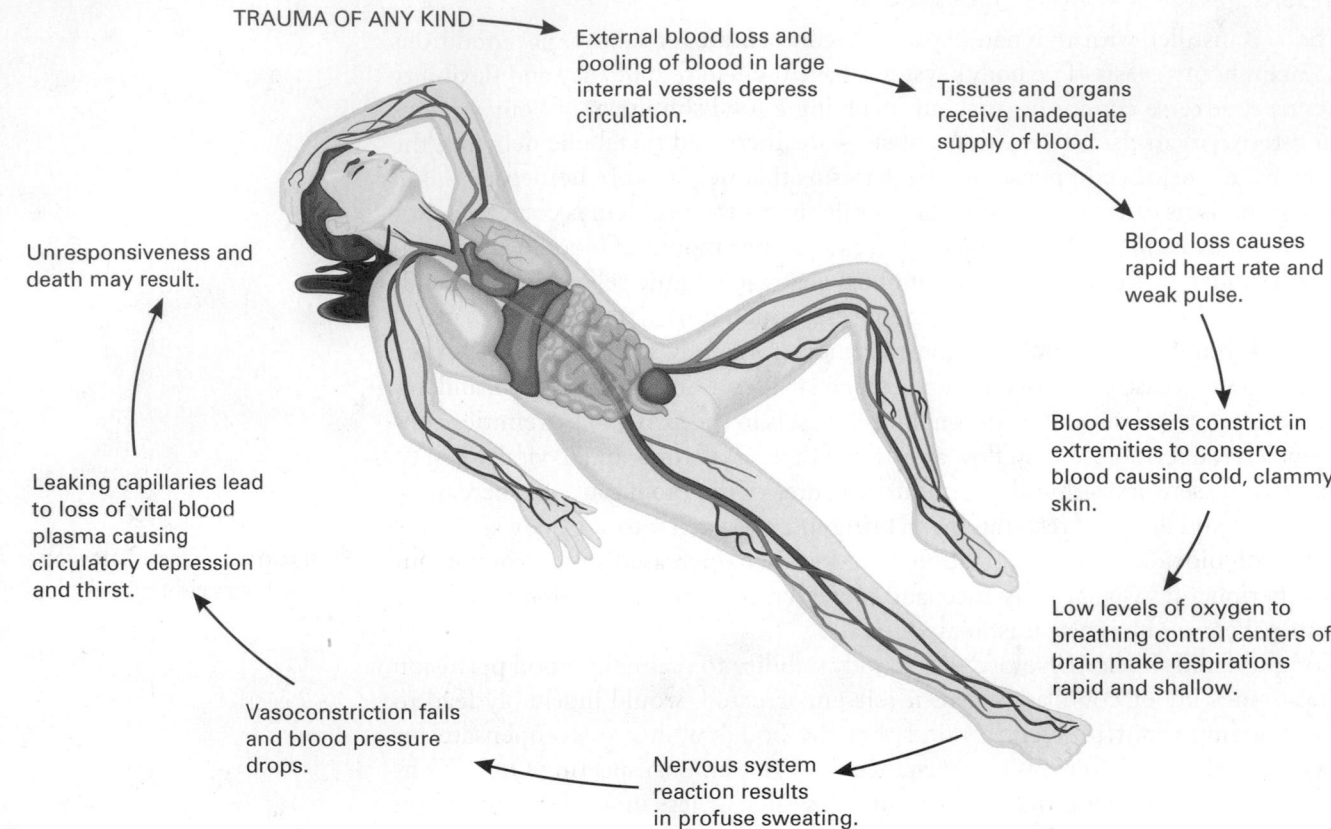

TRAUMA OF ANY KIND

External blood loss and pooling of blood in large internal vessels depress circulation.

Tissues and organs receive inadequate supply of blood.

Blood loss causes rapid heart rate and weak pulse.

Blood vessels constrict in extremities to conserve blood causing cold, clammy skin.

Low levels of oxygen to breathing control centers of brain make respirations rapid and shallow.

Nervous system reaction results in profuse sweating.

Vasoconstriction fails and blood pressure drops.

Leaking capillaries lead to loss of vital blood plasma causing circulatory depression and thirst.

Unresponsiveness and death may result.

**Figure 10-5** The cycle of shock.

organs die, resulting in organ system failure and eventually death. Despite even aggressive treatment, this form of shock is neither reversible nor survivable.

# Types of Shock

⊕ **10-6** List the four types of shock.

⊕ **10-7** Describe how the body compensates for shock.

As previously noted, shock occurs when one or more of the components of the cardiovascular system are adversely affected by disease or injury. These problems can be either volume related (e.g., involve the blood), container related (e.g., involve blood vessels), or pump related (e.g., involve the heart). With this firmly in mind, OEC Technicians must be familiar with four types of shock: hypovolemic shock, cardiogenic shock, distributive shock, and obstructive shock (Figure 10-6■).

## Hypovolemic Shock

Hypovolemic shock results from a critical decrease in circulating blood volume. It is a blood volume-related problem that is caused by either a loss of circulating blood or a loss of internal body water. Of the two, blood loss is more common and has more far-reaching effects (Figure 10-7■). Blood loss that results in shock, better known as hemorrhagic shock, can be caused by a variety of problems, including trauma, gastrointestinal bleeding, vascular disruption, vaginal bleeding, and when bleeding is a complication of pregnancy. Bleeding disorders and certain medications

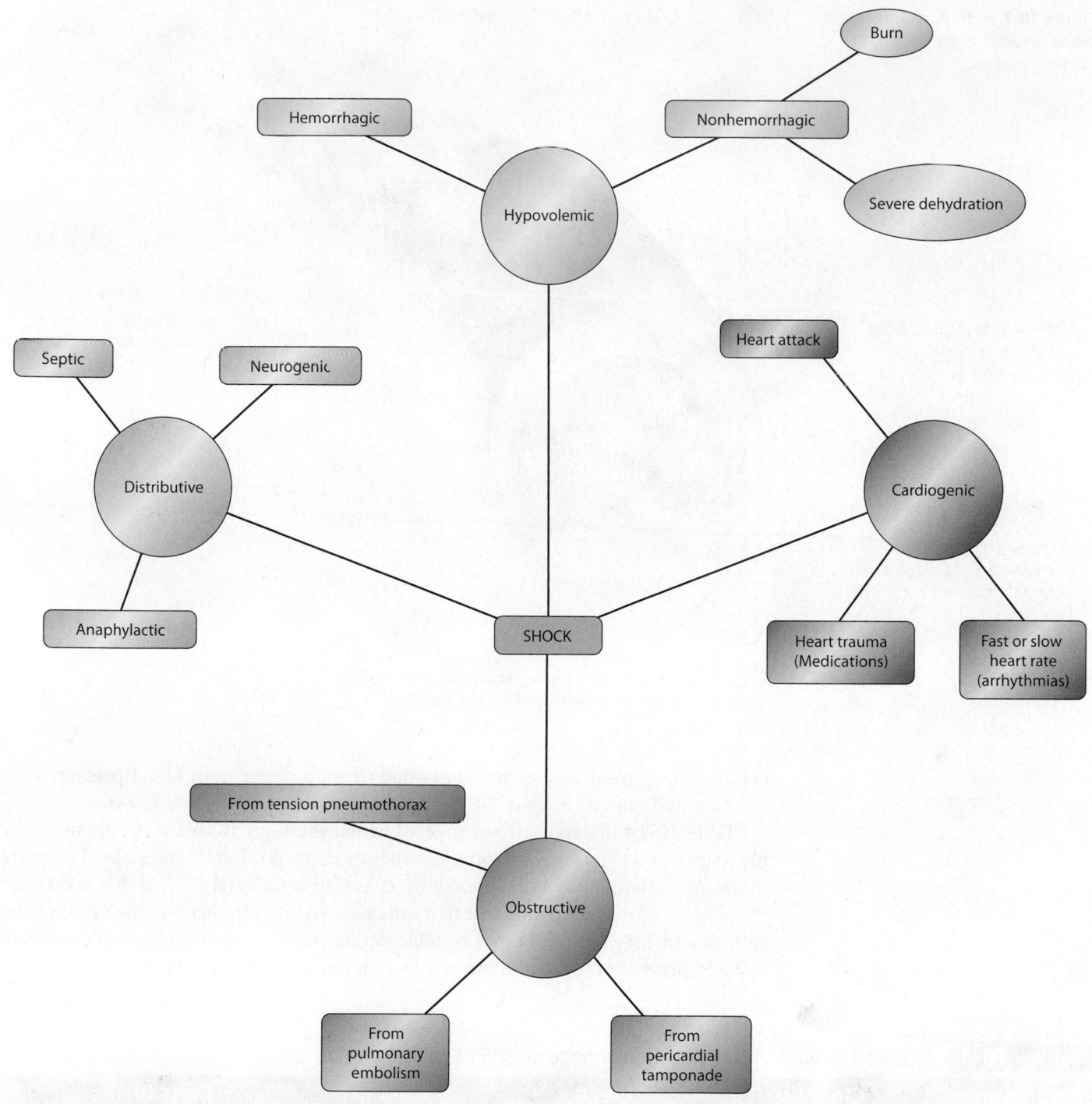

**Figure 10-6** The four types of shock.

(discussed later) may increase the severity of bleeding by preventing blood from clotting normally.

Blood loss can be external and obvious, or it can be **occult**—internal and hidden. The American College of Surgeons divides blood loss due to hemorrhage into four classes, ranging from class I, mild blood loss (less than 15 percent of total blood volume, or the equivalent of donating 1.5 units of blood) to class IV, extremely life threatening (blood loss of 40 percent of total blood volume or greater). Due to the

**occult** hidden.

**Figure 10-7** Hemorrhagic hypovolemia, the loss of blood, is one cause of hypovolemic shock.

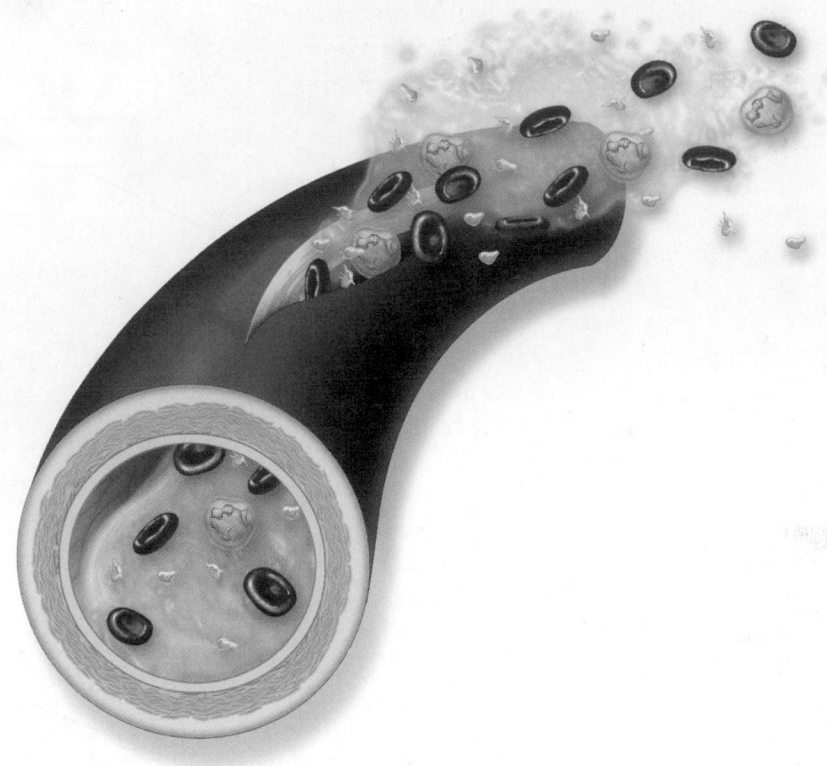

Hemorrhagic hypovolemia: loss of whole blood (plasma and formed elements)

compensating mechanisms previously described, a decrease in blood pressure may not be noted until more than 20–30 percent of total blood volume is lost.

Table 10-1■ illustrates the degree to which the body is able to compensate for blood loss, and that only with significant hemorrhage do alterations in blood pressure occur. An early indicator of hemorrhage is a relative tachycardia, but that is difficult to assess as significant in the context of someone who may be anxious due to pain from an injury or for other reasons. The table demonstrates that in some people a loss of up to 30 percent of blood volume may be required to begin to see a decrease in blood

**Table 10-1** American College of Surgeons Hemorrhage Classification System (for Adults)

| Parameter | Class I | Class II | Class III | Class IV |
|---|---|---|---|---|
| blood loss in mL | less than 750 mL | 750–1,500 mL | 1,500–2,000 mL | greater than 2,000 mL |
| blood loss as percent total blood volume | less than 15% | 15%–30% | 30%–40% | greater than 40% |
| pulse rate | above 100 | above 100 | above 120 | 140 or above |
| blood pressure | normal | normal | decreased | decreased |
| pulse pressure | normal or increased | decreased | decreased | decreased |
| capillary refill | normal | delayed | delayed | delayed |
| respirations | 14–20 | 20–30 | 30–40 | greater than 35 |
| urine output | less than 30 mL/h | 20–30 mL/h | 5–10 mL/h | minimal |
| mental status | slightly anxious | mildly anxious | anxious and confused | confused and lethargic |

pressure. Another way of looking at this is that if a person manifests signs of unmistakable shock immediately after an injury, it is very likely that the person has suffered very severe blood loss.

Hypovolemia due to excessive water loss (nonhemorrhagic hypovolemia, Figure 10-8■) can occur with severe burns, dehydration, excessive vomiting, diarrhea, sweating, and the use of diuretic medications such as furosemide (Lasix®). As water is lost from the body, compensatory mechanisms draw water away from the plasma and direct it to the spaces between the cells. This shift in fluid removes water from the bloodstream, thereby decreasing the circulating blood volume and lowering blood pressure.

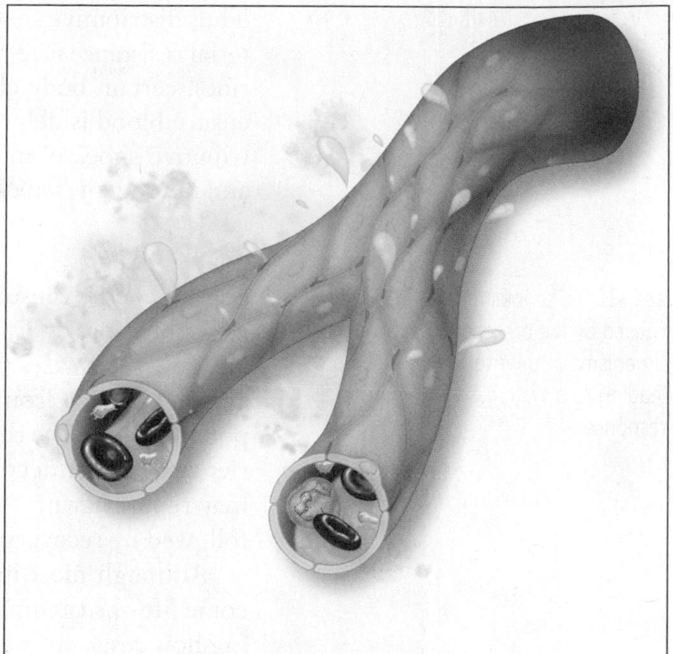

## Cardiogenic Shock

Cardiogenic shock is a condition in which the heart cannot adequately pump blood, resulting in poor cardiac output. It is a pump-related problem in which the defect occurs within the heart itself. Although the heart is a robust organ, it may fail for a variety of reasons, including valve problems, which prevent the heart from filling or emptying properly; heart attack, which results from heart muscle damage; slow or fast heart rates, which decrease cardiac output; medications; and trauma to the heart (Figure 10-9■).

## Distributive Shock

Distributive shock occurs when blood vessels lose their ability to constrict appropriately. The resulting decrease in arterial vascular resistance causes blood to pool within the capillary beds, producing a sudden drop in blood pressure and cellular hypoxia.

Nonhemorrhagic hypovolemia:
loss of plasma

**Figure 10-8** Nonhemorrhagic hypovolemia, a loss of plasma, is a second cause of hypovolemic shock.

**Figure 10-9** A heart attack, the most common cause of cardiogenic shock, occurs when the heart muscle is damaged from an artery to the heart becoming occluded.

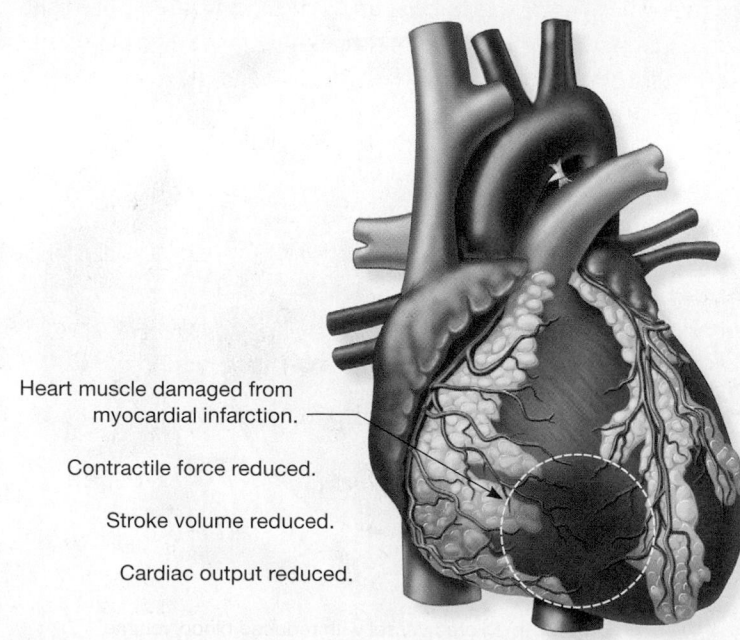

Heart muscle damaged from myocardial infarction.

Contractile force reduced.

Stroke volume reduced.

Cardiac output reduced.

Thus distributive shock is a container-related problem. Under normal conditions, arterial resistance is regulated by certain hormones (e.g., cortisol, vasopressin, epinephrine), certain body chemicals, the nervous system, and local receptors that help to ensure blood is delivered to where it is needed. Based on the underlying cause, distributive shock is subdivided into three subtypes: septic shock, anaphylactic shock, and neurogenic shock (Figures 10-10a■ and 10-10b■).

### Septic Shock

**sepsis** a serious medical condition caused by the presence of pathogenic organisms or thier toxins in the blood leading to a systemic inflammatory response.

Septic shock is caused by a severe systemic infection known as **sepsis** and is the most common cause of distributive shock. When functioning properly, the immune system typically recognizes the presence of an infection, attacks and destroys the pathogens, and clears them from the body. This is why circulating white blood cells are so important: they leave the capillaries to fight infection. Patients may describe their experience with an infection as "feeling poorly," "feeling sick," or "having the flu." They may report having a fever and complain of body aches and other symptoms. This is followed by recovery and resolution (Figure 10-11■).

Although most infections resolve quickly, others can progress to sepsis and become life-threatening. The reasons this occurs depend on a variety of factors, including how resistant the body is to the pathogens, how virulent the pathogens are, how well the immune system is functioning, and the overall health of the individual. Underlying medical conditions, which will be discussed in other chapters, may also affect one's ability to fight infection. Additionally, medications can adversely affect the immune system. Unless sepsis is corrected, the pathogens will multiply beyond control, causing profound vasodilation and cellular hypoxia.

### Anaphylactic Shock

Anaphylactic shock is caused by a severe allergic reaction to some substance to which an exposed person is susceptible. Common causes of anaphylaxis include insect bites

**Figure 10-10** (a) A normal blood vessel. (b) Blood vessel dilation shows reduced blood volume.

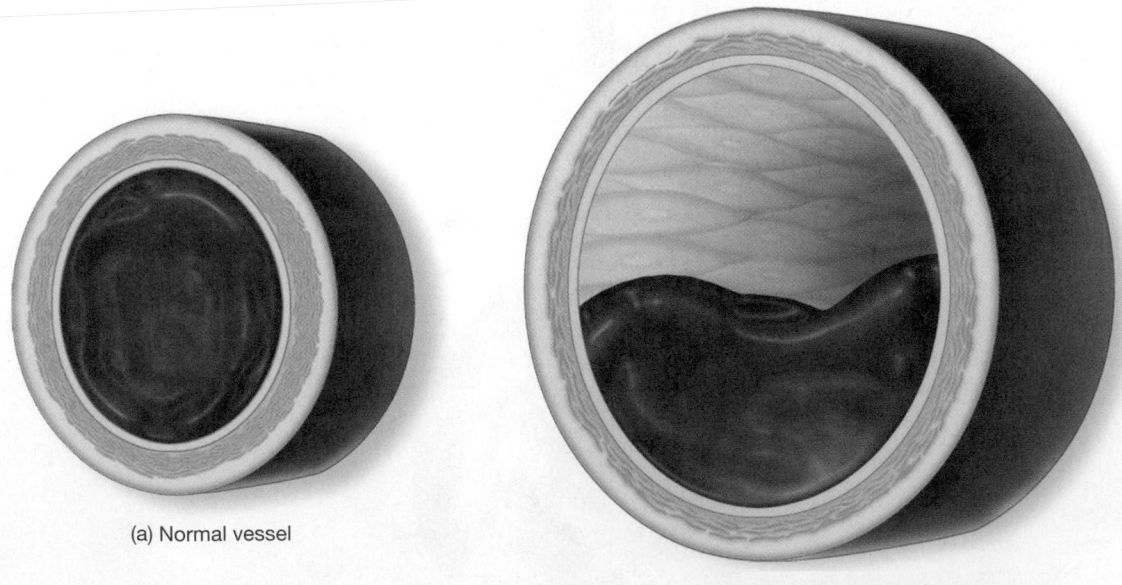

(a) Normal vessel

(b) Dilated vessel with reduced blood volume

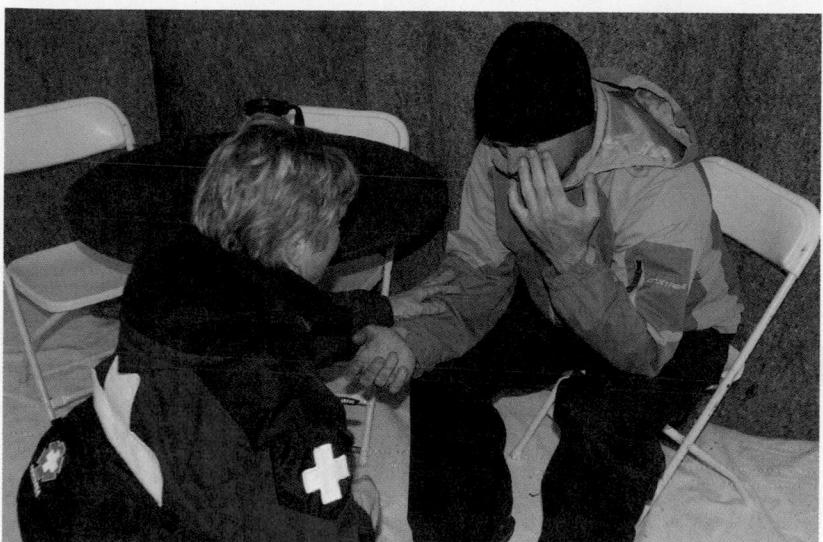

**Figure 10-11** A patient with septic shock, which is caused by a severe systemic infection, may complain of "feeling poorly."
Copyright Mike Halloran

or stings; shell fish, nuts, and other foods; and medications (Table 10-2■). Under normal conditions, such as when an offending source is introduced into the body, the immune system responds by releasing chemicals that aid the immune response. In a susceptible person, however, these chemicals cause generalized vasodilation and a host of other pathological problems. Without intervention, anaphylactic shock can quickly lead to respiratory arrest and death. A complete description of anaphylaxis, including causes, assessment, and treatment, is covered in Chapter 14, Allergies and Anaphylaxis.

## Neurogenic Shock

Neurogenic shock, the third type of distributive shock, is caused by disruptions of the central nervous system, most often resulting from spinal cord injury. When the spinal cord is damaged, normal neurological input to the blood vessels is disrupted, causing the vessels to dilate. The resulting marked drop in blood pressure is known as neurogenic (or spinal) shock. Fortunately, this process is not generally seen immediately after a spinal injury and usually occurs over a period of hours or even days. OEC Technicians should never attribute hypotension seen with a recent post-traumatic

## Table 10-2 Causes of Anaphylactic Shock

- Foods (peanuts, tree nuts, soy, milk, eggs, chocolate, shellfish)
- Environmental irritants (smoke, airborne particles)
- Pollen (weeds, grasses, trees)
- Molds (mildew, spores)
- Animal dander (skin flakes, fur)
- Medications (antibiotics, pain medications)
- Chemicals (latex)
- Other causes (blood transfusions, organ transplants, radiographic dyes)

spinal cord injury to neurogenic shock only. The most likely cause of the problem in trauma cases presenting with low blood pressure and signs and symptoms of shock is hemorrhagic shock due to blood loss.

## Obstructive Shock

Obstructive shock results when some type of blockage prevents oxygenated blood from reaching vital organs. The cause can be either external pressure being placed on the heart or a blockage within the arterial vasculature. Thus, the problem can be pump-related or container-related. The most common causes of obstructive shock are tension pneumothorax, pericardial tamponade, and pulmonary embolism.

### Tension Pneumothorax

As described in Chapter 6, Anatomy and Physiology, the inner chest wall is lined with a fibrous membrane known as the parietal pleura, whereas the lungs are covered by visceral pleura. Between these two membranes is a potential space known as the pleural space. This space is filled with a very small amount of pleural fluid, the lubricating properties of which allow the lungs to move freely while expanding and contracting during inhalation and expiration. If the integrity of the chest wall or lung is compromised (most often by trauma), air can seep into the pleural space causing tension pneumothorax (Figure 10-12a■). Spontaneous tears within the lung tissue also can cause air to leak into the pleural space. Unless the air is given a way to escape, pressure within the pleural space will rise, which can force the unaffected lung to compress the heart, impeding its ability to pump effectively. This loss of efficiency can significantly reduce the amount of blood that enters and exits the heart, causing a corresponding drop in blood pressure and shock. Thus, tension pneumothorax is a pump-related disorder. A complete description of tension pneumothorax, its causes, and treatment are covered in Chapter 23, Thoracic Trauma.

### Pericardial Tamponade

Obstructive shock can occur if fluid accumulates within the pericardium, the sac surrounding the heart. This fluid accumulation is called pericardial tamponade (Figure 10-12b■). As a result, the right side of the heart, which pumps blood to the lungs, can collapse, decreasing cardiac output and causing shock. The right side of the heart is more vulnerable to such collapse than the left side because the walls of the right side are thinner than those on the left side. Pericardial tamponade is thus a pump-related problem. Fluid that accumulates in the pericardium may be free blood caused by penetrating chest trauma, fluid that slowly accumulates from a medical condition, or pus resulting from a massive cardiac infection. Pericardial tamponade is covered in more detail in Chapter 23, Thoracic Trauma.

### Pulmonary Embolism

A pulmonary embolism is a condition caused when a blood clot becomes stuck in and blocks a pulmonary artery. This condition occurs when a blood clot called a thrombus becomes dislodged from a distant location, usually a vein in the legs or pelvis, travels through the right heart, and then becomes lodged in a pulmonary artery. The resulting blockage disrupts the flow of blood through the lungs and back to the heart and prevents gas exchange in the lungs (Figure 10-12c■). Pulmonary embolism is rapidly fatal if it occurs in a large pulmonary artery and is not treated immediately. A more detailed description of pulmonary embolism is presented in Chapter 13, Respiratory Emergencies.

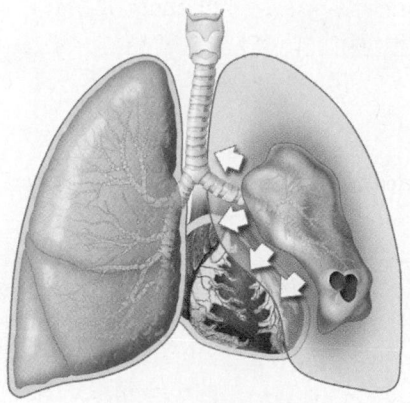
(a) Tension pneumothorax

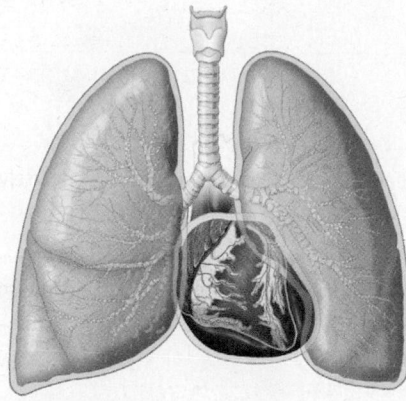
(b) Pericardial tamponade

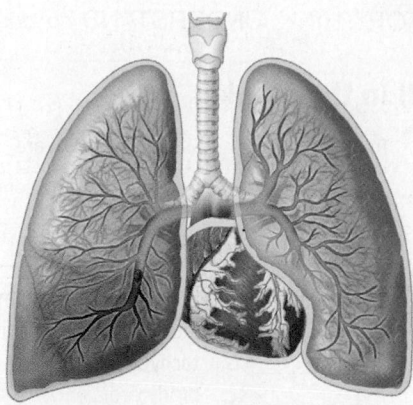
(c) Pulmonary embolism

**Figure 10-12** (a) In tension pneumothorax, air in the pleural space results in a collapse of the lung on the affected side and can compress the heart. (b) In pericardial tamponade, fluid fills the sac around the heart, compressing the heart and impairing its pumping action. (c) In pulmonary embolism, a blood clot in the pulmonary circulation reduces blood flow to lung tissue.

# STOP, THINK, UNDERSTAND

## Multiple Choice

Choose the correct answer.

1. Due to the body's ability to compensate, a drop in blood pressure may not be noticed until what proportion of blood volume has been lost?_____
   a. 10–20 percent
   b. 20–30 percent
   c. 30–40 percent
   d. 40–50 percent

2. A patient is showing signs and symptoms of severe shock immediately following an injury. What does this finding most likely indicate?_____
   a. cardiac failure
   b. severe blood loss
   c. a preexisting medical condition
   d. it is impossible for signs and symptoms of shock to develop this rapidly due to the body's compensatory mechanisms

## Matching

1. For each of the following descriptions, indicate which stage of shock applies.

   _____ 1. compensated shock
   _____ 2. decompensated shock
   _____ 3. irreversible shock

   a. decreased level of responsiveness; can be reversed but with possibly serious complications; cellular hypoxia; tachycardia; systolic BP less than 90 mmHg; shallow respirations; cool, moist, cyanotic skin; capillary refill delayed or not detectable
   b. cellular death, tissue death; not survivable
   c. brain signals body to release epinephrine; heart rate increases; ventricles contract more forcibly with each contraction; increase in stroke volume; constriction of blood vessels and redistribution of blood flow from skin and nonvital organs to vital organs; increased respiratory rate; survival of the patient without complications is possible

2. For each of the following descriptions, indicate the type of shock that applies.

   _____ 1. obstructive shock
   _____ 2. distributive shock
   _____ 3. hypovolemic shock
   _____ 4. cardiogenic shock

   a. occurs when blood moving from the heart to the arterial circulation is blocked
   b. results from a critical drop in circulating blood volume
   c. occurs when blood vessels lose their ability to constrict properly
   d. is often caused by a severe allergic reaction
   e. is caused by a loss of body water through vomiting or diarrhea
   f. is caused by heart failure
   g. is also known as "hemorrhagic" shock
   h. can be caused by latex, bee stings, or peanuts
   i. is caused by blood pooling in the pericardium
   j. has a slow onset and is associated with severe head or spinal trauma
   k. includes septic, anaphylactic, and neurogenic shock
   l. can be caused by tension pneumothorax

*continued*

STOP, THINK, UNDERSTAND *continued*

## Fill in the Blank

1. The three progressive stages of shock are_____, _____, and _____.

2. Shock occurs when one or more of the components of the cardiovascular system is adversely affected by injury or disease. The three primary components of this system are _____, _____, and _____.

3. The four types of shock are _____, _____, _____, and _____.

4. Place a check beside each sign or symptom that could indicate that a patient is going into shock.

   _____ **a.** lack of visible signs or symptoms

   _____ **b.** tachycardia

   _____ **c.** bradycardia

   _____ **d.** tachypnea

   _____ **e.** GCS less than 15

   _____ **f.** capillary refill slower than 2 seconds

   _____ **g.** normal blood pressure

# CASE UPDATE

You suspect that the man may be injured and tell your ski buddies to go ahead and ski while you evaluate the man further. You sit him down and then secure the area by placing both your skis and his in an "X" several yards above your location, where they can be seen by people traveling down the hill. When you return, you obtain a more complete history and assess the man. He tells you that his doctor recently put him on a "blood thinner" to prevent clots. He also tells you that he is taking a "beta blocker" for high blood pressure. As you are talking with him, the man appears slightly confused and says, "I don't feel very well." Soon after, two members of your patrol arrive.

***What do you think the problem is? What should you do next?***

# Factors Affecting Shock

Young and healthy individuals have the greatest capacity to compensate for shock, especially in its early stages, whereas very young and older individuals have less effective compensatory mechanisms and may abruptly decompensate after an initial period of *apparent* stability. In addition to the compensating mechanisms, other factors can influence how shock affects the body. Chief among these factors are age, concurrent illness or injury, preexisting medical conditions, and the use of mind-altering substances or medications, including prescription medications and over-the-counter (OTC) medications.

The presence of injury or illness, for example, can affect the severity of shock and can have cumulative effects. Preexisting medical conditions such as diabetes, heart disease, or anemia (a reduction in the number of circulating red blood cells) can hasten the effects of shock. Mind-altering substances can mask or mimic the signs of shock by altering vital signs or altogether eliminating the effects of pain, one of the tell-tale signs of injury. Even prescribed medications can alter the body's response to shock. OEC Technicians must be aware that these medications can mask the classic signs of shock or worsen shock by preventing the body's compensatory mechanisms from working properly.

One group of medications, known as "beta blockers," is used to treat heart disease and high blood pressure. Because beta blockers limit the heart's ability to beat faster, users of these medications may not be able to generate a faster heart rate even though the body is in shock. If the heart rate cannot go up, then the body's ability to compensate for shock by increasing cardiac output is limited. Among the most widely used beta blockers are Tenormin® (atenolol), Lopressor® (metoprolol) and Inderal® (propranolol).

Another group of medications of which you should be aware are **anticoagulants**, which inhibit the blood's natural ability to clot. The most notable members of this group of medications are Coumadin (warfarin) and Lovenox® (enoxaparin). Other medications that prolong blood clotting times include Plavix® (clopidogrel) and Aggrenox® (aspirin plus extended-release dipyridamole). Even some over-the-counter medications such as aspirin can reduce the blood's ability to clot properly. The implication for OEC Technicians is that anticoagulants can prolong bleeding, which can worsen hemmorhagic shock. Thus, even a seemingly minor injury can result in profound shock due to the body's inability to stop bleeding. Any patient who is taking one or more of these medications must be carefully assessed for any evidence of hemorrhaging, both external and internal, because bleeding may not be self-limiting.

**anticoagulant**   a medication that prevents blood from clotting; a "blood-thinner."

# Assessment

Assessment of patients in shock is no different than it is for any other patients. It begins with a scene size-up, during which potential threats to rescuer safety are identified and mitigated. Examine the scene and the patient for clues that could suggest possible causes of shock (Figure 10-13■). Try to identify the MOI or NOI, including evidence of trauma, heart attack, external or internal bleeding, allergy, or infection.

The scene size-up is followed by a primary assessment. If the patient is in shock, correct the ABCDs. Call for help and transport that includes ALS. Most patients in shock need correction of life-threatening conditions and immediate transport.

In the routine evaluation of any patient, you should do a secondary assessment, which includes a head-to-toe exam, a full set of vital signs, and a complete SAMPLE history. If during your routine evaluation of a patient who appears stable initially (as in our example of the case study in this chapter) you begin to suspect impending shock, you should immediately shift gears, correct the ABCDs, and arrange transport.

As you evaluate the patient, be ever vigilant for the signs and symptoms of shock (Figure 10-14■). Examine the patient carefully for any evidence of injury, both external and internal. Careful consideration of the mechanism of injury, paired with your knowledge of the locations of internal organs, could lead you to suspect internal bleeding. Assess the color and temperature of the patient's skin as well as capillary refill. Because shock often results in circulatory collapse, the skin may be pale or cyanotic and cool to the touch. Additionally, capillary refill may be delayed. These signs do not conclusively point to shock because cold weather can delay capillary refill or make the patient look pale. Likewise, the presence of sweating (**diaphoresis**) does not immediately denote the presence of shock because sweating commonly occurs among outdoor enthusiasts who are engaged in physically challenging activities, especially in warm weather. Conversely, hot dry skin, especially when combined with fever and low

⊕ **10-8**  List the classic signs and symptoms of shock.

**diaphoresis**   inappropriate excessive sweating.

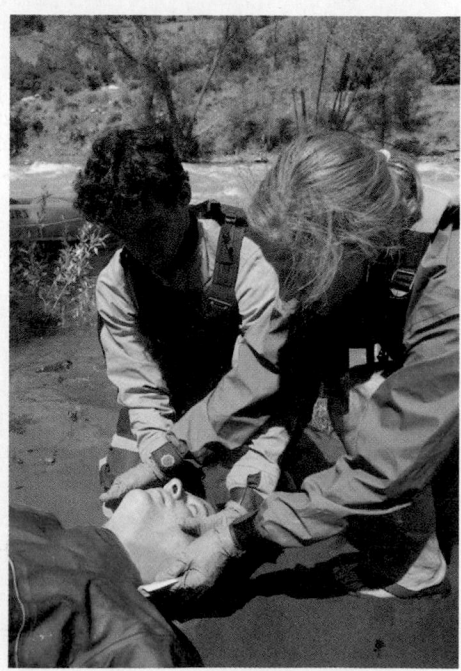

**Figure 10-13** Examine the scene and the patient for any signs of factors that could cause shock. Copyright Scott Smith

**Figure 10-14** The signs and symptoms of shock.

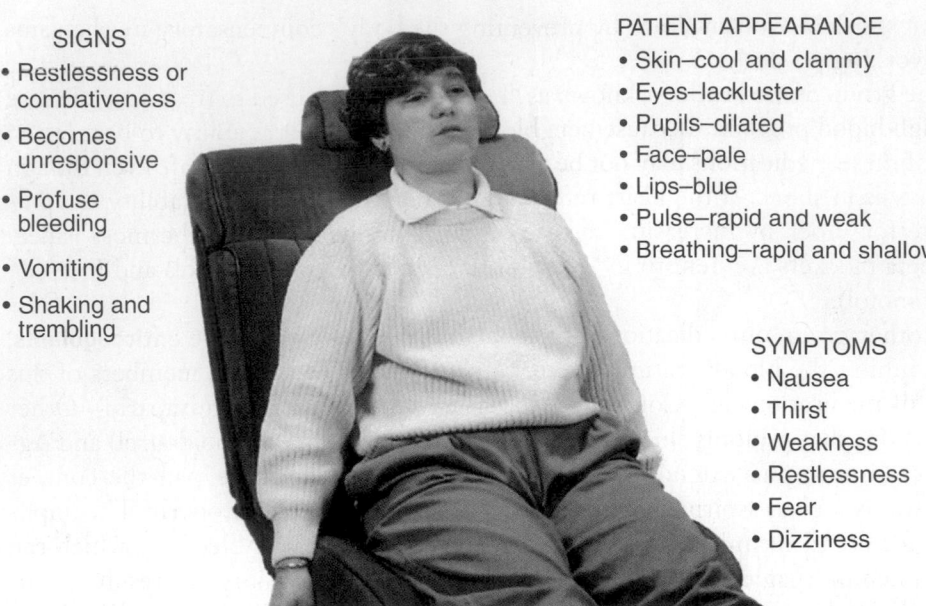

SIGNS
- Restlessness or combativeness
- Becomes unresponsive
- Profuse bleeding
- Vomiting
- Shaking and trembling

PATIENT APPEARANCE
- Skin–cool and clammy
- Eyes–lackluster
- Pupils–dilated
- Face–pale
- Lips–blue
- Pulse–rapid and weak
- Breathing–rapid and shallow

SYMPTOMS
- Nausea
- Thirst
- Weakness
- Restlessness
- Fear
- Dizziness

blood pressure, may indicate septic shock. When obtaining the history, pay close attention to known allergies, as they may have precipitated or contributed to the patient's condition. Determine if the patient is taking any medications that could alter the body's compensatory response to shock. Assess the patient's face and hands for evidence of swelling, which could indicate an anaphylactic reaction. Additionally, consider the patient's age and determine whether any mind-altering drugs have been taken.

Obtain vital signs and repeat them, noting each value; even subtle changes in the pulse rate, blood pressure, or respiratory rate could indicate an underlying shock state. Pay close attention to the pulse pressure (the difference between systolic and diastolic pressures) because a narrowing of pulse pressure is an early indicator of shock in cardiac tamponade. It is important to note that the presence of "normal" age-specific vital signs does not eliminate the possibility of shock because compensatory mechanisms can alter the clinical picture. When assessing the patient, be ever vigilant for the "classic" signs and symptoms of shock (Figure 10-15■):

- tachycardia
- hypotension (later)
- tachypnea
- pale, cool, diaphoretic skin
- altered mental status
- restlessness or combativeness
- thirst, weakness, and nausea

Although it is important to recognize this classic presentation pattern, remember that shock is a developing condition that may not be obvious when the patient is first examined due to the compensatory mechanisms previously described. It is also important to note that hypotension comes later in shock. Frequent reassessment of the patient is essential and should include monitoring the vital signs at regular intervals. When assessing a patient for shock, keep in mind the types of shock, the conditions with which they are associated, and whether the clinical picture you are seeing fits the situation. Neurogenic shock, for instance, typically presents with warm, dry skin as opposed to the more classic presentation.

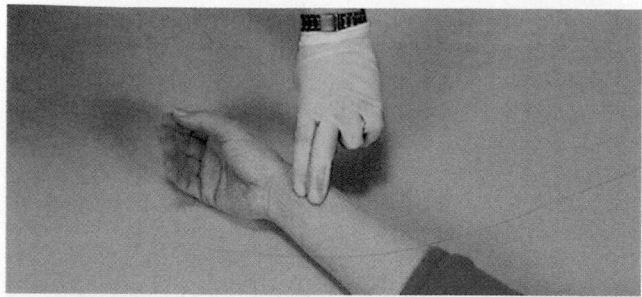

Increased pulse.

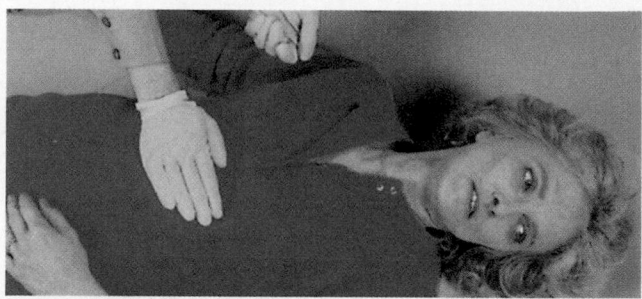

Increased respiratory rate.

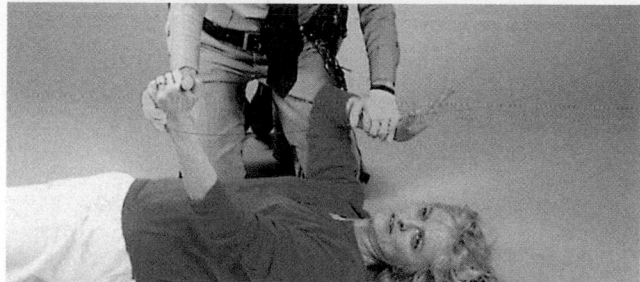

Restless or combative.

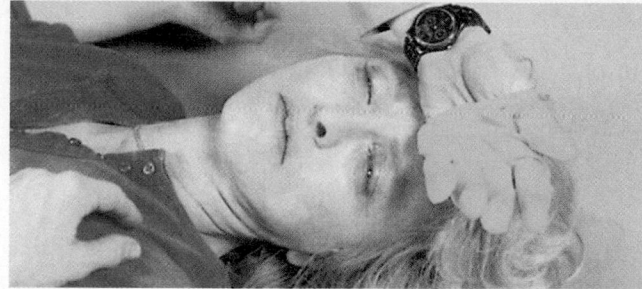

Skin changes and sweating.

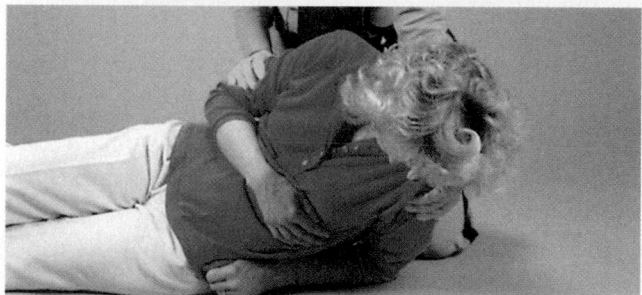

Thirst, weakness, and nausea.

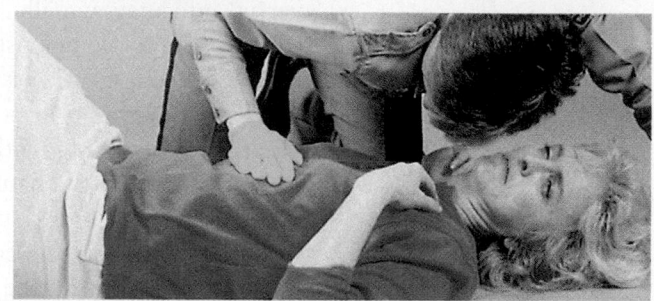

Loss of responsiveness.

**Figure 10-15** Assessing the classic signs and symptoms of shock.

# Management

Management of a patient in shock centers on returning the patient to a state of homeostasis. Given that shock is caused by inadequate tissue perfusion and oxygenation, initial treatment is focused on correcting any problems affecting the ABCDs that were identified during the primary assessment. Begin treatment by ensuring that the patient's airway is open and clear, using suction and gravity as necessary. Support the patient's ventilatory efforts as needed. If the patient is not breathing or if breathing is slow or shallow, assist ventilations using either a pocket mask or bag-valve mask connected to supplemental oxygen. If the patient has no pulse, immediately begin CPR. If a gag reflex is absent, insert a properly sized oropharyngeal airway or a nasopharyngeal airway. For all other shock patients, administer high-flow oxygen at 15 LPM via nonrebreather mask to maximize tissue oxygenation. Control external hemorrhage using the techniques presented in Chapter 18, Soft-Tissue Injuries.

If spinal injury is not suspected, place the person in a supine position with feet elevated 8–12 inches above the level of the heart, which may improve blood flow to the

10-9 Describe and demonstrate the management of shock.

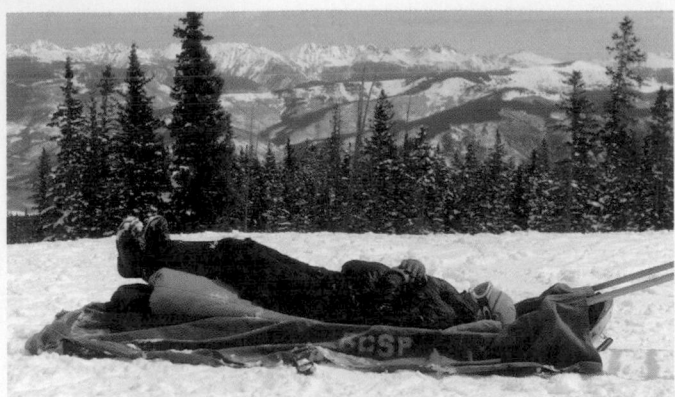

**Figure 10-16** If spinal injury is not suspected, place patient in a supine position with the feet elevated 8–12 inches above the heart.
Copyright Scott Smith

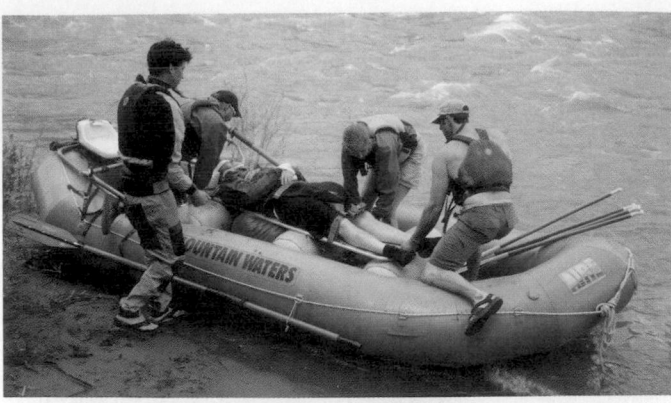

**Figure 10-17** Reevaluate the status of the patient once he is loaded into the transporation device.
Copyright Scott Smith

heart and stabilize blood pressure (Figure 10-16■). The use of a head-down, or Tren-delenburg position, which has historically been used by OEC Technicians, is contro-versial and may actually worsen the patient's condition by causing the abdominal organs to press up against the diaphragm, hindering the patient's ability to breathe. Unfortunately, terrain or other factors may make this unavoidable (Figure 10-17■). If it is necessary to transport a patient in a head-down position, reevaluate airway and breathing status frequently. Also, keep the patient warm and dry. Additional treat-ment depends on the nature of other problems that are present. The treatments for specific causes of shock, such as acute hemorrhage, anaphylaxis, heart attack, and ten-sion pneumothorax, are covered in other chapters.

Finally, transport the patient to a direct-care facility that has advanced care providers so that other therapies, such as intravenous therapy, blood, or medications, can be administered. In a field setting, rapid transportation is often life saving. Refer to OEC Skill 10-1■ for the treatment of a patient in shock.

## STOP, THINK, UNDERSTAND

### Multiple Choice
Choose the correct answer.

1. The most common cause of distributive shock is_____
   a. sepsis.
   c. cardiac failure.
   b. hypovolemia.
   d. neurosis.

2. Which of the following statements is false?_____
   a. Neurogenic shock results from a disruption of the CNS (central nervous system).
   b. In neurogenic shock, normal neurologic input to blood vessels is disrupted, causing vessel dilation.
   c. Neurogenic shock occurs rapidly and is generally seen in the immediate aftermath of spinal trauma.
   d. Neurogenic shock is a slow process, usually occurring over a period of hours or days in the aftermath of spinal trauma.

3. This type of prescription ($R_X$) medication can mask the signs and symptoms of shock by limiting the body's ability to increase heart rate. _____
   a. a narcotic
   b. a beta blocker
   c. an anticoagulant (a blood thinner)
   d. an analgesic

4. This type of prescription ($R_X$) can exacerbate shock by limiting or preventing the clotting of blood. _____
   a. a narcotic
   c. an anticoagulant
   b. a beta blocker
   d. an analgesic

*continued*

5. Which of the following factors can influence how shock affects the body?_____
   a. age
   b. a preexisting medical condition
   c. a prescription medication or substance abuse
   d. all of the above

6. Which of the following statements regarding shock is true?_____
   a. Tachypnea, hypotension, tachycardia, pale diaphoretic skin, and altered mental status are all classic signs/symptoms of shock.
   b. Compensatory mechanisms could mask or eliminate signs and symptoms.
   c. A 4-year-old is as likely to spiral rapidly into decompensated shock as is an 80-year-old.
   d. Signs and symptoms of shock could be masked by medications such as beta blockers, diuretics, or anticoagulants.
   e. All of the above are true.

7. Which of the following statements regarding the management of shock care is false?_____
   a. Care centers on returning the patient to a state of homeostasis.

   b. Any problems affecting the ABCDs should be corrected immediately.
   c. Care should be begun by ensuring that the patient's airway is open and clear using gravity or suction, as appropriate.
   d. Interventive care always takes priority over transport.

8. Which is the correct position in which to place a shock patient without suspected spinal trauma?_____
   a. Rothberg position
   b. supine position with elevation of the feet 8–12 inches above the heart
   c. a position in which the feet are elevated 6 inches above the heart
   d. modified COMA position
   e. none of the above

9. Which of the statements regarding shock is false?_____
   a. Shock is caused by inadequate tissue oxygenation.
   b. Shock is always a life-threatening condition.
   c. The longer shock goes uncorrected, the greater the chance for recovery.
   d. Early signs and symptoms of shock may be subtle due to compensatory mechanisms.

## Matching

Match the type of trauma or illness to the type of shock it could cause. (more than one answer may apply)

_____ 1. anaphylactic shock
_____ 2. neurogenic shock
_____ 3. cardiogenic shock
_____ 4. septic shock
_____ 5. hypovolemic shock

a. a head injury (concussion) that occurred three days ago
b. severe vomiting or diarrhea
c. a bee sting
d. exposure to latex gloves
e. cardiac tamponade
f. a massive infection in the bloodstream
g. tension pneumothorax

 CASE DISPOSITION

You inform the other patrollers that you believe the patient is suffering from hypovolemic shock due to internal injuries. The situation has been made worse because he takes an anticoagulant. Working with the other patrollers, you quickly put the man on high-flow oxygen and place him on a backboard with his feet elevated 8–12 inches. Covering him with blankets, you carefully load him into a toboggan. You ski down with the toboggan team and help them move the patient into the first-aid hut. Soon after, a helicopter arrives and transports the patient to a local trauma center. Several months later, you are in the ski area's cafeteria when someone taps you on the shoulder. It's the man and his granddaughter. He thanks you for "saving my life" and informs you that your suspicions were confirmed. Lifting up his sweater, he shows you an abdominal scar. His granddaughter tells you that the impact of the crash ruptured her grandfather's spleen. The doctor told her that had you not stopped and insisted that he be treated, he likely would have died.

# OEC SKILL 10-1 | Shock Management

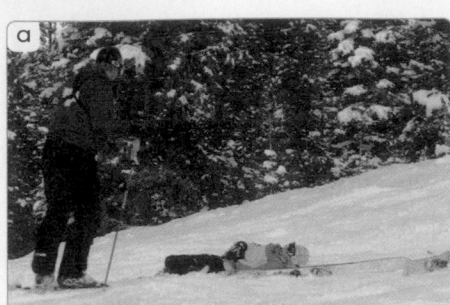

**a**

Assess scene safety and initiate Standard Precautions.
Copyright Scott Smith

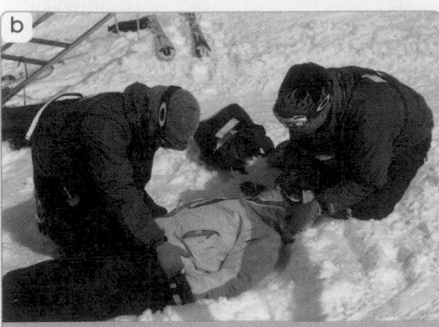

**b**

Perform a primary assessment. Assess ABCDs and correct any problems found.
Copyright Scott Smith

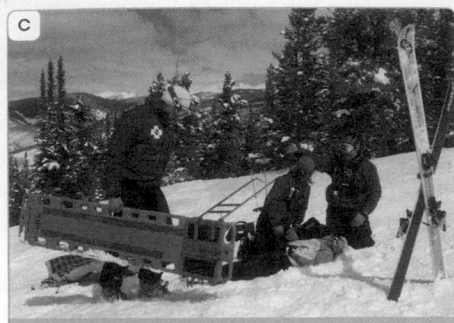

**c**

Call for help and arrange for transport that includes ALS.
Copyright Scott Smith

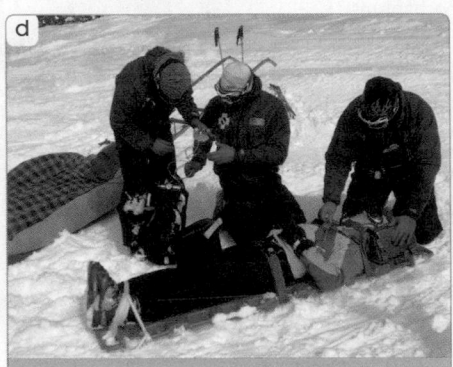

**d**

Monitor the airway and administer high-flow oxygen.
Copyright Scott Smith

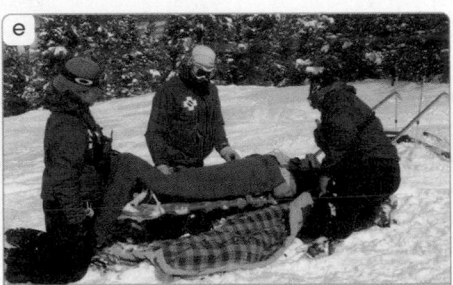

**e**

To prevent heat loss, keep the patient warm and dry.
Copyright Scott Smith

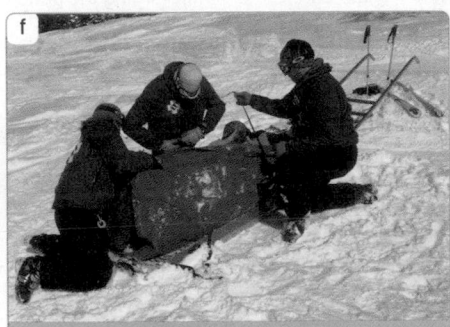

**f**

Place the patient with the head lower than the feet while maintaining spinal integrity.
Copyright Scott Smith

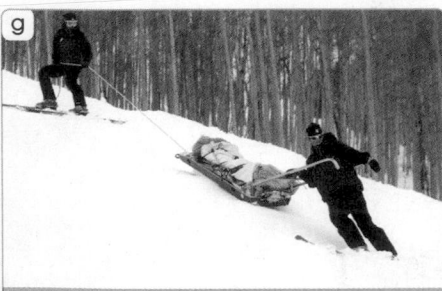

**g**

Provide for rapid transport.
Copyright Selko

## Skill Guide

Date:_____

(CPI) = Critical Performance Indicator

Candidate: _____

Start time: _____

End time: _____

## Shock Management

**Objective:** To demonstrate shock management.

| Skill | Max Points | Skill Demo | |
|---|---|---|---|
| Determine the scene is safe. | 1 | | (CPI) |
| Introduce self, obtain permission to treat/help. | 1 | | |
| Initiate Standard Precautions. | 1 | | (CPI) |
| Assess the ABCDs and treat as needed. | 1 | | (CPI) |
| Recognize patient is showing signs and symptoms of shock. | 1 | | |
| Apply high-flow oxygen. | 1 | | |
| Initiate steps to prevent heat loss from the patient. | 1 | | |
| Properly position the patient with the head lower than the feet, allowing for consideration of spinal integrity or any significant lower leg injury. | 1 | | |
| Provide for rapid transport. | 1 | | |
| Monitor vital signs regularly (every 3–5 minutes). | 1 | | |

Must receive 8 out of 10 points.

Comments: _____

Failure of any of the CPIs is an automatic failure.

Evaluator: _____ NSP ID: _____

PASS     FAIL

# ✚ Chapter Review

## Chapter Summary

Shock is a potentially lethal condition that results when inadequate blood circulation causes poor tissue perfusion. It is caused by factors that adversely affect the cardiovascular system. The resilient human body has compensating mechanisms that enable it to maintain life by responding quickly to compromised blood circulation. When these mechanisms fail, cells begin to die and organ systems fail, resulting in shock and, ultimately, death.

Shock is a problem that OEC Technicians will likely encounter when treating patients in outdoor environments. Although shock may be seen in isolation, it is more often observed in conjunction with other medical or traumatic disorders. OEC Technicians must be familiar with four types of shock: hypovolemic shock, cardiogenic shock, distributive shock, and obstructive shock. Of these, hypovolemic shock (or more

specifically, hemorrhagic shock) is the most common form of shock OEC Technicians will encounter.

Early recognition of the possibility of shock is essential in reducing the number of deaths from this condition. Although recognizing the classic signs of shock is important, careful examination of the mechanism of injury combined with subtle changes in the patient's level of responsiveness or blood pressure often provide early clues that the body is unable to meet its circulatory and metabolic needs.

With few exceptions, priorities for treating shock center on correcting problems affecting the ABCDs, delivering high-flow oxygen, and rapidly transporting the patient to a definitive-care facility. By following this stratagem, OEC Technicians will significantly help to reduce the number of shock-related deaths in outdoor settings.

## Remember...

1. Shock is caused by inadequate tissue oxygenation due to poor blood circulation.
2. There are four types of shock: hypovolemic shock, cardiogenic shock, distributive shock, and obstructive shock.
3. Shock is a life-threatening condition.
4. The longer shock goes uncorrected, the worse are the chances for recovery.
5. Early shock may be subtle due to physiological compensation.
6. A "normal" blood pressure does not exclude early shock.
7. The very young and the very old do not compensate well for shock.
8. Maintain a high index of suspicion for shock.

## Chapter Questions

### Multiple Choice

Choose the correct answer.

1. What is a common first sign of shock?_____
   a. an altered level of responsiveness
   b. a drop in BP
   c. a respiratory rate of 30
   d. vomiting

## Matching

**1.** Match each of the following conditions to its definition. (Conditions may be used more than once)

_____ **1.** tension pneumothorax

_____ **2.** cardiac tamponade

_____ **3.** pulmonary embolism

**a.** a breach in the integrity of the chest wall or lung

**b.** increased fluid within the pericardial sac can cause a complete blockage of blood flow from the right side of the heart to the left side of the heart

**c.** can be caused by spontaneous tears in lung tissue

**d.** characterized by air in the pleural space

**e.** caused by a clot

**f.** affects the pulmonary artery

**g.** can adversely affect both the heart and lungs

**h.** can be caused by penetrating chest trauma

**2.** Place the following actions a through d in order of priority for assessing a patient who may be going into shock.

_____ **1.**

_____ **2.**

_____ **3.**

_____ **4.**

**a.** Determine mechanism of injury and identify clues of possible causes of shock.

**b.** Initiate a primary assessment; assess the ABCDs.

**c.** Identify potential threats to rescuer(s) and/or to patient safety.

**d.** Immediately correct any life-threatening problems.

## Fill in the Blank

**1.** Which of the following individuals would have the best ability to compensate for shock? (check all that apply)

_____**a.** a 20-year-old track star

_____**b.** a healthy 40-year-old man

_____**c.** a healthy 4-year-old girl

_____**d.** a healthy, active 80-year-old woman

_____**e.** an athletic 50-year-old man with well-controlled diabetes

_____**f.** a normally healthy 12-year-old boy who has been vomiting for three days

_____**g.** a fit 50-year-old marathon runner who takes beta blockers

**2.** Which of the following signs and symptoms could be indicative of shock? (check all that apply)

_____**a.** pale skin

_____**b.** capillary refill longer than 2 seconds

_____**c.** diaphoresis/cool skin

_____**d.** hot dry skin, fever

_____**e.** swollen hands or feet

_____**f.** a change in vital signs

_____**g.** flatulence

_____**h.** a change in pulse pressure

_____**i.** tachycardia

_____**j.** diarrhea

_____**k.** tachypnea

_____**l.** hypotension

_____**m.** ringing in the ears

_____**n.** altered mental status

_____**o.** no initial signs or symptoms

## Scenario

*You receive a call to aid a teenager injured in the terrain park. At the scene, which you secure, you find a 14-year-old responsive male complaining of severe pelvic pain. The patient states that he failed to properly hit the ramp at this "rail" and hit his pubic area on the metal beam. You suspect internal bleeding.*

**1.** Internal bleeding can result in _____

**a.** hypovolemic shock.

**b.** cardiogenic shock.

**c.** distributive shock.

**d.** obstructive shock.

*The patient's radial pulse is 110, and the patient appears to be anxious.*

**2.** What stage of shock is this patient presenting?_____
- **a.** irreversible shock
- **b.** decompensated shock
- **c.** compensated shock
- **d.** post-trauma shock

**3.** When the body senses decreased blood circulation or oxygen, the brain releases_____ to speed up the heart.
- **a.** dopamine
- **b.** epinephrine
- **c.** insulin
- **d.** glucose

**4.** Which of the following conditions may constitute the initial evidence that the body may be in shock?_____
- **a.** Tachycardia (greater than 80 bpm)
- **b.** Tachypnea (10–18 rpm)
- **c.** delayed capillary refill (greater than 2 seconds)
- **d.** warm dry skin

**5.** Neurogenic shock is caused by_____
- **a.** internal bleeding.
- **b.** a severe allergic reaction.
- **c.** a reduction in cardiac output.
- **d.** a disruption of the central nervous system.

*After securing the scene, taking BSI precautions, introducing yourself to the patient, and obtaining permission to begin treatment, you start a primary assessment.*

*You find that the patient has spontaneous breathing and has a strong, rapid pulse. The patient is alert to time and place only. A secondary assessment finds unequal pupils and no tenderness or deformities. The patient is not wearing medical alert tags, and the SAMPLE history is vague. The patient's radial pulse is 120 beats per minute and respirations are 28 per minute.*

**6.** Upon the recognition of impending shock, you should_____
- **a.** correct the ABCDs and arrange transport.
- **b.** log roll the patient onto a backboard and transport the patient to base.
- **c.** insert an OPA and apply high-flow oxygen.
- **d.** attempt to locate the patient's parents.

## Suggested Reading

Landry, D. W., and J. A. Oliver. 2004. "Insights into shock." *Scientific American,* February.

Tintinalli, J. E., D. K. Gabor, et al. 2004. *Tintinalli's Emergency Medicine: Comprehensive Study Guide,* Sixth Edition, Section 4: Shock. American College of Emergency Physicians: New York, McGraw-Hill.

EXPLORE **myNSPkit** PEARSON

Please go to www.myNSPkit.com. Under Student Resources, you will find animations, videos, web links, and games related to this chapter—and much more. Look for information on types of shock, emergency care for shock, bleeding control by direct pressure, and other topics related to shock.

Register your access code from the front of your book by going to www.myNSPkit.com and selecting the appropriate links. If the in-cover access code has been redeemed, go to www.myNSPkit.com and follow links to **Buy Access.**

# Altered Mental Status

John S. Nichols, MD, PhD, FACS
Nici Singletary, MD, FACEP

## ⊕ OBJECTIVES

**Upon completion of this chapter, the OEC Technician will be able to:**

**11-1** Define altered mental status.

**11-2** List nine causes of altered mental status using the mnemonic AEIOU-TIPS.

**11-3** List and compare the four major types of diabetes.

**11-4** List the signs and symptoms and demonstrate the treatment of the following medical conditions:

   a. hypoglycemia        c. partial seizure
   b. hyperglycemia      d. generalized seizure

**11-5** Compare and contrast the three types of stroke:

   a. ischemic stroke       c. transient ischemic attack
   b. hemorrhagic stroke

**11-6** Describe how to assess a patient with altered mental status.

**11-7** Describe and demonstrate the treatment of a patient with altered mental status.

## ⊕ KEY TERMS

absence seizure, *p. 364*

altered mental status, *p. 356*

aura, *p. 364*

clonic activity, *p. 364*

coma, *p. 361*

delirium, *p. 359*

*continued*

## Chapter Overview

The body is a complex organism that constantly monitors its internal and external environment and rapidly adapts to changes. This process is controlled by the central nervous system (CNS), which regulates the functions of the other body systems. In order to function properly, the central nervous system requires a steady stream of data from all parts of the body. To preserve homeostasis, the CNS also requires a constant supply of fuel in the form of oxygen, **glucose**, and other nutrients. Should the data

*continued*

## HISTORICAL TIMELINE

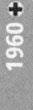

**1960** 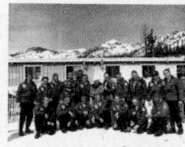 NSP volunteer ski patrollers cover winter Olympic Games at Squaw Valley.

**1962** 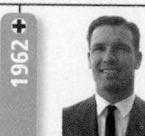 Charles W. Schobinger becomes National Director.

**1962** 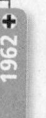 First NSP supply and equipment catalog.

dementia, *p. 362*
diabetes mellitus, *p. 366*
generalized seizure, *p. 364*
glucagon, *p. 358*

glucose, *p. 355*
glycogen, *p. 359*
hyperglycemia, *p. 368*
hypoglycemia, *p. 367*

insulin, *p. 358*
polydipsia, *p. 366*
polyuria, *p. 366*
tonic activity, *p. 364*

**glucose**   a simple sugar that is the end product of carbohydrate digestion in the body and the chief source of energy for most cells, especially neurons.

**altered mental status**   a condition in which a person's level of awareness or responsiveness has changed.

stream or the body's internal equilibrium be disrupted, the body will quickly lose its ability to sense and respond appropriately, resulting in a condition known as **altered mental status**.

Altered mental status (AMS) is a medical term used to describe an abnormal change in a person's level of awareness or responsiveness. AMS is a potentially serious problem that indicates that something is wrong within the central nervous system (Figure 11-1■). There are many causes of AMS ranging from the simple and easily treated to the complex and immediately life threatening. Signs and symptoms may be global, affecting many parts of the body, or they may be localized to one part of the body. To complicate matters, symptoms may vary widely and be subtle or even circumstantial in nature. This situation can present unique challenges to OEC Technicians who, without the benefit of diagnostic equipment, must be able to gather key information quickly, assess the patient and the surroundings for associated clues, differentiate among the various causes, and implement appropriate life-saving care. To accomplish this, OEC Technicians must first understand how the central nervous system and various internal factors affect responsiveness. Then, by learning a systematic approach, you will ensure that none of the major causes of AMS are overlooked.

## Anatomy and Physiology

Responsiveness is governed by a complex series of events that occur within the central nervous system, or more specifically, within the brain. In simple multi-celled organisms and humans, the purpose of the nervous system is to sense the environment and to react to it. Whether avoiding extremes in temperature or light, seeking oxygen or water, or finding nutrients to sustain life, this process helps to ensure the survival of individuals. Humans have an extremely complicated nervous system capable of such highly evolved functions as speech, locomotion, and intellect. In biological terms, these functions are known as higher cortical functions. When these functions are compromised, the result is that the body's ability to sense and react is altered, resulting in the condition known as AMS.

The components of the nervous system were described in Chapter 6, Anatomy and Physiology. There we saw that the central nervous system consists of the brain and spinal cord, whereas the peripheral nervous system consists of all the other portions of the nervous system.

The brain acts as a central processor that controls the rest of the body. It resides in the closed, nonexpandable skull and is surrounded by cerebrospinal fluid, which provides nutrients and a protective cushion. The brain consists of three major parts: the brain stem, which controls functions necessary for life such as breathing, swallowing, responsiveness, heart function, and blood pressure; the cerebellum, which controls balance and coordination; and the cerebrum, which controls emotion,

**Figure 11-1** Altered mental status is a potentially serious problem.
Copyright Edward McNamara

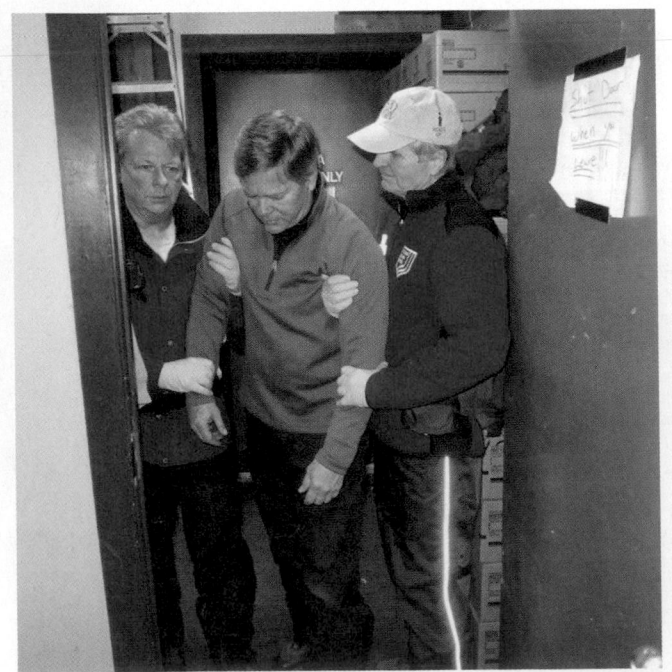

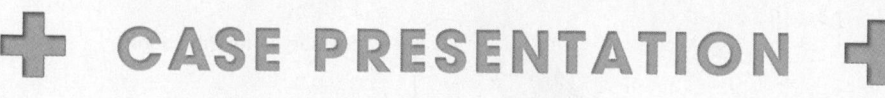

## CASE PRESENTATION

You are on your way to work and stop at a local convenience store. As you enter the store, you hear the manager yell at the clerk to "come quickly" because a customer is "really out of it" in the bathroom. Realizing that this phrase is often used to describe a person with an AMS, you identify yourself as an OEC Technician and immediately accompany the manager to the bathroom. When you arrive, you find a middle-aged man lying on the floor. He appears to be very confused and responds only to loud verbal stimuli. His radial pulse is fast and strong. His skin is pale and cool to the touch, and he appears diaphoretic.

**What should you do?**

thought, speech, integration, and memory as well as sensation and motor function (Figure 11-2■).

Within the central nervous system are nerve bundle pathways, known as tracts, that transmit information leading to and from discrete areas in the cerebrum and cerebellum. The simplest tracts are sensory and motor tracts (Figure 11-3■). The sensory pathways originate in receptors in the skin and continue through sensory nerves that connect to the spinal cord. From there, the tract continues to the cerebrum via tracts or nerves in the spinal cord and brain stem. These nerves connect to the opposite cerebral hemisphere's primary sensory area in the parietal lobe. Similarly, motor neurons within the parietal lobe transmit messages through the brain stem and spinal cord to peripheral nerves that control various muscles. Like sensory nerves, motor nerves originate on the opposite side of the brain from the muscles they control. Similar pathways can be found for vision, hearing, balance, taste, smell, and others. The pathways in the brain for these functions are less clearly understood.

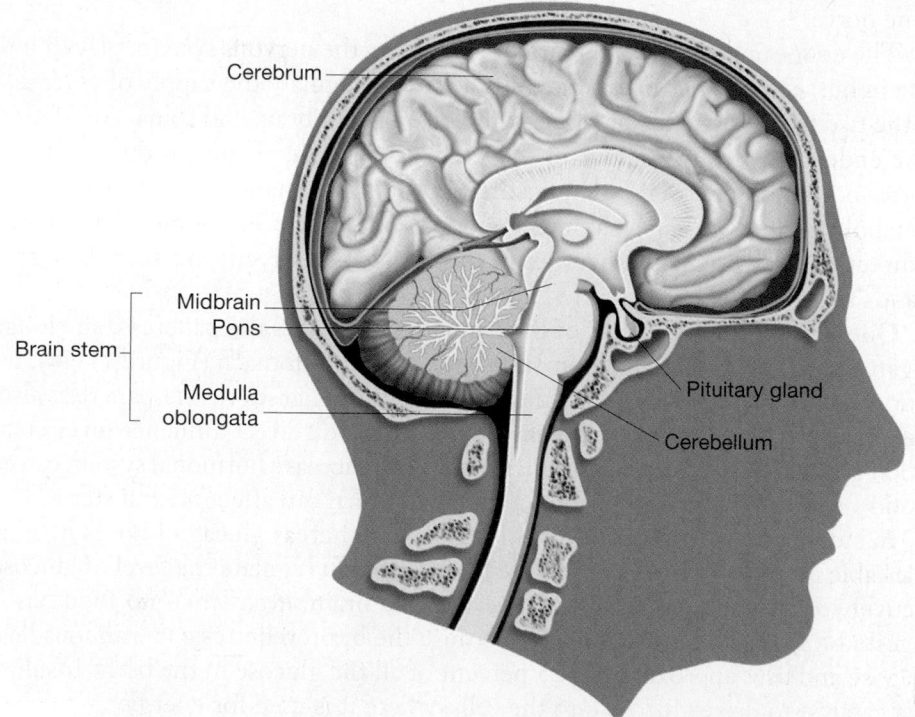

**Figure 11-2** The regions of the brain: the cerebrum, the cerebellum, and the brain stem, consisting of the pons and medulla oblongata.

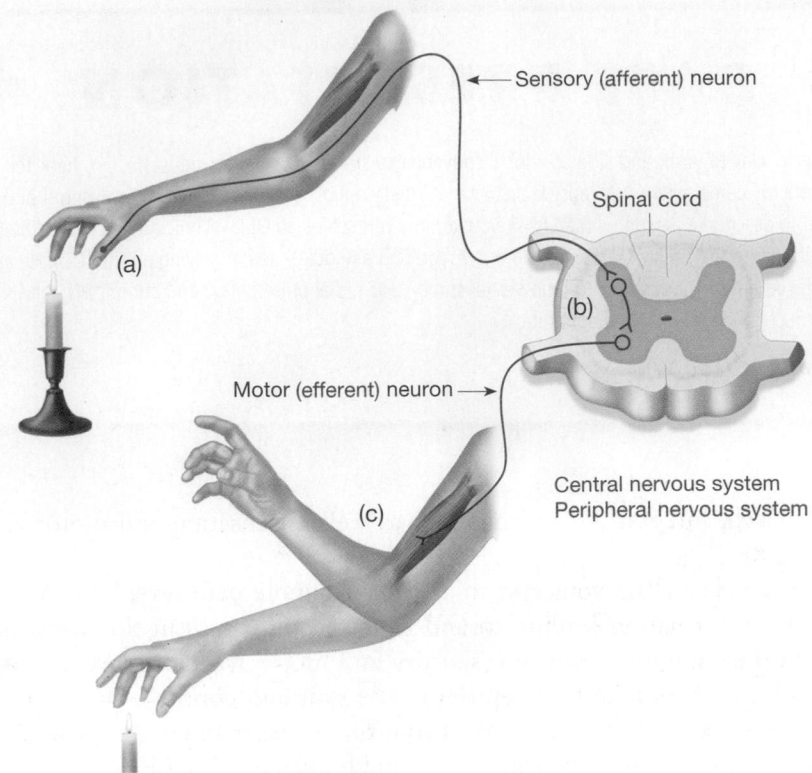

Sensory (afferent) neuron

Spinal cord

(a)

(b)

Motor (efferent) neuron

(c)

Central nervous system
Peripheral nervous system

**Figure 11-3** Some of the nerves of the peripheral nervous system.

Even less understood are the tracts involved in higher cortical functions such as memory, intellect, and ambition. In summary, the cerebral cortex receives signals from the sensory organs in the body through the peripheral nerves, acting on the signals, and then sends a message through the same peripheral nerves to the muscles, causing them to contract or relax. Both sensory and motor nerve fibers travel together in the same nerve.

The endocrine system, although distinct from the nervous system, plays a unique role in human responsiveness due to its ability to regulate the supply of glucose, one of the two main nutrients that are essential for proper brain and spinal cord function. The endocrine system consists of several organs whose glands produce and secrete hormones, the chemical messengers that transmit information that regulates growth, metabolism, and sexual development, among other functions. Some hormones cause a direct action, whereas others exert their effects indirectly by stimulating other glands to release other hormones.

One of the primary organs of the endocrine system is the pancreas, an elongated organ located in the upper abdomen, posterior to the stomach (Figure 11-4■). In addition to producing several enzymes necessary for digestion, the pancreas also secretes the hormones **insulin** and **glucagon**, which have a direct influence on circulating blood glucose (sugar) levels. Malfunction of the pancreas's hormonal system can cause blood sugar to be too high or too low, which in turn can affect mental status.

In simple terms, insulin lowers blood sugar, whereas glucagon raises it. In a remarkable example of homeostasis, the body is able to regulate the level of glucose effectively to maintain a constant delivery to the brain, even when no food has been ingested for days. This is important because the brain requires a continuous level of glucose and uses approximately 25 percent of all the glucose in the body. Insulin acts as a catalyst to drive glucose into the cells, where it is used for energy.

**insulin** a hormone produced in the pancreas that regulates blood sugar levels.

**glucagon** a hormone that stimulates the breakdown of glycogen, a storage form of glucose in the liver; is sometimes administered by injection to temporarily raise glucose levels in patients with symptomatic hypoglycemia.

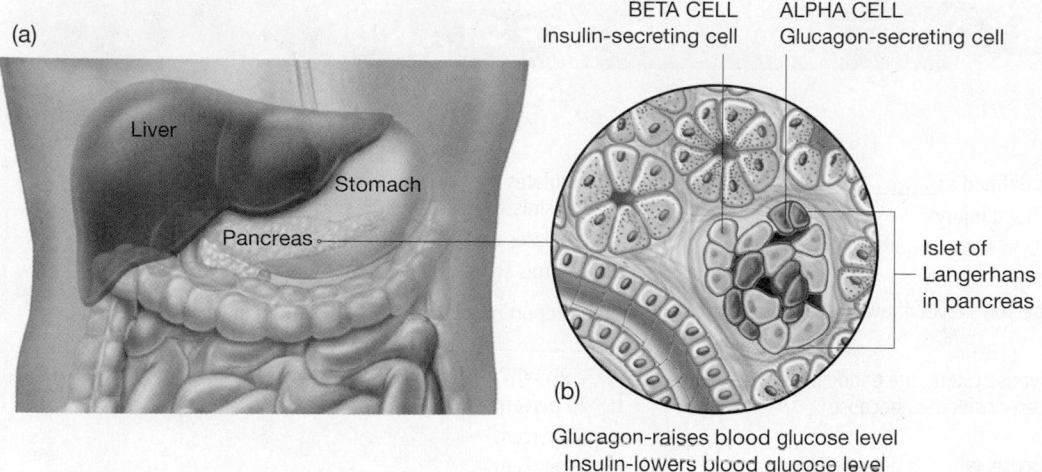

(a)

Liver

Stomach

Pancreas

BETA CELL
Insulin-secreting cell

ALPHA CELL
Glucagon-secreting cell

Islet of
Langerhans
in pancreas

(b)

Glucagon-raises blood glucose level
Insulin-lowers blood glucose level

**Figure 11-4** The pancreas produces digestive enzymes, plus the blood sugar-regulating hormones insulin and glucagon.

The pancreas constantly secretes insulin in low levels to maintain a constant level of sugar within the blood. However, after eating, blood sugar rises. In response, the pancreas secretes more insulin, which stimulates the muscles and other cells to absorb glucose from the blood and lowers blood glucose back to normal levels. Excess glucose is converted to **glycogen** in the liver or into fat and is stored for later use. Conversely, if the blood sugar level falls, as occurs during exercise or between meals, insulin secretion decreases, and the pancreas secretes glucagon. This hormone causes liver cells to release stored glycogen, which is then converted to glucose and released into the bloodstream. This ensures that the body has a constant supply of glucose even when food is not available. However, if the regulation of blood sugar by these hormones becomes ineffective or altered causing too high or too low a blood sugar, the result can affect the central nervous system causing alterations in the level of sensory awareness or responsiveness.

## Altered Mental Status

Malfunctions leading to AMS can affect all parts of the central nervous system equally, or it can be localized, affecting only a portion of the body. Global changes typically present as decreased levels of responsiveness, but may also include overly or abnormally stimulated states such as **delirium**, hallucination, combativeness, and delusions. Focal abnormalities resulting in AMS may cause motor weakness, balance problems, vision loss, or speech abnormalities. AMS is not a specific diagnosis or disease but is instead a descriptive term, indicating a general malfunction of the nervous system. The treatment an OEC Technician provides a patient with AMS depends on the suspected cause of AMS.

### Causes of Altered Mental Status

The myriad causes of AMS include metabolic disorders such as insufficient oxygen levels and low blood sugar; infections; nutrient imbalances; structural brain abnormalities such as trauma, tumors, and cerebral blood clots; toxic substances; and even behavior (Figure 11-5■). Regardless of the source, the exact cause may not be readily apparent. For this reason, OEC

**glycogen** a stored form of glucose or carbohydrate that is made by the body; located primarily in liver or muscle.

⊕ **11-1** Define altered mental status.

**delirium** a state of mental confusion and/or excitement characterized by disorientation with respect to time and place; may be associated with delusions and hallucinations.

⊕ **11-2** List nine causes of altered mental status using the mnemonic AEIOU-TIPS.

**Figure 11-5** Altered mental status (AMS) may stem from either metabolic or structural causes.

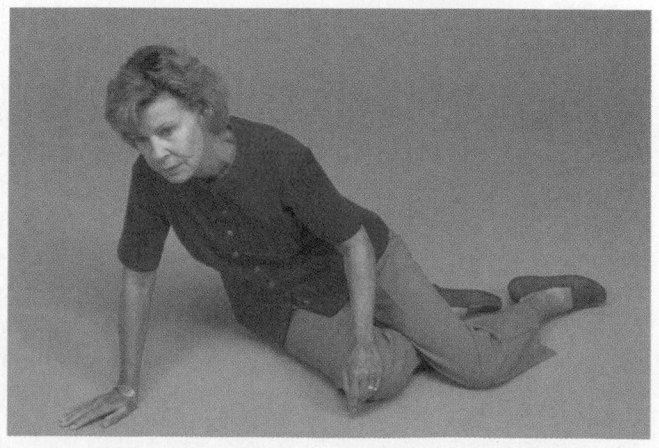

# STOP, THINK, UNDERSTAND

## Multiple Choice

Choose the correct answer.

1. Altered mental status (AMS) is defined as_____
   a. amnesia occurring after a head injury.
   b. unresponsiveness caused by a nontraumatic event.
   c. an associated motor sensory condition.
   d. an abnormal change is a person's level of awareness or responsiveness.

2. Although distinct from the nervous system, the endocrine system plays a unique role in human responsiveness because it_____
   a. regulates the supply of glucose, which is essential for proper brain and spinal cord function.
   b. regulates the production of cerebrospinal fluid, which allows transmission of sensory impulses through the brain.
   c. regulates motor tract transmissions.
   d. controls sensation and motor function.

3. What proportion of the body's circulating glucose does the brain use?_____
   a. 5 percent
   b. 25 percent
   c. 50 percent
   d. 75 percent

## Fill in the Blank

1. The brain consists of three major parts: the _____, _____, and _____.

2. The pancreas secretes enzymes necessary for digestion as well as _____ and _____, which regulate circulating blood sugar levels.

## Matching

Match each of the following components of the brain to its function.

_____ 1. controls emotion, thought, speech, integration, memory, sensation, and motor function

_____ 2. controls functions necessary for life such as breathing, heart function, blood pressure, and swallowing

_____ 3. provides nutrients and a protective cushion for the brain

_____ 4. controls balance and coordination

a. cerebral spinal fluid
b. brain stem
c. cerebellum
d. cerebrum

---

Technicians should be aware of the most common causes of AMS, which can easily be remembered using the acronym AEIOU-TIPS (Table 11-1■).

+ The A in AEIOU-TIPS stands for alcohol and acidosis.

   *Alcohol.* It is the most widely abused drug in the United States and is among the leading causes of AMS in nearly every patient population group ages 16 and older. This chemical depresses central nervous system function. A complete description of alcohol and its effects is presented in Chapter 12, Substance Abuse and Poisoning.

   *Acidosis.* This is a condition in which the body's pH falls below normal levels; the resulting reduced effectiveness of various body systems threatens homeostasis. Among the causes of acidosis are decreased respiratory or cardiac function, renal disease, severe hyperglycemia, and various gastrointestinal disorders.

+ The E in AEIOU-TIPS stands for epilepsy, environment, and electrolytes.

   *Epilepsy.* This potentially serious medical disorder results in sudden, recurrent seizures. It is described in greater detail later in this chapter.

   *Environment.* Changes in body temperature may also lead to AMS. The body must maintain a relatively constant internal temperature if neurons in the CNS are to function properly. Factors that cause core body temperature to rise above or fall below a tightly regulated temperature range can result in dramatic changes

**Table 11-1  Causes of Altered Mental Status: AEIOU-TIPS**

A—Alcohol and acidosis
E—Epilepsy, environment, and electrolytes
I—Insulin
O—Oxygen (hypoxia) and overdose
U—Uremia (kidney failure)
T—Trauma and tumors
I—Infection (CNS, sepsis)
P—Poisoning and psychiatric conditions
S—Seizures, stroke, and syncope

in a patient's level of responsiveness. Common conditions that can produce extreme temperature changes within the body are hypothermia and hyperthermia, both of which are described in Chapters 25 and 26, Cold-Related Emergencies and Heat-Related Emergencies, respectively. Other environment-related causes of AMS include exposure to insect bites and stings.

*Electrolytes.* These ionized molecules within the body maintain energy gradients and help transmit electrical impulses within neurons. To maintain homeostasis, the body requires that a careful balance of electrolytes be maintained at all times. Any imbalance involving one or more electrolytes can affect cellular function, resulting in AMS. Electrolyte levels are affected by various conditions, including diet, exercise, medication use, and overall health. Factors such as excessive sweating, vomiting, or diarrhea can rapidly deplete electrolytes such as sodium, chloride, or potassium, resulting in an imbalance and AMS.

✦ The first I in AEIOU-TIPS stands for insulin.

*Insulin.* Any condition that adversely affects the production and use of insulin or the regulation of blood glucose levels can produce AMS, both immediately and over longer periods of time.

✦ The O in AEIOU-TIPS stands for oxygen and overdose.

*Oxygen.* The brain requires an uninterrupted supply of oxygen to operate properly. Even minor decreases or short interruptions in cerebral oxygen levels result in an immediate decrease in global CNS functioning and overall responsiveness. Hypoxia is the most common cause of AMS.

*Overdose.* Overuse of drugs, whether prescription or illicit, is a cause of AMS that is frequently encountered by OEC Technicians. Overdoses involving opiates and depressant agents are especially problematic because both depress CNS function and respiration, resulting in decreased oxygenation and altered levels of responsiveness. Drug overdose is discussed in Chapter 12, Substance Abuse and Poisoning.

✦ The U in AEIOU-TIPS stands for uremia.

*Uremia.* This is a condition in which the kidneys are unable to effectively remove waste products from the body. Uremia causes lethargy, **coma**, and ultimately death unless the toxins are removed from the blood.

✦ The T in AEIOU-TIPS stands for trauma and tumors.

*Trauma.* Injury to the brain is an especially common cause of AMS and generally produces brain swelling and increased intracranial pressure (Figure 11-6■). The resulting structural damage to the brain can cause focal AMS changes or more global alterations in the level of responsiveness. Trauma may also disrupt blood flow to the brain by causing brain swelling or blood loss, both of which reduce the amount of oxygen that reaches the brain's vital control centers. Brain injury

**coma**  an abnormal loss of responsiveness during which the patient cannot be aroused by external stimuli.

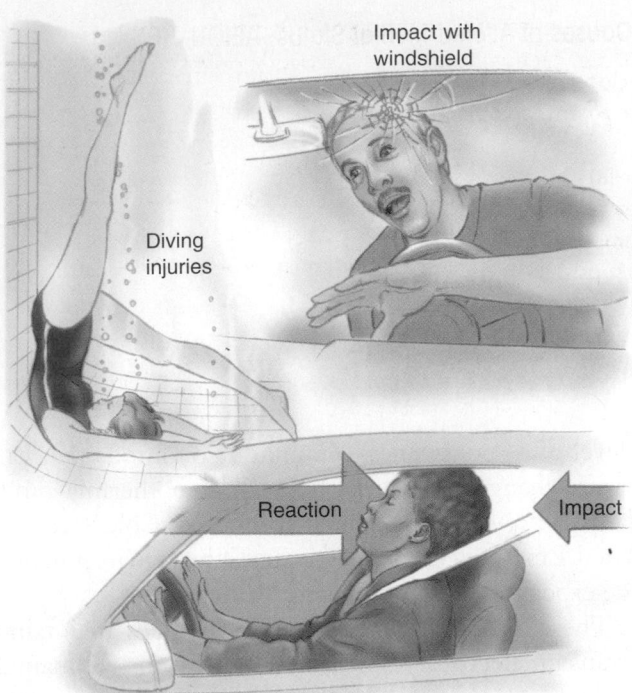

**Figure 11-6** Mechanisms of injury resulting in head and neck trauma may cause AMS.

is presented in more detail in Chapter 21, Head and Spine Injuries, whereas neurogenic shock from spinal cord trauma is addressed in Chapter 10, Shock.

*Tumors*. A tumor is an abnormal growth of cells that can be cancerous or malignant, or noncancerous or benign. Tumors that form within the brain can impair normal brain function, causing both global and focal changes.

✦ The second I in AEIOU-TIPS stands for infection.

*Infection*. An infection is the presence in the body of microorganisms that cause tissue damage. Even a small, localized infection resulting from a minor cut can spread throughout the body in the bloodstream, a condition known as sepsis. When associated with an infection, AMS is a grave sign that often results from sepsis or infections involving the brain and/or spinal cord (e.g., meningitis) and other major body structures.

✦ The P in AEIOU-TIPS stands for poisoning and psychiatric conditions.

*Poisoning*. A poison is a substance that, when taken into the body, can cause AMS and injury or death. Described in Chapter 12, Substance Abuse and Poisoning, poisoning can be caused by innumerable substances and may occur accidentally or purposefully.

*Psychiatric conditions*. A small percentage of patients with AMS may have a behavioral or underlying psychiatric disorder such as schizophrenia or manic-depressive disorder (Figure 11-7■). Other common behavior-related disorders that can cause AMS are depression and **dementia**. Older patients with conditions such as Alzheimer's disease or Parkinson's disease, especially during the diseases' later stages, may also exhibit AMS. Common psychiatric disorders are presented in Chapter 33, Behavioral Emergencies and Crisis Response, whereas Alzheimer's disease and Parkinson's disease are described in Chapter 31, Geriatric Emergencies.

✦ The S in AEIOU-TIPS stands for seizure, stroke, and syncope.

**dementia**　a broad impairment of intellectual function (cognition) that usually is progressive and that interferes with normal social and occupational activities.

*Seizure.* An electrical disturbance within the brain can be caused by various factors and may involve a portion of the body or the entire body.

*Stroke.* This generic term describes the loss of blood supply to part of the brain, resulting in neurological impairment. Depending on what part of the brain is affected, different neurological findings are present. The causes, signs, and symptoms of the three types of stroke are presented later in this chapter.

*Syncope* (fainting). This temporary loss of responsiveness is due to a disruption in blood flow to the brain. The causes and treatment of syncope are covered in Chapter 10, Shock.

## Conditions Associated with Altered Mental Status

### Epilepsy

Epilepsy is a chronic medical condition that causes recurrent seizures in an otherwise healthy individual. According to the Epilepsy Foundation, approximately 3 million Americans have some form of epilepsy, and 200,000 new cases of epilepsy are diagnosed each year. Although the cause of this disorder is still relatively unknown, research has revealed several factors, including head injury and brain trauma, brain tumors, genetic conditions, and chemical imbalances, that can induce recurrent seizure activity in susceptible individuals.

With early diagnosis and proper treatment, patients with epilepsy can participate in a wide range of physically demanding activities. Therapeutic management of epilepsy is generally preventive in nature and involves the use of medications known as anti-convulsants, which help control seizure activity.

### Seizures

A seizure is an electrical disturbance within the brain that causes alterations in awareness, attentiveness, responsiveness, behavior, or body movement. The signs and symptoms of seizures can be mild or severe depending on the part of the brain affected (Figure 11-8■). In its most dramatic form, a seizure results in violent, spasmodic movement of one or more opposing muscle groups and can cause a temporary loss of responsiveness. Seizures can last anywhere from seconds to hours, although most last 1–3 minutes. They usually end on their own and generally do not cause any long-term problems. Among the factors that may precipitate a seizure in susceptible individuals are pulsating lights or strobe lights and withdrawal from certain medications or alcohol. OEC Technicians should be familiar with two types of seizures: partial seizures and generalized seizures.

**Partial Seizures**   A partial seizure can be simple (responsiveness is not altered) or complex (responsiveness is altered) and may involve sensory changes, involuntary skeletal muscle activity, or any combination of the two. A simple partial seizure originates in one side of the brain but under certain conditions can quickly spread to the other side. Thus, a simple partial motor seizure may present as an involuntary jerking motion of a specific muscle group such as those in the hand, or it can spread to involve the entire arm, a condition known as a Jacksonian March seizure. Other signs associated with a simple partial motor seizure are grunting or in-

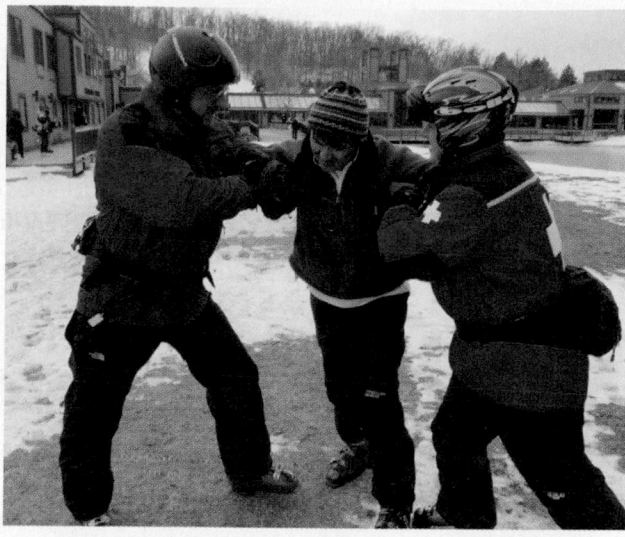

**Figure 11-7** Patients with behavioral or psychiatric disorders may present with AMS.
Copyright Edward McNamara

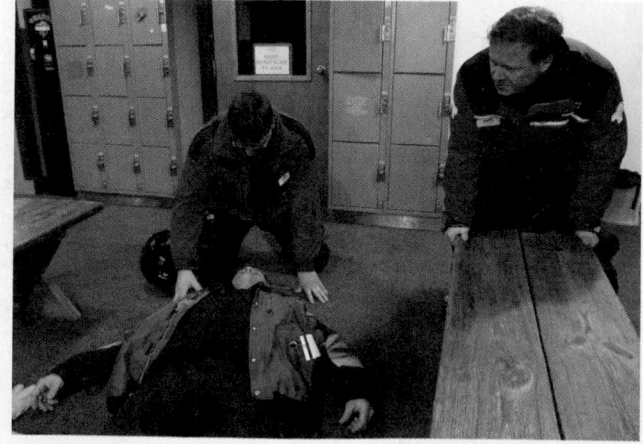

**Figure 11-8** Signs and symptoms of seizures may be mild or severe depending on the part of the brain that is affected.
Copyright Edward McNamara

comprehensible vocalizations, tensing of the torso muscles, and facial twitching, usually on one side only.

A patient experiencing a simple partial sensory seizure may complain of blurred vision, seeing spots or flashing lights, abnormal smells, buzzing noises, hot or cold sensations, tingling, numbness, or abnormal metallic tastes. These types of seizures generally do not result in a loss of responsiveness. By comparison, a complex partial seizure starts in one area of the brain and results in a loss of responsiveness. Sometimes, individuals undergoing a complex partial seizure display repetitive actions, known as automatisms, such as lip smacking, tugging at their clothes, head twisting, or body turning.

**Generalized Seizures**    Seizures that typically affect both sides of the body equally and result in a decreased level of responsiveness are considered **generalized seizures**. The mildest form, affecting mostly children and young adults, is called an **absence seizure**. This type of seizure, also called a petit mal seizure, is characterized by a vacant stare (i.e., "staring spells"), upward rolling of the eyes, or eyelid fluttering. An episode usually lasts less than 15 seconds and may not be noticed by others. The patient exhibits normal behavior immediately after and between episodes.

The most common type of generalized seizure, called a grand-mal seizure, may occur without warning and is characterized by muscle tensing and contraction, better known as tonic-clonic activity. During **tonic activity**, the muscles of the body tightly contract, causing the patient to forcefully stiffen. During **clonic activity**, the muscle groups spasm violently. The two types of muscle activity can occur independently or simultaneously. A generalized seizure can occur at any time and has three distinct phases: the pre-ictal, ictal, and post-ictal phases.

+ The pre-ictal phase occurs before the seizure and is sometimes preceded by a premonition of the impending seizure called an **aura,** a distinctive feeling or sensation that signals the patient that a seizure is about to occur (Figure 11-9■). Auras vary greatly among patients and are usually sensory in origin. They may present as a cognitive state such as déjà vu, a unique taste or smell, an auditory sensation or visual hallucinations. An aura usually lasts for only a few seconds but can last as long as several minutes.

+ The ictal phase usually begins with tonic muscle activity during which the patient may cry out and or fall stiffly to the ground (Figure 11-10a■). Clonic activity soon follows and may last for several minutes. During this phase the patient is unre-

**generalized seizure**   a seizure consisting of the sudden onset of unresponsiveness, tonic contraction of muscles, loss of postural control, and a cry caused by contraction of respiratory muscles that forces an exhalation; clonic contractions of muscles occur, followed by a period of somulence.

**absence seizure**   a sudden, temporary loss of mental awareness and physical activity lasting a few seconds to several minutes; also known as a petit mal seizure.

**tonic activity**   a general stiffening of the muscles.

**clonic activity**   the spasmodic jerking of muscles during a seizure.

**aura**   a subjective sensation that precedes a seizure.

**Figure 11-9** In the first or pre-ictal phase an aura may be experienced.

**Figure 11-10a** In the ictal phase the patient may first experience tonic movements.

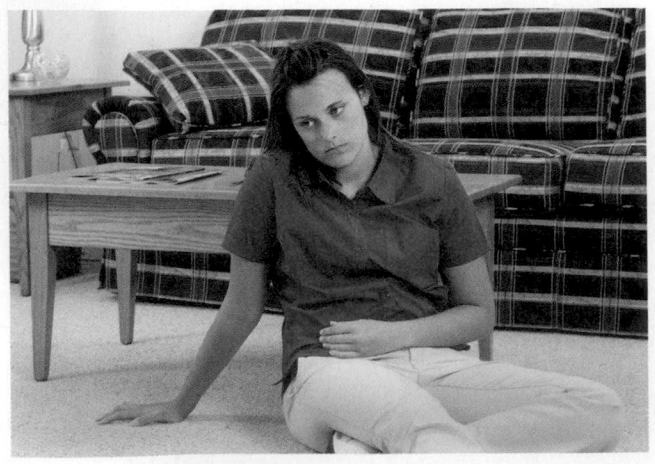

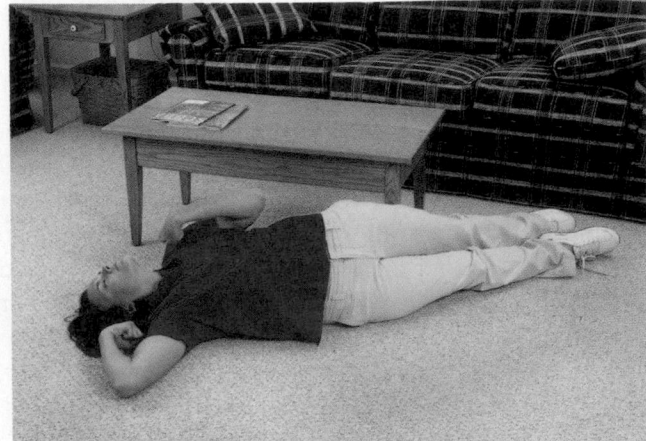

sponsive and may make grunting or gasping sounds. The jaw is usually clenched tightly, which can affect the patient's ability to breathe (Figure 11-10b■). In extreme cases, the patient may become slightly cyanotic, especially around the lips. The ictal phase typically lasts a very short time, usually 1 to 3 minutes. If the seizure lasts longer than 3 minutes, the cyanosis may become more pronounced.

✦ Post-ictal phase. Once tonic-clonic muscle activity stops, the post-ictal phase begins. During this phase, the patient is minimally responsive to voices or painful stimuli. The patient becomes limp and may unconsciously urinate or void the bowels due to relaxation of the urinary and anal sphincter muscles. The patient may exhibit snoring respirations or appear disoriented. With time, the patient becomes increasingly aware of the surroundings while becoming fully responsive and completely oriented. It is common for OEC Technicians to reach patients during this phase (Figure 11-10c■).

A condition known as status epilepticus is characterized by a seizure lasting longer than ten minutes, a prolonged post-ictal unresponsive state, or three or more seizures without regaining consciousness or becoming responsive. This is a medical emergency that can cause permanent brain injury, because the tremendous amount of energy expended during a prolonged seizure quickly depletes the brain of important energy substrates, thereby destroying delicate brain neurons.

### Seizure or Something Else?

Even though many people report having observed a seizure, often they saw some other medical condition that is unrelated to the brain. It is best to err on the side of caution: evaluate each report of seizure with the awareness that what you are seeing may be due to another medical condition and not a seizure.

**NOTE**

### Diabetes Mellitus

The body is normally very effective in maintaining a constant and appropriate supply of glucose in the blood. Normal blood sugar levels are between 70 and 110 mg/dL but may vary slightly depending on the individual's physiology and whether or not the person has recently eaten. When the body is no longer able to regulate the blood sugar level effectively and too much glucose is present in the blood, the patient is said to have diabetes mellitus, or simply "diabetes."

**◉ 11-3** List and compare the four major types of diabetes.

Diabetes is a chronic disease in which either the pancreas cannot produce enough insulin to meet metabolic needs, or the body's cells do not respond appropriately to insulin, or both. Normally, when a person eats a meal, glucose is absorbed from the small intestine into the bloodstream. The pancreas secretes insulin to facilitate the movement of glucose out of the bloodstream and into the cells, thereby providing the cells with the energy they need to function properly. If not enough insulin is

**Figure 11-10b** In the second or ictal phase of a grand mal seizure, the clonic muscle activity follows the tonic movements.

**Figure 11-10c** In the third or post-ictal phase of a grand mal seizure, the patient becomes flaccid and is minimally responsive.

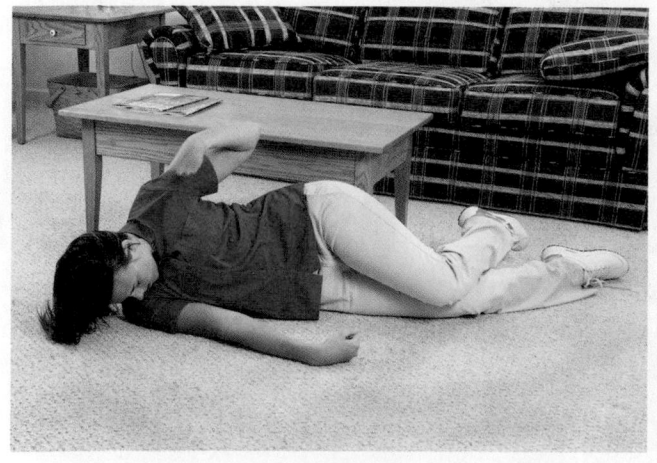

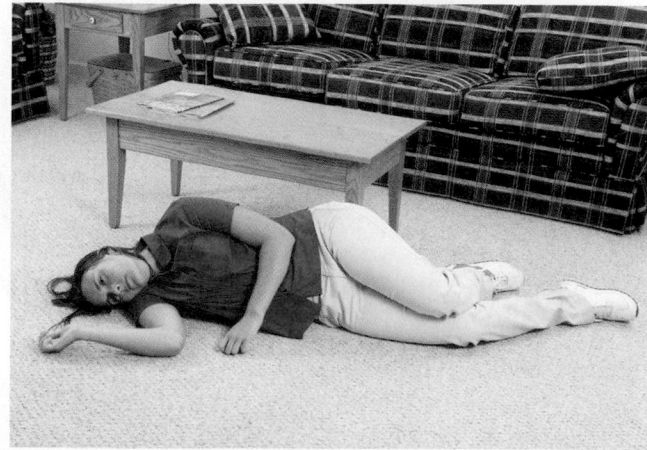

present, glucose cannot enter cells, so it accumulates in the bloodstream and raises circulating blood sugar levels.

Signs and symptoms of diabetes are numerous and vary with the duration of the disease (Figure 11-11a■).

**Polyuria**—an increased volume of urine—results when the kidneys attempt to excrete excess glucose from the bloodstream into the urine, and it is a common early sign of diabetes. An early symptom of diabetes is **polydipsia**, an abnormally increased thirst. This results in the body increasing the amount of fluids taken in orally, which in turn increases the volume of blood to dilute the glucose in it. Other symptoms may include increased appetite, unplanned weight loss or gain, fatigue, or dry mouth. Over time, diabetes can lead to a host of problems related to cellular damage.

It is estimated that over 6 percent of the U.S. population suffers from diabetes, and that the annual health cost of diabetes is over $100 million and growing. Diabetes also increases one's risk for developing other serious diseases and life-threatening infections. The long-term consequences of diabetes include damage or failure of various organs, including the eyes, kidneys, heart, blood vessels, and nerves.

There are four types of **diabetes mellitus**: Type 1, Type 2, gestational, and "other."

✦ Type 1 diabetes mellitus—previously known as insulin-dependent diabetes mellitus (IDDM) or juvenile-onset diabetes—accounts for 5–10 percent of all diabetes cases. Type 1 diabetes usually results from an autoimmune disorder in which cells of the immune system and antibodies attack the pancreas and destroy the cells responsible for producing insulin. The result is a high circulating blood glucose level, better known as hyperglycemia. Type 1 diabetes, which usually affects children and young adults, is treated with insulin that is usually self-administered via injection. Some patients use an insulin pump, a medical device that delivers

**polyuria**   excessive excretion of urine.

**polydipsia**   excessive thirst and fluid intake.

**diabetes mellitus**   a term that refers to a complex group of syndromes having in common a disturbance in the use of glucose; a condition that is often a result of a malfunction of the beta cells of the pancreas, whose function is the production and release of insulin.

**Figure 11-11a** Common signs and symptoms of a patient with low blood sugar and history of medication-controlled diabetes.

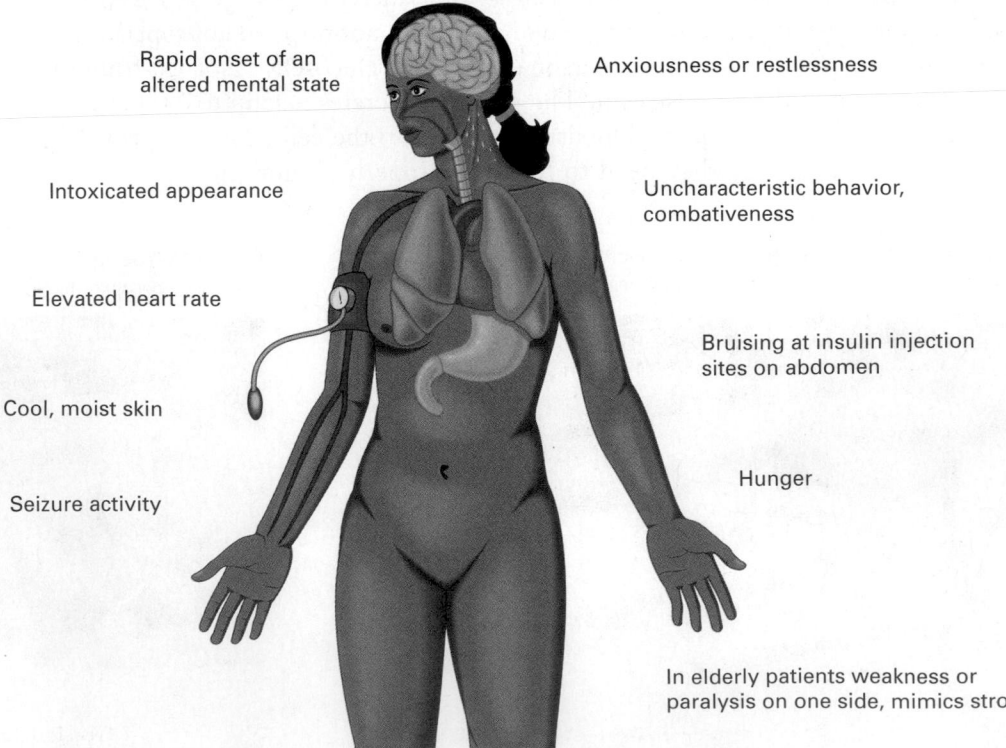

HYPOGLYCEMIC PATIENT, FROM UNCONTROLLED DIABETES
COMMON SIGNS AND SYMPTOMS

Rapid onset of an altered mental state

Anxiousness or restlessness

Intoxicated appearance

Uncharacteristic behavior, combativeness

Elevated heart rate

Bruising at insulin injection sites on abdomen

Cool, moist skin

Hunger

Seizure activity

In elderly patients weakness or paralysis on one side, mimics stroke smaller, more frequent doses of insulin. Some insulin pumps can monitor blood glucose levels and adjust the insulin dosage automatically.

✦ Type 2 diabetes mellitus. Previously referred to as adult-onset diabetes or non-insulin dependent diabetes mellitus (NIDDM), Type 2 is the most common form of diabetes and accounts for approximately 90–95 percent of all diabetes cases. Until recently, Type 2 diabetes was thought to affect only older individuals but is increasingly being diagnosed in young children, especially those who are obese. Unlike Type 1 diabetes, the problem is not solely related to insulin production, but instead to insulin's reduced effects on the body's cells. Thus, in Type 2 diabetes, the body's cells exhibit resistance to insulin, which prevents glucose from entering the cells (Figure 11-11b■). The reason for this is unknown, although studies show that the incidence of Type 2 diabetes is increased in people who are obese, particularly in the abdominal region. There may be a genetic predisposition to the disease. Most Type 2 diabetes patients do not initially require insulin injections and are treated through a regimen of weight loss, exercise, and "oral hypoglycemia agents," medications that lower blood glucose levels. Occasionally, as the patient gets older, low doses of insulin may be needed to regulate blood glucose levels.

✦ Gestational diabetes mellitus (GDM). Although this form of diabetes also affects insulin and blood sugar levels, it develops only during pregnancy. Gestational diabetes is further described in Chapter 34, Obstetric and Gynecologic Emergencies.

✦ "Other." The last type of diabetes includes other rare forms that are caused by genetic defects in the cells that produce insulin, the incorrect action of insulin, certain drugs or chemicals, and various hormone-related disorders.

Diabetic emergencies generally come to the attention of OEC Technicians only when the patient's circulating blood sugar level is either too low or too high. These conditions are known as hypoglycemia and hyperglycemia, respectively.

**Hypoglycemia** A circulating blood sugar level below 70 mg/dL is considered **hypoglycemia**, or low blood sugar. This condition most commonly occurs when the patient takes too much insulin or too much of an oral hypoglycemic medication (Table 11-2■). It may also occur if a diabetic takes a medication properly but either fails to eat a meal or to consume enough food. This is a common situation and is one that

⊕ **11-4** List the signs and symptoms and demonstrate the treatment of the following medical conditions:

a. hypoglycemia
b. hyperglycemia
c. partial seizure
d. generalized seizure

**hypoglycemia** an insufficient amount of glucose in the blood; may be associated with a myriad of signs and symptoms such as tremor, diaphoresis, drowsiness, headache, confusion, and lack of responsiveness.

**Figure 11-11b** Cellular response of a "normal" person vs a Type 1 diabetic in the production of energy.

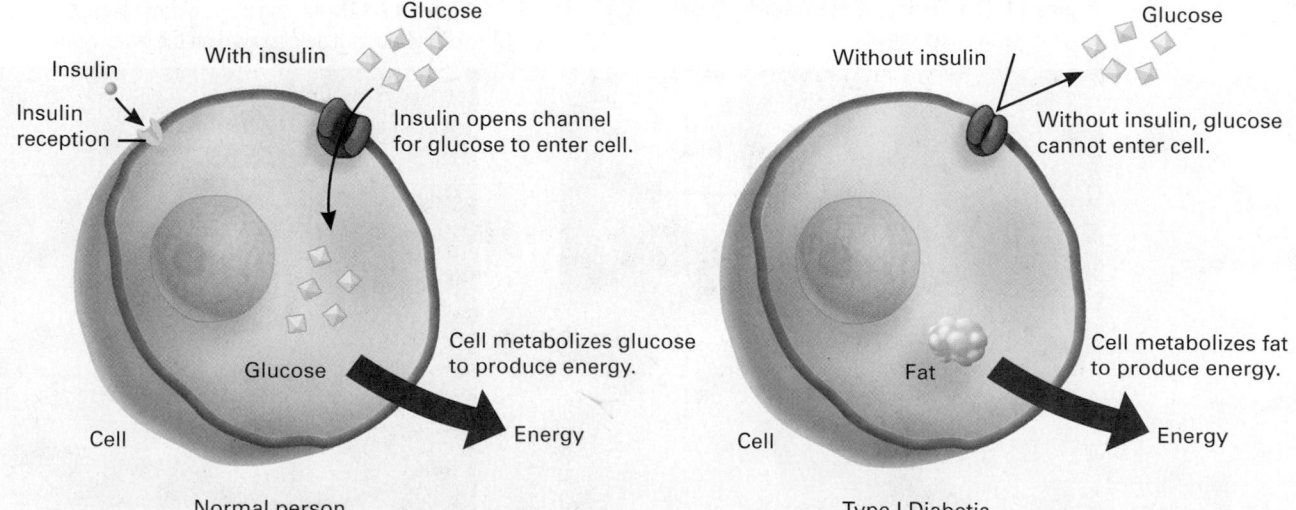

### Table 11-2 Causes of Diabetic Hypoglycemia

- An excessive dose of insulin
- An excessive dose or overdose of an oral hypoglycemic medication
- Too little food after taking diabetes medicine
- Overexertion, which exhausts glucose supplies
- Illness with vomiting (loss of glucose intake)
- Combinations of the previously listed causes

OEC Technicians will likely encounter in recreational settings. Outdoor enthusiasts who have diabetes may be at increased risk for hypoglycemia due to the natural increase in both metabolic rate and cellular glucose demands that accompany physical exercise.

There are many signs and symptoms of hypoglycemia. Early signs and symptoms are related to the release of epinephrine (adrenalin) by the adrenal glands and may include anxiety, dizziness, tachycardia, diaphoresis, tremor, headache, and mild confusion. The patient typically remains responsive and able to swallow. These symptoms, if recognized by the patient, are usually improved by ingesting a carbohydrate meal or supplemental glucose.

Blood sugar levels can fall very quickly in patients who take insulin. The brain depends on glucose to function, so if early hypoglycemia is not recognized and treated, neurologic symptoms will develop as hypoglycemia becomes more severe. The signs and symptoms of severe hypoglycemia—referred to in the past as insulin "shock"—include marked confusion, disorientation, lethargy and loss of responsiveness, slurred speech, seizures, and unilateral extremity weakness resembling a stroke. Irrational or combative behavior is especially common for some diabetics experiencing severe hypoglycemia. Fortunately, most diabetics monitor their blood glucose levels as often as four times a day to maintain therapeutic blood glucose levels and to prevent hypoglycemia (Figures 11-12a■ and 11-12b■).

**Hyperglycemia**    High blood sugar, or **hyperglycemia**, is defined as an elevated circulating blood sugar level that is higher than 180 mg/dL. In patients with known diabetes, the primary cause of hyperglycemia is failure to take one's diabetes medications, which can lead to a very high blood sugar level and polyuria, polydipsia, dry mouth, and fatigue. In some diabetics, escalating blood glucose levels lead to a

**hyperglycemia**   an excess of glucose in the blood; when severe, may be associated with confusion or changes in mental status.

**Figure 11-12a** Testing blood glucose level: first prick a finger to get a blood sample.

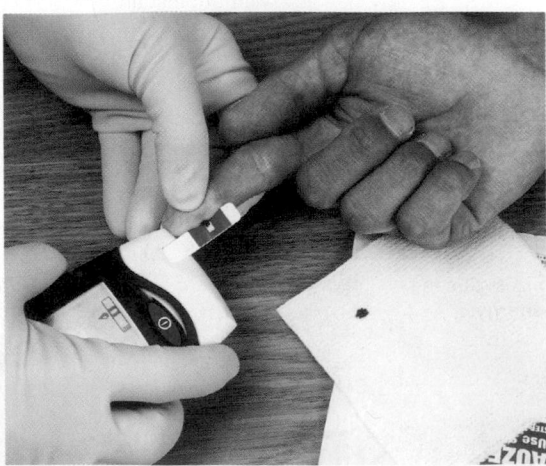

**Figure 11-12b** Testing blood glucose level: then read the blood glucose value displayed on the glucometer.

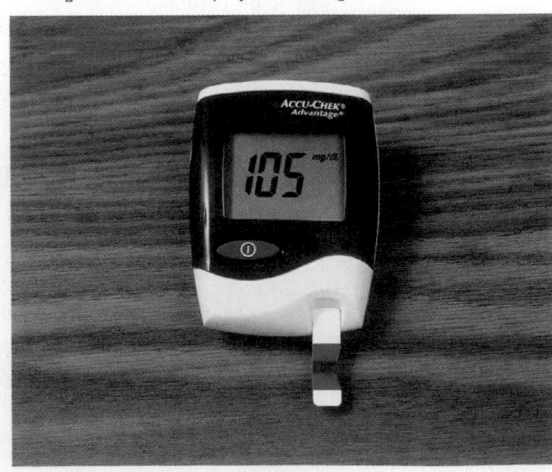

build-up of acids within the blood. These patients have associated nausea, vomiting, abdominal pain, and varying degrees of AMS. Unless treated, the combination of high blood sugar and acidosis can result in coma, brain damage, or death. Fortunately, this condition occurs far less often than does hypoglycemia and typically occurs over days to even months. Although potentially life threatening, hyperglycemia is unlikely to be encountered in outdoor recreational environments, with the noted exception of individuals who are stranded in a backcountry area and have either lost or run out of their diabetes medication. Individuals who do not know they have diabetes commonly present with signs and symptoms of hyperglycemia, but rarely with those of AMS.

# STOP, THINK, UNDERSTAND

## Multiple Choice

Choose the correct answer.

The causes of AMS can be remembered by the mnemonic AEIOU-TIPS, which stands for_____

a. AMS, Excitability/environment, Insulin level, Oxygen deprivation, Unresponsive, Trauma/tremors, Infection, Poisons, Seizures.

b. Allergy, Environmental, Insulin level, Ocular, Unresponsive, Tumor, Internal hemorrhage, Perforation, Syncope.

c. Alcohol/acidosis, Epilepsy/environment, Insulin, Oxygen/overdose, Uremia, Trauma, Infection, Poisoning, Seizure/stroke/syncope.

## Fill in the Blank

1. For each of the following signs or symptoms, indicate whether the CNS malfunction is global (G) or focal (F).

    _____ a. decreased level of responsiveness
    _____ b. delirium
    _____ c. motor weakness
    _____ d. hallucination
    _____ e. balance problems
    _____ f. vision loss
    _____ g. speech abnormalities
    _____ h. combativeness
    _____ i. delusions

2. Indicate for each of the following characteristic of diabetes whether it refers to Type 1, to Type 2, or to both.

    _____ a. insulin dependent
    _____ b. non-insulin dependent
    _____ c. 90-95 percent of all diabetes cases

    _____ d. 5–10 percent of all diabetes cases
    _____ e. cells exhibit resistance to insulin, which prevents glucose from entering cells
    _____ f. autoimmune disorder in which insulin-producing cells are destroyed
    _____ g. associated with obesity
    _____ h. not related to obesity
    _____ i. associated more commonly with younger patients
    _____ j. associated more commonly with older patients

3. Indicate whether each of the following characteristics relates to hypoglycemia or to hyperglycemia.

    _____ a. low blood sugar
    _____ b. high blood sugar
    _____ c. too much insulin
    _____ d. too little insulin

## Matching

Match each of the following terms with its definition.

_____ 1. alcohol

_____ 2. insulin

_____ 3. tumor

_____ 4. aura

_____ 5. polydypsia

_____ 6. acidosis

_____ 7. polyuria

a. an abnormal growth of cells that may be benign or malignant
b. a chemical that depresses CNS function
c. a decline in body pH below normal
d. a pancreatic hormone that regulates blood sugar levels
e. a subjective sensation that precedes a seizure
f. excessive excretion of urine
g. excessive thirst and fluid intake

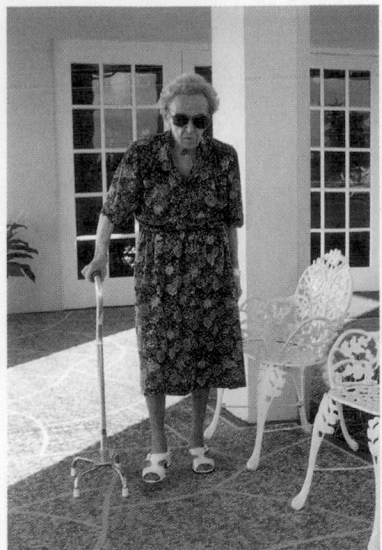

**Figure 11-13** Stroke patients often suffer impairment on one side of the body.

## Stroke

*Stroke* is a general term that describes neurological brain impairment resulting from low blood flow or a lack of blood flow to areas of the brain (Figure 11-13■). OEC Technicians should be familiar with three basic types of stroke and their signs and symptoms: ischemic, hemorrhagic, and transient (Figure 11-14■ and Figure 11-15■).

The most common type of stroke (80 percent of strokes) is an ischemic stroke, which is caused by a disruption of blood flow to a portion of the brain. The primary cause of an ischemic stroke is foreign material (an embolus) that travels through the bloodstream until it lodges in an artery in the brain, causing the condition called embolism. Examples of emboli that can cause an ischemic stroke include blood clots, fatty emboli from bone marrow fat in a long bone fracture and cholesterol plaques that break loose from the heart chambers or carotid arteries. Most emboli originate outside the brain. Once an embolus becomes lodged in the arterial cerebral circulation, blood flow to part of the brain may be reduced or completely stopped. Depending on the area affected, portions of the brain may cease to function properly, resulting in a variety of signs and symptoms. This type of stroke is also known as a "dry stroke" or "white stroke" because the cerebral blood vessels, although blocked, remain intact and do not bleed.

**Figure 11-14** A stroke can occur from bleeding into or around the brain or from an artery becoming occluded either temporarily or permanently.

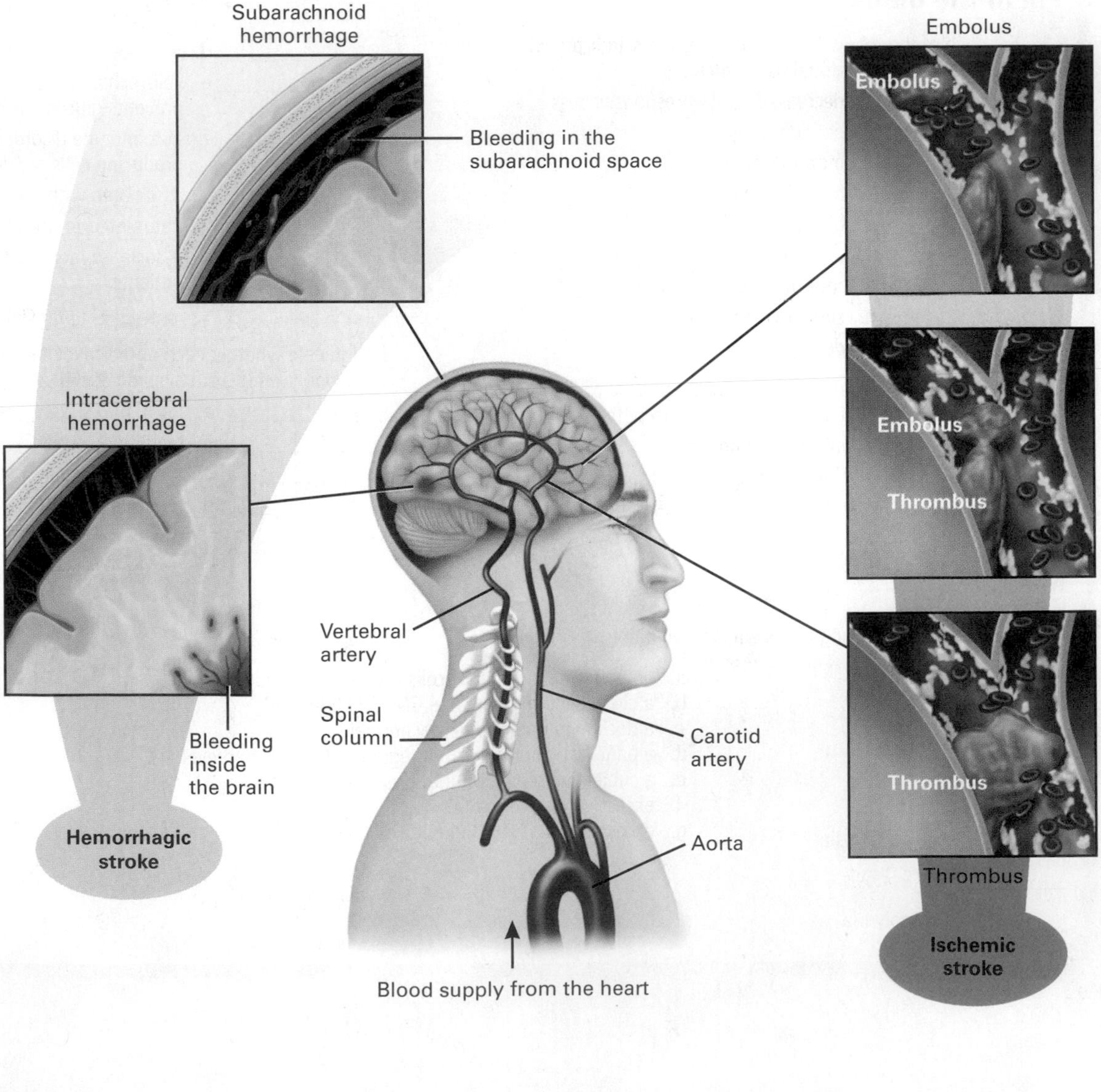

Subarachnoid
hemorrhage

Embolus

Embolus

Bleeding in the
subarachnoid space

Embolus

Thrombus

Intracerebral
hemorrhage

Vertebral
artery

Spinal
column

Bleeding
inside
the brain

Carotid
artery

Thrombus

Hemorrhagic
stroke

Aorta

Thrombus

Blood supply from the heart

Ischemic
stroke

The second type of stroke is a hemorrhagic stroke. This form, also known as an intracerebral hemorrhage or "wet stroke," or "red stroke" occurs when a blood vessel within the brain suddenly ruptures, releasing blood into the surrounding brain tissue. This not only reduces the amount of oxygen and nutrients available to the brain, but the resulting hematoma also places direct pressure on the delicate brain tissue confined within the skull. The most common cause of a hemorrhagic stroke is a structural weakness within the wall of a blood vessel within the brain. The constant force of blood pressing against the wall of the vessel can cause it to burst. The small, fragile "end arteries" located at the base of the brain are especially vulnerable to developing a weakness and rupturing. Depending on the size of the ruptured vessel and the extent of the brain affected, a hemorrhagic stroke can result in permanent neurologic problems or death.

The last type of stroke is a transient ischemic attack. Also known as a TIA or "ministroke," it is a reversible neurological deficit that is caused by a *temporary* interruption of blood flow to an area of the brain. No permanent brain injury results, and the signs and symptoms resolve completely within 24 hours. TIAs are typically caused by a small embolus that only temporarily blocks a small artery within the brain. Signs and symptoms of a TIA appear when an embolus becomes temporarily lodged in and blocks one of the cerebral arteries. However, once the embolus dissolves or no longer blocks the artery, the signs and symptoms quickly disappear. Although the symptoms often resolve spontaneously, a TIA serves as an early warning that a more serious stroke is likely to occur in the near future. It is for this reason that patients who exhibit signs or symptoms of a TIA should seek immediate treatment at a hospital.

**⊕11-5** Compare and contrast the three types of stroke:

  **a.** ischemic stroke

  **b.** hemorrhagic stroke

  **c.** transient ischemic attack

**Figure 11-15** Difficulty speaking and slurred speech, facial asymmetry, AMS, and impairment in motor function are among the most common signs and symptoms of strokes.

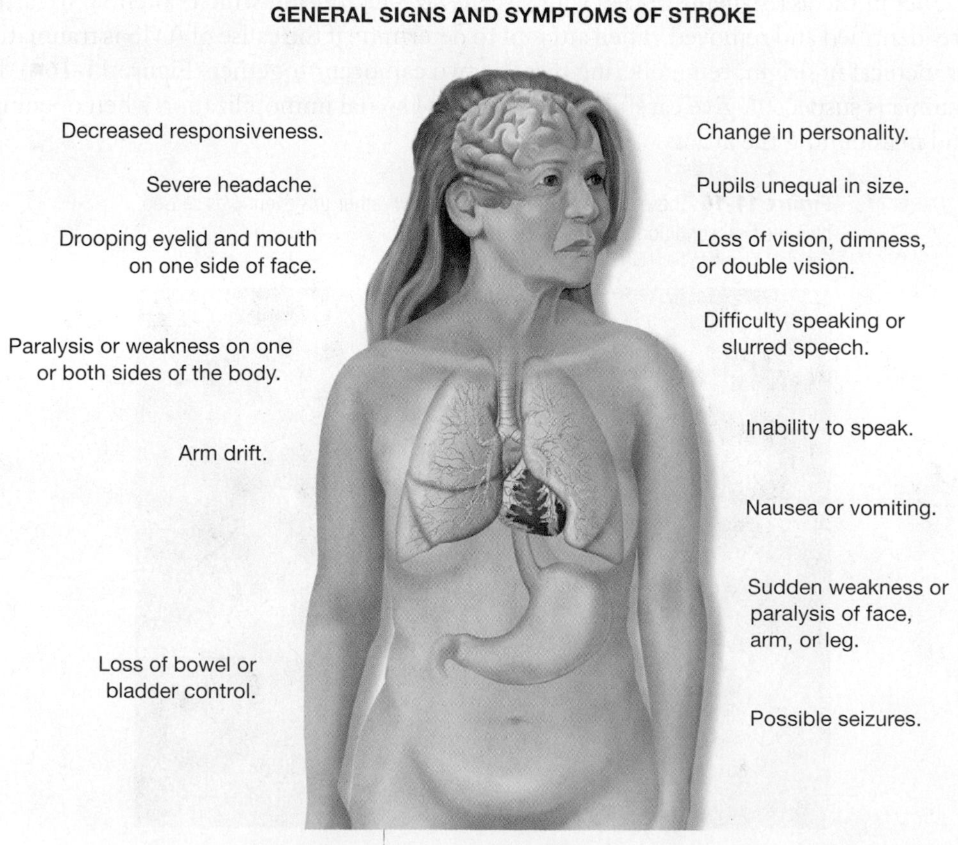

**GENERAL SIGNS AND SYMPTOMS OF STROKE**

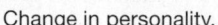

Decreased responsiveness.

Severe headache.

Drooping eyelid and mouth on one side of face.

Paralysis or weakness on one or both sides of the body.

Arm drift.

Loss of bowel or bladder control.

Change in personality.

Pupils unequal in size.

Loss of vision, dimness, or double vision.

Difficulty speaking or slurred speech.

Inability to speak.

Nausea or vomiting.

Sudden weakness or paralysis of face, arm, or leg.

Possible seizures.

# CASE UPDATE

You tell the store manager to hold the man's head and instruct the clerk to call for an ambulance. After introducing yourself to the patient, you begin to perform a secondary assessment, looking for any injuries or clues that might help you pinpoint the problem. Just as you are about to obtain a SAMPLE history, the man's eyes suddenly roll back, and then he makes a loud groaning sound, stiffens, and begins to shake violently. The manager yells, "He's having a fit! Quick, take his wallet and put it in his mouth before he dies!" He shoves the man's wallet into your hands.

*What should you do now?*

---

**11-6** Describe how to assess a patient with altered mental status.

## Patient Assessment

Determining the underlying cause of AMS can be challenging. In many instances the patient cannot communicate, making it more difficult to determine the cause. You may need to rely on circumstantial evidence such as interviews with family members or bystanders, or medic identification tags that list the patient's medications or illnesses. As a general rule, AMS in younger individuals is more likely to be caused by a toxic overdose or trauma, whereas the cause in older individuals is more likely to be a focal neurological insult such as a stroke. Diabetic and epilepsy-related emergencies can occur in any age group.

Some patients with psychiatric or behavioral illness may present a complicated picture of AMS. These patients should be considered to have a metabolic or structural lesion until proven otherwise at a definitive-care facility. Regardless of the underlying cause, AMS is considered an emergency until the cause can be determined and treated.

Begin the assessment process with a scene size-up, during which potential hazards are identified and removed. Then attempt to determine if the cause of AMS is traumatic or medical in origin, remembering that the two can occur together (Figure 11-16■). If trauma is suspected, give careful consideration of spinal immobilization when opening and maintaining the airway.

**Figure 11-16** These patrollers must determine whether this event was caused by a medical condition or a traumatic event.
Copyright Edward McNamara

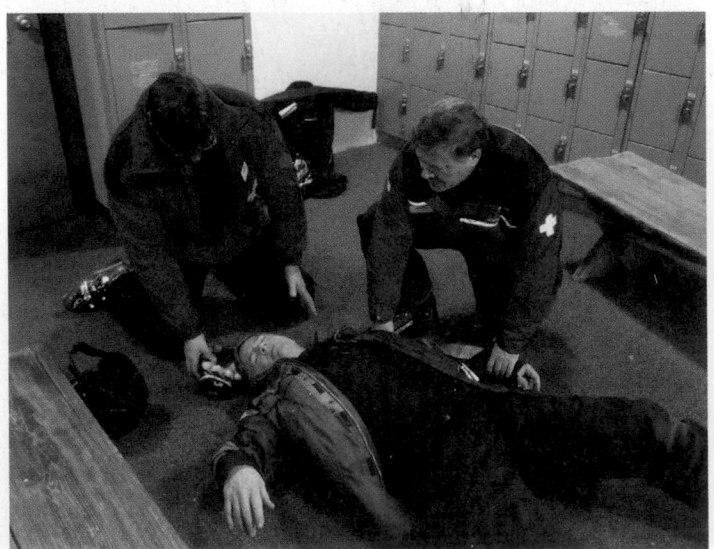

Once the scene size-up is complete, perform a primary assessment by carefully assessing the ABCDs to ensure that they are intact. Make sure the airway is open. Remember, the brain is very sensitive to even minor fluctuations in oxygen or blood glucose levels, and any problem affecting oxygenation or circulation must be identified and corrected quickly. If the patient is unresponsive, open the airway, and simultaneously check for breathing and a carotid pulse. If no pulse, begin CPR.

Hypoxia and hypoglycemia are the two most common causes of AMS that may be encountered by OEC Technicians. Be sure to evaluate the patient's level of responsiveness using the AVPU scale to determine the extent and severity of the AMS. If time permits, assess the LOR using the Glasgow Coma Scale. Monitor the level of responsiveness closely, performing serial assessments. Any patient who is initially disoriented but rapidly recovers may have suffered a seizure, syncope, or a temporary stroke. Next, assess the need for additional resources. This step is very important because early activation of advanced life-support procedures may be required for effective management of some of the more complex causes of AMS.

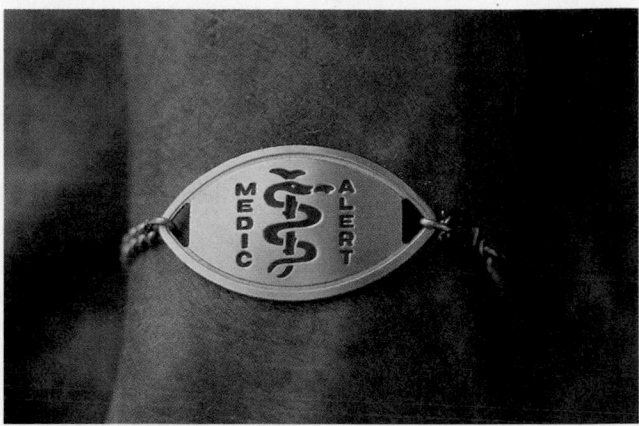

**Figure 11-17** Medical alert tags may provide medical information that is pertinent to the event.

Next, perform a secondary assessment by first obtaining a complete SAMPLE history (if possible) and vital signs. A relative who is present may help you with the history if the patient is unresponsive. Look for a medical identification tag on a bracelet or necklace or for a medical identification card in the patient's pocket, pack, wallet, or purse that may tell you of a medical condition, allergy, or medications the patient is taking (Figure 11-17■). Ask responsive patients if they have taken their medications as prescribed. Remember to use AEIOU-TIPS when assessing for AMS.

Attempt to determine the exact time when the symptoms began or were first noticed, noting whether the symptoms came on suddenly or more slowly. If the onset of symptoms is not known—if, for example, a patient awoke from sleep with the symptoms—attempt to determine when the patient was last known to be well. If the patient had a seizure, investigate whether or not the seizure began in one part of the body and how long the convulsions lasted. Note whether the patient's speech appears impaired, such as the slurring of words, the misuse of words, or incomprehensible speech, which may result from alcohol or drug intoxication, hypoglycemia, stroke, or a behavioral condition. Also note if the patient repeatedly asks the same question or says the same phrase over and over. If, for example, the patient repeatedly asks, "What happened?" or keeps saying, "I need to find my poles," this disoriented behavior may be a clue to an underlying brain injury or a diabetes-related problem.

Obtain a full accounting of the patient's signs and symptoms, including reports of increased thirst, increased appetite (polyphagia), and frequent urination, all of which are commonly reported by patients with diabetes. Complaints of increased fatigue, frequent headaches, and wounds that heal slowly are also associated with diabetes. Be especially attentive to reports of visual disturbances such as blurred vision or sudden blindness, which may be evidence of a stroke. Likewise, an impending seizure may be preceded by an aura such as "seeing spots or flashing lights."

Perform a thorough physical exam, using the DCAP-BTLS approach. Look closely at the pupils and inside the patient's mouth. Note pupil size and response. Pinpoint pupils are often associated with a narcotics overdose, whereas unequal pupils are an ominous sign that generally indicates a buildup of pressure within the brain, often due to trauma or stroke. Examine the mouth for cuts on the tongue or inside the cheeks, which commonly result from inadvertent biting that occurs during a convulsion following a seizure. Then check the patient's skin, noting its temperature and overall condition. Pale, moist skin may be due to shock or hypoglycemia; hot, dry skin may result from hyperglycemia or hyperthermia (Table 11-3■). Skin that is hot and moist may also be caused by an infection. Also check to see if the patient is incontinent of urine or feces, which may indicate that the patient had a seizure.

If the patient is unresponsive, ask friends or family if the patient has diabetes. If he has diabetes and has a blood glucose monitor, check the device for the time the level was last checked. If a reading has been taken within the last 30 minutes, compare its results to normal blood sugar values. Be aware, however, that the strips used to measure blood glucose levels have an expiration date, and that the use of outdated test strips may result in an inaccurate reading.

As part of the secondary assessment, you may wish to perform a more detailed assessment of the patient's neurological function by performing a mini-neuro exam consisting of the following components:

+ Level of responsiveness using the Glasgow Coma Scale
+ Pupillary exam
+ Motor-sensory exam
+ Higher cortical function exam
+ Vocal/speech exam

Proper use of the Glasgow Coma Scale and the procedures for performing the pupillary exam are described in Chapter 7, Patient Assessment.

The motor-sensory exam consists of assessing the ability of the limbs to move in unison and in a directed fashion, as well the patient's ability to sense and differentiate touch. This exam consists of two separate tasks. First, ask the patient to hold both arms straight out in front, with the palms turned upward for 10–15 seconds (Figure 11-18a■). If one

| Table **11-3** Comparison of Hypoglycemia and Hyperglycemia |
|---|
| **Findings in Progressively Severe Hypoglycemia** |
| Tremor |
| Anxiety |
| Headache |
| Diaphoresis |
| Dizziness |
| Confusion, disorientation |
| Slurred speech |
| Lethargy |
| Seizures |
| Weakness of one of more extremities |
| Irrational, combative behavior |
| Loss of responsiveness |
| **Findings in Progressively Severe Hyperglycemia** |
| Polyuria |
| Polydipsia |
| Dehydration |
| Warm, dry skin |
| Rapid weak pulse |
| Normal or low blood pressure |
| Sweet or fruity breath |
| Less than A (Alert) on AVPU scale |
| Rapid, deep respirations |

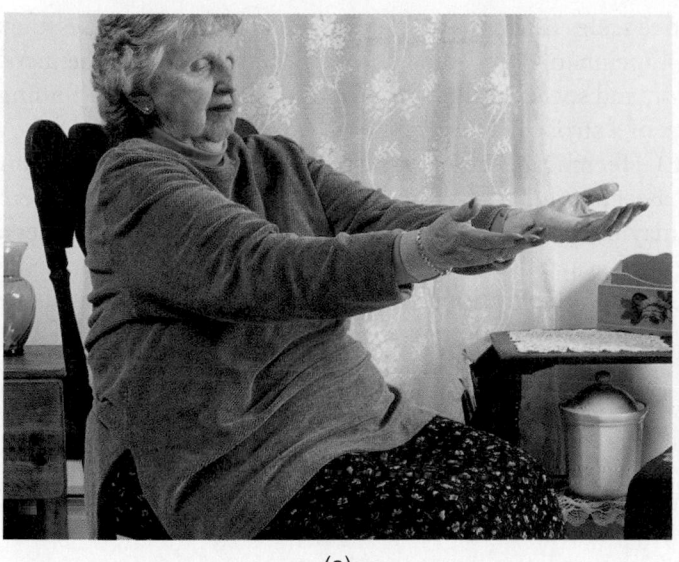 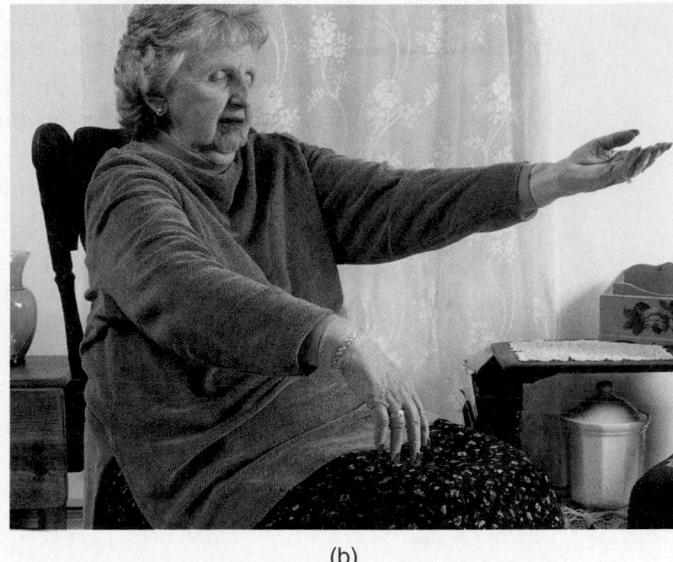

(a)                                                              (b)

**Figure 11-18** (a) Ask a potential stroke patient to extend the arms straight out in front with the palms facing up and the eyes closed. (b) Patients who have had a stroke are often unable to hold both arms extended in front; one arm may drift downward or the palm may rotate downward.

arm drifts downward, the patient has a documented motor deficit and may be experiencing a stroke (Figure 11-18b■). To assess sensation, ask the patient to close his eyes, and touch one of the patient's hands or feet. Then ask the patient to identify which hand or foot was touched. Repeat this test, touching a different hand or foot each time, until all the patient's extremities have been assessed.

Higher cortical function is checked by having the patient perform a task consisting of multiple steps. For instance, ask the patient to hold up two fingers on the right hand. This requires the brain to accurately process the request and to send the proper signal to the hand. The brain of a patient who is unable to perform the task accurately and quickly is not functioning properly, indicating an abnormality within the part of the brain that controls the higher cortical functions. The vocal-speech portion of the exam is assessed by having the patient repeat a phrase such as "The sky is blue and the sun is orange." A patient whose brain is not functioning properly cannot accurately repeat the phrase without such problems such as slurring the words (Figure 11-19■).

OEC Technicians must recognize the signs and symptoms of a stroke and recommend evaluation at a clinic or hospital. Signs and symptoms of a stroke include numbness and weakness or paralysis on one side of the body. A stroke may involve only the leg, the arm, or the face, or all of them. Speech and language may be affected as well. Sudden disorientation or inability to perform tasks such as buttoning a shirt, putting on a hat, or zipping a coat may be a sign of stroke. Visual problems, such as blurry vision or loss of vision for part of the visual field, may be a symptom. As a result, patients may walk into objects they might otherwise see. Patients may exhibit a sudden inability to walk, dizziness, or clumsiness. Any of these signs and symptoms and the complaint of a sudden and unusually severe headache should alert OEC Technicians to the possibility of a stroke. The patient may have experienced a TIA in which the signs and symptoms have resolved, or the signs and symptoms may be subtle.

**Figure 11-19** Ask a suspected stroke patient to repeat a simple phrase. The patient may have slurred speech, use incorrect words, or be unable to speak at all.

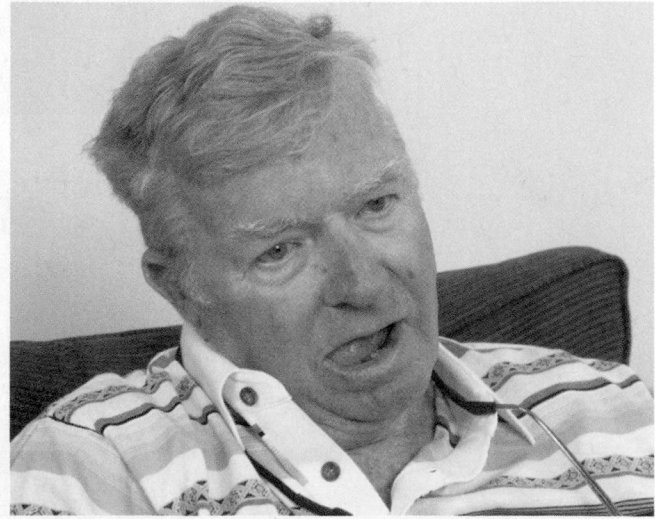

Among the several stroke scales that have been developed to aid in the assessment of a stroke patient is the Cincinnati Prehospital Stroke Scale. This assessment tool tests facial droop, arm drift, and speech. The presence of even one of these findings suggests a high probability of a stroke (Figure 11-20■).

It is important that OEC Technicians determine as near as possible the exact time of the onset of symptoms. Because the onset of symptoms may be painless and therefore silent, time of onset may be difficult to identify. Estimating the time of onset as accurate as possible is needed to establish a window for treatment, because treatment may be ineffective if therapy with medications (discussed later) is started outside the treatment window. If the time of onset of symptoms cannot be determined, the time of onset is considered to be the last time the patient was known to be normal.

In the early stages of a neurologic event such as a stroke, it is difficult to predict whether the symptoms will be reversible. Some conditions, such as a TIA, signal the potential for further episodes that may result in permanent injury. Thus, any patient

**Figure 11-20** Assessment parameters of the Cincinnati Prehospital Stroke Scale.

**Cincinnati Prehospital Stroke Scale**

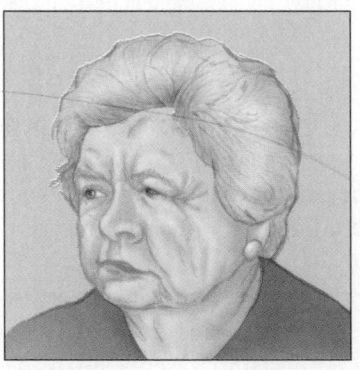

**Facial Droop**
Normal:    Both sides of face move equally
Abnormal:  One side of face does not move at all

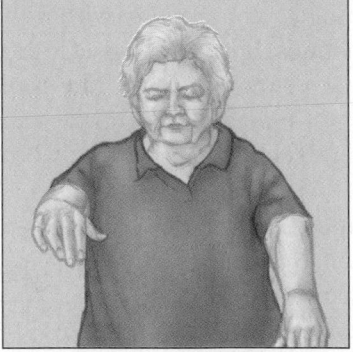

**Arm Drift**
Normal:    Both arms move equally or not at all
Abnormal:  One arm drifts compared to the other

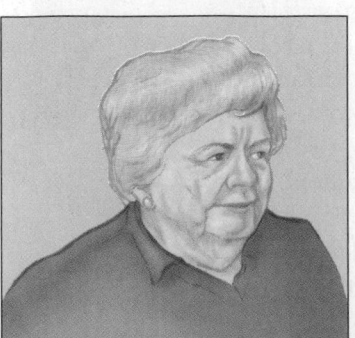

**Speech**
Normal:    Patient uses correct words with no slurring
Abnormal:  Slurred or inappropriate words or mute

presenting with AMS, including those with improving signs, should still be evaluated at a clinic or hospital. Early detection and rapid transport to an emergency care facility are the keys for improving the patient's survival after a stroke.

## Patient Management

The overall treatment of patients with an AMS is fairly straightforward and centers on correcting any problems affecting the ABCDs, providing oxygen, giving sugar to an awake diabetic, and rapidly transporting the patient to a definitive care facility (Figure 11-21■). As basic as this sounds, strict attention to these management priorities will significantly improve the patient's outcome. Once the patient's ABCDs have been appropriately managed, OEC Technicians may provide specific care, which should include adopting a "load and go" principle for life-threatening conditions.

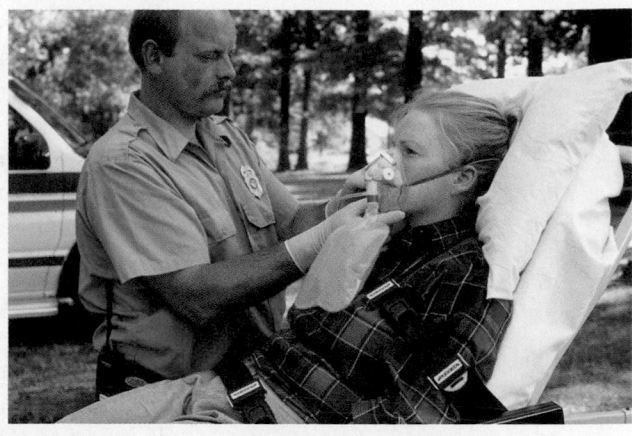

**Figure 11-21** Place a responsive patient for which no head or spinal injury is suspected in a supine position with the head and chest elevated.

All patients who exhibit an AMS should receive high-flow oxygen; use a nonrebreather mask for patients with effective, spontaneous respirations, and a bag-valve mask for patients whose respirations are either ineffective or absent. Check the patient's airway frequently, using suction as needed to ensure that it remains patent. Place a nasal or oral airway in the unresponsive patient to keep the airway patent.

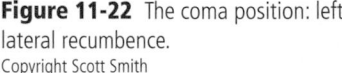

**11-7** Describe and demonstrate the treatment of a patient with altered mental status.

Spinal precautions should be taken for all unresponsive patients when the cause is unknown, because trauma may have produced a spine or other neurologic injury. The process for properly immobilizing the spine is presented in Chapter 21, Head and Spine Injuries. All other treatment is symptom based and is provided using the AEIOU-TIPS mnemonic as a guide.

### AEIOU-TIPS

To achieve symptom-based management of a patient with an AMS, use the AEIOU-TIPS mnemonic (described next) as a guide.

**A**—*Alcohol and Acidosis*. AMS due to alcohol intoxication can be a true emergency, especially if central nervous system function is impaired. Patients who are unconscious and unresponsive and have diminished respirations must be immediately transported to a hospital for evaluation by a physician. During transport, place the patient in the left lateral recumbent position to avoid the aspiration of vomit (Figure 11-22■). This

**Figure 11-22** The coma position: left lateral recumbence.
Copyright Scott Smith

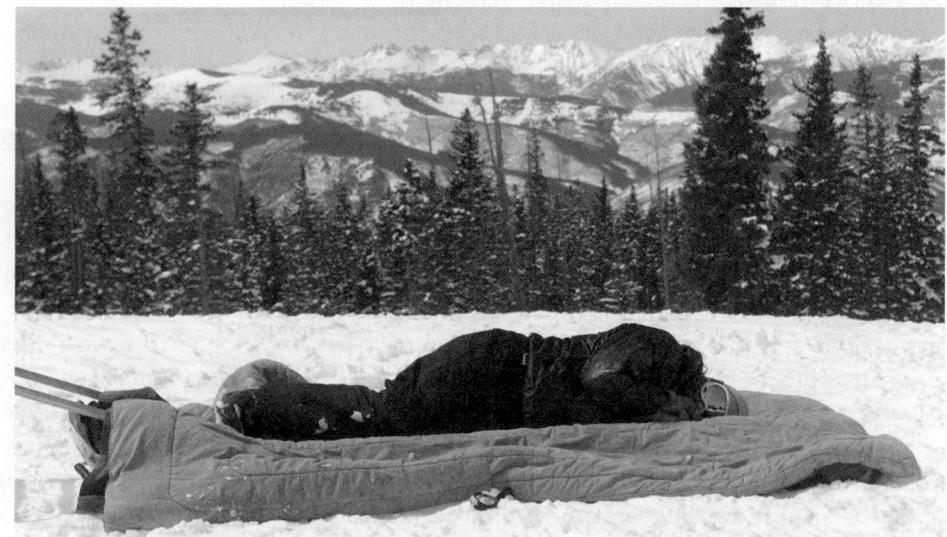

position may be particularly important for longer backcountry extrications. If respirations become shallow, it may be necessary to support the patient's ventilation efforts using either a nasopharyngeal airway or an oropharyngeal airway and a bag-valve mask.

Acidosis is a serious medical disorder that is best managed in a hospital by a physician. Hospital treatment of acidosis centers on identifying the underlying source of the acidosis and normalizing the body's pH, a process that can take several hours or days.

**E**—*Epilepsy, Environment, and Electrolytes*. Treatment of epilepsy is supportive. Any patient who is seizing must be protected from further traumatic injury. Treatment of seizures is described shortly. Careful suctioning may be needed to remove blood or mucus. Remove any broken teeth from the mouth to prevent their aspiration and to preserve any that may be salvageable.

The E in AEIOU-TIPS also stands for environment. Both hypothermia and hyperthermia are treated by correcting the core body temperature, whether by warming or cooling the patient. For information concerning how to manage temperature-related problems, see Chapter 25, Cold-Related Emergencies, and Chapter 26, Heat-Related Emergencies.

AMS associated with an electrolyte imbalance is a serious condition that warrants immediate referral to a hospital for electrolyte replacement therapy. Although complex sports drinks may provide some short-term benefit, especially when the symptoms are minor or the patient is in a remote setting that requires a long transport time, they typically lack the correct quantities or balance of electrolytes and often cannot be properly absorbed by the body.

**I**—*Insulin*. Any fully responsive diabetic who has AMS should receive oral sugar. In these cases, OEC Technicians should assume that the patient is hypoglycemic because hypoglycemia can quickly cause irreparable brain damage. If the patient was hyperglycemic, you will not cause further harm because the small amount of sugar that is administered will neither worsen the patient's condition nor alter the outcome. Administering sugar will, however, greatly benefit hypoglycemic patients, who constitute the largest percentage of diabetes patients in need of emergent care.

Before administering oral glucose, be sure the patient can follow simple instructions by asking the patient to hold an object such as cup of water. Ask the patient to drink a sip of the water to determine if the gag reflex is intact. Patients able to perform both tasks are candidates for oral glucose. Never place oral glucose into the mouth of an unresponsive patient because this can result in aspiration and serious pulmonary problems. An unresponsive diabetic patient requires IV glucose or subcutaneous glucagon, which can be provided only by an advanced care provider such as an IV-certified EMT or a paramedic. If an advanced provider is not immediately available, either summon one or rapidly transport the patient to a definitive-care facility. Check to see whether any family member present might be carrying an emergency glucagon kit and be trained in its use.

Only minimal absorption of "instant" glucose products occurs through the cheeks within the mouth. If the patient is responsive and has an intact gag reflex, the best way to treat early hypoglycemia is to have the patient swallow 15–20 grams of glucose (Figure 11-23■). This can be in the form of sucrose tablets, sugar cubes, or five packets of table sugar dissolved in water. Orange juice has been found to be less effective than any of these forms for raising blood sugar levels but can be used if several packets of table sugar are added to it. Commercially available glucose tablets are also effective, such as 3 BD glucose tablets (5 gm dextrose per tablet), or 4 Dex4 (4 gm per tablet) glucose tablets. If symptoms resolve (usually within 15 minutes of treatment), the patient should consume a small meal to prevent recurrent hypoglycemia. If symptoms do not

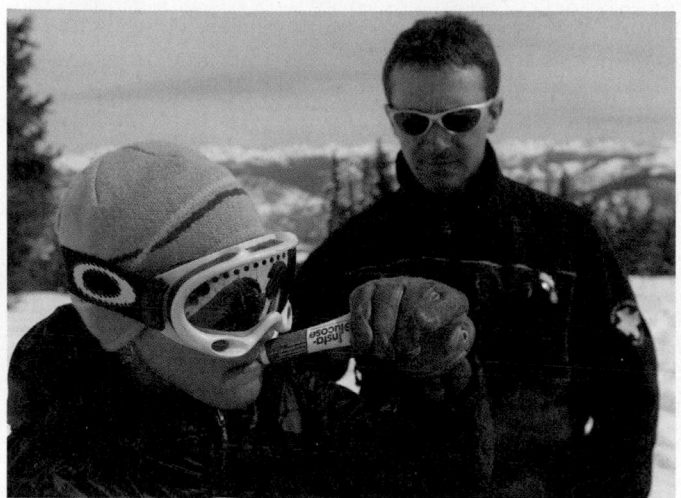

**Figure 11-23** Assist responsive hypoglycemic patients to insert glucose into their own mouth.
Copyright Scott Smith

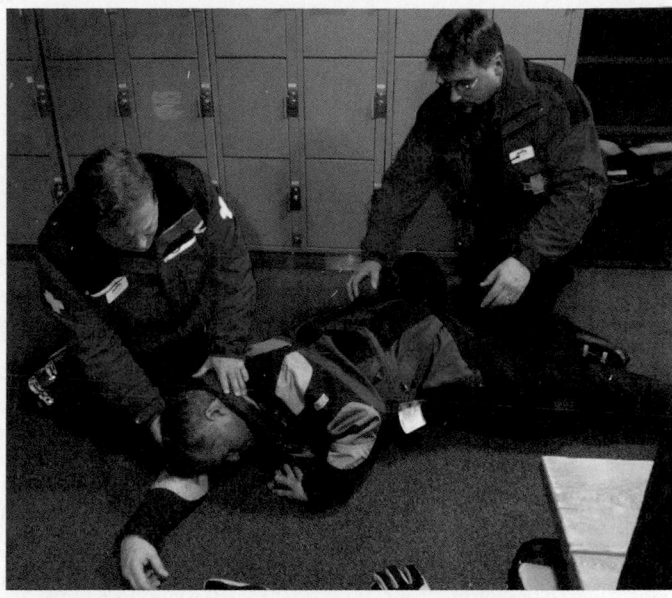

**Figure 11-24** If a patient's symptoms of hypoglycemia do not resolve, protect him from further injury. Look for another cause for his AMS.
Copyright Edward McNamara

resolve, there may be another cause for the patient's AMS, and the patient should be transported to an EMS access point or to a higher level of medical care (Figure 11-24■).

Patients often refuse further treatment or transportation to a hospital once their level of responsiveness improves. This is especially common among patients who have had diabetes for a long time. OEC Technicians should strongly recommend that such patients be evaluated by a physician for a treatable cause of the patient's low blood sugar. Diabetes patients who refuse additional treatment or transportation to the hospital should be advised of the implications of this decision and should be asked to sign a patient refusal form as indicated in Chapter 8, Medical Communications and Documentation.

**O**—*Oxygen and Overdose.* High-flow oxygen is recommended for all patients with AMS. Hypoxia is the most common cause of AMS and is the easiest problem to correct.

The mainstay of overdose management is to maintain the ABCDs and prevent aspiration of gastric contents. This is especially important with overdoses involving opiates or other sympathetic nervous system depressants, which can depress respiratory effort. Rapid transport to the hospital is warranted because some overdoses can be reversed by administering a specialized class of medications known as antagonists.

**U**—*Uremia.* When OEC Technicians encounter a patient in kidney failure resulting in uremia, they should try to make the patient comfortable, maintain the ABCDs, and urgently transport the patient to a definitive care facility, preferably one with the ability to perform emergent renal dialysis.

**T**—*Trauma and Tumors.* The treatment of trauma-related AMS is covered in Chapter 21, Head and Spine Injuries. In general, the management of severe trauma, especially brain injuries, focuses on diligent maintenance of the ABCDs and rapid transport to a trauma center. Treat for shock, if present, as described in Chapter 10, Shock, and ensure that the patient is well oxygenated. There is no specific prehospital treatment for a suspected tumor other than supportive care and rapid transport.

---

**Administering Oral Glucose to Pediatric Patients**

For patients under 10 years of age, administer half the adult dose (e.g., 10 grams, or 2–3 commercially available glucose tablets).

NOTE

**I**—*Infection*. Suspected infections, whether local or systemic, should be evaluated by a physician. Serious conditions such as sepsis, meningitis, or other infections involving the brain can be life threatening. In a remote setting in which the transport time is measured in hours to days, infected wounds should be cleaned as directed in Chapter 18, Soft Tissue Injuries. Fevers, if present, may be initially treated with cool compresses and self-administration of non-steroidal anti-inflammatory drugs (NSAIDs) such as acetaminophen or ibuprofen, if your local, regional, and state protocol allows. Treat septic shock as discussed in Chapter 10, Shock.

**P**—*Poisoning and Psychiatric Conditions*. The treatment of poisoning is varied and depends on the type, potency, and quantity of the toxin. In most instances, treatment is supportive in nature, with emphasis on preserving the ABCDs. If the cause is carbon monoxide, treat with high-flow oxygen. For other causes, refer to Chapter 12, Substance Abuse and Poisoning, or call the local poison center for specific treatment recommendations.

The field treatment of psychosis is also supportive in nature but is focused on preventing patients from harming themselves. Specific treatment recommendations may be found in Chapter 33, Behavioral Emergencies and Crisis Response.

**S**—*Seizures, Stroke, and Syncope*. Seizures are generally self-limiting and usually end without intervention by an OEC Technician. The primary goal is to protect the patient from further injury while letting the seizure run its course. OEC Technicians most often arrive during the post-ictal phase, during which care is generally supportive and emphasizes opening and maintaining the airway. Suction blood, mucus, and other secretions as necessary.

If the patient is actively seizing upon your arrival or begins to seize in your presence, protect the patient from falling, if possible. Move hard or sharp objects away from the patient to prevent injury. Use padding to protect the patient's head from hitting the floor or from striking objects that cannot be moved. If needed, instruct bystanders or other rescuers to stand in front of immovable objects to prevent the patient from striking them. Do not place anything in the mouth or between the teeth of a seizing patient, especially your fingers, as this action may result in a dental injury, mouth lacerations, laryngospasm, or the loss of a finger (yours!).

In the post-ictal stage, maintain the airway and deliver oxygen as needed. Use an oropharyngeal airway or a nasopharyngeal airway if there is evidence of prolonged unresponsiveness or airway compromise. In addition, if the seizure is associated with any type of fall, consider the possibility of trauma and treat accordingly. Halting a seizure in a patient who is in status epilepticus, which can permanently injure brain cells, requires a prescription medication. For this condition, ALS providers should be summoned. If ALS is not available, immediately transport these patients to a definitive-care facility. During transport, place seizing patients onto their side to allow blood and secretions to drain from the mouth. All first-time seizure patients also require further evaluation at a hospital.

The definitive treatment for a patient who has had a stroke must be provided in a hospital setting. OEC Technicians can, however, greatly improve the patient's chances of survival by providing high-flow oxygen, protecting the airway, and rapidly transporting the person to a definitive-care facility, preferably a stroke center. Even though stroke is a time-sensitive condition, new therapies may reverse the effects if administered soon after symptoms develop. New "clot busting" medications may reverse an ischemic stroke if given within an hour of onset. Do not delay transport unless spine trauma is highly suspected, in which case immobilize the spine as described in Chapter 21, Head and Spine Injuries and rapidly transport the patient.

If possible, notify the receiving clinic or hospital that a potential stroke patient is en route to their location.

The treatment for syncope is similar to that for hypovolemic shock and consists of oxygen therapy, elevating the patient's legs 8–12 inches above the level of the heart, and keeping the patient warm. Because the underlying cause of syncope is often a problem originating within the cardiovascular system, any syncopal patient should be transported for evaluation by a physician.

Be sure to protect patients against further injury of weak, paralyzed, or sensory-impaired extremities, because they may not be able to protect themselves. This is especially true for extremities, hands, and toes exposed to extremely hot or cold environmental conditions. Monitor and pad any areas that may come into contact with pressure points, sharp objects, or temperature extremes, especially when prolonged transport is involved. Continue to reassess the neurological findings for further deterioration or improvement. Document all findings and changes, including the time those findings were observed.

## Violent Behavior and Altered Mental Status

Any medically or traumatically brain-injured patient with AMS may exhibit violent, combative, or bizarre behavior. These patients can test your patience, as they are generally uncooperative and can endanger you and other rescuers if their behavior is not controlled. These patients are usually completely unaware of what they are doing and that their behavior is inappropriate. Many times you will not be able to reason with these patients. The most difficult situation arises when trauma dictates that the spine must be protected using a cervical collar and long spine board. In these instances, try to remain calm, and reassure patients to keep them calm. Whenever possible, avoid the use of force, because using force may be more harmful than trying to get patients to cooperate or to lie still.

 **CASE DISPOSITION**

You put the wallet in a safe place and tell the manager that nothing should ever be placed in the patient's mouth, as doing so only makes the situation worse. You instruct the manager to protect the patient's head from striking the floor during the seizure as you move a nearby trash can away from the patient. You time the seizure, which stops after approximately 45 seconds. You then place the man on his left side (left lateral recumbent position) and clear his airway of a small amount of blood. Next, you look in the patient's wallet and find a medical card that indicates that the man has diabetes.

After a few minutes, the patient becomes responsive. Although he is still slightly confused, he is able to tell you his name. The clerk returns and informs you that an ambulance will be arriving shortly. You ask the clerk to bring you a cup of water and five packets of pure sugar. You have the patient sip plain water first; then, after stirring the sugar into the cup, you instruct the patient to drink again, which he does. After a few minutes, he is fully oriented. He tells you that he was "running late" and did not eat breakfast that morning. The ambulance crew arrives, and you recognize the paramedic as a fellow patroller. You give her an oral hand-off report and help load the patient into the ambulance. As you are closing the doors, the patient thanks you for helping him.

# ✚ Chapter Review

## Chapter Summary

AMS, or altered mental status, is a generic term used to describe an abnormality in central nervous system function. The signs and symptoms of AMS may be global or focal, depending on the part of the brain that is affected. Global changes affect both sides of the body equally, whereas focal lesions may present as simple abnormalities in the sensory, motor, or visual tracts in the brain. More complex focal lesions may affect higher cortical functions such as language, speech, and the ability to accomplish multi-step tasks. Secondary injury to the brain can quickly result from a lack of oxygen or glucose, or from the buildup of pressure within the brain. These secondary injuries can compound the initial insult and result in permanent injury.

The causes of AMS may be metabolic, structural, toxic, or behavioral. Given the diversity of signs and symptoms, identifying the underlying cause of AMS can present unique challenges to even the most experienced OEC Technician. Because clues to the origins of AMS may be subtle, it is essential that you obtain a de-tailed patient history and perform a thorough physical assessment. When a patient is not able to provide a detailed history, bystanders or the patient's family or friends may be your only sources of information. The use of the AEIOU-TIPS mnemonic can be helpful in identifying potential causes of AMS that are readily treatable in the field and in recognizing those disorders that require emergent intervention and follow-up care in a hospital.

Even though the treatments of the specific causes of AMS in patients are diverse, the care that OEC Technicians provide is generally supportive in nature when provided in outdoor environments. In addition to maintaining the ABCDs, treatment priorities include ensuring that the patient is well oxygenated and is provided oral glucose when needed. Oxygen or glucose deficits can cause sudden and dramatic changes in the patient's level of responsiveness. By helping to preserve proper functioning of the central nervous system, OEC Technicians can minimize or even reverse the effects of AMS.

## Remember...

1. AMS describes an abnormality in brain function.
2. The causes of AMS are numerous and may result in global or focal changes.
3. The mnemonic AEIOU-TIPS can help determine the underlying cause of AMS.
4. Patients who exhibit AMS are considered "load and go" patients.
5. All patients with AMS need high-flow oxygen.
6. Diabetics with AMS need sugar, but only if they are able to follow commands and have an intact gag reflex.
7. Any patient with unwitnessed AMS should be treated for spinal injury until proven otherwise.
8. Seizures are usually self limiting. Treatment centers on protecting the patient from further harm.

## Chapter Questions

### Multiple Choice

Choose the correct answer.

1. A seizure can result in alterations in which of the following characteristics?_____
   a. awareness
   b. responsiveness
   c. body movement
   d. all of the choices

2. Status epilepticus is defined as _____
   a. the post-ictal phase of a seizure.
   b. a condition in which an epileptic patient is stabilized using an anticonvulsant medication.
   c. a seizure lasting more than 10 minutes, or three or more successive seizures without regaining responsiveness.
   d. a general tonic/clonic seizure.

3. Which of the following observations is indicative of a failed vocal/speech exam? _____
   a. slurred words
   b. inaccurate words
   c. Aphasia (inability to speak)
   d. all of the choices

4. Circle the following actions that are *not* part of an OEC Technician's care of a patient suffering from an AMS.
   a. maintaining the ABCDs
   b. administering high-flow $O_2$
   c. performing "load and go"
   d. taking spinal precautions if trauma is suspected
   e. administering oral glucose if the patient is responsive and able to swallow and a diabetes-related problem is suspected
   f. administering insulin if a diabetes-related problem is suspected
   g. placing the patient in a recovery position unless contraindicated by trauma

5. An OEC Technician's care of a seizing patient includes all of the following *except* _____
   a. maintaining the airway.
   b. suctioning as needed.
   c. placing a roller gauze or bite stick between the patient's teeth.
   d. protecting the patient from falling or striking a hard or sharp object.
   e. summoning ALS for a status epilepticus patient or for a first-time seizure patient.

6. Which of the following conditions is the most common cause of AMS? _____
   a. Diabetes
   b. Hypoxia
   c. drug overdose
   d. infection

## Fill in the Blank

1. Categorize each of the following descriptions as either post-ictal, pre-ictal, or ictal:
   _____ a. an aura or premonition
   _____ b. minimal responsiveness (V or P on AVPU), incontinence, encoporesis, disorientation
   _____ c. tonic muscle activity, falling, jaw clenching, cyanosis, unresponsiveness

2. The two most common, easily corrected causes of AMS are _____ and _____.

3. The stages of a mini-neuro exam are _____, _____, _____, _____, and _____.

4. The steps of a motor-sensory exam are _____ and _____.

5. An example of a higher cortical function exam is _____.

6. Place a check mark by each of the signs or symptoms that is indicative of a stroke.
   _____ a. numbness on one side of the body
   _____ b. weakness on one side of the body
   _____ c. paralysis on one side of the body
   _____ d. numbness or weakness of the right leg
   _____ e. a speech or language deficit
   _____ f. disorientation
   _____ g. inability to perform a task such as zipping up a coat
   _____ h. severe thirst
   _____ i. frequent urination
   _____ j. visual problems
   _____ k. inability to walk
   _____ l. dizziness

_____ **m.** headache

_____ **n.** a clear fluid dripping from the ears or nose

7. Which of the following pieces of information is important to gather when assessing a patient who may have had a stroke?

_____ **a.** the last time the patient appeared normal

_____ **b.** how recently the patient consumed an alcoholic beverage

_____ **c.** the time of onset of the signs and symptoms

8. The primary concern an OEC Technician should have when dealing with a patient suffering from an alcohol overdose is _____?

9. Describe how you would administer glucose to a responsive diabetes patient.

_____

_____

_____

## Matching

1. For each of the following type of stroke, indicate which description applies.

_____ **1.** ischemic stroke

_____ **2.** hemorrhagic stroke

_____ **3.** transient ischemic attack (TIA)

**a.** "wet" stroke

**b.** rupture of blood vessels

**c.** most common type of stroke

**d.** reversible neural deficit caused by temporary interruption of blood flow to brain

**e.** disruption of blood flow to brain

**f.** commonly caused by an embolus originating outside the brain

**g.** ministroke

**h.** structural weakness of blood vessels

**i.** can result in permanent neurological damage or death

**j.** typically caused by a small embolus that temporarily blocks small blood vessels in the brain

**k.** warns of likelihood of larger strokes in the future

2. Indicate whether each of the following signs/symptoms is associated with a partial seizure (P) or a generalized seizure (G).

_____ **a.** decreased level of responsiveness

_____ **b.** one-sided facial twitching

_____ **c.** incomprehensive vocabulary

_____ **d.** tonic/clonic activity

_____ **e.** automatisms

_____ **f.** complaint of abnormal smells

_____ **g.** incontinence

_____ **h.** grunting

_____ **i.** loss of responsiveness

_____ **j.** vacant stare

_____ **k.** cyanosis

_____ **l.** blurred vision

_____ **m.** numbness

## Scenario

*A collision between two skiers occurs at a busy intersection. Upon your arrival on scene you find patient 1 sitting up holding a shattered goggle lens and complaining of eye pain. Patient 2 is lying on his left side, mumbling with slurred speech and AMS. When you ask what happened, patient 1 responds that the two collided—that patient 2 was "flopping from side to side," and when patient 2 started to fall, his pole flew up and struck patient 1's goggle lens. And then patient 2 just dropped to the ground.*

*Thus patient 1 is responsive, alert, and oriented, whereas patient 2 is lying on their left side, mumbling with slurred speech and AMS.*

*MOI appears to be a skiing crash secondary to a medical emergency.*

1. Based on your initial findings, you suspect that patient 2 has had a/an _____
   a. heart attack.
   b. stroke.
   c. seizure.
   d. hypoglycemic episode.

*Remember a medical alert tag discovered during a secondary assessment could identify a patient with a history of diabetes.*

2. What mnemonic could you use during the assessment to assess altered mental status? _____
   a. SAMPLE
   b. AVPU
   c. SLUDGE
   d. OPQRST

3. An assessment tool available to OEC Technicians for identifying a potential cause of AMS is the _____
   a. Cincinnati Prehospital Stroke Scale.
   b. Boston Diabetic Scale.
   c. Denver Seizure Scale.
   d. Chicago Drug Scale.

*Treatment for patient 2 includes a call for an ALS transport, documentation of time of onset, high-flow O$_2$, monitoring of vitals, airway management, and rapid transport.*

## Suggested Reading

○○○○○○○○○○○○○○○○○○○○○○○○○○○○○○○○○○○○○○○○○○○○○○○○○○○○○○○○○○

American Diabetes Association Position Statement: Diagnosis and Classification of Diabetes Mellitus. 2008. *Diabetes Care 31*(1): S55–S60.

American Diabetes Association Position Statement: Standards of Medical Care in Diabetes. 2008. *Diabetes Care 31* (1):S12–S54.

Tomky, D. 2005. "Detection, Prevention, and Treatment of Hypoglycemia in the Hospital." *Diabetes Spectrum 18* (1):39–44.

EXPLORE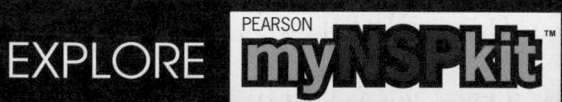

Please go to www.myNSPkit.com. Under Student Resources, you will find animations, videos, web links, and games related to this chapter—and much more. Look for information on stroke and seizure disorders.

Register your access code from the front of your book by going to www.myNSPkit.com and selecting the appropriate links. If the in-cover

# Substance Abuse and Poisoning

12

Maurus Sorg, MD, MPH

## ⊕ OBJECTIVES

**Upon completion of this chapter, the OEC Technician will be able to:**

**12-1** List and describe the four ways a drug enters and moves through the body.

**12-2** List the four routes of absorption.

**12-3** Define the following terms:

    a. poison                  c. substance abuse

    b. substance             d. toxin

**12-4** List and describe three commonly abused substances.

**12-5** List the signs and symptoms associated with commonly abused substances and with common poisonings.

**12-6** Describe and demonstrate the proper care of a patient who has abused a substance or been poisoned.

**12-7** List and describe two emergency sources for poison-related or chemical-related information.

## Chapter Overview

As an OEC Technician, you will undoubtedly encounter patients who are experiencing problems resulting from an exposure to a substance. Depending on the substance involved, an exposure may be accidental or intentional (Figure 12-1■). The effects of substances on the human body can vary greatly and can range from being medically therapeutic to producing minor distortions in perception and coordination to becoming immediately life threatening. The distinctions between the severity of effects are often slight and vary among individuals.

The use and misuse of a variety of substances in Western society, including the United States, are common. Any exposure, whether intentional or accidental, may

*continued*

## HISTORICAL TIMELINE

1962
First meeting of an advisory committee, the National Medical Committee was held.

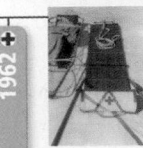
1962
National First Aid Committee was formed.

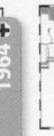 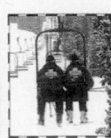
1964
Adopted the "gold cross" as its official emblem.

dermal poison, *p. 392*

designer drug, *p. 391*

ingested poison, *p. 394*

inhaled poison, *p. 400*

injected poison, *p. 394*

opiate, *p. 392*

poison, *p. 390*

substance abuse, *p. 390*

toxicological event, *p. 396*

toxin, *p. 390*

withdrawal, *p. 390*

pose direct risks to rescuers that must not be overlooked or ignored. Thus OEC Technicians must be alert when encountering a patient who has a suspected substance abuse or poisoning in order to reduce the chances of becoming harmed through accidental exposure. This can be challenging because the effects of some poisons, including carbon monoxide or organic pesticides, may not be immediately apparent but can still pose a severe threat to everyone in the immediate vicinity. One of the chief dangers posed by substance abusers is their false sense of reality and disturbed behavior and judgment. Sometimes the effects of the substance of abuse can mask or mimic other medical and psychological conditions.

This chapter provides an overview of substance abuse and poisoning. It includes the signs and symptoms that indicate that a toxicological exposure has occurred, a review of commonly abused substances and common poisons, and general guidelines for managing substance-abuse and poisoning patients.

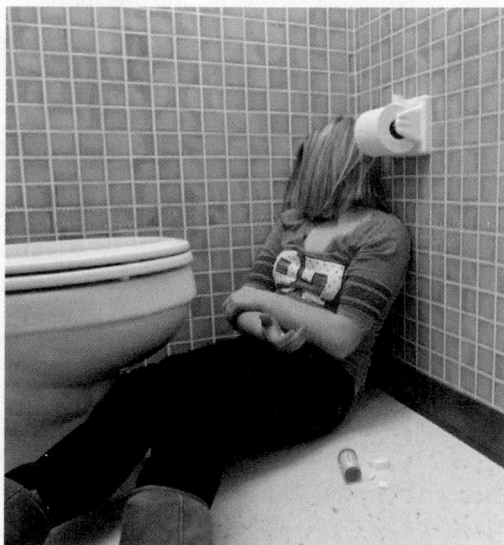

**Figure 12-1** Exposure to potentially harmful substances may be accidental or intentional.
Copyright Edward McNamara

## Anatomy and Physiology

Substances can exert many different effects on the body. Some, such as alcohol, act on multiple body systems; others, such as nerve agents, affect specific body systems or structures. In the broadest context, a substance is anything that has mass and occupies space. In the context of this chapter, a *substance* is any matter that can harm the body. It can be a solid (e.g., a pill, a plant part), a liquid (e.g., alcohol, a drain cleaner), or a gas (e.g., smoke, carbon monoxide).

### Physiologic Actions

Substances enter and affect and exit the body through four physiologic actions: absorption, distribution, metabolism, and elimination.

#### Absorption

Absorption is the way in which a substance or poison enters the body. The four routes of absorption are ingestion, inhalation, transdermal, and injection.

+ *Ingestion* involves the intake of a substance through the mouth and its absorption through the gastrointestinal tract (Figure 12-2a■). Some substances are easily absorbed across the mucous membranes of the mouth. Substances that are not immediately absorbed travel down the esophagus to the stomach. Depending on the nature and strength of the substance, the delicate mucosa lining the mouth, esophagus, and stomach may be damaged by contact with the substance. Once in the stomach, the substance mixes with the stomach contents, which may slow the rate of absorption. If the stomach is empty, the substance rapidly enters the intestines, which can quicken the rate of absorption. Little (if any) absorption occurs in the stomach; most absorption occurs within the small and sometimes the large intestines. Substances that are not absorbed are excreted from the body in

⊕ **12-1** List and describe the four ways a drug enters and moves through the body.

⊕ **12-2** List the four routes of absorption.

## ✚ CASE PRESENTATION ✚

You are doing some mountain biking in the fall at your ski area when you notice an unkempt middle-aged man coming down the trail toward you. He is stumbling as he walks, has slurred speech, and seems quite agitated.

**What should you do?**

the feces. Pills and liquids are commonly absorbed following ingestion. Some medications are extended release, which remain in the intestines for an extended period and then break down and release over a prolonged period.

✚ *Inhalation* is absorption through the lungs (Figure 12-2b■). Because the lungs have a rich vascular network, they are especially capable of absorbing many substances, including nicotine, carbon monoxide, and other gases. Some substances, however, are highly corrosive and when inhaled can damage the delicate lung tissue, causing swelling and bleeding. Other inhaled substances can travel through the bloodstream and affect other organs or body systems, such as the heart, and can cause excess fluid buildup in the lungs, inflammation, or even heart failure. Smoke from marijuana and tobacco and other gaseous substances are absorbed through the lungs.

✚ *Transdermal* is absorption through the skin (Figure 12-2c■). As the largest body system, the skin is highly vascular and is capable of absorbing a variety of substances. Scopolamine (anti-nausea), nitroglycerine (angina relief), and some narcotic pain patches work this way.

✚ *Injection* involves the use of a hypodermic needle or other sharp object to place a substance into the body's tissues, including into a muscle, beneath the skin, or directly into the bloodstream (Figure 12-2d■). Injectable medications are given this way, or a stinger from a bee or scorpion could inject toxic material into the body.

**Figure 12-2a** Ingestion is absorption through the gastrointestinal tract.

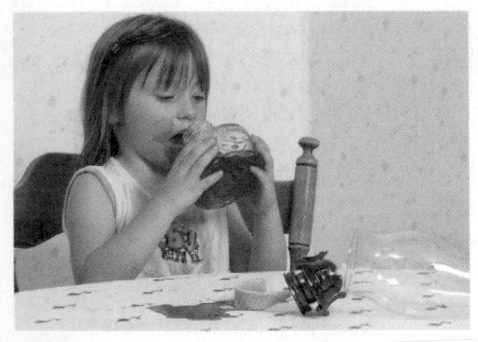

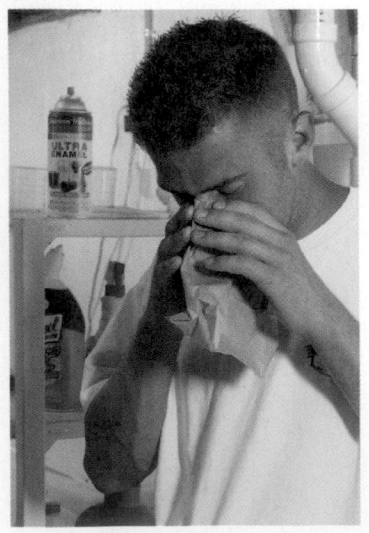

**Figure 12-2b** Inhalation is absorption through the lungs.

**Figure 12-2c** Transdermal absorption occurs through the skin, which is highly vascular and capable of absorbing a variety of substances.

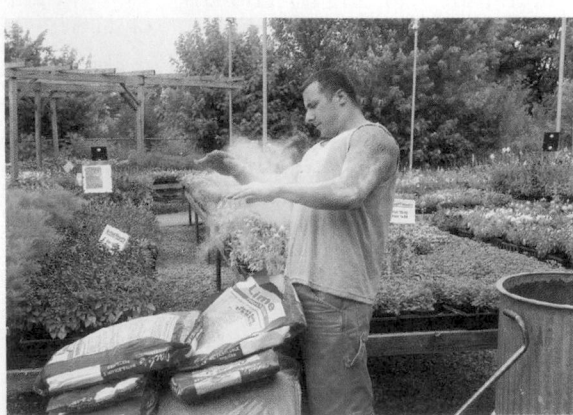

**Figure 12-2d** Injection is the placement of a substance into the body's tissues by use of a sharp object.

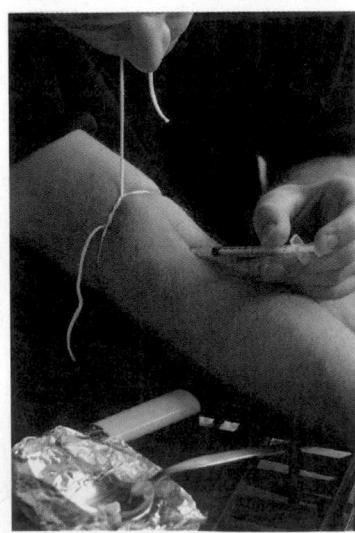

## Bodily Distribution

Once a substance is absorbed, it is transported to the site where it exerts its effects, a process known as distribution. Depending on the substance, the effects may be isolated to a single organ system, or may be systemic, affecting the entire body (Figure 12-3■). An overdose of acetaminophen, for example, causes an isolated effect on the liver, resulting in liver failure; whereas an overdose of heroin has wide-spread, systemic effects by depressing the central nervous system, which results in respiratory failure, loss of airway, and potentially cardiovascular collapse.

Distribution is affected by a number of factors. Certain body systems have barriers that either limit or prevent distribution to them. The most commonly discussed is the blood-brain barrier, which limits the types and amounts of substances in the blood which can cross into the brain. Also, substances, due to their properties, may:

+ enter the blood and bind to proteins
+ exist in the blood and in certain other tissues such as fat tissues
+ exist throughout the body outside of cells (extracellular fluid)
+ exist throughout the body but inside cells (intracellular).

Whether administered by injection into muscle or fat, inhaled or ingested, once the substance is in the bloodstream, it will circulate into the entire blood system quite rapidly.

## Metabolism

Metabolism, the third physiologic action, is the process by which the body breaks down a substance. The primary site of metabolism is the liver, although for some substances metabolism occurs within target cells. If the liver is diseased or injured, the time required for metabolism may be prolonged. Substances that are not completely broken down are recirculated through the liver, where further breakdown occurs through repeated metabolism. Some benign substances are metabolized in the body into ones that can harm the body.

## Elimination

Elimination, the fourth physiologic action, is a process by which the body purges itself of a substance through the urine, the gastrointestinal tract, the lungs, and/or the skin in sweat. Anything that impairs the proper functioning of these organ systems can reduce the rate of elimination.

## Body Systems Affected by Substance Exposure

Substances are used for a wide range of purposes in everyday life, including to cure disease and illness. Substances can affect individual tissues, organs, or entire organ systems. Some substances, such as alcohol, affect virtually every organ system in the body. The effects depend on many factors, including the strength of the substance, the amount absorbed, and the length of time the substance remains in the body. The following organs and body systems are most often affected by substances:

+ **The nervous system.** Substances can affect either the central nervous system (i.e., brain and spinal cord) or the peripheral nervous system (i.e., nerves), or both. Effects depend on which part(s) of the nervous system are affected and may be localized or general.

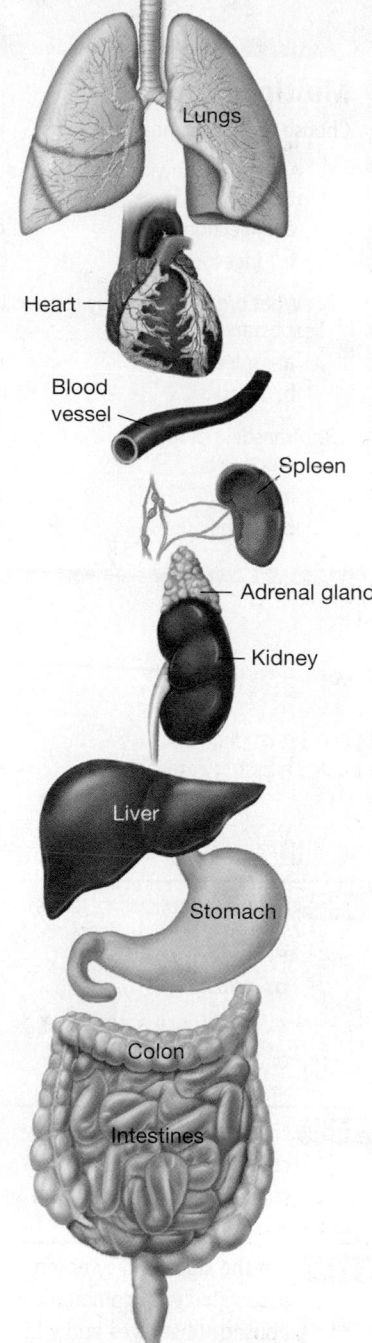

**Figure 12-3** When a substance is absorbed, a single organ or entire body systems may be affected.

# STOP, THINK, UNDERSTAND

## Multiple Choice

Choose the correct answer.

1. All of the following are routes of absorption except_____
   a. injection.
   b. ingestion.
   c. transdermal.
   d. myocardial.

2. What organ is primarily responsible for breaking down a substance?_____
   a. spleen
   b. liver
   c. kidneys
   d. gallbladder

3. Transdermal refers to the entry of a substance through which body structure?_____
   a. skin
   b. lungs
   c. bloodstream
   d. mouth

4. Inhalation refers to the entry of a substance through which body structure? _____
   a. skin
   b. lungs
   c. bloodstream
   d. mouth

5. The four physiological actions through which a substance enters, affects, and exits the body are _____
   a. absorption, ingestion, inhalation, and injection.
   b. absorption, ingestion, distribution, and metabolism.
   c. absorption, ingestion, distribution, and elimination.
   d. absorption, distribution, metabolism, and elimination.

+ **The heart.** Substances can affect the heart muscle, either increasing or decreasing its contractility. They also can affect heart rate or the conduction system of the heart, causing dysfunction and disturbances in cardiac rhythm. In severe cases, they can cause total cessation of heart activity.

+ **The eyes.** Substances can affect pupillary dilation or constriction, which can affect vision, and some substances affect the muscles responsible for coordinated eye movements.

+ **The blood.** Substances can affect the blood's ability to clot or carry oxygen, or they can affect the bone marrow, the site of red blood cell formation. Some substances can directly destroy blood cells; the effects of this type of exposure may take a long time to become apparent.

**12-3** Define the following terms:
   a. poison
   b. substance
   c. substance abuse
   d. toxin

**12-4** List and describe three commonly abused substances.

**12-5** List the signs and symptoms associated with commonly abused substances and with common poisonings.

**substance abuse** the intentional misuse of a substance that results in significant impairment.

**withdrawal** the physical and mental readjustment that accompanies the discontinued use of an addictive substance.

**poison** any substance that is injurious to health or dangerous to life.

**toxin** a noxious or poisonous substance produced by an organism.

# Commonly Abused Substances and Poison-Related Emergencies

**Substance abuse** is the intentional misuse of a substance that results in significant impairment or physical harm. Although teenagers and young adults may be particularly at risk for substance abuse, addictive dependence on substances can occur in individuals in any age group. Exposure at parties and social events often leads to the binge abuse of a substance, the occasional use of a substance out of proportion to the common norm. Addiction to a substance, a true medical/psychiatric illness, results when an individual's body craves the substance and when the absence of the substance results in some type of physical impairment due to **withdrawal**.

Drugs that are approved by the U.S. Food and Drug Administration have legitimate medical uses when taken as directed. These same drugs, however, can have toxic effects if misused or abused. An overdose occurs when a person takes a larger dose of a drug than is safe. Poisoning is a significant toxicological event that results in an injury, illness, or death secondary to exposure to a poison or toxin. A **poison** is a substance that causes harmful effects when introduced into the body; a **toxin** is a poison that comes from an organism. Overdoses and poisonings can be accidental or intentional. Often, the line between therapeutic benefit and toxic effect is a narrow one. In addition, any substance can have an unexpected and harmful effect unique to a specific person, referred to as an idiosyncratic reaction. The following list presents the chief categories of poisons and substances of abuse.

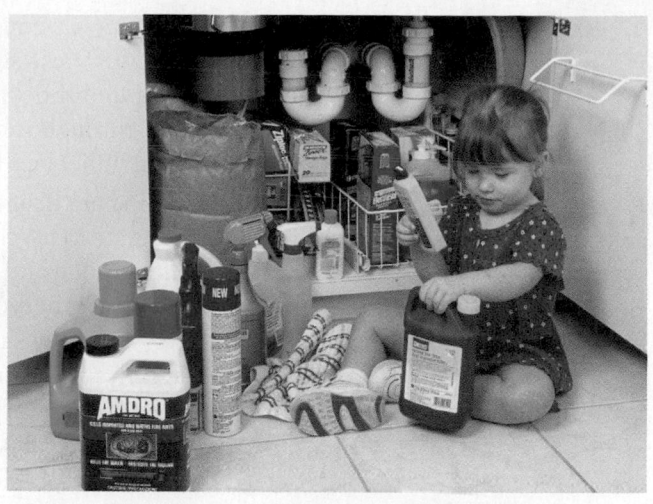

**Figure 12-4** Acids and bases are found in household cleaning solutions and pose grave risks to children.

+ *Acids and bases* are substances that are commonly used in the household for a variety of purposes, such as in cleaning solutions (Figure 12-4■). Acids (e.g., sulphuric, muiriatic, hydrochloric) and bases (e.g., sodium hydroxide, potassium hydroxide) can cause direct tissue damage, especially to the respiratory tract and the delicate mucosa of the mouth and GI tract.

+ *Antianxiety drugs and sedatives* are drugs that help relieve patients of anxious feelings. They are commonly prescribed for people with excessive emotions, panic disorders, or social disorders. Examples include diazepam (Valium), alprazolam (Xanax), and lorazepam (Ativan). *Sedatives* are drugs that help people relax. They are commonly used by patients with excessive emotions, panic disorders, or social disorders. Overdose and poisoning depresses the central nervous system, leading to decreased levels of responsiveness and depressed respirations.

+ *Antidepressants* are medicines used to treat depression. Some newer antidepressants also are used to treat anxiety and panic. Older antidepressants, known as tricyclics, are particularly toxic to the heart. Examples include sertraline (Zoloft), amitriptyline (Elavil), and fluoxetine (Prozac). Although newer drugs may be safer, overdosages can lead to arrhythmias, problems with perfusion, alterations in mentation, and seizures.

+ *Antipsychotics (tranquilizers)* are used to treat psychoses (i.e., thought disorders). Overdose can cause low blood pressure, disruption of the heart's conduction system. Both overdosage and normal dosages can cause dystonic reactions (abnormal muscle tone especially in the neck, changes in mentation and facial movements). Examples include haloperidol (Haldol) and chlorpromazine (Thorazine).

+ *Depressants* are a class of drugs that decrease central nervous system activity. Common depressants include alcohol, tranquilizers, opiates, antipsychotics, and antianxiety drugs. When used in combination, these drugs have increased toxicity and can cause excessive sedation, respiratory depression, and death.

+ *Designer drugs (club drugs)* are often used by teenagers and young adults. **Designer drugs** may impair brain function, causing seizures and coma. When combined with alcohol, some designer drugs can cause profound sedation and amnesia. Overdose can cause nausea and vomiting, respiratory difficulties, seizures, coma, and death. Some of these substances are made illegally, whereas others are prescription medications. Examples include Ecstasy (MDMA), GHB, rohypnol (a date rape drug), and ketamine (Special K).

+ *Hallucinogens* are drugs that distort sensory perceptions and impair emotion, judgment, and memory. Their chief danger lies in the loss of judgment by users and uncontrolled agitation and paranoia. Examples include LSD, PCP, and the plant toxin peyote.

+ *Inhalants* are the chemical vapors from common household products such as cleaning solvents, aerosols, spray paints, commercial adhesives, model glue, and freon. Inhaled substances can produce mind-altering effects similar to those of alcohol intoxication. Overdose can lead to the loss of sensation, unresponsiveness, shock, respiratory distress, and even death. Long-term effects can include permanent brain, lung, or heart damage.

**designer drug** a drug constructed by a chemist to produce unique and specific effects.

**opiate**  a narcotic drug that is derived from and has the same effect as opium.

**dermal poison**  a toxin absorbed through the skin.

◆ *Nerve agents* constitute a special class of chemicals used in warfare and acts of terrorism. These substances interrupt nerve impulses in the body, which can lead to profound shock, seizures, respiratory distress, and death. Poisoning typically occurs through inhalation or transdermal absorption. Examples include Sarin, Soman, Tabun, and VX.

◆ *Opiates* are drugs derived from opium or opium-like compounds. Sometimes referred to as narcotics, **opiates** are medically used to relieve pain; however, they can affect mood and emotion. Some opiates are synthetically designed. Opiates affect the central nervous system, causing a surge of euphoria, then alternating wakefulness and drowsiness with impairment of mental functioning. Overdose can cause significant respiratory depression and death. Examples of common prescription opiates are morphine, oxycontin, and oxycodone (Percocet™), acetaminophen and hydrocodone (Vicodin™), hydromorphone (Dilaudid™), and meperidine (Demerol™). Heroin is an illegal opiate.

◆ *Organophosphates* are chemicals used in insecticides, pesticides, and herbicides and are commonly found in household and commercial settings. Because of their broad application by agricultural spraying devices, the potential for many individuals to be simultaneously exposed is great. Poisoning most often occurs through inhalation, transdermal absorption, and ingestion (especially in children); a substance absorbed through the skin is called a **dermal poison**. The effects of organophosphate poisoning are similar to those caused by nerve agents.

◆ *Stimulants* are substances that increase central nervous system activity. Overdose with a stimulant speeds up vital body functions (heart rate, blood pressure, metabolic rate) and commonly causes excitement and agitation that can lead to erratic and dangerous behavior and even seizures, hypertension, and stroke. Examples include methamphetamine, cocaine, and crack.

◆ *Prescription drugs* are those drugs ordered by a licensed physician and are becoming increasingly misused by individuals of all age groups. Almost all prescription medications have potentially harmful effects if they are misused or not taken as directed. Many have toxic side effects if taken in excess. For some medications, the effective dose—sometimes called the therapeutic index— may be very close to the toxic dose. This is especially true for heart and blood pressure medications and for medications used to control seizures. Overdose is often accidental and can occur when a person shares a medication with a spouse or other family members. Prescription drug overdose is especially common among elderly patients.

A behavior known as polypharmacy, in which substances are taken in combination, is dangerous because the effects of the combination cannot always be accurately predicted. The effects of drugs taken in combination may be compounded, or one of the drugs may offset the effects of others. When the additive effects of polypharmacy produce a dangerous effect, the event is known as a multi-substance or polypharmacologic overdose. Drug combinations with the potential for polypharmacologic overdose include taking multiple prescription drugs, a prescription drug and an illegal drug together, using PCP and marijuana together (two illegal drugs), and consuming alcohol with any other substance. Polypharmacy is especially dangerous and common among the elderly, many of whom may be taking multiple medications prescribed by different health care providers.

◆ *Over-the-counter (OTC) medications* – Many people do not consider OTC medications dangerous because they are not prescribed by a physician and thus not thought of as a medicine by some. Overdosage or improper use, however, may have harmful side effects. Because of the easy access to these substances, they have become common drugs of abuse by some adolescents. Cough medicines have been identified as most commonly abused by adolescents. The ingredient used for nasal congestion and cough suppressant in overdosage can cause hallucination, which may be the desired effect. But they can also cause seizures, arrhythmias, hyperpyrexia, and CNS depression.

## Commonly Encountered Substances

OEC Technicians are often required to respond to events involving the following substances:

+ **Acetaminophen (Tylenol).** This over-the-counter drug is used to treat pain and help reduce fever. Acetaminophen is widely used and is a common ingredient in numerous combination medications such as over-the-counter "cold" medications. One may take plain Tylenol in addition to the combination medication, and thus ingest too much Tylenol. Overdose of acetaminophen is among the most common poisonings worldwide and can be life threatening. In toxic amounts, acetaminophen can cause irreversible liver damage.

+ **Alcohol.** Ethanol, the form of alcohol found in beverages, is the most commonly abused drug in the world. A disproportionate number of aircraft, motor vehicle, and recreational injuries are caused by the abuse of this mood altering, central nervous system depressant. Alcohol-related emergencies are relatively common and can be serious, even life threatening.

Alcohol has a wide range of effects and affects nearly every body system. Alcohol primarily inhibits central nervous system activity by slowing brain function, sensory input, and motor coordination. It also lowers one's inhibitions, which can lead to behavioral changes. Alcohol can depress the respiratory system, slowing both the rate and depth of respirations. It is also a diuretic (causes increase in urine output) possibly causing dehydration. In susceptible individuals, alcohol can lower blood sugar levels and enhance the effects of certain medications such as insulin and oral diabetes medications.

One of the most common alcohol-related emergencies that OEC Technicians may encounter is alcohol poisoning, a condition in which a person consumes too much alcohol and becomes severely impaired or even unresponsive. In severe cases, the person loses the gag reflex, aspirates his oral secretions or vomit, and stops breathing. Patients also can develop seizures or hypothermia as a result of alcohol poisoning.

Another condition that may be encountered is alcohol withdrawal. Most commonly, this is seen in people who have been drinking large amounts of alcohol over many years and then abruptly stop. Such sudden cessation can cause a variety of adverse effects, including muscle tremors, hallucinations, seizures, and even death.

+ **Aspirin (acetylsalicylic acid).** Used to relieve pain and swelling and to reduce fever, aspirin is a common ingredient in many combination drugs. Before the widespread use of child-proof caps, accidental aspirin overdose was relatively common and resulted in numerous deaths. Overdose, although less common today, can cause respiratory depression (although at first the victim becomes tachypneic), profound systemic acidosis, and death.

> ### Ethanol Percentages
>
> **NOTE**
>
> The percentage of ethanol (i.e., grain alcohol) in a drink is expressed by a somewhat obsolete measure called "proof," which is defined as twice the proportion of a drink (by volume) that is ethanol. For instance, a liquor that is 40 percent grain alcohol is said to be 80 proof. The maximum proof is 200 (i.e., 100 percent pure, scientific-grade grain alcohol). By contrast, blood alcohol content (BAC) is a measure of the mass of alcohol per volume of blood. For instance, if an individual's BAC is 0.10 percent, it means that there is one gram of alcohol per 1,000 milliliters of blood.

> ### Other Toxic Alcohols
>
> **NOTE**
>
> Other alcohols can also be toxic. Rubbing alcohol (isopropyl alcohol) and methanol can cause vomiting, confusion, slow breathing, seizures, low body temperature, pale or bluish skin, unresponsive, and death.

+ **Carbon monoxide (CO).** An odorless, colorless, and tasteless gas, carbon monoxide is a by-product of combustion. It impairs oxygenation of tissues by displacing oxygen molecules on red blood cells, thereby reducing the amount of oxygen in the blood. Effects of carbon monoxide poisoning range from mild to life threatening. Carbon monoxide poisoning is an extremely common cause of accidental death, especially in outdoor recreational settings involving stoves, vehicles, generators, and fires. It can occur in poorly ventilated tents, cabins, campers, and sheds. At high altitudes, where oxygen is less concentrated, the risks are even greater.

+ **Cocaine (coke, crack, snow, rock, nose candy).** A powerfully addictive drug that affects the nervous and cardiovascular systems, cocaine makes the user feel euphoric and energetic and may be inhaled, **ingested**, **injected**, or absorbed through the skin or mucosa. Cocaine constricts peripheral blood vessels and stimulates the central nervous system, increasing the heart rate, blood pressure, and body temperature. These changes can cause heart attack, seizure, stroke, and respiratory failure. Because of cocaine's toxic effects on the heart, sudden death can occur at any time during its use, even upon an individual's first exposure to it.

+ **Ethylene glycol.** Ingestion of this substance, which is a component of a variety of household and automotive products (including antifreeze), can cause organ damage, shock, and death.

+ **Iron supplements.** Iron supplements, including those in children's multivitamins, can be lethal if taken in large quantities. Death results primarily from liver and kidney failure. Like aspirin, iron overdoses were more common before child-proof caps were introduced.

+ **LSD (lysergic acid diethylamide, or "acid").** The effects of this powerful mood-changing drug are unpredictable and vary among individuals. Physical effects include elevated body temperature, heart rate, and blood pressure; sleeplessness; and loss of appetite. Large doses can cause delusions and visual hallucinations.

+ **Marijuana (pot, weed, cannabis, ganja, grass, Mary Jane).** The most commonly used illegal drug (which is becoming legalized in some states) in the United States, marijuana is smoked or ingested. The active ingredient in marijuana is tetrahydrocannabinol (THC). Marijuana distorts perceptions and affects thinking, memory, and learning. In some individuals it may be a "gateway drug," one that paves the way for the use of stronger substances of abuse. Marijuana is commonly used with other drugs such as alcohol or mixed with other drugs such as PCP. Hashish is a form of marijuana that contains a higher concentration of THC (Figure 12-5■).

+ **Methamphetamine (speed, meth).** The popularity of this drug, a powerful stimulant with a high potential for abuse and addiction, has grown significantly over the past decade. Methamphetamine produces a heightened state of arousal and physical activity and decreases appetite. Chronic use can lead to psychotic behavior, hallucinations, and stroke.

+ **Methane.** This highly flammable gas displaces oxygen if present in an enclosed space. In high concentrations, methane can cause profound hypoxia in the body. Although rare, death can occur.

+ **PCP (phencyclidine or angel dust).** This veterinary tranquilizer was initially developed for use as an anesthetic in humans. PCP blocks the perception of pain, and is commonly added to other drugs such as marijuana. Overdose can cause exceptionally violent or suicidal behavior and increases the user's risk of serious traumatic injury.

**ingested poison**   a toxin that enters the body through the mouth.

**injected poison**   a toxin injected into a vein or another tissue.

**Toxic Plants**

NOTE

The ingestion of toxic plants represents 5 percent of all exposures to toxins. As a whole, exposure to plant toxins is the least toxic of all accidental ingestion-related poisonings. The most common victims of this type of poisoning are curious children, foragers (i.e., hobbyists who look for natural foods), herbalists, pleasure seekers, and suicidal individuals. See Chapter 27, Plant and Animal Emergencies, for more information about the ingestion of toxic plants.

**Figure 12-5** Substance abuse can occur with a variety of drugs.

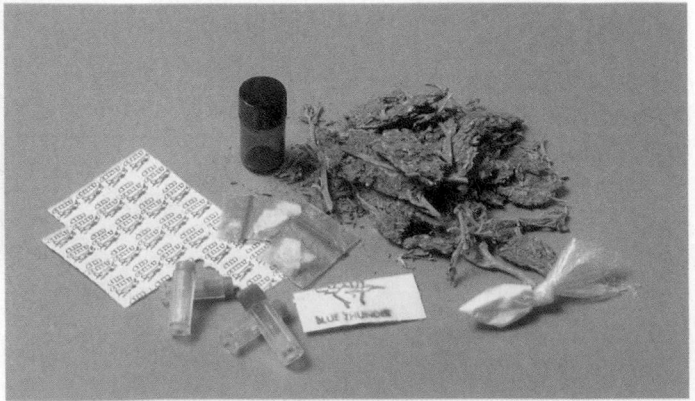

# STOP, THINK, UNDERSTAND

## Multiple Choice

Choose the correct answer.

1. What proportion of all exposures to toxins involves the ingestion of toxic plants?_____
   a. 5 percent
   b. 7 percent
   c. 10 percent
   d. 18 percent

2. Polypharmacy is common and especially dangerous in which of the following groups?_____
   a. recreational drug users
   b. teenagers
   c. alcoholics
   d. the elderly

3. Which of the following choices best describes a toxin? _____
   a. A poisonous substance that enters the body through injection.
   b. A poisonous substance that is made by humans.
   c. A poisonous substance that enters the body through ingestion.
   d. A poisonous substance that comes from organisms.

## Matching

Match the description on the left with the correct substance on the right. (some of the substances will not be used)

_____ 1. A highly flammable gas that displaces oxygen if encountered in an enclosed space.

_____ 2. The most commonly used illegal drug (in most states) in the United States; is smoked or ingested.

_____ 3. Use may cause seizures, impair brain function, and induce comas.

_____ 4. Is used in a variety of household automotive products, including antifreeze.

_____ 5. Is used to reduce fever and relieve pain and swelling.

_____ 6. A special class of chemicals used in warfare and acts of terrorism.

_____ 7. Tranquilizers used to treat thought disorders (psychosis).

_____ 8. The effects of this powerful mood-changing drug are unpredictable and vary among individuals.

_____ 9. Examples of this substance are Elavil (amitriptyline), Prozac (fluoxetine), and Zoloft (sertraline).

_____ 10. These drugs relieve pain and can effect mood and emotion; are sometimes referred to as narcotics.

_____ 11. This veterinary tranquilizer blocks the perception of pain.

_____ 12. These drugs or substances are used by people with excessive emotions, panic disorders, or social disorders; help people relax and include Valium, Xanax, and Ativan.

_____ 13. The chief danger of these drugs is the loss of judgment; they distort sensory perceptions and impair emotion, judgment, and memory.

_____ 14. This odorless, colorless, and tasteless gas is a by-product of combustion and is a common cause of accidental death, especially in outdoor recreational settings.

_____ 15. These drugs or substances increase central nervous system activity; examples include methamphetamine, cocaine, and crack.

_____ 16. Chronic use of this addictive stimulant with a high potential for abuse and addiction can lead to psychotic behavior, hallucinations, and stroke.

a. acetaminophen
b. alcohol
c. antianxiety drugs
d. antidepressants
e. antipsychotics
f. aspirin
g. carbon monoxide (CO)
h. cocaine
i. depressants
j. designer drugs
k. ethylene glycol
l. hallucinogens
m. inhalants
n. iron supplements
o. LSD (lysergic acid diethylamide)
p. marijuana
q. methamphetamine
r. methane
s. nerve agents
t. opiates
u. organophosphates
v. PCP (phencyclidine or angel dust)
w. sedatives
x. stimulants

# CASE UPDATE

Although the patient appears confused, you ask him some basic questions and determine that he is oriented to his name and situation only. The patient says he has been camping in the woods for the past week and has been drinking about a fifth of whiskey per day. He states that he ran out of alcohol about "two days ago" and went to find more. He declines to give any medical history. On examination, you find that his pupils are dilated, he feels warm, and has a moderately rapid pulse. He is very unsteady on his feet, and his hands are shaking.

**What should you do now?**

## Assessment

As for any incident, the very first action is to assess the scene. Pay careful attention to any potential hazards that may be present. Do not enter the scene if you suspect chemical poisoning. Instead, request assistance from the fire department and a Hazardous Materials (HazMat) team. If drugs are suspected, request law enforcement assistance. Requesting law enforcement assistance is especially important if the incident is a **toxicological event** that could involve public safety or require special handling of toxic chemicals or gases or designer poisons such as those used in terrorism situations. HazMat teams are specially trained and certified to handle these risks. Typical toxicological events include an overturned chemical tanker truck or a spill from a chemical storage site. If available, local police often provide crowd control and/or traffic control. Table 12-1■ lists the actions that OEC Technicians should take concerning toxicological events.

Once you are sure the scene is safe to enter, begin your primary assessment and correct any threats to life.

Chemical burns involving commercial cleaning agents can damage the oropharynx and can create enough swelling to cause airway obstruction. Inhalation exposures can cause swelling and inflammation of the respiratory system, resulting in difficulty breathing and hypoxia. Gases such as carbon monoxide can cause profound hypoxia. Narcotics and depressants can decrease respiratory drive, leading to hypoventilation. Many poisons have toxic cardiovascular effects that can significantly alter heart rate, heart rhythm, and blood pressure. Neurological abnormalities that result in confusion, seizures, and coma also are common.

Therefore, assess the ABCDs carefully and perform frequent reassessments to identify any changes. Carefully assess the patient's level of responsiveness using the AVPU scale. If time and conditions permit, consider assessing responsiveness using the GCS. Depending on the substance involved, the patient's condition can change quickly.

**toxicological event**  an event where a patient has been exposed to a harmful substance OR an incident in which the intentional or unintentional use of a substance or poison either endangers public safety and/or results in a medical emergency.

### Table 12-1 General Approach to a Toxicological Event

1. Ensure scene safety.
2. Practice Standard Precautions.
3. Determine that the incident involves poisoning or substance abuse.
4. Search the scene for evidence of a substance or poison (e.g., pill bottles, spray cans).
5. Examine the patient for evidence of exposure to a toxic substance.
6. Manage and transport the patient.

Next, perform a secondary assessment. Obtain a complete SAMPLE history, paying close attention to any mention of the use or misuse of any substances or exposure to a poison. Occasionally, the patient will volunteer this information. At the same time, carefully assess the scene for signs that suggest exposure to some harmful substance. Look for pill bottles, drug paraphernalia, suspicious containers or baggies, alcoholic beverage containers, or cans of spray paint or solvent. Be alert to peculiar odors such as gasoline, glue, or other chemicals. Collect all items, including pill bottles and commercial containers, because they can provide valuable information about the substance(s) involved. Bring them to the emergency department with the patient. Do not contaminate yourself or others with a suspected toxic substance. Try to determine the dosage of exposure and how long ago it happened. Determine whether the patient has other conditions (or injuries) that could complicate the situation. It is important for OEC Technicians to recognize that a poisoning or substance abuse situation has occurred.

Perform a physical exam using the DCAP-BTLS mnemonic, looking for any signs that indicate the patient may have been exposed to a poisonous substance. Many poisons depress the central nervous system, which can include blocking sensations of pain, so patients may be unaware that they sustained any injuries. Nausea and vomiting are common with exposure to poisons. Obtain a complete set of vital signs. The signs and symptoms of substances that may be toxic are presented in Table 12-2 ■.

## Table 12-2 Signs and Symptoms

| Substance | Signs and Symptoms |
|---|---|
| Acetaminophen | Nausea, vomiting |
| Aspirin | Nausea, vomiting, ringing in the ears |
| Acids and bases | Pain, tissue damage |
| Alcohol/depressants/sedatives | Altered mental status, confusion, poor coordination, abnormal gait, slurred speech, nausea, vomiting |
| Antipsychotics/antidepressants | Abnormal heart rate, abnormal heart rhythm, confusion |
| Carbon monoxide | Decreased level of responsiveness, lightheadedness, nausea, confusion, depressed mental status, reddened skin (late sign) |
| Cocaine | Agitation, chest pain, elevated heart rate and blood pressure; psychosis may also be observed |
| Ethylene glycol | Nausea, vomiting, altered level of responsiveness, elevated heart rate and blood pressure, seizure, coma |
| Hallucinogens (LSD) | Agitation, restlessness, psychosis, hallucinations, elevated heart rate, blood pressure, and skin temperature |
| Inhalants | Respiratory distress, confusion, hypoxia, respiratory failure, decreased level of responsiveness, shock, coma |
| Marijuana | Decreased level of responsiveness, confusion, drowsiness |
| Methane | Decreased level of responsiveness, confusion, drowsiness, nausea, vomiting |
| Narcotics | Euphoria, decreased level of responsiveness, respiratory depression |
| Organophosphates/ nerve agents | Excess salivation, tearing, coughing up mucus, respiratory depression, cardiovascular arrest due to respiratory failure, arrhythmias, headache, depressed mental status, coma |
| | The mnemonics SLUDGE and DUMBELS can help identify specific signs and symptoms associated with organophosphate poisoning or exposure to nerve agents: |

| SLUDGE | DUMBELS |
|---|---|
| **S**—Salivation | **D**—Defecation |
| **L**—Lacrimation (tearing) | **U**—Urination |
| **U**—Urination | **M**—Miosis (constriction of the pupils) |
| **D**—Defecation | **B**—Bronchorrhea (discharge of mucus from the airways) |
| **G**—GI irritation (vomiting) | **E**—Emesis (vomiting) |
| **E**—Eye (pupillary) constriction | **L**—Lacrimation (tearing) |
| | **S**—Salivation |

| Substance | Signs and Symptoms |
|---|---|
| PCP | Agitation, psychosis |
| Stimulants/methamphetamine | Agitation, psychosis, chest pain, elevated heart rate and blood pressure |

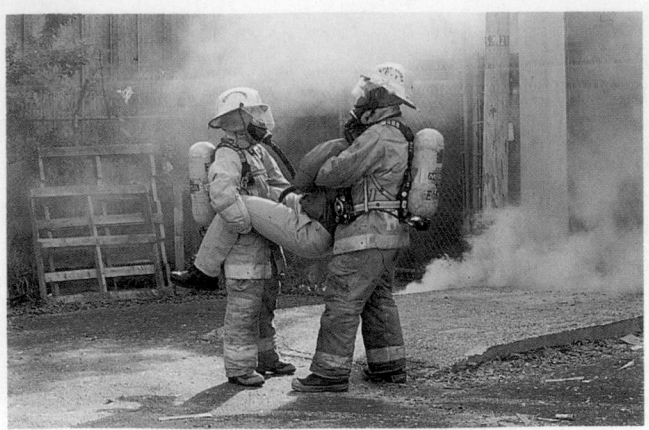

**Figure 12-6** Scene safety is an OEC Technician's primary concern. Request assistance from a HazMat team.

⊕ **12-6** Describe and demonstrate the proper care of a patient who has abused a substance or been poisoned.

# Management

Personal safety is of paramount importance (Figure 12-6■). The first step, then, is to secure the scene. You must ensure that your safety is protected first, and that further injury to the patient or yourself will not occur as you manage the patient. This is especially true with gaseous poisons (e.g., carbon monoxide and chlorine) and gaseous chemicals (e.g., insecticides and nerve agents). Do not enter the scene until it has been deemed safe by a Hazardous Materials team (HazMat), law enforcement officials, or both.

Treatment of a patient affected by a toxicological event is generally supportive in nature. It requires diligent attention to the patient's overall appearance, ABCDs, and vital signs. Perform the primary assessment and address any threats to life. Call early for transport and ALS if needed. The patient's respiratory status should be continually monitored for changes. Manage airway and breathing problems as necessary, using the techniques described in Chapter 9, Airway Management.

Only a relatively few toxicological emergencies can be effectively managed in the field. Beyond emergency interventions and normal supportive care, most toxicological emergencies require treatment in a definitive-care setting. High-flow oxygen is beneficial to all toxic exposures and is the primary treatment for events such as carbon monoxide poisoning and methane poisoning. Oxygen is also essential for patients exposed to any poisons that either stimulate or depress the central nervous system.

Beyond the initial assessment and stabilization of the patient, the care of the victim of a poisoning follows the following steps:

+ Reduce further exposure.
+ Reduce absorption.
+ Rapidly transport to a definitive-care facility.

## Reduce Further Exposure

For ingested poisons, dilute by having the patient drink water but only if instructed by your medical director or the local poison center, and if there are no contraindications. General contraindications for giving a poisoning patient water by mouth include nausea/vomiting, depressed level of responsiveness, or having ingested a substance that has the potential to depress level of responsiveness. Although the administration of an emetic (an agent that induces vomiting) was once recommended for cases involving certain ingested substances, subsequent studies have shown that inducing vomiting can be quite dangerous and does not significantly reduce absorption. Therefore, OEC Technicians should NEVER induce vomiting in a poisoning patient.

For dry topical poisons absorbed through the skin, brush off the particles with appropriate Personal Protective Equipment and rinse away any residue with water (Figure 12-7■). For wet poisons, thoroughly rinse with water. If ocular exposure occurred, immediately irrigate the eyes with copious amounts of sterile water or irrigation solutions as described in Chapter 22, Face, Eye, and Neck Injuries (Figure 12-8■). Remember to always protect yourself from becoming contaminated.

For inhaled poisons, immediately remove the patient from the source of poisoning (Figure 12-9■). Maintain the airway, administer high-flow oxygen via a nonrebreather mask, and consider transport with ALS if you observe a notable disturbance in coordination or balance, difficulty breathing, or altered mental status.

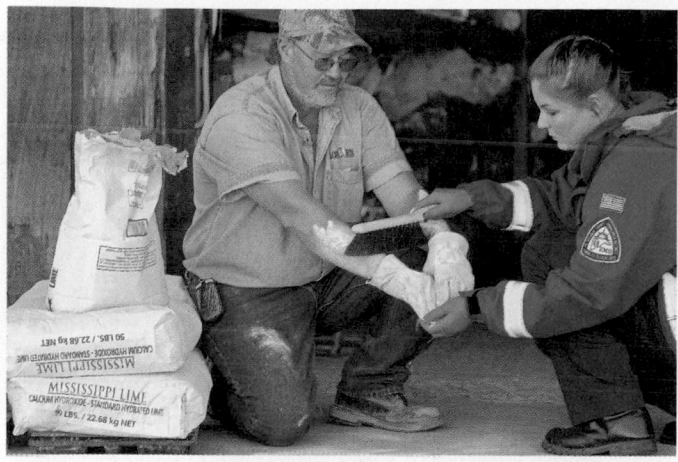

**Figure 12-7** Care for patients exposed to topical poisons involves brushing off any dry particles and rinsing the area with water.

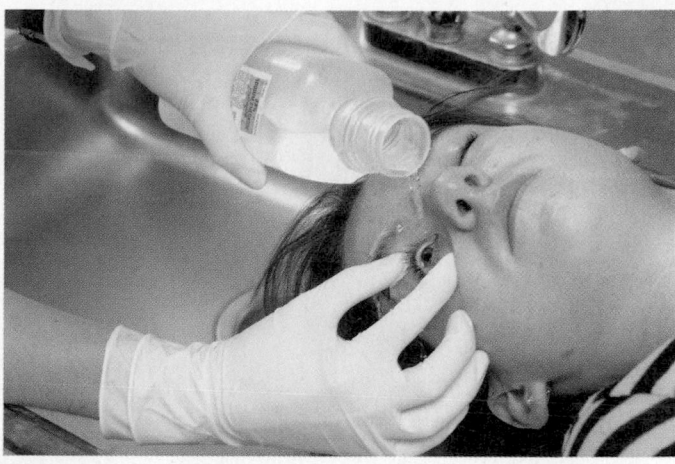

**Figure 12-8** If the substance contacted the eyes, immediately irrigate them with copious amounts of sterile water or appropriate irrigation solutions.

**Figure 12-9** Immediately remove the patient from the source of an inhaled poison.
Copyright Edward McNamara

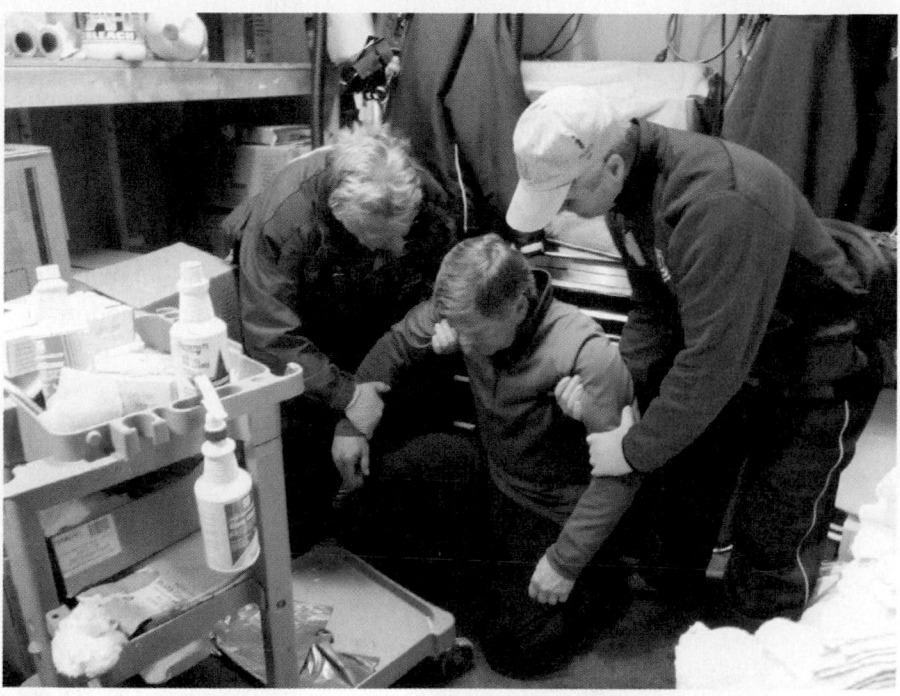

## Reduce Absorption

Activated charcoal absorbs and binds many poisons. It is a relatively safe medication that has been shown to be most effective in decreasing absorption if given within 60 minutes following ingestion of a poison (Figure 12-10■ and Table 12-3■). Charcoal may also be beneficial after 60 minutes in patients who have ingested extended release medications or have delayed emptying of the GI tract. Therefore, activated charcoal may be administered only if all of the following criteria are met:

+ You have been authorized by your medical advisor or local or state EMS authority to administer the medication.

+ You have been directed to administer charcoal by a poison control center or other approved medical direction for this specific patient.

+ The patient is awake, responsive, not nauseous and has not taken anything which will depress the mental status.

### When Charcoal is NOT Indicated

Because activated charcoal is very caustic to the respiratory system, it should *not* be given to any patient with a decreased level of responsiveness.

NOTE

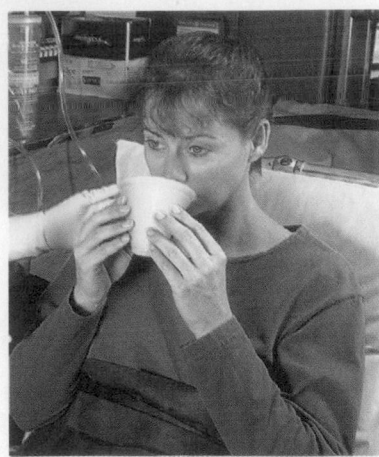

**Figure 12-10** Administer activated charcoal to absorb and bind many toxins.

**inhaled poison** a toxin that is absorbed through the lungs.

| Table 12-3 | Indications and Contraindications for the Use of Activated Charcoal in Poisoning Cases |
|---|---|

Indications
• Alcohols
• Arsenic
• Cyanide
• Iron
• Lithium

Contraindication
• Caustics

## Specific Interventions

✦ **Carbon monoxide poisoning.** Once the patient has been removed from the source of the CO gas, administer 100 percent oxygen via nonrebreather, if available. Sometimes hyperbaric oxygen (i.e., oxygen at high pressure) is necessary for severely poisoned patients.

✦ **Inhaled poisons such as dust, fumes, and aerosols. Inhaled poisons** may become deposited in the upper airways and cause damage at locations that depend on the size of the particles. Inhaled poisons include natural gas, or cyanide. Once again, 100 percent oxygen is the initial treatment of choice (Figure 12-11■).

✦ **Organophosphate poisoning (some insecticides and nerve agents).** In the event that you, a fellow rescuer, or a patient has been exposed to an organophosphate or a chemical nerve agent, administering the Mark I/Duodote antidote kit (discussed in Chapter 35, Special Operations and Ambulance Operations) can be life saving.

**Figure 12-11** For any poisoning incident, administer 100 percent oxygen as soon as possible.
Copyright Edward McNamara

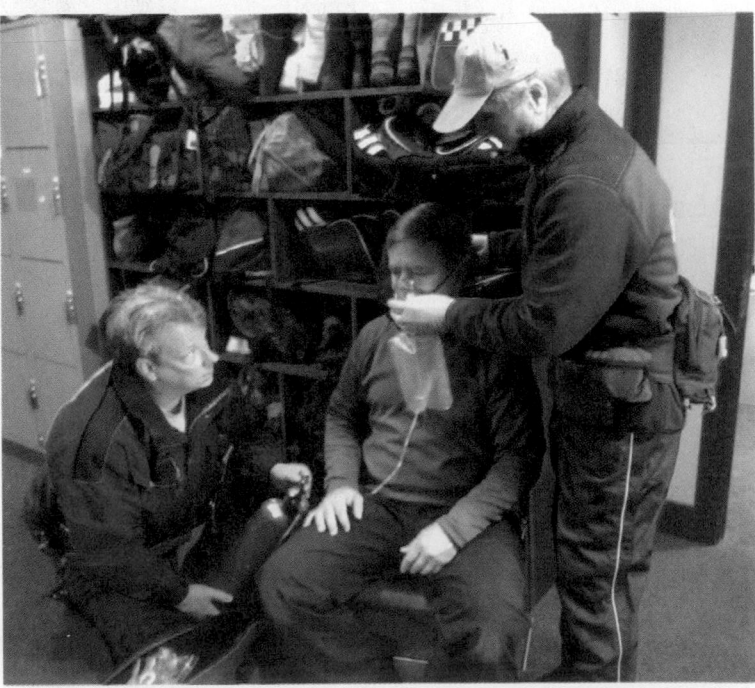

The approach to the ingestion of toxic plant material is similar to the approach used for other toxicological events. For more information about the treatment of toxic plant ingestions, see Chapter 27, Plant and Animal Emergencies. Specific treatments for other poisonings and toxic exposures are beyond the scope of training for OEC Technicians. When in doubt, support the patient's ABCDs and transport the patient to an acute-care facility.

## Help Is Only a Phone Call Away

Many times deciding on the best way to care for a patient is not easy, especially in outdoor environments, where transport times may be prolonged and treatment options are quite limited. Provided you have a radio or cell phone nearby, you may obtain immediate advice from a physician or toxicological specialist, by first contacting medical direction per your local protocols. You also may contact the National Capital Poison Center Help Hotline. The National Capital Poison Center operates 24 hours a day, 7 days a week, and can be reached at 1-800-222-1222, which serves as the phone number for every poison control center in the United States. The poison control center can give you up-to-date information about a poison and its treatment and give you recommendations concerning the necessity for additional medical care.

If you happen upon an accident scene involving the transportation of a toxic chemical, your first call should go to the Chemical Transportation Emergency Center (CHEMTREC). CHEMTREC is a service regulated by the National Oceanic and Atmospheric Administration (NOAA) of the U.S. Department of Commerce, but it is sponsored by the Chemical Manufacturers Association (CMA). Registration of a chemical allows CHEMTREC to perform its emergency-response function, which is to provide information concerning any of a registrant's products that may be involved in a transportation accident. A registered chemical is tagged with emergency information, including an emergency phone number, 1-800-262-8200, at which important information with regard to the product can be obtained.

**⊕ 12-7** List and describe two emergency sources for poison-related or chemical-related information.

## STOP, THINK, UNDERSTAND

### Multiple Choice
Choose the correct answer.

1. In what type of poisoning would you use the Mark 1/Duodote antidote kit?_____
   a. carbon monoxide poisoning
   b. aerosol poisoning
   c. organophosphate poisoning/nerve agent poisoning
   d. cyanide exposure

2. Activated charcoal is not indicated for use in which of the following substances?_____
   a. cyanide          c. iron
   b. aspirin          d. alcohols

3. What are three deadly poisons for children?_____
   a. aspirin, carbon dioxide, and iron
   b. ethylene glycol, carbon dioxide, and iron
   c. ethylene glycol, acetaminophen, and ibuprofen
   d. aspirin, acetaminophen, and iron

4. If chemical poisoning is suspected, what is your first concern?_____
   a. Secure the patient's airway.
   b. Assess the scene for evidence of a substance or poison.
   c. Secure the scene.
   d. Perform a physical exam to look for evidence of exposure to a toxin.

5. When is it safe to enter a scene at which a poisonous gas is present?_____
   a. When the scene is deemed safe by HazMat, law-enforcement officials, or both.
   b. When you determine that the scene is safe.
   c. After you have entered the scene and quickly moved the patient to a safe location.
   d. When all possible doors and windows have been opened and you have waited 15 minutes for the gas to dissipate.

**CASE DISPOSITION**

You suspect that the patient is exhibiting the signs of alcohol withdrawal. You place the patient in a position of comfort. Realizing that alcohol withdrawal is a true emergency and can result in seizures and even death, you contact a local rescue team to transport the patient to a definitive-care treatment facility. While waiting for help, you keep the patient calm.

You later learn that the patient had a seizure while being transported to the hospital. He makes a full recovery and is admitted to a substance rehabilitation clinic. Your medical advisor congratulates you for your actions, stating that the outcome would likely have been very different had the patient suffered an alcohol withdrawal seizure alone on the trail.

# Chapter Review

## Chapter Summary

Substance abuse or toxic exposures are common problems that OEC Technicians will likely encounter. Assessment centers on recognizing that a toxicological event has occurred and identifying signs and symptoms. Management centers on securing the scene, ensuring personal safety and safeguarding others, reducing the patient's exposure to toxic or poisonous substances, and providing supportive care. Diligent attention to the ABCDs is essential because the patient's condition can change quickly. These actions, combined with rapid transport to a definitive-care facility, will help increase the patient's chances of survival.

## Remember...

1. Personal safety is always the first priority.
2. Alcohol is the most commonly abused drug in the world.
3. Carbon monoxide poisoning is a silent killer.
4. Three deadly poisons for children are aspirin, acetaminophen, and iron.
5. Always try to identify the poison involved in an incident.
6. In the United States, poison-related information is available 24 hours a day, 7 days a week by calling the National Capital Poison Center 1-800-222-1222.

# Chapter Questions

## Multiple Choice

Choose the correct answer.

1. In caring for a poisoning victim after an initial assessment and stabilization, which of the following lists represents the order in which to act? _____
   a. Induce vomiting, reduce exposure to the poison, rapidly transport the patient to a definitive care facility
   b. Reduce exposure to the poison, induce vomiting, rapidly transport the patient to a definitive-care facility
   c. Reduce exposure to the poison, reduce absorption of the poison, rapidly transport the patient to a definitive-care facility
   d. Dilute the poison with water, induce vomiting, rapidly transport the patient to a definitive-care facility

2. What is the most commonly abused substance in the world?_____
   a. aspirin
   b. acetaminophen
   c. alcohol
   d. ecstasy

3. The body can eliminate a substance in each of the following ways *except*_____
   a. in urine.
   b. through absorption.
   c. in feces.
   d. in sweat.

4. When determining a patient's degree of exposure to a substance, you should try to quantify it according to_____
   a. quality and time.
   b. quantity and time.
   c. quality and quantity.
   d. time, quantity, and quality.

5. Which of the following choices lists two sources for emergency information concerning toxic chemicals and poisonings?
   a. CHEMTREC and The National Capital Poison Center
   b. The National Capital Poison Center and NOAA
   c. CHEMTREC and the CMA
   d. The CMA and NOAA

## Short Answer

1. List the four steps to managing a toxicological event. _____

   _____

2. Describe what activated charcoal does._____

   _____

3. What is the universal phone number for the National Capital Poison Center?_____

   _____

4. List the four routes by which substances are absorbed into the body._____

   _____

5. Describe the proper care for a patient who has experienced a toxicological event._____

   _____

## Matching

Match each of the following signs and symptoms with the substance that causes them.

_____  **1.** Abnormal heart rate, rhythm, confusion

_____  **2.** Euphoria, decreased level of responsiveness, respiratory depression

_____  **3.** Nausea, vomiting, ringing in the ears

_____  **4.** Decreased level of responsiveness, confusion, drowsiness

_____  **5.** Agitation, restlessness, psychosis, hallucinations, elevated heart rate/blood pressure and skin temperature

_____  **6.** Nausea, vomiting

_____  **7.** Decreased level of responsiveness, lightheadedness, nausea, confusion, depressed mental status, reddened skin (late sign)

_____  **8.** Altered mental status, confusion, poor coordination, abnormal gait, slurred speech, nausea, vomiting

_____  **9.** Agitation, chest pain, elevated heart rate and blood pressure; psychosis may also be observed

_____  **10.** Respiratory distress, confusion, hypoxia, respiratory failure, decreased level of responsiveness, shock, coma

**a.** acetaminophen
**b.** aspirin
**c.** alcohol/depressants/sedatives
**d.** antipsychotics/antidepressants
**e.** carbon monoxide
**f.** cocaine
**g.** hallucinogens (LSD)
**h.** inhalants
**i.** marijuana
**j.** narcotics

## Scenario

The park's office receives a request to help a teenager in the parking lot. There you find a 15-year-old patient who stares straight ahead and makes motions of grabbing objects out of the air. His friends inform you that he has been here before and has been acting strangely for several days and has gotten worse in the last hour. After securing the scene, you attempt to start an assessment of the patient. The patient keeps responding "the bugs won't go away."

You call the park office to notify the Park Police and to request an ALS ambulance for a patient with an AMS.

You begin a secondary assessment and find an elevated body temperature and an irregular pulse of 100. The respiratory rate is 24 and is not labored. His friends arrive and inform you that the patient has not slept in two days.

**1.** Based on your findings, you suspect that the patient has_____
  **a.** ingested alcoholic beverages.
  **b.** taken an antidepressant.
  **c.** ingested LSD.
  **d.** smoked marijuana.

Additional help arrives, and they obtain the names and addresses of the bystanders and friends. The interview of one of the teenager's friends reveals that the patient had consumed some small squares of paper with dots on them. The patient's blood pressure is 150/90, the pulse is reassessed at 100 and irregular, and the respiratory rate is 24 and not labored.

**2.** Which of the following drugs does *not* produce hallucinations?_____
  **a.** methamphetamine
  **b.** heroin
  **c.** PCP
  **d.** peyote

Substances and poisons enter and move through the body by four physiological processes: absorption, distribution, metabolism, and elimination.

**3.** Once a toxin has been absorbed through the GI tract, to what organ(s) does that toxin go next?_____
  **a.** the liver
  **b.** the kidneys
  **c.** the spleen
  **d.** the pancreas

## Suggested Reading

National Institute on Drug Abuse (NIDA) website: www.nida.nih.gov

Substance Abuse and Mental Health Services Administration (SAMHSA) website: www.samhsa.gov

Tintinalli, J. E., G. D. Kelen, and J. S. Stapczynski. 1999. *Emergency Medicine: A Comprehensive Study Guide*, 6th Edition. New York: McGraw-Hill.

EXPLORE **myNSPkit** PEARSON

Please go to www.myNSPkit.com. Under Student Resources, you will find animations, videos, web links, and games related to this chapter—and much more. Look for information on carbon monoxide poisoning, cocaine, activated charcoal use, and documentation tips.

Register your access code from the front of your book by going to www.myNSPkit.com and selecting the appropriate links. If the in-cover access code has been redeemed, go to www.myNSPkit.com and follow links to **Buy Access.**

# Respiratory Emergencies

Fred A. Severyn, MD, FACEP

## ⊕ OBJECTIVES

**Upon completion of this chapter, the OEC Technician will be able to:**

**13-1** Define the following terms:
- diffusion
- dyspnea
- respiration

**13-2** List the major anatomical structures of the lower airway.

**13-3** Identify the primary muscle of respiration.

**13-4** List the accessory muscles of respiration.

**13-5** Describe the physiology of breathing.

**13-6** Compare and contrast normal breathing and abnormal breathing.

**13-7** List the normal breathing rate for individuals in the following age groups:
- infant
- child
- adult

**13-8** Identify the most common cause of airway obstruction.

**13-9** List the signs and symptoms of acute respiratory distress.

**13-10** List the signs and symptoms of the following respiratory emergencies:
- asthma
- COPD
- spontaneous pneumothorax
- pulmonary embolism
- hyperventilation

*continued*

## Chapter Overview

OEC Technicians will encounter patients with breathing difficulties in outdoor settings. Problems can range from exercise-induced asthma or airway obstruction by a foreign body to severe respiratory distress from pulmonary embolism. Many patients can experience shortness of breath due to such medical conditions as heart attack, excessive blood loss, or conditions that have caused shock (Figure 13-1■).

*continued*

## HISTORICAL TIMELINE

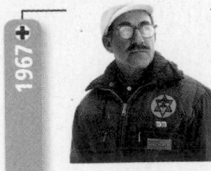

**1967**
First full-time Executive Director Eric Ericson hired.

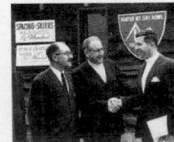

**1968**
Harry Pollard (National # 66) becomes National Director.

**13-11** Describe and demonstrate how to assess a patient who is having difficulty breathing.

**13-12** Describe and demonstrate the appropriate treatment of a patient in respiratory distress.

## ⊕ KEY TERMS

**accessory muscles of respiration,** p. 411

**airway patency,** p. 413

**alveoli,** p. 411

**anoxia,** p. 415

**bradypnea,** p. 418

**breath sounds,** p. 422

**bronchospasm,** p. 414

**chronic obstructive pulmonary disease (COPD),** p. 413

**crepitus,** p. 421

**dyspnea,** p. 410

**pleura,** p. 411

**pleural space,** p. 411

**pneumothorax,** p. 416

**pulmonary embolism,** p. 415

**ventilation,** p. 407

**wheezing,** p. 418

The oxygen supply to our tissues cannot be interrupted for more than 5–10 minutes without severe and possibly even irreversible consequences. Caring for patients with respiratory problems requires OEC Technicians to have a good understanding of the anatomy of the respiratory system, and of the mechanical and physiological mechanisms by which the lungs take in oxygen from the air and expel carbon dioxide, one of the body's waste products—a process called **ventilation**.

A comprehensive explanation of normal and abnormal respiration follows. Many important terms associated with respiration will be introduced and explained so that you will be able to communicate with peers and other medical personnel. By learning about the different diseases and conditions that cause respiratory compromise, and by understanding what you can do to correct acute medical breathing problems, you will have the resources to treat the second part of the primary (ABCD) assessment: breathing. Finally, by learning how to assess both the rate and quality of breathing, and how these values are different for children and adults, you will have the skills and knowledge you need to assist patients with respiratory emergencies. OEC Technicians do not *diagnose* breathing problems, but they can perform a rapid, thorough respiratory assessment, identify potential threats to life, and initiate life-stabilizing therapy that includes oxygen delivery and transport to a higher level of care.

Respiratory emergencies are a frequent complaint and are the source of many patient encounters in outdoor settings. It is estimated that 10–15 percent of the U.S. population has some type of underlying pulmonary disease such as asthma, emphysema, or chronic bronchitis. Now that new medications for treating breathing problems are available, individuals with respiratory problems who just 10 years ago could not visit remote areas are now actively participating in a variety of vigorous outdoor activities. As a result, the possibility that you will encounter a patient with a respiratory emergency has increased significantly.

Dyspnea—difficult or labored breathing accompanied by feeling short of breath—is one of the most common patient complaints that OEC Technicians encounter. The many causes of dyspnea range from the common cold to a potentially lethal blood clot in the pulmonary circulation. Attempting to determine the specific cause of dyspnea can be challenging even for experienced medical professionals. Fortunately, the basic assessment and treatment priorities remain the same for all health care settings.

**ventilation** the process by which air moves into and out of the lungs, so that oxygen can be exchanged for carbon dioxide in the alveoli.

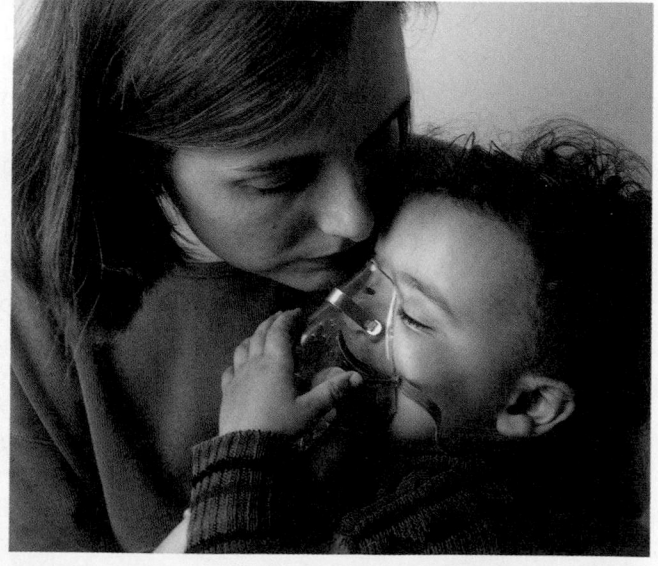

**Figure 13-1** More people than ever bring their children to ski areas even if they keep them in the lodge or nursery, increasing the chance that you will encounter children with respiratory emergencies.
Copyright Eddie Lawrence/Dorling Kindersley Media Library

## CASE PRESENTATION

You respond to the summit restaurant to evaluate a patient with "breathing problems." Upon arrival, you find a 62-year-old male complaining of severe shortness of breath, a cough, and chest pain. He is able to speak only a few words at a time and says, "I can't . . . catch . . . my breath." Additional questioning reveals that the man is from out of state and took the gondola to the top to see the view before the gondola stopped running. He hiked around the summit with his wife for about 30 minutes before he began to have breathing problems. The patient admits to a long history of cigarette smoking and appears to be in considerable distress.

**What should you do?**

This chapter begins by reviewing the major anatomical structures of the lower airway and the mechanics of breathing. It then discusses the most common types of respiratory emergencies that you will likely encounter, the signs and symptoms associated with each emergency, and their treatments.

## Anatomy and Physiology

**⊕ 13-1** Define the following terms:
- diffusion
- dyspnea
- respiration

The anatomical structures that make up the respiratory system are described in detail in Chapter 6, Anatomy and Physiology; now is a good time to review that material.

The airway begins at the lips and nostrils and terminates in the lung tissue. Traditionally, the airway is divided at the vocal cords into two parts, the upper airway and the lower airway. The upper airway is discussed in more detail in Chapter 9, Airway Management. The diaphragm and chest wall muscles mechanically expand the chest cavity, sucking outside air through the airway branches into the lung's many alveoli. These small "air sacs" are the sites at which oxygen in inhaled air is absorbed while carbon dioxide is released from the blood and exhaled (Figure 13-2■).

Air consists of 78 percent nitrogen, 21 percent oxygen, and 1 percent other gases. The relatively high oxygen concentration in air and the very low concentration of carbon dioxide drive the process of gas exchange at the alveolar level by a process called diffusion. Diffusion is a passive process whereby substances, in this case gases, move from an area of high concentration to an area of lower concentration until the concentrations equalize. Oxygen thus moves by diffusion into the blood in the capillaries in the alveoli while carbon dioxide diffuses out of the blood in the capillaries in the alveoli into the air that is exhaled. Once oxygen reaches the blood in the lung capillaries, it binds to hemoglobin in red blood cells and is carried throughout the body in the bloodstream. Carbonic acid, which is dissolved in the blood, is released from the capillaries as carbon dioxide.

Breathing rate, and depth, are controlled by the amount of the waste product carbon dioxide in the blood. The build-up of dissolved carbon dioxide in the blood produces carbonic acid, which changes the pH of the blood. Sensors located in the carotid arteries and in the aorta detect the changes in the pH and signal the brain to automatically control the rate and depth of breathing. When more carbon dioxide (carbonic acid) lowers the pH of the blood, the sensors in the carotid arteries tell the brain stem to send signals through the phrenic nerves to the diaphragm, and through the thoracic nerves to muscles in the chest wall, increasing the rate and depth of respiration in order to blow off (exhale) excess carbon dioxide. Although this is a complex process, the im-

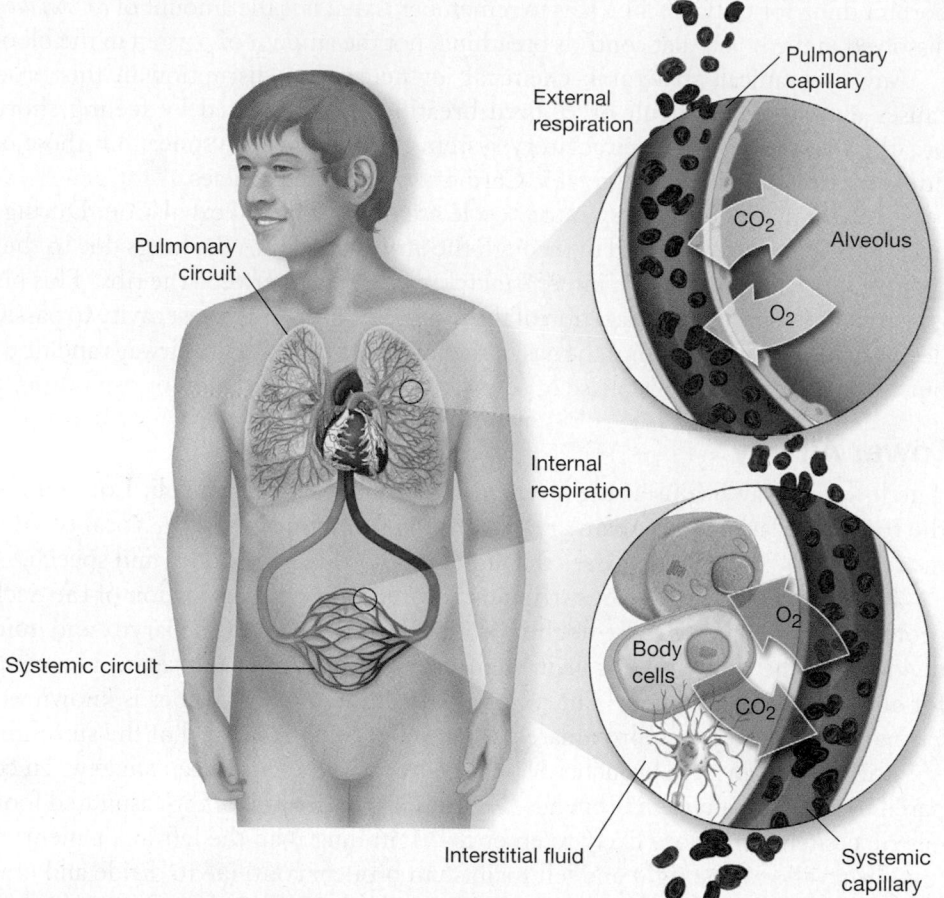

**Figure 13-2** Overview of ventilation and perfusion showing gas exchange at the alveolar level.

# STOP, THINK, UNDERSTAND

## Multiple Choice

Choose the correct answer.

1. Which of the following conditions are potential causes for nontrauma-related breathing difficulties in outdoor environments? (check all that apply)

    _____a. exercise-induced asthma

    _____b. an airway obstruction due to a foreign body

    _____c. pulmonary embolism

    _____d. heart attack (acute myocardial infarction, or AMI)

    _____e. hypoxia

    _____f. other medical conditions

2. Which of the following statements is true?_____

    a. An OEC Technician should be able to diagnose breathing problems and respond accordingly.

    b. It is beyond the scope of an OEC Technician to assess for, and intervene in, breathing problems.

    c. An OEC Technician must be able to perform a rapid, thorough respiratory assessment, identify potential threats to life, and initiate life-stabilizing therapy.

    d. An OEC Technician must be able to identify and evaluate breathing problems but may not treat them.

3. Which of the following statements about respiratory emergencies is true?_____

    a. A patient with asthma is rarely encountered by OEC Technicians because most patients suffering from this condition are not outdoor enthusiasts.

    b. Incidences of respiratory emergencies due to chronic health problems such as asthma are decreasing in wilderness settings due to better control and treatment.

    c. The possibility that an OEC Technician will encounter a patient in the wilderness who is suffering from a respiratory emergency has increased significantly in recent years.

    d. OEC Technicians may only transport, but not treat, a patient suffering from a respiratory emergency in the wilderness.

4. One of the most common patient conditions encountered by OEC Technicians is _____

    a. heart attack.

    b. pulmonary embolism.

    c. decreased level of responsiveness.

    d. dyspnea.

portant thing for OEC Technicians to remember is that it is the amount of *carbon dioxide* dissolved in the blood that controls breathing, not the amount of oxygen in the blood.

Any mechanical, structural, chemical, or neurologic disruption in this process causes **dyspnea**, or difficult or labored breathing accompanied by feeling short of breath. Disruptions in the circulatory system can also cause dyspnea, but these conditions are discussed in Chapter 15, Cardiovascular Emergencies.

The two phases of the respiratory cycle are inhalation and exhalation. During inhalation, air is actively sucked in through the airways and into the lungs due to the actions of the diaphragm and of intercostal muscles located between the ribs. This phase is also called inspiration. Relaxation of these muscles allows the chest cavity to passively decrease in size, which pushes the gas in the lungs out through the airways and into the outside environment. This phase of respiration is called exhalation or expiration.

## Lower Airway

The lower airway begins at the larynx and terminates at the alveoli. Located inside the top of the larynx (the Adam's apple) are folds of tissue called the vocal cords that move back and forth as air passes through them, producing sounds and speech.

The larynx is a cartilaginous structure located in the upper portion of the neck; it protects the vocal cords. The trachea originates at the base of the larynx and quickly divides into the right and left main stem bronchi, each of which serves as a conduit for air as it enters the lungs. The point at which the trachea divides is known as the carina and is located at approximately the level of the upper third of the sternum.

The right main stem bronchus leaves the trachea at a fairly steep angle when compared to the left main stem bronchus (Figure 13-3■). Because of this, aspirated food or gastric contents are more likely to enter the right lung than the left in a patient in an upright position. The right and left main stem bronchi continue to divide and branch into progressively smaller airways, much like the limbs and needles of an inverted evergreen tree. Eventually, each bronchiole divides into 2 alveolar ducts, which terminate at the alveoli (Figure 13-4■).

dyspnea   difficult or labored breathing accompanied by feeling short of breath.

+ **13-2** List the major anatomical structures of the lower airway.

+ **13-3** Identify the primary muscle of respiration.

+ **13-4** List the accessory muscles of respiration.

+ **13-5** Describe the physiology of breathing.

**Figure 13-3**  The bronchial tree: each primary (main) bronchus enters a lung, then branches into smaller and smaller secondary bronchi, tertiary bronchi, and bronchioles.

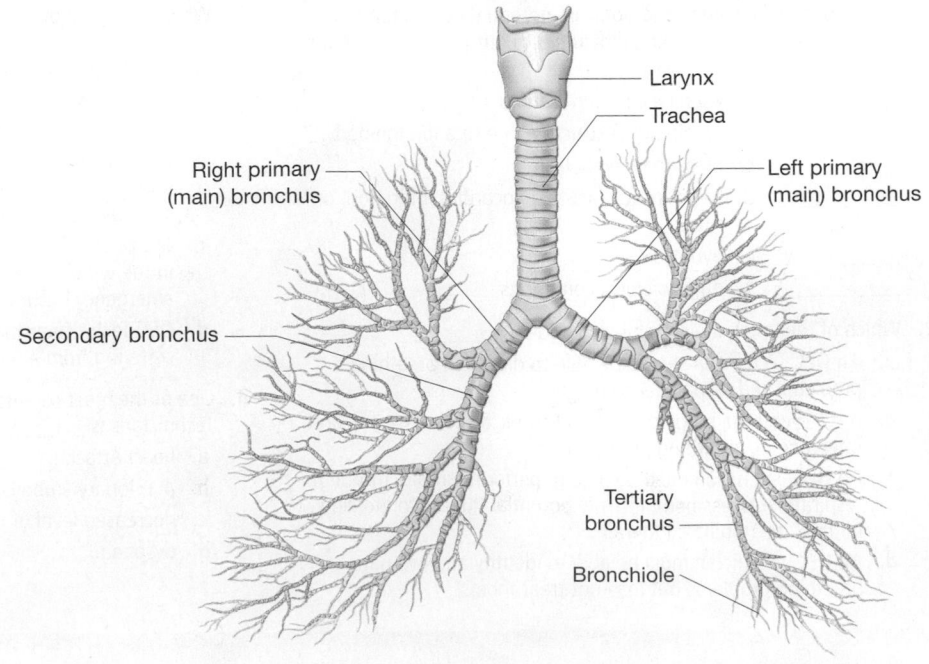

Larynx
Trachea
Right primary (main) bronchus
Left primary (main) bronchus
Secondary bronchus
Tertiary bronchus
Bronchiole

The tiny air sacs called **alveoli** are organized into grape-like clusters and are the functional units of the pulmonary system. Each of the approximately 700 million alveoli serve as the sites of gas exchange. It is here that a thin membrane separates each alveolus from individual red blood cells traveling through microscopic capillaries (Figure 13-5■). As the blood flows past the alveoli, oxygen diffuses into red blood cells while carbonic acid in the plasma diffuses as carbon dioxide into the alveoli for removal from the body during exhalation.

Between the exterior surface of the lung and the internal lining of the chest is a potential space known as the **pleural space**. Within this space is a small amount of fluid produced by the **pleura** that allows for efficient and painless movement of the lungs during inspiration and expiration. Under certain conditions, air or excess fluid may collect within this space, compromising normal expansion of the lung and thus respiration, and causing pain and dyspnea.

Breathing cannot occur without the muscles that actively expand the chest, increasing its volume and thus decreasing its internal pressure. The most important muscle in this process is the diaphragm. This dome-shaped muscular sheet, which divides the thoracic and abdominal cavities, is the primary muscle of respiration. Upon inhalation, the diaphragm tightly contracts and flattens, which expands volume of the chest, significantly lowering the pressure within the chest and sucking air into the lungs. During exhalation, the diaphragm relaxes and passively returns to its original position, reducing chest volume and increasing the pressure within the chest, which moves the air out of the body.

Other muscles, including those of the chest, shoulder, neck, and abdomen, help to bring air into the lungs but have a less important role than the diaphragm. Those muscles, collectively referred to as the **accessory muscles of respiration**, are recruited whenever the body's demand for oxygen exceeds the availability of oxygen. Chest muscles such as the pectoralis major, pectoralis minor, and intercostal muscles forcefully contract to expand the chest wall more fully and bring more oxygen-containing air into the body. Likewise, the sternocleidomastoid and scalene muscles, located on either side of the anterior neck, and the trapezius muscles, located on top of the shoulders, also contract upon inhalation, raising the top of the rib cage bringing more air

**alveoli** tiny air sacs within the lungs; the sites at which oxygen and carbon dioxide are exchanged between inhaled air and the bloodstream.

**pleural space** the potential space that lies within the pleura covering the outside of the lungs and the inside of the chest wall.

**pleura** the thin transparent membrane covering the outside of the lungs and the inside of the chest wall.

**accessory muscles of respiration** various muscles of the neck, chest, and abdomen that may become active when depth of respiration must be significantly increased.

**Figure 13-4** The bronchial tree ends at the alveoli (air sacs).

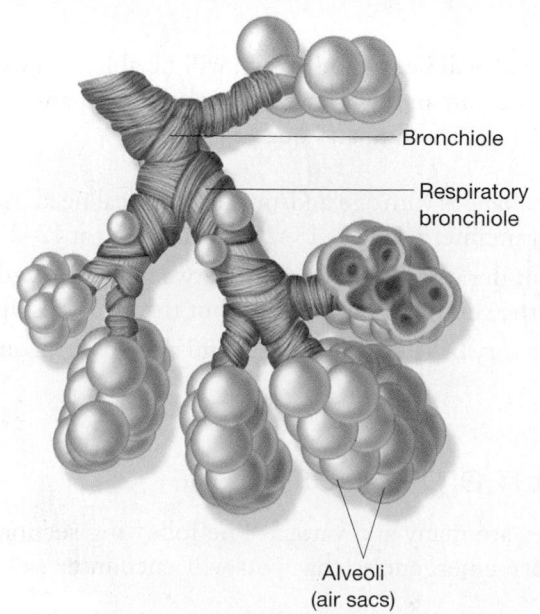

Bronchiole

Respiratory bronchiole

Alveoli (air sacs)

**Figure 13-5** Gas exchange between the air and the blood occurs within the alveoli.

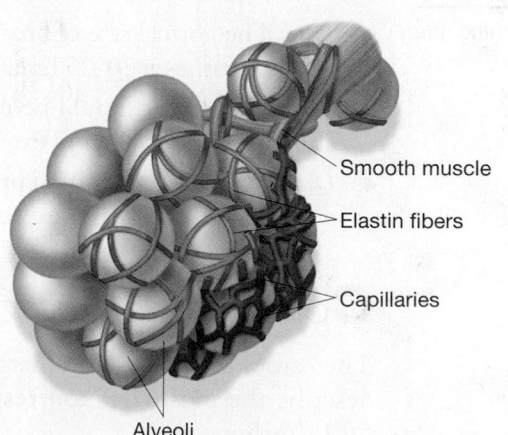

Smooth muscle

Elastin fibers

Capillaries

Alveoli

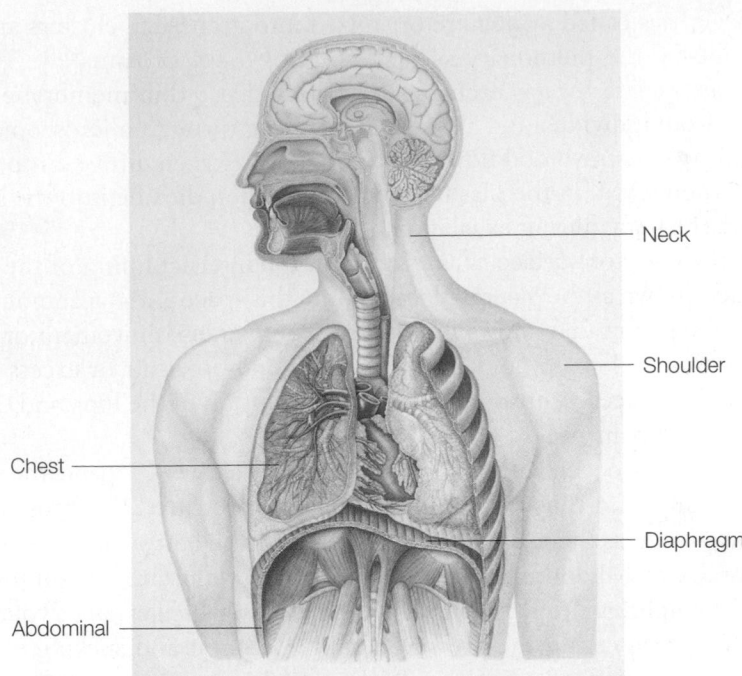

**Figure 13-6** The muscles in the structures shown are involved in the mechanics of respiration along with the Diaphragm.
Copyright Dorling Kindersley Media Library

into the lungs. The abdominal muscles also can help the diaphragm descend downward to further increase the internal volume of the chest cavity during inspiration (Figure 13-6■).

The circulatory system complements the respiratory system by pumping blood throughout the body, thereby transporting oxygenated red blood cells to body cells and removing carbon dioxide from the body via the lungs. Finally, the nervous system plays an important role in the breathing process as the brain controls the rate, depth, and regularity of respirations.

## Normal Breathing

⊕ **13-6** Compare and contrast normal breathing and abnormal breathing.

Individuals who have normal respirations will be in no distress, will be able to speak in full sentences, will have normal skin color, and will have normal chest expansion. Breathing is described according to its rate, rhythm, and quality:

⊕ **13-7** List the normal breathing rate for individuals in the following age groups:
- infant
- child
- adult

- *Rate*. The normal rate of breathing changes with age and/or physiological need. An infant breathes at 20–25 breaths per minute, a child at 15–20, and an adult at 12–20.
- *Rhythm*. Breaths should be equal in duration, and the time between each breath should be equal. During exercise, the rhythm remains equal but the rate goes up.
- *Quality*. All breaths should produce very little external sound and should be inconspicuous except during exercise.

## Common Respiratory Emergencies

The causes of respiratory emergencies are many and varied. The following sections describe the most common respiratory emergencies that you will encounter as an OEC Technician.

# STOP, THINK, UNDERSTAND

## Multiple Choice

Choose the correct answer.

1. Which of the following statements best describes the control of breathing?_____
   a. A lack of oxygen in the bloodstream drives the desire to breathe.
   b. A drop in the bloods pH due to a buildup of $CO_2$ as carbonic acid drives the desire to breathe.
   c. A low hematocrit drives the desire to breathe.
   d. Hypoxia drives the desire to breathe.

2. Diffusion is best described as_____
   a. a passive process whereby air, nutrients, or other products leach out of cells and tissues.
   b. an active process whereby air is forced out of the alveoli, through the bronchi, and out through the upper airway.
   c. a passive process whereby compounds move from an area of high concentration to an area of lower concentration until the concentrations equalize.
   d. a natural process by which an individual can override the drive to breathe.

3. The sensors that tell the brain to automatically control the rate, depth, and regularity of breathing are located in the_____
   a. brain stem.
   c. medulla oblongata.
   b. carotid arteries and aorta.
   d. bronchioles.

4. Which of the following statements about the bronchi is correct?_____
   a. Food or gastric contents cannot be aspirated into the lungs because the bronchi contain valves that prevent aspiration.
   b. The right and left bronchi are slanted equally, so aspirated food or gastric contents can enter either lung.
   c. A patient must be in a supine position in order to inadvertently aspirate food or gastric contents into the lungs.
   d. The right main bronchus leaves the trachea at a steeper angle than does the left bronchus, so food is more likely to be inhaled into the right lung by a patient in an upright position.

5. The sternocleidomastoid, scalene, pectoralis major, pectoralis minor, and intercostal muscles are collectively known as _____
   a. the accessory muscles of respiration.
   b. the diaphragmatic muscles of respiration.
   c. the bronchiolar carina.
   d. the passive muscles of respiration.

6. When assessing respirations, OEC Technicians describe breathing according to _____
   a. rate, rhythm, and quality.    c. rate only.
   b. rate, depth, and regularity.    d. rate and regularity.

7. An infant's normal respiratory rate is_____
   a. 20–25 breaths/minute.    c. 15–20 breaths/minute.
   b. 25–50 breaths/minute.    d. 12–20 breaths/minute.

8. Which of the following statements about respiration is true?_____
   a. All breaths should have clearly audible sounds.
   b. Breaths should be inconspicuous except during exercise.
   c. Exercise creates an irregular breathing rhythm.
   d. Respiratory rate is the most important thing to assess.

9. The exchange of oxygen ($O_2$) and carbon dioxide ($CO_2$) takes place in the_____
   a. alveoli.
   c. diaphragm.
   b. bronchus.
   d. epiglottis.

## Fill in the Blank

1. _____ are the grapelike clusters within the lungs where $O_2$ and $CO_2$ exchange occurs and are the functional unit of the respiratory system.

2. The primary muscle of respiration is the_____.

## Obstruction/Choking

For effective gas exchange to occur, **airway patency** must be maintained at all times. Any potential airway obstruction, whether due to the presence of a foreign body (e.g., food, vomit, debris) or to soft-tissue swelling (trauma or allergy/anaphylaxis), limits gas exchange and decreases oxygen levels. The tongue is the most common cause of airway obstruction. In a patient that is lying down, the relaxed tongue can fall across the posterior pharynx and block the upper airway. In addition, foreign bodies that get past the epiglottis may become lodged in the trachea, a bronchus, or one of the lower airways, resulting in a foreign body obstruction.

## Chronic Obstructive Pulmonary Disease

**Chronic obstructive pulmonary disease (COPD)** is a group of lung diseases that progressively block the lower airway passages. COPD is most often caused by long-term cigarette smoking, but it also may be caused by certain diseases or by prolonged exposure

⊕ 13-8 Identify the most common cause of airway obstruction.

**airway patency** a condition in which an airway is open and unobstructed.

**chronic obstructive pulmonary disease (COPD)** a condition in which the airways and alveoli become damaged, typically by long-term smoke exposure; its two most important forms are chronic bronchitis and chronic emphysema.

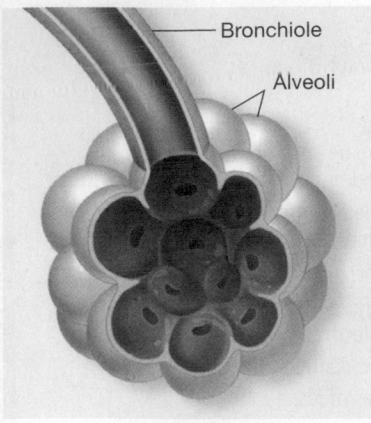

Normal

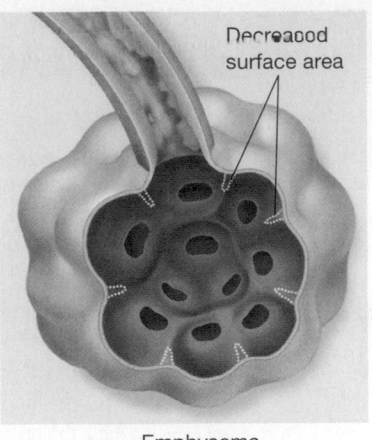

Emphysema

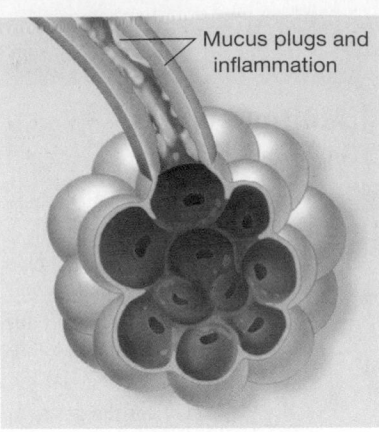

Chronic Bronchitis

**Figure 13-7** Two forms of chronic obstructive pulmonary diseases (COPD): emphysema and chronic bronchitis.

⊕ **13-10** List the signs and symptoms of the following respiratory emergencies:

- asthma
- COPD
- spontaneous pneumothorax
- pulmonary embolism
- hyperventilation

**bronchospasm** the involuntary contraction of the bronchioles.

to dust, chemicals, pollution, and other environmental irritants. According to a 2005 study by the Centers for Disease Control and Prevention, COPD is the fourth leading cause of death in the United States, claiming more than 125,000 lives each year.

OEC Technicians should be familiar with two forms of COPD: chronic bronchitis and chronic emphysema (Figure 13-7■). Chronic bronchitis is a persistent inflammation of the bronchial tubes that results in increased mucus production, thickening of the bronchial walls, and a persistent productive cough. Chronic emphysema is a condition in which destruction of the tiny alveolar sacs causes air to be trapped. The result is that these patients are unable to exhale adequate amounts of air from the lungs. Both forms of COPD develop gradually and result in permanent lung damage and hypoxia. Treatment of COPD centers on alleviating symptoms.

## Asthma

Asthma is a related form of chronic obstructive pulmonary disease (COPD) that is characterized by sudden, recurrent bronchiolar constriction and increased mucus production. However, unlike chronic bronchitis or emphysema, an acute asthma attack does not result in permanent lung damage and can be reversed by treatment. Although asthma is a common respiratory disorder, it can be life threatening and accounts for nearly 2 million visits to the emergency department each year

Although the exact cause of asthma is not known, researchers believe that genetics and environmental triggers such as pollen, mold, allergens, and cold air can stimulate an intense reaction within the lower airways, resulting in acute **bronchospasm**, inflammation, and mucus accumulation (Figure 13-8■). Strenuous physical activity also has been implicated as the cause of another, atypical variety of asthma, resulting in a condition known as exercise-induced asthma.

The condition called status asthmaticus involves a severe asthmatic attack that does not respond to either oxygen or inhaled medications. This condition requires the immediate dispatch of advanced life support and transport to the nearest hospital.

## Hyperventilation Syndrome

Hyperventilation syndrome (HVS) is a relatively common disorder that results in abnormally low levels of carbon dioxide in the blood. Excessive deep breathing, or hyperventilation, may be the body's response to some physiologic insult such as uncontrolled diabetes, or it may be induced by psychological factors. HVS is often preceded by anxiety or a panic attack. Although the condition is usually benign, it can mimic other forms of deep breathing that have a more serious origin, such as heart attack, a diabetic emergency, or a head injury. In its most severe form, HVS can cause peripheral tingling, spasms in the hands and feet, chest tightness, tachycardia, and a temporary loss of responsiveness. It has also been known to cause seizures in patients who have seizure disorders.

## Pulmonary Embolism

**Pulmonary embolism** (PE) is a serious, potentially life-threatening disorder. Specifically, a PE is a condition that occurs when a clot or other foreign material, called an embolus, travels in the bloodstream to the pulmonary artery or a branch of a pulmonary artery, resulting in the blockage of blood flow to a portion of one lung, a whole lung, or both lungs (Figure 13-9■). This interferes with normal blood flow to the lung tissues, eventually impairing gas exchange. In most cases, the source of blockage is a blood clot, although air bubbles, fat, and tumors are rare types of emboli.

Blood clots that often arise in the deep veins of either the lower legs or pelvis can break off and travel through the venous system through the right side of the heart and into the pulmonary circulation. The condition characterized by clots in these veins is called deep venous thrombosis (DVT). The causes of DVT are numerous and include prolonged sitting or immobilization, fracture of a long bone, recent surgery, heart disease, pregnancy, and certain inherited predispositions. A person who has had DVT previously is at an increased risk of a recurrence, especially if not undergoing chronic therapy to prevent recurrence.

Most cases of PE affect only small portions of the lung; however, large blockages can obstruct blood flow to the entire lung, causing severe **anoxia**, shock, and even

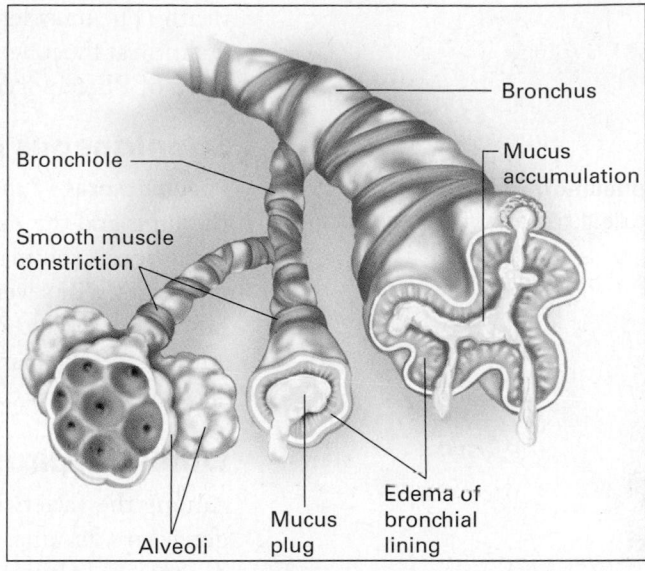

**Figure 13-8** Conditions that contribute to airflow resistance in asthma.

**pulmonary embolism**    a condition in which a clot or other obstruction (an embolus) partially or completely blocks a pulmonary artery.

**anoxia**    a condition characterized by the lack of an oxygen supply.

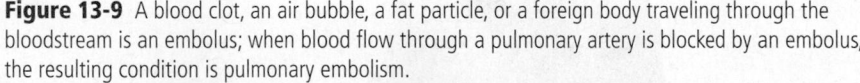

**Figure 13-9** A blood clot, an air bubble, a fat particle, or a foreign body traveling through the bloodstream is an embolus; when blood flow through a pulmonary artery is blocked by an embolus, the resulting condition is pulmonary embolism.

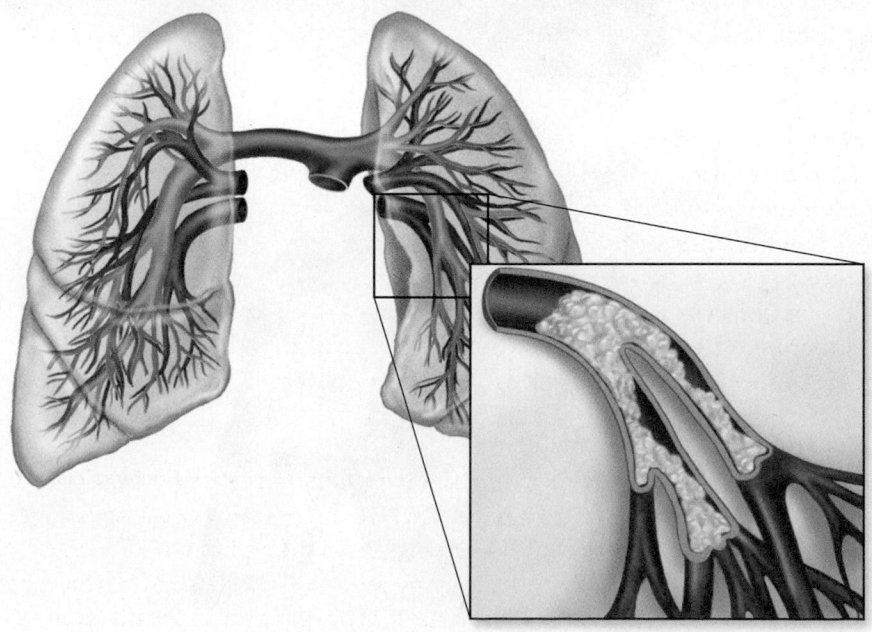

death. The most lethal type of PE is a "saddle embolus," which occludes the lung circulation at the junction between the right and left pulmonary arteries. Death from this form of PE can occur within minutes from acute right-sided heart strain and shock.

## Spontaneous Pneumothorax

**pneumothorax**    an abnormal collection of air within the pleural space.

**Pneumothorax** is an accumulation of air within the pleural space, the space between the lung and the inner chest wall (Figure 13-10■). The most common cause of this condition is traumatic injury to the chest wall, ribs, or lung itself. However, chronic emphysema or severe acute asthma can cause alveoli to rupture spontaneously, resulting in the escape of air from the lung into the pleural space. Depending on the amount of alveolar damage and subsequent air leakage, the problem may resolve spontaneously or cause profound hypoxia.

## Other Respiratory System-Related Conditions

Among the variety of other medical conditions that can result in a respiratory emergency are trauma, altitude illness, pneumonia, and carbon monoxide poisoning. Trauma and altitude illness are covered in Chapters 17 and 28, respectively.

Pneumonia, an infection of the lung tissue, is caused by bacteria, viruses, or fungi. These pathogens cause the alveoli to become filled with fluid or pus, which reduces gas exchange, resulting in hypoxia. It is usually accompanied by fever. Pneumonia is a common disease that affects approximately 3 million people in the United States each year.

Carbon monoxide, an odorless, colorless gas that is a by-product of incomplete combustion, binds to red blood cells more readily than does oxygen. As a result, it prevents oxygen in the lungs from being carried by red blood cells, causing anoxia and eventually death.

**Figure 13-10** Spontaneous pneumothorax, caused by a ruptured bleb (weakened area of lung tissue), causing air to enter the pleural cavity and eventually collapsing the lung.

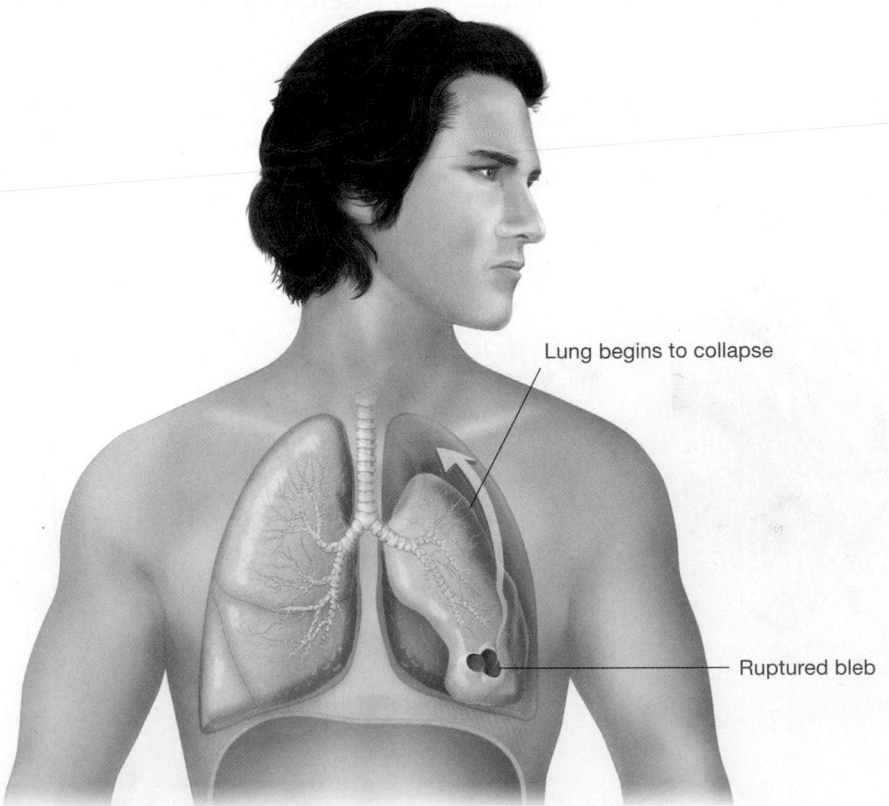

Lung begins to collapse

Ruptured bleb

# STOP, THINK, UNDERSTAND

## Multiple Choice

Choose the correct answer.

The most common cause of upper airway obstruction is _____

    **a.** food.          **c.** blood.

    **b.** vomit.         **d.** the tongue.

## Fill in the Blank

In order to get into the lower airway and cause a foreign body obstruction, a foreign body must get past the _____.

## Matching

1. Match each of the following respiratory emergencies to its description.

_____ **1.** asthma

_____ **2.** obstruction/choking

_____ **3.** COPD

_____ **4.** hyperventilation syndrome

_____ **5.** pulmonary embolism

_____ **6.** spontaneous pneumothorax

    **a.** a group of lung diseases that progressively block the lower airway passages, caused primarily by long-term smoking

    **b.** recurrent bronchiole constriction and increased mucus production

    **c.** an unresponsive patient's tongue blocking the posterior pharynx

    **d.** a serious, life-threatening disorder in which a clot travels from a part of the body to the pulmonary artery

    **e.** an accumulation of air in the pleural space

    **f.** abnormally low levels of $CO_2$ in the blood; may be caused by diabetes or psychological factors

2. Match each of the following conditions to its description.

_____ **1.** chronic bronchitis

_____ **2.** deep vein thrombosis

_____ **3.** emphysema

_____ **4.** pneumonia

_____ **5.** asthma

    **a.** a common respiratory disorder that can be triggered by exercise

    **b.** persistent inflammation of the bronchial tubes characterized by a productive cough

    **c.** a viral, bacterial, or fungal infection of the lungs

    **d.** the formation of clots in the lower legs and pelvis

    **e.** involves the destruction of alveoli

 # CASE UPDATE

You notify dispatch to have ALS awaiting the patient's arrival at the gondola base and then place the patient on a nonrebreather mask at 15 LPM of supplemental oxygen. The patient's wife relates that the patient has a history of asthma. He is diaphoretic, somewhat pale, and is sitting upright in a "tripod" position. You note audible wheezing during his single-word responses to your questions. His heart rate is 118, his respirations are 42 and shallow, and he has a blood pressure of 168/104. His wife tearfully relates that when he got this bad in the past, he had to use an inhaler and was placed on a ventilator. She removes the patient's inhaler from her purse and hands it to you.

***What do you think is wrong? What should you do?***

⊕ **13-9** List the signs and symptoms of acute respiratory distress.

⊕ **13-11** Describe and demonstrate how to assess a patient who is having difficulty breathing.

# Assessment

As always, you do a scene size-up and ensure that the area is safe. As you approach the patient, note whether any signs of acute respiratory distress are apparent, or whether the patient's breathing is absent or noisy. Conduct a primary assessment of the ABCDs, correcting any life-threatening conditions you identify, including opening and clearing the airway using any of the adjuncts identified in Chapter 9, Airway Management. If the patient has severe respiratory compromise, immediately summon ALS assistance. Assess the patient's circulation and level of responsiveness using the AVPU system or, if time permits, the Glasgow Coma Scale.

Note the patient's overall appearance and any revealing signs. Does the patient appear ill at ease, restless, agitated, or confused? Does he seem thin or obese? Chronic bronchitis patients are generally overweight, have a productive cough, appear slightly cyanotic, and use their accessory muscles to breathe, whereas chronic emphysema patients are usually quite thin, have a barrel-shaped chest due to the trapping of air, and breathe through pursed lips; they seldom have a productive cough. Asthma patients generally appear very anxious, have rapid shallow breathing, and may have audible **wheezing**. Patients with pulmonary embolism may be cyanotic, may be panicked due to hunger for air, and have rapid, deep respirations. They may even be unresponsive, depending on the severity of the embolism and any resulting shock. Patients who are hyperventilating also may appear panicked and exhibit rapid, deep respirations, but their color is usually normal.

The hallmark of any respiratory-related emergency is dyspnea. Because "difficulty breathing" is a subjective term, it is essential that OEC Technicians learn to recognize the signs and symptoms of acute respiratory distress, which provide valuable clues about the severity of the patient's condition and underlying hypoxia (Figure 13-11■). These signs, which often precede complete respiratory failure, include the following:

**wheezing** a high-pitched respiratory sound caused by a narrowing of the tubular airways.

- choking or gagging
- inability to speak
- open-mouthed breathing
- panting, gasping
- breathing through pursed lips
- tachypnea (greater than 30 rpm in adults)
- **bradypnea** (fewer than 10 rpm in adults)
- cyanosis
- nasal flaring
- sitting in an upright or tripod position
- changes in level of responsiveness

**bradypnea** a decreased respiration rate; in adults, less than 10 rpm.

In addition, patients who are having problems breathing will often assume a "tripod" position in which they sit upright while leaning forward with their hands near or gripping their thighs or knees (Figure 13-12a■). This position lets gravity pull the chest wall outward and downward, which allows the lungs to expand more fully. In severe cases, involuntary use of the accessory respiratory muscles will be evident, further aiding the patient's efforts to breathe. Collectively, these muscles forcefully expand the chest wall, maximizing the amount of air that is brought into the lungs during each inspiration. Finally, patients who are experiencing difficulty breathing, especially children, may exhibit abdominal breathing, in which the abdominal muscles forcefully expand the abdomen outward upon inspiration, which lowers the diaphragm

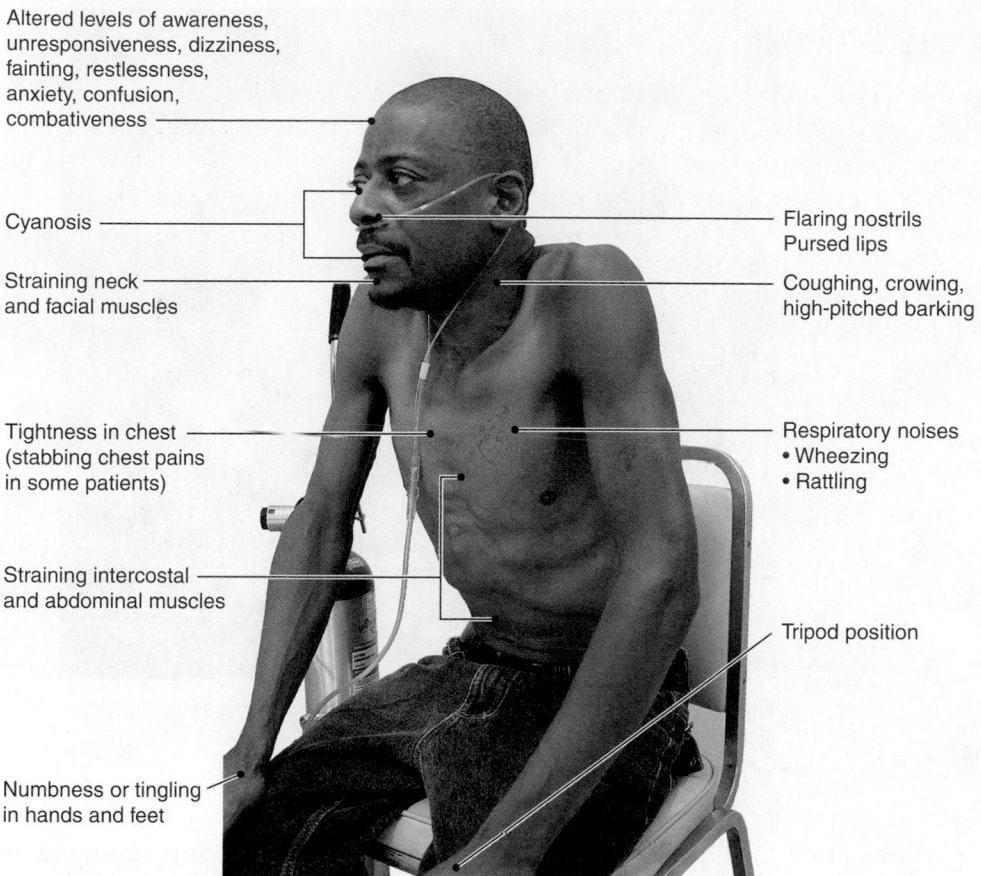

Altered levels of awareness, unresponsiveness, dizziness, fainting, restlessness, anxiety, confusion, combativeness

Cyanosis

Straining neck and facial muscles

Tightness in chest (stabbing chest pains in some patients)

Straining intercostal and abdominal muscles

Numbness or tingling in hands and feet

Flaring nostrils
Pursed lips

Coughing, crowing, high-pitched barking

Respiratory noises
• Wheezing
• Rattling

Tripod position

**Figure 13-11** Signs and symptoms of respiratory difficulty.

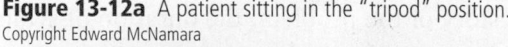

**Figure 13-12a** A patient sitting in the "tripod" position.
Copyright Edward McNamara

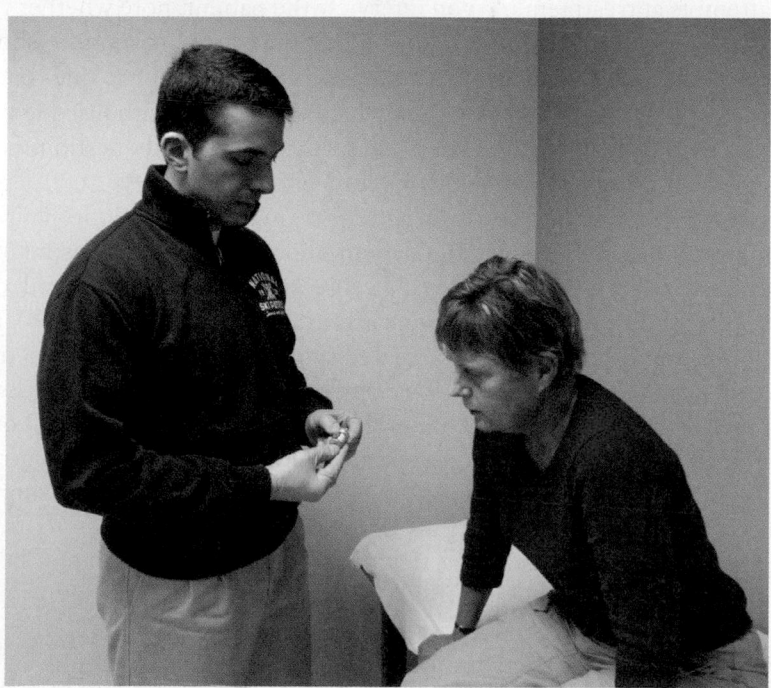

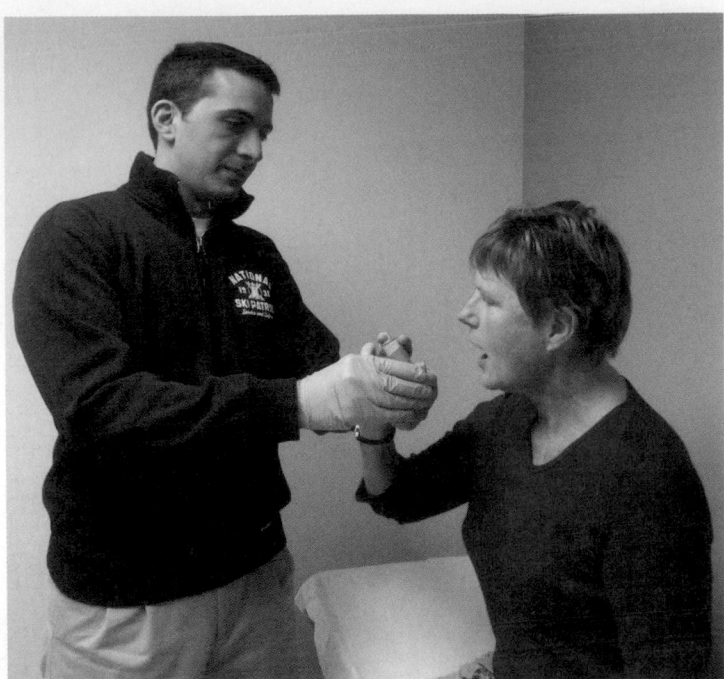

**Figure 13-12b** A patroller assisting a patient in administering medication from an inhaler.
Copyright Edward McNamara

and allows more air to enter the lungs, or they may exhibit expiratory grunting, in which the abdominal muscles force air out of the lungs at the end of each exhalation.

Next, perform a secondary assessment, which includes a medical history, physical assessment, and a check of the vital signs. Begin the secondary assessment by obtaining a chief complaint from the patient. If the patient's dyspnea is relatively mild, the patient will provide this information with minimal effort and may even offer other unsolicited information, such as history of the problem, the duration of symptoms, and previous attempts at treatment. As you interview the patient, note whether the person can speak in complete sentences, or whether responses are broken into short groups of words. Unfortunately, severe dyspnea often limits the patient to one- or two-word answers. Frame your questions so that they may be answered with just a few words, or as short yes-or-no questions. Do not ask too many open-ended questions because the patient may not be able to answer due to a hunger for air.

Obtain a SAMPLE history. Ask the patient if anything makes the symptoms better or worse, and be sure to query the patient about any medications he may be using, including over-the-counter drugs, herbs, and supplements. Find out if the patient uses an inhaler, and if so, whether it is available (Figure 13-12b■). As part of the history, attempt to identify any associated symptoms such as a productive cough, fever, chest pain, or swelling of the lower extremities. Also ask about past medical problems such as blood clots or any underlying lung disease (e.g., COPD or asthma).

If the patient's history includes a respiratory ailment, ask how the current problem compares to previous episodes. Ask the patient if he could walk a short distance without becoming short of breath. This is important because the ability to ambulate without respiratory difficulty suggests that the underlying condition may be relatively minor, whereas shortness of breath while at rest or when walking only a short distance indicates a potentially serious condition.

Observe skin color for pallor or cyanosis, looking closely at the inside of the patient's eyelids, around the lips and at the fingernail beds.

---

**NOTE**

## Common Medications for Respiratory Conditions

- Albuterol (Proventil, Ventolin)
- Ipratropium (Atrovent)
- Aminophylline
- Epinephrine
- Prednisone
- Terbutaline (Brethine)

Complete the rest of the physical examination in the usual fashion. For the chest exam, carefully palpate the skin of the patient's chest for the presence of any "crackling" or "Rice Krispies© feel" beneath the skin. This sign, known as subcutaneous emphysema or **crepitus**, is often due to a spontaneous pneumothorax and indicates that air or gas is present beneath the skin. Other potential causes of subcutaneous crepitus include penetrating trauma and severe skin and tissue infections.

Obtain a complete set of vital signs, including the rate, depth, and quality of respirations. Do not guess the respiratory rate; count the breaths for 30 seconds and multiply the count by 2 to determine breaths/minute. Because vital signs change over time, repeat the vital signs frequently (every 3–5 minutes), especially in patients exhibiting signs of acute respiratory distress (e.g., every 3–5 minutes). *Vital signs are dynamic and change over time.* It is for this reason that serial vital signs usually provide more information than a single, isolated measurement and can serve as a marker for progress, both favorable as well as unfavorable.

Respiratory rates less than 6–8 per minute or greater than 30 per minute in an adult are ominous and signify impending respiratory failure (remember that a normal respiratory rate for an adult is 12–20 per minute). Tachypnea and hyperventilation can have a variety of causes ranging from psychogenic in nature to a potentially lethal pulmonary embolism. Regardless of the underlying cause, a patient can sustain a rapid respiratory rate for only a short period of time. If the problem is psychogenic (e.g., hyperventilation), it will eventually go away. If the problem is more serious, compensatory mechanisms will eventually be lost, and sudden respiratory failure will then result, especially in children.

Patients who are hyperventilating may complain of tingling or a "pins and needles" sensation around the lips, hands, or feet, a condition known as paresthesia. Patients also may complain of not being able to open their hands due to excessive muscle cramping. Upon observation, the hands and fingers may appear contorted. Although alarming to the patient, these findings are benign and will disappear once the patient's respiratory rate slows. Such psychogenic hyperventilation is typically seen in very anxious patients.

An *advanced responder (Paramedic)* who auscultates the patient's lungs using a stethoscope can obtain valuable clues about the overall effectiveness of breathing efforts (Figure 13-13■). However, it is more important for OEC Technicians to assess whether

**crepitus** a "crackling" feel of the skin of the chest that is detected by palpation; is caused by the presence of air trapped beneath the skin.

**Figure 13-13** Stethoscope-aided auscultation of the patient's lungs makes breath sounds audible and can provide valuable clues to respiratory status.
Copyright Mike Halloran

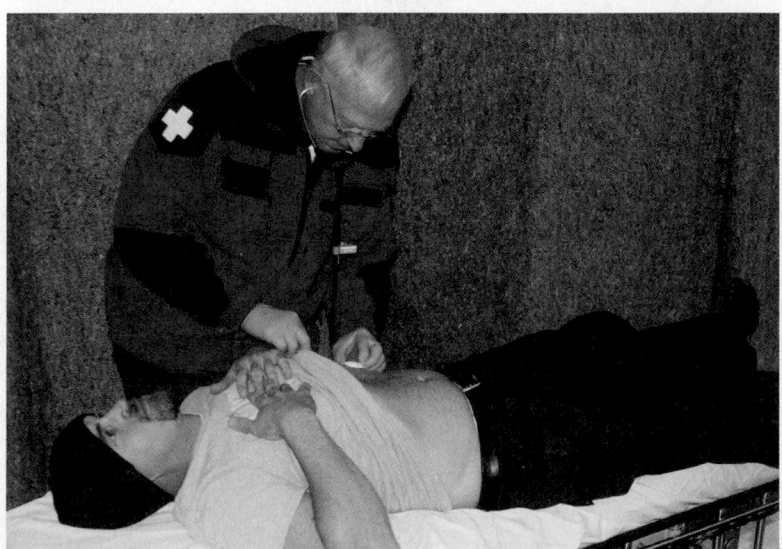

air is moving in and out of the lungs and to determine whether the patient is sufficiently oxygenated. This can be determined by assessing the patient's level of responsiveness, respiration quality and quantity, capillary refill, and skin color.

Normal breath sounds are regular, relatively quiet (like a sigh), and equal for the two lungs. Abnormal breath sounds are diminished or absent, noisy (wheezes, crackles, gurgles), or unequal between the two lungs. It is beyond the scope of competence for OEC Technicians to fully learn **breath sounds**, although, for advanced rescuers, breath sounds are addressed in Chapter 36, ALS Interface.

**breath sounds**   the noises produced by the pulmonary structures during respiration.

One of the most common abnormal lung sounds that OEC Technicians will likely encounter is wheezing, which indicates constriction of the lower airway passages. Wheezing is typically caused by asthma and is defined as a high-pitched respiratory sound that may be heard on inhalation, exhalation, or both. In most severe cases, wheezing can be heard without a stethoscope.

Again, when listening with a stethoscope, it is more important to recognize that a patient's breath sounds are absent or *abnormal* than to identify the cause of the abnormal sounds. Always tell the patient that you are going to listen to the lungs. When listening to breath sounds, place the patient in an upright position, preferably seated. The exception to this is when spinal injury is suspected, in which case the patient should remain in a neutral, supine position.

To avoid startling the patient with a cold stethoscope, warm it before use by vigorously rubbing it in a circular pattern on the palm of your hand. Also, place the stethoscope firmly against the patient's bare skin, not against clothing, as breath sounds may be subtle. Instruct the patient to breathe normally. If you are unable to hear the patient breathe, ask the patient to breathe through an open mouth or to breathe deeply. Using the large diaphragm of the stethoscope, listen at each location for approximately 15–30 seconds. As you listen, avoid unnecessary movement or talking, and do not allow the stethoscope tubing to rub against the patient's clothing or to bump into anything, because the resulting noise can make your assessment more difficult.

To assess lung sounds, see OEC Skill 13-1■.

1. *Upper lobes–anterior*: Place your stethoscope on the left side of the anterior chest approximately 1.5 inches below the middle of the clavicle (second intercostal space). Listen to the right upper lobe and compare the results.

2. *Lower lobes–anterior*: Place your stethoscope on the left side of the anterior chest at or below the level of the nipple line, over the anterior midaxillary line (fifth–sixth intercostal space). Listen to the right lower lobe and compare the results.

3. *Upper lobes–posterior*: Place your stethoscope on the patient's right upper back, between the top of the scapula and the spine, approximately 2 inches below the neck. Listen to the left upper lobe and compare the results.

4. *Lower lobes–posterior*: Place your stethoscope on the left lower back, below the bottom of the scapula. Listen to the right lower lobe and compare the results.

If you have a pulse oximeter and local protocol allows its use, assess the patient's blood oxygen concentration. Ideally, the patient's oxygen concentration should be 95 percent or higher. Any patient with a value below 90 percent should be aggressively treated with oxygen. Pulse oximetry is a useful tool for assessing oxygenation trends over time. Because the degree of dyspnea perceived by the patient does not correlate with the actual degree of hypoxia, this instrument provides valuable information for deciding when to increase oxygen therapy or when to expedite the patient's transfer to a higher level of medical care.

Note that pulse oximeters can give false readings, so if a patient with a pulse oximetry reading of 95 percent is cyanotic, breathing fast, and looks ill, trust your own observations and provide oxygen. Treat according to what the patient shows you, and not according to the number the pulse oximeter gives you.

# STOP, THINK, UNDERSTAND

## Multiple Choice

Choose the correct answer.

1. The uniform hallmark of respiratory-related emergencies is _____
   a. apnea.
   b. dyspnea.
   c. chest pain.
   d. anxiety.

2. Which of the following signs indicates impending respiratory failure in an adult?_____
   a. a respiratory rate less than 15 or greater than 24
   b. a respiratory rate less than 8 or greater than 30
   c. a respiratory rate less than 20 or greater than 30
   d. a respiratory rate of 28 coupled with a pulse rate of 110

3. Which of the following statements is correct?_____
   a. It is most important to determine the exact cause of abnormal breath sounds.
   b. It is not important for an OEC Technician to determine whether or not breath sounds are normal or abnormal, only to determine the depth, rate, and rhythm.
   c. It is more important to identify a patient's breath sounds as abnormal than to know the exact cause of the abnormal sounds.
   d. It is not within the scope of an OEC Technician's training to determine whether or not a breath sound is normal or abnormal.

4. A patient's pulse-oximetry reading is 88 percent. The patient is cyanotic, has a respiratory rate of 28, and appears ill. What is the correct determination based on this information?_____
   a. The patient is not critically ill because the pulse oximetry reading is comfortably within the normal range.
   b. The patient is critically ill and should be treated with oxygen and transported immediately.
   c. The patient is not immediately critical but should be observed because conditions could change.
   d. The patient's condition cannot be determined from the information provided.

## Matching

For each of the following five respiratory conditions, write the letter(s) of the signs, symptoms, or actions that apply for each condition. Signs and symptoms may be used more than once.

_____ 1. asthma
_____ 2. chronic bronchitis
_____ 3. chronic emphysema
_____ 4. pulmonary embolism
_____ 5. choking

a. anxiety
b. barrel-chested
c. breathing through pursed lips
d. breathing with accessory muscles
e. clutching at one's throat
f. slight cyanosis
g. moderate cyanosis
h. inability to speak
i. rapid deep respirations
j. rapid shallow respirations
k. overweight
l. thin
m. nonproductive cough
n. productive cough
o. wheezing
p. panic
q. unconscious/unresponsive

## Labeling

Categorize each of the following respiratory signs as either mild/moderate (M) or severe (S).

_____ a. respiratory rate of 22
_____ b. respiratory rate of 34
_____ c. respiratory rate of 8
_____ d. respiratory rate of 11
_____ e. panting
_____ f. nasal flaring
_____ g. can speak only 1–2 word sentences
_____ h. can speak full sentences
_____ i. choking
_____ j. coughing

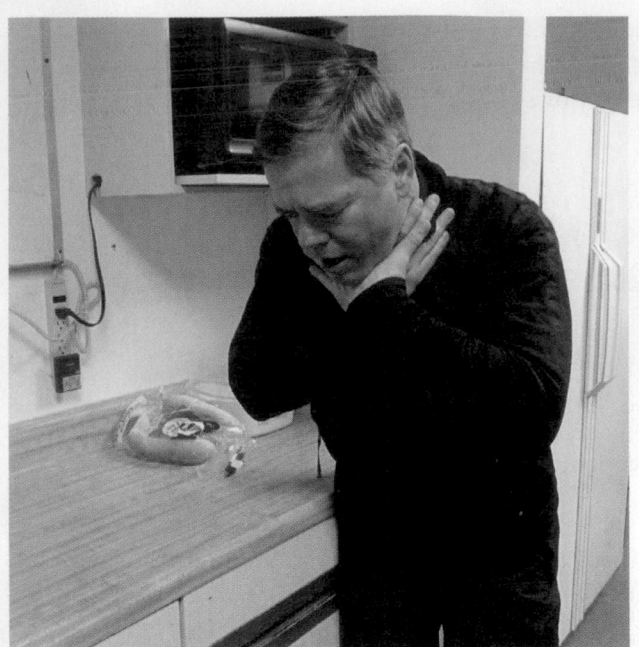

**Figure 13-14** This patient is choking; can he speak?
Copyright Edward McNamara

⊕ **13-12** Describe and demonstrate the appropriate treatment of a patient in respiratory distress.

# Management

The treatment of a respiratory emergency by OEC Technicians is fairly straightforward and centers on improving the patient's overall oxygenation. Because breathing is essential to life, treatment begins by ensuring that the airway is open and clear, which is typically accomplished using one or more of the techniques or adjuncts described in Chapter 9, Airway Management. In addition, assess and monitor the pulse and treat for shock if found.

If the patient is choking, determine whether the patient can speak (Figure 13-14■). If the person can speak, allow the patient to clear his airway on his own. If the patient is not able to speak, you must intervene quickly or the patient will soon die. To clear the airway of a patient who is choking, whether responsive or unresponsive, follow the current American Heart Association guidelines or American Red Cross guidelines for using the Heimlich maneuver.

If the patient is responsive and there is no indication of head or spine injury, allow the patient to assume a position of comfort that maximizes respiratory function. For most respiratory patients, this will be either a high-Fowler's position ("bolt-upright/90 degrees") or a "tripod" position, which helps keep the abdominal contents from pushing upward on the diaphragm and maximizes the actions of the accessory muscles of respiration. OEC Technicians should not place the patient in a supine position—unless signs of shock are present—because doing so will compromise the patient's breathing efforts and may even precipitate respiratory failure. When shock is not present and you are loading a patient into a ski toboggan for transport, place the patient's head uphill. A patient immobilized on a spine board may need the head of the board to be raised a foot or two.

Next, administer supplemental oxygen. All patients with a respiratory illness will benefit from this therapy, and it should never be withheld. As for whether to use a mask or a cannula, the simple answer is any patient with obvious respiratory distress, respiratory failure, cyanosis, diaphoresis (sweating), accessory muscle use, altered mental status, or inability to speak in complete sentences should be placed on a nonrebreather mask at 15 LPM. High-flow oxygen administration through a properly fitting facemask can dramatically improve oxygen delivery to the tissues and can be life saving. If the patient has very mild shortness of breath and can speak in complete sentences, and the rate, rhythm, and quality of respirations are normal, then a nasal cannula at 4–6 LPM may be used.

If pulse oximetry is used, adjust oxygen delivery to achieve an oxygen saturation level of 95 percent or greater. Remember that failure to provide adequate oxygen early only prolongs oxygen deprivation in the tissues. As a rule, start oxygen delivery high and gradually reduce it as necessary ("start high and titrate low"). If needed, assist the patient's ventilations using a bag-valve mask.

Occasionally you will encounter a patient who refuses to wear a mask, possibly from claustrophobia. Always encourage such patients to keep the mask on, but if they refuse, hold the mask as close to the face as possible, or use a nasal cannula at 6 LPM. This is better than no oxygen.

# The Use of Inhalers

Patients with a chronic respiratory illness such as asthma often carry a metered-dose inhaler, or "puffer," with them at all times. A metered-dose inhaler, or MDI, is a small pressurized canister containing a powerful medication that dilates the bronchioles, which opens the airways and allows the patient to breathe more easily (Figure 13-15■). A typical MDI consists of a medication canister, a plastic housing/mouthpiece, and an optional spacer.

Assuming that your local protocol allows it, you may need to *assist* patients who are having an asthma attack in the use of *their own* inhalers. Do not use someone else's inhaler, and make sure that the inhaler's expiration date has not passed. To assist patients with the self-administration of their own MDI, perform the following procedure (OEC Skill 13-2■).

1. Remove the protective cap from the mouthpiece.
2. Shake the inhaler vigorously for 3–5 seconds.
3. Instruct the patient to breathe out.
4. Holding the inhaler upright, instruct the patient to place his lips around the mouthpiece. (If the MDI includes a spacer, instruct the patient to place his lips around the open end of the spacer.)
5. Instruct the patient to breathe in slowly.
6. As the patient breathes in, depress the top of the inhaler once to administer a single dose of medication. Instruct the patient to hold his breath for at least 10 seconds after inhaling to ensure that the medication reaches the lower airways.
7. If needed, a second dose may be administered in 30–60 seconds by repeating steps 3–6.

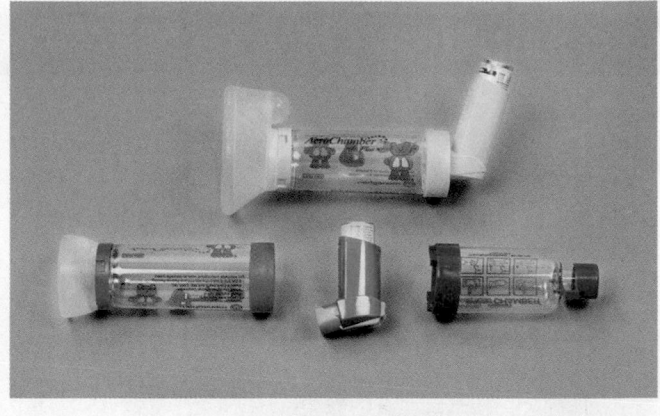

**Figure 13-15** Meter-dosed inhalers are small pressurized canisters containing a medication that improves breathing by opening the airways.

Among the most difficult conditions for OEC Technicians to assess is hyperventilation. Although it is not the responsibility of OEC Technicians to determine if a patient is hyperventilating, they do need to provide high-flow oxygen to any patient with respiratory distress.

All patients having a respiratory emergency should be encouraged to seek follow-up care in a hospital, regardless of the underlying cause. Throughout transport, continue oxygen therapy and monitor the patient's breath sounds and vital signs.

 **CASE DISPOSITION**

Your evaluation of the patient shows him to be in acute respiratory distress due to an asthma attack. You quickly obtain a SAMPLE history and perform a secondary assessment, which reveals shortness of breath and audible wheezing. You assist the patient in self-administering his albuterol inhaler as other team members prepare the patient for a trip down to the base.

Several team members accompany you during the trip down in case the patient stops breathing. You bring an airway bag that contains nasal and oral airways, a bag-valve mask, a portable suction unit, and an extra D cylinder of oxygen. During transport you continue administering supplemental high-flow oxygen with a nonrebreather mask and monitor the patient's vital signs and breath sounds. By the time you reach the base, the patient appears to be breathing much more easily. In addition, the patient's color has begun to return to normal, and he is no longer diaphoretic.

You give a quick hand-off report to ALS providers, who continue treatment and transport of the patient to a local hospital, where the patient is evaluated, placed on additional medication, and later discharged.

# OEC SKILL 13-1 | Auscultation of Breath Sounds

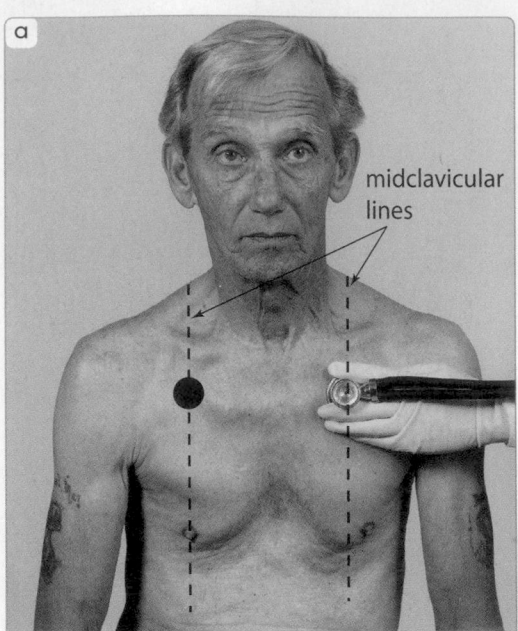

Upper lung lobes—Anterior: Place your stethoscope on the left side of the anterior chest, approximately 1.5 inches below the middle of the clavicle. Then listen to the right upper lobe and compare the results.

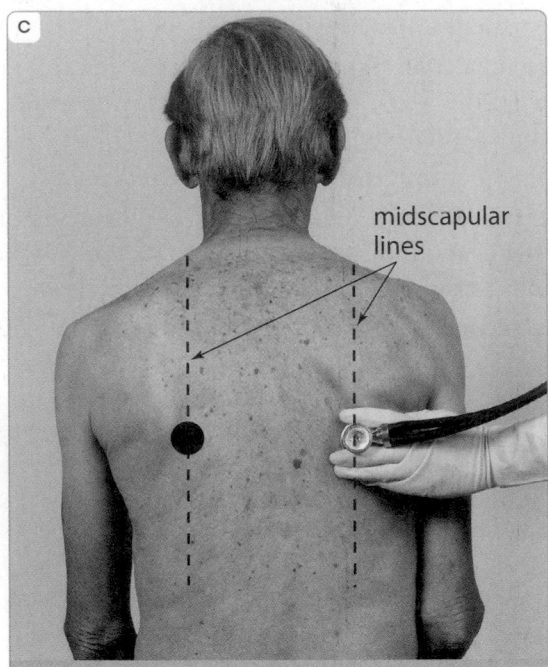

Upper lung lobes—Posterior: Place your stethoscope on the patient's right upper back, between the top of the scapula and the spine, approximately 2 inches below the neck. Then listen to the left upper lobe and compare the results.

Lower lung lobes—Posterior: Place your stethoscope on the left lower back, below the bottom of the scapula. Then listen to the right lower lobe and compare the results.

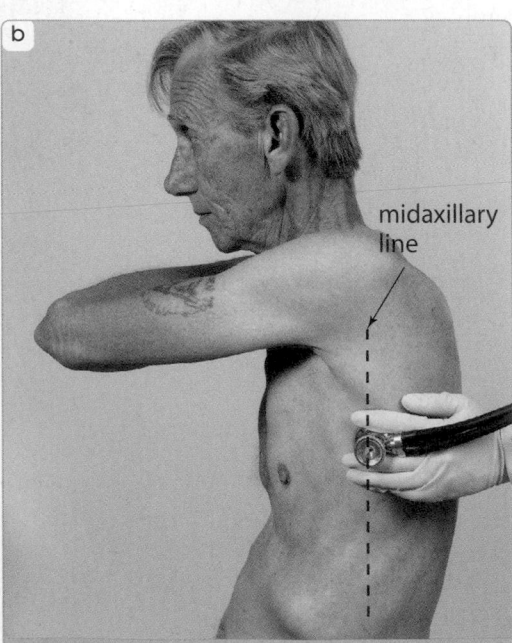

Lower lung lobes—Anterior: Place your stethoscope on the left side of the anterior chest, at or below the nipple line, over the anterior midaxillary line. Then listen to the right lower lobe and compare the results.

# OEC SKILL 13-2 | Assisting with a Metered-Dose Inhaler

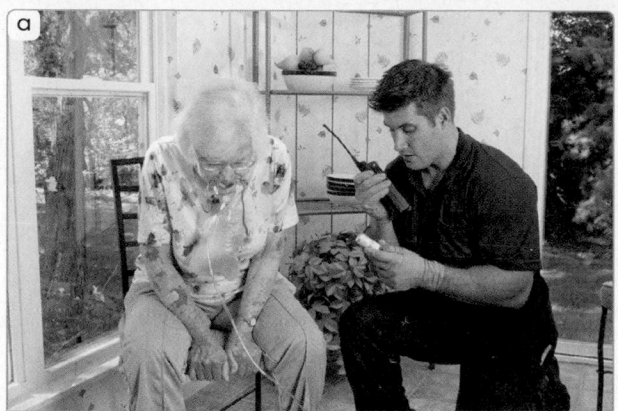

Check to see that the inhaler contains an appropriate medication, that it belongs to the patient, and that the expiration date has not passed. Remove the protective cap from the mouthpiece.

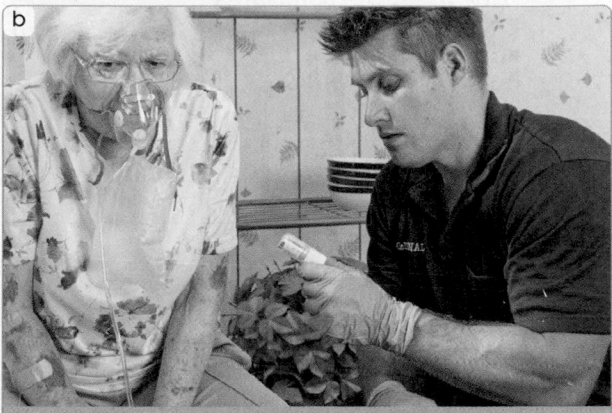

Shake the inhaler vigorously for 3–5 seconds.

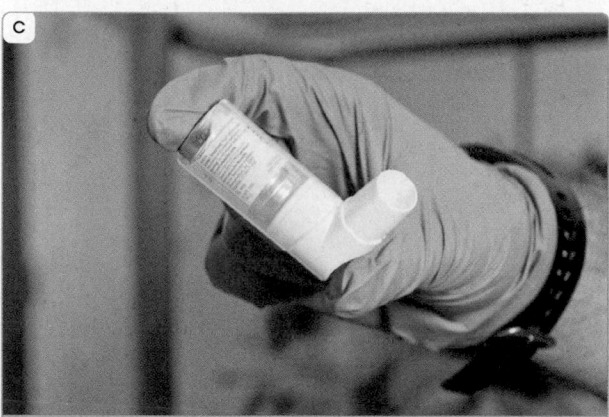

Instruct the patient to breathe out.

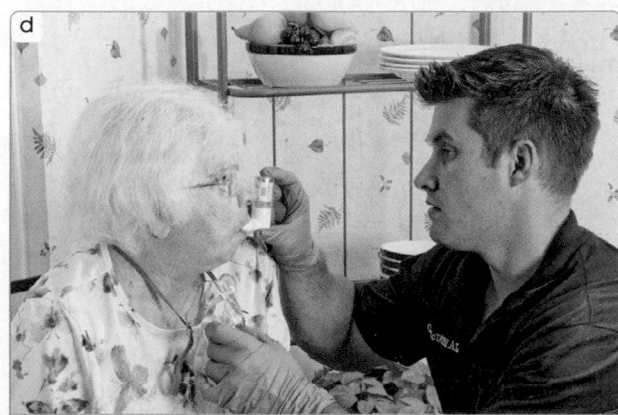

Holding the inhaler upright, instruct the patient to place their lips around the mouthpiece.

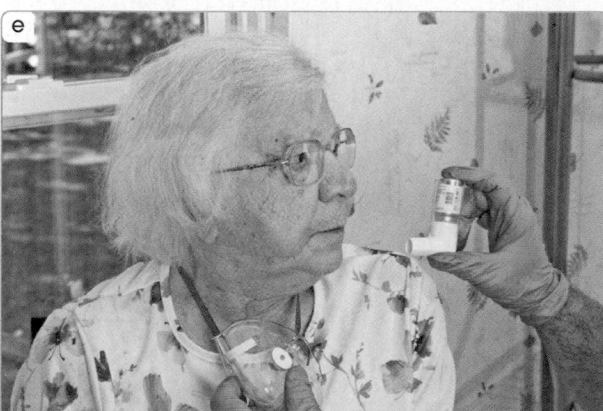

As the patient inhales, press the top of the inhaler once to administer a single dose of medication. Instruct the patient to hold their breath for at least 10 seconds after inhaling to ensure the medication reaches the lower airways.

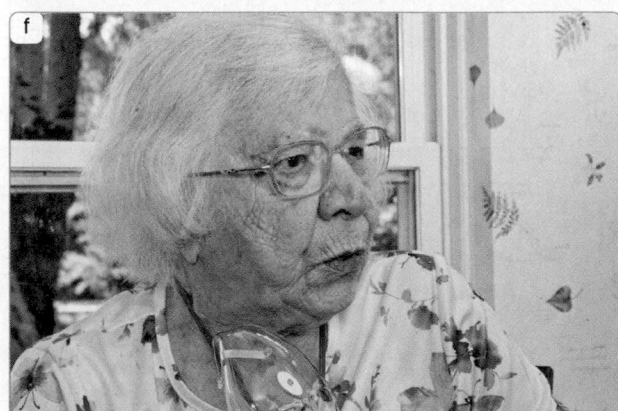

Instruct the patient to exhale slowly. If needed, a second dose may be administered in 30–60 seconds by repeating steps c–f.

## Skill Guide

Date: _____

(CPI) = Critical Performance Indicator

Candidate: _____

Start Time: _____

End Time: _____

## Auscultation of Breath Sounds

**Objective:** To demonstrate the ability to locate positions at which to listen for breath sounds.

| Skill | Max Points | Skill Demo | |
|---|---|---|---|
| Initiates Standard Precautions. | 1 | | (CPI) |
| Obtains permission from patient. | 1 | | |
| Warms stethoscope. | 1 | | |
| Upper Right Lobe Anterior: places stethoscope on right side of anterior chest 1–1.5" below the middle of the clavicle (2nd intercostal space). | 1 | | |
| Upper Left Lobe Anterior: places stethoscope on left side of anterior chest 1–1.5" below the middle of the clavicle (2nd intercostal space). | 1 | | |
| Lower Right Lobe Anterior: places stethoscope on the right side of chest 2" below the nipple line. | 1 | | |
| Lower Left Lobe Anterior: places stethoscope on the life side of the chest 2" below the nipple line. | 1 | | |
| Upper Right Lobe Posterior: places stethoscope on right upper back between top of the scapula and the spine 2" below the neck. | 1 | | |
| Upper Left Lobe Posterior: places stethoscope on left upper back between top of the scapula and the spine 2" below the neck. | 1 | | |
| Lower Right Lobe Posterior: places stethoscope on the right lower back below the bottom of the scapula. | 1 | | |
| Lower Left Lobe Posterior: places stethoscope on the left lower back below the bottom of the scapula. | 1 | | |
| Notes and verbalizes breath sounds—normal or abnormal. | 1 | | (CPI) |

| Must receive 10 out of 12 points. |
|---|

Comments: _____

Failure of any of the CPIs is an automatic failure.

Evaluator: _____    NSP ID: _____

PASS     FAIL

## Skill Guide

Date: _____

(CPI) = Critical Performance Indicator

Candidate: _____

Start Time: _____

End Time: _____

## Assisting with a Metered-Dose Inhaler

**Objective:** To demonstrate the process of assisting a patient in the use of a metered-dose inhaler.

| Skill | Max Points | Skill Demo | |
|---|---|---|---|
| Initiate Standard Precautions. | 1 | | (CPI) |
| Obtain patient's permission to assist. | 1 | | |
| Verify the correct medicine, the correct patient, the correct dose, and that the medication is not outdated. | 1 | | (CPI) |
| Vigorously shake the canister; remove the protective cap and apply spacer if available. | 1 | | |
| Assist patient by holding the device to the patient's mouth. | 1 | | |
| Encourage the patient to take a deep breath. Assist the patient by depressing the top of inhaler once to administer the spray. Instruct the patient to hold breath for approximately 10 seconds. | 1 | | |
| Repeat the treatment ONCE if no improvement according to the instructions on the inhaler, or in 30–60 seconds. | 1 | | |

Must receive 5 out of 7 points.

Comments: _____

Failure of any of the CPIs is an automatic failure.

Evaluator: _____  NSP ID: _____

PASS        FAIL

# Chapter Review

## Chapter Summary

Respiratory emergencies are among the most common emergencies that OEC Technicians will face. The causes of dyspnea are myriad and may be acute or chronic. Respiration has two phases: active for inhalation and passive for exhalation. The breathing process is complex and is made possible through the cooperation of several body systems, all of which are controlled by the central nervous system. Under normal conditions, breathing is an automatic process monitored by the brain through various sensors located in the aorta and carotids. Unfortunately, disease, illness, and injury can affect this process and reduce the delivery of oxygen to the tissues, creating hypoxia or anoxia.

Respiratory emergencies are among the most urgent conditions that you will care for as an OEC Technician. The ability to identify the signs and symptoms of acute respiratory distress quickly and provide life-saving interventions can truly save a person's life. OEC Technicians must ensure an open airway and administer oxygen when needed. Although respiratory emergencies can be very frightening for patient and rescuer alike, with early recognition and rapid intervention, OEC Technicians can dramatically reduce the morbidity and mortality associated with this common emergency.

## Remember...

1. The use of accessory muscles of respiration is a sign of acute respiratory failure.
2. Start oxygen therapy high and titrate low.
3. Check your local, state, or provincial protocols to determine whether you may assist a patient in the self-administration of a metered-dose inhaler.
4. In a patient with significant respiratory distress, use high-flow oxygen with a nonrebreather mask.
5. The most common cause of airway obstruction is the tongue.
6. Consult with your local medical advisor and mountain management and follow local, state, or provincial laws in establishing a protocol for providing oxygen to patients.

## Chapter Questions

### Multiple Choice

Choose the correct answer.

1. The first step in caring for a patient experiencing a respiratory emergency is to_____
   a. ensure that the airway is open and clear.
   b. ensure that the patient can speak in full sentences.
   c. administer oxygen before making any other determination.
   d. "load and go" without completing a full examination because any respiratory emergency is life threatening.

2. Unless contraindicated by injury, the best position in which to place a responsive patient suffering from a respiratory emergency is_____
   a. determined by the situation.
   b. in the supine position with the feet elevated to combat shock.
   c. in the patient's position of comfort that maximizes respiratory function.
   d. in the recovery position.

3. A patient that is wheezing and in a "tripod" position tells you that he is asthmatic. Which of the following actions may you take?_____
   a. Assist the patient with the use of an inhaler that is prescribed for him.
   b. The patient may administer his own inhaler, but you may not assist them beyond handing it to them as this constitutes practicing medicine without a license.
   c. You may assist the patient with an inhaler as long as it is the same type of medication (i.e., Albuterol) that the patient takes.
   d. You may not assist a patient with the administration of any medication.

4. The correct course of care for a patient who is hyperventilating is to_____
   a. comfort the patient and have him talk to you so the focus is on you and not on breathing fast.
   b. tell him he is causing the problem by being anxious and then instruct him to place a paper bag over the nose and mouth and breathe deeply.
   c. place him on a nonrebreather mask with high-flow oxygen.
   d. ignore him, because paying attention to this type of behavior only makes it worse.

5. For patients experiencing a respiratory emergency, which of the following pieces of information is the most important to obtain from the patients first?_____
   a. Their age, what and when they last ate, and whether they have a family history of similar problems.
   b. Whether or not they can speak in full sentences.
   c. What medication(s) they are on.
   d. Whether they are having any associated symptoms.

6. While auscultating the lungs of a patient complaining of shortness of breath, you notice a crackling sensation just beneath the skin where you press on it with the stethoscope. This finding could be indicative of_____
   a. asthma.
   b. pneumonia.
   c. subcutaneous emphysema.
   d. pulmonary embolism.

7. A patient who is hyperventilating tells you that he suddenly feels pins and needles in his fingers and toes and cannot unclench his hand. This finding is_____
   a. an ominous sign and warrants immediate transport to the nearest medical-care facility.
   b. a sign of impending anoxia, which should be treated with high-flow oxygen.
   c. benign and will resolve upon a decrease in the respiratory rate.
   d. benign and will resolve if the patient breathes rapidly for several minutes.

8. Which of the following statements regarding patients experiencing a respiratory emergency is false?_____
   a. All patients experiencing a respiratory emergency should be encouraged to seek follow-up care in a medical facility, regardless of the underlying cause.
   b. OEC Technicians should continue oxygen therapy and continually monitor breath sounds and vital signs throughout transport.
   c. OEC Technicians should assist patients experiencing an asthmatic attack with the use of their own inhaler per local protocols.
   d. OEC Technicians should discontinue oxygen therapy when a patient's pulse oximetry reading reaches normal levels of 92 percent or higher.

9. Which of the following statements about the administration of oxygen is true?_____
   a. Start oxygen therapy high and titrate low.
   b. Withhold oxygen from patients suffering from emphysema because oxygen therapy can cause them to stop breathing.
   c. Although oxygen therapy is comforting to the patient, it has little effect in reducing morbidity and mortality associated with respiratory emergencies.
   d. Administering oxygen is a difficult, complicated procedure that should be used only as a last resort.

## True or False

Indicate whether each of the following statements concerning the management of a respiratory emergency is true (T) or false (F).

_____ **a.** If the patient has very mild shortness of breath and can speak in complete sentences, you should not administer supplemental oxygen.

_____ **b.** If the patient has very mild shortness of breath and can speak in complete sentences, you should administer $O_2$ via a nasal cannula at 4–6 LPM.

_____ **c.** A patient with obvious respiratory distress should be placed on a nonrebreather mask at 15 LPM.

_____ **d.** A patient with altered mental status should be placed on a nonrebreather mask at 15 LPM.

_____ **e.** Administering oxygen to a patient who does not need it can cause respiratory complications and should thus be avoided.

_____ **f.** Failure to provide adequate oxygen early in care prolongs oxygen deprivation at the tissue level.

_____ **g.** The administration of oxygen is useful only if it is administered through a properly fitting mask.

# Scenario

*You are skiing and notice a snowboarder who is sitting on the slope and waving you over to her. Approaching the boarder, you meet a 14-year-old girl who tells you she can't breathe very well. She has asthma and has used her inhaler, but it's not working.*

*After removing your skis and securing the scene, you kneel down next to her. She is breathing fast and can talk to you in sentences, but she has to stop and breathe between each sentence. She appears anxious, and you note that her mucous membranes are pale.*

1. The patient requires two doses of medication from her metered-dose inhaler. What is the minimum time she should wait between administrations of her MDI?_____

   **a.** 30 seconds                    **c.** 5 minutes

   **b.** 2 minutes                     **d.** 10 minutes

*The nature of the patient's illness appears to be an asthma attack. She tells you that she is snowboarding with her friends and that her mom and dad are not at the ski area. You make a call to the base for a toboggan, some additional patrollers, an ALS ambulance, and $O_2$. You also ask base to attempt to contact the patient's parent(s).*

*As you advance from the primary assessment to a secondary assessment, you use the SAMPLE acronym to find out that in the past 5 minutes she has taken one dose from her inhaler.*

*Vital signs are as follows: Respirations are 28 and labored, with audible wheezes on exhalation; pulse rate is 120.*

2. Using a stethoscope, you auscultate for lung sounds and expect to hear_____

   **a.** normal respirations.                    **c.** whistling noises.

   **b.** coughing sounds.                        **d.** wheezing.

3. While you are assisting the patient in taking her MDI, which of the following instructions would be most appropriate just after she places her lips on the mouthpiece?_____

   **a.** "Please hold your breath and I will administer the medication."

   **b.** "Please inhale, then hold your breath, and I will give you the medication."

   **c.** "Please inhale slowly while I administer the medication. Then hold your breath for 10 seconds."

   **d.** "Please exhale, hold your breath, and I will administer the medication."

4. How many breaths per minute is a normal respiration rate for a child who is breathing adequately?_____

   **a.** 5–10                    **c.** 30–40

   **b.** 15–20                   **d.** 40–45

*Within minutes of assisting the patient with the administration of the second dose of Proventil (albuterol) through her MDI, she is breathing more easily and states that she feels much better.*

**5.** How does albuterol work within the body?_____

    **a.** It travels to the brain and stimulates the brain to send a signal to increase the respiratory rate.

    **b.** It is an anti-inflammatory medication that decreases lung swelling.

    **c.** It dilates the bronchioles, which opens the airways, allowing the patient to breathe easier.

    **d.** It opens up the throat to allow more oxygen to enter.

**6.** When auscultating breath sounds, you should_____

    **a.** have the patient take a deep breath and exhale before you listen for 15–30 seconds.

    **b.** listen to each lung lobe for 10 seconds.

    **c.** have the patient take a deep breath and then listen for 10 seconds during the patient's exhalation.

    **d.** listen for 10 seconds during the patient's inhalation.

*Your help arrives with the toboggan and $O_2$. You direct your helper to apply a nonrebreather mask with $O_2$ at 15 LPM. You bring the patient directly to the base.*

*After receiving the $O_2$ the patient presents with less respiratory distress but respirations of 28 per minutes and a productive cough.*

**7.** In what position should the patient be loaded in the toboggan?_____

    **a.** supine position, head downhill

    **b.** supine position, head uphill

    **c.** left lateral recumbent position, head uphill

    **d.** seated upright to reduce pressure against the diaphragm

EXPLORE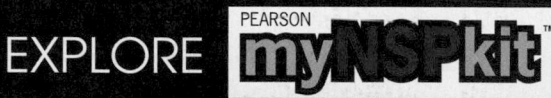

Please go to www.myNSPkit.com. Under Student Resources, you will find animations, videos, web links, and games related to this chapter—and much more. Look for information on spontaneous pneumothorax, asthma, oxygen delivery techniques, and other topics.

Register your access code from the front of your book by going to www.myNSPkit.com and selecting the appropriate links. If the in-cover access code has been redeemed, go to www.myNSPkit.com and follow links to **Buy Access.**

# Allergies and Anaphylaxis

Denis Meade, MA, EMT-P

14

## ⊕ OBJECTIVES

**Upon completion of this chapter, the OEC Technician will be able to:**

**14-1** Define the following terms:
- allergy
- allergic reaction
- anaphylaxis
- antigen
- hypersensitivity

**14-2** List four routes by which an antigen may enter the body.

**14-3** List four potential allergy sources.

**14-4** List the signs and symptoms of an anaphylactic reaction.

**14-5** Describe and demonstrate the steps for properly using portable epinephrine auto-injectors.

## ⊕ KEY TERMS

**allergen,** *p. 437*
**allergic reaction,** *p. 435*
**allergy,** *p. 434*
**anaphylaxis,** *p. 437*

**angioedema,** *p. 440*
**antibody,** *p. 436*
**antigen,** *p. 436*
**histamine,** *p. 437*

**hypersensitivity,** *p. 437*
**pruritus,** *p. 439*
**urticaria,** *p. 439*

## Chapter Overview

Stand in any of the world's countless national, provincial, state, or local parks and you will likely encounter beautiful sights. The same holds true for the innumerable ski areas and resorts that dot the planet. These settings are not as tranquil as they may appear, however, for in each are billions of microscopic particles that, for those who suffer from allergies, can turn an otherwise normal day into a sneezing, itching nightmare. Sadly, no place is safe for those who suffer from an **allergy** because these

*continued*

## HISTORICAL TIMELINE

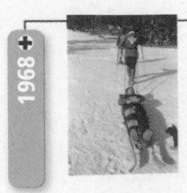

**1968** First Nordic ski patrollers course conducted.

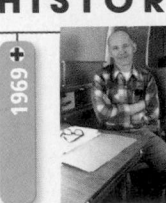

**1969** Walter Gregg appointed as national legal counsel. He served until his death in 1991.

**1969–1991** Attorney Gregg wrote NSP bylaws, negotiated statement of understanding with NSAA that clarified the role of patrollers at ski areas, and established the legal basis for the WEC program.

same particles are everywhere, including every allergy sufferer's own neighborhood and home.

Allergies are more than a simple nuisance; in their most severe form they can be deadly. Allergies are one of the most common medical conditions, affecting over 600 million people worldwide. Interestingly, people who live in developed nations are far more likely to have allergies than those who live in undeveloped nations. The reasons for this are unclear. What is clear is that the prevalence of allergies is rising at an alarming rate. Thus, OEC Technicians are increasingly likely to encounter patients who are experiencing an **allergic reaction**. In fact, you or someone you know probably has an allergy, because one American in three suffers from allergies. Allergy-related signs and symptoms can vary widely, from a simple runny nose to shortness of breath to life-threatening shock (Figures 14-1a■ and 14-1b■).

As an OEC Technician, you must be able to recognize the signs and symptoms of an allergic reaction and be ready to provide assistance at a moment's notice. This is especially true for severe allergic reactions, in which death can occur within minutes if the problem is not quickly treated. OEC Technicians are in a unique position to assist allergy patients because they are typically the first to arrive at the patient's side. Their proper and timely responses to the situation may lessen the overall effects of an allergic reaction and may even save the patient's life.

Upon completion of this chapter, you will have a basic understanding of the causes of allergies and their effects on the body. You also will be able to differentiate among the three degrees of allergic reactions based on the presenting signs and symptoms. Finally, you will learn how to assist patients in taking their emergency allergy medications in the event they are experiencing a severe allergic reaction.

## Anatomy and Physiology

The immune system is a complex collection of the body's cells, proteins, and organs that protect the body from foreign substances, including viruses, bacteria, and other microorganisms. Chief among the immune system's primary components are white

**allergy** an exaggerated immune response to a substance that does not normally cause a reaction.

**allergic reaction** a series of signs and symptoms that occur in response to exposure to an allergen.

⊕ **14-1** Define the following terms:

- allergy
- allergic reaction
- anaphylaxis
- antigen
- hypersensitivity

**Figure 14-1a** For people with allergies, any environment can trigger an allergic reaction.

**Figure 14-1b** Allergies are one of the most common medical conditions, affecting over 600 million people worldwide.

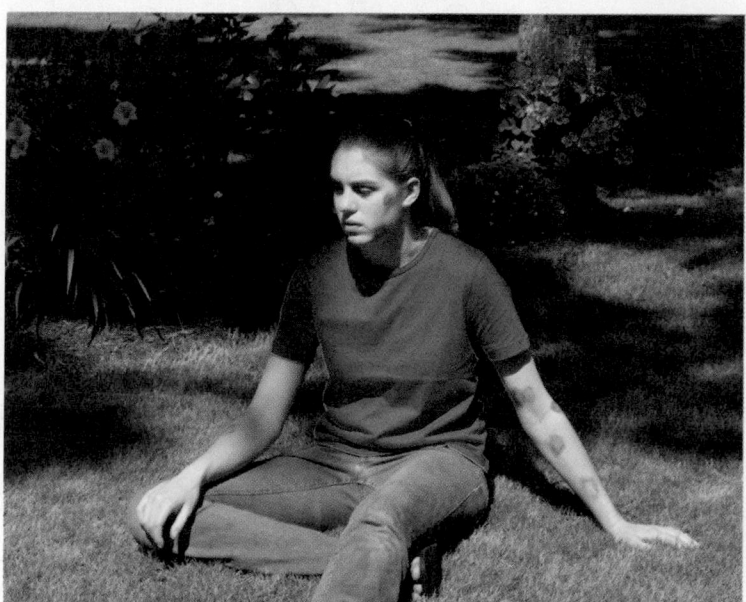

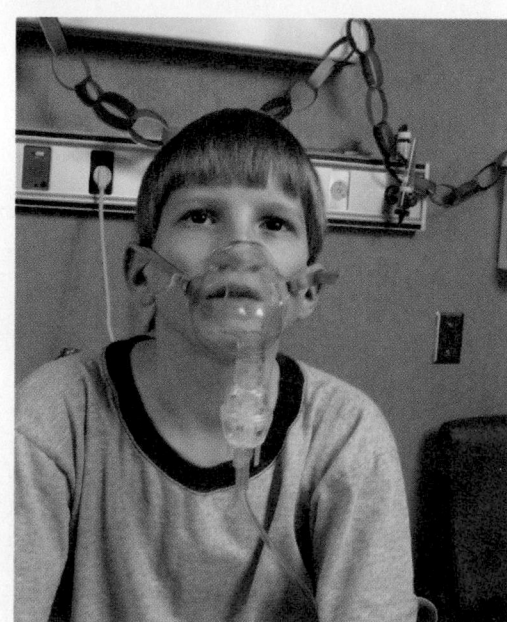

**antigen** a foreign substance that when introduced into the body stimulates the production of an antibody; can be a variety of substances, including toxins, bacteria, foreign blood cells, or the cells of transplanted organs.

**antibody** a protein that is produced by the body to neutralize or destroy specific antigens.

blood cells, hormones, lymph nodes, bone marrow, the thymus, and the spleen. The immune system is highly specialized and can distinguish between the body's normal cells and millions of foreign substances, known as **antigens**. Without the immune system, your body would be constantly invaded by pathogens that could easily harm or even kill you.

Under normal conditions, when an antigen is first introduced into the body, the immune system quickly responds by identifying the foreign substance and then developing antibodies against it. An **antibody** is a protein that helps destroy specific antigens. When mobilized, antibodies target the offending antigen, affixing themselves to it much like a key fits into a lock (Figure 14-2■). This triggers a chain of events, known as antigen-antibody reaction, which results in other components of the immune system attacking and destroying the antigen without harming normal body cells.

**Figure 14-2** The immune system forms antibodies that attach to antigens much as a key fits into a lock.

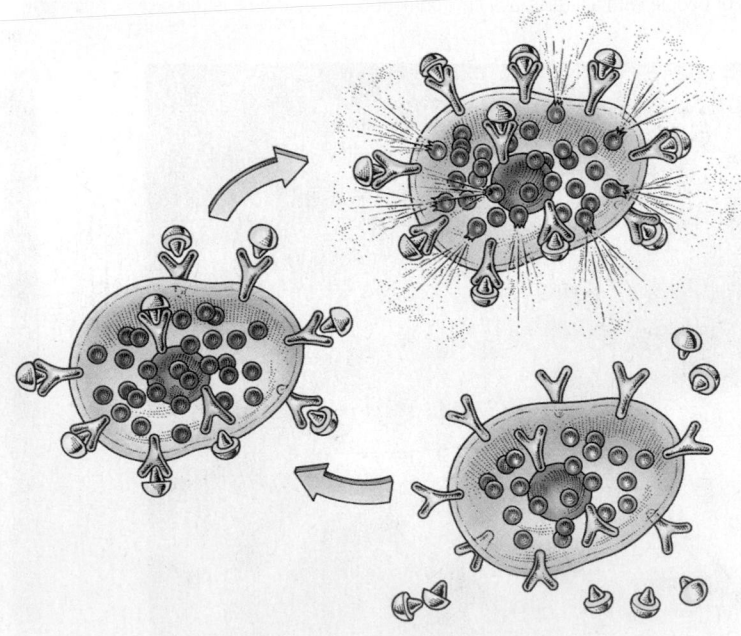

The antibodies produced in response to this initial exposure to the antigen are specific to that antigen, and those antibodies continue to be present in the body. That way, the next time that antigen enters the body, the immune system is ready. This explains why a person who contracts a disease such as measles enjoys life-long protection if reexposed to the disease again.

Occasionally, and for reasons unknown, the immune system overreacts to a substance that is otherwise harmless to humans (e.g., pollen) and develops a **hypersensitivity** to it. When this occurs, subsequent exposures cause the immune system to exaggerate its response by producing excessive amounts of antibodies. We know this hypersensitivity as an allergy, and the exaggerated response is better known as an allergic reaction. A severe allergic reaction, known as **anaphylaxis**, can result in life-threatening shock. Allergies can affect anyone and at any time, regardless of age (Figure 14-3 ■).

Any antigen that triggers an allergic response is known as an **allergen**. Allergens can enter the body via several routes. They can be inhaled, ingested, injected, or come in contact with the skin (topical). Once a person develops an allergy to a specific allergen, repeated exposure will always produce an allergic reaction. How the body responds to an allergen and how long the effects last depend on the body's sensitivity to the substance. A mild reaction typically causes skin-related effects, such as a rash or itching, whereas a severe antigen-antibody reaction stimulates a massive inflammatory response due to the release of **histamine** into the bloodstream, an event that can result in cardiovascular collapse and death.

Histamine is a protein produced by specialized cells in the immune system called mast cells. Histamine causes local and peripheral edema (swelling), bronchoconstriction (contraction of smooth muscles in the bronchi), vasodilation, hives, itching, and pain. It is the primary culprit in the production of an allergic reaction. Most allergic reactions occur within minutes to hours following the *second* exposure to the allergen. However, some allergic reactions occur much later, after repeated exposure to an allergen and once the body develops a hypersensitivity to the substance.

**hypersensitivity** an exaggerated immune response to an allergen, drug, or other foreign substance.

**anaphylaxis** a severe allergic reaction that can result in serious cardiac or respiratory compromise.

**allergen** a foreign substance (antigen) whose presence in the body stimulates an allergic reaction.

**histamine** a chemical that is released in the body as a result of an allergic reaction.

**14-2** List four routes by which an antigen may enter the body.

**Figure 14-3** Almost any substance can trigger an allergic reaction and allergies can affect anyone, regardless of age.

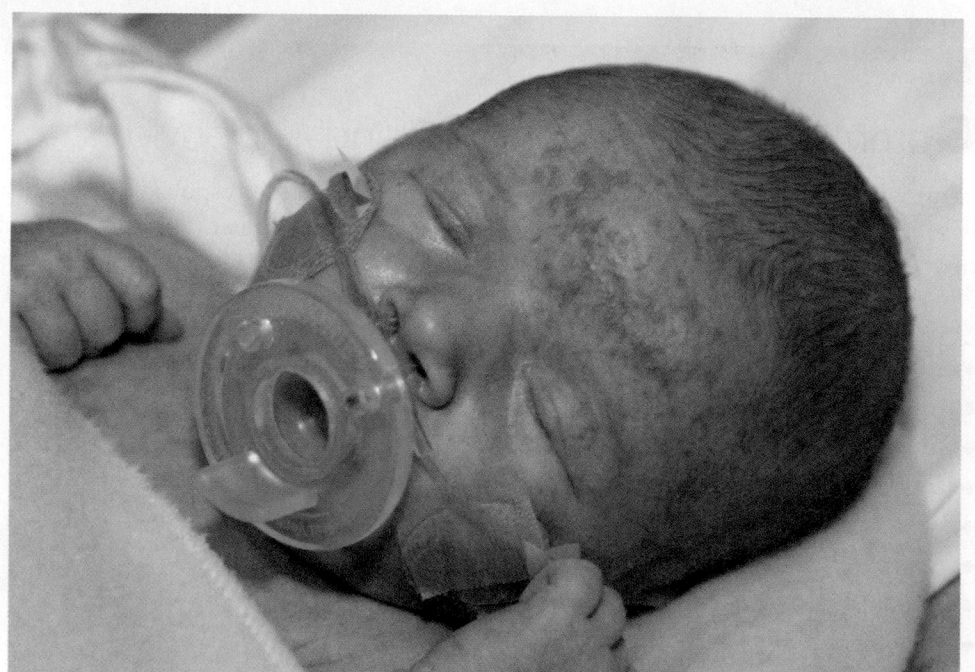

# STOP, THINK, UNDERSTAND

## Multiple Choice

Choose the correct answer.

1. Which of the following best describes an antigen?_____
   a. a normal body cell
   b. a substance foreign to the body
   c. a substance given to counteract a poison
   d. a substance produced by the spleen

2. An antibody is best described as_____
   a. a substance given to counteract a poison.
   b. a normal body cell.
   c. a protein that helps to destroy an antigen.
   d. a type of white blood cell that destroys bacteria.

3. Which of the following statements about the destruction of antigens is true?_____
   a. Components of the immune system are able to attack and destroy the antigen without harming other body cells.
   b. When an antigen is attacked by antibodies, healthy body cells are destroyed.
   c. Immunity to an antigen is a short-term phenomenon because once antigen-specific antibodies are produced, they quickly disappear from the body.
   d. None of the above statements are true.

4. An allergic reaction is best described as_____
   a. an under-reaction of the immune system that leaves the body vulnerable to irritating substances.
   b. an underproduction of antigens.
   c. red blood cells dying from antigens.
   d. an exaggerated response to a generally harmless substance.

5. Which of the following statements about allergies is true?_____
   a. They affect young, healthy individuals only.
   b. An allergic reaction to a substance can occur in minutes, hours, or even longer after exposure to the substance.
   c. Once hypersensitized to a substance, allergic reactions occur randomly, not consistently, to that substance.
   d. Anaphylaxis is the mildest type of allergic reaction.

6. A massive inflammatory response to a substance is caused by a protein known as_____
   a. a mast cell.
   b. a white blood cell.
   c. a leukocyte.
   d. histamine.

## Fill in the Blank

Which of the following are components of the body's immune system? (check all that apply)

_____ **a.** white blood cells
_____ **b.** hormones
_____ **c.** lymph nodes
_____ **d.** thymus
_____ **e.** spleen

---

⊕ 14-3 List four potential allergy sources.

# Common Causes of Allergies and Anaphylaxis

As previously described, an allergy is an exaggerated immune response to an otherwise harmless substance. Allergies can occur throughout the year (chronic allergies) or they can be seasonal, affecting an individual only during certain times of the year.

Allergies have a variety of causes, including the following substances (Figure 14-4■):

+ foods (e.g., peanuts, shellfish, nuts, soy, milk, eggs, chocolate)
+ insect bites and stings
+ environmental irritants (e.g., smoke, airborne particles)
+ pollen and plants parts (e.g., weeds, grasses, trees)
+ molds (e.g., mildew, spores)
+ animal dander (e.g., skin flakes, fur)
+ medications (e.g., antibiotics, pain medications)
+ chemicals (e.g., latex)
+ other causes (e.g., blood transfusions, organ transplants, radiographic dyes)

Peanuts are the number one cause of allergic reactions to food in the world (Figure 14-5■). The exact reason for this is unknown. In the United States, approximately 3 million people are allergic to peanuts. Studies indicate that children are more prone to peanut allergies than are adults. Dust mites, which are commonly found in household dust, are another leading allergen. Chemicals such as natural rubber and latex are also known to induce allergic reactions in people not previously diagnosed with any other allergic disorder. This explains why medical personnel, including OEC Technicians, are strongly encouraged to use latex-free medical supplies and equipment. Even severe stress can evoke an allergic reaction in susceptible individuals. Allergies may also have a genetic component. Allergic reactions are categorized according to their effects as mild, moderate, or severe. Unfortunately, most people do not realize they are allergic to a substance until they have a reaction.

## Mild Allergic Reactions

Mild allergic reactions typically result in local dermatologic changes. These skin reactions include a rash or hives, known as **urticaria**, which usually appears on the face and/or neck; flushed and/or itchy skin, known as **pruritus**; tingling in or around the mouth; swelling of the nasal mucosa, a runny nose, and nasal congestion; sneezing; watery reddened eyes; and a general feeling of being tired or "run down." Depending on the person's sensitivity to the allergen, signs and symptoms may take minutes, hours, or even days to develop. The effects usually disappear over time or with treatment.

**urticaria** hives or rashes that accompany an allergic reaction.

**pruritus** severe itching; frequently occurs in the skin during mild and moderate allergic reactions.

**Figure 14-4** Some of the many things that can cause an allergic reaction.

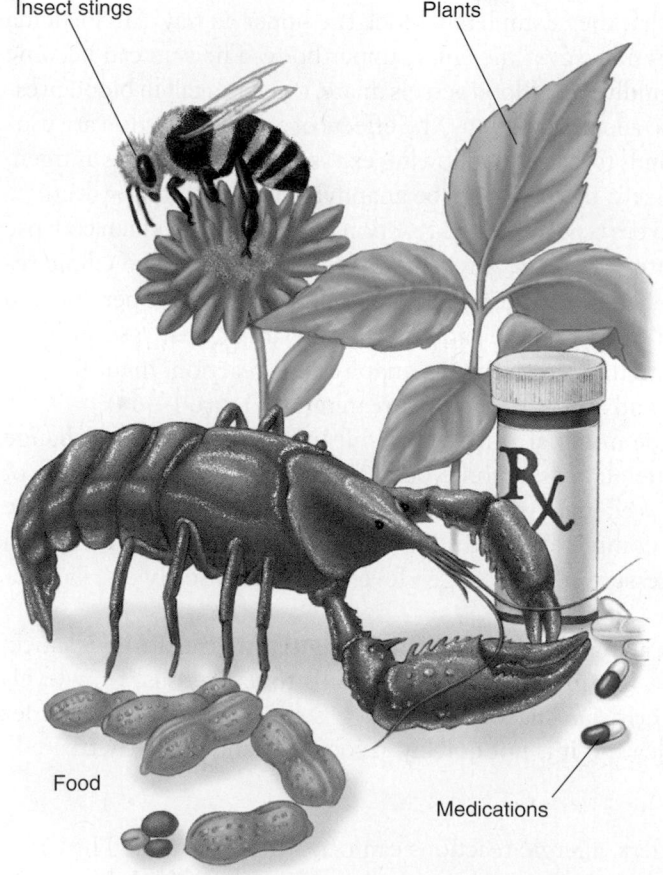

Insect stings

Plants

Food

Medications

**Figure 14-5** Peanuts are the most common allergy-causing food.

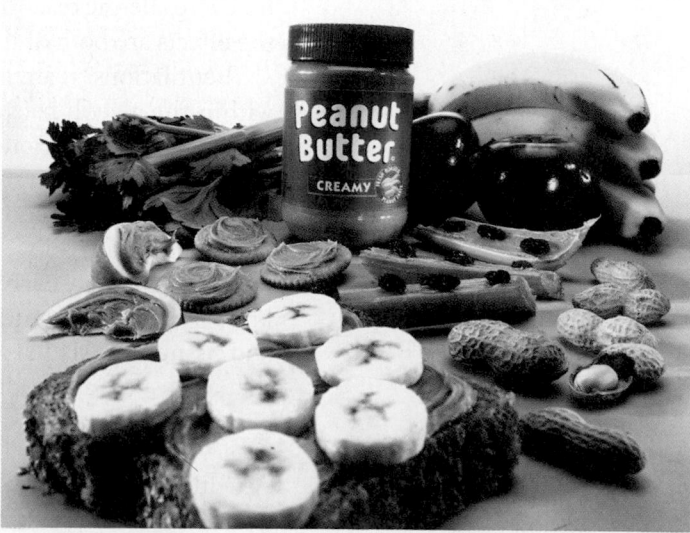

## Moderate Allergic Reactions

The effects of moderate allergic reactions include all those that occur in mild reactions, but they are more pronounced. Hives can appear on the chest and arms, and itching becomes increasingly difficult to endure. Additionally, the skin can become flushed or pale. **Angioedema**, the swelling of the tissues beneath the skin, is common around the eyes, mouth, and hands.

**angioedema**   swelling that occurs beneath the skin or mucosa as a result of an allergic reaction.

Moderate allergic reactions also affect the respiratory system. Breathing may become slightly compromised as the bronchioles constrict and secretions within them thicken. Wheezing is often present and may be pronounced. Swelling can become more pronounced in and around the face and lips. The tongue may also begin to swell, which can further hinder breathing. As breathing becomes compromised, the amount of oxygen reaching the brain may be reduced.

Gastrointestinal distress is common in moderate allergic reactions. This includes release of hydrochloric acid by the stomach's lining, creating heartburn, and contraction of intestinal wall smooth muscle, causing diarrhea. Also seen are intestinal cramping, nausea, and vomiting.

As with mild reactions, all these effects may appear within a few minutes after exposure to an allergen, or they may take several hours to become apparent. Depending on the person's individual physiologic makeup, including the effectiveness of the immunologic response, these effects may dissipate on their own or increase in severity.

## Severe Allergic Reactions

Severe allergic reactions cause major changes within the respiratory, integumentary, circulatory, and gastrointestinal systems due to the release of massive amounts of histamine. Within the respiratory system, the smooth muscles of the bronchioles tightly constrict, making wheezing severe and frequently audible. Additionally, the tongue and lips may become so swollen that they completely block the upper airway. Angioedema is very pronounced, and hives may cover the entire upper body. The skin can become increasingly flushed or profoundly pale. Blood vessels dilate, causing a fall in blood pressure. Unlike mild or moderate allergic reactions, the effects of a severe reaction are usually obvious within a few seconds to minutes following exposure to the eliciting antigen. If patients are not treated quickly, the result can be anaphylactic shock and/or death.

Anaphylaxis is the most severe type of allergic reaction and results in sudden collapse of the respiratory and circulatory systems. A recent study done at the Mayo Clinic reported that each year anaphylaxis is the cause of 50 emergency room visits per 100,000 individuals in the population. Many of these patients are unaware of their susceptibility to severe allergic reactions until they experience an anaphylactic reaction. In most cases, the effects are both dramatic and immediately life threatening (Figure 14-6■).

Ventilations, if any, may be minimal and often result in virtually no gas exchange within the alveoli because the airways become occluded due to the combination of tight bronchoconstriction and edema. Angioedema may progress to the point that the eyes and upper airway swell completely shut. Blood vessels dilate fully, resulting in a precipitous drop in blood pressure. Blood oxygen levels fall dramatically due to poor perfusion.

Unless quickly corrected, anaphylaxis can lead to a potentially lethal form of shock, known as anaphylactic shock, in which blood pressure falls to dangerously low levels and tissue hypoxia becomes critical. Anaphylactic shock is a serious medical disorder that almost always leads to death if it is not quickly recognized and properly treated.

## Prevention

As with many medical disorders, allergic reactions can often be prevented. This is especially true of a severe allergic reaction such as anaphylaxis. The method that physi-

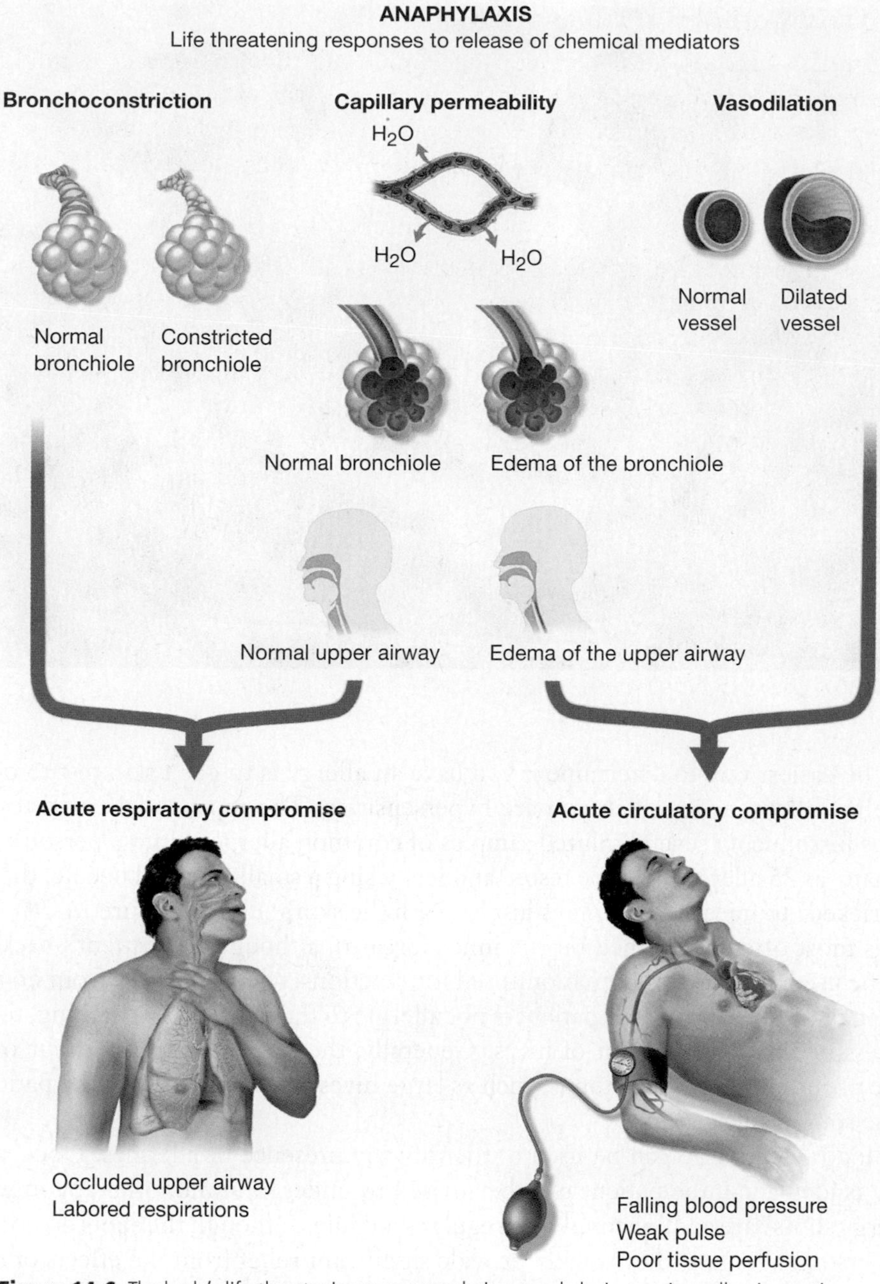

**ANAPHYLAXIS**
Life threatening responses to release of chemical mediators

**Bronchoconstriction**        **Capillary permeability**        **Vasodilation**

$H_2O$

$H_2O$        $H_2O$

Normal      Constricted
bronchiole  bronchiole

Normal     Dilated
vessel     vessel

Normal bronchiole      Edema of the bronchiole

Normal upper airway      Edema of the upper airway

**Acute respiratory compromise**        **Acute circulatory compromise**

Occluded upper airway
Labored respirations

Falling blood pressure
Weak pulse
Poor tissue perfusion

**Figure 14-6** The body's life-threatening responses during anaphylaxis, a serious allergic reaction that simultaneously affects the respiratory and circulatory systems.

cian allergists most commonly recommend for preventing an allergic reaction is called the "Triple A" approach, which centers on *Awareness*, *Avoidance*, and *Action*:

- *Awareness* involves both knowing that you have allergies and knowing the things that can trigger an allergic reaction. Awareness also includes having an emergency plan should an allergic reaction occur.

- *Avoidance* focuses on avoiding contact with known allergens.

- *Action* centers on what you should do if you have an allergic reaction. The actions involved generally include a combination of early activation of the emergency care system and self-treatment with one or more medications to combat any life-threatening effects.

**Figure 14-7** A skin test is a simple way to determine if an individual has an allergy.

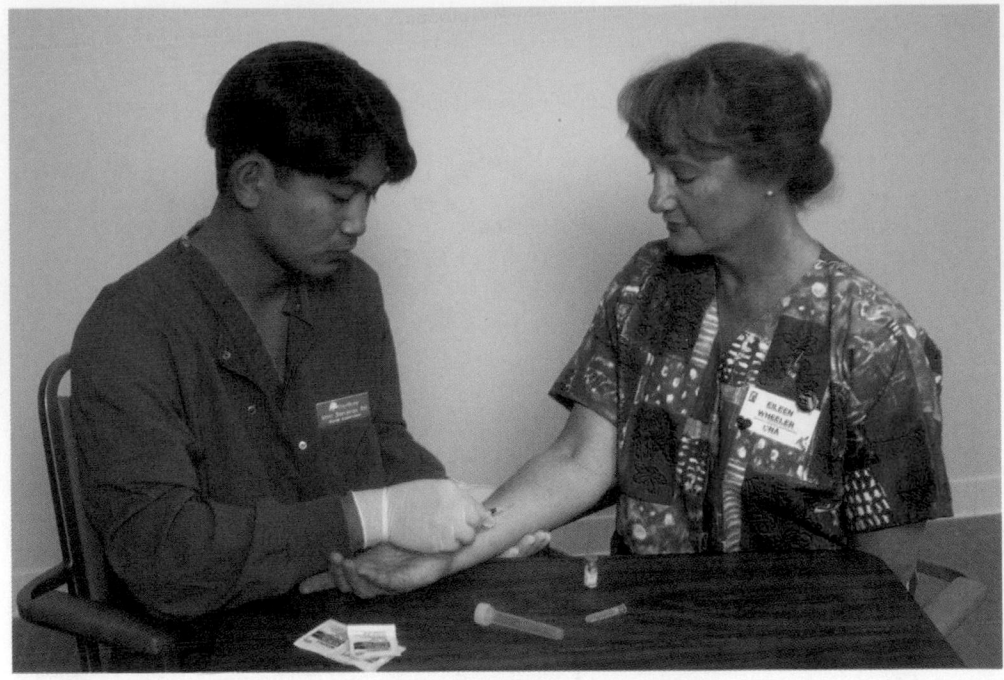

The easiest way to determine if you have an allergy is to get a skin test to determine the allergens to which you are hypersensitive. The most widely used test involves introducing several diluted samples of common allergens into a person's skin. As many as 25 allergens can be tested at once. Using a small pronged needle, the skin is "pricked" to inject the allergens just beneath the skin's surface (Figure 14-7■). This test is most often performed on the inner forearm, although the patient's back also may be used. The area is then monitored for reactions, which can vary from no reaction at all (in which case, the patient is not allergic to that allergen), to itching, to skin redness, to the development of hives. Generally, the faster the affects occur or the more pronounced the reaction is, such as large hives, the more allergic the patient is to the source allergen.

Blood testing also can be used to identify the presence of allergies. Once an allergy is identified, the patient may be advised to undergo immunotherapy in which "allergy shots" are administered on a regular schedule. Although the shots do not cure the person's allergies, they usually provide significant relief from the effects of allergic reactions.

 **CASE UPDATE**

After moving the patient to a safe area where there are no bees, you begin to assess her condition. She looks pale and appears to be in mild respiratory distress. Once you determine that the ABCDs are intact, you notify dispatch to send additional personnel with oxygen and an airway kit. You also request that an ALS provider respond. Secondary assessment reveals hives over the patient's neck and upper chest, and she has a slight wheeze. Respirations are 38 per minute and labored. The patient's face appears swollen.

***What should you do now?***

# Assessment

Assessment of a patient with a suspected allergic reaction is no different from the assessment of any other medical condition. Scene safety considerations still take precedence over care of the patient. As always, the scene must be carefully examined for any hazards to ensure that it is safe for rescuers to enter. This is particularly important if rescuers will be exposed to the suspected allergen, especially if those rescuers also have the same allergy as the patient. For instance, if a beehive has been disturbed and a swarm is present, it may be necessary to move the patient to another location before the assessment process can be initiated. To ignore an angry swarm is to invite unnecessary risk to rescuers and could quickly change the incident into a multi-patient situation. Any rescuer who has the same allergy as the patient should not risk exposure.

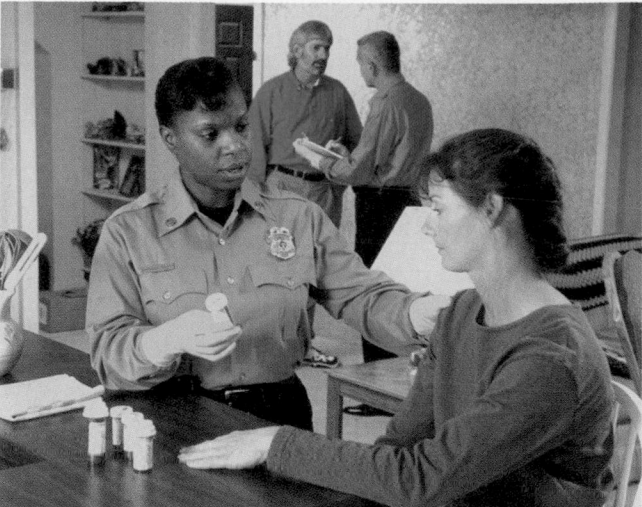

**Figure 14-8** When assessing patients suspected of having an allergic reaction, be sure to ask if they have taken any medications for their allergies.

The primary assessment is performed in the usual manner. See also Chapter 7, Patient Assessment. Treat any immediate threats to life. If an allergic reaction is suspected, continue to monitor the patient's ABCDs carefully because airway patency can change quickly and without warning! Depending on the severity of the patient's distress and available resources, OEC Technicians may need to focus attention solely on the ABCDs and forgo a secondary assessment until additional rescuers arrive. However, if no immediate threats to life are apparent, proceed with the secondary assessment. If you identify threats to life that cannot be controlled at the scene, immediate transport and call for ALS is paramount.

Obtain a SAMPLE history, paying close attention to any known allergies, the patient's use of allergy medications, and details of previous allergic reactions (Figure 14-8■). For patients with known allergies, specifically ask if they have ever had a severe allergic reaction or an anaphylactic reaction. Be sure to ask patients whether or not they have taken any medications to self-treat this current allergic reaction. Such self-treatment can range from taking an oral medication to self-injecting a powerful drug (see Table 14-1■).

Also ask if the patient has an epinephrine auto-injector with him, also known as a "crash kit." An auto-injector is a device that delivers a prescribed amount of medication to treat the effects of a severe allergic reaction. Patients who are highly allergic often are prescribed an epinephrine auto-injector in the event they experience a severe allergic reaction and are unable to reach a medical facility within a few minutes. In this situation, an auto-injector can be truly lifesaving.

**Table 14-1** Common Allergy Medications

| Brand Name | Generic Name |
|---|---|
| Allegra | fexofenadine |
| Astelin | azelastine hydrochloride |
| Benadryl | diphenhydramine |
| Clarinex | desloratadine |
| Claritin | loratadine |
| Chlor-Trimeton | chlorpheniramine |
| Dimetane | brompheniramine |
| Zyrtec | cetirizine |
| Tavist | clemastine |

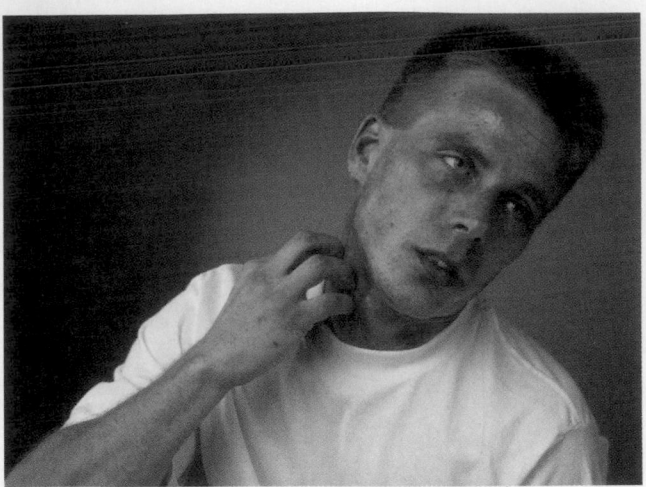

**Figure 14-9** Itching is one of the symptoms of an allergic reaction.

Physical findings will vary depending on the severity of the allergic reaction. As previously indicated, mild allergic reactions primarily affect the integumentary system (Figure 14-9■). By contrast, a moderate-to-severe allergic reaction affects multiple body systems, most notably the respiratory and circulatory systems.

Remember that the signs and symptoms of an allergic reaction are often evolving; they may not be immediately apparent and can change over time. As a rule, signs and symptoms associated with respiratory impairment (e.g., increasing dyspnea, difficulty swallowing, tongue swelling) are especially ominous and indicate a potentially serious reaction.

## Mild Allergic Reaction

The signs and symptoms of a mild allergic reaction include the following:

+ Itching/scratching
+ Flushed skin
+ Rash or hives over the face and neck
+ Watery, reddened eyes
+ Nasal congestion
+ Increased heart rate (over normal resting rate)
+ Tingling in/around the mouth
+ Fatigue

## Moderate Allergic Reaction

The signs and symptoms of moderate allergic reaction are the following and are more pronounced than in a mild reaction:

+ Anxiety, confusion
+ Tightness in the throat
+ Difficulty swallowing
+ Difficulty breathing
+ Wheezing
+ Rash or hives on the face, neck, chest, or arms
+ Persistent itching/scratching
+ Angioedema of the face or hands (patients often complain that rings feel tighter)
+ Abdominal pain or cramping
+ Nausea and/or vomiting
+ Elevated vital signs

## Severe Allergic Reaction

The signs and symptoms of a severe allergic reaction include the following:

+ Severe anxiety, feelings of impending doom
+ Decreased level of responsiveness (including coma)
+ Severe respiratory distress (e.g., "tripod" position, use of accessory muscles of respiration)

- Abnormal lung sounds (can vary from audible wheezing to a "silent chest" in which no breath sounds are heard)
- Severe angioedema of the tongue, face, and hands (eyes can swell shut, rings may not be able to be removed)
- Hives (may be located over the face, neck, chest, abdomen, and arms)
- Inability to swallow
- Tachycardia (significantly increased heart rate)
- Weak or absent peripheral pulses
- Hypotension (low blood pressure)
- Pallor
- Cyanosis around the lips and face

## Anaphylactic Shock

Anaphylactic shock is identified by the simultaneous presence of the signs of a severe allergic reaction and shock (hypovolemic shock), which include the following:

⊕ **14-4** List the signs and symptoms of an anaphylactic reaction.

- Systolic blood pressure below 90 mmHg
- Respirations greater than 20 rpm
- Heart rate greater than 110 bpm (in some cases, the patient may have a pulse rate less than 60 bpm)
- Level of responsiveness decreased, GCS less than 14

In addition, the patient's oxygen saturation levels as measured using a pulse oximeter are frequently less than 90 percent and may be less than 80 percent. Anaphylactic shock is a true emergency and must be treated quickly to prevent death.

# STOP, THINK, UNDERSTAND

## Multiple Choice

Choose the correct answer.

1. The number one cause of allergic food reactions worldwide is _____
   - a. peanuts.
   - b. grapes.
   - c. cheese.
   - d. wheat.

2. Which of the following statements about an allergic reaction is most correct?_____
   - a. Medical personnel can inadvertently cause a severe allergic reaction by touching a patient with a natural rubber (latex) glove.
   - b. Severe stress can evoke an allergic reaction.
   - c. Heredity may play a role in causing allergic reactions.
   - d. All of the above are true.

3. Anaphylaxis is best described as _____
   - a. a severe systemic skin rash due to an allergic response.
   - b. a severe allergic reaction that can result in cardiac or respiratory compromise.
   - c. a mild-to-moderate allergic reaction.
   - d. wheezing caused by an allergic response to some food such as a peanut.

4. Which of the following choices best describes the signs/symptoms of anaphylaxis?_____
   - a. decreased ventilations with airway occlusion
   - b. swollen eyes and airways
   - c. decreases in blood pressure and blood oxygen levels
   - d. all of the above

5. The Triple A approach refers to _____
   - a. allergy, antigen, and anaphylaxis.
   - b. antibody, airway, and alveoli.
   - c. awareness, avoidance, and action.
   - d. airway, assisted ventilations, and advanced life support.

6. Which of the following statements regarding allergies is true?_____
   - a. Scene safety is not as critical for patients having allergic reactions because it is highly unlikely that rescuers will be allergic to the same substance.
   - b. Airway patency can change quickly and without warning.
   - c. Regardless of the severity of an allergic reaction, the secondary assessment must be completed to help determine the cause of the reaction.
   - d. Allergic reactions are primarily psychological in nature.

*continued*

## STOP, THINK, UNDERSTAND *continued*

7. The signs and symptoms of allergic reactions are _____
   a. often evolving.
   b. largely psychogenic.
   c. almost always immediately apparent.
   d. not worrisome unless the patient tells you that he experienced a previous anaphylactic reaction.

## Fill in the Blank

The signs and symptoms of anaphylaxis are similar to those of hypovolemic shock. Fill in the typical values for vital signs that you might encounter for an anaphylactic patient.

a. BP: _____
b. Respiration: _____
c. Heart rate: _____
d. Level of responsiveness: _____
e. Pulse oximetry reading: _____

## Matching

Write the number for the degree of allergic reaction in the blank for each of the following signs and symptoms. There may be more than one answer for each.

1. mild
2. moderate
3. severe

_____ a. red, watery eyes
_____ b. nasal congestion
_____ c. feeling of impending doom
_____ d. pallor, cyanosis
_____ e. wheezing
_____ f. increased heart rate
_____ g. hives on neck, face, chest, and arms
_____ h. decreased level of responsiveness
_____ i. respiratory distress
_____ j. elevated vital signs
_____ k. nausea/vomiting

# Management

The initial management of an allergic reaction is similar to that for any kind of patient: take care of the ABCDs. Try to identify the allergen, as this knowledge might change care you provide. If during the primary assessment you find that the airway is open, breathing and circulation are normal, and no neurologic problems are apparent, then the patient needs to be treated symptomatically. If possible, remove the patient from the source of the allergen. Monitor the patient frequently, as the person may have only a mild rash at first and then over time go into a full blown anaphylactic reaction. Take vital signs frequently, and watch for changes that indicate a worsening condition. Any injuries or other medical problems should be treated in the usual manner (as described in future chapters). If the patient *appears* to be developing anaphylaxis, you should immediately treat the ABCDs and seek transport and ALS.

## Severe Allergic Reactions

Severe allergic reactions and anaphylaxis constitute a true emergency that must be treated immediately to prevent life-threatening shock. Begin treatment by correcting any ABCD-related problems. Open the airway. Oxygen should be given using a nonrebreather

### NOTE: Insect Stingers

If the source of an allergic reaction is a bee, hornet, or wasp sting, locate and remove the stinger as quickly as possible to prevent further injection of the venom. Use the flat edge of a credit card, fingernail, plastic knife, or similar object to scrape along the surface of the skin to dislodge the stinger (Figure 14-10■). If you decide to pull the stinger out using your thumb and index finger, pinch the area around the site to raise the stinger above the level of the skin before grasping the stinger as close to the skin as possible. Do not attempt to remove the stinger using tweezers because this can squeeze any venom remaining in the stinger's sac into the wound. Once the stinger is removed, apply ice, if available, to the site to minimize the pain.

mask at 15 LPM. If necessary, assist the patient's ventilations by giving high-flow oxygen using one or more of the techniques described in Chapter 9, Airway Management. Place the patient into a position of comfort. In most instances, this will be a seated and slightly forward position. This eases breathing efforts somewhat and allows maximum chest wall expansion. However, if the patient exhibits signs of shock or a decreased level of responsiveness, place the patient in a supine position with the feet elevated 8–12 inches (Figure 14-11■).

Once all ABCD issues have been addressed, arrange transport and notify advanced life support immediately. Severe anaphylaxis may require CPR. Remove any tight-fitting necklaces, scarves, or bandanas from around the neck. Additionally, remove tight-fitting watches, rings, and bracelets, all of which can restrict or occlude blood flow through swollen distal structures.

If an allergic reaction is suspected, determine whether the patient has a portable auto-injector. If he does, you may *assist* the patient in self-administering the medication. Do not use anyone else's epinephrine auto-injector.

## Epinephrine

Epinephrine is the drug of choice for managing severe allergic reactions. It promotes bronchodilation and vasoconstriction, thereby relieving dyspnea and hypotension. When used for this purpose, epinephrine comes prepackaged as a single-dose or dual-dose portable auto-injector sold under brand names such as Epi E-Z pen™, EpiPen™, and Twinject™ (Figures 14-12a■ and 14-12b■). A portable auto-injector administers the proper dose of epinephrine via an automatic needle-injection system. Most auto-injectors look like a fountain pen with a cap on it.

**Epinephrine** is available in adult and pediatric doses. The dose of epinephrine for an allergic reaction in an adult that weighs 30 kg (66 lb) or more is 0.30 milligrams (mg); the dose for children weighing 15–30 kg (33–66 lb) is 0.15 mg. To assist a patient in the use of a single-dose portable EpiPen™ epinephrine auto-injector, perform the following procedure (OEC Skill 14-1■):

1. Ensure that the medication is prescribed for the patient by checking the name on the medication.

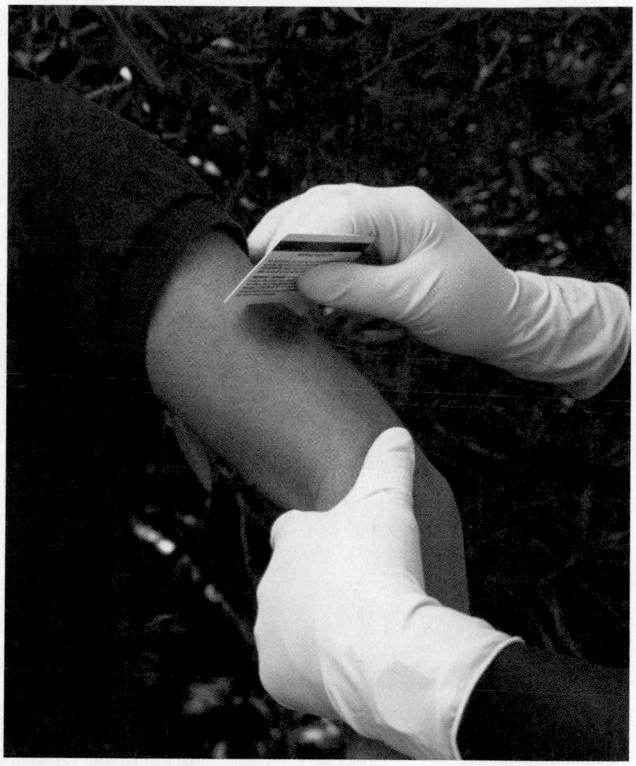

**Figure 14-10** One technique for removing a stinger, which prevents further injection of venom.

**✚ 14-5** Describe and demonstrate the steps for properly using portable epinephrine auto-injectors.

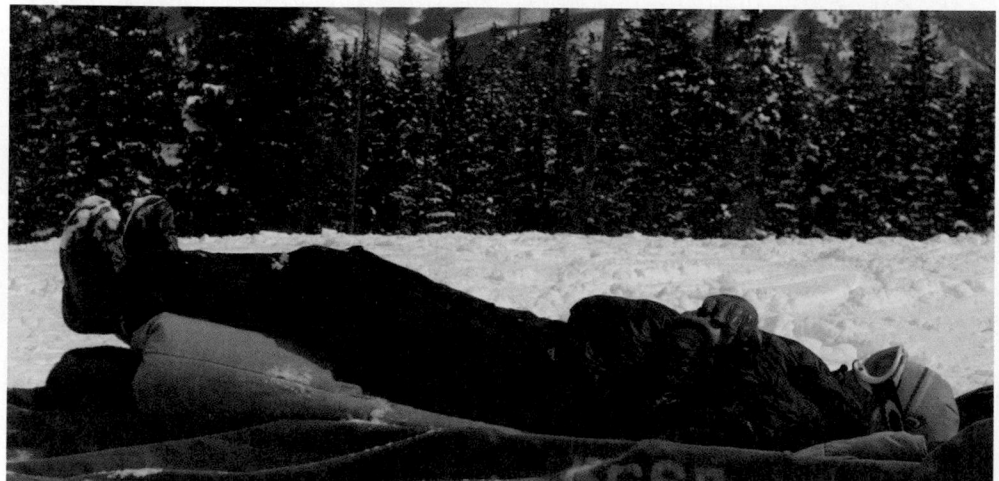

**Figure 14-11** Place any patient that shows signs of shock in a supine position with the feet elevated.
Copyright Scott Smith

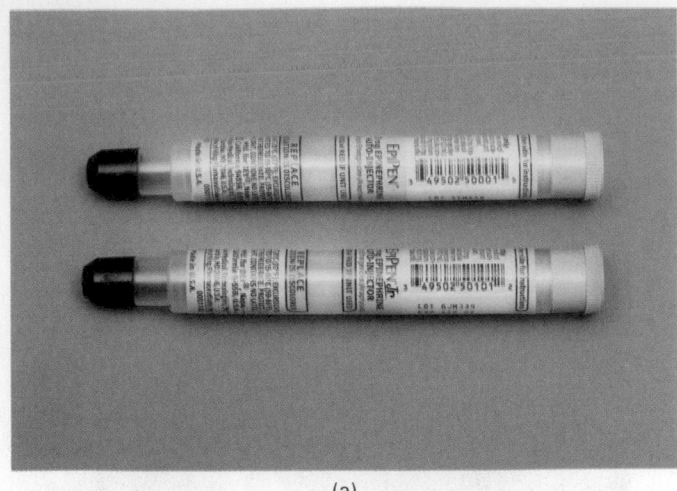 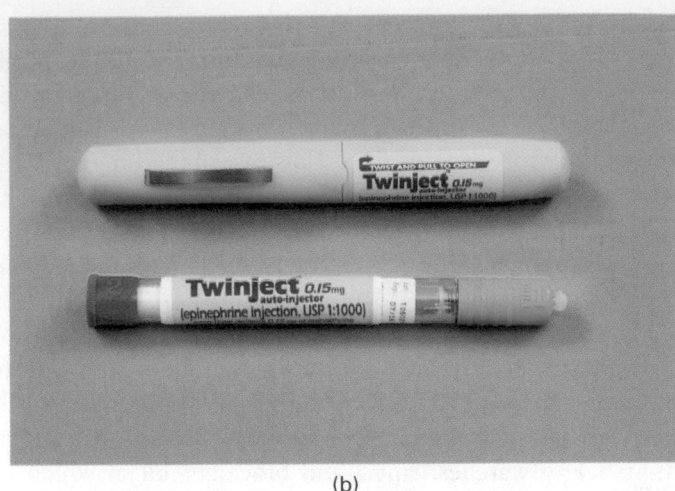

(a)                                                (b)

**Figure 14-12** Epinephrine pens: (a) EpiPen auto-injectors for infants/children and adults. (b) Twinject auto-injectors for infants/children and adults.

2. Assist the patient (as needed) in removing the medication from its protective package.

3. Check the expiration date of the medication.

4. Check the medication for any damage, discoloration (e.g., brown or pink), or particles in the fluid.

5. Remove the gray safety cap from the auto-injector. (The device will not function with the safety cap in place.)

6. Use your dominant hand to grasp the auto-injector firmly. Do not place your thumb over either end of the auto-injector, because doing so could result in the accidental injection of the medication into your thumb.

7. Help the patient place the black tip of the auto-injector against the patient's outer thigh muscle (halfway between the hip and knee). If possible, wipe the skin with an alcohol wipe first. If necessary, the EpiPen™ may be administered through clothing.

8. Help the patient firmly push the black tip against the thigh until the needle deploys. (You should hear an audible "click" as the medication is being injected into the thigh muscle.)

9. Hold the needle in place for a minimum of 10 seconds to allow the medication to be fully dispensed.

10. Assist the patient in removing the auto-injector, and then place it into a biohazard container. (If one is not available, place the device back in its protective package.)

11. Massage the injection site for 10–20 seconds.

12. Note the time at which the drug was administered.

To assist the patient in self-administering epinephrine using a Twinject™ auto-injector system, conduct the following procedure (OEC Skill 14-2■):

1. Perform steps 1–4 as described in the previous procedure.

2. Remove the green safety cap to expose the gray cap.

3. Remove the red end cap.

4. Perform steps 6 and 8–12 as previously described, pressing the gray tip firmly against the muscle of the outer thigh.

Epinephrine is a fast-acting drug. In most cases, a single dose will relieve the patient's symptoms within a few minutes. In severe cases, however, the patient may require additional doses of epinephrine; this is especially true for prolonged transport situations. A second dose of epinephrine is indicated if the patient's symptoms have not resolved within 10 minutes, or if they recur. If needed, a second dose of epinephrine may be administered using another EpiPen™. If using the Twinject™ system, a second dose may be administered manually using the enclosed pre-filled syringe (OEC Skill 14-3■). In most emergency care systems, a direct physician order is required to administer a second dose of epinephrine. If indicated, administer the second dose in the other thigh.

Monitor the patient's breathing, lung sounds, and vital signs every 3–5 minutes, noting any changes. Ideally, the patient's condition should rapidly improve following the administration of epinephrine. Evident improvement includes the patient being able to breathe more easily and an improvement in vital signs. Signs of shock also should quickly diminish as the vital signs begin to return to normal.

Any patient who experiences a moderate-to-severe allergic reaction or has received an epinephrine injection should always be transported to a hospital for further evaluation and follow-up. Likewise, anyone who accidentally injects epinephrine into a thumb or finger also should be transported to the hospital for a follow-up evaluation.

## STOP, THINK, UNDERSTAND

### Multiple Choice

Choose the correct answer.

1. The best first step in the management of any allergic reaction is to_____
   a. manage the ABCDs and remove the patient from the source of the allergen.
   b. immediately administer epinephrine and activate the EMS system by calling 911.
   c. manage the ABCDs and immediately administer epinephrine.
   d. immediately transport the patient to a definitive-care medical facility, because dealing with an allergic reaction is beyond the scope of an OEC Technician.

2. Which of the following statements describes the best method for removing a bee stinger?_____
   a. Grasp the stinger firmly with tweezers and pull swiftly.
   b. Scrape the stinger out of the skin using the side of a credit card or some other thin stiff object.
   c. Pull the stinger out with a commercial venom extractor.
   d. Stingers should be left in place because removing them could pose a hazard to rescuers.

3. The best first action for caring for a patient suffering from a severe allergic reaction or anaphylaxis is to_____
   a. administer epinephrine.
   b. place the patient into a "tripod" position.
   c. correct ABCD deficits.
   d. transport without delay.

4. What is the best course of action for maintaining the airway in a patient in severe or anaphylactic shock?_____
   a. Place the patient in the shock position and administer $O_2$ using a nonrebreather mask at 15 LPM.
   b. Place the patient in a prone position and administer $O_2$ using a nasal cannula at 6 LPM.
   c. Place the patient in a position of comfort and monitor the airway; do not administer $O_2$ unless the patient's respiratory rate is less than 10 breaths/minute.
   d. Place patient in a "tripod" position and immediately begin assist breathing with a BVM, regardless of the respiratory rate, because a patient in anaphylaxis will be unable to breathe well unassisted.

5. Which of the following statements regarding the care of a patient who is exhibiting signs or symptoms of an allergic reaction is true?_____
   a. An OEC Technician may assist a patient with the administration of injectable epinephrine following prescribed and local protocols.
   b. Only an RN, paramedic, or physician may assist with the administration of any medication, including injectible epinephrine.
   c. OEC Technicians may assist patients with taking any medication prescribed for allergic reactions, including Benadryl, Allegra, Epinephrine, and Solumedrol.
   d. OEC Technicians may carry and administer epinephrine per routine standing orders.

**CASE DISPOSITION**

Other OEC Technicians soon arrive with oxygen and a wheeled litter basket. You place the patient on a nonrebreather mask at 15 LPM. You then ask her if she has an epinephrine auto-injector. She points weakly at her camera bag. You locate her EpiPen™ and assist her in administering the medication in the lateral side of her thigh. Within a few minutes, she is breathing more easily, and her facial swelling begins to diminish. Shortly thereafter, an ALS provider arrives on scene. Together, you load the patient into the litter and transport her to the parking lot, where an ambulance takes her to a nearby hospital. She makes a full recovery and later presents your patrol with one of her scenic photographs of the area's mountains.

## OEC SKILL 14-1 | Administration with an Auto-injector: EpiPen™

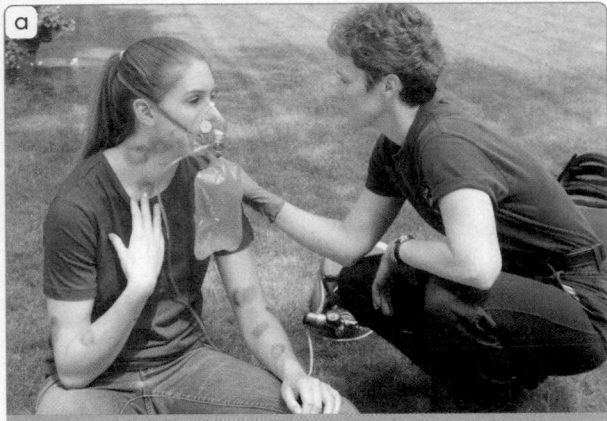

Perform a patient assessment and obtain a SAMPLE history.

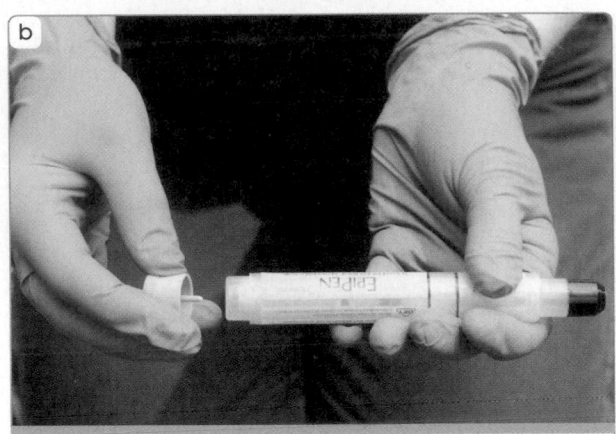

Remove the gray safety cap.

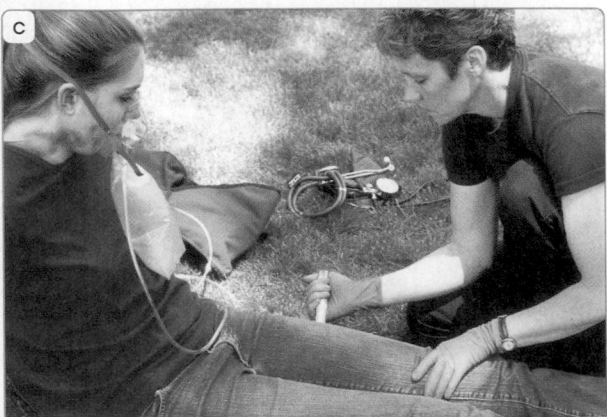

Assist the patient in placing the black tip of the auto-injector against the patient's outer thigh muscle and inject the dose of epinephrine into the patient.

## OEC SKILL 14-2 | Administration with an Auto-injector: Twinject™

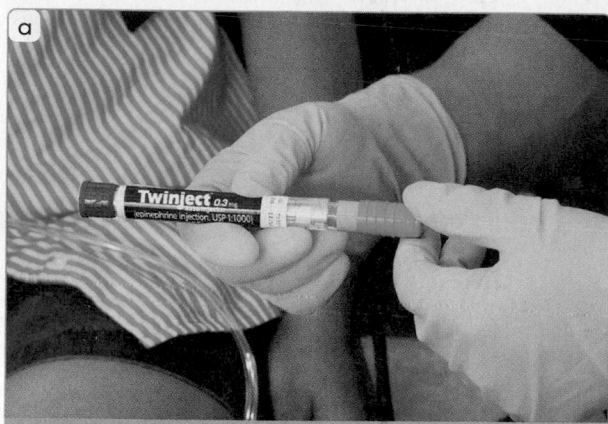

After ensuring that the medication is prescribed for the patient, remove the green cap from the device.

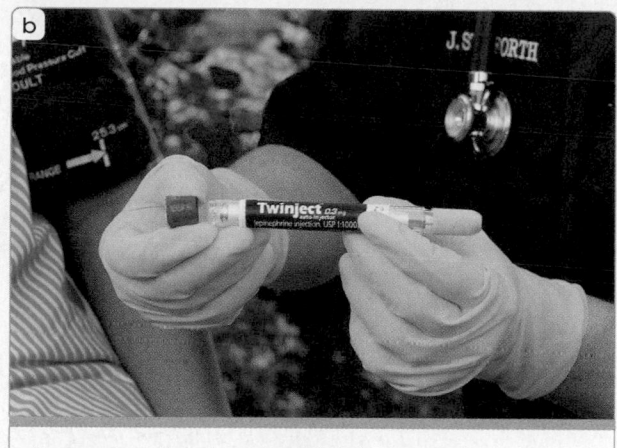

Remove the red cap from the end of the Twinject™.

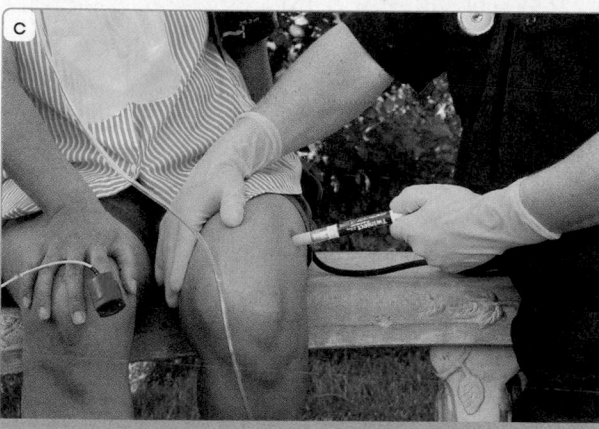

Assist the patient by holding the Twinject™ with the gray cap against the outside of the patient's thigh, halfway between the hip and the knee, and inject the dose of epinephrine.

# OEC SKILL 14-3    Administration with an Auto-injector: Twinject™ Additonal Dose

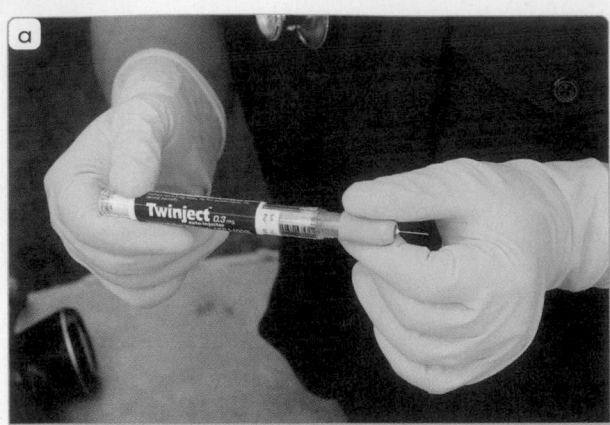

To administer a second dose using the Twinject™, start by removing the gray cap.

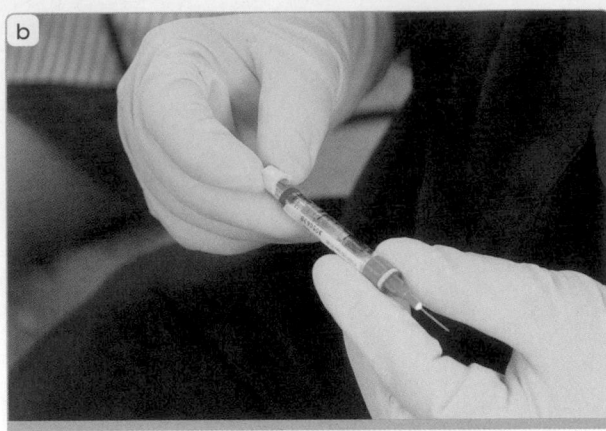

Remove the yellow safety collar from the needle plunger.

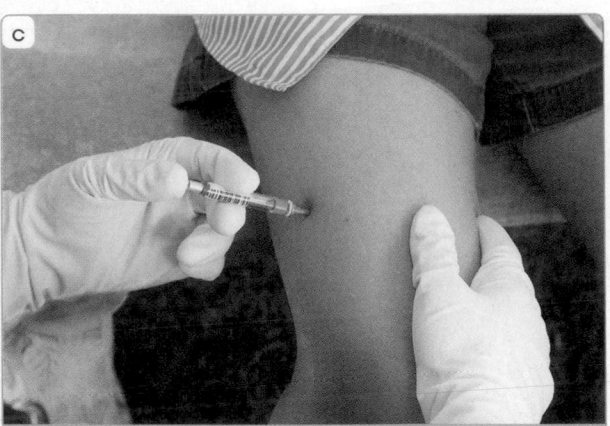

Assist the patient by injecting the second dose into the outside of the patient's other thigh.

## Skill Guide

Date: _____

(CPI) = Critical Performance Indicator

Candidate: _____

Start Time: _____

End Time: _____

## Administration with an Auto-Injector

**Objective:** To demonstrate assisting with the administration of a single dose auto injector.

| Skill | Max Points | Skill Demo | |
|---|---|---|---|
| Determines scene is safe. | 1 | | (CPI) |
| Initiates Standard Precautions. | 1 | | (CPI) |
| Obtains patient's permission to assist. | 1 | | |
| Verifies the correct medicine, the correct patient, the correct route, correct dose, and verifies medication is current. | 1 | | (CPI) |
| Ensures that patient meets the medical requirements for administration of auto injector. | 1 | | |
| Removes the pen from its protective case. Removes the cap with the black tip pointing to the thigh. Holds the pen in the middle keeping your digits from either end of the pen. | 1 | | |
| Assists the patient with administrating the pen by holding and firmly striking the outer thigh muscle between the knee and hip through the patient's clothing and holds for 10 seconds. If leg is exposed wipes area first with alcohol wipe. Listens for audible click to indicate needle was activated. Massages the injection site for 10–20 seconds after pen removal from the patient. | 1 | | |
| Records the event for type, quantity, and time. | 1 | | |
| Reassesses the patient vitals and lung sounds. | 1 | | |
| If applicable, and the patient has a second auto injector, assists with administration of a second dose. Records the type, quantity, and time. | 1 | | |
| Verbalizes proper disposal of the pens with exposed needle. | 1 | | |

Must receive 8 out of 11 points.

Comments: _____

Failure of any of the CPIs is an automatic failure.

Evaluator: _____ NSP ID: _____

PASS      FAIL

# Chapter Review

## Chapter Summary

Allergies are a common medical condition that affects millions of people worldwide. The dramatic rate at which this disorder is increasing makes it almost certain that OEC Technicians will encounter patients with allergy-related problems. By quickly recognizing the signs and symptoms of an allergic reaction, attending to the ABCDs, and assisting the patient in taking a medication such as epinephrine, OEC Technicians may be able to help reduce the morbidity and mortality associated with this disorder. Such actions, in combination with rapid transport to an emergency-care facility, will help ensure that patients who have had allergic reactions will be able to continue to explore the world in which they live and not be imprisoned by this very treatable condition.

## Remember...

1. An allergy is the body's overreaction to a foreign substance.
2. Allergies are caused by antigens called allergens.
3. Many people do not know they have an allergy until they suffer an allergic reaction.
4. Tongue swelling is an ominous sign of an allergic reaction.
5. Anaphylaxis can be fatal unless rapidly treated.
6. Peanuts are the number one food allergy in the world.
7. Allergic reactions may be prevented using the Triple A approach.

## Chapter Questions

### Multiple Choice

Choose the correct answer.

1. How does epinephrine help a patient having a severe allergic reaction?_____
   a. It causes tachycardia (a rapid heart rate), which improves tissue perfusion.
   b. It causes vasodilation (widening of the blood vessels), which calms the patient and improves tissue perfusion.
   c. It causes bronchodilation (widening of the bronchioles) and vasoconstriction (narrowing of the blood vessels), which help the patient breathe more easily, increases blood pressure, and improves tissue perfusion.
   d. It causes bradycardia (a slowed heart rate), which minimizes the amount of oxygen the body needs, and it reduces the production of mucus in the lungs, which improves ventilation.

2. Which of the following is true about allergies and anaphylaxis?_____
   a. Something as simple as a peanut can cause a fatal allergic reaction.
   b. Allergies are a psychological disorder.
   c. Allergic reactions diminish with exposure, which is why "allergy shots" work.
   d. It takes a large amount of allergen to cause an allergic reaction.

3. You are hiking with friends and stop to eat lunch. After one of the members of your party ate a peanut butter sandwich, she tells you that her throat is beginning to itch and that her chest feels tight. She denies ever having an allergic reaction before. What is your best course of action?_____
   a. Do nothing and simply observe her for a while because she is not known to be allergic to anything.
   b. Borrow an EpiPen™ from another member of your party and help her to administer it.
   c. Turn around with her and jog or walk briskly toward the trailhead, because doing so will produce natural adrenaline and endorphins, which can help stop an allergic reaction.

d. Help her into a position of comfort, observe her airway and vital signs, and call for assistance if within cell-phone range; otherwise, have two other members of your party hike out for help.

## Short Answer

A patient is having an anaphylactic reaction to a wasp sting and appears to be going into shock. What should you do?

_____

_____

_____

## Matching

Match each of the following terms to its definition.

_____ 1. allergen

_____ 2. allergic reaction

_____ 3. allergy

_____ 4. anaphylaxis

_____ 5. angioedema

_____ 6. antibody

_____ 7. antigen

_____ 8. histamine

_____ 9. pruritus

_____ 10. urticaria

a. a chemical that is released in the body in response to an allergic reaction

b. a series of signs and symptoms that occur in response to exposure to an allergen

c. swelling beneath the skin or mucosa that is caused by an allergic reaction

d. severe itching in the skin

e. a protein that is produced by the body to neutralize or destroy specific antigens

f. hives that accompany an allergic reaction

g. a foreign substance in the body

h. a substance (e.g., smoke, pollen, fungi) whose presence in the body causes an allergy

i. an exaggerated immune response to a substance that normally does not cause a reaction

j. a severe allergic reaction that can result in severe cardiac or respiratory compromise

## Scenario

*While you are on base duty early one morning, a family walks into Ski Patrol and asks for your help. The father states that his 14-year-old daughter is acting as if she may be allergic to something.*

*You invite the father and daughter into the treatment area. You note during a primary assessment that she is not in any respiratory distress, but she is scratching her chest area and has nasal congestion. Upon examination of her chest, you note a rash.*

1. Based on your initial findings, you suspect that the patient is experiencing a_____
   a. severe allergic reaction.
   b. moderate allergic reaction
   c. mild allergic reaction.
   d. minor allergic reaction.

*You attempt to reduce the number of possible causes of this allergic reaction.*

2. What mnemonic or acronym will help you identify the cause?_____
   a. OPQRST
   b. AVPU
   c. DCAP-BTLS
   d. SAMPLE

*As you interview the patient and her father, they indicate that she has no known allergies and has not been exposed to anything unusual, such as new bedding, soaps, foods, perfumes, and the like. When asked if this has happened before, the father said that she had congestion and itching during the early evening yesterday, but that it went away when she retired to bed. Yesterday the family had visited friends who have a long-haired dog, and the patient had played and petted the animal a lot over a four-hour period. When you ask if she is wearing the same clothing again today, the response is no, only the winter coat she is wearing is the same.*

*When asked when the reaction started today, the father stated it did not start until she put the coat on. You have the patient remove her coat, and within 10 minutes her congestion decreases.*

3. Based on the patient's improvement over the past 10 minutes, you ask if the patient's physician has recommended that the girl take an over-the-counter allergy medication such as_____
   a. aspirin.
   b. Benadryl.
   c. vitamin E.
   d. Servent.

## Suggested Reading

Krost, W. 2008. "Beyond the basics: The immune response." *EMS Mag.* 37(6): 70–75.

Hathaway, L. R. 2005. "Anaphylaxis." *Nursing 35*(1): 46–47.

Muelleman, R., and T. P. Tran. 2002. "Allergy, Hypersensitivity, and Anaphylaxis." In *Rosen's Emergency Medicine, Concepts and Clinical Practice*, Fifth Edition, edited by J. Marx and R. Walls. St. Louis, MO: Elsevier.

EXPLORE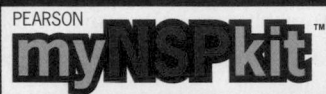

Please go to www.myNSPkit.com. Under Student Resources, you will find animations, videos, web links, and games related to this chapter—and much more. Look for information on anaphylaxis, using an Epipen, and causes of inadequate oxygenation in the blood.

Register your access code from the front of your book by going to www.myNSPkit.com and selecting the appropriate links. If the in-cover access code has been redeemed, go to www.myNSPkit.com and follow links to **Buy Access.**

# Cardiovascular Emergencies

**15**

John Latimer, MD
Roxanne Latimer, MD
Michael G. Millin, MD, MPH, FACEP
CPR Information:
Edward McNamara, BS, EMT-P
David Johe, MD

## ✛ OBJECTIVES

**Upon completion of this chapter, the OEC Technician will be able to:**

**15-1** List and describe the anatomical structures of the cardiovascular system.

**15-2** Describe the functions of the cardiovascular system.

**15-3** Describe the flow of blood through the cardiovascular system.

**15-4** Define the following:

- acute myocardial infarction
- atherosclerosis
- cardiovascular disease
- coronary artery disease
- hypertension

**15-5** List the signs and symptoms for each of the following cardiovascular disorders:

- acute myocardial infarction
- aortic aneurysm
- cardiogenic shock
- congestive heart failure
- pericardial tamponade
- pulmonary embolism

**15-6** List the arrhythmias associated with sudden cardiac death.

**15-7** Describe and demonstrate how to assess a patient with a cardiovascular emergency.

**15-8** Describe and demonstrate the proper care of a patient with a cardiovascular emergency.

*continued*

## Chapter Overview

Outdoor activities can provide a wealth of benefits to mind, body, and spirit. They also can be extremely rigorous and place tremendous demands on the body. To meet these demands, the cardiovascular system must work hard to bring oxygen and nutrients to the body's tissues and to remove the waste products of metabolism. At times, the cardiovascular system is unable to meet the demands placed on it by overexertion, underlying disease, and/or external factors. According to the National Center for

*continued*

## HISTORICAL TIMELINE

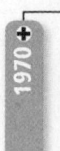

**1970** First NSP publication "National Notes" (later "National Patroller") was published.

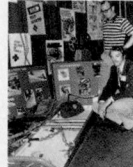

**1970** Largest percentage growth in history of NSP: added two new divisions and grew from 19,000 members to 22,629 members.

**15-9** List three common cardiac medications.

**15-10** Describe and demonstrate how to perform CPR on the following:

- an adult
- a child
- an infant

**15-11** Describe and demonstrate the proper use of an AED.

## ⊕ KEY TERMS

acute myocardial infarction (AMI), p. 466

advanced life support (ALS), p. 458

angina pectoris, p. 466

aorta, p. 459

aortic aneurysm, p. 475

arrhythmia, p. 467

arteriosclerosis, p. 464

asystole, p. 468

atherosclerosis, p. 464

automated external defibrillator (AED), p. 465

automatic implantable cardioverter defibrillator (AICD), p. 484

basic life support (BLS), p. 476

cardiac arrest, p. 485

cardiogenic shock, p. 468

cardiopulmonary resuscitation (CPR), p. 465

cardioversion, p. 482

congestive heart failure, p. 465

coronary artery bypass grafting (CABG), p. 485

coronary artery disease (CAD), p. 464

edema, p. 466

embolus, p. 468

hypertension, p. 465

infarction, p. 465

ischemia, p. 466

myocardium, p. 459

pacemaker, p. 482

perfusion, p. 472

pericarditis, p. 469

sudden cardiac arrest (SCA), p. 468

thrombus, p. 468

ventricular fibrillation, p. 468

ventricular tachycardia, p. 468

Health Statistics, cardiovascular disease (CVD) claimed 616,067 lives in 2007. CVD is the number one cause of death in the United States, accounting for more than one-fourth of all deaths each year.

When cardiovascular emergencies occur in outdoor settings, OEC Technicians are frequently the first emergency care providers to reach the patient (Figure 15-1■).

Because some cardiovascular disorders can be immediately life threatening, it is important that OEC Technicians are able to identify the signs and symptoms of these emergencies quickly, render appropriate care quickly, and summon **advanced life support (ALS)** assistance.

This chapter builds on the anatomy and physiology you learned in Chapter 6 by explaining how cardiovascular diseases occur and their effects. After studying this

**advanced life support (ALS)** a level of EMS care for which providers are trained and authorized to insert advanced airway devices, initiate intravenous lines, and give medications.

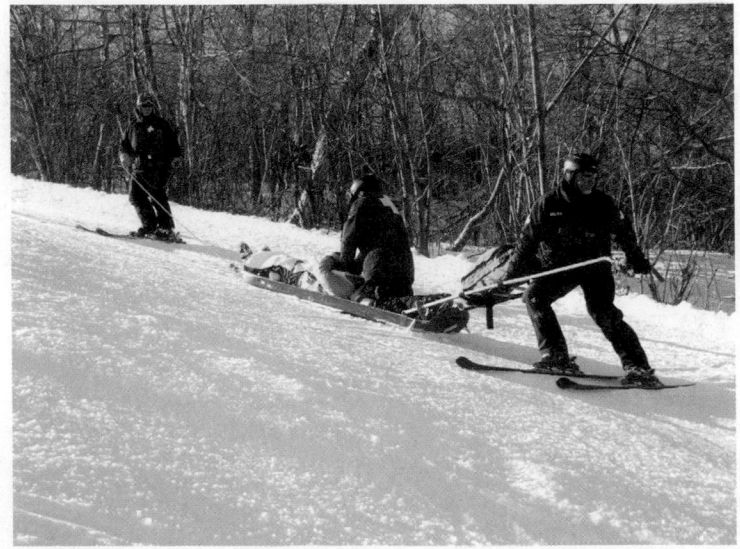

**Figure 15-1** When cardiovascular emergencies occur in outdoor settings, OEC Technicians are often the first to reach the patient.
Copyright Edward McNamara

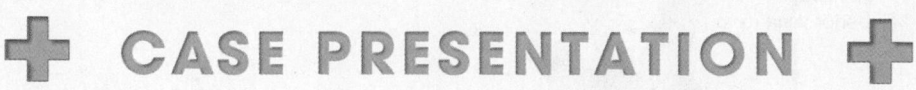

## CASE PRESENTATION

You are called to assist a 42-year-old man who is complaining of chest pain. Upon arrival, you find the patient sitting on a log. He appears to be in considerable distress. The patient tells you that he was hiking on snowshoes when he suddenly experienced a "crushing pain" in his chest that radiated down his left arm. He has a history of "heart problems" but has never experienced pain this bad before. He also complains of feeling weak and slightly nauseated. He is pale and is sweating profusely.

**What should be your first step in providing care?**

chapter, you will have a better understanding of common cardiovascular emergencies, the signs and symptoms associated with each, and how to manage these emergencies effectively in the field.

## Anatomy and Physiology

As described in Chapter 6, the cardiovascular system consists of three major components: the heart, blood vessels, and blood.

### The Heart

The heart is a thick muscular organ that pumps blood throughout the body. Located behind and just to the left of the sternum, the heart is approximately the size of a closed fist. It is enclosed within the tough, fibrous pericardial sac, which contains a small amount of pericardial fluid that allows friction-free movement of the heart within the sac.

The heart has four chambers and is commonly divided into a right side and a left side (Figure 15-2■). The right side receives deoxygenated blood from the body and pumps it to the lungs, whereas the left side receives oxygen-rich blood from the lungs and sends it to tissues throughout the body. Each side contains an atrium (upper chamber) and a ventricle (lower chamber). A thick muscular wall, known as the septum, divides the two sides of the heart. Separating the atria and ventricles are the atrioventricular valves (tricuspid and mitral). The semilunar valves (pulmonic and aortic) are located between the ventricles and the great arteries. These four valves direct blood forward and prevent backflow.

During an average day, the heart of an adult beats approximately 100,000 times and pumps about 2,000 gallons of blood. With each heartbeat, deoxygenated blood enters the right atrium from the superior and inferior venae cavae. When the right atrium contracts, the blood flows through the tricuspid valve into the right ventricle. From the right ventricle, it is pumped through the pulmonic valve into the pulmonary arteries and then to the lungs. Once in the lungs, oxygen enters the blood, and carbon dioxide (the waste product of tissue metabolism) leaves the blood by way of a process known as gas exchange. Blood then returns through the pulmonary veins into the left atrium. When the left atrium contracts, blood flows through the mitral valve into the left ventricle. From the left ventricle, blood is pumped through the aortic valve into the **aorta**. From there, blood is delivered to the rest of the body.

Imbedded within the heart muscle, or **myocardium**, is a vast array of electrical pathways that enables the heart to contract in a rhythmic, coordinated fashion

⊕ **15-1** List and describe the anatomical structures of the cardiovascular system.

⊕ **15-2** Describe the functions of the cardiovascular system.

⊕ **15-3** Describe the flow of blood through the cardiovascular system.

**aorta** the large muscular artery that originates at the heart and serves as the main trunk of the arterial system.

**myocardium** heart muscle tissue.

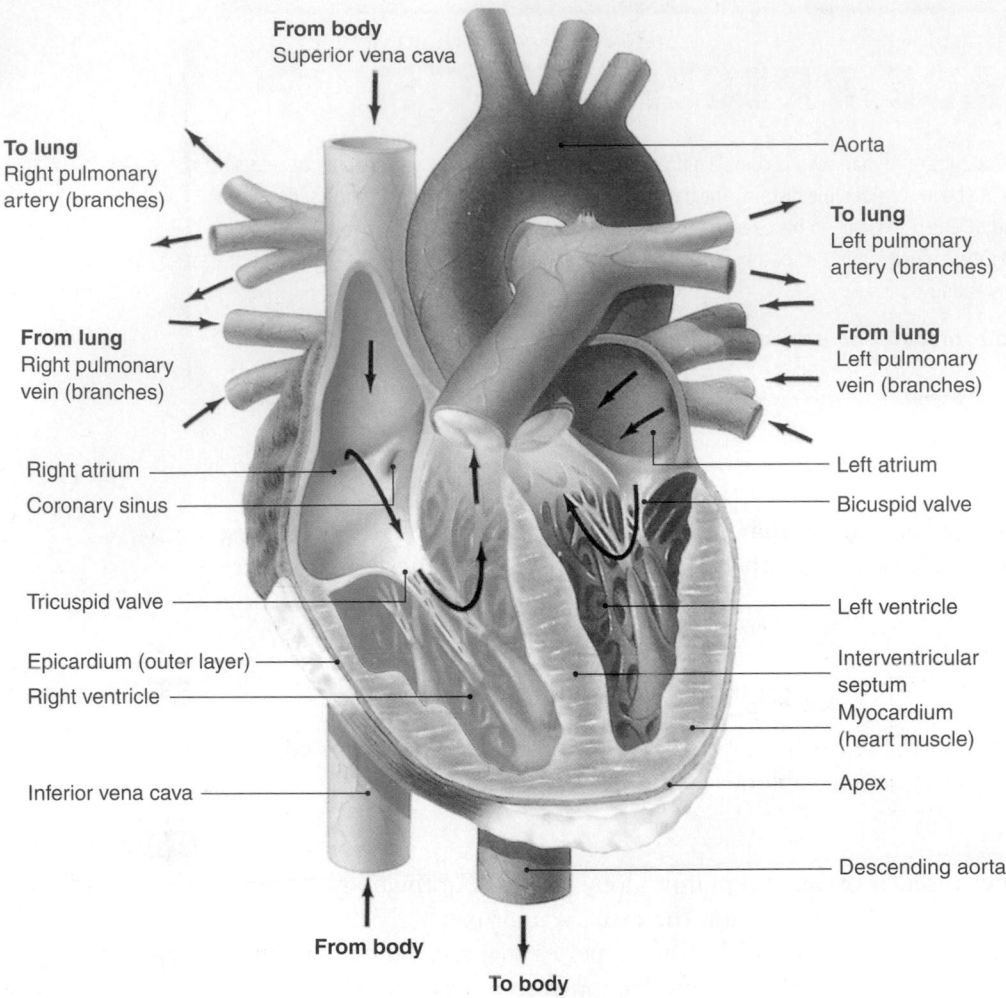

**From body**
Superior vena cava

**To lung**
Right pulmonary
artery (branches)

Aorta

**To lung**
Left pulmonary
artery (branches)

**From lung**
Right pulmonary
vein (branches)

**From lung**
Left pulmonary
vein (branches)

Right atrium
Coronary sinus

Left atrium
Bicuspid valve

Tricuspid valve

Left ventricle

Epicardium (outer layer)
Right ventricle

Interventricular
septum
Myocardium
(heart muscle)

Inferior vena cava

Apex

Descending aorta

**From body**

**To body**

**Figure 15-2** A cross section of the heart showing its internal structures and the paths of blood through the heart.

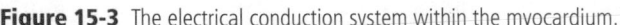

**Figure 15-3** The electrical conduction system within the myocardium.

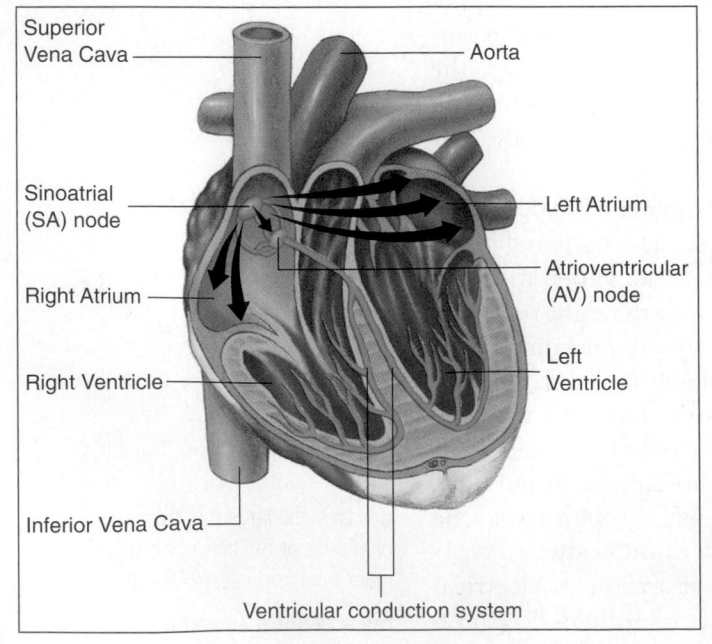

Superior
Vena Cava

Aorta

Sinoatrial
(SA) node

Left Atrium

Atrioventricular
(AV) node

Right Atrium

Left
Ventricle

Right Ventricle

Inferior Vena Cava

Ventricular conduction system

(Figure 15-3■). An electrical impulse starts in the right atrium and travels down the electrical pathways to both ventricles, stimulating forceful contractions of the ventricles.

## Blood Vessels

Blood vessels carry blood to and from the heart. There are three types of blood vessels: arteries, veins, and capillaries. Arteries transport blood away from the heart, veins bring blood to the heart, and capillaries connect the two. Except for the pulmonary arteries, arteries carry oxygen-rich blood. They have thick muscular walls that can constrict or dilate as needed.

The aorta, which leaves the heart at its superior border, is the largest artery in the body (Figure 15-4■). The coronary arteries, which carry oxygen-rich blood to the heart muscle, leave the aorta just above the heart. Next are the carotid arteries, which supply blood to the brain. The subclavian arteries supply the arms through the brachial, radial, and ulnar branches. In the torso, the aorta supplies the pelvis and legs through the iliac and femoral arteries. In the legs, the femoral arteries divide into the tibial and peroneal arteries.

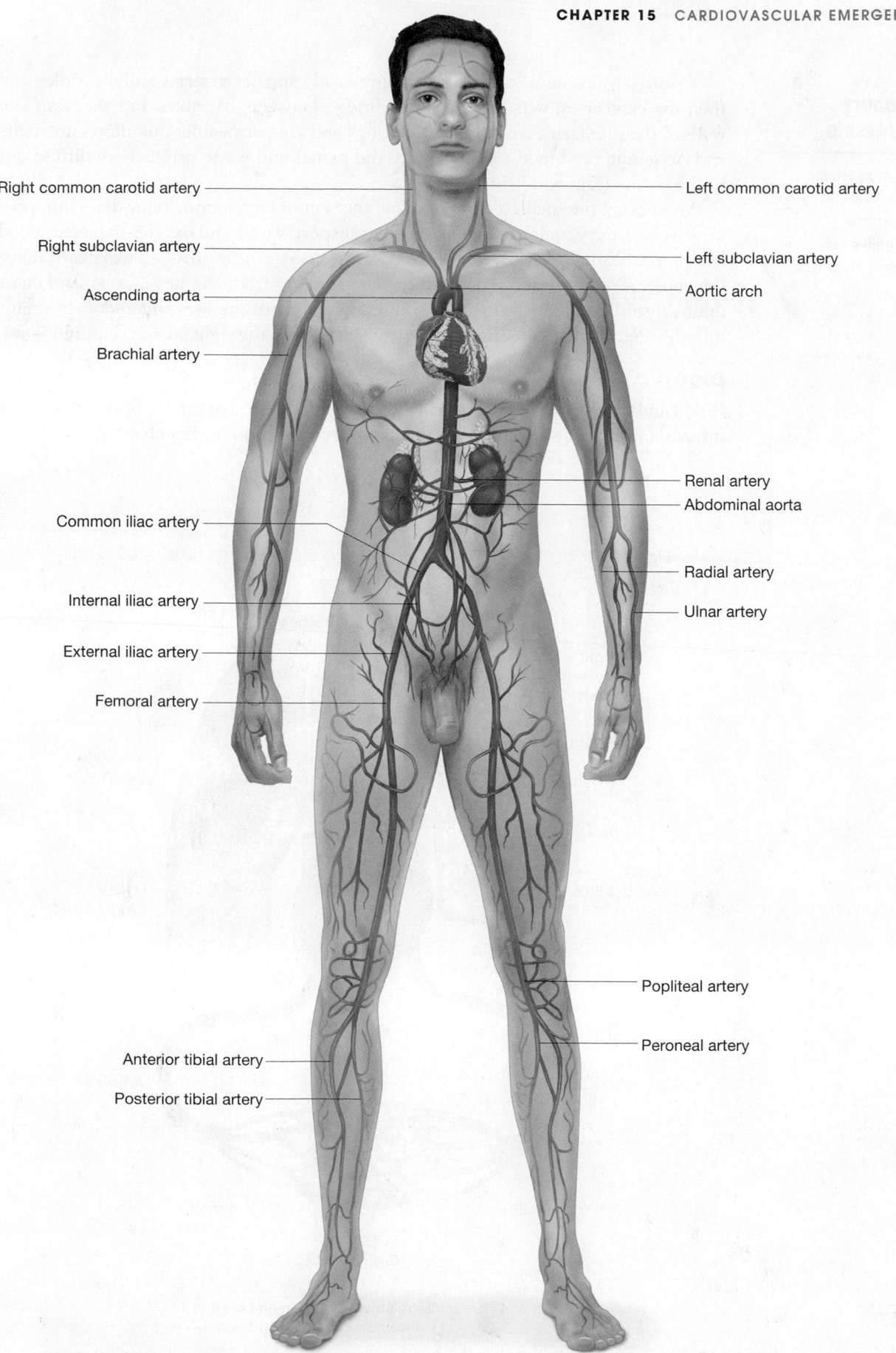

Right common carotid artery

Right subclavian artery

Ascending aorta

Brachial artery

Common iliac artery

Internal iliac artery

External iliac artery

Femoral artery

Anterior tibial artery

Posterior tibial artery

Left common carotid artery

Left subclavian artery

Aortic arch

Renal artery

Abdominal aorta

Radial artery

Ulnar artery

Popliteal artery

Peroneal artery

**Figure 15-4** The major arteries of the human body.

### Pulmonary Blood Vessels

The pulmonary arteries are the only arteries in the body that carry deoxygenated blood. The pulmonary veins are the only veins in the body that carry oxygenated blood.

Arteries continue to divide into progressively smaller arteries and arterioles and then the capillaries, which serve as the bridge between arterioles and venules. The walls of the capillaries are only one cell thick and are permeable; this allows nutrients and oxygen in the blood to diffuse into the tissues and waste products to diffuse out of the tissues (Figure 15-5■).

Venules are the smallest component of the venous circulation. They drain into progressively larger venules and veins, which transport wastes and oxygen-depleted blood back to the heart. Deoxygenated blood is returned to the heart through two major veins: the superior and inferior venae cavae. Venous blood from the head, arms, and chest drains into the superior vena cava, whereas blood from the legs and abdomen drains into the inferior vena cava. Both venae cavae drain into the right atrium (Figure 15-6■).

### Blood

Blood and its components were previously described in Chapter 10, Shock. For more information about blood, refer to the appropriate section in that chapter.

**Figure 15-5** The circulation and oxygen content of blood throughout the cardiovascular system.

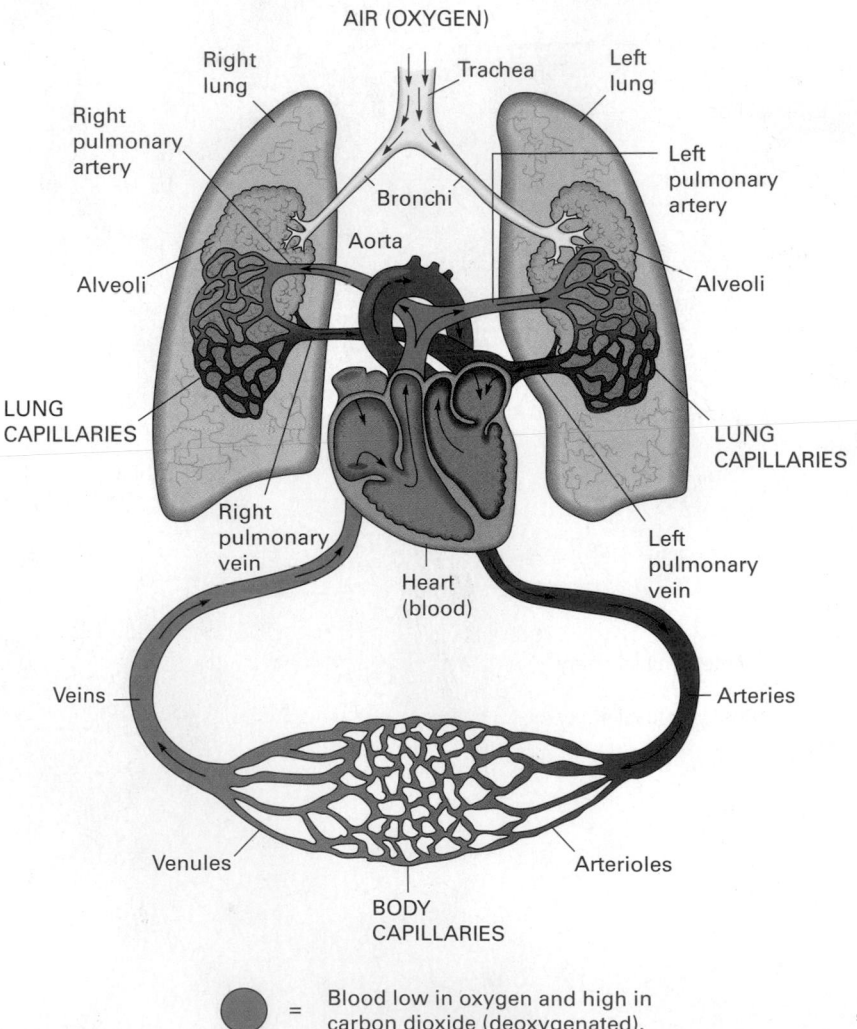

= Blood low in oxygen and high in carbon dioxide (deoxygenated).

= Blood high in oxygen and low in carbon dioxide (oxygenated).

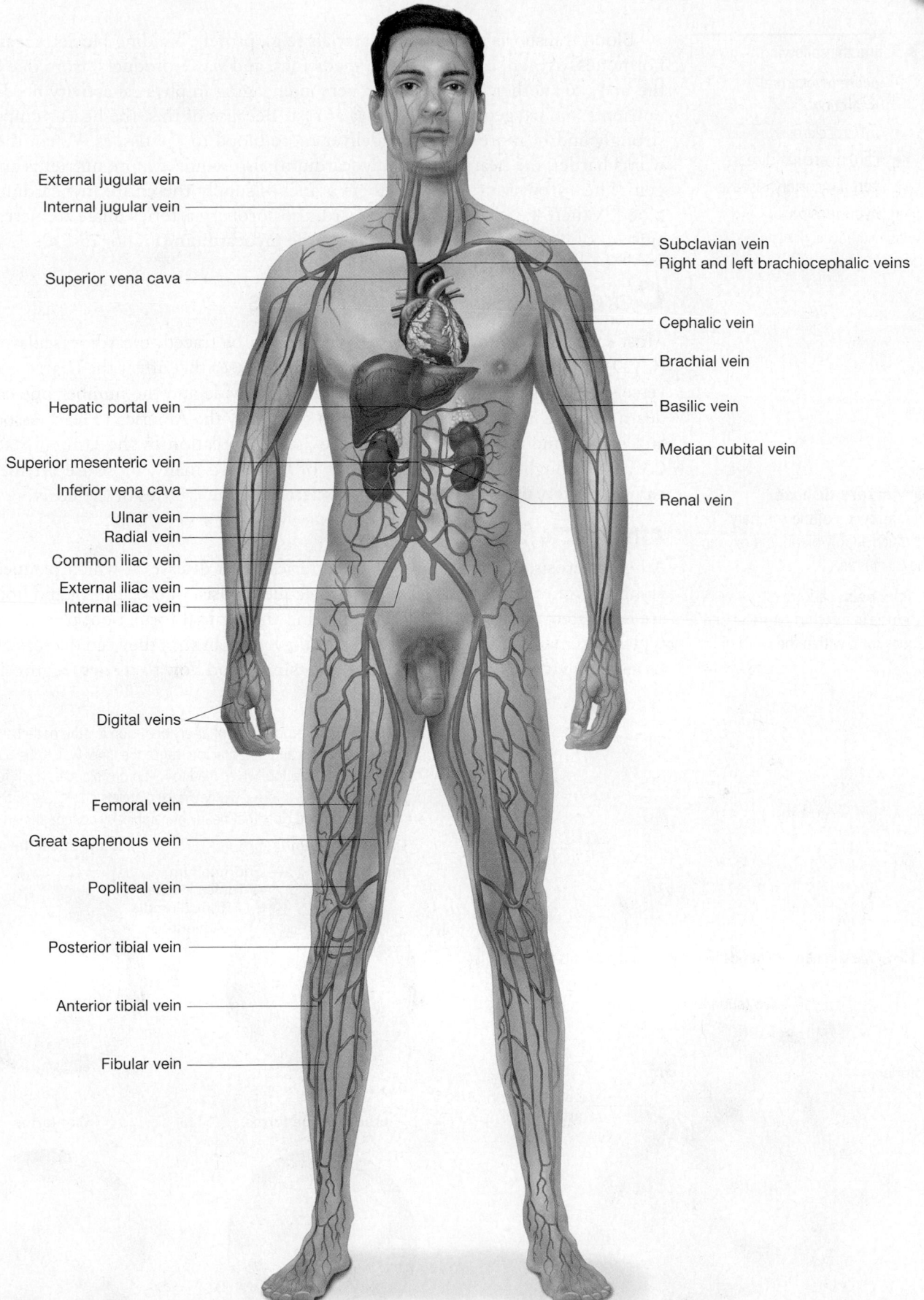

**Figure 15-6** The major veins of the human body, which return deoxygenated blood to the heart.

⊕ **15-4** Define the following:
- acute myocardial infarction
- atherosclerosis
- cardiovascular disease
- coronary artery disease
- hypertension

**coronary artery disease (CAD)**    narrowing of the coronary arteries, which supply blood and oxygen to the heart muscle.

**atherosclerosis**    a form of arteriosclerosis in which cholesterol and lipid plaques form within the walls of arteries.

Blood transports a variety of materials (e.g., protein building blocks, sugars, fats, hormones, oxygen, carbon dioxide, medicines, and waste products) from one area of the body to another. The body of a person engaging in physical activity needs more nutrients and oxygen than when it is at rest. Because of this, the heart pumps more strongly and/or more quickly to deliver more blood to the tissues. When the heart works harder, the heart muscle (myocardium) also requires more nutrients and oxygen. The coronary arteries and their branches supply the entire myocardium with blood. When the heart is pumping hard, the coronary arteries dilate to increase the amount of blood and oxygen supplied to the myocardium (Figure 15-7■).

# Cardiovascular Emergencies

Most causes of cardiovascular system failure can be traced to cardiovascular disease (CVD), a generic term that describes several diseases that affect the heart and blood vessels. CVD is the leading cause of death worldwide and the number one cause of death in the United States. According to studies by the American Heart Association and others, more than one-third of the adult population in the United States has CVD. Although the underlying causes of CVD are many, most are attributed to **coronary artery disease (CAD)**, or **atherosclerosis** of the arteries of the heart.

## Atherosclerosis

Atherosclerosis, or "hardening of the arteries," is a disease in which plaques form along the inner lining of arteries. These plaques consist of cholesterol and lipids and are deposited throughout a lifetime. During their initial formation, plaque deposits typically remain undetected. However, as they grow in size, they can decrease the internal diameter of an artery, thereby decreasing blood flow to tissues (Figure 15-8■).

**Figure 15-8** The progression of artery occlusion in atherosclerosis: (a) the patient's risk factors and other factors cause the inner wall to be damaged; (b) fatty deposits develop, which lead to (c) fibrous plaque, which further occludes the vessel's internal diameter; (d) platelets aggregate in these areas, forming blood clots that nearly or completely occlude the artery.

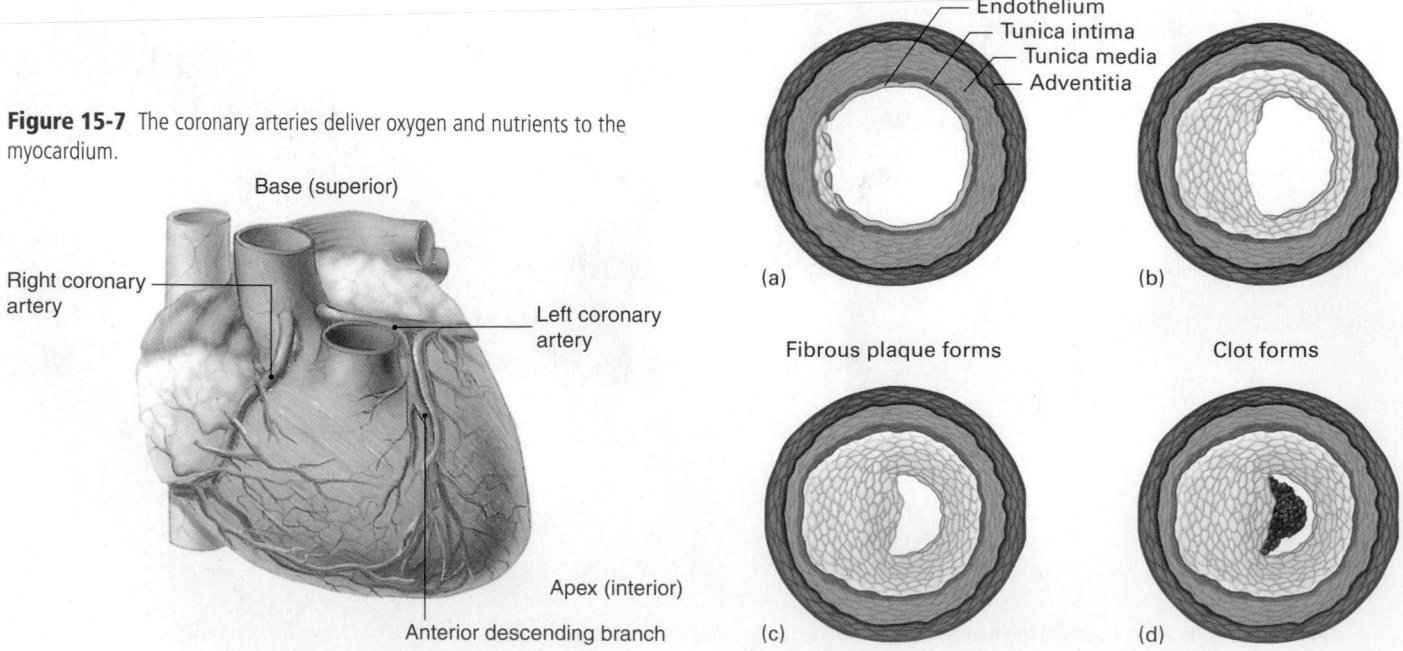

**Figure 15-7** The coronary arteries deliver oxygen and nutrients to the myocardium.

As plaques harden, the affected arteries cannot dilate properly as needed to increase the flow of nutrients and oxygen. When plaques build up within the coronary arteries, the heart may not receive the oxygen and nutrients it needs. The resulting decrease or lack of oxygen can cause portions of the heart muscle to die.

Cardiovascular disease can cause a host of problems, including high blood pressure, heart failure, acute myocardial **infarction** (AMI), and sudden cardiac death. A "heart attack" or AMI is more common in individuals 40–70 years of age. Young people in the United States are becoming increasingly at risk for CVD, **congestive heart failure (CHF)**, and AMI, primarily due to the combination of poor diet, inactivity, and obesity. Eating nutritious foods, staying active, quitting smoking, losing weight, and controlling hypertension and diabetes significantly reduce one's risk for CVD and can reduce deaths from CVD by up to 50 percent.

About 60 percent of unexpected cardiac-related deaths are treated by emergency medical services (EMS) providers. Therefore, it is likely that OEC Technicians will be called to attend to a cardiovascular emergency. Fortunately, early recognition and rapid treatment with critical interventions such as **cardiopulmonary resuscitation (CPR)** and the use of an **automated external defibrillator (AED)** can strongly improve the chances of survival.

## Hypertension

**Hypertension**, or an abnormally elevated blood pressure, is a common cardiovascular disorder that, according to the American Heart Association, affects nearly one billion people worldwide. In the United States, approximately 1 person in 3, or roughly 100 million people, is believed to have hypertension, although many cases are not reported until a problem occurs.

Hypertension is a condition in which the blood pressure within the arteries is abnormally elevated; clinical hypertension is defined as a systolic pressure greater than 140 or a diastolic pressure greater than 90. Hypertension occurs when the internal diameters of small arterioles narrow due to atherosclerosis or from other causes that restricts blood flow through the arteries. Vessel narrowing causes the pressure to build in these small vessels so that the same amount of blood can flow through the artery. Along with plaque buildup, the increased pressure damages small arteries in many of the body's organs. Even though many factors are related to hypertension, certain risk factors, including those associated with CVD, are believed to contribute to its occurrence. In addition to the risk factors previously described, high salt intake and chronic kidney disease also increase one's risk for hypertension.

Untreated, hypertension predisposes a person to heart disease because of the damage it causes to blood vessels over time. Fortunately, the condition can be treated through the combination of medications and eliminating controllable risk factors such as smoking and being overweight. Hypertension can also lead to other serious health problems, including stroke and kidney failure.

## Congestive Heart Failure

When the heart cannot adequately pump blood to body tissues, blood backs up into the major blood vessels leading to the heart, and subsequently certain organs. This condition is called congestive heart failure (CHF) and can occur in the right side of the heart, in the left side of the heart, or in both sides of the heart. Right-sided congestive heart failure results in the backup of blood in the systemic circulation, causing leakage of the fluid part of the blood into dependent tissues, most commonly the ankles and feet, and causes enlargement of the liver (Figure 15-9■).

**infarction** formation of an area of dead tissue due to inadequate blood flow.

**congestive heart failure** failure of the heart to efficiently pump blood to body tissues.

**cardiopulmonary resuscitation (CPR)** a procedure to revive a patient who is pulseless and not breathing.

**automated external defibrillator (AED)** a medical device used to deliver an electrical shock to a patient in an effort to restore an effective heart rhythm.

**hypertension** hypertension abnormally high blood pressure.

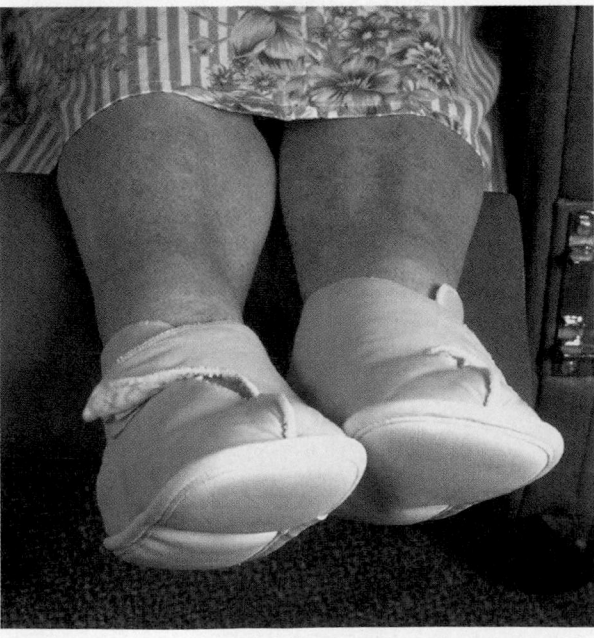

**Figure 15-9** Right sided congestive heart failure (CHF) typically causes edema in the lower extremities.

Left-sided congestive heart failure causes blood to backup in the lungs, resulting in pulmonary edema.

## Pulmonary Edema

Pulmonary **edema** is an accumulation of fluid in the lungs. It is caused by severe left-sided congestive heart failure resulting from acute myocardial infarction, direct trauma to the lung tissue, certain medical conditions (e.g., severe anemia), and certain drugs (e.g., heroin). When the left ventricle is no longer able to pump blood effectively, blood backs up into the lungs. This causes an increase in fluid pressure within the pulmonary capillaries. As a result, fluid seeps into the alveoli and prevents proper exchange of oxygen and carbon dioxide. This can lead to moderate-to-severe hypoxia with associated respiratory distress and even failure. To compensate for poor tissue perfusion, the respiratory centers within the brain signal the body to breathe faster.

As the lungs continue to fill with fluid, red blood cells leak into the alveoli, causing frothy, blood-tinged fluid to rise up the pulmonary tree. In severe cases, blood-tinged sputum may exit the mouth. As the condition worsens, the patient develops cardiogenic shock from profound hypoxia. Pulmonary edema also can be caused by altitude illness. For more information on this form of pulmonary edema, see Chapter 28, Altitude-Related Emergencies.

## Angina Pectoris

**Angina pectoris**, or simply angina, is chest pain or discomfort caused by **ischemia** of the myocardium (heart muscle), in which the oxygen demands of the heart muscle exceed the available supply (Figure 15-10■). Angina pectoris is a common occurrence among patients with coronary artery disease.

The most common cause is a narrowing of the internal diameter of the coronary arteries due to atherosclerotic plaque. During routine daily activities, a heart with a normal coronary arterial supply receives a sufficient amount of oxygen and nutrients. However, stressors such as physical activity and certain drugs place increased oxygen demands on the heart. If blood flow through the coronary arteries is reduced by plaque, the increased demand and insufficient blood supply overtaxes the heart, leading to ischemia of the myocardium. This is typically manifested as chest discomfort. When the stressor is eliminated, the pain usually subsides.

Another cause of angina is vasoconstriction or spasm of a coronary artery. If this artery is suddenly narrowed due to constriction, the amount of blood flowing through the vessel will not be sufficient to meet the heart's nutrient and oxygen needs. Coronary artery vasospasm may occur in response to certain drugs (e.g., methamphetamine and cocaine) or for unknown reasons. Table 15-1■ briefly describes three types of angina.

## Myocardial Infarction

A myocardial infarction (MI) or an **acute myocardial infarction (AMI)** is a blockage in one or more of the coronary arteries that results in ischemia and then in death of heart muscle supplied by the blocked artery(s) (Figure 15-11■). A blood clot is the most common source of the blockage, representing approximately 90 percent of all MI cases. After a small atherosclerotic plaque in the coronary artery has ruptured, a blood clot forms to repair the rupture, and the coronary artery can become completely blocked, preventing blood flow past the blockage. This is why an apparently healthy person with no known

**edema** abnormal buildup of fluid in body tissues.

**angina pectoris** sudden chest pain due to an inadequate supply of oxygen to the heart muscle; also called angina.

**ischemia** a deficiency in blood supply (and thus a deficiency of nutrients) to a tissue; if prolonged, may result in infarction.

**acute myocardial infarction (AMI)** the interruption of blood supply to part of the heart, causing death of heart muscle. Also known as a heart attack.

**Figure 15-10** Angina pectoris can result when an area of the myocardium becomes ischemic.

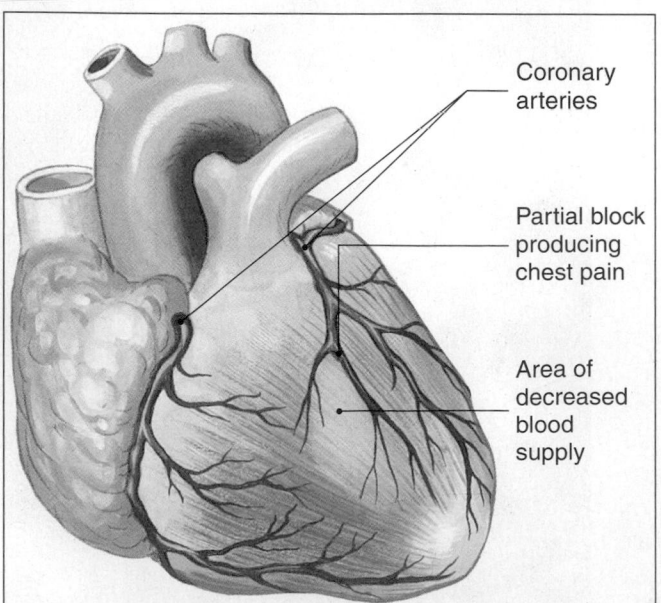

Coronary arteries

Partial block producing chest pain

Area of decreased blood supply

| Table **15-1** | Three Types of Angina |
| --- | --- |

- *Stable angina.* Occurs when the heart is forced to work harder than normal, as during rigorous physical activity. The onset is generally predictable, and the symptoms usually subside with rest or anti-angina medications such as nitroglycerin.
- *Unstable angina.* Can occur at anytime, including while at rest, and may not be relieved by anti-angina medications.
- *Prinzmetal's angina.* A form of angina in which the patient awakens with chest pain, which resolves with anti-angina medications. It is thought to be caused by spasm of a coronary artery.

heart disease or history of angina can have an acute myocardial infarction (Figure 15-12■). Another cause of MI is the gradual growth of plaques in coronary vessels until they completely prevent blood flow through the vessels.

When the heart tissue supplied by an obstructed coronary artery becomes oxygen starved, the tissue begins to die. This area of dead heart muscle is referred to as an infarct. If enough heart muscle is damaged, the heart cannot pump effectively, which can lead to a host of other life-threatening problems, including cardiac arrhythmias, congestive heart failure, cardiogenic shock, and sudden cardiac death.

## Cardiac Arrhythmias

The orderly, coordinated electrical stimulation of the myocardium is essential to healthy and efficient heart function. Any abnormality in this process, whether from an internal or external source, can lead to an irregular heart beat or heart rhythm, known as an **arrhythmia**, which can compromise normal heart function.

Some chronic arrhythmias are relatively benign, although they indicate a problem with the heart's electrical system. The primary cause of a life-threatening arrhythmia is ischemia of the heart muscle. Although the identification of cardiac arrhythmias is beyond the scope of this text, their effects are fairly straightforward: they either slow the heart rate to below 60 bpm (bradycardia), speed it up to above 100 bpm (tachycardia), or alter the regularity of the rhythm. Some arrhythmias can

### Acute Coronary Syndrome

NOTE

Acute coronary syndrome (ACS) is a group of conditions (including unstable angina and myocardial infarction) caused by a ruptured or eroded plaque within a coronary artery.

⊕ **15-6** List the arrhythmias associated with sudden cardiac death.

**arrhythmia** abnormal heart rhythm.

**Figure 15-12** A cross section of a heart showing normal tissue and infarcted tissue.

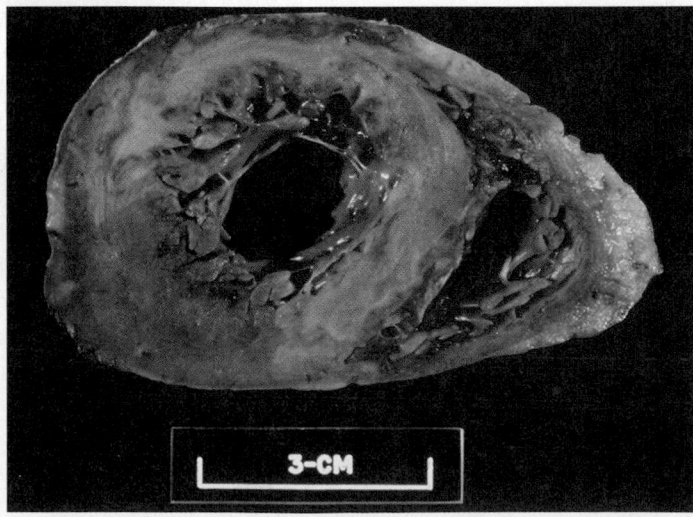

**Figure 15-11** A cross section of a myocardial infarction (MI).

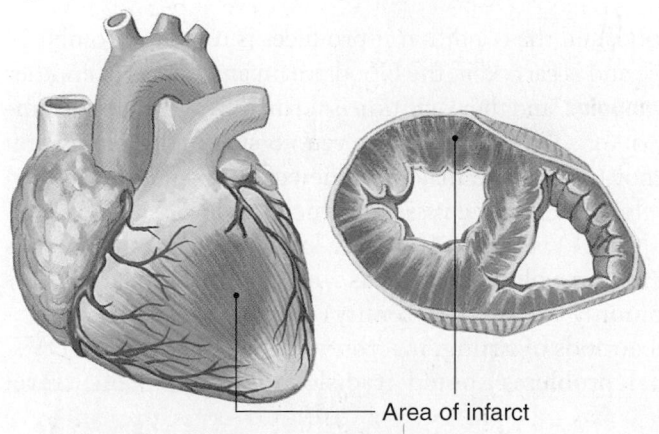

Area of infarct

**ventricular fibrillation**   chaotic and ineffective contraction of the ventricles that leads to cardiac arrest.

**ventricular tachycardia**   rapid contraction of the ventricles that can lead to ineffective blood flow to body tissues and eventually cardiac arrest.

**cardiogenic shock**   a condition whereby body tissues are oxygen deprived due to the heart's inability to adequately pump blood; may follow a large acute myocardial infarction.

**sudden cardiac arrest (SCA)**   the abrupt cessation of an effective heartbeat.

**asystole**   absence of a heartbeat due to lack of cardiac electrical activity.

**thrombus**   a clot in the blood.

**embolus**   a blood clot, fat, or other solid material in the venous system that breaks loose and is carried in the bloodstream, lodging in another site in the body.

affect the ability of the heart to pump blood, which can adversely affect blood pressure and lead to shock.

**Ventricular fibrillation** and pulseless **ventricular tachycardia** are two life-threatening arrhythmias that result in death if not rapidly treated. Cardiac arrhythmias also can cause blood to stagnate and clot within the heart. Such clots can break free and travel to the brain or elsewhere in the body, where they may block blood flow. A blood clot that ends up in the brain is likely to cause a stroke. This situation is discussed in greater detail in Chapter 11, Altered Mental Status.

## Cardiogenic Shock

If enough of the myocardium is suddenly and severely damaged, the heart may no longer pump effectively. This diminished pumping ability can cause blood pressure to fall resulting in **cardiogenic shock**. The most common cause of cardiogenic shock is myocardial infarction. Unless identified and treated quickly, cardiogenic shock has a potentially lethal outcome. As many as 70 percent of patients with cardiogenic shock secondary to AMI will die without prompt treatment in a definitive care facility.

## Sudden Cardiac Arrest

**Sudden cardiac arrest (SCA)** is the abrupt cessation of *effective* pumping of blood from the heart into the coronary arteries, the brain, and other vital organs. This condition is caused by either an abrupt cessation of cardiac electrical activity or an arrhythmia such as ventricular fibrillation or ventricular tachycardia. The condition occurs without warning. A patient that is affected by SCA (also known as sudden cardiac death or simply cardiac arrest) will not have a pulse. SCA is the leading cause of death in the United States, resulting in more than 325,000 deaths each year. Causes include myocardial infarction and the following three lethal arrhythmias:

+ *Ventricular fibrillation.* A condition in which the ventricles contract in a wildly chaotic manner that prevents the heart from pumping blood.
+ *Pulseless ventricular tachycardia.* A condition in which the ventricles contract at a markedly accelerated rate, dramatically decreasing cardiac output to the point at which a pulse is undetectable.
+ *Asystole.* A complete absence of a heartbeat due to a lack of electrical activity within the heart.

Whereas prompt treatment of pulseless ventricular tachycardia or ventricular fibrillation may result in restoration of an effective heartbeat, asystole is usually fatal, unless an underlying reversible cause or source is found.

## Thromboembolism

A **thrombus** is a clot in the blood, and the condition it produces is termed thrombosis. When a thrombus breaks loose and is carried in the bloodstream and lodges in another site in the body, it is called an **embolus**, and the condition is termed embolism. A thrombus can be a blood clot, fat, or other solid material in the venous system. Depending on its size, a thrombus that has not broken free may go undetected for months or even years before it disrupts blood flow through the vessel in which it is located.

Deep venous thrombosis (DVT) is the most widely known type of thrombosis and is a condition that occurs when a blood clot forms within one of the large veins of the extremities (more commonly the lower extremity) or the pelvis. Typically occurring following prolonged periods of sitting, inactivity, or immobilization, DVT can cause serious, even fatal problems should it dislodge from a vein, travel through the bloodstream, and cause embolism in the lungs. This condition is known as thromboembolism.

One of the most lethal forms of embolism is a pulmonary embolism (PE) (Figure 15-13■). In this condition, an embolus lodges in the pulmonary artery or one of its branches, blocking blood flow into the lung. This prevents oxygenation of blood at the alveoli distal to the site of the occlusion and also prevents blood from traveling from the lungs to the left side of the heart, and then to the vital organs, leading to shock. An embolus known as a "saddle embolus," which occurs where the main pulmonary artery splits into the right and left pulmonary arteries, disrupts blood flow to and gas exchange in both lungs, can be quickly fatal. The most common source of pulmonary embolism is thromboembolism originating in the pelvis or legs, although fat cells, plaque, and amniotic fluid also have been shown to cause this potentially lethal condition.

## Pericarditis and Pericardial Tamponade

**Pericarditis** is an inflammation of the pericardial sac. Among the numerous causes of pericarditis are myocardial infarction, bacterial and viral infections, and trauma. The inflammation can cause the layers of the pericardium to rub against one another, resulting in severe pain, especially upon deep inhalation or cough. In some cases, excess fluid may build up within pericardial sac, applying external pressure to the heart preventing adequate filling of the heart with blood, a condition known as pericardial tamponade, which restricts the heart's ability to pump effectively (Figure 15-14■). The symptoms of pericarditis can vary with its location and can last for hours or days, whereas pericardial tamponade is a life-threatening condition that requires emergency removal of the fluid from the pericardial sac. This procedure is typically performed by a trained physician only.

**pericarditis** inflammation of the pericardium or sac surrounding the heart, causing chest pain.

## Aortic Aneurysm/Aortic Dissection

An aneurysm is a localized dilation in a blood vessel that results from the degenerative weakening of the vessel wall over time. It is similar to a "bubble" that forms in an overinflated inner tube. The most common causes of an aneurysm are atherosclerosis and hypertension. An aortic aneurysm is an aneurysm that occurs anywhere along the length of the aorta (Figure 15-15■). Most aneurysms occur in the abdomen (known as an abdominal aortic aneurysm, or AAA) or in the chest (known as a thoracic aortic

**Figure 15-13** Pulmonary embolism.

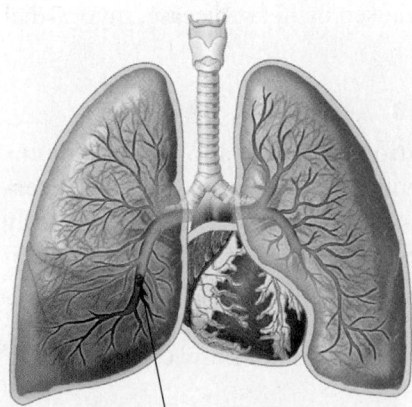

Pulmonary embolism

**Figure 15-14** Pericardial tamponade.

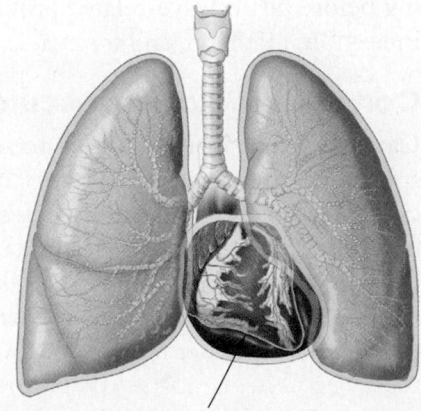

Pericardial tamponade

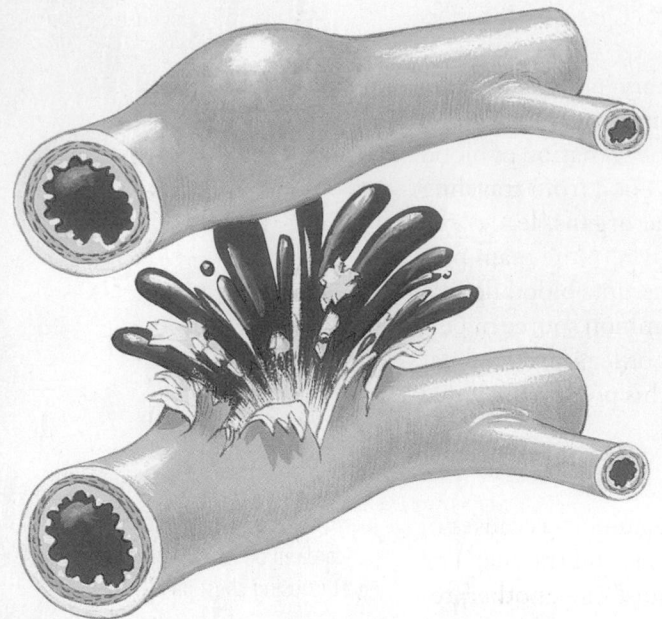

**Figure 15-15** An aortic aneurysm (bulge) can give way, causing an aortic rupture.

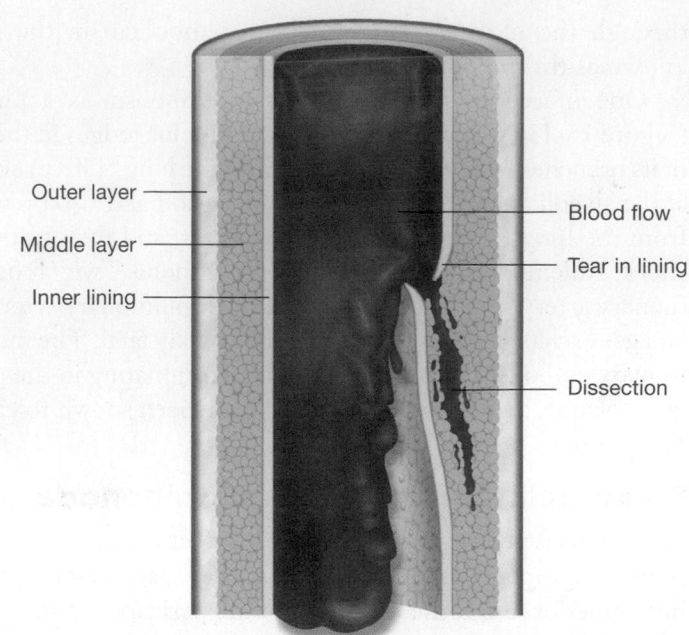

**Figure 15-16** The wall of this aorta has a dissection.

aneurysm). Aneurysms also may occur in blood vessels within the brain. Both types of aneurysms have a very high death rate should they rupture.

Aortic dissection is a condition in which the innermost lining of the aorta is disrupted and tears away from the wall of this large artery (Figure 15-16■). Due to the high pressure within the aorta, the tear grows in size and can penetrate the other layers of the vessel, weakening the vessel wall and making it susceptible to rupture. Should this occur, life-threatening internal bleeding ensues, and the patient can bleed to death within minutes.

## Heart Valve Disorders

The four heart valves help to ensure the timely, unidirectional flow of blood through and out of the heart. Occasionally, problems prevent one or more of these valves from functioning properly. When this happens, the heart may have to work harder, blood may leak backward, or blood may pool and/or clot within the heart. Most heart valve problems are congenital; that is, the valve formed improperly as the heart was forming before birth. Valve-related problems also are caused by heart disease, myocardial infarction, infection, and trauma.

## Concurrent Cardiovascular Diseases

Cardiovascular diseases often occur in combination with one another. If, for instance, a patient with a history of angina and hypertension overexerts while exercising, the heart may not receive enough blood and may become sufficiently ischemic to develop an arrhythmia and/or myocardial infarction. In turn, this can lead to congestive heart failure, pulmonary edema, and/or cardiogenic shock, which can cause sudden cardiac arrest. It is for this reason that *any* suspected cardiovascular disorder must be considered serious until evaluated by a physician.

# STOP, THINK, UNDERSTAND

## Multiple Choice

Choose the correct answer.

1. Antherosclerosis is best described as_____
   a. a deterioration of blood vessels due to aging.
   b. a buildup of cholesterol and calcium into plaque, which forms along the inner lining of arteries.
   c. heart failure.
   d. an arrhythmia that causes inadequate tissue perfusion.

2. Which of the following blood pressures is considered hypertensive?_____
   a. 100/70
   c. 130/86
   b. 120/80
   d. 140/90

3. Which of the following conditions can contribute to hypertension? (check all that apply)
   _____ a. atherosclerosis    _____ e. lack of exercise
   _____ b. high salt intake    _____ f. poor diet
   _____ c. chronic kidney disease    _____ g. smoking
   _____ d. artery narrowing    _____ h. obesity

4. Congestive heart failure is best described as_____
   a. a condition in which the heart muscle is starved for oxygen and slowly dies.
   b. the backing up of blood because the heart can no longer pump adequately.
   c. a sudden nonperfusing arrhythmia.
   d. cardiac death.

5. Pulmonary edema is best described as_____
   a. an accumulation of fluid in the lungs.
   b. swelling of the sac surrounding the lungs.
   c. a collapse of one or both lungs.
   d. a pooling of blood within the pulmonary artery.

6. Which of the following may cause pulmonary edema?_____
   a. direct trauma to lung tissue    c. diabetes
   b. anemia    d. all of the above

## Fill in the Blank

1. A(An) _____ is a localized dilation in a blood vessel that results from the degenerative weakening of the vessel wall over time.

2. _____ is a condition characterized as chest pain or discomfort caused by myocardial ischemia or a spasm of the coronary arteries and occurs when the oxygen demands of the heart muscle tissue exceeds the available supply.

## Matching

Match each of the following conditions to its description.

_____ 1. myocardial infarction
_____ 2. cardiac arrhythmias
_____ 3. cardiogenic shock
_____ 4. sudden cardiac arrest (SCA)
_____ 5. thromboembolism
_____ 6. pericarditis
_____ 7. pericardial tamponade
_____ 8. aneurysm
_____ 9. aortic dissection
_____ 10. ventricular fibrillation
_____ 11. asystole

a. a blood clot that breaks loose and is carried by the bloodstream until it lodges in another part of the body
b. the abrupt cessation of effective electrical activity within the heart
c. a complete absence of electrical activity within the heart
d. a blockage in one or more coronary arteries resulting in ischemia and then death of the heart muscle
e. irregular heart beat or rhythm; bradycardia or tachycardia
f. a life-threatening condition that occurs when the heart can no longer pump effectively
g. a sac formed by local dilation in a blood vessel
h. inflammation of the pericardial sac that surrounds the heart
i. a condition in which the innermost lining of the aorta tears away from the arterial wall
j. a buildup of fluid in the sac surrounding the heart that can restrict the heart's ability to pump blood effectively
k. a condition in which the ventricles contract in a wildly chaotic manner that prevents the heart from pumping effectively

## True or False

Indicate whether each of the following statements is true (T) or false (F).

_____ a. A cardiovascular problem is not considered serious until it causes signs and symptoms such as pain, nausea, or vomiting.
_____ b. Most cardiovascular problems are not serious and can be readily treated or controlled with diet, exercise, and medication.
_____ c. All suspected cardiovascular disorders must be considered serious until they are evaluated by a physician.
_____ d. Although potentially serious, most cardiac problems are not truly emergent, and thus transport need not be rushed.

**15-7** Describe and demonstrate how to assess a patient with a cardiovascular emergency.

## Note

### What Is Nitroglycerin?

Nitroglycerin is a medication that causes both arterial and venous dilation. Dilation of the coronary arteries during myocardial ischemia improves blood flow to the myocardium. Dilation of the peripheral blood vessels reduces the amount of blood that enters the heart, which also decreases the heart's overall workload. Nitroglycerin is commonly prescribed to patients who have a history of angina. It comes in several forms, including a paste or patch that is applied directly to the skin, a pill that is placed under the tongue, and a metered spray that is applied beneath the tongue.

**perfusion** the delivery of oxygen and nutrient-rich blood to tissues.

# Assessment

Begin your assessment as you would for any patient—by ensuring that the scene is safe. Next, perform a primary assessment in which any problems related to the ABCDs are addressed. Patients in SCA will be unresponsive, apneic, and pulseless, so immediately begin CPR as described later in this chapter.

Once the ABCDs are stable, begin a secondary assessment by obtaining a SAMPLE history, paying close attention to any complaints of chest pain and any medications that the patient may be taking, including nitroglycerin or aspirin. Patients experiencing a cardiovascular emergency may have difficulty communicating, so you may have to gather historical information from a relative at the same time you are performing an intervention to stabilize a patient.

If the patient complains of chest discomfort or pain, assess its nature and characteristics using the OPQRST mnemonic. Cardiac chest pain is usually described as either "heavy," "crushing," or "tight." Less commonly, patients with a cardiovascular emergency may describe the pain as "sharp," may indicate that the pain increases during inspiration, or may locate the pain in the chest wall or over the stomach. Be sure to ask patients if the pain stays in one location or radiates into the jaw or down the arm (Figure 15-17■) Such referred pain can indicate an AMI.

Patients with an aortic dissection often describe the pain as "tearing." Depending on the site of the dissection, the pain can be abdominal or acute severe back pain. Patients with pulmonary embolism may describe the pain as "sharp."

Ask patients whether the pain or other symptoms improve with rest or remain constant. Be sure to ask patients if they have taken any medication for the pain. If the answer is yes, ask what was taken and whether the symptoms then went away, diminished, or stayed the same. Also ask about a patient's medical history, including potential CVD risk factors: a previous history of cardiovascular disease, hypertension, diabetes, or smoking. Do not be afraid to ask about the use of street drugs—specifically, cocaine, because its use increases the risk for AMI.

Next, perform a detailed secondary physical exam. This exam may need to be done by another OEC Technician while the first OEC Technician is performing interventions for issues found during the primary survey. Patients with cardiac emergencies are usually short of breath. Carefully assess cardiac output by checking pulses, blood pressure (if you have a blood pressure cuff), the condition of the skin, capillary refill, and level of responsiveness, each of which provides evidence as to whether or not tissue **perfusion** is effective. Assess the skin for color, temperature, and profuse sweating or diaphoresis, which is a telling sign in conjunction with chest pain because it may indicate that the heart is ischemic. Be sure to auscultate the breath sounds to make sure they are present in each lung.

Reassess the patient and the vital signs at regular intervals—every 3–5 minutes if the patient is unstable, or every 10–15 minutes if the patient is stable—and compare the results to previous findings. Vital signs that are deteriorating indicate that a patient has a serious medical problem.

EARLY SIGNS OF ACUTE CORONARY SYNDROME (HEART ATTACK)

**Figure 15-17** Typical sites of chest discomfort and referred pain associated with cardiac emergencies.

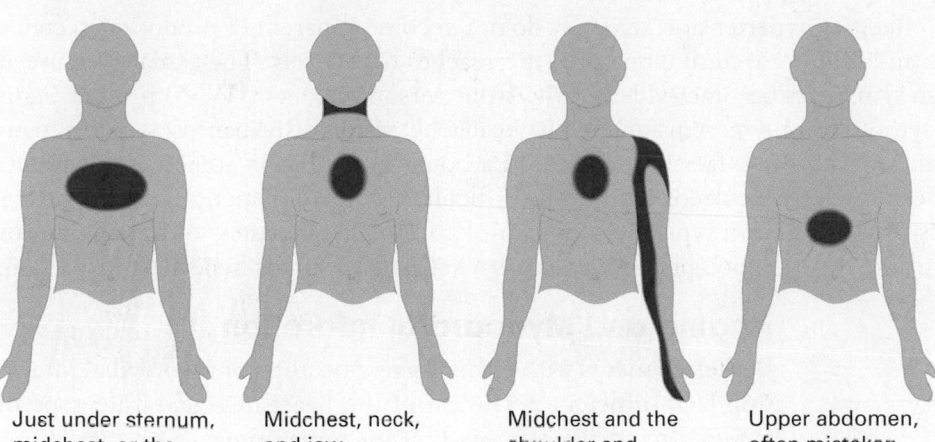

Just under sternum, midchest, or the entire upper chest.

Midchest, neck, and jaw.

Midchest and the shoulder and inside arms (more frequently the left).

Upper abdomen, often mistaken for indigestion.

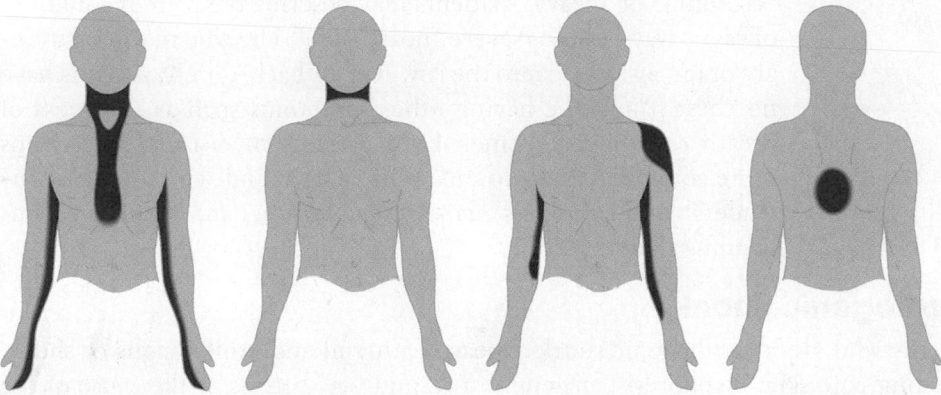

Larger area of the chest, plus neck, jaw, and inside arms.

Jaw from ear to ear, in both sides of upper neck, and in lower center neck.

Shoulder (usually left) and inside arm to the waist, plus opposite arm, inside to the elbow.

Between the shoulder blades.

# CASE UPDATE

After ensuring that the scene is safe, you summon ALS assistance and begin your assessment. You note a pulse of 128 beats per minute, respirations of 28 per minute and shallow, and blood pressure of 164/94. The physical exam reveals an overweight man who is short of breath and appears to be very anxious. He is diaphoretic. He describes the pain as a "9" on a scale of 1 to 10. Upon further questioning, you discover that he has a history of angina pectoris, but according to him, "This is the worst it's ever felt." He also says, "I feel like I'm going to die!"

**What should you do?**

**15-5** List the signs and symptoms for each of the following cardiovascular disorders:

- acute myocardial infarction
- aortic aneurysm
- cardiogenic shock
- congestive heart failure
- pericardial tamponade
- pulmonary embolism

## Hypertension

The effects of hypertension generally do not become apparent or produce detectable signs and symptoms until blood pressure reaches high levels. The actual pressure at which symptoms become evident varies from person to person. When present, signs and symptoms of hypertension include headache, vision disturbances, seizures, nausea and/or vomiting, facial flushing, and a bounding pulse. In some cases, patients may experience nosebleeds that can be difficult to control. Patients with dangerous levels of hypertension typically complain of chest pain, shortness of breath, and/or confusion. Take a blood pressure to assess whether a patient is hypertensive.

## Angina and Myocardial Infarction

Because patients with either angina pectoris or myocardial infarction lack sufficient perfusion of the heart muscle, either type of patient may present with the same signs and symptoms (Figure 15-18■). Patients may or may not complain of chest pain or chest discomfort. Although the chest pain is often described as "crushing" or "heavy," patients may describe the pain in a number of vague ways, even as severe "heartburn." The pain may be stationary or it may radiate into the jaw, arm, or back. Rarely, patients have no chest pain while having other symptoms such as shortness of breath or fatigue. Women have painless myocardial infarctions more commonly than do men. Other signs and symptoms may include anxiety, dizziness, nausea, diaphoresis, and feelings of impending doom or death.

> **NOTE**
>
> ### Silent MI
>
> Silent MI refers to a condition in which a patient is having AMI without chest pain. Although silent MIs are common in women, diabetics, and the elderly, they can (and often do) occur in any population. The term is actually a misnomer, because patients having an AMI will always have some symptoms. The two most common complaints in patients having AMI without chest pain are shortness of breath and fatigue. Other complaints include dizziness, abdominal pain, and nausea.

## Cardiogenic Shock

Patients who are in cardiogenic shock appear deathly ill and exhibit signs of shock, including pale skin, diaphoresis, anxiety, and respiratory distress. If the cause of the shock is AMI, the patient will likely be tachycardic and hypotensive. If the cause of

**Figure 15-18** Because both MIs and angina may present with similar symptoms, treat all causes of chest pain as a cardiac emergency.

### DISTINGUISHING ANGINA PECTORIS FROM MYOCARDIAL INFARCTION

|  | Angina Pectoris | Myocardial Infarction |
|---|---|---|
| Location of Discomfort | Substernal or across chest | Same |
| Radiation of Discomfort | Neck, jaw, arms, back, shoulders | Same |
| Nature of Discomfort | Dull or heavy discomfort with a pressure or squeezing sensation | Same, but maybe more intense |
| Duration | Usually 2 to 15 minutes, subsides after activity stops | Lasts longer than 10 minutes |
| Other symptoms | Usually none | Perspiration, pale gray color, nausea, weakness, dizziness, lightheadedness |
| Precipitating Factors | Extremes in weather, exertion, stress, meals | Often none |
| Factors Giving Relief | Stopping physical activity, reducing stress, nitroglycerin | Nitroglycerin may give incomplete or no relief |

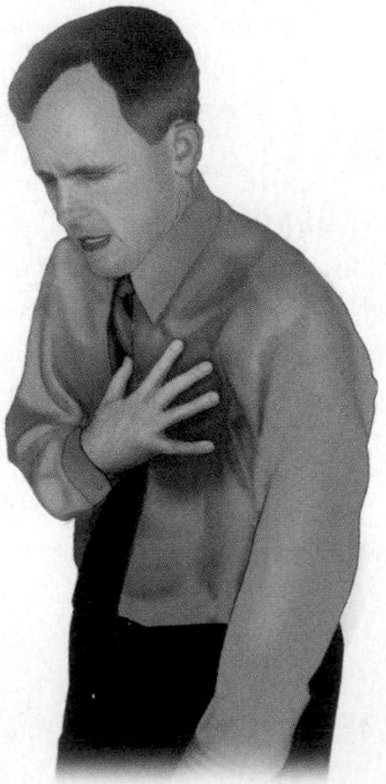

the shock is an abnormal heart rhythm, the patient may be bradycardic or tachycardic and hypotensive. Because MI is the primary cause of cardiogenic shock, any patient with suspected AMI should be evaluated for decreased perfusion and shock.

## Congestive Heart Failure

Patients with congestive heart failure (CHF) can display a wide range of signs and symptoms, depending on which side of the heart is affected (Figure 15-19■). For instance, right congestive heart failure causes edema in the lower extremities, manifested by swollen ankles that may or may not be painful to the touch. With time, the swelling can become severe and may progress up the leg. Pressing the swollen area gently pressed with a finger may leave an indentation. This sign, known as "pitting edema," is a common finding. The more pronounced the swelling, the more severe are the effects of heart failure. Because left congestive heart failure causes blood to back up into the lungs, patients may have shortness of breath that may be mild or a profound dyspnea with audible "bubbling" sounds or gasping breaths due to fluid in the lungs. Patients may have both right-sided and left-sided CHF at the same time.

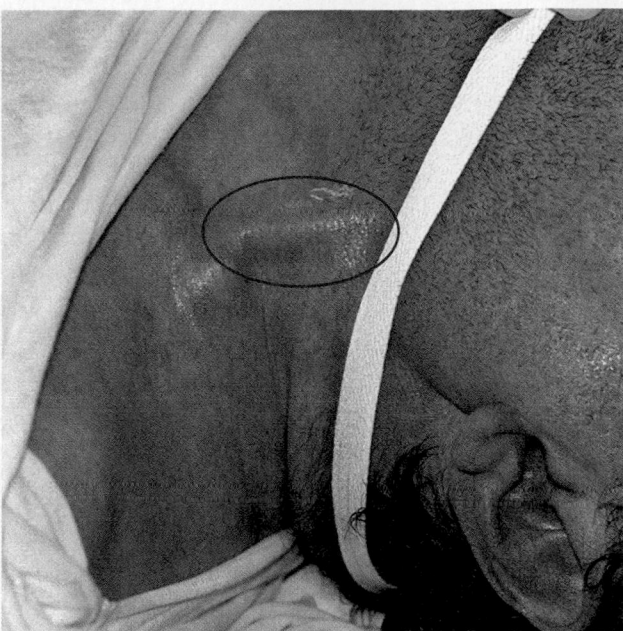

**Figure 15-19** A distended jugular vein is a late sign of congestive heart failure.
Copyright David Effron, MD

Congestive heart failure usually has a slow onset, developing over days, but rarely it can have a rapid onset, developing within minutes. A patient that has a rapid accumulation of fluid in the lungs due to congestive heart failure is often said to be in "flash pulmonary edema," a life-threatening emergency. Failure of the left ventricular muscle from a severe AMI to this part of the heart is the most likely cause.

## Pericardial Tamponade

As with cardiogenic shock, patients with pericardial tamponade appear gravely ill. Most are short of breath, appear anxious or restless, and have pale, cool, diaphoretic skin. Chest pain is common, as are tachycardia and hypotension due to decreased cardiac output. The hallmark signs of pericardial tamponade are hypotension, distended neck veins, and (for advanced responders) muffled or distant heart tones in which the heart beat is difficult to auscultate due to excessive fluid within the pericardial sac. Additionally, the pulse pressure narrows meaning the systolic and diastolic pressures get closer. This is because the left ventricle cannot force as much blood out, because the fluid in the pericardium limits the filling capacity of the left ventricle. Also, there may be a rise in diastolic pressure due to the external pressure on the heart. However, patients with gradual onset pericardial tamponade may initially present with fatigue and tachycardia only.

## Aortic Aneurysm/Dissection

A patient with a thoracic aortic dissection commonly complains of severe chest pain and occasionally back pain described as tearing, ripping, or stabbing. The pain frequently radiates to the back between the shoulders. Unless the dissection has ruptured, the patient may be hypertensive.

Abdominal **aortic aneurysms** often present with abdominal pain radiating to the groin or back pain. These patients also may complain of dizziness. On examination, the patient's abdomen may be tender and you may feel a large pulsatile mass in the abdomen. If the aneurysm ruptures, the patient goes into profound shock with hypotension and diaphoresis and is at great risk for dying. Be sure to assess vital signs and note any abnormalities.

**aortic aneurysm** an abnormal dilation, bulging, or ballooning of the aorta.

## Thromboembolism

The hallmarks of pulmonary embolism are a sudden onset of chest pain, shortness of breath, and tachycardia. The pain is often described as "sharp" and increases with deep breaths. The patient also may be cyanotic. If you have a pulse oximeter, you should find the patient to be hypoxic.

For patients you suspect have pulmonary embolism, look for the presence of deep venous thrombosis (DVT). The signs and symptoms of DVT typically affect only one leg and include severe pain, tenderness to touch, and swelling, usually in the calf. The most dangerous deep vein thrombi form in the larger pelvic veins and are often asymptomatic (without symptoms) until they break loose from within the vessel and cause pulmonary embolism. While finding a DVT will not affect your acute management, it can help support the diagnosis.

⊕ 15-8 ) Describe and demonstrate the proper care of a patient with a cardiovascular emergency.

# Management

Time is of the essence when caring for a patient with a suspected life-threatening cardiovascular problem. If the patient is having AMI, the more time that passes without medical intervention, the greater the extent of the myocardial infarction, the greater the heart damage, and the more likely this situation will proceed to sudden cardiac arrest. Studies also show that SCA occurs most often within the first hour of AMI. Accordingly, transport and ALS assistance should be requested immediately. Also call for oxygen and an AED as soon as possible. Initial care is directed toward correcting any problems related to the ABCDs. If the patient is having severe difficulty breathing, make sure the airway is open, assist the patient's breathing efforts, and provide high-flow oxygen with a nonrebreather mask.

## Care for Patients in Cardiac Arrest

During assessment, always evaluate the ABCDs and treat problems as they are found. However, for that small percentage of patients that are unresponsive, pulseless, and apneic, recognize the primary problem is lack of circulation and immediately begin CPR. Any *unresponsive* patient should be assessed following an ABCD approach.

After opening the airway, simultaneously check for breathing and a pulse. If a patient is in cardiopulmonary arrest as indicated by absent breathing and an absent pulse, begin **basic life support** measures immediately. If a patient is not breathing, or has no normal breathing (gasps), and after assessing the pulse, you are not sure about the presence of a pulse, assume the patient is in cardiac arrest. Effective cardiac resuscitation centers on implementing each of the following five interdependent life-saving links in the chain of survival:

**basic life support (BLS)** a basic level of EMS care for which providers are trained and authorized to provide basic interventions, including noninvasive airway devices, application of oxygen, CPR, and basic first aid.

1. Immediate recognition of cardiac arrest and activation of the emergency response system
2. Early CPR that emphasizes chest compressions
3. Rapid defibrillation if indicated
4. Early and effective advanced life support
5. Integrated post-cardiac arrest care

### Immediate Recognition of Cardiac Arrest and Activation of the Emergency Response System

Immediate recognition of cardiac arrest and activation of the emergency response system is the first link in the chain of survival, and focuses on recognizing the signs and symptoms of SCA and summoning trained medical personnel and appropriate

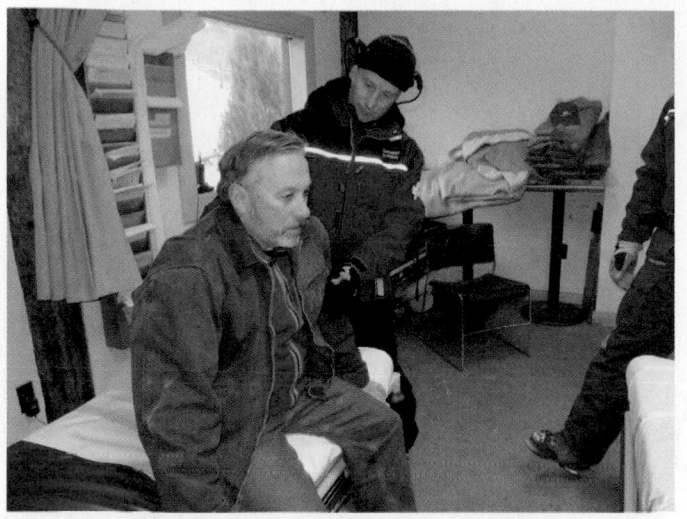

**Figure 15-20a** Early access is the key to survival; rescuers need to know the signs and symptoms of heart attacks.
Copyright Edward McNamara

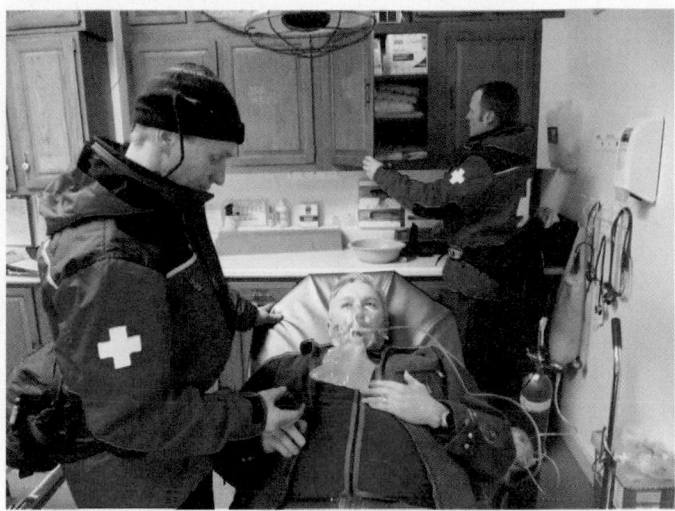

**Figure 15-20b** Early treatment and specialized medical equipment is a part of successful patient care.
Copyright Edward McNamara

specialized equipment (Figures 15-20a■ and 15-20b■). Delays in seeking assistance or providing needed care significantly decrease the patient's chances of survival. To assess for cardiac arrest in an unresponsive patient, rapidly open the airway and simultaneously check breathing and pulse for no more than 10 seconds.

### Early CPR Emphasizing Chest Compressions

Survival rates fall drastically when CPR is delayed. Because of this, CPR must be initiated as quickly as possible to anyone needing it. The goal of effective CPR is to pump oxygenated blood from the heart to other vital organs. The most critical step in the performance of CPR is the effective use of chest compressions, minimizing any interrupton of compressions. The current philosophy in cardiopulmonary resuscitation care is "Push hard, push fast" (at least 100 times a minute) while allowing time for full recoil of the chest to occur. Once begun, CPR should not be stopped unless:

+ The patient improves [Return of Spontaneous Circulation (ROSC)].
+ An AED has been attached to the patient and is ready to be used. The emphasis in the current approach is to not stop compressions until the AED is attached, powered on and ready to analyze.
+ Rescuers are too tired to continue.
+ Care has been transferred to another health care provider of equal or higher competency.
+ The patient is declared dead.

To perform one-rescuer CPR on an adult, take the following actions (Figures 15-21■, 15-22■; 15-23■):

1. Establish unresponsiveness by tapping the patient's shoulder and shouting, "Are you alright?" If spine injury is suspected, shout but do not shake the patient.

---

**CPR Technique**

NOTE

CPR technique for most age groups is the same. The exceptionis the newborn, listed separately below. Begin with 30 compressions, pushing one third the depth of the chest. Then give two breaths. Complete 5 cycles.

**Newborn:** *Start with 30 seconds of ventilation then compression to ventilation ration with be 3:1. 90 compressions and 30 rapid and very small breaths to achieve approximately 120 events per minute*

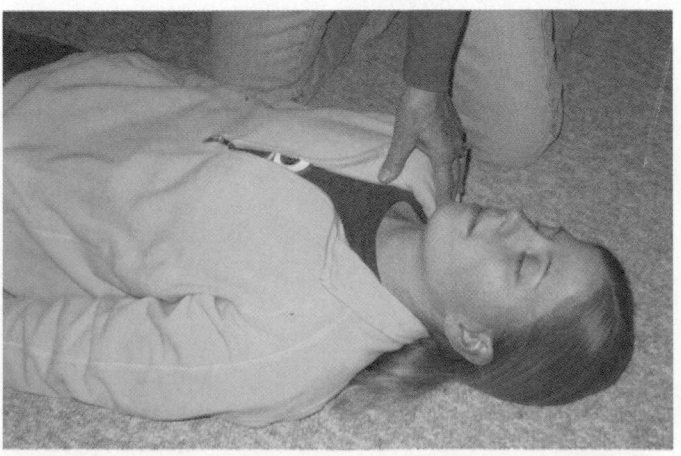

**Figure 15-21** One-rescuer CPR on an adult. Establish unresponsiveness by tapping the patient's shoulder and shouting, "Are you alright?"
Copyright Edward McNamara

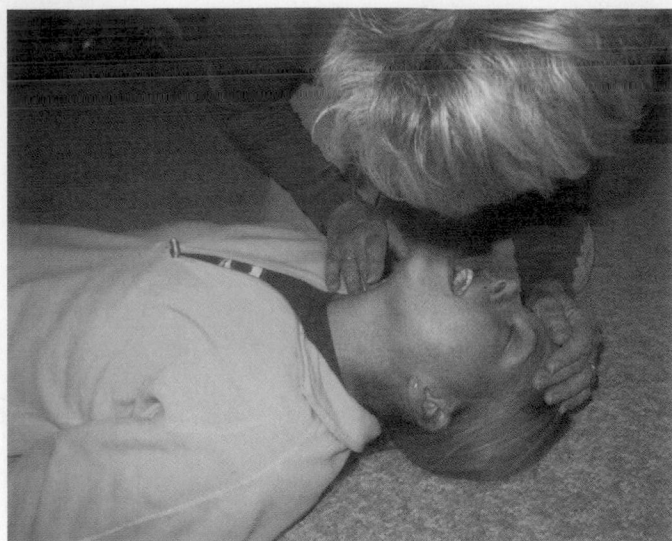

**Figure 15-22** Open the airway and simultaneously check for a carotid pulse and breathing for no longer than 10 seconds.
Copyright Edward McNamara

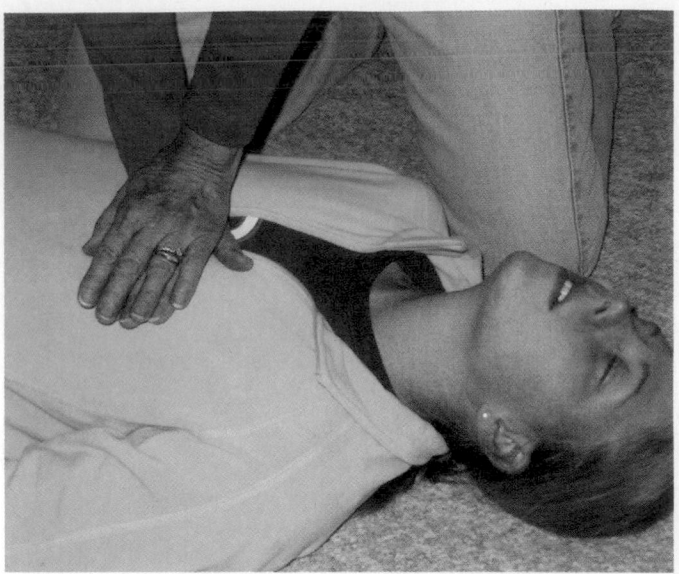

**Figure 15-23** Administer 30 chest compressions at a rate of at least 100 compressions per minute.
Copyright Edward McNamara

⊕ 15-10  Describe and demonstrate how to perform CPR on the following:

• an adult
• a child
• an infant

2. Open the airway and simultaneously check for a carotid pulse and breathing for no longer than 10 seconds. If there is no pulse or you are unsure there is a pulse, and apnea or gasping is present, immediately call for additional personnel, ALS, AED, transport, and oxygen.

3. If possible place the patient in a supine position on a hard, flat surface. Begin CPR using chest compressions prior to performing rescue breathing.

4. Administer 30 chest compressions at a rate of at least 100 compressions per minute. Place the heel of one hand on the center of the patient's chest (lower half of the sternum) and the heel of the other hand on top so that the hands are parallel and overlapped. Compression depth for the adult should be at least 2 inches, with compression and recoil times equal. Always allow the chest to completely recoil after each compression. For one-rescuer CPR, after 30 compressions open the airway and give two rescue breaths, then immediately continue chest compressions. Continue this technique in a 30 to 2 ratio (The combination of 30 compressions and two ventilations equals one cycle).

   The airway should be opened prior to giving breaths using the head tilt chin lift method unless there is a possibility of a cervical spine injury and then you should use the jaw thrust maneuver. Deliver each rescue breath over 1 second providing enough air to produce a visible rise in the chest. Allow complete chest recoil before the next breath is given.

5. Perform five cycles of CPR (approximately 2 minutes). If another rescuer is available, you can switch chest compressions (and respirations) with another rescuer.

6. If there is a pulse but there is no breathing, continue with rescue breaths at a rate of 1 every 5 seconds.

7. In some cases it may be necessary to briefly stop CPR, for example when an AED is delivering a shock or when moving from compressions to giving breaths. Attempt to keep these interruptions to a minimum and no longer than 10 seconds if possible. Interruptions in chest compressions for pulse check should be minimized even to determine if ROSC has occurred.

As other OEC Technicians arrive, continue performing CPR using two rescuers. To perform two-rescuer CPR on an adult, take the following actions:

1. Rescuer #1 (the rescuer actively performing CPR upon the arrival of Rescuer #2): Complete the current CPR cycle.
2. Rescuer #2:
   - Kneel beside the patient next to the chest (in preparation of performing chest compressions).
   - Assess the effectiveness of CPR while Rescuer #1 finishes the current cycle (check for the presence of a *carotid pulse*).
3. Rescuer #1: After completing the cycle of 30 chest compressions and two rescue breaths, remain positioned by the patient's head.
4. Rescuer #2: Administer 30 chest compressions at a rate of at least 100 compressions per minute. Place the heel of one hand on the center of the patient's chest (lower half of the sternum) and the heel of the other hand on top so that the hands are parallel and overlapped. Compression depth should be 2 inches. Count out loud, stopping momentarily after 30 compressions to allow Rescuer #1 to administer 2 rescue breaths.
5. Rescuer #1: Administer 2 rescue breaths.
   - Deliver each breath over 1 second.
   - Give enough air to produce a visible rise in the chest, allowing the chest to fully recoil between breaths.
6. Repeat steps 3–5 for approximately 2 minutes, then switch places and resume CPR; switch places every 2 minutes if the rescuer giving compressions tires.
7. If the patient has an adequate pulse but is not breathing, continue giving one rescue breath lasting 1 second every 5 seconds while further assessing circulation.

To perform CPR on a child who is one year to twelve years old (adolescence), follow these steps (Figures 15-24■, 15-25■; 15-26■):

1. Establish unresponsiveness by shaking the patient and shouting at him. If spine injury is suspected, shout but do not shake the patient.
2. Call for additional personnel, ALS, AED, transport, and oxygen.
3. Open the airway (The airway should be opened using the head-tilt, chin-lift method) and simultaneously check for a pulse *(carotid or femoral)* and breathing for no longer than 10 seconds. If no pulse or you are uncertain if you can find a pulse, and apnea (or ineffective gasps) Place the patient in a supine position on a hard, flat surface
4. Immediately begin CPR.
5. Administer chest compressions at a rate of at least 100 per minute. Push hard with at least enough force to depress one third of the diameter of the chest or approximately 2 inches.
   - Compress the lower half of the sternum.
   - Don't compress the ribs or xyphoid.

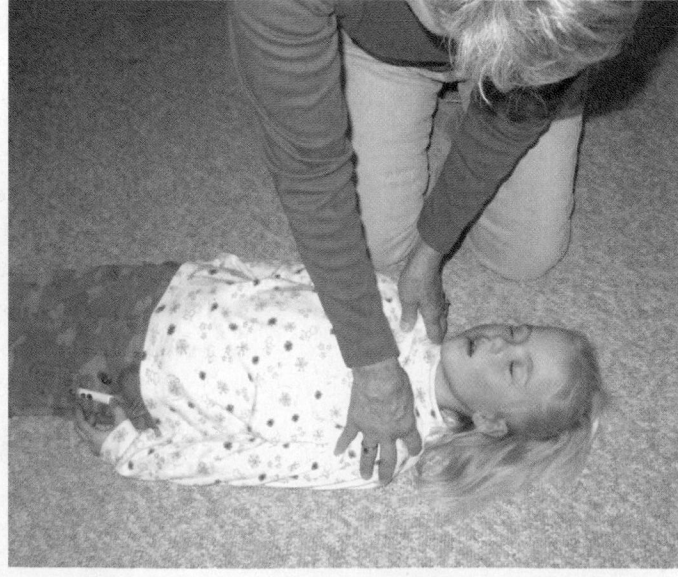

**Figure 15-24** Performing CPR on a child. Establish unresponsiveness by shaking the patient and shouting at her.
Copyright Edward McNamara

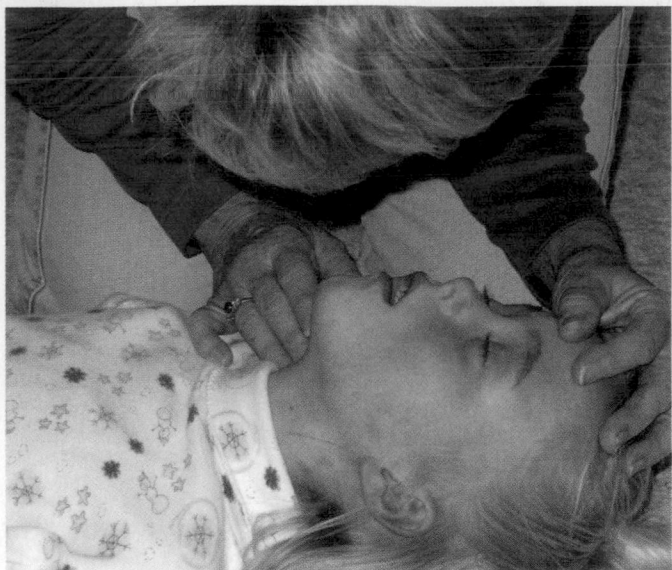

**Figure 15-25** Open the airway and simultaneously check for pulse (carotid or femoral) and breathing for no longer than 10 seconds.
Copyright Edward McNamara

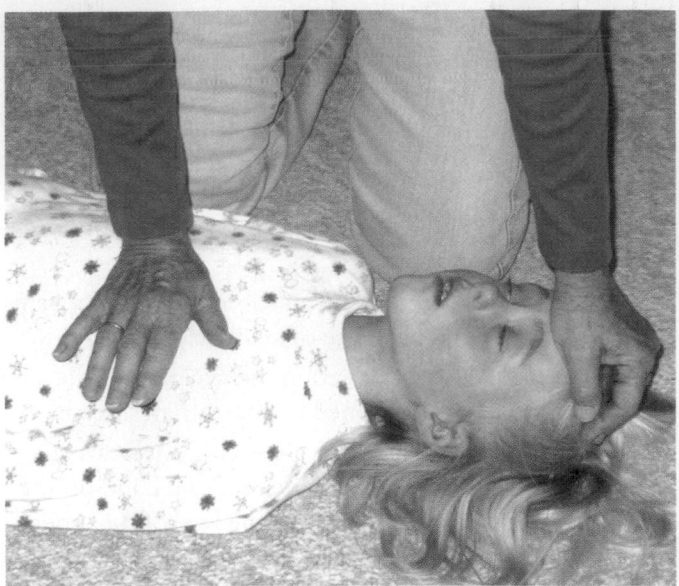

**Figure 15-26** Administer chest compressions at a rate of at least 100 per minute.
Copyright Edward McNamara

- Use the heel of one hand or two hands one on top of the other.
- Allow complete recoil after each compression.

**6.** For one-rescuer CPR, after 30 compressions give two rescue breaths. (The combination of 30 compressions and two ventilations equals one cycle).

When giving rescue breaths:

- Deliver each breath over 1 second.
- Give enough air to produce a visible rise in the chest and allow the chest to fully recoil before the second breath.
- CPR cycles should follow a 30 compressions to 2 breaths ratio.

**7.** If the patient has an adequate pulse (greater than 60 per minute) but is not breathing, continue giving one rescue breath every 3 to 5 seconds, or at a rate of 12 to 20 per minute.

To perform CPR on an infant, conduct the following steps (Figures 15-27■, 15-28■):

**1.** Open the airway using the head tilt chin lift method and simultaneously check for breathing and a *brachial* pulse for no longer than 10 seconds.

**2.** If there is no pulse and patient is apneic or has gasping respirations, call for additional personnel, ALS, AED, transport, and oxygen.

**3.** Place the infant in a supine position on a hard, flat surface.

**4.** Administer 30 chest compressions at a rate of at least 100 compressions per minute.

- Place two fingers on the sternum just beneath an imaginary line between the nipples. (For two rescuer, one rescuer should use the two thumb encircling technique).
- Compression depth should be approximately one-third the depth of the chest or 1 1/2 inches.
- Do not compress over xyphoid or ribs.

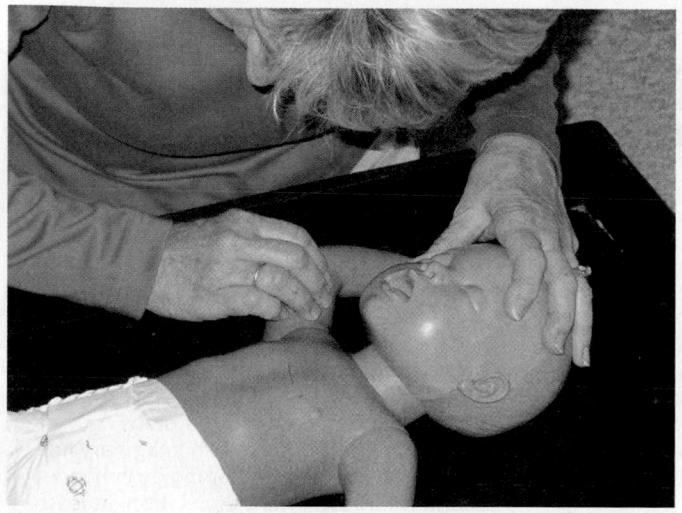

**Figure 15-27** CPR on an infant. Open the airway and simultaneously check for breathing and brachial pulse for no longer than 10 seconds.
Copyright Edward McNamara

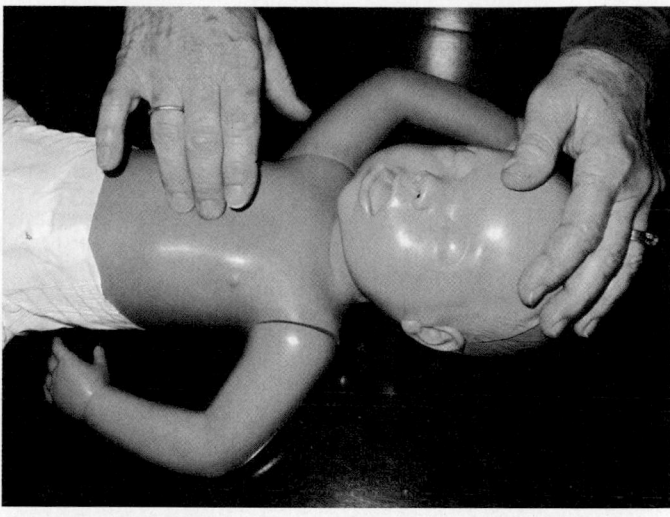

**Figure 15-28** Place two fingers on the sternum just beneath an imaginary line between the nipples.
Copyright Edward McNamara

**5.** Give two breaths.
  • Use a mouth-to-mouth or mouth-to-nose technique.
  • Each breath must be at least one second.
  • Insure that the chest rises and then recoils after each breath.
**6.** Repeat steps 3–5 for approximately 2 minutes, and then check for a pulse. If no pulse is present, continue performing CPR, rechecking the pulse every 2 minutes.
**7.** If two rescuers are present, one should handle the rescue breathing while the other performs the chest compressions.
**8.** If the patient has an adequate pulse but is not breathing, continue giving one rescue breath lasting 1 breath every 3 to 5 seconds, or 12–20 per minute.

Rarely the OEC Technician may be faced with performing CPR on a newborn who is in cardiac arrest. Compressions should be started in any neonatal patient who has a heart rate of less than 60 beats per minute. However, ventilations with supplemental oxygen, if immediately available, should be given first to the newborn, at least for thirty seconds. Compressions should be delivered to the lower third of the sternum, depressing the chest, one third of its front to back diameter. Use two fingers on the sternum supporting the neonate's back with the other hand, or circle the chest with both hands and use the two thumbs on the sternum. Following the initial 30 seconds of ventilation, compressions and ventilations should be coordinated to a 3:1 ratio, with 90 compressions and 30 rapid, very small breaths to achieve approximately 120 events per minute. Thus three compressions are followed by one ventilation, with exhalation occurring during the first of the next three compressions (Table 15-2■).

### Early Defibrillation
The third link in the chain of survival is to correct life-threatening arrhythmias such as ventricular fibrillation (VF) and ventricular tachycardia (VT) as soon as possible. While CPR is important to maintain circulation to vital organs, the key is to

> **Common Causes of Cardiac Arrest**
>
> The most common cause of cardiac arrest in children and infants is respiratory failure.
>
> **NOTE**

⊕ **15-11** Describe and demonstrate the proper use of an AED.

**Table 15-2** A Comparison of the CPR Procedures for Adults, Children, and Infants

| | Adult (older than 8 years) | Child (1–8 Years of age) | Infant (younger than 1 year old) |
|---|---|---|---|
| Airway (technique to open) | Head tilt-chin lift or jaw thrust for suspected cervical spine injury | | |
| Breathing (rescue breathing) | Two breaths (rate of one breath per second) | | |
| Circulation (compression landmark) | Center of sternum, between nipples | | Just beneath an imaginary line between the nipples |
| Circulation (compression method) "Push hard, push fast" | Two hands: (the heel of one hand on top of the other parallel and overlapped) | One or two hands: (if two hands, the heel of one hand on top of the other parallel and overlapped) | One rescuer: two fingers on sternum (just below an imaginary line between the nipples); two rescuers: place thumbs on center of sternum, directly below an imaginary line between the nipples, wrapping both hands around the chest. Infant Circulation: at least one third the depth of the chest, approximately 1 1/2 inches. |
| Circulation (compression depth) | 2 inches | Approximately 2 inches | |
| Circulation (rate of compressions) | At least 100 compressions per minute | | |
| Circulation (compression to ventilation ratio) | 30:2 | | |

**cardioversion** the restoration of a normal rhythm of the heart by electrical shock.

**pacemaker** a device that substitutes for the pace-making tissue of the heart; can be surgically implanted.

re-establish cardiac circulation. This is done by **cardioversion**, using a defibrillator. The device used in the field for cardioversion is called an automated external defibrillator (AED). It delivers an electric shock (defibrillation) to convert VT or VF to an effective heartbeat (Figure 15-29■). When an AED delivers a shock, it temporarily stops the heart's electrical activity, thereby allowing the heart's internal **pace-**

**Figure 15-29** An AED. Most AEDs have two capabilities: one for patients ages 8 to adult, and one with separate, smaller pads for children ages 1–8 years.
Copyright Scott Smith

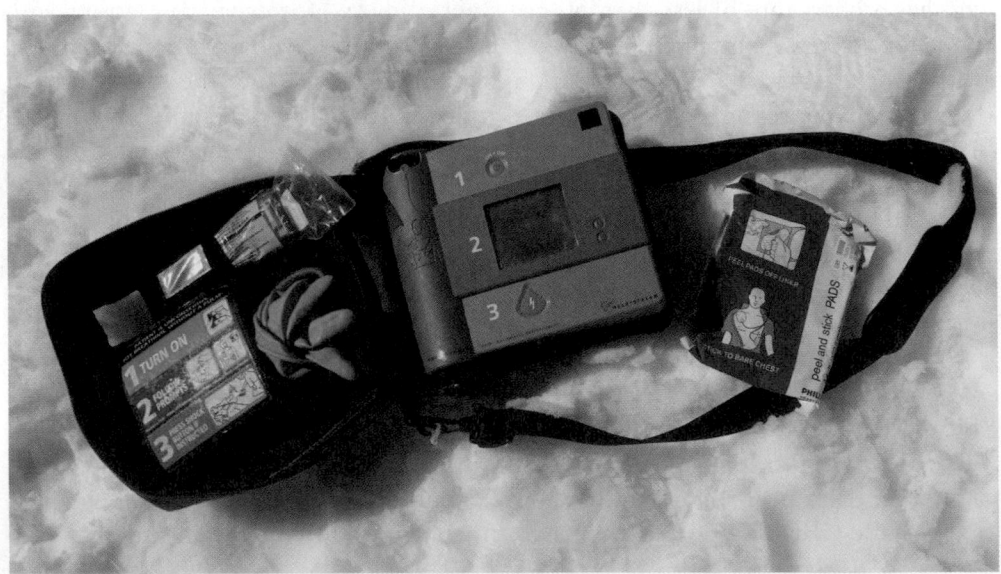

**maker** cells to reset and resume directing the heartbeat in an organized fashion. Since the institution of AED use by both trained and lay rescuers, patient survival from SCA has doubled. However, an AED must be applied quickly, as its effectiveness decreases very rapidly over several minutes. After 10 minutes of pulseless cardiac arrest due to VT or VF, the heart is nearly completely nonresponsive to electrical stimulation. Therefore an AED should be used as soon as it is available. When two trained rescuers are on scene with a patient who has SCA, one person CPR should be performed while the second rescuer seeks an AED.

If CPR is in progress and an AED is available, continue CPR until the AED is opened and the pads are applied. Stop CPR only when the machine is turned on and ready to analyze. Although originally designed for use on adults only, recent studies indicate that an AED may be safely used on cardiac-arrest patients of any age.

For adults and children 8 years and older, use standard adult-sized AED electrodes; for children less than 8 years old, a special energy dose-attenuating cable (which regulates the amount of electrical energy delivered) should be used. While the attenuating device is preferred, in its absence one should still use an AED on a child or infant of any age (Table 15-3■).

To use an AED, follow the AED manufacturer's recommendations. In general, the procedure for using an AED is as follows (OEC Skill 15-1■):

1. While CPR continues, expose the patient's bare chest. Dry the chest if it is wet. If the patient is wearing a nitroglycerin patch, remove it and completely wipe off any remaining nitroglycerin cream.

2. Open the AED case.

3. Remove the AED electrodes (use pediatric electrodes for children and infants <8 years of age when available) and affix them to the patient.

   - Remove the self-stick backing from each electrode.
   - Place the negative electrode (if marked) on the patient's upper right chest (or according to the manufacturer's recommendations). If the patient's chest is especially hairy and the electrode does not stick well, firmly apply the electrode, then rip the electrode away to remove excess hair. Once hair has been removed, affix a new set of electrodes to the chest.
   - Place the other electrode (the positive electrode) on the patient's lateral chest, just below the nipple and above the level of the diaphragm (or according to manufacturer's recommendations).
   - If in a child or infant both pads do not fit on the chest, use a chest and back placement instead.

**Table 15-3** Parameters of AED Use

| | **Adults (8 years and older)** | **Children (1–8 years old)** | **Infants (less than 1 year old)** |
|---|---|---|---|
| Indications | Pulselessness/apnea, ventricular fibrillation, ventricular tachycardia (pulseless) | | |
| AED use recommended? | Yes | Yes | Yes |
| Electrode/cable recommendations | Adult (standard) electrodes/cable | Energy dose-attenuating cable/electrodes | Energy dose-attenuating cable/electrodes |
| | | May use standard adult electrodes/cable | May use standard adult electrodes/cable |

## What Is an AED?

An AED is a portable device that identifies lethal arrhythmias (e.g., ventricular fibrillation or ventricular tachycardia) and tells you to press a button to deliver an electrical shock to restore an effective heartbeat. AEDs are increasingly available in public areas, and most provide step-by-step voice instructions. They are now used by people who have no formal medical training.

## Implantable Devices

Technology has enabled many cardiovascular disorders to be corrected, which has allowed many patients to resume an active lifestyle. For instance, a pacemaker helps the heart maintain a regular heartbeat. An **automatic implantable cardioverter defibrillator (AICD)** detects life-threatening arrhythmias and can apply a shock to the heart that restores a normal heartbeat. Both devices are surgically implanted beneath the skin, typically in the upper left chest. When activated, both devices deliver small electrical shocks that may be felt if you are touching the patient. However, they are very mild and pose no risk to rescuers. An AED may be used on a patient who has either of these implanted devices. The pads should not be placed over the location of the implantable device, which usually is visible as a raised area of skin where the device is located.

**automatic implantable cardioverter defibrillator (AICD)**   an implantable defibrillator that recognizes common lethal heart rhythms and then delivers an electrical shock to the heart to restore an effective heart rhythm.

4. Plug the cable into the appropriate connection port on the AED.
5. Turn the AED on.
6. Stop CPR and loudly instruct everyone to "Stand clear!"
7. Follow the instructions on the AED. In general, the AED should automatically:
   - Analyze the patient's heart rhythm. This may take a few seconds. Do not touch or allow anyone else to touch the patient while the AED is analyzing the patient's heart rhythm.
   - Indicate if an electrical shock is needed. If a shock is indicated, the AED will display or say "Shock Advised." The machine will then automatically charge to the appropriate energy dose. Once complete, the machine will display or say "Deliver Shock." (If the AED displays or says "No Shock Advised," resume CPR until it is time to once again to analyze, usually 2 minutes or five cycles.)
8. If the AED displays "Shock Advised," instruct everyone to "Stand clear!" several times. Look to make sure that no one is touching the patient.
9. Deliver the electrical shock by pressing the appropriate button on the AED.
10. If an acceptable rhythm is not detected, the machine will display or say, "Begin CPR." After approximately 2 minutes, the AED will instruct you to stop CPR.
11. Stop CPR and allow the AED to re-analyze the heart rhythm. If the AED indicates that a shock is advised, shock the patient following steps 8–9 above. If the AED indicates that no shock is advised, check the patient's pulse and treat accordingly.

### Early Advanced Care

The fourth link in the chain of survival is to call for an early response by paramedics. The initiation of IVs, the use of advanced airway techniques, and the administration of cardiac medications is critical to ensuring the survival of the patient.

## Hospital Care of MI Patients

As a result of technological advancements, the survival rate from an MI is high, provided the chain of survival (discussed shortly) is maintained. Once at the hospital, the following therapies may be used to restore effective circulation to the heart:

- *Thrombolytic therapy.* In this approach, medications commonly referred to as "clot busters" are injected into the patient to dissolve any blood clots or thrombi that may be occluding the coronary arteries.
- *Angioplasty.* In this surgical technique, a small balloon is inserted into a blocked coronary artery. Once positioned next to the site of the occlusion, the balloon is inflated, thereby restoring effective circulation.
- *Cardiac stent.* This device, a small wire-mesh tube, is surgically inserted into a formerly blocked coronary artery to keep the vessel open and to prevent its re-occlusion. Stents are commonly inserted following coronary angioplasty.

◆ *Coronary artery bypass grafting (CABG).* **Coronary artery bypass grafting (CABG)** is a procedure that involves taking a blood vessel from the patient's leg, arm, or chest and inserting it in such a way that it bypasses a blocked coronary artery.

**coronary artery bypass grafting (CABG)** an operation that uses grafts of healthy blood vessels to bypass diseased arteries that supply the heart tissue.

**cardiac arrest** cessation of a functional heartbeat.

## Cardiovascular Patients Who Are Not in Cardiac Arrest

Responsive patients with a suspected cardiovascular emergency may go into cardiac arrest at any time. Call immediately for assistance, oxygen, AED, and ALS. Attempt to keep patients calm because doing so will help reduce both anxiety and stress on the heart. Place the patient into a position of comfort. For patients with chest pain, this is usually either a semi-Fowler's or Rothberg position. Place *hypotensive* patients into a supine position and keep them warm. Elevate the feet 8–12 inches above the level of the heart to allow the venous blood in the legs to move into the pelvis and thorax, providing blood volume in the trunk to raise blood pressure. If CHF or pulmonary edema is suspected, the patient will likely prefer to be seated upright because this facilitates breathing. If possible, allow a CHF patient's legs to be in a dependent position (i.e., below the level of the heart), which allows excess fluid to pool in the lower extremities. This can also permit the patient to breathe more easily.

### Oxygen Therapy

Because respiratory distress and myocardial ischemia are commonly associated with cardiovascular-system disorders, it is important to maintain normal blood oxygen levels. In the prehospital environment it is difficult to measure blood oxygen levels, so when clinically indicated, oxygen therapy should be initiated as soon as possible. Administer high-flow oxygen at 15 LPM via a nonrebreather mask (Figure 15-30■). This treatment increases the amount of oxygen available to the heart muscle, which may help reduce the extent of myocardial damage. For CVD patients who are claustrophobic when an oxygen mask is used, continue to calm them as you render care, to avoid worsening their anxiety and increasing oxygen demands on the heart. You may have to weigh the relative risks and benefits of using a mask compared to a nasal cannula. If an agitated patient continues to remove the mask, administering oxygen at 4–6 LPM by nasal cannula is better than no oxygen, but the use of a mask is preferred. In a patient needing CPR, the use of a mask or BVM with high-concentration oxygen attached is highly recommended.

### Nitroglycerin

Some patients with angina pectoris may carry their own nitroglycerin, a medication used to relieve chest pain. As with all prescribed medications, this drug may be used only by the patient for whom it has been prescribed. If the *patient's own* nitroglycerin is available, you may need to assist him in taking this medicine (Figure 15-31■). Check your area, state, or provincial protocols to determine if you are permitted to assist a patient in taking nitroglycerin. Nitroglycerin should be given only to a patient with chest pain who is awake and responsive. It should NOT be given to patients if any of the following contraindications pertain:

◆ the nitroglycerin is expired
◆ systolic blood pressure is less than 100 mmHg

**15-9** List three common cardiac medications.

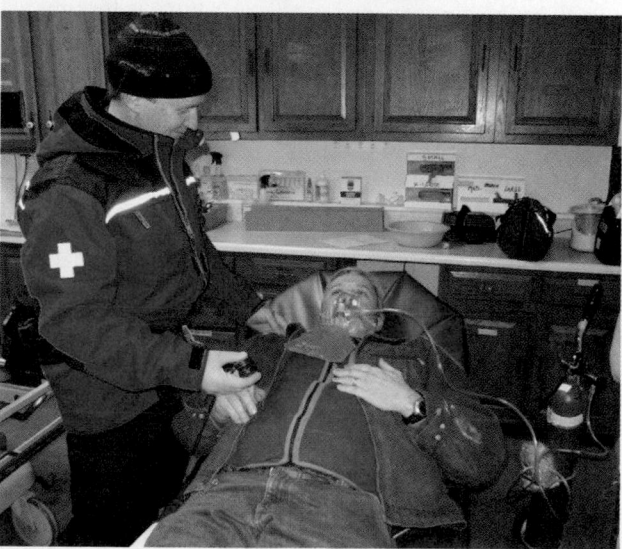

**Figure 15-30** Oxygen therapy may help reduce cardiac pain, cardiac arrhythmias, and damage to the heart muscle.
Copyright Edward McNamara

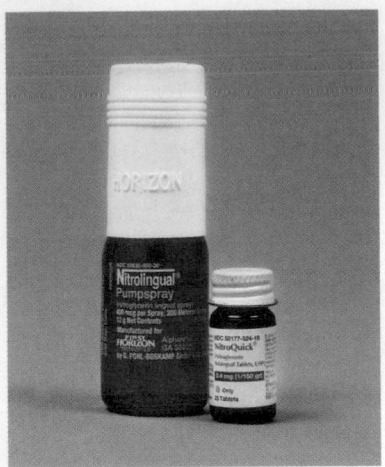

**Figure 15-31** Nitroglycerine may be delivered as a spray or as sublingual tablets for angina pectoris.

+ the patient has taken three does of nitroglycerin for this episode of chest pain
+ the patient has used a medication for erectile dysfunction (e.g., Viagra®, Levitra®, Cialis®) within the past 24 hours
+ chest pain is due to trauma (is not cardiac in origin)
+ the patient admits to taking cocaine

To assist patients in taking their own nitroglycerin tablets, follow these steps:

1. After checking systolic blood pressure to ensure it is over 100 mmHg, contact Medical Direction if that is required by your agency to get permission to administer the nitroglycerine.
2. Check to make sure the medication is prescribed for this patient. Check the drug's expiration date; do not administer if the drug has expired.
3. Put on your disposable gloves, and then remove one tablet from the bottle and place the tablet in the patient's hand.
4. Instruct the patient to place the medication under his tongue and to allow it to dissolve completely. Tell the patient not to chew or swallow the tablet. If necessary, assist the patient by putting the medication in place once the patient has lifted his tongue.

To assist the patient in taking his own nitroglyccrin sublingual spray, follow these steps:

1. After checking systolic blood pressure to ensure it is over 100 mmHg, contact medical direction if that is required by your agency to get permission to administer the nitroglycerine.
2. Check the medication to ensure it is prescribed for the patient. Check the drug's expiration date; do not administer if the drug has expired.
3. Do NOT shake the metered dose spray.
4. Instruct the patient to lift his tongue.
5. Apply one spray beneath the patient's tongue.

If the patient is still experiencing chest pain, you may administer two more doses of nitroglycerin, for a total of three doses, at 5-minute intervals. This total of three doses includes any nitroglycerin the patient may have taken immediately before your arrival on scene. Recheck the patient's blood pressure after each dose. If systolic pressure is less than 100 mmHg, do not give more nitroglycerin.

After taking nitroglycerin, the patient will likely experience a burning sensation beneath the tongue and may get a headache. Both symptoms are normal and indicate that the medication is working properly. Reassure the patient that these are commonly occurring symptoms with this type of medication. Document in the prehospital care report the date, time, and dosage (if known) at which the drug was administered. Reassess the patient frequently for signs of improvement (e.g., decreased severity of pain) and recheck the vital signs at regular intervals.

### Aspirin

Because AMI is caused by a blood clot in a coronary artery, AMI is typically treated with medications, including aspirin that prevents the development of blood clots. Aspirin is not only a very effective medication for preventing the development of blood clots; it is proven to be safe to administer in during myocardial infarction. Therefore, if you suspect a patient is having AMI and you are authorized by your local medical advisor to assist the administration of aspirin, do so. Do not give aspirin to anyone who is either allergic to or sensitive to salicylates (e.g., aspirin, wintergreen). Give aspirin only to patients who are fully responsive and can swallow.

To assist a patient in taking aspirin, follow these steps:

1. Select the proper dosage of aspirin. Use either one adult buffered aspirin (325 mg per tablet) *or* four chewable baby aspirin (81 mg per tablet for total of 324 mg).
2. Check the expiration date of the aspirin; do not use the medication if it has expired.
3. Instruct the patient to chew the aspirin before swallowing it.

As before, document the date, time, and dosage administered. Reassess the patient frequently, including the vital signs.

Whenever possible, minimize the patient's physical exertion because exertion increases the oxygen demand on the heart. This may be difficult, however, in back-country settings, especially if resource availability requires the patient to self-evacuate under his own power. If available, use one of the transportation methods described in Chapter 5, Moving, Lifting, and Transporting Patients.

Conditions such as aortic aneurysm, aortic dissection, pulmonary embolism, and pericardial tamponade all have high mortality rates if life-saving interventions are not rendered quickly. Unfortunately, the field care for these threats to life is limited to treating the patient for shock and providing rapid transportation. Therefore, as soon as conditions permit, transport these or any other cardiovascular patients emergently to a definitive-care facility. Table 15-4■ summarizes some important information concerning common cardiac medications.

So, to summarize, most cardiovascular emergencies need rapid primary assessment, correction of threats to life that may include CPR and the use of an AED, the administration of oxygen, and rapid transport. Always arrange for ALS. If the patient is stable, proceed by gathering a more detailed medical history and conducting a secondary assessment.

## What Does Aspirin Do?

Aspirin blocks the clumping of platelets, components of blood that clump together and stimulate the formation of a clot that repairs a ruptured blood vessel. During acute myocardial infarction, platelets tend to clump together to repair a ruptured plaque within a coronary artery. However, in this case the repair of the ruptured plaque is harmful, because it leads to the formation of a thrombus that can occlude the artery, causing the cardiac muscle distal to the artery to become ischemic and die. Therefore, by blocking the clumping of platelets, aspirin also blocks thrombus formation, thereby preventing the development of a myocardial infarction and if an AMI has occurred, decreasing its level of severity. Aspirin also blocks pain impulses in the CNS and dilates peripheral blood vessels.

**Table 15-4** Common Cardiac Medications

| Drug Name (generic name) | Drug Type | Mechanism of Action |
|---|---|---|
| Plavix (clopidogrel), aspirin | anti-platelet | Prevents clumping of platelets, thereby preventing the formation of clots |
| Nitroglycerin | vasodilator | Causes dilation of both arteries and veins |
| Tenormin (atenolol), Toprol/Lopressor (metoprolol) | beta blocker | Lowers blood pressure, slows the heartbeat |
| Prinivil/Zesteril (lisinopril) | ACE inhibitor | Lowers blood pressure |
| Lipitor (atorvastatin) | statin | Lowers harmful cholesterol levels |
| Lasix (furosemide), HCTZ (hydrochlorothiaizide) | diuretic | Removes excess fluid from the body |
| Cordarone (amiodarone) | anti-arrhythmic | Used to treat certain arrhythmias, makes heartbeat more regular |
| Coumadin/Jantoven (warfarin) | blood thinner | Oral blood thinner, used to treat blood clots, CHF, and certain arrhythmias |

## STOP, THINK, UNDERSTAND

### Multiple Choice

Choose the correct answer.

1. A patient who presents with frothy blood-tinged sputum and hypoxia is most likely suffering from_____
   a. angina pectoris.
   b. acute hypertensive syndrome.
   c. pulmonary edema.
   d. pericardial tamponade.

2. After you have assisted a patient in taking a prescribed dose of nitroglycerin, the patient begins to complain of a burning sensation beneath the tongue and a headache. What is your best course of action?_____
   a. Immediately place the patient into the shock (recovery) position because these symptoms are indicative of an adverse reaction to the medication.
   b. Administer a second dose of nitroglycerin; the headache indicates that the initial dose is not working.
   c. Do not permit the patient to take any more nitroglycerin, because these symptoms indicate an adverse reaction to the medication.
   d. Remind and reassure the patient that these symptoms are a normal occurrence.

3. You have just assisted a patient in self-administering a metered-dose spray of nitroglycerin to a patient who is having chest pains. Five minutes later, the patient is still complaining of chest pains. What is your best course of action?_____
   a. Take the patient's blood pressure. If the systolic BP is greater than 100 mmHg, you may help the patient administer a second dose of nitroglycerin.
   b. Transport the patient immediately to the nearest medical facility because the nitroglycerin has obviously not been effective.
   c. Immediately administer another dose of nitroglycerin because this patient is most likely having an AMI.
   d. Reassure the patient that it takes a few minutes for nitroglycerin to take effect and continue monitoring the patient.

4. A 51-year-old woman you encounter on a hiking trail is complaining of suddenly feeling extremely tired, a little bit nauseous, and "tight" in her chest. She has no significant medical history, takes no medications, and is trim and physically fit. What is your best course of action?_____
   a. Suggest that she "take it easy" for a few minutes because she is probably just fatigued from the hike.
   b. Suggest that she call her doctor when she gets home.
   c. Have her sit down, begin a SAMPLE assessment, and check her vital signs because she may be having an AMI.
   d. Have her sit down, eat a granola bar, and drink some water because she is most likely hypoglycemic and dehydrated.

5. You are assessing a patient who is complaining of chest pains and shortness of breath and whose friends tell you that they were "partying pretty hard last night." What is your best course of action?_____
   a. Have the patient sit down and evaluate for a possible AMI.
   b. Ignore the remark because a patient's personal habits are none of your business.
   c. Tell the patient that he is probably just hung over and to go home and "sleep it off."
   d. Suggest that the patient dissolve two aspirins under his tongue as this will most likely relieve his symptoms.

6. A 45-year-old male patient who is complaining of severe abdominal pain suddenly exhibits the signs and symptoms of profound shock. Even though you are not qualified to diagnose a patient, what is most likely wrong with this patient?_____
   a. He is probably suffering from appendicitis.
   b. He is most likely suffering an AMI.
   c. He may have suffered a ruptured abdominal aortic aneurysm.
   d. You do not yet have enough information to make a determination.

### Short Answer

1. The five links of the American Heart Association's chain of survival are:

   _____

   _____

   _____

   _____

   _____

2. What is the meaning and significance of the expression "Push hard, push fast"?

   _____

   _____

   _____

*continued*

3. A patient suffering from apparent cardiac chest pain refuses to allow you to place a nonrebreather oxygen mask on his face. What is your best course of action?

_____

_____

4. You respond to a request for medical assistance on a long overseas flight. The flight attendant directs you to a 37-year-old male passenger who is complaining of chest pain, shortness of breath, and tachycardia. He states that the pain is "very sharp" and gets worse when he takes a deep breath. You notice that he appears to be somewhat cyanotic. What do you think is going on with this patient? What should you do?

_____

_____

## Matching

Match each of the following signs/symptoms with the cardiac emergency of which it is most likely indicative. (signs/symptoms may be used more than once)

_____ 1. angina

_____ 2. acute myocardial infarction/heart attack

_____ 3. hypertension

_____ 4. deep vein thrombosis

_____ 5. aortic dissection

_____ 6. abdominal aortic aneurysm

_____ 7. right-sided congestive heart failure

_____ 8. left-sided congestive heart failure

_____ 9. pulmonary embolism

_____ 10. pericardial tamponade

_____ 11. cardiogenic shock

a. crushing or heavy chest discomfort
b. pain radiating into jaws, down an arm (referred pain), or into the back
c. "tearing" chest pain; additional pain in the abdomen, or severe back pain, or pain between the shoulders
d. abdominal pain radiating to the groin; dizziness
e. sharp pain, headache, visual disturbances, nausea/vomiting, facial flushing, bounding pulse
f. shortness of breath, anxiety, dizziness, nausea, diaphoresis
g. deathly ill appearance, signs and symptoms of shock
h. swollen ankles or legs
i. shortness of breath, audible "bubbling" breath sounds
j. hypotension, distended neck veins, muffled hearttones/beat, narrowing pulse pressure (drop in systolic BP, rise in diastolic BP)
k. sharp chest pain of sudden onset, shortness of breath, tachycardia
l. recurrent chest pain relieved by nitroglycerin
m. severe leg pain

 # CASE DISPOSITION

You administer oxygen by nonrebreather mask at 15 LPM. Using a rolled-up jacket, you place the patient in the semi-Fowler's position. Soon after ALS personnel arrive, you assist them in transporting the patient to an ambulance waiting at the trailhead. Later, you learn that the patient had a myocardial infarction. He underwent a procedure to open up the blocked coronary vessel and is expected to make a complete recovery.

# OEC SKILL 15-1 | AED Use

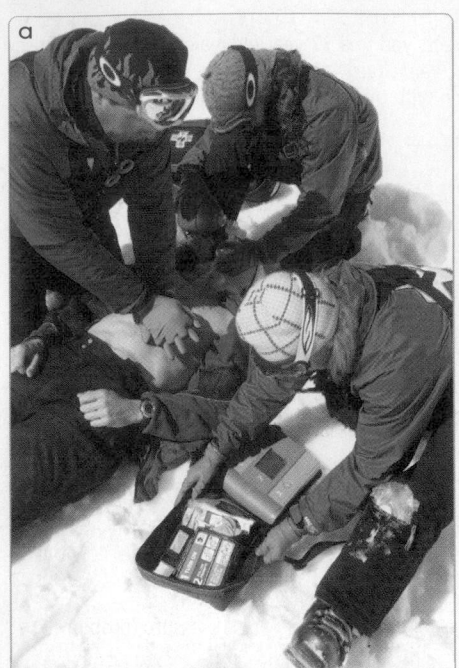

While continuing CPR, expose the patient's bare chest. Dry the chest if it is wet. Remove any nitroglycerin patch and completely wipe off any remaining nitroglycerine cream. Open the AED case.
Copyright Scott Smith

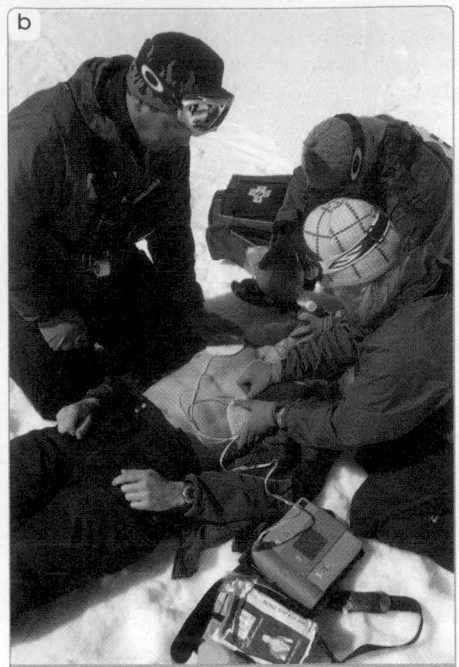

Turn on the AED. Remove the AED electrodes and attach them to the patient's chest. Plug the cable into the appropriate connection port on the AED. Attempt to do this without stopping CPR if possible.
Copyright Scott Smith

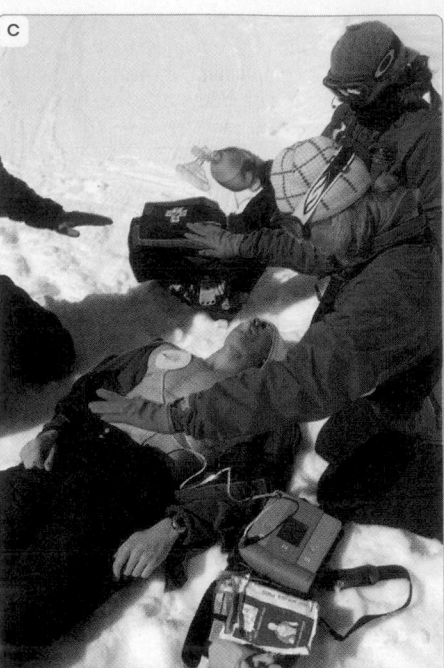

Stop CPR and loudly instruct everyone to "Stand clear!" Follow the instructions on the AED, which should automatically lead you through the steps.
Copyright Scott Smith

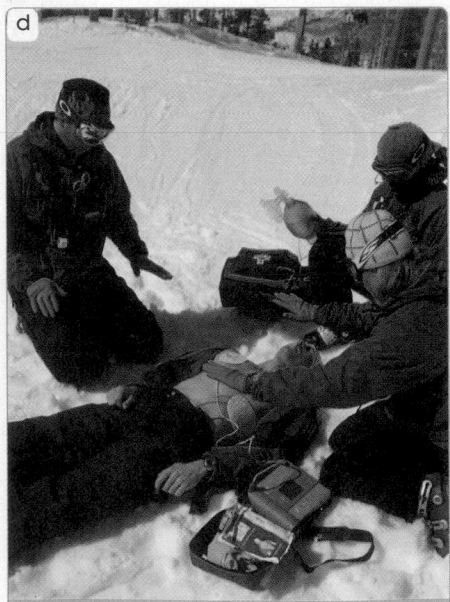

Before you deliver the electrical shock, look to make sure that no one is touching the patient.
Copyright Scott Smith

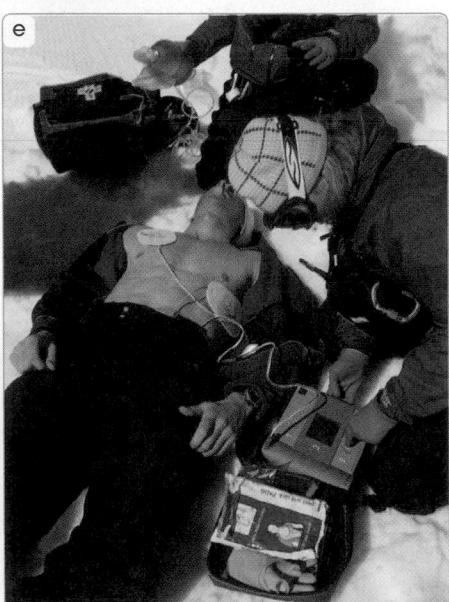

Deliver shock by pressing the appropriate button on the AED. If an acceptable rhythm is not detected, the machine will display, "Begin CPR." After approximately 2 minutes, the AED will instruct you to stop CPR so it can reanalyze. Follow the AED's instructions.
Copyright Scott Smith

# Chapter Review

## Chapter Summary

Cardiovascular disease (CVD) is a common problem that affects millions of people around the world, and it may not be apparent until an emergency occurs. Physical exertion, such as that experienced when engaging in outdoor activities, places increased demands on the heart. If the heart is unable to meet those demands, it can become ischemic and begin to fail. Risk factors such as obesity, smoking, and poor diet all contribute to the occurrence of CVD. So, too, do untreated medical disorders such as uncontrolled hypertension and diabetes, as well as the use of certain illegal drugs.

Given the prevalence of CVD, it is highly likely OEC Technicians will encounter a patient experiencing a cardiovascular-related emergency. As part of the chain of survival, it is essential that OEC Technicians recognize the signs and symptoms associated with SCA and other common CVD-related emergencies early, initiate care quickly, and summon advanced assistance. These actions, in combination with early defibrillation, ALS intervention, and rapid transportation to a definitive-care facility, can significantly improve the survival rate from cardiovascular disease.

## Remember...

1. Cardiovascular disease is the number one cause of death worldwide.
2. If a cardiovascular emergency is suspected, immediately summon ALS assistance.
3. Chest pain and shortness of breath are serious symptoms that may indicate a life-threatening problem.
4. Shortness of breath or fatigue may be the only indications that a patient is having a cardiovascular emergency.
5. Administer high-flow oxygen to any patient complaining of chest pain or shortness of breath.
6. Any patient with chest pain, shortness of breath, or fatigue should be encouraged to seek medical care at a hospital.
7. A responsive patient experiencing presumed cardiac chest pain should be given an aspirin as soon as possible if permitted by local protocol.
8. When performing CPR, "Push hard, push fast" (greater than 100 times a minute), allowing full chest recoil and minimize any interruptions in compressions.
9. AEDs may be used on patients of any age.

## Chapter Questions

### Multiple Choice

Choose the correct answer.

1. The number one cause of death in the United States is_____
   a. motor vehicle accidents.
   b. influenza.
   c. cardiovascular disease.
   d. HIV.

2. How much blood does the average adult heart pump each day?_____
   a. 500 gallons
   b. 1,000 gallons
   c. 1,500 gallons
   d. 2,000 gallons

3. A common finding in someone who is having a "heart attack" is _____
   a. diaphoresis.
   b. a swollen calf.
   c. difficulty swallowing.
   d. all of the above.

4. If a second dose of nitroglycerin is not helpful for a patient with AMI, and you cannot detect his pulse, the first thing you should do is _____
   a. give a third dose of nitroglycerin rapidly.
   b. assess the patient's breathing.
   c. administer oxygen.
   d. start compressions.

**5.** Right-sided congestive heart failure is best described as_____
  **a.** a condition in which the heart muscle is starved for oxygen and slowly dies.
  **b.** blood backing up due to failure of the right side of the heart, which can no longer pump adequately.
  **c.** a sudden nonperfusing arrhythmia.
  **d.** blood backing up from failure of the left side of the heart.

**6.** The most common cause of cardiac arrest in children is _____
  **a.** trauma.
  **b.** blood loss.
  **c.** respiratory failure.
  **d.** septic shock.

**7.** The proper procedure for the oral administration of nitroglycerin is _____
  **a.** to place the medication under the tongue.
  **b.** to chew the medication and then swallow it.
  **c.** to swallow the medication whole.
  **d.** to dissolve the medication in one-quarter cup of warm water.

**8.** The proper procedure for administering a metered-dose nitroglycerin spray is _____
  **a.** to have the patient exhale, then have him inhale while you spray the medication into his mouth.
  **b.** to spray the medication directly into the patient's mouth and instruct him to swallow.
  **c.** to spray the medication under the patient's tongue.
  **d.** to spray the medication into the patient's nostril.

**9.** You suspect a patient may be having a heart attack. Your medical advisor permits you to administer aspirin. How should aspirin be administered to a patient having chest pains?_____
  **a.** It should be placed under the tongue.
  **b.** It should be chewed, then swallowed.
  **c.** It should be swallowed whole.
  **d.** It should be dissolved in a quarter cup of warm water and then drunk.

**10.** A patient who is having "heavy" chest pain tells you that she is allergic to wintergreen. This is particularly important to know in this situation because _____
  **a.** identifying allergies is an important part of the SAMPLE assessment.
  **b.** this patient could be having an allergic reaction to a wintergreen-flavored mint.
  **c.** giving this patient aspirin could cause an allergic reaction.
  **d.** all of the above are true.

**11.** A patient that presents with frothy blood-tinged sputum and hypoxia is most likely suffering from _____
  **a.** angina pectoris.
  **b.** acute hypertensive syndrome.
  **c.** pulmonary edema.
  **d.** pericardial tamponade.

**12.** In the resort's restaurant you encounter a 72-year-old woman who is complaining of suddenly feeling extremely tired and a little bit nauseous, and of a pain in her calf. She has no significant medical history, takes no medications, and is trim and physically fit. What is your best course of action?_____
  **a.** Suggest that she "take it easy" for a few minutes because she is probably just fatigued from skiing too much.
  **b.** Suggest that she call her doctor when she gets home.
  **c.** Have her sit down, begin a SAMPLE assessment, and check her vital signs.
  **d.** Have her sit down, eat a granola bar, and drink some water because she is probably hypoglycemic and dehydrated.

## True or False

Indicate whether each of the following statements is true (T) or false (F).

_____ **a.** A cardiovascular problem is not considered serious until it causes symptoms such as pain, nausea, or vomiting.

_____ **b.** Hypertension can be treated or controlled with diet, exercise, and medication.

_____ **c.** All suspected cardiovascular disorders must be considered serious until they are evaluated by a physician.

_____ **d.** Although potentially serious, most cardiac problems are not truly emergent, and so transport need not be rushed.

# Scenario

*Down at the waterfront you see a small crowd of people gathering around a 60-ish male who is sitting on the ground holding his chest. You identify yourself as an OEC Technician and request permission to help, examine, and treat the man. The scene is safe and you have just one patient.*

*The man informs you that he is having severe chest pain, 8 out of 10 on the pain scale. He has a history of angina and takes nitroglycerine to relieve the pain. This time the patient reports getting no relief after taking one nitroglycerin tablet.*

1. Which of the following symptoms does not typically accompany an angina episode?_____
   a. difficulty breathing
   b. jaw pain
   c. pain radiating down the arm
   d. tearing, ripping, or stabbing pain

*The man reports during the secondary assessment that he did not exert himself, has undergone no trauma, and first noticed the onset of symptoms within the last hour.*

2. You encourage the patient to take another nitroglycerine tablet and assist him in administering it _____
   a. if the patient has taken fewer than three doses of nitroglycerine.
   b. if the patient has taken an erectile-dysfunction medication within 24 hours.
   c. if the nitroglycerine's expiration date has passed.
   d. if it is his wife's nitroglycerine.

*From a secondary assessment and using the OPQRST mnemonic, you learn that the patient is experiencing "tearing" pain radiating from his chest to his back.*

3. Based on the symptoms, you suspect that the patient is experiencing _____
   a. pulmonary embolism.
   b. congestive heart failure.
   c. an aortic aneurysm/dissection.
   d. pericardial tamponade.

4. For a patient who is experiencing chest pain that is not related to trauma and who is not allergic or sensitive to salicylates, OEC Technicians may assist the patient, if authorized by their local medical advisor, in taking _____
   a. 10 mg Prinivil.
   b. one 325-mg adult buffered aspirin.
   c. one 81-mg chewable baby aspirin.
   d. 10 mg Coumadin.

# Suggested Reading

American Heart Association. 2001. *BLS for Healthcare Providers.* Dallas, TX, American Heart Association.

American Red Cross, 2010. *CPR for the Professional Rescuer.* Washington, DC, American Red Cross.

Marx, J., MD, et al. 2002. *Rosen's Emergency Medicine Concepts and Clinical Practice,* Seventh Edition. St. Louis, MO, Elsevier.

Vander, A. J., J. H. Sherman, and D. S. Luciano. 2008. *Human Physiology: The Mechanisms of Body Function,* Eleventh Edition. St. Louis, MO, Elsevier.

# Gastrointestinal and Genitourinary Emergencies

Denis Meade, MA, EMT-P
Michael G. Millin, MD, MPH, FACEP

## ⊕ OBJECTIVES

**Upon completion of this chapter, the OEC Technician will be able to:**

**16-1** List at least six possible causes of emergencies involving the gastrointestinal and genitourinary systems.

**16-2** List the signs and symptoms of emergencies involving the gastrointestinal and genitourinary systems.

**16-3** Compare and contrast visceral pain and parietal pain.

**16-4** Describe and demonstrate how to assess the abdomen.

**16-5** Describe and demonstrate the management of a patient with a severe GI/GU emergency.

## ⊕ KEY TERMS

**guarding,** *p. 500*
**hematemesis,** *p. 504*
**hematochezia,** *p. 504*

**melena,** *p. 504*
**peritonitis,** *p. 500*
**referred pain,** *p. 500*

**sensory nerves,** *p. 500*
**visceral nerves,** *p. 500*

## Chapter Overview

The solid and hollow organs that make up the gastrointestinal and reproductive systems are located within the abdominal and pelvic cavities; however the urinary system is located both posterior to the abdominal cavity in the flanks and within the pelvic cavity. The function of these organs includes digesting food, regulating water balance, eliminating wastes, and reproduction. Because of their relative proximity to each other, their interrelated tasks, and their common nerve pathways, problems affecting one organ or system can seriously affect the others. This explains why the signs and symptoms associated with gastrointestinal and genitourinary problems are

*continued*

## HISTORICAL TIMELINE

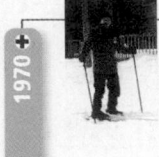

**1970** Warren Bowman becomes NSP National Medical Advisor.

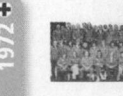

**1972** Geneva Basin ski patrol won outstanding patrol from 1972–1973.

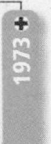

**1973** NSP accepted the 81-hr EMT course as a substitute for ARC training.

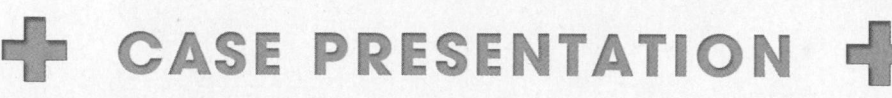

# ✚ CASE PRESENTATION ✚

You are working first-aid duty in the patrol room when a 35-year-old man slowly walks in complaining of severe abdominal pain. You steer the patient to the nearest exam table and begin to assess his condition. Moments later, he vomits. The vomit is clear and does not appear to contain blood. The patient apologizes and states that he started feeling ill this morning but decided to come skiing anyway to be with his family. He has not suffered any recent trauma, and is not currently taking any medications. There is nothing pertinent in the patient's past medical history. He says that he has never experienced anything like this before and describes his abdominal pain as "intense."

***What should you do?***

---

often similar. Understanding the location and basic function of the major organs within the abdominal and pelvic cavities will greatly assist OEC Technicians in identifying common gastrointestinal and genitourinary disorders.

Patients with acute abdominal or pelvic pain can present unique challenges to OEC Technicians. A patient's symptoms may be vague, overlapping, or misleading; patients often do not seek care until their symptoms are unbearable; and severe pain or embarrassment may make patients reluctant to allow a thorough exam. Additionally, assessment of the abdominal and pelvic cavities in outdoor environments can be complicated by external factors such as inclement weather or overly curious bystanders. Transporting a patient with acute abdominal or pelvic pain over uneven or rough terrain for even short distances can be traumatic, for patient and rescuers alike.

Fortunately, caring for patients with an acute abdominal or pelvic problem need not be difficult. With a basic understanding of the anatomy and physiology of abdominal and pelvic structures and of the types of medical conditions that could be encountered, OEC Technicians can effectively manage most GI/GU problems. The goal is not to diagnose the *exact* cause of the problem but to rapidly identify any potentially serious emergency, to render emergency care, and to move the patient quickly toward definitive care (Figure 16-1■).

## GI/GU Anatomy & Physiology

A detailed description of the anatomy and physiology of the abdomen and the pelvic cavity was presented in Chapter 6, Anatomy and Physiology. Several anatomic diagrams are included in this chapter to further your understanding concerning the locations of structures within the four quadrants of the abdomen. These quadrants are formed by two imaginary perpendicular lines that intersect at the umbilicus (Figure 16-2■).

The abdominal and pelvic cavities contain several hollow and solid organs. The hollow organs—the stomach, gallbladder, small and large intestines, appendix, ureters, and urinary bladder—contain materials such as food, bile, feces, and urine. When those materials leak out of one of these structures, due to either a rupture or a laceration during trauma, the result is peritonitis, or inflammation of the peritoneum.

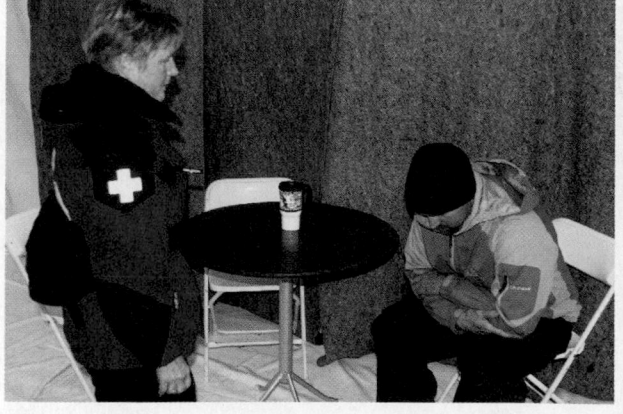

**Figure 16-1** A thorough medical assessment and a good SAMPLE history are important when treating a patient who has abdominal pain.
Copyright Mike Halloran

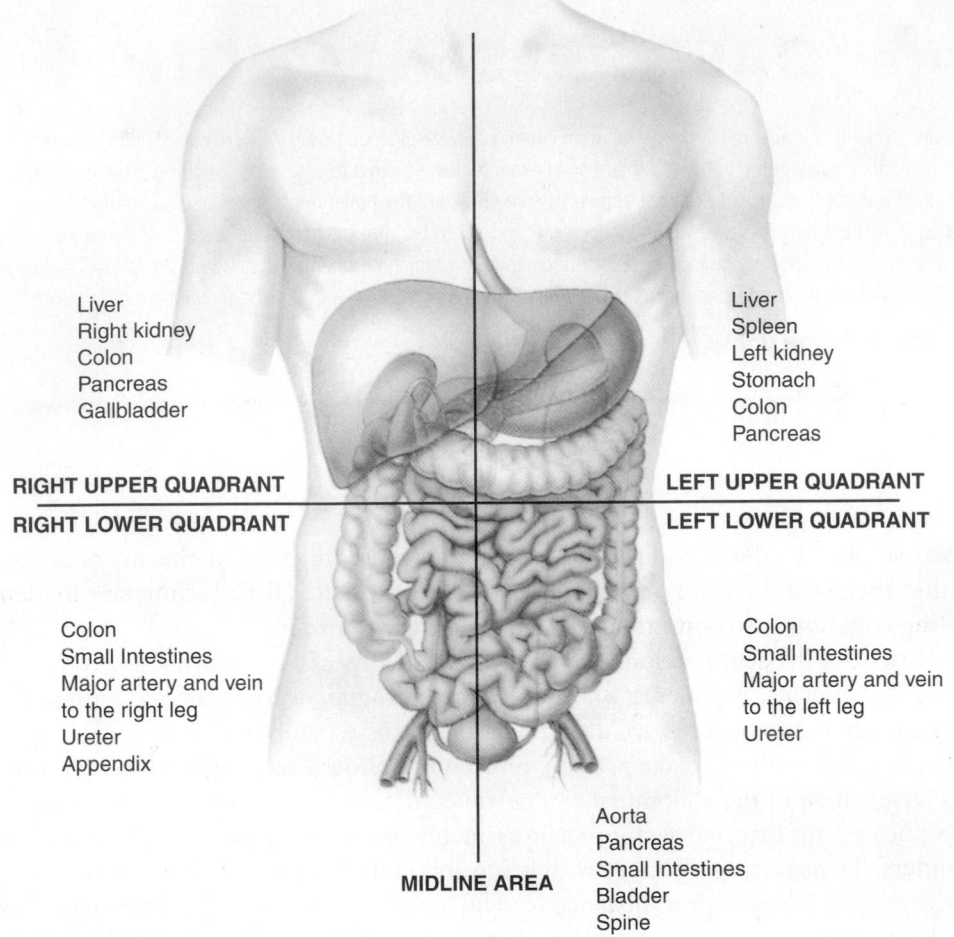

Liver
Right kidney
Colon
Pancreas
Gallbladder

**RIGHT UPPER QUADRANT**

**RIGHT LOWER QUADRANT**

Colon
Small Intestines
Major artery and vein
to the right leg
Ureter
Appendix

Liver
Spleen
Left kidney
Stomach
Colon
Pancreas

**LEFT UPPER QUADRANT**

**LEFT LOWER QUADRANT**

Colon
Small Intestines
Major artery and vein
to the left leg
Ureter

**MIDLINE AREA**

Aorta
Pancreas
Small Intestines
Bladder
Spine

**Figure 16-2** Knowing the structures within the four quadrants of the abdominal cavity is useful when treating a patient who has abdominal pain.

Peritonitis can cause intense abdominal pain, nausea, vomiting, fever, and septic shock. Refer to Chapter 10, Shock, for more detailed information on shock.

The solid organs within the abdomen are the liver, pancreas, spleen, and ovaries. The liver is a chemical powerhouse that makes proteins, synthesizes blood clotting chemicals, and produces bile to aid in the digestion of fat. The pancreas produces digestive enzymes and hormones to regulate blood sugar. The spleen stores blood cells and helps to make antibodies for fighting infections. The ovaries produce eggs that are essential for reproduction. Because the solid organs are highly vascular, damage to them can result in profuse internal bleeding that can lead to hemorrhagic shock.

The kidneys and ureter, which are just outside the posterior abdominal cavity in the flanks, filter and excrete liquid waste and transport it into the bladder in the pelvis. Because they are not inside the abdomen, they are located in the "retroperitoneal" (behind the peritoneum or abdomen) space.

Large blood vessels are also found within the abdominal cavity. The two largest however, are the abdominal aorta and inferior vena cava, which are retroperitoneal and located just in front of the spine (Figures 16-3a■ and 16-3b■). The pelvic cavity contains numerous vascular structures that are generally well protected by the pelvic bones but can be injured during pelvic trauma. Disorders affecting any of the blood vessels within the abdominal, pelvic, or retroperitoneal cavities can quickly lead to life-threatening blood loss, shock, and even death.

**Figure 16-3a** The major arteries of the body.

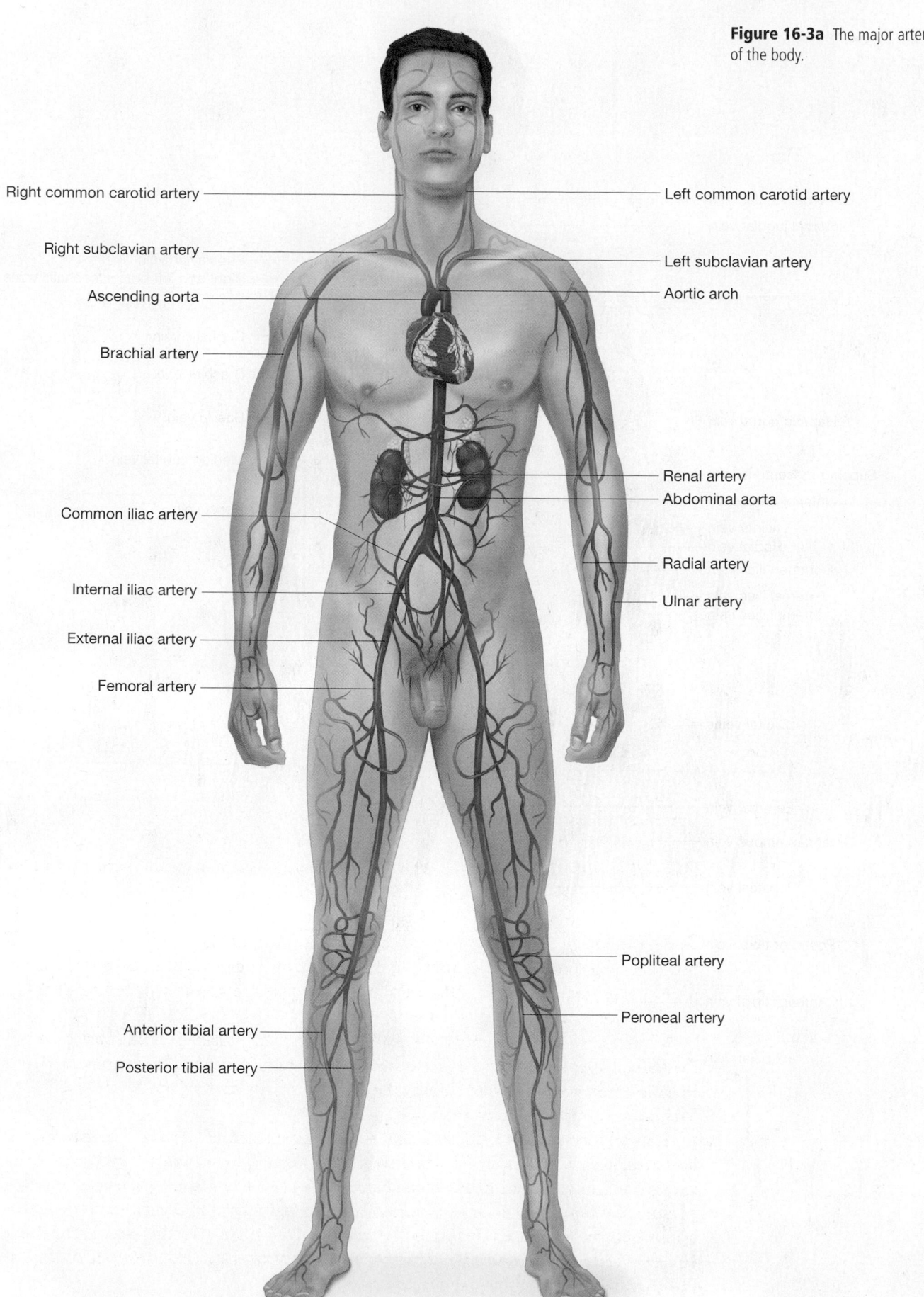

Right common carotid artery

Right subclavian artery

Ascending aorta

Brachial artery

Common iliac artery

Internal iliac artery

External iliac artery

Femoral artery

Anterior tibial artery

Posterior tibial artery

Left common carotid artery

Left subclavian artery

Aortic arch

Renal artery

Abdominal aorta

Radial artery

Ulnar artery

Popliteal artery

Peroneal artery

**Figure 16-3b** The major veins of the body.

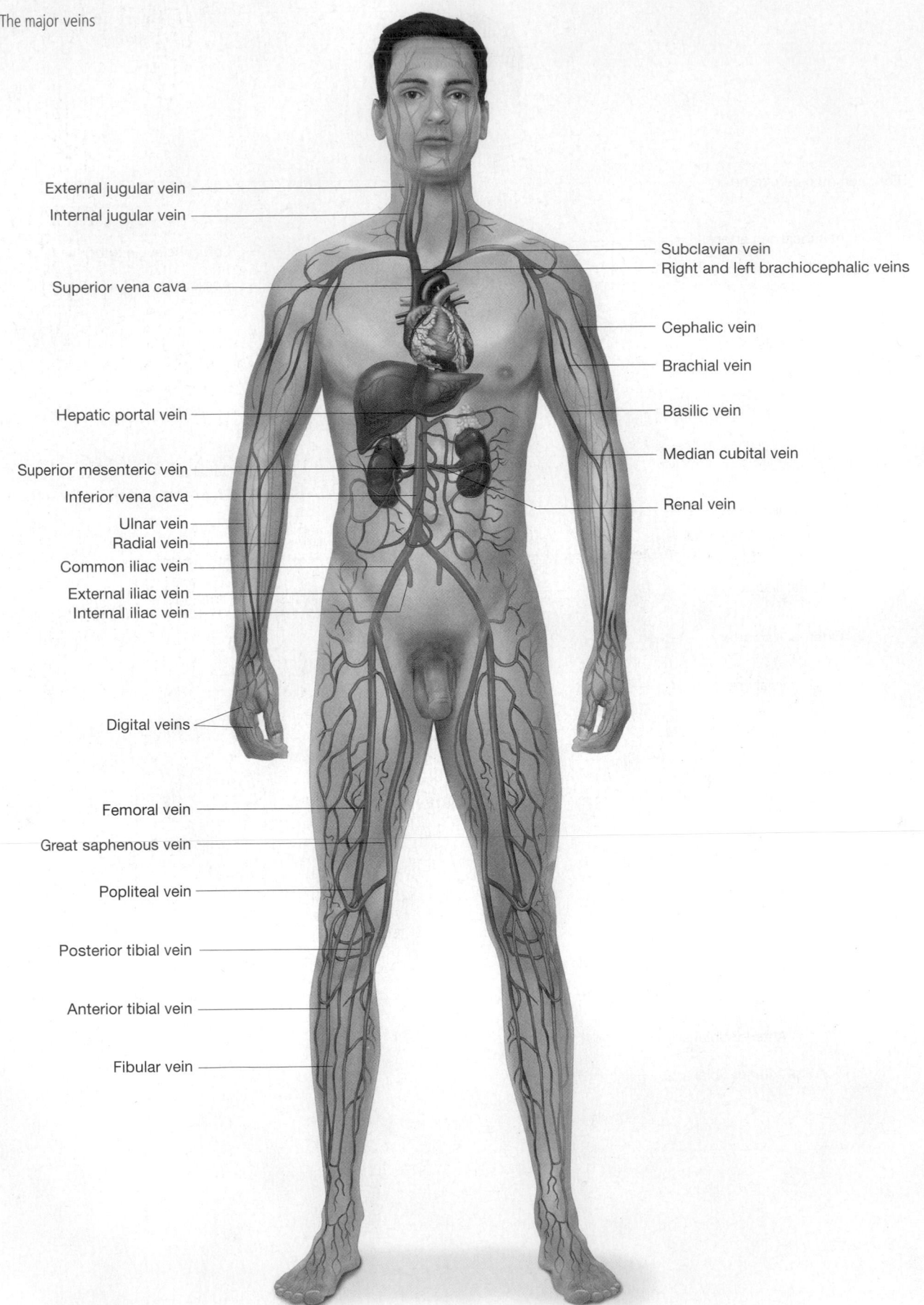

External jugular vein

Internal jugular vein

Superior vena cava

Hepatic portal vein

Superior mesenteric vein

Inferior vena cava

Ulnar vein

Radial vein

Common iliac vein

External iliac vein

Internal iliac vein

Digital veins

Femoral vein

Great saphenous vein

Popliteal vein

Posterior tibial vein

Anterior tibial vein

Fibular vein

Subclavian vein

Right and left brachiocephalic veins

Cephalic vein

Brachial vein

Basilic vein

Median cubital vein

Renal vein

# STOP, THINK, UNDERSTAND

## Multiple Choice

Choose the correct answer.

1. Which of the following statements regarding assessing the abdomen is false? _____
   a. Assessing abdominal complaints can be difficult because the nerve pathways for the gastrointestinal, urinary, and reproductive systems are in relative proximity to each other.
   b. Problems affecting one organ can seriously affect other organs because of the proximity of the organs to one another.
   c. Assessing abdominal complaints is straightforward because abdominal organs are specifically located and easily palpated.
   d. One of the problems encountered in assessing abdominal complaints is a patient's reluctance to allow the exam due to embarrassment or pain.

2. Which of the following statements about the location of the kidneys is true?_____
   a. They lie anterior to the liver and spleen, in the superior region of the peritoneum.
   b. They are located retroperitoneally.
   c. They lie inferior to the pubis symphysis, bilaterally.
   d. They are attached to the diaphragm.

3. Which of the following groups consists of hollow organs?_____
   a. the stomach, bowel, appendix, and ureters
   b. the stomach, gallbladder, kidneys, and ovaries
   c. the liver, pancreas, and spleen
   d. the pancreas, appendix, and urethra

4. Which of the following statements is incorrect?_____
   a. Part of the colon is in the right upper quadrant.
   b. The stomach is in the left upper quadrant.
   c. The ureters are in the abdomen.
   d. The appendix is in the right lower quadrant.

## Short Answer

1. List the four abdominal quadrants, and identify the major organs that are present in each quadrant.
   a. _____
   b. _____
   c. _____
   d. _____

2. What are the two large blood vessels just posterior to the abdominal cavity?

## Matching

Match each of the following organs to its primary function.

_____ 1. liver
_____ 2. pancreas
_____ 3. kidneys
_____ 4. ovaries
_____ 5. urinary bladder
_____ 6. ureters
_____ 7. spleen

a. stores blood cells and makes antibodies for fighting infection
b. stores urine until it can be excreted from the body
c. a chemical powerhouse that makes protein, synthesizes blood clotting chemicals, and produces bile to aid in the digestion of fat
d. produces digestive enzymes
e. filter and excrete liquid waste
f. produce eggs for reproduction
g. transport urine from the kidneys to the urinary bladder

# The Acute Abdomen

Sudden, severe, unexplained pain in the abdomen is referred to as an "acute abdomen" and encompasses many different maladies that occur in the abdominal or pelvic cavities. Rapid recognition of this condition is of paramount importance because more-advanced medical care is often urgently needed. Although many intra-abdominal conditions can result in an acute abdomen, correctly identifying the source of the problem is often difficult. In fact, studies show that upon first examination, physicians accurately diagnose the exact cause of acute abdomen only 50 percent of the time. Thus, as stated previously, it is more important that OEC Technicians are able to recognize that

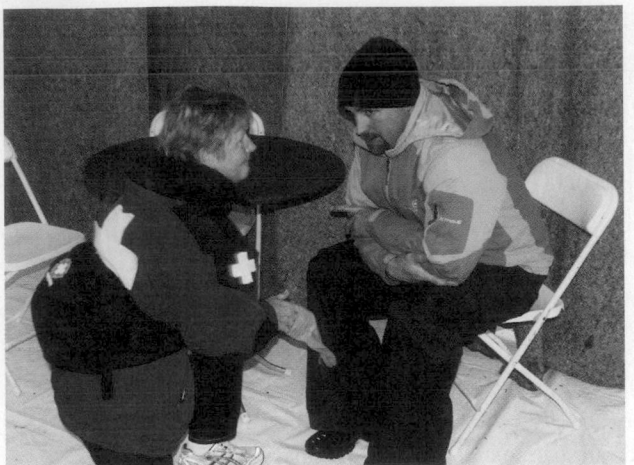

**Figure 16-4** OEC Technicians must recognize the signs and symptoms of an acute abdomen.
Copyright Mike Halloran

**peritonitis** an inflammation (irritation) of the peritoneum, the thin tissue that lines the inner wall of the abdomen and covers most of the abdominal organs.

**sensory nerves** nerves that send signals to the brain for perception of touch, pressure, heat, cold, and pain.

**visceral nerves** a collection of nerves that convey impulses between a part of the central nervous system and a viscus, such as an internal organ in the chest or abdomen.

**referred pain** pain that originates in one part of the body but is felt in another part of the body.

**guarding** an involuntary action in which the abdomen becomes rigid upon examination.

---

**⊕ 16-1** List at least six possible causes of emergencies involving the gastrointestinal and genitourinary systems.

---

**⊕ 16-2** List the signs and symptoms of emergencies involving the gastrointestinal and genitourinary systems.

---

**⊕ 16-3** Compare and contrast visceral pain and parietal pain.

---

a patient is very ill and needs to go to the hospital than it is to pinpoint the source of the problem (Figure 16-4■).

The two hallmarks of acute abdomen are severe pain and inflammation of the peritoneum, known as **peritonitis**. As described in Chapter 6, the peritoneum is a thin membrane that lines the abdominal cavity and contains both **sensory** and **visceral** nerves. When contacted by blood or contaminants (e.g., gastric contents, urine, or feces), these nerve endings become irritated, resulting in pain. The severity of pain depends on the structures involved and whether the affected nerves are **sensory nerves** or **visceral nerves.**

Sensory nerves, which enable one to perceive touch, pressure, heat, cold, and pain, are located in the skin over the abdominal wall and within the peritoneum. When sensory nerves become irritated, the location of the pain can be precisely pinpointed (i.e., the patient *can* point to the exact location of the pain). This is known as "parietal pain." In contrast, visceral pain is caused by irritation of visceral nerves and is described as diffuse, or spread over a large area (the patient *cannot* point to the exact location of the pain). Additionally, distention or contraction of the peritoneum stimulates various visceral stretch receptors that can cause pain to be perceived at a distant location, such as the back or shoulder; this condition is known as **referred pain** (Figure 16-5■).

## Causes of Acute Abdomen

### Appendicitis

Appendicitis is an inflammation of the appendix, a small, wormlike appendage in the right lower quadrant that comes off the cecum, the first part of the colon. Appendicitis is caused by obstruction of the hollow tubular appendix due to infection, hard stools, undigested nuts, or parasites. This condition requires urgent surgical intervention and can cause serious complications and even death if surgery is delayed. Rupture of the appendix can result in peritonitis and internal bleeding. Patients with appendicitis often present with generalized periumbilical (around the navel) or upper abdominal pain that may initially be dismissed as a cramp or a muscle spasm. With time, the pain grows in severity and typically moves to the right lower quadrant. The pain is often accompanied by abdominal **guarding**, nausea, vomiting, and fever, but rarely diarrhea.

### Pancreatitis

Pancreatitis is an inflammatory condition in which digestive juices become trapped within the pancreas and the organ begins to digest itself (undergo auto-digestion). Pancreatitis can be mild or life threatening and can occur suddenly or recur throughout one's life. Causes include excessive alcohol consumption (the number one cause), gallstones (which block the pancreatic duct), medications, trauma, viral infections (e.g., hepatitis), and pancreatic tumors or cancer (Figure 16-6■).

Pancreatitis is either acute or chronic. Acute pancreatitis is a serious emergency that can result in death if not treated quickly. Patients present with a sudden onset of moderate-to-severe parietal pain in both upper quadrants, often with referred pain to the back or left shoulder. The pain is usually constant and worsens with movement, coughing, or deep inspiration, or if the patient is placed in a supine position. The abdomen is usually distended and is very tender to palpation. Guarding is present. Nausea and vomiting are common and may be accompanied by a low-grade fever. The vital signs may be elevated. In severe cases, the patient may present with shock-like

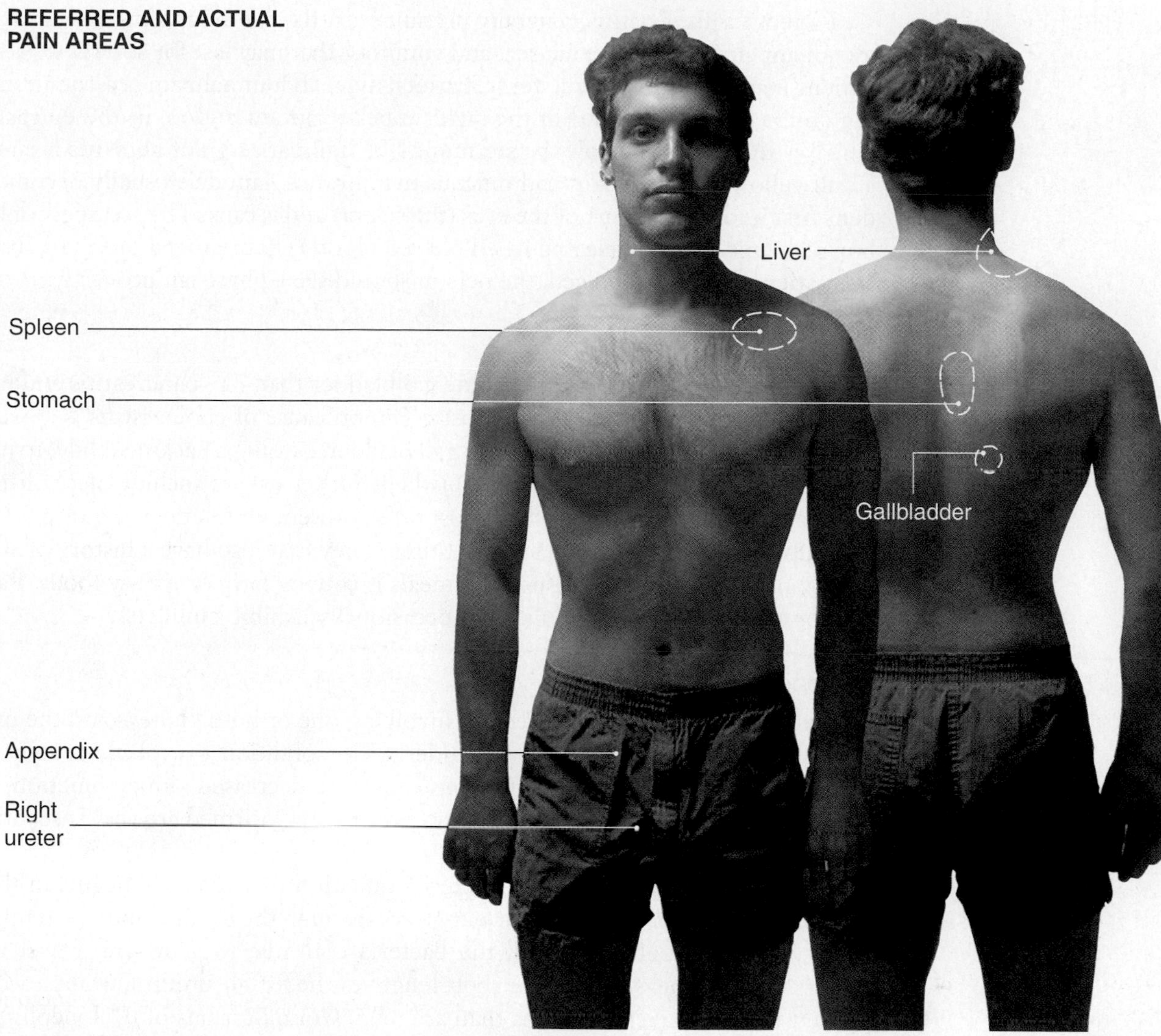

## REFERRED AND ACTUAL PAIN AREAS

Liver

Spleen

Stomach

Gallbladder

Appendix

Right
ureter

**Figure 16-5** Pain within the abdominal cavity can be accompanied by referred pain.

signs (e.g., rapid pulse and breathing, low blood pressure, sweating), which may result from multiple organ failure; this is considered a life-threatening situation.

Chronic pancreatitis is an ongoing condition that causes scar tissue to form within the pancreas, which results in decreased pancreatic function. This condition typically develops after years of alcohol abuse but can be caused by many of the same factors that cause acute pancreatitis. Signs and symptoms are similar to acute pancreatitis, may be present for days, and often worsen after eating a meal or drinking alcohol. Untreated, pancreatitis can lead to decreased pancreatic function and even to diabetes if a sufficient number of pancreatic cells are destroyed.

**Figure 16-6** The location of the pancreas in relation to the stomach and liver. The pancreas spans the left and right upper quadrants.

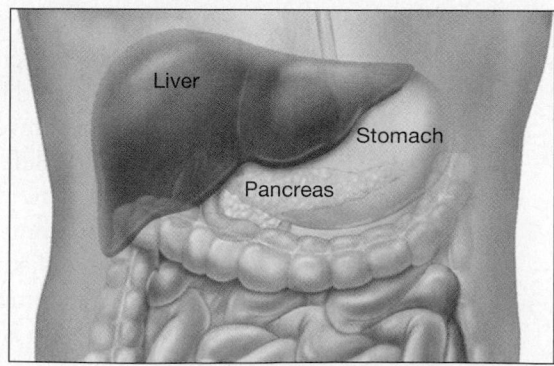

Liver

Stomach

Pancreas

## Hepatitis

Hepatitis is inflammation of the liver. Untreated, it can result in decreased liver function and a host of related problems. Hepatitis can be acute, but certain types of hepatitis may become chronic (persist for more than 6 months). The most common cause of hepatitis is a viral infection, although bacteria, alcohol, medications (e.g., acetaminophen, birth control pills), chemicals, and autoimmune disorders can also result in liver inflammation.

Patients with hepatitis generally present with flu-like symptoms such as fatigue, loss of appetite, headache, nausea, and vomiting that may last for several weeks. The patient may have a low-grade fever. Parietal-type abdominal pain is a common finding and is typically located in the right upper quadrant and/or in the epigastrium, which is the area just below the sternum. The hallmark sign of hepatitis is jaundice, a dull yellowing of the skin and mucous membranes. Jaundice usually becomes evident first in the white part of the eyes (the sclera) and is caused by an excess of bilirubin, a chemical that is released when old red blood cells are metabolized by the liver. If a patient appears jaundiced, the person should see a physician promptly.

### Cholecystitis

Cholecystitis is an inflammation of the gallbladder that, like pancreatitis and hepatitis, can be acute or chronic. The most common cause of cholecystitis is a gallstone that is blocking the duct that exits the gall bladder, causing a backup of bile, irritation, and sometimes infection of the gallbladder. Other causes include alcoholism and trauma. Patients with cholecystitis most often present with tenderness or pain in the right upper quadrant, nausea, and vomiting. They may also have a history of abdominal pain following a meal, especially meals involving fatty or greasy foods. Patients may or may not have a fever and may occasionally exhibit jaundice.

### Pyelonephritis

Pyelonephritis is a bacterial infection involving one or both kidneys and the ureters, the tubes leading to the urinary bladder. The condition can occur acutely or be chronic. Over time, repeated infections can cause decreased kidney function, shock and even death in rare cases. The young, elderly, and infirmed are very susceptible to kidney infections.

Pyelonephritis is caused by a bacterial infection that typically begins in the urinary bladder. Bacteria enter the urinary tract through the urethra and travel up to the urinary bladder. Left untreated, the bacteria continue to grow and travel up the ureters to the kidneys. Due to the short length of the female urethra, women are more prone to urinary tract infections than are men. Complications of pyelonephritis can include infection throughout the body, known as sepsis, kidney stones, and kidney failure.

Patients with a kidney infection appear ill and present with a variety of signs and symptoms, including severe abdominal, flank, or back pain; fever; warm or hot skin; chills and shivering; nausea and vomiting; pain or increased frequency of urination; or abnormal urine (discolored urine, blood in the urine, foul-smelling urine).

### Nephrolithiasis

Nephrolithiasis is the presence of kidney stones, which are formed when mineralized salts within the kidneys crystallize into small, hardened deposits that grow in size over time. Stones may travel out of the kidney and become trapped within one or both ureters. When this occurs, urine flow may become blocked, causing pressure, spasm and intense pain within the affected ureter. Causes of kidney stones include increased levels of stone forming chemicals within the kidney, dehydration, congenital kidney defects, and certain medical conditions such as high blood pressure, diabetes, and gout.

Patients with a kidney stone that has become lodged within a ureter are usually in severe distress and are generally in excruciating pain. The pain may be localized in the abdomen or (more commonly) in the flank, and it may radiate into the groin area. The pain is often described as "tearing" or "stabbing," and often the patient is unable

**Table 16-1**  Causes of Bowel Obstruction

*Previous abdominal surgery* resulting in the development of scar tissue
*Structural problems* such as twisting, herniation, and the presence of foreign bodies or impacted feces
*Diet-related problems* such as a low-fiber diet, failure to adequately chew solid foods, and insufficient water intake (dehydration)
*Medications* such as oxycodone (a narcotic pain medication) and loperamide (an anti-diarrhea medication
*Chronic medical conditions* such as Crohn's disease or diverticulitis
*Cancers* that form tumors that obstruct the lumen of the intestines

to sit still due to the intensity of the pain. Other signs and symptoms include pain upon urination, blood in the urine, nausea, and vomiting.

## Bowel Obstruction

Bowel obstruction, or ileus, is a serious medical emergency in which a segment of either the small intestine or the large intestine becomes partially or completely blocked. As a result, solids and/or liquids cannot move normally through the digestive tract. The causes of bowel obstruction are listed in Table 16-1■.

Patients with bowel obstruction commonly present with a history of constipation, visceral abdominal pain, guarding, profound nausea, and vomiting. Fever may or may not be present. The patient's abdomen may be bloated or grossly distended. Vital signs may initially be elevated, indicating severe distress, but can quickly fall, leading to shock and even death if the condition is not recognized and treated rapidly.

## Perforated Bowel

A perforated bowel is a true emergency in which a hole or tear develops in the intestines, resulting in the contents leaking into the abdominal cavity. This can rapidly lead to peritonitis, sepsis, and death if the problem is not rapidly corrected by surgery. The causes of perforated bowel include bowel obstruction, excess stomach acid, ulcerative disease, trauma, and chronic weakness of the intestinal wall. Patients with a perforated bowel present with intense, visceral abdominal pain that worsens with movement or deep inspiration and is accompanied by guarding, high fever, severe nausea, and intense vomiting.

## Peptic Ulcerative Disease, GERD, and Gastrointestinal Bleeding

Peptic ulcerative disease (PUD) is a condition in which excess stomach acid creates a defect of the lining of the esophagus, stomach, or duodenum (the first section of the small intestine) (Figure 16-7■). Specific bacteria that may grow in the lining of the stomach also lead to PUD. Gastritis, or esophagitis, inflammation of the stomach or esophagus can occur causing "heartburn" type symptoms. Esophagitis is caused by gastro-esophageal reflux disease (GERD), a condition in which stomach contents mixed with hydrochloric acid flow back into the esophagus.

The many factors that can cause excessive acid production in the stomach include fatty foods, caffeine, smoking, and alcohol. Patients with PUD may present with chest pain, upper abdominal pain, nausea, or a complaint of a sour taste in the mouth. The pain is often described as "gnawing." At times, it may be difficult to differentiate pain from peptic ulcerative disease from pain resulting from acute heart disease. OEC Technicians should assume that the pain is of a serious nature until proven otherwise.

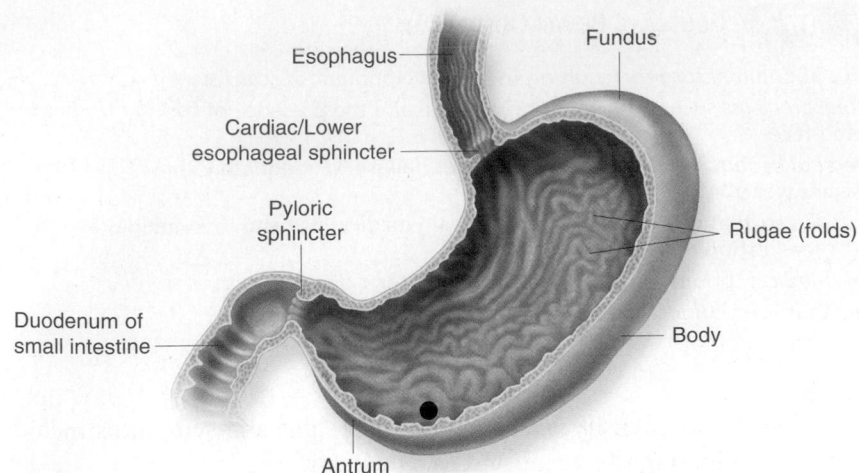

**Figure 16-7** Peptic ulcer disease occurs when excess stomach acid penetrates through the wall of the stomach, esophagus, or duodenum. Note the stomach ulcer in black.

In severe cases of peptic ulcer disease, erosions can penetrate a blood vessel within the upper gastrointestinal tract, causing a life-threatening hemorrhage known as a "GI bleed." GI bleeding, which can occur in any part of the gastrointestinal tract, can also be caused by medication (e.g., aspirin), alcohol, tears within the esophagus or intestines, or ruptured blood vessels.

Upper GI bleeding can present as blood-tinged vomit, known as **hematemesis**, that is either bright red or has a "coffee grounds" appearance. GI bleeding can also present as **hematochezia**, which are bright red stools. Stool that contains bright red blood typically indicates that bleeding is occurring within the lower GI tract, most commonly from a hemorrhoid or from the colon. Hematochezia could also result from a serious upper GI bleed with rapid evacuation of the stool. Tarry, black, foul-smelling stools, known as **melena**, indicate bleeding that originates within the upper GI tract. OEC Technicians should recommend hospital care for any patient who presents with blood or "coffee grounds" in the vomit, or significant bright red blood or melena in the stool.

**hematemesis**   vomiting up blood.

**hematochezia**   the passage of bloody stools.

**melena**   black, tarry stools.

### Abdominal Aortic Aneurysm (AAA)

Over time, the abdominal aorta can become weakened and develop a bulge formed by a localized dilatation of the wall of the aorta, a condition known as an aneurysm. Typically due to chronic, uncontrolled hypertension and arteriosclerosis, aneurysms can become so large that (rarely) they cause pain or dizziness upon standing. Rupture of an aneurysm is a true emergency that can rapidly lead to massive blood loss and sudden death. Patients with an abdominal aortic aneurysm typically present in shock and may complain of flank, lower back, or abdominal pain, weakness, and/or dizziness. The medical history often includes recent fainting spells, and the skin may be cool and pale. Patients with AAA often have unequal femoral pulses.

### OB/GYN-Related Conditions

The abdominal and pelvic cavities contain the structures of the female reproductive system which, when affected by disease, can cause signs and symptoms similar to those of acute abdomen. Common causes of OB/GYN-related conditions are ectopic pregnancy, ovarian cysts, bladder infections, and pelvic inflammatory disease. Refer to Chapter 34, Obstetric and Gynecologic Emergencies, for more information.

# Common Gastrointestinal Ailments

OEC Technicians will also likely encounter a variety of less urgent GI/GU-related ailments ranging from mild stomach discomfort or GI upset to intermittent, unexplained abdominal pain, profound diarrhea, or constipation. While seemingly benign in nature, many of these ailments are highly concerning for patients and may actually be early signs of a more serious underlying problem. Many of the patients who exhibit these problems should be referred to a hospital for a more comprehensive examination by a physician.

## Gastroenteritis

Gastroenteritis, an inflammatory condition involving the stomach lining and/or intestines, is one of the most common GI problems that OEC Technicians will encounter. It is typically caused by a bacterial, viral, or parasitic infection but may also result from noninfectious sources such as excessive alcohol use or prolonged aspirin/ibuprofen use. Patients with gastroenteritis present with cramping abdominal pain, bloating, nausea, vomiting, and/or diarrhea. Fever may or may not be present depending on the cause of the inflammation. Patients may become dehydrated due to a combination of vomiting and diarrhea. Pain may be localized to the upper quadrants or may be diffuse. Generally, gastroenteritis is not life threatening, and the symptoms resolve fairly quickly. If symptoms persist for over 24 hours, the patient could become dehydrated. If blood appears in vomit or stool, the condition may be due to undiagnosed GI bleeding. In either case the patient should be encouraged to seek follow-up care at a medical facility.

## Indigestion

The upper GI tract, which includes the esophagus, stomach, and duodenum, can become inflamed due to stress, a viral illness, rich or spicy foods, or excessive alcohol consumption. This inflammation can result in nausea and/or vomiting. Indigestion usually presents with dull or cramping pain in the upper abdominal quadrants but may be located as high as the center of the chest. The latter case is caused by stomach acid that ascends into the lower esophagus (GERD), resulting in pain that is more commonly known as heartburn. Due to its relative proximity to the heart, this type of pain can often mimic a heart attack. Vomiting usually relieves the pain, at least for a while. Generally, indigestion is self-limiting, dissipates with time, and does not require evaluation by a physician. Persistent or severe indigestion, however, warrants examination by a doctor to rule out the possibility of other, more serious medical conditions.

## Nausea and Vomiting

Noxious stimuli can cause the muscles in the wall of the stomach to violently contract, sending stomach contents (partially digested food and digestive acid) up the esophagus and out the mouth. Vomiting is usually preceded by a feeling of impending vomiting, more commonly referred to as nausea. Common causes of nausea and vomiting include motion sickness, altitude, food poisoning, viral or bacterial infections, irritating drugs or chemicals (aspirin, alcohol), ulcers, tumors, and abdominal trauma.

Vomiting that is excessive or occurs over time without fluid replacement can cause a host of other problems, most notably profound dehydration. Vomiting that occurs in an unresponsive patient is especially serious because the person can develop significant complications if the vomit is aspirated into the trachea and lungs. Aspiration can lead to a lung infection, a potentially life-threatening condition. Therefore, quickly clean or suction vomit out of the upper airway of an unresponsive patient to prevent aspiration pneumonia.

## Colic

Colic is intermittent, severe abdominal pain caused by the obstruction and distention of a hollow organ. It is caused when strong muscular contractions within the wall of a hollow organ such as the gallbladder, bowel, or ureter are unsuccessful in forcing the organ's contents past the obstruction. Gallstones, tumors, a twisted bowel, trapped gas, or a mass of hard stool within the bowel, and kidney stones are all common sources of colic. Colicky bowel pain is generally first experienced around the navel but can be located anywhere within the abdominal and pelvic cavities and can move over time. When a ureter is blocked by a kidney stone, colicky pain occurs in the flank and radiates to the groin.

## Diarrhea and Bloody Stool

Diarrhea is defined as the passage of frequent, liquid stools. It is caused by viruses, bacteria, protozoa, chemicals, and other gastric irritants, and by medical conditions such as bowel disease, intestinal tumors, and food allergies. Untreated, some of these conditions can become chronic. Like vomiting, excessive or prolonged diarrhea can lead to profound dehydration.

In outdoor environments, most cases of acute diarrhea are caused by contaminated water or food. In urban settings, modern sanitation has largely eliminated most causes of diarrhea. However, bowel infections with adenovirus and rotavirus commonly cause diarrhea in urban population centers and on cruise ships.

## Viruses, Protozoa, and Bacteria

Several viruses, protozoa, and bacteria warrant mention because they can also cause diarrhea. Depending on the causative microorganism, some illnesses are self-limiting, lasting generally less than 24 hours, whereas others can be deadly, especially within in the young, elderly, or infirmed. Prominent among the bacterial, protozoan, and viral agents of gastrointestinal ailments are the following organisms:

- Staphylococci are bacteria of the genus *Staphylococcus* that grow everywhere in the environment. When people eat foods such as mayonnaise that have not been refrigerated for several hours and have unknowingly been contaminated with certain strains of "staph," acute diarrhea (and vomiting) can occur.

- Bacteria in the genus *Salmonella*, which are often present in undercooked poultry, can cause the same problems as *Staphylococcus* food poisoning. Although salmonellosis is usually self-limiting, it lasts longer than food poisoning with *Staphylococcus*.

- *Giardia lamblia* and *Cryptosporidium* are protozoa that are present in untreated surface water, usually in outdoor environments. Infections with either can cause chronic diarrhea and mild, chronic dehydration. Fortunately, several medicines are available to treat both infections.

- *Escherichia coli* (E. coli) is a common bacterial species that is a normal resident in all human colons. Although these bacteria typically aid in digestion by breaking down food, certain strains can cause deadly diarrhea. When travelers are exposed to strains of these bacteria that are not present in their colon, the result can be what is commonly referred to as "traveler's diarrhea" or "Montezuma's revenge."

Left untreated, encounters with any of the aforementioned microorganisms can cause dehydration, loss of electrolytes, starvation, shock, and even death. Hospitalization with intravenous therapy is recommended.

## Constipation

Constipation is the inability to excrete feces, a condition that nearly everyone suffers occasionally. Manifested by unusually large, hard, and dry stools that are passed in-

### NOTE

### Preventing Traveler's Diarrhea

Traveler's diarrhea can be prevented by meticulous attention to personal cleanliness. Wash your hands before preparing and eating food, protect food from spoilage or flies that carry bacterial contamination, and treat drinking water either by filtering, boiling, or chemically decontaminating it. Avoidance of eating raw or undercooked meat and seafood, vegetables, or fruit is imperative. Peeling vegetables or fruit can significantly reduce one's chances of becoming sick. Ice and water used to wash food can also be contaminated, so drink bottled water or bottled beverages whenever possible.

frequently, constipation can occur due to physical inactivity, dehydration, lack of dietary fiber, or a more urgent condition such as a tumor blocking the intestinal canal. Outdoor enthusiasts who do not eat enough fiber or don't drink enough water over several days are especially vulnerable to constipation.

## STOP, THINK, UNDERSTAND

### Multiple Choice
Choose the correct answer.

1. Which of the following statements regarding acute abdomen is false?_____
   a. OEC Technicians should be able to pinpoint the source of an acute abdomen.
   b. Upon first examination, physicians accurately diagnose the source of an acute abdomen approximately 50 percent of the time.
   c. OEC Technicians need not make a specific diagnosis and need only recognize that a patient is ill enough to warrant transport to a hospital.
   d. An acute abdomen can rapidly lead to septic or hypovolemic shock.

2. A patient who says he is having heartburn presents with persistent signs and symptoms that resemble a heart attack (substernal pain, nausea, and vomiting). Which of the following is your best course of action?_____
   a. The patient is most likely suffering from indigestion; suggest that he follow up with his physician as soon as possible.
   b. Immediately arrange transport with ALS because this patient could be having a heart attack.
   c. Monitor the patient until you can be certain whether this condition is indigestion or a heart attack.

   d. Suggest that the patient take some over-the-counter antacids to see if that helps relieve the symptoms.

3. Colic is best described as_____
   a. an inflammatory condition involving the lining of the stomach.
   b. intermittent, severe abdominal pain caused by obstruction and distension of a hollow organ.
   c. a violent contraction of the stomach muscles due to noxious stimuli.
   d. persistent, abdominal pain caused by inflammation of a solid organ.

4. Vomiting in an unresponsive patient is especially serious because_____
   a. it could signify that the patient has an allergy to something he ate.
   b. the patient could become dehydrated.
   c. this could indicate that they are suffering from potentially life-threatening gastrointestinal problems, including a ruptured bowel.
   d. the patient could aspirate vomitus.

### Matching
Match each of the following terms to its definition or description.

_____ 1. sensory nerve
_____ 2. parietal pain
_____ 3. visceral pain
_____ 4. referred pain
_____ 5. peritonitis

a. pain perceived at a distant location such as the back or shoulder caused by stretching of the peritoneum
b. severe inflammation of the peritoneum that causes abdominal pain
c. perceives touch, pressure, cold, heat, pain; is located in the skin over the abdomen and in the peritoneum.
d. pain spread over a large area such that a patient cannot pinpoint its exact location
e. pain that a patient can easily and precisely pinpoint

 **CASE UPDATE**

On examination of the patient, you notice that he is pale, sweating, and feels warm to the touch. He relates that his pain was originally near his navel but has now "moved down and to the right." Examination of the abdomen reveals severe tenderness in the right lower quadrant. He tells you that every bump in the road on the way to the ski hill felt like he was "being stabbed in my gut." The patient has a heart rate of 116, blood pressure is 132/88, and respirations are 20 and shallow.

*What do you think is wrong with the patient?*

⊕ 16-4 Describe and demonstrate how to assess the abdomen.

# Assessment

Due to the number and complexity of gastrointestinal and genitourinary organs, there are many possible causes of acute abdominal and pelvic pain in addition to those just described (Table 16-2■). As previously indicated, this can make assessment of the abdomen and the pelvic region extremely difficult. Because emergent conditions involving the GI/GU systems rarely present without pain, it is important to examine patients to identify the nature and extent of their pain. Again, the role of OEC Technicians is not to diagnose the underlying cause but to recognize the signs and symptoms associated with an emergent condition and initiate life-saving care if needed (Table 16-3■). If shock exists, life-saving care should be initiated in lieu of performing a complete physical examination while simultaneously referring these patients to a higher level of care.

## ABCDs

After ensuring that the scene is safe, begin the assessment process with a careful examination of the patient's ABCDs and vital signs. Then gather a thorough medical history and perform a physical exam. OEC Technicians should ask patients about their medical history and pain symptoms using the SAMPLE and OPQRST mnemonics, respectively. Attempt to determine if pain is constant or intermittent, how long the pain has been present, and whether the pain has moved since its initial onset. The patient should also be queried about any factors that aggravate or relieve the condition, such as motion, coughing, breathing, belching, or urination. Finally, determine whether any associated signs and symptoms, such as nausea, vomiting, diarrhea, bloody stool, fever, or loss of appetite, are present.

**Table 16-2**   Causes of Acute Abdominal Pain

| |
|---|
| Abdominal aortic aneurysm |
| Appendicitis |
| Bowel obstruction |
| Gastritis and GI bleeding |
| Pancreatitis |
| Perforated bowel |

**Table 16-3**   Signs and Symptoms of Acute Abdomen

| Signs and Symptoms | Description |
|---|---|
| Pain and tenderness | Pain that is sharp, dull, localized, generalized, or rigid, and pain referred to another location |
| Nausea and vomiting | Stomach upset with regurgitation |
| Anorexia | Lack of desire to eat |
| Fever | Increased core body temperature |
| Jaundice | Yellow skin and mucous membranes |
| Tachycardia | Rapid heart rate |
| Hypotension | Low blood pressure |
| Hematemesis | Blood in vomit; may be red or black and resemble coffee grounds |
| Hematochezia | Blood in stool; may be red or black and tarry |
| Hematuria | Blood in the urine |

## Physical Exam

Begin your physical examination of patients with acute abdominal or pelvic pain by calming the patients to allay their anxiety. OEC Technicians should ask permission to examine the abdomen and should explain to patients what they are going to do before starting any examination. Place the patient into a position of comfort; a supine position with the knees slightly flexed allows the abdominal and pelvic muscles to relax. If possible, move the patient to a warm location, as this will make the exam much easier.

Examination of the abdomen and pelvic region in indoor settings is typically a two-step process involving inspection and palpation. During the inspection step, the area is exposed and observed for clinical signs such as trauma, distention, bulging, or discoloration. Note whether the patient is motionless or is unable to sit still, as well as how the abdominal wall moves with the patient's respirations. If pain is present, ask the patient to use one finger to point to the site at which the pain is most intense (Figure 16-8a■). If the pain is diffuse, ask the patient to use a finger to draw a circle indicating the boundaries of the pain.

The second step, palpation of the abdomen, is a systematic process that involves physically compressing each of the four quadrants to determine the presence or absence of pain, masses, tensing, guarding, or rigidity. OEC Technicians should not be afraid to palpate the abdomen, because even deep palpation should not cause further injury. Before palpating the abdomen, OEC Technicians should ensure that their hands are warm, because placing cold hands on the abdomen of unsuspecting patients can cause the patients to tense their abdominal muscles, which can complicate the exam process.

Begin palpating the abdomen in the quadrant farthest away from the site of the pain; examine the painful quadrant last. Place one hand atop the other and gently place them on the patient's abdomen (Figure 16-8b■). Rest your hands in this position for a moment to allow the patient to become comfortable. Then, moving slowly, apply firm but gentle downward pressure; note the patient's response and whether the abdominal muscles suddenly tense in response. Slowly release the pressure, gently gliding your hands from one quadrant to the next, and then repeat the process for each quadrant. Note any evidence of tenderness upon examination. Lastly, palpate gently just above the pubic bone in the midline, where the bladder is located.

A sudden release of pressure during an examination of the abdomen may result in severe pain to the patient, a finding that denotes inflammation of the peritoneum. This sign, known as "rebound tenderness," usually indicates the presence of a serious intra-abdominal problem. Even though OEC Technicians may inadvertently evoke rebound tenderness during an examination, this finding is not useful in prehospital settings, and thus OEC Technicians should not intentionally elicit it.

**Figure 16-8a** Ask the patient to point with one finger where the pain is.

**Figure 16-8b** Start palpating the abdominal quadrant farthest away from the site of pain, with one hand placed on top of the other.

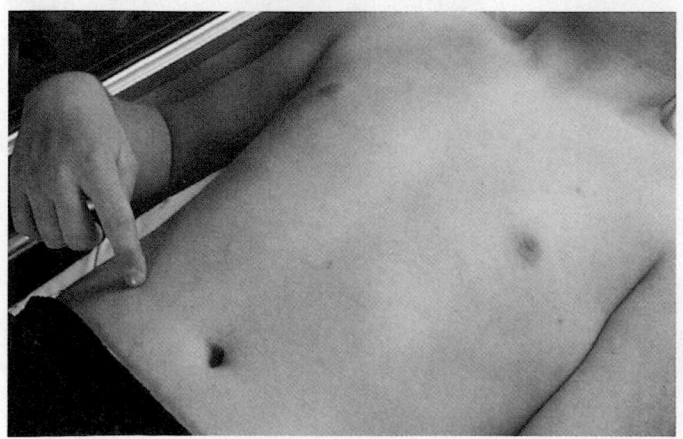

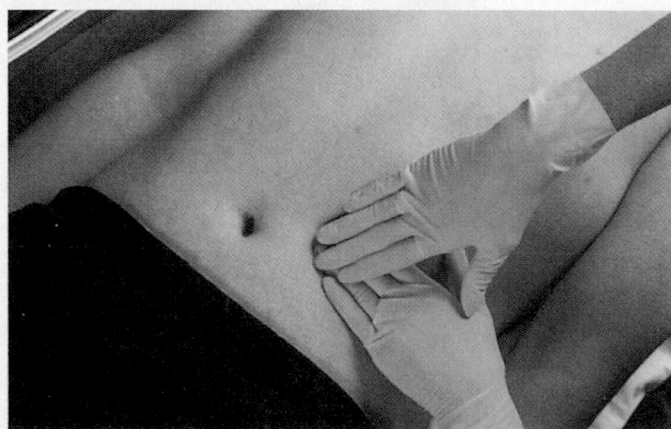

Check the right and left flank areas individually, noting any tenderness or discoloration. Continue the rest of the physical exam in the usual manner. You may wish to obtain orthostatic vital signs if the patient will tolerate it.

**16-5** Describe and demonstrate the management of a patient with a severe GI/GU emergency.

# Management

The treatment of patients with a suspected GI/GU problem in outdoor settings generally involves supportive care. Many conditions require an in-depth evaluation by a physician, and surgical correction and/or long-term care are often required. Despite this, OEC Technicians can do many things to improve a patient's overall comfort and the subsequent outcome. If possible, move the patient to a location that has a comfortable temperature.

Initial treatment includes correcting any problems involving the ABCDs (Figure 16-9■). During the physical exam you already placed the person into a position of comfort. For most GI/GU patients, this is either a supine position with the knees slightly flexed, or a seated position with the head raised 45–60 degrees (Figure 16-10■). Patients may be restless, so be empathetic to their discomfort and help them remain calm. Keep patients warm by using jackets, blankets, reflective blankets, or sleeping bags as needed. Given that many GI/GU problems frequently present with flu-like symptoms, patients often experience hot and cold cycles. Thus, the process of applying and removing blankets may need to be repeated many times.

Provide supplemental oxygen as needed, typically using a nonrebreather mask at 12–15 LPM. Anticipate vomiting and be ready to clear the airway by removing the oxygen mask and turning the patient onto his side. Suction the airway as needed to prevent aspiration. Despite their requests, do not give patients anything to eat or drink because many abdominopelvic conditions require surgical intervention. The presence of food or liquids in the stomach can worsen some GI/GU problems, can cause the patient to vomit, and can make surgery more dangerous.

Continue to monitor the patient's vital signs, because they can change rapidly. Anticipate shock and treat accordingly if the patient exhibits the characteristic clinical signs (e.g., fast pulse, rapid breathing, low blood pressure). With few exceptions, patients with significant abdominopelvic pain require further evaluation. Transfer these patients to a higher level of care or encourage them to seek physician evaluation and definitive treatment.

**Figure 16-9** Correct any problems involving the ABCDs.
Copyright Mike Halloran

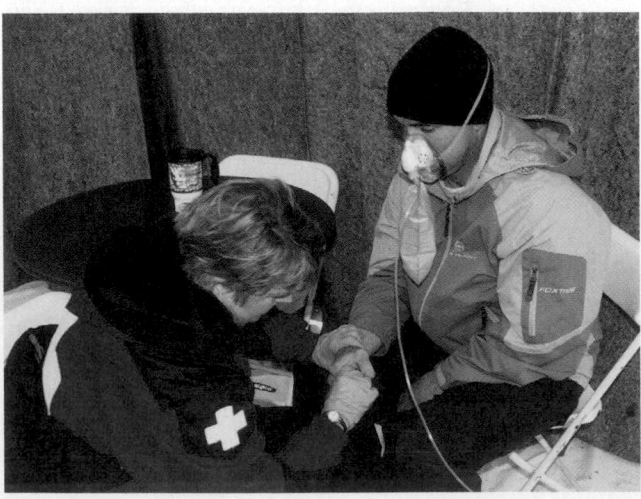

**Figure 16-10** This patient has been placed in a position of comfort.
Copyright Edward McNamara

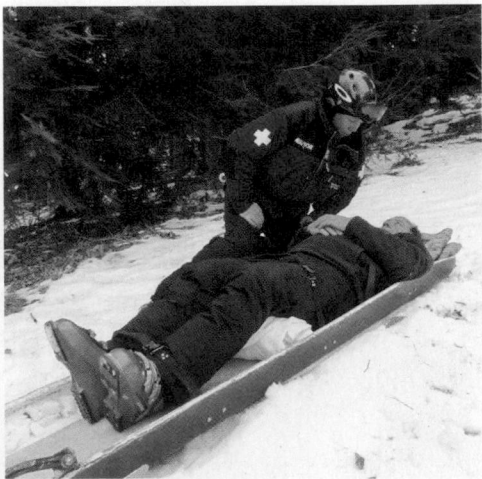

# STOP, THINK, UNDERSTAND

## Multiple Choice

Choose the correct answer.

1. Which of the following statements regarding gastrointestinal and genitourinary complaints is true?_____
   a. Emergent conditions involving the GI/GU systems often present without pain.
   b. GI/GU emergencies can lead to hemorrhagic or septic shock.
   c. GI/GU emergencies are rarely seen by OEC Technicians.
   d. OEC Technicians should diagnose the underlying cause of GI/GU problems.

2. When assessing a patient with a GI/GU complaint, which of the following actions is important?_____
   a. monitoring/evaluating the ABCDs, SAMPLE, OPQRST, and vital signs
   b. determining if the pain is constant or intermittent
   c. identifying the presence of aggravating or relieving factors
   d. all of the above are important

3. The proper sequence for examining the abdominal quadrants of a patient complaining of lower right abdominal pain is_____
   a. RLQ, LUQ, RUQ, and then LLQ.
   b. the peri-umbilical area, the diaphragmatic region, and then the pelvic region.
   c. to palpate the quadrant farthest from the pain first, palpate the painful quadrant last, and make sure you palpate all four quadrants.
   d. to palpate the painful quadrant first, then move in a clockwise sequence.

4. Rebound tenderness is best described as_____
   a. vague, nondescriptive pain that occurs when a patient moves.
   b. a severe pain in a patient when the pressure of palpation is suddenly released during an abdominal examination.
   c. a type of pain that is initially relieved by vomiting but returns within a short period of time.
   d. pain that radiates into a location other than the point of origin.

5. What is generally the most comfortable position for a responsive patient suffering from a GI/GU complaint?_____
   a. Supine with the knees slightly flexed
   b. The recovery position
   c. The Trendelenburg position
   d. Supine with the feet elevated 8–12 inches

6. Which of the following statements regarding care of the patient with a GI/GU problem is false?_____
   a. You may need to apply and remove blankets continually.
   b. You should provide oxygen with a nonrebreather mask at 12–15 LPM, and you must be prepared to clear the airway due to vomiting.
   c. You must anticipate that the patient may spiral into shock.
   d. You may permit the patient to eat a small amount of food because doing so may help combat nausea.

## Short Answer

You suspect that a patient may be suffering from an abdominal aortic aneurysm. Check all the actions that you should take.

_____ a. Do a full assessment, including SAMPLE and OPQRST.
_____ b. Take a set of initial vital signs, and record another full set every 5 minutes.
_____ c. Treat for shock.
_____ d. Check both femoral pulses.
_____ e. Call for a BLS (basic life support) unit and transport the patient.

_____ f. Administer high-flow oxygen.
_____ g. Take a set of initial vital signs, and record another full set every 15 minutes.
_____ h. Call for an ALS (advanced life support) unit.
_____ i. Transport the patient rapidly to the nearest definitive medical/surgical care facility.

 CASE DISPOSITION

As you examine the patient and listen to his story, you become concerned that the patient may have an acute abdomen. You place the patient on oxygen, keep him comfortable, and have him transported to the hospital. A week later the patient's wife comes to the patrol room to thank you and the other patrollers for taking such great care of her husband. She reports that he had surgery for acute appendicitis and is now doing well.

# Chapter Review

## Chapter Summary

Acute abdominal or pelvic pain can be a trying experience, for patients and rescuers alike. The condition causing it can also be deadly. Even though the causes of an acute abdomen are myriad, the focus of the examination need not be complicated. The ultimate goals are to recognize those patients whose signs and symptoms suggest the presence of a potential acute abdomen, to implement life-saving measures, and to rapidly transport the patients to a definitive-care facility for evaluation by a physician.

By having a fundamental understanding of the locations of various abdominal and pelvic structures and knowing the basic causes of common GI/GU problems, OEC Technicians will be prepared to quickly and effectively manage most GI/GU-related disorders that they will encounter.

## Remember...

1. The abdominal and pelvic cavities contain solid and hollow organs, major blood vessels, and nerves. The aorta, abdominal vena cava, kidneys, and ureters are just posterior to the abdominal cavity.
2. The abdomen can be divided into four quadrants.
3. Patients with abdominopelvic pain may not present until their signs and symptoms are unbearable.
4. Abdominal pain may be the first indication of a life-threatening emergency.
5. Abdominal assessment includes an examination of all four abdominal quadrants. All patients with abdominal pain should be taken seriously and either referred to a physician or transported to a hospital.
6. Do not give a patient complaining of abdominal pain anything by mouth.
7. A heart attack (AMI) can present with abdominal pain.
8. Acute abdominal pain may be a symptom of some intra-abdominal trauma (such as a ruptured spleen or a renal injury) suffered the previous day.

## Chapter Questions

### Multiple Choice

Choose the correct answer.

1. Which of the following statements regarding assessing the abdomen is false?_____
   a. Assessing abdominal complaints can be difficult because the nerve pathways for the gastrointestinal, urinary, and reproductive systems are in relatively close proximity to each other.
   b. Because abdominopelvic organs are close to each other, problems affecting one system or organ can seriously affect organs in another system.
   c. Assessment of abdominal complaints is straightforward because the abdominal organs are specifically located and easily palpated.
   d. One of the problems encountered while assessing abdominal complaints is a patient's reluctance to allow the exam due to embarrassment or pain.

2. Abdominal pain could indicate which of the following conditions?_____
   a. an acute myocardial infarction
   b. a urinary tract infection
   c. constipation
   d. all of the above

3. Colic can be caused by_____
   a. obstruction and distension of the colon.
   b. drinking too much water.
   c. a violent contraction of the stomach muscles due to noxious stimuli.
   d. passing a bloody stool.

**4.** A generally healthy male patient presents with recent signs and symptoms of nausea and vomiting but very little abdominal pain. Which of the following is your best course of action?_____

    **a.** The patient most likely is suffering from indigestion; suggest that he follow up with his physician.

    **b.** You determine that the patient may be having a silent heart attack and call for ALS and transport.

    **c.** Have the patient urinate in a cup and look for blood in the urine.

    **d.** Suggest that the patient take some over-the-counter antacids to see if they help relieve the symptoms.

**5.** You would advise a patient who complains of sudden right lower quadrant pain to_____

    **a.** go to the hospital by ambulance.

    **b.** purchase an over-the-counter antacid such as Tums or Maalox.

    **c.** drink some milk to settle the stomach, and if that does not help to follow up with a physician.

    **d.** urinate in a cup and look for blood in the urine.

**6.** Which of the following statements regarding acute abdomen is true?_____

    **a.** OEC Technicians need to be able to pinpoint the source of an acute abdomen.

    **b.** Rarely is there nausea and vomiting.

    **c.** OEC Technicians should not make a specific diagnosis but instead need only recognize that the patient is ill enough to warrant transport to a hospital.

    **d.** An acute abdomen can never result in septic or hypovolemic shock.

**7.** Which of the following organs is *not* inside the abdomen? _____

    **a.** stomach          **c.** pancreas

    **b.** kidney           **d.** small intestine

## Matching

**1.** Match each of the following terms to its definition.

_____ **1.** appendicitis

_____ **2.** abdominal aortic aneurysm

_____ **3.** bowel obstruction

_____ **4.** cholecystitis

_____ **5.** guarding

_____ **6.** hematemesis

_____ **7.** hematochezia

_____ **8.** hepatitis

_____ **9.** melena

_____ **10.** nephrolithiasis

_____ **11.** pancreatitis

_____ **12.** perforated bowel

_____ **13.** pyelonephritis

_____ **14.** referred pain

**a.** an involuntary action in which the abdomen becomes rigid on examination

**b.** also known as kidney stones; causes excruciating pain that is localized in the abdomen or may either be referred to the flank or radiate into the groin

**c.** blockage of the large or small intestine; patients typically present with constipation, visceral abdominal pain, guarding, nausea, and vomiting

**d.** vomiting up blood

**e.** inflammation of a small, wormlike appendage in the RLQ; patients initially present with peri-umbilical or upper abdominal pain that grows in severity and moves to the RLQ

**f.** inflammation of the gallbladder; typically causes pain in the RUQ, nausea, and vomiting

**g.** inflammatory condition in which digestive juices become trapped and the organ begins to auto-digest

**h.** condition caused by chronic, uncontrolled hypertension; patients typically present in shock, may complain of flank or abdominal pain, weakness, dizziness, and fainting spells and has unequal femoral pulses

**i.** pain that originates in one part of the body but is felt in another part of the body

**j.** a kidney infection; patients have excruciating abdominal pain radiating into the flank or groin

**k.** a hole or tear in the intestines that causes peritonitis; patients have intense, visceral abdominal pain that worsens with movement or inspiration, fever, guarding, nausea, and intense vomiting

**l.** the passage of bloody stools

**m.** black, tarry stools

**n.** inflammation of the liver; is characterized by jaundice; patients present with flu-like symptoms, fatigue, loss of appetite, headache, nausea, and vomiting

**2.** Match each of the following microorganisms to its description:

_____ **1.** *Escherichia coli* (*E. coli*)

_____ **2.** *Giardia lamblia*

_____ **3.** *Salmonella*

_____ **4.** *Staphylococcus*

**a.** commonly present in undercooked poultry; causes acute diarrhea and vomiting

**b.** grow everywhere in the environment; typically ingested in unrefrigerated foods such as mayonnaise

**c.** found normally in all human colons, where it aids in the digestion of food; certain strains can cause "traveler's diarrhea" or "Montezuma's revenge"

**d.** is present in untreated surface water, usually in outdoor environments; can cause chronic diarrhea and mild chronic dehydration

## Short Answer

Explain the difference between a solid organ and a hollow organ, and explain the concerns you would have if organs of either type were to rupture.

_____

_____

_____

_____

# Scenario

*You are dispatched to the mountain to assist a 16-year-old female who is not feeling well. The patient is sitting on the side of the trail and complains of severe abdominal pain. The outside temperature is 15°F; with the wind chill factor, the perceived temperature is −10°F. The scene is safe, so you begin a primary assessment. A crowd of patrons gathers and asks you if you need help.*

**1.** For any female of child-bearing age that presents with severe abdominal pain, OEC Technicians should suspect _____

**a.** pulmonary embolism.

**b.** AIDS.

**c.** appendicitis.

**d.** pelvic inflammatory disease.

*Assessment of abdominal complaints can be complicated in outdoor environments by cold temperatures and bystanders. Your plan of action is to call for transport and quickly move her to the base, where a more detailed examination can be performed.*

**2.** Sudden unexplained abdominal pain is referred to as_____

**a.** abdominal quad pain.

**b.** abdominal pain disorder.

**c.** chronic abdominal pain.

**d.** acute abdomen.

*The patient is delivered to the base, where a secondary assessment is started using the SAMPLE and OPQRST mnemonics. The patient informs you that the pain is located in both lower quadrants of the abdominal cavity. She has no allergies, is not taking any prescribed medications, and has no past medical history. She ate lunch today, and no trauma has occurred that could account for the pain. When asked whether she could be pregnant, she replies that she is not sexually active.*

**3.** Generalized abdominal pain that cannot be pinpointed by the patient is referred to as_____

**a.** abdominal quad pain.

**b.** eviscerational pain.

**c.** peritoneal cavity pain.

**d.** visceral pain.

*The patient reports that her pain is non-radiating, is 6 out 10 on the pain scale, and is intermittent. She reports that she has been urinating frequently with some slight pain. She is seven days late with her menstrual cycle; past cycles have not been painful. Her forehead is warm to the touch. You make a call to the young woman's parents.*

**4.** Based on your findings, you suspect the patient has_____

**a.** an inflamed appendix.

**b.** a urinary tract infection.

**c.** a kidney stone.

**d.** a gallstone.

*Later evaluation of the patient's vital signs are pulse 120 and regular, and respirations 24 and shallow and temperature of 104°F.*

5. Your treatment for this patient should be to_____

   a. place her in a position of comfort, monitor for vomiting, apply $O_2$ via nasal cannula, and monitor vital signs.

   b. lay her in the supine position with elevated feet, apply $O_2$ with a nonrebreather mask, and monitor vital signs.

   c. lay the patient in the right lateral recumbent position, apply $O_2$ with a nonrebreather mask, and monitor vital signs.

   d. apply $O_2$ via nasal canal, monitor vital signs, and prepare the patient to walk to a waiting ambulance.

## **S**uggested Reading

Boey, J. H. 1994. "The Acute Abdomen." In *Current Surgical Diagnosis and Treatment,* Tenth Edition, edited by L. W. Way. Norwalk, CT: Appleton & Lange.

Murphy, P., and D. M. Meade. 1997. "Assessing and Managing Abdominal Pain." *JEMS* 22(4): 69–84.

Slasar, M. H., and E. Goldberg. 2006. "Acute Abdominal Pain." *Medical Clinics of North America* 90(3): 481–503.

EXPLORE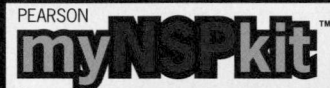

Please go to www.myNSPkit.com. Under Student Resources, you will find animations, videos, web links, and games related to this chapter—and much more. Look for information on gastrointestinal and renal system overviews and other topics.

Register your access code from the front of your book by going to www.myNSPkit.com and selecting the appropriate links. If the in-cover access code has been redeemed, go to www.myNSPkit.com and follow links to **Buy Access**.

# Principles of Trauma

Seth C. Hawkins, MD, FAWM

## ⊕ OBJECTIVES

**Upon completion of this chapter, the OEC Technician will be able to:**

**17-1** Define the following terms:
- kinematics
- mechanism of injury
- index of suspicion

**17-2** Compare and contrast high-velocity injuries and low-velocity injuries.

**17-3** Compare and contrast the five mechanisms of injury.

**17-4** Describe the role of a trauma center in improving the survival of a trauma patient.

**17-5** Describe and demonstrate the management of a trauma patient in outdoor or wilderness settings.

## ⊕ KEY TERMS

**golden hour,** *p. 526*
**index of suspicion,** *p. 526*
**injury pattern,** *p. 517*

**kinematics,** *p. 517*
**kinetic energy,** *p. 518*
**trauma,** *p. 517*

**trauma center,** *p. 526*
**trauma surgeon,** *p. 527*

## Chapter Overview

In the past few decades, the number of people who participate in outdoor activities has risen dramatically. Thanks in part to advances in outdoor gear and improved fitness, people of all ages and varying athletic ability are enjoying the outdoors in record numbers. Many are particularly healthy individuals who engage in activities that entail a high risk of injury. Because of this, traumatic injuries are disproportionately more common among outdoor sports enthusiasts when compared to other medical conditions. Injuries that would often be considered survivable after rapid transport to

*continued*

## HISTORICAL TIMELINE

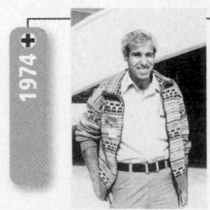

**1974** National pilot program is established for Nordic patrollers under the leadership of David Hodgdon.

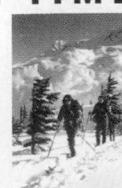

**1975** NSP Board votes to modify the NSP emergency care course to better address the needs of patrollers.

# ✚ CASE PRESENTATION ✚

A skier is moving through an expert mogul field at a high rate of speed when he loses control and falls, careening into and over several large moguls before sliding to a stop more than 50 feet down the slope. Upon your arrival on scene, you find the patient lying on his back, responsive, and alert. His skis are off and he is complaining of pain in his right hip and right flank area. Bystanders state the fall was "spectacular" and that the crash "looked like it really hurt!" The patient says, "I think I'll be all right. I just want to go to my condo."

**What should you do?**

a trauma center are complicated by remote locations and environmental factors. Indeed, even in areas with access to sophisticated care, **trauma** is the leading cause of death in patients ages 40 and under. Therefore, because trauma is the most common emergency that OEC Technicians will encounter, it is essential that ski patrollers and other OEC Technicians have a firm understanding of the pathophysiology and basic management principles of trauma.

This chapter will serve as a primer for the chapters that follow. It begins with a discussion of the forces involved in trauma, beginning with an overview of basic physics and moving on to the mechanisms of injury. The chapter discusses the common patterns of injury so that OEC Technicians can rely on their ability to accurately assess the extent of injuries and avoid missing injuries that might otherwise be overlooked. The chapter will also build upon the basic principles introduced in Chapter 7, Patient Assessment by covering the principles of systematically evaluating trauma patients, so that OEC Technicians can avoid distractions and panic and follow a clear and organized assessment plan. Finally, the chapter concludes with the basic principles of trauma management, which will be discussed in greater detail in subsequent chapters.

## Kinematics

Gauging the extent of an injury requires a basic understanding of physics, specifically the roles of mass, speed, and energy, and the relationship among them. Understanding these relationships will enable OEC Technicians to identify potentially serious injuries, whether or not tell-tale clinical signs are evident. This understanding is possible because energy, when applied to the human body, causes the body and its parts to move in abnormal ways that result in identifiable injury patterns (Figure 17-1■). An **injury pattern** is a set of problems associated with a specific source of trauma. To understand the relationship between physics and trauma, we will consider a fundamental concept known to all snow sports enthusiasts—motion.

**Kinematics** is the branch of mechanics that studies the movement of body segments without consideration given to its mass or the forces making it move. The concepts involved are

**trauma** physical injury caused by an external force.

**injury pattern** a combination of injuries commonly seen in a patient based on the mechanism of injury.

**kinematics** the branch of mechanics that studies the movement of body segments without consideration given to its mass or the forces making it move.

**Figure 17-1** To evaluate injuries, rescue personnel must understand the relationship between the possible expected injuries and the roles that speed, mass, and energy play.
Copyright Scott Smith

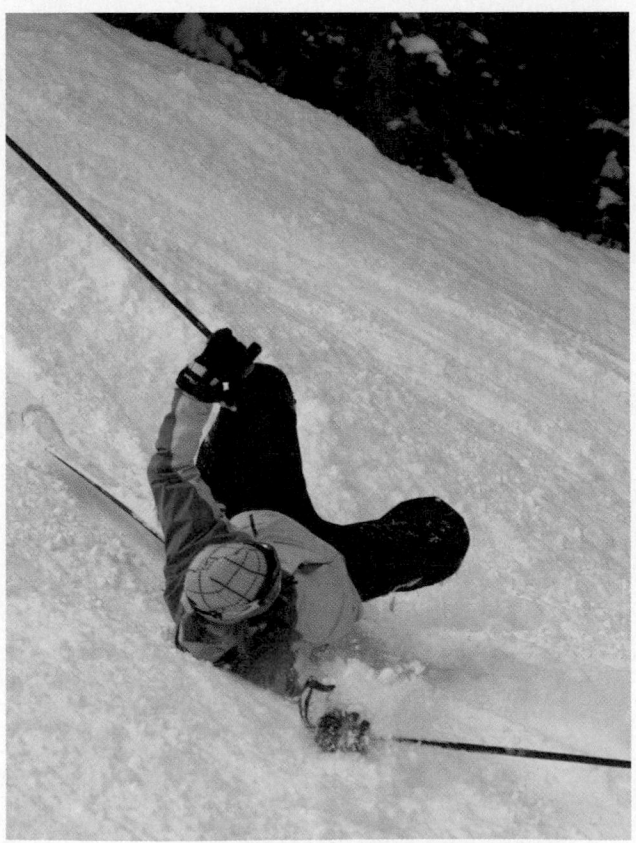

**17-1** Define the following terms:
- kinematics
- mechanism of injury
- index of suspicion

best illustrated by Sir Isaac Newton's first law of motion, which states that "a body in motion will remain in motion unless acted upon by an outside force." The law also states that "an object at rest will remain at rest unless acted upon by an outside force."

The significance of this law is best illustrated by the following situation. According to Newton's first law, a snowboarder moving down a slope (an object in motion) will continue to move downhill unless acted on by some outside force (Figure 17-2a■). Similarly, a skier who has stopped in the middle of the slope (an object at rest) will not move unless acted upon by some outside force. If the skier has stopped in the path of the snowboarder such that the snowboarder hits the skier, the snowboarder's energy of motion would be transferred to the skier, stopping the snowboarder and causing the skier to abruptly move (Figure 17-2b■). This brings to mind Newton's third law of motion, which states that "For every action there is an equal and opposite reaction." Similarly, when a skier hits a large tree, the skier's motion is abruptly halted (Figure 17-3■).

Another law of physics is the "law of conservation of energy," which helps explain why injury patterns can be predicted. According to this law, energy can be neither created nor destroyed but can only be changed in form or transferred between objects. In the case of the skier who crashed into a tree, a certain amount of energy, aided by gravity, was required to start the skier moving down the mountain. As she accelerated down the slope, energy in the form of downhill motion increased. When her forward motion was abruptly stopped by hitting the tree, the energy—known as "**kinetic energy**"—was just as abruptly transferred into her body.

Physicists use the following equation to calculate kinetic energy:

$$\text{kinetic energy (KE)} = \frac{\text{mass} \times \text{velocity}^2}{2}$$

In this equation, mass (m) equals the weight mass × velocity$^2$ of an object (in kilograms, or kg), whereas velocity (v) is the speed at which the object is traveling (mea-

**kinetic energy**   the energy generated by a body in motion; mathematically expressed as mass × velocity.

**Figure 17-2a** Newton's first law: This snowboarder will continue to move downhill unless acted upon by some outside force (perhaps some stationary object).
Copyright Scott Smith

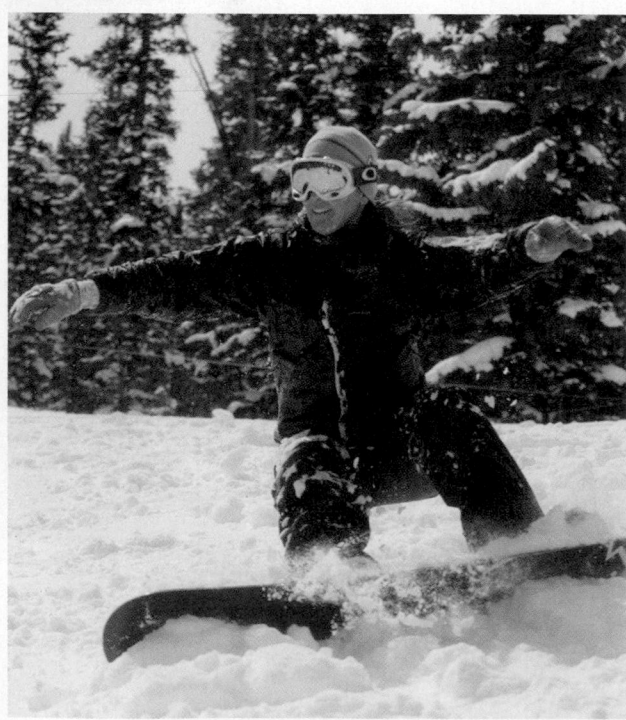

**Figure 17-2b** This snowboarder is stopping after hitting a skier and transferring energy to the skier who was thrown farther down the slope.
Copyright Scott Smith

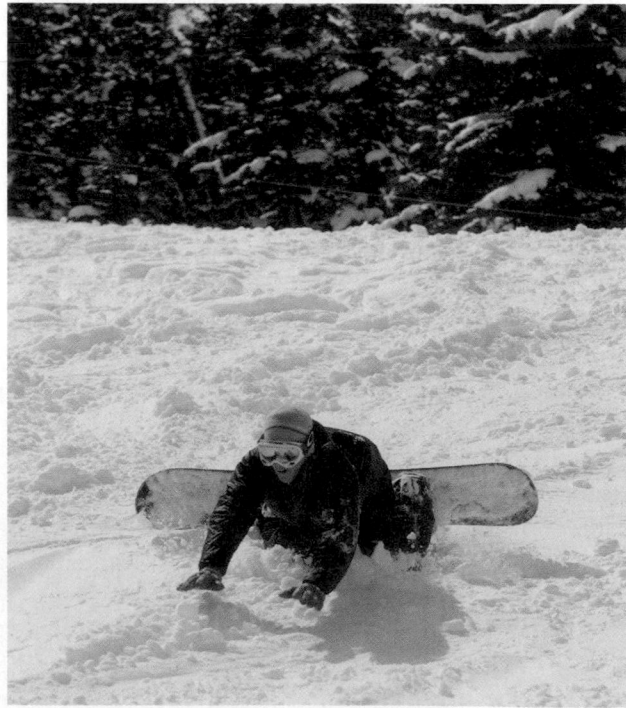

sured in meters per second, or mps). Using this equation, it is easy to see that speed is much more important than weight in determining the amount of kinetic energy (measured in joules) that is transmitted to a body (Figure 17-4a■). Thus, a very large snowboarder will experience less transmitted force when hitting the ground at a low speed than will a smaller snowboarder who is moving at a very high speed (Figures 17-4b■ and 17-4c■).

Another physics concept that is relevant to injury patterns is "stopping distance," or the amount of space necessary for kinetic energy to dissipate during an impact. Imagine if instead of hitting a tree, a snowboarder struck a pliable net that could stretch to absorb her impact (Figure 17-5■). Once she had completely stopped, the amount of kinetic energy transferred to her would be the same, but the distribution and severity of injury would be vastly different because of the flexibility of the object she struck spread the transfer of the energy over both distance and time. So both speed and stopping distance are key factors that dramatically affect both injury potential and the severity of injuries that actually occur.

Just as the type of material the body strikes can influence injury severity, so does the composition of the body's internal structures. Put another way, because different body parts have different densities, they absorb kinetic energy differently (Figure 17-6■). Hollow organs such as the lungs and intestines are filled with air, whereas solid organs such as the kidneys and muscles are filled with fluid, which is much denser than air. Still other body parts, such as bone and cartilage, are more rigid and have even greater

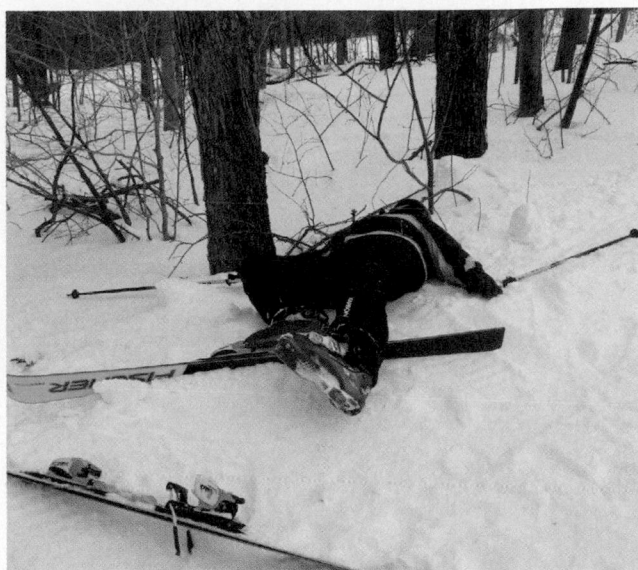

**Figure 17-3** Newton's third law: for every action there is an equal and opposite reaction. When this skier collided with the tree, the energy of motion was transferred to the skier's body.
Copyright Edward McNamara

**Figure 17-4a** Speed is a much more important factor than mass when considering potential injuries from collisions.
Copyright Scott Smith

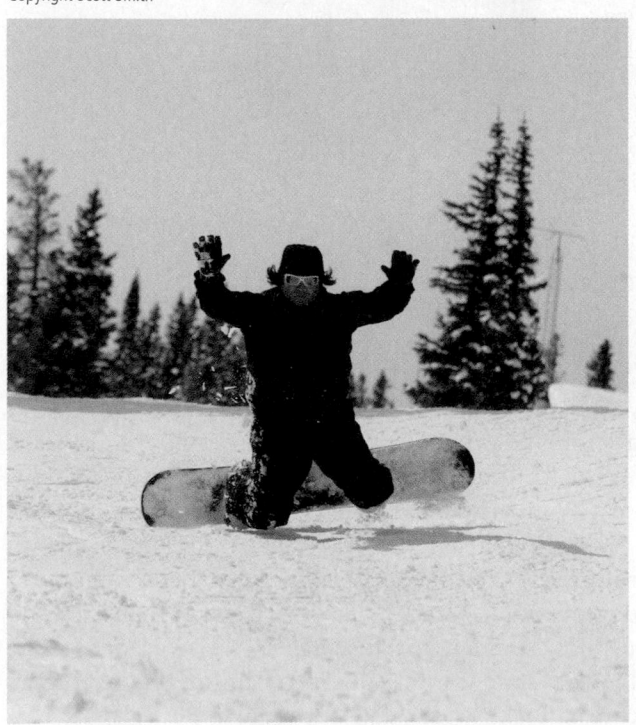

**Figure 17-4b** A large person going slowly has less kinetic energy, and thus is likely to experience less injury, than a smaller person going very fast.
Copyright Scott Smith

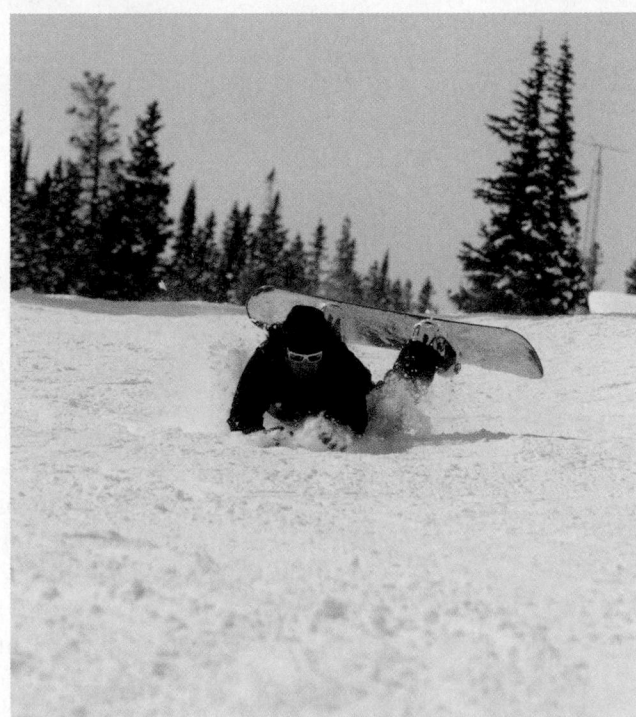

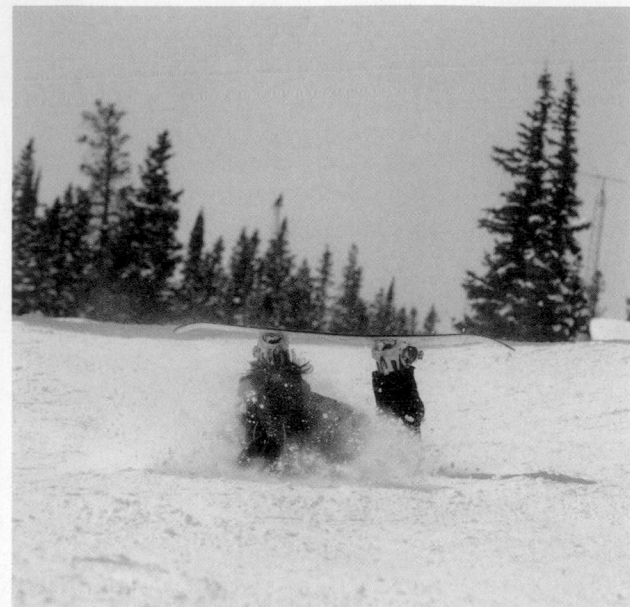

**Figure 17-4c** When a snowboarder falls forward, the potential for knee and wrist injury is great.
Copyright Scott Smith

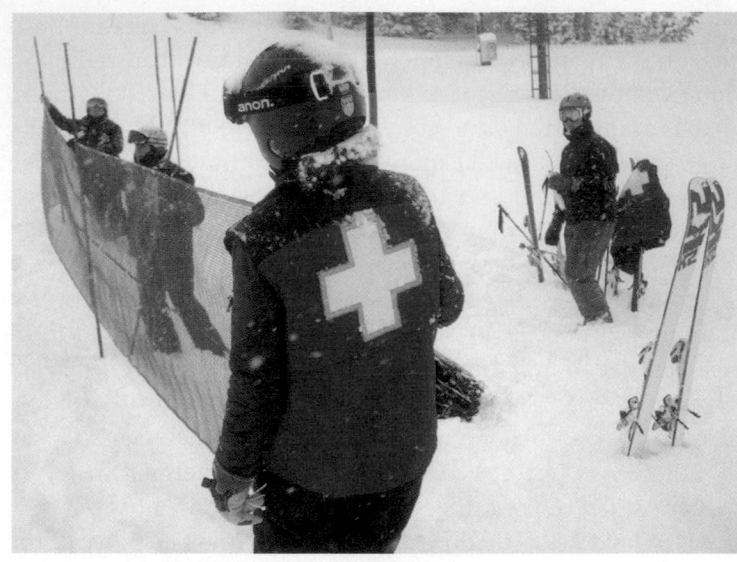

**Figure 17-5** Impacting a soft, pliable surface allows the energy to be dissipated over a longer distance and a longer time, so you would expect fewer injuries to be incurred.
Copyright Scott Smith

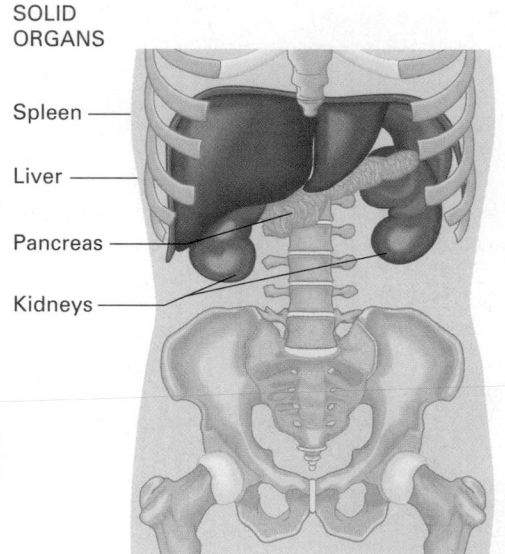

SOLID ORGANS

Spleen
Liver
Pancreas
Kidneys

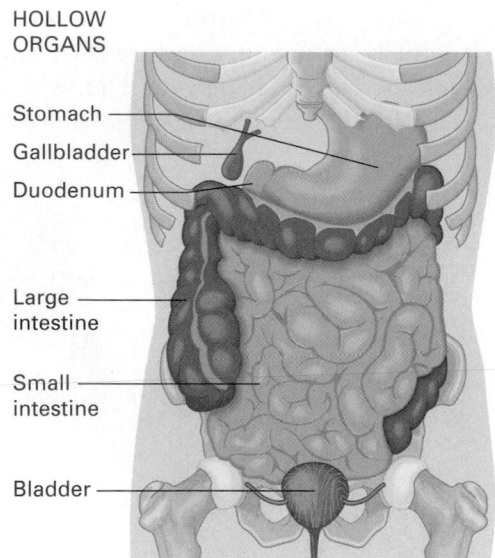

HOLLOW ORGANS

Stomach
Gallbladder
Duodenum

Large intestine

Small intestine

Bladder

**Figure 17-6** Solid organs (left) are denser than hollow organs (right) and thus are more likely to rupture upon impact.

density. Because each of these structures absorbs and transmits energy differently based on their densities, they have different "thresholds of injury."

Bone is well suited to protecting underlying structures because it is more resistant to cuts and punctures than is skin. When a bone breaks, it absorbs kinetic energy and reduces the amount of energy available to be transmitted to less-dense structures that lie beneath. Hollow ("air-dense") organs are less likely to rupture than are solid ("water-dense") organs. The urinary bladder, for instance is considered an "air-dense" organ when empty, and in that state it is less likely to rupture due to trauma than is a full bladder, which is considered a "water-dense" organ.

# Pathophysiology and Mechanisms of Injury

The severity of bodily injury is directly related to three factors: the amount of kinetic energy absorbed, the direction the energy travels through the body, and the density of the body structures impacted. Taken together, these three factors result in different types of injuries, referred to as "mechanisms of injury" or MOI (Figure 17-7■). In different situations, each of these factors can have greater or lesser influence on the locations and severity of the injuries incurred.

OEC Technicians should be familiar with the following five major MOIs:

1. Blunt injury
2. Penetrating injury
3. Rotational injury
4. Crush injury
5. Blast injury

> ### Kinetic Energy
>
> A 100 kg/220 lb person is traveling at 4 meters per second and a 60 kg/132 lb person traveling at 8 meters per second (different speeds). The patient who weighs less has more kinetic energy, and therefore more force when striking a fixed object. Speed is more important than weight, when calculating kinetic energy.
>
> $$KE = \frac{100 \text{ kg} \times 4 \text{ mps}^2}{2} \quad KE = \frac{1,600}{2} \quad KE = 800 \text{ joules}^*$$
>
> $$KE = \frac{60 \text{ kg} \times 8 \text{ mps}^2}{2} \quad KE = \frac{3,840}{2} \quad KE = 1,920 \text{ joules}^*$$
>
> *a joule is the standard metric unit of energy

**Figure 17-7** Mechanisms of injury (MOI) are determined by the force that produced the injury, and the direction and intensity of the injury.

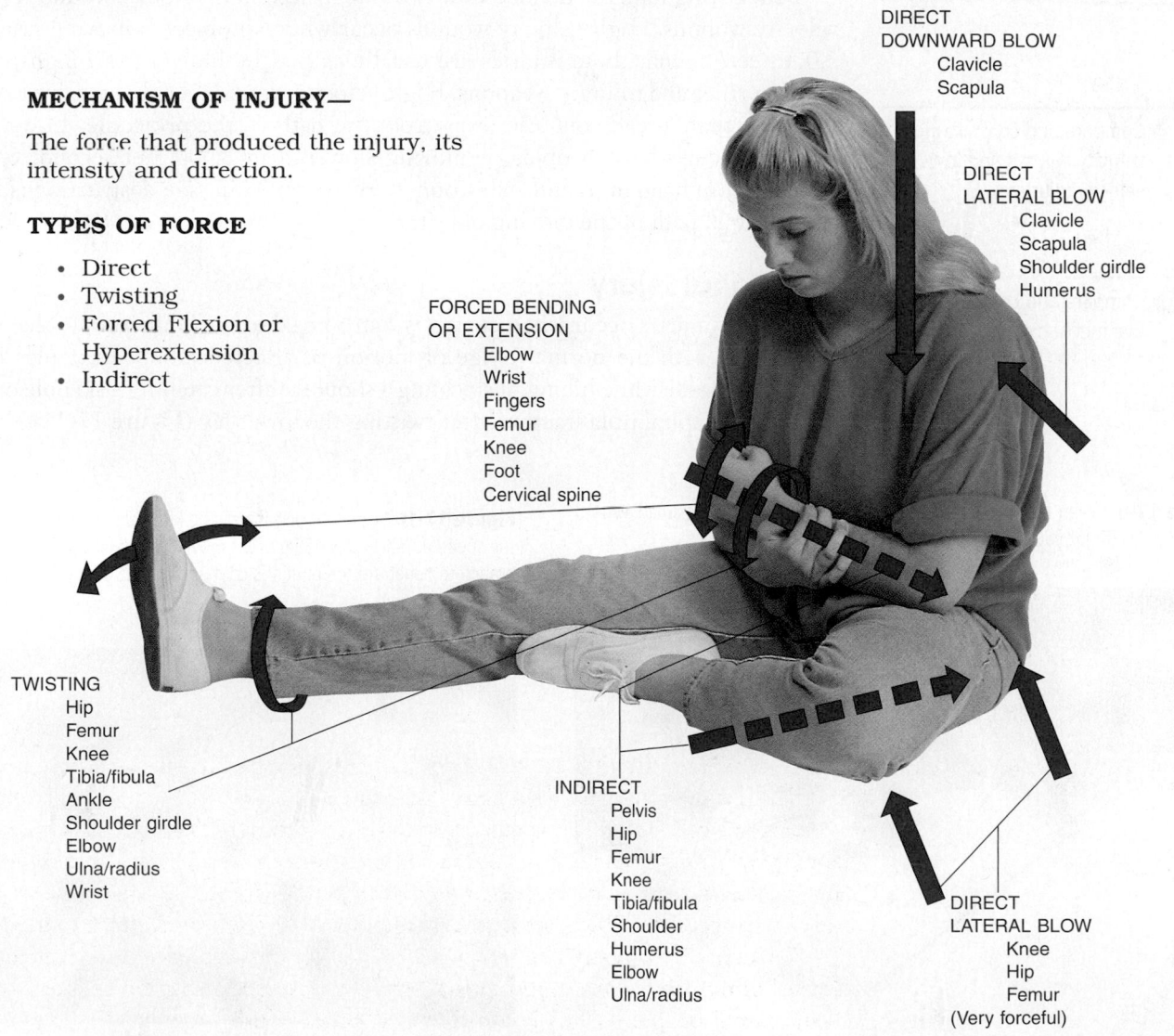

**MECHANISM OF INJURY—**

The force that produced the injury, its intensity and direction.

**TYPES OF FORCE**

- Direct
- Twisting
- Forced Flexion or Hyperextension
- Indirect

FORCED BENDING OR EXTENSION
Elbow
Wrist
Fingers
Femur
Knee
Foot
Cervical spine

DIRECT DOWNWARD BLOW
Clavicle
Scapula

DIRECT LATERAL BLOW
Clavicle
Scapula
Shoulder girdle
Humerus

TWISTING
Hip
Femur
Knee
Tibia/fibula
Ankle
Shoulder girdle
Elbow
Ulna/radius
Wrist

INDIRECT
Pelvis
Hip
Femur
Knee
Tibia/fibula
Shoulder
Humerus
Elbow
Ulna/radius

DIRECT LATERAL BLOW
Knee
Hip
Femur
(Very forceful)

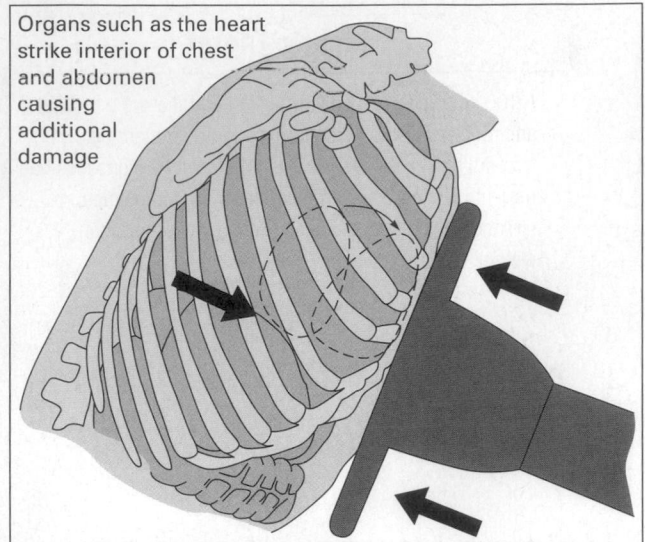

Organs such as the heart strike interior of chest and abdomen causing additional damage

**Figure 17-8** In blunt injuries, the kinetic energy is transmitted through the skin to underlying bones, tissues, and organs, which may become damaged upon impact.

⊕ **17-2** Compare and contrast high-velocity injuries and low-velocity injuries.

⊕ **17-3** Compare and contrast the five mechanisms of injury.

## Blunt Injury

A blunt, or "closed," injury is one in which kinetic energy is transmitted through, but does not break, the skin. Instead, it is transmitted to underlying structures, resulting in injuries such as bruised tissues, internal bleeding, broken bones, and organ damage (Figure 17-8■). Blunt injuries are commonly seen in falls, ski slope collisions, snow machine accidents, and as a result of physical assault (Figure 17-9■). Generally a blunt injury affects a larger portion of the skin's surface than does a penetrating injury.

## Penetrating Injury

A penetrating, or "open" injury, is one that breaks the skin and damages underlying structures. A smaller surface of the skin is affected when an object in motion, such as an ice tool, a knife, or a bullet, strikes the body with enough kinetic energy to pierce the skin. It can also occur when the body is moving with enough kinetic energy to impale itself upon an object such as a tree branch, a ski pole, an ice axe, or a bicycle handle bar (Figure 17-10■).

Penetrating injury is divided into two categories: high-velocity wounds and low-velocity wounds. High-velocity wounds occur when an object is moving faster than 2,000 feet/second; these injuries are usually caused by bullets from high-powered hunting rifles and military weapons. High-velocity wounds cause extensive tissue destruction that spreads out and away from the path of the projectile. Low-velocity wounds occur when an object is moving slower than 2,000 feet/second. Gunshot wounds from hand guns and stab wounds are examples. Tissue destruction is limited to the actual path of the moving object.

## Rotational Injury

Rotational injuries occur when energy is transmitted to the body in ways that are not compatible with the normal range of motion of affected joints. Examples include turning an ankle while hiking, dislocating a shoulder after catching a ski pole on a tree branch, or a spiral tibia fracture after twisting the lower leg (Figure 17-11■). In each

**Figure 17-9** When this skier went into this wall, blunt injuries resulted. What other injuries might you expect to find?
Copyright Edward McNamara

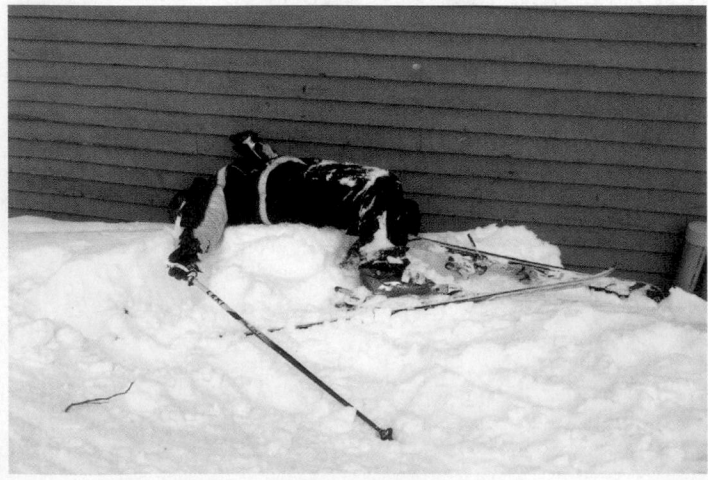

**Figure 17-10** A penetrating injury. The kinetic energy associated with the speed at which this patient was moving was enough for this tree branch to penetrate the patient's coat and skin and lodge within underlying tissues.
Copyright Charles Stewart, M.D. and Associates

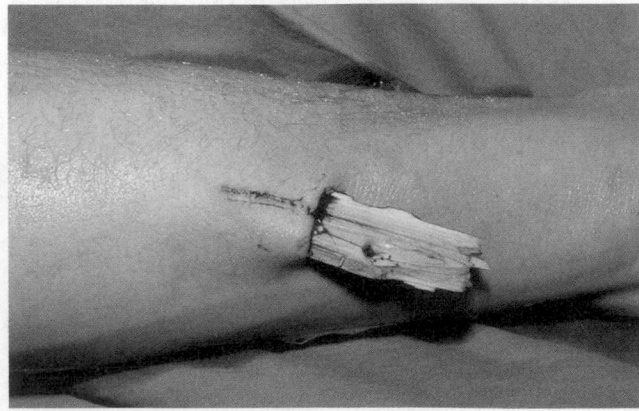

of these examples, the resulting trauma can be as significant as with other mechanisms of injury. However, the primary factor in a rotational injury is the direction the energy is traveling through the body, as opposed to the amount of kinetic energy absorbed in the impact of an object that strikes the body.

## Crush Injury

A crush injury occurs when a body part is caught between two or more heavy objects and is subjected to significant compressive force or pressure. This type of injury can produce devastating wounds that include penetrating trauma, blunt trauma, or both. Such injuries are common in river sports, backcountry skiing, and mountaineering and occur, for example, when an extremity is pinned between a large rock and a tree for an extended period of time (Figure 17-12■). Avalanche victims can also suffer from crush injuries.

## Blast Injury

Blast injuries are caused by an explosive force and are divided into four categories: primary, secondary, tertiary, and miscellaneous (or quaternary) injuries.

Primary blast injuries are due to a massive pressure wave that strikes the body following the rapid release and expansion of gases. Solid and water-dense tissues (such as the liver or urinary bladder) are minimally affected, whereas air-dense tissues (such as the lungs, ears, or intestines) can be contused or ruptured.

Secondary blast injuries are caused by airborne objects that strike the body. Tertiary blast injuries occur when the body is forcibly thrown and strikes other objects such as a wall or the ground.

Tertiary blast injuries are usually seen only in high-energy explosions (Figure 17-13■). Miscellaneous, or quaternary, injuries are caused by other blast-related factors such as ex-

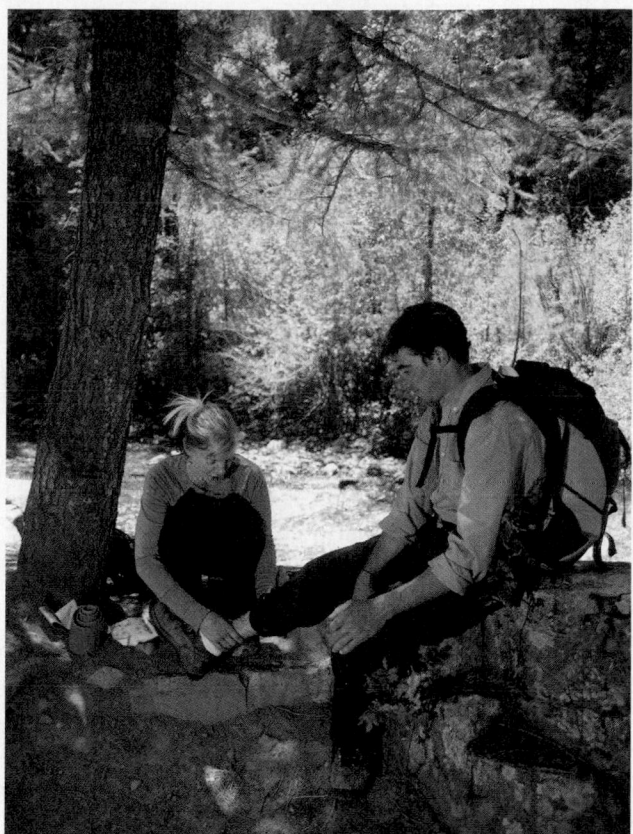

**Figure 17-11** In a rotational injury, the direction of the force applied to a joint is often a more important factor than the amount of kinetic energy absorbed.
Copyright Scott Smith

**Figure 17-12** A crush injury (or compression injury) results when soft tissues and bones are trapped and squeezed between two heavy objects, such as a rock and a tree.
Copyright Edward McNamara

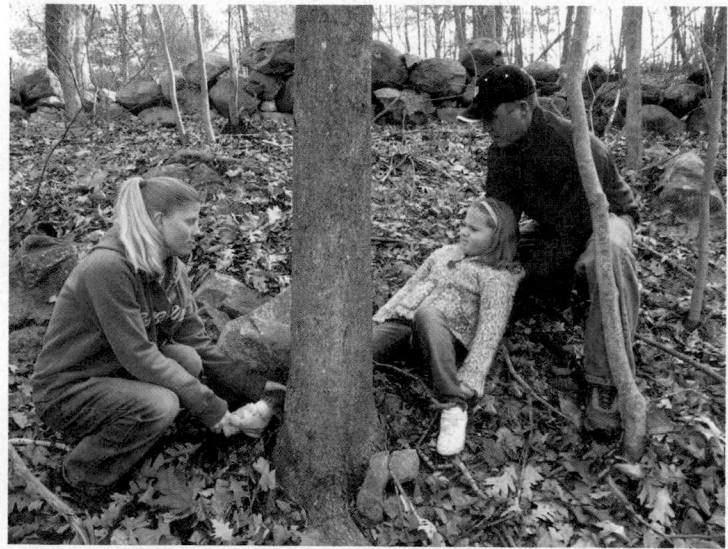

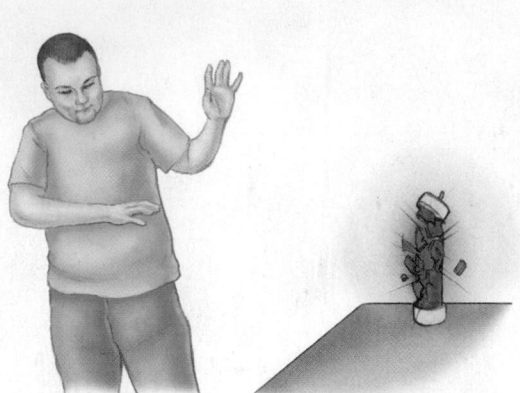

**(a) Explosion**
Instantaneous combustion of the explosive agent creates superheated gases. The resulting pressure blows the bomb casing apart.

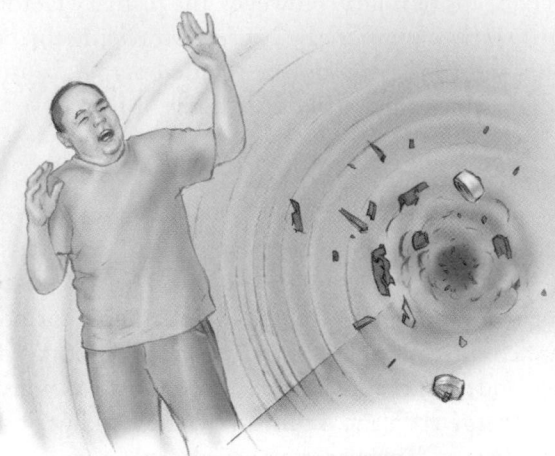

**(b) Pressure Wave/Primary Injury**
Air molecules slam into one another, creating a pressure wave moving outward from the blast center, causing pressure injuries.

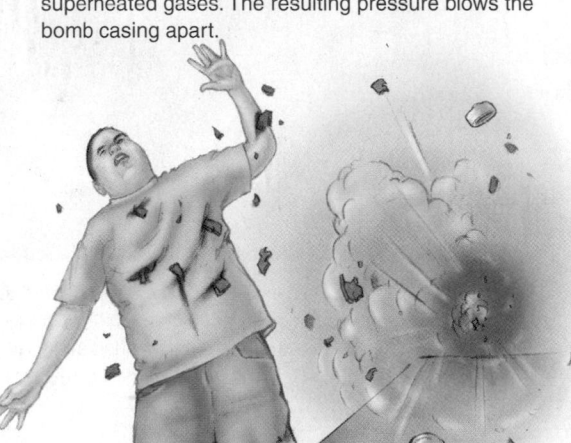

**(c) Blast Wave/Secondary Injury**
Instantaneous combustion of the explosive agent creates superheated gases. The resulting pressure blows the bomb casing apart. Pieces of the bomb become projectiles that cause injuries by impacting the victim.

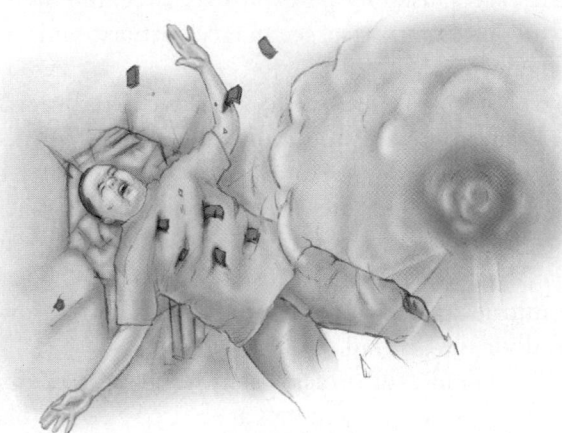

**(d) Victim Displacement/Tertiary Injury**
The blast wind may propel the victim to the ground or against objects, causing further injuries.

**Figure 17-13** Blast injuries: injury can result from the initial blast, from the patient being struck by debris, and/or from the patient being thrown by the blast.

posure to steam or burning materials, inhalation of toxins, or impact by debris from a collapsing building. Illnesses that are aggravated by a blast, including asthma, angina, hypertension, and anxiety, are also considered quaternary injuries.

Blast injuries are more commonly associated with an industrial accident or a military/terrorist event, but they could be encountered in backwoods environments. Examples include a camp stove explosion, a mountain lodge or gas/oil rig explosion an accidental explosion during avalanche control measures, and setting off land mines while traversing terrain in a previously war-torn country. During the initial stages of blast injuries, patients often exhibit a reflex response, termed a "blast pattern triad," which consists of initial apnea, bradycardia, and hypotension. Fortunately, these abnormal vital signs usually return to preblast values within a relatively short time unless other significant injuries are present.

# The Three Phases of Injury

The events surrounding injuries and the actions that health care providers can take with respect to injury management are often divided into three stages:

1. the pre-injury phase
2. the injury phase
3. the post-injury phase.

## Pre-Injury Phase

The pre-injury phase consists of the events and conditions leading up to an injury and can include medical predispositions such as alcohol intoxication, hypoglycemia, or hypothermia. It can also include mechanical predispositions such as a ski binding that fails to release, or environmental conditions such as the heights to which rock climbers ascend (Figure 17-14■). It is to this phase that risk management and injury prevention efforts, such as "Ski Safe" and helmet awareness programs, are directed. Preventive interventions, such as those implemented by the NSP Safety Team or ski areas, can be as important to overall trauma care as the successful management of actual traumatic injuries.

## Injury Phase

The injury phase is the brief period during which energy is transferred through a patient's body, resulting in physical injury from one of the various mechanisms previously described (Figure 17-15■). When assessing a trauma patient, it is important to

**Figure 17-14** In the pre-injury phase, factors such as predisposing health conditions and environmental conditions affect the likelihood of injury.
Copyright Scott Smith

**Figure 17-15** During the injury phase, a force or energy is transferred to the body, causing injury—in this case, to the patient's leg. This patient has also entered the beginning of the post-injury phase.
Copyright Scott Smith

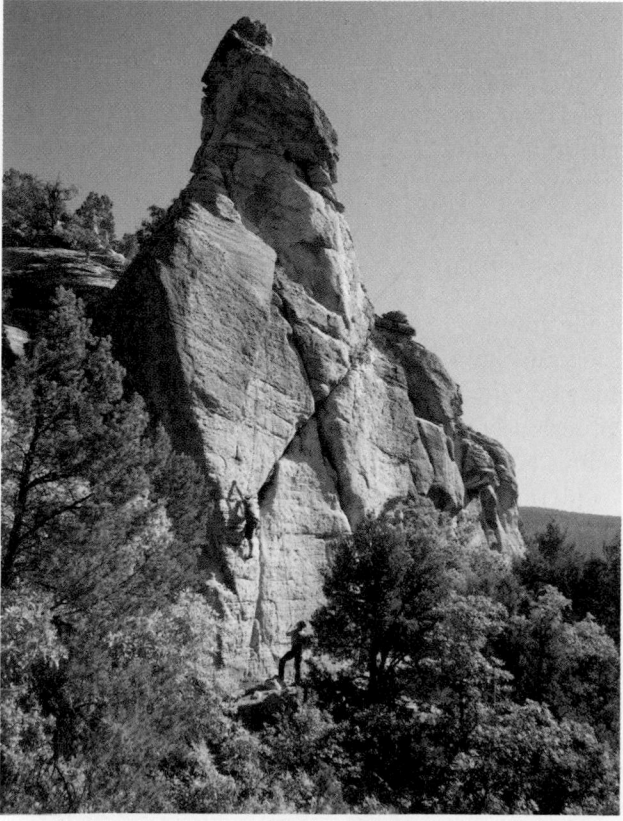

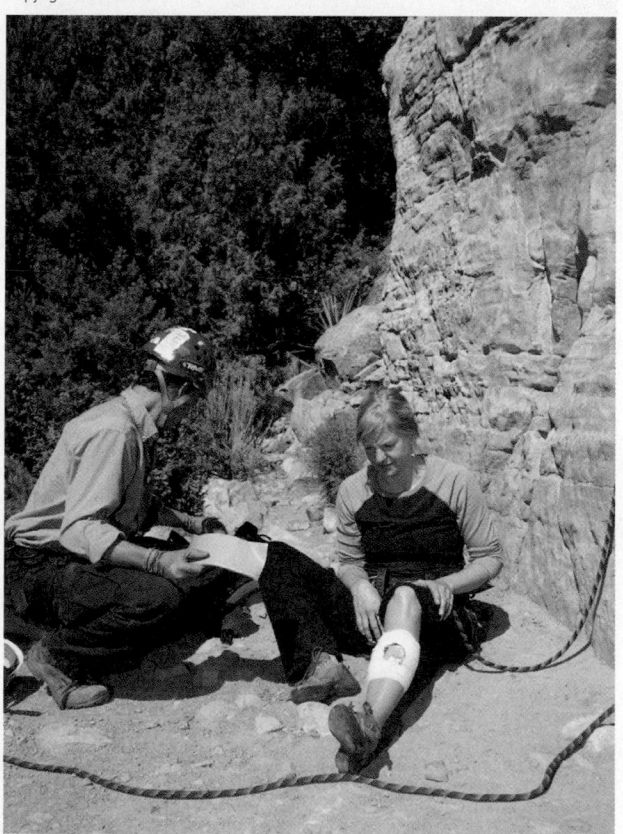

**index of suspicion** when evaluating a patient who has sustained trauma, the initial impression of what could be injured and how bad the injury is, based on the mechanism of injury.

**golden hour** the first 60 minutes following a serious traumatic event, during which prompt medical treatment may prevent death.

---

⊕ **17-4** Describe the role of a trauma center in improving the survival of a trauma patient.

**trauma center** a specialized hospital providing 24-hour trauma care, including stabilization, critical care, subspecialty care, and nursing care.

**Figure 17-16** This patient's initial care and rescue are occurring during the post-injury phase; in this case, the post-injury phase will likely last weeks or months.
Copyright Scott Smith

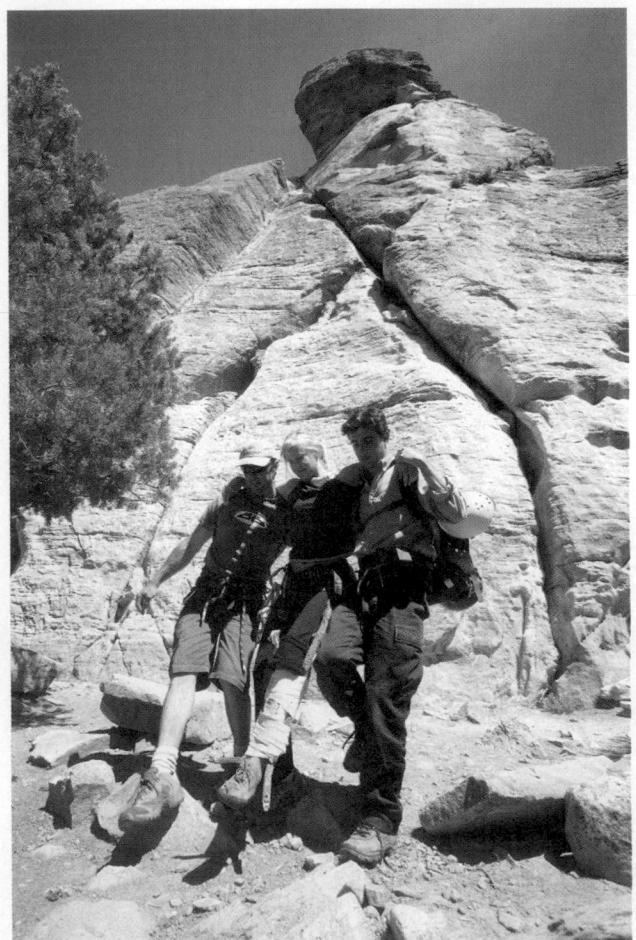

consider the direction in which energy has traveled, the amount of energy that was transferred, and the effect that the energy could have on the person's body, as each influences the types of injuries likely to be sustained. OEC Technicians must use this information to develop an **index of suspicion** to identify both the probability and likely severity of specific injuries. As previously mentioned, this index of suspicion and a physical examination are often all you will have to assess and treat an injury, because x-rays, blood tests, and other diagnostic tools will not be available.

### Post-Injury Phase

The post-injury phase begins as soon as energy transfer is complete (Figure 17-16■). This phase includes three times, or "peaks," when traumatic death generally occurs. The first peak occurs in the first few seconds to minutes following a catastrophic injury such as a massive brain injury, an injury to the upper spinal cord, or trauma to the heart. The second peak occurs in the first minutes to an hour following a critical injury such as a collapsed lung or massive bleeding. The third peak occurs in the days to weeks after the initial injury and is usually due to complications that arise from the traumatic incident, such as an infection or organ failure.

Deaths that occur in the first peak are often difficult to prevent in wilderness settings, although rapid intervention with procedures such as airway management and control of arterial bleeding can be life saving. Likewise, prompt initiation of ABCD-related procedures is especially important during the first 60 minutes of trauma care. Often referred to as the "**golden hour**," this first hour following injury is a crucial period during which survival rates may theoretically be enhanced if critical injuries are identified and properly managed (Figure 17-17■). In backcountry or wilderness settings, these actions can be difficult, and thus immediate evacuation to a specialized definitive-care facility, known as a trauma center, becomes a prime consideration for any patient with serious injuries. In the backcountry definitive care may not be available for many hours or even days, well past the second peak. In these cases, focus your care on preventing death during the third peak by providing meticulous wound care, preventing dehydration and malnutrition, and lessening the risk of complications resulting from immobility (e.g., pressure ulcers, pulmonary embolism).

## Trauma Systems

The role of the trauma system is especially relevant for OEC Technicians because awareness of the location of the nearest **trauma center** may affect the plans they make concerning the evacuation of seriously injured patients.

OEC Technicians such as ski patrollers, climbing and rafting guides, and wilderness medical teams should remain aware of the relative distances to hospitals that are designated trauma centers, and to those hospitals that are not so designated. Given an equal travel time, a designated trauma center will almost always be the preferred destination for critically injured, multi-system trauma patients. On occasion, injury severity or great distance may dictate that a trauma patient is not transported to a designated trauma center. If available, air evacuation should be considered if it will enable a severely traumatized victim to reach a designated trauma center more quickly (Figure 17-18■).

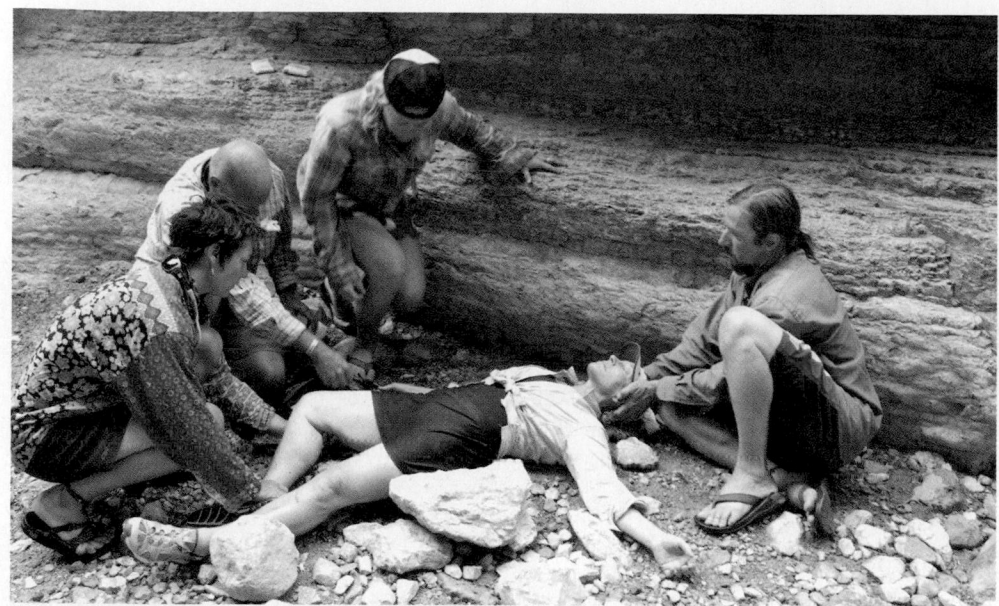

**Figure 17-17** In the backcountry, immediate extrication and evacuation, especially within the golden hour, may not be a realistic goal. Focus on the third peak of the post-injury phase: the prevention of death from complications.
Copyright Craig Brown

As mentioned in Chapter 2, a system of designated trauma centers has been established in the United States to provide specialized care to injured patients. Trauma centers are equipped to provide care to trauma patients at any time and are specifically designed to manage patients whose injuries involve two or more body systems, a condition known as "multi-system trauma." Examples of patients with multi-system trauma are a patient with fractures and a ruptured urinary bladder, who requires both orthopedic and urology management, and a patient with a serious head injury and a penetrating chest wound, who requires neurologic, thoracic, and vascular management. Definitive trauma care is coordinated by a **trauma surgeon**, who is a physician with specialized training in the treatment of severely injured patients (Figure 17-19■).

**trauma surgeon** a physician who specializes in trauma care.

The American College of Surgeons designates each trauma center at one of five levels based on the specialization, complexity, and availability of care that the facility can accommodate.

**Figure 17-18** Severely injured trauma patients should be transported to a designated trauma center as quickly as possible.
Copyright Mark Ide

## Level I

A Level I trauma center is the highest designation; it has 24-hour, in-house general/trauma surgeons as well as prompt availability of all major surgical subspecialties, anesthesia, specialized equipment, and specific other resources. Additionally, a Level I trauma center must maintain a certain volume of admitted trauma patients and have ongoing research and surgical residency programs.

## Level II

A Level II trauma center has the same surgical availability requirements as a Level I facility. It, however, is not required to conduct research or to have a surgical residency program.

## Level III

A Level III trauma center has a designated trauma surgeon available at all times but does not have every subspecialist available. In addition, a Level III facility can provide emergency resuscitation, surgery, and intensive care services and has transfer agreements with Level I or Level II centers to provide ongoing care for trauma patients whose medical needs exceed the Level III center's resources.

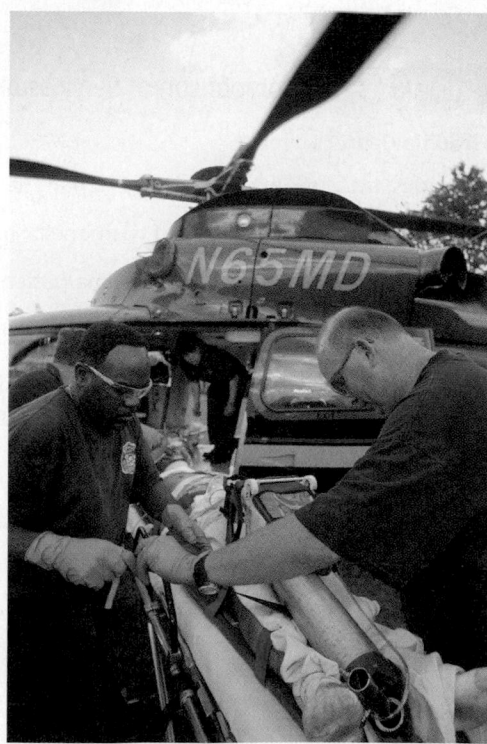

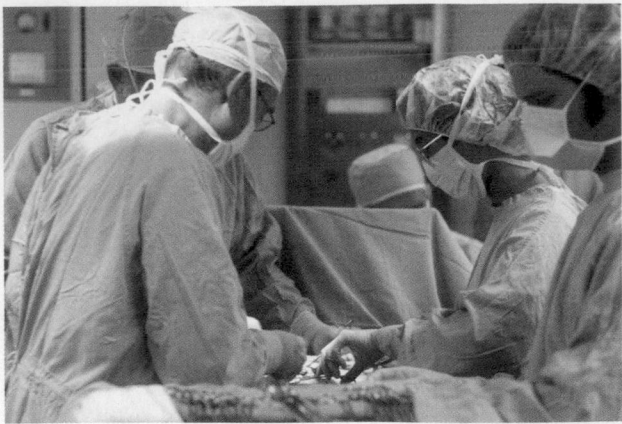

**Figure 17-19** In a trauma center, a trauma surgeon coordinates the critical medical interventions severely injured patients need to survive.

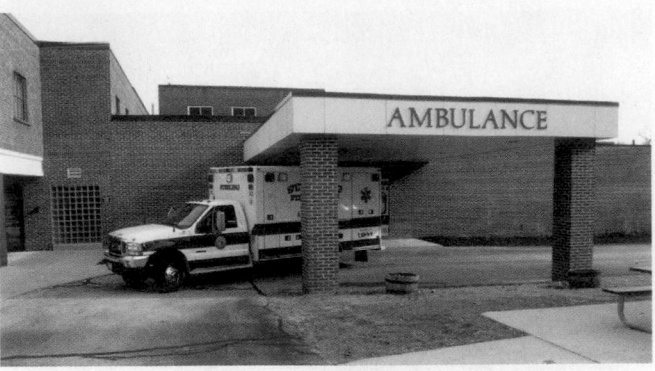

**Figure 17-20** Trauma centers are designated according to the level of care they are able to deliver. Community hospitals such as this one are not able to provide the level of trauma care that is available at Level I trauma centers. Copyright Edward McNamara

## Levels IV and V

Level IV and V trauma centers have a trained trauma nurse available at all times and have access to a physician who can be available upon the patient's arrival. These facilities provide basic resuscitative measures for trauma patients and have formal transfer agreements with Level I or II trauma centers to ensure quick access to definitive trauma care. Level I, II, and III trauma centers are typically located in densely populated areas, whereas Level IV and V centers are typically located in more sparsely populated regions (Figure 17-20■). Table 17-1■ compares the services available at the various levels of trauma centers.

## Pediatric Trauma

Level I and II pediatric trauma centers are also available to treat younger trauma patients. As their name implies, these centers focus exclusively on the needs of pediatric trauma patients. The differences between these two levels are identical to those of the Level I and II trauma centers just described.

## Table 17-1  Comparison of Services at Different-Level Trauma Centers

| Trauma Center Level | I | II | III | IV | V |
|---|---|---|---|---|---|
| Provides initial evaluation of trauma patient | x | x | x | x | x |
| Has formal transfer agreement with one or more higher level trauma centers | x | x | x | x | x |
| Provides initial stabilization of trauma patients | x | x | x | x | |
| Provides 24-hr availability of trauma equipment | x | x | x | | |
| Has a designated trauma nurse coordinator | x | x | x | | |
| Has a trained, in-house trauma staff | x | x | x | | |
| Has 24-hr sub-specialty coverage | x | x | | | |
| Meets minimum number of critical trauma patients seen annually | x | x | | | |
| Has trained, 24-hr in-house surgeon | x | x | x | | |
| Provides 24-hr comprehensive trauma care | x | x | | | |
| Performs trauma research | x | | | | |
| Has formal education and prevention programs | x | | | | |

# STOP, THINK, UNDERSTAND

## Multiple Choice

Choose the correct answer.

1. Kinetic energy is expressed by the equation KE = mass $\times$ velocity$^2$/2. What does this mean to you as a patroller?_____
   a. It means that body mass is more important than velocity when analyzing an accident.
   b. It means that speed is more important than body mass when analyzing an accident.
   c. It means that body mass and velocity should be given equal consideration when analyzing an accident.
   d. It means that if a large individual falls at a slow speed, he won't get hurt.

2. Another way to describe kinetic energy as it relates to an accident scene is_____

   a. that a large snowboarder will experience less transmitted force when hitting a tree at a slow speed than will a smaller snowboarder traveling at a higher speed.
   b. that a small individual who is traveling at a high speed and hits a tree is less likely to be injured than a larger individual traveling at a slower speed who hits the same tree.
   c. that if a large snowboarder hits a tree at a slow speed, first aid will not be necessary.
   d. that smaller individuals can't get hurt unless they are going fast.

3. What are the first 60 minutes of trauma care called?_____
   a. the desperate hour        c. the critical hour
   b. the vital hour            d. the golden hour

## List

List two key factors that dramatically affect both the potential and the severity of an injury.

_____

_____

_____

## Matching

1. Match each of the following MOIs with the following descriptions.

   _____ 1. blast injury
   _____ 2. blunt injury
   _____ 3. crush injury
   _____ 4. penetrating injury
   _____ 5. rotational injury

   a. A snowboarder falls and slides into a tree, impaling his thigh on a branch.
   b. While climbing in a river valley, a heavy rock tips over and pins your left leg between the fallen rock and another boulder.
   c. While skiing down a mogul field, you fall spread eagle into a mogul and come to a jarring stop with painful ribs and abdomen.
   d. A bike racer runs into a parked car.
   e. While skiing through the trees, a skier catches his pole in some low branches, dislocating his shoulder.
   f. A river guide is thrown from his raft and bounces through the rapids, receiving multiple injuries.
   g. While walking back to your condo after a long day of skiing, your husband slips on a patch of ice, twisting his knee.
   h. A camp stove explodes, injuring a fellow camper.
   i. A police officer is shot in the line of duty.
   j. A skier twists his leg, fracturing his tibia and fibula.

2. Match each of the levels of trauma center with the following descriptions. (some descriptions may have more than one answer)

   _____ 1. Level I trauma center
   _____ 2. Level II trauma center
   _____ 3. Level III trauma center
   _____ 4. Level IV trauma center
   _____ 5. Level V trauma center

   a. is typically located in sparsely populated regions
   b. is the highest designation of trauma center
   c. has a designated trauma surgeon available at all times, but does not have every subspecialist available
   d. has the same requirements as a Level I center but is not required to conduct research
   e. is typically located in densely populated areas

# CASE UPDATE

You are concerned that the mechanism of injury—slamming into hard, compacted snow at a high rate of speed—may have caused internal injuries. Your suspicions are soon confirmed, because even though no external trauma is apparent, the patient's condition begins to deteriorate. The patient's initial pulse and respirations were 92 beats/min and 18 breaths/min; they are now 140 beats/min and 26 breaths/min. You suspect that this deterioration in condition is due to internal bleeding caused by blunt trauma. You notify the dispatcher to send assistance and to activate the local trauma system, including ALS transport. The pain in the patient's right hip area is significant, and you know that any mishandling could accelerate the deterioration of the patient's general condition.

*What should you do now?*

# Assessment

The general principles for assessing patients, which were discussed extensively in Chapter 7, hold true when assessing a trauma patient. The process begins, as always, with a scene size-up in which potential hazards are identified and addressed, and by donning appropriate protective gear. Because traumatic injuries often include the presence of body fluids such as blood, urine, and cerebrospinal fluid, OEC Technicians must take precautions following Standard Precautions to safeguard themselves from these and other hazards.

The scene size-up includes an assessment of the mechanism of injury, which can yield valuable clues regarding how seriously the patient may be injured and the type of injury (Figure 17-21■). If the MOI has produced severe injuries, assess the need for spinal stabilization and, if indicated, manually immobilize the neck as described in Chapter 21, Head and Spine Injuries (Figure 17-22■). Determine as well whether the incident involves multiple patients, or whether the injuries incurred require immediate ALS intervention or rapid evacuation to a trauma center.

A trauma assessment should include a quick evaluation of the patient's level of responsiveness followed by a primary assessment of the ABCDs, with initial emphasis on identifying the need for life-saving interventions. This should take no more than

**Figure 17-22** If the MOI has produced serious injuries, spinal immobilization may be indicated.
Copyright Scott Smith

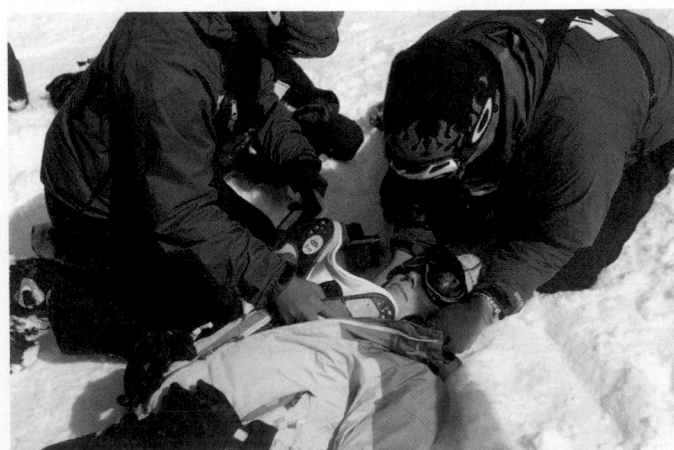

**Figure 17-21** The scene size-up and an assessment of the MOI for the potential and severity of injury can yield important clues to a patient's injuries.
Copyright Scott Smith

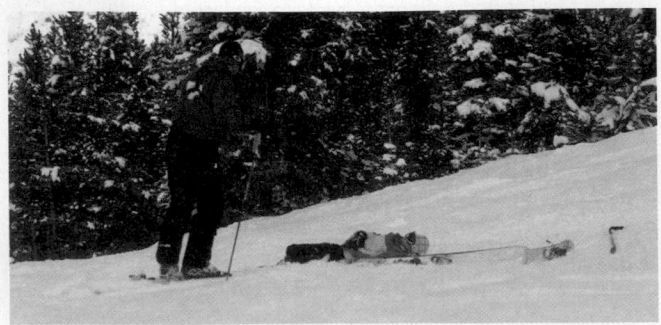

30 seconds to complete. Once immediate threats to life have been corrected, perform a head-to-toe secondary assessment in which the head, neck, chest, abdomen, pelvis, upper legs, back, and finally the extremities are checked for other injuries. The DCAP-BTLS mnemonic, which was discussed in Chapter 7, is a very helpful tool that can facilitate this process, all of which should take two minutes or less.

Obtaining a complete medical history is a critical part of the secondary assessment. If the patient is unresponsive and there were no witnesses to the incident, a good history may not be attainable. You must then base your assessment of what happened on what the scene tells you. For example, if you find an unresponsive patient with an oddly angled thigh lying beneath a cliff, he most likely fell off the cliff. Also, check patients for a medic alert tag. In addition to a standard SAMPLE history, described in Chapter 7, gather the following trauma-specific information:

+ The forces involved. Assessment of many suspected trauma injuries may be based only on a good understanding of basic physics and pathophysiology. Any apparent injury to a body part, even based solely on the mechanism of injury and without any initial objective findings, should prompt a thorough evaluation of that body part, as serious trauma may not be initially apparent.

+ Treatment rendered prior to your arrival. Well-meaning bystanders often attempt to render aid to an injured person. Unfortunately, their actions may include remedies that could have unintended consequences or even cause additional injury. Examples include moving a patient with a spinal injury, blocking the airway by placing a jacket under the patient's head, inserting an object into the mouth of a seizing patient, or applying an inappropriate tourniquet.

As part of the history gathering process, use the organized approach for assessing pain provided by the OPQRST mnemonic. Obtain a set of vital signs during the secondary assessment (Figure 17-23■). Take the pulse and respirations; blood pressure may be approximated by finding a carotid, femoral, or radial pulse as described in Chapter 7.

The information obtained through the trauma assessment should enable you to decide if the patient's injuries require immediate transport and to formulate a treatment plan (Figure 17-24■). When making a transport decision, consider whether or not evacuation is necessary because this may warrant the mobilization of a helicopter, an extrication vehicle, or a specialized wilderness search and rescue team. Likewise,

**Figure 17-23** Obtaining a set of baseline vital signs is an important component of a secondary assessment.
Copyright Scott Smith

**Figure 17-24** The trauma assessment should enable you to decide if the patient's injuries require immediate transport and to formulate a treatment plan.
Copyright Scott Smith

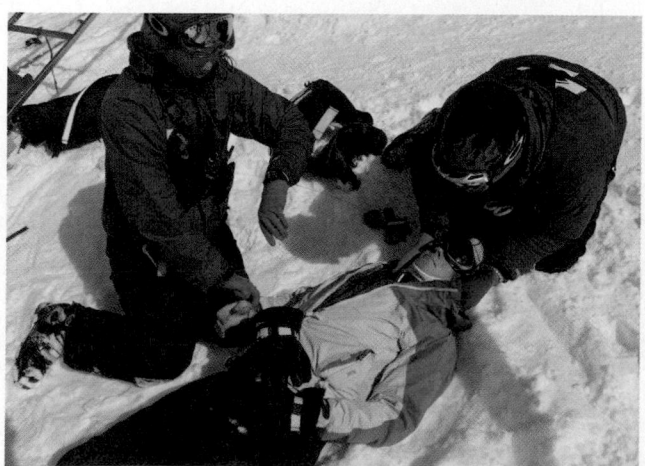
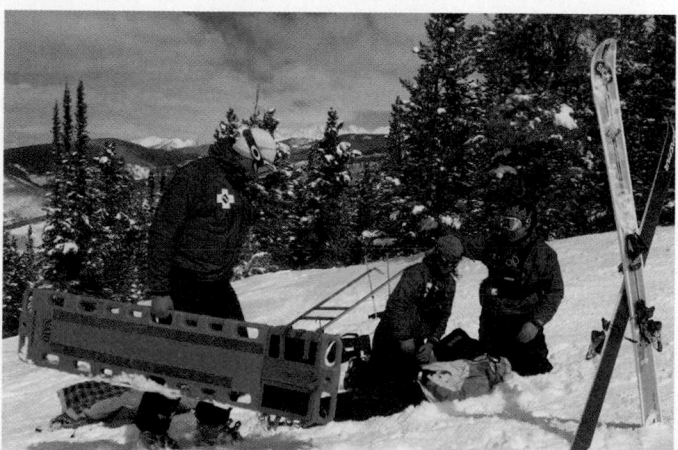

environmental factors such as current weather conditions, expected weather changes, terrain, temperature, time of day, altitude, tide changes, and the availability of survival gear must also be considered.

Monitor and reassess the patient frequently by taking vital signs every five minutes for critical patients, and every 15 minutes for noncritical patients. Reassess the area of injury frequently to ensure that, for example, bleeding that had been controlled has not started again.

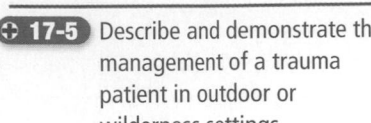

⊕ **17-5** Describe and demonstrate the management of a trauma patient in outdoor or wilderness settings.

# Management

Management of trauma patients varies greatly and depends on the kinematics involved, the mechanism of injury, injury severity, available resources, and distance to a medical facility. The treatment of specific injuries is covered in the chapters that follow.

As for any patient, the first step in managing a person who has been injured is to mitigate any hazards that may be present. In outdoor settings, this can be extremely difficult, if not altogether impossible. Next, assess the ABCDs and correct any immediate threats to life. If the patient is unresponsive, it is important to first open the airway, simultaneously assess breathing, and take a carotid pulse for a maximum of 10 seconds. If the patient is not breathing and there is no pulse, immediately begin CPR. See also Chapter 15, Cardiovascular Emergencies. In some cases, such as those involving active bleeding within the upper airway or an arterial bleed, you may not be able to proceed past this step until other rescuers arrive to assist. Stabilize the patient's spine, if indicated, by applying manual stabilization to the head and neck. This process, which must be maintained until replaced with mechanical stabilization, is covered in detail in Chapter 21, Head and Spine Injuries. Once all life threats have been managed in severely injured patients, administer oxygen at 12–15 LPM, by nonrebreather mask (Figure 17-25■). Monitor patients for shock and treat accordingly, being careful to keep them warm because hypothermia can hasten the effects of shock.

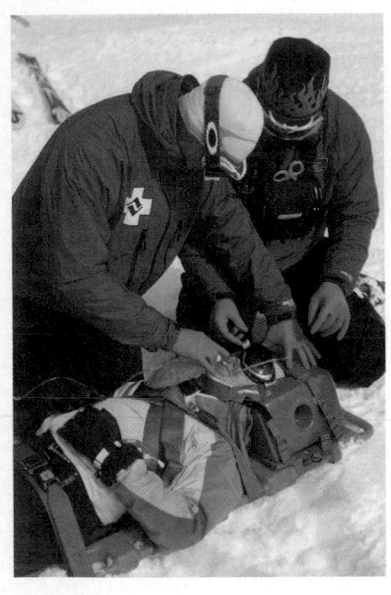

**Figure 17-25** Administer oxygen at 12–15 LPM by nonrebreather mask to severely injured patients to treat for shock.
Copyright Scott Smith

For patients who are stable and do not require "load and go" transport, turn your attention to any less critical injuries or problems that may exist, such as stabilizing long-bone fractures by applying splints. Then, prepare patients for transport to a medical care facility or, when appropriate, to a trauma center. The mode of transportation largely depends on your findings during the assessment. In general, protect trauma patients who exhibit evidence of neurologic compromise or a severe MOI from the elements and secure them either to a long spine board or in a basket-style litter (Figure 17-26■). Base your additional treatment decisions on reassessment findings. Finally, document your assessment findings and the treatments you provided on a patient care report, a copy of which should accompany the patient to the hospital.

**Figure 17-26** In general, keep patients warm and load them for transport with the most severe injury uphill.
Copyright Scott Smith

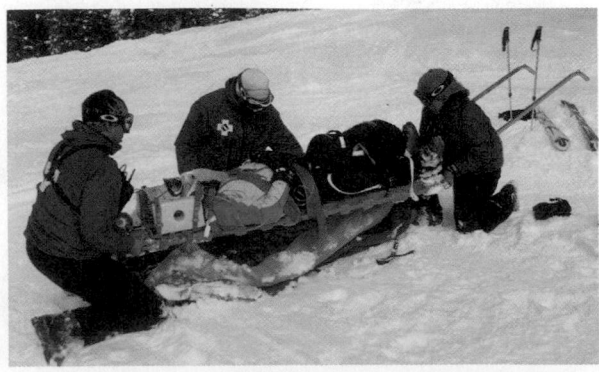

## CASE DISPOSITION

As other patrollers arrive, you inform them that you believe the patient is suffering from blunt trauma and has a high potential for serious internal injury. Given the mechanism of injury, the patient's deteriorating state, and your assessment findings, you suspect a fractured pelvis and internal bleeding.

Recognizing that this is a load-and-go situation, you place the patient on high-flow oxygen by nonrebreather mask and prepare to evacuate him from the slopes as expeditiously as possible. The patrollers use a sheet/blanket wrap to stabilize the pelvis, immobilize the spine and rapidly secure him to a backboard. (This is discussed in Chapter 24, Abdomen and Pelvic Trauma.) By radio, you notify the base clinic of your impending arrival. After delivering the patient, you assist the ALS provider start an IV. Soon after, a helicopter crew arrives and begins administering blood to the patient. They transport him past the local community hospital, which is only a few miles away, in favor of a Level II trauma center just a few air miles farther.

Later that day, the clinic physician joins you during a break in the patroller hut. He shakes your hand and tells you that he received a call from a trauma surgeon congratulating him and his staff on the rapid and comprehensive field care of the patient, who broke his pelvis in four places and is now stable and expected to make a full recovery.

# Chapter Review

## Chapter Summary

Trauma is an all-encompassing term used to describe a wide variety of injuries ranging from minor scrapes, bumps, and bruises, to broken bones and internal injuries, to life-threatening, multi-system injuries. Trauma is a common occurrence among outdoor recreationalists and an emergency that OEC Technicians will frequently encounter.

Many factors influence how trauma affects the human body, chief of which are kinematics, the mechanism of injury, and pathophysiology. Careful assessment of each of these factors forms the basis for the index of suspicion that OEC Technicians use to identify injury potential and severity, and to address patients' needs for initial care, equipment, and transportation.

Regardless of cause, effective serious trauma management in outdoor environments has three goals: early recognition of injury potential by assessing the mechanism of injury, quick correction of immediate threats to life, and rapid evacuation to a trauma center for definitive care, which may include surgical intervention.

A basic understanding of the forces associated with trauma provides OEC Technicians the information they need to understand the five mechanisms of trauma. This knowledge, when combined with an organized and rapid approach to trauma assessment, enables ski patrollers and OEC Technicians to recognize and treat potentially serious injuries quickly. These actions, in turn, help reduce the incidence of trauma-related deaths in our nation's outdoor recreational areas.

## Remember...

1. Trauma prevention is as important as trauma management.
2. Injuries can be divided into three phases: pre-injury, injury, and post-injury.
3. The five mechanisms of trauma are penetrating injury, blunt injury, crush injury, rotational injury, and blast injury.

4. A trauma center is a specialized medical facility geared toward addressing the specific needs of trauma patients.

5. Whenever possible, multi-system trauma patients should be taken to a trauma center.

6. When indicated by the MOI, early immobilization of a trauma patient's spine is essential.

7. The three goals of serious trauma management are early recognition, correction of threats to life, and rapid transportation to a trauma center.

# Chapter Questions

## Multiple Choice

Choose the correct answer.

1. How long should a primary assessment of a trauma patient take? _____
   a. 30 seconds
   b. 1–2 minutes
   c. 2–3 minutes
   d. 3–4 minutes

2. Which one of the following phases is not one of the three phases of injury? _____
   a. the post-traumatic phase
   b. the post-injury phase
   c. the pre-injury phase
   d. the injury phase

3. How often should you reassess critically ill patients? _____.
   a. every 2 minutes
   b. every 7 minutes
   c. every 15 minutes
   d. every 5 minutes

4. How often should you reassess patients with noncritical conditions? _____
   a. every 2 minutes
   b. every 7 minutes
   c. every 15 minutes
   d. every 5 minutes

5. Which one of the following is *not* a goal of trauma management in outdoor environments? _____
   a. quick corrections of immediate threats to life
   b. rapid evacuation to a trauma center
   c. avoiding taking time to care for the spine
   d. early recognition of injury potential

## List

1. List three tasks conducted during a scene size-up for a traumatic injury.

   _____

   _____

   _____

2. What does MOI stand for?

   _____

   _____

3. A complete history, including a SAMPLE history, should be obtained (if possible) at a trauma scene. What other trauma-specific information should be obtained?

   _____

   _____

   _____

**4.** What does the mnemonic OPQRST stand for?

_____

_____

_____

_____

_____

## Short Answer

**1.** To what hospital does your patrol usually send patients, and what level trauma center is it?

_____

_____

_____

**2.** What is the fastest way to access a Level I trauma center at your patrol?

_____

_____

_____

## Scenario

*You receive a call to go to the ski area's parking lot, close to the main chalet, to help someone with an unknown problem. There you locate a 22-year-old male, who appears restless, anxious, and complains of stomach pain. When asked what happened, the patient responds that about 12 hours ago he got into a fight with another male over a past girl friend. The patient reports that while he was on the ground he was punched in the stomach and kicked just below the ribs on his left side.*

**1.** The initial contact of the assailant's foot to this man's skin constitutes the_____
  **a.** contact phase.              **c.** impact phase.
  **b.** post-injury phase.          **d.** injury phase.

**2.** The mechanism of trauma that applies to this incident is_____
  **a.** crush injury.               **c.** secondary injury.
  **b.** blunt injury.               **d.** primary injury.

*After getting permission to do a secondary assessment, you find tenderness in the patient's upper left flank. The patient denies any head, back, or neck pain. The mechanism of injury leads you to believe that cervical stabilization is not required.*

*Palpation of the patient's upper left flank results in his rating his pain at 5 out of 10 on the pain scale. The patient also reports pain in his left shoulder even though he was neither struck nor fell on that shoulder.*

**3.** The patient's pain rating can be identified during a secondary assessment using the _____
  **a.** SAMPLE acronym.            **c.** SOAP acronym.
  **b.** DCAP-BTLS mnemonic.        **d.** OPQRST mnemonic.

*As you continue your assessment, the patient's pulse is 90 and weak, and his respirations are 26 per minute and shallow. The patient's skin is cool and moist. You determine that this is a "load and go" transport.*

*The SAMPLE interview confirmed that the patient's injuries occurred 12 hours ago. You reexamine the left shoulder and find no injuries that would explain the pain. Your knowledge of the mechanism of injury and the recognition that the shoulder pain is referred pain will help you confirm the suspected injury.*

**4.** The suspected injury in this incident is_____

    **a.** a ruptured appendix.

    **b.** an injured kidney.

    **c.** internal bleeding from a ruptured/damaged spleen.

    **d.** a dislocated shoulder.

## Suggested Reading

American Academy of Orthopaedic Surgeons 2008. "Action at an Emergency" and "Victim Assessment and Urgent Care." In *Wilderness First Aid: Emergency Care for Remote Locations*, edited by B. Gulli. Sudbury, MA: Jones & Bartlett Publishers.

Collier, B. R., et al. 2007. "Wilderness Trauma, Surgical Emergencies, and Wound Management." In *Wilderness Medicine*, Fifth Edition, edited by P. S. Acerbic. Philadelphia: Mosby-Elsevier.

Forgey, W. 1999. *Wilderness Medicine: Beyond First Aid*, Fifth Edition, Chapter 3. Merrillville, IN: ICS Books.

National Association of EMTs. 2007. *Prehospital Trauma Life Support*, Sixth Edition. St. Louis: Mosby JEMS Elsevier.

 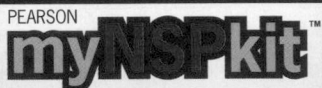

# Soft-Tissue Injuries

David Johe, MD

## ⊕ OBJECTIVES

**Upon completion of this chapter, the OEC Technician will be able to:**

**18-1** List four functions of the skin.

**18-2** List the layers of the skin.

**18-3** List and describe three types of closed soft-tissue injuries.

**18-4** List and describe nine types of open soft-tissue injuries.

**18-5** Describe the emergency care for the following injuries:
- closed soft-tissue injury
- open soft-tissue injury
- amputation
- impaled object

**18-6** Describe and demonstrate three methods for controlling external bleeding.

**18-7** Compare and contrast a dressing and a bandage.

**18-8** Demonstrate the proper procedure for applying each of the following:
- dressing
- bandage
- compression dressing
- tourniquet

## ⊕ KEY TERMS

**amputation,** *p. 547*
**bandage,** *p. 559*
**burn,** *p. 549*

**closed injury,** *p. 542*
**compartment syndrome,** *p. 545*
**compression dressing,** *p. 556*

**crush injury,** *p. 548*
**dermis,** *p. 540*
**dressing,** *p. 552*

*continued*

## Chapter Overview

Soft-tissue injuries are common occurrences in outdoor recreation and are an inherent risk of nearly every outdoor sport and activity. They are among the most common emergencies that OEC Technicians will encounter (Figure 18-1■). Identifying various soft-tissue wounds, controlling external bleeding, and caring for these injuries are essential skills.

*continued*

## HISTORICAL TIMELINE

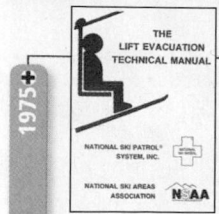

**1975** NSP publishes first "Lift Evacuation Technical Manual".

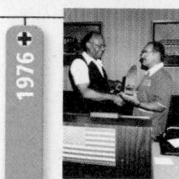

**1976** Charles Haskins becomes National Director.

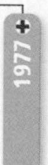

**1977** Patrollers required to complete the American Red Cross CPR course.

ecchymosis, *p. 543*
epidermis, *p. 539*
exsanguination, *p. 554*
extravascular, *p. 543*
hematoma, *p. 543*
hemorrhage, *p. 552*

hemostatic dressing, *p. 561*
impaled object, *p. 547*
inciscion, *p. 546*
occlusive dressing, *p. 561*
open injury, *p. 546*
pressure dressing, *p. 553*

puncture, *p. 547*
subcutaneous tissue, *p. 538*
subungual hematoma, *p. 543*
tourniquet, *p. 552*
universal dressing, *p. 558*

**subcutaneous tissue**  tissue between the dermis and the fascia overlying the muscle; contains fat, nerves, and blood vessels.

Soft-tissue injuries encompass wounds of the skin, the **subcutaneous tissue**, and muscle, and include everything from uncomplicated bumps to simple lacerations and bruises to life-threatening bleeding and major amputations (Figure 18-2■). In addition to the primary soft-tissue trauma caused by those injuries, underlying blood vessels, nerves, bones, and organs also may be damaged. Soft-tissue injuries can be serious and if not treated immediately can result in major organ injury and failure.

The skin has several functions, the most important of which is to serve as a protective barrier to external contaminants. In addition to its protective functions, the skin contains millions of tiny nerves that continually send sensory information to the brain. Although it is flexible and resilient, the skin is not impervious to injury and is easily damaged when exposed to abrasive or sharp objects or to heat, cold, or caustic substances. When penetrated, the skin's underlying structures and organs may be exposed to a variety of bacteria that can establish infections.

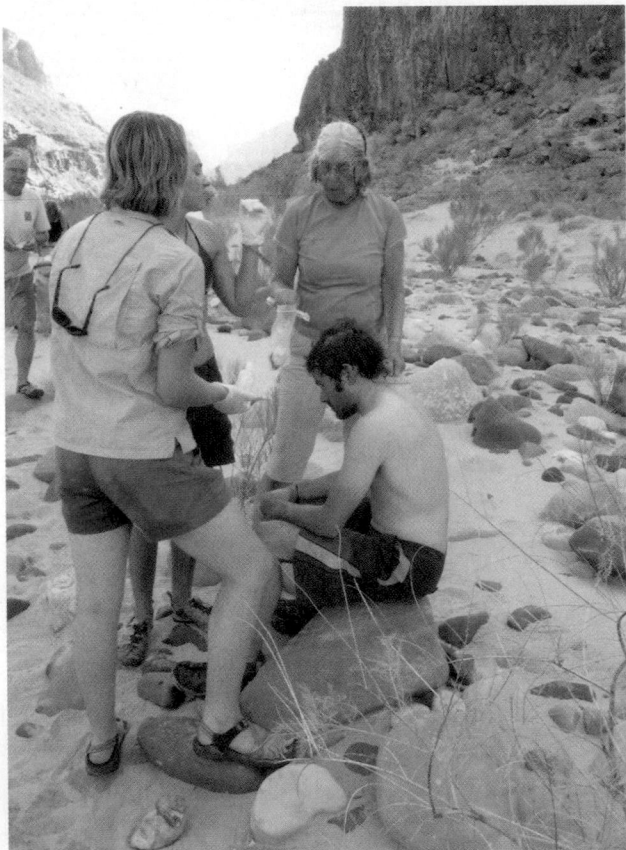

**Figure 18-2** Soft-tissue injuries such as this scalp laceration are very common in outdoor environments.
Copyright Brigitte Schran Brown

**Figure 18-1** The anatomy of soft tissues.

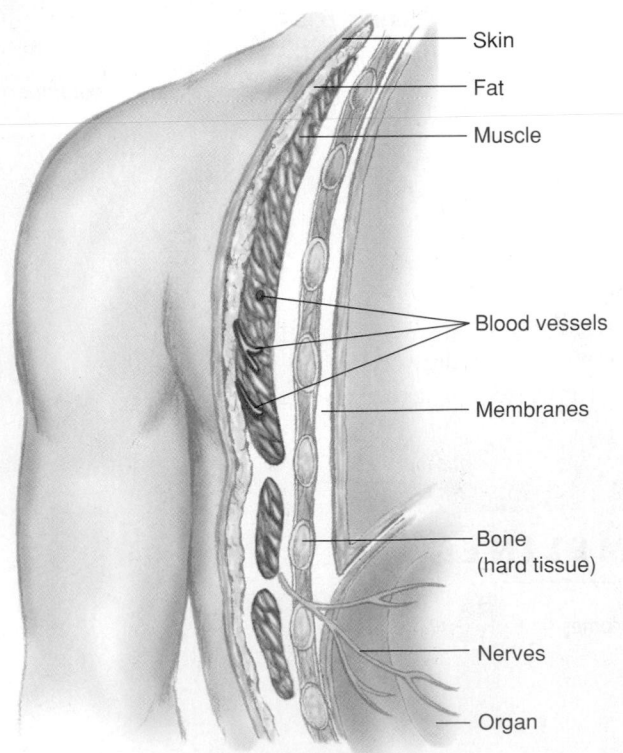

Skin
Fat
Muscle

Blood vessels

Membranes

Bone
(hard tissue)

Nerves

Organ

**CASE PRESENTATION**

As a member of your area bike patrol, you are called to assist a participant in a summer bicycle race who apparently lost control on the curve of a steep gravel road. As you approach the patient, you can see that his left arm and leg are covered with blood. He is responsive and alert but in obvious pain. When you introduce yourself and ask him what happened, he says, "I ate it big time." The patient is wearing a helmet and denies striking his head. He denies any neck or back pain. You note a deep, actively bleeding laceration over the cyclist's left bicep and multiple abrasions on his left arm and legs.

*What should you do?*

# Anatomy and Physiology of Skin

The skin is the body's largest organ and covers its entire external surface. It serves many purposes, including acting as a protective barrier, regulating body temperature, maintaining water balance, and synthesizing vitamin D.

## Skin Anatomy

As described in Chapter 6, Anatomy and Physiology, the skin consists of two layers: the **epidermis**, which lies on the surface and is several layers thick, and the dermis, which lies beneath the epidermis and contains several unique structures. Beneath the dermis are the subcutaneous tissue, muscles, bones, and other underlying structures (Figure 18-3■).

⊕ **18-1** List four functions of the skin.

⊕ **18-2** List the layers of the skin.

**epidermis** the outer layer of skin that act as a watertight protective covering.

**Figure 18-3** The anatomy of the skin.

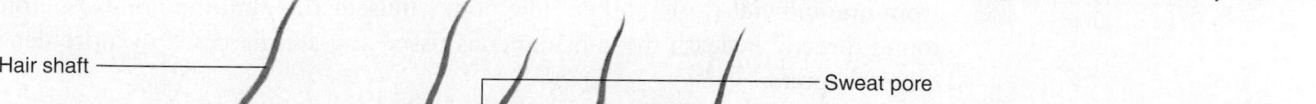

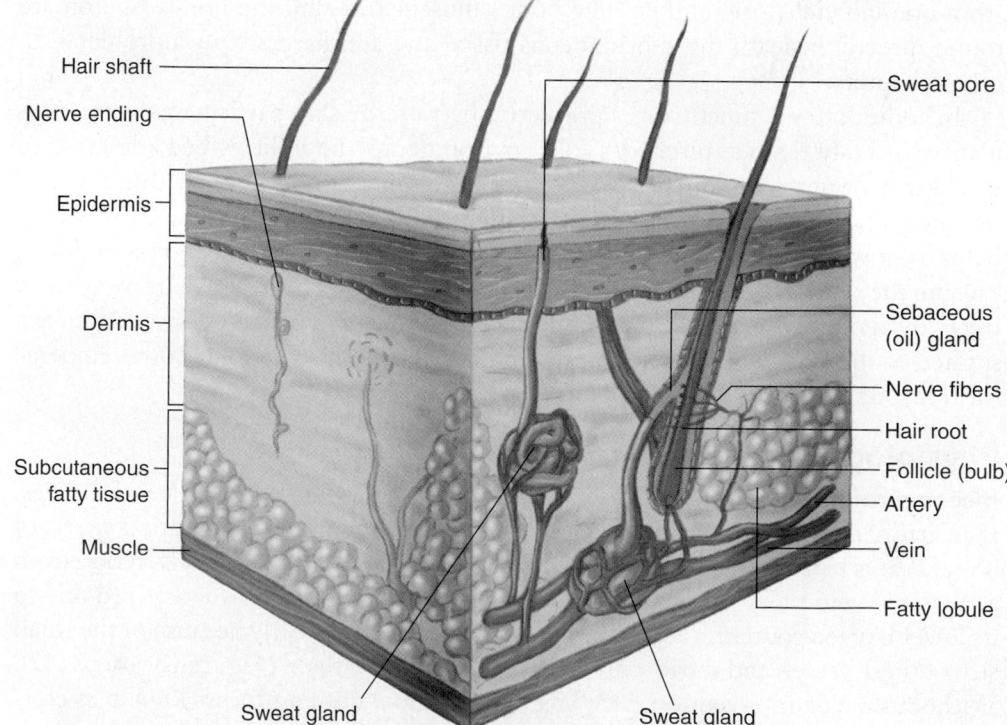

The epidermis grows from a germinal (basal) layer and continuously produces new cells that steadily migrate toward the surface. As these cells become more superficial, they are bonded securely together by an oily material to form a watertight, protective layer that helps the body retain water and prevents bacteria and other organisms from entering the body. The outermost epidermal cells are continually being rubbed away by normal daily activities and bathing and are replaced by new cells from below. The epidermis is very thick on the soles of the feet, the palms of the hands, the back, and the scalp, but it is very thin in other areas of the body, such as the back of the hand. Pigment granules in the deepest cells of the basal layer, along with small blood vessels in the dermis, combine to produce skin color.

**dermis** the inner layer of the skin; contains hair follicles, sweat glands, nerve endings, and blood vessels.

The **dermis** is the layer of the skin deep to the epidermis, and it contains several important structures, including hair follicles, sebaceous (oil) glands, sweat glands, blood vessels, and specialized nerve endings.

Hair follicles are the structures that produce hairs. Adjacent to each follicle are both a sebaceous gland and a very small muscle. Sebaceous glands secrete an oily substance, known as sebum, onto the skin surface. In addition to its waterproofing function, sebum helps keep the skin supple and prevents it from cracking. The adjacent muscle fibers cause the hair to stand on end when a person becomes cold or frightened. Hair grows continuously and is either cut off, sheared away by pressure or contact with clothing, or falls out.

Sweat glands secrete a liquid that helps cool the body. Sweat is released from the dermis onto the surface of the skin through small pores, or ducts, that pass through the epidermis. Blood vessels that provide nutrients and oxygen to the skin are found in the dermis and send small branches up to the basal layer of the epidermis.

Specialized nerve endings found within the dermis detect and then transmit to the brain data concerning heat, cold, body position, external pressure, and painful and pleasurable stimuli.

The subcutaneous tissue lies beneath the dermis and is composed almost entirely of fat, which insulates the body and stores energy. The amount, thickness, and composition of subcutaneous tissue vary greatly from one area of the body to another and from one individual to another. The body's musculature and the bony skeleton are found directly beneath the subcutaneous tissue and are discussed in more detail in other chapters.

In addition to its function as a protective barrier, the skin participates in the regulation of body temperature. In a cold environment, hair follicles become erect to trap warm air near the skin's surface. At the same time, blood vessels within the dermis and subcutaneous tissue constrict to shunt blood away from these areas, which helps to slow heat loss. Conversely, in a hot environment, dermal blood vessels dilate, causing the skin to become warm and flushed, which allows heat to radiate away from the body and into the environment. Additionally, sweat glands secrete sweat onto the surface of the skin, where it evaporates and thus cools the skin (and body temperature) through the process of evaporation.

## Physiology of Bleeding and Clotting

Bleeding results from a leak or breakage in an artery, a vein, and/or tissue capillaries. If an artery is damaged, the high arterial pressure within produces pulsating spurts of blood that is bright red because of its higher oxygen content. Conversely, blood from a lacerated vein flows freely and evenly under less pressure and is darker red due to its lower oxygen content. Capillary bleeding tends to ooze slowly because of the small size of these vessels and the low pressure of blood within them (Figure 18-4■, p. 542). Without outside intervention, bleeding will continue until a process known as clotting, or coagulation, seals off the damaged blood vessel

# STOP, THINK, UNDERSTAND

## Multiple Choice

Choose the correct answer.

1. Which of the following statements about the skin is false?_____
   a. It is the largest organ of the body.
   b. External cells are continually being rubbed off and replaced.
   c. The outermost layer, the dermis, contains multiple layers of pigment.
   d. The epidermis retains water and keeps out bacteria.

2. What is the function of subcutaneous fat?_____
   a. It produces glucose needed for energy.
   b. It has no real purpose and if thick is unhealthy and detrimental to human survival.
   c. It produces vitamin D.
   d. It insulates the body and stores energy.

## True or False

Indicate whether each of the following statements about the epidermis is true (T) or false (F).

_____ a. It is the second, or inner, layer.
_____ b. It continually produces new cells.
_____ c. Old epidermal cells migrate to the surface to form a watertight layer.
_____ d. The epidermis helps the body retain water and prevents bacteria and other organisms from entering the body.
_____ e. It varies in thickness in different locations in the body.

## Matching

Match each of the following components of the dermis to its description.

_____ 1. cause hair to stand on end when a person is cold or frightened

_____ 2. are sources of nutrients and oxygen to skin

_____ 3. produce sebum, the substance that waterproofs the skin and keeps it supple

_____ 4. senses variations in temperature, body position and monitors external stimuli and pressure

_____ 5. produce hairs

a. hair follicles
b. blood vessels
c. sebaceous glands
d. small muscles
e. nerve endings

## Short Answer

1. Name the top two layers of the skin.

_____

_____

2. Describe the mechanism by which the skin regulates body temperature in a cold environment.

_____

_____

_____

3. Describe the mechanism by which the skin regulates body temperature in a warm environment.

_____

_____

_____

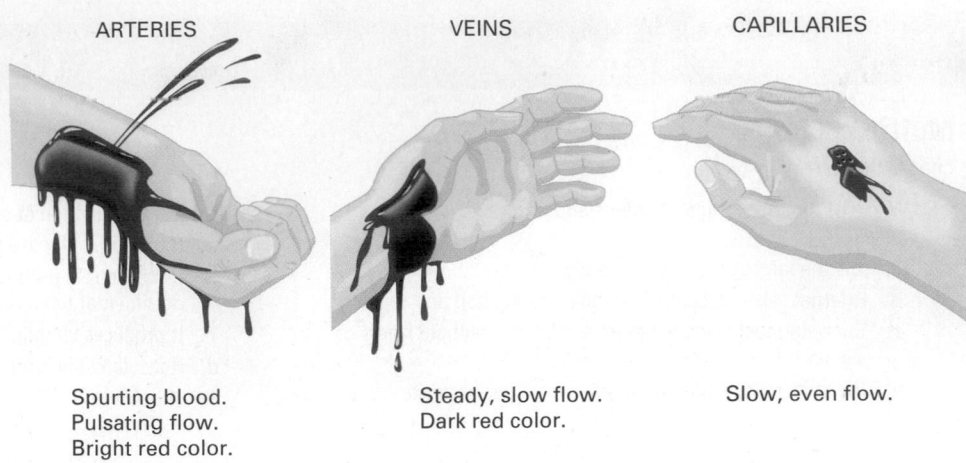

| ARTERIES | VEINS | CAPILLARIES |
|---|---|---|
| Spurting blood. Pulsating flow. Bright red color. | Steady, slow flow. Dark red color. | Slow, even flow. |

**Figure 18-4** The characteristics of bleeding from arteries, veins, and capillaries.

Clotting and skin repair are parts of a complex process that involves several body systems working together. First, blood vessels within the affected area constrict to minimize blood loss. Next, circulating platelets and plasma proteins bind together along the inner wall of the damaged vessel to form a temporary "plug," thereby sealing the hole in the vessel. At the same time, an inflammatory response causes swelling in the area, pushing the sides of the wound closer together. Additional platelets and plasma proteins bind at the periphery of the wound, forming a scab, which acts as a temporary barrier that keeps out bacteria and other contaminants. White blood cells migrate to the wound to fight infection. Within a few days, the scab is replaced underneath by epidermal cells that have quickly multiplied. Depending on the size and depth of the wound, complete tissue replacement may take several days to weeks.

Some patients take prescribed "blood thinning" medications. These medications, called anticoagulants, do not really thin the blood; instead, they therapeutically slow the normal clotting process in patients with certain medical conditions, such as a heart arrhythmia or a history of a blood clot in the leg, lungs, heart, or brain. Bleeding is more difficult to control in these patients. Ask patients if they take a "blood thinner" such as aspirin, Coumadin, Pradaxa, or Plavix.

**⊕ 18-3** List and describe three types of closed soft-tissue injuries.

# Types of Soft-Tissue Injuries

The soft tissues are commonly injured because they are located in the more superficial layers of the body and are therefore the first to be exposed to environmental stresses and/or traumatic events. OEC Technicians should be familiar with three types of soft-tissue injuries:

+ closed injuries
+ open injuries
+ burns

## Closed Injuries

**closed injury** damage beneath the skin or a mucous membrane from trauma while the overlying skin remains intact.

Closed soft-tissue injuries result in damage to structures beneath the skin or mucous membranes while the overlying skin surface remains intact. These injuries run the gamut from mild to severe, depending on the mechanism of injury. OEC Technicians most commonly encounter the following three types of closed soft-tissue injuries:

+ contusions
+ hematomas
+ crush injuries

## Contusions

In contusions, the outer layer of skin is not disrupted, but cells within the dermis are injured and small blood vessels are torn. Contusions are typically produced when a blunt force strikes the body or when the body strikes an immovable surface (Figure 18-5■). The extent and severity of the injury depends on the amount of energy absorbed by the soft tissue. As a result of the force of the impact, cellular fluid and blood leak into the injured area, causing tenderness, pain, and localized swelling. The breakdown of blood cells that leak out of capillaries beneath the dermis eventually produces a characteristic blue or black skin discoloration known as a bruise, or **ecchymosis**. As the injury heals, the bruise will change in color from black or purple to yellow or green. Eventually, a bruise will disappear as the leaked blood is reabsorbed by the body.

## Hematomas

A **hematoma** is an **extravascular** collection of blood that is confined to a localized area within an injured tissue or body cavity, usually as the result of a blunt soft-tissue injury (Figure 18-6■). Hematomas are produced when an injured blood vessel bleeds, bone marrow leaks out of a broken bone, or a highly vascularized solid organ is damaged. In severe cases, a hematoma can contain enough blood to cause hemorrhagic shock.

A **subungual hematoma** is a special type of hematoma that occurs beneath a nail bed. This type of hematoma, which also is caused by blunt trauma, can be very painful due to the buildup of pressure within the affected area.

## Crush Injuries

A crush injury is produced when an extensive force strikes the body suddenly or when a force is continuously applied to the body over an extended period of time (Figure 18-7■). The resulting degree of tissue damage depends on several factors, including the magnitude of the forces involved, the severity of the crushing, and the duration of the force applied. In addition to causing immediate direct soft-tissue injury, sustained compression eventually interrupts circulation within the tissues,

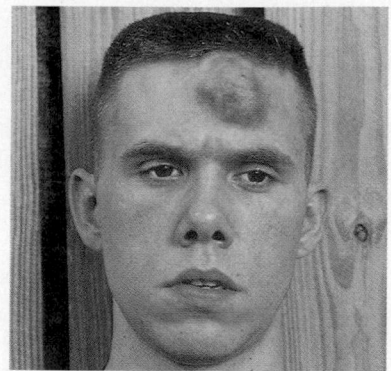

**Figure 18-5** An example of a contusion.

**ecchymosis** a bruise; discoloration of the skin associated with a closed wound; signifies bleeding within the skin.

**hematoma** an extravascular collection of blood within the body's tissues or in a body cavity.

**extravascular** outside of a blood vessel.

**subungual hematoma** a painful extravascular collection of blood under a nail.

**Figure 18-6** A hematoma underlying an abrasion.

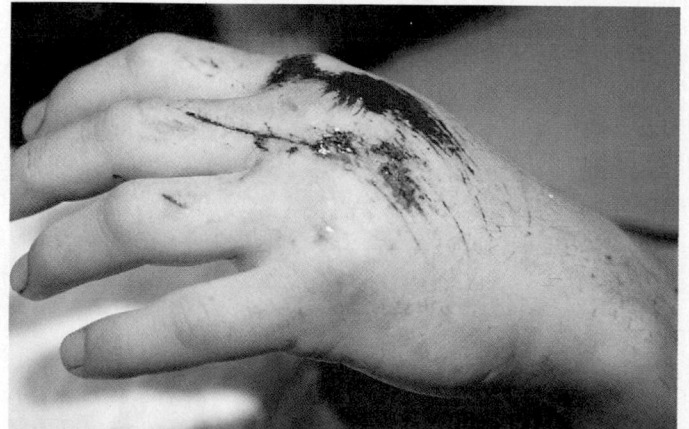

**Figure 18-7** An example of a crush injury. Note the extreme swelling resulting from compression of the soft tissues.
Copyright E.M. Singletary, MD

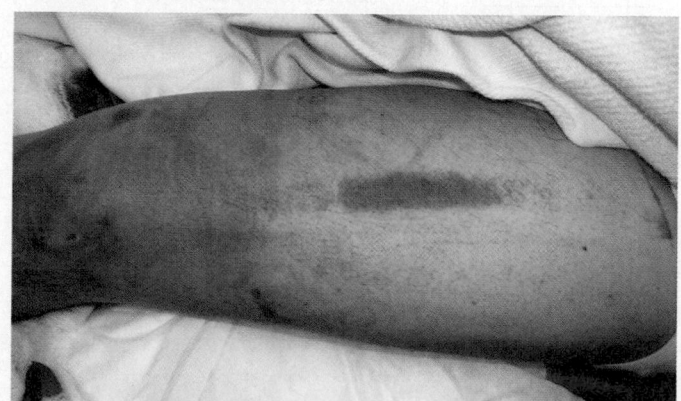

# STOP, THINK, UNDERSTAND

## Multiple Choice
Choose the correct answer.

1. Coagulation is defined as_____
   a. a constriction.
   b. a process by which oxygen molecules are attached to red blood cells.
   c. the clotting or the sealing of a break in a damaged blood vessel.
   d. the sloughing off or replacement of dead skin cells.

2. Which of the following best describes a closed tissue injury?_____
   a. A wound that has scabbed over or healed.
   b. A wound in which platelets and plasma proteins have formed a plug.
   c. A wound with no obviously visible opening, such as a needle stick.
   d. A wound in which underlying tissues are damaged but the overlying skin remains intact.

## Matching

1. Identify each of the following descriptions as indicative of bleeding from a capillary (C), an artery (A), or a vein (V).

   _____ 1. blood flows freely and continually

   _____ 2. blood flows in pulsating spurts

   _____ 3. blood is bright red

   _____ 4. blood is dark red

   _____ 5. blood is lower in oxygen content

   _____ 6. blood is higher in oxygen content

   _____ 7. blood oozes slowly from the wound

2. Match each of the following injuries to its definition or description.

   _____ 1. a collection of blood that is confined to a localized area within an injured tissue or body cavity

   _____ 2. a bluish discoloration under the skin, with pain, tenderness, and localized swelling, that results from blunt trauma

   _____ 3. a true emergency requiring immediate transfer to a trauma center to prevent limb loss

   _____ 4. an injury caused by extensive force or a force that is applied continuously over an extended period of time

   _____ 5. a hematoma under the nail bed, caused by blunt trauma

   a. contusion
   b. hematoma
   c. crush injury
   d. compartment syndrome
   e. subungual hematoma

## Sequence
Number the following six events in the process by which bleeding is stopped in the order in which they occur.

   _____a. An inflammatory response causes swelling, which push the sides of the wound together.

   _____b. Platelets and plasma proteins within the wound bind together to form a scab.

   _____c. The scab is replaced by epidermal cells.

   _____d. Blood vessels within the area constrict to minimize blood loss.

   _____e. White blood cells migrate to the wound site to fight infection.

   _____f. Circulating platelets and plasma proteins bind together on the inside wall of the damaged vessel to form a "plug."

## List
Name the three types of soft-tissue injuries.

_____

_____

_____

thereby producing further cell damage and/or tissue death. If, for example, a tree trunk has fallen on and trapped a patient's legs, the sustained damage to leg tissues due to crushing (compression) will continue until the weight of the tree is removed.

Another injury resulting from significant trauma to the tissues of a limb, usually from compression, is called **compartment syndrome**. In this type of injury, damaged cell walls begin to leak fluid into the potential space that lies between them. If this resultant swelling, or edema, continues to expand within a large muscle's connective tissue covering, the pressure within the tissues may increase to dangerous levels. Eventually blood vessels servicing the edematous area become compressed, thereby diminishing or even interrupting blood flow to the injured soft tissue. Compartment syndrome is a true emergency that requires rapid transport to a trauma center to prevent the loss of the limb.

## Open Injuries

Open soft-tissue injuries involve disruption of the skin and possibly damage to the soft tissue underneath (Figure 18-8■). These injuries can result in extensive external bleeding. Because the integrity of the epidermal layer is compromised, the wound may be exposed to microorganisms or become contaminated by foreign bodies such as

### Relieving the Pressure of a Subungual Hematoma

In the rare instance when emergency care is more than a few hours away, it may become necessary to relieve the pressure of a subungual hematoma. To decompress this type of painful injury, follow these steps:

1. Gently wash the finger tip. Heat a paper clip or the blunted end of a needle or pin with a lighter, a match, or an open flame until the metal is red hot.

2. Touch the hot tip of the paper clip in the center of the darkened nail bed and gently push down to allow the paper clip to burn through the nail. The trapped blood will suddenly escape as the pressure is released, providing immediate relief from severe pain.

3. Immediately remove the paper clip to prevent it from penetrating the nail bed.

4. Dress and bandage the wound.

**compartment syndrome** a condition in which the swelling of injured muscles within their connective tissue coverings causes pressure that can damage tissue and cut off blood flow.

⊕ **18-4** List and describe nine types of open soft-tissue injuries.

**Figure 18-8** Six of the nine types of open soft-tissue injuries.

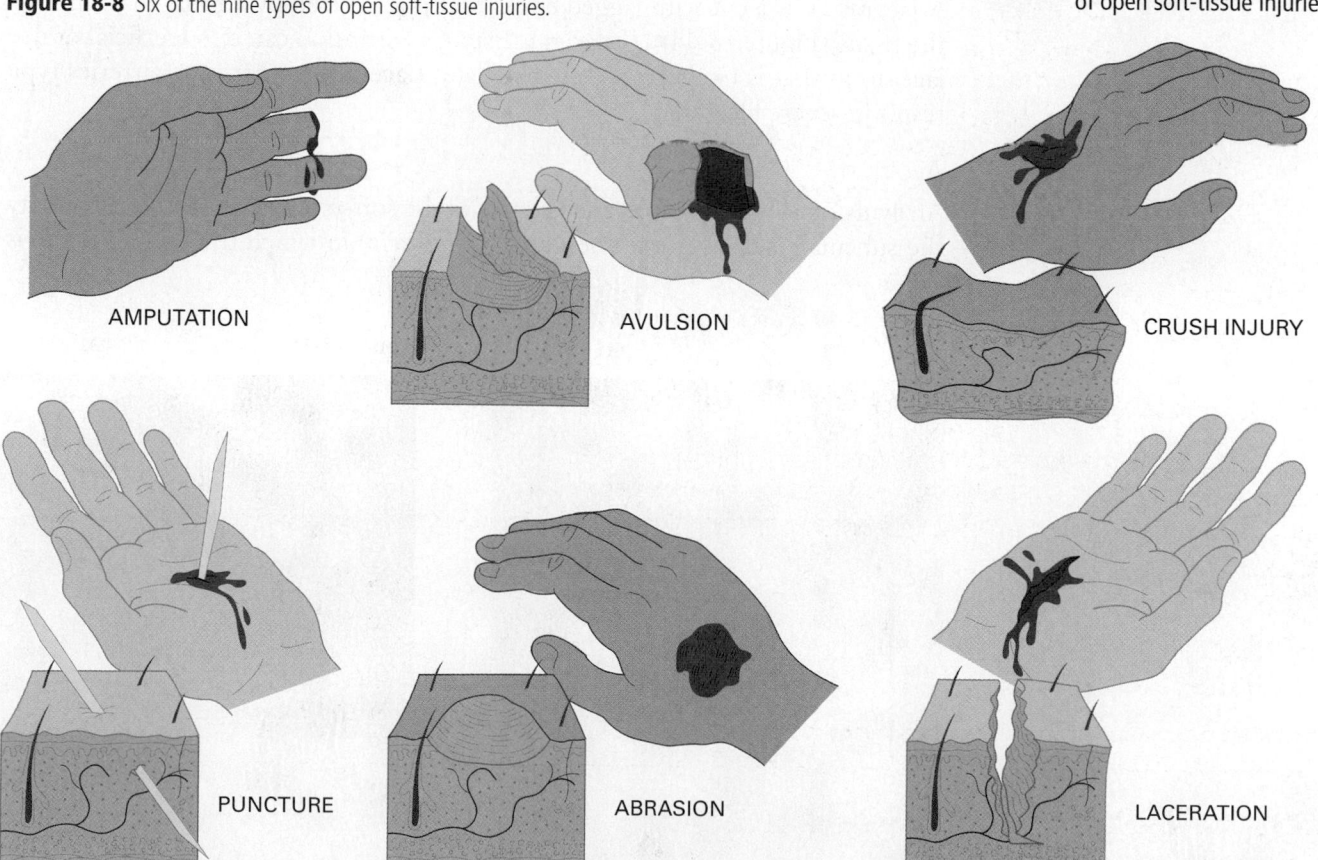

AMPUTATION

AVULSION

CRUSH INJURY

PUNCTURE

ABRASION

LACERATION

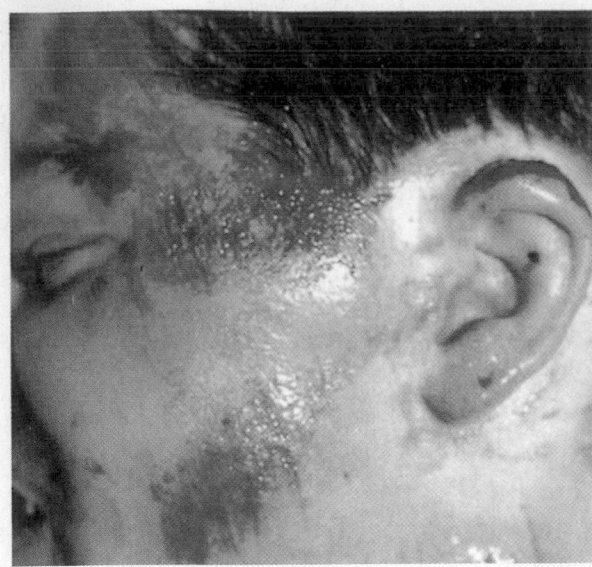

**Figure 18-9** An abrasion.

dirt, rocks, or other debris. There are nine types of open soft-tissue wounds:

- Abrasion
- Incision
- Laceration
- Avulsion
- Amputation
- Puncture
- Open crush injuries
- High-pressure injection
- Mechanical tattooing

### Abrasions

An abrasion is an **open injury** involving the outermost layer of skin (Figure 18-9■). It is caused when a body part scuffs or grates across a rough, abrasive surface such as a gravel road, a rocky protrusion, corn snow, or some other rough surface. It is unusual for an abrasion to extend through the dermis, although blood may seep outward from injured capillaries in the dermis. These injuries, called a variety of slang names such as a strawberry, road rash, and road burn, may be extremely painful.

### Incisions

An **incision** is a cut that has clean, smooth edges (Figure 18-10■). This type of injury can be superficial, extending only through the skin and subcutaneous tissue, or it can be deep, involving underlying muscle and adjacent nerves and blood vessels. A knife or other sharp object causes incisions.

### Laceration

A laceration is a cut with jagged edges that is produced by a force that rips or tears the tissue (Figure 18-11■). Like an incision, a laceration can be superficial or deep. A laceration that is irregular is called stellate. Lacerations that sever arteries typically result in severe bleeding.

### Avulsion

An avulsion is the incomplete separation of the soft-tissue layers (most often between the subcutaneous layer and the underlying fascia) in which the injured tissue is left

**Figure 18-10** An incision, which has smooth, straight edges.

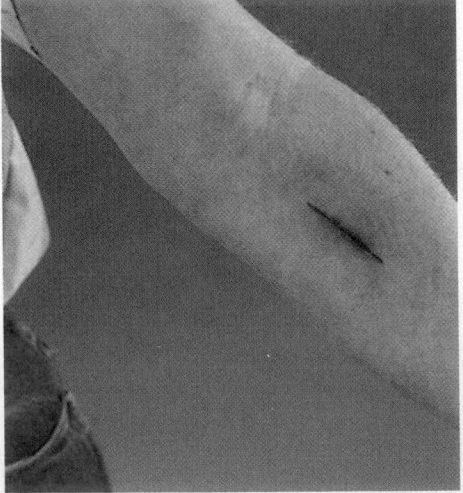

**Figure 18-11** A laceration, which has jagged edges.

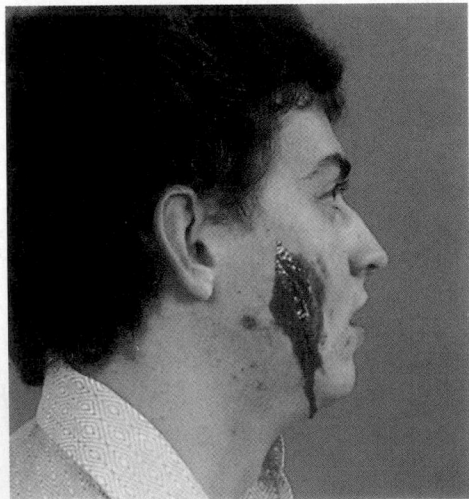

dangling as a flap (Figure 18-12■). Because the soft tissue is torn, the resultant skin edges are irregular. Significant bleeding usually accompanies this type of injury. If the avulsed tissue is hanging by only a small bridge of skin, circulation in the avulsed segment may be compromised.

## Amputation

An **amputation** is the complete or nearly complete separation of a body part or limb. Amputations are serious injuries that may involve an entire extremity (e.g., an arm or a leg), an appendage (e.g., a hand, foot, finger, or toe), or some other anatomical part (e.g., an ear, a nose, or the lips). Bleeding from this type of wound can be severe, even life threatening (Figures 18-13a■ and 18-13b■).

## Puncture

A **puncture** is an injury involving the penetration of soft tissue. Pointed objects, such as sticks, nails, tree limbs, ski poles, tent stakes, or ice tools, are common causes of this type of injury. Bullets or knives may also cause puncture wounds. Even though the entrance wound may be small, serious damage to underlying structures can occur. If the puncture penetrates the chest, abdomen, or a major artery, it can cause severe, potentially fatal bleeding (Figures 18-14a■ and 18-14b■).

An object that causes a puncture wound and remains embedded in the patient's body is known as an **impaled object** (Figure 18-15■). Objects may be impaled in any part of the body and can occur accidentally or intentionally. Common impaled objects include knives, sticks, tree limbs, fence posts, rebar, glass shards, ski poles, fishhooks, arrows, and nails. As with any puncture wound, an impaled object can cause serious damage to underlying tissues. The impaled object may effectively seal the wound, thereby preventing life-threatening bleeding. Impaled objects are not removed in the field unless they hinder rescue efforts or compromise the patient's airway (Figure 18-16■).

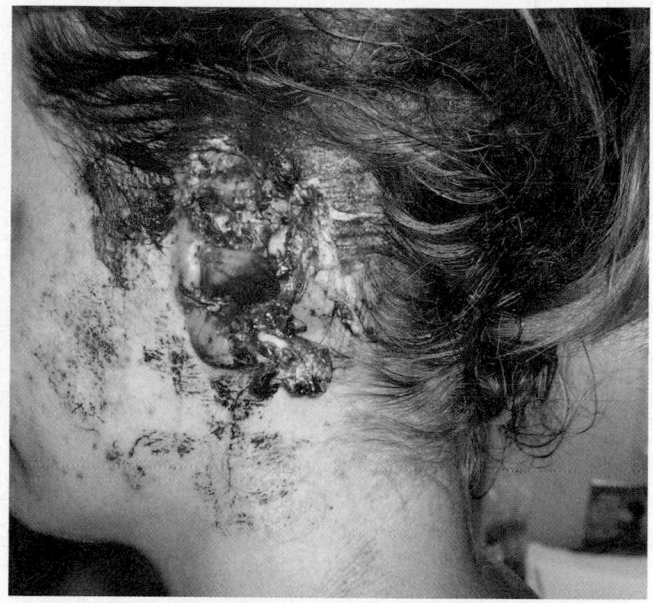

**Figure 18-12** An avulsion involving the ear.
Copyright E. M. Singletary, MD

**amputation**   the complete or nearly complete separation of a body part or limb.

**puncture**   a penetrating wound resulting from a sharp, pointed object.

**impaled object**   a foreign object that remains in the body in a puncture wound.

**Figure 18-13b** Wrap an amputated part in saline-moistened gauze.
Copyright E. M. Singletary, MD

**Figure 18-13a** An amputation of the thumb.
Copyright E. M. Singletary, MD

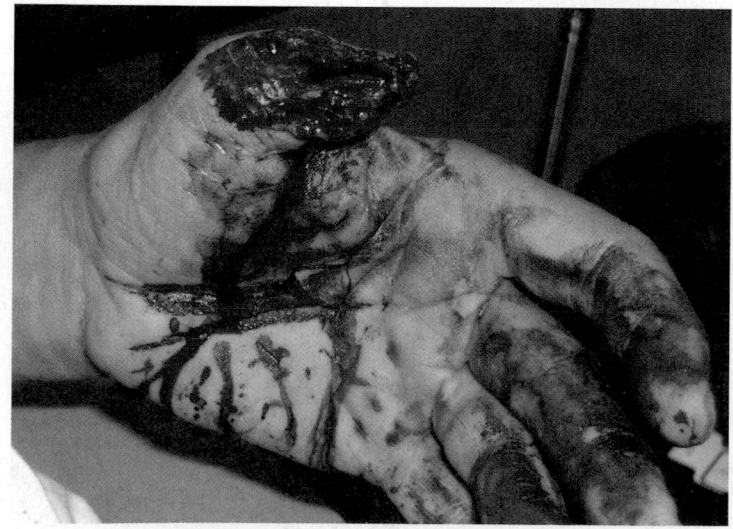

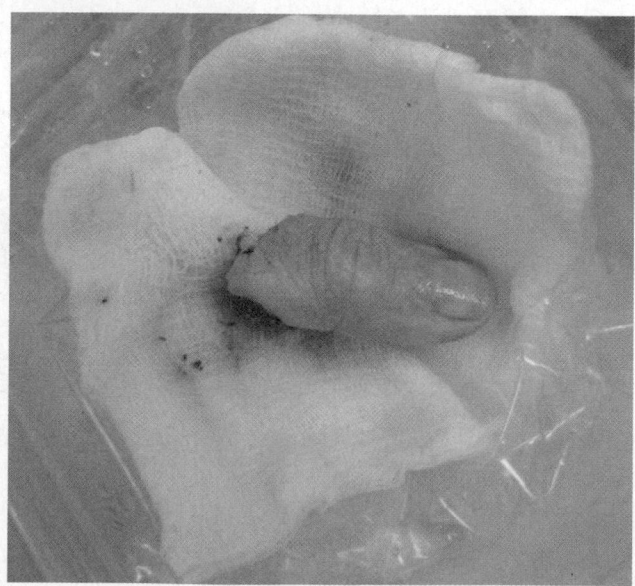

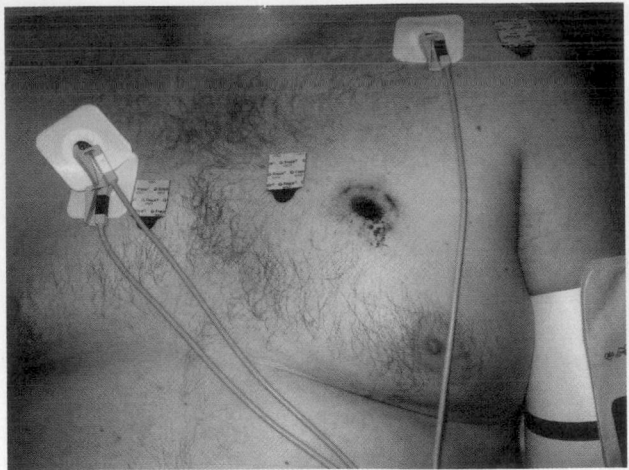

**Figure 18-14a** A puncture wound in the chest.
Copyright E. M. Singletary, MD

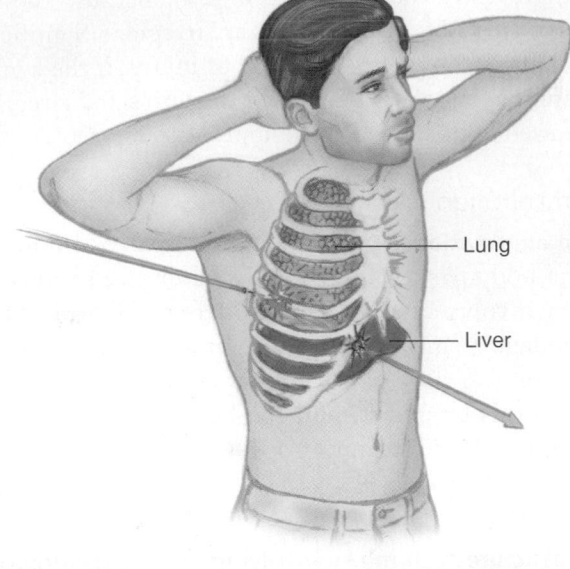

**Figure 18-14b** Bullet wounds can take unpredictable paths and can cause serious damage to structures deep within the body.

Lung

Liver

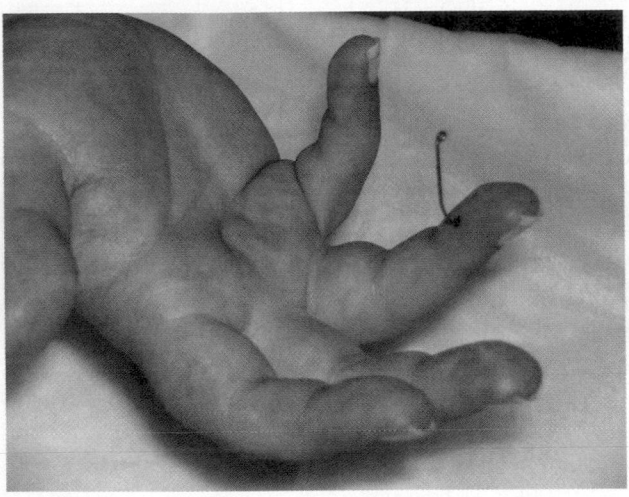

**Figure 18-15** An impaled object in a finger.
Copyright E. M. Singletary, MD

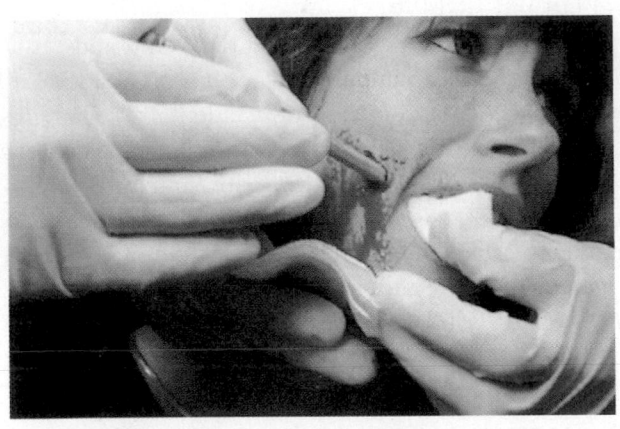

**Figure 18-16** It is safe to remove an impaled object from the cheek, only if the object is obstructing airflow.

**crush injury** compression injury in which a great amount of force is applied to the body.

### Open Crush Injury

Open **crush injuries**, as with closed crush injuries, may damage underlying internal organs, fracture adjacent bones, and/or generate widespread soft-tissue damage (Figure 18-17■). Even if the external bleeding caused by such an injury appears negligible, internal bleeding may be extensive and can produce life-threatening hypovolemic shock. If the patient survives a massive crush injury, the result is often a permanently painful and deformed area.

### High-Pressure Injection

A high-pressure injection injury involves the introduction of a liquid or gas into the body from a pressurized source (Figure 18-18■). In many instances, the presenting wound is very small and may initially be passed off as minor. High-pressure injection injuries can cause severe damage to underlying tissues, blood vessels, and nerves. Because the substance is injected into the tissues with great force, high-pressure injec-

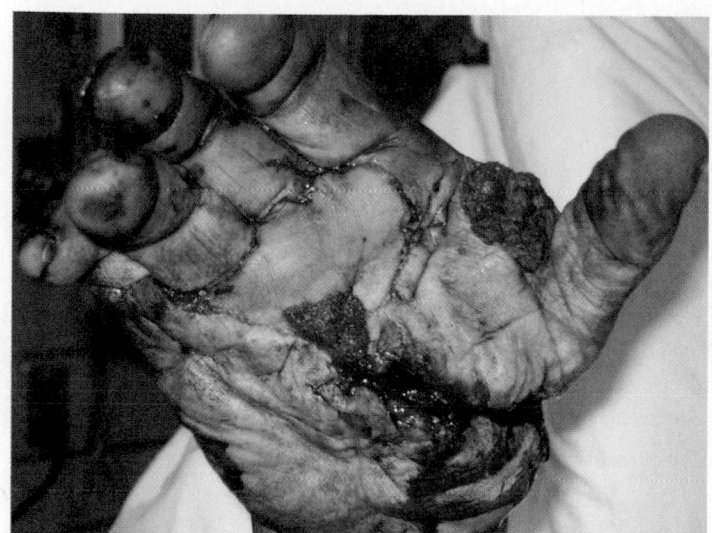

**Figure 18-17** An open crush injury.
Copyright E. M. Singletary, MD

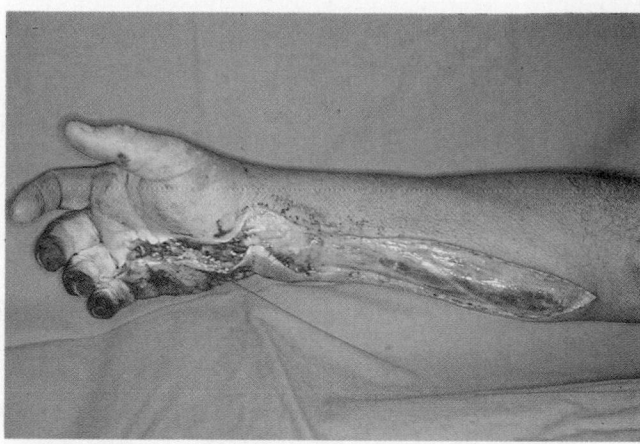

**Figure 18-18** A high-pressure injection injury resulting from the injection of pressurized grease.

tion injuries must be considered serious until proven otherwise. These injuries may result in surgical amputation of the affected part. Common sources of high-pressure injection injuries include high-pressure water sprayers, grease guns, paint sprayers, and pneumatic tools. Most injuries involve the hands, arms, or legs.

## Mechanical Tattooing

Mechanical tattooing is a form of open soft-tissue injury that occurs when foreign debris such as dirt, rocks, or tar is ground into a wound or the adjacent skin. Such injuries can leave indelible marks on the skin. Powder residue from a gunshot wound suffered at close range also can result in mechanical tattooing.

## Burns

A **burn** is a unique type of soft-tissue injury that is caused by exposure to excessive energy. Burns, which are covered in depth in Chapter 19, Burns, may be caused by thermal heat, heat resulting from friction, chemicals, electricity, or nuclear radiation.

**burn**   a lesion of the skin caused by thermal or frictional heat, chemicals, electricity, or nuclear radiation.

# STOP, THINK, UNDERSTAND

## Multiple Choice
Choose the correct answer.

1. The type of injury that involves a breech in the skin and damage to soft tissue underneath is called_____
   a. a hematoma.
   b. an open injury.
   c. a closed injury.
   d. compartment syndrome.

2. Which of the following statements about impaled objects is false?_____
   a. The penetrating object has been left embedded in the body.
   b. In general, the object should be left in place by OEC Technicians.

   c. This type of wound typically bleeds profusely.
   d. This type of wound often causes serious underlying tissue damage.

3. Which of the following statements about a high-pressure injection injury is false?_____
   a. The presenting wound is typically large.
   b. The injury involves the introduction of a liquid or gas into the body from a pressurized source.
   c. The injury often requires surgical amputation of the injured part.
   d. The injury typically involves the limbs.

*continued*

STOP, THINK, UNDERSTAND *continued*

4. Mechanical tattooing is defined as _____
   a. a form of body art In which dye is injected under the skin.
   b. a type of self-mutilation requiring psychiatric follow-up for the patient.
   c. the result of foreign debris such as dirt, gunpowder, or small rocks being ground into the skin.
   d. none of the above.

## Matching

Match each of the following types of open wound to its definition or description.

_____ **1.** a clean cut with smooth edges; can be deep or superficial and is caused by a knife or other sharp object

_____ **2.** an incomplete separation of tissue layers in which tissue is left dangling as a flap

_____ **3.** an injury that is characterized by a small entrance wound but almost always involves damage to underlying structures

_____ **4.** a wound that occurs when outermost layer of skin is scuffed or grates across a rough surface; also known as "road rash"

_____ **5.** a cut with jagged edges produced by a force that rips or tears tissue; can be superficial or deep, linear or stellate, and often occurs in conjunction with other soft-tissue injury

_____ **6.** a complete or nearly complete separation of a body part or limb

_____ **7.** a wound that may impair underlying internal organs, fracture bones, and generate widespread tissue damage; damage may be permanent

_____ **8.** a wound caused by exposure to excessive energy

a. avulsion
b. abrasion
c. amputation
d. burn
e. incision
f. laceration
g. puncture
h. open crushing

## Short Answer

A laceration is usually characterized as either linear or stellate. Explain what each of these terms means in relation to a laceration.

_____

_____

_____

 # CASE UPDATE

You instruct a race official to close the site to ensure that no other cyclists crash into the scene. The patient can speak to you normally, so he has an airway and is breathing, and his heart is pumping blood. Using Standard Precautions, you apply direct pressure to the arm laceration using a sterile dressing and bandage. The deep laceration over the patient's left bicep is no longer bleeding. A large bruise over the superior-lateral aspect of the patient's left shoulder is tender to the touch, and multiple abrasions are apparent over the lateral aspect of the patient's left arm and leg. Many of the abrasions contain dirt and small stones that appear to be ground into the skin and are slowly oozing blood. The cyclist also has large abrasions on the palms of both hands. He is able to rotate his left arm in all directions without an increase in pain. All extremities have normal motor and sensory function. The patient's pulse is 88/min, and his respirations are 16/min.

***What should you do now?***

# Assessment

Soft-tissue injuries often look very impressive, especially when they are associated with significant external bleeding. When they are encountered, it is easy to focus only on the obvious damage and to overlook other, potentially more serious injuries. To avoid this common pitfall, the assessment of soft-tissue injuries must be approached like any other medical or traumatic emergency: it begins with a scene size-up. Start by donning appropriate personal protective equipment (PPE) and ensuring that the scene is safe to enter. Do not enter any scene involving guns, knives, suspected violence, or criminal activity until local law enforcement has secured the scene.

Once the scene is secured, perform a primary assessment of the patient's ABCDs to identify potential threats to life, correcting any that may be present (Figure 18-19■). Control external bleeding using the techniques described in the next section of this chapter. Assess the patient's level of responsiveness using the AVPU scale. If spinal injury is suspected, ensure manual stabilization of the cervical spine.

Upon completion of the primary assessment, perform a secondary assessment using DCAP-BTLS, and obtain a thorough medical history. Collect a SAMPLE history, making sure to ask if the patient is taking an anticoagulant, especially if bleeding is difficult to control. As you assess the patient, remember that the forces that produce closed soft-tissue injuries also can damage underlying structures, bones, and internal organs. Maintain a high index of suspicion and presume that any patient who has an obvious soft-tissue injury, regardless of whether it is closed or open, has other more serious hidden injuries (Figure 18-20■). For example, a patient who has an obvious puncture wound in the chest may have internal bleeding and a lung injury.

When assessing penetrating injuries such as a gunshot or stab wound, try to determine the caliber of the gun and how many rounds were fired, or the maximum length of the knife or other penetrating object. This will help you determine the extent of possible injuries.

**Figure 18-20** A patient with an obvious injury may have more serious, less-apparent injuries.
Copyright Craig Brown

**Figure 18-19** Once the scene is safe, perform a primary assessment and control any bleeding.
Copyright Craig Brown

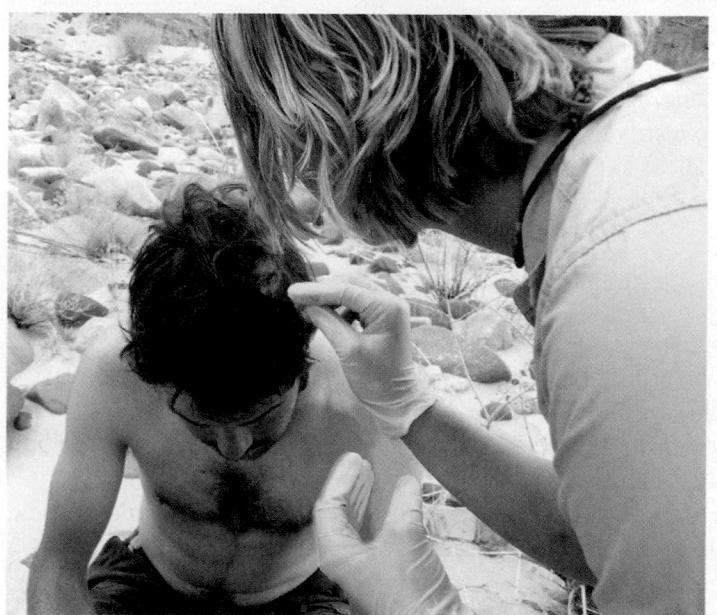

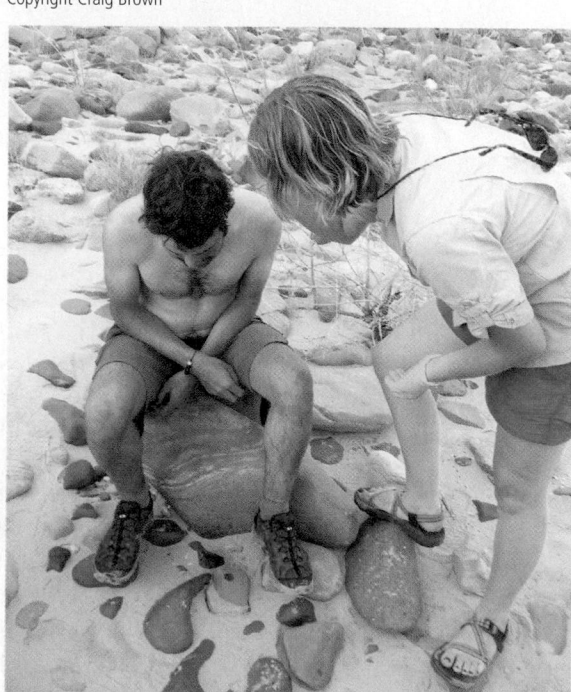

# STOP, THINK, UNDERSTAND

## Multiple Choice
Choose the correct answer.

1. Which of the following statements regarding soft-tissue injuries is true?_____
   a. Because they can bleed heavily and look awful, soft-tissue injuries can distract a rescuer from other, more insidious injuries.
   b. Rescuers should follow the typical ABCD progression of assessment and intervention when dealing with this type of wound.
   c. There could be a significant injury under a contusion.
   d. All of the above are true.

2. A patient has been stabbed in the chest with a 6-inch-long ice pick. When you assess the wound, you find it to be very small and insignificant in appearance, with minimal bleeding. What assumptions can you make about this injury?_____
   a. The wound is most likely superficial.
   b. The wound is probably severe.
   c. You do not have enough information to make any assumption about this wound.
   d. OEC Technicians should never make any assumptions about any wound.

3. Which of the following statements about patients with stab or gunshot wounds is true?_____
   a. The worst part of the injury is visible to the rescuer.
   b. These types of wound do not require you to check distal circulation, movement, and sensation (CMS).
   c. There is a good chance that you, as the initial caregiver, could end up testifying in court at a later date.
   d. You do not need to document this type of incident on a patient care report because the pertinent information will be recorded in a police report.

4. Which of the following pieces of information should you provide to the emergency department regarding a gunshot or stabbing injury?_____
   a. The caliber bullet and other information about the gun involved in the incident.
   b. The type and length of weapon that caused the stab wound(s).
   c. An ongoing report of the patient's vital signs.
   d. All of the above.

## Short Answer

Explain how to remove blood that is under a nail. _____
_____

---

+ **18-6** Describe and demonstrate three methods for controlling external bleeding.

**hemorrhage** the escape of blood from the vessels; bleeding.

**dressing** any material (preferably sterile) used for covering and protecting a wound.

**tourniquet** an instrument that when tightened around an arm or leg temporarily arrests the flow of blood through a large artery.

Carefully assess the patient for signs of shock. Be sure to check distal circulation, movement and sensation (CMS) in all extremities (even with seemingly minor soft-tissue injuries), and obtain a complete set of vital signs. Thoroughly document the circumstances surrounding the injury, the patient's general condition, and your assessment findings on a patient care report.

Many shooting- or stabbing-related incidents end up in court. The initial caregiver could be required to testify in court at a later date. Ensure that your written report accurately reflects all of the assessment performed and all of the treatment rendered.

# Management

Management of soft-tissue injuries is fairly straightforward. Once problems affecting the patient's airway and breathing have been corrected and you are sure the heart is adequately circulating blood, subsequent treatment is focused on controlling external **hemorrhage** and preventing further contamination of the wound. Controlling bleeding, especially life-threatening hemorrhage, is a fundamental OEC skill and is performed during the primary assessment. Under most conditions, external bleeding, whether arterial, venous, or capillary, can usually be controlled by applying direct pressure, using a pressure **dressing**, or *rarely* using a **tourniquet**.

## Direct Pressure

Direct pressure, the primary method used to control external bleeding, is performed by placing a dressing (e.g., a 4×4 or a 4×8) on the wound and then applying firm pressure directly over the wound using gloved fingers and/or palm (Figure 18-21■). This technique occludes underlying blood vessels until normal clotting mechanisms can seal them. When applying direct pressure to a wound, always observe Standard Precautions by wearing appropriate PPE.

## Dressings

A dressing is a piece of material, usually cloth or a cloth-like fabric, that is placed directly on a wound. Ideally, the dressing should be sterile, come prepackaged, and be large enough to extend at least one inch beyond all wound edges. To control external hemorrhage using a dressing, place the dressing over or into the wound and apply firm downward pressure with your gloved hand. If necessary, add additional sterile dressings over the initial dressing. Once applied, do not remove the original dressing. Instead, add to the base layer, because stripping off the primary dressing will disrupt any clotting that has occurred and cause additional bleeding.

If the situation is urgent and a sterile dressing is not available, use any clean soft material or even the palm of your gloved hand to apply direct pressure. If you have been using the pressure of your gloved hand and a dressing becomes available, apply the dressing and maintain direct pressure once the bleeding has slowed significantly or stopped. Most external bleeding, including arterial bleeding, can be controlled with direct pressure. This includes bleeding for people who are on anticoagulants, but pressure will need to be applied for a much longer time, sometimes 30 minutes.

Direct pressure also may be applied using a **pressure dressing** or the addition of a hemostatic dressing in which the bandage compresses the dressing directly over the wound. Commercially available hemostatic bandages have been used successfully by the military and some EMS agencies over the past several years. Insure that your mountains Management and Medical Director have approved of the use of these agents prior to adding them to your treatment protocols. See OEC Skill 18-1■.

Some authors advocate the elevation of extremities. This technique has not been shown to help control bleeding and will distract providers from the proven technique of direct pressure. Elevating an injured body part may also cause further injury if there is an underlying injury such as a fracture that has not been splinted.

## Tourniquet

The use of tourniquets to control bleeding was once highly controversial but in recent years has gained greater acceptance for use in severe bleeding in an extremity. A tourniquet is now considered an effective method for controlling bleeding and completely stops blood flow distal to the area of application. These devices are applied only when hemorrhaging from an extremity cannot be controlled by other methods (Figure 18-22■). Two situations that might warrant use of a tourniquet are when a major artery is squirting blood and the application of several pressure dressings fails to stop the bleeding, and when extensive bleeding occurs in an extremity that is significantly

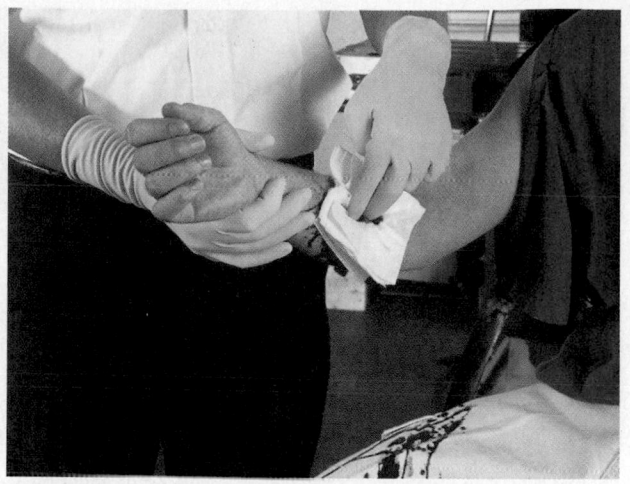

**Figure 18-21** Most bleeding can be controlled by applying direct pressure to the wound.

### Geriatric Considerations

As members of our aging population spend more time outdoors, OEC Technicians are increasingly likely to encounters patients who are taking Coumadin (e.g., warfarin sodium), Plavix (clopidogrel bisulfate), or aspirin (acetylsalicylic acid) to reduce their chances of blood-clot related cardiovascular problems. Because these medications prolong bleeding time, they can result in life-threatening hemorrhage from seemingly innocuous internal and external wounds.

**NOTE**

**pressure dressing**   a dressing that closes bleeding blood vessels by compressing the wound.

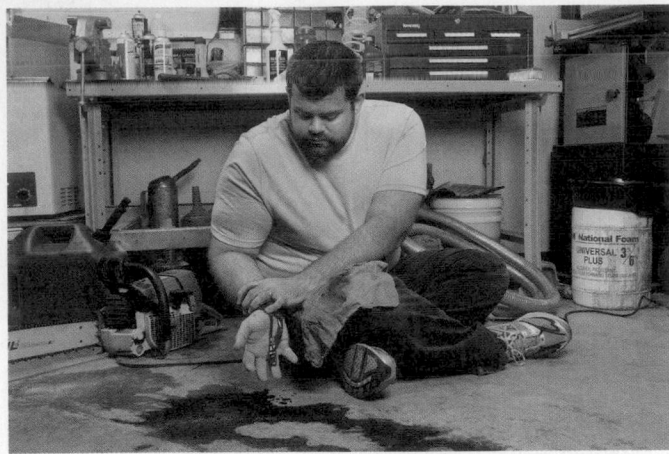

**Figure 18-22** A tourniquet is used only when bleeding cannot be controlled using any other method.

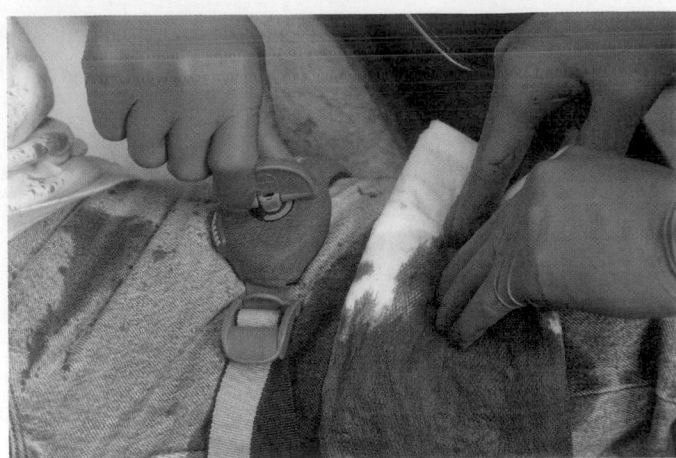

**Figure 18-23** Tourniquets are often commercially produced but can be made from a cravat.

**exsanguination**    massive blood loss resulting in death; the process of bleeding to death.

disrupted without clean lacerations making clotting and vascular constriction at the site less effective and bleeding unlikely to be controlled. An additional use of a tourniquet may be when you have a patient with multiple severe extremity injuries with significant bleeding and other issues for example airway problems. The use of the tourniquet will allow you to stem the bleeding from that extremity while you are dealing with other higher priority life saving issues. Use of a tourniquet always is accompanied by the risk of losing the patient's limb. If the bleeding is severe and places the patient at great risk for bleeding to death, an event known as **exsanguination**, a tourniquet can be life saving and should be applied. When using tourniquets there is some evidence that cooling the extremity can minimize potential damage from the tourniquet.

Tourniquets can be purchased commercially (e.g., Combat Application Tourniquet®, Delfi® EMT) or fashioned from available materials such as a cravat or a folded triangle bandage. It is important to note that the commercial tourniquets have proven to be more effective and safer than the home made variety and are recommended (Figure 18-23■).

To create a tourniquet, fold a triangle bandage into a long band about 3 inches wide. Wrap the band around the patient's extremity once or twice, positioning it as distally as possible but at least several inches proximal to the wound and more than 3 inches distal to either the elbow or the knee. Tie the ends together with an over-handknot. Place a 6- to 8-inch stick on the knot and then tie a square knot. Twist the stick only until the tourniquet is tight enough to stop the bleeding. Secure the stick in place with another cravat. Write the time the tourniquet was applied on a piece of tape and stick it to the patient's forehead. Also record the time on a patient care report. Leave the tourniquet in plain view. Never use wire, rope, extension cords, or other thin materials to create a tourniquet because these materials can concentrate the pressure in too narrow an area and cause serious local tissue damage. See OEC Skill 18-2■.

**Figure 18-24** A blood pressure cuff can be used as a tourniquet.

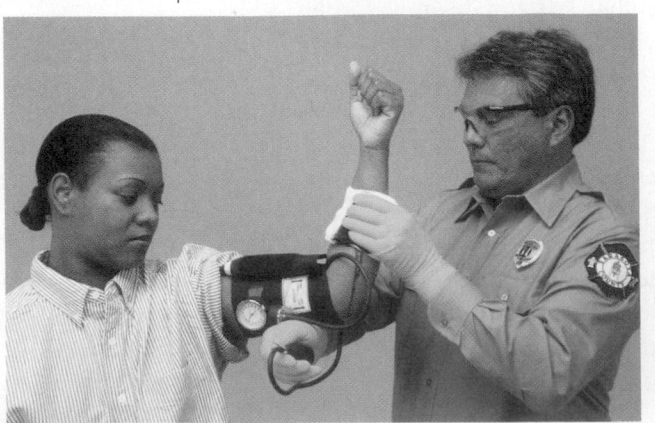

Other techniques may prove useful in helping to control external hemorrhage from an extremity wound, including use of an air splint, a technique called splint immobilization, or a blood pressure cuff (Figure 18-24■) which act as a modified pressure dressing. Although less effective than the previously described techniques, these methods can help reduce blood loss, especially when used in combination with a dressing.

An air splint, or a pneumatic counter-pressure device, is an inflatable device that slows bleeding by providing constant pressure to the entire extremity to which it is applied (Figure 18-25■). Air splints become stiff, unwieldy, and difficult to apply in cold environments due to their plastic construction. They also are vulnerable to puncture by sticks, rocks, and other sharp objects. Splint immobilization, which will be covered in Chapter 20, Musculoskeletal Injuries, decreases motion at the injury site, which facilitates clot formation at the bleeding site, especially in injuries involving a broken long bone.

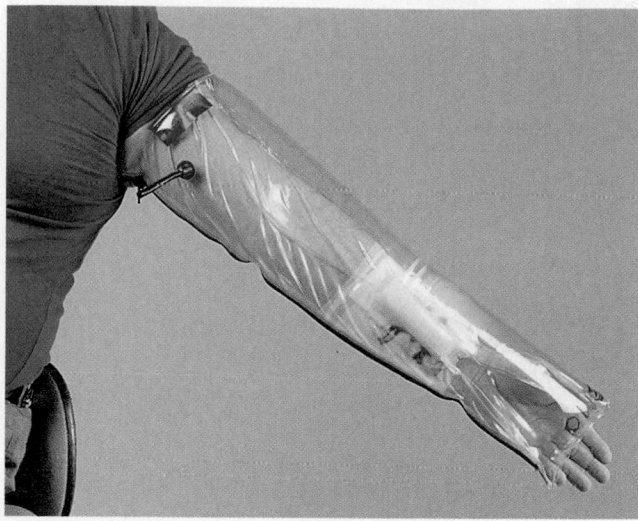

**Figure 18-25** An inflatable air splint.

## Treatment for Specific Soft-Tissue Injuries

### Contusions

Most contusions do not require emergency assistance other than the application of an ice pack. However, it is important to remember that there may be a significant internal injury under a large contusion. Under most circumstances, cold therapy should be applied in 20-minute increments (e.g., 20 minutes on, then 20 minutes off) with a bandage or cloth between the ice and skin so that the skin does not freeze. For more complex closed soft-tissue injuries, treat according to the acronym RICES:

**R—Rest:** Cease activity or the use of the affected limb. Inactivity helps to reduce swelling.

**I—Ice:** Place ice or snow in a plastic bag and wrap the bag in a folded cloth. Cold therapy slows down bleeding in the tissues (by causing blood vessels to constrict), reduces swelling, and helps to diminish the pain.

**C—Compression:** Apply a compression bandage to the injury site. The resulting pressure helps reduce tissue bleeding by closing off injured blood vessels.

**E—Elevation:** Elevate the injured area above heart level to reduce blood flow and swelling in the area.

**S—Splint:** Immobilize the injured part using either a commercial splint or one fabricated from available materials. Splinting helps to slow bleeding and decrease pain. See OEC Skill 18-3■.

⊕ **18-5** Describe the emergency care for the following injuries:

- closed soft-tissue injury
- open soft-tissue injury
- amputation
- impaled object

### Open Injuries

Open soft-tissue injuries require a different approach in order to reduce the risk of wound contamination and infection. In general, most open soft-tissue injuries that are minor—that is, abrasions, cuts that do not require suturing, and small lacerations—and that have not had significant bleeding or contamination can be treated in a definitive-care facility within several hours.

Treat any open soft-tissue injury in the following manner:

1. Control bleeding while observing Standard Precautions.
2. Once bleeding is controlled, provide wound care. If the wound is superficial irrigate with water to clean the wound and if deep leave the wound to be cleaned at the hospital. For dirty and grossly contaminated wounds when definitive medical care is more than 90 minutes away, carefully expose the wound and control initial active bleeding in the usual fashion (Figure 18-26■). Then, carefully wash around all open wounds with soap and water, and *gently* irrigate all open wounds copiously with a 20–30 cc syringe if available containing sterile water or saline solution. If sterile water or saline is not available use tap water (Figure 18-27■).

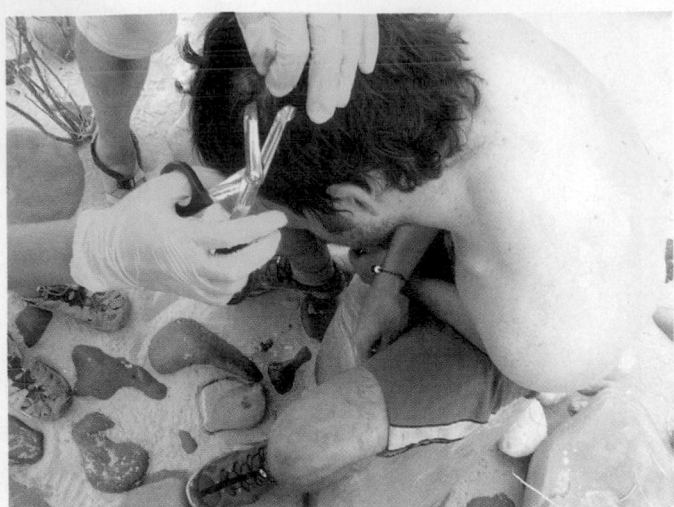

**Figure 18-26** When treating a patient in a remote location, carefully expose the wound.
Copyright Craig Brown

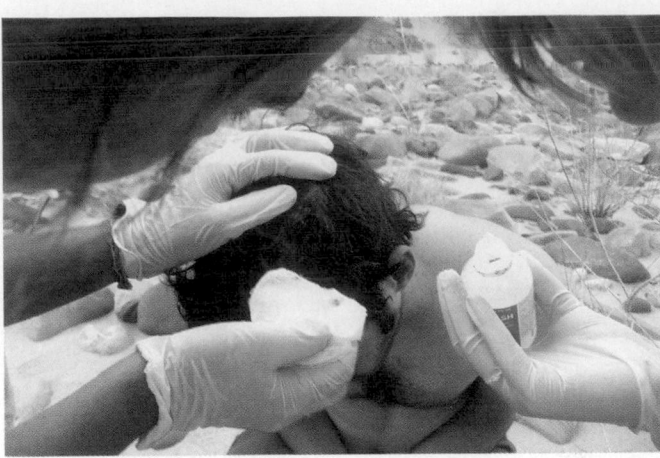

**Figure 18-27** Irrigate all wounds with sterile water.
Copyright Craig Brown

**3.** Cover the wound with a dressing.

**4.** Secure the dressing using a bandage.

**5.** Splint all wounds in extremities and elevate the injured area above the level of the heart to reduce swelling.

### Complex Soft-Tissue Injuries

Complex soft-tissue injuries such as avulsions, amputations, and impaled objects require specialized treatment.

**Avulsions**   Control bleeding. Cleanse the injury site as previously described to remove any debris. Replace the flap in its original position and apply a sterile compression bandage to help reduce blood loss and contamination, and possibly to restore blood flow to the avulsed tissue.

**Amputations**   Control bleeding. For any amputation with associated severe bleeding, directly apply several pressure bandages; if that is not effective, apply a tourniquet as previously described. Additional treatment will vary slightly depending on whether the amputation is incomplete or complete.

With an incomplete amputation, immobilize the injured part with a bulky **compression dressing** and a splint above and below the affected area to protect against further injury or further tissue separation. Never detach any partial amputation.

If the amputation is complete, preserve all amputated parts, no matter how damaged they may appear to be. Thanks to advances in microsurgical training and techniques, today's surgeons can reattach many amputated limbs, even those that have been without a blood supply for several hours. The key to success is appropriate care of the amputated part, both at the incident scene and en route to the hospital.

Wrap the amputated part in a couple of layers of saline-moistened (not soaked) gauze, and place it in a plastic bag. Seal the plastic bag and place it in a container with ice. The amputated part should not be placed directly on the ice because this could result in a frostbite injury to the tissues. The objective is to keep the detached part cool without allowing it to freeze. Do not submerge an amputated part in water because this will damage the tissue. Always ensure that the amputated part is transported with the patient.

**compression dressing**   an occlusive dressing that applies some pressure to a bleeding wound; it should not compromise circulation, movement, or sensation distal to the wound.

# STOP, THINK, UNDERSTAND

## Multiple Choice

Choose the correct answer.

1. Which of the following statements regarding patient management is true?_____
   a. Managing soft-tissue injuries is complex.
   b. Controlling bleeding takes precedence over correcting airway or breathing problems.
   c. External arterial bleeding can usually be controlled in the field by OEC Technicians.
   d. External arterial bleeding can rarely be controlled in the field by OEC Technicians.

2. Elevation should be used for which of these injuries?_____
   a. a laceration to the flank
   b. a sprained ankle
   c. an abrasion to the lower back
   d. a puncture wound to the abdomen

3. Which of the following statements concerning how to stop bleeding is true?_____
   a. Elevation of the injured extremity is considered a priority to stop bleeding.
   b. Tourniquets may be used on patients with numerous significant extremity injuries with severe bleeding.
   c. Pressure on a bleeding wound should always be accompanied with the use of ice to speed clotting.
   d. Always remove the initial soiled dressing and add more when attempting to stop a wound from bleeding.
   e. All of the above are true.

4. Which of the following statements about the use of a tourniquet is true?_____
   a. A tourniquet should be placed as distal as possible and at least several inches proximal to the wound.
   b. A tourniquet can be used on any part of the body except the neck.
   c. On an arm or leg, a tourniquet should be placed 1 inch from either the elbow or the knee.
   d. Tourniquets are the initial choice to stop major bleeding, not controlled by pressure.

5. Which of the following materials are appropriate for use as a tourniquet? (check all that apply)
   _____ a. a commercial product such as a military combat dressing
   _____ b. a triangular bandage folded such that it is 3 inches wide
   _____ c. a 4-inch-wide roller gauze
   _____ d. a short piece of 9-mm climbing rope
   _____ e. a 1-inch-wide roller gauze

6. The most effective method for treating a contusion is the application of_____
   a. a pressure dressing.
   b. a tourniquet.
   c. a bandage.
   d. an ice pack.

7. Cold therapy achieves which of the following? (check all that apply)
   _____ a. decreases bleeding
   _____ b. decreases swelling
   _____ c. decreases pain
   _____ d. causes blood vessels to dilate

8. RICES stands for _____
   a. regulate, inspect, compress, elevate, splint.
   b. routinely ice, contuse, elevate, sew up.
   c. rapid inspection for circulation and extremity stability.
   d. rest, ice, compression, elevation, splint.

9. If definitive medical care is more than 90 minutes away, which of the following actions constitutes appropriate field care?
   a. Attempt to close small wounds with steri-strips (commercial bandages used to close small wounds), butterflies, or band-aids.
   b. Leave larger wounds open.
   c. Cover all wounds with a sterile dressing.
   d. All of the above are correct.

## True or False

Indicate whether each of the following statements regarding the use of direct pressure to control bleeding is true (T) or false (F).

_____ a. It is performed by applying firm localized finger/palm pressure directly to the wound site.

_____ b. A sterile dressing and a gloved hand should be used.

_____ c. Because direct pressure causes underlying vessels to collapse, it should only be used as a "last resort."

_____ d. The edges of the dressing should not extend beyond the wound's edges.

_____ e. Once a dressing is applied, OEC Technicians should not remove it.

_____ f. Venous bleeding, but not arterial bleeding, can be controlled by direct pressure.

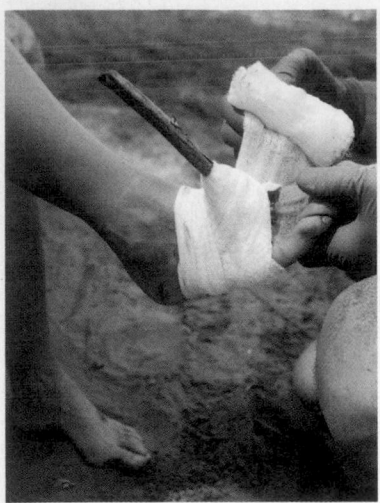

**Figure 18-28** Control the bleeding and stabilize the impaled object in the position you found it.
Copyright Edward McNamara

**⊕ 18-8** Demonstrate the proper procedure for applying each of the following:

- dressing
- bandage
- compression dressing
- tourniquet

**⊕ 18-7** Compare and contrast a dressing and a bandage.

**universal dressing**   sterile, soft, highly absorbent, individually wrapped dressing that provides superior padding and protection for major wounds; usually measures 12 inches by 30 inches; also called *trauma dressing*.

Replantation of an amputated part is ideally performed within 4 to 6 hours after injury, but success has been reported up to 24 hours after the injury if the amputated part has been kept cool. See OEC Skill 18-4■.

**Impaled Objects**   After controlling bleeding, the primary goal of treatment for a patient with an impaled object is to stabilize the object in the position you found it (Figure 18-28■). If you need to quickly move the impaled patient for safety reasons, do so in a slow and gentle fashion so as not to cause additional injury. An impaled object should be removed only by a physician in an operative setting (in an emergency department or in surgery). Attempting to remove the item at the injury scene may damage important contiguous structures, and more importantly, may initiate uncontrollable bleeding.

To stabilize an impaled object, follow this procedure:

1. Manually stabilize the object so that it cannot move and damage surrounding and underlying tissues while you perform the next steps in this procedure.
2. Remove or cut off all clothing surrounding the impaled object.
3. Control bleeding by direct pressure.
4. Apply a bulky dressing around the object. If the object is long or unwieldy, it may be necessary to shorten it by cutting off some of the exposed portion.
5. Keep the object from being nudged or moved during transport by stabilizing it with tape or bandages. If available, consider securing a plastic cup, a bowl, or half of a plastic water bottle over the object after it has been stabilized.

Do not manipulate or attempt to remove the object unless it interferes with the patient's airway or breathing. If it interferes with breathing, maintaining or restoring an effective airway takes priority over stabilizing the object.

Make every attempt to leave an impaled object in the patient. If the object is large (e.g., a long rod, a pole, or a bar), it should be cut off before the patient is transported. In very rare instances an impaled object might have to be removed, but this should be done only as a last resort because it may result in severe, life-threatening bleeding. If, for example, a backcountry hiker has become impaled through the abdomen by a heavy steel bar embedded in the ground, trying to cut through the bar or waiting for a cutting torch would take too much valuable time, and the patient might bleed to death. In such a case, extricate the patient from the impaled object as efficiently as possible, apply a large dressing with direct pressure, and transport the patient emergently. Similarly, an impaled object that obstructs the airway (e.g., cheek, mouth, or throat) may also need to be removed.

A knife that is embedded in a homicidal, suicidal, or combative patient poses an immediate danger to the safety of the patient, rescuers, and bystanders. Based on local protocols, you may need to restrain the patient, allowing the weapon to remain in the patient. See OEC Skill 18-5■.

## Dressing and Bandaging

Conventional sterile 4×4 and 4×8 gauze pads, soft self-adherent roller dressings, and assorted small adhesive-type dressings (Curads®, Band-Aids®) are sufficient to cover most wounds that you will encounter (Figures 18-29a■ and 18-29b■). The **universal dressing**, sometimes called the trauma dressing, which measures 9 inches by 36 inches and is made of a thick, absorbent cotton material, is well suited for covering large open wounds and also works well to pad rigid splints (Figure 18-29c■). All these dressings are commercially available in compact, individually wrapped sterile pack-

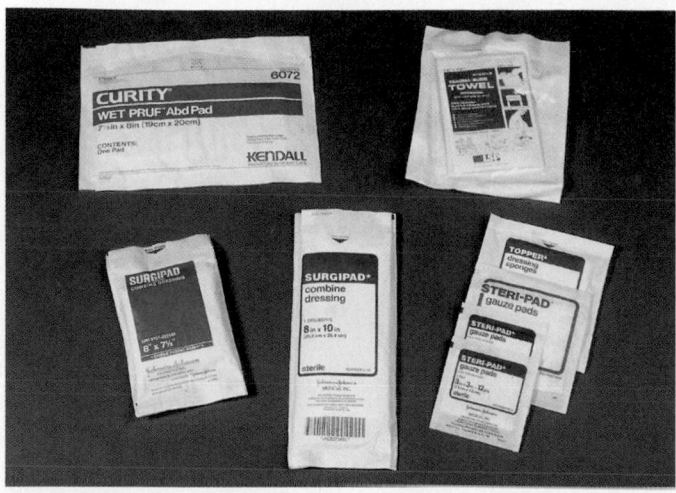

**Figure 18-29a** Sterile gauze pads.

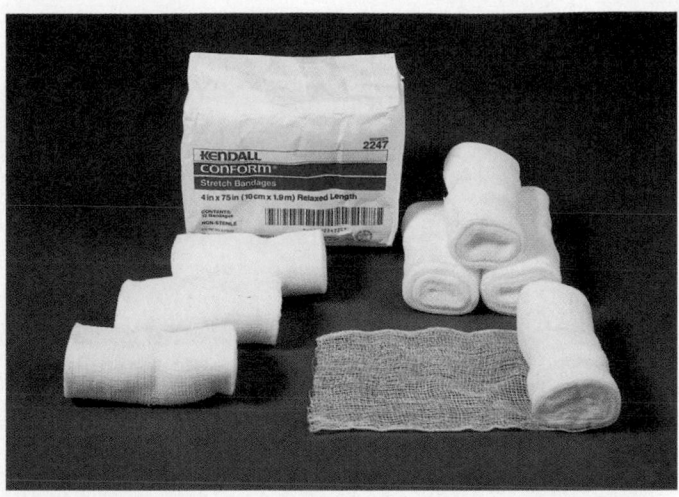

**Figure 18-29b** Nonelastic, self-adhering dressing and roller bandages.

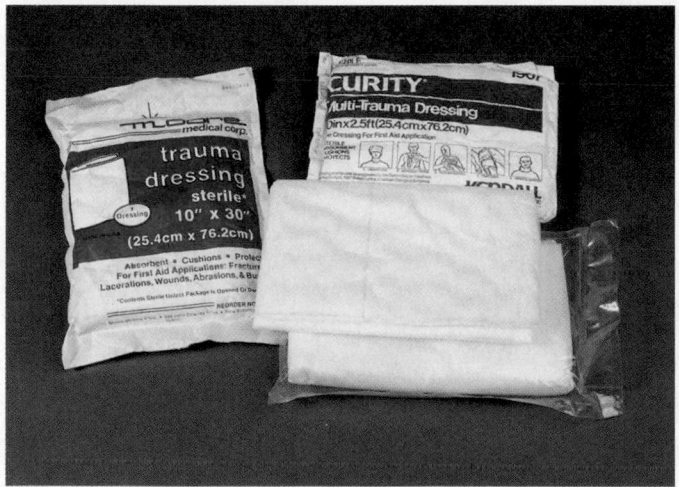

**Figure 18-29c** Multi-trauma dressings.

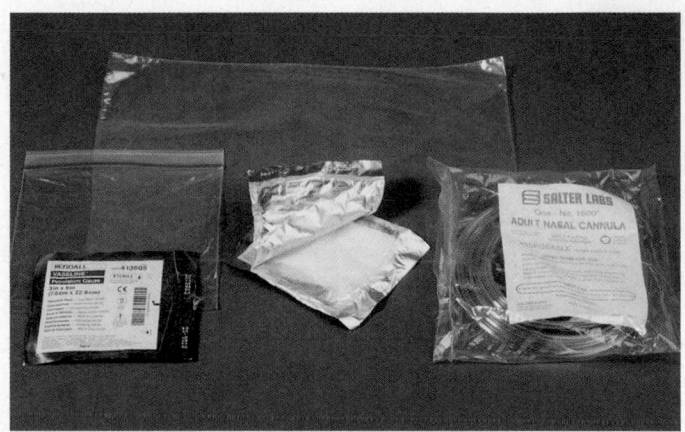

**Figure 18-29d** Materials that can be used as occlusive dressings.

ages. Gauze pads such as 4×4s can be used on smaller wounds. Adhesive-type dressings (Band-Aids®) are appropriate for minor wounds, whereas occlusive dressings (e.g., Vaseline® gauze, aluminum foil, plastic cling wrap) are used in special situations in which the wound requires an occlusive dressing (Figure 18-29d■).

A **bandage** is a piece of material that is used to hold a dressing or splint in place. The term *bandaging* usually refers to the process of applying both a dressing and bandage. Most wounds require dressings and bandages to prevent further contamination and to absorb blood and wound secretions. Become familiar with the indications, functions, and proper application of each of the many types of bandages.

Self-adhering roller bandages (e.g., Kerlix™), rolls of soft gauze (e.g., Kling®), triangular bandages folded into 2- to 3-inch wide strips, or adhesive tape are used to secure dressings in place. Kerlix™ is a commercial self-adherent roller bandage that is available in multiple widths and is considered by many to be the most effective because its elasticity makes it easy to apply. Kling® is a commercially available, tightly woven, light gauze wrap that also may be used to secure a dressing in place but is less elastic than Kerlix™, which is a loosely woven gauze wrap.

**bandage** a strip or roll of gauze or other material used for wrapping or binding a body part.

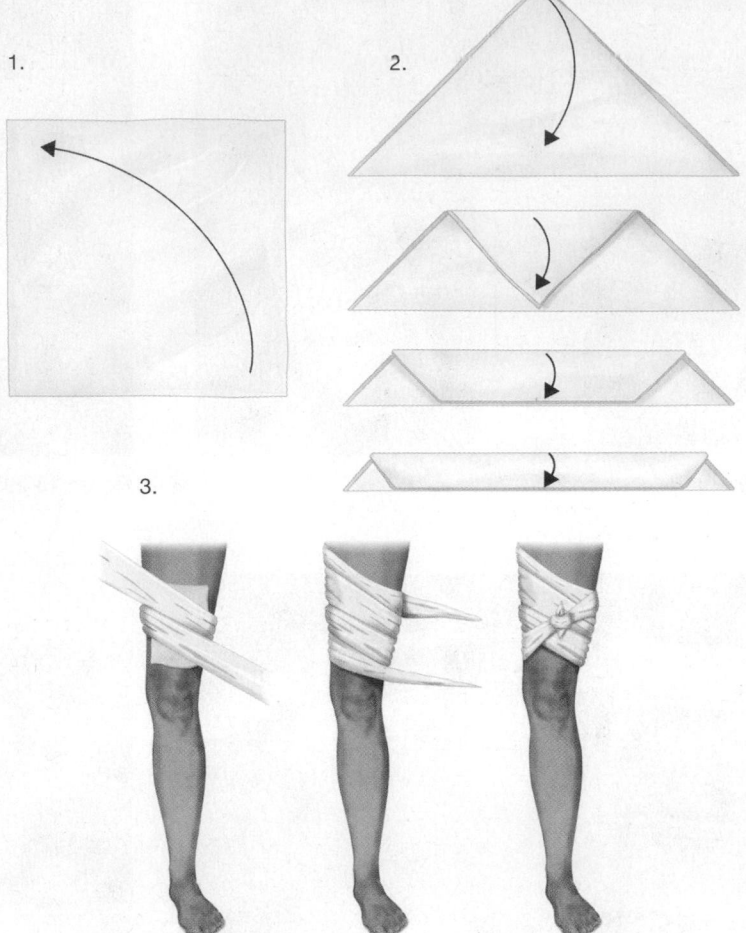

**Figure 18-30** Triangular bandages can be used to secure dressings in place.

## Principles of Bandaging

Most bandages that are placed on an extremity are wrapped entirely around the body part, which introduces the danger of restricting circulation if the bandage is too tight (Figure 18-30■). For this reason, always leave fingers and toes exposed so that you can perform CMS checks distal to any bandage that has been applied. In addition, you should be able to insert two fingers between the patient and the bandage.

Do not use elastic bandages, because they tend to tighten on the injured part. In some instances, an Ace® wrap may even function like a tourniquet and subsequently cause additional tissue damage or loss of limb.

Adhesive tape can be used to secure small dressings (4×4s) in place and is helpful in closing/securing larger dressings. Remember that allergies to adhesive tape are common. (The allergy is generally not to the tape, but to the adhesive itself, which contains latex.) If you discover during your SAMPLE history that the patient has this allergy, use latex-free tape. See OEC Skill 18-6■. Other general treatments for soft-tissue injuries may include providing supplemental oxygen, treating for shock, and splinting suspected musculoskeletal injuries.

## Special Types of Dressings and Bandages

OEC Technicians must be able to provide emergency care for all types of soft-tissue injuries. A necessary skill for treating soft-tissue injuries is the ability to tie a square knot (left over right, then right over left), which is essential for successful bandaging and splinting.

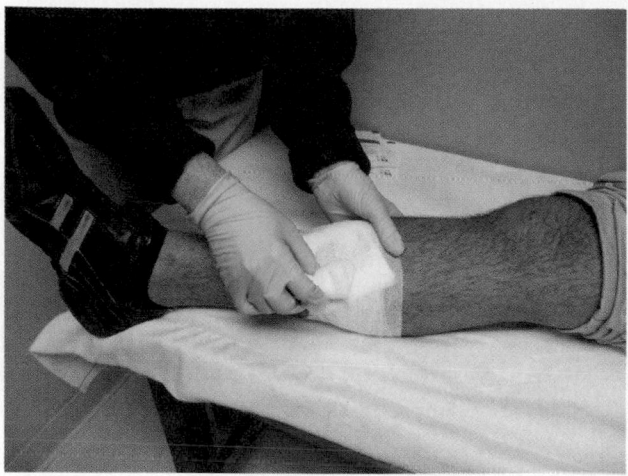

**Figure 18-31a**  After placing several sterile dressings over the wound, begin distal to the injury and wrap the roller bandage over the dressing in a proximal direction.
Copyright Edward McNamara

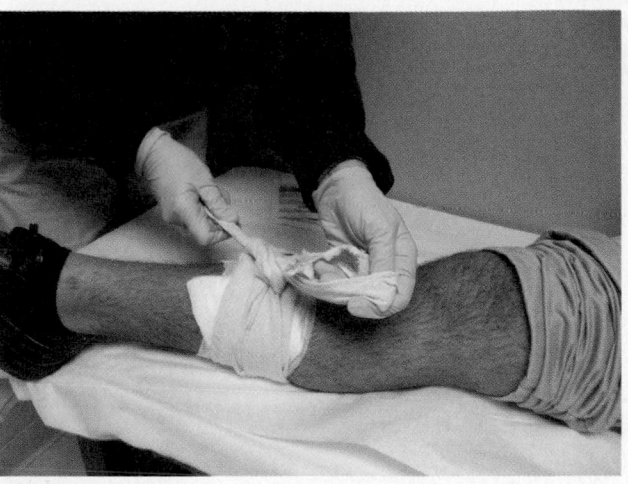

**Figure 18-31b**  If necessary to stop bleeding secure the roller bandage in place with a cravat knotted over the wound to add pressure.
Copyright Edward McNamara

The dressings and bandages that are used to treat wounds that require special emergency care include pressure dressings, occlusive dressings, stabilizing dressings, and hemostatic dressings.

**Pressure Dressings**  A pressure dressing is used to maintain direct pressure on a bleeding wound. It consists of several sterile dressings secured in place by a firmly applied self-adhering roller bandage. If a self-adhering roller bandage is unavailable, then a folded triangular bandage will suffice (Figures 18-31a■ and 18-31b■). To apply a pressure dressing, begin distal to the injury and wrap the roller bandage over the dressing, all the time moving proximally. If needed, a cravat can then be applied to add more pressure. Check circulation, motor function, and sensation (CMS) distally after applying the pressure dressing.

**Occlusive Dressings**  **Occlusive dressings** cover sucking chest wounds and open neck wounds with an airtight layer of sterile Vaseline® gauze, plastic cling wrap, or aluminum foil. Commercially available sterile occlusive dressings are packaged individually wrapped. One of these used for chest wounds is the Asherman® chest seal.

These dressings prevent air and liquids from entering (or exiting) the wound. Add a sterile 4×4 gauze pad on top, and the four edges of this airtight covering securely to the skin with adhesive tape. (Sealing all four edges might worsen the problem if used for a chest wound so for chest wound seal only three sides.) Use a sterile universal dressing moistened with sterile saline to cover open abdominal wounds in which organs are exposed. Secure with a dry universal dressing taped to the abdomen. For all other puncture-type wounds to the head, neck, or abdomen, seal all four sides of the occlusive dressing to prevent wound contamination. See OEC Skill 18-7■.

**Stabilizing Dressings**  A stabilizing dressing is used to secure an impaled object in place. It consists of several layers of a thick sterile dressing that are wrapped around the object and held in place by tape or a self-adhering roller bandage (Figures 18-31a and 18-31b). Fully stabilizing the object may require wrapping several layers of folded cravats around the object to form a doughnut (Figure 18-32■). If you do not have a stabilizing dressing, stabilize the object with several cravats and secure it with a square knot (Figure 18-33■).

**Hemostatic Dressings**  The newly developed **hemostatic dressings** are dressings which contain a topical hemostatic agent that promotes clotting. Marketed under

**occlusive dressing**  dressing made of Vaseline® gauze, aluminum foil, or plastic wrap that prevents air and liquids from entering or exiting a wound.

**hemostatic dressing**  a surgical gauze/mesh impregnated with a material that stops arterial and venous bleeding in seconds.

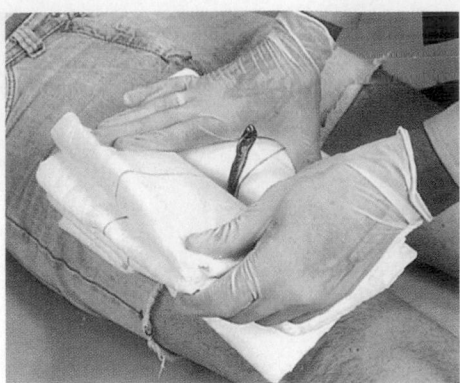

**Figure 18-32** Stabilizing an impaled object with a bulky dressing or several layers of cravats.

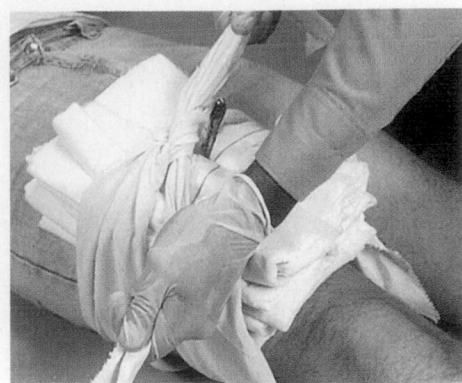

**Figure 18-33** Anchoring an impaled object with cravats to keep it from moving.

such names as the HemCon® Bandage or Quickclot® Bandage, this type of dressing has been extensively tested by the U.S. armed forces on the battlefields of Afghanistan and Iraq.

Hemostatic bandages are a latex-free fabric mesh that has been impregnated with a topical hemostatic agent, which is a bio-compatible substance. When placed directly on a wound, the bandage sticks to surrounding tissue. These bandages reduce clotting time because red blood cells and platelets carry a negative electrical charge and are attracted to substances like chitosan, which is impregnated in it and bears a positive charge. The red blood cells thus create a very tight, coherent seal as they are drawn into the bandage.

A variety of sizes of hemostatic bandages are sold individually wrapped in a vapor barrier pouch, and they are expensive. If permitted by state, provincial, or local protocols and you have access to this type of bandage, consider using them in situations of bleeding which cannot be controlled by direct pressure. Otherwise, a combination of a standard, sterile dressing and a pressure bandage will suffice.

## Bandaging Problem Areas

Moveable joints and irregularly shaped areas of the body require special bandaging techniques, as do spherical and conical anatomical regions. Because bandages tend to loosen when the joints beneath them move, choose a 3- to 6-inch self-adherent roller bandage to secure a sterile dressing applied to wounds near joints (Figure 18-34■). Begin applying the bandage from below the joint, and move diagonally in a figure-eight pattern to above the joint and then back down, overlapping the wrap as you go. Either tuck in the free end or secure it with adhesive tape. If roller bandage is not available, multiple 3- to 6-inch wide strips made from cravats may be used.

Conical regions such the arm, forearm, thigh, and leg are also best bandaged using a self-adherent roller bandage (Figures 18-35■, 18-36■, and 18-37■). Make several turns below the dressing, and then continue up, over, and above the dressing, overlapping the edges as you wrap. Anchor the loose end either under an edge of the bandage or with a strip of tape.

It is difficult to keep a dressing in place on the head. Either secure the dressing using a 2- to 3-inch self-adherent roller bandage as a compression band, or create a bandana wrap using a triangular bandage (Figure 18-38■). See OEC Skill 18-8■.

Because hands are always moving, even after being injured, bandages tend to work loose easily. An effective technique for

**Figure 18-34** When dressing an elbow, secure it with a roller bandage in a figure-eight pattern.

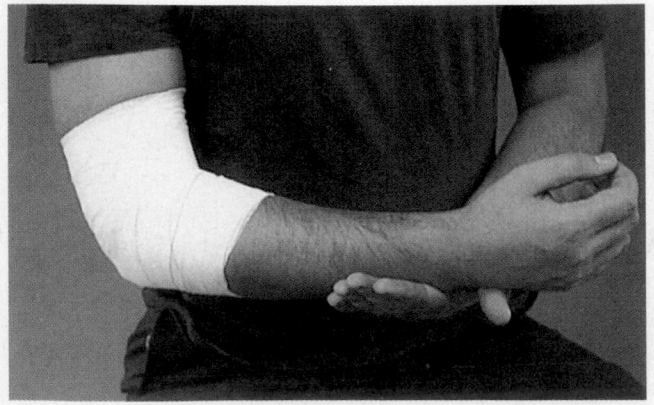

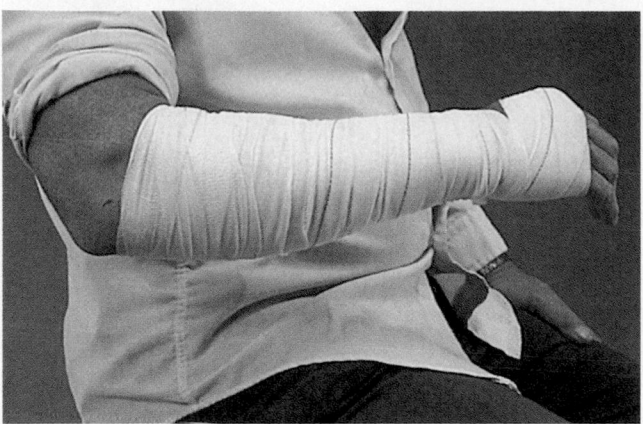

**Figure 18-35** In bandaging a forearm, start distally by making several turns below the dressing, then continue up and over the dressing, overlapping the edges.

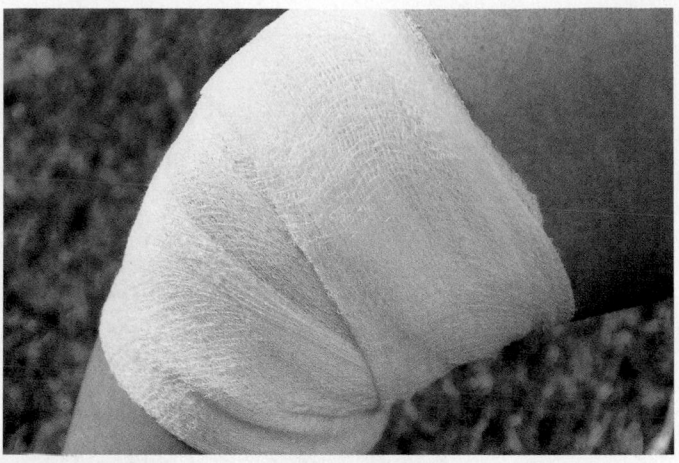

**Figure 18-36** In bandaging a knee, start below the joint and move in a figure-eight pattern above the joint and back down, overlapping as you go.

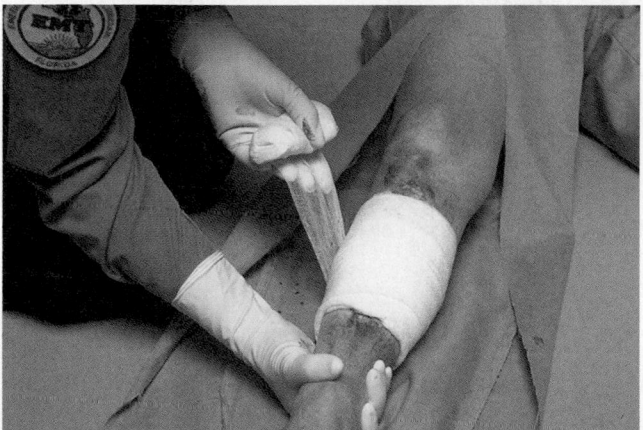

**Figure 18-37** For bandaging conical body parts, dress and firmly bandage the wound, so the dressing will not move or slip from the wound.

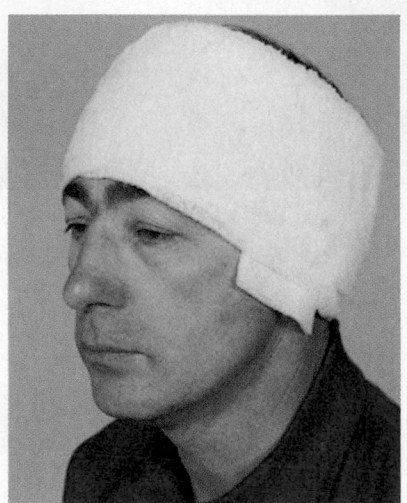

**Figure 18-38** A head and/or ear bandage.

bandaging wounds involving the palm or the back of the hand is to immobilize the entire hand. This is accomplished by placing small sterile pads (2×2) between the fingers and a roller gauze in the palm, putting the hand into the "position of function" (Figures 18-39a■ and 18-39b■). Next, wrap the hand with nonelastic bandage, elevate it above heart level, and sling and swathe it into place. When wrapping the gauze, try to leave the thumb and the finger tips exposed to facilitate CMS checks (Figure 18-40■). When the patient's fingers must be left relatively free so the hand can be used during rescue, use a suitable alternate bandaging technique for palm and dorsal hand wounds. Employ a modified figure-eight bandage or apply a short splint to the hand and distal forearm.

A finger is a difficult structure to bandage because of its cylindrical shape and ability to move in multiple directions. If at all possible, use 1-inch roller gauze for smaller wounds, and a bulky hand bandage for large finger wounds. An alternative finger bandage is the modified figure-eight hand bandage, in which the finger is wrapped in an overlapping circular fashion with 1/2- or 1-inch roller gauze, which is then brought diagonally through the palm and around the wrist several turns (Figure 18-41■). The free end is secured with adhesive tape. Do not wrap bandages around a finger too tightly, because doing so can compromise capillary refill. See OEC Skill 18-9■.

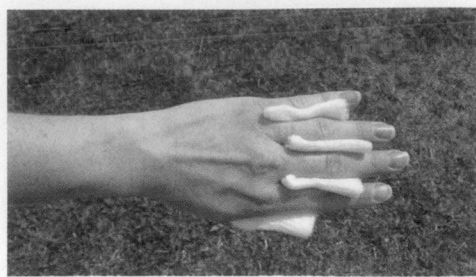

**Figure 18-39a** For an injury involving the palm or the back of hand, place sterile pads between fingers.
Copyright Edward McNamara

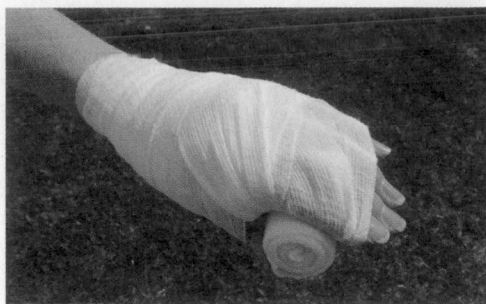

**Figure 18-39b** Wrap the entire hand with a non-roller bandage.
Copyright Edward McNamara

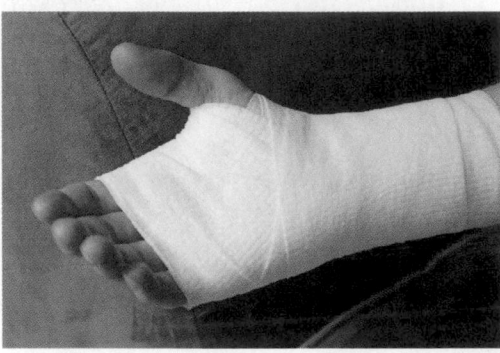

**Figure 18-40** Leave the fingers and thumb exposed for checking on circulation, motor, and sensation (CMS) function.

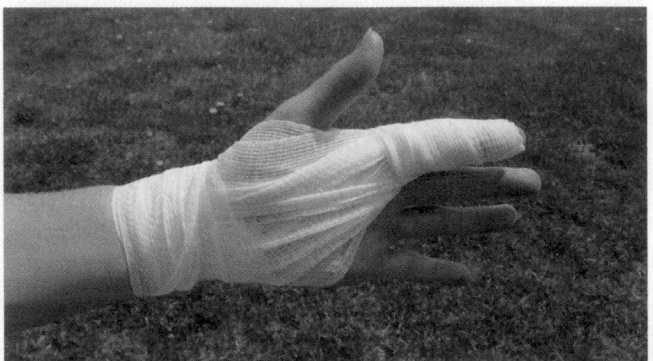

**Figure 18-41** An example of a finger bandage.
Copyright Edward McNamara

## STOP, THINK, UNDERSTAND

### Multiple Choice

Choose the correct answer.

1. Care of an avulsed injury includes all of the following except_____
   a. cleansing the injury site and removing any visible debris.
   b. replacing the avulsed flap into its original position.
   c. bandaging the avulsed flap in any position that protects it.
   d. applying a sterile compression bandage.

2. Which of the following statements about amputations is true?_____
   a. An amputation involves only completely severed parts.
   b. A badly mangled or damaged amputated part should not be preserved or sent to the hospital with the patient because it cannot be reattached.
   c. Surgeons can reattach an amputated part only if it has been without a blood supply for less than 1 hour.
   d. All amputated parts should be preserved and sent to the hospital with the patient.

3. Which of the following statements about an impaled object is true?_____
   a. The primary treatment goal for OEC Technicians is to stabilize the object in the position found.

   b. The primary treatment goal for OEC Technicians is to remove the object without causing further bleeding or causing as little bleeding as possible.
   c. Only objects impaled in extremities may be removed by OEC Technicians.
   d. Only objects impaled in the chest or abdomen may be removed by OEC Technicians.

4. Which of the following statements about an impaled object is false?_____
   a. Maintaining or restoring an effective airway takes priority over stabilization of the object.
   b. It is acceptable to remove an immoveable object (i.e, a steel guard rail) to facilitate transport of a patient.
   c. It is acceptable to remove a large object if the patient is to be evacuated by helicopter or the object is too large for an ambulance.
   d. A dangerous impaled object such as a knife should never be removed in the field.

*continued*

5. A patient has received a penetrating wound to the chest. You can hear air whistling when the patient inhales or exhales. What type of dressing would you apply?_____
   a. a pressure dressing
   b. an occlusive dressing
   c. a stabilizing dressing
   d. a homeostatic dressing

6. During your secondary assessment of a patient with a stab wound to the abdomen, he tells you that he is taking Coumadin (Warfarin), a blood thinner. What implication could this have for this patient?_____
   a. Nothing; it would not affect the patient or your care of him.
   b. The medication would cause this patient's blood to clot more quickly, thereby minimizing any bleeding he might have.
   c. The medication could cause your patient to bleed more profusely and less controllably.
   d. The medication would drop the patient's blood pressure, so he would not bleed as profusely.

7. Which of the following statements about bandaging are true? (check all that apply)
   _____ a. Bandages placed on an extremity should be wrapped entirely around that body part.
   _____ b. Fingers and toes should be left exposed.
   _____ c. CMS checks distal to any bandage should be performed.

   _____ d. Adhesive tape or the glue on it can cause allergic reactions.
   _____ e. You should not be able to insert a finger between the patient and the bandage.

8. Which of the following statements about pressure dressings are true? (check all that apply)
   _____ a. They should be wrapped snugly enough that you cannot insert a finger between the dressing and the patient's skin.
   _____ b. They should be wrapped loosely enough that you can insert two fingers between the patient's skin and the dressing.
   _____ c. They should be wrapped distally to proximally.
   _____ d. They should be wrapped proximally to distally.
   _____ e. CMS should only be checked after wrapping the wound.
   _____ f. CMS should be checked before and after wrapping the wound.
   _____ g. The injury should be splinted after dressing to minimize movement and further tissue damage.
   _____ h. Fingers and toes should be left exposed to facilitate observing CMS.

## Matching

Match each of the following terms to its definition.

_____ 1. a self-adhering roller bandage brand name available in multiple widths

_____ 2. a type of bandage that OEC Technicians should never use to secure a dressing

_____ 3. used to close a small wound

_____ 4. a piece of gauze (2×2, 3×3, 4×4, 4×8, trauma pad) that is placed directly over a wound

_____ 5. used to hold a dressing in place

_____ 6. a roll of soft gauze

a. dressing
b. bandage
c. elastic bandage
d. Kling®
e. Kerlix™
f. butterfly bandage

 **CASE DISPOSITION**

You apply dressings over the extremity abrasions that are contaminated with dirt and small stones and secure them in place with Kling®, removing larger contaminants with sterile forceps. Next, you bandage the patient's hands to prevent further contamination. You then recheck the distal circulation, motor function, and sensation to ensure that the bandages are not too tight. Finally, you place an ice pack over the hematoma on the patient's left shoulder, securing it in place with a loose Kerlix™ wrap. An ambulance arrives shortly thereafter and transfers the patient in a sitting position to a nearby definitive-care facility.

# OEC SKILL 18-1 | Controlling Bleeding

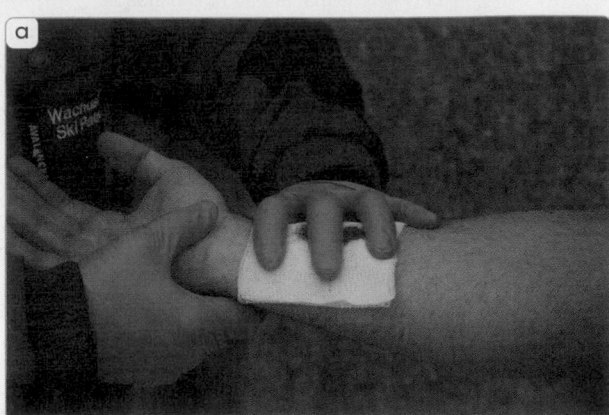

Place a sterile dressing over the wound and apply direct pressure.
Copyright Mike Halloran

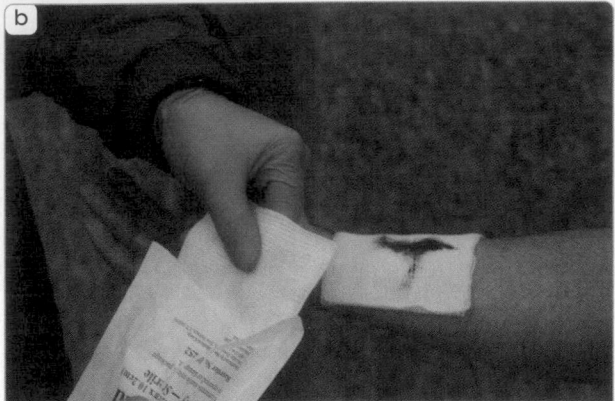

If the bleeding does not stop, add other sterile dressings over the first dressing and again apply direct pressure.
Copyright Mike Halloran

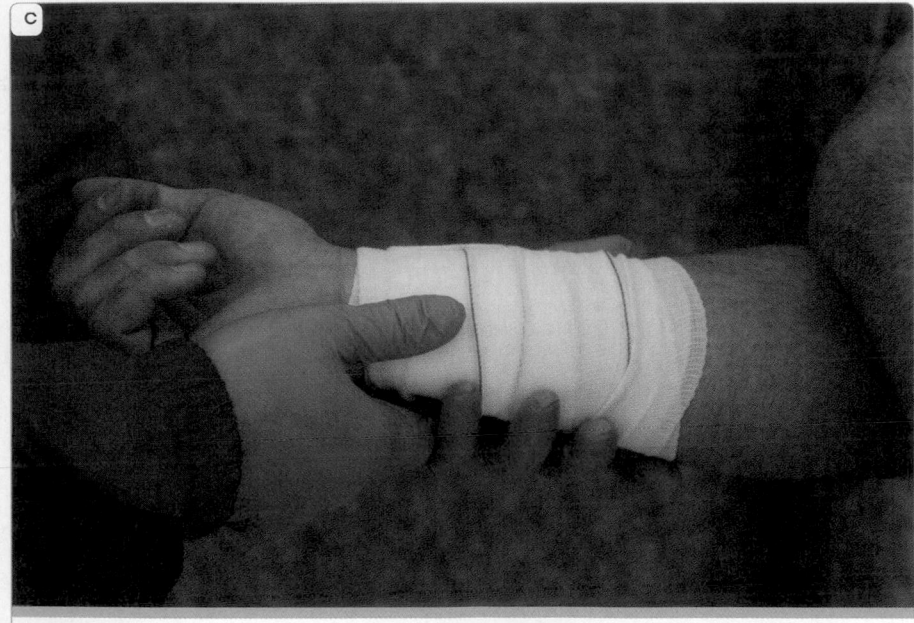

Bandage extremity.
Copyright Mike Halloran

# OEC SKILL 18-2 | Applying a Tourniquet

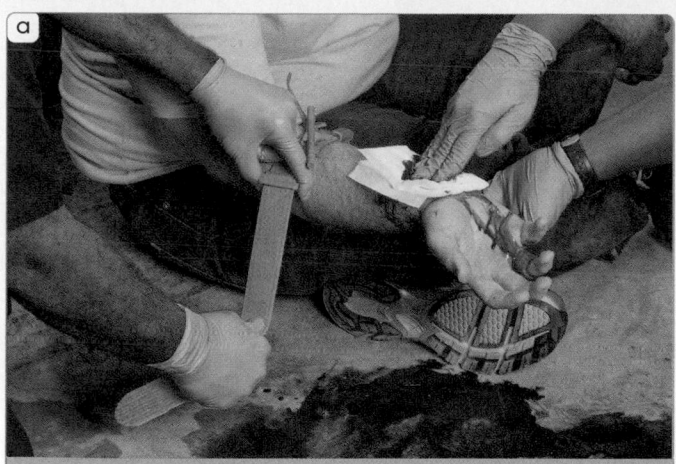

a

While preparing the tourniquet, apply direct pressure to a dressing placed over the wound.

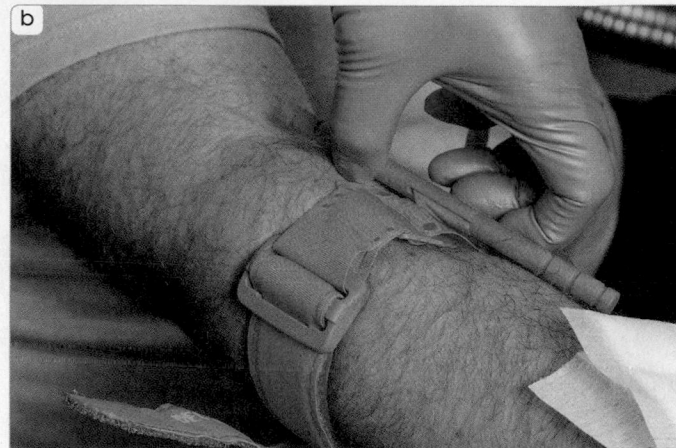

b

Tie the tourniquet around the injured extremity several inches above (proximal to) the injury but not over a joint.

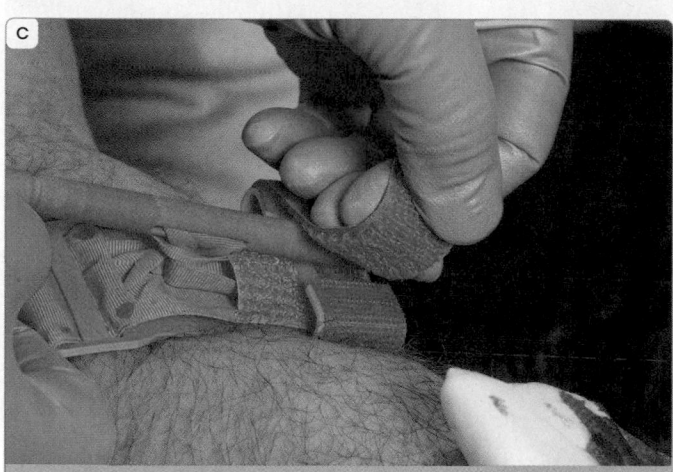

c

Pack large wounds with gauze. Twist the rod to tighten the tourniquet only to the extent needed to control the bleeding.

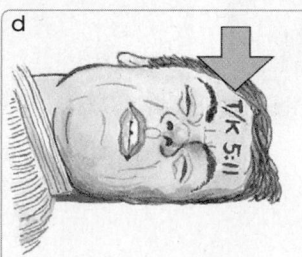

d

Write the time at which the tourniquet was applied either directly on the patient's forehead or on a piece of tape applied to the patient's forehead.

# OEC SKILL 18-3    Treating Closed Soft-Tissue Injuries

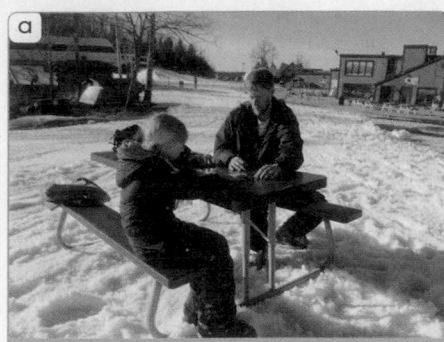

**a**

R stands for rest.
Copyright Edward McNamara

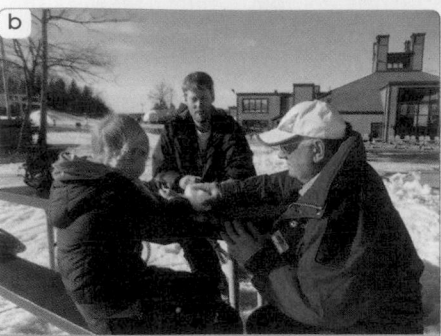

**b**

I stands for ice.
Copyright Edward McNamara

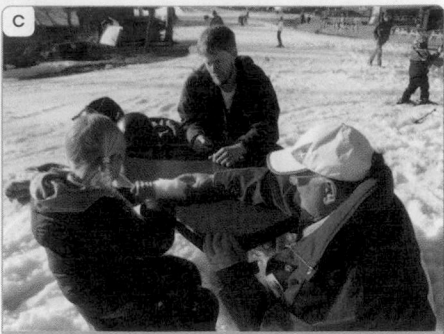

**c**

C stands for compression.
Copyright Edward McNamara

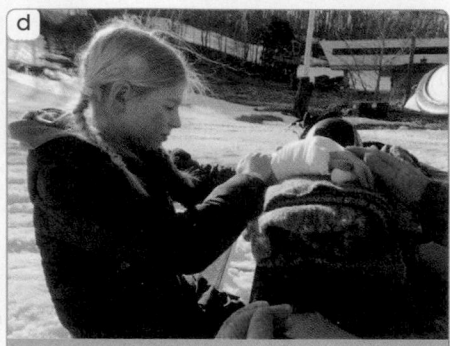

**d**

E stands for elevation.
Copyright Edward McNamara

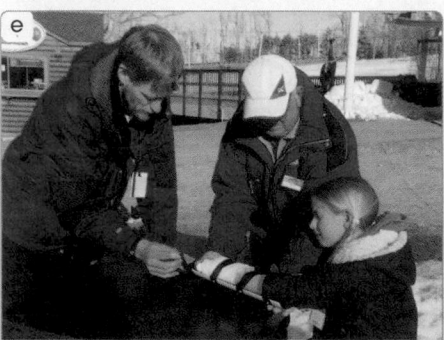

**e**

S stands for Splinting.
Copyright Edward McNamara

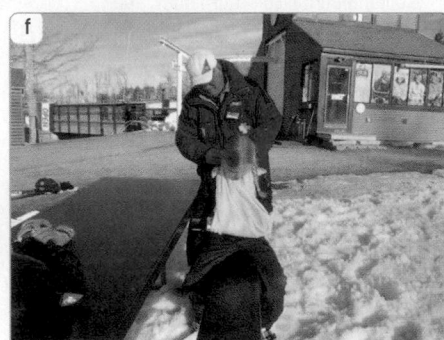

**f**

Always apply a sling and swathe after splinting an upper extremity.
Copyright Edward McNamara

# OEC SKILL 18-4 | Emergency Care for an Amputated Part

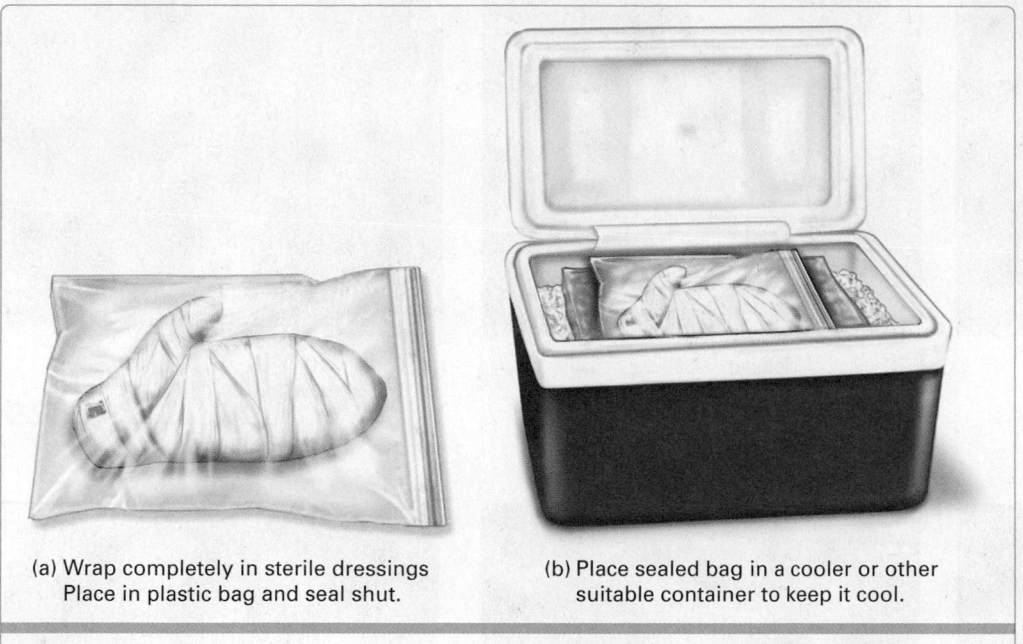

(a) Wrap completely in sterile dressings
Place in plastic bag and seal shut.

(b) Place sealed bag in a cooler or other
suitable container to keep it cool.

Wrap all amputated parts in sterile dressings moistened with sterile saline, place them in plastic bags, and seal the bags.
Place the sealed plastic bags in an ice-filled container, but do not place the bags directly on the ice.

# OEC SKILL 18-5 | Stablizing an Impaled Object

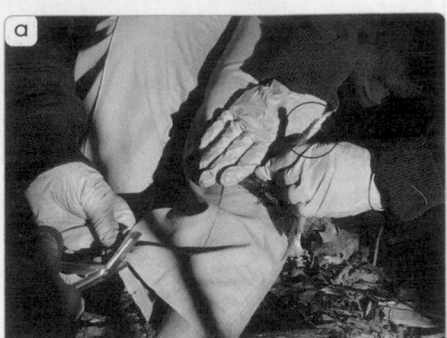

Manually stabilize the impaled object to minimize its movement.
Copyright Edward McNamara

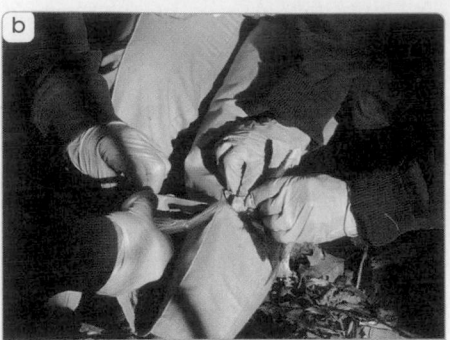

Remove all clothing around the impaled object.
Copyright Edward McNamara

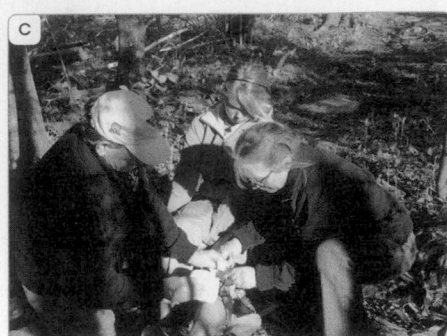

Control the bleeding.
Copyright Edward McNamara

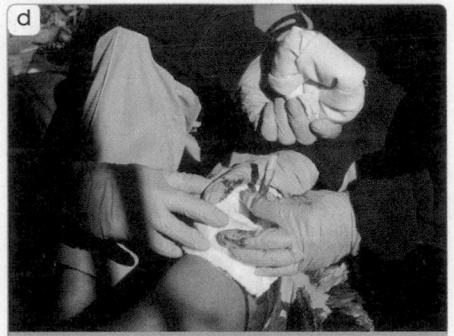

Apply a donut dressing around the impaled object.
Copyright Edward McNamara

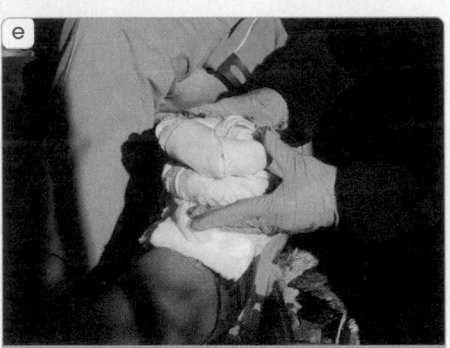

Stabilize the impaled object against the body.
Copyright Edward McNamara

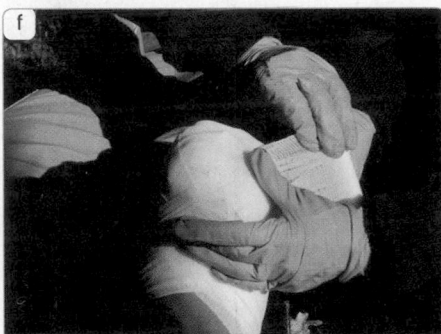

Apply a large, bulky dressing.
Copyright Edward McNamara

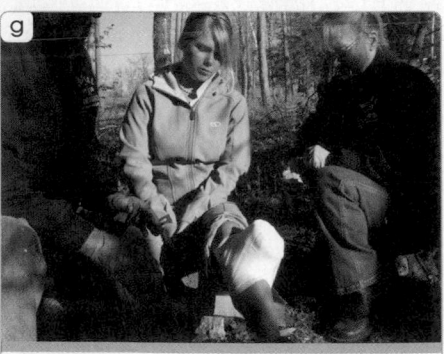

Keep the object from being moved during transport.
Copyright Edward McNamara

## OEC SKILL 18-6 — Using a Self-Adhering Roller Bandage

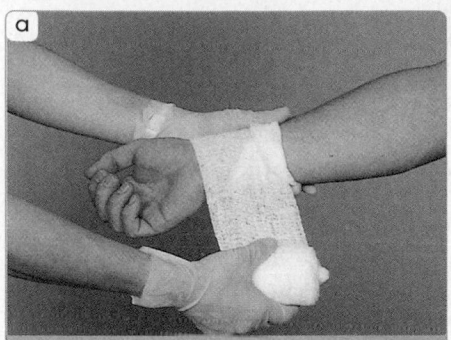

a

Use your hand to hold the dressing in place and secure the roller bandage with several wraps around the wound.

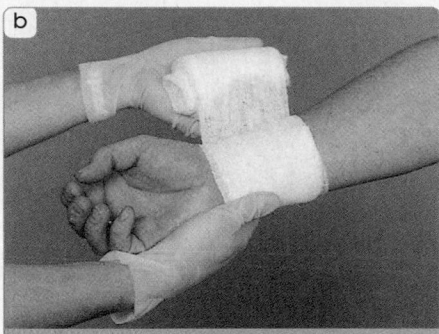

b

After the dressing and bandage are anchored, continue to wrap the bandage around the wound, overlapping it and keeping it snug.

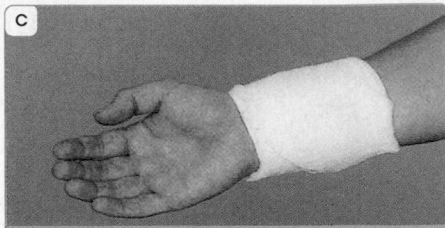

c

After covering an area larger than the wound, tie the bandage in place or secure it with tape.

## OEC SKILL 18-7 — Using an Occlusive Dressing

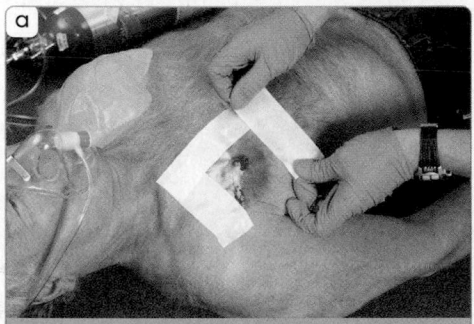

a

For an open chest wound, seal three sides of the occlusive dressing.

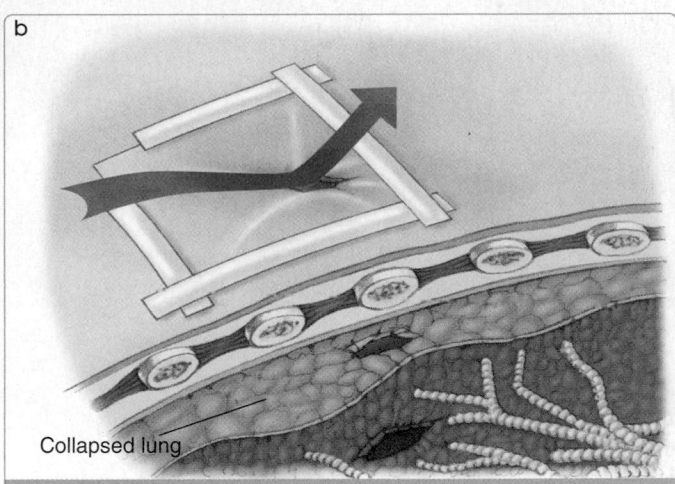

b

Collapsed lung

On inspiration, an occlusive dressing seals the wound, preventing air or liquids from entering.

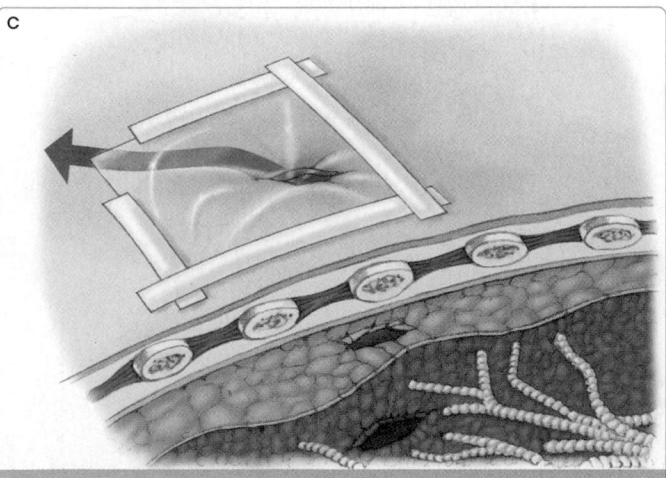

c

On expiration, trapped air escapes through the untaped section of the dressing.

# OEC SKILL 18-8 | Using a Triangular Bandage Bandana Wrap

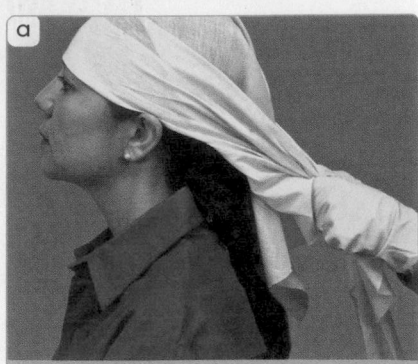

**a**

Fold the bandana to make a 2 inch hem. Position the bandage on the head with the folded edge facing out. Let the point of the bandana hang behind the patient's head.

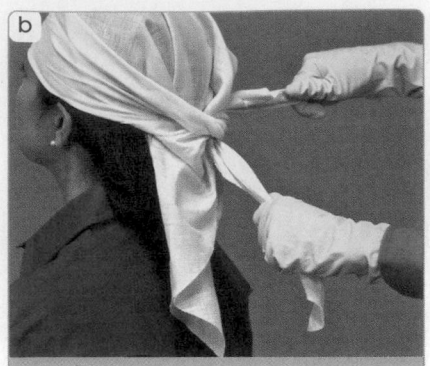

**b**

Draw the ends of the bandana behind the patient's head.

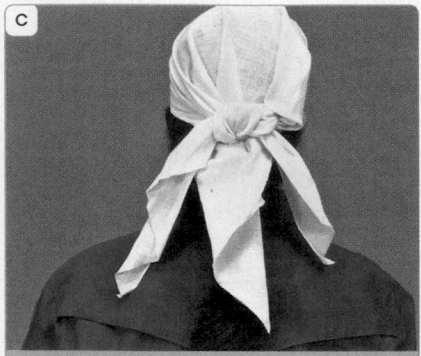

**c**

Tie the ends over the point of the bandana.

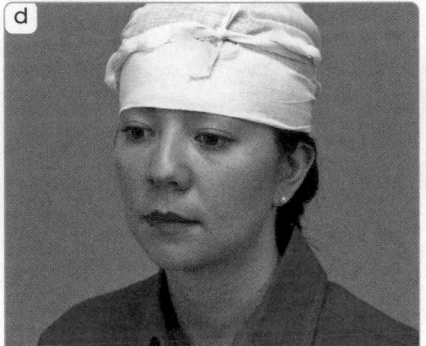

**d**

Pull the ends to the front of the head and tie them together. Take the point of the bandana and tuck it into the crossed fold.

## OEC SKILL 18-9 | Bandaging a Finger

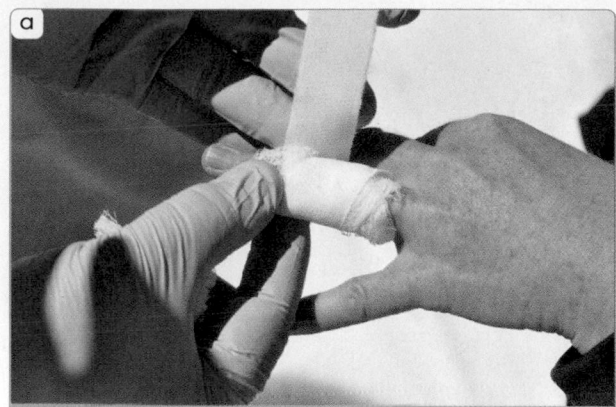

While supporting the injured finger, secure the dressing and begin to wrap the finger with a roller bandage.
Copyright David Johe, MD

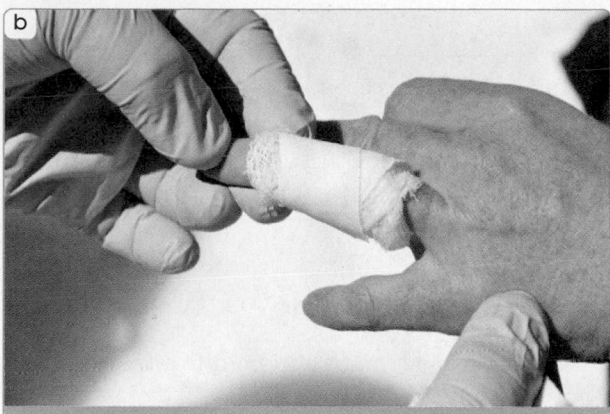

Secure the bandage with adhesive tape.
Copyright David Johe, MD

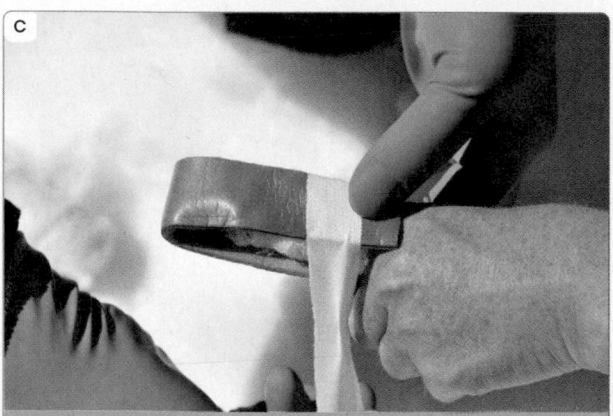

If appropriate, apply a splint to the finger.
Copyright David Johe, MD

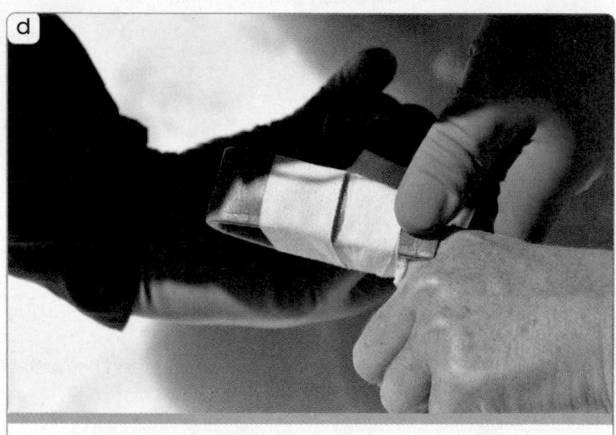

Secure the splint to the finger.
Copyright David Johe, MD

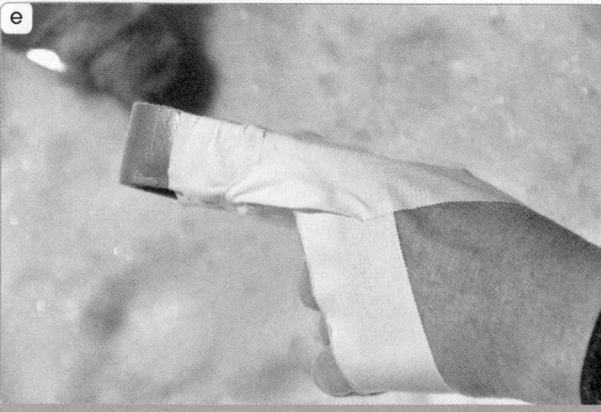

Use either a roller bandage or tape to secure the bandage to the hand.
Copyright David Johe, MD

## Skill Guide

Date: _____

(CPI) = Critical Performance Indicator

Candidate: _____

Start Time: _____

End Time: _____

## Controlling Bleeding

**Objective:** To demonstrate control of bleeding in an open soft-tissue wound.

| Skill | Max Points | Skill Demo | |
|---|---|---|---|
| Determines scene is safe. | 1 | | (CPI) |
| Introduces self, obtains permission to help/treat. | 1 | | |
| Initiates Standard Precautions. | 1 | | (CPI) |
| Exposes the wound site. | 1 | | (CPI) |
| Identifies the severity of the bleeding. | 1 | | |
| Applies sterile dressing and direct pressure. | 1 | | (CPI) |
| Maintains direct pressure; applies additional dressing if needed. | 1 | | |
| If bleeding continues, remove dressing and apply a hemostatic bandage (if authorized). | 1 | | (CPI) |
| If bleeding continues despite direct pressure and hemostatic bandage, Verbalizes application of a tourniquet and mark forehead. | 1 | | (CPI) |
| Bandages the wound and immobilizes as appropriate. | 1 | | (CPI) |
| Treats for shock as indicated. | 1 | | |
| Prepares patient for transport. | 1 | | |

Must receive 10 out of 12 points.

Comments: _____

Failure of any of the CPIs is an automatic failure.

Evaluator: _____   NSP ID: _____

PASS      FAIL

## Skill Guide

Date: _____

(CPI) = Critical Performance Indicator

Candidate: _____

Start Time: _____

End Time: _____

## Stabilizing an Impaled Object

**Objective:** To demonstrate how to stabilize an impaled object.

| Skill | Max Points | Skill Demo | |
|---|---|---|---|
| Determines scene is safe. | 1 | | (CPI) |
| Introduces self, obtains permission to help/treat. | 1 | | |
| Initiates Standard Precautions. | 1 | | (CPI) |
| Manually stabilizes object, ensuring that no movement or additional damage occurs to surrounding/underlying tissue. | 1 | | |
| Exposes the wound site. | 1 | | |
| Applies direct pressure using a dressing to control bleeding. | 1 | | (CPI) |
| Does not remove the object unless it interferes with airway. Stabilizes the object and body part using bulky dressings around object. If airway is blocked/compromised, removes the object. | 1 | | (CPI) |
| Secures the object with the appropriate materials. Shortens object if it is too long or unwieldy. | 1 | | |
| Secures the patient to a long board for stabilization. | 1 | | |
| Assures that the object cannot move during transport. | 1 | | |

Must receive 8 out of 10 points.

Comments: _____

Failure of any of the CPIs is an automatic failure.

Evaluator: _____ NSP ID: _____

PASS    FAIL

# ⛨ Chapter Review

## Chapter Summary

As the largest organ of the body, the skin is susceptible to a wide variety of soft-tissue injuries ranging from minor to severe. These injuries are often accompanied by external bleeding which, on occasion, can be life threatening, especially if the injury involves amputation of a limb or arterial damage. Identifying, assessing, and effectively treating soft-tissue injuries include the abilities to control external hemorrhage and apply a proper field dressing and bandage. Determine whether structures under wounds are damaged, and care for these "hidden" injuries. By applying these skills, you will help to significantly reduce morbidity and mortality, reduce the incidence of infection, and facilitate the overall healing of the skin.

## Remember...

1. The skin is the largest organ in the body, and it serves three purposes: it provides a protective barrier, it functions in the control of body temperature, and it acts as a sensory organ.
2. The three types of soft-tissue injuries are closed injuries, open injuries, and burns.
3. External bleeding is controlled using direct pressure, a pressure dressing, or rarely a tourniquet.
4. When applying a dressing to control bleeding, do not remove it because doing so can disrupt clots and cause more bleeding. Instead, add additional dressings.
5. Hemostatic bandages contain a substance that helps stop external bleeding.
6. Do not use elastic bandages to secure dressings.
7. Splinting a soft-tissue injury helps decrease bleeding and reduces pain.
8. Applying an effective field dressing and bandage is an important skill for OEC Technicians.

## Chapter Questions

### Multiple Choice

Choose the correct answer.

1. You are called to a restroom where a man has been stabbed with a knife. Which of the following actions should you take?_____
   a. To ensure your safety, be sure the alleged perpetrator has left the scene before approaching the patient.
   b. Enter the rest room immediately and order everyone but the victim to leave the room.
   c. Notify law enforcement before approaching the scene.
   d. Do not enter the room or approach the scene; OEC Technicians may not enter a potential crime scene.

2. Using inappropriate material for a tourniquet can cause_____
   a. serious tissue damage.
   b. inadequate pressure to control bleeding.
   c. worse bleeding.
   d. venous pooling.

3. Which of the following statements regarding cold therapy is correct?_____
   a. Ice should be applied continually to the affected area until pain and swelling has stopped.
   b. Ice should be applied in 20-minute increments (20 minutes on, and 20 minutes off) over a bandage or cloth.
   c. Cold therapy can cause underlying tissue damage and should not be implemented by OEC Technicians.
   d. None of the above are correct.

4. Your exam reveals that a patient has a 3-inch long, broken-off piece of a tree branch protruding from his upper thigh. A medical facility is less than an hour away. Which of the following actions constitutes correct patient care?_____

   a. Maintain Standard Precautions, stabilize the branch in place with bulky gauze and bandages, cover the branch and the dressings with a plastic bowl if available, secure the bowl to the upper thigh, recheck CMS, and transport.

   b. Maintain Standard Precautions, carefully but swiftly remove the branch, then staunch any bleeding with direct pressure, dress the wound with a 4×4 dressing, cover the dressing directly with a pressure dressing, splint the wound, recheck CMS, and transport.

   c. Maintain Standard Precautions, place a trauma pad directly on top of the branch and secure the pad with a pressure dressing, splint the wound, recheck CMS, and transport.

   d. Maintain Standard Precautions, carefully but swiftly remove the branch, flush the wound with sterile saline or clean water, staunch any residual bleeding with direct pressure, dress the wound with a 4×4 dressing, cover the dressing directly with a pressure dressing, splint the wound, recheck CMS, and transport.

## Matching

1. For each of the following descriptions of wounds, indicate the correct bandaging to use.

   _____ 1. a knife impaled in a patient's abdomen

   _____ 2. a sucking chest wound

   _____ 3. a patient on a river trip with a 9-hour hike-out time, suffering from a moderate 1-inch laceration on the back of the hand

   _____ 4. a hiker who suffers a 1/4″ incision to the thumb from a Swiss Army knife

   _____ 5. an ice skater who suffers a deep, 4-inch gash to the calf that will not stop bleeding

   _____ 6. a snowboarder who did a "scorpion" and lacerated the back of his head

   _____ 7. a shoulder laceration

   _____ 8. a motorcyclist who suffers an amputation of his foot just above the ankle

   a. occlusive dressing

   b. pressure dressing

   c. a figure-eight pattern using a 3- to 6-inch self-adhering roller

   d. bulky gauze and rollers

   e. steri-strip

   f. commercial band-aids

   g. tourniquet

2. Indicate which of the following actions you would take if the patient were less than 90 minutes away (L) or greater than 90 minutes away (G) from a higher level of care. Some actions may apply for both.

   _____ a. control bleeding

   _____ b. do not wash or irrigate an open wound

   _____ c. wash around the wound with soap and water

   _____ d. remove loose dirt and visible foreign material

   _____ e. irrigate the wound with a 20–30 cc syringe containing clean water or saline

   _____ f. secure the dressing with a choice of bandage

   _____ g. secure the dressing with a self-adhering roller

   _____ h. splint an extremity wound

   _____ i. elevate an extremity wound above heart level

## Short Answer

Describe the correct method for the field preservation of a completely amputated body part. _____

_____

_____

# Scenario

*The "over-seventy" club is skiing at your area. You are dipatched for a member who is down and injured. Upon arrival you find an 84-year-old male sitting and guarding his right forearm. His clothing is torn, the wound is actively bleeding and bright red blood is on the snow.*

*After securing the scene you ask the patient what happened and he responds that he fell and caught his arm between the steel edge of the ski and the ground. The patient is responsive, alert, and oriented based on his response.*

*After applying PPE, you grab some 4×4s and hand them to the patient to place on the wound. The patient is asked to hold pressure on the bandages. A rapid trauma assessment is made and you rule out any head, neck or back injury. You call for a toboggan, O2 and ALS ambulance based on the blood loss.*

**1.** This wound is classified as _____

    **a.** contusion.

    **b.** avulsion.

    **c.** hematoma.

    **d.** laceration.

*The secondary assessment is started and during the SAMPLE interview the patient informs you that he is taking Coumadin for deep vein thrombosis.*

**2.** With this information you call the base and request that a snowmobile come to the scene with _____

    **a.** occlusive dressing.

    **b.** hemostatic dressing.

    **c.** burn dressing.

    **d.** an ACE bandage.

# Suggested Reading

Finley, J. M. 1981. *Practical Wound Management: A Manual of Dressings*. Chicago: Year Book Medical Publishers.

Hughey, M. J. 2001. http://www.bbrooksidepress.org/Projects/OperationalMedicine/DATA/operationalmed/ Manuals/Standard1stAid/chapter5.html

Mistovich, J. J., B. Q. Hafen, and K. J. Kamen. 2004. *Prehospital Emergency Care*, Seventh Edition. Upper Saddle River, NJ: Prentice Hall.

 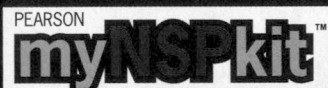

# Burns

Jane Lee Fansler, MD

## ⊕ OBJECTIVES

**Upon completion of this chapter, the OEC Technician will be able to:**

**19-1** List four types of burns.

**19-2** List the signs and symptoms for each type of burn.

**19-3** Compare and contrast the methods for classifying burns.

**19-4** Describe the clinical significance of a voice change in the setting of a thermal burn.

**19-5** Compare and contrast direct current and alternating current.

**19-6** Describe how to assess burn severity using the "Rule of Nines" system.

**19-7** Describe and demonstrate the management of a burn patient.

## ⊕ KEY TERMS

**alternating current (AC),** *p. 583*
**amp (A),** *p. 583*
**chemical burn,** *p. 582*
**direct current (DC),** *p. 583*
**electrical current,** *p. 583*

**first-degree burn,** *p. 585*
**fourth-degree burn,** *p. 585*
**full-thickness burn,** *p. 585*
**partial-thickness burn,** *p. 585*
**scald,** *p. 581*

**second-degree burn,** *p. 585*
**superficial burn,** *p. 585*
**thermal,** *p. 581*
**third-degree burn,** *p. 585*
**volt (V),** *p. 583*

## Chapter Overview

The skin, the largest organ of the human body, performs a myriad of critical functions. It provides an excellent barrier that protects the delicate tissues and structures that lie beneath it and helps regulate body temperature. With minimal care, the skin can adapt to a wide variety of environments and is constantly replenishing itself while lasting a lifetime. Unfortunately, this organ is not impervious to injury and is easily damaged when exposed to conditions such as excessive heat, corrosive substances, or friction. Even the sun's harmful rays can damage unprotected skin. The result is a soft-tissue injury known as a burn.

A burn is defined as an injury caused by excessive exposure to thermal, chemical, electrical, or radioactive agents. Each year burns account for approximately 700,000

*continued*

## HISTORICAL TIMELINE

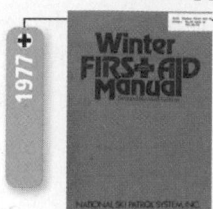

**1977** Warren Bowman writes the second revised edition of the NSP's *Winter First Aid Manual*, which sold for $1.25.

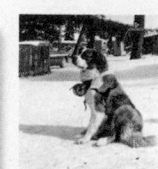

**1977** NSP adopts "Rusty" (a St. Bernard wearing a first-aid belt) as mascot.

# CASE PRESENTATION

You are walking into the lodge on a cold winter afternoon when a woman rushes up to you with her four-year-old son, who is crying in anguish. The mother explains that she had been cooking instant noodles in the cafeteria microwave and had walked just a few steps away to answer her cell phone. She ran back when she heard her son scream and found that he had pulled the boiling-hot dish out of the microwave and onto himself. The child has no past medical history, is not taking any medications, and has no allergies.

*What should you do?*

emergency department visits, nearly 45,000 hospitalizations, and more than 3,000 fatalities. Burns affect individuals of all age groups and can occur virtually anywhere and at anytime.

For the OEC Technician, a patient with burns is a medical emergency that is especially challenging when encountered in a non-urban, outdoor environment. Burns can be extremely painful and may very quickly result in massive tissue loss. In severe cases, the body can lose large quantities of fluid, resulting in profound shock or even death. Reducing the prevalence of serious injury and long-term complications involves burn management, which requires rapid field intervention and timely treatment. Burn patients often require rapid transportation to a specialized care facility. If backcountry evacuation is required, even a moderate burn can become a difficult problem.

Outdoor environments, despite their beauty and serenity, present numerous burn hazards, from prolonged exposure to the sun, to campfire flames, to contact with hot rocks, sand, or soil. Even resort and backcountry lodge settings are not immune to the risks posed by burns, because high-energy equipment, hot grease in kitchens, cleaning solutions, and other super-heated surfaces are common in these settings. Employees in the maintenance facilities at ski areas can be exposed to gasoline and other petroleum products. OEC Technicians must be vigilant regarding any potential burn hazards in the environment and be prepared to act quickly if summoned to a burn-related emergency.

This chapter will prepare OEC Technicians to assess and care for burn patients. Patrollers will learn how to differentiate burns by their source, assess and classify burns by depth, and estimate the extent of a burn. Because burn management is based on both the cause and the severity of the burn, the chapter also describes treatment principles for each type of burn. Although most burns are not life threatening, those that are must be managed quickly. Using the combination of a systematic approach to burn injuries and basic trauma resuscitation principles, OEC Technicians will be able to deliver high-quality care and reduce morbidity and mortality among burn patients.

## Anatomy and Physiology

The skin is composed of two primary layers: the epidermis and the dermis. Beneath these layers lies the subcutaneous tissue, which attaches the skin to other, underlying structures (Figure 19-1■). As the largest organ in the body, the skin has the following important functions:

+ Protection of underlying structures
+ Defense against invading pathogens

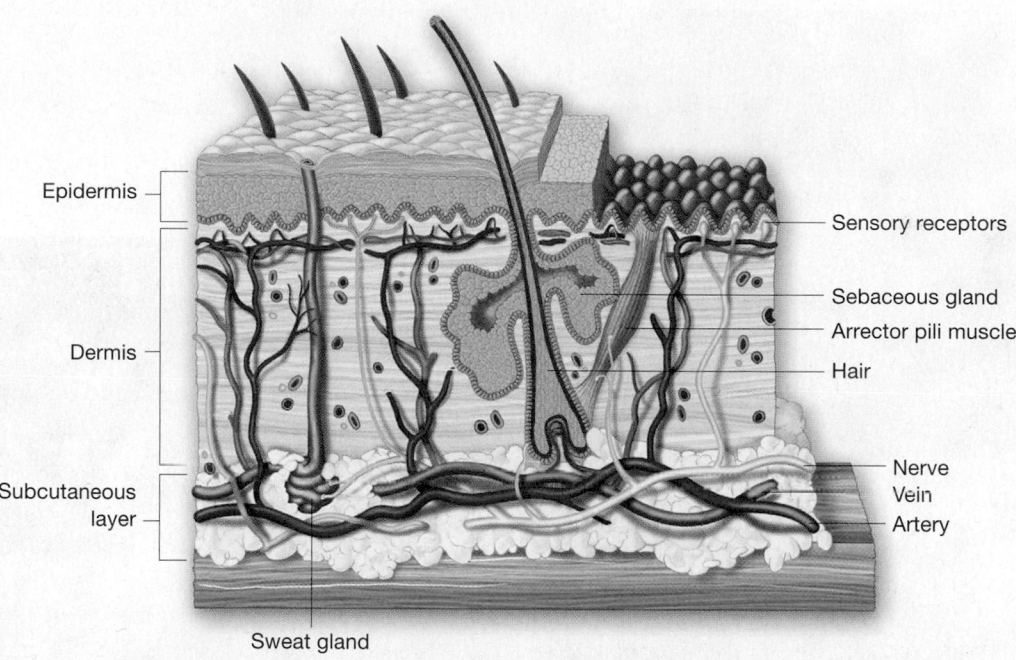

**Figure 19-1** The anatomy of the skin.

+ Sensation
+ Temperature regulation
+ Prevention of fluid loss
+ Synthesis of vitamin D
+ Excretion

The epidermis, the outermost layer of the skin, serves as a protective barrier. This layer is thicker in abrasion-prone areas such as the heels of the feet and the palms of the hands. The epidermis does not contain any blood vessels and depends on the dermis for its nourishment.

The dermis lies beneath the epidermis and is tightly connected to it by a basal membrane. It contains important structures, including nerve endings, hair follicles, sweat glands, and blood vessels.

The dermis contains two types of glands: sweat glands and sebaceous glands. Sweat glands help keep the body cool, whereas sebaceous glands lubricate the skin, preventing cracking and drying. Although the skin provides protection from everyday bumps, scrapes, and external pathogens, it is not impenetrable and is vulnerable to damage when exposed to extreme temperatures, caustic substances, and other hazardous sources.

⊕ **19-1** List four types of burns.

⊕ **19-2** List the signs and symptoms for each type of burn.

# Types of Burns

OEC Technicians should be familiar with four different types of burns: thermal burns, chemical burns, electrical burns, and radiation burns.

## Thermal Burns

The most common type of burn suffered is a **thermal burn**, caused when heat comes directly into contact with the skin. Temperatures greater than 46°C (115°F) are sufficient to inflict a thermal burn. Common causes of thermal burns include open flames; hot water, hot steam, or superheated air, which cause a **scald**; and physical contact with

**thermal**   pertaining to heat.

**scald**   an injury caused by a hot liquid or a hot, moist vapor.

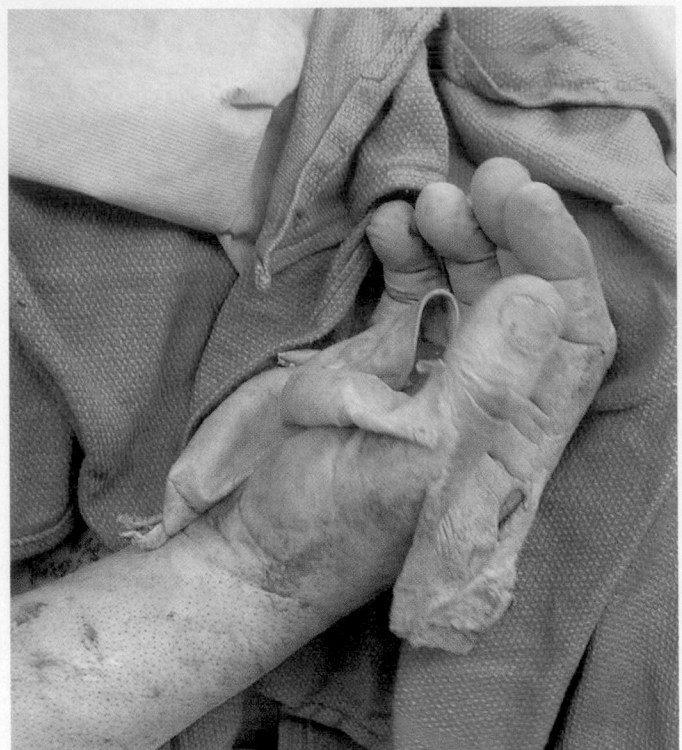

**Figure 19-2a** A thermal burn on the hand (note the remaining half of a glove) of a commercial painter who was injured when a spark ignited the vapors from a spray-paint gun he was using in an enclosed area.
Copyright Charles Stewart M.D. and Associates

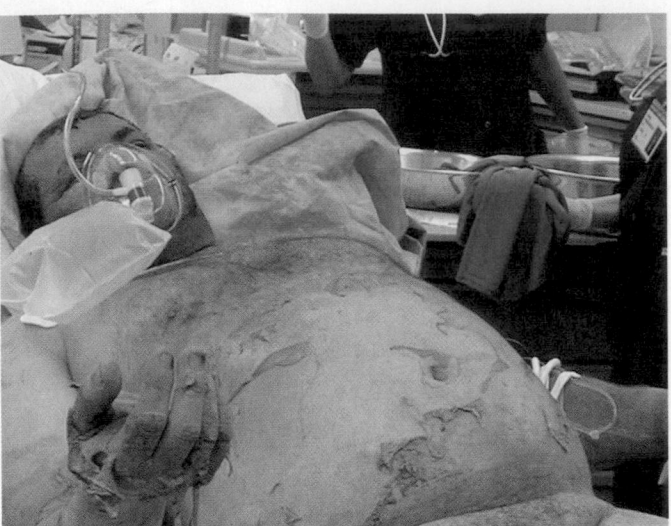

**Figure 19-2b** This commercial painter may also have inhalation injuries from hot air or steam.
Copyright Charles Stewart M.D. and Associates

a hot object such as an iron, molten tar, or a light bulb. While most thermal burns occur on the skin surface, they also can also occur inside the body under certain circumstances. For example, patients who breathe heated air or hot steam into their lungs may receive an inhalation burn that causes extensive damage to delicate lung tissue (Figures 19-2a■ and 19-2b■).

## Chemical Burns

**chemical burn** a burn caused by a caustic substance, such as an acid or a base.

**Chemical burns** result from exposure to caustic substances, which are called acids or bases depending on the substance's potential of hydrogen (pH)—the concentration of hydrogen ions in solution. The pH scale ranges from 1 (strong acid) to 14 (strong base); a pH of 7 is considered neutral because it is neither acidic nor basic. Each whole number on the pH scale represents a tenfold difference from the next whole number. For instance, a solution with a pH of 6 is ten times more acidic than a solution with a pH of 7, whereas a solution with a pH of 5 is 100 times more acidic than a solution with a pH of 7.

The extent of injury resulting from exposure to caustic substances varies with the concentration of the chemical, the amount of chemical involved, and the duration of contact. Alkaline (or basic) chemicals tend to cause more extensive chemical burns than acids because they penetrate the skin more deeply. Mucous membranes, especially in the mouth, can be burned if the patient has ingested a caustic chemical.

Acidic and alkaline solutions are commonly found in commercial settings such as a mountain resort or backcountry lodge, often in cleaning solutions (Table 19-1■). Unlike most household equivalents, commercial cleaners are typically in concentrated forms that require dilution before use. In addition to acids and bases, chemical burns can be caused by substances such as mustard gas, a powerful vesicant (blister-producing agent).

## Table 19-1   Common Acids and Bases

**ACIDS (pH <7)**
Sulfuric acid
Hydrochloric acid
Hydrofluoric acid
Muriatic acid
Carbolic acid (phenol)
Phosphoric acid
Nitric acid
Acetic acid

**BASES (pH >7)**
Sodium hydroxide (caustic soda)
Potassium hydroxide (caustic potash)
Lye
Lime
Calcium carbonate
Magnesium
Chlorine bleach

## Electrical Burns

A burn that occurs when the body comes into contact with an **electrical current** is called an electrical burn. Many factors determine the severity of an electrical burn, including the amount and type of electricity contacted, where the electricity enters and exits the body, and the duration of contact. Under normal conditions, electricity flows from some electrical source to an electrical ground following the "path of least resistance"—that is, the pathway that has the highest conductivity and the least resistance. The importance of this to OEC Technicians is that skin is a relatively poor conductor with high resistance. When it becomes wet or oily, the body's conductivity increases and its resistance markedly decreases. Internal structures such as blood vessels and nerves are highly conductive and have low resistance, which is why electrical injuries traveling through the body produce severe internal injuries.

OEC Technicians should always consider internal injuries whenever a patient has been exposed to a significant electrical current, which can pass into and burn (essentially cook) any organ in the body. The heart can be significantly damaged or can stop altogether when a significant electrical current travels through it.

An electrical current is categorized by its direction of flow and its power or voltage. Current can be unidirectional, which is commonly referred to as **direct current (DC)**, or it can be bidirectional, better known as **alternating current (AC)**. Of the two, alternating current is more dangerous because the energy pulses 60 times per second in the United States (50 times per second in Europe). Pulsations in the current can cause the victim to remain in contact with the energy source for longer periods of time, resulting in more significant damage. The unit by which electrical current is measured is the **amp (A)**.

The unit by which the power of an electrical current is measured is the **volt (V)**. High-voltage power (greater than 1,000V AC or 1,500V DC) is commonly found in power lines and in commercial settings, whereas low-voltage power (50–1,000V AC, or 120–1,500V DC) is found in most residential settings. Both types can produce lethal injuries (Figure 19-3■). An electrical shock as little as 100mA can be lethal if the current passes through critical areas of the body such as the brain, heart, or lungs. Energy levels between 500 and 1,000 volts can produce significant internal burns.

⊕ **19-5** Compare and contrast direct current and alternating current.

**electrical current**    a stream of electricity that moves along a conductor.

**direct current (DC)**    electrical current that flows in one direction only.

**alternating current (AC)**    electrical current that periodically flows in opposite directions.

**amp (A)**    a unit of current produced by 1 volt acting through the resistance of 1 ohm.

**volt (V)**    a unit of electric potential or electromotive force, equal to 1 watt per ampere or 1 joule per coulomb.

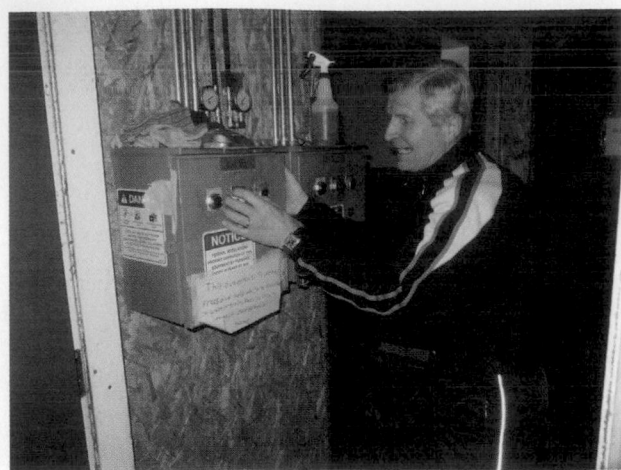

**Figure 19-3** Electrical burns may happen unexpectedly and can be lethal.
Copyright Edward McNamara

Electricity passing through the body typically produces a surface burn where it entered and where it exited the body, and the current may affect all tissues in between (Figure 19-4■).

Lightning is another form of electrical injury and is covered in detail in Chapter 26, Heat-Related Emergencies.

## Radiation Burns

Following exposure to an object, substance, or element that emits radiation, a radiation burn may occur. Depending on the source, exposure may be brief or prolonged. Radiation is transmitted in the form of rays or particles and may be transmitted by a variety of sources, including tanning beds, plant and grow lights, heat lamps, black lights, medical X-rays, welding equipment, and other industrial or military equipment. The sun is another source of radiation; it transmits ultraviolet (UV) light, which can burn the skin. At higher altitudes, sunburn occurs upon shorter exposure to sunlight because the less-dense atmosphere at greater elevations provides less protection against UV rays.

Radioactive decay of substances produces three types of natural radiation: alpha, beta, and gamma radiation. Gamma radiation, which includes X-ray radiation, is by far the most dangerous and penetrates the skin the deepest. At a dose used for a chest X-ray, gamma rays appear to be safe. At higher doses or for longer exposures, gamma radiation causes catastrophic burns. Fortunately, this form of radiation is generally encountered only in health care settings, laboratories, and industrial environments. Gamma radiation is produced by nuclear weapons and some other weapons of mass destruction. Of the four types of burns, radiation burns—with the exception of UV-related sunburns or burns associated with welding equipment—are the least likely to be encountered by OEC Technicians.

**Figure 19-4** Electricity passing through an individual may cause a variety of injuries in addition to entrance and exit burns.

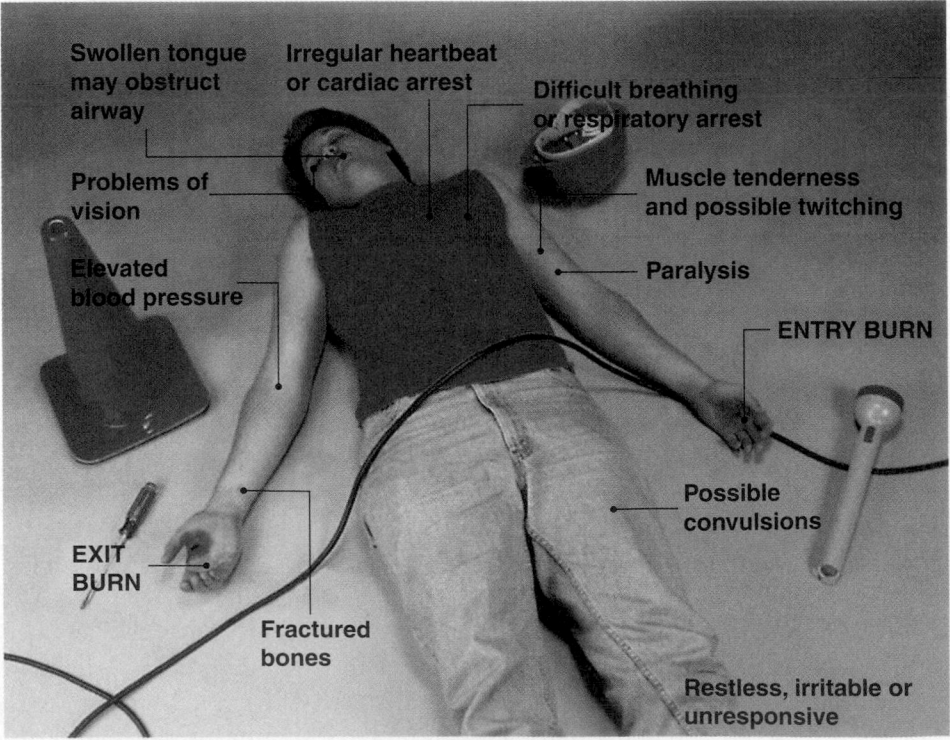

# The Classification of Burns

Burns are classified according the depth of skin damage using two methods: the thickness-based method, which classifies burns as **superficial burns**, **partial-thickness burns**, or **full-thickness burns**, and the degree-based approach, which classifies burns as **first-degree burns**, **second-degree burns**, **third-degree burns**, and **fourth-degree burns**. Both methods are commonly used in emergency and burn medicine, often in conjunction with one another (Figure 19-5■).

Accurately classifying burn injuries is an important skill for OEC Technicians to learn because this information is used to determine initial treatment, subsequent therapy, and whether hospitalization should occur in a specialized burn center. In the sections that follow we consider the classification of burns.

## Superficial Burns

A superficial burn (a first-degree burn) is the mildest form of burn and affects the epidermis only (Figure 19-6■). It is characterized by skin that is hot, dry, and reddened. Although the epidermis remains intact, mild swelling due to internal fluid shifts may occur (Figure 19-7■). Pain and tenderness is mild to moderate due to intact but irritated nerve endings. Healing is usually spontaneous, occurs within a few days, and may be accompanied by superficial sloughing of the epidermal layer ("peeling"). Too much exposure to the sun and remaining too long in a tanning bed are the most common sources of superficial burns.

**⊕ 19-3** Compare and contrast the methods for classifying burns.

**superficial burn** a first-degree burn.

**partial-thickness burn** a second-degree burn.

**full-thickness burn** a third-degree or fourth-degree burn.

**first-degree burn** a burn that affects the epidermis only, causing reddening of the skin and mild edema but no blisters.

**second-degree burn** a burn that affects the epidermis and the dermis and results in blisters.

**third-degree burn** a burn that destroys the epidermis and the dermis and extends into the subcutaneous tissue.

**fourth-degree burn** a burn that extends into muscle and bone.

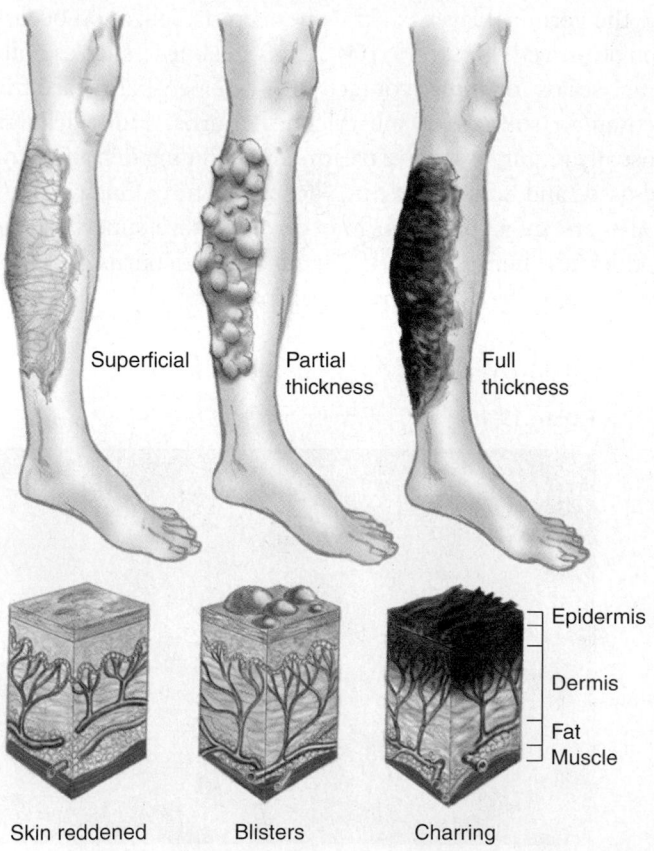

**Figure 19-5** The classification of burns by depth.

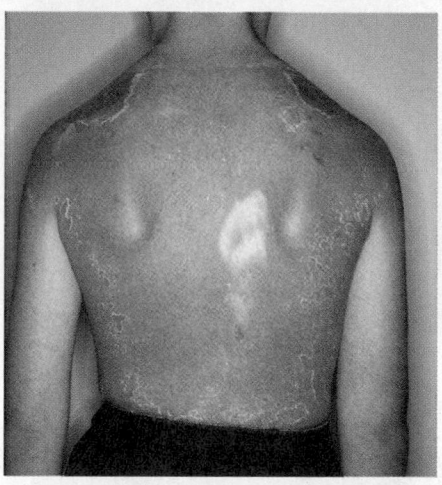

**Figure 19-6** Superficial (or first-degree) burns.
Copyright Charles Stewart M.D. and Associates

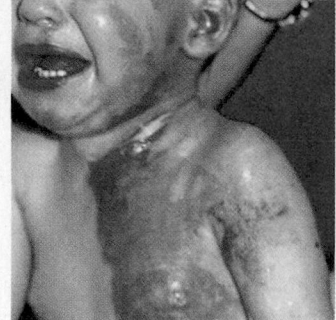

**Figure 19-7** A pediatric patient with superficial (first-degree) burns.

## Partial-Thickness Burns

A partial thickness burn (a second-degree burn) affects both the epidermis and dermis but does not exceed the regenerative capabilities of the skin. This category of burn is characterized by reddened skin and blisters that form as a result of plasma leaking into the spaces surrounding epidermal cells (Figure 19-8■). Unless the blisters break, the skin is dry and reddened. Ruptured blisters give the area a wet, oily appearance, again due to leaking plasma. Nerve endings remain intact but are inflamed and irritated. As a result, the skin is painful to the touch, with the pain described as moderate to severe. OEC Technicians should consider calling for ALS to provide intravenous pain medication for patients with extensive partial-thickness burns. A partial-thickness burn may be surrounded by patches of superficial burns.

Healing time depends on the extent of the burn, the stability of blisters, and how long it takes for the plasma to be reabsorbed. Scalding is the most common cause of partial thickness burns, although caustic chemicals frequently result in this category of burn.

## Full-Thickness Burns

A full-thickness burn (third-degree burns) is a devastating injury that destroys all layers of the skin and can extend into the underlying structures (fourth-degree burn) (Figure 19-9■). Fourth-degree burns can be extensive, including muscle and bone. When full-thickness burns cover a large surface area of the body, the mortality rate is high.

In a full-thickness burn, the skin takes on a white or charred "leathery" appearance and is usually dry. Pain is usually absent due to complete destruction of nerve endings, although the site may be surrounded by partial-thickness and superficial burns that are painful. Healing time is usually protracted and depends on the extent of the burn area and on the extent and seriousness of other concurrent injuries. Skin does not grow back, because the germinal layer of skin where epithelialization occurs has been destroyed (Figure 19-10■). Thermal burns, such as boiling water, scalds, or direct contact with an open flame, are the most common sources of full-thickness burns. Full-thickness burns usually require extensive treatment, including debridement of dead tissue and skin grafting in a hospital setting. Such serious burns also are more prone to infection than are superficial or partial-thickness burns. Table 19-2■ summarizes burns as classified according to the degree-based approach.

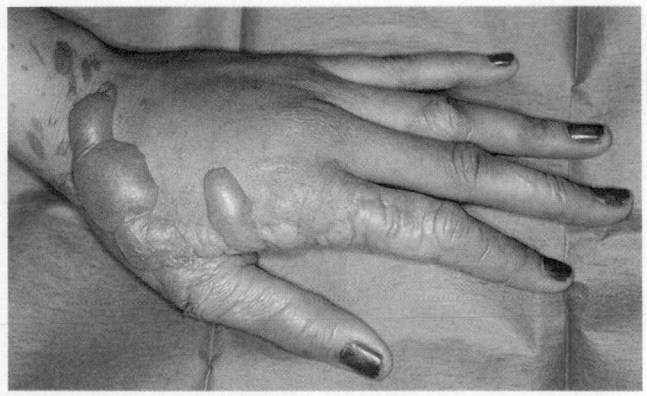

**Figure 19-8** A partial-thickness burn; note redness and blisters.
Copyright Charles Stewart M.D. and Associates

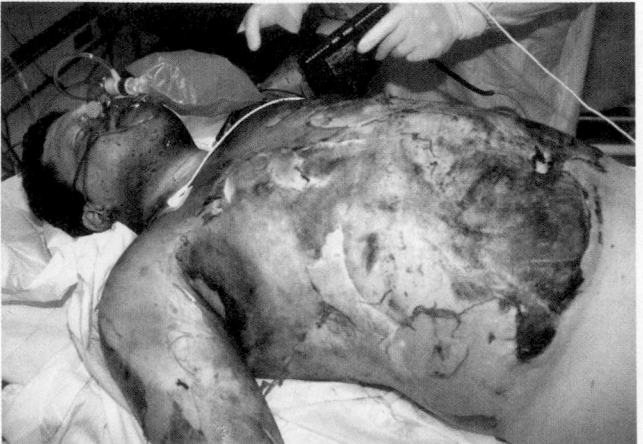

**Figure 19-9** A full-thickness burn.
Copyright Edward Dickinson, M.D.

**Figure 19-10** This full-thickness burn is an electrical burn.

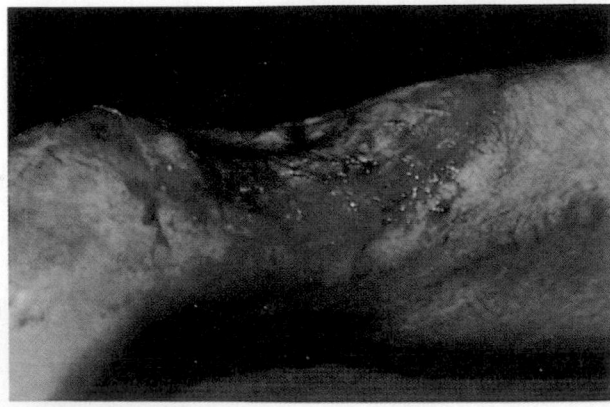

**Table 19-2** Burn Classification

| Burn | Appearance of Skin | Skin Layers Affected |
|---|---|---|
| First-degree burn | Red, no blisters | Epidermis |
| Second-degree burn | Blisters, wet appearance | Epidermis and dermis |
| Third-degree burn | Charred or white, dry | Epidermis, dermis, and underlying soft tissues |
| Fourth-degree burn | Blackened | Epidermis, dermis, and underlying tissues, including muscle and bone |

# STOP, THINK, UNDERSTAND

## Multiple Choice

Choose the correct answer.

1. In what layer of the skin are nerve endings located?_____
   a. epidermis
   c. germinal layer
   b. dermis
   d. keratin stratum

2. Which of the following functions does the skin not perform?_____
   a. synthesis of vitamin C
   c. excretion
   b. prevention of fluid loss
   d. sensation

3. What type of burn can be caused by grow lights, tanning beds, and medical X-rays?_____
   a. thermal burns
   c. electrical burns
   b. chemical burns
   d. radiation burns

4. What type of burn is usually caused by physical contact with objects, scalding liquids, or a flame?_____
   a. thermal burns
   c. electrical burns
   b. chemical burns
   d. radiation burns

5. Which type of burn is characterized by reddened skin and blisters?_____
   a. superficial burns
   c. full-thickness burns
   b. partial-thickness burns
   d. third-degree burns

## Fill in the Blank

1. A partial-thickness burn is equivalent to a _____ degree burn.

2. A superficial burn is equivalent to a _____ degree burn.

3. A full-thickness burn is equivalent to a _____ degree burn.

 # CASE UPDATE

You don gloves and immediately remove the four-year-old's clothing, including his underpants. After confirming that the ABCDs are intact, you call for assistance on the radio and then begin a secondary assessment. Upon examination of the patient, you note that the boy's chin and the front of his neck for a distance of about twice as long as his palms are bright red and are surrounded by larger areas of redness in a splash-like pattern. Blisters appear to be forming on the front of his chest. The child is still shrieking and claws frantically at his mother. He is breathing rapidly and his heart rate is 110 and regular at the brachial artery pulse point.

***What should you do now?***

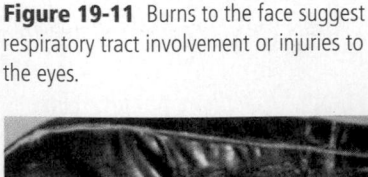

**19-4** Describe the clinical significance of a voice change in the setting of a thermal burn.

> **Protect Yourself**
>
> Caution! When treating a burn patient, ensure your own safety by protecting yourself from sources of heat, chemicals, and electricity. Wear protective gear as indicated.

# Assessment

The first priority when assessing a burn patient is to ensure that the scene is safe to enter. Put out any fires, turn off the electricity, and remove any chemicals. Call a Haz-Mat team if the scene contains any chemicals or radiation that could harm you or others. The function of a HazMat team is discussed in Chapter 35, Special Operations and Ambulance Operations. Touching a patient who is still in contact with a live electric wire can be dangerous, perhaps even fatal. Only after all potential dangers have been abated may you begin the assessment process. If the source of the burns is not obvious, attempt to identify it as part of the scene size-up because this information may be useful in both the assessment and in making treatment decisions.

As soon as you are aware that a toxic substance or bodily fluids may be present, use Standard Precautions, and use personal protective equipment (PPE). At a minimum, use eye, face, and hand protection. For chemical burns, consider using chemical-resistant gloves and a protective gown or over-garment. Do not overlook this critical step; some chemicals may not be readily apparent, and failure to adequately protect yourself increases your risk of injury. Some chemicals give off toxic gases that can cause damage to the eyes and lungs, and burns can expose structures beneath the skin to potential contaminants and pathogens. Observe Standard Precautions to reduce the risks to you and to your patient.

The next step is to assess the ABCDs, beginning with evaluating the patency of the airway. Patients who are exposed to thermal sources or caustic chemicals, especially those involving inhaled substances such as smoke or acid vapors, are at high risk for serious airway injuries (Figure 19-11■). Burn injuries to the upper airway caused by inhaled steam usually require prompt ALS intubation. The soft mucosa in the upper airway above the vocal cords is especially vulnerable to heat and caustic vapors and can swell significantly, resulting in airway obstruction and the inability to breathe. The lower airway, although better protected by the larynx from direct heat, can still suffer inhalation injuries, which may not be immediately apparent but can cause sudden respiratory compromise. Signs and symptoms associated with an inhalation injury include the following:

+ Obvious burns involving the head, face, or neck
+ Singed hair, including the eyebrows, nose hairs, and facial hair
+ Soot and other by-products of combustion on the face, in the mouth, or around the nostrils
+ Hoarseness or voice changes
+ Airway swelling
+ Darkened oral or nasal discharge known as carbonaceous sputum

**Figure 19-11** Burns to the face suggest respiratory tract involvement or injuries to the eyes.

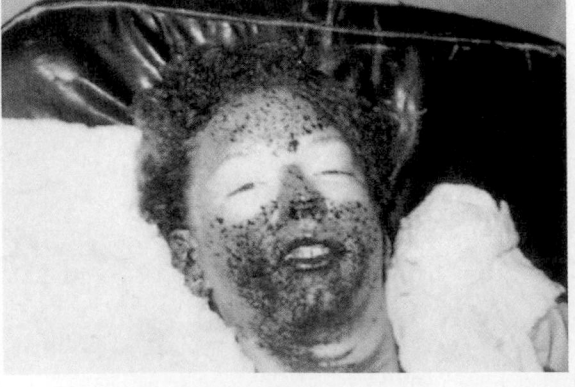

Upon recognizing these signs and symptoms, OEC Technicians must begin immediate treatment and activate the emergency care system. Maintaining the airway, giving oxygen as indicated, and arranging for rapid transport are the priorities of care for patients with inhalation injuries. Whenever inhalation injuries are suspected, immediately arrange ALS transport to a burn or trauma center. The window of time during which patients can be intubated by an ALS provider before airway swelling becomes too great is typically narrow. Finish the primary assessment by assessing circulation and correcting any external bleeding, and by determining the patient's level of responsiveness and distal neurologic function.

Perform a thorough secondary assessment (as described in both Chapter 7, Patient Assessment and Chapter 17, Principles of Trauma) and take vital signs. Use the SAMPLE acronym to obtain a medical history, which can reveal valuable clues regarding the mechanism of injury and may help to identify other possible injuries and preexisting medical conditions such as diabetes, prior myocardial infarction, or pulmonary disease, which can be exacerbated by the stress of burn injuries. Obtain information regarding the patient's medications and tetanus immunization status.

If the source of the burn involves flames that occurred in an enclosed area, assume that the patient may have carbon monoxide (CO) poisoning. Symptoms of elevated CO levels include headache, nausea, and altered mental status. Even though cherry-red skin is often described as a feature of CO poisoning, it is rarely observed in pre-hospital environments and occurs only after significant exposure. In this situation, skin redness is probably the result of burns. If exposure to CO is expected, give the patient high-flow, high-concentration oxygen through a nonrebreather mask.

If the source of the burn is a hot liquid, attempt to determine how long the liquid was in contact with the skin. Find out if the burn was irrigated with water or if a cream or lotion was applied to the burn before your arrival.

If you suspect the burn results from exposure to a chemical, attempt to identify the chemicals involved by examining the container, paying particular attention to the identities and concentrations of the active ingredients. Do not expose yourself or others to the chemical.

If the burn source is electricity, attempt to determine which body part was in direct contact with the electrical source and for how long. Attempt to identify the source of the electricity (e.g., an electrical outlet in the lodge, or the power supply to the lift motor). In injuries involving electricity, the patient's burns are usually more extensive than is first apparent, because the greatest injuries are often internal and involve deep tissues or organs. Moreover, the patient is at greater risk for cardiac-related injury or arrest when electricity is involved. Determining the path of the electrical current through the patient's body (as indicated by the sites of entrance and exit burns) and applying your knowledge of human anatomy can help you identify which internal structures may have been affected.

Once the initial threats to life have been mitigated, the history obtained, and the secondary assessment completed, the next step is to evaluate the severity of the burns by classifying them using either the degree-based or thickness-based methods. Next, calculate the total area of skin that has partial-thickness or full-thickness burns; superficial burns should be described and noted but are not included in this calculation. This calculation is accomplished using the Rule of Nines (Figure 19-12■). In this method, the surface of the body is divided into the following 11 sections, each of which represents approximately 9 percent of total body surface area (TBSA):

**⊕ 19-6** Describe how to assess burn severity using the "Rule of Nines" system.

- Head (front and back)
- Chest
- Abdomen
- Upper back
- Lower back
- Right arm
- Left arm
- Front of right leg
- Back of right leg
- Front of left leg
- Back of left leg

For children and infants, the percentages are the same with the exception of the head (18 percent) and the legs (14 percent). This difference is because compared to adults, the head of a child or an infant is proportionally larger, while the legs are proportionally shorter. The genital area, regardless of the person's age, represents 1 percent of TBSA.

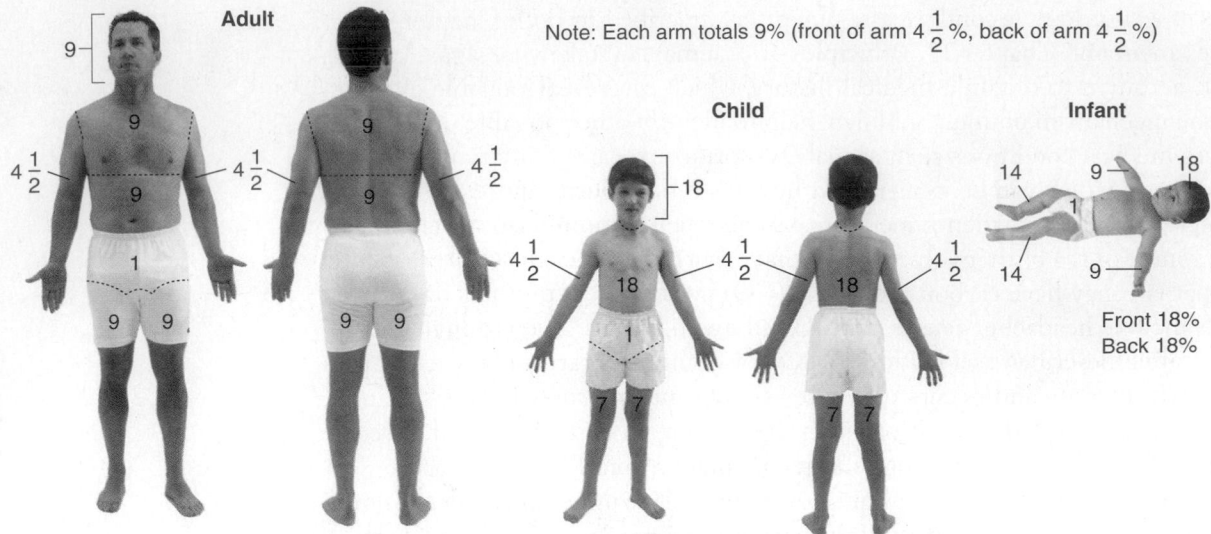

**Figure 19-12**  The Rule of Nines for estimating the proportion of the body surface affected by burns.

For burns that cover a large area, body sections can be combined. For instance, a burn involving the entire back covers 18 percent of TBSA, as does a burn involving all of the chest and abdomen. Similarly, a burn involving the entire right leg, front and back, covers 18 percent of TBSA.

Another simple way to estimate the total percentage of body area that is burned is the palm approach. This technique is especially useful for estimating the extent of relatively small burns. With this technique, the palm of the *patient's* hand represents approximately 1 percent of TBSA. The TBSA of the burns is thus estimated by the number of the patient's palms required to cover the burns.

The area of the body with partial-thickness and full-thickness burns (or second-degree and higher burns) is important in determining the care of a patient. The more severe the burns and the greater the amount of TBSA involved, the more difficult it is to manage the injuries, and the higher the mortality rates. Thus OEC Technicians must be able to quickly identify burn patients whose injuries are considered critical and require immediate treatment and rapid transportation (Figure 19-13■). According to the American Burn Association, patients who meet any of the following criteria are considered critical and should be taken to one of the nation's 125 designated burn centers:

+ Burns to a child under 10 years old or to an adult over 65 years old
+ Burns involving more than one body part (e.g., torso and leg)
+ Burns involving the head, neck, hands, feet, genitals, or major joints
+ Inhalation injury or burns
+ Burns associated with difficulty breathing or hoarseness
+ Chemical or electrical burns (including lightning injury)
+ Partial-thickness (second-degree) burn greater than 10 percent of TBSA
+ Any full-thickness (third- or fourth-degree) burn
+ Burns associated with trauma
+ Burns with a serious underlying medical disorder (e.g., diabetes, heart disease)
+ Burns in a patient who has special social, emotional, or physical needs
+ Exposure to radioactive materials

---

**NOTE**

### Potential Airway Injury

A hoarse voice can be a sign of injury to the airway, so always assess patients with hoarseness for potential respiratory compromise.

---

**NOTE**

### Pediatric Considerations

When treating pediatric burn patients, always consider the possibility that the injuries were not accidental. Given the high index of suspicion for child abuse, determine whether the injuries you observe are consistent with the circumstances of the incident as reported to you.

**CRITICAL BURNS**

- Burns to a child <10 years old or to an elderly person >65 years old

- Burns involving more than one body part (e.g., torso and leg)

- Burns involving the head, neck, hands, feet, genitals, or major joints

- Inhalation injury or burns

- Burns associated with difficulty breathing or hoarseness

- Chemical or electrical burns (including lightning injury)

- Partial-thickness (2nd degree) burn >10% TBSA

- Any full-thickness (3rd or 4th degree) burn

- Burns associated with trauma

- Burns with a serious underlying medical disorder (e.g., diabetes, heart disease)

- Burns in a patient who requires special social, emotional, or physical needs

- Exposure to radioactive materials

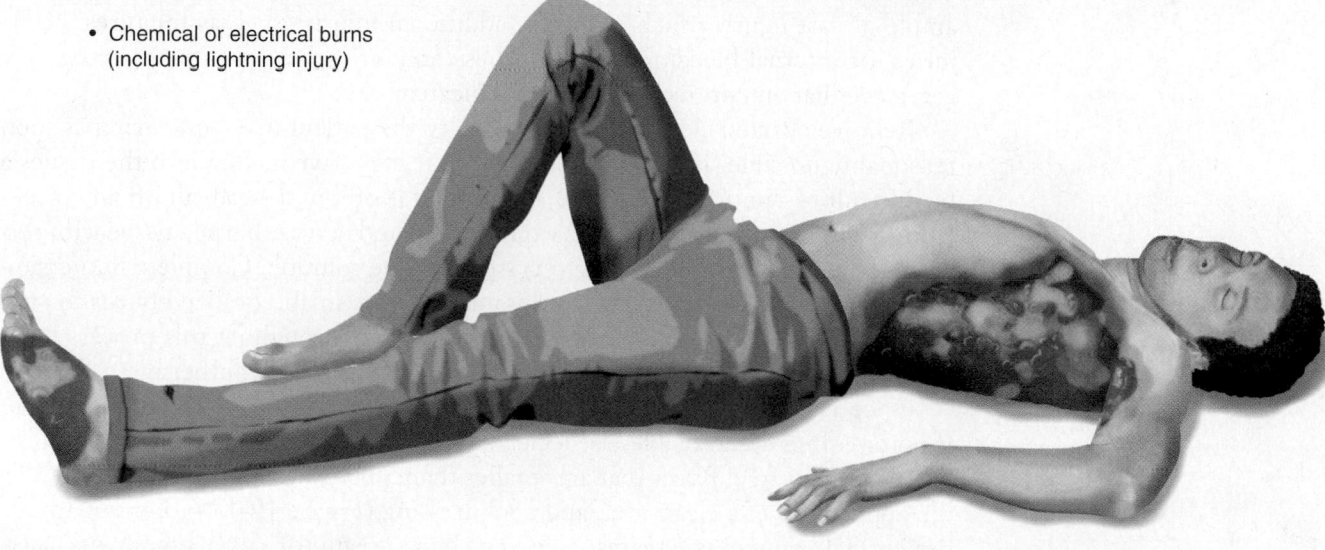

**Figure 19-13** The criteria for designating burns as critical.

# Management

⊕ 19-7 Describe and demonstrate the management of a burn patient.

Continue to ensure your safety and that of other rescuers, which take precedence over the treatment of patients. OEC Technicians should wear special chemical-resistant gloves that provide protection from strong acids or bases when touching patients whose skin is still contaminated with such chemicals. Do not go near a patient who is contaminated by radioactivity; instead, wait for specially clothed and equipped personnel to arrive. Do not allow sloppy hazard mitigation or decontamination practices to decrease a patient's chances of survival because rescuers have become injured.

The primary focus of initial burn care is to stop the burning process to prevent further injury (Figure 19-14■). Only after this is accomplished can the second goal begin: treating the patient's injuries. The first step is to separate the patient from the burn source. A patient on fire needs to be rolled on the ground or covered with a blanket or jacket to put out the fire. Obviously such actions are performed during the scene size-up and before any assessment is begun.

In general, treatment of burn patients, like that for any patients, starts with correcting any ABCD-related problems. Ensure that the airway is open and that the patient is breathing

**Figure 19-14** The first goal of initial burn care is to stop the burning process.

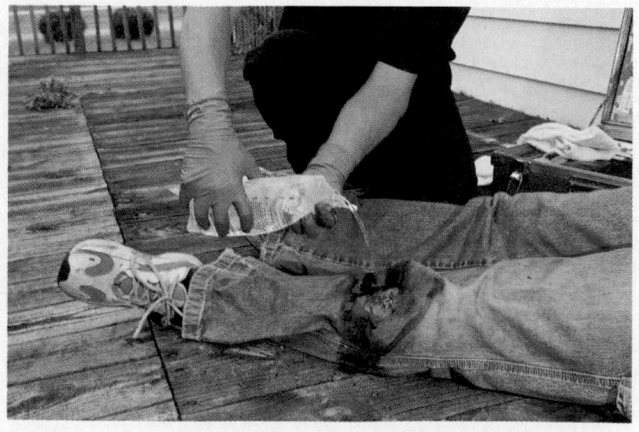

adequately. Burns that affect the chest wall, especially full-thickness burns and burns that encircle the trunk, can compromise chest wall expansion, leading to restricted breathing. In such cases, assist the patient's respirations, as needed, using appropriate airway adjuncts and supplemental oxygen. Apply high-flow oxygen at 15 LPM via a nonrebreather mask to patients who are able to breathe on their own. This will not only help reduce the likelihood of shock, but also may provide some measure of pain relief. Remember that oxygen is highly flammable, and its use near an open flame is extremely dangerous.

Electrical burns are associated with heart conduction problems, so initiate CPR if the patient is pulseless.

Control external bleeding using the techniques described in Chapter 18, Soft-Tissue Injuries. Patients with burns often have another mechanism of injury, for example a blast injury, which can cause additional injuries such as fractures, head injuries, or internal bleeding. Care for these and any other injuries as needed. Use a cervical collar and protect the spine if indicated.

Remove charred clothing and any jewelry the patient may be wearing as soon as reasonably possible. If clothing is synthetic, it may have melted into the tissues and be difficult to remove; in that case, do not pull it off but instead cut off any pieces of cloth that are not imbedded in the wound. Cool and irrigate burned tissue with room-temperature tap water or (better yet) sterile saline solution. Complete immersion of the burned body part in water is advisable only for small, localized burns for which the patient still has sensation. Monitor the patient throughout this process because cooling with water in outdoor environments can result in hypothermia.

Once a larger burn has been sufficiently cooled, cover it with dry, sterile dressings. If no dressings are available, use a clean, cotton-based article of clothing, preferably one that is lint free. Burns that are smaller than 5 percent of TBSA may benefit from the application of a clean, wet, and cool dressing (Figure 19-15■). Do not apply antimicrobial ointments, creams, aloe vera burn cream, or other emollients because their use complicates future hospital care.

**Figure 19-15** Emergency supplies needed to care for burns.

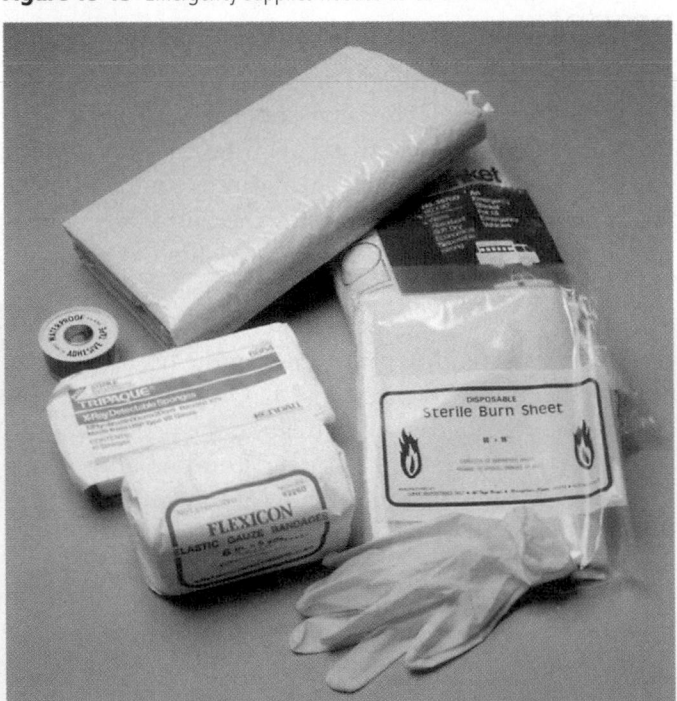

Keep patients warm by covering them with a clean sheet or blanket. Applying clean linens can also decrease pain severity by reducing air movement over burned tissue. Continuously monitor the patient and treat for shock, which can occur even with burns that are less than 5 percent of TBSA.

For significant upper body burns, elevate the patient's head and chest 20–30 degrees to minimize upper body edema. If the burn is accompanied by suspected spinal injury, secure the patient on a long spine board with full spinal immobilization and elevate the head end of the board. Be prepared to provide considerable emotional support to the patient.

Additional treatment for specific types of burns follows.

# Thermal Burns

The first priority, as previously indicated, is to extinguish any burning or smoldering clothing using the National Fire Protection Association's time-honored practice of "Stop, Drop, and Roll." With this technique, a person on fire is instructed not to run, but to drop to the ground immediately and then roll back and forth or be rolled by rescuers until the flames are extinguished. At the same time, rescuers can cover the patient with a coat or blanket to smother the flames if water or a $CO_2$ fire extinguisher is not immediately available. Do not use a chemical fire extinguisher. Do not swat at the flames with a blanket or jacket; doing so only fans the flames and makes them larger. Extinguish the flames and then remove any clothing that is burned, singed, or smoldering (Figure 19-16■).

If thermal burns are due to a hot liquid, remove all wet items of clothing (especially diapers) because they can hold the hot liquid against the skin, increasing the duration and thus the severity of the burns. Additionally, some fabrics, especially those used in outdoor athletic apparel, melt when sufficiently heated and may leave a hot adherent residue on the patient's skin. Do not attempt to pull this material from the skin because doing so may cause additional damage.

Do not break any blisters that are present because this action increases the risk of infection. Do not apply cold compresses because their use may precipitate hypothermia.

## Chemical Burns

For burns resulting from contact with a caustic substance, quickly remove all of the patient's clothing (including undergarments and socks) and jewelry—regardless of whether or not they appear contaminated—to ensure full removal of the chemical and to minimize tissue damage. In the process, use PPE to protect yourself, especially

> **Stop the Burn**
>
> - Stop the burning process.
> - Remove clothing and jewelry near the affected area.
>
> NOTE

**Figure 19-16** Extinguish any burning or smoldering clothes before removing them.

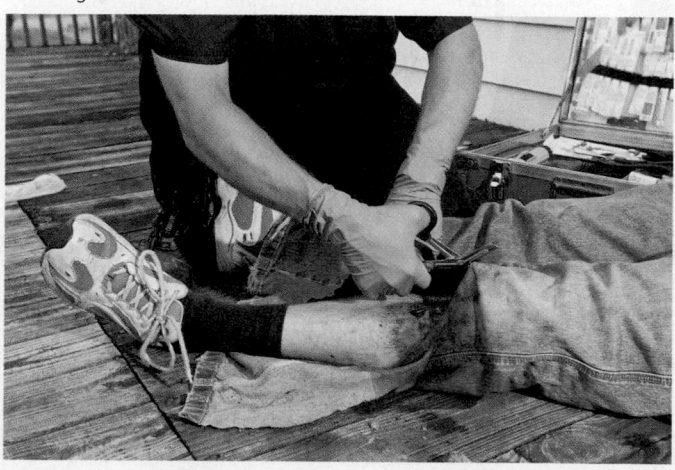

Chemical burn—flood area with water.

Dry lime—brush from skin and clothing.

**Figure 19-17** Some of the basics of the emergency care of chemical burns.

your hands, from the caustic substance. If large amounts of the chemical are present, consider mobilizing a HazMat team for achieving full decontamination.

Because some dry chemicals become even more caustic when activated by water, brush off any dry chemical residues that may remain on the patient (Figure 19-17■).

Immediately irrigate the chemically burned areas with large amounts of tepid water for at least 15 minutes, or until the burning sensation ceases. This includes the eyes, which should be bandaged after irrigation is complete (Figures 19-18a■ and 19-18b■). Because alkali burns penetrate more deeply than acid burns, they may require longer irrigation times to completely clear the chemical. During irrigation, avoid extending burns to uninjured areas by turning the patient so that the irrigating water flows away from unaffected skin. Avoid causing further tissue injury by not forcefully directing water onto the injury. Do not rub the injured tissue because doing so will likely result in massive tissue sloughing. (Figures 19-18a and 19-18b).

If you are in an outdoor environment in which tap water is not available, remember that your first objective in treating any burn is to stop the burning. Therefore, even though the chances of infection are increased if you rinse a patient's burns in water from a stream or pond, the burning must be stopped. Use the cleanest water available.

Once irrigation is complete, cover all burned areas in the manner previously described. If at any time you are unsure about the specific chemical you are dealing with or have treatment-related questions, you can obtain emergency information 24-hours a day by calling **Chemtrec**, the national emergency chemical information center, at **1-800-262-8200**.

## Electrical Burns

The first step in managing a patient with an electrical burn is to *make sure the power source is turned off.* This cannot be overstated; fatal injuries can occur if you or anyone else comes into contact with the electrical current or with a patient who is still in contact with the electrical current. If available, have specially trained personnel separate the patient from the power supply.

**Chemical Burn Alert**

N O T E

Caution! When managing chemical burns, do not apply a neutralizing agent because this may cause a thermal reaction, worsening the injury. Dust off any dry chemicals and irrigate the area with room-temperature water. Note as well that the application of water to some chemicals also produces heat.

**Figure 19-18a** Flush chemical substances from the eyes.

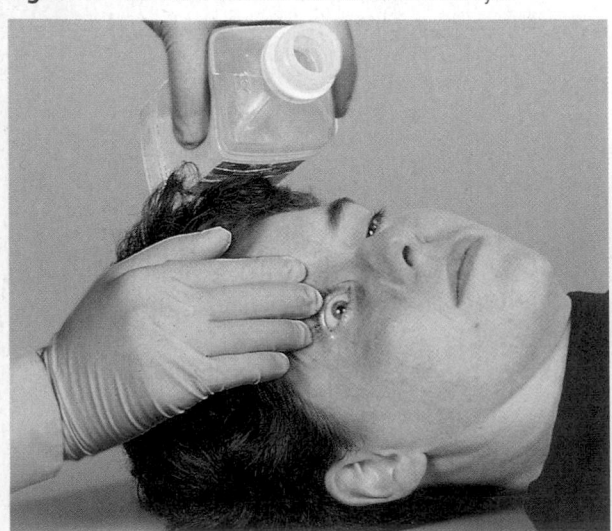

**Figure 19-18b** After flushing, apply sterile gauze pads to both eyes.

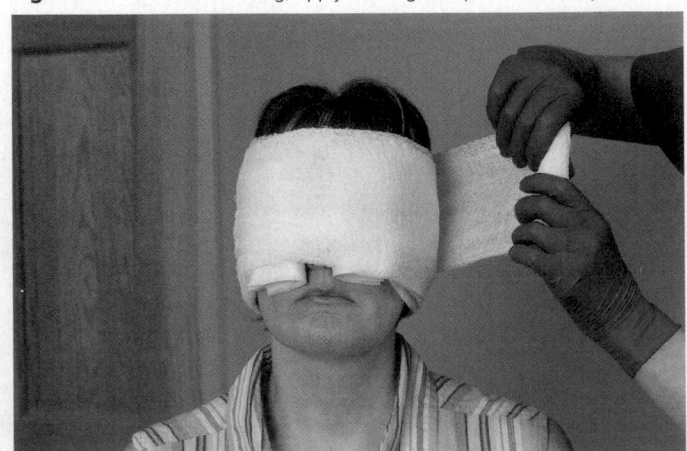

All patients who have been electrically shocked should be fully immobilized on a backboard. Move the patient to a safe area, protecting the spine by manually stabilizing the neck. Maintain the airway and give supplemental oxygen. Evaluate for shock and treat appropriately. Cardiac arrest resulting from electrical injury is fairly common. If the patient goes into cardiopulmonary arrest, treat in the usual manner by beginning CPR and attaching an AED, if available.

During the secondary assessment of a patient with electrical burns, look for the points of entry and exit, which can help you determine which underlying structures may have been affected by the current (Figure 19-19■). Whereas entrance wounds are often small, exit wounds are usually extensive and deep. Cover all wounds in the usual manner. (See OEC Skill 19-1■.)

## Radiation Burns

Radiation burns other than those resulting from exposure to UV light require specialized equipment and management techniques that are beyond the scope of this text. Patients can become contaminated by radioactive material with or without direct contact with the source. Patients who have been contaminated by radiation should be approached only by HazMat team members wearing special protective gear. If radiation injury resulted from an industrial accident or a terrorist attack, do not enter the area; instead, notify a team that specializes in such incidents. UV-related burns are typically treated in the same manner as first-degree burns.

# Further Care and Transport

Although most burns are minor, severe burns can develop numerous complications, including shock, sepsis, ARDS (acute respiratory distress syndrome), and cardiac arrest. Patients that have all but the most minor burns must be transported to a definitive-care facility, preferably a designated burn center, because of the likelihood of extensive tissue damage, underlying injuries, and the need for long-term care. If a burn center is not available, transport the patient to the nearest trauma center.

If possible, summon advanced care providers to transport the patient, because they are able to administer pain medications and other advanced therapies that can make the patient significantly more comfortable and lessen the incidence of shock.

Transport burn patients on a clean, dry sheet to prevent the person from sticking to the backboard, toboggan, litter, or stretcher. Provide the transporting crew or hospital staff a complete oral hand-off report that includes the source of the burn, any pertinent history, clinical findings and treatment administered, and the patient's responses to the treatment.

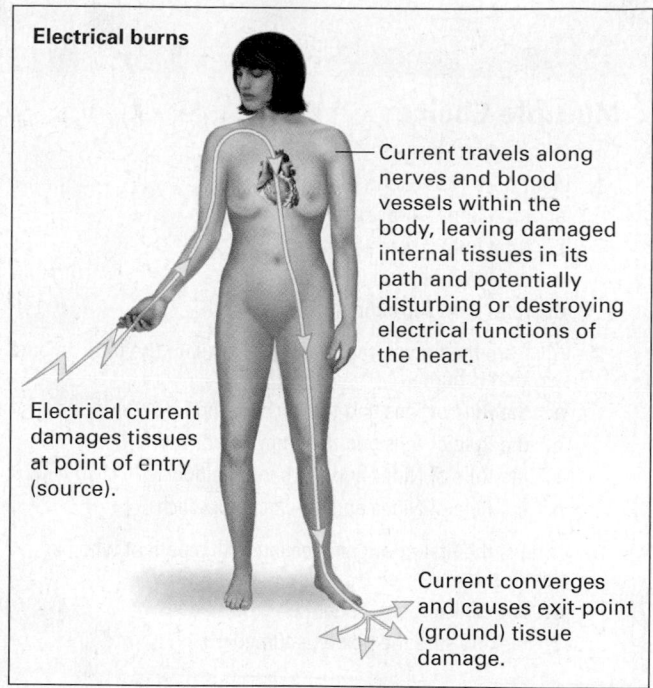

**Electrical burns**

Current travels along nerves and blood vessels within the body, leaving damaged internal tissues in its path and potentially disturbing or destroying electrical functions of the heart.

Electrical current damages tissues at point of entry (source).

Current converges and causes exit-point (ground) tissue damage.

**Figure 19-19** Look for entry and exit burns when electricity is the cause of the injury.

## Entrance and Exit Wounds

Remember that patients injured by electricity often appear to be much better off than they actually are because many of their burns are beneath the surface. Take vital signs frequently and be prepared for extensive resuscitation (CPR and AED).

NOTE

## Extensive Burns

Remember that with extensive burns, patients lose the ability to thermoregulate. Make sure they do not become hypothermic by wrapping them in warm, dry sheets.

NOTE

# STOP, THINK, UNDERSTAND

## Multiple Choice

Choose the correct answer.

1. What does TBSA stand for?_____
   a. total body surface area
   b. total burn surface area
   c. total body surrounding area
   d. total burn surrounding area

2. What are the two methods used to calculate the total amount of skin that is burned?_____
   a. the Rule of Tens and the hand method
   b. the Rule of Tens and the palm approach
   c. the Rule of Nines and the hand method
   d. the Rule of Nines and the palm approach

3. What is the first priority in dealing with a patient who has electrical burns?_____
   a. immobilizing the patient on a backboard.
   b. making sure the power is turned off.
   c. applying high-flow oxygen via a nonrebreather mask.
   d. removing the patient's clothing.

4. Which of the following actions for managing significant burns is correct?_____
   a. elevate the patient's head 20–30 degrees to minimize upper body edema.
   b. elevate the patient's feet 12 inches to minimize upper body edema.
   c. keep the patient flat to minimize upper body edema.
   d. elevate the patient's feet 12 inches to treat for shock.

5. For which two things should you treat burn patients?_____
   a. shock and hypoglycemia
   b. shock and hyperglycemia
   c. shock and hyperthermia
   d. shock and hypothermia

## Short Answer

1. List four signs and symptoms associated with an inhalation injury. _____, _____, _____, and _____

2. What takes precedent over the treatment of any patient?

   _____

   _____

 CASE DISPOSITION

After examining the child, you determine that his injuries consist of first- and second-degree burns due to thermal scalding. Using the palm approach, you calculate that the patient's burns cover 4 percent of TBSA and that he has no airway involvement. With assistance from the mother and other patrollers, you gently irrigate the burns with room-temperature sterile saline and then lightly cover the second-degree burns with sterile gauze. You summon an ambulance, which transports the patient and his mother to a local hospital for further treatment.

# OEC SKILL 19-1 | Caring for Burns

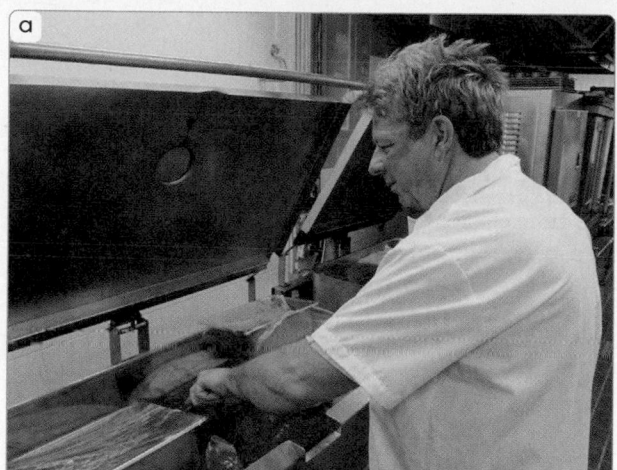

Burns can happen unexpectedly.
Copyright Edward McNamara

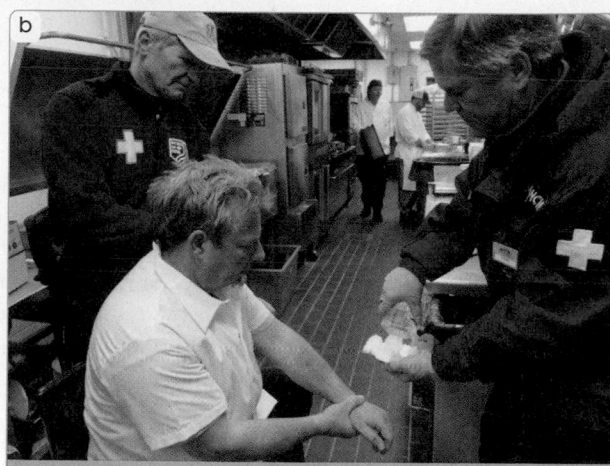

Remove any affected clothing, stop the burning process, and cool the burn.
Copyright Edward McNamara

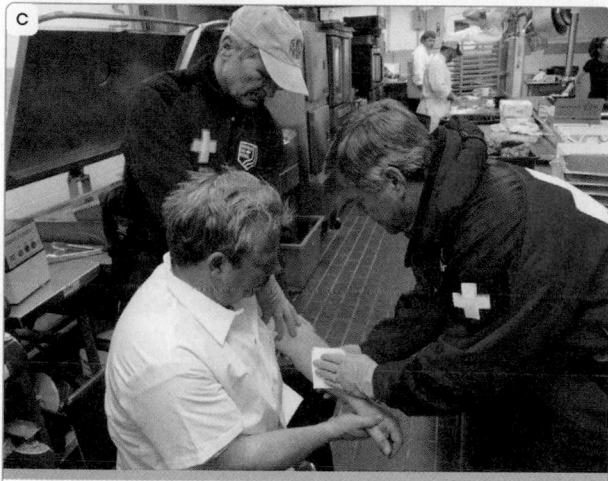

Apply a sterile gauze dressing to the wound. Wet the dressing only if the wound is less than 5 percent of TBSA.
Copyright Edward McNamara

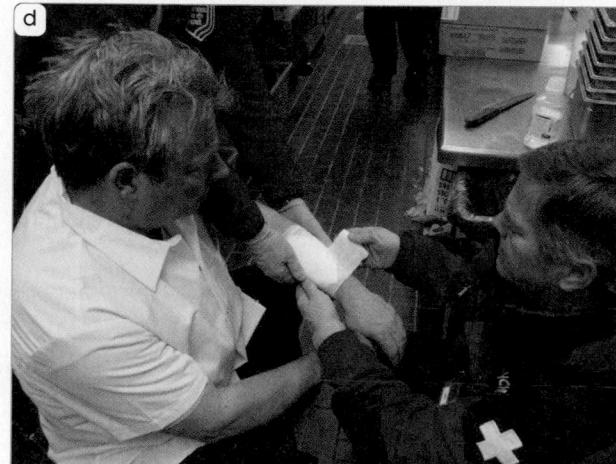

Bandage the wound to keep the dressing securely in place. Then prepare to assist the patient to find further medical treatment.
Copyright Edward McNamara

# Chapter Review

## Chapter Summary

The skin is a remarkable organ that performs several key functions in preserving homeostasis. Although resilient and durable, the skin is easily damaged when exposed to flames, hot liquids, hot surfaces, caustic substances, electricity, or radiation. Once the skin's protective barrier is breached, the body becomes vulnerable to a host of problems that include hypothermia, massive fluid loss, and infection. Unchecked, these problems can lead to organ or system failure, shock, and even death.

Burn-related trauma causes potentially devastating injuries that affect the lives of hundreds of thousands of people each year. Burns can cause intense pain and may result in massive tissue loss and disfiguring injury. Even with prompt treatment, the effects of a moderate-to-serious burn can be life altering.

Because burns can occur any time and in any place and are among the more challenging emergencies that OEC Technicians may face, patrollers must be mentally and physically prepared to address the unique needs of this patient population.

By understanding the basic anatomy and physiology of the skin, and by learning to accurately assess the cause and severity of a burn, OEC Technicians can implement an appropriate burn-specific course of treatment. By acting quickly and arranging rapid transportation to an appropriate emergency care facility, OEC Technicians may be able to decrease the potentially devastating effects and reduce the mortality of burn-related injuries.

## Remember...

1. Rescuer and bystander safety is the top priority when treating a burn patient.
2. The four types of burns are thermal burns, chemical burns, electrical burns, and radiation burns.
3. The focus of treatment is stopping the burning process.
4. Brush off dry or powdered chemicals first.
5. Irrigate chemical burns with water for a minimum of 15 minutes.
6. Inhalation injuries are often associated with facial burns and vocal hoarseness.
7. Burns are classified by the depth of the injury.
8. Use the Rule of Nines to calculate the extent of burns.
9. Do not delay transport of patients with significant burns.
10. Treat burn patients for shock and hypothermia.
11. Transport burn patients to a burn center or trauma center, whenever possible.

## Chapter Questions

### Multiple Choice

Choose the correct answer.

1. What is the largest organ of the human body?_____
   a. heart
   b. brain
   c. spleen
   d. skin

2. Which of the following burns is the most painful?_____
   a. a superficial burn
   b. a partial-thickness burn
   c. a full-thickness burn
   d. a third-degree burn

3. Which of the following types of burn follows the path of least resistance?_____
   a. thermal burns
   b. chemical burns
   c. electrical burns
   d. radiation burns

**4.** Which of the following burns produces a charred leathery appearance of the skin?_____

   **a.** a first-degree burn

   **b.** a superficial burn

   **c.** a partial-thickness burn

   **d.** a full-thickness burn

**5.** What is your first treatment priority for a patient with second- and third-degree burns over 30 percent of the body?_____

   **a.** Cool and irrigate the burned tissue with room-temperature tap water.

   **b.** Remove burned clothing.

   **c.** Secure the patient's airway.

   **d.** Administer high-flow oxygen at 15 LPM via a nonrebreather mask.

## Short Answer

List six burn criteria that are considered critical and would send a patient to the burn center.

_____

_____

_____

_____

_____

_____

## Labeling

On the following figure, label the percentage of body surface area assigned to each of the following anatomical sections: head, chest, abdomen, upper back, lower back, right arm, left arm, front of right leg, back of right leg, front of left leg, and back of left leg.

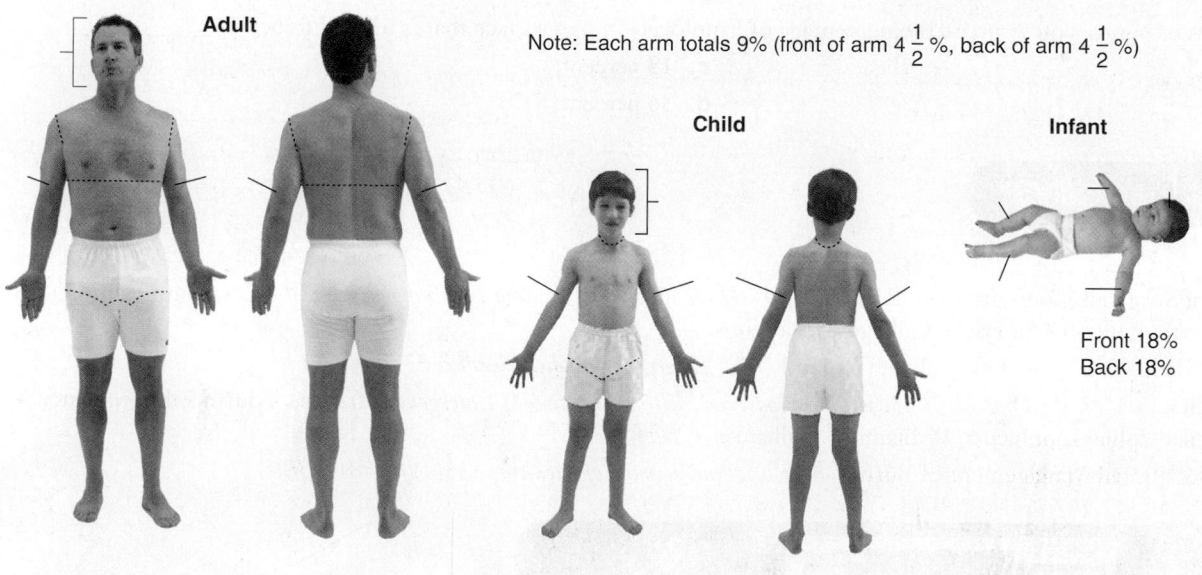

**Adult**

Note: Each arm totals 9% (front of arm 4 $\frac{1}{2}$ %, back of arm 4 $\frac{1}{2}$ %)

**Child**

**Infant**

Front 18%
Back 18%

# Scenario

*While two employees were making emergency repairs to the low-pressure steam boiler in the power house, a valve is accidently snapped off and a plastic line severed. You get the call and upon arrival find the two injured employees outside the building. The two report that the emergency shutoff was activated after the incident, and that the boiler is now shut down. With the scene secured, you start to evaluate the two injured employees.*

1. Which of the following is *not* a source of burns?_____
   - **a.** thermal heat
   - **b.** chemicals
   - **c.** electricity
   - **d.** high-frequency radio signals

*Employee 1 had an unknown liquid sprayed on his face. Employee 2 received steam burns to his arms. Both employees are responsive and alert to person, place, and time. Neither demonstrates difficulty breathing, has a medical history, or takes any prescription drugs.*

*Another employee appears and retrieves the MSDS (Material Safety Data Sheet) sheet for the liquid in the plastic line that was severed. The MSDS indicates that the liquid has a pH of 7.*

2. This liquid material should be considered to be_____
   - **a.** alkaline.
   - **b.** acidic.
   - **c.** neutral.
   - **d.** a hydrochloric solution.

*You call for additional patrollers, $O_2$, and the burn treatment kit, and for an ambulance for both employees. Your helpers start to flush the eyes of employee 1 to remove any debris that could have been in the plastic line. Employee 2 has second-degree burns to the underside of his forearms only.*

3. Second-degree burns are characterized by_____
   - **a.** dry skin.
   - **b.** reddened skin.
   - **c.** blisters.
   - **d.** both b and c

4. To inflict a thermal burn, the temperature of the burn source must be greater than_____
   - **a.** 115°F.
   - **b.** 115°C.
   - **c.** 25°C.
   - **d.** 100°F.

5. Using the Rules of Nines, you estimate the percentage of Employee 2's skin surface that is burned to be_____
   - **a.** 4.5 percent.
   - **b.** 9 percent.
   - **c.** 18 percent.
   - **d.** 36 percent.

# Suggested Reading

American College of Surgeons Committee on Trauma. 2004. *ATLS: Advanced Trauma Life Support for Doctors*, Seventh Edition (Student Course Manual). Chicago: American College of Surgeons.

DeBoer, S., C. Felty, and M. Seaver. 2004. "Burn Care in EMS." *Emergency Medical Services* 33(2): 69–76.

Haro, L. H., S. Miller, and W. W. Decker. 2005. In *Harwood-Nuss' Clinical Practice of Emergency Medicine*, Fourth Edition, edited by A. B.Wolfson. Philadelphia: Lippincott, Williams & Williams.

Monafo, W.W. 1996. "Initial Management of Burns." *New England Journal of Medicine* 335(21): 1581–1586.

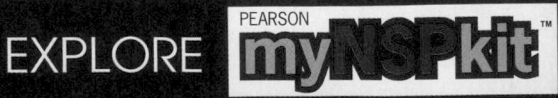

EXPLORE PEARSON **myNSPkit**™

# Musculoskeletal Injuries

David Johe, MD

## SECTION 1
## Anatomy and Physiology

### + OBJECTIVES

**Upon completion of this section of this chapter, the OEC Technician will be able to:**

**20-1.1** Describe the functions of the following structures:

a. bones
b. cartilage
c. joints
d. muscles
e. synovium
f. tendons

**20-1.2** Describe the physiology of human movement.

**20-1.3** Describe how musculoskeletal tissues heal.

**20-1.4** List the six types of musculoskeletal injuries.

**20-1.5** Compare and contrast sprain and strain.

**20-1.6** Describe two classifications of fractures.

**20-1.7** List the signs and symptoms of sprains and fractures.

**20-1.8** Define the following terms:

a. dislocation
b. fracture
c. sprains

## Chapter Overview

This chapter has three sections. Section 1 includes general information about the musculoskeletal (MS) system, including anatomy, physiology, and common injuries. It is important to understand these concepts before proceeding to Section 2, which explains how to assess the MS system, both in a general way and then for each specific part of the arm or leg. Section 3 details how OEC Technicians care for MS injuries. This section includes important skill guides that need to be practiced using a "hands on" approach.

*continued*

## HISTORICAL TIMELINE

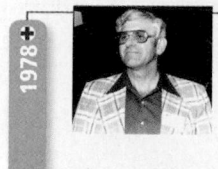

**1978** Donald Williams becomes National Director.

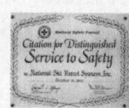

**1979** NSP awarded National Safety Council Distinguished Service to Safety Award.

## ⊕ KEY TERMS

abduction, *p. 607*
acromioclavicular (A/C) joint, *p. 623*
adduction, *p. 607*
angulation, *p. 625*
appendicular skeleton, *p. 604*
articular cartilage, *p. 604*
articulation, *p. 633*
axial, *p. 604*
axial skeleton, *p. 604*
bone crepitus, *p. 621*
callus, *p. 610*
cardiac muscle, *p. 608*
cartilage, *p. 602*
cortex, *p. 604*
dislocation, *p. 602*
dorsal, *p. 628*

dorsiflex, *p. 630*
fracture, *p. 610*
immobilization, *p. 610*
"jams and pretzels," *p. 673*
joint, *p. 602*
joint capsule, *p. 606*
ligament, *p. 602*
meniscus, *p. 633*
musculoskeletal system (MS), *p. 602*
palmar, *p. 613*
periosteum, *p. 604*
plantarflex, *p. 630*
popliteal fossa, *p. 633*
skeletal muscle, *p. 608*
sling and swathe, *p. 640*

smooth muscle, *p. 608*
splint, *p. 602*
sprain, *p. 602*
stabilized extrication, *p. 674*
strain, *p. 602*
subluxation, *p. 616*
synovium, *p. 606*
tendon, *p. 602*
tension, *p. 610*
traction, *p. 644*
traction splint, *p. 644*
valgus, *p. 632*
varus, *p. 632*
volar, *p. 656*
zone of injury, *p. 612*

**musculosketetal system (MS)** the combination of the bony skeleton, the voluntary muscles, and other supporting structures that gives the body form and enables movement.

**joint** a site at which two or more bones meet.

**cartilage** a tough, elastic, fibrous connective tissue found in various parts of the body, including the joints, outer ear, and end of the nose.

**ligament** tissue that connects a bone to another bone; connective tissue that provides structure for a joint.

**tendon** the non-contractile continuation of a muscle that gives it a mechanical advantage.

**strain** a stretched or torn muscle or tendon.

**sprain** a stretched or torn ligament.

**dislocation** a separation or displacement of the bones of a joint.

**splint** a mechanical device used to prevent a part of the body from moving, protecting it from further injury.

The human body includes a complex collection of integrated systems. The body's **musculoskeletal system (MS)** allows the body to perform organized movement and to stand and walk upright. The system's primary components are the voluntary muscles and the bony skeleton, but the system also includes **joints**, the **cartilage** on the ends of bones at joints, fluid that lubricates the joints, **ligaments**, **tendons**, and the interface between the nervous system and the muscles. The MS system enables us to use our legs for walking and our arms for performing tasks. Without the MS system, we would be a mass of tissue without structure or form.

The bones and muscles also protect vital organs within the body's cavities. This protection can occur directly, as when the vertebrae of the spinal column protect the spinal cord, or indirectly, as when one holds up a forearm to prevent an object from striking the body.

This chapter provides a review of the anatomy of the various components of the MS system. It is important that you know the names of the major bones, muscles, and joints, as well as how ligaments, tendons, and joints work. The chapter also discusses the physiology of movement, and how the MS system repairs itself. Common musculoskeletal injuries, including **strains**, **sprains**, **dislocations**, ruptures of tendons, and fractures are discussed with respect to both assessment and management, as are **splints** and other adjuncts used in treatment. And because OEC Technicians may need to perform emergent maneuvers to correct neurologic and vascular injuries to the extremities, these procedures are discussed as well.

OEC Technicians will see a variety of musculoskeletal injuries, so it is important that they understand the presentation and care of each, as described in the last part of this chapter. Whereas the many details presented can deepen the knowledge of seasoned OEC Technicians, new OEC Technicians should strive to understand and apply the principles relevant to the care of MS injuries.

## Anatomy and Physiology

The various components of the skeleton are crucial to the makeup and function of the MS system. OEC Technicians need to have a good understanding of the parts of the MS

**CASE PRESENTATION**

On a great day for spring skiing, a call comes over the radio for someone to respond to Moonshadow for a possible leg injury. Getting off the top of the lift, you cut across and find a helmeted teenager on twin-tipped skis, just below a jump, sprawled out on the snow. He is complaining that his right thigh hurts "very bad." You notice that his right forearm is positioned at an unnatural angle. His buddies standing nearby say that he landed "hard."

***What should you do?***

system, including the names of major bones, muscles, and joints. For a more in depth review of these elements, refer to Chapter 6, Anatomy and Physiology.

## The Skeleton

The skeleton functions as a rigid framework to protect the internal organs, provides the body form we recognize as human, and produces blood cells. The skeleton consists of bones, connective tissue, and cartilage (Figure 20-1■).

**⊕ 20-1.1** Describe the functions of the following structures:

a. bones
b. cartilage
c. joints
d. muscles
e. synovium
f. tendons

**Figure 20-1** The human skeleton.

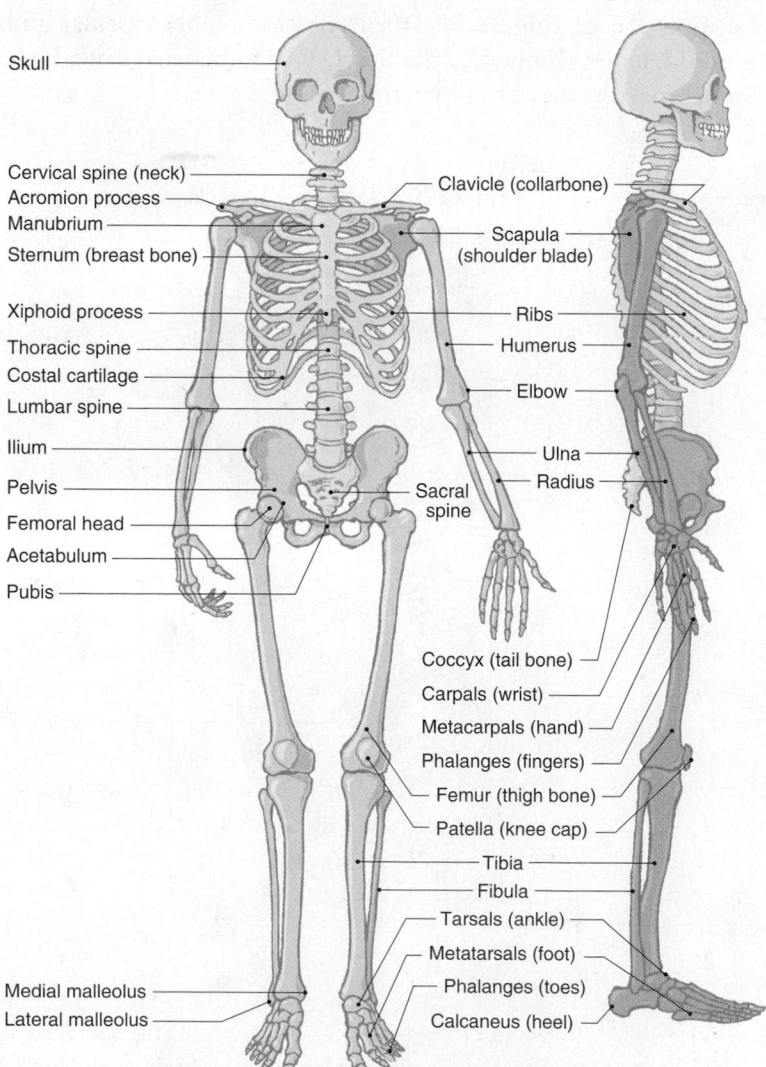

**axial skeleton** the central core of the bony skeleton, consisting of the skull, spine, and supporting thoracic bones.

**appendicular skeleton** the periphery of the skeleton; the bones of the arms and legs.

**axial** pertaining to the axis of a body part.

**articular cartilage** the cartilage that is affixed to the end of a bone within a joint.

**periosteum** the thin outer covering of a bone.

**cortex** the hard outer layer of a bone.

The skeleton is divided into two major parts, the **axial skeleton** and the **appendicular skeleton**. The **axial** skeleton has 80 bones and consists of the skull, vertebrae, and thoracic cage (Figure 20-2a■). It transfers weight from the head, trunk, and upper extremities to the lower extremities at the pelvis. These bones are responsible for the upright position of the human body. The appendicular skeleton has 126 bones and consists of the bones of the shoulders, arms, pelvis, and legs (Figure 20-2b■). These bones are responsible for manipulating objects (the shoulder and the upper extremities) and for locomotion (the pelvis and the lower extremities).

The body contains three major types of bones based on shape: long bones, flat bones, and irregular bones (Figure 20-3■). Long bones include the humerus, radius, and ulna of the two upper extremities, and the femur, tibia, and fibula of the two lower extremities. Flat bones protect internal organs and include the skull, the scapula of the upper extremities, the ribs, the sternum, and the pelvic bones. Irregular bones have multiple functions and include the vertebrae, and the bones of the wrists, hands, ankles, and feet.

Long bones consist of two parts: the epiphysis or bone ends, and the diaphysis or shaft (Figure 20-4■). Bone ends are covered with **articular cartilage**, which provides a nearly friction-free surface that allows bone ends to move smoothly against one another. Children's bones grow longer near the ends, along the epiphyseal line. Fractures at this line, especially during early childhood, can affect bone growth and development.

The outer part of a bone is a tough lining known as **periosteum**. Beneath the periosteum is the hard **cortex**. Within the cortex is the bone marrow, a less-dense region where blood cells are made (Figure 20-5■). Bones are highly vascular and receive 10–20 percent of the blood pumped by the heart. When the cortex of a bone breaks, the highly vascular marrow may bleed severely.

**Figure 20-2** (a) The appendicular skeleton. (b) The axial skeleton.

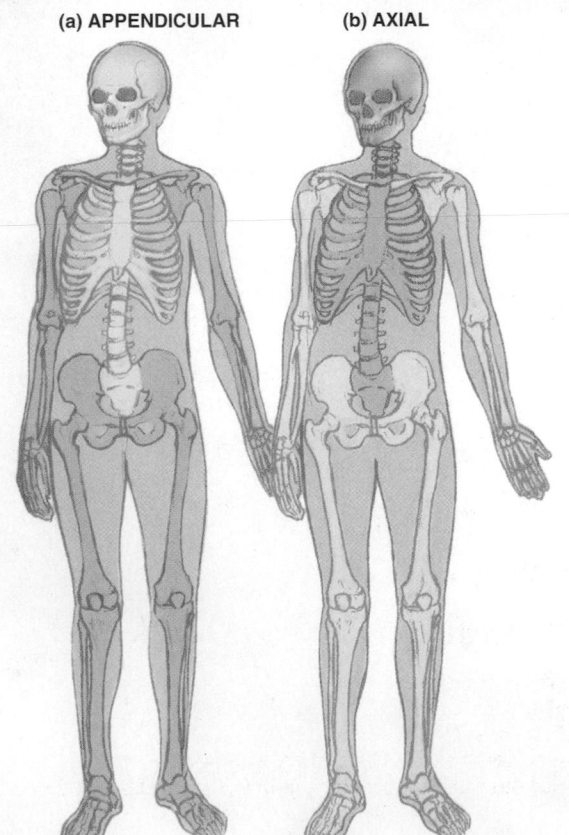

**(a) APPENDICULAR**     **(b) AXIAL**

**Figure 20-3** Three major types of bones according to shape.

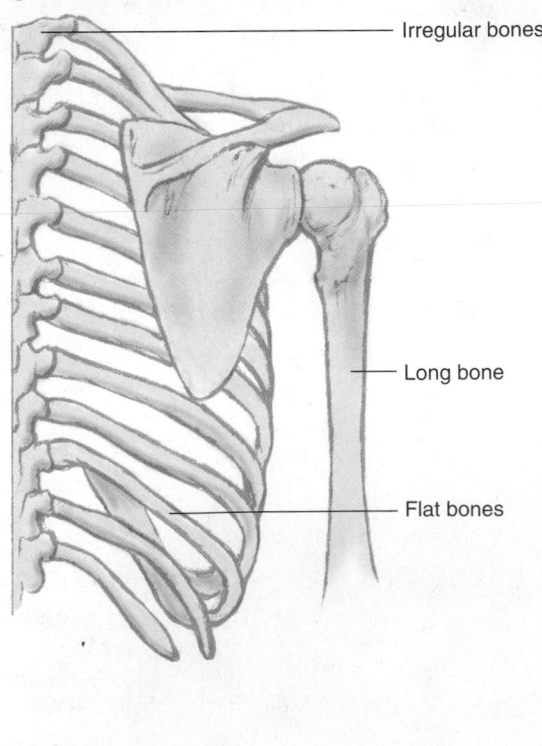

Irregular bones

Long bone

Flat bones

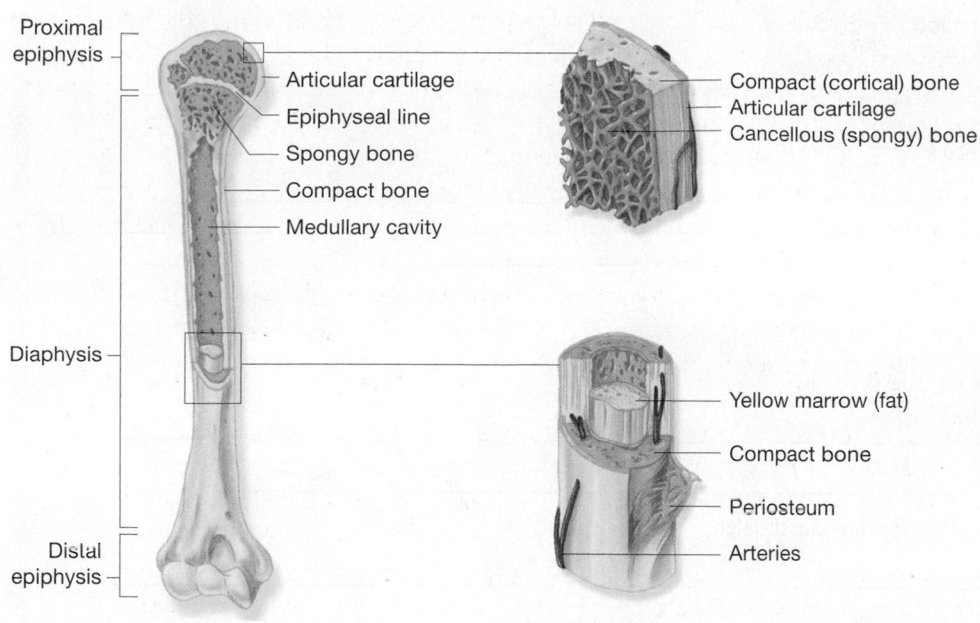

**Figure 20-4** The components of a long bone.

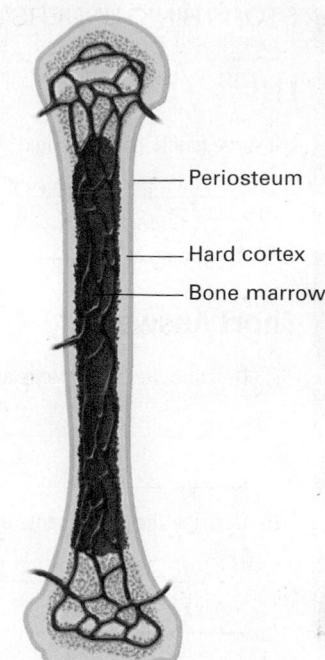

**Figure 20-5** The internal anatomy of a long bone.

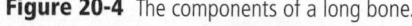

# STOP, THINK, UNDERSTAND

## Multiple Choice

Choose the correct answer.

1. The purpose of the articular cartilage is to_____
   a. provide structure.
   b. provide stability.
   c. increase red blood cell production by one-third.
   d. allow smooth movement between bones within a joint.

2. The function of the epiphyseal line in children is_____
   a. bone growth.          c. white blood cell production.
   b. skeletal stability.   d. bone flexibility.

3. Bones receive what percent of all blood pumped by the heart?_____
   a. 5–10 percent
   b. 10–20 percent
   c. 20–30 percent
   d. Bones do not receive blood because they make blood cells.

## Matching

1. Match each of the three parts of a bone to its description.

   _____ 1. cortex
   _____ 2. marrow
   _____ 3. periosteum

   a. hard layer located just beneath the bone's surface
   b. tough, outer lining of bone
   c. less-dense part of bone; site of blood cell production

2. Match each of the shapes of bones to its description.

   _____ 1. long bones
   _____ 2. flat bones
   _____ 3. irregular bones

   a. examples are the humerus, radius, ulna, tibia, and fibula
   b. bones that protect the internal organs (include the skull, ribs, scapula, and sternum)
   c. multi-function bones that include the vertebrae and the bones of the wrist, hand, ankle, and foot

*continued*

## STOP, THINK, UNDERSTAND *continued*

### List

List three functions of the rigid skeletal framework.

1. _____
2. _____
3. _____

### Short Answer

1. Describe the components and actions of the axial skeleton.

   _____

   _____

2. Describe the components and functions of the appendicular skeleton.

   _____

   _____

### Fill in the Blank

1. The end of a bone is called the_____; the shaft is called the _____.
2. The skeleton is divided into two major parts: the _____ and the _____.

## Joints

**joint capsule** a sheet of fibrous connective tissue enclosing a synovial joint.

**synovium** the inner layer of the joint capsule whose cells make a viscous fluid that lubricates joints.

The site at which two or more bones make contact is known as a joint. Joints enable the body to bend, straighten, and produce all body movements. A joint consists of two or more bones and the connective tissues that surround, stabilize, and support the joint, called the **joint capsule**. This capsule contains a slippery lubricant known as synovial fluid made by the **synovium**. This fluid, along with the bones' articular surfaces, allows the bones to move freely within the joint capsule. The names of some joints come from the bones that form them. For example, the radiohumeral joint at the elbow is where the radius and the humerus meet. Other joints have unique names, such as the knee or the hip.

Joints provide different degrees of movement. Many joints, such as the knee, hip, elbow, and shoulder joints, are essentially *freely movable* (Figure 20-6■). A few joints, such

**Figure 20-6** Types of movable joints.

Slightly movable

Freely movable

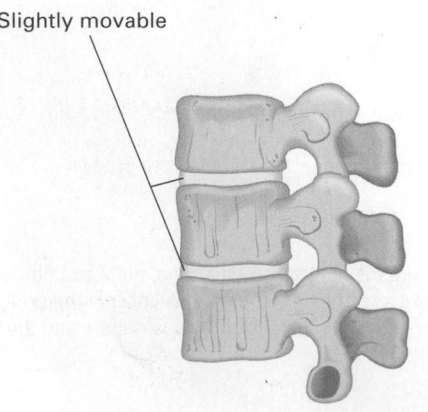
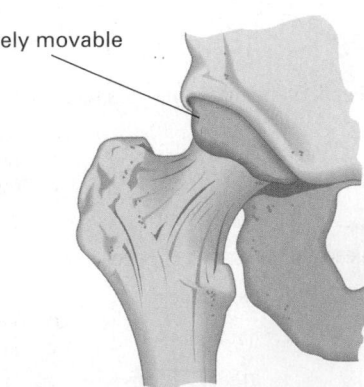

as those between vertebrae, are *slightly movable*. Other joints permit *minimal movement* because thickened fibrous ligaments firmly stabilize the bone ends. The acromioclavicular joint of the shoulder is one example. Some joints are present during childhood but later fuse to form a solid, immoveable, bony structure (e.g., joints of the skull).

OEC Technicians should be familiar with five structural types of joints:

+ *Ball and socket joints* allow movement in multiple planes, including flexion, extension, **abduction**, and **adduction**. The shoulder and hip are examples.
+ *Hinge joints* allow movement in one plane only: flexion and extension. The elbow, knee, and finger joints are examples.
+ *Gliding joints* permit bones to slide or glide over one another. The wrist and ankle are examples.
+ *Pivot joints* allow one bone to rotate on another. The joint at the base of the thumb and the radioulnar joint of the elbow are examples.
+ *Suture joints* (sometimes called fixed joints) permit little to no motion. Examples include the sacroiliac and symphysis-pubic joints in the pelvis, and the joints in the skull that closed after infancy (Figure 20-7■).

**abduction**   to move away from the midline of the body.

**adduction**   to move toward the midline of the body.

## Ligaments

Ligaments are thick bands of tissue that connect two bones together. Composed of strong connective tissue, ligaments resist stretching, thereby restricting joint movement to the range of normal motion. By holding one bone to another bone, ligaments provide structure and stabilize the skeleton (Figure 20-8■).

In the knee, ligaments located on each side connect the femur to the tibia medially, and the femur to the tibia and fibula laterally. This forms a stable hinge joint allowing

**Figure 20-7** An example of a suture joint.

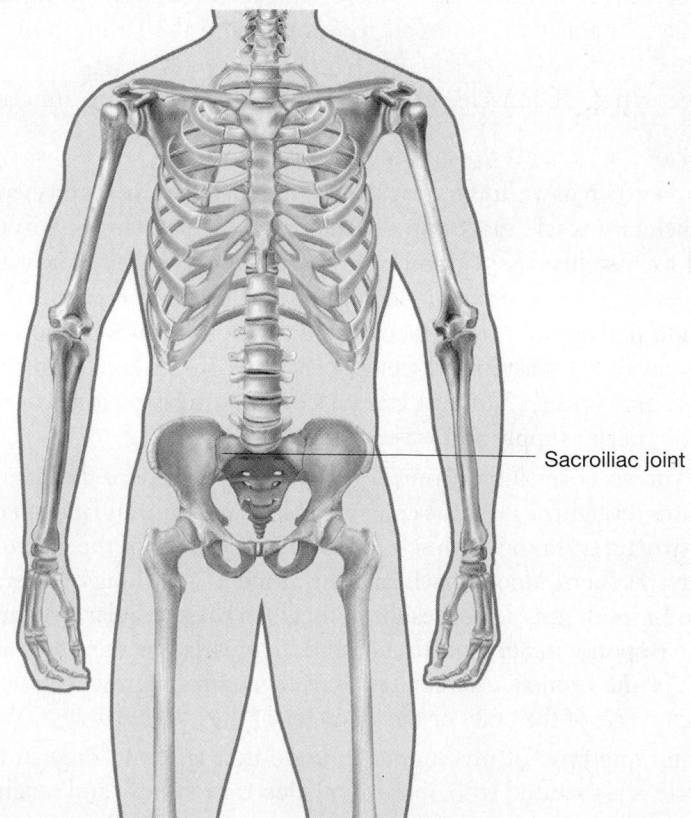

**Figure 20-8** The anatomy of the knee. Ligaments connect bone to bone and are an essential part of the skeletal system.

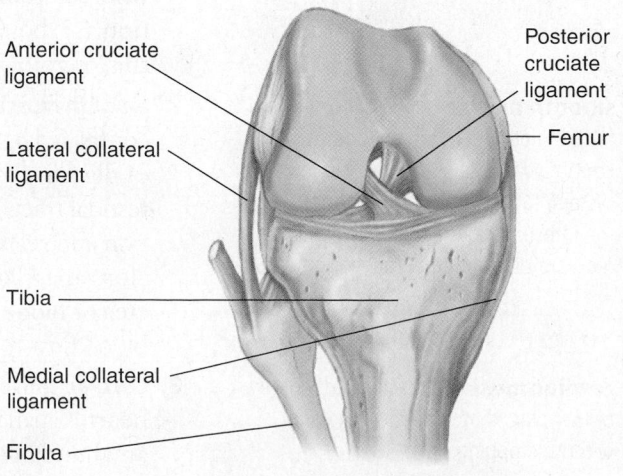

Sacroiliac joint

Anterior cruciate ligament

Posterior cruciate ligament

Femur

Lateral collateral ligament

Tibia

Medial collateral ligament

Fibula

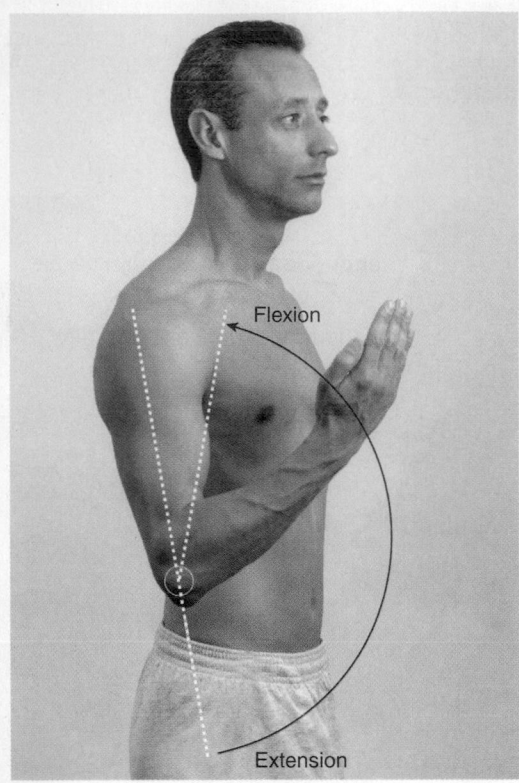

**Figure 20-9** Flexion and extension are the two main movements of the elbow.

motion only in the anterior/posterior plane. Conversely, the shoulder joint, with only a few restrictive ligaments, is able to move in almost any direction.

The extent to which a joint can move is determined by the degree of tightness or laxity of the ligaments and capsule that hold the bone ends together, and by the orientation of the bone ends to each other. Therefore, although the amount and type of motion differs from joint to joint, all joints restrict motion to some degree. When a joint is pushed beyond this limit, damage occurs. The supporting ligaments can overstretch or tear, or the capsule can tear open. Regardless, the joint becomes unstable, which can limit function.

## Muscle

Muscle is a unique type of tissue that, when stimulated, has the ability to contract. Muscle tissue shortens when two proteins, actin and myosin, "ratchet" on each other during the active phase of contraction. After a muscle has contracted, it passively returns to its original length during the relaxation phase. The combination of contraction and relaxation enables the body to move the extremities, walk, and perform normal daily activities. Muscles respond to chemical and electrical signals that travel from the brain and through the spinal cord and peripheral nerves to initiate the movement of a specific body part. If the signal from the nerve cannot reach the muscle because of disease or injury, the muscle can no longer contract, and muscle function is reduced or lost.

Most of the more than 600 muscles in the muscular system are divided into complementary pairings. For instance, the biceps and triceps are paired muscles: contraction of the biceps muscles enables us to flex the elbow, whereas contraction of the triceps muscles enables us to extend the elbow (Figure 20-9■). These complementary pairings are essential for effective movement and for the manipulation of objects. Damage to either muscle in a pairing will impair movement and the strength of the affected extremity or area.

The body has three types of muscle, each of which has a unique function (Figure 20-10■).

**skeletal muscle**   type of muscle that attaches to the bony skeleton and is controlled voluntarily by the nervous system; functions to move joints to perform physical activities.

1. **Skeletal muscle** (also known as voluntary muscle) is under direct voluntary control of the brain. Skeletal muscle makes up the major visible muscle mass in the body and is named for its close association with the skeleton. As with most tissues, skeletal muscles have a generous blood supply, and they are controlled by nerves. Arterial blood delivers oxygen, glucose, and other nutrients to muscles, whereas veins carry away the waste products associated with muscular contraction (carbon dioxide and water). Muscles cannot continue to function without this ongoing cycle of energy supply and waste removal.

**smooth muscle**   type of muscle found in organs of the body; is controlled by the autonomic nervous system; functions to push food through the intestine, contract blood vessels, and regulate other internal functions.

2. **Smooth muscle** (also known as involuntary muscle) performs most actions that are not controlled by conscious thought, such as the control of blood pressure and movement of digestive system structures. Smooth muscle is found in the walls of the gastrointestinal tract, the urinary system, blood vessels, and the bronchi of the lungs. Contraction and relaxation of smooth muscle pushes the contents of these tubular structures along their course. In response to nervous stimuli, smooth muscle can alter the diameter of blood vessels or the bronchi, thereby respectively controlling the volume of blood flow to different parts of the body or the diameter of the lower airways.

**cardiac muscle**   specialized muscle of the heart that contracts regularly without stopping.

3. **Cardiac muscle** is a unique type of involuntary muscle that is found only in the heart. Cardiac muscle is associated with an internal electrical system and receives an abundant blood supply.

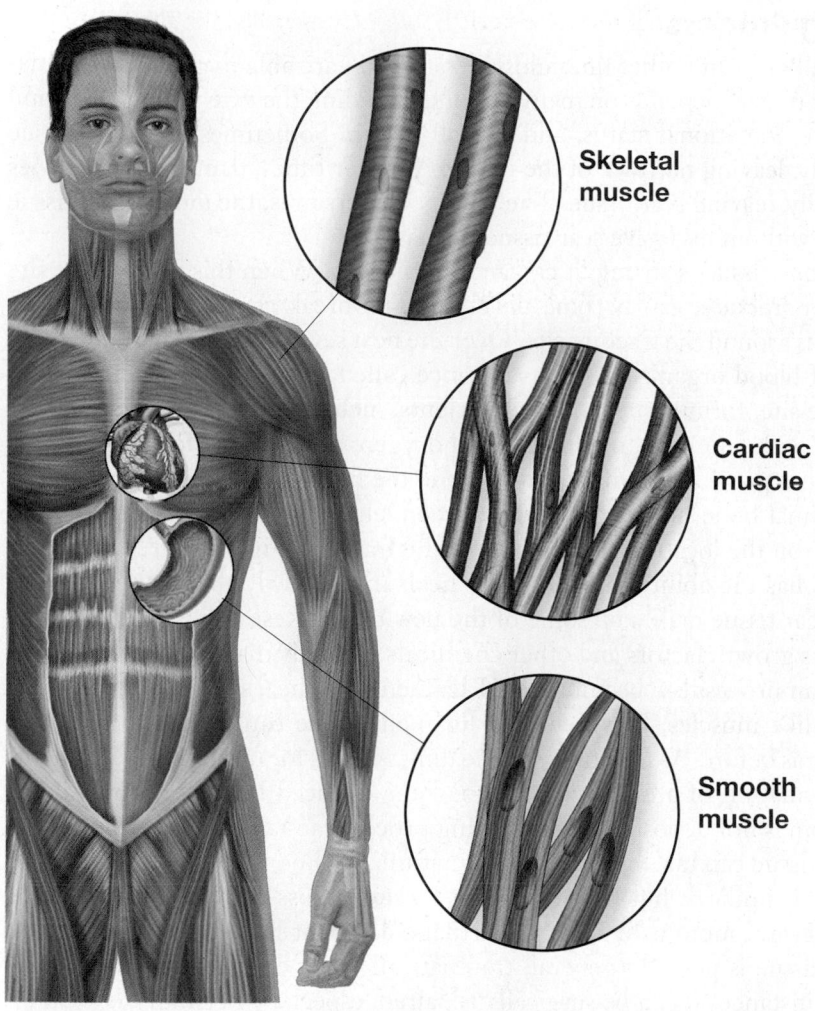

**Figure 20-10** The three types of muscle.

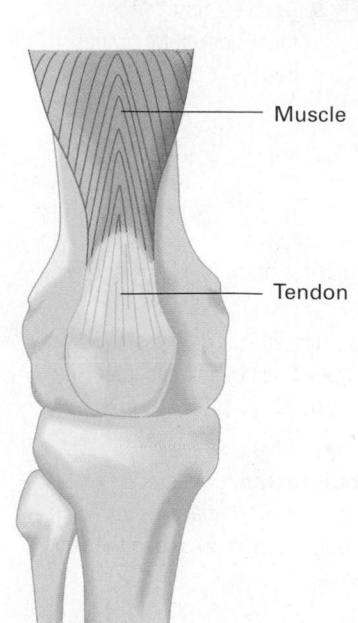

**Figure 20-11** Tendons attach muscles to bone.

Smooth muscle and cardiac muscle are structurally distinct from skeletal muscle and are not part of the MS system; they are presented here to highlight their differences from skeletal muscle.

## Tendons

Tendons are the straplike continuations of a muscle that connect a muscle to a bone. This tissue is very strong and transmits the force of a contracting muscle to the bone. Like ligaments, tendons can be damaged through overstretching and tearing. When a tendon is damaged, the effectiveness of a muscle is significantly reduced (Figure 20-11■).

## The Physiology of Movement

Body movement is a coordinated process in which skeletal muscles receive a signal from the brain to contract. This signal may produce voluntary movement, such as when you lift an object, or it may produce involuntary movement, such as when you quickly pull your hand away from an open flame. The contraction of muscles causes flexion or extension of a joint; the bones to which the muscles are attached act as levers. As these muscles relax, opposing muscles contract, moving the joint in the opposite direction. When repeated, this process results in sustained body movement, such as walking.

> **The Difference Between a Ligament and a Tendon**
>
> Ligament: a tissue that connects one bone to another.
> Tendon: a tissue that connects a muscle to a bone.

**NOTE**

**20-1.2** Describe the physiology of human movement.

**⊕ 20-1.3** Describe how musculoskeletal tissues heal.

**fracture**    a break in a bone's cortex.

**callus**    material at a fracture site that forms from a hematoma and later becomes bone.

**immobilization**    the process of holding an object in place, as for a fracture by a cast or internal orthopedic hardware.

**tension**    the amount of force necessary to stretch something; when used to refer to aligning a fractured long bone, the force required to straighten out the affected limb (usually 7–8 pounds).

## The Healing Process

Once damaged, bones and other musculoskeletal tissues are able to generate new tissue. The ability to heal depends on many factors, including the extent of damage and the person's age, nutritional status, and overall health. Sometimes damaged tissue heals completely, leaving no trace of the injury. At other times, damaged tissue does not heal normally, leaving scar tissue. The younger a person is, the more likely tissue will regenerate without excessive scar tissue formation.

Although bone tissue is strong, it can and does break. When this occurs, the site of the break, or **fracture**, can become unstable. The break causes bleeding, and a hematoma forms around the fracture site. Over the next several weeks, this hematoma or collection of blood organizes into a substance called **callus**. Later, calcium is deposited into the site, forming new bone. Nutrients, including proteins, calcium, and vitamins, along with energy from glucose, and oxygen, are essential for proper bone healing. Oxygen is provided from arteries close to the fracture site. Also important to promoting optimal bone healing is **immobilization**, either by surgical hardware or a cast, depending on the location and severity of the fracture (Figure 20-12■).

Muscle also has the ability to heal, but it heals more slowly than bone. In most cases, fibrous scar tissue makes up some of the new tissue. Researchers are currently studying various growth factors and other chemicals the body makes following injury to see if the repair process can be improved. Ligaments also heal slowly and with some scar tissue. Unlike muscles, however, new ligament tissue can make the structure nearly as strong as before. As for bones, the healing process for muscles and ligaments involves the formation of a hematoma that is later replaced by new fibrous tissue; however, calcium is not deposited. This healing process can take six weeks or longer. New ligament tissue can take up to a year to mature.

Tendons heal similarly, but because of the **tension** across them, they need to be protected for several months or longer. Cartilage does not heal, because the blood supply to this tissue is poor. In general, traumatically torn cartilage is removed, although in rare instances it can be surgically repaired, especially in children.

### Smoking and Healing

NOTE

Cigarette smoking drastically slows healing in soft tissues and bone. In a person who smokes even one cigarette a day, a fractured bone may take much longer to heal.

**Figure 20-12** An X-ray of a lower leg showing surgical hardware and a surrounding cast.
Copyright Nancy Pitstick

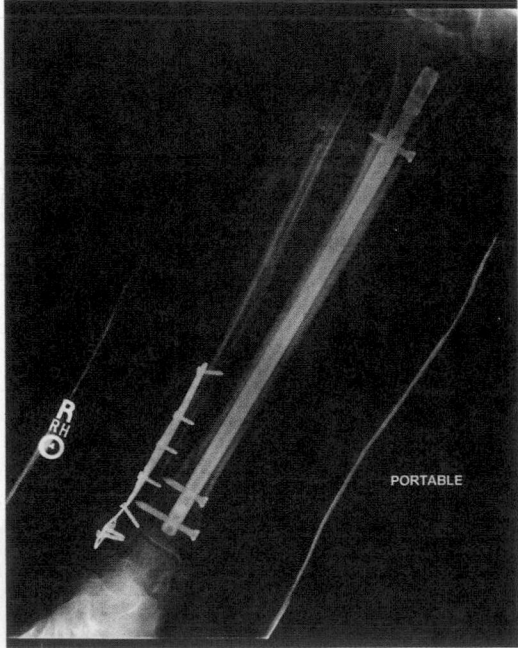

# STOP, THINK, UNDERSTAND

## Multiple Choice
Choose the correct answer.

1. Which of the following statements about joints are true? (check all that apply)

    _____ a.  A joint is a location where a long bone bends.

    _____ b.  A joint is a location where two or more bones make contact with each other.

    _____ c.  Joints contain a slippery lubricant known as articulum.

    _____ d.  Different joints provide different degrees of movement.

    _____ e.  Joints allow the body to bend, straighten, and move.

    _____ f.  A joint capsule lubricates the joint.

2. An example of a freely movable joint is_____

    a.  the hip.
    b.  the vertebrae.
    c.  an acromioclavicular joint.
    d.  a suture.

3. Ligaments connect_____

    a.  bone to bone.
    b.  bone to muscle.
    c.  bone to tendon.
    d.  tendon to joint.

4. The extent to which a joint can move is determined by_____

    a.  the strength of the muscles that support it.
    b.  the amount of synovium it contains.
    c.  the directional angle of the bone end relative to the articular cartilage.
    d.  the degree of tightness or laxity of the ligaments, and the orientation of the bone ends to each other.

5. Which of the following statements about skeletal muscle tissue are true? (check all that apply)

    _____ a.  Muscle tissue has the ability to contract.

    _____ b.  Muscle tissue lengthens when actin and myosin ratchet on each other.

    _____ c.  Muscle tissue passively returns to its original length during the relaxation phase.

    _____ d.  Muscle tissue is controlled by the nervous system.

    _____ e.  Even if signals from the central nervous system are interrupted, muscles can still contract due to muscle memory.

6. Muscle pairing is best defined as_____

    a.  comparing the size and shape of the muscles on one side of the body to the other.

    b.  the combination of a muscle and a tendon that work together to move a joint.

    c.  two muscles that work together to extend or flex a joint by contracting at different times.

    d.  a muscle that is directly connected to two bones.

7. Tendons connect _____

    a.  bone to bone.
    b.  muscle to bone.
    c.  ligament to joint.
    d.  muscle to muscle.

8. Which of the following statements about the healing process is true?_____

    a.  Children are more likely than adults to develop scar tissue.
    b.  Tissue heals faster in adults than in children.
    c.  The younger one is, the more likely damaged tissue will regenerate with minimal scarring.
    d.  Wounds in elderly patients do not heal.

9. Which of the following sequences correctly lists the events in bone healing?_____

    a.  callus formation, bone, hematoma, calcium deposition
    b.  hematoma, calcium deposition, callus formation, bone
    c.  hematoma, callus formation, calcium deposition, bone
    d.  calcium deposition, callus formation, hematoma, bone

10. Which of the following statements regarding bone and ligament healing is false?_____

    a.  To heal, a bone requires nutrients, proteins, calcium, vitamins, and energy from glucose.
    b.  Oxygen is a vital component of bone growth and is provided by nearby arteries.
    c.  Immobilization is necessary for optimal bone healing.
    d.  Bone growth and healing are slower than muscle growth and healing.

11. Which of the following statements about muscle and ligament repair is true?_____

    a.  Healed ligaments can be as strong as they were before the injury.
    b.  Muscle heals more quickly than bone.
    c.  A hematoma interferes with ligament or muscle healing.
    d.  The healing process usually takes 2–3 weeks.

12. Which of the following statements about cartilage and tendon healing is true?_____

    a.  Tendons heal faster than either bones or muscles.
    b.  Tendons can take months to heal.
    c.  Cartilage heals well.
    d.  Cartilage heals faster than either bone or muscle.

## Matching

1. Match each of the following types of joints with its description.

    _____ 1.  ball and socket joint
    _____ 2.  fixed joint
    _____ 3.  gliding joint
    _____ 4.  hinge joint
    _____ 5.  pivot joint

    a.  allows little or no motion; examples are the sacroiliac and symphysis pubis and sutures in infants' skulls
    b.  allows movement in multiple planes such as flexion, extension, abduction, and adduction; an example is the shoulder
    c.  allows movement in one plane only (flexion and extension); examples are a finger, the elbow, or the knee
    d.  the wrist and ankle have this type of joint
    e.  located at the thumb or the radial ulnar joint, this type allows one bone to rotate on another

*continued*

STOP, THINK, UNDERSTAND *continued*

2. Match each of the following terms with its description. Terms may be used more than once.

_____ 1. muscle

_____ 2. tendon

_____ 3. smooth muscle

_____ 4. skeletal muscle

_____ 5. cardiac muscle

_____ 6. ligament

a. a ropelike continuation of a muscle that connects a muscle to a bone
b. an involuntary muscle that is associated with an internal electrical system and an abundant blood supply
c. this type of muscle is technically not part of the musculoskeletal system
d. also known as "involuntary" muscle; controls functions such as blood pressure and digestion, and alters the diameter of blood vessels
e. connects bone to bone
f. is under voluntary control

---

⊕ **20-1.7** List the signs and symptoms of sprains and fractures.

⊕ **20-1.8** Define the following terms:
  a. dislocation
  b. fracture
  c. sprain

⊕ **20-1.4** List the six types of musculoskeletal injuries.

**zone of injury** the area that is close to or surrounding an injury of an extremity, such as a sprain or fracture.

⊕ **20-1.5** Compare and contrast sprain and strain.

# Common Musculoskeletal Injuries

OEC Technicians may encounter the following types of MS injuries:

+ strains
+ sprains
+ ruptured tendons

+ fractures
+ dislocations
+ multiple simultaneous MS injuries

In nearly all cases, bone and joint injuries are accompanied by injury of or damage to the surrounding soft tissues, nerves, and blood vessels. This area, known as the **zone of injury**, can be large or small depending on the amount of kinetic energy that caused the trauma (Figure 20-13■).

## Sprains

A sprain is an injury involving the stretching or tearing of a ligament. This type of injury occurs when a joint is displaced beyond its normal range of motion. Sprains typically affect the ligaments on one side of a joint and may occur with other MS injuries. Mild ligament sprains heal relatively quickly, usually in several weeks, whereas completely torn ligaments often need surgical repair. In outdoor sports, sprains most often involve the shoulder, wrist, knee, or ankle, but a sprain can affect any joint.

## Strains

A strain is a stretched or torn muscle. Commonly referred to as a "pulled muscle," a strain is often caused by overexertion and poor body mechanics. Strains affect mus-

**Figure 20-13** Two zones of injury. One is at femur fracture site, and the other is at the tibial fracture site.

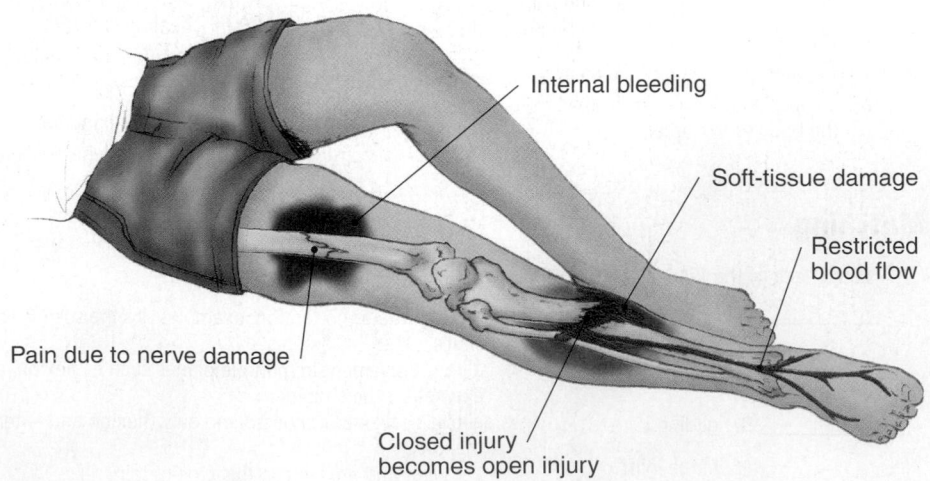

Internal bleeding

Soft-tissue damage

Restricted blood flow

Pain due to nerve damage

Closed injury becomes open injury

cle tissue only and do not result in bone, ligament, or joint damage. A strain can be mild, requiring only a few days to heal, or it can be severe, requiring surgical repair and months of healing. Muscles that are commonly strained include the hamstring muscles, the biceps, and the muscles of the back.

## Ruptured Tendons

Sudden and forceful contraction of a muscle can damage either the muscle tissue or a tendon. This injury results in a reduction or a complete loss in the movement of the associated joint upon muscle contraction. Poor body mechanics can increase the likelihood of tendon rupture. Diseased or fatigued tendons are also prone to rupture. Common tendons that rupture are the Achilles tendon in the ankle, the biceps tendon at the shoulder or elbow, and the flexor tendons in the fingers (on the **palmar** side of the hand). Other tendons that rupture less frequently include the quadriceps tendon above the patella (knee cap) and a tendon that is part of the rotator cuff in the shoulder.

## Fractures

A fracture is a break in a bone. Although most fractures are caused by trauma, they may also result from bone disease. A fracture may occur anywhere along a bone and can affect any bone. OEC Technicians must be familiar with a variety of types of fractures; the most common categories are closed fractures and open fractures.

A closed fracture is one in which the overlying skin surface has not been disrupted (Figure 20-14a■). An open fracture is one in which the overlying skin has been opened. Also known as a compound fracture, this injury occurs when either an external force penetrates the skin and fractures the underlying bone, or when the sharp ends of a broken bone penetrate the surface of the skin (Figure 20-14b■). Open fractures are a true emergency because the opening in the skin allows contaminants to enter the body. Bacteria entering the wound may cause infection of the bone and local tissues. In severe cases, infection can later spread to other parts of the body.

Fractures may be further classified according to whether or not the broken bone remains in normal anatomical alignment. In a *nondisplaced* fracture, the ends of a fractured bone remain in alignment. An extremity with a nondisplaced fracture might appear normal except for swelling at the fracture site. Nondisplaced fractures are often difficult to detect, even for experienced physicians, so X-rays are required to identify many of these injuries. A *displaced* fracture causes the affected extremity to appear bent, crooked, short, or rotated (Figure 20-15■). This abnormal appearance is caused by the ends of a fractured bone being anatomically misaligned.

Fractures are often categorized by whether or not the injured bone is broken all the way across. In a *complete fracture*, the bone surfaces are completely separated (Figure 20-16a■). In an *incomplete fracture* (sometimes called a hairline or torus fracture),

---

**Strain versus Sprain**

You *strain* a muscle or tendon and *sprain* a ligament.

NOTE

**palmar** on the palm side of the hand.

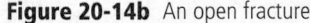

**20-1.6** Describe two classifications of fractures.

---

**Figure 20-14a** A closed fracture.

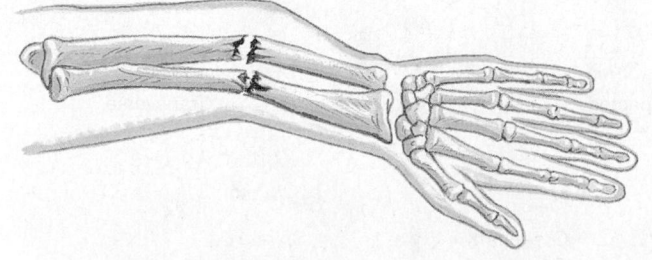

**Figure 20-14b** An open fracture.

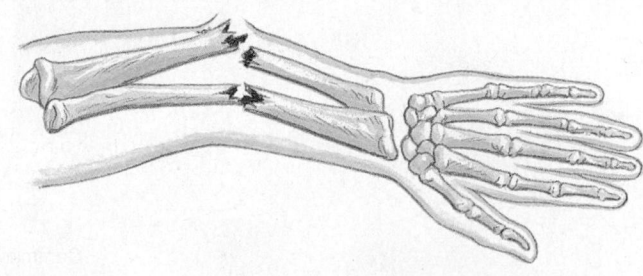

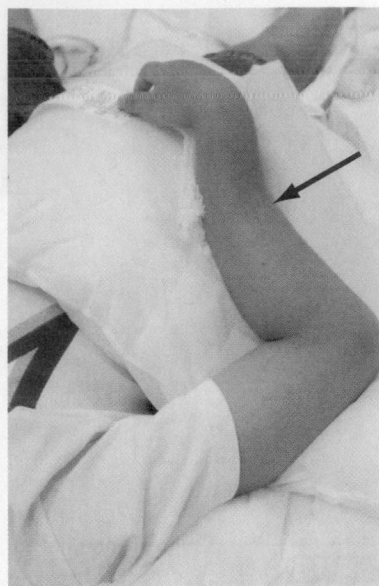

**Figure 20-15** A displaced fracture of the forearm.
Copyright E. M. Singletary, M.D.

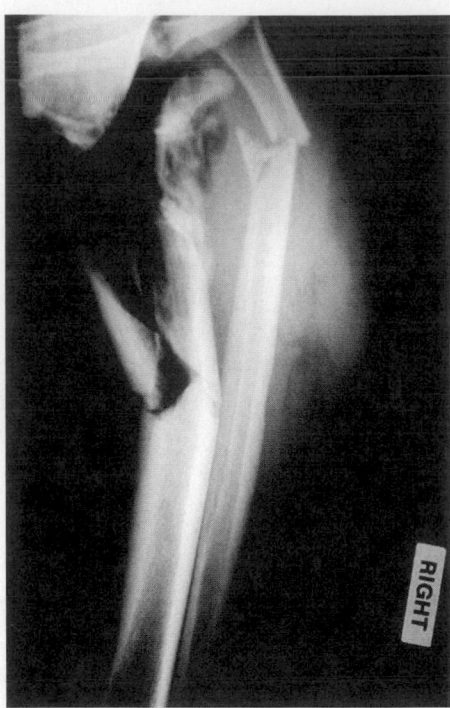

**Figure 20-16a** A complete fracture.
Copyright Charles Stewart, M.D.

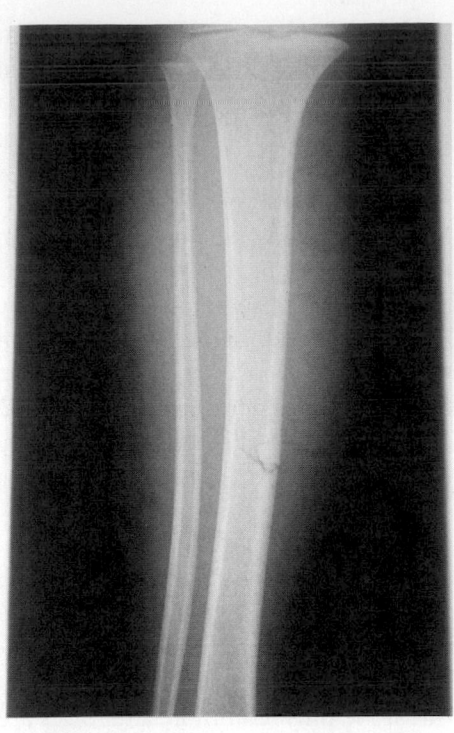

**Figure 20-16b** An incomplete fracture of the tibia.
Copyright Charles Stewart, M.D.

the fracture line does not completely penetrate the entire bone, leaving one side of the bone intact (Figure 20-16b■). Incomplete fractures are nondisplaced. X-ray studies are generally needed to determine whether a fracture is complete or incomplete.

Some fractures are named according to either the specific mechanism of injury or the shape of the fracture line (Figures 20-17■). Table 20-1■ also lists and describes some types of fractures.

**Figure 20-17** Types of fractures.

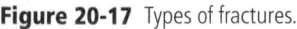

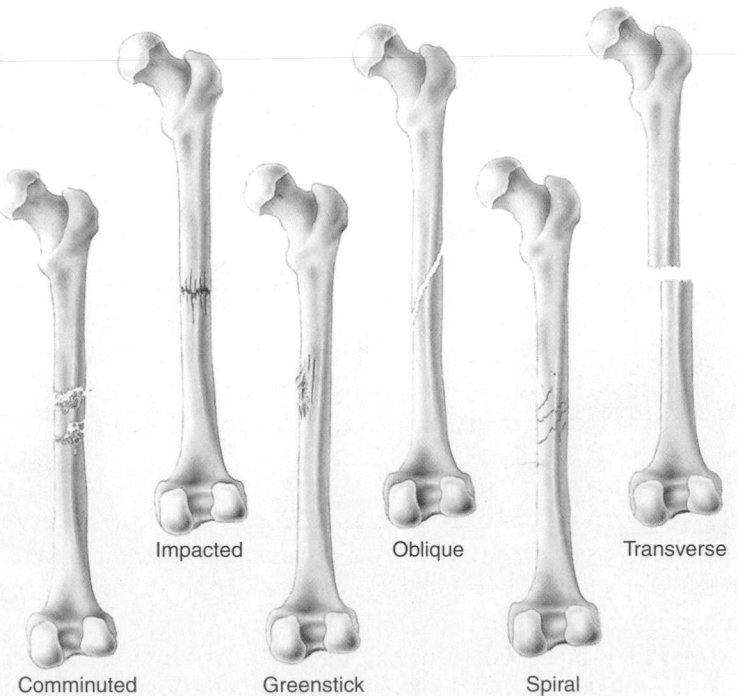

Comminuted

Impacted

Greenstick

Oblique

Spiral

Transverse

**Table 20-1**   Types of Fractures

| Fracture Type | Description |
|---|---|
| Butterfly fragment | A fracture that occurs upon direct trauma to a long bone, in which a third piece of broken bone that looks like a butterfly's wing is on the side opposite the trauma; seen in fractures of the tibia and humerus. |
| Comminuted | A fracture that has three or more fragments; may be seen in any long bone. |
| Compression | A fracture in which a bone becomes shortened into itself; results when an axial load is put on the bone; occurs in the vertebrae. |
| Epiphyseal | A fracture of the bone's growth plate, near the end of the bone; occurs in children who are still growing. |
| Greenstick | An incomplete fracture in which the bone "bends" like a stick from a young tree branch; most commonly occurs in children. |
| Impacted | A fracture in which one of the bone ends is embedded into each other. |
| Oblique | A fracture that runs through the bone at an angle. |
| Pathologic | A fracture in an area of diseased or damaged bone; seen in cancerous bone or in a bone that is weakened by age. |
| Spiral | A fracture in which a twisting force causes a spiral-shaped injury in a long bone, especially the tibia. |
| Transverse | A fracture that runs straight across the bone. |

**Table 20-2**   Potential Internal Blood Loss in Closed Fractures*

| Site of Fracture | Blood Loss |
|---|---|
| Pelvis | 1,300–1,500 mL |
| Femur | 500–1,000 mL |
| Humerus | 300–500 mL |
| Tibia/Fibula | 150–250 mL |
| * Losses may be greater in open fractures. | |

Due to the vascular nature of bones and surrounding tissues, certain fractures can result in significant internal and/or external blood loss (see Table 20-2■). Closed fractures are associated with internal blood loss, which generally stops due to the limited space available for blood to accumulate. If the space for blood to accumulate inside the body is large, as is the case for the thigh with a femur fracture, a significant amount of blood can be lost internally. Open fractures may result in a greater loss of blood because local soft tissues do not restrict the bleeding.

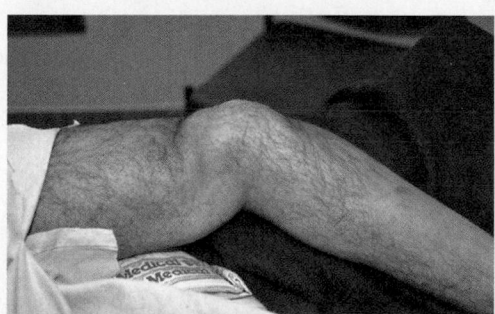

**Figure 20-18**  A dislocation of the knee.
Copyright Edward T. Dickenson, M.D.

## Dislocations

A dislocation is a separation or displacement of the bones of a joint (Figure 20-18■). This injury usually requires forceful trauma. In some people who have previously dislocated a joint, minimal force may be all that is necessary to dislocate that joint again.

When a joint dislocates, the joint capsule and surrounding ligaments can stretch or tear. Additionally, the soft tissues, blood vessels, and nerves

**subluxation**   an event in which a joint dislocates partially and returns to its normal anatomical position.

surrounding the joint are often damaged. A joint can partially dislocate and then return to its normal anatomical position, a condition known as **subluxation**, or it can be completely dislocated or "locked" out of normal anatomical position. When the bone ends remain out of position, joint movement can be dramatically, often completely restricted. Both partial and complete dislocations are very painful. The most commonly dislocated joints are the shoulders, elbows, fingers, hips, knees, and ankles.

## Multiple Simultaneous MS Injuries

As stated previously, injuries involving the MS system often damage more than one structure. For instance, dislocations are nearly always associated with some type of sprain. Likewise, open fractures are commonly associated with muscle, tendon, and/or ligament damage. One of the more prevalent multiple MS injuries that OEC Technicians encounter is a fracture-dislocation, in which a fractured bone is accompanied by a joint dislocation. Any joint in the body can sustain a fracture-dislocation, although most occur in the shoulders, elbows, fingers, and ankles. As one can imagine, these injuries are very painful. Fracture-dislocations may be accompanied by neurologic or vascular damage and are true medical emergencies.

# STOP, THINK, UNDERSTAND

## Multiple Choice
Choose the correct answer.

1. The zone of injury is _____
   a. the geographical location where an accident occurred and 10 feet circumference.
   b. the pinpointed location of a bone fracture.
   c. the area the patient identifies as being painful.
   d. the soft tissue, nerves, and blood vessels adjacent to a bone or joint injury.

2. A sprain is best defined as_____
   a. an injury that results in the stretching or tearing of a ligament.
   b. a stretched or torn muscle.
   c. a tendon that is stretched beyond its normal range of motion.
   d. a hairline crack in a bone that is caused when a ligament is stretched beyond its normal limits.

3. Which of the following statements is true?_____
   a. You strain a muscle and sprain a ligament.
   b. You strain a ligament and sprain a muscle.
   c. You tear a muscle and rupture a ligament.
   d. You rupture a ligament and sprain a muscle.

4. Which of the following statements is false?_____
   a. Poor body mechanics can increase the likelihood of tendon rupture.
   b. Disease or fatigue has little or no bearing on the likelihood of tendon rupture.
   c. A ruptured tendon can cause a complete loss of the associated joint's motion.
   d. The ankle, elbow, and fingers are common locations for tendon injuries.

5. A mid-humeral fracture in a six-year-old in which the bone "bends" is called_____
   a. a branch fracture.
   b. an epiphyseal fracture.
   c. a greenstick fracture.
   d. a nightstick fracture.

6. Which bone, when fractured, has the greatest potential for blood loss? _____
   a. tibia/fibula
   b. humerus
   c. pelvis
   d. femur

7. A dislocation is best described as_____
   a. a complete tear of a ligament.
   b. a separation or displacement of the bones of a joint.
   c. a broken joint bone.
   d. an epiphyseal fracture.

8. A subluxation is best defined as a _____
   a. bone that telescopes into itself.
   b. ligament that stretches but does not tear.
   c. displaced vertebra.
   d. joint that partially dislocates and then returns to its normal anatomical position.

9. One of the most commonly encountered musculoskeletal injuries is_____
   a. a vertebral-pelvic fracture.
   b. a fracture-dislocation.
   c. a strain-dislocation.
   d. an open fracture-laceration.

# CASE UPDATE

After making sure that the scene is safe, placing crossed skis above the site, and taking Standard Precautions, you perform a primary assessment. The patient states that he caught "way too much air and crashed." The patient's respiratory rate is 16 and his left radial pulse is 100 and strong, but the radial pulse in his injured right arm is absent. You immediately call for assistance, a long spine board, a splint for the femur and transportation to the first aid room. Because of the mechanism of injury, the lack of a right radial pulse, and the fact that ground transport to definitive care will take over 2 hours, you radio for air transport.

***What should you do next?***

# SECTION 2
# Assessment of Musculoskeletal Injuries

## ⊕ OBJECTIVES

**Upon completion of this section of this chapter, the OEC Technician will be able to:**

**20-2.1** Describe the general assessment of MS injuries.

**20-2.2** Describe the signs and symptoms of MS injuries.

**20-2.3** List specific injuries involving the arm and leg.

**20-2.4** Describe and demonstrate how to assess each specific arm or leg injury.

## Assessment

The general assessment of a musculoskeletal injury is the same for any type of injury and begins with a scene size-up. Identify potential safety hazards, paying careful attention to where the patient is located, especially whether the patient is visible to others coming into the area. Potentially dangerous situations include a mountain bike racer injured on a blind curve or an injured skier lying just beyond a jump (Figure 20-19■).

⊕ **20-2.1** Describe the general assessment of MS injuries.

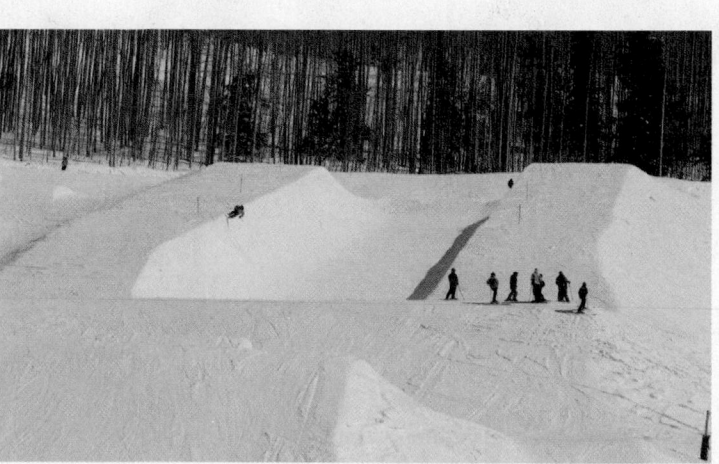

**Figure 20-19** Scene size-up is an especially important part of a primary assessment when patients may be out of view of oncoming skiers.
Copyright Scott Smith

Whenever possible, mark the scene's location or place a bystander or fellow OEC Technician a short distance from the scene to direct people away from the patient's location. Determine how many patients are present, because some incidents, such as collisions, result in more than one patient and various MS injuries. Request assistance immediately if the incident involves multiple patients.

Next, assess the patient's ABCDs and correct any threats to life. Carefully examine the patient for external bleeding, which may not be apparent, especially if the patient is wearing bulky clothing or multiple layers. Control severe bleeding using the techniques described in Chapter 18, Soft-Tissue Injuries. Assess responsiveness using the AVPU scale. If time and conditions permit, obtain a Glasgow Coma Score. Following the primary assessment, manually stabilize the head and spine if neurologic injury is suspected. Be sure to assess the mechanism of injury, which may provide helpful clues that can help you better understand the patient's *possible* injuries. As a

**Figure 20-20** For some mechanisms of injury, multiple injuries could be possible.

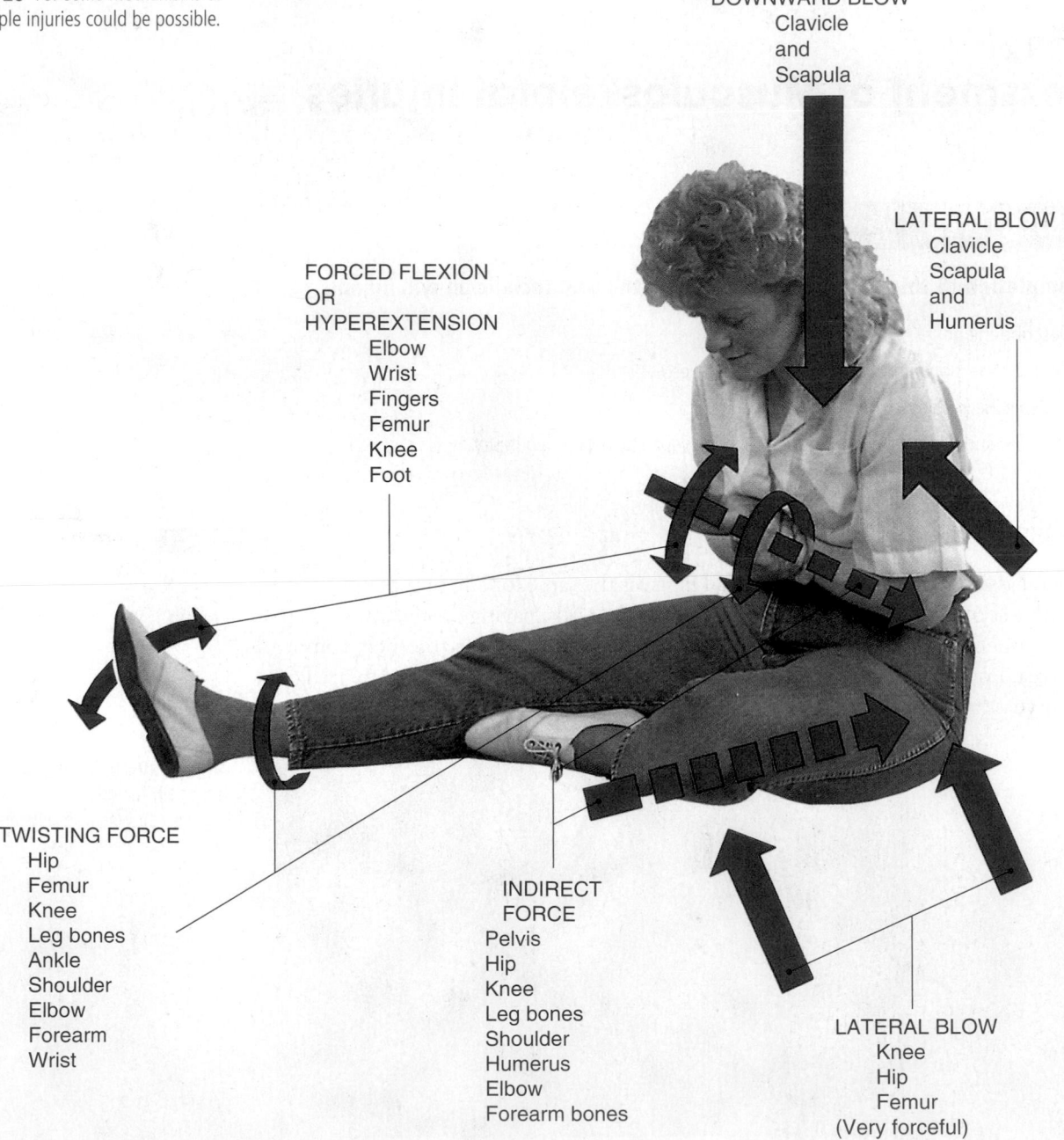

DOWNWARD BLOW
Clavicle
and
Scapula

LATERAL BLOW
Clavicle
Scapula
and
Humerus

FORCED FLEXION
OR
HYPEREXTENSION
Elbow
Wrist
Fingers
Femur
Knee
Foot

TWISTING FORCE
Hip
Femur
Knee
Leg bones
Ankle
Shoulder
Elbow
Forearm
Wrist

INDIRECT
FORCE
Pelvis
Hip
Knee
Leg bones
Shoulder
Humerus
Elbow
Forearm bones

LATERAL BLOW
Knee
Hip
Femur
(Very forceful)

rule, any patient who has a potential threat to life, or is unstable, unresponsive, or has suspected multiple fractures, is considered a high priority and should receive immediate care and rapid transport. If the patient is unresponsive immediately open the airway and simultaneously check for breathing and a pulse. If no pulse, start CPR.

Some MOIs may result in more than one injury (Figure 20-20■). Any mechanism with enough force to break bones can also damage other body systems. The type, extent, and severity of injury depend on several factors, which include the following:

+ Mode, direction, and magnitude of the forces that produced the injury
+ Patient's age
+ Quality and uniqueness of any sports equipment involved
+ Position of the extremity in relation to the body at impact
+ Characteristics of the surface(s) with which the patient came into contact

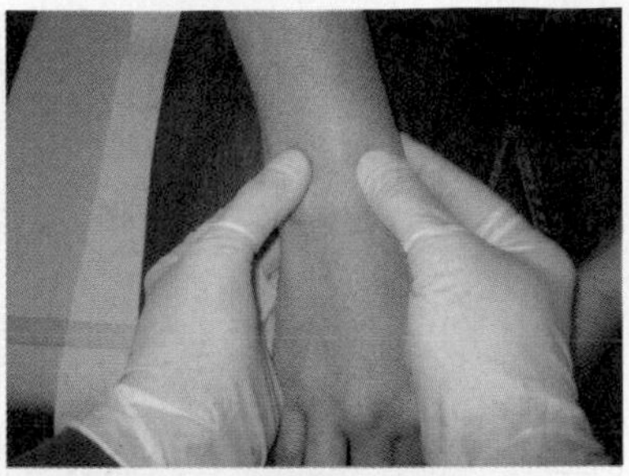

Once the ABCDs have been managed, perform a secondary assessment. Begin by obtaining a SAMPLE history. The most common symptom of a musculoskeletal injury is pain. If the patient presents with pain, ask the person to point with one finger to where it hurts. Pain on gentle palpation to this site is known as point tenderness (Figure 20-21■). If the area of pain or tenderness is quite large, ask the patient to draw a circle around the site with a finger. Assess the nature and quality of the patient's pain.

Perform a physical exam using DCAP-BTLS. Make sure you perform a full body assessment, looking for head, chest, and abdominopelvic injuries as well as extremity injuries. Avoid focusing on only a single obvious MS injury. For instance, focusing your attention on a leg that is bent at an unnatural angle may cause you to overlook a serious head or internal abdominal injury. Unless severe bleeding or vascular compromise is associated with a musculoskeletal injury, note its presence and assess injuries in the standard order of assessment: head, neck, chest, abdomen, pelvis, and then the extremities.

Another common finding that generally indicates musculoskeletal injury is deformity an area of the body that is misshaped or bulging in appearance (Figure 20-22■). Mild deformity is generally caused by swelling or internal bleeding, whereas gross deformity usually results from a fracture or a dislocation.

Patients who suffer an MS injury often try to protect the site from further injury. For instance, a person with a sprained wrist, a posterior shoulder dislocation, or a broken radius bone will typically hold their forearm close to their body and be reluctant to move it. This sign is known as guarding (Figure 20-23■).

Swelling is a common sign of MS injury and is usually due to localized damage to surrounding soft tissues (Figure 20-24■). Swelling that occurs quickly is considered serious

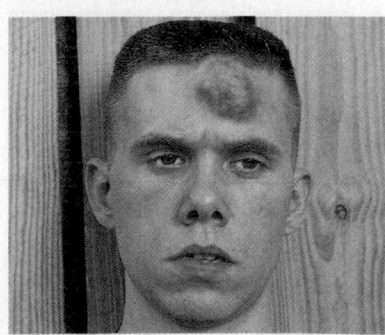

**Figure 20-21** An important aspect of a secondary assessment is locating the point of tenderness.
Copyright E. M. Singletary, MD

**Figure 20-22** Deformity often indicates a musculoskeletal injury.

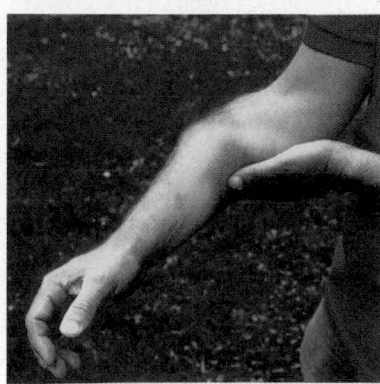

**Figure 20-23** The presence of MS trauma is often indicated by a sign called guarding.
Copyright E. M. Singletary, MD

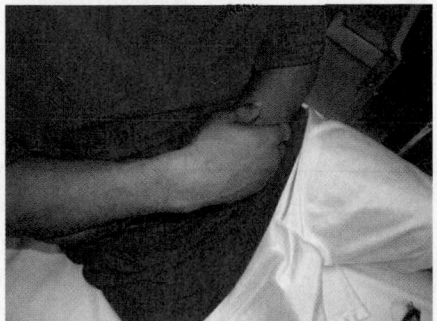

**Figure 20-24** Swelling and ecchymosis are signs of underlying hemorrhage.

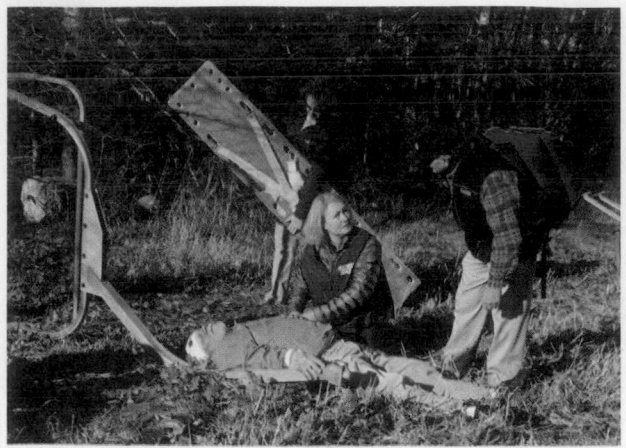

**Figure 20-25** As part of the assessment, the lead patroller formulates a plan concerning treatment and transport needs.
Copyright Mike Halloran

and signals internal bleeding. Swelling accompanied by ecchymosis indicates that underlying blood vessels have been ruptured.

Extremities that are crooked, grossly misaligned, or otherwise deformed are generally obvious. Examine these and other suspected MS injuries by assessing the distal neurovascular status first. Commonly referred to as "CMS," this process involves checking for a pulse (circulation), whether or not the patient can move the fingers or toes (movement), and whether or not the patient can feel a touch distal to the injury site (sensation). If the injury involves the axial spine, assess distal CMS in all limbs. These findings should be documented on an NSAA, a PCR, or other relevant report form.

Examine the rest of the extremity before examining the zone of injury. Do not palpate the zone of injury first, because the patient is likely to pull away due to pain, making further examination more difficult. This is especially true in young children, who are often fearful as well as in pain. Attempt to expose the injury site as soon as possible. Use judgment, however, in preserving the patient's modesty, whenever possible. In cold, rainy, or windy weather, cover all exposed skin immediately after examination and/or rendering emergency care to prevent cold injury. Similarly, in sunny weather, cover suspected MS injuries to prevent prolonged exposure to the sun's harmful rays.

Unless bleeding is profuse, it is not always wise to expose the zone of injury or to cut off an expensive jacket on scene. In these instances, briefly look or feel under the patient's clothing, assessing for pain, deformity, or blood on your gloved hand. Ensure that external bleeding is controlled. If transport time is minimal and there is no bleeding, it may be better to stabilize the extremity without exposing the injury and then move the patient to a more controlled environment.

Compare any injuries discovered to the mechanism of injury while keeping in mind that other, potentially more serious, injuries may be present. If the trauma *appears* minor, such as a laceration that is no longer bleeding, make sure you perform a complete assessment so that you do not miss a broken bone under the laceration or a life-threatening pneumothorax beneath a fractured rib.

During the assessment, begin formulating a plan concerning what you will do to manage the injured part(s), which mode of transport to use, and any special considerations (e.g., displaced fractures, patient care needs, uneven terrain, and so on) (Figure 20-25■). As part of this process, determine what equipment, including splints, may be needed, and request that these items be brought to the scene. If a toboggan, litter, ambulance, or other mode of transport will be needed, notify dispatch as soon as possible. Call for ALS if required, and remember that ALS can be very beneficial in pain control.

Reassess the patient frequently, including the vital signs and distal CMS. Document any changes on the appropriate form(s).

**⊕ 20-2.2** Describe the signs and symptoms of MS injuries.

## Signs and Symptoms of Common MS Injuries
Next we consider the signs and symptoms of some common MS injuries.

**1.** The signs and symptoms of sprains:
- Point tenderness over the injured ligaments
- Swelling and bruising within the zone of injury
- Joint instability, which is characterized by abnormal motion of the affected joint (especially in the knees and ankles) but may be masked by major joint swelling, severe tenderness, and/or guarding

- Decreased motion due to pain, swelling, and/or ligament instability
- Difficulty bearing weight on the injured joint (in the lower extremities)

2. The signs and symptoms of strains:
   - Point tenderness over a muscle or a portion of a muscle
   - Pain when using the injured muscle to flex or extend an extremity
   - Bruising over a muscle
   - Swelling or hematoma over a muscle

3. The signs and symptoms of ruptured tendons:
   - A noticeable "gap" under the skin where the tendon has ruptured (this is a hall-mark sign for this type of injury)
   - Minimal pain due to minimal nerve involvement
   - Little bruising or swelling (tendons contain few blood vessels)
   - Lack of joint movement because the tendon no longer connects the muscle to the bone

4. The signs and symptoms of fractures:
   - Pain at the fracture site that worsens upon movement of the affected bone
   - Tenderness to palpation
   - Swelling due to internal bleeding from the fracture site
   - Ecchymosis
   - Decreased motion due to pain, and lack of bone continuity
   - Deformity due to bone misalignment
   - Any wound over a suspected broken bone is always considered a sign of an open fracture
   - **Bone crepitus**

   Open fractures are characterized by the presence of a laceration near the fracture, a bone sticking through the skin, or exposed bone fragments (Figure 20-26■).

5. The signs and symptoms of dislocations:
   - Pain
   - Swelling
   - Deformity
   - Reduced joint motion
   - Joint "locking" or "freezing" (a complete inability to move the joint)

**bone crepitus** a noise or palpable feeling of crackling when fractured bone ends rub together.

### Signs and Symptoms of a Fracture

**NOTE**

Two clear signs of a fracture are feeling or hearing bone ends moving or grating against one another, known as bone crepitus, and false motion that occurs when a portion of an extremity moves where it should not move.

**Figure 20-26** An open fracture.

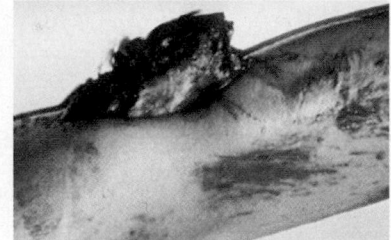

# STOP, THINK, UNDERSTAND

## Multiple Choice

Choose the correct answer.

1. An unresponsive patient is found lying below a terrain park feature. His respirations are shallow and labored, and he has an open, bleeding fracture of the femur. What is the *first* thing you should do? _____
   - **a.** secure his airway
   - **b.** stop the bleeding
   - **c.** apply a traction splint
   - **d.** secure scene safety

2. Which of the following statements is false? _____
   - **a.** A significant MOI could be indicative of a multi-system injury.
   - **b.** Any MOI with enough force to break a bone can also damage other body systems.
   - **c.** The mode and direction of force have little effect on an injury.
   - **d.** A patient's age can influence the severity of an injury.

3. The most common sign or symptom of a musculoskeletal injury is _____
   - **a.** pain.
   - **b.** bleeding.
   - **c.** deformity.
   - **d.** swelling.

4. If a patient complains of knee pain, your next question should cover _____
   - **a.** OPQRST.
   - **b.** SAMPLE.
   - **c.** AVPU.
   - **d.** ABCD.

*continued*

STOP, THINK, UNDERSTAND *continued*

5. A mild deformity of the knee is most likely caused by
   _____
   a. swelling or internal bleeding.
   b. a fracture.
   c. a dislocation.
   d. a complete rupture of a tendon.

6. A gross deformity of the wrist is most likely due to _____
   a. swelling or internal bleeding.
   b. a ruptured tendon.
   c. a fracture or a dislocation.
   d. a sprain or a strain.

7. CMS stands for _____
   a. circulation, mechanism, shock.
   b. crepitus, motion, splint.
   c. circulation, movement, sensation.
   d. correction, manipulation, straighten.

8. When assessing a patient with an obviously deformed limb, in which order should you check the limb? _____
   a. first, before you assess the head or neck
   b. in the normal assessment sequence
   c. last, unless there is obvious bleeding or a concern for compromised CMS
   d. further assessment is not necessary because the deformity is an obvious indicator of injury

## Matching

Match each of the following probable injuries to the assessment finding that indicates it.

_____ 1. fracture

_____ 2. sprain

_____ 3. strain

_____ 4. ruptured tendon

_____ 5. dislocation

a. pain over the site that increases with movement
   tenderness, swelling, ecchymosis
   decreased range of motion, deformity, crepitus
b. point tenderness over a ligament
   swelling and bruising, joint instability
   decreased range of motion
   inability to bear weight
c. point tenderness over a muscle
   pain upon extension and flexion
   bruising, swelling/hematoma over muscle
d. minimal pain
   minimal bruising or swelling
   lack of joint movement
   noticeable "gap" can be felt under skin
e. pain
   swelling
   visible deformity
   reduced joint motion
   locking/freezing of the joint

**20-2.3** List specific injuries involving the arm and leg.

**20-2.4** Describe and demonstrate how to assess each specific arm or leg injury.

## Assessment of Upper Extremity Injuries

Upper extremity injuries are commonly encountered in participants of outdoor activities. Most are caused by falling onto an outstretched hand, an elbow, or a shoulder.

The pain associated with an upper extremity injury is almost always increased by movement of the extremity. In many instances, this pain causes patients to guard the injury in a characteristic manner: they rotate their shoulder internally, flex their elbow, and hold their arm against their chest wall while supporting the forearm with the opposite hand (Figure 20-27■).

When assessing a suspected upper extremity injury, follow a standard approach that includes neurovascular assessment (CMS), inspection, and palpation. This approach increases the likelihood that injuries will not be overlooked, an important consideration when an arm has multiple injuries. Also assess capillary refill to evaluate distal blood supply, realizing that refill times may be delayed in outdoor environments, especially in cold settings.

Begin the assessment by evaluating each upper extremity individually. Do not palpate both arms at once, because if there is a pain response, you will not know which arm hurts and will need to repeat the exam, which can cause further pain. Identify the zone of injury first, and examine it last unless a threat to life such as bleeding is associated with the zone.

Examine and palpate the scapula, the most proximal part of the arm. Next, palpate the sternoclavicular joint, the entire length of the clavicle, the **acromioclavicular (A/C) joint**, and the acromion process. Using both hands, palpate the anterior and posterior aspects of the shoulder, and proceed with gentle but firm palpation down the humerus to the elbow. Gently press on the inside, the outside, and the "point" of the elbow. Continue palpating down the length of the radius and ulna to the wrist. Palpate each of the bones of the hand and fingers. Be sure to go back and *gently* palpate the zone of injury at the end of the upper extremity exam.

Evaluation of movement of an extremity should be attempted only if it does not cause pain, because excess movement can cause additional damage to surrounding tissues, bones, blood vessels, and nerves. If movement is assessed, proceed carefully and stop at the first indication of increased pain.

The assessment of specific upper extremity injuries is described in the sections that follow.

## Clavicle and Shoulder Injuries

The clavicle, or collarbone, is located on the superior portion of the anterior chest wall (Figure 20-28■). This bone has a joint on either end, and it is the only bone of the arm

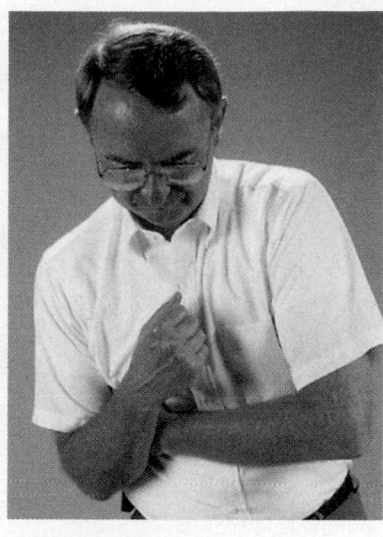

**Figure 20-27** A patient with an upper extremity or rib injury often exhibits guarding to protect the injury.

**acromioclavicular (A/C) joint** joint of the shoulder in which the acromion (top of the scapula) and the clavicle articulate.

**Figure 20-28** The shoulder girdle, which includes the clavicle and the scapula.

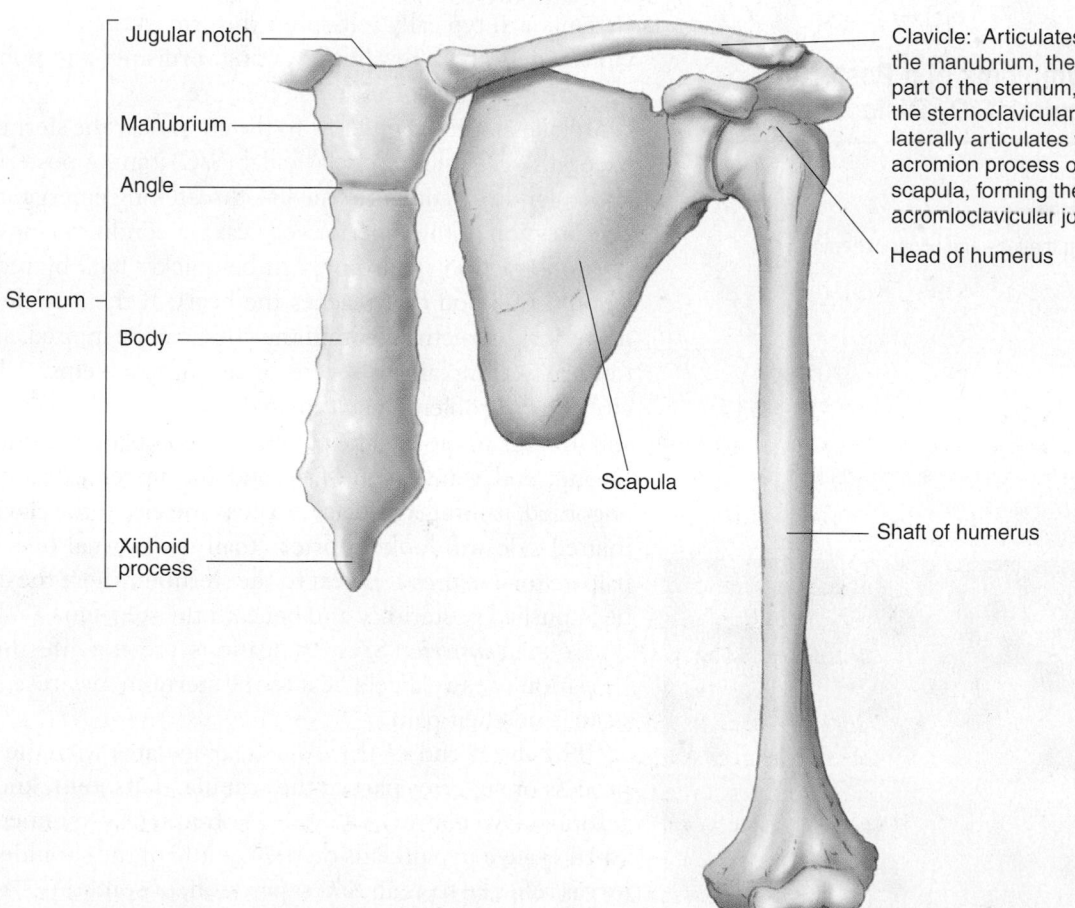

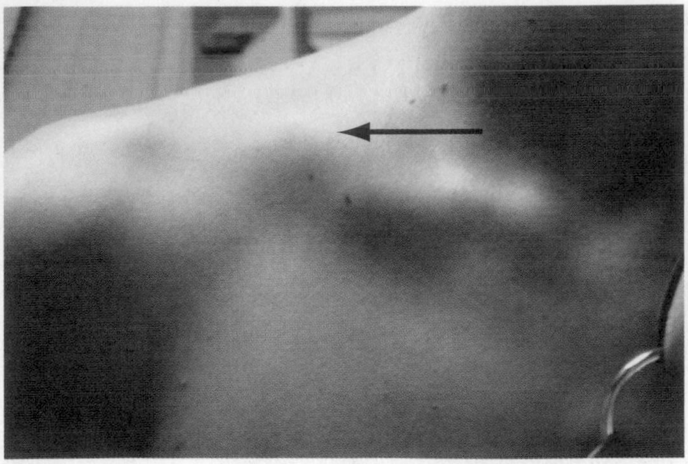

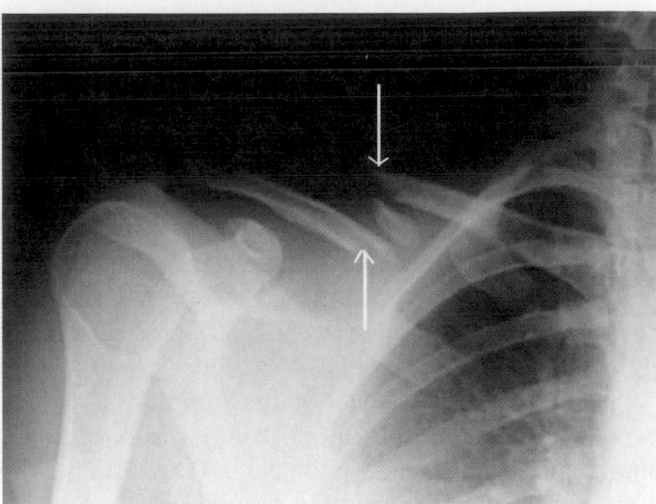

**Figure 20-29a** The "tenting up" of the skin over a fractured clavicle.
Copyright E. M. Singletary, MD

**Figure 20-29b** An X-ray of a fractured clavicle.
Copyright E. M. Singletary, MD

to articulate with the chest wall. The sternoclavicular joint attaches this bone to the sternum, whereas the acromioclavicular joint attaches this bone to the acromion of the scapula. The clavicle is the most frequently fractured bone in the body.

The clavicle commonly fractures in the middle or distal portions of the bone. As a result, the skin may "tent" over the fracture site due to the fractured end protruding up, resulting in deformity (Figures 20-29a■ and 20-29b■). This injury can be quite painful, and any movement of the arm hurts. Young children may say that the entire arm hurts. Patients will typically self-splint the arm to the chest wall as previously described. Swelling, tenting, bruising, and point tenderness are hallmarks of a clavicle fracture.

It takes a significant blow to the chest near the sternum to sublux or dislocate the sternoclavicular (S/C) joint. A posterior sternoclavicular dislocation is a true life-threatening emergency because compression of the superior vena cava, a condition known as vena cava obstruction syndrome, can be quickly fatal by reducing the amount of blood that reaches the heart. If the clavicle is pushed posteriorly, structures within the chest can be injured, and the patient may complain of severe breathing problems. Additionally, circulatory problems resulting in decreased cardiac output may result in signs of shock. The patient will complain of difficulty swallowing, and veins in the face and the upper extremity will be engorged, causing a red face. Expose the chest; the clavicle on the injured side will look "shorter" than the normal one. Look and palpate for a depression next to the sternum where the clavicle has been pushed posteriorly and beneath the sternum.

Isolated *anterior* S/C dislocations are not life threatening. Palpation of the clavicle next to the sternum may reveal a prominence and elicit pain.

The distal end of the clavicle articulates with the acromion process or superior part of the scapula. This joint, known as the acromioclavicular or A/C joint, is frequently sprained or dislocated when a person falls on the "point" of the shoulder. This injury is referred to as an A/C separation, or sometimes a "shoulder *separation*" (Figure 20-30■). This is different from a true shoul-

> **NOTE**
>
> ### Signs and Symptoms of a Posterior Sternoclavicular (S/C) Dislocation
>
> - Severe breathing problems
> - Difficulty swallowing
> - Engorged veins in the face and upper extremity
> - Reddened face
> - Shock

**Figure 20-30** An A/C separation (a separated shoulder). The patient is pointing to his normal shoulder.
Copyright John Dobson

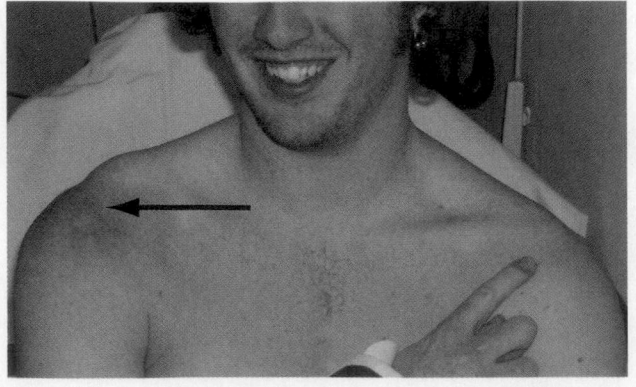

der *dislocation* between the glenoid cavity (socket) and the humeral head (ball). A skier who falls forward or a biker who goes over the handlebars may incur this injury by landing on the shoulder. Point tenderness is present over the A/C joint and just medial and inferior to the joint, where the ligaments that hold the clavicle down are located (and injured). If a mild deformity at the distal end of the clavicle is present, then a more serious A/C separation has occurred. Rarely, the clavicle will protrude significantly upward.

The shoulder or glenohumeral joint has a very lax capsule, and the ligaments that hold the shoulder in position are not very strong. Because of this, the shoulder can easily dislocate, especially if forces are applied from certain directions. This type of injury is especially prevalent in contact sports such as hockey, lacrosse, and football; it can also occur in violent falls during skiing or snowboarding and may be seen in kayaking and mountain-biking related accidents. This joint is the most frequently dislocated large joint in the body. Over 95 percent of shoulder dislocations are anterior. If an OEC Technician suspects a shoulder dislocation, the mechanism of injury may help identify the direction in which the humeral head is dislocated.

The mechanism for anterior dislocation is forceful abduction and external rotation of the arm at the shoulder. The arm usually "locks" in this position, making an OEC Technician's job of packaging the patient somewhat difficult. Patients guard the dislocated shoulder aggressively, usually by sitting, holding the shoulder up and out with the other hand, and not allowing you to lower the arm. Exposing the shoulder will reveal a skin "dent" under the acromion, where the humeral head has dislocated down and anteriorly. Any dislocated shoulder is very painful, and occasionally you may see some numbness of the outside of the shoulder or in the fourth and fifth fingers.

Posterior dislocations are rare and are most commonly seen in vehicle collisions in which a person reaches out and puts his hand on the dash just before impact, causing the humeral head to be forced in a directly posterior direction. The same mechanism of injury is seen when someone falling forward "breaks his fall" using an arm in which the elbow is locked, which pushes the humeral head out posteriorly.

Fracture of the scapula on the posterior chest wall is rare and usually indicates a severe MOI. Injuries to the chest wall (rib), internal chest, and spine are common when the scapula is fractured due to large forces. The socket part of the shoulder, or glenoid process, which is part of the scapula, can be fractured when significant force is applied to the outside of the shoulder, pushing the humeral head in and fracturing the underlying glenoid. Patients with a fractured scapula hold the arm very still and resist any movement of the limb.

**angulation**  a sharp bend in a broken bone; a broken bone that is visibly crooked.

## Humerus Fractures

Like all long bones, the humerus may fracture anywhere along its length. The ball of the humerus can be broken, although the "neck" just below the ball is more frequently fractured, especially in children and older adults. Generally, the cause is an intense direct blow to the shoulder. The top of the humerus can break into several pieces. The patient complains of pain directly over the fracture site. Deformity is uncommon because the large muscles over the proximal humerus hide the fracture, even if it is angulated.

Fractures involving the shaft of the humerus are common. Signs such as point tenderness, swelling, and **angulation** halfway between the shoulder and the elbow suggest the presence of a mid-shaft humerus fracture. Such fractures can be very unstable and often result in false movement of the bone. Humerus fractures can be significantly angulated, and because the radial nerve spirals around the

### Detecting Injury Type

Patients with A/C injuries, clavicle fractures, scapular fractures, and humeral head and neck fractures generally hold their arm against their abdomen; patients with posterior shoulder dislocations hold their arm against their abdomen and will not let you bring the arm away from the abdomen (external rotation). By contrast, patients with anterior dislocated shoulders hold their arm out and up. Thus the position in which a patient holds the injured arm can help you identify the possible injury.

NOTE

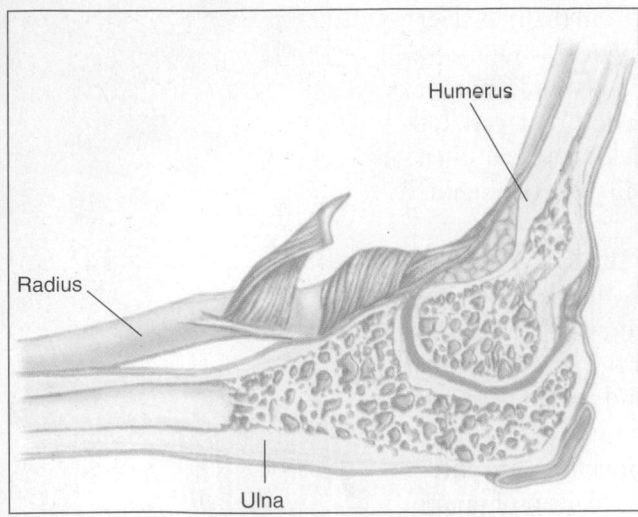

**Figure 20-31** The bones that form the elbow.

back of the humeral in mid-shaft, bone fragments can damage this nerve, resulting in loss of extension of the wrist and fingers.

### Elbow Injuries

Fractures, dislocations, and fracture-dislocations of the elbow are not uncommon in outdoor environments. The elbow joint is composed of three bones: the radius, the ulna, and the humerus (Figure 20-31■). Elbow injuries are very painful, can present with gross deformity at the elbow, and can have significant neurologic and/or vascular complications.

The elbow is surrounded by many veins and large nerves and by the brachial artery, all of which can be injured. Adults, and more commonly children, fracture the distal humerus just above the elbow, because the bone there is not very thick. This fracture, called a supracondylar fracture of the elbow, can have disastrous early and late complications in children, including nerve damage, arterial interruption, crooked healing, or muscle damage from loss of blood supply. This injury is most often caused by falling directly onto the elbow. Signs and symptoms can include gross deformity, severe pain, swelling, and possible CMS deficits.

Fractures can also occur to the olecranon process or to the radial head. The olecranon or "point" of the elbow can be fractured by falling directly on it. Signs include swelling over the tip of the elbow, and possibly a gap between the fractured bone ends. Additionally, the patient will not be able to extend the arm at the elbow. A radial head fracture occurs when the radius is forced up into the distal end of the humerus. The most common source of this injury is falling on an outstretched hand. Pain will be present on the lateral side of the elbow. Movement, especially turning the palm down or up (pronation/supination), is very painful.

An elbow dislocation may occur if a patient falls on an outstretched hand with the elbow in partial flexion. As a result, the joint becomes locked, usually at about 40–50 degrees of flexion (Figure 20-32■). This injury is more common in adults than in children. Pain is severe and is aggravated by movement. Swelling develops rapidly, and CMS function can be compromised.

Nursemaid's elbow, an injury seen in toddlers younger than 5 or 6 years old, results when an adult, who is walking beside the child and holding her hand, impatiently jerks the child's hand to hurry her, thereby dislocating the head of the radius in the elbow joint. Nursemaid's elbow can also be caused by "swinging" a young child by the hands. Symptoms include self-splinting (holding the arm against the body), slight flexion of the arm, and pain. Often, the child will cry if you touch or move the arm. Because elbow injuries involving young children can result in permanent damage if not managed in a timely manner, all elbow injuries should be examined by a physician.

### Forearm Injuries

Direct or indirect trauma to the arm between the elbow and wrist can cause a variety of injuries, including fractures. Sometimes it is difficult to differentiate between a fracture and a soft tissue injury such as a contusion.

Fractures of the shaft of the radius and/or ulna can occur from direct trauma or when an individual falls onto an outstretched hand (Figure 20-33■). This type of injury is common among snowboard-

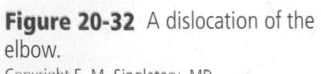

**Figure 20-32** A dislocation of the elbow.
Copyright E. M. Singletary, MD

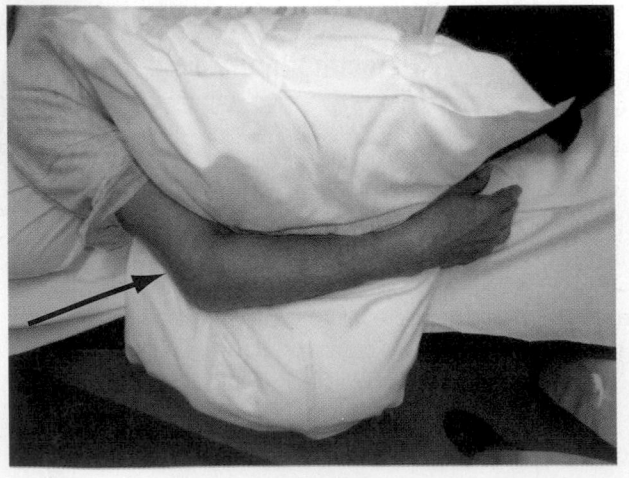

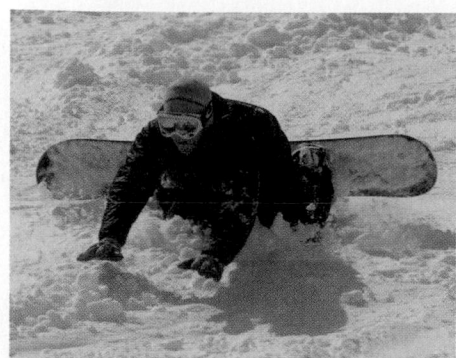

**Figure 20-33** Injuries to the forearms often occur when falling onto outstretched hands.
Copyright Scott Smith

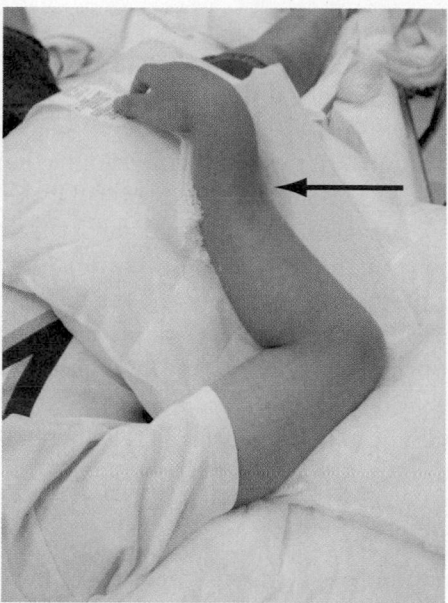

**Figure 20-34a** A forearm injury.
Copyright E. M. Singletary, MD

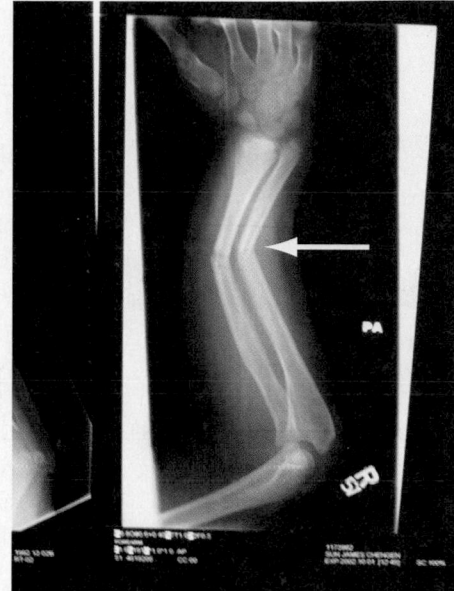

**Figure 20-34b** An X-ray showing a fractured radius and ulna.
Copyright E. M. Singletary, MD

ers and bicyclers who have fallen forward or backward. If both bones are fractured, the limb may be angulated and exhibit false movement. Swelling, point tenderness, and deformity may also be seen (Figures 20-34a■ and 20-34b■). As with elbow injuries, CMS can be compromised.

A fracture to the distal end of the ulna can result from falling on this bone. Another mechanism of injury is a direct blow to the distal ulna. This type of injury, commonly referred to as a "nightstick" fracture, can occur when individuals raise their arms to protect themselves from striking or being struck by a solid object. A large tree branch, a hockey stick, or a snowboard rail is commonly involved in this type of injury.

## Wrist Injuries

Falling forward on the palm of the hand can result in fractures to the distal radius and ulna. This injury, known as a Colles' fracture or "silver fork" fracture, results in a characteristic injury pattern in which the displaced bones resemble an overturned fork. The distal end of the fractured radius is pushed in the direction of the back of the hand. Deformity, pain, swelling, and false movement are common. A Colles' fracture is a common snowboard injury. Rarely, one can fall on the dorsum (back) of the hand, causing a reverse Colles' or "Smith's" fracture in which the fractured end of the radius is displaced toward the palm.

The most commonly fractured of the eight carpal bones is the scaphoid, also known as the navicular bone. Like other upper extremity injuries, this injury is caused by falling on an outstretched hand and is a rather common injury among snowboarders who fall forward on the toe side of their board, a fall known as a "mousetrap." It can also result from falling off a horse or while rock climbing. Among the symptoms are pain in the lateral side of the wrist joint in the "snuff box," the area distal to the end of the radius and proximal to the base of the thumb's metacarpal. Other carpal bones may also fracture. Dislocation or fracture-dislocation of the carpal bones results in a deformed wrist, severe pain, swelling, and reduced motion. The patient is often found cradling the injured wrist in the opposite hand.

Hand and Finger Injuries

A common skiing injury to the upper extremity is a sprain of the ulnar collateral ligament of the thumb. This injury, called skier's thumb, occurs when a ski pole catches on the snow and bends the thumb laterally and **dorsally**, disrupting the ligament at the base of the thumb next to the web between the thumb and index finger (Figure 20-35 ■). This injury can also occur in hikers who fall while using walking poles.

Any of the bones of the hand may be fractured or dislocated. If the first metacarpal (the bone at the base of the thumb) is fractured, the thumb may appear dislocated where it attaches to the hand. One of the most common hand injuries is a "boxer's fracture," a fracture of the fifth metacarpal bone that is caused by punching any hard object or falling on your hand when it is clinched in a fist.

Other hand and finger injuries can involve damaged tendons, creating severe disability. Symptoms include pain, swelling, and loss of motion. Depending on the forces involved, the fingers may be angulated and deformity may result. A good way to assess the neurologic function of the hand's three nerves (median, radial, and ulnar) is shown in Table 20-3 ■.

Amputations involving the fingers may be partial, in which the finger is still attached to the hand by a tendon or skin, or it may be complete, in which case the finger is entirely separated from the hand.

One of the worst injuries to the hand can result from trying to remove a stuck object from a running snowblower. When an object gets stuck, the blades stop spinning, so the tendency is to reach into the blade area and pull the object out. If you have not turned off the machine, the blades will immediately start turning again once the object is free, potentially severely damaging the hand. *Always shut off the snowblower first, and use a stick or pole to push out the stuck object.*

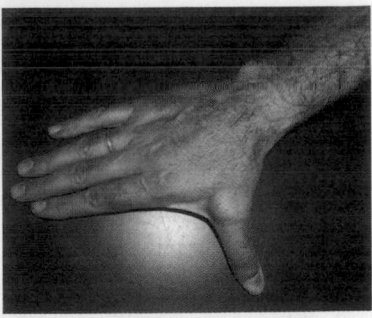

**Figure 20-35** Skier's thumb.
Copyright Edward McNamara

**dorsal**    toward the back of the body or of a body part.

### Pole and Strap Injury

NOTE

It is important to learn and remember the proper way to hold a ski pole with straps. If you hold it the wrong way when you fall, the strap of the pole may torque the thumb, causing the injury known as skier's thumb.

| Table 20-3 | Sensation and Motor Assessment of Three Nerves of the Hand | |
|---|---|---|
| **Nerve** | **Motor Action that Results** | **Location of Sensation** |
| Median | makes a fist or flexes the fingers | present on the volar (palm side) of thumb |
| Radial | extends the fingers | present on the the volar (palm side) of pinkie |
| Ulnar | spreads the fingers apart | present on the back of thumb |

## STOP, THINK, UNDERSTAND

### Multiple Choice

Choose the correct answer.

1. Which of the following statements describes the correct way to assess an injury to an upper extremity? _____
   a. The injured arm should be examined first.
   b. The uninjured arm should be examined first.
   c. Both arms should be examined at the same time.
   d. Only the uninjured arm should be examined.

2. The evaluation of movement of an injured extremity should _____
   a. never be done, because it exacerbates the injury.
   b. always be done, so that the extent of injury can be determined.
   c. be done only if movement does not cause pain.
   d. be done whenever a compromise in CMS is suspected.

3. The only upper extremity bone that articulates with the chest wall (the ribs) is the _____
   a. humerus.
   b. radius.
   c. ulna.
   d. clavicle.

4. The most commonly fractured bone in the human body is the _____
   a. humerus.
   b. femur.
   c. clavicle.
   d. scapula.

*continued*

5. Falling onto the "point" of the shoulder frequently causes what type of injury? _____
   a. An A/C joint sprain or dislocation
   b. A shoulder dislocation
   c. A fracture of the humeral head
   d. A fracture of the sternum

6. Which of the following statements about shoulder dislocations is true? _____
   a. Most shoulder dislocations are superior.
   b. Most shoulder dislocations are inferior.
   c. Most shoulder dislocations are anterior.
   d. Most shoulder dislocations are posterior.

7. A patient who presents holding her arm up and out, away from her body, and refuses to let you move it closer to her torso to splint it, is most likely suffering from what type of injury? _____
   a. a posterior shoulder dislocation
   b. an anterior shoulder dislocation
   c. a supracondylar clavicular fracture
   d. too little information was given to make such a determination

8. Besides pain, another common complaint associated with a shoulder dislocation is that the_____
   a. entire arm is numb.
   b. outside of the shoulder or the fourth and fifth fingers are numb.
   c. patient cannot move the thumb.
   d. patient is unable to flex or bend the wrist.

9. The most common place for a humeral fracture is _____
   a. in the middle of the shaft.
   b. at the epiphysis.
   c. at the neck, just below the ball.
   d. at the proximal end.

10. Which of the following statements about humeral fractures is false?_____
   a. Deformity associated with a fracture of the humeral neck is the most common sign.
   b. Humeral fractures are generally caused by an intense, direct blow to the shoulder.
   c. The ball of the humerus can break into multiple pieces.
   d. Humeral shaft fractures can be significantly angulated and can damage the radial nerve in the arm.

11. A supracondylar fracture of the elbow in children is _____
   a. rare and not very worrisome.
   b. potentially disastrous.
   c. rare but is common in adults.
   d. generally caused by falling onto an outstretched elbow.

12. Where is the olecranon process located?_____
   a. the distal end of the thumb    c. the tip of the elbow
   b. the distal end of the fibula    d. the apex of the wrist

13. Nursemaid's elbow is most commonly caused by _____
   a. repetitive bending of wrist and elbow.
   b. wrenching an arm behind a back.
   c. repetitive motion or overuse of the elbow.
   d. pulling a child by the hand.

14. Which of the following upper extremity bones is/are most frequently injured by snowboarders?_____
   a. radius and ulna    c. olecranon process
   b. humerus    d. metacarpals

15. A nightstick fracture is best described as a _____
   a. fracture of the humerus caused by falling onto the shoulder.
   b. fracture of the ulna caused by a direct blow from a hard object.
   c. radial-ulnar fracture caused by falling onto an outstretched hand.
   d. rare wrist fracture caused by falling onto the top of the hand.

16. To OEC Technicians, a "mouse trap" is_____
   a. an item used to catch rodents.
   b. a common snowboard injury.
   c. an uncommon digital injury.
   d. a rare type of finger injury.

17. A "boxer's fracture" is a_____
   a. fracture of the scaphoid bone.
   b. thumb dislocation.
   c. wrist fracture.
   d. fracture of the fifth metacarpal bone.

18. What is "skier's thumb"? _____
   a. a fracture of the scaphoid bone just above the thumb
   b. a sprain of the ulnar collateral ligament of the thumb
   c. a very uncommon digital injury
   d. a fracture of both the carpals and phalanges

## Short Answer

1. Describe the position in which you are most likely to find a patient who has an upper extremity injury.

2. Why is fracturing the scapula dangerous?

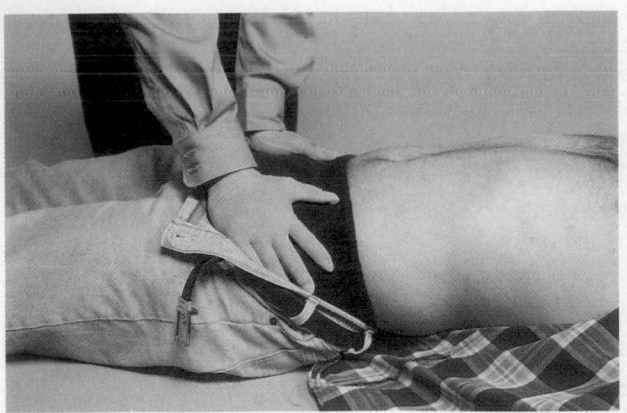

**Figure 20-36** Assess the pelvic bones by pressing gently medially on the iliac crests.

# Assessment of Lower Extremity Injuries

The process for evaluating a leg is similar to that for an arm. As before, assess the MOI, check distal CMS, then inspect, and palpate the entire extremity. Assess each leg systematically. Avoid touching the zone of injury, unless exposure reveals bleeding, until after you have examined the entire leg. Always control bleeding first.

Because patients with fractures or dislocations in one or both legs do not want to move the affected limb(s) and are very sensitive to any movement, try not to move the extremity unnecessarily as you examine it. If conditions permit, inspect the area being examined before palpating it.

Begin the exam by palpating the pelvis. Although the pelvis is not really part of the leg, the ball of the femur fits into the acetabulum or socket of the pelvis. Although a more detailed description of a pelvic exam is described in Chapter 24, Abdominal and Pelvic Trauma, a brief explanation of a pelvic exam is presented here.

Assess the stability of the pelvic bones by gently pressing medially (inward) on the iliac crests (Figure 20-36■). Then, assess each hip by gently pushing medially (inward), feeling for tenderness and bone stability.

Next, examine each leg individually. Using two hands, one on the inside of the leg and one on the outside of the leg, start near the groin and gently but firmly palpate down the femur to the knee (Figure 20-37■). Palpate the knee over the patella, at the back, and both medially and laterally. If pain is present, perform a more detailed knee exam in a controlled environment. Continue palpating down the lower leg (tibia and fibula) to the ankle. If the patient is wearing a ski boot or other heavy footwear, consider leaving it on until the patient has been moved indoors. After the boot has been removed using the method described in OEC Skill 20-14, palpate the ankle on each side. Palpate the foot, paying particular attention to the heel, arch, and outside of the foot.

Assess distal neurovascular status of each leg. In the event of serious leg injury, inclement weather, or heavy clothing/footwear, it may not be possible to perform a complete neurovascular exam until the patient is moved indoors. In such cases, assess movement by simply having patients wiggle their toes up and down (**dorsiflex** and **plantarflex** respectively). Determine whether patients can feel the toes wiggling inside the boot. Assess distal pulses as soon as possible after the removal of the patient's footwear (Figure 20-38■).

Next consider the assessment of specific lower extremity injuries.

## Hip and Pelvis Injuries

The hip joint is a ball-and-socket joint with strong ligaments that hold the bones in position. Significant force is required to dislocate the hip, which can occur anteriorly or posteriorly. Both injuries are extremely painful and are aggravated by movement of the affected leg.

**dorsiflex** to move a part of the body dorsally (toward the back).

**plantarflex** movement of the foot or toes downward, toward the sole of the foot.

**Figure 20-37** Assess the leg from the femur to the knee.

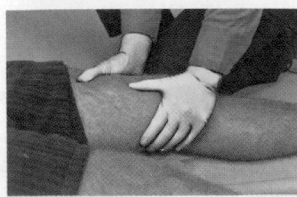

**Figure 20-38** Check distal pulses in the foot. Posterior Tibialis on the left and Dorsalis Pedis on the right.

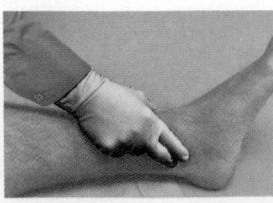
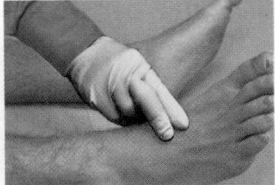

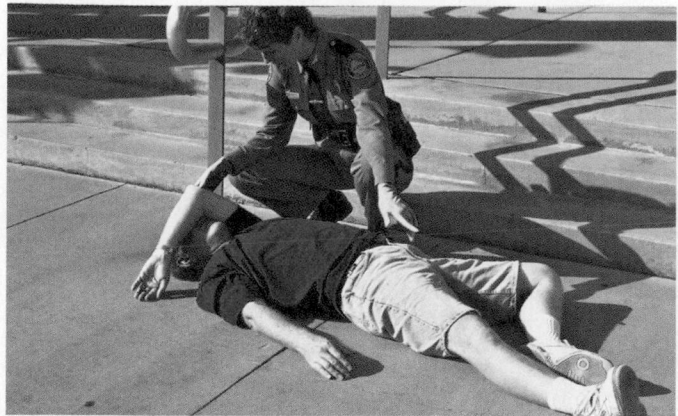

**Figure 20-39a** An anterior hip dislocation.

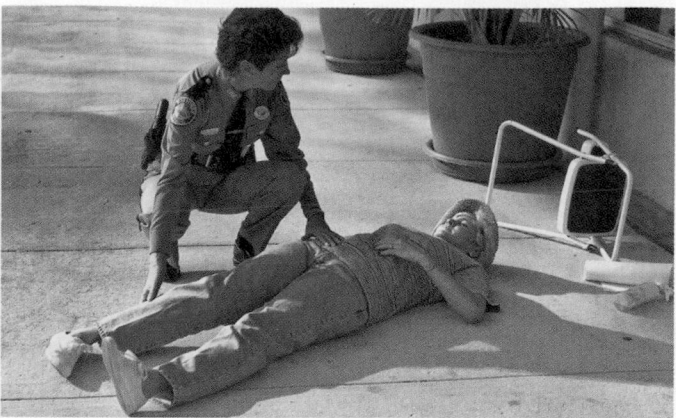

**Figure 20-39b** A posterior hip dislocation.

Signs of the less common anterior hip dislocation include abduction of the thigh and external rotation of the knee (Figure 20-39a■). Over 90 percent of hip dislocations are posterior dislocations (Figure 20-39b■). The mechanism of injury for this hip dislocation is a significant force applied to the knee of a person who is sitting. In this position, the *flexed* hip is pushed out the back of the socket (acetabulum). This type of injury is most commonly seen in an unrestrained person in a car collision whose knee hits the dashboard, forcing the hip backward. Fracture of either the acetabulum or the femoral head may occur as the hip dislocates. Signs of a posterior hip dislocation include internal rotation of the knee and shortening of the affected leg.

The sciatic nerve can be injured in a dislocated hip, possibly resulting in temporary partial paralysis or complete paralysis of the ankle and foot. Additionally, the major blood vessels supplying the hip joint cross the anterior portion of the joint's capsule and can be compromised if the capsule is stretched or torn. The longer the hip remains dislocated, the more damage can occur to the head of the femur. If blood does not reach the femoral head for some time (usually several hours), the bone cells in the femoral head die, resulting in very painful arthritis later in life. This is the main reason why a dislocated hip is considered a true orthopedic emergency. Once a hip has dislocated, the joint is usually "locked" out of position until it is put back into place by a physician.

Fractures of the pelvis are discussed in Chapter 24, Abdominal and Pelvic Trauma. Pelvic fractures can cause serious internal bleeding leading to shock, and injuries to the genitalia are commonly associated with pelvic fractures.

## Femur Fractures

Femur fractures are usually seen only in high-energy trauma. As for any long bone, the femur can fracture anywhere along its length. The femur is commonly divided into three parts: the proximal femur, the shaft, and the distal femur. Fractures involving the proximal femur are commonly referred to as "hip fractures" and are not frequently encountered in snow sports, unless there is excessive speed and direct trauma involved. Older individuals, whose bones are more brittle, experience these fractures much more commonly, often from simple falls.

Most patients with a *displaced* proximal femur fracture present with signs similar to a posterior hip fracture: the affected leg is shortened and externally rotated. Pain is extreme and is generally located in the groin or inner aspect of the thigh. Occasionally pain is referred to the knee, even though the knee is not injured. Movement makes the pain worse.

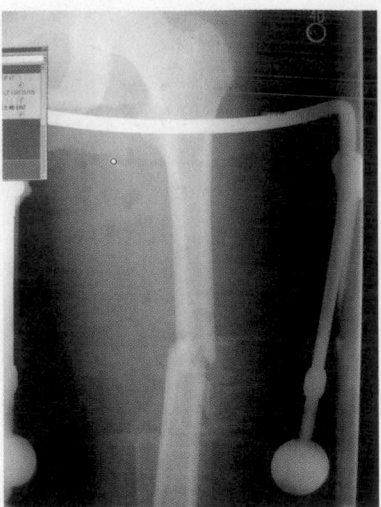

**Figure 20-40**  An X-ray of a mid-shaft fracture of the femur.
Copyright E. M. Singletary, MD

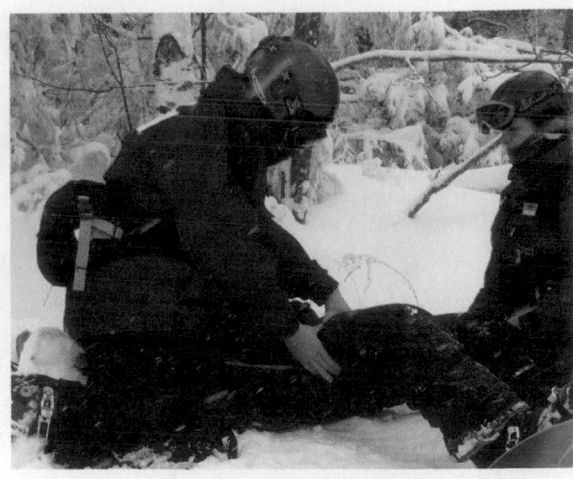

**Figure 20-41**  Information concerning the mechanism of injury and a thorough assessment of the patient provide clues about the nature of a thigh injury.
Copyright Edward McNamara

Fractures of the middle third of the femur (known as the "shaft") are caused by direct and forceful trauma to the thigh, a fall, or intense twisting of the thigh (Figure 20-40■). Assessment of the mechanism of injury generally provides clues concerning the forces involved (Figure 20-41■). Direct trauma results in a transverse fracture, whereas twisting results in a spiral fracture or an oblique fracture. Falls from a height often result in a comminuted fracture. Signs and symptoms of a femur fracture include intense pain, deformity, thigh swelling, and false movement. The bone may also be angulated.

The distal end of the femur has two large flared ends known as the medial and lateral condyles. A fracture occurring just above or between the two is called a supracondylar femur fracture. Fractures involving this area are characterized by severe pain and swelling just above the knee, deformity, inability to move the knee, and spasm of the thigh muscles. In addition, just behind the distal end of the femur are the large popliteal artery and its branches, the popliteal veins, and the major nerves to the lower leg. These structures can be damaged by jagged bone ends produced by a distal femur fracture. If this occurs, distal CMS may be compromised, resulting in poor perfusion, decreased motor function, and decreased sensation in the lower leg.

## Knee Injuries

Knee injuries constitute 30 percent of all ski injuries and are a common occurrence in many other outdoor activities, especially those involving twisting of the knee during running and jumping. Most knee injuries are sprains involving the four main ligaments that support the knee joint. Return to Figure 20-8. The medial collateral and lateral collateral ligaments act as hinges on each side of the knee. Inside the joint are the anterior and posterior cruciate ligaments, which prevent forward and backward motion of the femur on the tibia. Depending on the mechanism of injury, one or more of these ligaments can be stretched or torn.

The most common ski injury is a medial collateral ligament sprain. This injury occurs when the knee is stressed while in a **valgus** position (when the knee is forced medially into an extremely "knock-kneed" position). Symptoms of this injury include point tenderness above, below, or over the joint line on the inside of the knee. Much less frequent is an injury to the lateral collateral ligament, which can occur if the knee is stressed in the opposite or **varus** position, in which the knee is forced laterally (as if the

**valgus**   medial (inward) angulation of a bone or joint (toward the midline).

**varus**   lateral (outward) angulation of a bone or joint (away from the midline).

limb were suddenly made bow-legged). With this injury, pain is localized to the lateral part of the knee. The anterior cruciate ligament can be torn when a skier "sits back" and falls, or when someone is running and stops abruptly. Typically, the patient will report feeling or hearing a "pop" and has immediate pain in the knee. This common injury is the bane of all outdoor recreationalists and athletes, as it usually requires surgical repair and lengthy rehabilitation.

Cartilage injuries are also common. The articular cartilage on the ends of the femur and tibia where they come together to form the knee joint can be damaged when the knee is injured. Additionally, on the medial side of the knee is a C-shaped cartilage, known as the medial **meniscus**, whereas on the lateral side is an O-shaped cartilage called the lateral meniscus. These menisci cushion the knee and help stabilize the joint by increasing the depth of the "dish" on each side of the knee where each round femoral condyle articulates with the tibia. The menisci can be damaged or torn when the knee joint is compressed or twisted. Injuries often cause the cartilage to become torn, causing pain, swelling or fluid in the knee joint, and reduced mobility.

Fractures near the knee may involve the distal end of the femur, the proximal end of the tibia or fibula, the patella, or a combination of these bones. The patella, or "knee cap," is a large bone on the anterior portion of the knee that is connected to the quadriceps muscle's tendon superiorly. Inferiorly, a ligament connects the patella to the top front of the tibia. Trauma can fracture the patella, rupture the quadriceps tendon or the patellar ligament, or dislocate the patella.

Fracture of the patella is typically caused by either falling directly on the front of the knee or receiving a significant direct or blunt force on the anterior knee. The amount of force necessary to fracture the patella is great, as it is a dense bone. Patella fractures may be open, so expose the zone of injury to assess for bleeding.

Dislocation of the patella is fairly common, and most busy ski patrollers will see a patellar dislocation sometime during their career. This injury occurs more frequently in teens and in women because their knees are more likely to be in a valgus position, in which the insides of the knees are closer together than are the inside of the ankles. The common mechanism of injury involves twisting the knee in a slightly flexed position while forcefully contracting the quadriceps muscle. Excessive direct force to one side of the patella or the other can also dislocate it. Once a patella dislocates, the risk for future dislocations is great. Nearly all patella dislocations are *lateral* because the tissue holding the patella in place is disrupted on the medial side of the knee. This results in a knee that is flexed and has a large firm bulge (the patella) on the lateral side of the knee. The isolated deformity is significant and characteristic, but it is not limb threatening. Often, the patella will "pop" back into place spontaneously as the leg is straightened. If this occurs before an OEC Technician has examined the knee, the medial aspect of the knee will be tender to touch, and both ecchymosis and swelling may be present.

A patella dislocation should not be confused with a *dislocated knee*, which is a very serious problem. Refer to a patella that is out of place as a dislocated patella, not as a dislocated knee.

A knee dislocation is a true but very rare orthopedic emergency (Figure 20-42■). However, once an OEC Technician has seen one, it will never be forgotten. The injury is associated with massive trauma in which at least three (if not all four) of the ligaments of the knee are completely torn. This allows the actual knee joint, not merely the patella, to move into an abnormal anatomical position. There is gross deformity, in which the proximal tibia is in front or behind the femur. Additionally, the leg may be severely angulated at the knee joint. Because there is no longer any true **articulation** in this portion of the leg, important neurovascular structures in the **popliteal fossa** are frequently damaged, resulting in severe neurovascular compromise. The most important

**meniscus** a specialized cartilage found in some joints; such as the knee and the acromioclavicular (A/C) joint.

**articulation** the site at which the ends of two or more bones come together to form a joint.

**popliteal fossa** posterior part of the knee.

**Figure 20-42** A dislocation of the knee.

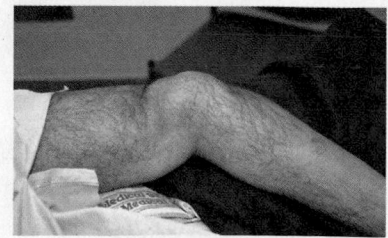

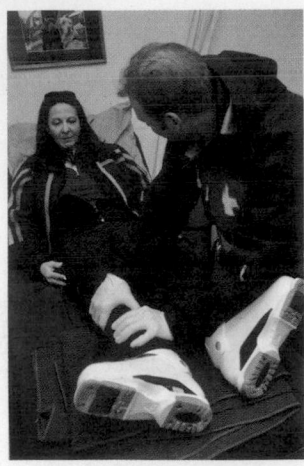

**Figure 20-43** In a controlled environment, expose the knee and further assess for possible injuries.
Copyright Studio 404

of these structures is the popliteal artery, which can be lacerated or compressed, causing a pulseless, pale, and cold foot. The pain with this injury is severe. Since the mechanism of injury for this injury is severe, a complete patient assessment is needed to ensure that no potential threats to life are present.

Rupture of the quadriceps tendon or patellar ligament is another knee-related injury that OEC Technicians may encounter. This injury may be caused by an excessively forceful contraction of the quadriceps muscle that rips the quadriceps tendon off the top of the patella. The same MOI can cause the patellar ligament to rip below or off the bottom of the patella. This injury is more common in weight lifters and in individuals with chronic disease such as diabetes. With either injury, the patient will likely report hearing a "pop." A palpable "gap" is present in the extensor mechanism where the tendon or ligament ruptured, and the patient will be unable to straighten the affected leg at the knee. Swelling from internal bleeding occurs in the zone of injury.

Assessment of a knee injury at the accident scene should be brief. It is not necessary to diagnose the injury in the field; instead, try to establish a mechanism of injury; attempt to isolate the part of the knee that is injured; assess injury severity, deformity, and CMS; and make a decision concerning immobilization and transport.

Further assessment of the knee is best performed in a controlled environment such as a warm aid room (Figure 20-43■). Expose the leg from mid-thigh to the toes. Look for swelling, point tenderness, bruising, or deformity. Ask the patient to point with one finger where it hurts the most. Tenderness along the outside or the inside of the joint usually indicates a ligament or cartilage injury, whereas pain over the distal femur, patella, or proximal tibia suggests a possible fracture (Figure 20-44■). It is not the OEC Technician's responsibility to perform a full orthopedic exam, but if you suspect any one of these injuries, recommend further evaluation by a physician.

Most knee injuries are characterized by localized tenderness, joint swelling (usually resulting from blood in the joint), bruising, deformity, reduced movement, and pain that can be intense. As with other orthopedic injuries, movement intensifies the pain. Often, patients will be unable to stand or walk on their own. Distal CMS is usually intact.

> **N O T E**
>
> ### Knee Joint Trauma
>
> Following trauma, the knee joint can fill up with blood, synovial fluid, or both. In all cases, a large, swollen knee joint usually means that something is seriously wrong with the knee. Rapid swelling of the knee joint usually indicates a buildup of blood and a more serious injury. A buildup of excessive synovial fluid in the knee takes longer, usually hours, resulting in gradual swelling.

## Tibia and Fibula Injuries

The two bones between the knee and the ankle are the larger, weight-bearing tibia and the smaller, nonweight-bearing fibula. The two bones are connected to the femur and the ankle/foot by muscles and ligaments. The tibia articulates with the femur to form the knee joint, whereas the ankle joint is a "mortise" joint formed where the talus bone fits into the space created by the tibia and fibula.

Proximal tibia fractures can be extremely painful and may occur when someone falls from a height or simply lands flat when performing a jump in a terrain park. In this injury, the bottom of the femur is forced into the top of the tibia, compressing the tibia and causing a compression fracture of the top of the bone just below the joint line. This injury is becoming increasingly frequent in older skiers (Figure 20-45■).

Fractures to the shafts of these bones can occur anywhere along the bone. Tibia and fibula fractures are often seen in skiers, especially those using snow-blades that do not have release bindings. The incidence of this injury is lower in snowboarders. Frequently, both lower bone shafts in the same leg will break at the same time, a condition known as a "tib-fib"

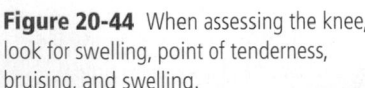

**Figure 20-44** When assessing the knee, look for swelling, point of tenderness, bruising, and swelling.

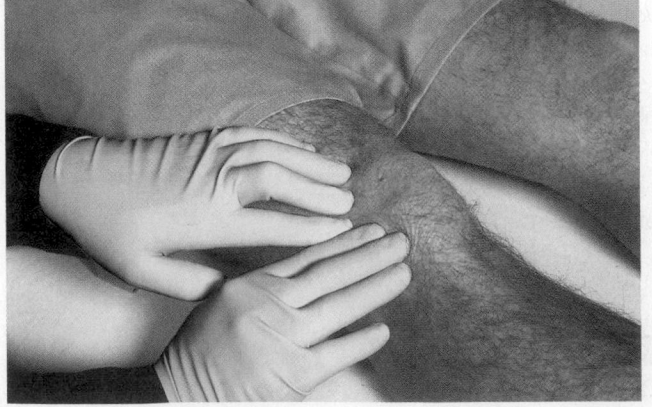

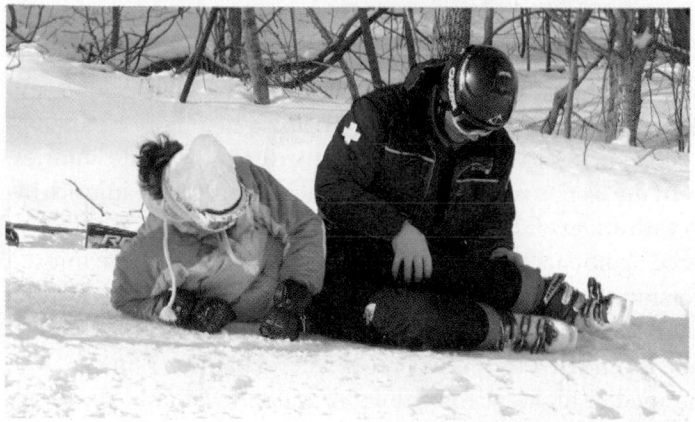

**Figure 20-45** A compression fracture of the proximal tibia is a common injury among skiers.
Copyright Edward McNamara

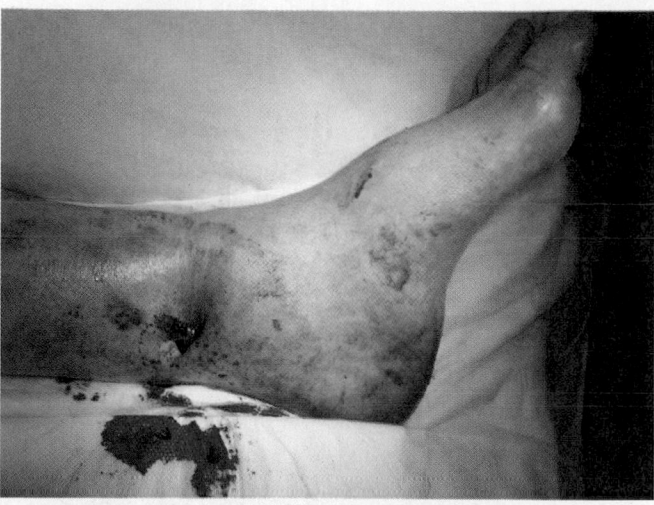

**Figure 20-46** An open fracture of the tibia.
Copyright E.M. Singletary, MD

fracture. Less often, direct trauma or other infrequent MOIs can break the shaft of one bone only. Open fractures involving the tibia can easily occur because the entire anterior bone is just under the skin (Figure 20-46■).

Injuries that occur while skiing include a *boot top* fracture, in which the fibula or the tibia and fibula undergo a transverse fracture; a *spiral* fracture, in which the tibia is broken in the middle and the fibular shaft is broken above or below the tibial fracture; and a *direct blow* fracture, in which either bone is broken across and may have a "butterfly" fragment (Figure 20-47■).

## Ankle Injuries

Ankle injuries are common among outdoor enthusiasts, especially those who traverse rough or uneven terrain (Figure 20-48■). OEC Technicians see a gamut of injuries, from a mild sprain to a deformed, open fracture-dislocation. Sneakers, soft snowboard boots, soft alpine boots, and low-top cross-country ski boots give little support to the ankle, allowing it to twist or bend sideways. Most ankle injuries are due to "rolling" the joint, which typically occurs in one of two ways: either stepping on the outside of the foot and turning the arch up (a condition known as *inversion*), or by coming down on the inside

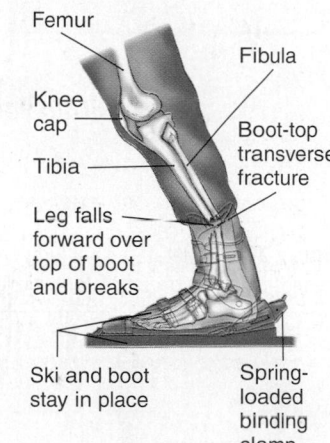

**Figure 20-47** A boot top fracture can involve the tibia, the fibula, or both bones.

**Figure 20-48** Ankle injuries commonly occur on rough or uneven terrain.
Copyright Scott Smith

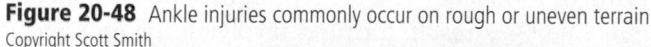

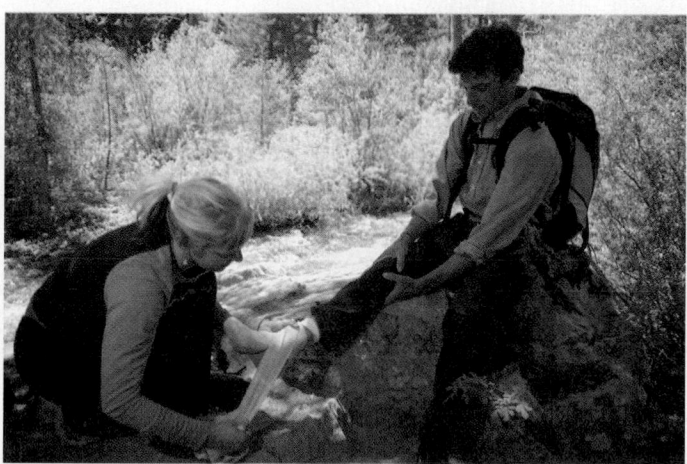

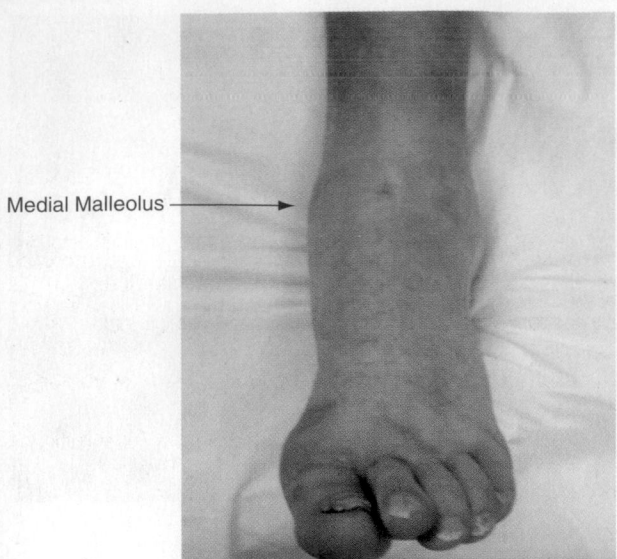

**Figure 20-49** A fracture of the medial malleolus of the ankle.

Medial Malleolus

**Figure 20-50** Metatarsal fractures are the most common traumatic foot injuries.

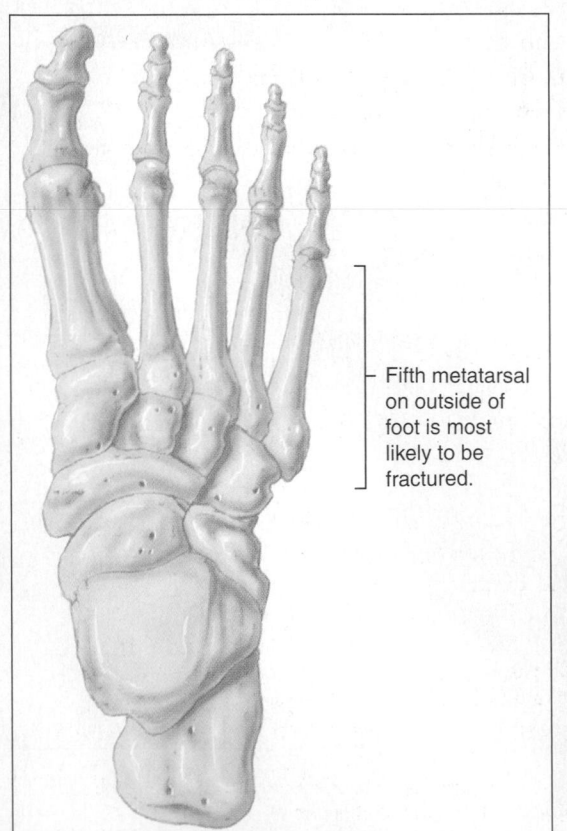

Fifth metatarsal on outside of foot is most likely to be fractured.

of the foot and flattening the arch (known as eversion). Of the two injury types, inversion is more common and results in a sprain or fracture to the outside of the ankle. High lace-up hiking boots and plastic-shelled alpine ski boots hold the ankle in a more rigid position, reducing both the incidence and severity of ankle injuries. However, the likelihood of tibial shaft fractures and knee injuries increases with stiffer or higher boots.

Three ligaments on the lateral side of the ankle may be injured by inversion. One symptom of this injury is tenderness *below* the lateral ankle bone, known as the lateral malleolus of the fibula. If the bone is tender, a fracture is more likely than a sprain.

The medial malleolus is the large bulge located at the distal end of the tibia on the medial side of the ankle. One large wide ligament located there may be injured when the ankle everts (turns outward). Tenderness above this ligament suggests the presence of a medial malleolus fracture (Figure 20-49■).

Snowboarders have recently begun to experience a unique ankle injury that appears to be a sprain but is actually a fracture that, left untreated, can result in serious disability. A bone in the middle of the ankle, the talus, is broken beneath the lateral ankle ligaments when the snowboarder jumps and lands on a "flat," severely dorsiflexing the ankle (shoving the foot up toward the shin). X-rays may not show this injury, and a CAT scan is needed to detect it. Surgery may be needed to prevent future disability, so any snowboarder with lateral ankle pain should see an orthopedist.

Other mechanisms that cause ankle injury include axial compression due to a fall from a height, twisting, or shearing. When combinations of forces are involved, more severe injuries result.

Ankle injuries can range in severity from mild to severe. Additionally, one side of the ankle could be fractured, the other side sprained, or both sides could be broken. Determining whether an ankle injury is a sprain or a fracture requires an X-ray. Most ankle injuries present with point tenderness, swelling, ecchymosis, and reduced motion of the joint. Patients may or may not be able to bear weight on the joint. It is a fallacy that individuals can walk on a sprained ankle but cannot walk on a fractured one.

## Foot and Toe Injuries

In snow sports, the foot is usually held to a flat surface (e.g., a ski, snowboard, or snowshoe), and the type of boots worn generally holds the foot immobile. As a result, fractures involving the foot and toes are uncommon. However, they do occur in other winter sports (e.g., tubing and ice skating). Foot injuries occur more frequently in recreational activities and sports in which the shoes worn are soft and the foot is allowed to twist. Toe and metatarsal fractures are common, as are sprains of the mid-foot and great toe joint. Toe injuries most commonly occur when a person kicks a fixed object. The calcaneus (heel bone) is broken more often than any other tarsal bone. Landing on the heel during a jump or fall from height is the most common mechanism of injury for a calcaneal fracture. Metatarsal fractures occur frequently in jumping sports such as basketball or volleyball. The fifth metatarsal on the lateral side of the foot is most likely to be fractured (Figure 20-50■). Participants in marching, running, or other activities that continually load the bottom of the foot are subject to stress or fatigue fractures. Repetitive, slight bending (or repetitive stress) of the bone eventually causes it to crack or break.

# STOP, THINK, UNDERSTAND

## Multiple Choice

Choose the correct answer.

1. The components of a proper pelvic bone examination include _____
   a. pressing in medially on the iliac crests, palpating each buttock, and pushing inward on each hip.
   b. pressing downward on each iliac crest separately, assessing the femur, and gently and slightly lifting and extending each leg.
   c. asking patients whether or not they are able to walk.
   d. placing patients in a supine position and assessing the lower extremities for injury; if none are found, assisting patients to draw their knees up and then let them fall apart.

2. Which of the following statements regarding hip dislocation is true?_____
   a. The majority of hip dislocations occur posteriorly.
   b. Sitting while the knee is forced back is a primary cause of an anterior dislocation.
   c. Signs of an anterior hip dislocation include a knee that is internally rotated and a leg that is shorter than the other.
   d. Signs of a posterior hip dislocation include abduction of the thigh and external rotation of the knee.

3. Which of the following statements about hip dislocations is false?_____
   a. A hip dislocation is generally not a true orthopedic emergency.
   b. A hip dislocation can cause complete paralysis of the ankle and foot.
   c. The longer a hip is dislocated, the more damage will likely occur to the ball of the femur.
   d. Hip dislocations can result in debilitating arthritis later in life.

4. Which of the following statements about femur fractures is false?_____
   a. They are usually seen only in high-speed trauma in younger people.
   b. Proximal femur fractures are often referred to as "hip fractures."
   c. Femoral neck fractures occur only in younger patients.
   d. Hip fractures present with a shortened, rotated leg.

5. The most common ski injury is a_____
   a. boot-top (tib/fib) fracture.
   b. humeral dislocation.
   c. medial-collateral ligament sprain.
   d. mid-shaft femur fracture.

6. A patient's knee cap has "popped out." A correct description on the patient report would note that the patient has _____
   a. dislocated her knee cap.      c. dislocated her patella.
   b. dislocated her knee.         d. a knee deformity.

7. A patient presents with gross deformity of the knee; the proximal tibia is displaced in front of the femur, and her foot is pale and cold. This patient is suffering from what type of injury? _____
   a. a dislocated patella
   b. a dislocated knee

   c. a tibial condylar rupture
   d. a tibial-fibular supracondylar rupture

8. Which of the following statements about knee injuries is true? _____
   a. It is important to diagnose the injury in the field so that proper treatment can be rendered.
   b. It is important to do a very thorough evaluation of the knee at the accident scene.
   c. The assessment of a knee injury at the accident scene should be brief and to the point.
   d. It is important that an OEC Technician conduct a full orthopedic exam.

9. To OEC Technicians, "rolling a joint" refers to _____
   a. an activity with an illegal substance.
   b. testing the range of motion of a joint.
   c. dislocating the knee or another hinge joint.
   d. inverting or everting an ankle.

10. A hiker's complaint of pain *above* the medial malleolar ligament probably indicates the presence of a_____
    a. patellar dislocation.      c. fibular fracture only.
    b. medial malleolar fracture.  d. tib-fib fracture.

11. The best advice to give a snowboarder with lateral ankle pain is _____
    a. ice it and rest.
    b. walk it off.
    c. go see an orthopedist.
    d. OEC Technicians should not give advice.

12. Which of the following statements is true? _____
    a. A patient can walk on a sprained ankle, but not on a fractured ankle.
    b. The ability to walk is not a good indication of whether or not an ankle is fractured because patients can often walk on a fractured ankle.
    c. Patients generally cannot walk on either a fractured ankle or a sprained ankle.
    d. Patients cannot walk on a combination sprain-fracture of the ankle.

13. The most commonly fractured bone in the foot is/are the _____
    a. talus.      c. calcaneus.
    b. patella.    d. phalanges.

14. Which of the following statements about axial skeletal injuries is true?_____
    a. There are four ligaments on the lateral side of the ankle that can be potentially injured due to an inversion.
    b. The incidence of tib-fib fractures is higher in snowboarders due to the failure of their bindings to release during a fall.
    c. Rapid swelling of a knee joint is most often due to the buildup of blood.
    d. Due to the nature of knee injuries, it is critical that they be exposed and fully evaluated on scene.

*continued*

STOP, THINK, UNDERSTAND *continued*

## Matching

1. Match each of the following injuries to its MOI, description, or signs and symptoms.

   _____ 1. displaced fracture of the proximal femur

   _____ 2. mid-shaft fracture of the femur

   _____ 3. fracture of the patella

   _____ 4. proximal tibial fracture

   _____ 5. supracondylar femur fracture

   a. this fracture incidence is increasing in older skiers

   b. presents with a shortened and externally rotated leg; extremely painful, and pain may be referred to the knee

   c. characterized by severe pain, swelling just above the knee, deformity, inability to move the knee, and thigh muscle spasm; can also damage the large popliteal artery and veins and various nerves

   d. caused by direct and forceful trauma to the thigh, such as a fall or twisting injury; intensely painful, appears deformed with thigh swelling and false movement

   e. extreme force is needed for bone to fracture

2. Match each of the following injuries to its description.

   _____ 1. boot top fracture

   _____ 2. spiral fracture

   _____ 3. direct blow fracture

   _____ 4. tib-fib fracture

   a. a concurrent break of the shafts of both the tibia and the fibula

   b. a fracture in which the bone is broken transversely and may have a "butterfly" fragment

   c. a common skiing injury in which the tibia or the fibula suffers a transverse fracture

   d. an injury in which the tibia is broken in mid-shaft and the fibular shaft is broken above or below the tibial fracture

## Short Answer

1. A hip joint is what type of joint?

   _____

   _____

2. What is the valgus position?

   _____

   _____

3. List some of the causes of fractures of the metatarsals.

   _____

   _____

# Axial Skeleton Injuries

Evaluation and care for trauma to the head, neck, and spine are described in Chapter 21, Head and Spine Injuries. Significant axial injuries generally take precedence over injuries to an extremity unless severe bleeding in a limb must be managed. A patient can have both spinal trauma and an extremity injury at the same time. As a result, OEC Technicians must be able to rapidly evaluate and care for the extremity while simultaneously managing significant spinal trauma or other life-threatening problems. Injuries to the axial skeleton are associated with numerous outdoor activities, including skiing, snowboarding, snowmobiling, tubing, sledding, white-water rafting, mountain biking, and climbing. Injuries to the axial skeleton are covered in Chapter 21, Head and Spine Injuries, whereas fractures involving the sternum and ribs are covered in Chapter 23, Thoracic Trauma.

SECTION 3
# Treatment of Musculoskeletal Injuries

## ⊕ OBJECTIVES

**Upon completion of this section of this chapter, the OEC Technician will be able to:**

**20-3.1** Explain the general management of a patient with an MS injury.

**20-3.2** List and demonstrate the use of the following types of splints:

    a. sling and swathe
    b. Quick Splint
    c. soft splint
    d. rigid splint
    e. traction splint

**20-3.3** Demonstrate how to care for specific injuries to the arm or leg.

**20-3.4** Demonstrate how to remove a boot, including a ski boot.

**20-3.5** Describe and demonstrate placing a patient in the anatomical position using the principles of "jams and pretzels."

# Management

⊕ **20-3.1** Explain the general management of a patient with an MS injury.

The management of musculoskeletal injuries is the same for other injuries. Begin with a scene size-up, eliminating any hazards that may be present. Next, manage any life-threatening problems and assess ABCDs in a primary assessment. Bleeding is common with MS injuries and can be severe, especially with open fractures. Control external bleeding using the techniques described in Chapter 18, Soft-Tissue Injuries. Be sure to observe Standard Precautions. Bandage wounds appropriately, using sterile dressings that completely cover the wound. Cover exposed bone ends to keep them from becoming contaminated. When appropriate, call for ALS personnel, especially for open fractures, severely angulated extremities, and dislocations. If available, apply high-flow oxygen as needed.

The ability to differentiate one MS injury from another is difficult in the field. The general care of sprains, dislocations, and fractures is essentially the same and involves the following actions:

1. Use Standard Precautions to avoid contaminating yourself or others.
2. Formulate a plan of action early, get the right equipment for the patient's injuries, and summon EMS transport if needed. Call for ALS if there are threats to life or if pain medication may be needed.
3. Expose the zone of injury to look for abrasions, lacerations, contusions, punctures, swelling, deformity, or bleeding.
4. Bandage any wound appropriately, applying a pressure bandage if it is bleeding. Use sterile dressings, and completely cover the wound. Make sure bleeding is controlled, and check the wound frequently for additional bleeding.
5. Use the correct splint or other immobilization device for the injury. When a fracture is immobilized, it hurts less. Avoid letting an injured extremity move uncontrollably, as this may cause more tissue damage and pain. Check CMS prior to splinting.

6. Use some cooling method (e.g., ice or snow in a plastic bag) early to treat bruising or swelling. Cover the ice with a cloth or a bandage so that the skin is cooled but is not allowed to freeze.

7. Make sure the patient is comfortable during transport, especially if an extremity is immobilized in an unusual position.

8. Reassess neurovascular status of the limb frequently, and if it worsens, readjust bandages, splints, or other dressings.

9. Provide oxygen if appropriate.

10. Transport as soon as is practical to a higher level of care.

## Splinting

Splinting is a skill that all OEC Technicians should practice and master. A splint is a piece of equipment—whether commercially made, homemade, or improvised on scene—that is used to safely immobilize an extremity or other body part.

### Reasons for Splinting

Splints are used for the following reasons:

- To decrease the movement of the ends of broken bones and to allow a hematoma at the fracture site to clot. This prevents further blood loss (and for a broken femur, prevents shock).
- To decrease pain at the fracture site
- To reduce muscle spasms, by placing the limb in better anatomical alignment
- To prevent a sharp bone end from penetrating the skin and making a closed fracture an open fracture
- To prevent any further damage to soft tissues, including muscles, nerves, and blood vessels
- To allow easier transport because the body is in better anatomical alignment
- To prevent paralysis in spinal injuries (by using a back board) by limiting fractured vertebrae from moving, preventing spinal cord damage

### Types of Splints

⊕ **20-3.2** List and demonstrate the use of the following types of splints:

a. sling and swathe
b. Quick Splint
c. soft splint
d. rigid splint
e. traction splint

**sling and swathe** a soft splint used to immobilize many upper extremity injuries.

OEC Technicians have a variety of types of splints at their disposal (Figure 20-51■). Most splints may be used for a variety of injuries, although some are designed for a specific type of injury. Knowing when and how to use each type of splint effectively is one of the hallmarks of a highly trained OEC Technician.

There are four main types of splints: soft, rigid or semi-rigid, traction, and improvised.

**Soft Splints: Sling and Swathe Splints**   A **sling and swathe**, a splint that is fashioned from two triangle-shaped cravats, is the splint that OEC Technicians use most commonly. This device is used primarily to immobilize upper extremity injuries, including clavicle fractures, shoulder separations, humerus and elbow injuries, and wrist injuries (Figure 20-52■). A sling and swathe provides a stable platform for the arm and can be used to either immobilize just the arm or the arm with a separate splint in place. Properly applied, a sling and swathe holds the arm close to the body, thereby preventing further movement. It is the most commonly used splint by OEC Technicians. There are two ways to apply a sling and swathe. Depending on the injury one method may be better than the other.

**Air Splints**   An air splint is a dual-walled, tube-shaped device used to temporarily immobilize a long bone. Constructed of clear, soft plastic, an air splint is applied around an

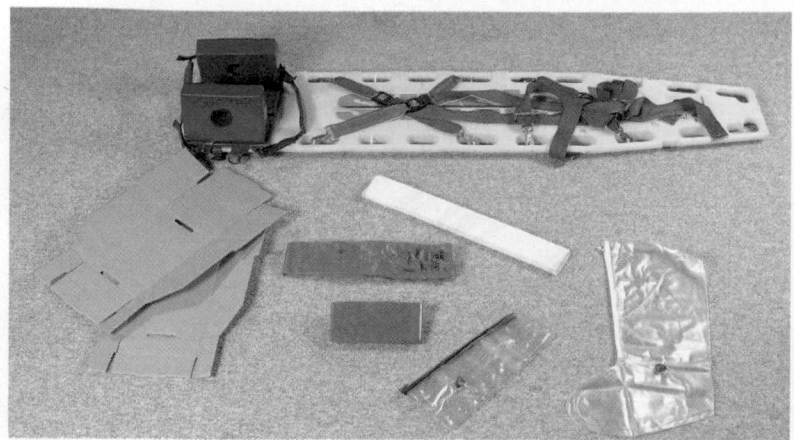

**Figure 20-51** Some examples of the many different types of commercial splints.
Copyright Edward McNamara

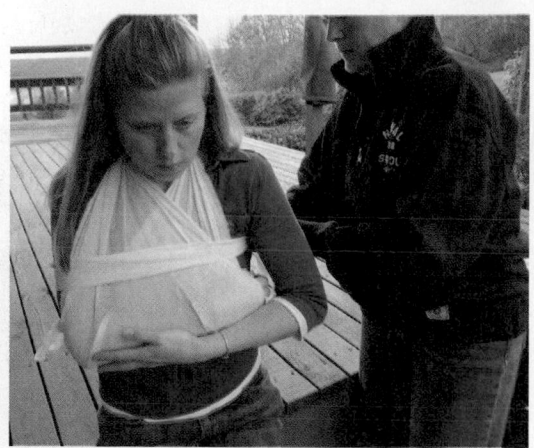

**Figure 20-52** A sling and swathe is used primarily to immobilize injured upper extremities.
Copyright Edward McNamara

extremity and secured in place, usually by a zipper. It is then inflated with air to form a rigid splint around the injured extremity. By applying constant external pressure to a wound, it also helps control bleeding. Air splints are most often used to immobilize injuries below the elbow or knee. Some air splints are specially shaped like an extremity so they can be applied to an elbow or ankle; others can splint an entire leg or arm. Air splints are commonly used within emergency care systems, where they are simple to use, inexpensive, and easier to clean than other splints (Figure 20-53■).

Despite these advantages, their use and applications in outdoor settings is limited for several reasons. First, because they are made of plastic, they can be easily punctured by sharp or abrasive objects, rendering them unusable. Second, they are affected by temperature and altitude. In very cold weather, the plastic can become stiff or brittle, making the splint difficult to use. Additionally, changes in temperature and altitude cause the air inside the splint to contract or expand, which can cause the splint to become too loose or too tight.

**Vacuum Splints** A vacuum splint is a device that consists of a closed, airtight plastic bag that contains thousands of small plastic pellets. Following its application to the injured extremity, the air is sucked out of the splint with a special pump, forming a rigid enclosure around the limb (Figure 20-54■). Vacuum splints are available in a variety of sizes, ranging from small ankle or forearm splints to full-body splints used to immobilize the spine. Vacuum splints provide excellent insulation in cold weather. Conversely, they can cause heat retention in warm or hot weather. Also, it is not possible to apply an ice or other cold compress over the splint, because the cold cannot penetrate this splint. And like air splints, vacuum splints can be easily punctured. Despite this, vacuum splints are widely used in Europe and are becoming more widely used in North America, including by ski patrols.

**Blanket Roll/Pillow Splint** A blanket can be fashioned into a splint to fit around or beside nearly any joint, whether large (e.g., shoulder, knee) or small (e.g., elbow, ankle). When fashioned into a tight roll, a blanket is especially effective for injuries in which patients will not allow their arm to be brought to their side, such as a shoulder dislocation.

For shoulder injuries that need to be held firmly with the elbow away from the body, fashion a blanket into a special splint known as a blanket roll splint. A blanket roll can also be used under a knee as a splint. Creation of this splint and its application is described in detail later in this chapter. Pillows and other soft materials can also be used effectively to splint various joint injuries, most notably elbow and ankle injuries, especially when these joints are severely deformed (Figure 20-55■).

**Figure 20-53** Air splints are easier to use within the emergency care system.

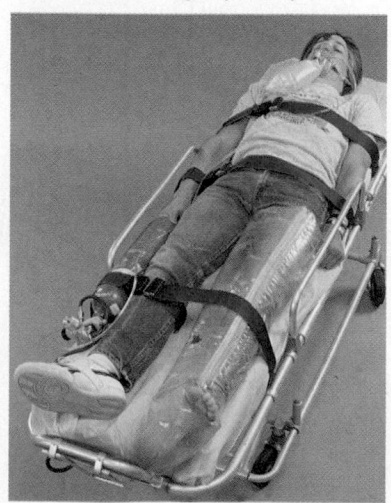

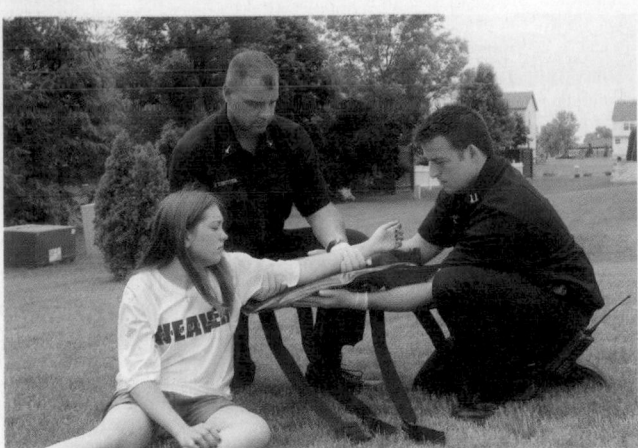

**Figure 20-54** A vacuum splint in use on an injured arm.

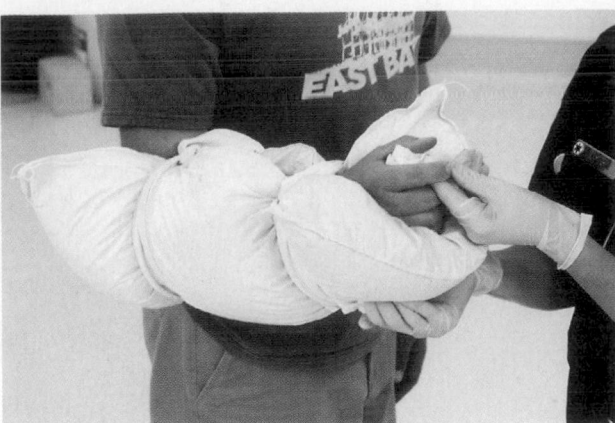

**Figure 20-55** A pillow splint can be used on wrist and hand injuries when rigid splints are not available.

**Pelvic Binders**   Because fractures of the pelvis often cause life-threatening blood loss, they are among the most devastating musculoskeletal injuries. Similar to fractures of the spine, pelvic fractures should be stabilized emergently in the field, if possible before the patient is transported. Two methods of pelvic binding are commonly used to manage these injuries: a sheet wrap and a commercial pelvic sling (Figure 20-56■). Refer to Chapter 24, Abdominal and Pelvic Trauma for details regarding how to apply a pelvic binder.

### Rigid or Semi-Rigid Splints

**Cardboard, Wood, or Metal Splints**   As the name implies, rigid splints are constructed of stiff materials such as heavy cardboard, wood, or metal. OEC Technicians commonly use these splints because of their reliability, low cost, effectiveness in all weather and altitude conditions, and ease of use. Some are available commercially, whereas others may be fashioned from readily available materials and are just as effective (Figure 20-57■). Rigid splints are applied to the sides, front, and/or back of an injured limb and are generally held in place by roller gauze (bandage) or cravats (Figure 20-58■). Cardboard splints are used primarily to splint an arm or leg

**Figure 20-56** A SAM™ pelvic sling.
Copyright Candace Horgen

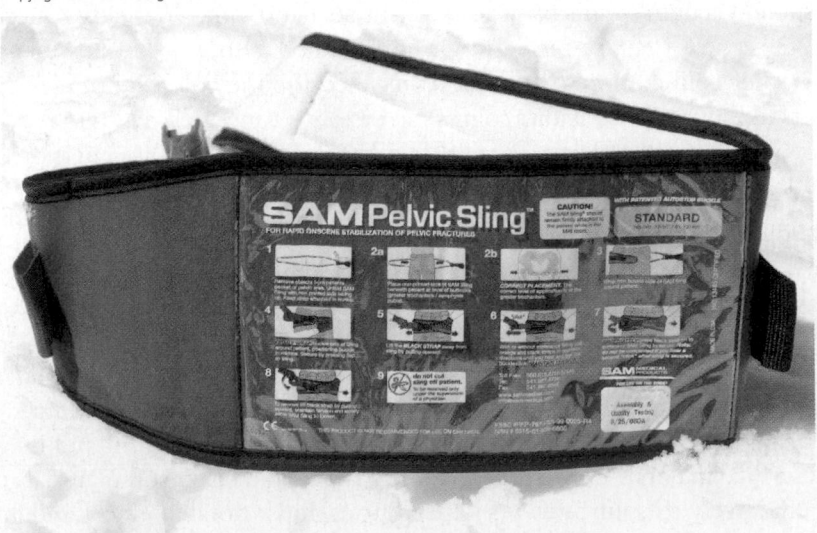

(Figure 20-59a■). Cardboard splints are best used in dry environments unless they are specially treated with a water-resistant coating (Figure 20-59b■).

Although cardboard splints are commercially available, they are easy to make using corrugated cardboard. The most useful splint to hold a lower leg firmly is 15 inches by 42 inches, with folds and cuts placed in the correct places. For an elbow or a forearm, a double thickness of cardboard 3 inches by 12 to 15 inches is effective.

Wood splints are more rigid than cardboard and provide very effective immobilization. Like cardboard splints, wood splints are available commercially or can be homemade. Some commercial wood splints are padded and are enclosed in a water-resistant shell. Homemade splints should be sanded smooth on all sides and sealed to prevent splintering. Wood splints are available in a variety of sizes; they may be constructed of quarter-inch exterior-grade plywood, 3 inches wide and 12 to 15 inches long. Some are as long as 36 inches. Wood splints are commonly used to immobilize long bones (radius, ulna, humerus, tibia, and fibula) and joints (elbow, knee, and wrist).

**Quick Splint** The Quick Splint has been used by ski patrols for many years. Made of lightweight plastic or plywood, they are the mainstay of care for lower leg injuries among ski patrollers. They are especially effective for knee, tibia, or fibula injuries. A Quick Splint is easy to use and may be applied rapidly by one or two people. Its compact design allows it to easily fit on a fully loaded toboggan.

**Airplane Splint** An airplane splint is a special-purpose rigid splint fabricated from two 4-inch by 12-inch wooden boards that are held together with a hinge that allows the device to be adjusted to different angles. The splint is secured into position with cravats. It may be used in conjunction with a Quick Splint to secure an injured knee in the bent position (Figure 20-60■). It may also be used in place of a blanket roll to hold an arm up in a shoulder injury.

**Malleable Metal Splints** These splints are made of lightweight aluminum or wire mesh. As their name implies, malleable splints can be molded to fit the injured

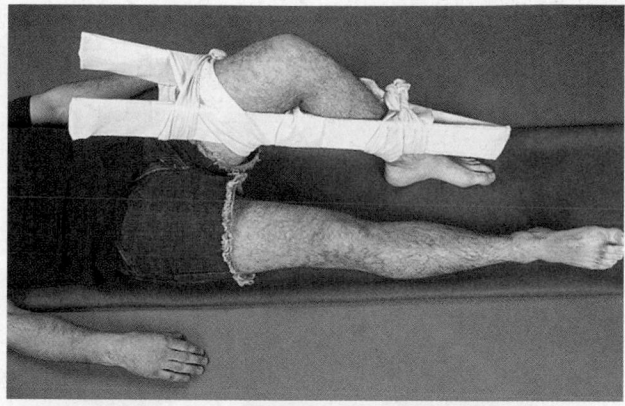
**Figure 20-57** An example of a rigid splint.

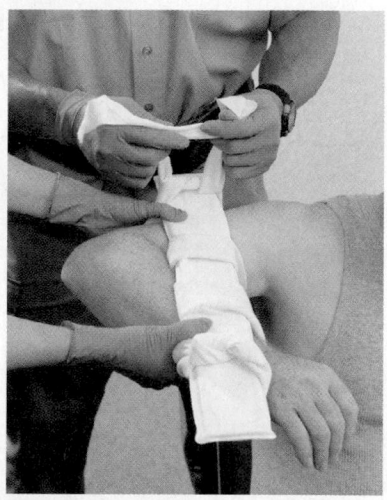
**Figure 20-58** Rigid splints are held in place with roller gauze or cravats.

**Figure 20-59b** Cardboard splints are used in dry environments to splint an arm or leg.
Copyright Edward McNamara

**Figure 20-59a** A cardboard splint.
Copyright Edward McNamara

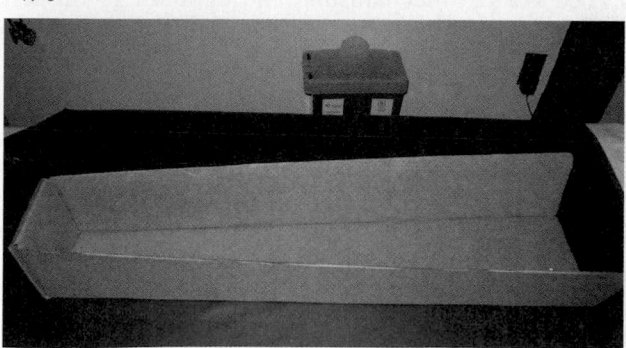

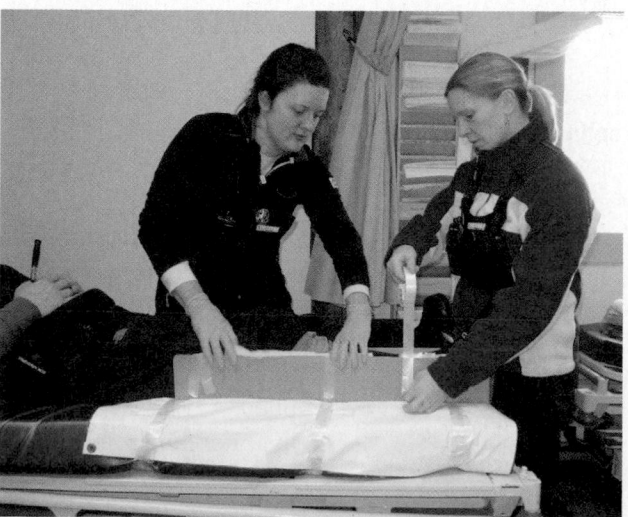

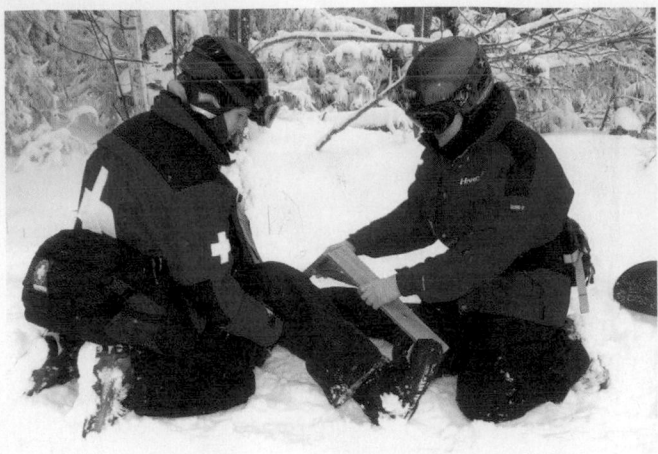

**Figure 20-60** An airplane splint being applied.
Copyright Edward McNamara

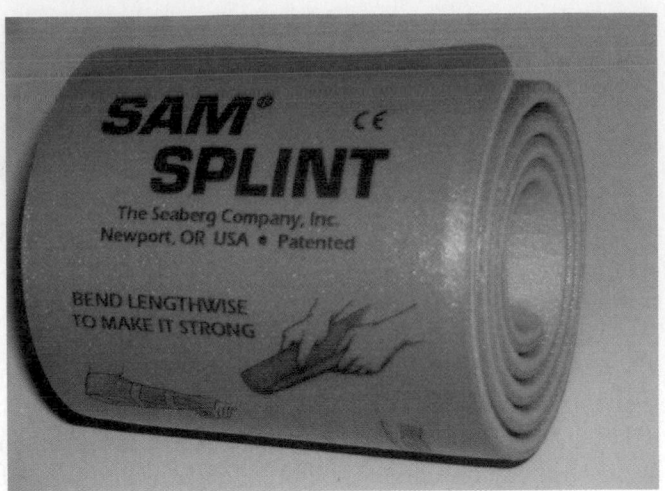

**Figure 20-61** A SAM™ splint.
Copyright John Dobson, M.D.

extremity. Wire, ladder, and padded aluminum splints are commercially available. You can also fabricate a ladder or wire splint from wire mesh obtained from a hardware store. These splints can be shaped to fit precisely around an elbow or ankle joint in a *sugar tong* configuration. They can also immobilize a body part in either the position it was found or a position of function. Once applied, a roller bandage or several cravats hold the splint in place. Wire and ladder splints generally come in 3-inch by 30- or 36-inch sizes and can be folded to fit in a backpack. Metal splints should be padded for the patient's comfort.

The SAM™ Splint is a 4-inch by 36-inch piece of malleable aluminum that is covered on both sides by a thin layer of foam (Figure 20-61■). Developed by orthopedic surgeon Sam Scheinberg upon his return from the Vietnam War, the SAM™ (Structural, Aluminum, Malleable) splint is used by the U.S. military and is very popular among emergency and rescue professionals worldwide. It can be easily shaped to better conform to the patient's anatomy or position and comes packaged as a 3-inch cylinder for easy transportation. If one looks at the original scheme of how to apply a SAM™ Splint, it involves creasing the splint for its entire length in the middle, making a short "T" of the splint, with the bottom of the "T" doubled, so it is rigid. Without the "T", when applied it takes the shape of a "U" and is less rigid. Applying a SAM™ Splint involves folding and molding the material into shapes that are rigid and firmly immobilize the injured extremity.

### Traction Splints

A **traction splint** is a device that applies longitudinal traction to a fractured long bone. In emergency care, **traction** is defined as a safe mechanism for straightening a broken bone. *Longitudinal* traction is the placement of an in-line force to a fractured long bone in the direction of its normal alignment for the purpose of regaining bone length and reducing pain. Traction aligns the limb in a more anatomically neutral position, preventing further soft-tissue damage. By immobilizing the fracture site, the splint also helps to reduce blood loss. Because excessive traction is harmful to an injured limb, OEC Technicians should set and control the amount of traction being applied. A traction splint does not reduce a fracture, but it does align the fractured bone in a more anatomically favorable position.

Many different types of femoral traction splints are commercially available, including splints made by Sager, Kendrick, and Hare (Figure 20-62■). Although each

**traction splint**   a splint used on a lower extremity to align a fracture, such as a mid-shaft fracture of the femur.

**traction**   the amount of force required to straighten a limb and keep it in alignment; for a fractured femur, typically 10 percent of the patient's body weight, or approximately 15 pounds.

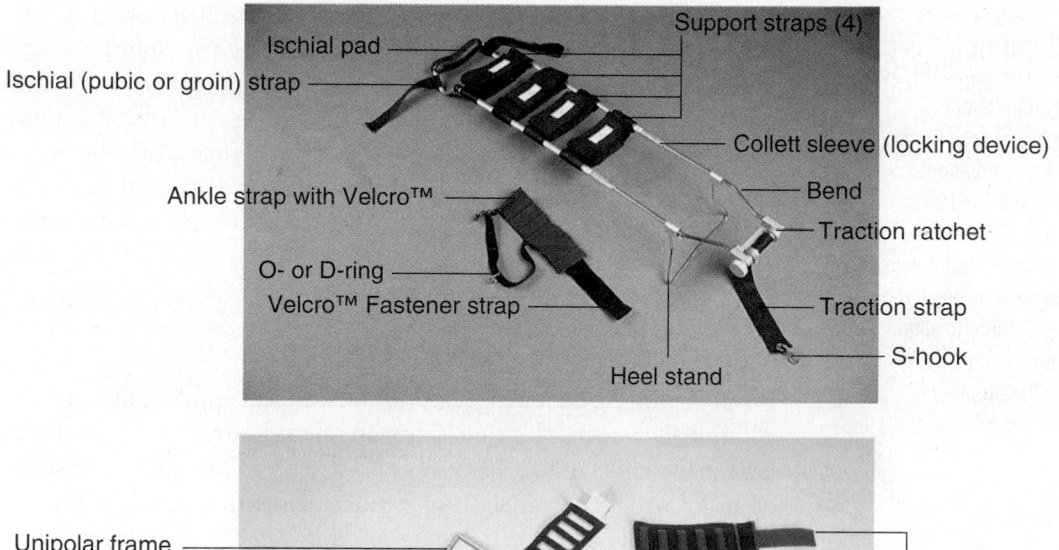

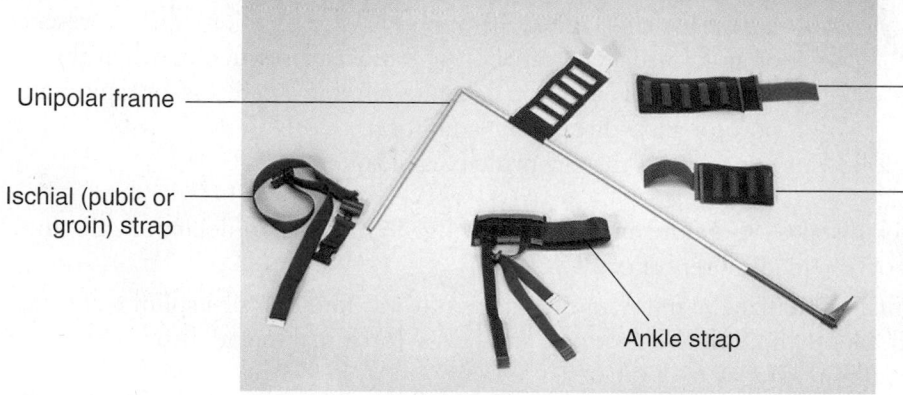

**Figure 20-62**  Commercially available traction splints.

has its own advantages and "ease of use," they work in a similar fashion by splinting the femur exerting mild traction (Figure 20-63■).

Traction splints are used primarily for fractures involving the middle third of the femur. Recently, some EMS authors and traction splint manufacturers (Sager) have advocated the use of these devices, *using tension*, for proximal femur fractures, including classical hip fractures. In fact, they now encourage this splint's use for these injuries, especially if the fractures were produced by high-energy forces (frequently seen in extreme velocity snow sports accidents). Check with both your local medical advisor and the manufacturer of your traction device to determine if your equipment may be used in this manner. Traction splints are contraindicated in fractures of the distal third of the femur, as is its use on any upper extremity fracture.

The Hare splint has also been reported to have been used successfully with less tension applied for tibial shaft fractures. In this setting, the Velcro™ attachments applied below the knee and above the ankle (but not over the fracture site) help hold the tibia in position. If no other device is available, a traction splint could be used in this fashion. However, a Quick Splint is a better choice for a tibia fracture. A femoral traction splint with stabilizing rods on either side can be used in a "floating knee" (a fracture of the femur and tibia in the same leg), as discussed later.

## Improvised Splints

Occasionally, you may need a splint but find that one is not readily available. In these instances, an effective splint may be fashioned from available materials. For instance, a magazine can be made into

### Thomas Splint

The original lower extremity traction splint was developed by British surgeon Dr. Hugh Owen Thomas in 1875 and dubbed "The Knee Appliance" (Figure 20-64■). It received great reviews for its use in helping wounded soldiers during World War I. When applied, this device prevented hypovolemic shock by allowing the hematoma from a femur fracture to stabilize.

**Figure 20-63**  A Hare traction splint.
Copyright E. M. Singletary, MD

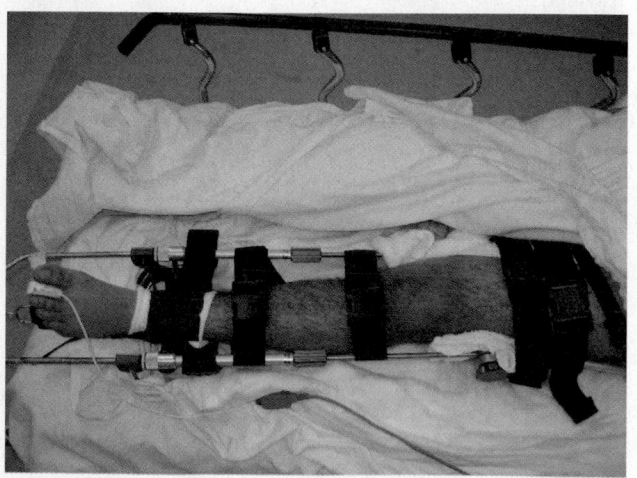

### Traction versus Tension

When applying a traction splint for certain femur fractures, OEC Technicians must apply *traction* to align the leg. This requires pulling on the foot with about 15 pounds of force. The force of traction should be no more than 10 percent of total body weight. When alignment is necessary for other long bone fractures, *tension* is used. Tension involves pulling with less force, generally 7 to 8 pounds, or only enough force to align the bone. If the patient complains that you are pulling too hard, release some tension. After the proper application of traction or tension, patients will generally tell you that the limb feels better.

a splint for a forearm, a foot, or an ankle (Figure 20-65a■). A plastic cooking utensil or a Popsicle™ stick can be used to splint a finger when a tongue blade is not available. Larger splints can be made from ski poles, tree branches, oars, or any other long, stiff object (Figure 20-65b■). There are countless ways to splint an extremity. Imaginative OEC Technicians who understand the principles of splinting, both for immobilization and traction, can treat nearly any extremity injury they encounter. Use an improvised splint only if the one commonly used for the injury is not available.

### Principles of Splinting

Proper splinting requires a careful, methodical approach to prevent additional damage. As a rule, splint an injured extremity before moving the patient (Figures 20-66a–e■). The exceptions are the presence of an immediate hazard to the patient or rescuer, or when the patient's general condition demands *immediate* care and/or rapid transport for a life-threatening condition.

The following list presents the key principles of splinting:

+ Check distal CMS before and after splinting. Remember to document the findings on the medical report or PCR.
+ Manually stabilize the injury in the position it was found until a splint can be applied. Gently hold the bones above and below (proximal to and distal to) the suspected injury site.
+ Select an appropriate splint.
+ Properly size the splint. Ideally, the splint should span the joint above and the joint below the injury. If the fracture involves a long bone such as the radius, size the splint using the uninjured arm as a guide. If both arms are injured, use your judgment in sizing the splint. Malleable splints should be shaped to match the injured extremity (make all adjustments away from the injury so as not to accidently move the injured area).
+ Pad the splint (if needed) to maximize the patient's comfort. This is especially important if the patient will be moved over rough or uneven terrain.
+ Position the splint. Place the splint next to the injured area or gently slide the splint under or around the extremity.

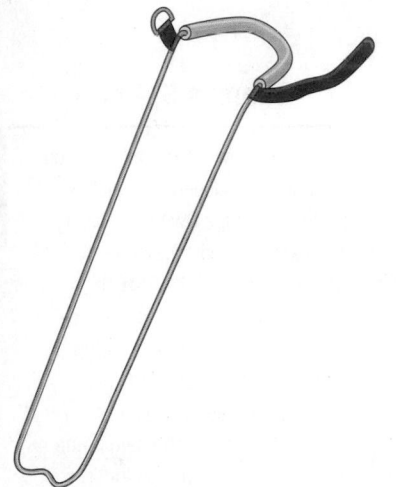

**Figure 20-64** A Thomas splint.

**Figure 20-65a** The use of a magazine as a splint.

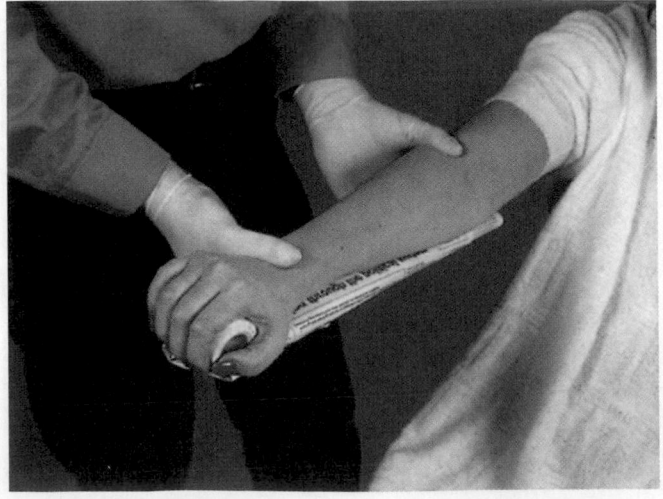

**Figure 20-65b** A variety of items can be used as splints.

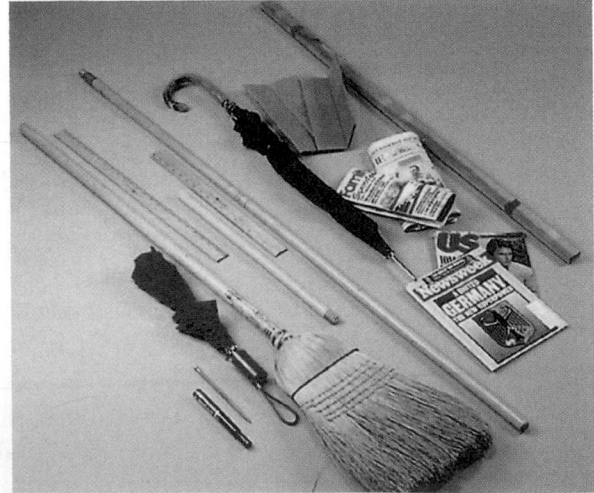

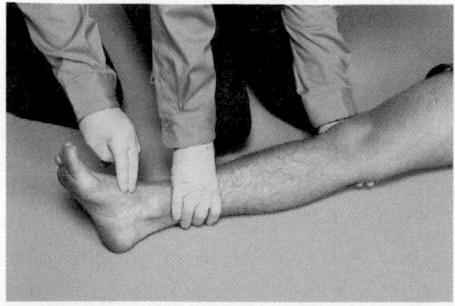

**Figure 20-66a** Assess circulation, motor, and sensory functions.

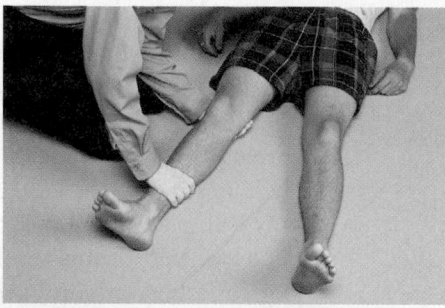

**Figure 20-66b** Manually stabilize the injured limb.

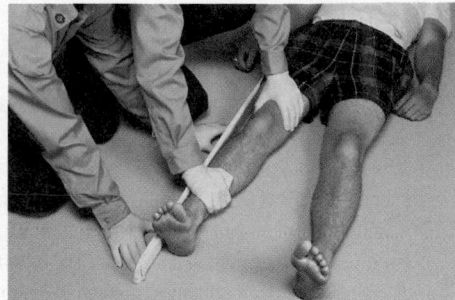

**Figure 20-66c** Measure the splint.

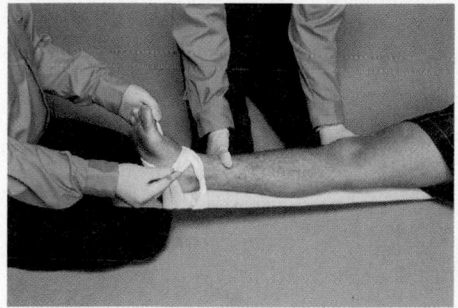

**Figure 20-66d** Position the splint by sliding it next to or under the limb and then immobilize the joint above and below the injury.

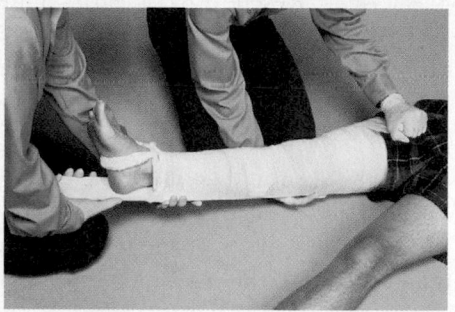

**Figure 20-66e** Secure the splint with gauze or roller bandage. Recheck CMS.

+ Secure the splint. Use roller gauze, cravats, or tape to secure the injured body part(s) to the splint. Be careful not to make the splint too tight because doing so can affect distal neurovascular status.
+ Again assess CMS, and adjust the splint if now compromised. Record your findings.

For fractures of a long bone shaft with obvious deformity, follow this procedure:

1. Use gentle longitudinal *tension* to align the upper arm or the lower leg for angulated/rotated injuries so that a splint may be applied.
2. Use gentle in-line *traction* to align femur fractures so that a traction splint can be applied. Alignment is important whenever the extremity is in a state of vascular or neurologic compromise (Figure 20-67■).

If the patient exhibits signs and symptoms of significant shock, quickly attempt to align the injured limb(s) as close to normal anatomical position as possible. Place an injured arm to the chest and splint it anatomically, or an injured leg to the other leg and put the patient on a spine board (total body immobilization), and then treat for shock and provide rapid transport.

At times, placing an injured extremity into anatomical position before splinting may be difficult if not impossible. These circumstances include patients with open fractures, severely angulated fractures, dislocations, or fracture-dislocations close to a joint; patients or children who will not let you move the injured limb; and patients with an impaled object in the injured extremity. Elbow, shoulder, hip, and knee injuries with deformity may need to be immobilized using some creativity. When faced with

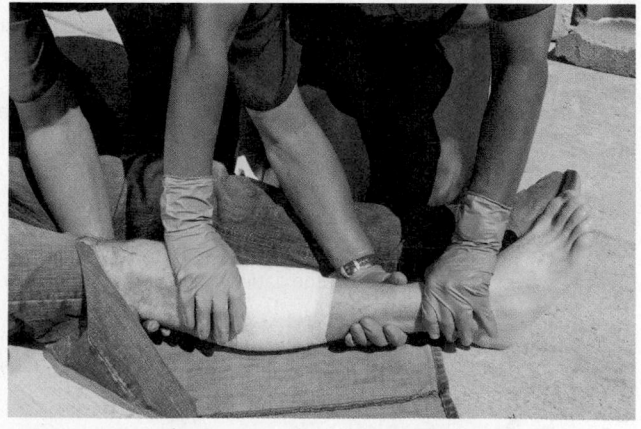

**Figure 20-67** Use gentle longitudinal tension to align an extremity.

### Wilderness Rescue Tip

If you will be unable to get a patient with a bone end protruding through the skin to a higher level of care for more than 8 hours, attempt to place the bone back into the body. The cells of a bone end that remain outside the body for too long will die. Wash the fracture site with sterile water or saline and then put the bone back into the body using gentle axial tension. If a sterile solution is not available, use clean water, boiled (and cooled) water, or disinfected water. Never use water from a pond or creek. This course of action may also be necessary on a cruise ship that is hours from port or hours outside of rescue helicopter range.

these situations, remember the previously described principles, place the limb in the most comfortable, best immobilized position possible, and transport the patient.

OEC Technicians should neither attempt to set (reduce) a fracture nor *force* exposed bone fragments of an open fracture back into their normal anatomic alignment, especially when the injury involves the femur. These procedures are the physician's responsibility. However, if bone ends do go back into the wound below the skin, as is a common occurrence with the proper application of a traction splint, leave the bones where they are and communicate to the EMS personnel that the fracture was open. See the Wilderness Rescue Tip to learn about an exception to this guideline.

If you cannot apply a splint before moving the patient, such as one impaled on a fixed object, maintain manual traction or manual immobilization until the patient is free from the object, and then splint the injury. As described in a previous chapter, impaled objects should generally be left in place.

If ecchymosis or local edema is present, control bruising and swelling early on by applying cold packs or ice or snow in a plastic bag, if available. Be sure to place a cloth or bandage between the ice and skin to avoid local cold injury. Make the patient as comfortable as possible during transport, especially when an immobilized extremity is in an unusual position.

Reassess neurovascular status of the limb frequently, and if it worsens, readjust bandages, splints, or other dressings as needed.

## STOP, THINK, UNDERSTAND

### Multiple Choice
Choose the correct answer.

1. In assessing a trauma patient who complains of severe ankle pain, your appropriate course of care is_____
   a. to assess the injury and determine whether or not the ankle is sprained or fractured, and treat it based on this determination.
   b. ask the patient to walk on it to help you determine what type of care you should provide.
   c. treat a sprain, a dislocation, or a fracture the same.
   d. treat a fracture or dislocation the same but differently from a sprain.

2. While realigning an open, protruding fracture, the exposed bone fragment slides back under the skin. Which of the following actions should you take? _____
   a. Complete the splinting, extrication, and transportation, and communicate to EMS personnel during handoff that the fracture was open.
   b. Immediately stop realigning the limb, splint as it is, and transport the patient immediately.
   c. Return the limb to the position in which you originally found it, splint it, transport the patient immediately, and notify EMS of the open fracture.
   d. Apply immediate tension or increased traction to the limb, transport the patient rapidly, and notify EMS of the situation.

3. You are sailing in the Caribbean on a friend's boat when a member of your group falls and suffers an open tibial fracture from which the bone end is obviously protruding. Given that it may take you 12 hours to reach help, what is your best course of action?_____
   a. Gently clean the wound/bone end with sterilized water, apply gentle tension until the bone end is pulled back under the skin, and then bandage and splint the limb.
   b. Gently clean and bandage the wound, and then splint it in the position found so as not to disturb the bone end.
   c. Cover the wound and bone with a moist, sterile dressing, then apply traction and splint.
   d. Bandage (but not splint) the injury until after medics arrive.

4. Which of the following statements correctly describes the next correct action to take immediately after splinting an injury?_____
   a. Document the type, time, and location of the splint onto your IRF (incident report form).
   b. Remember to loosen and retighten the splint every 15 minutes to increase circulation and prevent tissue damage.
   c. Apply an ice pack.
   d. Check distal CMS.

*continued*

5. When should you check CMS on an injured extremity?

_____

a. before and after splinting
b. after splinting only
c. if the patient complains of parasthesia
d. only if you feel you need to

6. Which of the following describes the purpose of a traction splint? (check all that apply)

_____ a. to apply longitudinal traction to a bone
_____ b. to apply in-line force to a fractured bone

_____ c. to regain bone length
_____ d. to reduce pain
_____ e. to place a limb in a more anatomically correct position
_____ f. to contain blood loss
_____ g. to reduce a fracture
_____ h. to produce stabilization of a humeral fracture
_____ i. to reduce tension for a proximal femur fracture
_____ j. to produce tension for a patellar fracture
_____ k. to produce traction for a distal femur fracture

## Short Answer

1. For each of the following injuries, list the type or types of splint you would use.

a. wrist fracture_____
b. femur fracture_____
c. ankle fracture_____
d. vertebral fracture_____
e. clavicular fracture_____

f. hip or pelvic fracture_____
g. humeral fracture_____
h. shoulder dislocation_____
i. finger fracture_____

2. List six items you could use to make an improvised splint, and explain the type of injury for which each improvised splint could be used.

_____

_____

_____

_____

_____

_____

3. List three of the seven key principles of splinting.

_____

_____

_____

## Fill in the Blank

1. Traction means applying approx. _____ lb of force.

2. Tension means applying _____ lb of force.

## Caring for Specific Extremity Injuries

Although there is some overlap in the care of extremity injuries, certain fractures, dislocations, or MS injuries require unique care. The methods described in this section, although commonly used by OEC Technicians and other emergency medicine professionals around the world, may differ slightly from area to area due to local protocols or a medical director's guidance. Remember, when faced with significant trauma with life-threatening injuries, the first priority of OEC Technicians is to get the patient to a higher level of care rapidly without causing any further harm.

⊕ 20-3.3 Demonstrate how to care for specific injuries to the arm or leg.

### Upper Extremity Injuries

When providing emergency care to any patient with an injured upper extremity, *be sure to remove rings, bracelets, and any other jewelry from the wrist or fingers* early in the process, before significant swelling occurs. (If possible, put jewelry on the *other*, uninjured arm or hand.) Be sure to document this on the patient care report and keep the jewelry safe.

### Shoulder, Clavicle, and Scapula Injuries

Nearly all of these injuries can be treated with a sling and swathe. During transport, patients may wish to remain sitting or may prefer lying on the unaffected side. To apply a sling and swathe, follow this procedure (OEC Skill 20-1■):

1. Assess CMS.
2. Rescuer #1: Support the patient's elbow while it is bent to about a 90 degree angle.
3. Rescuer #2:
   - Place a triangle bandage on the patient's chest, under the injured arm.
   - Position the long edge of the bandage so that it lies opposite the mid-clavicular line and just medial to the fingertips of the injured arm. The upper corner should pass over the opposite shoulder, and the apex of the triangle should be just beyond the elbow of the injured arm.
   - Fold the lower corner of the bandage anteriorly around the forearm, and then up and over the shoulder on the injured side.
   - Raise or lower the arm to an appropriate level at which it will remain.
   - Tie the two long ends of the sling together at *the side of the neck* (to prevent pressure on the back of the neck); if the knot is placed over the midline of the neck, pad it for the patient's comfort.
   - Bring the apex forward and pin it to the front of the sling, or tie a knot in the apex.
   - Reassess CMS.

Make sure the tips of the fingers are visible to allow for CMS checks. Properly applied, the forearm should be cradled in the sling, with its weight evenly distributed.

To make the swathe:

1. Fold a second triangular bandage to form a cravat that is 2–4 inches wide (or wider, for humerus fractures).
2. Wrap the cravat around the patient's chest, with the middle of the swathe over the injured arm that is resting on the side of the chest. Place the two ends of the swathe under the opposite arm.
3. Tie the two ends snugly with a square knot.

The following alternate method of applying a sling avoids placing any pressure on the injured shoulder or a fractured clavicle (Figures 20-69a■ and 20-69b■). Always check CMS before and after applying the sling.

1. Rescuer #1: Support the patient's elbow while it is bent to just under a 90 degree angle.
2. Rescuer #2:
   - Lay the long corner of the triangle bandage across the patient's chest and over the uninjured shoulder in the mid-clavicular line, as before.

---

### How to Tie a Square Knot?

**NOTE**

A square knot is a very useful knot for securing a cravat. To tie a square knot, follow these instructions (Figures 20-68a-d■):

1. Cross End A over End B to form an "X."
2. Wrap End A around End B.
3. Cross End A over End B again.
4. Wrap End A around End B.
5. Pull on both ends at the same time to tighten.

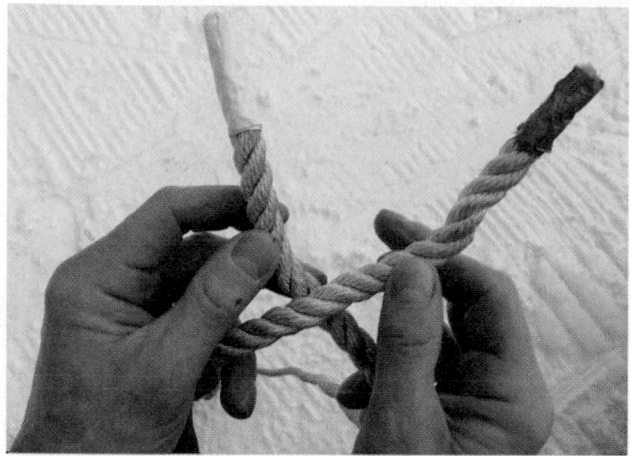

**Figure 20-68a** Cross End A over End B to form an "X."
Copyright Edward McNamara

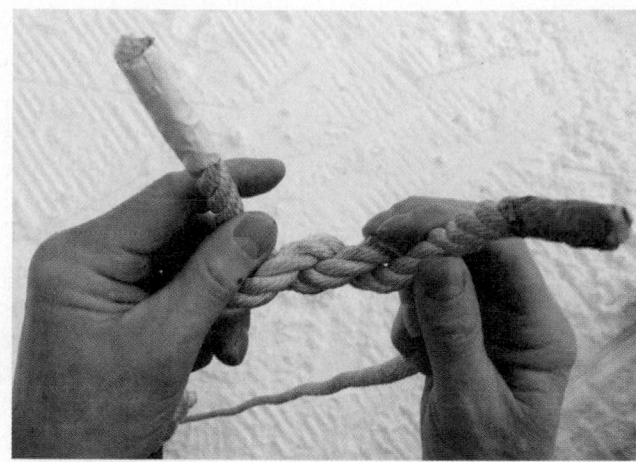

**Figure 20-68b** Wrap End A around End B.
Copyright Edward McNamara

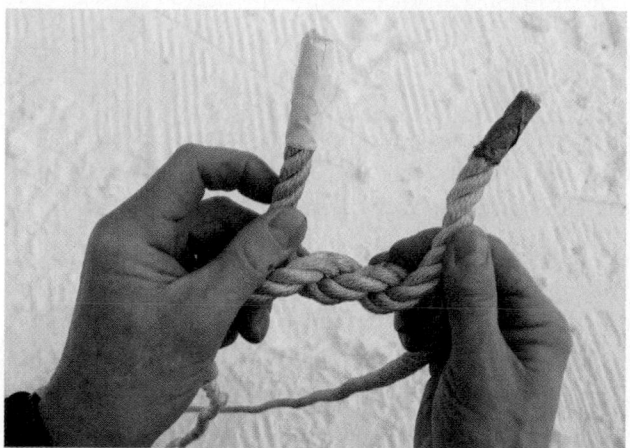

**Figure 20-68c** Cross End A over End B.
Copyright Edward McNamara

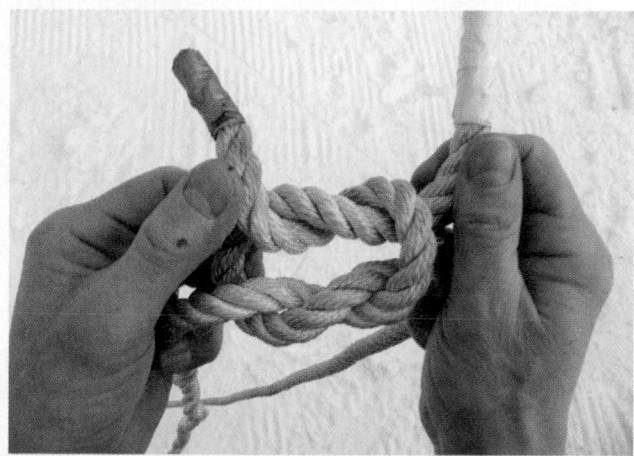

**Figure 20-68d** Wrap End A around End B and pull on both ends to tighten.
Copyright Edward McNamara

**Figure 20-69b** Bring the other end of the cravat up around the forearm and under the axilla. Tie the corner to the opposite upper corner behind the patient's back.
Copyright Edward McNamara

**Figure 20-69a** Lay one end of cravat across the patient's chest.
Copyright Edward McNamara

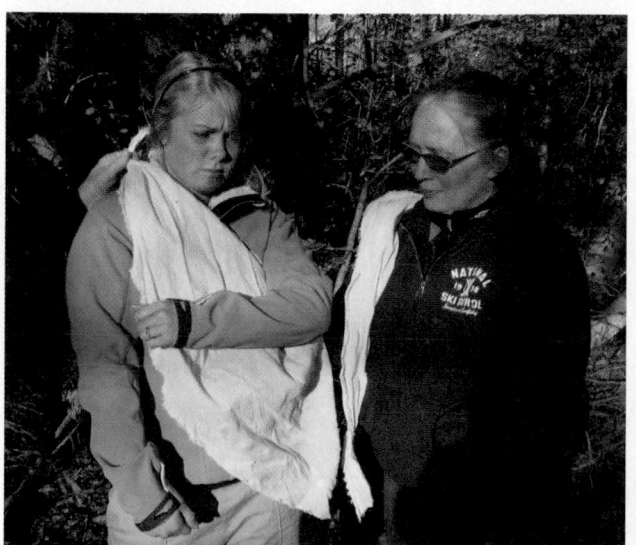

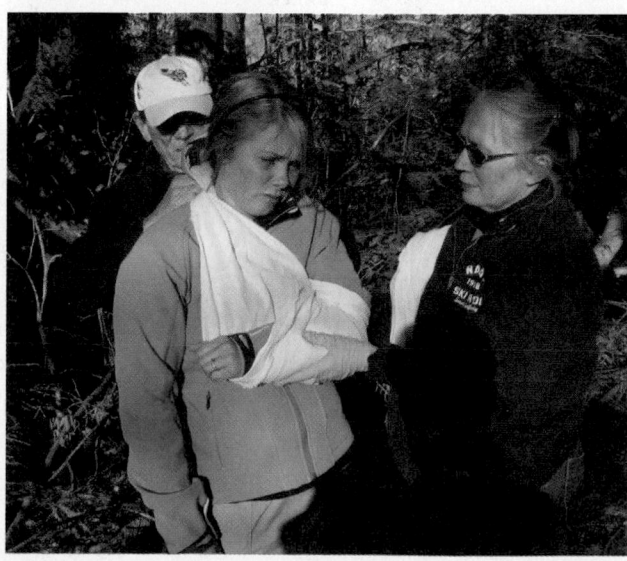

- Bring the other corner of the sling up and around the forearm and under the near axilla.
- Tie this corner to the opposite upper corner *behind the patient's back* to keep pressure off of the injured clavicle.

**3.** Tie the swathe around the patient's chest and forearm rather than around the injured part of the upper arm.

Another method for immobilizing a clavicle fracture is a figure eight splint. This device can be purchased commercially or made using two cravats. This method is used to immobilize fractures of the proximal and middle thirds of the clavicle. It should not be used for fractures of the distal third of the clavicle because the cravat could be placed directly over the fracture site, causing additional pain. The figure eight splint may actually immobilize the clavicle better and provide more pain relief, and it should normally be used in conjunction with a sling and swathe. However, a figure eight splint is not used for acromioclavicular (A/C) injuries.

To create and apply a figure eight splint (OEC Skill 20-2■):

**1.** Place the patient in a sitting position.
**2.** Check CMS.
**3.** Place one cravat around each shoulder (over and under the armpit). The ends to be tied should be placed behind the patient. Make sure the front of the cravat has a wide band. Do not place the band directly over the fracture site.
**4.** Cross the ends of the cravats that are behind the patient to make a "figure eight."
**5.** Tighten the cravats, and tie the ends together using two square knots, so that the positions of the shoulders are the same as if the patient were sitting normally.
**6.** Tighten the figure eight until the patient's shoulders are in normal posture and are not pulled too far back.
**7.** Check CMS.

For management of a posterior sternoclavicular (S/C) dislocation without severe vascular compromise or breathing difficulty, use a sling and swathe. When a vascular or respiratory threat to life is present, OEC Technicians should attempt to reduce the clavicle, or the patient could die rapidly. Although this practice is controversial, it is taught in most comprehensive wilderness texts and should be initiated without delay.

Follow this procedure to reduce a posterior S/C dislocation (see OEC Skill 20-3■):

**1.** Place the patient in a supine position.
**2.** Check CMS.
**3.** Place a tight blanket roll between the patient's shoulder blades to elevate the thorax off the ground.
**4.** Using two rescuers, apply simultaneous traction/counter-traction:
- Rescuer #1: Apply traction to the arm on the affected side by holding the wrist and pulling the arm out from the body and toward the ground (posteriorly).
- Rescuer #2: Apply counter-traction by pulling on the other side of the body using a broad cravat placed across the upper chest and upper back.
- Check CMS.

An alternative one-person method for reducing a posterior S/C dislocation involves placing the rescuer's knee in the center of the patient's upper back while the patient is sitting. The rescuer applies force by pulling back hard on the shoulders to get the proximal end of the clavicle to slip out from behind the sternum and off the trachea, esophagus, and vena cava. Following reduction, apply a figure eight splint holding the clavicle out from behind the sternum, and then apply a swathe. The patient will probably want to sit up for transport. If the posterior S/C dislocation does not reduce, provide oxygen and rapidly transport the patient to a higher level of care.

Anterior S/C dislocations require minimal care and are best managed using a sling and swathe applied in the manner previously described.

Care of an anterior dislocated shoulder requires OEC Technicians to use patience and sometimes creativity. As a rule, OEC Technicians do not attempt to reduce a dislocated shoulder. If you encounter patients who have a history of dislocated shoulders and ask you to assist in reducing their shoulder, do not do so. Instead, immobilize the patient's shoulder in a position of comfort using a blanket roll or airplane splint and encourage the person to seek medical attention for reduction.

To apply a blanket roll splint to a shoulder, perform the following steps (OEC Skill 20-4■):

1. Rescuer #1:
   - Place an open blanket on a flat surface. Fold it longitudinally in thirds or fourths lengthwise according to how large a splint you need based on the deformity of the injured shoulder.
   - Place four cravats crosswise on one end of the folded blanket. For identification purposes later you may tie knots in the ends of cravats (i.e., one in #1, two in #2 etc.) so that you will be able to identify the corresponding ends of the cravats when you go to tighten and then tie them.
   - Roll the blanket firmly, including the cravats.
   - Check CMS.
   - Position/place the roll snugly up in the axilla (armpit) of the dislocated shoulder. Hold the roll in place.
2. Rescuer #2:
   - Tie one of the cravats over the opposite shoulder and around the neck.
   - Tie the other cravat around the patient's waist.
   - Stabilize the hand and forearm on the blanket with the other two cravats.
3. Reassess CMS.

In the rare situation in which the patient's arm is unable to be brought down onto the blanket roll, stabilize the injured arm with cravats in the best way possible to avoid movement. The latter is best accomplished in a toboggan or on a litter with the patient in a semi-sitting position, sometimes with another OEC Technician sitting behind the patient.

## Humerus Fractures

Fractures involving the humeral shaft often need to be realigned by applying *gentle longitudinal tension* before they can be splinted. Tell the patient to expect some discomfort before applying tension, a splint, and a sling and swathe. If the patient resists your alignment effort, or if any movement to restore normal anatomical alignment is too painful, splint the arm in the position you found it using a rigid splint.

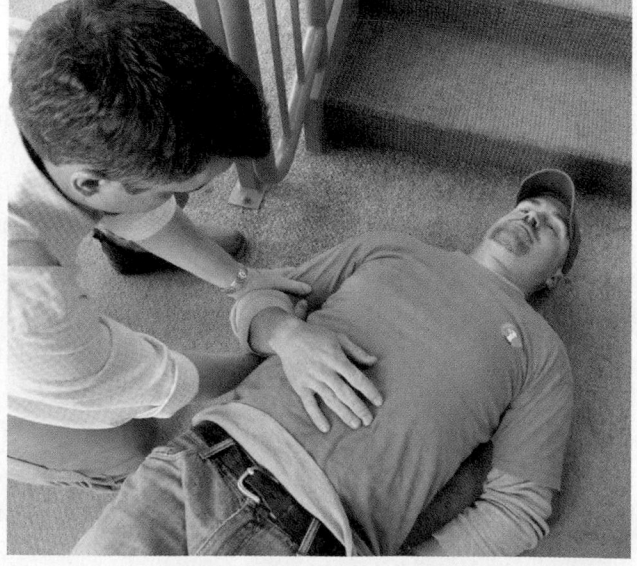

**Figure 20-70** To align the humerus, place the patient in a supine position and apply gentle longitudinal tension.
Copyright Edward McNamara

To realign a displaced fractured humerus (Figure 20-70■):

1. Place the patient in a supine position.
2. Assess CMS.
3. With the flattened palm of one hand, support the humeral shaft along the posterior surface of the humerus, just above the elbow.
4. Grasp the anterior surface of the distal humerus, just above the elbow, with the other hand.
5. Apply gentle longitudinal tension (not traction) down from the shoulder in line with the normal axis of the humerus while the upper arm is held along the side of the patient's body. The patient's forearm should be placed with the elbow at a 90 degree angle in contact with the patient's abdomen. You are not reducing the fracture, but aligning it for better pain control and packaging.
6. Once normal length and improved alignment of the arm are achieved, continue to stabilize the limb by holding it in place with a sling and swathe using a rigid splint along the humeral shaft and forearm for stabilization.
7. Reassess CMS.

Follow these steps to splint a fractured humerus using a rigid splint (OEC Skill 20-5■):

1. Select an appropriate splint (e.g., a wire, ladder, or malleable splint).
2. Measure and form the splint using the opposite arm as a guide. The splint should be bent to hold the elbow at approximately a 90 degree angle and should be long enough to continue down the forearm to the distal palm crease, thereby immobilizing the wrist.
3. Assess CMS.
4. Gently place the splint under the arm.
5. Secure the arm to the splint with roller gauze or cravats. The wrap should be "snug" but not tight. Never use elastic material, which can constrict blood flow.
6. Gently place the upper arm against the patient's chest and the forearm on the patient's abdomen, and then apply a sling and a wide swathe, as previously described.
7. Reassess CMS.

If there are no contraindications, place the patient in a High-Fowler position or lying on the patients uninjured side during transport.

### Elbow Injuries

In the field, it is difficult to differentiate among elbow injuries, especially in children (Figure 20-71■). Due to the abundance of blood vessels and nerves in the area, it is best to splint elbow injuries in the position found, apply a sling and swathe, and rapidly transport the patient to definitive care. Most elbow injuries are found in a bent position.

To immobilize an elbow injury, follow these steps:

1. Rescuer #1: Stabilize the injury above and below the elbow. Do not allow the elbow to bend more.
2. Rescuer #2:
   - Check CMS.
   - Select the appropriate splint (e.g., SAM™ or wire splint).
   - Fold or bend the splint into the correct configuration to match the elbow's position.

**Figure 20-71** Splint elbow injuries in children in the position the injury was found.

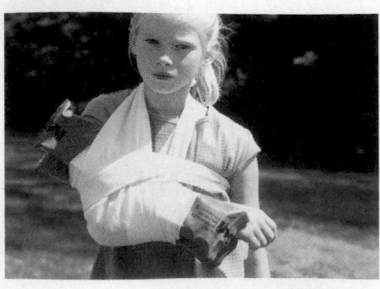

- Place the splint along the posterior aspect of the arm from the axilla to the hand (past the wrist).
- Secure the splint to the arm with cravats or a rolled bandage, without putting pressure on the elbow. Do not use an elastic bandage.
- Place the entire arm against the chest and abdomen.
- Apply a sling and swathe.
- Reassess CMS.

For alternate technique to immobilize an elbow, (OEC Skill 20-6■):

1. Rescuer #1: Stabilize the injured arm.
2. Rescuer #2:
   - Assess CMS.
   - Apply wooden splints to the medial and lateral aspects of the arm, extending past the wrist and past the upper third of the humerus.
   - Secure splints in place using three roller bandages or cravats:
     - Cravat 1 is applied around the splints and the upper arm.
     - Cravat 2 is applied around the splints and the forearm.
     - Cravat 3 is applied around both splints (but not the arm) in the hollow of the elbow.
   - Apply a sling and swathe.
   - Reassess CMS.

If distal CMS is worsened by applying the splint or a sling and swathe, loosen them and reapply them with less pressure, or extend the elbow slightly. If CMS is still compromised, do not try to readjust again; instead rapidly transport the patient.

Splinting the arm of a patient who presents holding the injured elbow straight is a relatively easy task. Simply apply a malleable or other rigid splint from the axilla to the hand, along the entire length of the posterior arm, and secure the arm to the splint with roller gauze (Figures 20-72a–c■). Do not place pressure over the zone of injury. Then, splint the arm to the side of the body for transport supine on a litter or in a toboggan.

If during your assessment of a deformed elbow injury you become sure that the limb distal to the injury has a CMS deficit, it may be appropriate to gently attempt axial alignment to improve blood supply or neurologic function to the distal arm by restoring normal anatomical appearance of the elbow. Always follow local protocol, preferably under medical direction, and do not attempt axial alignment unless final definitive care by a physician is more than two hours away. Most commonly the position of the elbow following gentle longitudinal tension to the arm is extended just

**Figure 20-72a** Application of a splint for a straight arm in a child.

**Figure 20-72b** Application of a splint for a straight arm in an adult.

**Figure 20-72c** A vacuum splint applied to a straight arm.

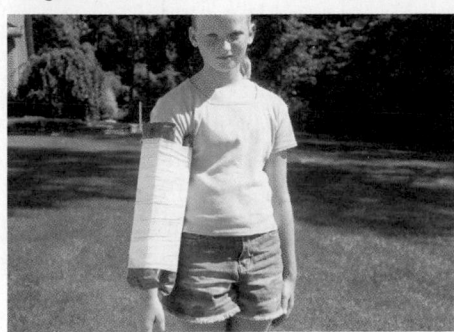

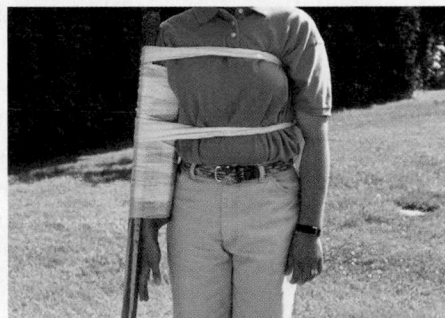

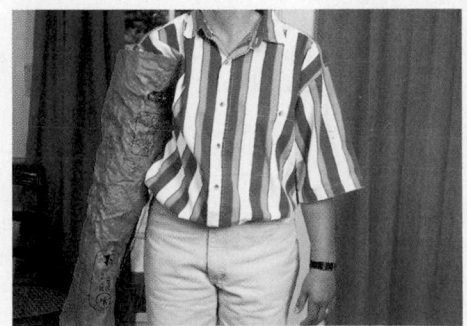

past 90 degrees. Have a finger on the radial pulse, and when it returns, splint the arm in this position. This maneuver may or may not restore a radial pulse.

OEC Technicians must be gentle and careful throughout this procedure because rough handling or excessive manipulation of the elbow joint may worsen neurologic or vascular compromise. If the pulse is restored after a single realignment attempt, splint the limb in the position where the distal pulse was restored. If no pulse returns after a single attempt, splint the arm in the position most comfortable to the patient. If possible, place the arm in a sling and swathe. Rapidly transport. If the elbow is straightened too much for a sling, secure the arm to the body with swathes.

### Forearm Injuries

For fractures of the shafts of the radius and ulna, immobilize the elbow and the wrist. When the forearm is severely deformed (especially when there is CMS compromise), gently realign the arm if the patient will allow it; if not, splint the arm in the position found.

A sugar tong splint or long arm splint is best for this type of fracture because it prevents *rotation* of the forearm at the elbow, allowing less movement at the fracture site and therefore causing less pain. A sugar tong splint is made using a malleable splint wrapped around a joint and covering both sides of the extremity, thereby preventing rotation of the joint.

To splint a forearm fracture, following these steps (see OEC Skill 20-7■):

1. Rescuer #1: Stabilize the fracture.
2. Rescuer #2:
   - Assess CMS.
   - Select the appropriate splint (malleable, wire, or ladder splint).
   - Form the splint into the shape of a sugar tong.
   - Gently move the splint into position. Apply the splint from where the fingers attach to the palm, then along the **volar** (palm-side) forearm, around the elbow so that rotation of the forearm is limited, and then on the dorsum of the forearm back to where the fingers attach to the back of the hand.
   - Secure the forearm to the splint using roller gauze or cravats.
   - Apply a sling and swathe.
   - Reassess CMS.

**volar** on the front of the body.

Alternatively, to immobilize a forearm fracture, use a *long* arm splint such as a ladder splint that starts at the axilla and proceeds posterior along the arm down to the palm crease along the arm.

### Wrist Injuries

Generally, patients are most comfortable when an injured wrist and hand are placed in the "position of function." If the patient resists this position, splint the injury in the most comfortable position.

Fractures of the distal radius and/or ulna can be managed by placing a SAM™, cardboard, or wooden splint on the palm side of the forearm and securing it with roller bandage or a cravat (Figure 20-74■). Alternatively, use a sugar tong splint or place splints on both the dorsum and palm side of the forearm and secure these in place with appropriate bandage. Place padding in the palm to help immobilize the hand (Figure 20-75■). A palm-side splint should extend beyond where the fingers attach to the hand. Leave the fingertips exposed to facilitate assessment of distal CMS.

Other injuries to the wrist (including carpal bone injuries) are treated the same way as a distal radius fracture: place the hand in a position of function, splint the in-

---

**NOTE**

### Position of Function

The position of function, in which the wrist is slightly dorsiflexed (positioned upward) with the fingers slightly curled down, can be achieved by placing a soft roller bandage in the patient's palm (Figure 20-73■). It can be used in conjunction with any method of splinting of the forearm or wrist for patient comfort.

jury, and apply a sling and swathe. Encourage the patient to seek prompt, follow-up care by a physician.

## Hand and Finger Injuries

Splint a suspected fracture involving a metacarpal in a manner similar to that used for a wrist injury. Whenever possible, keep the hand in a position of function. For a fracture of the thumb or of the first metacarpal at the base of the thumb, immobilize the thumb and wrist as a unit. For suspected skier's thumb, splint the entire thumb (from tip to base) with a tongue blade, or use a small splint on the back of the thumb. Gently secure the thumb to the index finger with roller gauze or tape to prevent the thumb from moving.

Splint other finger fractures using a tongue blade (or other small, stiff object) and tape (Figures 20-76a■ and 20-76b■). Do not apply tape too tightly. Do not attempt to reduce dislocated fingers; instead, use a small splint to immobilize dislocated fingers in the position found and recommend prompt follow-up care with a physician. Impaled objects that penetrate the hand or fingers should be stabilized in place. Amputated fingers should

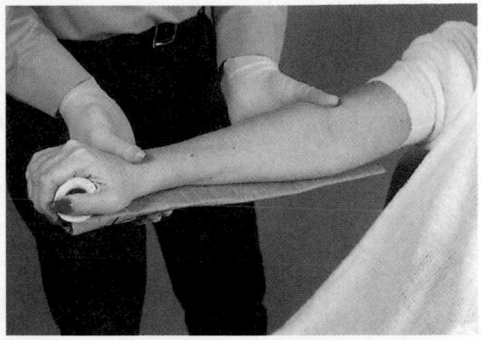

**Figure 20-73** Splinting a wrist in the position of function.

**Figure 20-74** A blanket roll splint for a wrist and forearm injury.

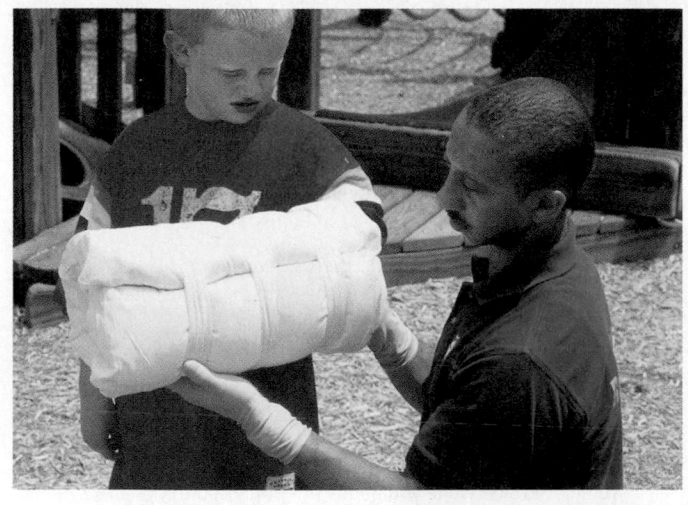

**Figure 20-75** Padding placed in the palm helps to immobilize the hand.
Copyright Edward McNamara

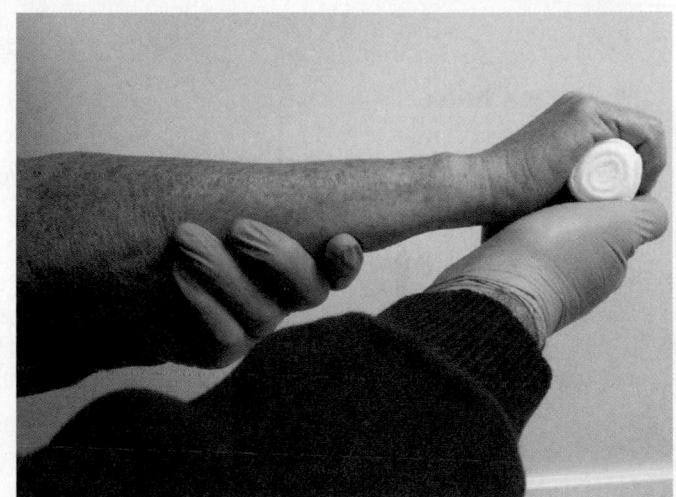

**Figure 20-76a** Splint an injured finger to an adjacent finger.

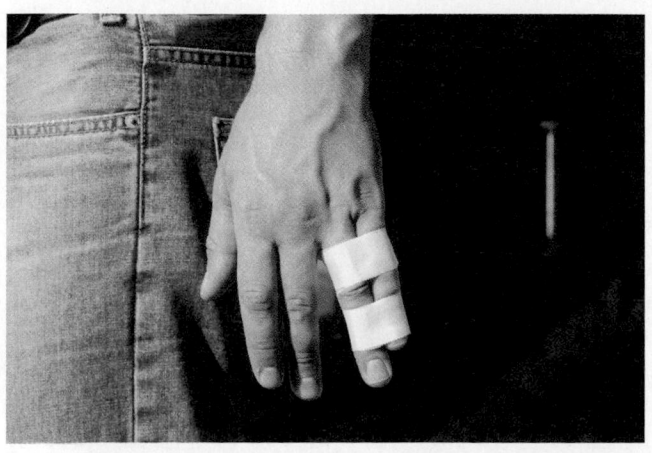

**Figure 20-76b** Use of a tongue depressor as a splint.

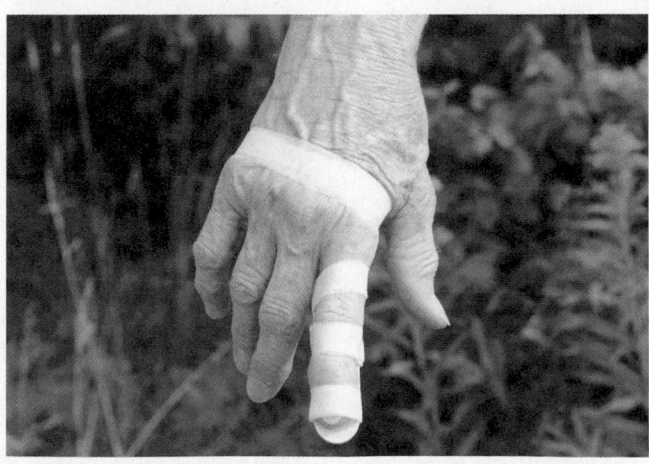

be managed as described in Chapter 18, Soft-Tissue Injuries and transported with the patient. Obviously these patients should also seek prompt, follow-up care.

To immobilize the hand using a forearm/hand splint, perform the following procedure (OEC Skill 20-8■):

1. Rescuer #1: Stabilize the bones above and below the injury.
2. Rescuer #2:
   - Assess CMS.
   - Select an appropriate splint.
   - Size the splint.
   - Gently place the hand and fingers in a position of function.
   - Place an unrolled roller gauze in the palm of the hand to maintain the position of function.
   - Place the palm side of the forearm, wrist, and hand on a cardboard, wooden, or SAM™ splint (the wrist should be slightly dorsiflexed). Secure the wrist and hand to the splint using soft roller gauze or cravats. Do not use elastic wrap. Leave the fingertips exposed.

## STOP, THINK, UNDERSTAND

### Multiple Choice
Choose the correct answer.

1. Which of the following instructions is the correct action to take for a patient with a wrist fracture who is wearing jewelry on the injured hand?_____
   a. Leave the jewelry in place, check CMS frequently, and document the situation.
   b. Remove the jewelry (if possible, replace it on the opposite hand), check CMS, and document the situation.
   c. Tape the rings securely in place, check CMS, and document the situation.
   d. Remove the jewelry from the ring finger and replace it onto the pinkie of the same hand to accommodate for swelling, check CMS, and document the situation.

2. Which of the following splints is appropriate for a patient with an acromioclavicular injury? _____
   a. figure eight splint
   b. aling and swathe splint
   c. rigid or SAM™ splint
   d. pillow splint

3. Which of the following actions is appropriate for managing a patient with a posterior sternoclavicular dislocation who has vascular compromise and is having difficulty breathing?
   _____
   a. Sling and swathe the patient's arm on the affected side and transport.
   b. Sling and swathe the patient's arms, bilaterally.
   c. Attempt to reduce the fracture immediately either by using two-rescuer traction and counter-traction or by placing a knee in the center of the patient's upper back and simultaneously pulling back hard on the shoulders.
   d. There is nothing you can do beyond arranging for immediate transport by the fastest route to the nearest trauma center.

4. A skier has fallen and suffered an anterior shoulder dislocation. He tells you that "it pops out all the time" and asks you to help him "put it back in."

   Your best course of action is to _____
   a. accommodate the patient's wishes and follow his instructions for relocating the shoulder carefully.
   b. firmly grasp the wrist and elbow on the patient's injured side and hold tightly while the patient, not you, provides the counter pull to slide the bone back into the socket.
   c. have your partner secure a swathe around the patient's chest, below the armpit on the injured side, and pull from the uninjured side while you gently but firmly counter pull by grasping the patient's wrist on the injured side and applying firm downward traction.
   d. explain that it is not within your protocols to perform a reduction maneuver; then offer to immobilize the arm and transport the patient.

5. Which of the following statements regarding upper extremity splinting are true? (check all that apply)
   _____ a. Generally a sling and swathe is the splint of choice for a posterior shoulder dislocation.
   _____ b. Generally a blanket roll and sling is the splint of choice for an anterior shoulder dislocation.
   _____ c. A posterior sternoclavicular dislocation must often be treated with immediate reduction/relocation.
   _____ d. A shoulder that dislocates repeatedly is best treated by relocating it before slinging and swathing it.

*continued*

_____ e. The best splint for a fractured or dislocated elbow is a rigid splint from elbow to wrist, and slinging/swathing the forearm with the elbow bent carefully to 90 degrees against the chest.

_____ f. If medical care is farther than 2 hours away and a patient with an elbow fracture exhibits reduced CMS in the affected hand, one attempt at restoring normal anatomic appearance of the elbow or arm is an appropriate action for an OEC Technician to take.

_____ g. Gently attempt to replace dislocated fingers in anatomical position using gentle axial tension. Once in place, splint the fingers in a position of function.

6. The position of function for the hand is best described as _____
   a. the wrist positioned slightly dorsal, with the fingers slightly curled.
   b. the wrist straight, palm down, with the fingers straight.
   c. a wrist cocked with the fingers straight.
   d. the wrist bent, palm down, with fingers gently balled into a fist.

7. Which of the following is the correct procedure for splinting fractures of the shafts of the radius or ulna? _____
   a. Immobilize the wrist and forearm with a SAM™ or other rigid splint.
   b. Immobilize the elbow and wrist with a SAM™ or other rigid splint.
   c. Apply a sling and swathe only.
   d. Allow the patient to self-splint the injury against their chest, and then secure with gauze or cravats.

8. When should you attempt to realign a shaft fracture of the forearm?_____
   a. Whenever possible, if the patient allows it.
   b. When the forearm is significantly deformed especially if there is CMS compromise.
   c. Only if you cannot splint the arm any other way.
   d. An OEC Technician should never attempt to realign a fracture.

9. To appropriately care for a dislocated finger,_____
   a. gently attempt to relocate the finger, then tape it to the finger next to it.
   b. place a rolled cravat or rolled gauze in the patient's palm, then wrap the hand securely in gauze until all the fingers are immobilized; apply a sling and swathe.
   c. do not attempt to relocate the finger; tape it as is onto the finger or fingers on either side.
   d. do not attempt to relocate the finger; secure it in place with a tongue blade and tape or roller.

## Short Answer

1. Why should a figure eight splint not be used for a fracture of the lateral third of the clavicle (the third closest to the shoulder)?

2. Where should you tie the knot for a sling, and why?

3. When dealing with an upper extremity injury, why should the fingertips be left exposed?

- Apply a sling and swathe.
- Reassess CMS.

## Lower Extremity Injuries

Lower extremity injuries occur in any outdoor activity, but OEC Technicians encounter them especially frequently among snow sports enthusiasts.

### Pelvis Fractures

Splint pelvic fractures using a pelvic binder, a sheet splint, or a SAM™ pelvic splint, as described in detail in Chapter 24, Abdominal and Pelvic Trauma. The patient should then be immobilized using a long spine board or full-body air splint. Due to the highly vascular nature of the pelvis and the potential for life-threatening bleeding, all patients with pelvic injuries should be transported to a hospital for evaluation by a physician. Pelvic binding is the treatment of choice for this injury.

### Hip Dislocations

Care for a dislocated hip centers on stabilizing the affected leg and gently lifting and transferring the patient to a long spine board. Do not try to reduce the hip; most patients will not let you move it. Splint the hip in the position found by stabilizing the affected hip (and leg) with rolled blankets, pillows, or backpacks. Secure the patient to the long spine board.

Remember, pelvis and hip injuries often involve significant mechanisms of injury and require full spine immobilization. Place the patient in the most comfortable position and transport rapidly to a medical facility for definitive care.

### Femur Fractures

Immobilize hip injuries, including fractures involving the proximal third of the femur, using a long spine board, a full-body vacuum splint, or a double pole splint. The most commonly used method for immobilizing and transporting a patient with a hip fracture involves placing the patient gently on a long spine board, padding voids (especially the one under the knee), and strapping the patient to the board. Alternatively, place a full-body vacuum splint under the patient, wrap it around the torso, pelvis, and legs, and remove the air to form a rigid structure. A double poled femur splint may be used for a hip fracture, applying approximately 7–10 lbs of longitudinal *tension*, which is less than is used for a mid-shaft femur fracture. Have helpers stabilize the affected leg, and apply the device according to the manufacturer's recommendations. Place the patient on a long spine board for lifting and transport. Because these injuries are sometimes associated with other serious injuries, immobilize the spine.

Immobilize mid-shaft femur fractures with a traction splint, unless the patient has multisystem trauma and is rapidly deteriorating into a load-and-go situation (Figure 20-77■). In that case, place several cravats around both legs, place the patient on a long spine board, and consider rapid transport the top priority. Because a large amount of blood (500–1,000 mL) can bleed into the thigh from a femur fracture, *anticipate* shock, especially if there are other significant injuries. Although the patient may develop shock, exsanguination from a closed femur fracture only is highly unlikely. Accordingly a tourniquet is indicated only for *severe* external bleeding that cannot be controlled by direct pressure and is not indicated for a closed femur fracture.

Treat a suspected mid-shaft femur fracture as soon as is reasonably possible using manual stabilization and the application of in-line traction. In a snow sport setting, several factors should be considered before in-line traction is applied:

1. If the ski or snowboard is still attached to the injured leg, leave it in place until "all is ready." A ski or snowboard can be a great "stabilizer" of the fracture site until the appropriate equipment and personnel are on scene.

2. If the ski/snowboard is no longer on the injured leg, leave the leg alone, perform a scene size-up and a primary assessment, and call for equipment/additional help.

3. Because the application of in-line traction can be very tiring, it should be performed for as short a time as is possible. Leave the ski in place, ensure that adequate personnel are present,

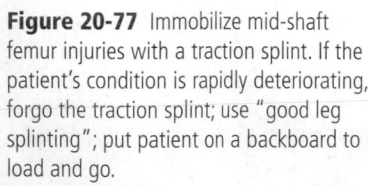

**Injury to an Artificial Joint**

If you encounter an injury to a limb that has an artificial joint, care for the injury the same way you would for a limb that has natural joints.

**Figure 20-77** Immobilize mid-shaft femur injuries with a traction splint. If the patient's condition is rapidly deteriorating, forgo the traction splint; use "good leg splinting"; put patient on a backboard to load and go.
Copyright Edward McNamara

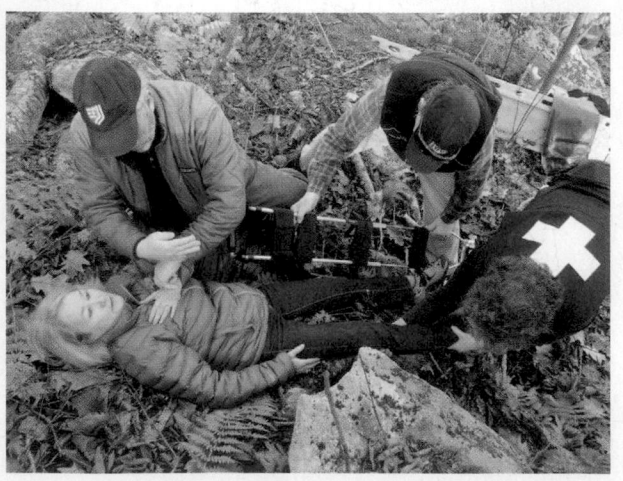

expose the injury site, and have the traction equipment out and ready to be applied.

**4.** When all is ready, apply the splint.

Adhere to the following principles concerning the initial application of all traction splints, regardless of manufacturer: have sufficient resources available, fully prepare the splint for application, use proper axial alignment, provide continuous traction once traction is applied, avoid unnecessary movement of the injured leg, and secure the patient and splint to a long spine board.

Ideally, two or more rescuers should be used to apply a traction splint. Depending on the terrain or slope angle, an additional rescuer or bystander may be needed to stabilize patients to keep them from sliding in the direction that the traction is being pulled. Stabilize a patient by kneeling above the patient's head and grasping beneath both armpits. If bystanders provide assistance, OEC Technicians must instruct them regarding what they should do.

Among the most popular and effective commercial traction devices available to OEC Technicians are the Hare, Sager, KTD, and Thomas half ring splints. Learn the proper use of each device that is available to you.

Follow these basic steps to apply a traction splint on a femur (see OEC Skill 20-9■):

**1.** Rescuer #1: Use Standard Precautions. Expose and assess the injury to determine its proximity to the hip or knee joint. Check for bleeding and treat it if present. Remove overlying clothing by cutting or ripping along a seam. (Many ski pants have zippers that run the length of each leg.) Manually stabilize the fracture site both above and below the injury.

**2.** Rescuer #2:
- Use Standard Precautions. Check on distal CMS on the injured leg indirectly (tap on boot, ask the patient to wiggle the toes); remove the boot only when environmental conditions do not present additional hazards to the patient and your local protocols say you should do this.
- Prepare a traction splint and adjust it to the proper size according to the manufacturer's instructions; use the uninjured leg to measure the splint.
- Remove the ski or snowboard if present and then apply the ankle hitch while Rescuer #1 continues to manually stabilize the fracture site.
- Firmly grasp the ankle hitch with one hand; place the other hand under the calf and cooperate with Rescuer #1 in using manual traction to straighten the leg into anatomical alignment. Maintain traction while Rescuer #1 releases the manual stabilization of the fracture site.

**3.** Rescuer #1:
- Position the splint snugly against the patient's ischial tuberosity.
- Secure the groin strap around the patient's upper thigh.
- Connect the ankle strap of the hitch to the end of the splint and turn the crank/knob gradually to replace the manual traction of the splint with mechanical traction; as the mechanical traction is being applied, Rescuer #2 releases the manual traction. It may take some time for muscle spasms to ease off before the patient feels relief.

**4.** Rescuers secure Velcro™ support straps per the manufacturer's instructions. (Cravats can be used in place of Velcro straps.) Ensure that the limb is securely held in the splint.

5. Reassess CMS in the injured leg. Treat for shock by keeping the patient warm and by providing high-flow oxygen.

6. Prepare the patient for transport on a long spine board and then hand the patient off to EMS personnel.

**Traction Hitch**

N O T E

If the need arises, you can always improvise a traction hitch from cravats (Figure 20-78■).

After the splint is applied, consider placing loosely rolled blankets or pillows between the patient's knees, and if the patient permits, splint the affected leg to the non-affected leg with folded cravats. Log roll the patient onto the uninjured side or gently lift and secure the patient onto a long spine board. This immobilizes the hip and helps with lifting the patient from the ground into the toboggan or onto a litter. Do not allow the patient to move to a sitting position because most traction splints will slide up the buttocks, rendering the splint ineffective. Place a folded blanket under the knee of the *uninjured* leg to keep it partially flexed to relieve the muscle tension on the same side of the body as the broken femur.

It is best to use a traction splint for *any* fracture of the middle third of the femur. If jagged bone ends sticking out of an open femur fracture cause additional pain as traction is applied, place a sterile bandage over any exposed bone, apply tension (not traction), and rapidly transport the patient. If the bone ends retract into the skin, leave it inside the body.

As a general rule, a traction splint should be removed by a physician or other qualified hospital staff only. OEC Technicians might be involved in removing or readjusting a traction splint under two conditions: when mechanical traction is ineffective because of loosening or incorrect application, and when assisting those EMTs who are required to remove the boot and assess CMS prior to transport to a hospital. If it becomes necessary to remove or replace the splint, provide and maintain manual sta-

**Figure 20-78** The use of a cravat to make an ankle hitch.

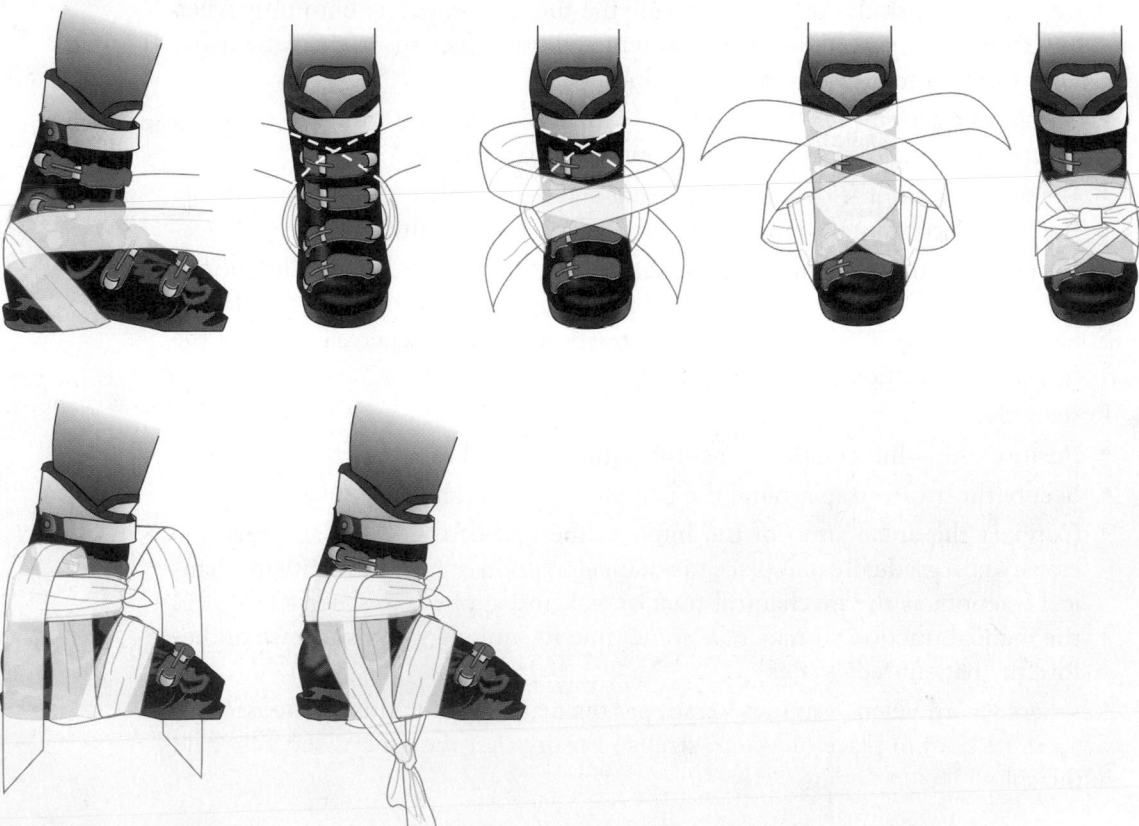

bilization and axial traction below the fracture site until mechanical traction is again established with the splint.

A traction splint should *not* be used for a distal femur fracture because the splint can force jagged bone ends into the popliteal space, damaging the nerves and blood vessels there. The best splint for this injury is a rigid splint such as Quick Splint (sometimes in conjunction with an airplane splint) or a long, flexible ladder splint bent at the knee. The splint should extend from the groin to the foot. Attempt to splint the leg in the position that is most comfortable for the patient. If the patient exhibits signs of distal CMS impairment and the total transport time to a definitive care facility is greater than 2 hours, a single attempt to realign the leg (keeping the knee slightly bent) is appropriate (Figure 20-79■).

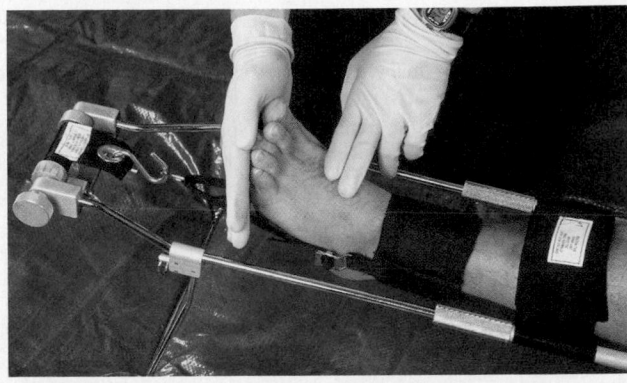

**Figure 20-79** Recheck CMS once the traction splint has been applied.

Any of the following findings of impaired CMS in a traumatized leg require immediate attention:

1. Impaired circulation presenting as a cold, pale foot
2. Absent dorsalis pedis *and* posterior tibialis pulses
3. Numbness of the foot or loss of motor function in the lower leg

To realign a femur fracture with distal CMS compromise, follow these steps (Figure 20-80■):

1. Rescuer #1: Stabilize the thigh.
2. Rescuer #2:
   - Firmly grasp the posterior aspect of the top of the calf, just below the knee. (If a distal injury is also present, the ankle may be used instead of the calf.)
   - Keeping the knee slightly bent, apply gentle but steady longitudinal traction to align the posterior angulation of the femur distal to the fracture. Attempt this *once only*.

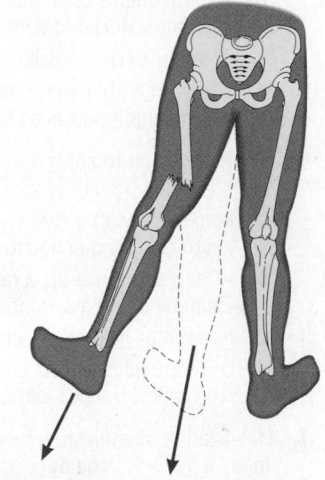

**Figure 20-80** Apply gentle traction to align the femur.

---

## STOP, THINK, UNDERSTAND

### Multiple Choice

Choose the correct answer.

1. The correct type of splint for a pelvic fracture would be _____
   - **a.** traction splint.
   - **b.** pelvic distraction sling.
   - **c.** pelvic binder.
   - **d.** Thomas half ring.

2. Which of the following methods for caring for a patient with a dislocated hip is correct? _____
   - **a.** Using long-axis tension, carefully realign the hip; then roll the patient onto a long spine board and immobilize as per usual protocol.
   - **b.** Reduce the fracture, if possible, through long-axis traction; either secure the patient's foot to the base of the long spine board to maintain traction or (if the patient will tolerate it) use a traction splint.
   - **c.** Stabilize the affected leg, gently lift the patient onto a long spine board, splint the hip in the position found, and stabilize the patient with rolled blankets, pillows, or packs.
   - **d.** Stabilize the affected leg with a traction splint or a rigid splint, roll the patient onto a long spine board, and secure the patient in a position of comfort.

3. How should an OEC Technician splint the injury of a patient with an apparent hip fracture? _____
   - **a.** On a long spine board, with full spinal precautions, including a C-collar and a head stabilizer.
   - **b.** On a long spine board with a C-collar but without a head stabilizer.
   - **c.** On a long spine board with neither C-collar nor head stabilizer.
   - **d.** With a full-length Quick Splint; then secure both legs (including the splint) with 4-inch to 6-inch swathes.

*continued*

STOP, THINK, UNDERSTAND *continued*

4. Which of the following methods of stabilization is correct for a patient with a fracture of the proximal femur?_____
   a. The application of a traction splint.
   b. The use of a traction splint with 7–10 lbs of tension, then placement onto a long spine board with spinal immobilization.
   c. The use of a traction splint in conjunction with a long spine board.
   d. Careful reduction of the fracture, then stabilization on a long spine board with the patient's legs tied together with wide cravats.

5. Which of the following statements regarding blood loss from a femur fracture is true?_____
   a. Exsanguination is a possibility, so OEC Technicians should work as quickly as possible to stabilize and transport the patient.
   b. A tourniquet is often indicated for internal and external bleeding associated with a femur fracture.
   c. Bleeding, while a possibility, is rare with a closed femur fracture.
   d. A patient with a femur fracture may develop shock, but exsanguination from a closed femur fracture alone is unlikely.

6. When preparing to apply a traction splint to a mid-shaft femur fracture, when should traction be applied?_____
   a. Immediately after reaching the patient to avoid further neurovascular damage to the limb.
   b. After a scene size-up, a rapid assessment, and a request for equipment and assistance.
   c. As soon as help and traction splint have arrived on scene.
   d. Once the traction splint has been secured to the leg and mechanical traction can be applied via the device.

7. Stabilization of a midshaft femoral fracture site prior to applying an ankle hitch is done by_____
   a. supporting the fracture site above and below the injury using your forearm on either side of the femur.
   b. supporting the fracture site by placing one hand directly below the fracture site and the other directly above.
   c. placing one hand firmly on each side of the knee and applying traction.
   d. grasping the ankle firmly with both hands and applying tension.

8. Bandaging an open femur fracture should be done_____
   a. before splinting.         c. after splinting.
   b. during splinting.         d. at no time ever.

9. Under which of the following circumstances should manual *traction* (as opposed to stabilization or tension) be applied by two rescuers before applying a traction splint? _____
   a. Any time a traction splint is to be applied.
   b. Only if there is no obvious angulation or deformity.

c. To replace protruding bone fragments when it will take 8 hours or more for a patient to reach definitive medical care.
d. To reduce an angulated femur fracture.

10. Which of the following statements about boot removal and the use of traction splints is correct?_____
    a. Always remove a ski or other sport boot prior to applying a traction splint.
    b. Always leave a ski or other sport boot on when applying a traction splint.
    c. The removal of a ski or sport boot in conjunction with traction splinting is completely up to the discretion of the first OEC Technician on scene.
    d. The removal of a ski or sport boot in conjunction with traction splinting is generally determined by local protocols and individual circumstances.

11. A patient with a traction splint on her right leg begins to complain that her ski boot is "uncomfortable." What is your next course of action?_____
    a. Gently remove the boot and traction splint, and then switch to a rigid stabilization splint.
    b. Reapply manual stabilization, remove the boot, and then reapply the traction splint.
    c. Gently remove the traction splint, loosen the boot but leave it on for stabilization, and then apply a rigid stabilization splint instead.
    d. Explain to the patient that this is a normal occurrence with traction splints, encourage her to wiggle her toes to improve circulation.

12. When you apply traction to an open mid-shaft femur fracture, the patient screams, "Stop, you're making it worse!" What is your best course of action?_____
    a. Have the patient take a deep breath in through the nose and out through the mouth, and reassure the patient that the pain will soon stop.
    b. Reduce the traction by 2–5 lbs and then secure the splint.
    c. Gently increase the traction until the pain stops and patient expresses relief.
    d. Switch from traction to tension, and then rapidly transport the patient.

13. A patient with a distal femur fracture exhibits signs of distal CMS impairment. Transport time to definitive medical care is longer than 2 hours. What is your best course of action?_____
    a. Make a single attempt to realign the leg, keeping the knees slightly bent.
    b. Make a single attempt to realign the leg, keeping the knees straight.
    c. Attempt to realign the leg until CMS is restored.
    d. Apply a traction splint.

## Short Answer

Describe two acceptable reasons for removing a traction splint once it has been applied.

_____

_____

_____

If distal pulses, sensation, or motor function return, or if the color of the foot improves, splint the extremity in the position where the improvement(s) are first observed. If the realignment attempt is unsuccessful, causes too much pain, or is met with resistance by the patient, splint the leg in the position of maximum comfort and transport rapidly.

## Knee Injuries

As a rule, splint knee injuries in the position found because the patient will usually not want to straighten the knee. Allow the patient to keep the knee slightly bent, and splint the knee using either a Quick Splint (with or without a properly angled airplane splint under the knee), two rigid board splints placed on each side of the knee with cravats, or a wire/ladder splint (Figure 20-81■). If severe angulation is present, OEC Technicians may need to use various types of padding and straps or cravats to immobilize the leg on a long spine board. Angulated knee injuries may also be immobilized using a vacuum splint or blanket roll.

For a patella dislocation, even if the patella spontaneously reduces itself, splint the extremity and encourage the patient to go to the hospital for follow-up care. Inform receiving emergency personnel that the patella reduced spontaneously. Always apply cold packs to this injury because significant swelling (usually internal bleeding around the patella) can occur.

A dislocated knee that has a distal pulse should also be splinted in the position it was found, because moving the joint could cause sudden distal neurovascular compromise (most notably, interruption of the blood supply to the foot). If there is no distal pulse and gross deformity, you may perform *one* attempt to axially align the knee joint with the help of other OEC Technicians. If toboggan transport time to an aid room is short, spend a brief time splinting the leg outdoors and then attempt alignment indoors. Apply manual stabilization and move the limb slowly, reassessing the pulse after moving the leg a few inches only. Stop if you palpate a pulse in the foot, and splint the leg in that position (usually straight in the frontal plane, with slight knee flexion). If the foot remains pulseless after alignment, splint the extremity and transport. All dislocated knees, even if they spontaneously reduce and have normal neurovascular findings, require immediate evaluation at a hospital because the popliteal artery can occlude several hours after the initial injury. Air transport may be appropriate for this injury in cases that involve prolonged transport.

To apply an airplane splint, perform the following procedure (OEC Skill 20-10■):

**1.** Rescuer #1: Manually stabilize the extremity.
**2.** Rescuer #2:
  - Check CMS.
  - Adjust the splint to the approximate correct angle.

> ### Gross Deformity
>
> If a distal pulse is detected, do not attempt to align any major knee injury with gross deformity. Instead, splint the leg as found.
>
> NOTE

**Figure 20-81** Splint an injured knee in the position found.

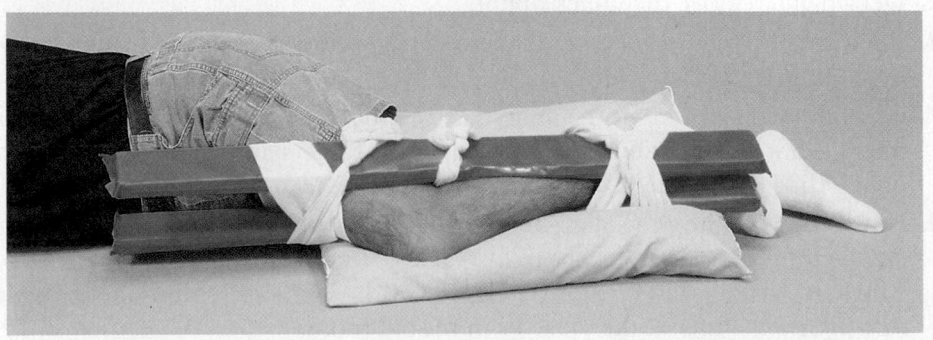

- Turn the knob to lock the splint at the appropriate angle.
- Apply the splint to the extremity, and adjust the angle, if necessary.

**3.** Rescuer #1: Hold the splint and leg in place.

**4.** Rescuer #2: Use cravats to attach the splint to the extremity (not over the zone of injury).

If splinting a bent knee: put the airplane splint behind the knee, attach it to the leg with cravats, and place both in a Quick Splint. This allows the knee to be placed in the Quick Splint without bending it.

If splinting a bent elbow: place the splint on the inside of the elbow, attach with cravats, and apply a sling and swathe.

If splinting a shoulder: place the splint against the side of the chest and upper arm, and fasten with cravats.

To apply a Quick Splint, follow these steps (OEC Skill 20-11■):

**1.** Rescuer #1: Open the splint flat, either parallel to the patient's injured extremity or in line with/distal to the foot.

**2.** Rescuer #2: Take a position opposite Rescuer #1 if the splint is at the side of the patient's leg, or on either side of the leg if the splint is distal to the foot.
- Grasp the patient's foot with one hand and apply slight longitudinal *tension*; place the other hand just below the knee or under the lower thigh to support the extremity. (The "pant leg pinch lift" is another useful method for lifting and supporting the injured extremity into a Quick Splint.)
- On the count of three, lift the extremity.

**3.** Rescuer #1: Slide the splint underneath the leg from the bottom to the top or from the side.

**4.** Rescuer #2: Gently lower the extremity into the center of the splint.

**5.** Rescuer #1: Close the sides of the Quick Splint like a clamshell, thereby holding the leg snuggly with the splint.

**6.** Rescuer #2: Firmly secure the splint straps, rope, or webbing.

A Quick Splint that has been applied at the accident scene is often replaced by a disposable cardboard splint before sending the patient to the hospital. However, OEC Technicians must use caution when considering the removal of a Quick Splint when there are serious multiple injuries, a very unstable fracture, a bandaged open fracture, or a fracture that is accompanied by advancing hypovolemic shock. In such cases, rapid transport takes precedence.

To perform the procedure for replacing a Quick Splint with a cardboard splint, follow these steps (OEC Skill 20-12■):

**1.** First manually stabilize the injury site.

**2.** Detach and remove the Quick Splint.

**3.** Remove the patient's boot in your emergency facility if appropriate and required by local protocol.

**4.** Carefully support and lift the injured extremity and then slide a preformed cardboard splint into position under the leg, in the same manner as you did when applying the Quick Splint.

**5.** Lower the leg into the splint, and pad all voids between the extremity and the cardboard. Pad under the knee to keep it slightly flexed. Tape the top of the pre-bent sides to hold the leg in place. Check CMS. Cardboard splints do not replace *traction splints* either at the scene or in the aid room.

Many knee injuries ultimately require surgical repair and rehabilitation. For this reason, any patient with a suspected knee injury should be advised to seek further medical care by a physician or orthopedist.

## Tibia and Fibula Injuries

All suspected tib-fib fractures should be rapidly immobilized to prevent further injury. Expose the zone of injury if above the boot, control bleeding (if necessary), and cover the skin to prevent cold injury (if applicable). Cover open wounds with a sterile dressing to prevent contamination. Generally, the boot is left on until the patient is moved inside (see the discussion of boot removal in a later section). CMS can be assessed by tapping on the boot and asking patients if they can move their toes. Once the patient is inside, the boot can be removed using the technique described later in the chapter. Additionally, the pulses, skin color, sensation, and movement of the foot and toes can be assessed, if not already done.

If the leg is angulated, it may need to be realigned before placement into a splint. As described previously, this procedure is best done with two rescuers. The principles of realigning a tib-fib fracture are similar to those used to realign a humerus fracture. If the patient will not allow you to move the injured leg, splint the angulated extremity in the position found. Often, this will require patience and ingenuity.

Tib-fib fractures are best managed using a long ladder splint, two rigid splints, or a Quick Splint, which is the most widely used device for this type of fracture. If the fracture is nondisplaced, an air splint or vacuum splint may be used.

To immobilize a tib-fib fracture with two rigid splints, follow this procedure (OEC Skill 20-13■):

1. Rescuer #1: Stabilize the bones above and below the injury.
2. Rescuer #2:
   - Place one long padded splint on the *medial* aspect of the patient's leg such that it is above the knee and below the ankle.
   - Place a second long padded splint on the *lateral* aspect of the patient's leg in the same relationship to the knee and the ankle.
   - Thread a cravat near the top of the splints, and tie the two splints together. (Roller gauze may be used if cravats are not available.)
   - Thread a second cravat just above the knee (above the injury) and tie the two splints together.
   - Thread a third cravat below the injury, and tie the two splints together.
3. Both Rescuers: Help the patient onto the stretcher or toboggan; use a long spine board as a lifting device, if needed.

Alternatively, perform the following steps to splint a tib-fib fracture using a vacuum splint (this is best accomplished with two rescuers):

1. Rescuer #1: Stabilize the bones above and below the injury.
2. Rescuer #2:
   - Prepare the vacuum splint according to the manufacturer's instructions.
   - Place the splint next to the patient's leg.
3. Rescuer #1: Gently lift the patient's leg.
4. Rescuer #2: Slide the vacuum splint under the patient's lower leg.
5. Rescuer #1: Gently lower the patient's leg onto the vacuum splint.

6. Rescuer #2: Remove air from the splint following the manufacturer's instructions.

7. Both Rescuers: gently lift the patient and place on a long spine board. Secure the patient's leg to the board.

If a Quick Splint or other commonly used splint is not available, as a last resort a Hare or other double pole traction splint may be used to cradle the fractured tibia. Support the fractures with Velcro straps and apply *tension* to the bones using the ankle hitch. Do not place straps over the zone of injury. This procedure is not appropriate for an ankle injury.

### Femur/Tibia Fracture in the Same Leg

Fractures involving the femur and tibia in the same leg disrupt the stability of the bones between the fractures, causing the knee to "float" between the two fractures (Figure 20-82■). Patients with this type of injury often have other ABCD-related injuries that require attention first. While caring for the patient's more significant injuries, try to keep the affected leg axially aligned.

Immobilize a "floating knee" injury by applying a Quick Splint over the entire length of the leg. Another rescuer should provide tension and alignment, similar to the method used for an isolated tibia fracture. Some ski patrols effectively use a Quick Splint that incorporates a trombone slide for a floating knee. If available, place the Quick Splint/trombone slide splint around the femur. Extend the trombone slide with enough tension to align the fractures above and below the knee. Place cravats above and below the tibia injury to act as slings to stabilize the bones. The trombone part of the splint is kept off the ground or backboard.

Alternatively, apply a traction splint using only tension. Even though immobilizing this injury with a traction splint was once discouraged, a recent study in England showed that a double pole traction device such as a Thomas splint (or a Hare traction device with tension, not traction) may be used successfully.

### Ankle Injuries

Ankle deformity generally indicates either a dislocation or (more frequently) a fracture-dislocation. OEC Technicians should not attempt to align or reduce ankle deformities when CMS is intact. (Doing so is extremely painful.) If distal CMS is compromised or if the bone appears ready to come through the skin, *one* attempt to reduce the ankle may be tried. As with reducing other bones, apply *gentle* but firm tension by

**Figure 20-82** A Quick Splint can be used when injuries involve both the femur and the bones of the lower leg.

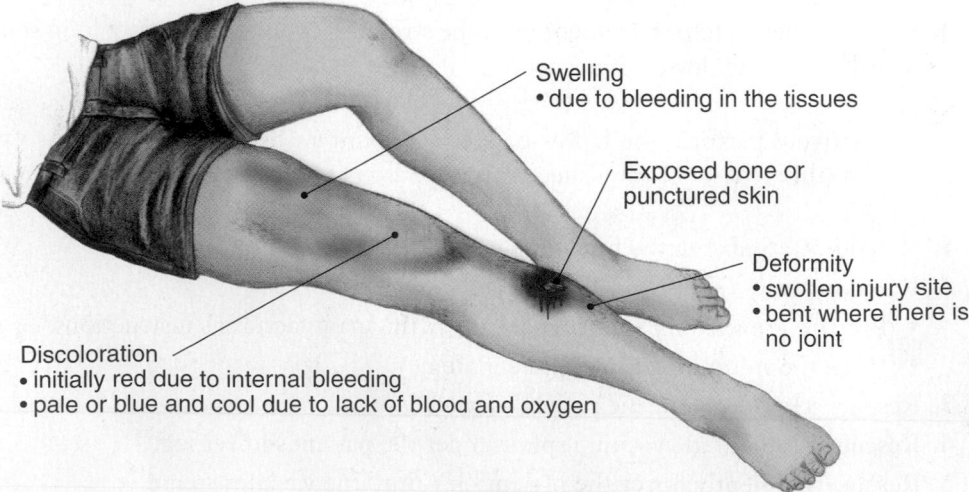

Swelling
• due to bleeding in the tissues

Exposed bone or punctured skin

Deformity
• swollen injury site
• bent where there is no joint

Discoloration
• initially red due to internal bleeding
• pale or blue and cool due to lack of blood and oxygen

pulling on the heel (and the top of the foot) and put the ankle back into normal anatomical position. Regardless of whether or not the ankle is realigned, do not let go of it until it is immobilized. Because ankle sprains may be difficult to differentiate from ankle fractures, management of ankle injuries should include immobilization, splinting, and follow-up evaluation by a physician. A blanket roll or a pillow splint wrapped around the ankle is often best (Figure 20-83■). Other splints such as a Quick Splint, a cardboard box splint, an air splint, or a malleable splint, may also be used but may be difficult to apply if the ankle is dislocated.

To apply a pillow splint, follow this procedure:

1. Rescuer #1: Stabilize the ankle above and below by holding the foot and the tibia at mid-shaft.
2. Rescuer #2:
   • Position a soft pillow under the ankle such that the foot rests in the middle of the pillow.
   • Gently bring the corner of the pillow over the dorsum (top) of the foot, molding the pillow to the shape of the foot. Leave the tip of the toes exposed to facilitate CMS reassessment.
   • Secure the pillow in place with roller gauze or tape.

Even though an air splint designed for use on ankle injuries is usually difficult to apply to a deformed ankle, an air splint may be effective for a non-displaced ankle injury. To apply an air splint, perform these steps (Figure 20-84■):

1. Rescuer #1: Stabilize the ankle above and below the joint.
2. Rescuer #2:
   • Remove the air splint from its protective case.
   • Unzip or unfasten the splint.
   • Place the splint into position according to the manufacturer's instructions (if possible leave the toes exposed to facilitate CMS reassessment).
   • Zip the splint up or fasten the securing straps.
   • Inflate the splint to the pressure recommended in the manufacturer's instructions. (You may need to blow into the inflation port or connect the splint to a hand pump.)

**Figure 20-83** A pillow splint can be applied to an injured ankle.

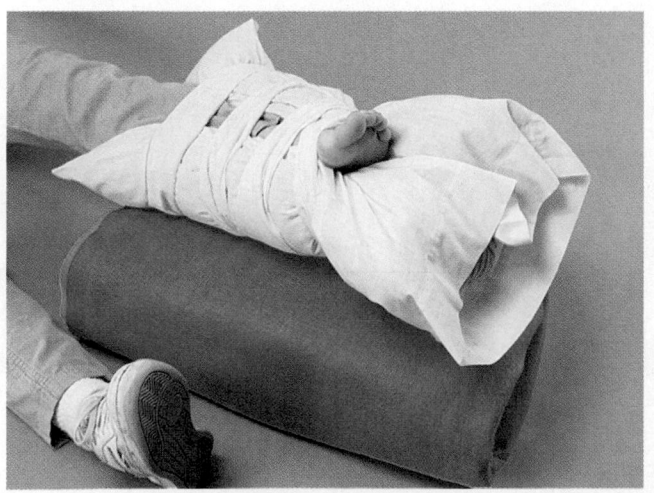

**Figure 20-84** Immobilization of an injured ankle using an air splint.

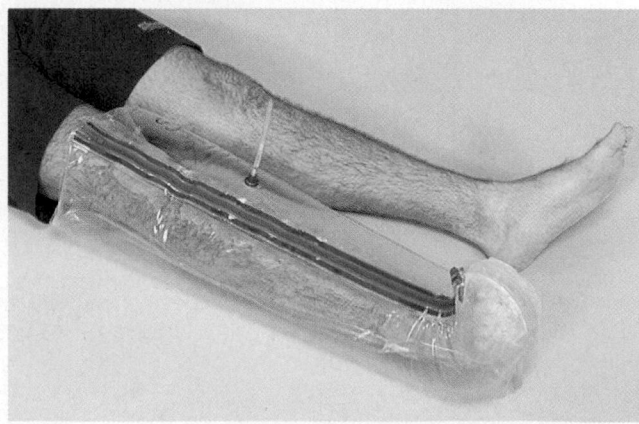

In wilderness settings, people with ankle injuries may need to self-evacuate. In this instance, it is important to firmly stabilize the zone of injury. Help patients walk by applying either cloth bandages, cravats, or tape wrapped in a figure eight pattern (Figure 20-85■). Check CMS to the toes frequently because cravats or tape may become too tight as the foot swells.

Boot removal may be very difficult in ankle injuries. During inclement weather, it is generally best to leave the boot on until the patient is inside, the ankle is elevated on an exam table, and more assistance is available. The procedure to remove a boot is discussed in the next section of this chapter.

### Foot and Toe Injuries

Splint these injuries using a blanket roll, a pillow splint, or a rigid, well-padded splint. Be sure to leave toes slightly exposed so that distal CMS may be assessed. Foot and toe injuries, especially open injuries and puncture wounds, have a high rate of infection. For this reason, the patient should be encouraged to seek follow-up care.

**20-3.4** Demonstrate how to remove a boot, including a ski boot.

# Boot Removal

When a lower extremity injury occurs in snow sports, the decision whether or not to remove the individual's boot on the hill or in the aid room remains the subject of considerable discussion. The current recommendation of the National Ski Patrol is to leave the boot on in outdoor environments, unless local treatment protocols dictate otherwise. Previously, some local medical directors recommended removing the boot, either on scene in the outdoors or once inside the aid room. Because most transport times are relatively short, leaving the boot on for femoral traction splinting makes sense because the boot can be removed at the hospital following the administration of intravenous pain medication.

Each resort area should develop a local protocol regarding boot removal. The formulation of this protocol must include input from the patrol medical advisor and should take into consideration the injury, environmental conditions at the time of the incident (temperature, precipitation, and wind), and transport times from the acci-

**Figure 20-85** Using a bandage or a cravat to support an injured ankle.

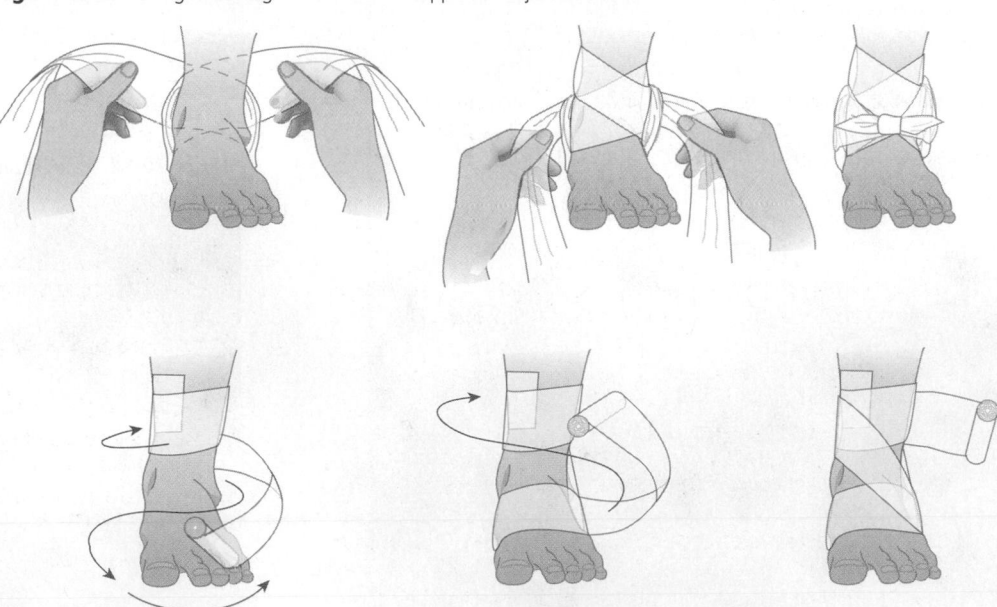

dent scene to the aid room and from the aid room to the hospital. Protocol considerations should also include the type of splint needed, probable or actual CMS status in the extremity distal to the injury, and the patient's comfort. Obviously, boot removal in the aid room, where extra help is available, is easier.

If the boot is unfamiliar to you, remove the opposite boot first to learn how best to proceed. In general, do not use a saw on a ski boot. Hiking boots and other lace-up boots can be removed by completely undoing the laces.

To remove a boot, perform the following procedure (OEC Skill 20-14■):

1. Rescuer #1: Stabilize the boot that is to be removed.
2. Rescuer #2:
   - Unbuckle or unlace the boot completely.
   - Spread the boot shell, pulling the tongue forward as far as it can go, or open a rear entry boot's back as far as it can go. (An alternate method is to place a hand on each side of the ankle.)
3. Rescuer #1: Stabilize the leg/ankle either by placing one hand on the front of the ankle and one hand on the back of the ankle, or by holding both sides of the ankle. Hold this position firmly as the boot is removed.
4. Rescuer #2:
   - Gently remove the boot by sliding its heel away from the foot, followed by the toe.
   - Assess distal CMS.
   - Prepare and apply a splint.
   - Reassess distal CMS.

It is important to monitor the patient's perception of pain throughout this procedure. If resistance is met, stop and attempt to further loosen the boot. If necessary, stop the procedure and splint the ankle with the boot in place.

## STOP, THINK, UNDERSTAND

### Multiple Choice

Choose the correct answer.

1. As a rule, knee injuries should be splinted_____
   a. into the correct anatomical position with the knee straight, the toes up, and the heel down.
   b. bent, with the knee rotated either medially or laterally, depending on patient's comfort and the best CMS.
   c. in the position found.
   d. with the knee as straight as possible and in alignment with the femur and pelvis.

2. A patient tells you that her patella "popped out" but went back in when she tried to move the leg. Your next course of action is to_____
   a. apply tension because the patella will most likely pop out again and cause neurovascular damage.
   b. apply ice, splint the extremity with a rigid splint or a Quick Splint, arrange for transport to the emergency department, and notify the department that the patella reduced spontaneously.
   c. apply ice and encourage the patient to see her doctor as soon as possible.
   d. do nothing because the situation has resolved itself.

3. When you assess a football player who has dislocated his knee and find a strong distal pulse, you should use _____
   a. a fixed splint in the position found.
   b. a fixed splint after axially aligning the knee using two-person tension.
   c. a traction splint after axial alignment.
   d. a traction splint with only a tension setting to align the leg.

4. A patient with a grossly deformed, dislocated knee has no palpable distal pulse. What is your best course of action?_____
   a. Splint the knee in the position found and transport the patient rapidly.
   b. Apply a traction splint and transport the patient rapidly.
   c. Make one attempt to axially align the knee joint, moving only an inch at a time.
   d. Gently rotate the knee into a flexed position and then secure it with a fixed splint.

*continued*

STOP, THINK, UNDERSTAND *continued*

5. Which of the following statements about transferring a patient from a Quick Splint to a cardboard splint is true?_____
   a. It is generally safe to do as long as the fracture is stable, there are not multiple injuries, the fracture is closed, and there is no evidence of hypovolemic shock.
   b. Switching from a Quick Splint to a cardboard splint is advisable because the cardboard splint need not be removed to X-ray the limb.
   c. Once a Quick Splint is in place, it is inadvisable to replace it with a cardboard splint because doing so can exacerbate the injury.
   d. Contrary to popular belief, cardboard splints generally do not provide adequate support and should not be used.

6. When is it acceptable to use a cardboard splint in place of a traction splint?_____
   a. never
   b. always
   c. only when a traction splint is unavailable
   d. only when the fracture involves the femur

7. A "floating knee" is caused by what?_____
   a. a direct blow that dislocates the patella
   b. a distal femur fracture
   c. a fracture involving the femur and the tibia in the same leg
   d. a torn meniscus

8. Which of the following splints are best for a "floating knee"?_____
   a. A full-leg Quick Splint, a Quick Splint with a trombone slide, or a traction splint.
   b. A long spine board, with the patient's legs tied together for additional stability.
   c. A full-length rigid splint or a vacuum splint.
   d. Two SAM™ or other malleable splints.

9. After one attempt to reduce the ankle fracture of a patient without a distal pulse, the distal pulse remains absent. Your best course of action is to_____
   a. make another attempt; if this fails, splint the ankle in the position found with a rigid splint.
   b. do not make another attempt; splint the ankle but do not let go of it until it is immobilized in the splint.
   c. immediately release tension and wrap the ankle in a pillow or blanket splint.
   d. apply a traction splint.

10. Which of the following courses of care is generally correct for a patient with a probable ankle sprain?_____
    a. Immobilize, splint, and ice the ankle, and arrange for transport to a medical facility.
    b. Apply a soft elastic wrap, elevate and ice the injury, and encourage the patient to stay off of it for at least 24 hours.
    c. Encourage the patient to gently flex the ankle periodically, and then ice it between flexation exercises.
    d. Encourage the patient to "walk it off."

11. As a general rule, the National Ski Patrol makes which of the following recommendations about removing ski boots in conjunction with traction splinting?_____
    a. Remove the boot.
    b. Leave the boot on.
    c. Leave the boot on if transportation time is short and the patient can get to definitive medical care and pain management quickly.
    d. The NSP does not make a recommendation about ski boot removal.

12. While attempting to remove a boot from a patient with a fractured femur, the patient screams in pain. At this point rescuers should_____
    a. work more quickly and efficiently to remove the boot.
    b. stop temporarily to allow the patient's pain to subside before continuing.
    c. encourage the patient to breathe in through the nose and exhale through the mouth to minimize the pain until the removal is complete.
    d. stop the procedure and leave the boot on.

13. Which of the following statements regarding sport boot removal is false?_____
    a. Avoid using saws on ski boots.
    b. If unfamiliar with a boot, remove the boot from the uninjured leg first.
    c. Never remove a sports boot once a leg has been placed in a traction splint.
    d. A sports boot should be removed if a patient complains of CMS compromise.

14. For any fracture, distal CMS should be checked_____
    a. before applying the splint.
    b. after applying the splint.
    c. before and after applying the splint, and periodically thereafter.
    d. when you get around to it.

## Short Answer

1. Describe the steps you would take to relocate a dislocated knee that has CMS compromise.

   _____

   _____

2. Why must *all* dislocated knees, even those that reduce spontaneously and have normal neurovascular findings, be evaluated at a hospital?

   _____

   _____

## Stabilized Extrication and Transfer: "Jams and Pretzels"

Patients who incur serious MS injuries in the field often are found in a contorted position with severely angulated limbs. To effectively immobilize and transport these patients, it is often necessary to move them into an anatomically correct supine position so that they may be fully immobilized on a backboard.

Rescuers encounter injured patients in one of six basic anatomical positions: three primary positions (1, 2, and 3) and three variations (1a, 2a, and 3a). These positions were popularized by Warren Bowman, M.D. and were introduced to the NSP in *Outdoor Emergency Care*, Third Edition under the general topic of "jams and pretzels." The following descriptions of positioning and the methods of moving patients are adapted from his descriptions (Figures 20-86a–f■).

**Position 1:** Patients are supine, in a neutral anatomical position with the back straight and the eyes facing forward. The extremities are straight, with the palms against the thighs. Ideally, patients should be aligned in this position before transfer to a long spine board.

**Position 1a:** Patients are supine but their head, neck, back, and/or extremities are rotated, bent, or in some position other than an anatomically correct position.

**Position 2:** Patients are on their side, but in a neutral anatomical position with the back straight, the eyes facing forward, the extremities straight, and the palms against the sides of the thighs. Patients in this position should be rolled in one direction to the other to Position 1 by using a log roll.

**Position 2a:** Patients are on their side, with the head, neck, back, and extremities in any position except a normal anatomical position.

**Position 3:** Patients are prone but in a neutral anatomical position, except that the head is usually turned to the side.

**Position 3a:** Patients are prone, with the head, neck, back, and extremities in any position except a neutral anatomical position.

The goal of positioning an injured patient is to move the person, especially one with a suspected spinal injury, into Position 1, either on the ground or on a spine board, without causing any damage to the spinal cord or further neurologic injury.

⊕ **20-3.5** Describe and demonstrate placing a patient in the anatomical position using the principles of "jams and pretzels."

**"jams and pretzels"** a phrase that refers to the process by which someone who is injured and an awkward position is returned to normal supine anatomical position while maintaining spinal alignment.

**Figure 20-86a** Position 1.

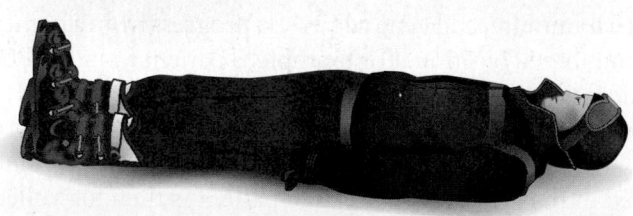

**Figure 20-86b** Position 1a.

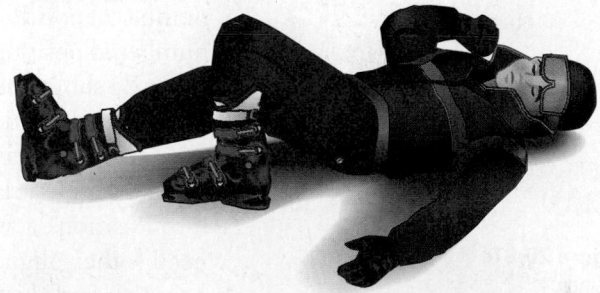

**Figure 20-86c** Position 2.

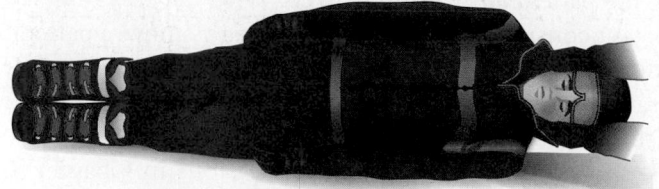

**Figure 20-86d** Position 2a.

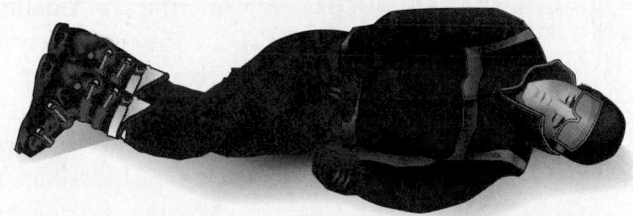

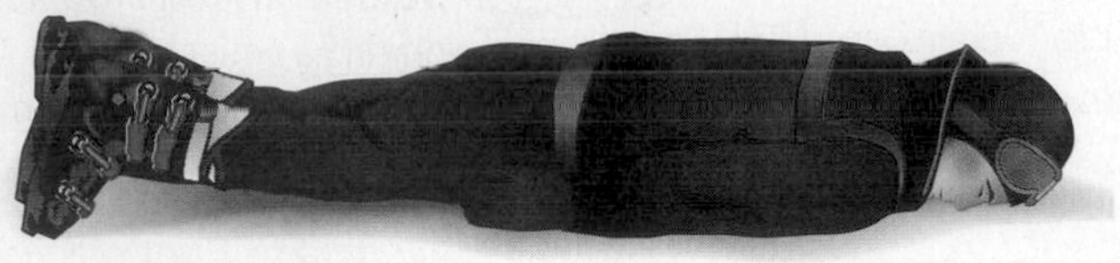

Figure 20-86e Position 3.

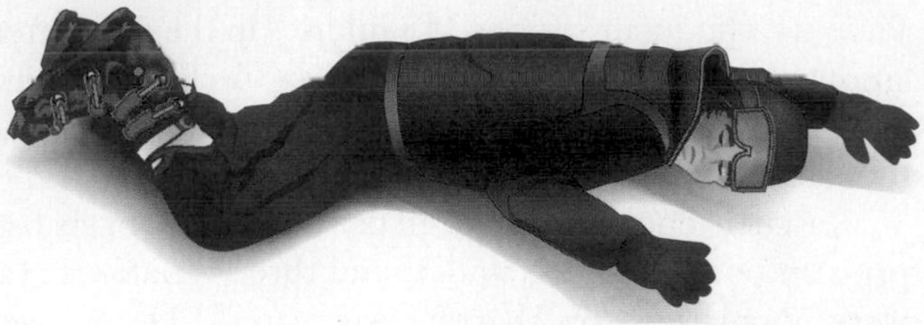

Figure 20-86f Position 3a.

When a patient lies supine in the anatomical position, the back of the person's head (occiput), shoulders, buttocks, calves, and heels are all in the same line. In this position, the three important posterior reference points are the head, shoulders, and hips, and the three important anterior reference points are the nose, naval, and toes.

**stabilized extrication** keeping a patient's spine anatomically aligned during removal from an accident, therefore preventing any neurologic damage.

The process of placing a patient into anatomical alignment is termed **stabilized extrication**. The goal of stabilized extrication is to align the patient such that the three posterior reference points remain aligned in both the vertical and horizontal planes. The key to performing stabilized extrication, then, is to keep these three reference points both aligned and in the same plane while the patient is being moved. When this is accomplished, the spine will be stabilized and little or no motion will occur in the spinal segments. When properly positioned, the three anterior points should also form a straight line.

Four rescuers are usually needed to move (align) a patient into Position 1 (supine): one at the patient's head, one at the shoulders, one at the hips, and one at the legs. All movements should be coordinated by a lead OEC Technician who, ideally, observes and directs the actions of the other rescuers. If needed, the leader can assist the team, positioning himself at the patient's head. Rescuers should move the patient smoothly, without hesitation, and in unison following the leader's directions. The team must manually stabilize the three posterior reference points *at all times*.

Move the patient axially (by sliding) or vertically (by lifting and/or lowering), but never move the patient sideways. All movements should be in increments of 6–12 inches and should be started and stopped at the leader's command. When the patient's limbs, head, or neck need to be straightened, move only one joint at a time in only one plane at a time while manually stabilizing the three posterior reference points.

Align all body parts into Position 1, 2, or 3 as early as possible, unless major pain or resistance occurs. Begin with the head and neck so that the airway can be protected. Perform all maneuvers with confidence but not in a hurried manner. Try to keep the number of positions selected at a minimum, and generally try to progress from a higher numbered position to a lower numbered position. For example, a patient found in Position 2a should be manually aligned into Position 2, then log rolled into Position 1.

Moving a patient found in Position 3a with the head turned to the side is more complex. In this instance, the body and extremities are aligned into Position 3 while the head and neck are stabilized in the position found. The patient is then log rolled into Position 2a, with the head maintained as is until the body reaches Position 2. The head is then aligned to Position 2. Finally, the patient is log rolled into Position 1 on a spine board (Figures 20-87a–c■). If the patient is located in a confined area or is positioned awkwardly (for example, jammed against a tree), try to align the patient using the same method moving the patient *away* from the tree.

**Figure 20-87a** When only two rescuers are available, align the patient to Position 3 while stabilizing the head and neck.
Copyright Scott Smith

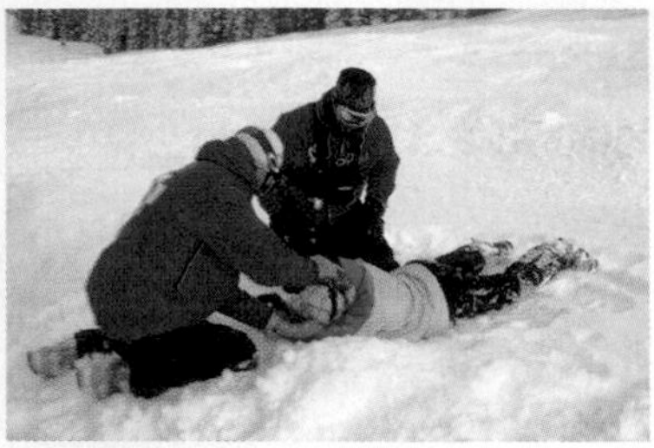

**Figure 20-87b** Roll the patient from Position 2a to Position 2.
Copyright Scott Smith

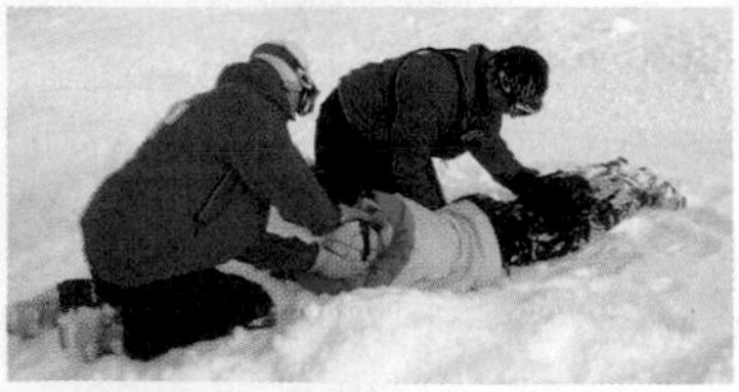

**Figure 20-87c** Roll the patient into Position 1.
Copyright Scott Smith

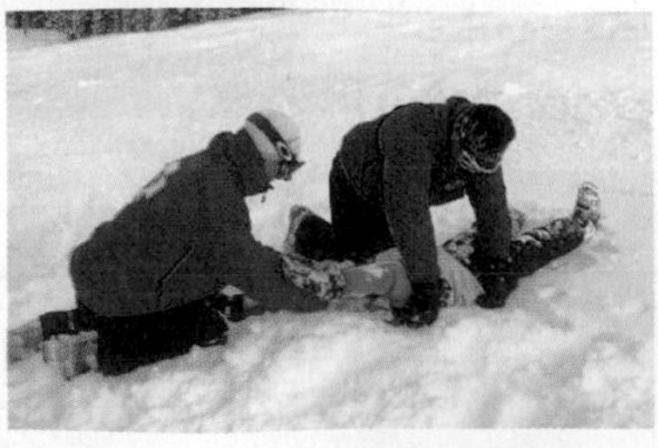

Rescuer safety is an important consideration when attempting to move a patient. To avoid injuring one's back or another body part, every rescuer should remember to lift with the hips and legs rather than with the back. Keep the back straight. Don't twist or bend forward or to the side, and hold the load (the patient) as close to the body as possible. You may wish to review the appropriate sections in Chapter 5, Moving, Lifting, and Transporting Patients.

# STOP, THINK, UNDERSTAND

## Multiple Choice

Choose the correct answer.

1. "Jams and pretzels" refers to_____
   a. a snack.
   b. an extrication procedure.
   c. a method of setting up a rescue pack.
   d. realigning of a patient found in a contorted position with angulated limbs.

2. The positioning goal of "jams and pretzels" is to _____
   a. place the patient in anatomical Position 1 without causing damage to the spinal cord or further neurologic injury.
   b. secure a patient into a side-lying recovery Position 3 to maintain the airway.
   c. maintain the patient in a prone, neutral Position 2 without exacerbating spinal cord damage.
   d. transport the patient in the anatomical position found.

3. The three important posterior reference points that must be kept in alignment and the same plane are the_____
   a. neck, torso, and lower extremities.
   b. head, shoulders, and hips.

   c. torso, the upper extremities, and the lower extremities.
   d. head, shoulders, and lower extremities.

4. Which of the following statements about moving a patient in the correct anatomical position is correct? _____
   a. Use three rescuers: one stationed at the head, one at the torso, and one at the lower extremities; move the patient sideways and vertically in 6-inch to 12-inch increments.
   b. Use anywhere from two to four rescuers stationed at the head, neck, shoulders, and hips, and move each patient slowly and carefully in any necessary direction.
   c. Use four rescuers (at the head, shoulders, hips, and legs) and move in short increments of 6 inches to 12 inches while manually stabilizing the three posterior reference points.
   d. Follow the head rescuer's lead and directions to stabilize the patient in whatever manner is necessary because no two patients are ever positioned exactly alike.

## List

The five anatomical parts of a supine patient that are in contact with an imaginary flat spinal plane are:

a. _____
b. _____
c. _____
d. _____
e. _____

# CASE DISPOSITION

You perform a secondary assessment, which reveals a mid-shaft right arm injury with displacement and no distal pulse, and a possible mid-shaft right femur fracture with no external bleeding. Other OEC Technicians soon arrive. Because of the lack of a distal pulse and the long transport time to the hospital, you explain to the teen that you need to straighten his arm, that it will hurt, and that you need to get blood flowing to his fingers. Gently, you apply tension to his right hand, feeling the location where the radial pulse is located, while your partner holds the elbow. Upon straightening the arm, the radial pulse becomes strong. You expose the arm, find no bleeding, cover it back up, and splint it with a long SAM™ arm splint in a "sugar tong" configuration, and secure the splint with a roller bandage. You then apply a sling and swathe. He lies in a supine position, covered in a blanket your partner has provided. His right radial pulse remains strong.

With assistance from the other rescuers, you apply a Sager splint for the possible mid shaft femur fracture, leaving the ski boot on the foot. You then log roll the patient onto his left (uninjured) side and place him on a long spine board so that you can lift him into the waiting toboggan, where he can lie with his feet uphill. You again assess CMS of both affected extremities and vital signs before rapid transfer to the patrol room. The ALS ambulance arrives, and he is transported to the hospital.

You learn the next day that he had surgery on both his arm and leg, that both have normal CMS, and that he will make a full recovery.

# OEC SKILL 20-1    Applying Sling and Swathe

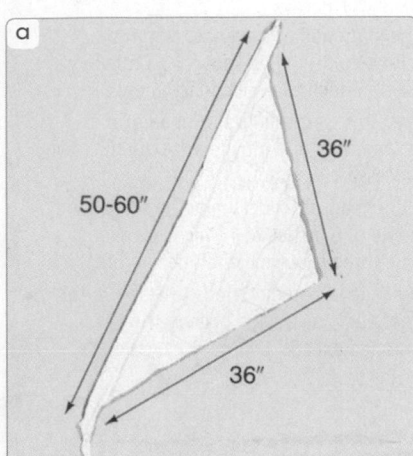

Prepare the sling with a cravat or by folding a cloth into a triangle.

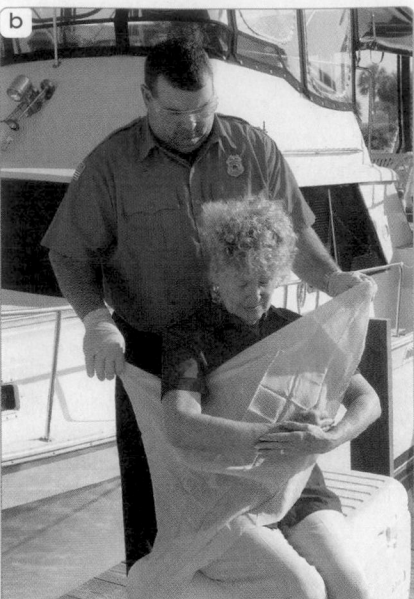

After assessing CMS, place the sling on the chest under the injured arm. Have the patient support the arm, or if there are two rescuers, have the second

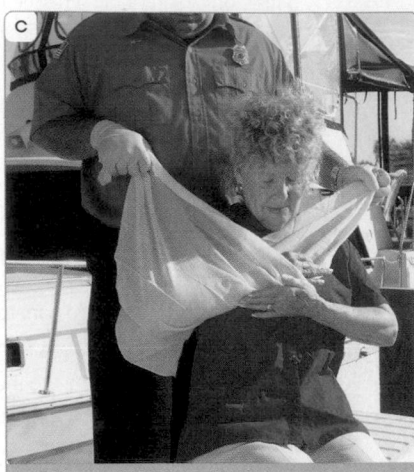

Fold the lower half up and over the injured arm, then up and over the shoulder on the injured side. Raise or lower the arm to the appropriate level.

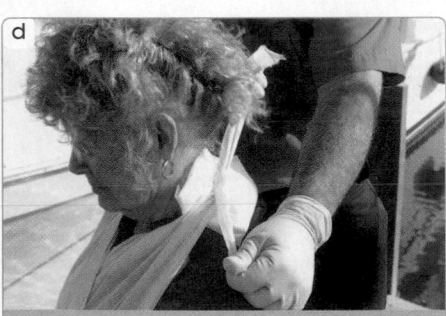

Tie the two ends at the side of the neck and place a pad under the knot.

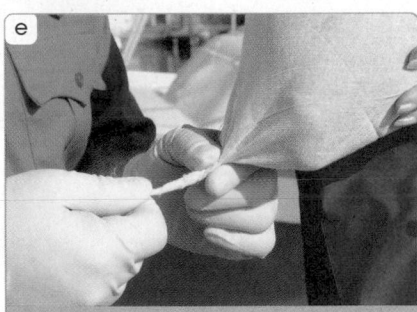

Secure the point of the sling and either pin it to the front or tie a knot.

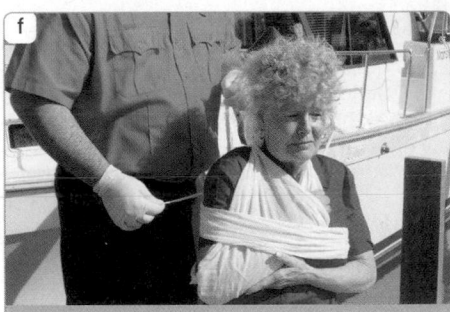

For the swathe: Fold a second triangular bandage to form a cravat that is 2–4 inches wide. Wrap around the patient's chest with the middle of the cravat over the injured arm, and tie the two ends under the opposite arm. Reassess CMS..

# OEC SKILL 20-2 | Creating and Applying a Figure Eight Splint

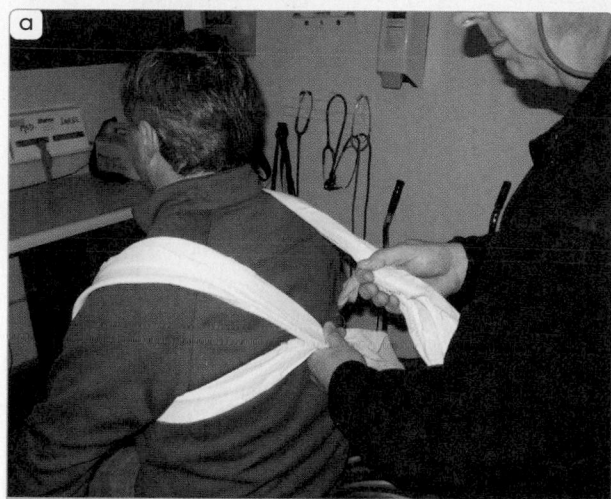

On a seated patient, take two cravats and place one around each shoulder.
Copyright Edward McNamara

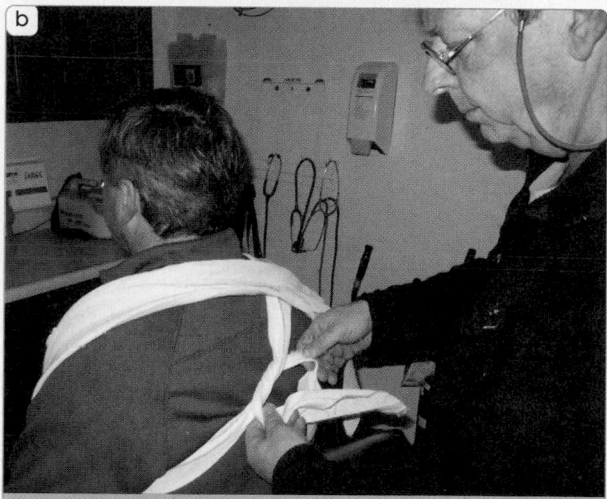

Cross the ends of the cravats behind the patient to make a figure eight.
Copyright Edward McNamara

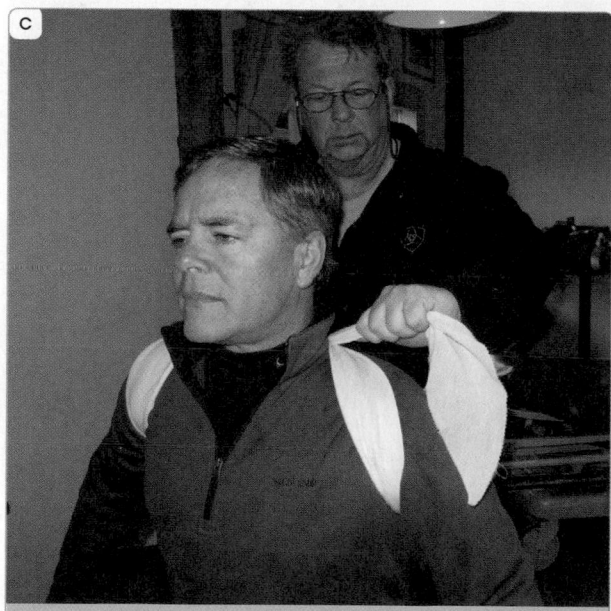

Tighten the cravats and tie the ends together.
Copyright Edward McNamara

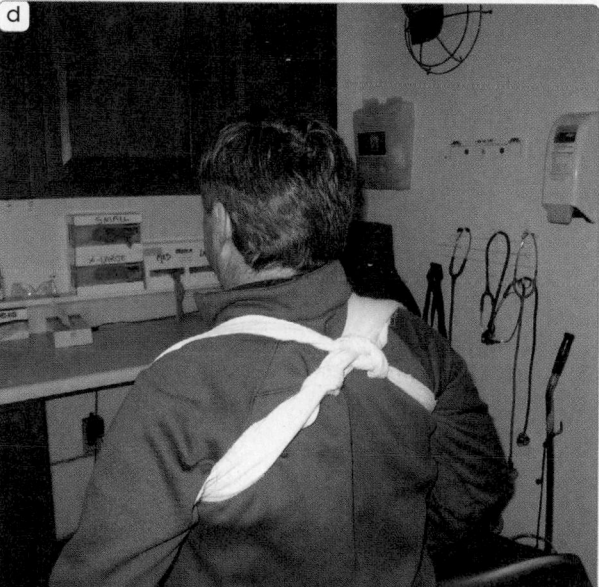

Tighten the figure eight until the patient's shoulders are in a normal position, not pulled back.
Copyright Edward McNamara

## OEC SKILL 20-3 Reducing a Posterior Sternoclavicular (S/C) Injury

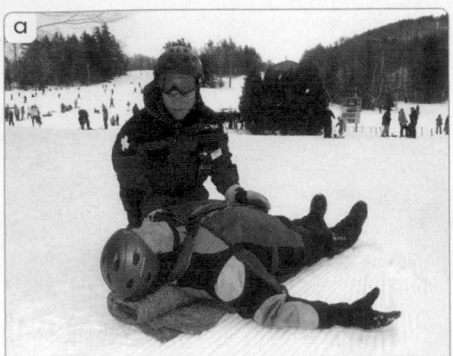

a

Place a blanket roll between the shoulder blades to elevate the thorax.
Copyright Edward McNamara

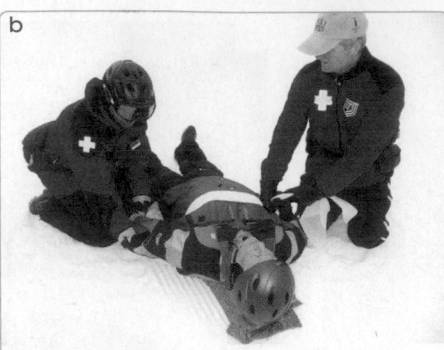

b

Apply traction to the arm on the affected side by pulling the arm at the wrist.
Copyright Edward McNamara

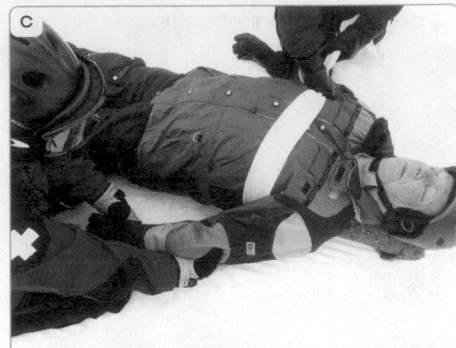

c

Apply counter-traction by pulling on the other side near the axilla with a long broad cravat.
Copyright Edward McNamara

## OEC SKILL 20-4 Applying a Blanket Roll Splint to a Shoulder

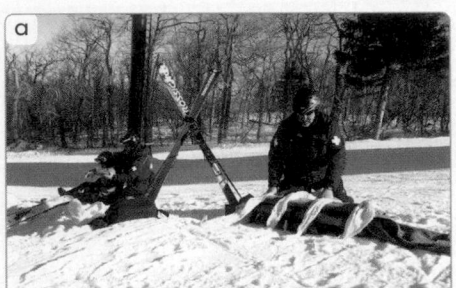

a

Fold a blanket lengthwise into thirds or fourths and lay four cravats crosswise onto the blanket. Knots can be tied in the cravats for differentiating ties.
Copyright Edward McNamara

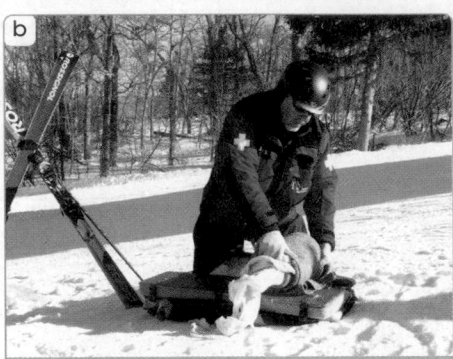

b

Roll or fold the blanket into the appropriate size to fit the patient.
Copyright Edward McNamara

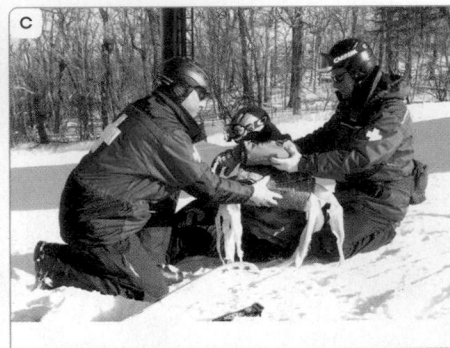

c

Place the blanket roll snugly up into the patient's armpit and hold in place.
Copyright Edward McNamara

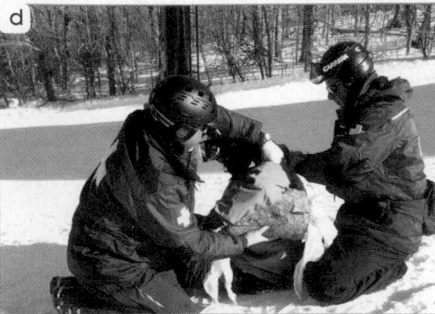

d

Tie one of the cravats from the blanket roll under the opposite shoulder and another around the neck.
Copyright Edward McNamara

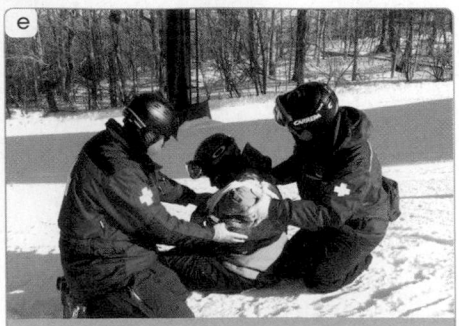

e

Stabilize the hand and forearm with the other two cravats and then reassess CMS.
Copyright Edward McNamara

## OEC SKILL 20-5 | Splinting a Humerus Fracture Using a Rigid Splint

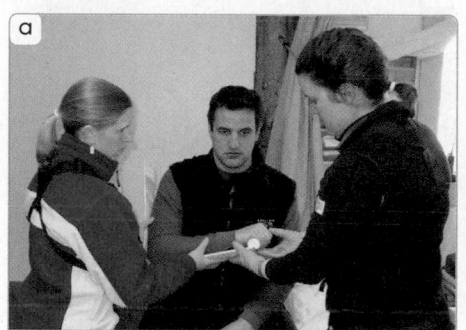

a

Select an appropriate splint. Form the splint such that it will hold the elbow at a 90 degree angle.
Copyright Edward McNamara

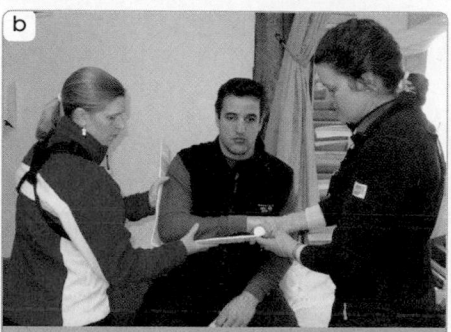

b

Assess CMS and gently place the splint under the arm.
Copyright Edward McNamara

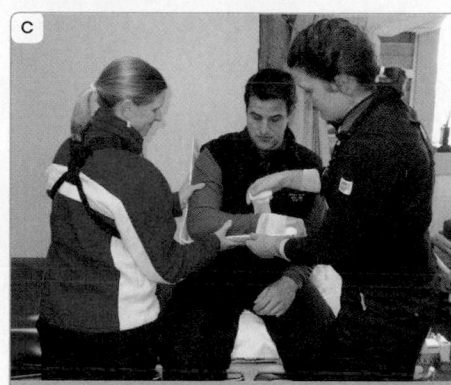

c

Secure the arm snugly to the splint. Reassess CMS.
Copyright Edward McNamara

## OEC SKILL 20-6 | Rigid Splint Fixation of an Injured Elbow

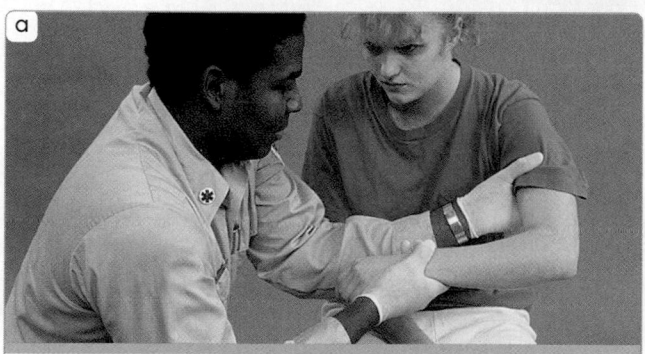

a

Stabilize the arm and assess CMS.

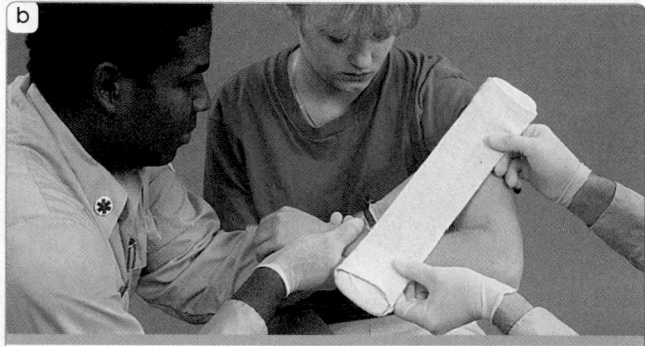

b

Apply a rigid splint that extends past the wrist and past the upper third of the humerus.

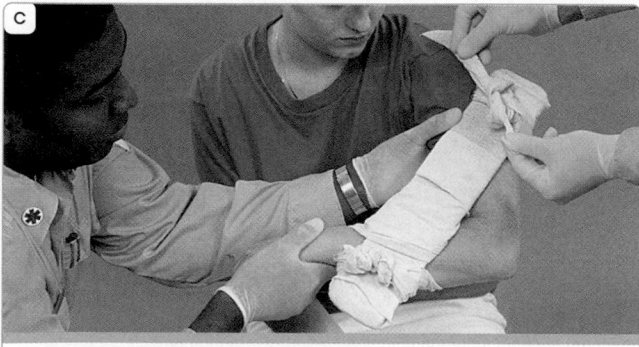

c

Secure the splint in place using a roller bandage or cravats.

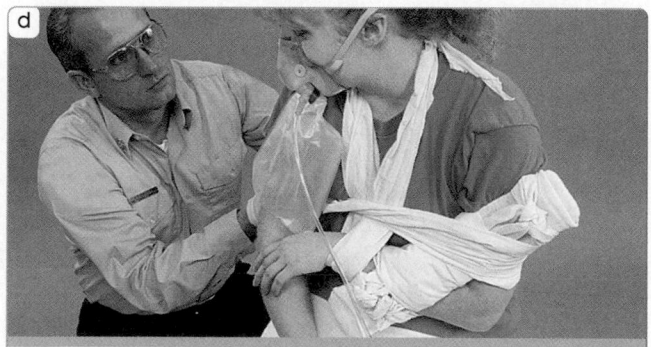

d

Apply a sling and swathe. Reassess CMS.

## OEC SKILL 20-7 | Splinting a Forearm Fracture

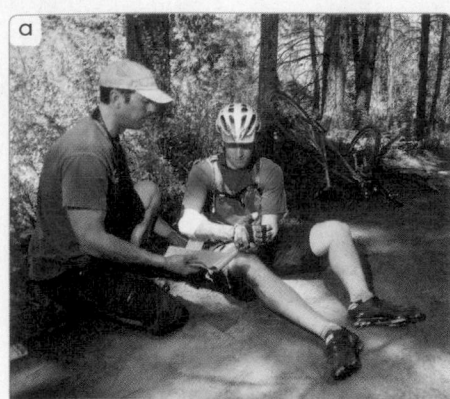

**a**

Select an appropriate splint and form it into the desired shape so that it extends from the palm to above the elbow.
Copyright Scott Smith

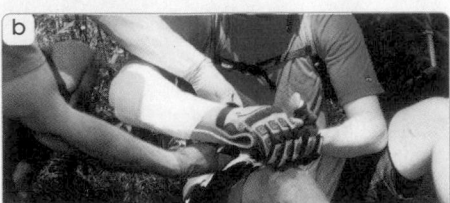

**b**

Secure the forearm to the splint with roller gauze.
Copyright Scott Smith

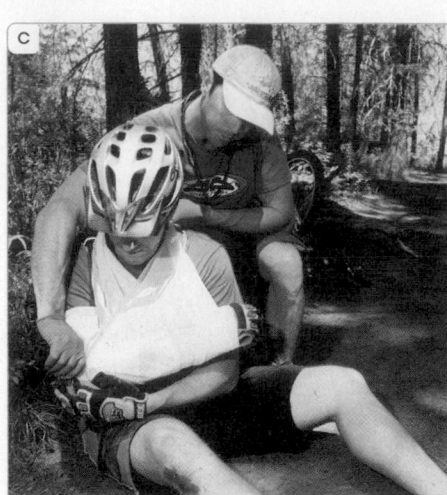

**c**

Apply a sling and swathe and reassess CMS.
Copyright Scott Smith

## OEC SKILL 20-8 | Splinting to Immobilize the Hand

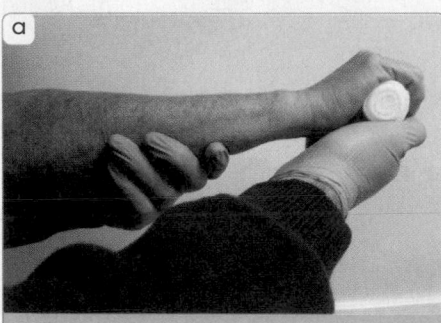

**a**

With the hand stabilized, place a roll of gauze in the palm.
Copyright Edward McNamara

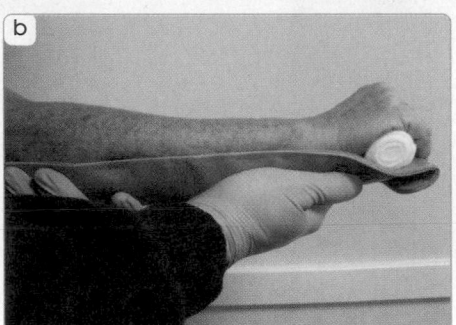

**b**

Place the palm side of the arm on a splint.
Copyright Edward McNamara

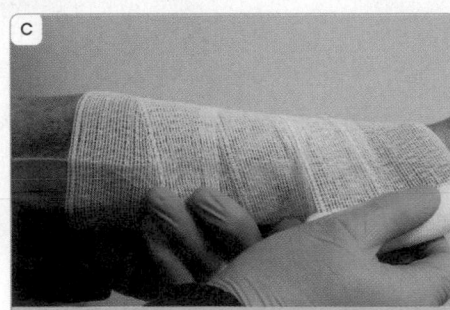

**c**

Secure the arm to the splint using soft roller gauze. Reassess CMS.
Copyright Edward McNamara

# OEC SKILL 20-9 | Applying a Traction Splint to a Femur

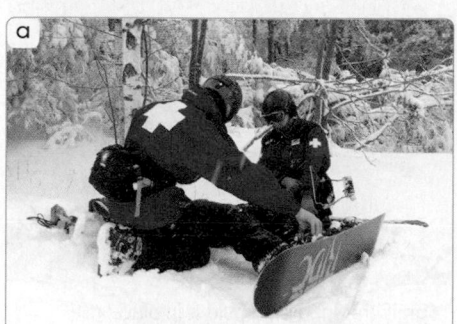

Assess the injury and remove clothing if necessary. Stabilize the fracture site.
Copyright Edward McNamara

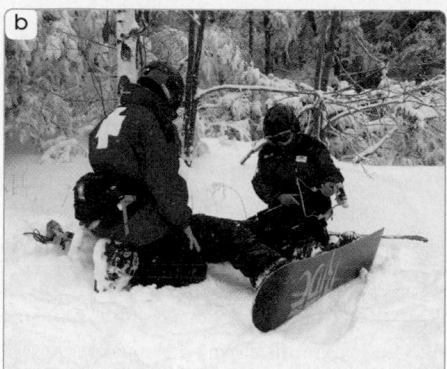

Prepare the traction splint.
Copyright Edward McNamara

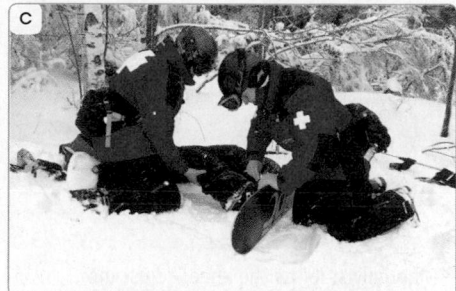

With a person stabilizing the patient's legs, remove the skis or snowboard.
Copyright Edward McNamara

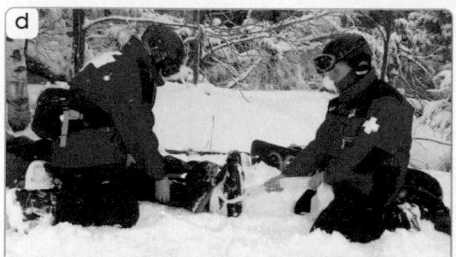

Apply the ankle hitch. Pull on the ankle hitch to straighten the leg into anatomical alignment and maintain slight traction.
Copyright Ed McNamara

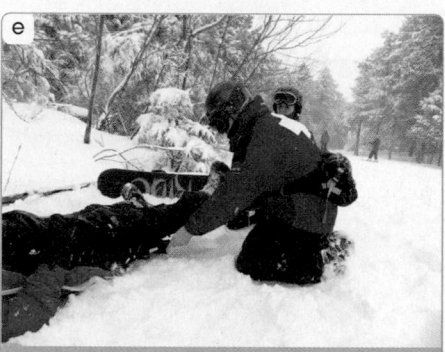

Position the splint so that it is snug to the ischial tuberosity.
Copyright Edward McNamara

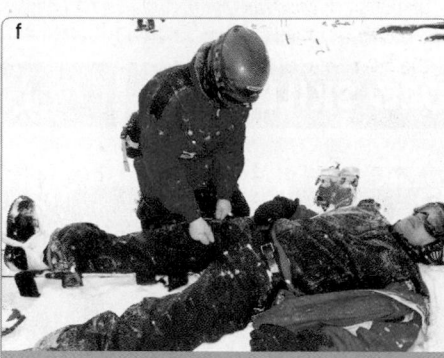

Secure the groin strap.
Copyright Edward McNamara

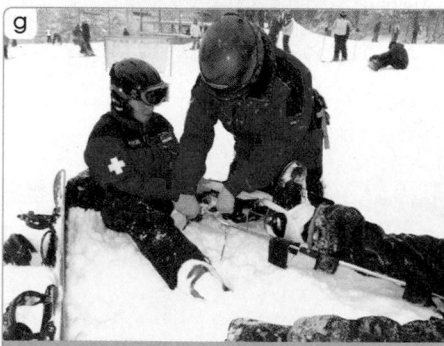

Connect the ankle strap of the hitch and crank slowly so that the manual traction is gradually replaced by mechanical traction.
Copyright Edward McNamara

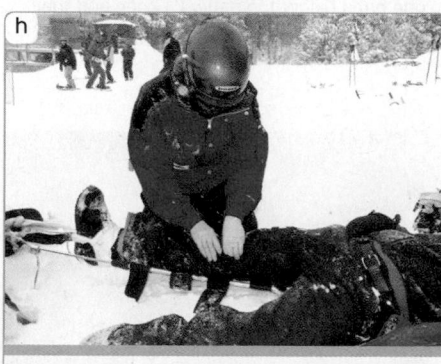

Secure the straps: two above the knee and two below the knee. Reassess CMS.
Copyright Edward McNamara

## OEC SKILL 20-10 | Applying an Airplane Splint

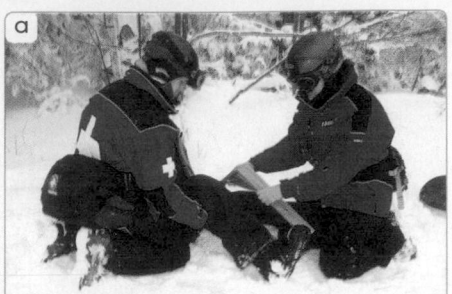

**a**

Manually stabilize the knee. Adjust the splint to the correct angle and lock it.
Copyright Edward McNamara

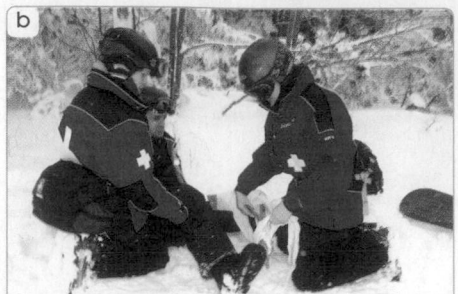

**b**

Wrap two cravats around the upper part of the splint and two cravats around the lower part of the splint.
Copyright Edward McNamara

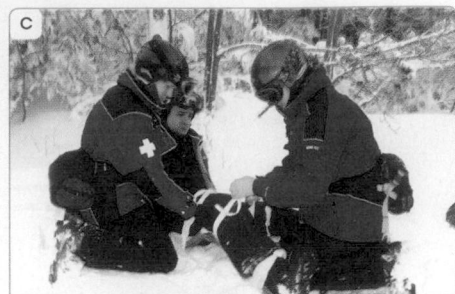

**c**

Apply the splint and hold it in place; use cravats to attach the splint to the leg. Reassess CMS.
Copyright Edward McNamara

## OEC SKILL 20-11 | Applying a Quick Splint

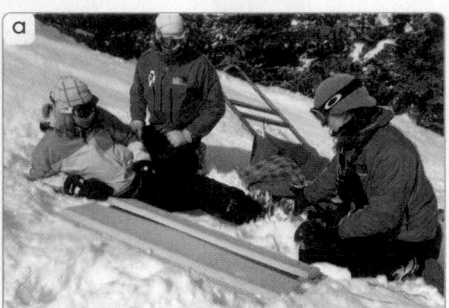

**a**

Assess the injury. Open the splint flat and place it either alongside or distal to the area to be splinted.
Copyright Scott Smith

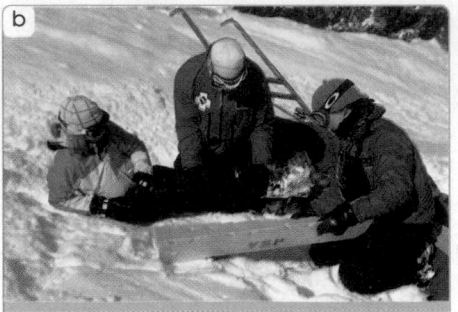

**b**

Place one hand under the patient's foot and one hand below the patient's knee and then lift the leg.
Copyright Scott Smith

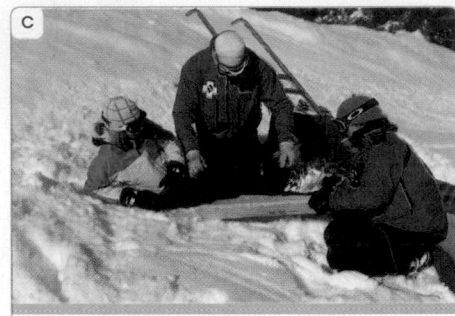

**c**

Another option for lifting the leg is to use the pant leg pinch lift.
Copyright Scott Smith

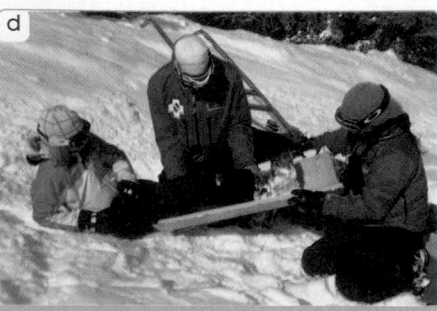

**d**

Slide the splint underneath the leg, either from bottom to top or from the side, and gently lower the extremity into the center of the splint.
Copyright Scott Smith

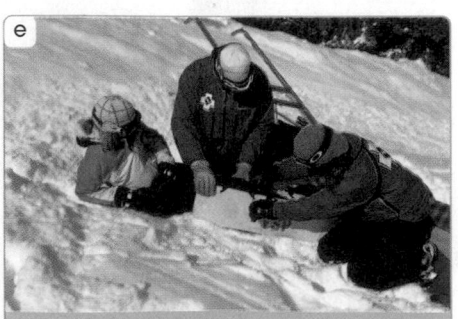

**e**

Close the sides of the Quick Splint, holding the leg snugly, and then secure the splint straps, rope, or webbing. Reassess CMS.
Copyright Scott Smith

## OEC SKILL 20-12 — Replacing a Quick Splint with a Cardboard Splint

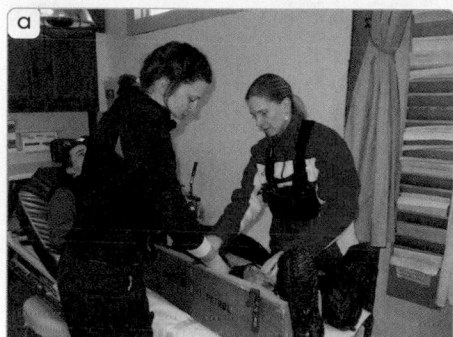

Stabilize the leg and unclip the splint.
Copyright Edward McNamara

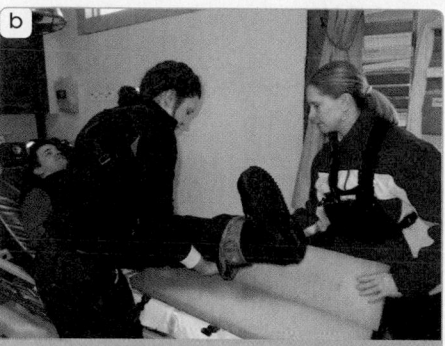

Raise the leg and remove the splint.
Copyright Edward McNamara

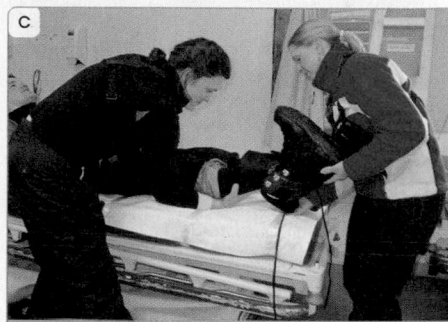

Remove the patient's boot.
Copyright Edward McNamara

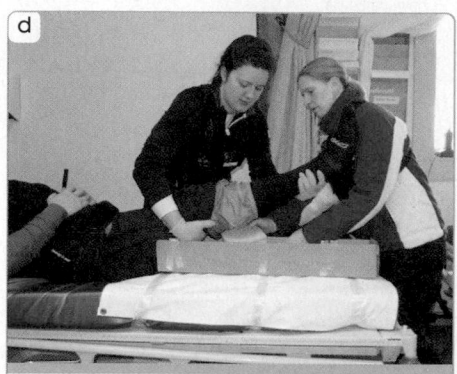

Support and lift the injured extremity and then slide the preformed cardboard splint into position under the leg.
Copyright Edward McNamara

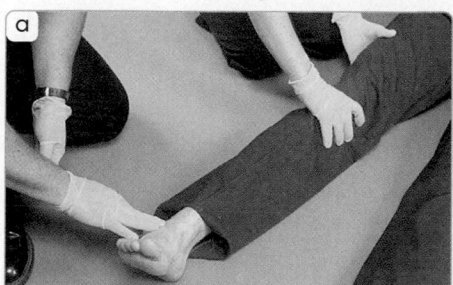

Lower the leg into the splint, and then pad all voids between the extremity and the cardboard. Place tape over the sides of the splint together to hold the leg in place. Reassess CMS.
Copyright Edward McNamara

## OEC SKILL 20-13 — Immobilizing a Tib-Fib Fracture with Two Rigid Splints

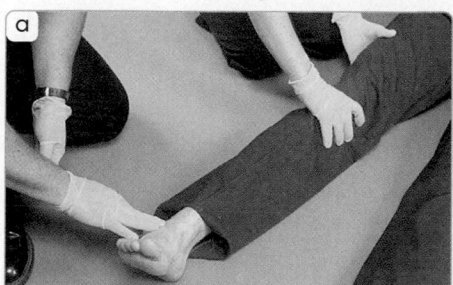

Check the CMS and stabilize the leg. Measure for splint size using the uninjured leg.

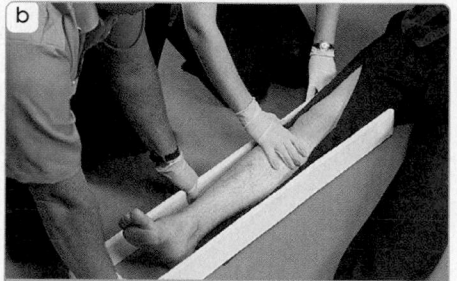

Place the splints on either side of the leg such that they extend above the knee and below the ankle.

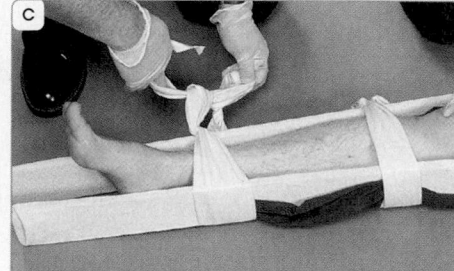

Tie the splints together with gauze or cravats. Reassess CMS.

## OEC SKILL 20-14    Removing a Boot

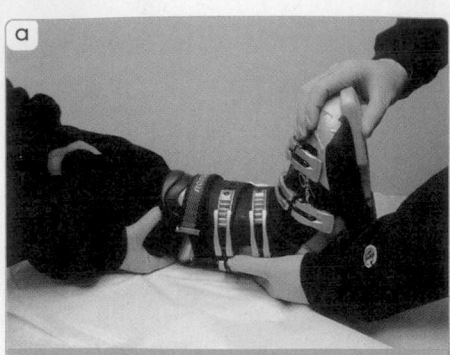

**a** Stabilize the leg from which the boot is to be removed.
Copyright Edward McNamara

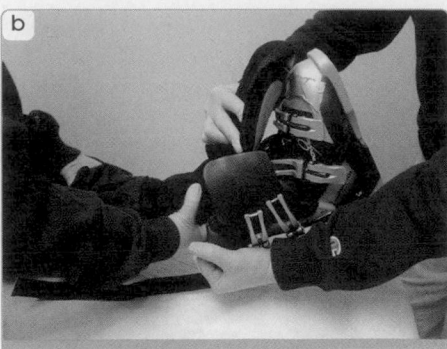

**b** Unbuckle or unlace the boot and pull the boot open.
Copyright Edward McNamara

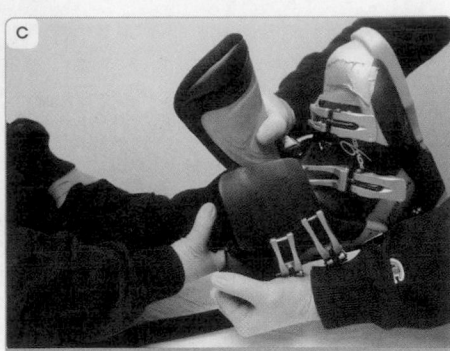

**c** Stabilize the leg by putting one hand on the front of the leg and the other hand on the back of the ankle. Slowly remove the boot.
Copyright Edward McNamara

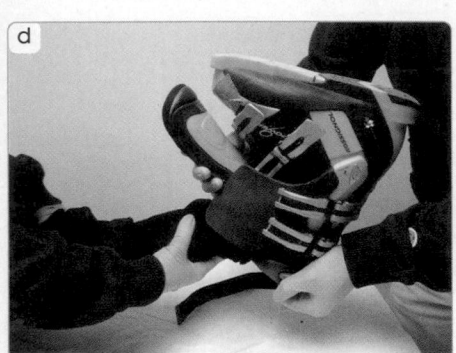

**d** Remove the boot by sliding the heel of the boot away from the sole of the foot.
Copyright Edward McNamara

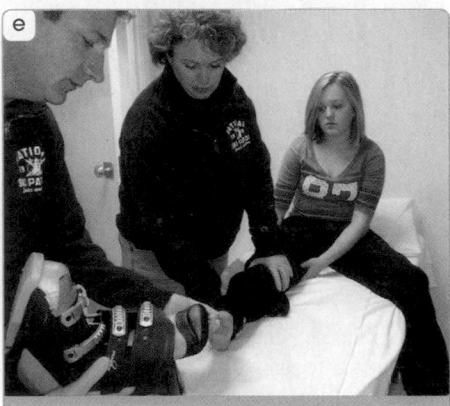

**e** While still stabilizing the leg, reassess CMS.
Copyright Edward McNamara

## Skill Guide

Date:_____

(CPI) = Critical Performance Indicator

Candidate: _____

Start time: _____

End time: _____

## Figure Eight Application

**Objective:** To demonstrate application of a figure eight splint.

| Skill | Max Points | Skill Demo | |
|---|---|---|---|
| Determines that scene is safe. | 1 | | (CPI) |
| Introduces self, obtains permission to treat/help. | 1 | | |
| Initiates Standard Precautions. | 1 | | (CPI) |
| Exposes/visualizes injured area to determine that a figure eight is appropriate. | 1 | | (CPI) |
| Places patient in a sitting position. | 1 | | |
| Assesses CMS. | 1 | | (CPI) |
| Places one cravat around each shoulder (over and under the armpit); ensures that the cravat is not directly over the fracture site and that front of cravat has wide band. | 1 | | |
| Crosses ends of cravats that are behind patient to make a figure eight. | 1 | | |
| Tightens cravats so that the position of the shoulders is the same as if the patient were sitting normally (shoulders should not be pulled all the way back). | 1 | | |
| Ties cravats with square knots, ensuring that the shoulders are in normal position. | 1 | | |
| Reassesses CMS. | 1 | | (CPI) |
| Treats for shock if appropriate. | 1 | | |
| Prepares patient for transport. | 1 | | |

Must receive 10 out of 13 points.

Comments: _____

Failure of any of the CPIs is an automatic failure.

Evaluator: _____ NSP ID: _____

PASS      FAIL

## Skill Guide

Date:_____

(CPI) = Critical Performance Indicator

Candidate: _____

Start time: _____

End time: _____

## Splinting an Upper Extremity Injury

**Objective:** To demonstrate the proper management and splinting of an upper extremity injury.

| Skill | Max Points | Skill Demo | |
|---|---|---|---|
| Determines scene is safe. | 1 | | (CPI) |
| Introduces self, obtain permission to help/treat. | 1 | | |
| Initiates Standard Precautions. | 1 | | (CPI) |
| Exposes injury to assess and manage the ABCDs. | 1 | | (CPI) |
| Bandages any wounds as necessary. | 1 | | |
| Directs helper to stabilize abouve and below the injury site. | 1 | | (CPI) |
| Assesses for CMS. | 1 | | (CPI) |
| Technician chooses the correct device/material for splinting/stabilization. | 1 | | |
| Sizes splint properly; pading as needed and positions splint. | 1 | | |
| Rotates extremity if necessary and as tolerated by patient. | 1 | | |
| Extremity is splinted and stabilized with minimal movement. | 1 | | (CPI) |
| Sling and swathe correctly applied and restricts movement of injured extremity. | 1 | | |
| Reassesses CMS. | 1 | | (CPI) |
| Applies cooling method to help reduce swelling/bruising. | 1 | | |
| Prepares patient for transport. | 1 | | |
| Provides oxygen/treat for shock if appropriate. | 1 | | |

Must receive 13 out of 16 points.

Comments: _____

Failure of any of the CPIs is an automatic failure.

Evaluator: _____ NSP ID: _____

PASS     FAIL

## Skill Guide

Date:_____

(CPI) = Critical Performance Indicator

Candidate: _____

Start time: _____

End time: _____

## Blanket Roll Splint for Shoulder

**Objective:** To demonstrate the appropriate use of a blanket roll for shoulder splinting/stabilization.

| Skill | Max Points | Skill Demo | |
|---|---|---|---|
| Determines that scene is safe. | 1 | | (CPI) |
| Introduces self, obtains permission to treat/help. | 1 | | |
| Initiates Standard Precautions. | 1 | | (CPI) |
| Exposes injury; assesses and manages the ABCDs. | 1 | | (CPI) |
| Places blanket on flat surface, sizing the roll by folding the blanket to fit the size needed. | 1 | | |
| Places four cravats crosswise on one end of folded blanket; rolls blanket firmly, including cravats. | 1 | | |
| Assesses CMS. | 1 | | (CPI) |
| Positions rolled blanket and cravats snugly in the axilla (armpit) of the dislocated shoulder. | 1 | | |
| While helper holds blanket roll in place, ties one set of cravats over the opposite shoulder around the neck. | 1 | | |
| Secures second cravat around the patient's waist. | 1 | | |
| Stabilizes hand and forearm on the blanket with the remaining two cravats. | 1 | | |
| Reassesses CMS. | 1 | | (CPI) |
| Applies cooling method to help reduce swelling/bruising. | 1 | | |
| Prepares patient for transport. | 1 | | |
| Provides oxygen/treats for shock, if appropriate. | 1 | | |

Must receive 12 out of 15 points.

Comments: _____

Failure of any of the CPIs is an automatic failure.

Evaluator: _____ NSP ID: _____

PASS    FAIL

## Skill Guide

Date:_____

(CPI) = Critical Performance Indicator

Candidate: _____

Start time: _____

End time: _____

## Posterior S/C Dislocation Reduction

**Objective:** To demonstrate how to reduce a posterior S/C dislocation.

| Skill | Max Points | Skill Demo | |
|---|---|---|---|
| Determines that scene is safe. | 1 | | (CPI) |
| Introduces self, obtains permission to treat/help. | 1 | | |
| Initiates Standard Precautions. | 1 | | (CPI) |
| Assesses CMS. | 1 | | (CPI) |
| Ties wide cravat around upper chest, under armpits. | 1 | | |
| Forms a tight blanket roll. | 1 | | |
| Places patient in supine position, with blanket roll under shoulder blades. | 1 | | |
| Rescuer #1 applies traction to the wrist on affected side by pulling arm out and downward toward ground. | 1 | | (CPI) |
| Rescuer #2 simultaneously places counter-traction on the other side of body by pulling on cravat tied around upper chest. | 1 | | (CPI) |
| Reassesses CMS. | 1 | | (CPI) |
| Applies figure-eight splint and then applies a swathe. | | | (CPI) |
| Treats for shock. | 1 | | |
| Arranges for transport of patient. | 1 | | |

Must receive 10 out of 13 points.

Comments: _____

Failure of any of the CPIs is an automatic failure.

Evaluator: _____ NSP ID: _____

PASS    FAIL

## Skill Guide

Date:_____

(CPI) = Critical Performance Indicator

Candidate: _____

Start time: _____

End time: _____

## Splinting a Lower Extremity Injury

> **Objective:** To demonstrate the proper management and splinting a lower extremity injury.

| Skill | Max Points | Skill Demo | |
|---|---|---|---|
| Determines that scene is safe. | 1 | | (CPI) |
| Introduces self, obtains permission to help/treat. | 1 | | |
| Initiates Standard Precautions. | 1 | | (CPI) |
| Exposes injury to assess and manage the ABCDs. | 1 | | (CPI) |
| Bandages any wounds, as necessary. | 1 | | |
| Directs helper to stabilize above and below the injury site by grasping the boot/shoe with one hand and grasping below the knee with the second hand. | 1 | | (CPI) |
| Assesses for CMS. | 1 | | (CPI) |
| Removes boot/shoe per local protocol. | 1 | | |
| Chooses the correct device/material for splinting/stabilization. | 1 | | |
| Sizes splint properly; uses pads as needed and positions splint. | 1 | | |
| Applies gentle traction/tension as needed, rotating extremity if necessary and if tolerated by patient. | 1 | | |
| Splints and stabilizes extremity with minimal movement. | 1 | | |
| Reassesses CMS. | 1 | | (CPI) |
| Applies cooling method to help reduce swelling/bruising. | 1 | | |
| Prepares patient for transport. | 1 | | |
| Provides oxygen/treats for shock, if appropriate. | 1 | | |

| Must receive 13 out of 16 points. |
|---|

Comments: _____

Failure of any of the CPIs is an automatic failure.

Evaluator: _____ NSP ID:_____

PASS      FAIL

## Skill Guide

Date:_____

(CPI) – Critical Performance Indicator

Candidate: _____

Start time: _____

End time: _____

# Traction Splinting

**Objective:** To demonstrate the ability to apply a traction splint.

| Skill | Max Points | Skill Demo | |
|---|---|---|---|
| Determines that scene is safe. | 1 | | (CPI) |
| Introduces self, obtains permission to treat/help. | 1 | | |
| Initiates Standard Precautions. | 1 | | (CPI) |
| Exposes and assesses the injury to determine the location and proximity to hip or knee joint; checks for bleeding and treats bleeding if present. | 1 | | |
| Rescuer #1 manually stabilizes the fracture site above and below the injury. | 1 | | (CPI) |
| Rescuer #2 stabilizes the boot/shoe or the ski/snowboard if the equipment is still in place. | 1 | | |
| Rescuer #3 assesses CMS. | 1 | | (CPI) |
| Rescuer #3 prepares traction splint and adjusts to proper size according to manufacturer's instructions; rescuer uses uninjured leg to measure splint. | 1 | | |
| Rescuer #2 removes ski or snowboard if present and then applies the ankle hitch. | 1 | | |
| Rescuer #2 firmly grasps ankle hitch with one hand and places other hand under the calf and moves the injured leg in a coordinated fashion with Rescuer #1 to straighten leg into anatomical alignment using manual traction; maintains traction as Rescuer #1 releases manual stabilization. | 1 | | |
| Rescuer #3 positions the splint according to manufacturer's directions and secures the groin strap around upper thigh. | 1 | | |
| Rescuer #3 connects ankle strap if needed and turns crank/knob, gradually replacing manual traction with mechanical traction. | 1 | | |
| Rescuers secure Velcro support straps or cravats. | 1 | | |
| Secures patient to a backboard. | 1 | | (CPI) |
| Reassesses CMS. | 1 | | (CPI) |
| Treats for shock/provides oxygen. | 1 | | (CPI) |
| Prepares patient for transport, activates EMS. | 1 | | (CPI) |

Must receive 13 out of 17 points.

Comments: _____

Failure of any of the CPIs is an automatic failure.

Evaluator:_____ NSP ID:_____

PASS     FAIL

## Skill Guide

Date:_____

(CPI) = Critical Performance Indicator

Candidate: _____

Start time: _____

End time: _____

## Boot Removal

**Objective:** To demonstrate ability to remove snow sports boot on injured lower llmb.

| Skill | Max Points | Skill Demo | |
|---|---|---|---|
| Determines that scene is safe. | 1 | | (CPI) |
| Introduces self, obtains permission to treat/help. | 1 | | |
| Initiates Standard Precautions. | 1 | | (CPI) |
| Rescuer #1 stabilizes the boot to be removed. | 1 | | |
| Rescuer #2 unbuckles/unlaces the boot completely. | 1 | | |
| Rescuer #2 spreads the boot open. | 1 | | |
| Rescuer #1 stabilizes injured area of leg/ankle by placing one hand on front of ankle and one hand on back of the ankle, holding this position firmly as the boot is removed. | 1 | | (CPI) |
| Rescuer #2 gently removes boot by sliding heel away from foot, followed by the toe portion; monitors patient for indications of excessive pain; stops or modifies procedures as appropriate. | 1 | | |
| Assesses CMS. | 1 | | (CPI) |
| Prepares and applies splint, keeping movement of injured extremity to a minimum. | 1 | | |
| Reassesses CMS after splint is applied. | 1 | | (CPI) |
| Treats for shock, if appropriate. | 1 | | |
| Prepares patient for transport. | 1 | | |

Must receive 10 out of 13 points.

Comments: _____

Failure of any of the CPIs is an automatic failure.

Evaluator:_____ NSP ID:_____

PASS     FAIL

# 🛡 Chapter Review

## Chapter Summary

The most common situation facing OEC Technicians involves injuries to an extremity. These are the "bread and butter" injuries that require an extensive amount of skill because no two are ever alike in outdoor environments. Inclement weather, unusual body positioning, the presence of other severe injuries, damage to vessels and/or nerves, and bleeding makes each injury unique. Each long bone can break in many different ways.

OEC Technicians need to become adept in assessing the entire musculoskeletal system and identifying the various types of musculoskeletal injuries. Although the standard, generally used methods for splinting or immobilizing the various extremity in-

juries are described in this chapter, OEC Technicians may need to improvise, all the while remembering the principle of "first do no harm." Immobilization decreases pain, slows bleeding, prevents further injury, and makes transport easier.

During the assessment of extremity injuries, it is best to ask patients to point with one finger to exactly where it hurts. When immobilizing an extremity, OEC Technicians need to remember to assess CMS, both before and after the procedure.

When caring for musculoskeletal injuries, OEC Technicians must not cause injury to themselves or to others. Proper lifting is especially important in avoiding back injuries.

## Remember...

1. The musculoskeletal system allows movement and protects internal structures.
2. The human skeleton has 206 bones.
3. The upper extremity includes the shoulder, arm, elbow, forearm (lower arm), wrist, hand, and fingers.
4. The lower extremity includes the hip, thigh, knee, leg, ankle, foot, and toes.
5. Skeletal muscles facilitate movement under direct voluntary control of the brain.
6. A fracture is a disruption in the continuity of a bone.
7. A dislocation is the disruption of a joint in which the bone ends no longer remain in normal contact with each other.
8. A splint is a soft or rigid device applied to an injured extremity.

9. The four basic types of splints are soft, rigid or semi-rigid, traction, and improvised.
10. The most frequent injury in skiing is a knee sprain.
11. The most frequent injury while snowboarding is a distal radius fracture.
12. A common upper extremity injury among skiers is skier's thumb.
13. The clavicle is the most commonly broken bone in the body.
14. For extremity injuries, remove all rings, bracelets, or other jewelry from the hand or foot immediately, before swelling occurs.
15. Treat all threats to life first, and then manage musculoskeletal injuries.

## Chapter Questions

### Multiple Choice

Choose the correct answer.

1. The thigh of a patient who has suffered an apparent femur fracture is swelling rapidly. Which of the following statements regarding this injury is correct? _____
   a. Fractures typically cause localized swelling, so this swelling does not cause great concern.
   b. The swelling is most likely caused by the displaced femur pushing the large vastus muscle upward.
   c. The swelling could be indicative of serious internal bleeding and may be life threatening.
   d. Some internal bleeding occurs with all fractures; concern should be raised only if signs and symptoms of shock develop.

**2.** A 5-year-old patient complains that "my whole arm hurts." Which of the following injuries is this complaint most likely indicative of? _____

    **a.** a wrist fracture

    **b.** a fracture of the clavicle

    **c.** a fracture of the radius and ulna

    **d.** all of the above

(For questions 3 and 4) A patient has suffered a blow to the chest near the sternum and exhibits the following signs and symptoms:

- Difficulty swallowing
- Engorgement of facial and upper extremity veins
- Respiratory distress
- Signs/symptoms of shock
- Clavicle on one side looks shorter than the other

**3.** What condition could this patient be suffering from? _____

    **a.** a posterior sternoclavicular dislocation

    **b.** an anterior sternoclavicular dislocation

    **c.** a fracture of the clavicle

    **d.** a fracture of the scapula

**4.** This injury described is _____

    **a.** insignificant.

    **b.** relatively minor.

    **c.** fairly major.

    **d.** potentially life threatening.

**5.** A hiker trips over a rock and falls directly onto her shoulder. What is the least likely injury to occur with this MOI? _____

    **a.** a humeral fracture

    **b.** an acromioclavicular separation

    **c.** a fracture of the scapula

    **d.** an anterior shoulder dislocation

**6.** The classic MOI for an anterior shoulder dislocation is _____

    **a.** forceful adduction and internal rotation of the arm and shoulder.

    **b.** forceful abduction and external rotation of the arm and shoulder.

    **c.** a point fall directly onto the shoulder.

    **d.** a fall onto an outstretched arm.

**7.** A snowboarder forcefully dorsiflexes his ankle when landing big air. An injury you should consider from this is a _____

    **a.** fractured talus bone.

    **b.** medial-lateral ankle sprain or dislocation.

    **c.** foot fracture.

    **d.** tibial-fibular fracture.

**8.** Which of the following injuries should an OEC Technician attempt to reduce? _____

    **a.** An anterior shoulder dislocation on a patient whose shoulder "pops out" frequently.

    **b.** An anterior sternoclavicular dislocation with intact CMS.

    **c.** A posterior sternoclavicular dislocation with accompanying vascular or respiratory compromise.

    **d.** None of the above because it is not within the scope of practice for an OEC Technician to reduce dislocations.

**9.** Regardless of the type of traction splint used, which of the following general principles apply to all types of traction splints? (check all that apply)

    _____ **a.** Have sufficient resources available.

    _____ **b.** Ensure that at least two rescuers are available to apply the splint.

    _____ **c.** Have the splint at hand, prepared, and ready to apply.

    _____ **d.** Ensure proper axial alignment.

    _____ **e.** Provide intermittent traction.

    _____ **f.** Move the limb only as much as is absolutely necessary.

    _____ **g.** Prior to splinting tie the patient's legs together for extra stability.

    _____ **h.** Secure the patient and traction splint to a long spine board.

**10.** At which point after applying tension to realign a dislocated ankle should you release tension? _____

    **a.** as soon as the ankle realigns into the correct anatomical position

    **b.** just before the splint is applied

    **c.** after the ankle is immobilized

    **d.** once tension is applied, you may not release it.

## Short Answer

**1.** Why can a supracondylar fracture of the elbow have disastrous consequences for a patient?

_____

_____

_____

**2.** Why is a hip dislocation considered a true medical emergency?

_____

_____

_____

**3.** A trauma patient with an obviously broken humerus and ankle exhibits signs and symptoms of shock. Describe what you should do.

_____

_____

_____

**4.** While on a hike in a remote wilderness, a member of your party falls and suffers an open tibial fracture with the bone end protruding from the skin. You are out of cell phone range and ten hours from the trailhead. Describe how you would treat this injury.

_____

_____

_____

**5.** You are in a remote wilderness setting caring for a patient with a non-dislocated ankle injury. You have securely immobilized the injury with a SAM™ splint and cravats. The patient tells you she thinks she can walk out. What should you do?

_____

_____

_____

## Matching

**1.** Match each of the following injuries to the assessment findings.

_____ **1.** fracture

_____ **2.** strain

_____ **3.** sprain

_____ **4.** dislocation

_____ **5.** ruptured tendon

**a.** pain
swelling
visible deformity
reduced joint motion
locking/freezing joint

**b.** point of tenderness over ligament
swelling and bruising
joint instability
decreased range of movement
inability to bear weight

**c.** minimal pain
minimal bruising or swelling
lack of joint movement
noticeable "gap" under skin

**d.** pain over site; increases with movement
tenderness
swelling
ecchymosis
decreased range of movement
deformity
crepitus

**e.** point of tenderness over muscle
pain with extension and flexion
bruising
swelling/hematoma over muscle

**2.** Match each of the following terms to its definition.

_____ **1.** impacted fracture

_____ **2.** strain

_____ **3.** spiral fracture

_____ **4.** dislocation

_____ **5.** compression fracture

_____ **6.** ruptured tendon

_____ **7.** displaced fracture

_____ **8.** comminuted fracture

_____ **9.** sprain

_____ **10.** incomplete fracture

_____ **11.** closed fracture

_____ **12.** non-displaced fracture

_____ **13.** open fracture

_____ **14.** complete fracture

_____ **15.** butterfly fragment

_____ **16.** transverse fracture

_____ **17.** epiphyseal fracture

_____ **18.** greenstick fracture

**a.** a separation or displacement of the bones of a joint

**b.** an injury in which a third piece of broken long bone that is located on the opposite side of the fracture; common with tibial and humeral fractures

**c.** a long bone fracture caused by twisting

**d.** a bone being shortened into itself; common in vertebrae

**e.** a fracture in which the skin above a fractured bone is breached; also called a compound fracture

**f.** caused by simultaneous muscle contracture and stretching

**g.** a simple fracture in which the overlying skin is not damaged or disrupted

**h.** a fracture that is often difficult to detect because the bone remains in correct anatomical alignment

**i.** includes total separation of the bone surface

**j.** a fracture in which one side of the bone remains intact; also called a hairline or torus fracture; swelling may be its only sign

**k.** an injury that results in the stretching or tearing of a ligament

**l.** a stretched or torn muscle

**m.** a fracture with two or more parts

**n.** a fracture in which bone ends are anatomically misaligned

**o.** a fracture in which the bone ends are imbedded into each other

**p.** a fracture in a child's growth plate

**q.** a fracture in a straight line across a bone

**r.** an incomplete fracture commonly seen in children

# Scenario

*You are part of a group of OEC Technicians that are providing emergency medical services at a Motorcross race. The track is a large oval with many corners and jumps. Your position is on the backside of a 15-foot-high dirt jump. During an elimination heat a biker loses control while in flight and crashes to the ground on the back side of the jump and in the path of other riders.*

*You make a radio call to race officials to stop the race to secure the scene. Once the red flag has been waved, the race is stopped. Now that the scene is safe, you approach the injured biker. Having observed the crash, you suspect serious injuries.*

1. Whenever the _____ appears significant, there may be more than one injury.

   a. SAMPLE
   b. AVPU
   c. MOI
   d. MCI

*The patient is responsive, alert, and oriented to person, day, time, and place. You complete a primary assessment and start a secondary assessment. Because you suspect a possible spinal injury, you check CMS.*

2. For a musculoskeletal injury, checking CMS involves checking_____

   a. cough, movement, and lung sounds.
   b. contact, memory, and sensation.
   c. capillary refill, muscle tone, and sensation.
   d. circulation, movement, and sensation.

*You make a call for a long board, $O_2$, and a paramedic ambulance to treat traumatic injuries. On secondary assessment you identify a possible pelvic fracture. No external bleeding is evident.*

3. Treatment for a suspected pelvic fracture involves_____

   a. placing the patient on the injured side of the body using a log roll.
   b. applying a sheet splint or a pelvic binder.
   c. placing the patient in a seated position for transport.
   d. placing the patient in a supine position with the head elevated.

# Suggested Reading

Duthie, R., and G. Bentley (Editors). 1996. *Mercer's Orthopedic Surgery*, Ninth Edition. New York, NY: Oxford University Press: A Hodder Arnold Publication.

Pollak, N. A. (Editor). 2008. *Nancy Caroline's Emergency Care in the Streets*, Sixth Edition. Sudbury, MA: Jones and Bartlett.

Simon, R., C. Sherman, and S. J. Koenigsknecht. 2006. *Emergency Orthopedics: The Extremities*, Fifth Edition. New York, NY: McGraw-Hill Medical.

EXPLORE 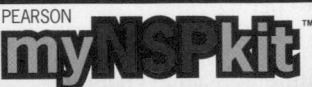 PEARSON myNSPkit™

Please go to www.myNSPkit.com. Under Student Resources, you will find animations, videos, web links, and games related to this chapter—and much more. Look for information on types of joints, interactive skeletal anatomy, and various splitting demonstrations.

Register your access code from the front of your book by going to www.myNSPkit.com and selecting the appropriate links. If the in-cover access code has been redeemed, go to www.myNSPkit.com and follow links to **Buy Access**.

# Head and Spine Injuries

John S. Nichols, MD, PhD, FACS
Michael Bateman, EMT-B, OEC Technician

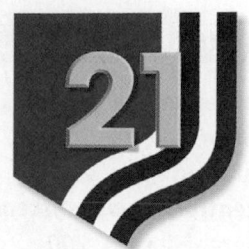

## ⊕ OBJECTIVES

**Upon completion of this chapter, the OEC Technician will be able to:**

**21-1** Correctly identify the major anatomical components of the central nervous system.

**21-2** Define traumatic brain injury.

**21-3** Describe common traumatic injuries involving the head, neck, and back.

**21-4** Describe the signs and symptoms of potential head injuries involving the brain.

**21-5** Describe the signs and symptoms of potential spinal injuries.

**21-6** Describe how to properly assess a patient with a suspected neurologic injury, including neck and spine injuries.

**21-7** List the signs and symptoms of increased intracranial pressure.

**21-8** Demonstrate how to properly treat a patient with a head, neck, spine, or back injury.

**21-9** Demonstrate how to maintain proper spinal alignment while placing a patient onto a long spine board from the following positions:
- lying
- sitting
- standing

**21-10** Describe and demonstrate how to remove a helmet.

## Chapter Overview

Outdoor activities provide participants unique opportunities for exercise, camaraderie, and adventure. However, biking, climbing, rafting, skiing, and snowboarding carry inherent risks for injuries, including serious injuries involving the head, neck, spine, or back that range from relatively minor to immediately life threatening. Some have life-altering consequences. This chapter covers traumatic injuries to the nervous system. Stroke and other medical conditions that affect the CNS are discussed in other chapters.

*continued*

## HISTORICAL TIMELINE

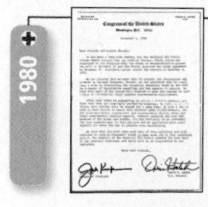

**1980** President Jimmy Carter signs legislation providing a federal charter to NSP.

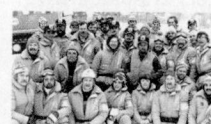

**1980** NSP patrollers provide coverage for 1980 Winter Olympic Games in Lake Placid, NY (the first volunteer Nordic patrol at a major international event).

## ⊕ KEY TERMS

antegrade amnesia, *p. 707*
axon, *p. 700*
brain stem, *p. 700*
central nervous system (CNS), *p. 698*
cerebellum, *p. 700*
cerebrospinal fluid, *p. 700*
cerebrum, *p. 700*

diffuse axonal injury, *p. 704*
epidural hematoma, *p. 709*
intracranial pressure, *p. 703*
lucid period, *p. 710*
neural ischemia, *p. 712*
neuron, *p. 700*

peripheral nervous system, *p. 700*
recurrent traumatic brain injury, *p. 708*
retrograde amnesia, *p. 707*
spinal cord, *p. 700*
subdural hematoma, *p. 710*
traumatic brain injury, *p. 698*

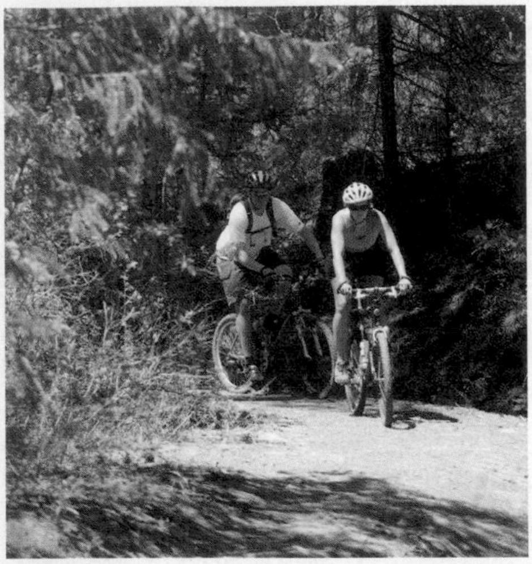

**Figure 21-1** Your central nervous system is constantly reacting to environmental and sensory input.
Copyright Scott Smith

**central nervous system (CNS)**   the part of the nervous system that includes the brain and spinal cord.

**traumatic brain injury**   physical trauma to the brain; can be localized or diffuse.

⊕ **21-2** Define traumatic brain injury.

A person's ability to sense and react to the external environment depends on the coordinated functioning of the **central nervous system (CNS)** (Figure 21-1■). Injuries that interrupt this functioning can dramatically affect homeostasis and can result in permanent disability if they are not managed properly. When engaging in outdoor activities, trauma to the CNS is an ever-present potential hazard. CNS injuries are among the most serious that OEC Technicians encounter.

CNS trauma is associated with high mortality and morbidity rates, significant economic consequences, and serious effects on victims' quality of life. One of the most severe forms of CNS trauma is **traumatic brain injury** (TBI), a leading cause of traumatic death in individuals under age 45 that occurs approximately every 15 seconds in the United States.

The U.S. Consumer Product Safety Commission noted that during 2007, hospital emergency rooms treated the following numbers of sports-related head injuries:

- Cycling: 64,993
- Football: 36,412
- Baseball and softball: 25,079
- Basketball: 24,701
- Powered recreational vehicles (ATVs, dune buggies, go-carts, mini bikes, off-road): 24,090
- Skateboards/scooters (powered): 18,542
- Soccer: 17,108
- Skateboards/scooters: 16,477
- Winter sports (skiing, sledding, snowboarding, snowmobiling): 16,120
- Water sports (diving, scuba diving, surfing, swimming, water polo, water skiing): 12,096
- Horseback riding: 11,759
- Health club (exercise, weightlifting): 11,550
- Golf: 8,417
- Trampolines: 7,075
- Hockey: 5,483
- Gymnastics/dance/cheerleading: 5,459
- Ice skating: 3,703
- Fishing: 3,560
- Rugby/lacrosse: 3,281
- Wrestling: 2,640

# CASE PRESENTATION

You are dispatched to an accident in which a skier has collided with a tree. Upon your arrival, you find an unresponsive male skier, approximately 30 years old, lying on his side at the base of a large tree. You immediately open the airway and simultaneously check for breathing and for a carotid pulse for no longer than 10 seconds in accordance with the 2010 Emergency Cardiac Care (ECC) recommendations. You note that the patient is breathing and has a pulse. He is wearing a helmet, but it is cracked in two places. You note blood leaking from the patient's nose and ears. The ski tracks indicate that the patient went straight into the tree.

***What should you do?***

An estimated 5.3 million people in the United States have long-term or lifelong deficits resulting from TBI, including the following:

- Memory loss
- Reduced problem-solving capacity
- Stress and anger-management issues
- Emotional upset, including depression
- Job skill impairment
- Chronic seizure disorders
- Functional changes in thought, speech, learning, emotions, behavior, and sensation
- Increased risk of Alzheimer's, Parkinson's, and other brain disorders that become more prevalent with age

The direct (medical) and indirect (lost productivity) costs of TBI are astronomical and total an estimated $60 billion annually. According to the U.S. Centers for Disease Control and Prevention (CDC), approximately 1.7 million people suffer TBI each year in the United States, and over 50,000 of them die. The numbers for spinal cord injury (SCI) are lower than those for TBI. The CDC reports that 11,000 people sustain SCI annually in the United States, and approximately 200,000 citizens live with an SCI-related disability. In individuals under age 65, motor vehicle accidents are the leading cause of SCI, whereas in those over age 65, falls are the leading cause. Approximately 18 percent of spinal cord injuries are caused by sports and recreational activities. The annual cost of treating SCI is estimated to be $9.7 billion.

It is clearly imperative that OEC Technicians understand the mechanisms responsible for traumatic CNS injuries and are able to quickly recognize the signs and symptoms of specific CNS injuries. They also must be able to safely manage patients with traumatic head, neck, and back injuries and minimize additional injury. In so doing, OEC Technicians can help to reduce the morbidity and mortality associated with this devastating form of trauma.

## Anatomy and Physiology

The axial skeleton in humans consists of a skull and 33 vertebrae in the spine (Figure 21-2■).

Inside the skull is the brain, which has three parts: the cerebrum, cerebellum, and brain stem. See Chapter 6, Figure 6-18. The brain has gray and

 **21-1** Correctly identify the major anatomical components of the central nervous system.

**axon** long, slender projection of a nerve cell (neuron) that conducts electrical impulses away from the neuron's cell body.

**spinal cord** tubular bundle of nervous tissue and support cells that extends from the brain downward to the sacrum within the vertebral canal; part of the central nervous system.

**cerebrospinal fluid** serum-like fluid that functions in shock absorption for central nervous system structures; circulates through passages within the brain and within the meninges surrounding the brain and spinal cord.

**Figure 21-2** The axial skeleton: the skull and the bones of the spinal column.

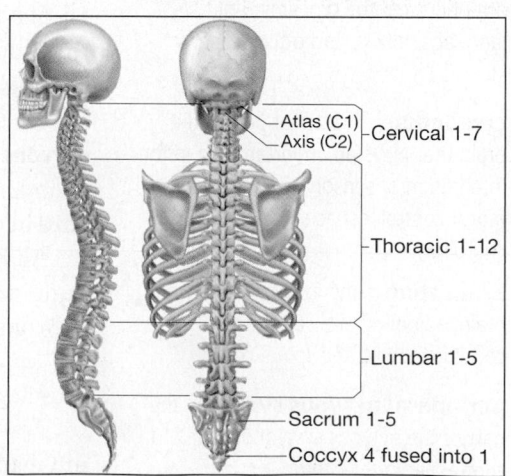

Atlas (C1)
Axis (C2)
Cervical 1-7
Thoracic 1-12
Lumbar 1-5
Sacrum 1-5
Coccyx 4 fused into 1

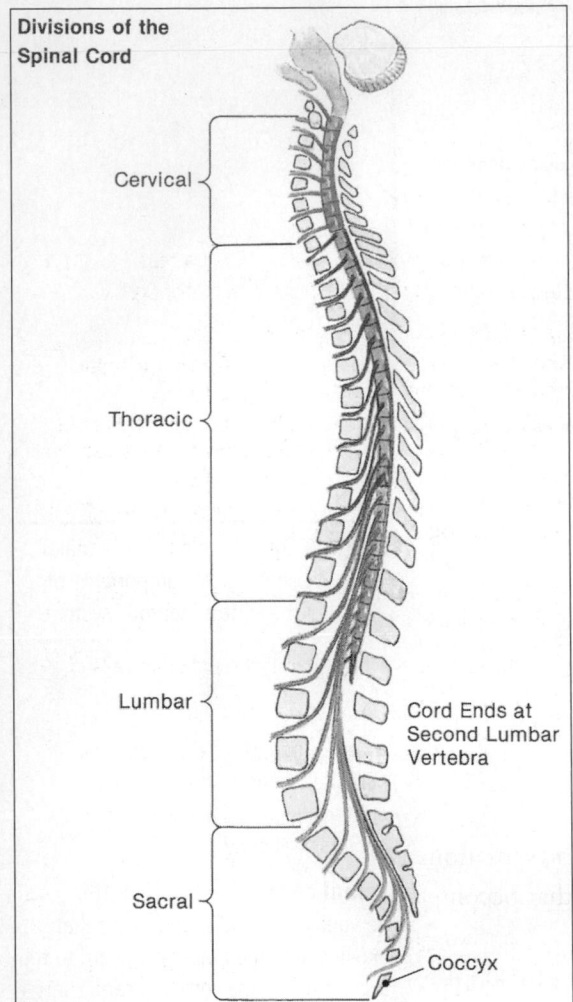

**Divisions of the Spinal Cord**

Cervical

Thoracic

Lumbar

Cord Ends at Second Lumbar Vertebra

Sacral

Coccyx

**Figure 21-3** Divisions of the spinal cord.

**neuron**   nerve cell.

**cerebrum**   region on the top of the brain that integrates sensory perception and motor control and is involved in attention and the processing of language, music, and other sensory stimuli.

**cerebellum**   posterior part of the brain that plays an important role in the integration of sensory perception and motor control, especially for coordination.

**brain stem**   the lower part of the brain, adjoining and structurally continuous with the spinal cord.

**peripheral nervous system**   the part of the nervous system outside the central nervous system.

white matter. The gray matter of the brain consists of regions of closely packed neuron cell bodies that are involved in muscle control, sensory perceptions (such as seeing and hearing), memory, emotions, and speech. White matter consists of neuronal tissue mainly containing the long nerve cell processes called **axons**. Situated between the brain stem and the cerebellum, the white matter includes structures at the core of the brain such as the thalamus and hypothalamus. The structures of the white matter called nuclei are involved in relaying sensory information from the rest of the body to the cerebral cortex and in regulating autonomic functions such as body temperature, heart rate, and blood pressure. Certain nuclei are involved in the expression of emotions, the release of hormones from the pituitary gland, and the regulation of food and water intake.

Even though the brain constitutes only about 2 percent of an average adult's body weight, it receives 15 percent of the blood supply and consumes 20 percent of the circulating oxygen and glucose. The **spinal cord** originates at the base of the brain and enters the spinal column through the foramen magnum, a hole in the base of the skull. The spinal cord extends within the vertebrae of the spinal column down to the lower back; from there, nerves continue to the coccyx (Figure 21-3■). The brain and spinal cord, which together make up the central nervous system, are covered by a three-layered membrane called the meninges. Circulating inside these protective membranes is **cerebrospinal fluid (CSF)**.

A highly specialized cell called a **neuron** is the functional unit of the nervous system. The body's millions of neurons transmit signals throughout the body and collectively function as an organized and very complex wiring system. The largest collection of neurons, located within the brain, directs the functions of the other neurons.

The parts of the brain shown in Chapter 6, Figure 6-18 perform various functions. The uppermost part, called the **cerebrum**, consists of an outer part, or cortex, which controls higher functions such as sense perception, voluntary movement, speech, thought, and memory, and an inner part, or hypothalamus, which is the major control center for the autonomic nervous system and controls body temperature, hunger, thirst, and fatigue (sleep). The **cerebellum** controls balance, motor coordination, movement, posture, and muscle tone. The **brain stem** is made up of the pons, thalamus, and medulla oblongata. The brain stem controls basic body functions such as cardiac, respiratory, and other brain-processing functions.

The spinal cord, which contains thousands and thousands of neurons, resembles an old-fashioned telephone cable containing many, many wires. It serves as a cable that runs to and from the body and brain. If severed, both sensory and motor function below the level of interruption is lost.

The nerves that connect the rest of the body to the spinal cord make up the **peripheral nervous system**. The peripheral nerves that connect to the spinal cord within the neck go to and from the shoulders and arms, whereas the peripheral nerves that attach to the spinal cord in the low back and sacrum (tailbone) go to and from the buttocks, legs, and genitalia.

All humans are "wired" by the peripheral nerves in the same way. Each of us has the same nerves in our arms and legs in generally the same anatomical location. Sensory neurons in these nerves send messages from the body to the spinal cord and then on to the brain. The brain sends signals through the spinal cord to motor neurons to make muscles work. Sensory and motor neurons exist together inside each peripheral nerve.

For a more detailed description of the nervous system, review the neurology section in Chapter 6, Anatomy and Physiology.

# STOP, THINK, UNDERSTAND

## Multiple Choice

Choose the correct answer.

1. A person's ability to function depends primarily on_____
   a. strength and endurance.
   b. the coordinated function of the central nervous system.
   c. his or her personality.
   d. his or her inherent intellect.

2. One of the most serious forms of CNS trauma is_____
   a. stroke.      c. TBI.
   b. AMI.      d. CNS.

3. The leading cause of death in individuals younger than 45 years of age is_____
   a. TBI.      c. CVA.
   b. AMI.      d. CSF.

4. A traumatic brain injury can result in which of the following? (check all that apply)
   _____ a. memory loss
   _____ b. reduced problem-solving capability
   _____ c. stress and anger-management issues
   _____ d. euphoria
   _____ e. job skill impairment

   _____ f. epilepsy
   _____ g. behavioral disorders
   _____ h. decreased risk of Parkinson's disease
   _____ i. increased risk of Alzheimer's disease

5. Which of the following statements is true?_____
   a. The care provided by OEC Technicians in the field can reduce the morbidity and long-term effects of CNS injuries.
   b. Although care provided by OEC Technicians in the field can be life saving, initial basic life-support measures cannot affect the disabilities that may occur with CNS injuries.
   c. There is very little OEC Technicians can do to render any meaningful aid to an individual with a head or spinal cord injury.
   d. The care of a patient with a spinal cord injury is beyond the scope of OEC Technicians.

6. The nervous system cell that directs the function of other cells of this type is the_____
   a. cerebrum.      c. pons.
   b. foramen magnum.      d. neuron.

## Matching

Match each of the following nervous system structures to its primary function.

_____ 1. brain stem
_____ 2. cerebrum
_____ 3. cerebellum
_____ 4. hypothalamus
_____ 5. neuron

a. functions in motor coordination, balance, posture, and muscle tone
b. is made up of the pons, thalamus, medulla oblongata; controls basic life-support functions such as breathing and cardiac function
c. controls higher functions such as senses, perception, voluntary movements, speech, thought, and memory
d. controls heart rate, blood pressure, temperature, sleep, and memory acquisition
e. sends messages to and from body parts via the spinal cord and brain

## Labeling

Place each of the following labels in its correct location in the accompanying illustration. Go to Chapter 6, Figure 6-18.

1. cerebrum
2. cerebellum
3. brainstem
4. hypothalamus
5. spinal cord

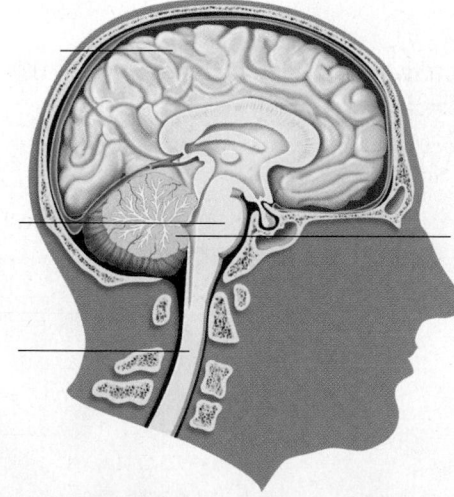

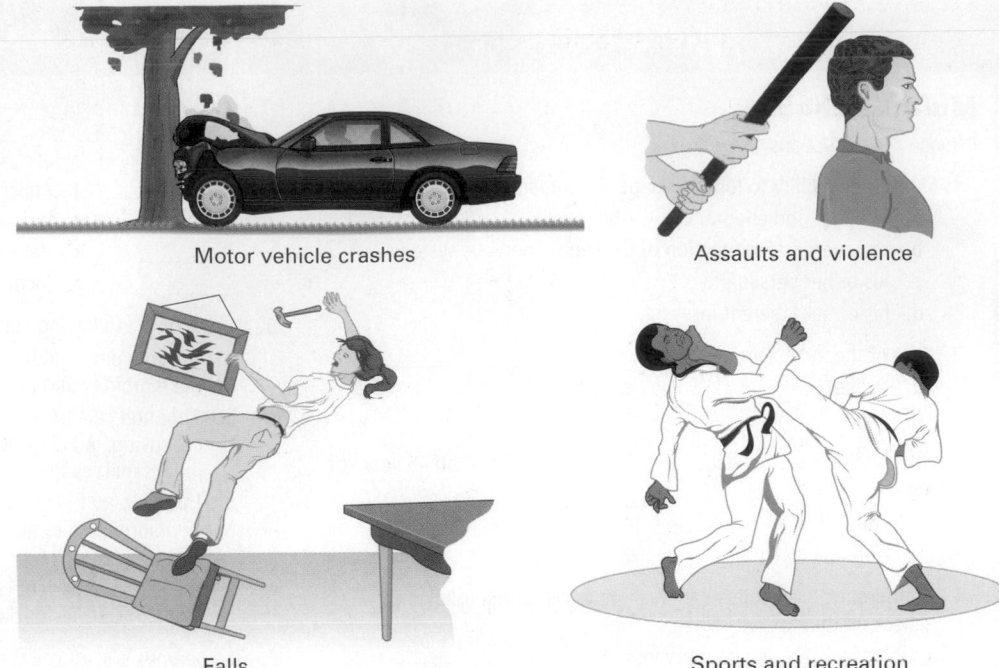

Motor vehicle crashes

Assaults and violence

Falls

Sports and recreation

**Figure 21-4** Different mechanisms of head injury.

**⊕ 21-3** Describe common traumatic injuries involving the head, neck, and back.

# Common Mechanisms of Injury

Although the components of the central nervous system are generally well protected within their bony enclosures, they are not impervious to injury if subjected to significant forces (Figure 21-4■). Among the most common mechanisms of injury to the head, neck, and back are:

+ Rapid deceleration (impact-related trauma)
+ Rapid acceleration
+ Compression injury to the spinal column (from a falling object or a diving accident) (Figure 21-5■)
+ Penetrating or impaled object (Figure 21-6■)
+ Near drowning

**Figure 21-5** A compression injury.

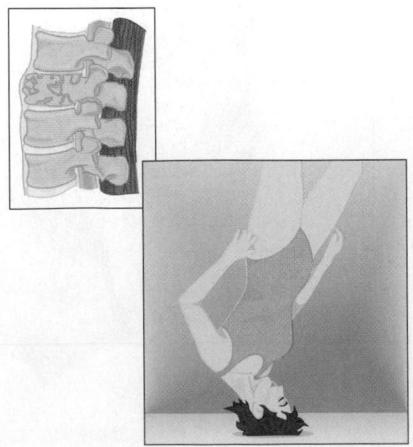

**Figure 21-6** A penetration injury or impaled object.

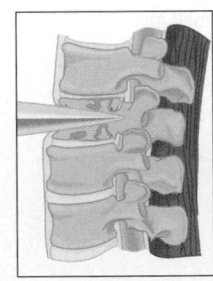

- Hypothermia and hyperthermia
- Electrical injury, including lightning strike

Primary CNS injuries occur from external trauma, whereas secondary injuries result from inadequate brain perfusion, increased **intracranial pressure**, or hypoxia. Many times a secondary CNS injury is a delayed reaction to a primary injury.

## Increased Intracranial Pressure (ICP)

Maintaining the very narrow range of pressure that the circulating cerebrospinal fluid (CSF) exerts on the inside of the skull and on the structures of the brain is essential for preserving homeostasis. Because the volume within the skull is fixed, any increase in volume within the skull, whether due to bleeding or edema (swelling), increases the intracranial pressure. The result is compression of brain tissue, reduction in brain function, and ultimately death.

## Coup-Contrecoup Injury

The brain "floats" in the small volume of CSF between the inside of the skull and the brain tissue. Although this fluid cushions and protects the brain, a blow to the head of sufficiently large force can cause the brain to strike the inside of the skull, resulting in a unique injury known as a coup-contrecoup injury. *Coup-contrecoup* is a French term meaning "blow-counter blow."

A coup-contrecoup brain injury is caused by rapid deceleration of the head, as can occur when a skier or a mountain biker strikes a tree or some other immovable object (Figure 21-7■). Upon impact with the object, the brain keeps moving forward and strikes the inside of the skull ("coup"), which can damage structures large and small within the brain. The "contrecoup" portion of the injury occurs when the brain rebounds and strikes the inside of the skull on the side opposite the "coup" injury (Figure 21-8■).

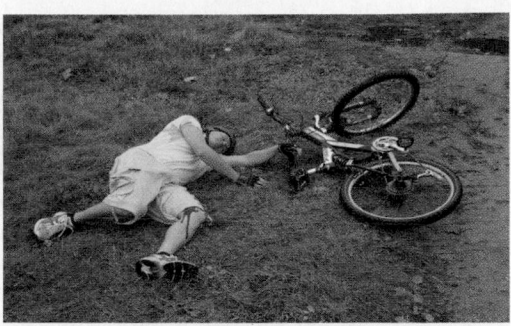

**Figure 21-7** This mountain biker has hit his head during a crash.
Copyright Mike Halloran

**intracranial pressure** the pressure within the skull; can also be exerted on the brain tissue and cerebrospinal fluid.

**⊕ 21-7** List the signs and symptoms of increased intracranial pressure.

### Geriatric/Pediatric Considerations

An infant's incompletely developed brain is small compared to the skull, and the brain of elderly individuals may have become smaller with age. In both situations, the brain has more room to move within the skull. As a result, both geriatric and pediatric patients experience *more severe coup-contrecoup injuries* due to the increased distance the brain can travel.

**Figure 21-8** The forces involved in a coup-contrecoup injury.

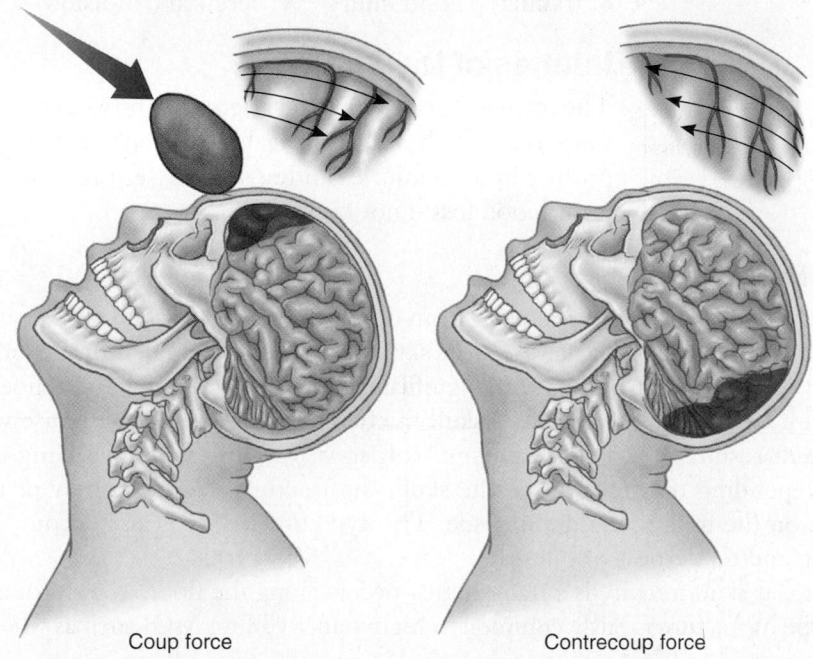

Coup force                Contrecoup force

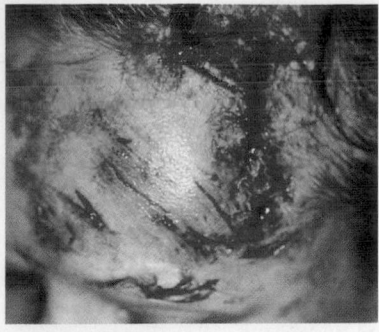

**Figure 21-9** In closed head injuries, the skull remains intact.

**Figure 21-10** Presentations of some closed head injuries.

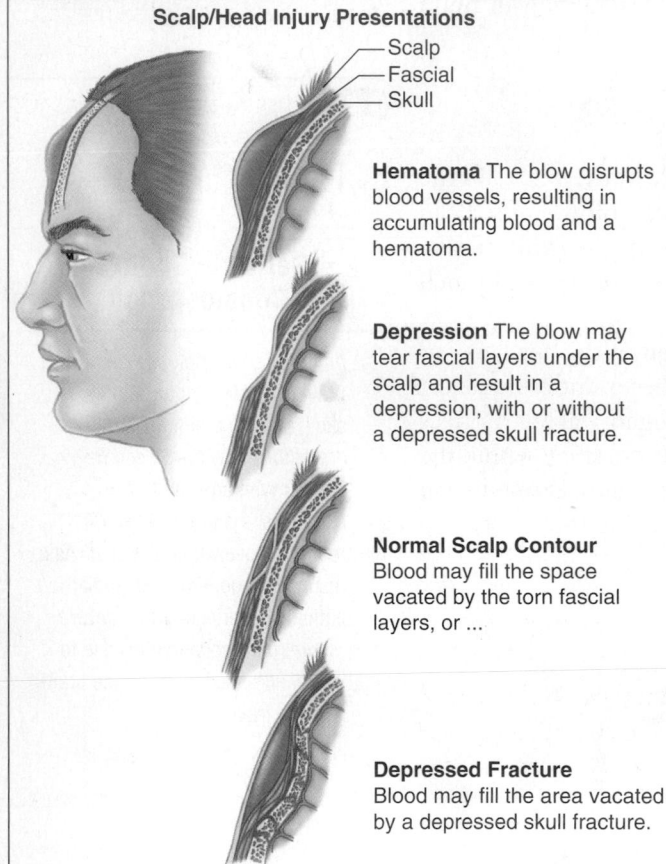

**Scalp/Head Injury Presentations**

— Scalp
— Fascial
— Skull

**Hematoma** The blow disrupts blood vessels, resulting in accumulating blood and a hematoma.

**Depression** The blow may tear fascial layers under the scalp and result in a depression, with or without a depressed skull fracture.

**Normal Scalp Contour** Blood may fill the space vacated by the torn fascial layers, or ...

**Depressed Fracture** Blood may fill the area vacated by a depressed skull fracture.

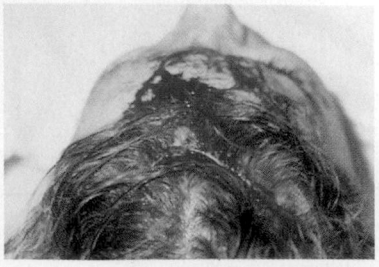

**Figure 21-11** An open head injury.

In many instances, a coup-contrecoup injury is not immediately apparent because no external signs of trauma may be evident. Depending on the forces involved, coup-contrecoup injuries can result in severe intracranial bleeding, swelling, and can compromise normal brain function.

Many older people are now taking anticoagulants, which are medications that delay blood clotting to prevent heart attacks and strokes. Thus, in individuals who take Coumadin (warfarin), Plavix, or aspirin, bleeding in the brain resulting from head trauma lasts longer and can quickly result in life-threatening intracranial bleeding.

## Common Injuries

Injuries to nervous system structures, including the head, neck, back, and spine, can be divided into two broad categories: closed injuries and open injuries.

Closed CNS injuries are those in which the integrity of the cranium and spinal column is not compromised. Closed injuries include contusions; hematomas; lacerations not associated with an underlying fracture; fractures of the skull, spine (vertebrae), scapula, and posterior ribs; epidural and subdural hematomas; and **diffuse axonal injury** (DAI) (Figures 21-9■ and 21-10■). Open CNS injuries are those in which brain matter or bone fragments are exposed, or in which CSF is leaking from a wound or a cavity such as the nose or ears (Figure 21-11■). Additionally, CNS injuries may be accompanied by muscle strains or soft tissue injuries to the face or scalp.

## Head and Brain Injuries

Common injuries to the head and brain include the following conditions:

+ injuries of the scalp
+ skull fractures
+ traumatic brain injury
+ concussion
+ recurrent traumatic brain injury
+ cerebral contusion

### Injuries of the Scalp

The scalp is susceptible to a variety of soft tissue injuries. Because the scalp has a generous blood supply, bleeding can be profuse in head injuries and in some cases can lead to significant blood loss if not treated quickly.

### Skull Fractures

Open or closed skull fractures result from blunt trauma to the skull and are classified as linear, depressed, or basilar. A linear skull fracture has a single nondisplaced fracture line and usually presents with significant soft-tissue swelling and tenderness of the scalp. Conversely, a depressed skull fracture is a comminuted fracture with displacement resulting in a characteristic "soft spot" or depression overlying the fracture. Depending on the force to the skull, the fracture fragments may or may not intrude on the underlying brain tissue. This type of fracture is also accompanied by swelling and tenderness of the scalp.

A basilar skull fracture is a fracture that occurs along the floor, or base, of the skull. This type of fracture is fairly common in high-velocity blunt MOI such as when a skier

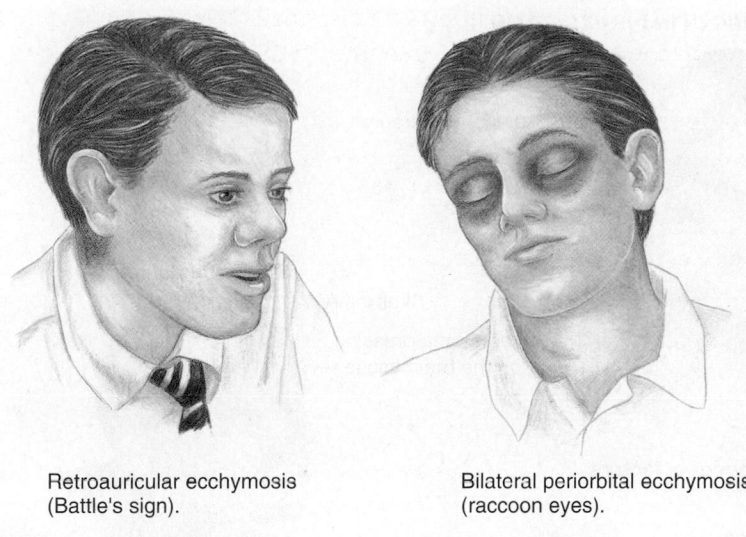

Retroauricular ecchymosis (Battle's sign).

Bilateral periorbital ecchymosis (raccoon eyes).

**Figure 21-12** Battle's sign (on the neck behind the ear) and raccoon eyes.

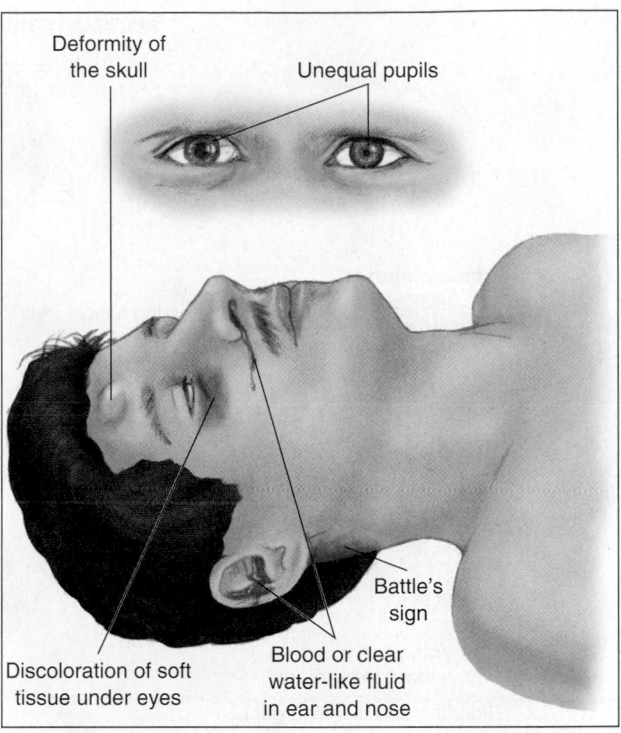

**Figure 21-13** Battle's sign and other signs of brain injury.

strikes a tree, when a climber strikes his head during a fall, or when a mountain biker crashes into a large stationary object. Fractures in this area may allow cerebral spinal fluid to leak out of the cranial vault and into the ear canals, nasal passageway, or mouth. Over several hours patients may develop one or both of the classic findings of a basilar skull fracture: "raccoon eyes" and Battle's sign, or ecchymosis behind the ear (Figures 21-12■ and 21-13■).

## Traumatic Brain Injury

Traumatic brain injury (TBI) is defined as a mechanical injury to the brain that results in short-term and/or long-term neurologic deficit (Figure 21-14■). Males are twice as likely to suffer TBI than are females, and four times as likely to be killed by a TBI, because males are more likely than females to be involved in high-risk activities. See Table 21-1■.

TBI is most commonly associated with high-speed acceleration/deceleration forces, rotational forces such as those incurred in a collision or fall, and penetrating forces of high-velocity missiles such as bullets (Figure 21-15■). TBI-related injuries include concussions, cerebral contusions, cerebral hematomas, diffuse axonal injury, and intracerebral hemorrhages (Table 21-2■).

## Concussion

A concussion is a temporary disruption of coordinated brain function caused by trauma (Figure 21-16■). Different scales are used to determine the severity of a concussion, but in general they are classified as mild, moderate, or severe. Mild concussion involves minor disruption of brain function and no loss of responsiveness but may include such signs and symptoms as confusion, dizziness, nausea, vomiting, headache, and visual and auditory disturbances. A moderate concussion is a head injury involving a loss of responsiveness that lasts less than five minutes and more pronounced disruption of brain function. A severe concussion is a head injury involving a loss of responsiveness that lasts longer than five minutes and significant disruption of normal brain function. In both moderate and severe concussions, other signs and symptoms of brain injury are usually present.

Many patients who suffer a concussion exhibit some measurable memory loss, known as amnesia. The severity of amnesia depends on the extent of the concussion and

**diffuse axonal injury** the most common and devastating types of traumatic brain injury; results when damage occurs over a more widespread area than in focal brain injury.

### The Two Phases of Brain Injury

Injury to the brain usually involves two temporal events: a primary injury, such as a collision with a tree, a rock, or the ground, and a secondary (or delayed) injury, caused by hypoxia and exacerbated by increasing intracranial pressure and altered cerebral blood flow.

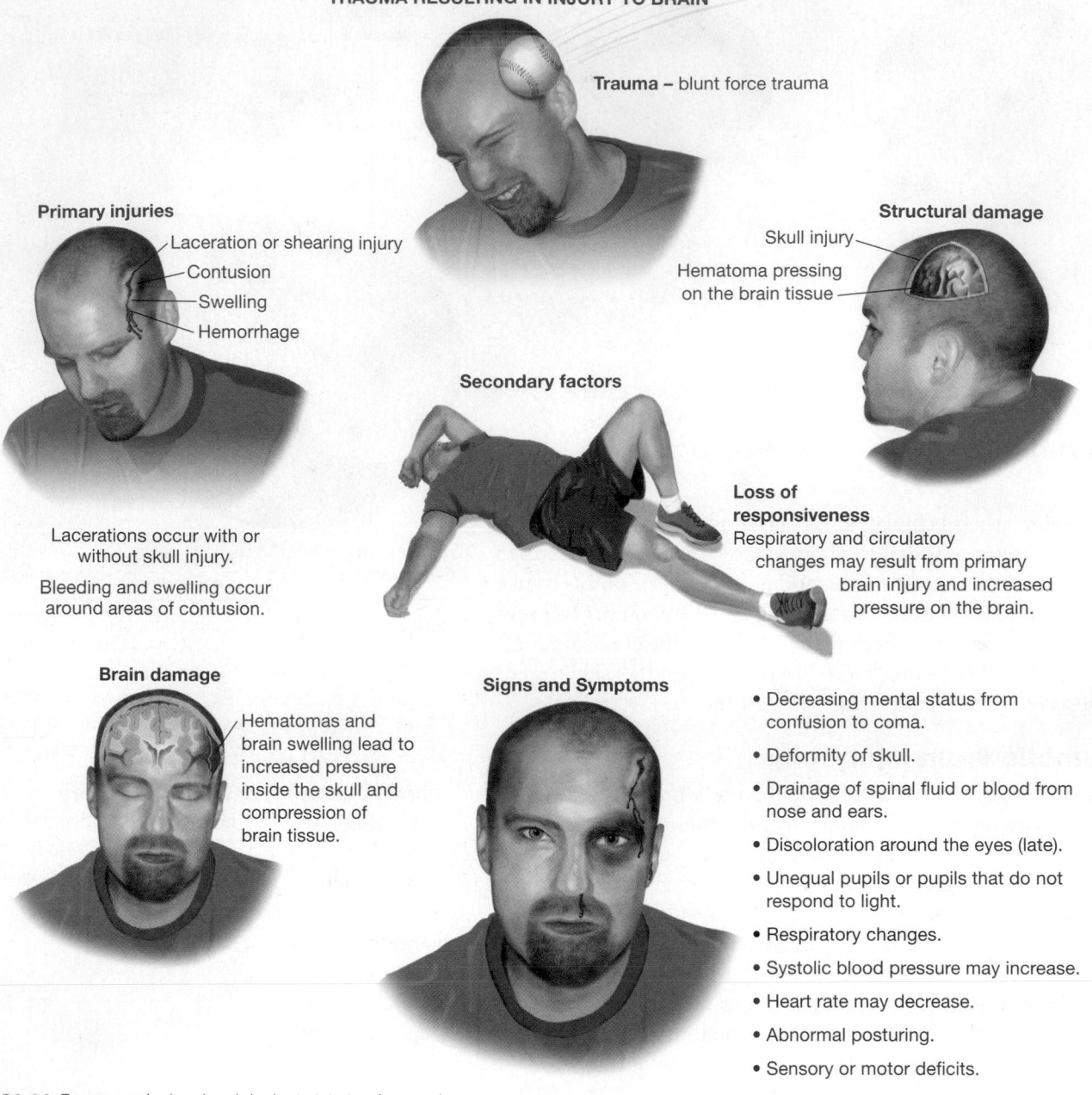

**TRAUMA RESULTING IN INJURY TO BRAIN**

**Trauma** – blunt force trauma

**Primary injuries**
- Laceration or shearing injury
- Contusion
- Swelling
- Hemorrhage

Lacerations occur with or without skull injury.

Bleeding and swelling occur around areas of contusion.

**Structural damage**
- Skull injury
- Hematoma pressing on the brain tissue

**Secondary factors**

**Loss of responsiveness**
Respiratory and circulatory changes may result from primary brain injury and increased pressure on the brain.

**Brain damage**
Hematomas and brain swelling lead to increased pressure inside the skull and compression of brain tissue.

**Signs and Symptoms**
- Decreasing mental status from confusion to coma.
- Deformity of skull.
- Drainage of spinal fluid or blood from nose and ears.
- Discoloration around the eyes (late).
- Unequal pupils or pupils that do not respond to light.
- Respiratory changes.
- Systolic blood pressure may increase.
- Heart rate may decrease.
- Abnormal posturing.
- Sensory or motor deficits.

**Figure 21-14** Trauma to the head and the brain injuries that result.

## Table 21-1   The Demographics of TBI

- Males are about twice as likely as females to sustain a TBI.
- The two age groups at highest risk for TBI are children under 4 and teens ages 15–19.
- Adults 75 years of age or older have the highest rates of TBI-related hospitalization and death.
- African Americans have the highest death rate from TBI.
- TBI hospitalization rates are highest among African Americans and American Indians/Alaska Natives (AI/AN).

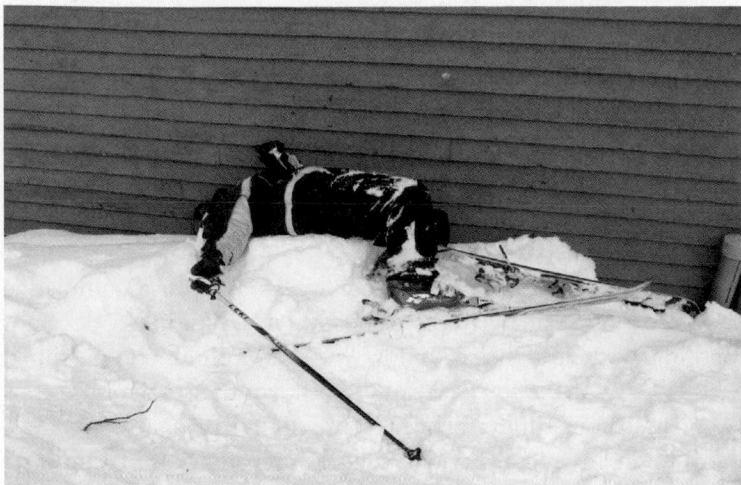

**Figure 21-15** For this skier, the primary head injury resulted from a collision with the building; the nature of the secondary injuries remains to be seen.
Copyright Edward McNamara

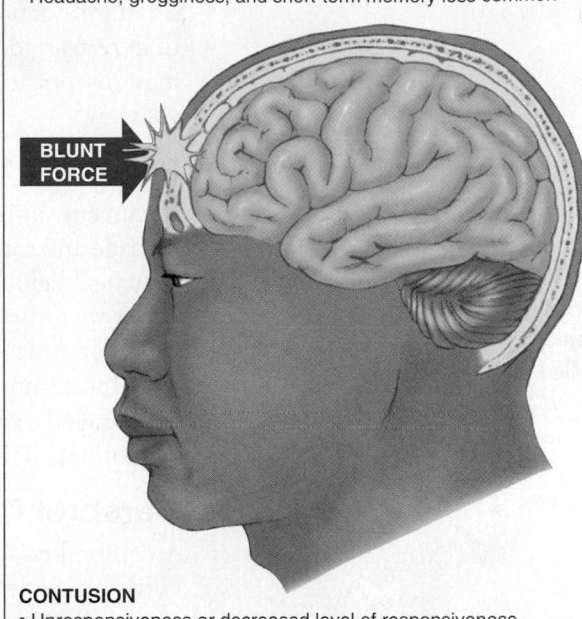

**CONCUSSION**
• May have brief loss of consciousness or unresponsiveness
• Headache, grogginess, and short-term memory loss common

**BLUNT FORCE**

**CONTUSION**
• Unresponsiveness or decreased level of responsiveness
• Bruising of brain tissue

**Figure 21-16** Concussion, a type of closed head injury.

can be classified as either retrograde or antegrade amnesia. Patients with **retrograde amnesia** have no recollection of events *before* the injury, including the injury itself. **Antegrade amnesia** is characterized by no recollection of events occurring *after* the injury. Patients with amnesia often present with a distinctive speech pattern in which they repeatedly ask questions such as, "What happened?" or "Where am I?" or "Who are you?" sometimes for hours following the injury. This condition, known as perseveration, is indicative of both the confusion experienced by these patients and of antegrade amnesia.

**retrograde amnesia** loss of memory of events that occurred before a traumatic event to the brain; an inability to recall old information.

**antegrade amnesia** loss of memory of events that occurred *after* a traumatic event to the brain; an inability to recall new information.

| Table 21-2 | Signs and Symptoms of Traumatic Brain Injury |
| --- | --- |

• Initial period of unresponsiveness
• Altered mental status
• Headache
• Nausea, vomiting
• Slurred speech
• Pupillary dilation or unresponsiveness
• Rise in systolic blood pressure and pulse pressure
• Slow pulse
• Lucid period
• Leakage of CSF from ears, nose, open wounds
• Slow or irregular respirations
• Amnesia
• Dizziness
• Seizures
• Incontinence
• Numbness, tingling, or paralysis in one or more extremities
• Posturing
• Paralysis
• Raccoon eyes (a late sign, if seen at all)
• Battle's sign (a late sign, if seen at all)

Post-concussive syndrome (PCS) is a complex set of symptoms ranging from permanent memory loss (usually limited to the event) to difficulty focusing and problem-solving to depression and behavioral disturbances. If antegrade amnesia lasts longer than retrograde amnesia, the prognosis is worse. Over time, many of these symptoms may disappear as the brain heals, although full recovery can take months or even years.

## Recurrent Traumatic Brain Injury

Recurrent, mild TBIs that occur within hours, days, or weeks can cause cumulative damage and can lead to severe long-term disability or death. If the first injury does not fully heal before a second injury occurs, the second injury, even if mild, may be much worse than the first. A University of Pittsburgh study has shown that to avoid serious subsequent head injury, a patient must fully recover from a first TBI before being allowed to resume participation in any sport. Patients who exhibit signs of TBI must be encouraged to cease the activity that caused the injury and to seek medical care. Always ask patients if they have had any other recent head injury (brain trauma).

## Cerebral Contusion

A cerebral contusion is a bruise involving the brain. This type of injury typically involves the rupture of small, superficial blood vessels and generally affects localized areas of the brain. A cerebral contusion is more serious than a concussion but may present with identical signs and symptoms.

⊕ **21-4** Describe the signs and symptoms of potential head injuries involving the brain.

**recurrent traumatic brain injury** a condition in which the head suffers multiple, successive injuries before a previous injury has fully healed; subsequent injuries can be much more severe due to the occurrence of previous injuries.

# STOP, THINK, UNDERSTAND

## Multiple Choice
Choose the correct answer.

1. Which of the following statements about TBI (traumatic brain injury) is true?_____
   a. Females are twice as likely as males to suffer from it.
   b. Males are four times as likely as females to die from it.
   c. The primary cause is internal, such as a stroke or an aneurism.
   d. Mild concussions are the easiest type of TBI to identify and diagnose.

2. A concussion is best defined as _____
   a. a brief loss of consciousness or unresponsiveness.
   b. a form of altered mental state due to internal causes.
   c. a temporary disruption of coordinated brain function caused by trauma.
   d. a permanent, disabling, or fatal type of brain injury.

3. Post-concussive syndrome is best defined as _____
   a. a condition in which the patient repeats the same question over and over.
   b. a rapid swelling of the brain stem that can result in permanent disability or death.
   c. the physical signs or symptoms of a TBI, including prolonged vomiting, headache, and visual disturbance.
   d. a complex set of symptoms ranging from permanent memory loss of the event to depression or behavioral disturbances.

## Labeling

Label each of the following descriptions as indicative of a mild concussion (MI), a moderate concussion (MO), or a severe concussion (SC).

_____ a. a patient who is reported to have been unresponsive for 4 minutes following a blow to the head

_____ b. a patient who was reported to have been unresponsive for about a minute following a blow to the head

_____ c. a patient who was reported to have been unresponsive for 7–8 minutes following a blow to the head

_____ d. a patient who appears confused after a blow to the head but did not lose responsiveness

_____ e. a patient who did not lose responsiveness but has a bad headache and is nauseated after a blow to the head

_____ f. a patient who wanders into an aid room, is confused and disoriented, vomits and perseverates, and is suffering from retrograde amnesia

*continued*

## Fill in the Blank

1. A patient with _____ amnesia has no recollection of events before an injury or of the injury itself.

2. A patient with _____ amnesia has no recollection of events after the injury event.

## List

List three common causes of head, neck, and back injuries.

_____

_____

_____

_____

## Matching

Match each of the following terms to its definition.

_____ **1.** coup-contrecoup injury

_____ **2.** increased intracranial pressure

_____ **3.** linear skull fracture

_____ **4.** depressed skull fracture

_____ **5.** basilar skull fracture

    **a.** a condition caused by brain swelling or a hematoma

    **b.** a fracture along a single line in which the bones remain in alignment

    **c.** a fracture occurring on the floor of the cranium in which cerebrospinal fluid may leak out

    **d.** a condition caused when the brain strikes the inner wall of the skull twice; a type of injury that may not initially be apparent to rescuers

    **e.** a comminuted fracture that presents as a soft spot on the skull

## Cerebral Hematoma

A hematoma, as described in Chapter 18, Soft-Tissue Injuries, is an accumulation of blood outside the vascular system. Because the cranium is an enclosed space, a hematoma within this space can compress the brain and result in serious damage. OEC Technicians must be familiar with three types of cerebral hematomas: an epidural hematoma, a subdural hematoma, and an intracerebral bleed (Figure 21-17■).

An **epidural hematoma** is a TBI that results in arterial bleeding between the skull and the dura mater. In most cases, the source of bleeding is the middle meningeal artery, generally as a result of blunt trauma that causes a skull fracture. A hematoma can rapidly increase the pressure within the skull, which can further compress the brain and

**epidural hematoma** a traumatic brain injury in which a buildup of blood occurs between the dura mater and the skull.

**Figure 21-17** Three types of cranial hematomas.

**CRANIAL HEMATOMAS**

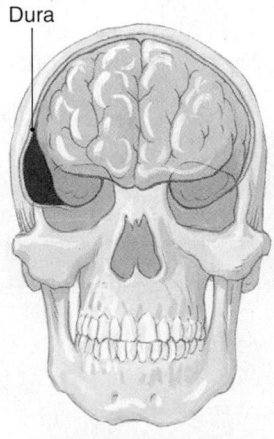
Dura

Subdural
(under the dura)

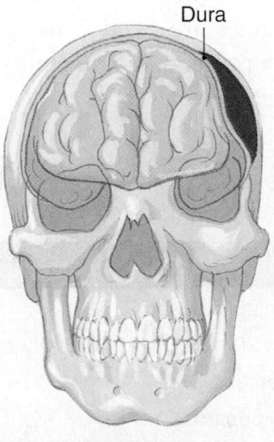
Dura

Epidural
(outside the dura)

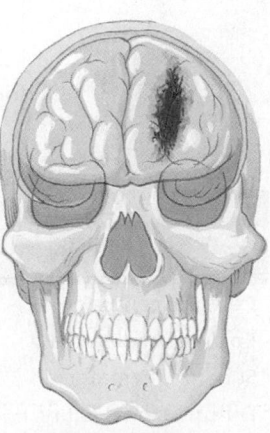
Intracerebral
(inside the brain tissue)

**lucid period** a short period during which the condition of a patient with a traumatic brain injury temporarily improves before again deteriorating.

**subdural hematoma** an accumulation of blood between the outer covering of the brain (dura mater) and the surface of the brain.

compromise vital brain functions. The onset of signs and symptoms is rapid and consists of an initial period of unresponsiveness followed by a "**lucid period**" in which the patient is relatively alert and then becomes increasingly less responsive and eventually comatose. Without rapid treatment, the patient can quickly die.

A **subdural hematoma** is a collection of venous blood between the dura mater and the brain. This type of injury is generally caused by rapid deceleration injuries such as skier-skier or skier-object collisions, falls from height, and violent shearing forces such as might occur if one becomes caught in an avalanche. A subdural hematoma is often associated with underlying cerebral contusions and may resemble the signs and symptoms of an epidural hematoma, with the noted exception of the lucid period, which does not occur with subdural hematoma. Because the source of bleeding is venous in origin and progresses more slowly, the onset of symptoms may not be appreciated for hours, days, or even weeks after the initial insult.

All types of cerebral hematoma are potentially life threatening and require surgical correction. OEC Technicians are not expected to be able to differentiate between different types of neurosurgical emergencies, or among any serious brain injuries. It is, however, crucial that OEC Technicians be able to identify patients with signs and symptoms of significant head injuries and arrange appropriate transport to a trauma center capable of managing such injuries.

### Pediatric Considerations

**NOTE**

Fontanelles are soft spots on a baby's head that allow the bony plates of the skull to flex during the infant's passage through the birth canal. The flexibility of the skulls of infants allows intracranial volume to expand significantly. As a result, 25–30 percent of an infant's blood volume can accumulate inside the skull due to hemorrhage resulting from head trauma, and the infant may become hypotensive before the signs and symptoms of increasing ICP become apparent.

### Diffuse Axonal Injury

Diffuse axonal injury (DAI) is a devastating TBI that results in widespread brain damage. It is caused by high-velocity rotational acceleration/deceleration mechanisms such as those experienced in high-speed ski, snowmobile, and white-water crashes (Figure 21-18■). Although the exact pathophysiology of this injury is not completely understood, two events are believed to occur. First, severe rotational forces cause the axons of the white matter to shear away from the denser neuron bodies of the gray matter. This destruction causes widespread suppression of electrical activity within the brain. Patients with DAI may be unresponsive at the time of injury or become unresponsive later.

Following this injury patients remain in a chronic vegetative state without significant improvement. As many as 90 percent of patients with DAI never recover from their injury. Advanced radiologic studies are needed to determine if DAI has occurred. Table 21-3■ presents the mortality rates for specific TBIs in outdoor environments.

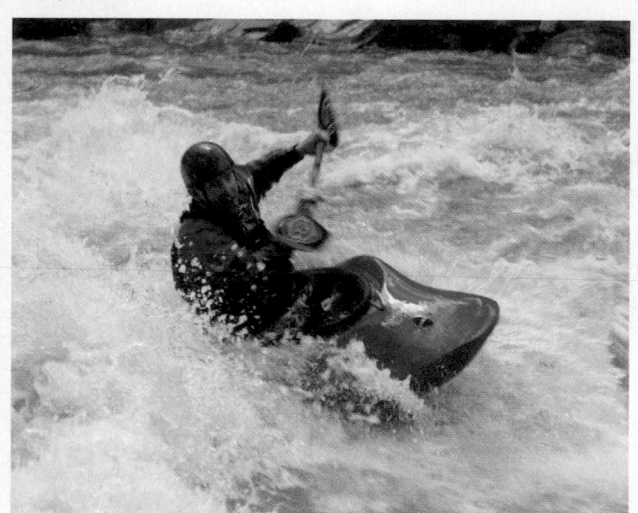

**Figure 21-18** Diffuse axonal injury can be caused by white-water crashes.
Copyright Scott Smith

| Table 21-3 | Mortality Rates for Specific Traumatic Brain Injuries in Outdoor Environments |
| --- | --- |
| **Brain Injury** | **Mortality Rate** |
| Cerebral contusion | Less than 20 percent |
| Epidural hematoma | Less than 20 percent if surgically removed within 1 hour |
| Subdural hematoma | 40–60 percent |
| Diffuse axonal injury | Up to 90 percent |

## Intracerebral Hemorrhage

Because the brain is a highly vascular structure, bleeding within the brain due to trauma can infiltrate the brain tissue, disrupting normal cerebral function. Such intracerebral bleeding can be life threatening because it can cause a rapid rise in intracranial pressure. The prognosis is very poor for individuals who take anticoagulants.

## Spinal Injuries

The bony spine and the spinal nerves are divided into the *cervical* or neck division, the *thoracic* or upper back division, the *lumbar* or lower back division, and the *sacral/coccygeal* or tailbone division. Spinal cord injuries (SCIs) can occur in any of these sections of the spine, especially during activities associated with high speeds, heights, and rapid acceleration or deceleration. As with TBI, males are more likely to sustain an SCI than are females. More specifically, males ages 15–29 years represent more than 50 percent of all SCI cases.

Common neck and back injuries include soft-tissue injuries, muscle or ligament strains, and fractures. Muscle strains of the neck and back are common sports injuries and are likely to be encountered by OEC Technicians on a fairly regular basis. The neck and back muscles protect the spinal cord by limiting movement, but they are susceptible to injury when subjected to twisting and translational forces. Injuries involving the paraspinal musculature are quite painful due to muscle spasms. Hyperflexion or hyperextension of the neck muscles may result in whiplash, a painful injury involving overstretching or tearing of the neck muscles and ligaments. Whiplash can occur when the head is suddenly thrown backward, as might occur during a rear-end crash, a sudden acceleration, or when a skier is struck by another skier.

Fractures of the vertebrae are among the most frequent spine-related injuries. They may occur from blunt, penetrating, compression, twisting, or distraction forces. Because of the spine's flexibility in the cervical and lumbar regions, those vertebrae are more susceptible to hyperflexion, hyperextension, and rotational injuries. The more rigid thoracic vertebrae are more prone to blunt and compression trauma, as are the sacral and coccygeal vertebrae.

Because the cervical vertebrae are thinner than other vertebrae, they are more prone to fracture. These fractures can occur with any of the mechanisms previously described. Diving sports pose an especially high risk for cervical injuries. Fracture of the first vertebra ($C_1$), often referred to as a Jefferson fracture, is most often caused by severe axial loading of the spine in which a weight or force is transmitted along the spinal column. Other common sources of this type of fracture are falling or receiving a downward blow to the head, as might occur from falling ice or rocks.

Fractures of the second cervical vertebra ($C_2$) are often referred to as a Hangman's fracture (Figure 21-19■). This fracture is generally caused when the face forcibly strikes an object, causing the neck to snap violently backward. The name refers to the MOI from hanging, during which the neck also abruptly snaps backward.

Fractures and fracture-dislocations involving both $C_1$ and $C_2$ vertebrae, known as atlas-axis injuries, may occur following rapid deceleration and most often occur when the neck is forcibly hyperextended. The causes of this type of fracture are similar to those in Jefferson and hangman's fractures and are regularly encountered in serious injuries involving rapid deceleration. Fractures that occur to cervical vertebrae $C_3$–$C_5$ can damage the

21-5 Describe the signs and symptoms of potential spinal injuries.

**Figure 21-19** Hangman's fracture.

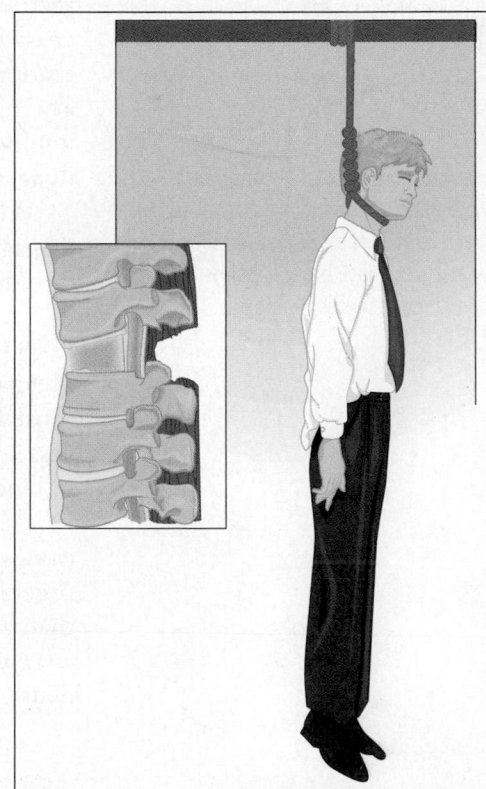

phrenic nerves that innervate the diaphragm, resulting in a patient who is unable to breathe on his own. One easy way to remember this is the phrase "$C_3$, $C_4$, $C_5$, keep the diaphragm alive."

The bones that make up the thoracic vertebrae and the posterior thoracic cage also may be damaged. The thoracic vertebrae, ribs, and scapula form a semi-rigid cage that protects the spine and underlying organs. Upper thoracic spine fractures are less common than fractures involving the cervical, lower thoracic, or lumbar spine.

The scapula is a thick bone that is rarely injured. Fractures of the scapula usually occur as a result of significant blunt trauma delivered directly to the bone and are often associated with rib and spine fractures and other internal thoracic injuries. Always look for internal chest injuries when the scapula appears to be fractured.

Rib fractures are painful injuries that involve a single rib in a single location or multiple ribs in multiple places. The posterior ribs near the spine are protected by the paraspinal musculature. Because they are less flexible than the anterior ribs due to their connection to the thoracic vertebrae, they are more prone to injury due to blunt trauma.

The most common fractures of the spine occur in the lower-thoracic (mid-back) and lumbar (lower back) areas, or at the junction of the two (the thoracolumbar junction). Men experience fractures of the thoracic or lumbar spine from trauma four times more often than do women. Injuries involving the lumbar vertebrae are due to twisting forces and sudden axial loading, which can violently compress the vertebrae. Such injuries can also result from acceleration-deceleration forces, as when deceleration flexes the lumbar spine in an individual restrained by a seatbelt. Injury of the sacral vertebrae is rare, whereas fracture of the coccyx is common and occurs when a person falls on the buttocks.

Neurologic injuries involving the neck and back may result from direct or indirect injuries to the spinal cord. Direct or primary injury to the spinal cord can be caused by a broken or displaced vertebra putting pressure on the cord or by a laceration of cord nerve fibers by sharp bone ends. In most cases, indirect or secondary injury is caused by pressure from bleeding within the spinal canal, which can impinge on the spinal cord, or from traumatic swelling of the spinal cord resulting in **neural ischemia**.

**neural ischemia**    a condition in which part of the brain or spinal cord receives too little oxygenated blood; damage to these organs results after only a few minutes of anoxia.

When a patient with spinal trauma is moved without taking spinal precautions, damage also can occur when unstable vertebrae or vertebral bone fragments intrude into the spinal canal and place direct pressure on the spinal cord.

## Neurogenic Shock

Neurogenic shock, covered in detail in Chapter 10, Shock, is a form of shock that is caused by disruption of the autonomic nervous system. As a result, peripheral blood vessels dilate, trapping blood in the capillary beds, which causes a precipitous drop in blood pressure. The most common cause of neurogenic shock is spinal cord injury, although it may also be caused by TBI. In addition to a low blood pressure, the condition is characterized by bradycardia and often a normal respiratory rate. Neurogenic shock is a potentially life-threatening complication of head or spine trauma that, although rare, must be considered. OEC Technicians should always consider *other* causes of shock, especially hypovolemic shock, before attributing shock to neurogenic causes.

# STOP, THINK, UNDERSTAND

## Multiple Choice

Choose the correct answer.

1. A cerebral contusion is best defined as_____
   a. a rupture of small, localized blood vessels causing a bruise in the brain.
   b. a rapid movement of the brain within the skull caused by rapid acceleration or deceleration.
   c. a secondary insult to the brain in the aftermath of an initial concussion.
   d. rapid brain swelling.

2. The signs and symptoms of a cerebral contusion are often _____ those of a concussion.
   a. worse than
   b. the same as
   c. not as severe as
   d. better than

3. Which of the following statements about a diffuse axonal injury (DAI) is true? _____
   a. It is a high-velocity injury from which a patient rarely recovers.
   b. It is a low-velocity, blunt-trauma injury with a high recovery rate.
   c. Unresponsiveness associated with this injury is short term.
   d. OEC Technicians can determine if a patient is suffering from a DAI by performing a simple neurological test in the field.

4. Because of the fontanels in their skulls, infants can bleed what percentage of their blood volume into their skull before signs of hypotension are evident?_____
   a. 5–10 percent
   b. 10–20 percent
   c. 25–30 percent
   d. 45–50 percent

5. Which of the following statements regarding spinal injuries is false?_____
   a. Males ages 15–29 years have the highest percentage of spinal cord injuries.
   b. The cervical and lumbar vertebrae are more susceptible to hyperflexion, hyperextension, and rotational injuries.
   c. The thoracic vertebrae are more prone to blunt and compression trauma.
   d. Because they are fused, the sacral and coccygeal vertebrae cannot be fractured.

## Matching

1. Match each of the following injuries with the vertebral damage it causes.

   _____ 1. $C_1$ or Jefferson fracture

   _____ 2. $C_2$ or hangman's fracture

   _____ 3. atlas-axis fracture

   _____ 4. $C_3$–$C_5$ (or any spinal cord injury above these levels)

   a. caused by compression of the top of the head such as occurs by diving into shallow water or being struck on the head by a falling rock
   b. a highly unstable fracture caused when the face strikes an object and the neck is snapped violently backward, such as occurs when a passenger strikes the inside of a car windshield
   c. involves both $C_1$ and $C_2$ vertebrae, usually caused by deceleration trauma
   d. can result in patients' inability to breathe on their own

2. Identify each of the following descriptions as referring to either a subdural hematoma (S), an epidural hematoma (E), or both (B).

   _____ a. an arterial bleed between the skull and the dura mater

   _____ b. an accumulation of venous blood between the brain and the dura mater

   _____ c. usually caused by deceleration or violent shearing-force trauma

   _____ d. compresses the brain, which compromises vital brain function

   _____ e. generally caused by blunt trauma

   _____ f. the onset of signs and symptoms is usually very rapid

   _____ g. may not be apparent for hours, days, or even weeks after the injury

   _____ h. involves a decreased level of responsiveness, unresponsiveness without a lucid period, and slow onset of signs/symptoms

   _____ i. typical progression of signs or symptoms involves unresponsiveness followed by a lucid period, secondary unresponsiveness, and death

## Short Answer

Why is a subdural hematoma a serious injury?

# CASE UPDATE

You quickly ensure safety by securing the scene, and then you summon assistance. You instruct rescuers to bring a long spine board, a C-collar, oxygen, and a trauma pack. You also request a toboggan and a helicopter for transport. The patient's pulse is 92 and regular. As you await help, you make sure the patient's airway remains open by using a jaw-thrust maneuver that maintains cervical spinal alignment, and you make sure he continues to breathe. At the same time, you begin to visually assess the patient's injuries. He has contusions on his right facial cheek and his forehead. Soon, several other OEC Technicians arrive on scene.

**What should you do now?**

---

**⊕ 21-6** Describe how to properly assess a patient with a suspected neurologic injury, including neck and spine injuries.

# Patient Assessment

After securing the scene, you begin an assessment of any patients with a head, neck, back, or nervous system injury by determining the mechanism of injury. Among the situations that have a significant potential for neurologic injury are the following:

+ A fall greater than 2.5–3 times the patient's height.
+ A moderate- to high-speed motor vehicle collision in which:
  • One or more occupants were killed.
  • The patient was unrestrained and/or was ejected from the vehicle.
  • The vehicle was a bicycle, a motorcycle, a snowmobile, or an all-terrain vehicle (ATV), especially if no helmet was worn.
+ A pedestrian or bicyclist was struck by a motor vehicle.
+ A skier/snowboarder/cyclist collided with another skier/snowboarder/cyclist or a fixed object such as a tree or lift tower.
+ A gunshot wound to the head, neck, chest, back, abdomen, or pelvis or that is proximal to the elbow or knee.
+ Burial in an avalanche or cave-in.
+ An impact by a rock, tree, or other falling object.
+ A high-voltage electrical shock, including a lightning strike.

Once the scene size-up is complete and you have considered the mechanism of injury, immediately perform a primary assessment and correct any immediate threats to life (Figure 21-20■). Make sure the patient has an airway, is breathing, and has a good pulse. Note: If the patient is unresponsive, follow the 2010 ECC guidelines and open the airway while simultaneously checking for breathing and a carotid pulse for no longer than 10 seconds. If necessary begin CPR, if not then assess the "D" in ABCD. Mental status is established by asking simple questions to responsive patients. Ask: What is your name, where are you, what day of the week is it, and what happened to you? Also assess mental status using the mini-neurologic exam, including AVPU, pupillary exam, and (if there is time) the Glasgow Coma Scale. Also assess distal neurologic motor and sensory function in all four extremities.

If the patient is unresponsive or you suspect a spine injury, maintain spinal alignment while caring for threats to life. If an emergency maneuver is required to establish an airway in an unresponsive patient or if rescue

**Figure 21-20** This rescuer is sizing up the scene and the patient.
Copyright Mike Halloran

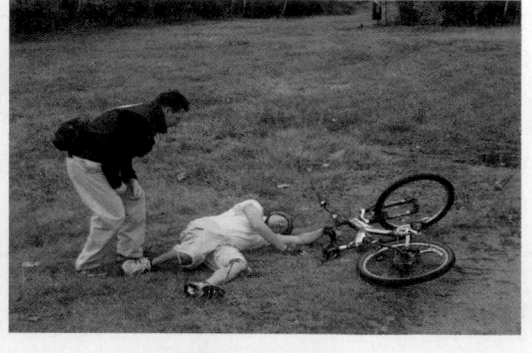

breathing or CPR is required, maintain cervical spine stabilization manually and open the airway using the jaw-thrust maneuver. Apply a cervical collar and perform life-saving interventions such as CPR as needed.

Once manual stabilization is initiated in a responsive patient, continue to hold the patient's head in a neutral position until the person is fully immobilized on a long spine board. Do not allow the patient to move.

Manually stabilize the neck and spine of any patient with a significant mechanism for potential head or spinal cord injury. To stabilize the spine, perform the following procedure (OEC Skill 21-1■):

1. Kneel next to the patient's head, either to the side or at the top of the head.
2. Place your hands on either side of the patient's head, with the palms adjacent to the ears and the fingers supporting the jaw and the back of the head.
3. Gently move the head so that the patient's eyes are looking forward and the patient's nose and chin are aligned with the sternum. *Never force the head into alignment.* If the patient has muscle spasms in the neck; if your movement causes increased pain in the neck or numbness, tingling, or weakness in the extremities; or if alignment compromises airway or breathing, stop what you are doing and stabilize the patient in the position found.
4. Do not allow the patient to move.

Remember that the ABCDs take precedence in your assessment. Once the airway, breathing, and circulation are established, if there is any concern for spinal injury, immobilize the entire spine. If the patient is unresponsive or in shock, immediately transport; otherwise begin the secondary assessment.

## Mini-Neurologic Exam

The assessment of a patient with a suspected head or spinal injury should include a thorough exam of the nervous system. Many responders now use the Glascow Coma Scale, which is somewhat more difficult to use than is the AVPU scale. A hybrid of these is known as the mini-neurologic exam (Table 21-4■), which consists of the following three components:

+ level of responsiveness
+ **A**lert, **V**erbal (responses to), **P**ain (responses to), **U**nresponsive (AVPU)
+ pupillary exam (PERRL)
+ best motor response (from the Glascow Coma Scale)

> ### Documentation Tip
>
> When using the AAO × 4 scale for evaluating mental status (patient is alert and oriented to person, place, time, and situation), be sure to indicate which questions the patient is oriented to, instead of just stating a number. For example, instead of writing "The patient is alert and oriented × 2," write, "The patient is alert and oriented only to person and place, but not to time and situation."

**Table 21-4** Components of the Mini-Neurologic Exam

- Level of responsiveness (AVPU)
- Pupillary exam
- Best motor response (Glascow Coma Scale)
  - Patient follows commands
  - Localized pain
  - Withdrawal from pain
  - Flexor posturing (pain)
  - Extensor posturing (pain)
  - No response (flaccid paralysis)

During the assessment, determine the patient's level of responsiveness (LOR) based on the AVPU scale. Patients who have suffered neurologic insult may appear normal, confused, agitated, combative, or comatose. Assessment of the LOR must be ongoing because it can change rapidly.

The **pupillary exam** is performed as described in Chapter 7, Patient Assessment. Pay close attention to any abnormal findings such as pupils that are unequal, dilated, or unresponsive.

Assessment of the patient's **best motor response** is taken directly from the motor response section of the Glasgow Coma Scale and should be performed as follows:

1. Ask the patient to hold up two fingers on the left hand and two fingers on the right hand. If he complies, this is the best motor response.
2. If the patient is unable to follow your command, grasp his index finger between your penlight and thumb and gently squeeze. If after an initial withdrawal from this painful stimulus, the patient reaches for the penlight, he is localizing pain. Repeat on the opposite side.
3. If the patient continues to withdraw from the painful stimulus, his best motor response is "withdraws from pain."
4. If upon a painful stimulus the patient does not localize or withdraw but instead exhibits flexor posturing (flexion of the arms and legs and dorsiflexion of the feet), the best motor response is "flexor posturing" (Figure 21-21■).
5. If instead of flexor posturing, the patient exhibits extensor posturing (extension of the arms and legs and plantar flexion of the feet), record the response as "extensor posturing" (Figure 21-22■).
6. If the patient does not respond to a painful stimulus but exhibits a flaccid paralysis (slack, immobile limbs), he has no motor response (Figure 21-23■).

Record your findings for the mini-neurologic exam according to your observations. You might write, for example, "Verbal on AVPU; can respond to questions and his answers make sense; responds to pain; pulls away from painful stimuli."

**Figure 21-21** A patient exhibiting flexor posturing.

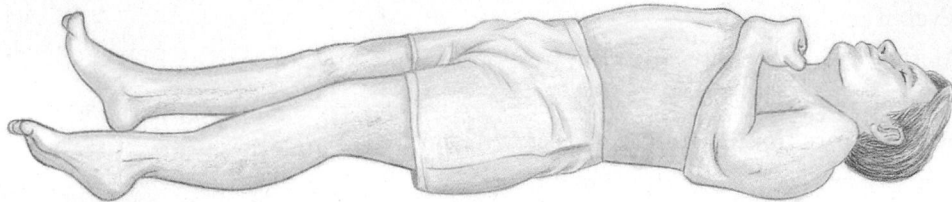

**Figure 21-22** A patient exhibiting extension posturing.

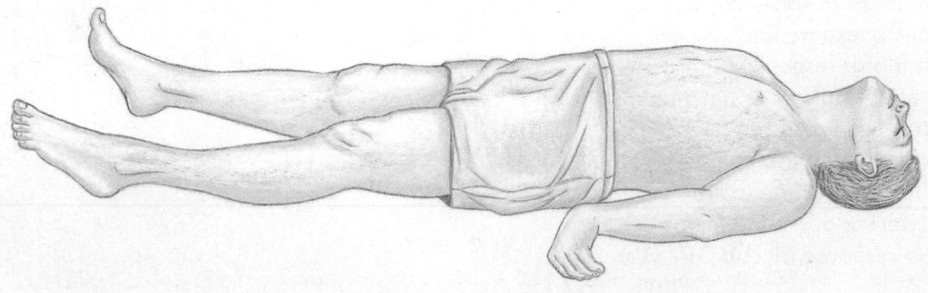

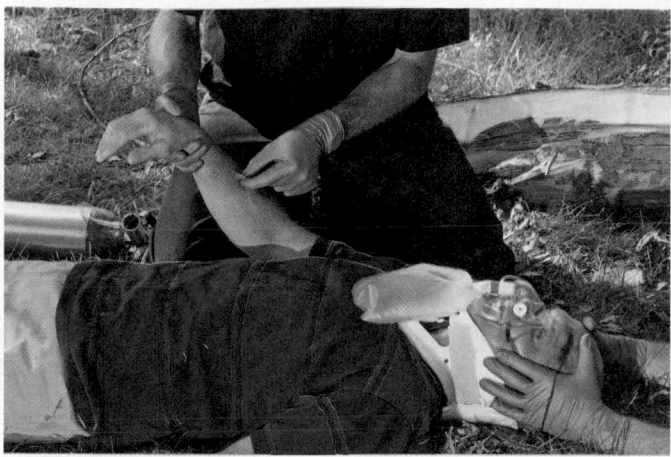

**Figure 21-23** Assessing neurological, motor. and sensory function.

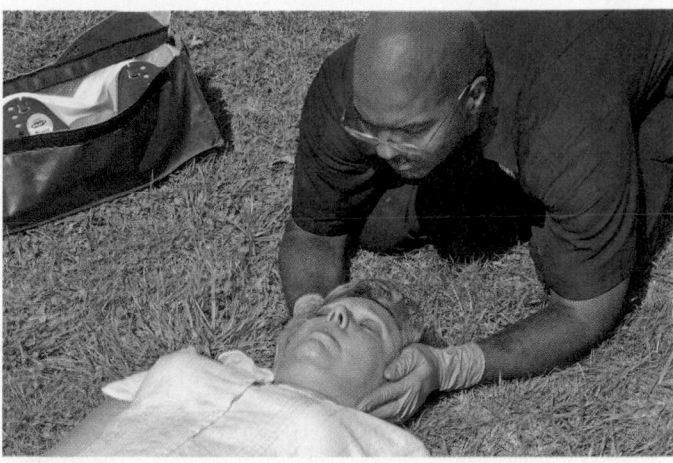

**Figure 21-24** Maintain manual stablization throughout the assessment of the patient.

Secondary assessment consists of a combination of observation and palpation. Because of the possible catastrophic consequences of spinal cord injury, manual stabilization of the C-spine should be maintained at all times during the assessment and treatment of these patients (Figure 21-24■). One OEC Technician can manually stabilize the C-spine, as previously described, while another performs the assessment.

Begin your secondary assessment in the usual fashion by palpating the bony structures of the face, cranium, and neck, and by looking and feeling for any evidence of trauma using the DCAP-BTLS mnemonic.

Examine the ears, nose, and mouth for leakage of CSF, which is an indicator of a skull fracture. All skull fractures suggest a high-impact mechanism of injury, and almost always occur in combination with traumatic brain injury. By itself, CSF appears clear and colorless and may be mistaken for sweat, rain, or melted snow. In the setting of neurologic trauma, CSF will likely be mixed with blood and may leak from the ear canals, nostrils, or mouth.

To determine if CSF is present, perform a "halo test" (Figure 21-25■). Place a small amount of the leakage onto a piece of sterile gauze. If CSF is present, it will diffuse faster than blood and leave a distinctive "bull's eye" formation in which a red center (blood) is surrounded by a pinkish ring (a CSF and blood mixture). If a patient with a head injury is exhibiting an abnormal neurological exam (decreased GCS, or focal weakness in a limb), then *do not* waste time performing a "halo test."

As you are performing your assessment, obtain a SAMPLE history and take vital signs. Attempt to determine the forces involved and whether the patient was rendered unresponsive, even if only momentarily. Be sure to ask the patient (or a friend or relative) if the patient has diabetes or a history of seizures, or if he used any mind-altering substances, including alcohol and illicit drugs, because these can also alter neurologic findings. You may need to care for the patient for both the medical problem and the neurologic trauma.

Complete a head-to-toe exam following the procedure described in Chapter 7, Patient Assessment, noting any non-neurologic injuries, especially fractures of the scapula and posterior ribs. Because of the forces involved, the proximity of the scapula to the spine, and the frequency of multiple associated injuries, all patients with a suspected scapula or posterior

**Figure 21-25** The "halo test" can detect the presence of cerebrospinal fluid.

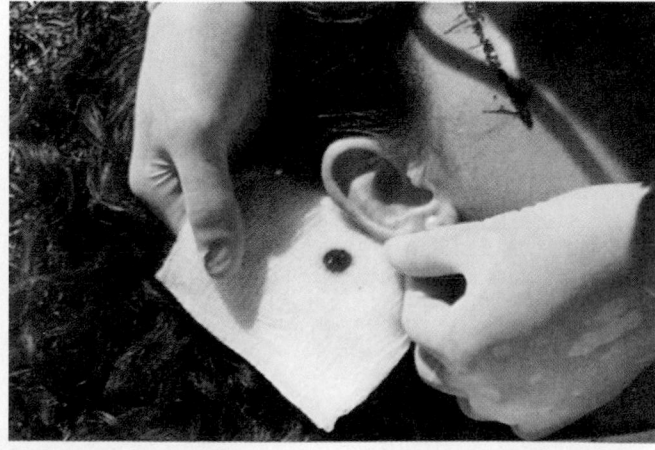

rib fracture should be assumed to have a spine injury until proven otherwise. Next, reassess the vital signs and carefully evaluate each value. TBI with increased intracranial pressure is associated with the following changes in vital signs:

+ Increased systolic blood pressure
+ Decreased diastolic blood pressure
+ Tachypnea (abnormal respiratory rate and pattern)
+ Bradycardia (abnormally slow heart rate)

Posturing is an abnormal neurologic finding that indicates that the central nervous system has suffered a serious injury. Assessment of a suspected neurologic injury is not considered complete without a check of the patient's distal circulation, movement and sensation (CMS). Besides having loss of sensation and motor function below the injured level of the spinal cord, patients with a spinal cord injury often display a characteristic sign in which the skin below the level of the injury is flushed, whereas above the level of the injury the skin color is normal or pale. This response results from disruption of the nerve pathways. In most cases the impairment will be present on both sides of the body, but in rare instances it can be on one side only. As indicated previously, spontaneous breathing may be absent in a patient with a spinal cord injury at or above the level of $C_5$. Males may have a persistent erection, called a priapism, due to CNS damage.

After you have completed your initial assessment, continue to monitor the patient's ABCDs, level of responsiveness (LOR), distal CMS, and vital signs, documenting any changes you observe.

## STOP, THINK, UNDERSTAND

### Multiple Choice
Choose the correct answer.

1. When approaching a scene in which a patient may have sustained a neurologic injury, the second-most important thing (after establishing scene safety) for rescuers to establish is_____
   a. the mechanism of injury (MOI).
   b. the age and sex of the patient.
   c. the patient's history of prior injuries.
   d. any allergies the patient might have.

2. When caring for a patient with a suspected spinal cord injury, which of the following actions should take priority?_____
   a. manually stabilizing the patient's neck and spine
   b. assessing and caring for the ABCDs while protecting spine
   c. calling for a long spine board
   d. arranging for transportation to the nearest trauma center

3. When a patient shows evidence of raccoon eyes and Battle's sign several hours following a trauma, this finding could be indicative of_____
   a. an occluded airway.
   b. a $C_4$ fracture.
   c. a skull fracture.
   d. an epidural hematoma.

4. CSF leaking from a patient's nose could be indicative of _____
   a. a vertebral fracture.
   b. a DAI.
   c. a severe concussion.
   d. a skull fracture.

5. The observation that a patient's systolic and diastolic blood pressure values are moving increasingly farther apart could suggest that_____
   a. the patient may be having a heart attack or may be suffering from some other coronary insult.
   b. the patient has suffered a traumatic brain injury with increasing intracranial pressure.
   c. the patient is slipping into hypovolemic shock.
   d. you do not have enough information to properly assess the patient's condition.

6. A mini-neurologic exam consists of which of the following components?_____
   a. assessing the ABCDs, grip strength, and level of responsiveness
   b. assessing the SAMPLE and AVPU
   c. assessing the AVPU, PERRL, and best motor response from the GCS
   d. checking the pupils, tapping the patient's feet, and asking the patient to squeeze your fingers

# Management

The goals of emergency management of traumatic brain and spinal cord injuries are to adequately maintain the patient's vital signs and to avoid secondary injury (especially to the nervous system) while transporting the patient (Figure 21-26■). This is accomplished by caring for threats to life following the ABCDs while not allowing any spinal movement, and reducing ischemia of neural tissue. As a general rule, treatment of patients with head or spine injuries consists of the following steps:

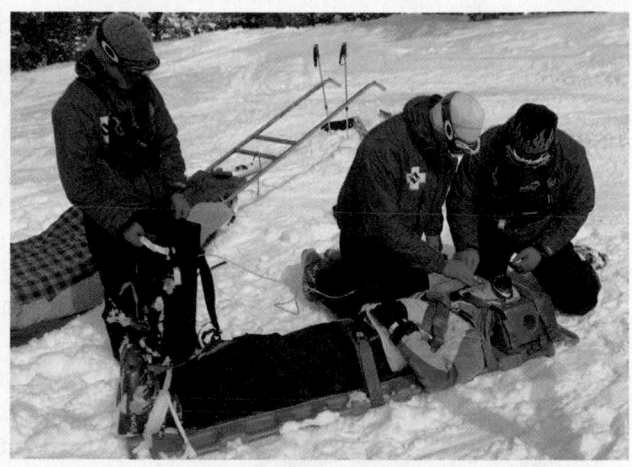

**Figure 21-26** Head and spinal immobilization is crucial in limiting the potential of further nervous system injuries.
Copyright Scott Smith

1. Correct any threats to life that may be present while protecting the spine, especially the C-spine. Perform CPR, if necessary. Establish and maintain an adequate airway using the jaw-thrust maneuver and any of the adjuncts described in Chapter 9, Airway Management. If the patient is unresponsive and has no gag reflex, insert an OPA (oropharyngeal airway) or NPA (nasopharyngeal airway). Suction the airway as needed.

2. Ensure adequate respirations and provide supplemental oxygen. If the patient is breathing, administer oxygen via nonrebreather mask at 15 LPM. If the patient is not breathing or is breathing less than eight times per minute, ventilate the patient using a BVM (bag-valve mask) and supplemental oxygen at a rate of one breath every six to eight seconds.

3. Control external bleeding and maintain blood flow to body tissues.

4. Following assessment of mental status, determine if any care is needed for other medical problems, particularly problems that could also involve compromised mental status (e.g., diabetes).

5. Protect the spine using manual stabilization until spinal immobilization equipment becomes available. Many patients with TBI also have a spine injury, especially of the cervical spine. Because of the potential catastrophic consequences of spinal cord injury, all patients with a head injury should be treated as if they also have a spine injury. Patients who are walking and say "I don't remember falling" or "I don't know where I am" should be considered to have a traumatic brain injury and require spinal immobilization unless there is a *clear* medical reason for the change in mental status. If the patient is lying on the ground, keep the person still and lying down, or if sitting or standing, stabilize the spine in the position found. Once spinal equipment is made available, immobilize the patient's entire spine using the appropriate technique described on the following pages.

6. Treat other injuries. Treat localized soft-tissue injuries as described in Chapter 18, Soft-Tissue Injuries, but note that unlike comparable injuries of the extremities, simple lacerations involving the scalp can cause profuse bleeding and shock. Because of this, dress and bandage all scalp wounds using a roller gauze or Kling style of wrap to help maintain pressure and control bleeding. If CSF is leaking from the ears or nose, do not attempt to stop the flow.

   In the setting of multiple rib fractures or a scapula fracture, assume that the patient has a spine injury and treat accordingly. Patients with a significant MOI should be fully immobilized to a long spine board and given supplemental oxygen, regardless of the chief complaint or signs and symptoms.

7. Continually monitor the patient. Check the patient's level of responsiveness and other vital signs every five minutes and record any changes.

8. Transport the patient with the head uphill to prevent worsening of an intracranial head injury. Transport the patient to a definitive care facility as soon as possible.

⊕ **21-8** Demonstrate how to properly treat a patient with a head, neck, spine, or back injury.

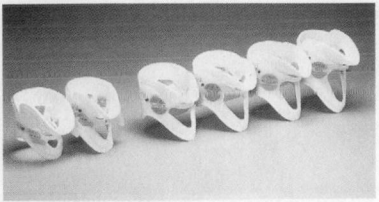

**Figure 21-27a** Different sizes of Stifneck cervical spine immobilization collars.

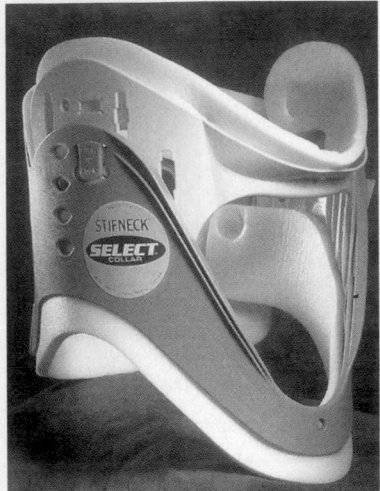

**Figure 21-27b** The Stifneck Select collar can be adjusted to fit all sizes.

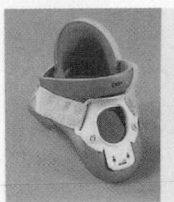 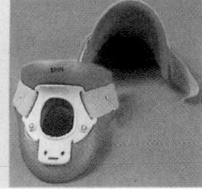

**Figure 21-27c** The Philadelphia Cervical Collar.
Copyright Philadelphia Cervical Collar Company

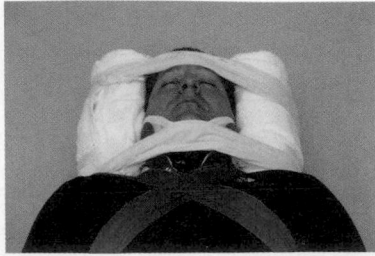

**Figure 21-28** Head stabilization using rolled towels or blankets placed on either side of the patient's head.
Copyright Mike Halloran

## Sizing and Applying a Cervical Collar

Manual, in-line stabilization of the head and C-spine is the first step in properly immobilizing a patient with a spine injury. Because it is impractical to continue manual, in-line stabilization during transport, use an adjunct device. Rigid cervical collars (also called C-collars or extrication collars) are designed to provide support for the head and C-spine during transport, but they provide only partial protection. Therefore, always use these devices in conjunction with a long spine board (LSB), and be sure to maintain manual stabilization even after the C-collar is applied and until the patient is fully secured to the LSB (Figures 21-27a–c■).

To be effective, a C-collar must be properly sized to the patient. When properly sized, a C-collar should rest on the shoulder and provide firm support under the chin, along both sides of the mandible, and at the occiput on the back of the head, without obstructing the airway. OEC Technicians should always follow the manufacturer's directions.

In general, to properly size and apply a C-collar, follow these steps (OEC Skill 21-2■):

1. Maintain or establish manual stabilization of the head and C-spine using the technique previously described.
2. Measure the patient and C-collar. Be sure to follow the manufacturer's specifications for sizing for each of the different collar types. An improperly sized or applied C-collar can compromise airway patency and C-spine stability, and cause further injury. Therefore, if the appropriate size is not available, or if the C-collar cannot be applied appropriately for any reason, do not use it. Instead, place a tightly rolled towel against each side of the head as a modified head block, or place a horseshoe-shaped blanket over the top of the head, and then secure the patient's head to the LSB using cravats (Figure 21-28■).
3. Apply the C-collar.
   - Open the patient's coat or shirt.
   - Move any bulky clothing out of the way. Do not put the collar on over clothing.
   - Slide the posterior neck portion of the collar behind the patient's neck.
   - Swing the chin portion of the collar up over the patient's chest until it cups the chin.
   - Secure the C-collar using the Velcro™ closure and ensure a proper fit.

In general, a properly sized C-collar will stabilize the head and C-spine in neutral alignment without hyperextending the neck, and the chin will rest flush with the edge of the chin cup. A collar that is too small can apply pressure to the throat and obstruct the airway; one that is too big can allow flexion of the neck and compromise C-spine stabilization. See OEC Skill 21-2 for sizing and applying a cervical collar.

## Placing a Patient on a Long Spine Board

Even though the spine consists of 33 vertebrae, for splinting purposes it is treated as a single long bone with joints above (at the neck) and below (at the hips). As described in Chapter 20, Musculoskeletal Injuries, to be properly splinted a long bone must be immobilized beyond the joints proximal and distal to the bone. In patients with spine injuries, this is accomplished by applying a rigid cervical collar (C-collar), placing the patient onto an LSB, and securing the patient's torso, pelvis, extremities, and (last) the head to the board (Figures 21-29a■ and 21-29b■). The patient must be log rolled onto the LSB due to the fact that he has a possible spine injury.

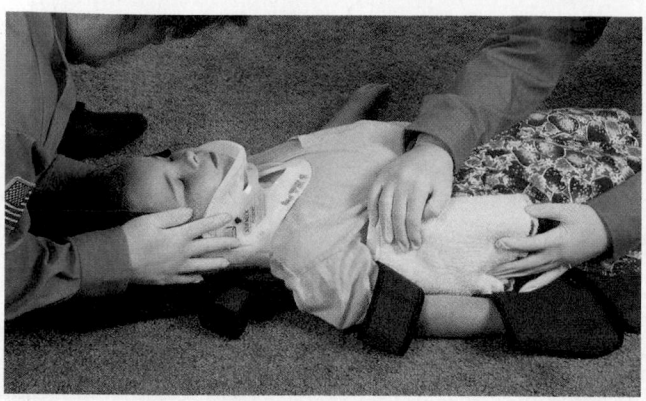

**Figure 21-29a** After the patient has been placed on the board, apply padding to both sides of the torso.

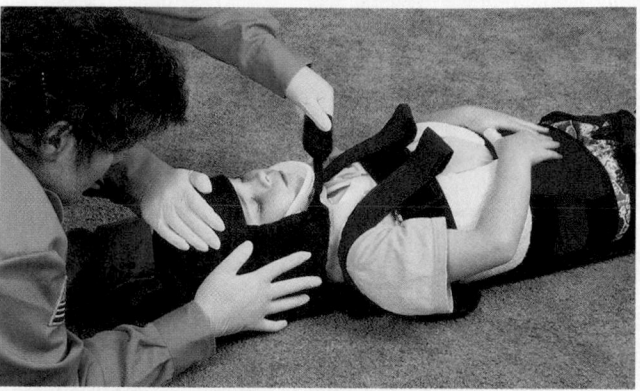

**Figure 21-29b** Another rescuer provides head stabilization.

## Supine Patient

For patients who are log-rolled, the procedure must be carefully executed to prevent any twisting or excessive bending of the spine. Ideally, a log roll should be performed using at least four rescuers. To log roll a supine patient onto an LSB, perform the following procedure (OEC Skill 21-3 ■):

**21-9** Demonstrate how to maintain proper spinal alignment while placing a patient onto a long spine board from the following positions:

- lying
- sitting
- standing

1. Rescuer #1 kneels above the patient's head and manually stabilizes the cervical spine, as previously described.
2. Rescuers #2, #3, and #4 kneel along one side of the patient.
3. Rescuer #2:
   - Assesses the patient's circulation, sensation, and movement in each extremity and later documents the findings on the PCR.
   - Kneels beside the patient's shoulder/upper chest.
   - Grasps the patient's shoulder and hip.
4. Rescuer #3:
   - Positions the board beside the patient.
   - Kneels beside the patient's hip.
   - Grasps the patient's hip (consider overlapping hands with Rescuer #2) and grasps the patient above the knee.
5. Rescuer #4:
   - Kneels beside the patient's knee/lower leg.
   - Grasps the patient's upper thigh (consider overlapping hands with Rescuer #3) and grasps the patient below the knee.
6. Rescuer #1 instructs Rescuers #2, #3, and #4 to roll the patient onto his side on the count of three.
7. Rescuers #2, #3, and #4 gently and simultaneously roll the patient toward them as one unit.
8. Rescuer #2 checks the patient's upper and lower back for injuries by both inspection and palpation and then slides the backboard into position next to the patient, tilting the board at a 45-degree angle to the patient's back. (If available, another rescuer may move the LSB into position.)
9. Rescuer #1 instructs Rescuers #2, #3, and #4 to lower the patient onto the LSB on the count of three.
10. Rescuers #2, #3, and #4 lower the patient as one unit onto the LSB.

As the rescuers continue to hold the patient, Rescuer #2 checks to make sure the patient is properly centered on the LSB. If the patient is not, the patient must be centered by performing an axial drag (OEC Skill 21-4■).

To center the patient on the LSB, follow these steps:

1. Rescuer #1 instructs Rescuers #2, #3, and #4 to slide the patient toward the foot of the board (toward the rescuers) on the count of three.
2. Rescuers #2, #3, and #4 slide the patient as one unit (keeping the patient's toes, navel, and nose in the same line) toward the foot of the LSB.
3. Rescuer #1 instructs rescuers to slide the patient into the proper position on the count of three.
4. Rescuers #2, #3, and #4 slide the patient into position as one unit.

This procedure may be repeated as necessary until the patient is properly positioned on the LSB. Alternatively, at the start of the procedure place the board with about a foot and a half of it extending *above* the patient's head and then do an axial drag to center the patient.

Once properly positioned on the LSB, the patient is secured using straps, cravats, tape, or a commercial device. To secure the patient onto the LSB, perform the following procedure (OEC Skill 21-5■):

1. Secure the torso. Cross the straps from over the shoulder to just above the opposite hip and tighten smoothly as the patient takes a deep breath. Do not tug or overtighten. (An appropriately tight strap should allow you to fit one finger between the strap and the patient and should never compromise the patient's ability to breathe.) If you are using a commercial device, follow the manufacturer's directions. Pad any voids using towels, blankets, or clothing to prevent movement or twisting of the spine and to improve the patient's comfort.
2. Secure the pelvis and the extremities. Beginning where the torso straps end to prevent gaps, cross the pelvis straps from above the iliac crests (the patient's hips) to just below the level of the greater trochanter of each femur (the upper thigh). This ensures that the entire weight of the pelvis is contained within the straps and is properly immobilized. (Alternatively, a single strap can be placed across the pelvis at the level of the pubis bone.) An additional strap should be placed across the mid-thighs between the end of the pelvis straps and the knees. Place another strap across the lower legs. If the patient has a possible pelvis or hip fracture or an abdominal injury, you may need to place the straps just above or below the injury, but never place them tightly across the abdomen. Pad all voids.
3. Secure the head last. If you are using a commercial head immobilization device, follow the manufacturer's directions. If you are using towels rolls:
   - Roll two standard towels and securely tape each roll.
   - Place one towel on each side of the patient's head.
   - Secure the head by placing a large piece of tape or a cravat over the patient's forehead. Be sure not to cover the eyelids. Place a second piece of tape over the C-collar just below the chin.

   An alternative method is to place a rolled-up (horse-collar shaped) blanket around the patient's head and secure it at the chin and forehead.
4. Reassess the patient's airway and breathing. Also reassess distal circulation, sensation, and movement in each extremity. Document these CMS findings on the PCR. Monitor the patient throughout transport. Given that vomiting is common

with traumatic brain injury, have suction available and be prepared to roll immobilized patients onto their sides while they remain strapped to the board.

## Sitting Patient

Not every spine injury patient you encounter will be lying down. Some will be wedged against a rock or tree; some will sit down following their accident. Manage these patients in much the same way you would a patient who is supine: by manually stabilizing the head and C-spine and by placing the patient on a short spine-immobilization device—preferably a short board or a vest-type immobilization device—before transitioning to an LSB. If your patrol does not use either of these devices, place the patient supine and then move him to an LSB.

To immobilize the spine of a patient who is sitting, follow these steps (OEC Skill 21-6■):

1. **Rescuer #1:** Manually stabilize the head and cervical spine by kneeling next to or behind the patient's head and establish manual in-line stabilization of the head and C-spine. Continue this until the patient is strapped onto the board.
2. **Rescuer #2:** Assess circulation, movement and sensation (CMS) in each extremity. Document CMS findings on the PCR at a later time.
3. **Rescuer #2:** Size and apply the cervical collar in the manner previously described.
4. **Rescuers #2 and #3:** Apply the immobilization device.
   - If you are using a short board, place the device behind and directly against the patient's back, aligning the top of the device with the top of the patient's head. Then cross the torso straps over the patient's shoulders and secure the patient to the board. Pad behind the patient's head, filling any gaps that are present, and secure the head using a cravat tied around the board and the patient's forehead, over the eyebrows. Tie a second cravat over the C-collar.
   - If using a vest-type immobilization device, follow the manufacturer's directions.
   - If your patrol does not use these devices, skip this step and go directly to step 5.
5. **Rescuers #2 and #3:** Move the patient to the LSB. Place the LSB next to the patient's buttocks and lift the patient onto it. With Rescuer #1 maintaining manual in-line stabilization of the head and C-spine, lift the patient from the armpits and hips and lower the person onto the LSB.
6. Lower the patient into a supine position on the LSB, sliding the patient axially. If present, secure the short board or vest-type immobilization device to the LSB. Otherwise, secure the patient directly to the LSB as previously described.
7. Reassess the patient's distal pulse, sensation, and motor function. Record both these CMS findings and the earlier findings on the PCR.

## Standing Patient

You may arrive on scene to find a patient who is standing or walking around with a possible TBI or spinal injury. Such patients should be fully immobilized. At least three rescuers, preferably four, are required to perform this procedure. To immobilize the spine of a standing patient, follow these steps (OEC Skill 21-7■):

1. **Rescuer #1** stands beside or behind the patient and manually stabilizes the patient's head and C-spine. It is helpful for this rescuer to be tall.
2. **Rescuer #2** checks distal pulse, sensation, and movement in each extremity and then sizes and applies a cervical collar.
3. **Rescuer #3** prepares and positions an LSB behind the patient.

+ 21-10  Describe and demonstrate how to remove a helmet.

4. Rescuers #2 and #3 stand next to the patient, one on either side.
   - Rescuer #2 (standing next to the patient's right side) places his right arm under the patient's right armpit and grasps the LSB slot above the patient's shoulder. Rescuer #2's left hand grasps the patient's right elbow, holding the arm in place. (This prevents the patient from sliding when being lowered to the ground.)
   - Rescuer #3 (standing next to the patient's left side) places his left arm under the patient's left armpit and grasps the LSB slot above the patient's shoulder, directly opposite Rescuer #2. Rescuer #3's right hand grasps the patient's left elbow, holding the arm in place.

5. Lower the patient to the ground.
   - Rescuer #1 instructs Rescuers #2 and #3 to lower the LSB to the ground on the count of three while maintaining in-line stabilization of the head and spine until the patient is secured to the LSB.
   - Rescuers #2 and #3 slowly drop their knee closest to the LSB and lower the patient and backboard to the ground. Keep the patient centered on the LSB. (If available, a fourth rescuer or bystander can hold the patient's feet against the board during this step.) Move slowly to allow Rescuer #1 to move his hands over the LSB while maintaining manual, in-line stabilization of the head and spine. When ready, Rescuers #2 and #3 slowly lower the patient and backboard to the ground while keeping the patient centered on the LSB.

6. Secure the patient to the LSB in the usual manner.

7. Reassess the distal pulse, sensation, and movement in each extremity.

## Procedure for Removing a Helmet (Lying Patient)

As a result of effective injury prevention efforts, most cyclists, ATV riders, snow machine riders, rafters, climbers, and an increasing number of skiers and snowboarders now wear helmets while participating in their chosen sports (Figures 21-30a–c■). In fact, the National Medical Committee of the NSP recommends that anyone who participates in a snow sport wear a helmet to reduce the severity of injuries to the head. Even though the presence of a helmet can complicate the management of the patient, you do not always need to remove the helmet. If a helmet fits properly, does not obstruct the airway or interfere with assessment and management of the airway, and can be incorporated into proper immobilization of the spine, it may be left on.

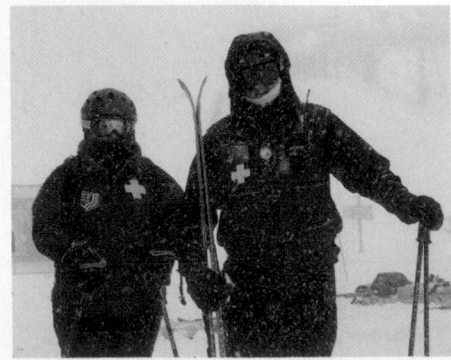

**Figure 21-30a** Ski patrollers wearing helmets for protection.
Copyright Studio 404

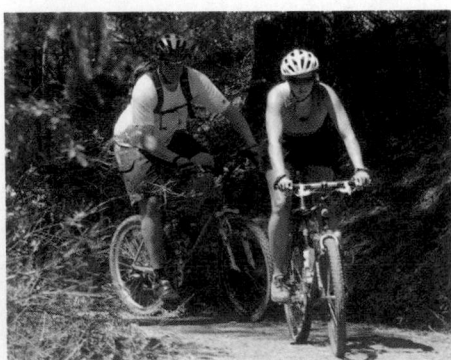

**Figure 21-30b** Cyclists wearing helmets for protection.
Copyright Scott Smith

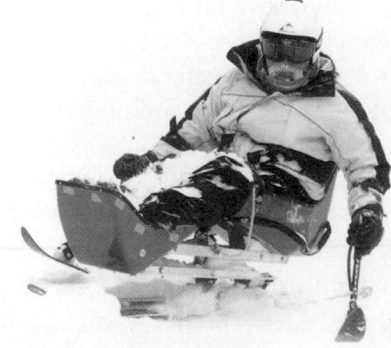

**Figure 21-30c** Adaptive skiers wearing helmets for protection.
Copyright Greg Bala

It is recommended that you remove a helmet only if:

✦ The patient does not have a patent airway, is not breathing adequately, and the helmet prevents you from managing these problems.

✦ The helmet is too big or otherwise allows the patient's head to move while it is left in place.

✦ The helmet prevents you from properly immobilizing the spine.

✦ The patient is in cardiac arrest.

✦ The helmet is broken and thus does not allow proper head and neck immobilization.

To remove a helmet, follow these steps (OEC Skill 21-8■):

**1.** Align the patient axially.

**2.** Rescuer #1: manually stabilize the head and C-spine by placing one hand on either side of the helmet.

**3.** Rescuer #2: carefully open the face shield and/or remove goggles (if present). Unfasten the chin strap and place one hand at the occiput and the other at the chin. If blood is suspected, use Standard Precautions.

As an alternative method, Rescuer #2 places one hand along either side of the patient's head at the bottom edge of the helmet, so that the fingers are in position to support each side of the face up over the ears.

**4.** Remove the helmet.

• Rescuer #1 grasps the helmet straps or sides of the helmet and pulls them apart, spreading the helmet, then pulls the helmet axially away from the patient's head, providing forward rotation of the helmet to ease passage of the chin guard (plastic device that protects the mouth and chin area on some types of ski and other sports helmets) off the face.

• Rescuer #2 slides the fingers up to the occiput and chin (or on both sides of the head over the ears), ensuring that the patient's head and C-spine remain immobilized.

**5.** Apply a cervical collar:

• Rescuer #1 places the helmet aside and takes over manual in-line stabilization of the head and C-spine.

• Rescuer #2 sizes and applies the cervical collar in the fashion previously described.

> ### Removing a Player's Shoulder Pads
>
> **NOTE**
>
> If removing the shoulder pads from an injured football, lacrosse, or hockey player, do not pull them off over the head; instead, remove them by untying/unlacing/cutting them. This approach applies to any sports equipment, including helmets, whose removal causes hyperextension of the neck (Figure 21-31■).

**Figure 21-31** Depending on the type of injury, a helmet need not always be removed.

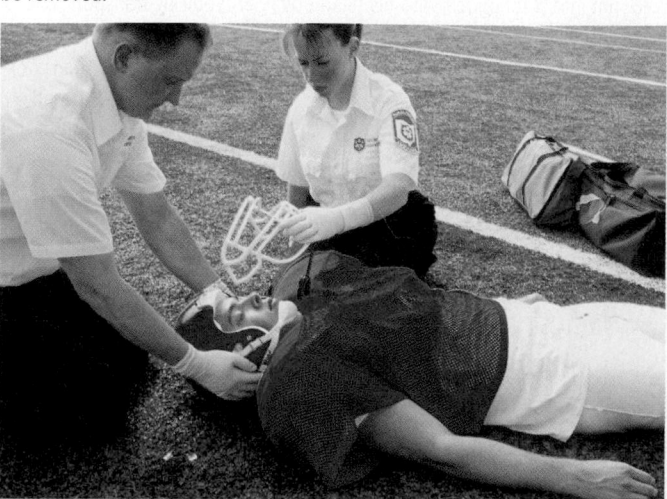

# STOP, THINK, UNDERSTAND

## Multiple Choice

Choose the correct answer.

1. The correct sequence for immobilizing a patient on a long spine board_____
   a. is to apply a C-collar, then secure the torso, pelvis, extremities, and head.
   b. is to apply a C-collar, then secure the head, torso, pelvis, and extremities.
   c. is to secure the torso, then apply a C-collar and secure the head, pelvis, and extremities.
   d. depends on the patient's situation.

2. When should you check CMS in a patient with a spinal cord injury? _____
   a. Before placing the patient on the spine board.
   b. Before and after placing the patient on the spine board, and periodically thereafter.
   c. Only after handing the patient over to the transporting agency.
   d. Only after placing the patient on a spine board.

3. Under which of the following circumstances should a helmet be removed? (check all that apply)
   _____ a. Whenever a patient is immobilized on a long spine board

   _____ b. All helmets should be left in place until the patient reaches the hospital.
   _____ c. Whenever a patient does not have a patent airway or is not breathing adequately
   _____ d. Whenever the helmet is too large and allows the patient's head to move
   _____ e. Whenever the helmet prevents you from properly immobilizing the spine
   _____ f. Whenever the patient is in cardiac arrest
   _____ g. Whenever the patient complains of nausea and may vomit

4. When a patient is an athlete wearing shoulder pads in conjunction with a helmet, the shoulder pads should be_____
   a. left in place.
   b. pulled off over the patient's head.
   c. cut/untied straps to be removed.
   d. cut off so they aren't removed over the patient's head.

---

#  CASE DISPOSITION

You instruct one OEC Technician to take over manually stabilizing the patient's cervical spine and maintaining the airway with the jaw-thrust maneuver, and you instruct another to place the patient on high-flow oxygen. You palpate the entire body and find no other injuries. You place a C-collar on the patient, and with the assistance of other patrollers carefully log-roll him onto a long spine board. His vital signs remain stable. After securing the patient to the LSB, you load him into a toboggan with his head uphill, and quickly transport him to a nearby landing zone, where his care is transferred to a helicopter's medical crew after giving them a brief but pertinent hand-off report. The patient is then flown to the nearest trauma center.

During your monthly patrol meeting later that week, you learn that the patient had a linear skull fracture with an epidural hematoma and a fractured vertebra at $C_6$. Although the patient's condition is serious, he appears to be making progress and reportedly has a good chance of returning to a normal life. The neurosurgeon was very impressed with the care the patient received in the field and commends you and your team for recognizing the severity of the brain injury, protecting the patient's spine, and getting him to the hospital so quickly.

## OEC SKILL 21-1 | Manual Spine Stabilization

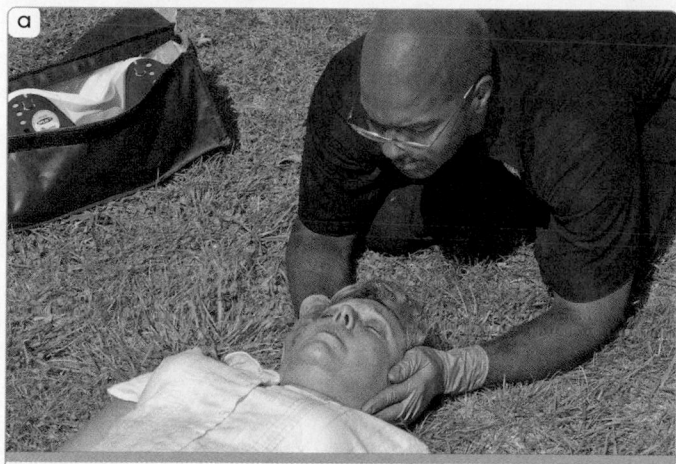

Position your hands on either side of the patient's head by his ears. Position your hands near the patient's ears.

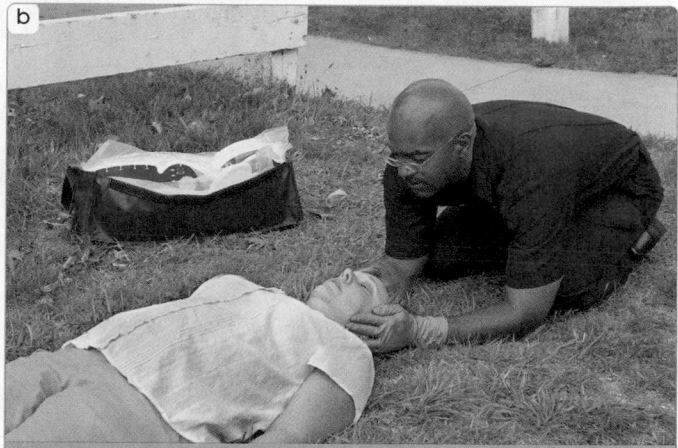

Keep the patient's head in a neutral position, and align the patient's nose and navel.

## OEC SKILL 21-2 | Sizing and Applying a Cervical Collar

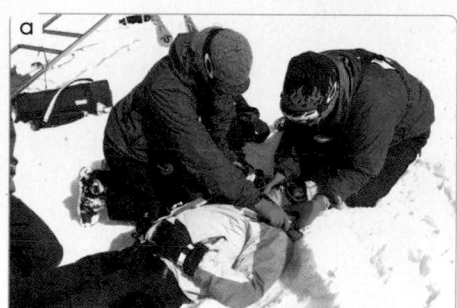

Before applying the collar, open the patient's jacket widely for ease of collar placement.
Copyright Scott Smith

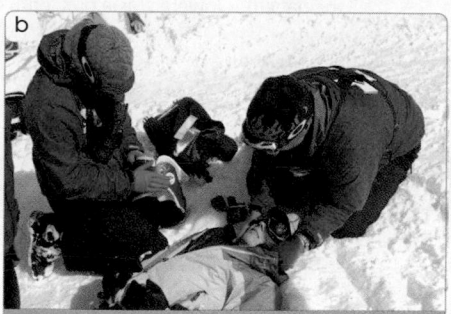

Follow the manufacturer's directions for determining the correct size of the collar.
Copyright Scott Smith

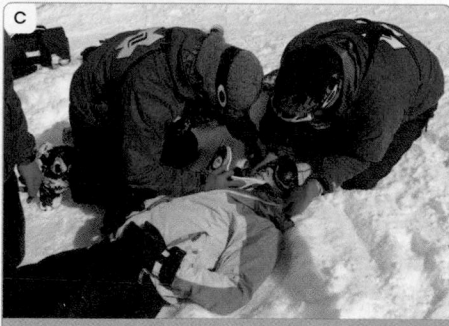

Applying the cervical collar: start by sliding the posterior portion behind the neck, then move the chin portion so that it cups the chin, and finally secure the collar tightly.
Copyright Scott Smith

## OEC SKILL 21-3 | Supine Patient: Log Roll onto a Long Spine Board

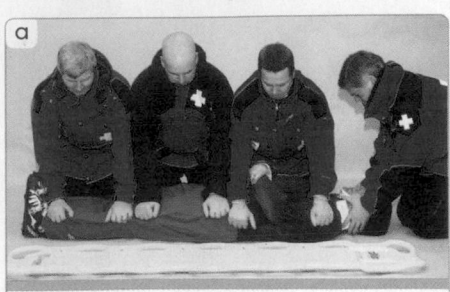

**a**

The rescuer at the patient's head holds the head and calls the commands.
Copyright Mike Halloran

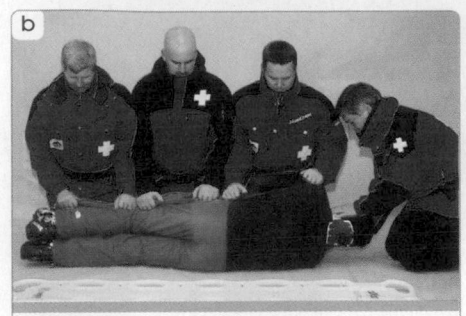

**b**

In unison, the rescuers roll the patient toward themselves.
Copyright Mike Halloran

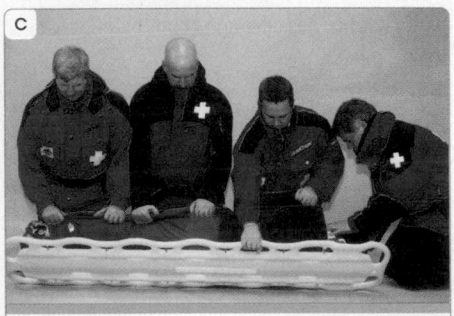

**c**

Rescuer #2 evaluates the patient's back and puts the board in place.
Copyright Mike Halloran

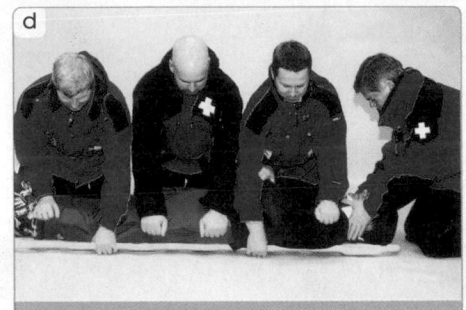

**d**

Rescuer #1 calls out the count of three, and the patient is lowered, as a unit, onto the board.
Copyright Mike Halloran

## OEC SKILL 21-4 | The Axial Drag

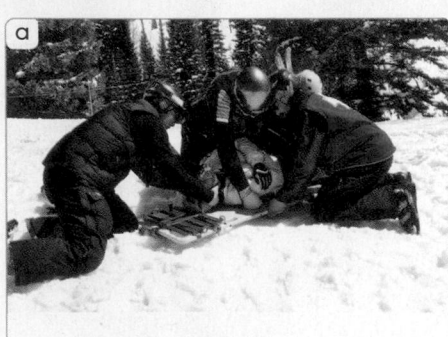

**a**

Using a log roll, roll the patient onto the board.
Copyright NSP

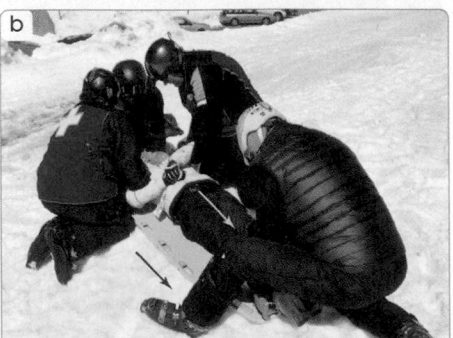

**b**

Reposition the patient on the board by sliding the patient down the board as a unit. Remember: *never push or pull the patient laterally*; always use the slide up or down and over technique.
Copyright NSP

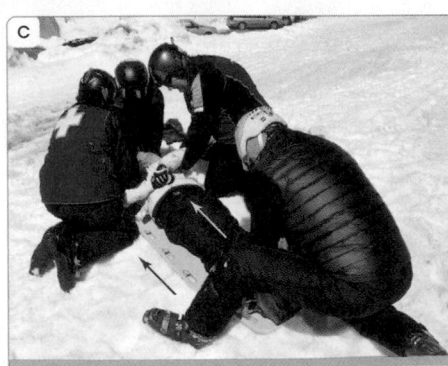

**c**

Slide patient up into position on the board as a unit.
Copyright NSP

## OEC SKILL 21-5 | Securing the Patient onto a Long Spine Board

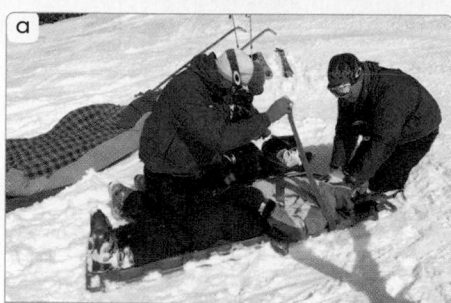

a

This patient's chest and pelvis is being strapped to the board.
Copyright Scott Smith

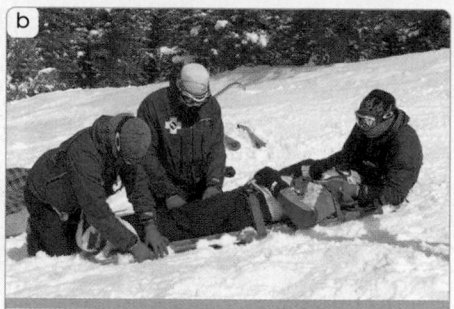

b

Secure the legs and feet.
Copyright Scott Smith

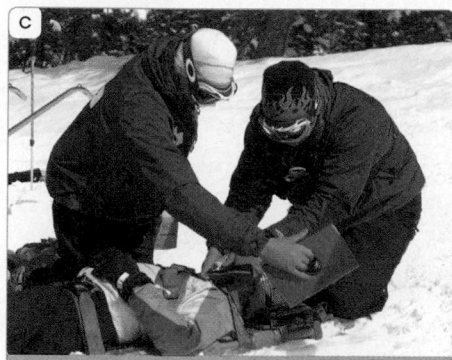

c

Stabilize the head using blocks.
Copyright Scott Smith

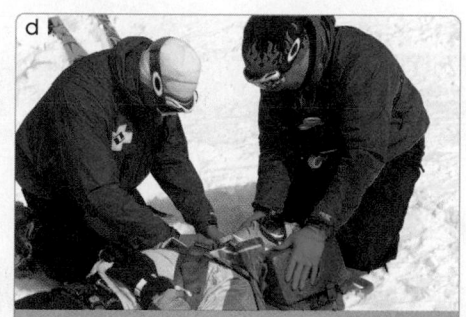

d

Secure the blocks in position.
Copyright Scott Smith

## OEC SKILL 21-6 | Immobilizing a Seated Patient

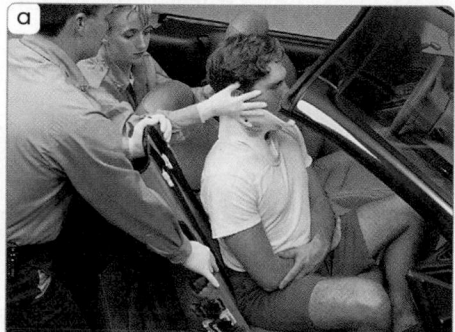

a

Manually stabilize the head and C-spine, apply the cervical collar, and then slip the immobilization device behind the patient.

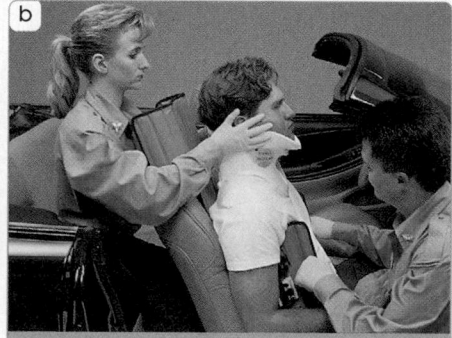

b

Align the immobilization device for proper positioning.

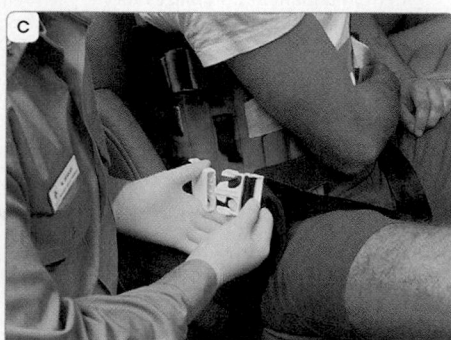

c

Secure the chest and leg straps.

## OEC SKILL 21-6    Immobilizing a Seated Patient *continued*

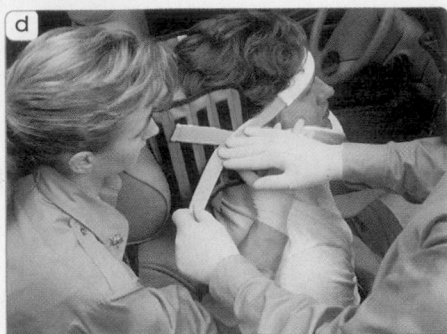

Secure the patient's head with the head straps.

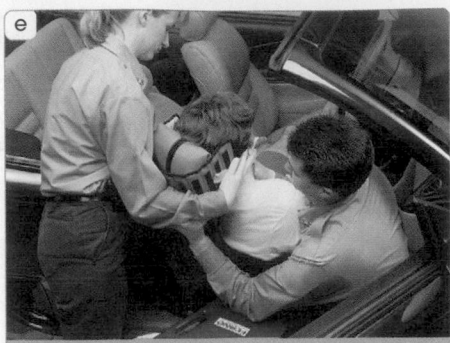

Tie the patient's hands together and pivot the patient onto the long spine board while maintaining in-line stabilization.

## OEC SKILL 21-7    Immobilizing a Standing Patient

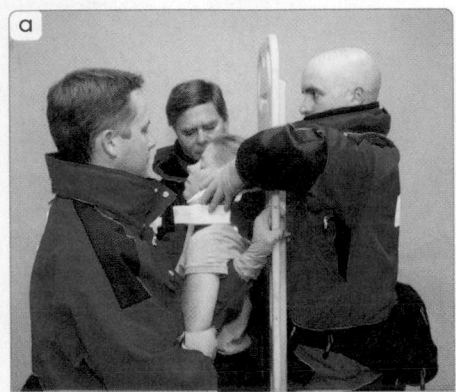

Rescuer #1 stands behind (or beside) the patient and manually stabilizes the patient's head and C-spine.
Copyright Mike Halloran

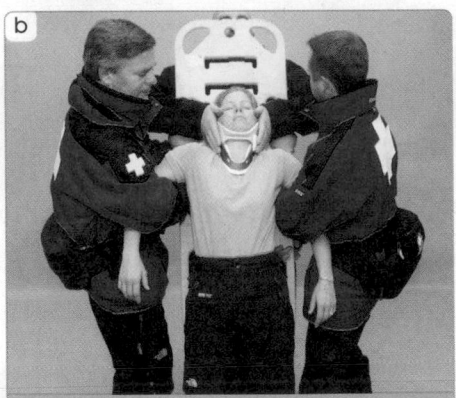

Rescuer #2 checks distal pulse, sensation, and movement in each extremity and then sizes and applies a cervical collar.
Copyright Mike Halloran

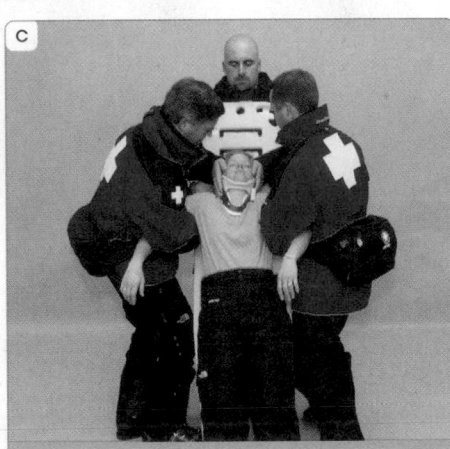

Rescuer #3 prepares and positions the LSB behind the patient.
Copyright Mike Halloran

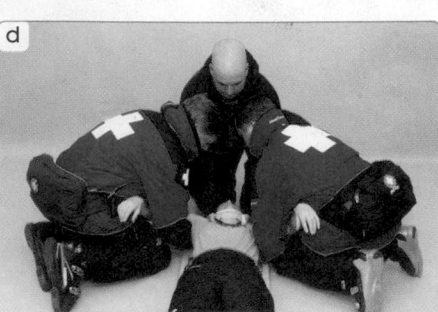

Rescuers #2 and #3 stand next to the patient, one on either side, and lower the patient to the ground. The patient is then secured to the backboard.
Copyright Mike Halloran

## OEC SKILL 21-8 | Removing a Helmet from a Lying Patient

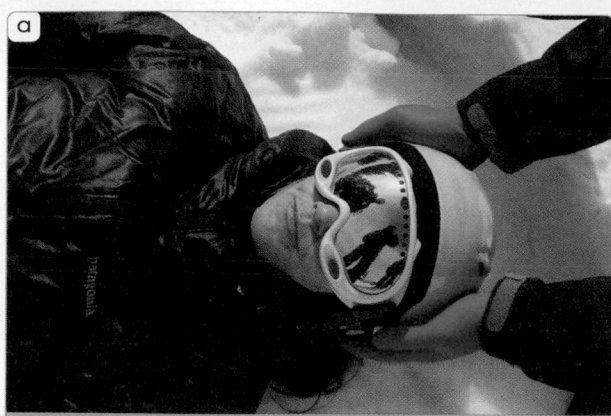

**a**

Align the patient axially and manually stabilize the head and C-spine.
Copyright Scott Smith

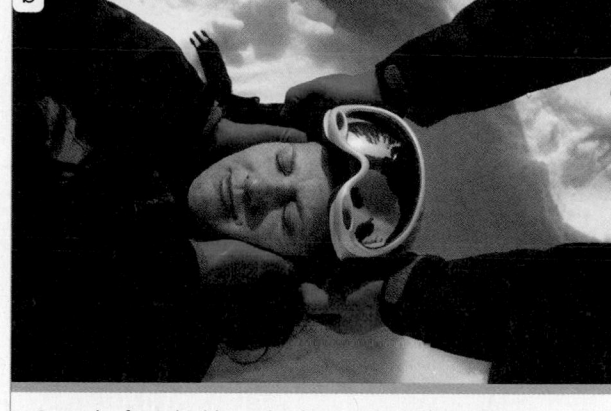

**b**

Open the face shield or take the goggles off the patient's eyes.
Copyright Scott Smith

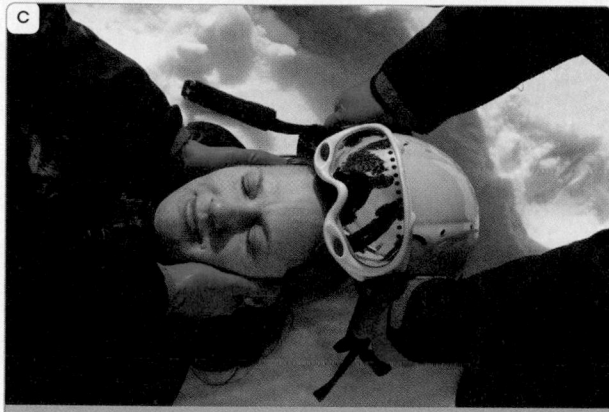

**c**

Stabilize the patient's head as the helmet is removed.
Copyright Scott Smith

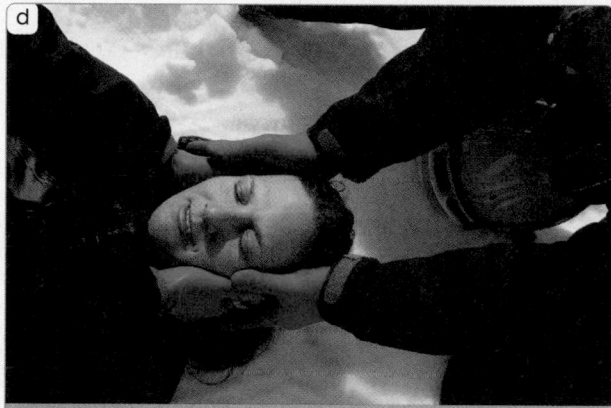

**d**

Continue to stabilize the head until the cervical collar is applied.
Copyright Scott Smith

## Skill Guide

Date:_____

(CPI) = Critical Performance Indicator

Candidate: _____

Start Time: _____

End Time: _____

## Manual Spine Stabilization

**Objective:** To demonstrate the ability to manually stabilize the cervical spine.

| Skill | Max Points | Skill Demo | |
|---|---|---|---|
| Determines scene is safe. | 1 | | (CPI) |
| Introduces self, obtains permission to treat/help. | 1 | | |
| Initiates Standard Precautions. | 1 | | (CPI) |
| Kneels beside or above the patient's heads. | 1 | | |
| Places hands on either side of the patient's head with the palms adjacent to the ears, the fingers supporting the jaw and the back of the head. | 1 | | |
| Gently moves the patient's head so that the eyes are looking forward; the patient's nose and chin are aligned with the sternum. | 1 | | |
| Continues manual stabilization until the patient is secured to a backboard. | 1 | | (CPI) |

Must receive 6 out of 7 points.

Comments: _____

Failure of any of the CPIs is an automatic failure.

Evaluator: _____    NSP ID:_____

PASS    FAIL

## Skill Guide

Date:_____

(CPI) = Critical Performance Indicator

Candidate: _____

Start Time: _____

End Time: _____

## Sizing and Applying a Cervical Collar

**Objective:** To demonstrate ability to properly measure and apply a cervical collar.

| Skill | Max Points | Skill Demo | |
|---|---|---|---|
| Determines scene is safe. | 1 | | (CPI) |
| Introduces self, obtains permission to treat/help. | 1 | | |
| Initiates Standard Precautions. | 1 | | (CPI) |
| Establishes or maintains manual stabilization of head and C-spine. | 1 | | |
| Measures patient for C-collar per manufacturer's recommendations. | 1 | | |
| Opens coat or shirt and removes any bulky clothing around neck/shoulder area. | 1 | | (CPI) |
| Slides posterior neck portion of the collar behind the patient's neck. | 1 | | |
| Swings the chin portion of the C-collar up the patient's chest until it cups the chin. | 1 | | |
| Secures the C-collar using Velcro closures, ensuring a proper fit. | 1 | | (CPI) |

Must receive 7 out of 9 points.

Comments: _____

Failure of any of the CPIs is an automatic failure.

Evaluator: _____   NSP ID:_____

PASS       FAIL

Date: _____

(CPI) = Critical Performance Indicator

Candidate: _____

Start Time: _____

End Time: _____

## Supine Patient: Log Roll onto a Long Spine Board

**Objective:** To demonstrate the ability to log roll a patient onto a backboard.

| Skill | Max Points | Skill Demo | |
|---|:---:|:---:|:---:|
| Determines scene is safe. | 1 | | (CPI) |
| Introduces self, obtains permission to treat/help. | 1 | | |
| Initiates Standard Precautions. | 1 | | (CPI) |
| Rescuer #1 kneels above patient's head and takes/maintains spinal stabilization. | 1 | | (CPI) |
| Rescuers #2, #3, and #4 kneel along one side of the patient. | 1 | | |
| Rescuer #2 assesses CMS, kneels beside the patient's shoulder/upper chest, and grasps the patient's shoulder/hip. | 1 | | (CPI) |
| Rescuer #3 positions backboard beside the patient and kneels at the patient's hips; grasps the patient's hips, overlapping hands with Rescuer #2 and above the knee. | 1 | | |
| Rescuer #4 kneels beside the patient's knee/lower leg; grasps the patient's upper thigh, overlapping with Rescuer #3. | 1 | | |
| Rescuer #1 directs the roll, ensuring that all rescuers are ready to roll the patient toward them as a unit. | 1 | | |
| Rescuer #2 slides backboard into position, tilting the backboard, and then palpates the patient's spine for any injuries. | 1 | | |
| Rescuer #1 directs other rescuers in lowering the patient onto the backboard as a unit. | 1 | | (CPI) |
| Rescuer #2 ensures that the patient is centered on the backboard; if needed, the patient is recentered on the board using axial movements. | 1 | | |
| Secures the patient on the backboard in the usual method. | 1 | | |
| Reassesses CMS. | 1 | | (CPI) |

Must receive 11 out of 14 points.

Comments: _____

Failure of any of the CPIs is an automatic failure.

Evaluator: _____ NSP ID: _____

PASS      FAIL

## Skill Guide

Date:_____

(CPI) = Critical Performance Indicator

Candidate: _____

Start Time: _____

End Time: _____

## Short Board Immobilization

**Objective:** To demonstrate ability to secure a sitting patient to a short board.

| Skill | Max Points | Skill Demo | |
|---|---|---|---|
| Determines scene is safe. | 1 | | (CPI) |
| Introduces self, obtains permission to treat/help. | 1 | | |
| Initiates Standard Precautions. | 1 | | (CPI) |
| Manually stabilizes the head/cervical spine, kneeling next to the patient; establishes in-line stabilization. | 1 | | (CPI) |
| Assesses CMS in each extremity. | 1 | | (CPI) |
| Correctly sizes and applies cervical collar. | 1 | | |
| Places board behind the patient's back, aligning the top of the device with the top of the patient's head. | 1 | | |
| Crosses torso straps over the patient's shoulders and secures to board; pads behind the patient's head, filling voids; secures the patient's head to the board using two cravats (forehead and chin). | 1 | | |
| Moves the patient to a long board by placing the long board next to the patient's buttocks; lifts the patient onto the long board, maintaining C-spine stabilization. | 1 | | (CPI) |
| Lowers the patient into a supine position on the long board, securing the patient and the short board to the long board in the usual fashion. | 1 | | |
| Reassesses CMS in each extremity. | 1 | | (CPI) |

Must receive 9 out of 11 points.

Comments: _____

Failure of any of the CPIs is an automatic failure.

Evaluator: _____ NSP ID:_____

PASS     FAIL

## Skill Guide

Date: _____

(CPI) = Critical Performance Indicator

Candidate: _____

Start Time: _____

End Time: _____

# Removing a Helmet from a Lying Patient

**Objective:** To demonstrate the proper way to remove a helmet.

| Skill | Max Points | Skill Demo | |
|---|---|---|---|
| Determines scene is safe. | 1 | | (CPI) |
| Introduces self, obtains permission to help/treat. | 1 | | |
| Initiates Standard Precautions. | 1 | | (CPI) |
| Stabilizes the cervical region in a neutral, in-line position. (Aligns patient axially.) | 1 | | (CPI) |
| Rescuer #1 manually stabilizes head/C-spine by placing hands on either side of the helmet. | 1 | | |
| Rescuer #2 opens/removes the face shield or goggles. | 1 | | |
| Rescuer #2 removes the chin strap and places one hand at the patient's occiput (base of helmet) and the other at the patient's chin to ensure head/C-spine immobilization. | 1 | | (CPI) |
| Rescuer #1 grasps the helmet straps and pulls apart, spreading the helmet. | 1 | | |
| Rescuer #1 pulls the helmet axially from the patient's head with forward rotation of the helmet. | 1 | | |
| Rescuer #1 continues to gently remove the helmet. | 1 | | |
| Rescuer #2 slides the fingers up to the patient's occiput, ensuring no loss of stabilization. | 1 | | |
| Rescuers exchange immobilization without loss of stabilization. | 1 | | (CPI) |

Must receive 9 out of 12 points.

Comments: _____

Failure of any of the CPIs is an automatic failure.

Evaluator: _____    NSP ID:_____

PASS     FAIL

## Skill Guide

Date:_____

(CPI) = Critical Performance Indicator

Candidate: _____

Start Time: _____

End Time: _____

## Immobilizing a Standing Patient

**Objective:** To demonstrate ability to perform a standing backboard.

| Skill | Max Points | Skill Demo | |
|---|---|---|---|
| Determines scene is safe. | 1 | | (CPI) |
| Introduces self, obtains permission to treat/help. | 1 | | |
| Initiates Standard Precautions. | 1 | | (CPI) |
| Rescuer #1 stands beside or behind the patient; manually stabilizes the patient's head/C-spine. | 1 | | |
| Rescuer #2 checks CMS in each extremity; sizes and correctly applies cervical collar. | 1 | | (CPI) |
| Rescuer #3 prepares and positions backboard behind the patient. | 1 | | |
| Rescuers #2 and #3 stand next to the patient, one on either side; Rescuer #2 stands on the right side of the patient, places one hand on the patient's elbow and the other under the patient's armpit and grasps the backboard slot above the patient's shoulder. Rescuer #3 does the same on the other side of the patient. | 1 | | |
| Moving as a unit and maintaining spinal stabilization, the rescuers lower the patient to the ground. | 1 | | (CPI) |
| If necessary, realigns/recenters the patient on the board using axial movements. | 1 | | |
| Secures the patient to the backboard in the usual manner. | 1 | | |
| Reassesses CMS. | 1 | | (CPI) |

Must receive 9 out of 11 points.

Comments: _____

Failure of any of the CPIs is an automatic failure.

Evaluator: _____  NSP ID:_____

PASS    FAIL

# ⛨ Chapter Review

## Chapter Summary

Traumatic injuries to the head, neck, and back, especially those involving the brain and spinal cord, are potentially life-threatening or life-altering events. The central nervous system, although fairly well protected, is not impervious to injury and can become damaged as a result of various mechanisms of injury. Effective management of patients with neurologic injuries depends on your understanding of the anatomy of the nervous system, performing an accurate assessment, and providing careful support of the integrity of the spine. The ability of OEC Technicians to properly assess and treat these serious head and spine injuries can make the difference between life and death, between short-term recovery and long-term deficit, and between independence and a life of dependence on others.

## Remember...

1. Brain and spinal cord injuries are potentially life altering or life threatening.
2. Spine injury should be assumed in the setting of serious head injury.
3. TBI is the leading cause of traumatic death in patients under age 45.
4. "$C_3$, $C_4$, $C_5$, keep the diaphragm alive."
5. The treatment goals for neurologic injuries are preserving the ABCDs, eliminating spinal movement, and limiting neural ischemia.
6. All patients with a significant MOI or head, neck, and back injuries should be immobilized on an LSB and given supplemental oxygen.

## Chapter Questions

### Multiple Choice

Choose the correct answer.

1. What should you assume about a climber who has fallen and suffered a fractured scapula?_____
   a. He probably has a spinal injury.
   b. He probably has a skull fracture.
   c. He will most likely develop a subdural hematoma.
   d. An OEC Technician should never make any assumptions about a patient.

2. When you palpate the spine of a patient who has been thrown from a horse and landed on her head, you discover a gross deformity of $C_4$ and $C_5$. What additional concern should you immediately have? _____
   a. that the patient may vomit
   b. that the patient may immediately go into neurogenic shock
   c. that the patient may no longer be able to breathe spontaneously
   d. that the patient may develop an epidural hematoma

3. After an initial assessment, you continue to monitor the patient's condition by checking the _____
   a. ABCDs, LOR, distal CMS, and vital signs.
   b. ABCDs, SAMPLE history, and DCAP-BTLS.
   c. vital signs every 15 minutes.
   d. vital signs and pulse oximetry readings.

**4.** What type of assumption should you *first* make about a patient who approaches you and tells you that he does not know where he is and cannot remember what happened to him?_____
- **a.** He is possibly under the influence of alcohol or another substance.
- **b.** He is possibly suffering from a metabolic problem such as low blood sugar.
- **c.** He is possibly suffering a stroke.
- **d.** He has possibly suffered a traumatic brain injury and requires spinal immobilization.

**5.** The best way to treat a head-injury patient who has clear fluid leaking from his ears is to_____
- **a.** place the patient in the recovery position.
- **b.** bandage the patient's head, including the ears, with a roller gauze.
- **c.** not bandage the ears and allow the fluid to flow out.
- **d.** gently insert cotton or a rolled sterile $2 \times 2$ into the outer ear canal.

**6.** Which of the following mechanisms of injury have significant potential for neurologic injury? (check all that apply)
- **a.** _____ choking on a piece of steak
- **b.** _____ a fall greater than a patient's height
- **c.** _____ a pedestrian stuck by a vehicle traveling 5 mph or faster
- **d.** _____ a collision between a snowboarder and a tree
- **e.** _____ a kayaker who is wearing a helmet and takes a swim through a rapid
- **f.** _____ a gunshot wound to the abdomen
- **g.** _____ a gunshot wound to the pelvis or chest
- **h.** _____ a burial in an avalanche or snow cave
- **i.** _____ a golfer struck by lightning
- **j.** _____ a climber who is wearing a helmet and is struck by a falling rock

## Matching

Match each of the following CNS-related terms to its description.

_____ **1.** arachnoid mater
_____ **2.** spinal cord
_____ **3.** cerebellum
_____ **4.** cerebrospinal fluid (CSF)
_____ **5.** cerebrum
_____ **6.** brain stem
_____ **7.** diffuse axonal injury (DAI)
_____ **8.** dura mater
_____ **9.** epidural hematoma
_____ **10.** meninges
_____ **11.** neural ischemia
_____ **12.** neuron
_____ **13.** peripheral nervous system (PNS)
_____ **14.** pia mater

**a.** a condition in which part of the brain or spinal cord is without oxygen from the blood; damage to these parts results after only a few minutes of anoxia

**b.** a tubular bundle of nervous tissue that connects to the brain

**c.** the middle layer of the three meninges, the membranes that cover the brain and spinal cord

**d.** the part of the brain, lying posterior to the pons and medulla oblongata and inferior to the occipital lobes of the cerebral hemispheres, that is responsible for the regulation and coordination of complex voluntary muscular movement as well as the maintenance of posture and balance

**e.** lower part of the brain continuous with the spinal cord

**f.** any of the impulse-conducting cells that constitute the brain, spinal column, and nerves, consisting of a nucleated cell body with one or more dendrites and a single axon; also called a nerve cell

**g.** the large rounded part of the brain occupying most of the cranial cavity, divided into two cerebral hemispheres that sits on top of the rest of the brain; controls and integrates motor, sensory, and higher mental functions, such as thought, reason, emotion, and memory

**h.** an accumulation of blood between the skull and the dura mater, usually caused by trauma or rupture of an artery

**i.** the part of the nervous system constituting the nerves outside the central nervous system, including the cranial nerves, spinal nerves, and sympathetic and parasympathetic nervous systems

**j.** an insult to the spinal cord resulting in a change, either temporary or permanent, in its normal motor, sensory, or autonomic function

_____ **15.** spinal cord injury (SCI)

_____ **16.** subdural hematoma

**k.** the tough fibrous membrane covering the brain and the spinal cord and lining the inner surface of the skull

**l.** an accumulation of blood between the outer covering of the brain and the surface of the brain

**m.** one of the more common and devastating types of traumatic brain injury in which damage occurs over a more widespread area than occurs in focal brain injury

**n.** the membranes that cover the brain and spinal cord, specifically the arachnoid mater, pia mater, and dura mater

**o.** a watery fluid that flows around the surface coverings of the brain and spinal cord

**p.** the fine vascular membrane that closely envelops the brain and spinal cord under the arachnoid mater and the dura mater

# Scenario

_You have day duty in July at your resort and receive a call reporting that a small child is unresponsive under the jungle-gym at the playground. You respond with another OEC Technician, a backboard, $O_2$, and a trauma bag. The child, who is about 5 years old, is lying prone, has a patent airway, is breathing, and has a radial pulse of 120._

_A bystander tells you that he called 9-1-1 and that an ambulance is coming._

**1.** After checking the ABCDs, the next step would be to_____

   **a.** apply a cervical collar and roll the patient on his back.

   **b.** start a secondary assessment.

   **c.** apply a cervical collar and log roll the patient onto the backboard.

   **d.** measure and insert an OPA if the patient has no gag reflex and apply $O_2$ with a nonrebreather mask at 12 LPM.

_The bystander tells you that he did not see what happened, and there are no other witnesses. A check of the patient's pupils finds the right pupil at 2 mm and the left pupil at 6 mm._

**2.** The difference in pupil size is caused by _____

   **a.** one eye receiving more sunlight than the other.

   **b.** nothing unusual; differences in pupil size can be normal.

   **c.** an abnormal intracranial pressure.

   **d.** all of the above.

**3.** The best practice for placing a child on an adult-sized backboard is to_____

   **a.** use the basic setup and place a blanket roll on either side of the patient to fill the void.

   **b.** remove the head block base, use a blanket roll around the patient's head, place a small pad under the patient's shoulders, and place a blanket roll on either side of the patient.

   **c.** use a head block base, place a blanket roll around the patient's head, and fill the voids on the sides with blanket rolls.

   **d.** use a head block base and place a small pad under the patient's head and neck.

_Falls that result in landing head first, such as diving accidents, can lead to fractures to the cervical vertebrae._

**4.** This type of fracture usually _____

   **a.** occurs to $C_2$ and is called a Washington fracture.

   **b.** occurs to $C_3$ and is called a Kennedy fracture.

   **c.** occurs to $C_1$ and is called a Jefferson fracture.

   **d.** occurs to $C_5$ and is called an Adams fracture.

_Based on the patient's unresponsive status, unknown down time, the height of the fall, and the vital signs, you recognize that this is a load and go situation. A head and cervical injury is suspected. While waiting for the ALS crew to arrive, you monitor the patient's vitals and breathing and remain prepared for vomiting should responsiveness return. The pulse remains at 120 and the respiratory rate is 28 and nonlabored._

# Suggested Reading

*Advanced Trauma Life Support for Doctors,* Eighth Edition, 2008. Chicago: American College of Surgeons.

Greenberg, M. S. 2006. *Handbook of Neurosurgery,* Sixth Edition. New York: Thieme.

Harken, A. H., and E. E. Moore. 1996. *Abernathy's Surgical Secrets,* Third Edition. St. Louis, MO: Elsevier.

*Management and Prognosis of Severe Traumatic Brain Injury.* 2000. Brain Trauma Foundation and the American Association of Neurological Surgeons. Rolling Meadows, IL: The American Association of Neurological Surgeons.

Rengachary, S. S., and Ellenbogen, R. G. 2005. *Principles of Neurosurgery,* Second Edition. St. Louis, MO: Elsevier Mosby.

"Traumatic Brain Injury in the United States: A Report to Congress," Atlanta: Centers for Disease Control and Prevention.

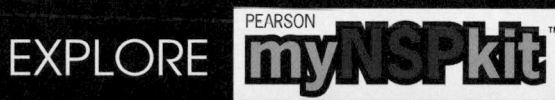

EXPLORE

PEARSON **myNSPkit**™

Please go to www.myNSPkit.com. Under Student Resources, you will find animations, videos, web links, and games related to this chapter—and much more. Look for information on helmet removal, c-spine stabilization, and other topics.

Register your access code from the front of your book by going to www.myNSPkit.com and selecting the appropriate links. If the in-cover access code has been redeemed, go to www.myNSPkit.com and follow links to **Buy Access.**

# Face, Eye, and Neck Injuries

Bruce Evans, MD

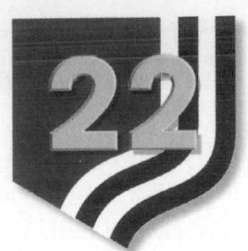

22

## ⊕ OBJECTIVES

**Upon completion of this chapter, the OEC Technician will be able to:**

**22-1** Describe the function of the iris.

**22-2** List possible causes of eye injuries.

**22-3** Describe and demonstrate how to assess eye injuries.

**22-4** Describe and demonstrate the management of a patient with a penetrating injury to the eyeball.

**22-5** Identify the important structures of the anterior and posterior neck.

**22-6** List the signs and symptoms of emergencies of the neck and upper airway.

**22-7** List the functions of the following:
- facial bones
- lacrimal glands
- neck muscles

**22-8** List the signs and symptoms of emergent injuries to the face, eyes, and neck.

**22-9** Describe and demonstrate how to assess face, eye, and neck injuries.

**22-10** Describe and demonstrate the proper care of a face, eye, or neck injury.

## ⊕ KEY TERMS

**anisocoria,** *p. 745*
**blowout fracture,** *p. 749*

**cornea,** *p. 745*
**epistaxis,** *p. 749*

**external auditory canal,** *p. 749*
**hyphema,** *p. 751*

*continued*

## Chapter Overview

Face and neck injuries are common in outdoor environments. When they are severe, these injuries can be life threatening and demand all the skills of OEC Technicians. Such injuries may be the result of blunt or penetrating trauma. They also can result from environmental exposure, as seen with chemical burns or cold weather injuries. Traumatic injuries involving the face or neck may bleed profusely due to the generous

*continued*

## HISTORICAL TIMELINE

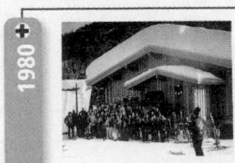

**1980** Oldest active ski patroller, Henry Collins (age 84), retires.

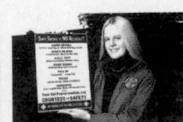

**1985** Ad hoc committee drafts the curriculum for a patrol-oriented medical course to be called Winter Emergency Care.

lacrimal gland, *p. 746*
mandible, *p. 743*
maxilla, *p. 743*

orbit, *p. 744*
retinal detachment, *p. 760*

sternocleidomastoid muscle, *p. 747*
subcutaneous emphysema, *p. 756*

blood supply in these areas of the body. Pain can be severe due to the abundance of nerves and the relative sensitivity to injury, especially injuries involving the eyes.

A patient's fear of vision loss requires a high degree of professional composure from rescuers. Even minor facial and neck injuries may cause patients to become anxious because of associated bleeding, pain, or fear of permanent disability.

Facial and neck emergencies often result from mechanisms of injury that should alert OEC Technicians to the possibility of coexisting injuries. An examination of patients for closed head and cervical-spine injuries should be included in the assessment of these patients. Successful management of these injuries depends on the rescuer's solid understanding of the injuries and a strict adherence to the priorities in assessment: airway, breathing, circulation, and disability.

# Anatomy and Physiology

The anatomical structures of the face and neck are confined to a relatively small area. Because of their close proximity, trauma to one sensory or vascular structure may be accompanied by injury to other structures. Understanding these anatomical relationships helps OEC Technicians better evaluate the extent of injuries when caring for patients.

## Facial Structures

The face constitutes the anterior portion of the head. It contains numerous structures essential not only for sensing the environment, but also for survival. The sensations of sight, sound, smell, and taste all originate within the sensory systems of the face. The nose, mouth, and pharynx are parts of the upper airway. Sensory systems in the face are partially protected by the facial bones, whereas vital structures in the neck are relatively vulnerable. The trachea and great vessels of the neck are protected only by the relatively thin layers of skin and muscle.

The face consists of 14 bones. The forehead, the most superior aspect of the face, is supported by the frontal bone, which protects the front of the brain. The zygomatic bones connect to the frontal bone to form the cheeks and the inferior rims of both eye sockets. These bones, along with the nasal bones and the maxillae (singular: **maxilla**) combine at the middle of the face to support the cartilage and soft tissues of the nose.

The maxillae, which are the largest bones of the face, form the upper jaw, the hard palate of the mouth, the floor of the nose, and the lower portion of each eye socket. The U-shaped **mandible**, or lower jaw bone, hinges on both sides with the temporal bones at the temporomandibular joints (TMJ), making the lower jaw the only movable bone of the face. The teeth are anchored in either the maxillae or the mandible. When brought together, the alignment of the teeth form the bite or occlusion. The tongue, lips, gums, and palate constitute the rest of the oral structures (Figure 22-1■).

The face and mouth are highly vascular, which explains why injuries to this region of the body typically involve significant external bleeding, and entail the risk of internal bleeding that forms a hematoma.

**maxilla** the bone of the mid-face; the cheek bone.

**mandible** the jaw bone.

**Figure 22-1** The cranium and facial bones.

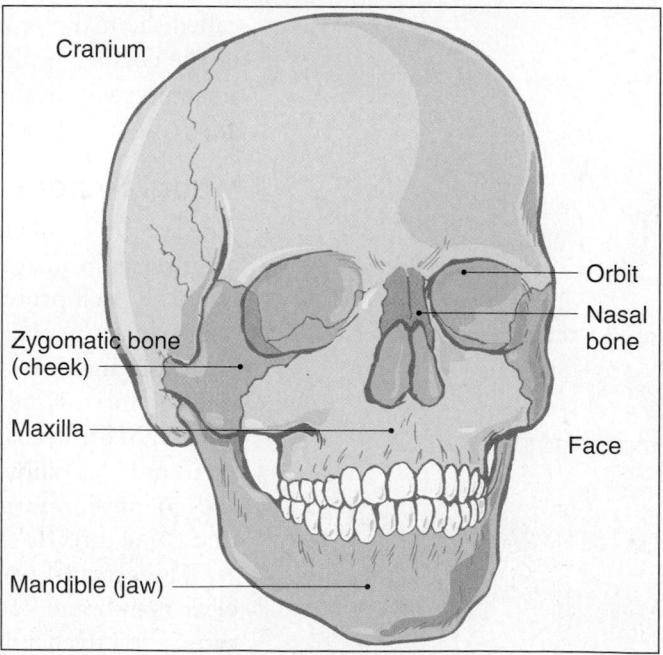

## CASE PRESENTATION

You are checking boundary and trail closures when you see a snowboarder lying in the snow several feet beyond a yellow closure rope. As you approach, you notice that the rider's track goes underneath the closure rope. The rider is lying on his back, holding his neck with both hands. He appears to be in considerable distress.

*What should you do?*

The face contains cartilage that combines with the facial bones to provide overall structure to the face. The nasal septum is made of cartilage, as is the pinna, the underlying structure of the external ear.

The face is interlaced with 43 muscles that control voluntary movement of the eyes and mouth and are responsible for facial expressions such as smiling and frowning. The facial muscles also are responsible for nasal flaring, which helps to bring more oxygen-containing air into the body in times of severe respiratory distress. The mastoid muscles connect to the mandible and facilitate the opening and closing of the mouth and chewing. The skull and facial bones have small openings, known as foramina, through which nerves and blood vessels pass to more superficial soft-tissue structures. Control of both the facial muscles and the sensory organs is provided by a vast network of nerves. One of the largest nerves, the facial nerve, traverses the zygomatic bones and controls the muscles of facial expression.

### Auditory and Balance System

The external parts of the ear known as the pinna, tragus, lobules (lobes), and helix are positioned over the temporal bone on each side of the skull. Each temporal bone is penetrated by a large foramen through which sound waves for hearing pass. Sound waves entering the auditory canal cause the thin tympanic membrane that covers the opening to the auditory foramen to vibrate, transmitting sound signals to the ear's inner structures. Within this specialized system are three tiny auditory ossicles—bones called the malleus, incus, and stapes—that convert sound waves into signals that go to the cochlea or organ of hearing, then on to the brain via auditory nerves. Other structures within the inner ear, collectively called the vestibular system, control balance (Figure 22-2■).

### Visual System

The sense we call vision begins when light enters the globe-shaped eyeball. The eye captures light images that are then sent to the brain via the optic nerve. The eye is relatively well protected within a bony socket formed by the skull and facial bones. This socket, known as the **orbit**, protects much of the fluid-filled eyeball while simultaneously anchoring the muscles that control voluntary eye movement. Although significant force is needed to injure the bones that make up the orbit, the anterior portion of the eyeball is relatively unprotected and therefore susceptible to injury. Six small muscles, known as extraocular muscles, attach to each eye and enable the two eyes to move in various directions in unison. These muscles are controlled by nerves that come directly from the brain.

The external part of the eye and the inner lining of the eyelids consist of a thin clear membrane known as the conjunctiva, which contains small blood vessels. Located directly behind the conjunctiva in the anterior portion of the globe is the

**orbit**   the bony socket of the eyeball.

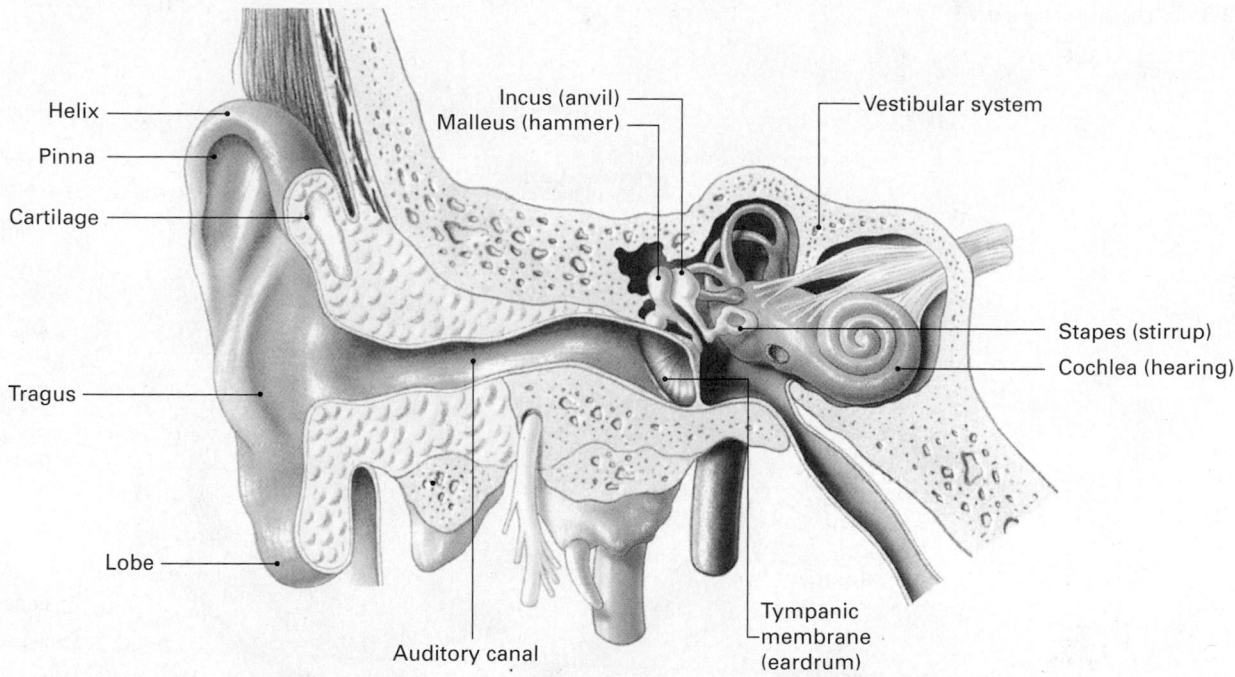

**Figure 22-2** The anatomy of the ear.

**cornea**, which is surrounded by the sclera. The round, transparent cornea bends or refracts light as it enters the eye. The white portion of the eye, called the sclera, is composed of a thick, fibrous material that gives the eye its characteristic globe shape (Figure 22-3■).

The eye has two fluid-filled chambers: an anterior chamber and a posterior chamber. The anterior chamber is filled with a thin watery substance known as aqueous humor. This clear fluid can leak out of the eye in the event of a penetrating injury, but it is regenerated over time following repair of the eye. The anterior chamber begins deep to the cornea and ends at the circular iris.

The iris works like a camera shutter to adjust the amount of light entering the eye. Pigment in the iris accounts for the color of the eye. In the center of the iris is the pupil, visible as a black circle. Constriction of the iris narrows the pupil and allows less light to pass through the lens of the eye, whereas dilation of the iris widens the pupil and allows more light to enter the eye.

Under normal conditions, the pupil very quickly becomes smaller in response to bright light. This is called the direct response. If you shine a light into only one eye, the other eye's iris will also constrict if the visual system is functioning properly (indirect response). Unequal pupil size, a condition known as **anisocoria**, may be caused directly due to an insult to the eye, or indirectly due to a problem in the brain. In a small percentage of the population, the pupils are normally unequal in size.

Between the iris and the lens is the posterior chamber. The lens of the eyeball is used to fine-tune the focusing of light at the back of the eye. Depending on the distance an object is from the eye, certain small muscles within the eye change the shape of the lens so that light is focused on the retina, which is analogous to the film in a camera. When the muscles contract, the lens becomes flatter; when they relax, the lens becomes rounder. Light then passes into the vitreous humor, a jelly-like fluid. Unlike aqueous humor, vitreous humor cannot be regenerated by the body if it is lost due to injury. It is the volume of these two fluids that fills the eyeball with enough pressure to maintain its globe-like shape.

**cornea** the clear but highly sensitive surface of the eye that refracts light entering into the visual system.

⊕ **22-1** Describe the function of the iris.

**anisocoria** unequal size of the pupils.

**Figure 22-3** The anatomy of the eye.

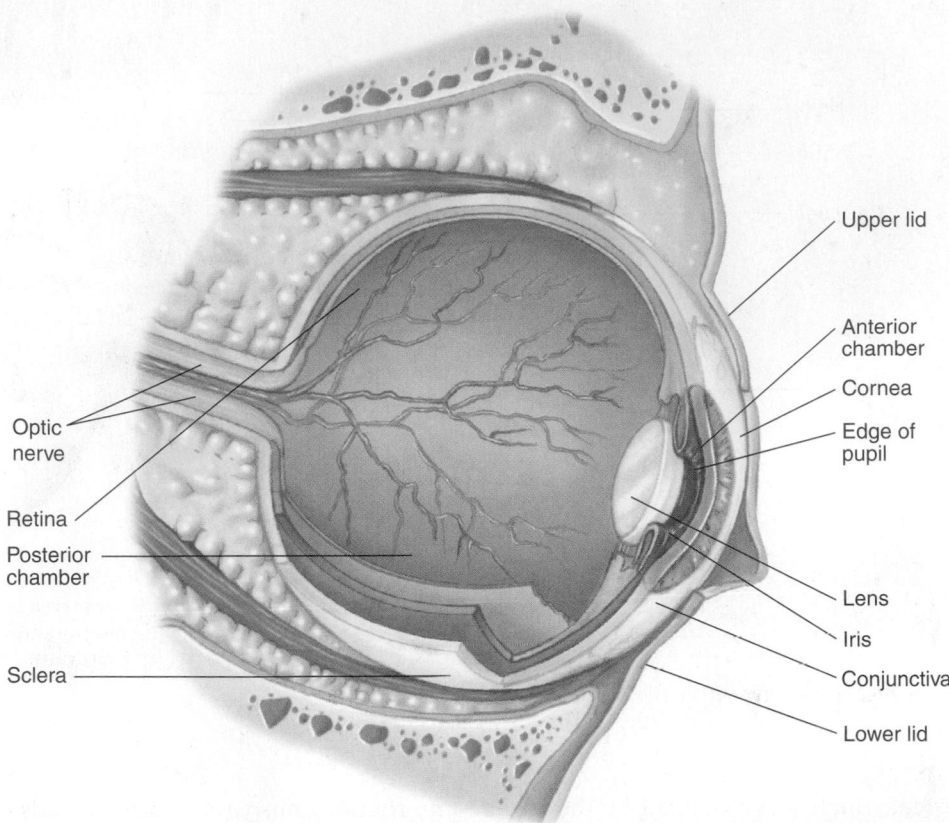

Upper lid

Anterior chamber

Cornea

Edge of pupil

Optic nerve

Retina

Posterior chamber

Lens

Iris

Conjunctiva

Sclera

Lower lid

---

🟦 **22-7** List the functions of the following:

- facial bones
- lacrimal glands
- neck muscles

**lacrimal glands** glands that produce tears, which irrigate the surface of the eye.

Light entering the eye then strikes the retina, a sheet of light-sensitive nerve endings located on the inside curve at the back of the globe. These nerve endings transmit signals stimulated by light through the optic nerve to the brain, which then formats the information as a visual image. The sensation of depth perception is created because the brain receives slightly different signals from each eye when looking at a given object, especially objects in our near field of vision.

**Lacrimal glands,** also called tear glands, are positioned above each eye and provide constant irrigation in the form of tears (Figure 22-4■). Tears and blinking flush away

**Figure 22-4** The anatomy of the lacrimal apparatus.

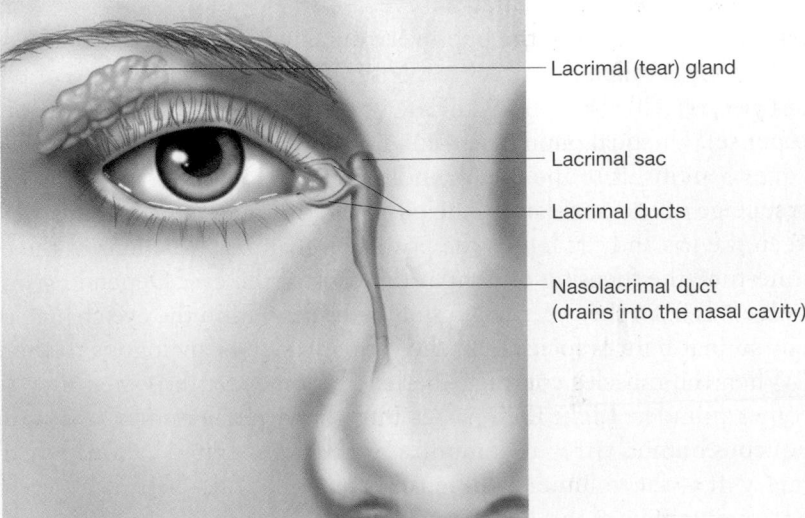

Lacrimal (tear) gland

Lacrimal sac

Lacrimal ducts

Nasolacrimal duct (drains into the nasal cavity)

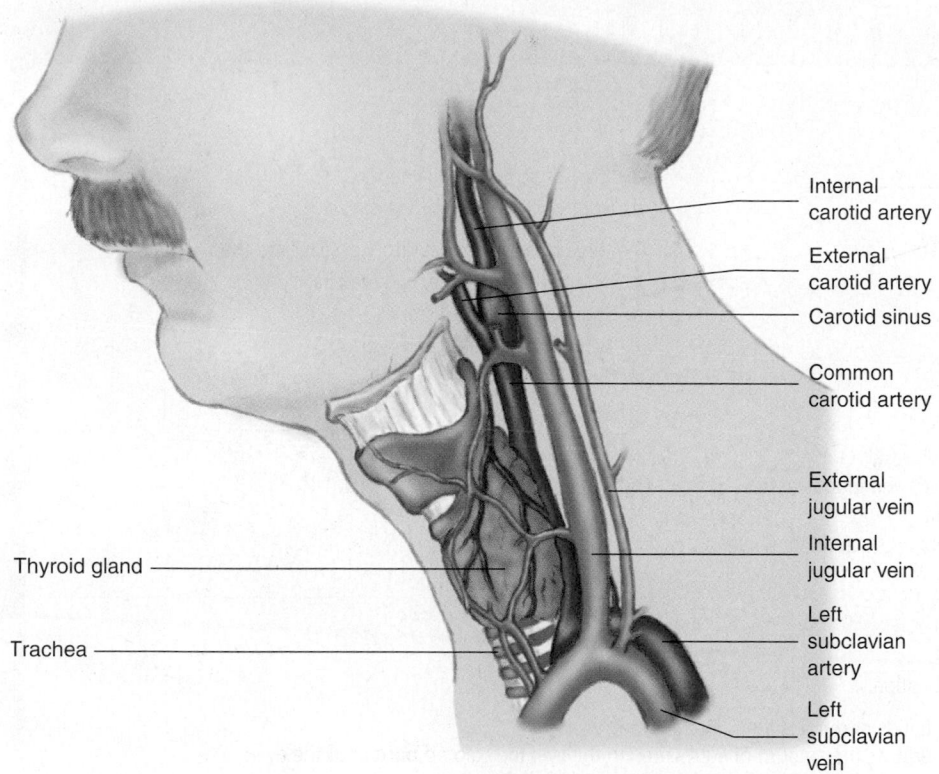

**Figure 22-5** The anatomy of the neck.

- Internal carotid artery
- External carotid artery
- Carotid sinus
- Common carotid artery
- External jugular vein
- Internal jugular vein
- Left subclavian artery
- Left subclavian vein
- Thyroid gland
- Trachea

surface debris and clean the exposed surface of the eye. Tears drain toward the inner side of each eye and into the lacrimal (tear) ducts.

## Neck Anatomy

The anterior part of the neck contains a number of relatively unprotected vital structures: the carotid arteries, jugular veins, esophagus, trachea, and thyroid gland (Figure 22-5■). Trauma to these structures can result in significant bleeding, swelling, and loss of support to the airway.

In the midline of the anterior neck, palpable just beneath the skin, is the thyroid cartilage of the larynx (Figure 22-6■). This cartilage is more prominent in men than it is in women or children. Inferior to the larynx is the trachea; the esophagus is situated directly posterior to the trachea. Approximately 1–2 cm on either side of the larynx are the carotid arteries, which supply blood to the neck and head. The large jugular veins, which drain blood from the head, lie just beneath the skin in the anterior neck.

In the posterior neck are the cervical vertebrae and several muscles. The **sternocleidomastoid muscles** are on the sides of the neck. Within the vertebrae is the spinal cord. The cervical spine and spinal cord are discussed in Chapter 21, Head and Spine Injuries.

⊕ **22-5** Identify the important structures of the anterior and posterior neck.

**sternocleidomastoid muscle** the powerful muscle at the sides of the neck that facilitate turning of the head.

**Figure 22-6** The structure of the larynx.

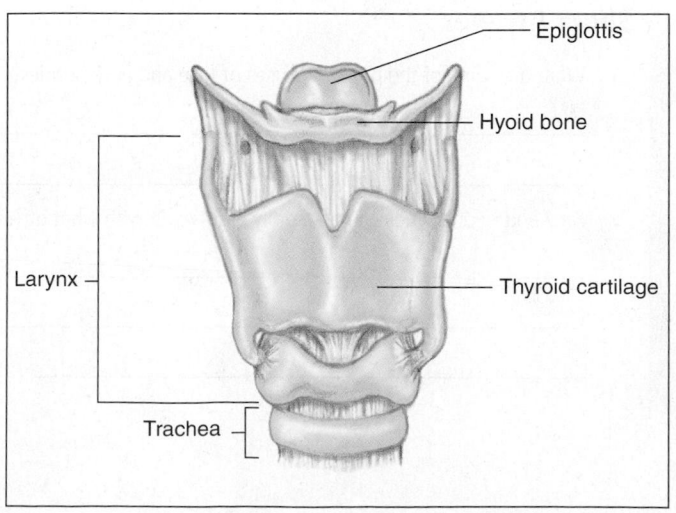

- Epiglottis
- Hyoid bone
- Thyroid cartilage
- Larynx
- Trachea

# STOP, THINK, UNDERSTAND

## Multiple Choice

Choose the correct answer.

1. The main blood vessels of the neck are the_____
   a. carotid arteries and the jugular veins.
   b. sternocleidoid vein and the carotid artery.
   c. subclavian and carotid arteries.
   d. occular and auditory arteries and veins.

2. The face consists of how many bones?_____
   a. 4          c. 14
   b. 8          d. 24

3. The function of the auditory ossicles is to_____
   a. serve as an opening through which nerves and blood vessels pass.
   b. convert sound waves into signals carried by the auditory nerve to the brain.
   c. provide structure for the face.
   d. control movement of the eyes.

4. The three bones of the auditory ossicles are the_____
   a. foramena, mandible, and maxilla.
   b. malleus, incus, and stapes.
   c. frontal, zygomatic, and orbit.
   d. temporomandibular, occlusion, and palate.

5. The face has how many muscles?_____
   a. 12         c. 33
   b. 23         d. 43

## Matching

Match each of the following structures to its description.

_____ 1. optic nerve

_____ 2. extraocular muscles

_____ 3. conjunctiva

_____ 4. cornea

_____ 5. sclera

_____ 6. iris

_____ 7. pupil

_____ 8. lens

_____ 9. lacrimal gland

_____ 10. vitreous humor

_____ 11. retina

_____ 12. sternocleidomastoid muscle

a. bends or refracts light entering the eye
b. adjusts the amount of light entering the eye; the colored portion of the eye
c. the small opening of the eye through which light enters
d. a thin membrane covering the external surface of the eye and lining the inside of the eyelid
e. the white of the eye
f. produces tears
g. collects light and transmits images
h. a jelly-like substance that helps give the eyeball its shape
i. fine-tunes the focusing of light onto the back of the eye
j. transmits light signals to the brain
k. enable eye movement
l. enables neck movement

## Short Answer

1. What are some of the primary causes of face and neck injuries?

_____

_____

2. Face and neck injuries can be readily associated with what other types of injury?

_____

_____

_____

*continued*

3. Name the four senses that originate within the structures of the face.

_____

_____

_____

4. Why do facial lacerations tend to bleed profusely?

_____

_____

_____

5. Why are the trachea and great vessels of the neck vulnerable to injury?

_____

_____

_____

# Common Face, Eye, and Neck Injuries

In individuals participating in outdoor recreational activities, the face and neck are typically exposed and thus are especially susceptible to direct trauma and environmental injuries such as frostbite or sunburn (Figure 22-7■). The most important structures of the face and neck are those that are part of the airway. Thus an OEC Technician's knowledge of specific injuries to this region is crucial in ensuring that a patient's airway remains open.

## Face Injuries

The face is vulnerable to a variety of soft-tissue injuries, most of which affect the lips, mouth, and tongue. Due to the vascular nature of the face and the proximity of major nerves to the surface of the skin, bleeding can be severe and may on occasion be accompanied by nerve damage (Figure 22-8a■).

Other facial injuries seen by OEC Technicians include lacerations from sharp objects or fractures from blunt or penetrating trauma. Blunt trauma with significant force to the front of the face can lead to multiple fractures involving the maxilla and other bones in the face. These fractures often result in airway obstruction due to significant bleeding and swelling of nasal and oral structures (Figure 22-8b■). When fractured, the mandible may break in multiple locations, which can result in significant bleeding inside the mouth.

Fractures that involve the bony socket of the eye, or **blowout fractures**, may either injure the eye or cause the muscles that attach to the eye to become trapped within the fracture, thereby affecting the eye's ability to move (Figure 22-8c■). This type of injury can result in double vision.

Direct trauma to the nose may result in a fracture of the nasal bone (Figure 22-9■). While nasal bone fractures do not typically require emergent treatment, they may be associated with airway compromise and/or bleeding from the nose, a condition known as **epistaxis**. Additionally, epistaxis can result from drying of the mucous membranes due to cold air or a patient picking the nose.

The exposed location of the external ear makes it susceptible to lacerations and contusions (Figure 22-10■). Additionally, a foreign body lodged in the **external auditory**

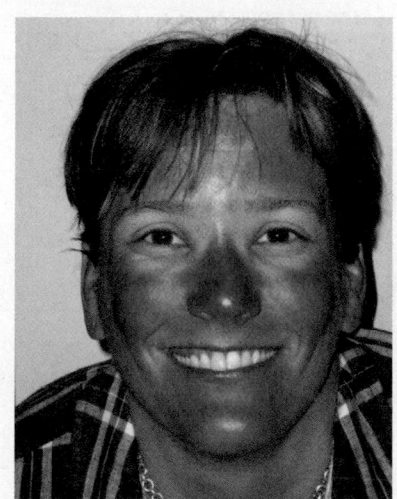

**Figure 22-7** Because they are exposed, the face and neck are especially vulnerable to direct trauma and environmental injuries such as this sunburn.
Copyright David Johe, MD

---

⊕ **22-6** List the signs and symptoms of emergencies of the neck and upper airway.

**blowout fracture** an injury caused by direct trauma to the eye or face that fractures the bony eye socket; can entrap the muscles that enable normal eye movement.

**epistaxis** nosebleed.

**external auditory canal** the passageway through the outer ear that ends at the tympanic membrane.

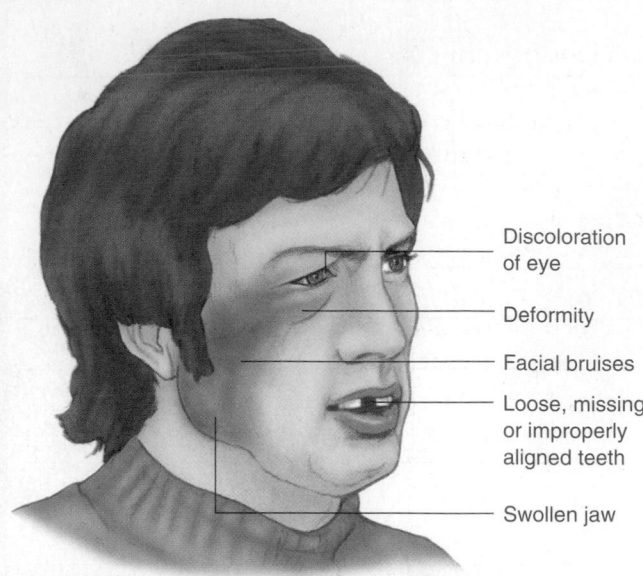

Discoloration of eye

Deformity

Facial bruises

Loose, missing or improperly aligned teeth

Swollen jaw

**Figure 22-8a** Signs of a facial fracture.

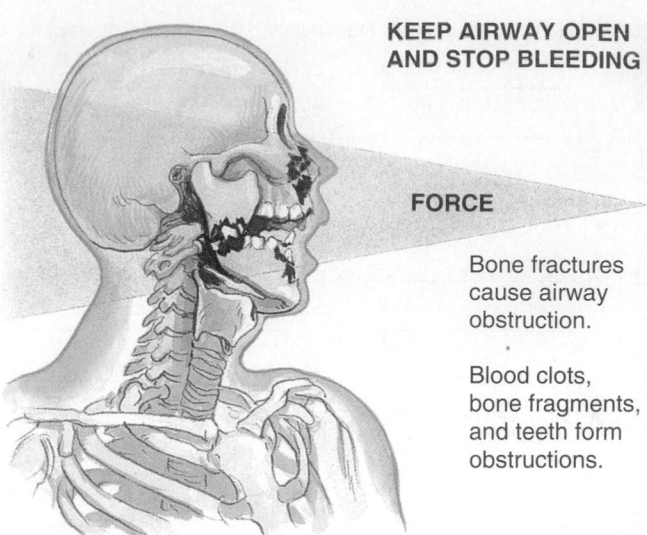

KEEP AIRWAY OPEN AND STOP BLEEDING

FORCE

Bone fractures cause airway obstruction.

Blood clots, bone fragments, and teeth form obstructions.

**Figure 22-8b** Monitor the airway when treating facial fractures.

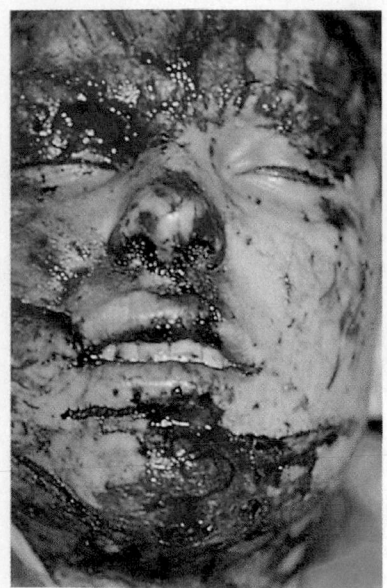

**Figure 22-8c** Injuries to the face. In this case the right cheek has a depressed fracture.

**canal** can be extremely painful and anxiety provoking. The tympanic membrane may be injured or may rupture from loud noises, such as those associated with an explosion, or can rupture from pressure buildup within the ear, as seen in inner-ear infections. The buildup of fluid within the ear is painful, but rupture of the tympanic membrane provides relief. Tympanic membrane rupture can also result from barotrauma incurred during deep-sea diving, as discussed in Chapter 29, Water Emergencies.

Injuries to the teeth occur in outdoor activities, especially those involving speed, the potential for projectiles, or direct physical contact with others or with a hard surface. Chipping a tooth is the most common dental injury encountered, whereas a complete avulsion (a tooth knocked out) is the most serious dental injury. Teeth also may be fractured, leaving a jagged piece of tooth at the gum line. When a tooth is bleeding, the nerves inside the tooth have been exposed, resulting in significant pain and an increased risk of infection. If a loose tooth becomes dislodged and is not removed from the mouth, airway obstruction can result. Direct trauma to the mouth can cause a dental appliance (e.g., dentures, a bridge, a retainer) to break, which can lacerate the gum or possibly obstruct the airway.

**Figure 22-9** A nose injury.

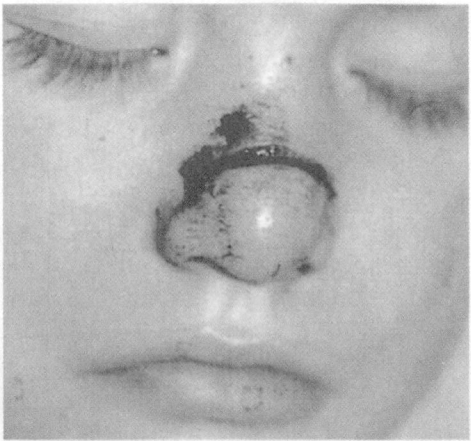

**Figure 22-10** An injury to the ear.

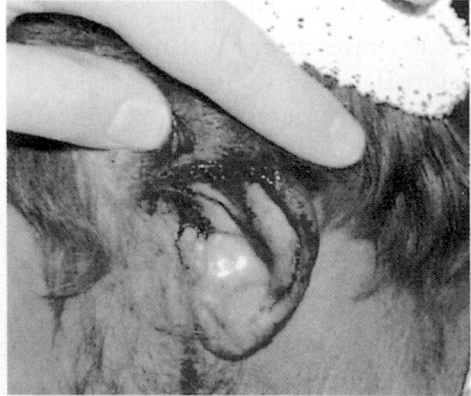

## Eye Injuries

Light-related injuries are one of the most frequent sources of eye injury, especially if eye protection is not worn. Exposure to UV rays (from the sun or welding), chemicals, and various gases can cause eye damage. Injuries from overexposure to UV light, as commonly occur in snow sports, can range from a superficial burn to permanent damage to the conjunctiva or cornea. Often known as snow blindness, these injuries may not become apparent until several hours after the exposure. UV light from an arc-welding lamp, a sun lamp, or sunlight reflected off a snow field or water may cause severe pain in association with conjunctivitis, swelling, and excessive tear production.

The eyes are especially vulnerable to abrasive and penetrating injuries, including impaled objects (Figure 22-11■). Small particles such as blowing sand can get beneath the eyelid, abrading or scratching the surface of the eye. Patients may have the sensation that there is a foreign body in the eye and will likely be sensitive to bright light. In severe cases, particles can penetrate an unprotected eye. Work-related activities, such as grinding metal, operating a drill, performing high-speed sanding, or working around debris kicked up from helicopters, also can result in penetrating eye injuries from small particles. Objects such as tree branches, ice tools, ski poles, darts, and other pointed objects can also easily penetrate the globe. A ball or other smooth object can directly strike the globe, resulting in blunt trauma.

Regardless of the mechanism, globe laceration or rupture should be considered anytime the eye has suffered direct trauma or suspected penetration. Globe ruptures—conditions in which the integrity of the eyeball has been compromised—are a leading trauma-related cause of blindness (Figure 22-12■).

Direct trauma to the eye can disrupt the lens of the eye, so that light cannot be focused correctly on the retina. Trauma can also cause the retina to detach, or peel off the inside of the eyeball, resulting in blindness. Lacerations to the upper or lower eyelid need attention by a properly trained physician. In both blunt and penetrating injuries to the eye, blood may accumulate in the aqueous fluid (anterior chamber) of the eye, resulting in **hyphema**. Usually seen in penetrating injuries, blood in the vitreous fluid (posterior chamber) is a very serious problem.

## Neck Injuries

Injuries involving the structures of the neck can be immediately life threatening and are frequently associated with severe swelling or formation of a hematoma that can compromise the airway. Blunt trauma is a leading cause of neck and throat injuries that may damage not only the vital structures in the anterior neck but also the cervical spine. Direct blows to the anterior neck and "clothesline" or ligature-type injuries can be deadly because the concentrated force can crush the larynx or trachea. This type of injury also can cause deep lacerations and open wounds.

These injuries are usually difficult to manage in the field. Penetrating neck injuries are especially concerning because they often damage multiple structures, including the trachea and major blood vessels. Neck and throat injuries can be deceptive: although they may initially appear benign they are frequently associated with grave underlying trauma.

Open neck injuries are among the most serious injuries OEC Technicians may encounter (Figure 22-13■). Lacerations involving either a carotid artery or a jugular vein produce profuse bleeding that can result

⊕ **22-2** List possible causes of eye injuries.

⊕ **22-8** List the signs and symptoms of emergent injuries to the face, eyes, and neck.

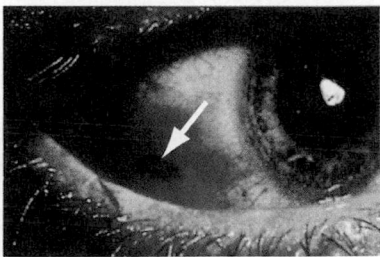

**Figure 22-11** Unprotected eyes are susceptible to impaled foreign objects, which in this case has been removed; note hole.

**hyphema** blood in the anterior chamber of the eye.

**Figure 22-12** A globe rupture caused by a penetrating object.

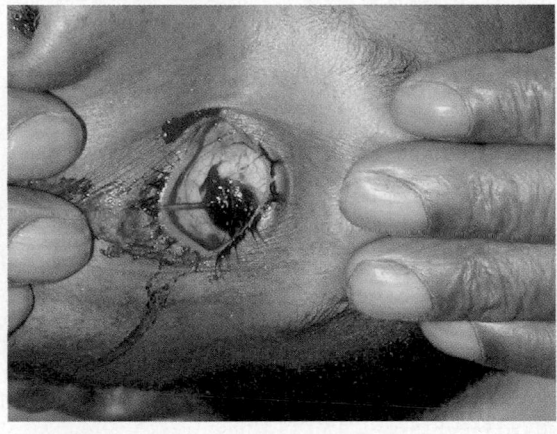

**Figure 22-13** An open neck injury.

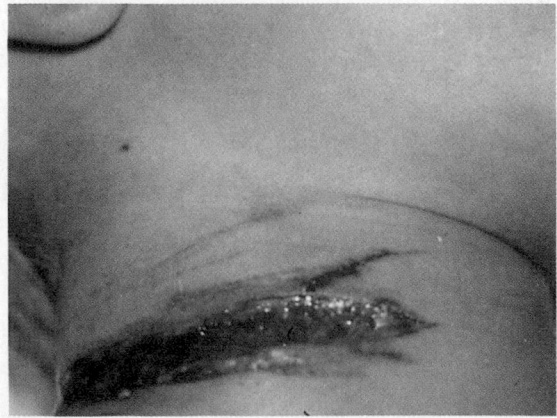

in life-threatening shock if not immediately controlled. In some instances, air may be sucked into the venous system through the damaged vessel, producing an air embolus. If large quantities of air reach the right atrium and right ventricle, cardiac air embolism causing cardiac arrest may follow. If the air passes through the heart, it can lodge in the lungs, causing pulmonary air embolism. Penetrating injuries to the trachea and esophagus can result in profound hypoxia, aspiration of gastric contents, and a host of other problems.

# STOP, THINK, UNDERSTAND

## Multiple Choice
Choose the correct answer.

1. A blow-out fracture is best described as_____
   a. bursting of the auditory ossicles and the ear drum.
   b. a fracture of the bony socket of the eye.
   c. a mandibular or maxillary fracture that dislocates the jaw.
   d. a fracture of 75 percent or more of the facial bones.

2. Double vision can be caused by_____
   a. a detached retina.
   b. a burst auditory ossicle.
   c. an orbit fracture that entraps the muscles that move the eye.
   d. inflammation of the conjunctiva.

3. The primary concern with a mandible fracture is_____
   a. the inability to chew.
   b. a loss of taste sensation.
   c. airway compromise.
   d. paralysis.

4. Epistaxis is another word for_____
   a. a blow-out fracture.
   b. a dislocated jaw.
   c. a nosebleed.
   d. vitreous humor leaking from the eye.

5. The most common source of eye injury is_____
   a. UV light.
   b. impaled objects.
   c. heat.
   d. blunt trauma.

## Matching
Match each of the following terms or structures to its description.

_____ 1. anisocoria
_____ 2. pinna
_____ 3. foramina
_____ 4. blowout fracture
_____ 5. cornea
_____ 6. epistaxis
_____ 7. external auditory canal
_____ 8. hyphema
_____ 9. lacrimal gland
_____ 10. mandible
_____ 11. maxilla
_____ 12. orbit
_____ 13. retinal detachment
_____ 14. sternocleidomastoid muscle
_____ 15. subcutaneous emphysema

a. the structure that produces tears that irrigate the eye surface
b. a nosebleed
c. the clear but highly sensitive surface of the eye that allows light into the visual system
d. air-filled bubbles that are palpable underneath the skin and indicate injury to an airway structure
e. small openings in a bone
f. the bony socket of a facial bone that contains an eyeball
g. blood in the anterior chamber of the eye
h. an injury caused by direct trauma to the eye or face that fractures the bones in the floor of the orbit; the injury may entrap the muscles that enable normal eye movement
i. a condition characterized by an unequal size of the pupils
j. the bone of the upper jaw and mid-face
k. a powerful muscle at the sides of the neck that facilitates turning of the head
l. the lower jaw bone; makes up the lower portion of facial structures
m. the outer part of the ear
n. separation of the retina from the inner eye wall at the posterior aspect of the eyeball
o. the outer canal of the ear which ends at the tympanic membrane

*continued*

## Short Answer

1. List three possible causes of epistaxis.

_____

_____

_____

2. List three possible causes of tympanic membrane rupture.

_____

_____

_____

3. Why are injuries of the neck potentially life threatening?

_____

_____

4. Why is a "clothesline" injury to the neck potentially lethal?

_____

_____

# CASE UPDATE

Evaluating the scene as you approach the injured snowboarder, you look for fixed objects other than the closure rope that the patient may have hit. Evaluating the likely mechanism of injury, you suspect that the snowboarder could have serious neck trauma.

Upon examination, you notice that the patient is clearly anxious and is having difficulty breathing. His respiration rate is 24 per minute with shallow inspirations, and as he tries to respond to your questions he can speak only in a hoarse whisper. You note as well that the snowboarder cannot swallow his saliva and is drooling from his mouth. His pulse is 100 bpm. His face lacks any visible signs of injury or asymmetry, and his pupils appear equal. No trauma is apparent around his ears or scalp. When you examine the patient's neck, you notice a dark red abrasion and underlying swelling on the right anterior portion of his neck. Palpation of the posterior neck reveals no tenderness or deformities.

**What should you do?**

⊕ 22-9 Describe and demonstrate how to assess face, eye, and neck injuries.

# Assessment

Pain and anxiety are commonly associated with facial and neck injuries. Any injury that makes breathing difficult produces great anxiety. Trauma to the face may injure highly sensitive structures such as the lips, nose, or eyes. Copious bleeding from facial and neck injuries is likely to cause apprehension, for the patient and any bystanders alike.

Any facial injury mandates that the assessment process begin with a careful assessment of the airway. The rich vascular supply to the head and neck can result in profuse bleeding. Disability from trauma to the brain or cervical spinal cord is likely. Responsiveness and neurologic function of all extremities must be assessed. In a patient who has a significant head injury, the chances that there is also a significant injury to the cervical spine are greater than 10 percent.

OEC Technicians should continue to monitor the ABCDs, because over time the airway may become obstructed, bleeding can recur, or the patient's mental status or neurologic function may change.

If the primary assessment is unremarkable, OEC Technicians should begin a secondary assessment by asking patients about their symptoms and their medical history in the normal fashion, using the SAMPLE acronym and the OPQRST mnemonic, respectively.

The physical examination already began with any observations made during the primary assessment. Continue the assessment by looking at the entire scalp and the face and neck for lacerations, abrasions, punctures, or other injuries. Look for facial asymmetry, such as a depressed cheek bone from a fracture.

⊕ 22-3 Describe and demonstrate how to assess eye injuries.

## Assessment of the Eye

Begin the ocular exam by asking patients if they can see normally, and if they can see normally with each eye. Ask if there is double vision. Next, look at each eye. Does each pupil appear round, or irregular? Patients who have had lens replacement surgery or cataract surgery may have irregularly shaped pupils, so be sure to ask about past eye surgery. If only one eye is injured, start the assessment by examining the other eye, noting its reaction to light. Then assess the injured eye by comparing it to the uninjured eye. Conducting an eye exam may be somewhat difficult, because patients may be reluctant to open a severely injured eye. Never force someone to open an injured eye.

Gently attempt to open swollen eyelids to assess the pupillary reaction to light. Any visible differences in the size or response of the pupils may indicate an injury to either the eye or the brain (Figure 22-14■). Check extraocular motions of the eyes.

To examine extraocular motions of the eyes:

1. Face the patient's face.
2. Hold up one finger and have the patient focus on the finger with both eyes. Tell the patient to follow the finger.
3. Move your finger up, down, to the right, and to the left watching the patient's eyes to make sure both eyes follow your finger in a coordinated manner.

Move your finger toward the patient's nose and the patient's eyes should become slightly "crossed."

Examine injured or painful eyes for the presence of foreign bodies, blood, or clear fluid. An injured eye that does not react to light should raise your suspicion of potential globe damage or rupture. If you are unable to assess pupil reactions, assume the globe has been injured until proven otherwise.

The eyelids may reflexively close, making examination difficult. The presence of a clear fluid may represent tears, which can make visualization of a small foreign body

**Figure 22-14** Check the pupils for size, equality, and reactivity to light.

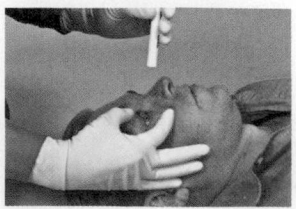

difficult, but such fluid may also be fluid leaking from inside the globe as a result of a puncture wound.

Be aware that some patients will have different findings in each eye. A patient with a prosthetic or glass eye, for instance, may have matching iris color but will lack a pupillary response in the prosthetic eye. Likewise, patients with naturally occurring anisocoria will have unequal pupils. Patients with this condition generally know about it, so be sure to ask patients with unequal pupils if this is normal for them (Figure 22-15■).

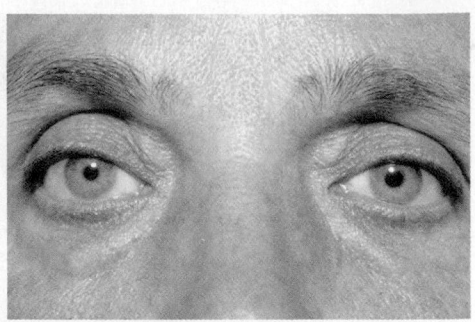

**Figure 22-15** A patient with unequal pupils.

## Assessment of the Mid-Face and Nose

Examine the nose for bleeding, asymmetry, and obstruction. Assess the cheeks for symmetry and equality in appearance. The maxilla could be fractured on one or both sides, causing the cheek to look deformed or depressed. Assess bone stability by gently pressing down on the zygomatic bones and maxillae on both sides of the nose (Figure 22-16■). Then, gently press down on the maxilla just beneath the nares on the upper lip. Any detected instability is cause for concern.

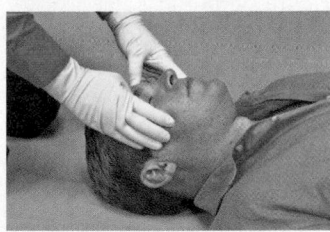

**Figure 22-16** Thoroughly palpate the face during the assessment.

## Assessment of the Mouth

Examine the lips and the inside of the mouth for bleeding. Pale or bluish lips could indicate hypothermia, hypoxia, or significant blood loss. Check for loose or missing teeth and lacerations of the tongue. Gently palpate the face, jaw, and neck for tenderness or crepitus that could indicate a fracture.

Assess the clarity of the voice and see if the patient is swallowing normally. If possible, have the patient open and close the mouth and ask if the teeth "close properly." If there is a malocclusion due to a jaw fracture (mandible or maxilla), the patient will either not be able to bite or will say that the teeth "do not make contact correctly."

## Assessment of the Ear

Examine each ear for obvious evidence of trauma. If bleeding is present, try to determine whether the source is the external part of the ear, the ear canal, or a nearby site from which blood has flowed into the external auditory canal. Look for *clear* fluid coming out of the ear; it may be cerebrospinal fluid leaking from a basal skull fracture (Figure 22-17■). Look for swelling or ecchymosis over the bony prominence of

**Figure 22-17** Cerebrospinal fluid (in this case, mixed with blood) leaking from the ear of a trauma patient.

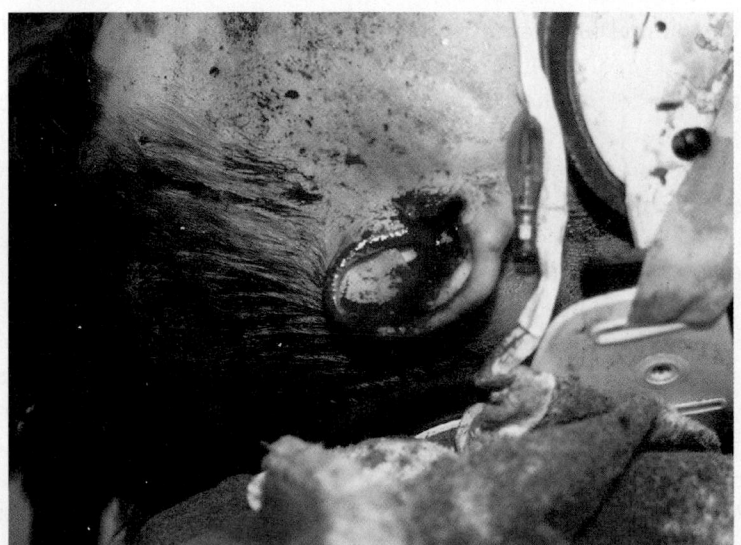

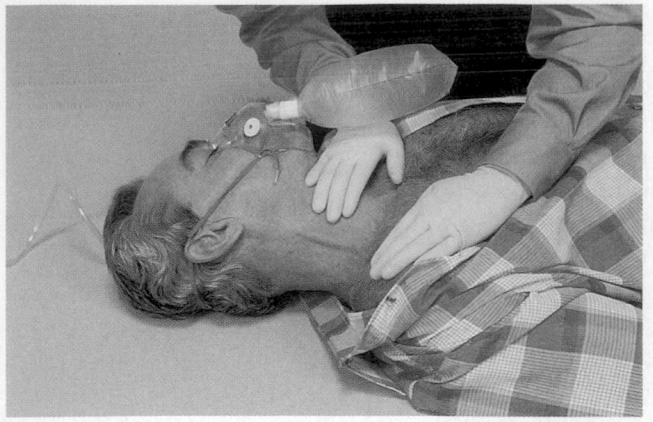

**Figure 22-18** Inspect the neck for jugular vein distention, tracheal deviation, and Medic Alert tags.

**subcutaneous emphysema**　air-filled bubbles that are palpable underneath the skin; indicates an injury to an airway structure.

> ### Significant Facial Injury
>
> **N O T E**
>
> A significant facial injury may be associated with a significant injury to the brain or cervical spine.

**⊕ 22-10**　Describe and demonstrate the proper care of a face, eye, or neck injury.

the mastoid process behind each ear; bruising to this area hours after head trauma, known as Battle's sign, may indicate local trauma to the mastoid process or a fracture of the base of the skull. Examine the external canal of the ear for a foreign body, especially small toy parts in children and insects in both adults and children. Look for gray or green material leaking from the ear, which may indicate an infection. Next, assess the patient's hearing by talking directly into each ear; use the same pitch and amplitude for each ear and then ask if your voice has the same quality and loudness in both ears.

### Assessment of the Neck

Perform a DCAP-BTLS inspection of the anterior and posterior aspects of the neck. Look for symmetry between the two sides and assess the color of the overlying skin. Listen to the patient breathe and talk, noting any changes in voice quality, hoarseness, or audible breath sounds. Ask the patient to swallow and observe the results. Difficulty or pain upon speaking or swallowing are causes for concern and may indicate impending airway compromise. Gently palpate the larynx and trachea for stability, and look for such abnormalities as distention of the jugular vein (Figure 22-18■).

Look to see if any midline structures appear to have shifted or if there is swelling, bruising, or **subcutaneous emphysema**. Anteriorly located swelling or solid masses (hematomas) may signify a ruptured carotid artery or jugular vein, which can cause profuse bleeding and rapidly lead to airway obstruction. Palpate the posterior neck for tenderness and deformity, which may indicate a cervical-spine injury. As a rule, cervical-spine injury should be suspected for any face, eye, or neck injury because the pain and anxiety these injuries cause often distract the patient when you examine the posterior neck.

Because neck injuries can have far-reaching effects, provide inline manual stabilization of the head and neck. Also assess CMS in all extremities. As for all trauma patients, complete the secondary exam and obtain a complete set of vital signs. Reassess the patient frequently because airway compromise and swelling may not be immediately apparent.

## Management

Following your initial impression and management of any safety issues, field management of face, eye, and neck injuries may warrant rapid assessment and frequent reevaluation. Even during short transports, these injuries can rapidly progress to life-threatening situations. As for any patient, problems that affect the airway, breathing, circulation, or disability (neurologic deficit) take precedence over secondary management concerns. Manage the airway as needed, using the techniques and equipment described in Chapter 9, Airway Management. If the airway is compromised, use the jaw-thrust maneuver to protect the cervical spine, not the head-tilt method. Suction the patient's mouth and nose as needed to keep the airway patent.

Because the face, mouth, and neck are highly vascular and bleeding can be significant, it is essential that Standard Precautions be observed at all times. Control bleeding of the scalp or face. External bleeding usually can be managed with direct pressure. If facial fractures are suspected, be careful not to press too hard. If significant face or neck trauma is present, immobilize the patient's spine. If spinal injury is not suspected, lean the patient forward to prevent blood from draining into the airway and from being swallowed.

High-flow oxygen should be provided to all patients with face, eye, or neck trauma, especially in the presence of airway compromise or external bleeding. Advanced life support personnel should be notified to provide assistance when appropriate.

## Management of Facial Injuries

The primary goal when managing a patient with a facial fracture is to keep the airway open and clear. These patients often need aggressive airway management, including appropriate positioning, suctioning, oxygen, and occasionally ventilatory support.

Regardless of whether epistaxis is mild or severe, direct pressure is the best way to control this type of bleeding. The nares (nostrils) should be pressed together just below the bony prominence of the nose (Figure 22-19■). Hold pressure up to 15 minutes before evaluating ongoing bleeding. Lean the patient forward to allow blood and other secretions to drain out of the nose and mouth. The most common mistake in the management of epistaxis is to remove the pressure too soon. If you are unable to control the bleeding with direct pressure, place a cloth- or bandage-wrapped ice pack on the bridge of the nose.

The focus of care for a mouth injury is ensuring a patent airway. Tongue lacerations are controlled with direct pressure. Remove any broken teeth that may be present. Even though a tooth that is displaced but still in its socket is at risk for avulsion and could cause airway obstruction, leave it in place, if possible.

Pick up any tooth that has been completely knocked out of its socket (an avulsed tooth) by its crown. Avoid touching the root (the part that was below the gum). DO NOT WASH OR SCRUB AN AVULSED TOOTH. If the patient is alert and you do not anticipate that you will be transporting the patient over especially bumpy terrain, (if available rinse gently with sterile saline or tepid tap water) place the tooth back in the socket or have the patient keep the tooth against the inside of the cheek. Remind the patient to not swallow or aspirate the tooth.

If a patient cannot safely keep an avulsed tooth in the socket or against the cheek, it should be preserved using other means. Ideally, the tooth should be placed in Hank's solution, a product designed for tooth preservation. If this product is not available, place the tooth in either milk or sterile saline.

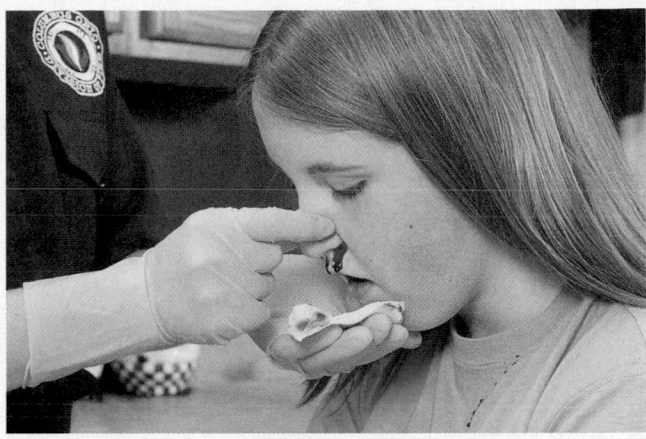
**Figure 22-19** To control a nosebleed, have the patient sit down and lean forward, and pinch the nostrils together.

### An Avulsed Tooth

If a patient has altered mental status or is unable to clear his own secretions, never place an avulsed tooth back in the socket because of the significant risk that the patient will swallow or aspirate it during transportation.

**NOTE**

## STOP, THINK, UNDERSTAND

### Multiple Choice
Choose the correct answer.

1. When assessing an injured eye, which of the following actions are incorrect?_____
   a. Assessing the uninjured eye first.
   b. Not attempting to elicit a response to light.
   c. Attempting to open a swollen eyelid (if the patient allows it).
   d. Assuming damage or rupture to the globe if you cannot elicit a pupillary reaction.

2. When you observe clear liquid dripping from an eye that has suffered a puncture wound, what should you assume about this injury?_____
   a. The fluid is vitreous or aqueous humor unless proven otherwise.
   b. The fluid is most likely tears.
   c. The fluid is probably cerebrospinal fluid.
   d. OEC Technicans should never assume anything.

*continued*

## STOP, THINK, UNDERSTAND *continued*

**3.** While examining a patient complaining of a possible ankle fracture, you notice that one pupil responds to light while the other pupil does not respond at all. The patient denies hitting his head. These findings may indicate_____

   **a.** a closed head injury.     **c.** a prosthetic eye.

   **b.** anisocoria.     **d.** a blowout fracture.

**4.** When a patient with a traumatic throat injury complains of difficulty swallowing and talking, this finding could be indicative of_____

   **a.** an impending cold or upper respiratory infection.

   **b.** an allergic reaction.

   **c.** an impending airway compromise.

   **d.** a muscle spasm.

**5.** What is the best position in which to place a patient with no suspected spinal trauma who is bleeding profusely from severe epistaxis? _____

   **a.** in a supine position

   **b.** in the Trendelenberg position

   **c.** in a prone position

   **d.** sitting, leaning forward

**6.** The primary goal when caring for a patient suffering from a facial fracture is_____

   **a.** keeping the airway open and clear.

   **b.** spinal immobilization.

   **c.** managing bleeding.

   **d.** rapid extrication and transportation.

**7.** The best first course of treatment for epistaxis is _____

   **a.** ice.     **c.** pressure.

   **b.** elevation.     **d.** packing.

**8.** Which of the following actions are correct actions when caring for an avulsed tooth? (check all that apply)

_____ **a.** Pick the tooth up by the crown.

_____ **b.** Avoid touching the tooth's roots.

_____ **c.** Wipe or wash the tooth gently and carefully to remove debris.

_____ **d.** Always make at least one attempt to replace the tooth in the socket.

_____ **e.** It is acceptable for responsive patients to hold the tooth in their cheek.

_____ **f.** Place the tooth in sterile water.

_____ **g.** Place the tooth in milk.

## Short Answer

**1.** Swelling or solid masses in the anterior part of the neck could signify what?

_____

_____

_____

**2.** Why should you assess a patient with a neck or throat injury frequently?

_____

_____

_____

**3.** Tongue lacerations are best controlled by what type of pressure?

_____

_____

_____

## Management of Ear Injuries

Bleeding from a lacerated external ear and ear avulsions are controlled using direct pressure, a dressing, and a bandage. In both cases, the applied dressing should include bulky support between the pinna and the scalp. If the external ear is completely amputated, preserve the part as described for an amputated finger in Chapter 18, Soft-Tissue Injuries. Most pinna-related injuries can be successfully repaired if they are attended to quickly. Any patient with a severe external ear injury should be transported to a physician for cosmetic repair.

Manipulation of a foreign body stuck in the external auditory canal can cause injury to the tympanic membrane and can be very irritating to the patient. When faced with this situation, turn patients onto their side with the affected ear down to see if the object will fall out on its own. If it does not, the patients should be evaluated in a medical facility for removal and follow-up treatment. Tympanic membrane rupture, whether from trauma or infection, does not require an occlusive or pressure dressing. Instead, allow secretions to drain by having patients tilt their head toward the affected side. If there are no other injuries, patients may be transported in this position to a medical facility for further treatment, which may include antibiotic therapy to minimize the risk of long-term hearing loss.

Part of the inner-ear system controls balance. Symptoms of inner-ear balance problems are usually associated with chronic illness but may be caused by more serious problems such as a recent stroke. For this reason, any patient who reports dizziness, sudden balance problems, or a rapid onset of severe nausea should be evaluated by a physician.

Facial injuries may be associated with a variety of soft-tissue injuries, which can be significant or relatively minor. Often, these injuries bleed profusely. Most soft-tissue injuries around the nose, mouth, and ears respond well to direct pressure and an appropriate dressing. When applying a dressing, make sure you keep the airway open. Because of the potential for permanent scarring, soft-tissue injuries involving the face should be evaluated in an emergency department as soon as possible.

## Management of Eye Injuries

Because eye injuries can result in blindness, any patient with an eye injury should be transported for physician evaluation. Soft-tissue injuries around the eye should be managed with the utmost care to avoid applying pressure to the eyeball. Obvious penetrating injuries, massive orbital trauma, and suspected globe rupture require emergent referral to an eye specialist.

Small foreign bodies on the surface of the eye are a common problem. If the patient allows, carefully retract the upper and lower eyelids to examine for the presence of a superficial foreign body. Inflammation—reddening of the conjunctiva, known as conjunctivitis—may be readily apparent. Pain may be aggravated by bright light.

Foreign bodies that have adhered to the inner surfaces of the eyelids may also be removed with a cotton-tipped applicator. To examine the inside surface of the upper eyelid, pull the lid forward and up over a cotton swab (Figures 22-20a–d■).

Objects that have adhered to the conjunctiva may penetrate the surface of the eyeball, especially when the injury involves metalwork, such as filing or hammering. These injuries require urgent consultation with an ophthalmologist. Larger

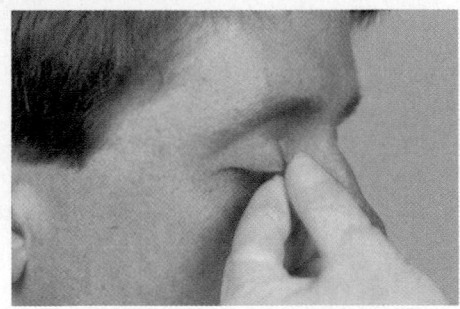
**Figure 22-20a** To remove a foreign body from the eye, grasp the eyelashes between the thumb and forefinger and instruct the patient to look down.

**Figure 22-20b** Place a swab along the center of the upper eyelid.

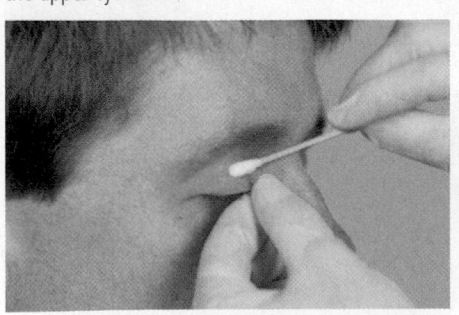

**Figure 22-20c** Pull the eyelid forward and up over the swab.

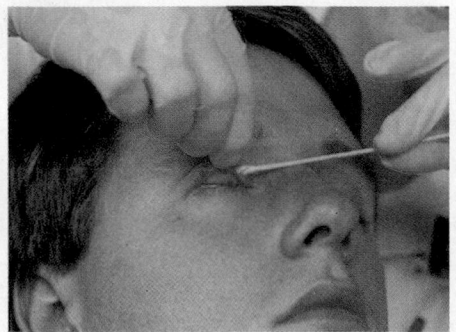

**Figure 22-20d** Once the underside of the eyelid has been exposed, use a clean, moistened swab to remove the foreign object.

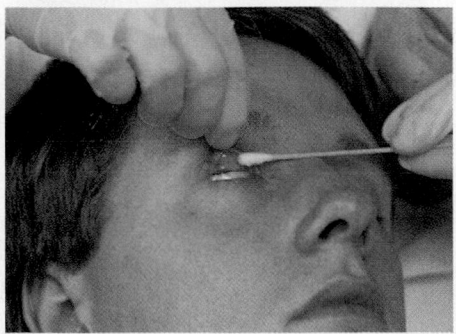

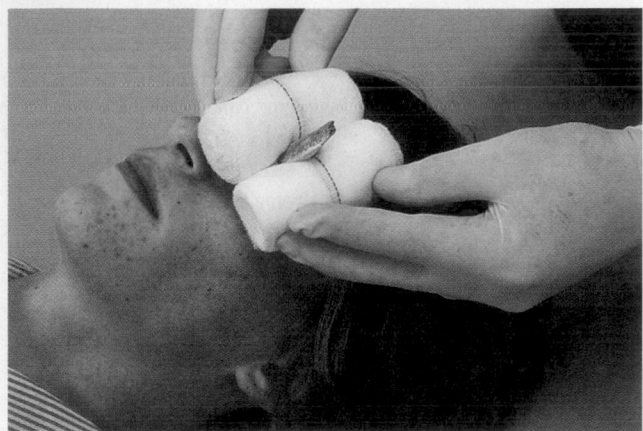

**Figure 22-21** Secure an object impaled in the eye to prevent movement.

⊕ **22-4** Describe and demonstrate the management of a patient with a penetrating injury to the eyeball.

**retinal detachment** separation of the retina from the inside of the posterior wall of the eyeball.

foreign bodies impaled in the eye require eye stabilization prior to transport. Use a circular or ring dressing or cup to protect the eye, and use a gauze bandage to stabilize the impaled object (Figure 22-21■). Great care must be taken not to move the impaled object during transport. See OEC Skill 22-1■.

### Eyelid and Eyeball Lacerations

Eyelid lacerations, which may bleed profusely because of the blood supply to this part of the face, are commonly controlled with gentle direct pressure. Because the eyeball itself also may be injured, do not apply pressure to the eye itself to avoid causing leakage of the vitreous humor. The eye or globe should never be manipulated. If the eyeball is out of the socket, it should be covered with a moistened, sterile dressing to prevent drying. Do not attempt to put the eyeball back in the socket.

When one eye is injured, cover both eyes to decrease synchronous movement of the injured eye when the uninjured eye moves. Note that bandaging both eyes will make the patient unable to see at all, which can be extremely frightening to some people. Therefore, stay with such patients and talk to them, guide them, and reassure them.

### Blunt Trauma

Direct trauma to the eye or surrounding soft tissue can cause bleeding within the eye. If the bleeding fills the anterior chamber of the eye, the result is a hyphema (Figure 22-22■). Patients with a hyphema should be transported in a sitting position, if possible.

Any blunt trauma to the eye may also cause **retinal detachment**, the symptoms of which are seeing specks, flashing lights or "floaters" in the visual field, or decreased vision in that eye. Patients reporting any of these symptoms require emergent evaluation by an ophthalmologist. Cover both of the patient's eyes without pressure and transport.

### Burns to the Eye

Exposure to chemicals, heat, and UV or intense light can burn the surface of the eye. Such exposure often injures both of the patient's eyes. Quick assessment and treatment of these injuries may allow OEC Technicians to prevent further damage to the eyes.

**Figure 22-22** Blood in the anterior chamber of the eye is called a hyphema. (The white ring was caused by the camera's flash.)

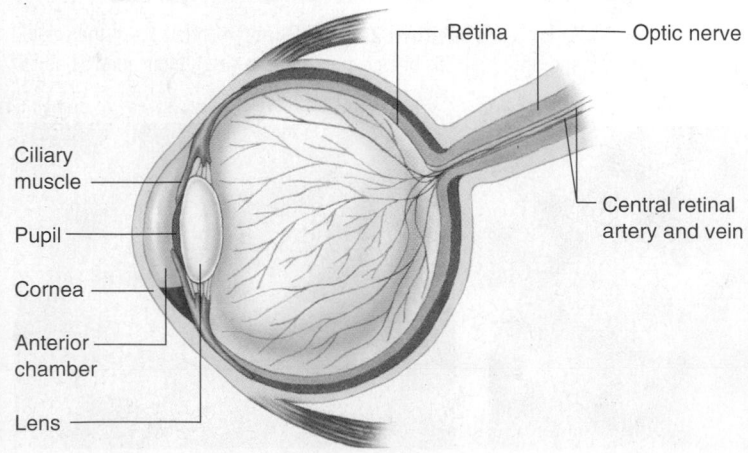

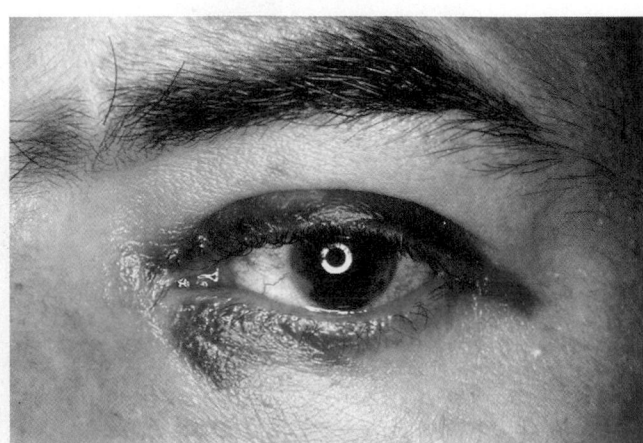

**Chemical Burns** Exposure to any chemical strong enough to irritate the eyes should be presumed to be an emergency (Figure 22-23■). To minimize the injury, immediately and gently irrigate the eye with tepid sterile saline solution (or tepid tap water, if saline is not available). Medical irrigation faucets may be available in commercial or industrial settings. In the absence of specialized equipment in outdoor environments, directly irrigate the eye with saline or clean water from a bag or bottle by pouring into the medial corner of the eye. If available, a gently running shower or faucet also may work. Regardless of the flushing technique used, take care not to contaminate the unaffected eye.

To be effective, irrigation requires the use of copious fluids. Irrigate the affected eye for at least 5 minutes. If the burn was caused by a strong chemical, irrigate the eye for 20–30 minutes. If pain persists, continue the irrigation. It may be difficult for patients to keep their eyelid(s) open during irrigation, so they may require your assistance.

Damage from strong acids or strong bases can continue even after copious irrigation. Such patients should be referred for emergency care. Assume that if the patient still has pain, then damage from the chemical remains ongoing. You may be able to reduce damage to the eye by continuing irrigation during transport. Be sure to note the chemical(s) involved using the MSDS sheet, and include that information in your hand-off report to subsequent rescuers or care providers.

Patients that require eye irrigation will naturally want to keep their eyes closed, especially if they are experiencing pain. To facilitate irrigation, use gloved hands and if needed use gauze to help keep the slippery eyelids open (Figure 22-24■). To irrigate the eyes, follow these steps:

+ Attach irrigation solution to intravenous tubing. (If intravenous solution is not available, use *tepid* tap water. Place the water in a clean plastic bag and poke a small hole in the corner or pour slowly from a medicine bottle.)
+ Gently hold the patient's eye open.
+ Direct the solution into the affected eye, so that it flows from the medial (nasal) side of the eye to the lateral (cheek) side of the eye.

**Thermal Burns** When the eyelids or the surface of the eye is burned by the heat of a thermal accident, take immediate action to stop the burning. Then cover both eyes with a moist sterile dressing and immediately transport the patient for definitive care. Regardless of whether the burn is to the eyelid or the eye, specialist care and follow up are required.

**Figure 22-23** Treat chemical burns to the eye by irrigating the eye with copious amounts of water.

**Figure 22-24** Flushing a foreign particle from the eye.

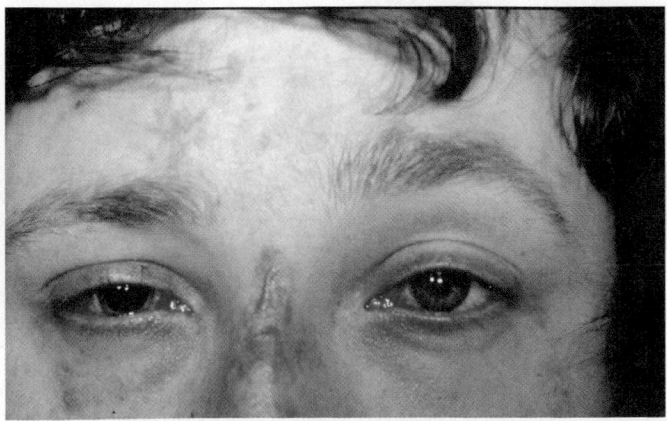

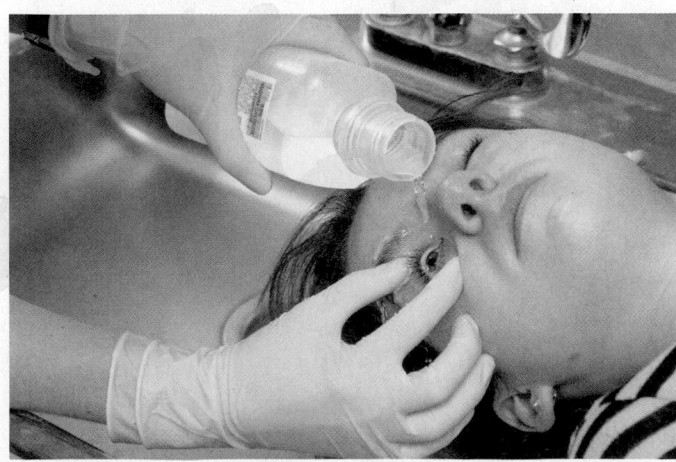

### Removing Contact Lenses

Put on gloves.

1. Removing a soft contact lens: Always remove the lens from the uninjured eye first. Instruct the patient to look up and then pull the lower lid down. Place your index finger on the lens and slide it down to the white of the eye. Squeeze the lens lightly with your thumb and index finger and remove it gently.

2. Removing a hard contact lens: Remove the lens from the right eye first. Put an index finger on the center of the upper lid and a thumb on the center of the lower lid. Press the thumb and index finger together to force the patient to blink. The contact lens will pop out. You may also use a small commercial suction device in order to remove the hard contact lens.

**Light Burns**    Different sources of light burn different parts of the eye. Light from welders, UV light, and "black lights" can cause damage. Depending on what part of the eye is injured, the patient may or may not have pain associated with the injury. Treat superficial burns to the cornea by applying a moist sterile dressing and an eye shield, and transport the patient for evaluation by a specialist as soon as possible. If you suspect a light injury as the cause of a loss of vision in the absence of pain, manage the injury as a retinal burn, which requires evaluation by a specialist.

### Dealing with Contact Lenses

Contact lenses may be difficult to see upon physical exam. When evaluating patients for an eye injury, always ask them if they wear contact lenses. Attempt to remove a contact lens only when a patient has suffered a chemical burn to the eye, when irrigating the eye, or when assisting someone who has requested your assistance in the removal of a lens (Figures 22-25■ and 22-26■). In other situations, the manipulation required to remove the lens may cause further damage to the eye. If the patient wore contact lenses during your eye exam, relay this information to the EMS provider who assumes care of the patient from you.

### Dealing with Artificial Eyes

It may be difficult to distinguish a patient's prosthetic eye from a natural eye. The patient may have some ability to move the prosthetic eye using extraocular muscles, making any visible difference between the two eyes very subtle. A prosthetic eye will not have direct or consensual papillary response. If you have any doubt about the ability of the pupil to react to light, do not hesitate to ask the patient if the eye is a prosthesis. Doing so may well allow you to provide better care for the patient.

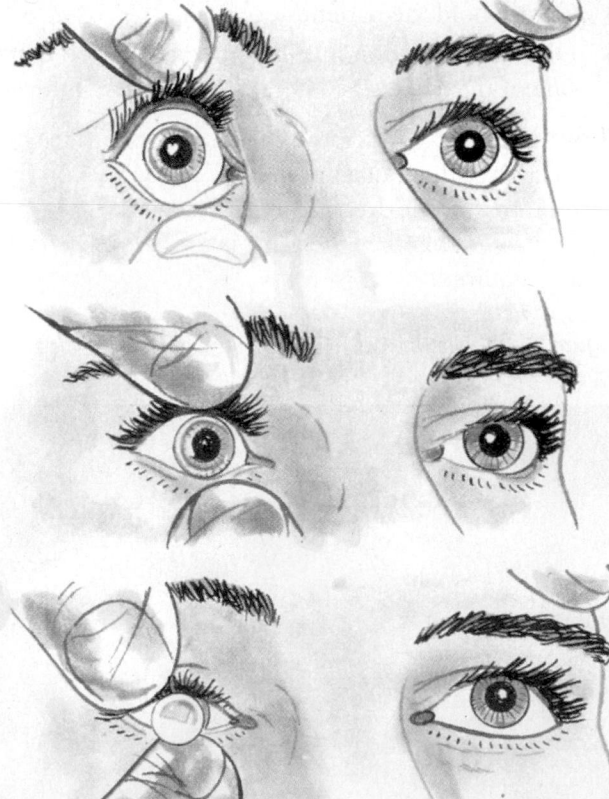

**Figure 22-26** Removing a hard contact lens.

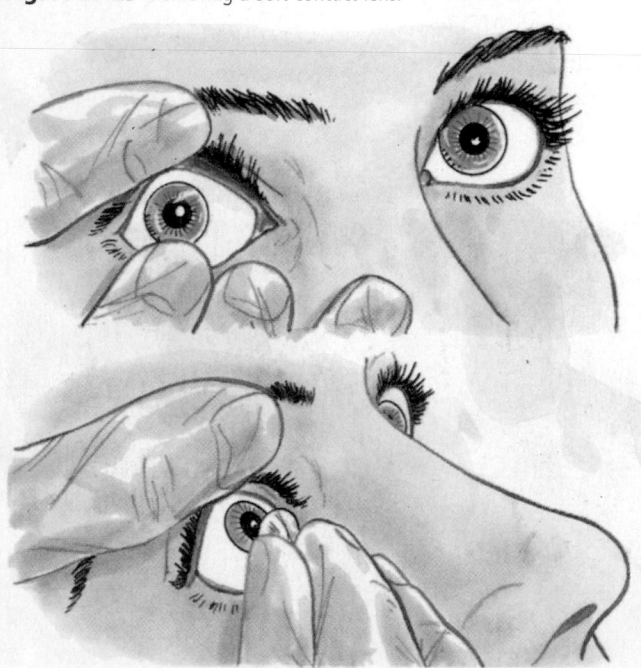

**Figure 22-25** Removing a soft contact lens.

## Management of Neck Injuries

Injuries to the anterior neck can be life threatening, may be associated with cervical-spinal injuries, and should be considered an emergency by OEC Technicians. Manage the ABCDs and the spine accordingly. Open neck injuries with severe bleeding usually can be controlled using the combination of an occlusive dressing and then sterile dressings and direct pressure. Keep patients with anterior neck bleeding lying down to help reduce the chances of air embolism. If the patient sits up, air can enter a large vessel in the neck.

Be careful not to apply direct pressure to both sides of the neck simultaneously because doing so can reduce blood flow to the brain. Likewise, do not wrap bandages around the neck because this can compromise both the airway and circulation. Instead, place an occlusive dressing over the wound and then secure a pressure dressing over the wound by wrapping roller gauze in a figure-eight pattern around the neck and around the arm and armpit of the opposite shoulder (Figures 22-27a –d■).

Immobilize impaled objects in place unless they compromise the airway.

Blunt trauma to the anterior neck can be more difficult to manage than penetrating neck trauma because structural damage may completely occlude the airway. Aggressively manage the airway, summon advanced life-support assistance, and urgently transport the patient to the nearest medical facility.

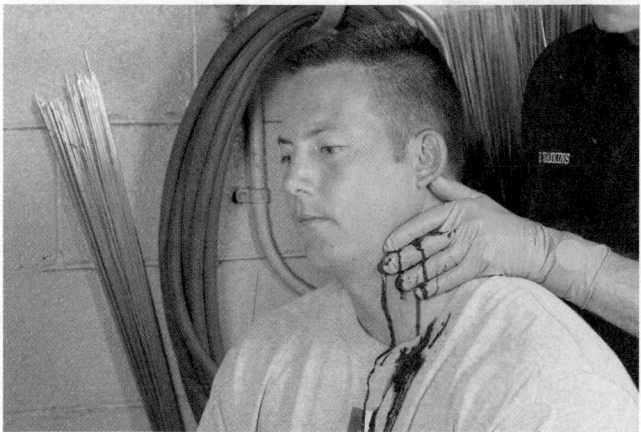

**Figure 22-27a** Treatment of a severed blood vessel in the neck begins with placing a gloved hand over the wound to control bleeding. Apply only enough pressure to control bleeding.

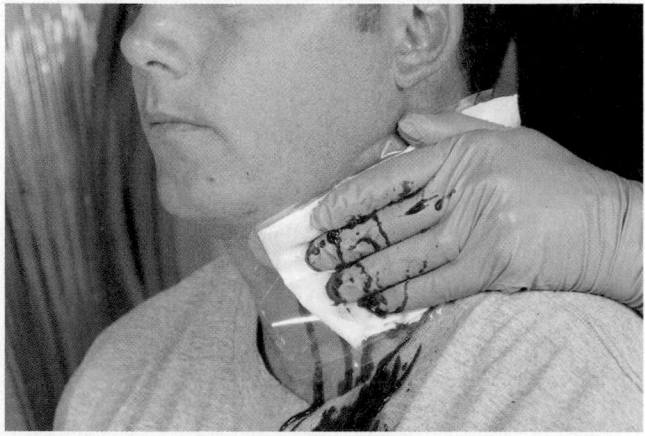

**Figure 22-27b** Apply an occlusive dressing that extends beyond the wound; then cover with a regular dressing.

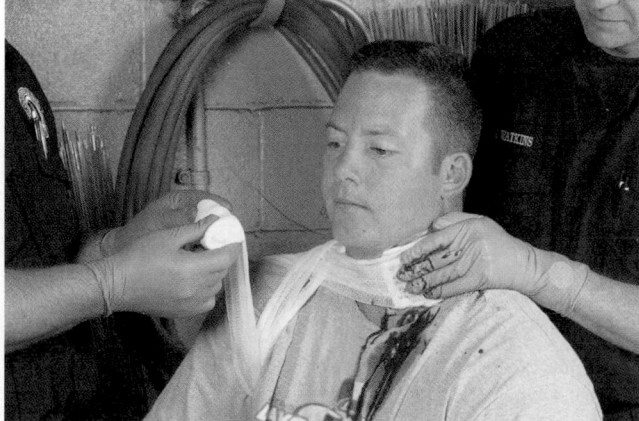

**Figure 22-27c** Once the bleeding is controlled, apply a pressure dressing that does not go circumferentially around the neck.

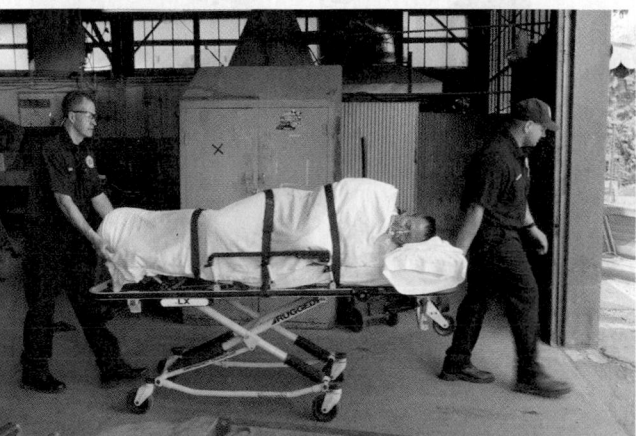

**Figure 22-27d** If no spinal injury is suspected, place the patient on the left side with the head tilted down. Apply $O_2$ and treat for shock.

# STOP, THINK, UNDERSTAND

## Multiple Choice

Choose the correct answer.

1. The correct care for a foreign body stuck in an ear is to_____
   a. gently irrigate the ear with normal saline.
   b. carefully pull the object out with tweezers; stop if resistance is met.
   c. have the patient lie on the same side as the affected side of the head.
   d. do nothing; most foreign bodies will work their way out on their own.

2. The correct care for bleeding lacerations around the eye is to _____
   a. apply direct pressure and bandage.
   b. bandage with minimal pressure.
   c. irrigate only.
   d. allow the wound to clot on its own.

3. Which of the following statements regarding a foreign body in the eye is correct?_____
   a. Resulting corneal abrasion can cause ongoing pain and discomfort even after the object is removed.
   b. Gently attempt to lift the foreign body off the eye with a cotton-tipped applicator.
   c. Foreign bodies adhered to the inner surface of an eyelid may not be removed with a cotton-tipped applicator.
   d. Foreign bodies imbedded in the eye do not need to be evaluated by a physician/ophthalmologist.

4. Why should both eyes be covered when only one eye is injured?_____
   a. to minimize movement of the injured eye
   b. to enable movement of the injured eye
   c. to enable the injured eye to close
   d. to minimize movement of both eyes

## True or False

Indicate whether each of the following statements is true (T) or false (F).

_____a. Exposure to any chemical strong enough to irritate the eye should be presumed to be an emergency.
_____b. Assume that ongoing pain after chemical exposure means ongoing damage.
_____c. Damage from strong acids or strong bases can be halted quickly with a saline rinse.
_____d. When irrigating an eye contaminated with a chemical, avoid getting the irrigant in the other eye.
_____e. A thermal burn to the eyelid generally means the eye itself was protected from injury.
_____f. Different sources of light burn different parts of the eye.

 # CASE DISPOSITION

As you wait for backup to arrive at the scene of the accident, you reassure the snowboarder while stabilizing his head and neck. Upon the arrival of additional patrollers and equipment, you have an assistant maintain cervical alignment while you apply high-flow oxygen using a nonrebreather mask and affix a C-collar. You give clear instructions to your partners regarding your assessment and the need for rapid transportation to the emergency department. Your team maintains spinal alignment while placing the patient on a backboard and into a toboggan using C-spine precautions. During the brief transport you reassess the patient's condition several times.

You give the ALS provider your hand-off report, which includes your concern for a progressively worsening compromise of the patient's airway. The ALS provider intubates the patient, as he is concerned that the airway could become obstructed. Following transport to the hospital, vascular studies show that the patient did not injure his carotid arteries, his jugular veins, or his C-spine. His airway problem resolved over the first 24 hours of his two-day hospital stay.

One month later, the snowboarder stops at the patrol hut to thank you for the quality of care he received from you.

## OEC SKILL 22-1 | Stabilizing an Impaled Object in the Eye

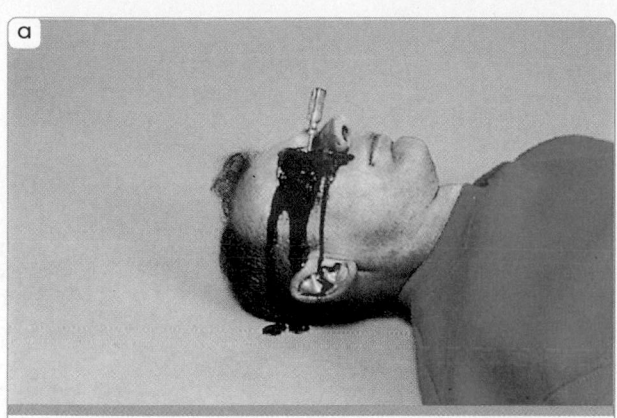

**a**

Do not remove the impaled object from the eye.

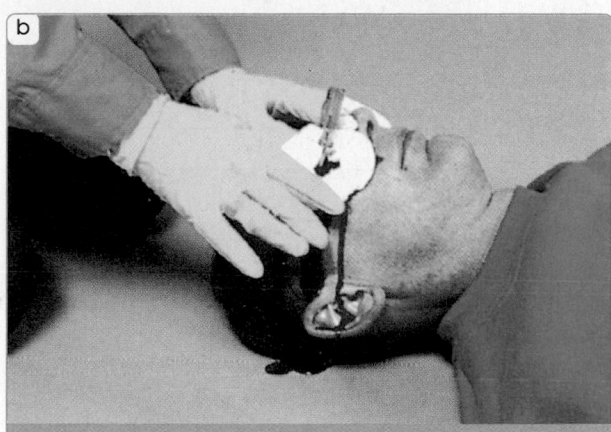

**b**

Place padding around the eye.

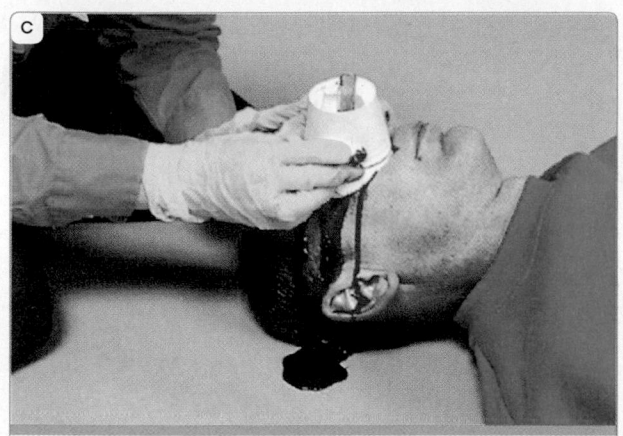

**c**

Place a paper cup over the impaled object to aid in stabilizing the injury.

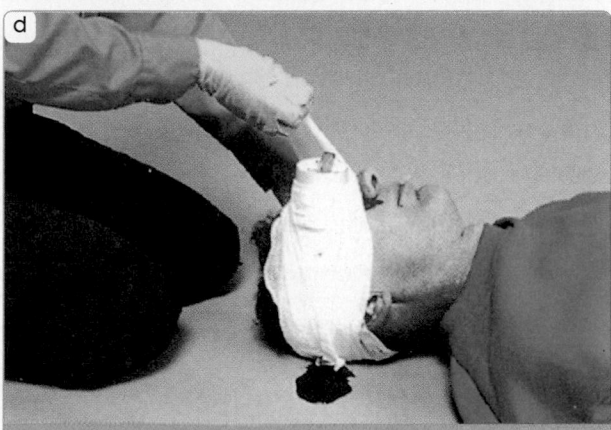

**d**

Use a roller bandage to secure the cup in place.

## Skill Guide

Date: _____

(CPI) = Critical Performance Indicator

Candidate: _____

Start Time: _____

End Time: _____

## Stabilizing an Impaled Object in the Eye

**Objective:** To demonstrate the proper stabilization of a foreign or impaled object in the eye.

| Skill | Max Points | Skill Demo | |
|-------|------------|------------|---|
| Determines scene is safe. | 1 | | (CPI) |
| Introduces self, obtains permission to help/treat. | 1 | | |
| Initiates Standard Precautions. | 1 | | (CPI) |
| Creates a stabilizing device (use a handmade cravat donut or a paper cup). | 1 | | |
| Covers the injured eye with a moist sterile dressing. | 1 | | |
| Applies the stabilizing device to stabilize the object from movement. | 1 | | (CPI) |
| Secures the object with the appropriate materials covering both eyes. | 1 | | |
| Communicates to the patient the procedure you will perform. | 1 | | |

Must receive 5 out of 8 points.

Comments: _____

Failure of any of the CPIs is an automatic failure.

Evaluator: _____ NSP ID: _____

PASS      FAIL

# ⛉ Chapter Review

## Chapter Summary

OEC rescuers will encounter face, eye, and neck injuries in outdoor environments. Whereas many of these injuries will be minor, some may be severe, and a few may even be life threatening. Always evaluate and care for the ABCDs first. Knowing the anatomy and the locations of structures such as the carotid arteries or trachea will help the rescuer assess the potential severity of these injuries. Environmental exposures of the face are also common.

Traumatic injuries can result in profuse bleeding from facial and neck wounds. A patient's fear of suffocation or loss of vision will require a high degree of professional composure from rescuers. Even minor facial and neck injuries may stimulate a patient's anxiety.

Finally, serious facial and neck emergencies are often associated with injuries to other systems. Assessing for closed head and cervical-spine injuries must be part of the initial assessment and all subsequent evaluations.

## Remember...

1. Facial and neck injuries can be associated with severe pain and anxiety.
2. Facial and neck injuries can rapidly become life threatening.
3. Assess the stability of the patient's airway by listening to the patient talk.
4. Direct pressure applied to an injured globe of the eye may worsen the injury.
5. Facial and neck asymmetry is a clue to traumatic injury.
6. Facial fractures require a significant mechanism of injury, so associated closed head or cervical-spine injuries must be considered as well.
7. Facial and neck injuries are likely to increase your chance of exposure to the patient's bodily fluids.
8. Face and neck injuries require frequent assessment.
9. Any significant face, neck, or head injury requires cervical (and spinal) immobilization.

## Chapter Questions

### Multiple Choice

Choose the correct answer.

1. Anisocoria is_____
   a. a hearing deficit.
   b. vitreous or aqueous humor leaking from the eye.
   c. unequal pupils.
   d. teeth and jaws that do not align properly.

2. An eyelid laceration_____
   a. is superficial and warrants little or no follow-up.
   b. requires medical follow-up.
   c. is serious only if it involves the eye itself.
   d. can ultimately cause a permanent loss of vision.

3. Under what circumstance are OEC Technicians permitted to pack a nostril to control a nosebleed?_____
   a. An OEC Technician may not pack a nostril under any circumstances.
   b. When the OEC Technician cannot control bleeding with direct pressure and ALS is more than 60 minutes away.
   c. Any time the OEC Technician feels packing is the appropriate course of action.
   d. If a fracture prevents applying direct pressure.

**4.** The correct care for a patient with a ruptured tympanic membrane is_____

 **a.** an occlusive dressing.                                 **c.** a pressure dressing.

 **b.** small amounts of packing in the outer ear canal.       **d.** allowing it to drain by tilting the head to the affected side.

**5.** Which of the following is the correct procedure for caring for an eyeball that has been knocked out of its socket?_____

 **a.** Make one attempt only at replacing the eyeball, and then cover both eyes with moist, sterile dressings.

 **b.** Gently bandage both eyes with dry, sterile dressing, securing the eyeball in place while taking care not to compress it.

 **c.** Cover the eyeball with a moist, sterile dressing and leave it in the place you found it.

 **d.** Replace the eyeball carefully into the socket, and then gently apply a pressure dressing over both eyes.

## Short Answer

**1.** A patient has suffered a major neck laceration involving the jugular vein and the carotid artery. Besides possible hypovolemic shock, what other life-threatening complications could occur?

_____

_____

_____

**2.** What maneuver should an OEC Technician use when opening the airway of a patient who has suffered a clothesline injury to the throat and is not breathing?

_____

_____

_____

**3.** A patient who has not experienced trauma complains of sudden-onset dizziness, a lack of balance, severe nausea, and other symptoms of an inner-ear problem. What much more serious condition could actually be occurring?

_____

_____

_____

# Scenario

On a crisp fall day you are manning a checkpoint a quarter mile from the end of a mountain bike race. A frantic woman comes running up from the adjacent campground, screaming, "My husband's had his face burned by an explosion!"

You call to base to report that an adult male has received burns from a campfire. When you arrive on scene, you find a man in his early 50s sitting at a picnic table, hunched over and breathing hard. His face, upper chest, and upper arms are badly burned. His shirt is charred and appears to be sticking to his skin. His hands and arms are shaking. A gasoline can sits nearby.

**1.** The primary safety concern for this scene is_____

 **a.** keeping bystanders away.

 **b.** managing the patient's airway.

 **c.** putting out the fire and securing the gasoline can before attempting to treat the patient.

 **d.** calming the wife, who is hysterical.

You secure the scene by using a fire extinguisher to put out the fire in the fire pit. You take the gasoline can and direct the wife to move it farther from the scene. After identifying yourself, getting permission to treat the man, and using Standard Precautions, you remove the patient's shirt and pour a jug of drinking water over the patient's burns to cool them and prevent further burning. The man's radial pulse is 100 per minute and weak. Respirations are counted at 26 and labored, as the patient is having difficulty breathing. His vision appears to be normal.

*You call to base requesting additional help, O₂, and an ALS unit to report to campsite #12 to aid a male patient with severe burns and difficulty breathing. You take a blanket from the campsite and cover the patient, being careful not to put it on the patient's burned areas.*

2. The treatment for singed eyelids and eyebrows is _____
    a. affixing sterile moist dressings over both eyes with cling wrap around the head.
    b. affixing sterile dry dressings over both eyes with cling wrap around the head.
    c. applying sterile dry dressings with an ice pack on top.
    d. constant flushing of the face and no dressings.

*You begin a secondary assessment by gathering SAMPLE information as you start to apply dry dressings to his burns. A med alert bracelet found on his wrist reads, "heart disease, hypertension, on Coumadin." Because his wrist is not burned, you leave the alert tag on him. He is not allergic to any medication and has eaten two hours before the incident. He also has consumed three cans of beer. The patient is not sure whether he was ever unresponsive or not.*

*When questioned about the events leading up to the burns, the patient tells you that the fire was going out, so he poured gasoline on it, and it exploded.*

*Other OEC Technicians arrive, and you verify that all of the fires in the immediate area have been extinguished. You direct your helpers to supply oxygen to the patient via a nonrebreather at 15 LPM.*

*A recheck of the vital signs as the ALS unit arrives with the O₂ has the pulse at 90 and respirations at 28 and labored.*

3. The patient has sustained partial-thickness burns to the neck, head, and face after pouring gasoline on a smoldering campfire. Which one of the following statements indicates that the OEC Technician is properly caring for him? _____
    a. "While waiting for the ambulance, I am going to make sure the patient's airway remains open."
    b. "I am going to apply a special antibiotic lotion to the burned areas to prevent scarring."
    c. "I am going to put ice packs on your chest to cool the burn."
    d. "I need to clean the dirt from the burned areas to prevent infections."

*You place the patient in full C-spine immobilization because the force from the explosion remains unknown. The patient is taken to the nearest trauma center and is then flown via helicopter to a burn center.*

## Suggested Reading

Chapeau, W., and P. Pons. 2007. *Emergency Medical Technician: Making the Difference.* St. Louis, MO: Mosby JEMS, Elsevier Publishers.

Markovchick, V., and P. Pons. 2003. *Emergency Medicine Secrets,* Third Edition, Philadelphia, PA: Hanley and Belfus Publishers.

Sanders, M. J. 2007. *Mob's Paramedic Textbook,* Revised Third Edition. St. Louis, MO: Mosby JEMS, Elsevier Publishers.

EXPLORE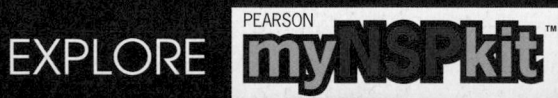

# Thoracic Trauma

James Geiling, MD, FACP, FCCM
Matthew Fulton, BA, NREMT-P

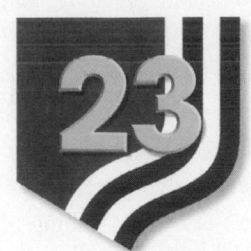

## ⊕ OBJECTIVES

**Upon completion of this chapter, the OEC Technician will be able to:**

**23-1** List the major anatomical structures of the thoracic cavity.

**23-2** Describe the basic physiology of thoracic structures.

**23-3** Describe the pathology of the following thoracic injuries:

- flail chest
- pneumothorax
- hemothorax
- tension pneumothorax
- sucking chest wound
- pericardial tamponade

**23-4** List the signs and symptoms of various thoracic injuries.

**23-5** Describe and demonstrate how to assess the chest for trauma, using the L.A.P. method.

**23-6** Describe and demonstrate the emergency management of a sucking chest wound.

## ⊕ KEY TERMS

aneurysm, *p. 780*
aortic rupture, *p. 779*
closed chest injury, *p. 774*
commotio cordis, *p. 780*
flail chest, *p. 775*
hemoptysis, *p. 783*

hemothorax, *p. 778*
myocardial contusion, *p. 774*
open chest injury, *p. 774*
paradoxical motion, *p. 775*
pericardial tamponade, *p. 778*
pneumothorax, *p. 777*

pulmonary contusion, *p. 774*
pulse pressure, *p. 779*
sucking chest wound, *p. 777*
tension pneumothorax, *p. 777*
traumatic asphyxia, *p. 781*

## Chapter Overview

Many outdoor activities carry inherent risks that can expose participants to serious bodily injury, including chest trauma. Patients do not experience chest trauma as often as they experience injuries to the extremities. Patients with chest trauma may appear to be stable at first, but if the injury is not recognized and treated quickly, severe consequences that can rapidly lead to death are possible. In outdoor settings, even

*continued*

## HISTORICAL TIMELINE

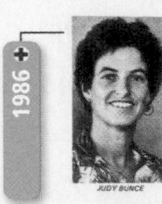

1986 — NSP hires first National Education Director.

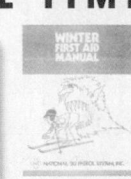

1986 — Field trials of new WEC program begin.

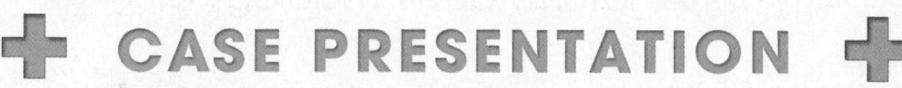

## CASE PRESENTATION

You are riding the chair lift above the terrain park when you observe a snowboarder entering the half pipe. He launches off the lip and rotates backward in the air. Miscalculating his position, he slams into the rail on the top deck and slides down the wall. When he comes to a stop, you can see that he is lying motionless on the snow. You radio your partner to respond with a toboggan. Upon reaching the summit, you hear your partner, who is now at the scene, requesting a trauma pack, an ambulance, and ALS. Grabbing the pack that includes oxygen from the summit hut, you proceed to the scene. Upon your arrival, the patient is sitting up and is complaining of difficulty breathing. He is resisting your partner's attempts to maintain manual spinal stabilization.

*What should you do?*

seemingly minor chest injuries can present numerous challenges because they can complicate other injuries or aggravate underlying medical conditions. For example, a nondisplaced rib fracture could make breathing difficult for someone who had to self-evacuate from the backcountry. The care for serious chest injuries includes addressing the ABCDs, caring for the specific condition, providing oxygen, and transporting rapidly to a higher level of care.

The chest (or thorax) contains such vital organs responsible for sustaining life as the heart, lungs, and great vessels. Protected by the bony rib cage and the thoracic spine, the thoracic cavity can withstand considerable force. Despite its resilient nature, the thorax is not impervious to injury. It can be damaged via the various mechanisms of injury previously described in Chapter 17, Principles of Trauma. Trauma can cause superficial injuries that affect only the chest wall, or it can cause internal injuries to the organs and structures within the chest. Due to quick compensation by normal systemic mechanisms, serious thoracic injuries may initially seem minor or go undetected. Repeated assessment of the patient and the vital signs over time may reveal that the injury is quickly becoming life threatening.

Chest injuries account for approximately 25 percent of all traumatic deaths in the United States. In winter sports, snowboarders suffer a higher rate of chest injuries than do skiers (6 percent vs. 3 percent) and are more likely to sustain rib fractures (55 percent vs. 41 percent), most often because of failed freestyle maneuvers. As more skiers enter terrain parks, this statistic may change. Snowmobilers, off-piste travelers, rafters, alpine climbers, and those who traverse avalanche-prone terrain are also at increased risk for chest trauma. Up to 10 percent of blunt thoracic injuries and 15–30 percent of penetrating chest injuries require urgent surgical intervention. Even when surgery is not indicated, intensive in-hospital supportive care is often required while injuries heal.

OEC Technicians should be familiar with the anatomy and physiology of the thorax and its internal organs. Review the appropriate sections of Chapter 6, Anatomy and Physiology before proceeding, or refer to those sections as you read this chapter. Being familiar with the different accident mechanisms that can produce a chest injury and the signs and symptoms of specific thoracic injuries will enable you to make better decisions regarding the petient's treatment and the need for urgent transportation, both of which will help significantly in reducing morbidity and mortality from thoracic trauma.

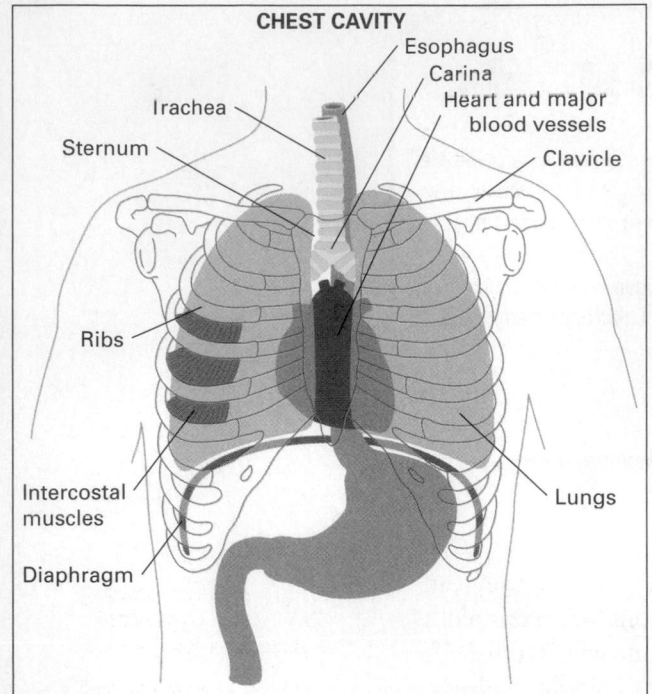

**CHEST CAVITY**

Esophagus
Carina
Trachea
Heart and major
blood vessels
Sternum
Clavicle

Ribs

Lungs

Intercostal
muscles

Diaphragm

**Figure 23-1** The anatomy of the chest cavity.

**23-1** List the major anatomical structures of the thoracic cavity.

**23-2** Describe the basic physiology of thoracic structures.

# Anatomy and Physiology of the Chest

The thorax extends from the base of the neck to the lower edge of the rib cage or costal margin (Figure 23-1■). It is enclosed by the bony rib cage, sternum, thoracic spine, and diaphragm. The ribs protect the thoracic organs and provide structural support through their connections to the thoracic vertebrae in the back and to the sternum through flexible cartilages in front. The thoracic cavity contains two major organs necessary for life: the lungs, which take in oxygen and excrete gaseous waste products, and the heart, which pumps the blood. The heart lies near the center of the chest beneath the sternum. Between the lungs is the area known as the mediastinum, which contains the heart, aorta, vena cava, trachea, esophagus, thymus gland, and several nerves.

Each lung is divided into vertically arrayed lobes. The right lung has three lobes, whereas the left has only two lobes because the apex of the heart slightly intrudes into the left side of the chest. The trachea divides into two bronchi at a point known as the carina, located just behind the top of the sternum. Each bronchus divides into progressively smaller branches until the air passages reach the aveoli, where gas exchange occurs.

The diaphragm, the primary muscle of respiration, separates the thoracic and abdominal cavities. This dome-shaped sheet of muscle attaches anteriorly at the xiphoid process, posteriorly at the lumbar vertebrae, and laterally at the lower ribs. During inhalation, the diaphragm contracts and descends into the abdomen, enlarging the thoracic cavity and creating a negative pressure within the chest, which draws oxygen-containing air into the lungs. During exhalation the diaphragm passively relaxes and returns to its resting position. This reduces the volume of the thoracic cavity and raises the internal pressure, expelling unused gases and carbon dioxide from the body.

The diaphragm is controlled by two "phrenic" nerves that connect to the spinal cord at levels $C_3$, $C_4$, and $C_5$ in the neck and travel to the diaphragm. Spinal cord injury at or above this level impairs respiration because the loss of signals through the phrenic nerves affects diaphragmatic function. This is why a patient will suffocate if the spinal cord is transected at or above $C_3$. The diaphragm is assisted in the work of breathing by the intercostal muscles, which are located between the ribs. Embedded within these muscles under each rib are the intercostal arteries, veins, and nerves.

The thoracic cavity contains two types of pleura: the visceral pleura, which surrounds the lungs, and the parietal pleura, which lines the inside wall of the chest. Between the visceral and parietal pleurae is a small amount of serous fluid, which acts as a lubricant that allows the lungs to move freely while they expand and contract. Normally there is no space between the two pleural layers, but trauma and various disease processes can change this and create breathing problems.

The heart is contained within a sac called the pericardium. As is the case for the pleurae, a small amount of serous fluid within the pericardium allows the heart to move freely inside the pericardium with each beat. Normally, little space exists between the sac and the heart, but injuries or other conditions that allow fluid or blood to accumulate within the pericardial sac can compromise heart function and reduce cardiac output.

The thoracic cavity is unusual in that its overall size changes during each respiration. Its size also can change due to the relative positions of the diaphragm or of the body as a whole. For instance, when a person is in a supine position, the diaphragm may rise as high as the level of the nipples. Thus, what appears to be a chest injury by the external location of a wound may actually be an abdominal injury, and vice versa.

# STOP, THINK, UNDERSTAND

## Multiple Choice

Choose the correct answer.

1. Which of the following statements regarding chest injuries is true?_____
   a. The internal structures of the thoracic cavity are frequently injured because they are poorly protected by overlying bony structures.
   b. Severe chest injuries may initially be asymptomatic due to the body's excellent compensatory mechanisms.
   c. Because it takes a large amount of force to cause thoracic injury, most chest injuries are obvious and quickly apparent.
   d. There is little OEC Technicians can do for patients suffering from thoracic injuries beyond administering oxygen and providing rapid extrication to definitive medical care.

2. The large muscle that does much of the work of breathing and separates the thoracic and abdominal cavities is the_____
   a. vena cava.
   b. vastus lateralis.
   c. mediastinum.
   d. diaphragm.

## Fill in the Blank

1. The superior anatomical boundary of the chest cavity is the _____, and the inferior boundary is the _____.

2. The left lung has _____ lobes, whereas the right lung has _____ lobes.

3. The diaphragm attaches anteriorly at the _____, posteriorly at the _____, and laterally at the _____.

## Labeling

1. Label the following components of the thoracic cavity on the accompanying figure: clavicles, sternum, xiphoid process, and lungs.

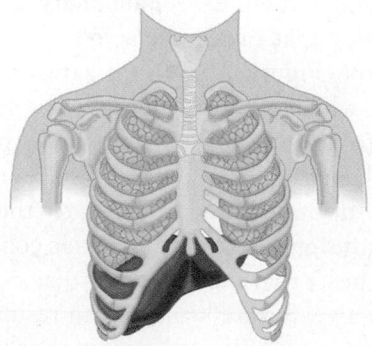

2. Label the following components of the lungs on the accompanying figure: oral pharynx; nasal pharynx; lungs; carina; pleura; trachea; epiglottis.

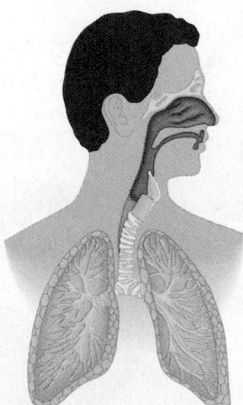

**closed chest injury** a chest injury without penetration of the chest cavity.

**open chest injury** a chest injury that involves penetration of the chest wall.

⊕ **23-3** Describe the pathology of the following thoracic injuries:

- flail chest
- pneumothorax
- hemothorax
- tension pneumothorax
- sucking chest wound
- pericardial tamponade

⊕ **23-4** List the signs and symptoms of various thoracic injuries.

**pulmonary contusion** a bruise of the lung tissue.

**myocardial contusion** a bruise of the heart muscle.

**Figure 23-2** A pulmonary contusion is a bruise on the lung tissue that causes the alveoli to fill with fluid and blood.

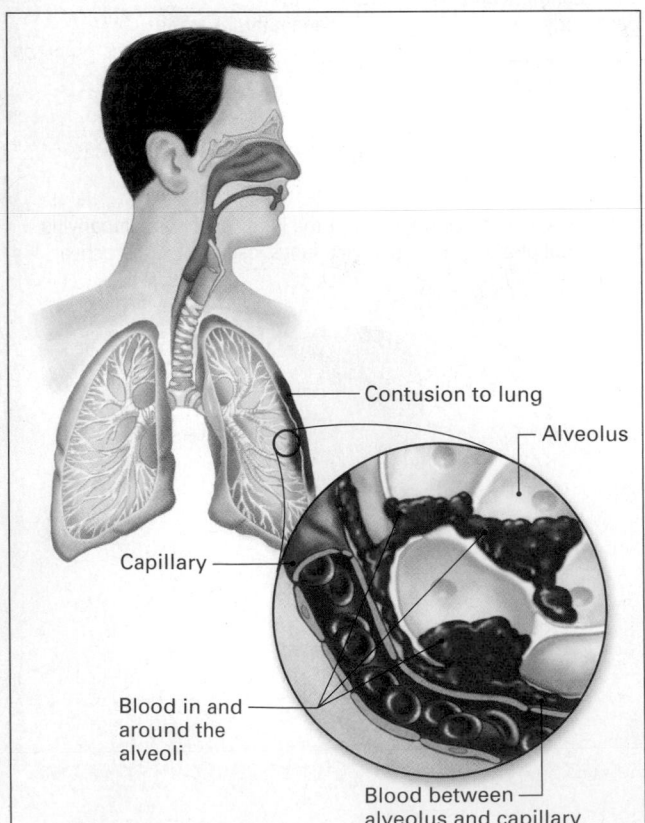

Contusion to lung

Alveolus

Capillary

Blood in and around the alveoli

Blood between alveolus and capillary

# Chest Injuries

## Mechanisms of Injury

Injuries to the chest are normally described as either closed or open. A **closed chest injury** is typically caused by blunt trauma and frequently occurs as a result of a fall or collision with a large object, such as a tree. An **open chest injury** is caused by physical penetration of the chest cavity by an object such as a tree branch, ski pole, or knife. Compression is another common mechanism of injury for chest trauma. Internal damage of thoracic structures can occur directly due to applied force to the heart or lungs, or it can occur indirectly such as when a fractured rib lacerates a nearby structure. Thoracic damage can also be caused by inertia, as when sudden deceleration of the body after a fall or a vehicular crash causes tissues such as the ascending aorta to violently tear away from their attachments. Regardless of the source, internal chest injuries are more difficult to assess, and sometimes to manage, than are more obvious external injuries, and they almost always require advanced care.

## Types of Chest Injury

OEC Technicians may encounter several thoracic injuries, including the following:

- contusions
- fractures and dislocations
- flail chest
- pneumothorax/hemothorax
- pericardial tamponade
- aortic tear or rupture

In addition, OEC Technicians may encounter other forms of chest trauma such as commotio cordis or traumatic asphyxia. Although less common, the potential for these injuries in recreational settings is real, and they can be rapidly fatal if they are not recognized and treated quickly.

### Contusions

Like any body part, the chest is susceptible to a variety of soft-tissue injuries. Minor blunt trauma may result in a simple contusion of the chest wall that is accompanied by localized swelling, bruising, and pain. More significant mechanisms of injury can cause internal organ contusions and can occur even when the skin over the rib cage has not been penetrated. In such cases, forcible compression of the chest wall causes damage to underlying structures. A **pulmonary contusion** is a bruise of the lung tissue that causes the alveoli to become filled with fluid and blood (Figure 23-2■). As a result, gas exchange is compromised, which can cause hypoxia, the severity of which is proportional to the size of the contusion. A pulmonary contusion commonly occurs in patients who suffer rib fractures, even if the bones do not directly lacerate the lung tissue. A **myocardial contusion**, also called a cardiac contusion, is a bruise involving the heart that may cause cardiac contractions to become less effective. Severe bruising can result in an arrythmia, reduced cardiac output, or cardiogenic shock.

### Fractures and Dislocations

Impact-type injuries are the most common cause of fractures of the bones of the anterior and lateral chest wall, including the ribs, clavicle, and sternum. Crushing injuries can also cause fractures.

The thoracic cage is an anatomical marvel that can withstand relatively high amounts of energy while remaining intact. When fractures occur, OEC Technicians must have a high index of suspicion for internal damage because energy that is great enough to fracture a bone may be transmitted to underlying structures. Clavicle and rib fractures are among the most common thoracic injuries and are an inherent risk in many outdoor activities. Clavicle fractures are discussed in Chapter 20, Musculoskeletal Injuries.

## Rib Fractures

Rib fractures can impair breathing due to intense pain that is usually centered over the fracture site. Breathing is often shallow because deep respirations increase movements of the fractured bone, intensifying the pain. To lessen discomfort, patients may "self-splint" or apply direct pressure over the injured site to keep the fractured bone ends from moving. In some instances, the sharp end of a displaced fractured rib can lacerate underlying lung tissue, blood vessels, or both, causing additional problems that will be described later in this section.

The elderly are at high risk for fractured ribs because their bones are more brittle than those of younger individuals. If multiple ribs are broken, a flail chest (discussed next) can occur.

## Flail Chest

A **flail chest** is defined as two or more adjacent ribs, each of which is fractured in two or more places (Figure 23-3■). Alternatively, two or more ribs could be separated from the spine posteriorly, or from the sternum anteriorly, and be broken in a separate place, and still be considered a flail chest. The resulting thoracic instability causes the injured segment of the chest wall to move independently of the rest of the rib cage. The isolated segment, or "flail" segment, moves inward upon inspiration and outward upon expiration, which is the opposite movement from that of the rest of the chest, a condition known as **paradoxical motion**.

Patients with a flail chest usually complain of severe chest wall pain and shortness of breath. They may attempt to self-splint the injured area by firmly holding the flail segment in place as they breathe.

Be alert for other associated injuries, because the forces required to produce a flail chest are sufficient to cause more serious internal injuries. The lung tissue directly beneath the flail segment is often contused and may not expand properly. Even though patients self-splint the injury site, shallow breathing, and underlying lung contusion can quickly result in the patient becoming hypoxic.

## Scapula Fracture

Scapula fractures are associated with severe trauma and serious internal injury. For more information about scapula fractures, refer to Chapter 20, Musculosketelal Injuries.

## Sternum Fracture

Fractures of the sternum, although uncommon, can be life threatening because the significant force required to break this very hard bone can cause underlying organ damage. A serious myocardial or pulmonary contusion should always be suspected with a fractured sternum. Rarely, the entire sternum can become a flail segment should the ribs on both sides become fractured or separated from the sternal cartilage. The most common source of

**flail chest** a condition in which two or more adjacent ribs are fractured in two or more places, causing a free-floating segment of the chest wall.

**paradoxical motion** inward movement of a flail chest segment upon inhalation.

**Figure 23-3** A flail chest is when each of two or more adjacent ribs are fractured in two or more places.

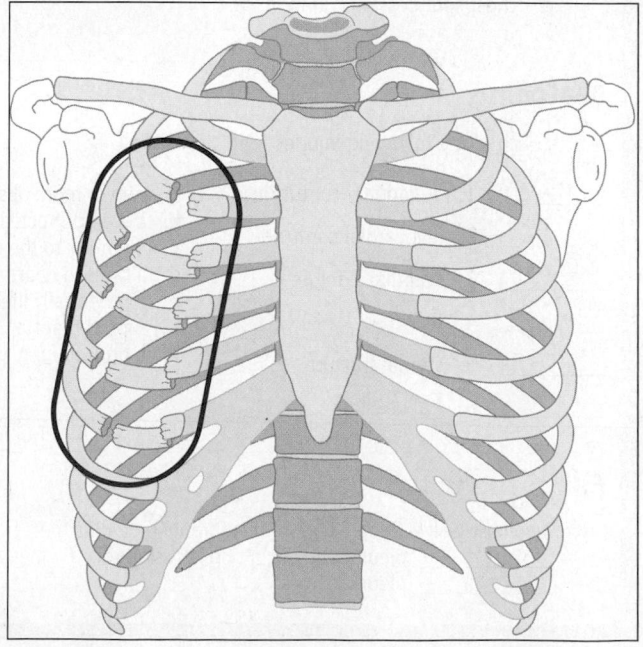

this is external chest compressions applied during CPR, even when performed properly. High-speed blunt chest trauma also can produce this type of injury. Seat belts help prevent this injury by preventing drivers from hitting the center of the steering wheel. If a patient has a sternal injury resulting from a very rapid deceleration, suspect an associated rupturing or tearing of the aorta, which is life threatening.

### Sternoclavicular Joint Injury

The sternoclavicular joint, which is formed where the clavicle inserts onto the sternum, can become dislocated. If a patient complains of pain at the sternoclavicular joint, palpation may demonstrate a posterior clavicle dislocation under the sternum, with a skin depression next to where the clavicle attaches to the sternum. The medial clavicle should normally be immediately under the skin. In this situation the medial clavicle has dislocated posteriorly and can put pressure on the great vessels, trachea, esophagus, and structures around it, causing a true emergency. This is discussed in more detail in Chapter 20, Musculoskeletal Injuries.

## STOP, THINK, UNDERSTAND

### Multiple Choice

Choose the correct answer.

1. Which of the following statements about a flail chest is true?_____
   a. Paradoxical motion occurs whenever a rib is fractured.
   b. Paradoxical motion is characterized by the flail segment moving outward with inspiration and inward with expiration.
   c. A patient with a flail chest can become hypoxic very quickly.
   d. Unlike other fractures, a flail chest can be difficult to diagnose because it is relatively painless.

2. The most common cause of a sternum fracture is_____
   a. blunt trauma such as a collision with a tree.
   b. penetrating trauma such as being impaled by a tree branch.
   c. a spontaneous fracture, which is most common among elderly individuals.
   d. chest compressions during CPR.

3. A space between the pleural layers is_____
   a. normal.
   b. caused by exhalation.
   c. caused by inhalation.
   d. caused by trauma.

4. The mediastinum contains which of the following structures? (check all that apply)
   _____ a. Spleen
   _____ b. Liver
   _____ c. Heart
   _____ d. Lungs
   _____ e. Great vessels
   _____ f. Diaphragm
   _____ g. Pancreas

### Matching

Match each of the following injuries to its description.

_____ 1. pulmonary contusion

_____ 2. myocardial contusion

_____ 3. scapular fracture

_____ 4. flail chest

_____ 5. sternal fracture

_____ 6. fractured rib

a. two or more ribs fractured in two or more places
b. a well-protected bony structure which is usually fractured only by severe force trauma
c. an injury to the thoracic cavity that may result in internal injuries as well
d. a bruised heart muscle that can no longer maintain a regular beat, resulting in cardiogenic shock
e. a potentially life-threatening fracture which can result in myocardial or pulmonary contusion or a ruptured aorta
f. a bruised lung, which can result in the alveoli filling with fluid and blood, causing hypoxia

### Fill in the Blank

1. The chest wall is lined by a thin membrane known as the _____ pleura, and each lung is surrounded by the _____ pleura.

2. A substance known as _____ fluid acts as a lubricant between the two layers of the thoracic cavity.

## Lower Rib Cage Injury

Cartilage along the bottom of the anterior rib cage can be torn, stretched, or separated from the bone, mimicking the signs and symptoms of rib fracture. This condition is usually benign but can be quite painful and may hinder breathing. In the field it is difficult to differentiate from a broken rib.

## Pneumothorax

Under normal conditions, each lung lies very close to the inside of the thoracic cavity. Between the surface of the lung and the inside of the chest wall is the (potential) pleural space. Trauma or a leak in the lung can cause air to collect in the pleural space, a condition known as a **pneumothorax**. This condition is manifested by shortness of breath or hypoxia because air in the pleura space prevents the lung from fully expanding.

**pneumothorax** air in the pleural space.

A pneumothorax can be caused by either blunt or penetrating trauma, or it can occur spontaneously due to underlying disease such as asthma, sudden changes in altitude, or other causes. It can also be caused by compressive forces on the chest and by blast injuries.

The most common source of pneumothorax is penetrating trauma in which a hole in the chest wall allows external air to enter the pleural space. With each inspiration, the difference between the pressure within the thorax and the pressure in the external environment causes air to be sucked into the pleural space, particularly when the size of the hole is three-fourths the diameter of the trachea or greater (Figure 23-4a■). If enough air enters the pleural space, the lung may partially collapse, resulting in decreased gas exchange and hypoxia. With this type of injury, OEC Technicians may hear a sucking noise each time the patient breathes as air enters the pleural space. This situation is known as a "**sucking chest wound**" and requires rapid treatment and transport to prevent serious complications.

**sucking chest wound** a chest wound that penetrates the pleura or lung, allowing air to be "sucked" into the pleural space upon each inspiration.

Pneumothorax also may occur as a result of blunt trauma. A direct blow that covers a large area of the thoracic wall at the peak of the inspiratory cycle can cause one or both lungs to burst. If air continues to accumulate within the pleural space, it can lead to an even more dangerous condition known as a tension pneumothorax.

A **tension pneumothorax** is defined as an accumulation of pressurized air within the pleural space. Left untreated, this build-up of intrathoracic pressure can cause the organs within the thoracic cavity to become compressed, resulting in reduced lung capacity, severe respiratory distress, and eventually decreased cardiac output. With sufficient pressure, one lung will completely collapse. As more pressure builds, the heart, great vessels, and trachea within the mediastinum are pushed into the opposite side of the chest, sometimes collapsing the other lung. A rapid reduction in blood volume being pumped to the lungs occurs because the vena cava collapses, so no blood is returned to the right side of the heart (Figure 23-4b■). The development of tension pneumothorax in both lungs is likely rapidly fatal.

**tension pneumothorax** the accumulation of pressurized air within the pleural space; causes the displacement of the great vessels, tracheal deviation, distention of the jugular veins, and compression of the other lung.

Tension pneumothorax can also develop in closed chest trauma when a sharp bone fragment of a fractured rib punctures a lung or bronchus. Air leaks out of the hole in the lung or bronchus and into the pleural space. Pressure can build within minutes to a few hours, creating the same life-threatening situation. Finally, a tension pneumothorax can develop, or be made *worse*, by the application of positive pressure such as occurs in rescue breathing using a bag-valve mask. With each breath, more air passes through any internal airway hole into the pleural space, thereby changing a stable pneumothorax into an unstable tension pneumothorax.

The hallmarks of a tension pneumothorax are shortness of breath, distended neck veins (known as jugular venous distention or JVD), tachycardia, low blood

**OPEN PNEUMOTHORAX**        **TENSION PNEUMOTHORAX**        **HEMOTHORAX**

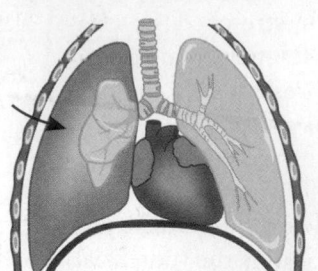 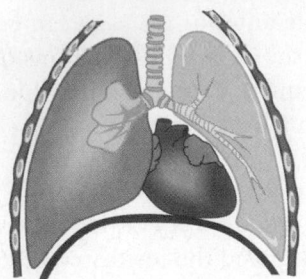 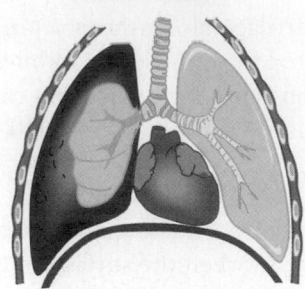

(a) Air enters the chest cavity through an open chest wound or leaks from a lacerated lung. The lung cannot expand.

(b) Air continuously fills pleural space, lung collapses, pressure rises, and the trapped air compresses the heart and other lung.

(c) Blood leaks into the chest cavity from lacerated vessels or the lung itself and the lung compresses.

**Figure 23-4** Three complications of chest injuries. (a) Open pneumothorax. (b) Tension pneumothorax. (c) Hemothorax.

pressure, and cyanosis. Decreased lung sounds are detected in the lung that has deflated. Tracheal deviation, in which the trachea shifts away from the side of the tension pneumothorax, may be observed, but this is a very late sign.

Tension pneumothorax can lead to subcutaneous emphysema, or "sub-Q air." In this condition, pressurized air leaks out of the pleural cavity into the soft tissues and becomes trapped under the skin, causing a Rice-Krispies®-like "crackling" sensation of the skin when pressed with the fingers. This condition is generally exhibited in the neck first but can spread to the shoulders, chest, or back, depending on the patient's position. Because air rises, subcutaneous emphysema is typically found in the highest point of the thoracic cavity. This condition is usually benign, but the pneumothorax causing it can be life threatening.

Rarely, pneumothorax can occur spontaneously, typically in young adults. In this situation, no trauma occurs; however, a small air pocket (or bleb) on the lung surface ruptures, allowing air to escape into the pleural space. The signs and symptoms of this type of pneumothorax are identical to those previously described and can advance to become a tension pneumothorax should enough air enter the space. Patients experience sharp pain in the chest and back.

### Hemothorax

**hemothorax** an accumulation of blood in the pleural space.

A **hemothorax** is similar to a pneumothorax except that instead of air, blood accumulates within the pleural space (Figure 23-4c■). This condition is caused by disruption of one or more blood vessels within the chest and can be due to either blunt or penetrating trauma. Hemothorax can also occur spontaneously as a result of a thoracic aneurysm, although this is very rare. Hemothorax due to arterial bleeding can be potentially lethal; because the pleural space can hold 3–4 liters of blood, profound hypovolemic shock can quickly ensue. The pathology of hemothorax is likewise similar to pneumothorax in that blood can compress or collapse one or both lungs, resulting in hypoxia and shock. As with other types of chest trauma, pain and shortness of breath are common complaints.

In some instances both air and blood can leak into the pleural space simultaneously, producing a condition known as a hemopneumothorax. The mechanisms of injury that can produce hemopneumothorax are associated with multi-system trauma and have a high morbidity and mortality.

### Pericardial Tamponade

**pericardial tamponade** the accumulation of blood or other fluid within the pericardial sac.

Blunt or penetrating chest trauma can cause bleeding of the heart or the great vessels into the pericardial sac, causing the condition known as **pericardial tamponade**

(Figure 23-5■). The rupture of a cardiac vessel or a small hole in the heart's wall can also cause this problem. Pericardial tamponade also may be caused by various nontraumatic medical conditions in which fluid other than blood accumulates within the pericardial sac. In bacterial sepsis, pus may be the source of the tamponade. Viral infections around the heart can cause serous fluid to compress the heart.

As blood or other fluid accumulates within the fibrous pericardial sac, pressure builds on the heart. Because the left ventricular wall is thicker than the right, the right ventricle collapses first. This prevents the walls of the right side of the heart from expanding, impairing venous return of blood from the venae cavae. At the same time, blood backs up into the jugular veins in the neck. With less blood being pumped to the lungs for oxygenation, cardiogenic shock and death occur rapidly.

Pain, shortness of breath, and distended neck veins are early signs of pericardial tamponade. If the problem is not immediately resolved, muffled heart sounds and a decrease in the **pulse pressure** develop. The combination of findings—distended neck veins, muffled heart sounds, and a pulsus paradoxus—is known as Beck's Triad.

## Aortic Rupture and Dissection

Rapid deceleration injuries are common sources of injury in many outdoor activities and can cause a host of potentially serious problems that may not be immediately apparent. **Aortic rupture** is the most lethal of these hidden injuries.

When the moving human body dramatically slows or stops rapidly when the chest hits a fixed object, the structures within the chest remain in motion for a short period of time. This inertia and the sudden stop inflict a tremendous shearing force on the

### What Is Pulsus Paradoxus?

During every inspiration, blood pressure becomes noticeably reduced; during every exhalation, BP increases. Pulsus paradoxus is a clinical sign in which a decrease in systolic blood pressure of 10 mmHg or more occurs upon inspiration. Pulsus paradoxus is caused by a variety of thoracic injuries, including cardiac tamponade, and by such medical disorders as emphysema, pulmonary embolism, and left ventricular failure.

**pulse pressure**   the difference between the maximum (systolic) and minimum (diastolic) blood pressures during a single heartbeat.

**aortic rupture**   development of a leak in the largest blood vessel in the body; results in massive bleeding that is usually fatal.

**Figure 23-5** The physical findings of pericardial tamponade.

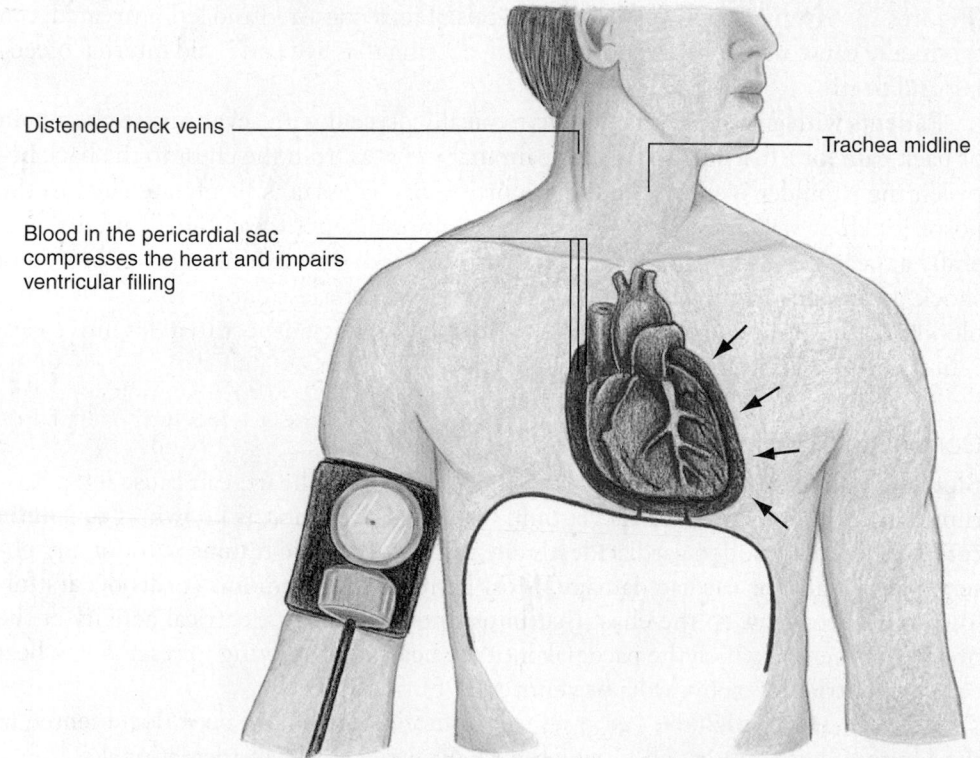

Distended neck veins

Trachea midline

Blood in the pericardial sac compresses the heart and impairs ventricular filling

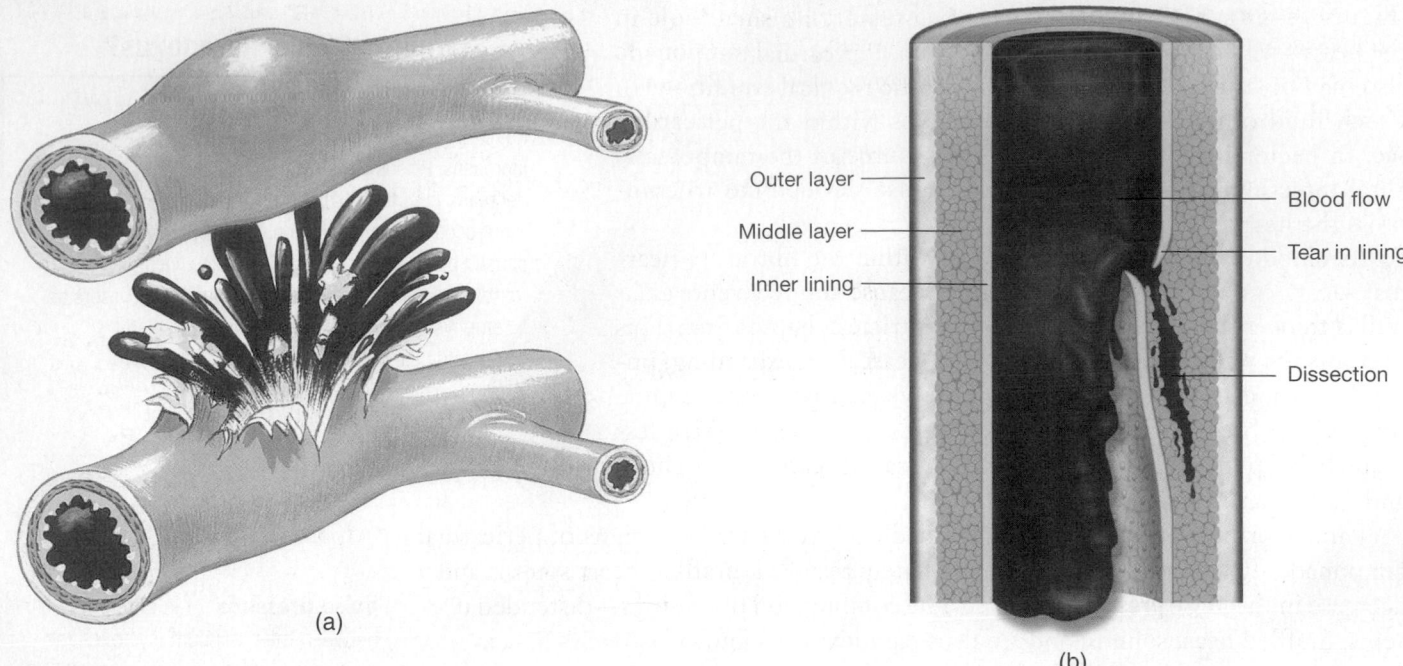

**Figure 23-6**   (a) The progression of an aortic aneurysm to aortic rupture. (b) Aortic dissection.

**aneurysm**   ballooning of an artery that weakens it and predisposes it to rupture.

internal organs and on the tissues that hold them in place. The aorta is especially vulnerable to deceleration injuries; the resulting rupture or tearing is usually followed by rapid internal hemorrhage, hypovolemic shock, and death. A tear in the aorta may occur when only part of the thickness of the vessel's wall is disrupted. This condition is not always immediately fatal, but it can cause other conditions, most notably an **aneurysm** (ballooning of the less dense outer layer of the wall of the aorta) or aortic dissection, in which blood leaks out between the layers of the wall of the aorta (Figures 23-6a■ and 23-6b■). Both conditions, if unrecognized and left untreated, can eventually cause the vessel to rupture, again causing massive and rapid internal bleeding and death.

Patients with an aorta-related injury typically present with severe acute chest pain or back pain, or a tearing or stabbing pain that radiates from the chest to the back between the shoulder blades. The upper portion of the aorta is firmly attached to the posterior chest wall and thus this is where it is most likely to tear. Such patients generally appear gravely ill, and if the aorta has ruptured, they exhibit signs of profound shock. If the tear in the aorta is between the large arteries that go to each arm the blood pressure can be different in the two arms. Rapid transport to a definitive care center is necessary to prevent a lethal outcome.

### Commotio Cordis

**commotio cordis**   sudden cardiac death due to blunt thoracic trauma without any observable thoracic or cardiac damage.

Blunt trauma to the chest, especially to the area over the heart, can cause lethal disruptions in the heart's electrical rhythm. One such condition is known as **commotio cordis,** defined as sudden cardiac death due to blunt thoracic trauma without any observable thoracic or cardiac damage. Most commonly, commotio cordis occurs following a direct blow to the chest that interrupts the heart's electrical activity at the precise moment in which the pacemaker of the heart is attempting to reset after a beat causing ventricular tachycardia or ventricular fibrillation.

Between 1998 and 2009, 128 cases of commotio cordis have been documented in the United States, almost all of which have occurred in urban recreational settings.

The condition most often affects young, healthy individuals, with more than 90 percent of cases occurring in children less than 16 years of age. Of concern to OEC Technicians is that as more young children flock to our nation's snow terrain parks and BMX bicycle parks, the potential for this injury is increasing. Although most reported cases involve direct anterior chest trauma from a baseball, a softball, or a lacrosse ball, one case involved a snowball, and in another case a child was hit in the chest by a snow sliding saucer.

## Traumatic Asphyxia

**Traumatic asphyxia**, or crush asphyxia, is an injury in which external pressure on the chest wall prevents normal chest expansion for breathing, resulting in profound hypoxia or anoxia (Figure 23-7■). This injury involves compression that is typically caused by entrapment under a heavy object, such as a vehicle or avalanche debris. It also can result from massive thoracic cage fractures that render the chest wall unable to expand.

Traumatic asphyxia may result in ruptured blood vessels, particularly in the face and neck, which can cause bulging eyes, ruptured blood vessels in the eyes, and an overall purplish discoloration of the face.

**TRAUMATIC ASPHYXIA**

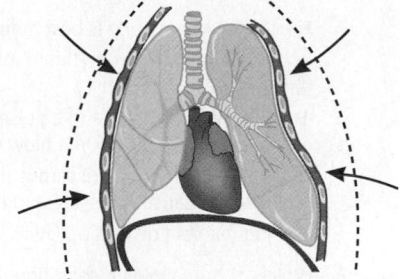

Severe chest compression puts pressure on heart and forces blood back into vein of the neck. It may cause severe lung damage.

**Figure 23-7** Traumatic asphyxia.

**traumatic asphyxia** the inability to breathe and hypoxia that results from the inability of the chest wall to expand due to external pressure or massive crushing trauma.

# STOP, THINK, UNDERSTAND

## Multiple Choice
Choose the correct answer.

1. Which of the following statements about lungs is false? _____
   a. They normally fill up the entire thoracic cavity.
   b. The pleural space between the lungs and chest wall is normally filled with air.
   c. Negative pressure causes air to rush into the lungs.
   d. Small air sacs known as alveoli allow air to enter into the visceral pleural space.

2. Which of the following conditions or situations can cause a pneumothorax? (check all that apply)
   _____ a. prolonged shortness of breath
   _____ b. blunt trauma
   _____ c. penetrating trauma
   _____ d. asthma
   _____ e. traveling rapidly from sea level to an altitude of 9,000 feet
   _____ f. a compression injury
   _____ g. an allergic reaction

3. Which of the following statements about a tension pneumothorax is true?_____
   a. Due to a mediastinal shift, it can result in no blood returning to the right side of the heart.
   b. A tension pneumothorax is caused by blunt trauma, whereas a hemothorax is caused by penetrating trauma.
   c. You cannot make a tension pneumothorax worse by ventilating a patient with a positive pressure breathing device such as a bag-valve mask.
   d. All of these statements are true.

4. Which of the following are possible signs or symptoms of a tension pneumothorax? (check all that apply)
   _____ a. shortness of breath
   _____ b. distended neck veins (JVD)
   _____ c. tachycardia
   _____ d. cyanosis
   _____ e. tracheal deviation
   _____ f. Rice-Krispies™-like crackling sensation of the skin
   _____ g. bradycardia
   _____ h. hypertension

5. Which of the following statements about a hemothorax is true?_____
   a. It occurs when air accumulates in the pleural space.
   b. It can cause aortic rupture.
   c. It can be caused only by penetrating trauma.
   d. It can result in 3–4 liters of blood accumulating in the pleural space.

6. The pericardial sac contains which of the following organs?_____
   a. the lungs
   b. the heart and the bases of the great vessels
   c. the bronchioles and alveoli
   d. the mediastinum

continued

## STOP, THINK, UNDERSTAND *continued*

7. Pericardial tamponade is best defined as _____
   a. an irregular heart rhythm due to a disruption in the heart's electrical conductivity.
   b. a complete absence of a pulse (a heartbeat) due to a disruptive blunt-trauma blow to the heart muscle.
   c. a collection of blood, serous fluid, or pus within the pericardial sac that causes pressure and interferes with blood flow.
   d. jugular vein distension (JVD).

8. Which of the following conditions could cause pericardial tamponade? (check all that apply)
   _____ a. blunt-force chest trauma
   _____ b. penetrating chest trauma
   _____ c. bacterial sepsis
   _____ d. a buildup of serous fluid due to a viral infection

_____ e. a violent fit of coughing
_____ f. prolonged, violent vomiting

9. One of the most common causes of traumatic asphyxia during outdoor activities is_____
   a. being trapped beneath an avalanche.
   b. inhaling carbon monoxide.
   c. a sucking chest wound.
   d. bleeding from a myocardial contusion.

10. A potentially fatal blunt trauma injury that primarily affects young, healthy children in urban recreational settings is_____
    a. cardiac myopathy.
    b. commotio cordis.
    c. traumatic asphyxia.
    d. pericardial tamponade.

## Environmental Factors

High altitude can complicate a thoracic injury due to the decreased partial pressure of available oxygen and the lower barometric pressure (which expands gas volumes). Increased altitude may cause a pneumothorax to worsen. In one case report, a woman who had sustained an apparently mild chest injury boarded a commercial airliner. Even though the aircraft cabin maintained an atmospheric pressure equivalent to 8,000 feet, the relative change in air pressure caused a slight pneumothorax to worsen, resulting in severe difficulty breathing. A return to sea level relieved the patient's distress.

Descent in elevation may improve breathing and oxygenation for many chest injuries. When you have a patient with a pneumothorax, take them to a lower altitude rapidly. The effects of altitude have direct implications for OEC Technicians when considering the use of aeromedical evacuation of a patient with a suspected pneumothorax or other internal thoracic injury.

 **CASE UPDATE**

You calm the patient and convince him to allow your partner to maintain cervical spine stabilization while you perform an assessment. The patient's airway is open, there is no external bleeding, and circulation to all extremities is normal. The patient's mental status is also normal. He appears to be having moderate difficulty breathing and is holding his right upper chest and side with both hands. He has shallow respirations at 28 per minute that are unrelieved with high-flow oxygen via a nonrebreather mask. His pulse is 102 beats a minute. When you palpate the patient's rib cage, he winces in pain. He states that his chest hurts "real bad" and that it is painful to breathe. Other patrollers arrive to assist.

***What should you do now?***

# Assessment

Assessment of patients with a suspected thoracic injury is no different than for any other trauma patient. Begin with a scene size-up, evaluating and mitigating any hazards that may be present. Assess the mechanism of injury to determine the forces involved.

Upon completing the scene size-up, use appropriate Standard Precautions and begin a primary assessment. Carefully assess the ABCDs to ensure that they are intact. Open and clear the airway as necessary. Next, assess the patient for adequate breathing and oxygenation, paying particular attention to the rate and quality of respirations. A patient with a chest injury may exhibit rapid breathing or other signs of respiratory distress, including the use of accessory muscles. Next, control bleeding. Check the patient's pulse: is it fast, normal, or slow? Is it bounding or weak? Are the pulses equal on both sides of the body? Assess the patient's mental status and neurologic condition. Now mobilize additional resources as needed, including requesting advanced providers if the patient's condition warrants it.

Once the primary assessment is complete, quickly move on to a secondary assessment. Note the patient's overall appearance and skin color. Does the person appear anxious? Is the patient pale or cyanotic? Quickly check the head, face, and neck. Do the patient's eyes appear bloodshot or bulge outward, which could indicate traumatic asphyxia? Are the neck veins distended, which could suggest pericardial tamponade or tension pneumothorax? Is the trachea deviated to one side? Is there **hemoptysis**?

Ask the patient to take a deep breath and then exhale, and observe for any signs of discomfort such as wincing or self-splinting. Also observe the chest for equal and symmetrical movement. If you have a stethoscope, listen to each lung to make sure breath sounds are present bilaterally.

If major thoracic injuries are present or suspected, do not waste precious time identifying each individual injury. Instead, correct any life-threatening situations and prepare the patient for rapid evacuation to a definitive care facility.

When examining the thorax, use the systematic approach described in Chapter 7, Patient Assessment. Being systematic helps reduce the chance of overlooking potentially serious problems involving vital thoracic structures.

Environmental or other conditions can make it impractical to perform a detailed chest assessment in the field. One approach that is often used is the L.A.P. method, which divides the thoracic examination process into three parts:

+ **L**—Look
+ **A**—Auscultate
+ **P**—Palpate

To perform an L.A.P. exam, inspect the thorax, chest, upper back, and axillae (armpits) for obvious trauma using the DCAP-BTLS acronym. **Look** for contusions, deformity, and potentially serious injuries such as a sucking chest wound, an impaled object, or an obvious flail segment. As the patient breathes, see if both sides of the chest expand fully and symmetrically. Look for paradoxical motion of the chest in which a portion of the chest wall moves inward during inspiration. If present, suspect a flail chest and impending shock.

**Auscultate** the lungs both anteriorly and posteriorly to ensure that breath sounds are present, equal, and clear bilaterally. If breath sounds are absent or if any abnormal sounds are detected, suspect an internal injury to the pulmonary system or some

---

⊕ **23-5** Describe and demonstrate how to assess the chest for trauma, using the L.A.P. method.

**hemoptysis**  coughing up blood.

---

### Assessment

The patient's upper back and armpits are a part of the chest wall and should be thoroughly assessed. If penetrating trauma is suspected and it becomes necessary to move oversized or pendulous breasts or folds of fatty tissue out of the way to properly assess the chest wall, do so with diligent attention to the patient's comfort and dignity.

NOTE

underlying respiratory disease. OEC Technicians need not understand all of the different pathologic breath sounds. *Seasoned* OEC Technicians will become familiar with normal breath sounds and should be able to identify abnormalities, such as diminished (difficult to hear) breath sounds, which may indicate the presence of a pneumothorax.

**Palpate** the entire chest, axillary regions, and upper back for tenderness and deformity. Be sure to "walk" the patient's clavicles with your fingertips, because a displaced clavicle fracture may cause a pneumothorax. Fractures involving the scapula are especially ominous because tremendous force is usually required to break this bone. Many scapular and sternal fractures are associated with internal chest injuries.

Next, assess the integrity of the sternum, again using your fingertips and then the flat side of your hand. As you palpate the chest, be alert for subcutaneous emphysema or any flail segments. If you do not detect any obvious injuries, use both hands to apply moderate inward pressure on the lateral walls of the rib cage and ask the patient to take a deep breath. Then, apply moderate downward pressure on the sternum, again asking the patient to take a deep breath. If the patient experiences pain with either of these tests, stop. These two tests are very helpful in identifying thoracic cage instability or rib fractures that may not be readily apparent.

Complete the remainder of your secondary assessment in the usual fashion and obtain a complete set of vital signs. Reassess the patient frequently, including vital signs and breath sounds. Document your findings on the patient care report. Serial vital signs are essential in any case involving suspected thoracic trauma because changes may be subtle and could indicate internal bleeding and decompensated shock. Pay close attention to the pulse pressure. Narrowing of the pulse pressure may indicate the presence of a pericardial tamponade. Table 23-1■ summarizes the signs and symptoms of chest trauma.

---

⊕ **23-6** Describe and demonstrate the emergency management of a sucking chest wound.

---

# Management

Thoracic injuries are often associated with multi-system trauma and can very quickly progress to a life-threatening condition. Any thoracic injury that is associated with respiratory distress or hypotension is considered a "load and go" situation: correct any life-threatening conditions, provide oxygen, immobilize the spine if necessary, and rapidly evacuate the patient to a definitive care facility, preferably a designated trauma center.

Patients who have suffered commotio cordis will present in cardiac arrest and must be treated aggressively using current cardiopulmonary resuscitation techniques, including defibrillation. Likewise, patients with traumatic asphyxia must have the external pressure relieved from the thoracic cage quickly and then should be given aggressive ventilatory support.

If the patient has been caught in an avalanche, quickly remove snow or other avalanche debris from around the patient's chest. Ensure that the airway is open and clear, and that breathing efforts are effective. Use suction as necessary to ensure airway patency. If you suspect serious problems such as traumatic asphyxia, tension pneumotho-

| Table **23-1** | Signs and Symptoms of Chest Trauma |
|---|---|

- Pain at site of injury that can be aggravated by breathing
- Abnormal chest wall findings: punctures, contusions, unusual chest wall motion
- Dyspnea
- Tachypnea
- Cyanosis
- Hemoptysis
- Tachycardia
- Falling blood pressure

rax, or cardiac tamponade, summon additional assistance immediately. Call for transport and advanced care providers.

Apply high-flow oxygen via a nonrebreather mask if the patient's breathing efforts are spontaneous and effective. If necessary, assist ventilations using a bag-valve mask and supplemental oxygen. Again, if the patient worsens while bagging, think of tension pneumothorax. Control external bleeding using the procedures described in Chapter 18, Soft-Tissue Injuries.

Any obvious sucking chest wound should be treated immediately to prevent the development or worsening of an underlying pneumothorax. Begin by covering the wound with a gloved hand to occlude the opening. Next, cover the wound with an occlusive dressing. Even if there is no obvious "sucking" sound, it is appropriate to cover any penetrating thoracic wound with an occlusive dressing. Among the several commercial products available for this purpose are Vaseline® gauze, a Bolin™ chest seal, and an Asherman™ chest seal. If none of these products are available, an occlusive dressing may be improvised using plastic wrap, a plastic bag, aluminum foil, or other impermeable material. Tape the occlusive dressing in place on three sides, which will prevent air intake through the wound upon inspiration but will allow pressurized air within the thoracic cavity to escape. Monitor the patient closely for signs of tension pneumothorax, and readjust the dressing so that air can escape if there is evidence of air buildup (Figure 23-8■).

Remember that serious thoracic injuries are load and go situations. However, if a spinal injury is suspected, apply manual cervical spine stabilization and rapidly immobilize the entire spine using conventional procedures and equipment.

Treat other soft-tissue injuries of the chest in the usual manner using standard bandages and dressings. Bulky pressure dressings may be needed to help control heavy bleeding.

Rib fractures can be very painful, especially upon inspiration or movement. Carefully splint the affected area using soft, bulky dressings, and secure them to the chest to minimize the movement of fractured bone ends. Do not splint the chest if doing so will impair breathing or delay other needed care and transportation. It is best to avoid placing a

---

### Use of a Bag-Valve Mask

**NOTE**

Use caution when using a bag-valve mask in patients with a suspected lung tissue injury, and observe the results of your treatment closely. When there is a tension pneumothorax, using a bag-valve mask for ventilation may make the condition worse by forcing more air into the pleural space. In this situation, it may be better to allow patients who are still breathing on their own to breathe 100 percent oxygen using a high-flow rebreather mask without assistance. If the patient's respiration rate and depth are not adequate, you may have no choice but to continue ventilations.

---

### Advanced Life Support for Tension Pneumothorax

**NOTE**

In most areas, Advanced Life Support providers can provide needle chest decompression for tension pneumothorax in the field. The insertion of a needle into the pleural space allows the pressurized air in the chest to escape. Needle thoracostomy is *not* part of the OEC curriculum but is described in Chapter 36, ALS Interface.

---

**Figure 23-8** Taping an occlusive dressing on three sides of a sucking chest wound helps prevent a tension pneumothorax.

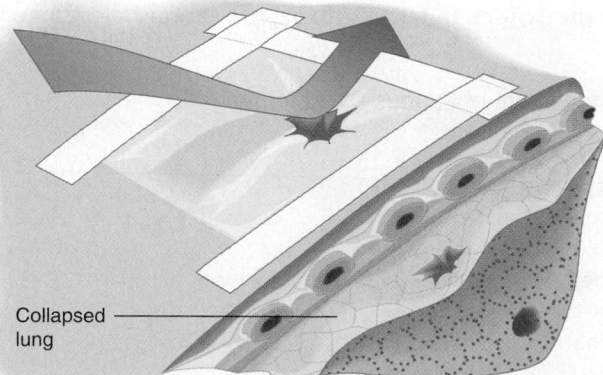

On inspiration, dressing seals wound, preventing air entry

Collapsed lung

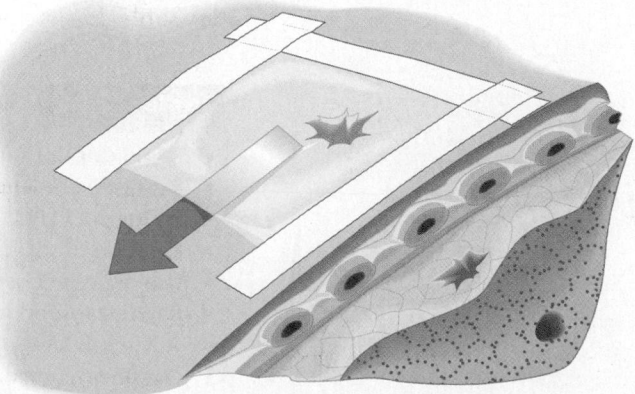

Expiration allows trapped air to escape through untaped section of dressing

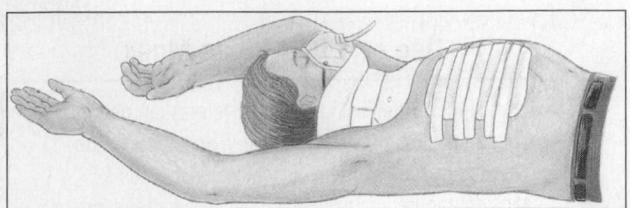

**Figure 23-9** Treat flail chest by administering oxygen and gently splinting the flail segment with a blanket, pillow, or pad.

tightly constrictive bandage around the circumference of the chest because it can inhibit chest wall expansion during inhalation.

Splint flail segments above and below the fractured section in the same manner as for an isolated rib fracture. If the flail segment is especially large, a large trauma dressing, pillow, folded clothing, magazine, or other material is often more effective in stabilizing the bones than are traditional dressings (Figure 23-9■). If the patient is able to hold the splint in place, encourage him to do so and then secure the splint and dressing against the chest wall. If the flail segment causes severe pain or respiratory distress, it may be helpful to assist the patient's respirations using a bag-valve mask and oxygen. The positive pressure from the bag-valve mask will reduce the paradoxical motion of the flail segment. If the patient will not tolerate the bag-valve mask, it may be better to minimize distress by using a high-flow nonrebreather mask and allowing the patient to sit quietly.

Impaled objects should be left in place. Objects such as a tree branch, ski pole, or knife should not be removed because the object may be preventing hemorrhage, pneumothorax, or exsanguination. If the impaled object is large, you may need to shorten it (e.g., trimming a tree branch) to facilitate safe, efficient transport.

When shortening an impaled object, avoid causing further injury due to excessive movement of the object. If using a cutting torch, be careful that the metal does not get hot enough to cause a thermal injury to the patient. Remove the impaled object from patients with rapidly deteriorating conditions *only* if the object is fixed (immovable) or if bringing in cutting equipment will take too long. In this situation, be ready to care for excessive bleeding, pneumothorax, or other threats to life once the object has been removed. It is always best to leave an impaled object in the patient if you can do so.

Give careful consideration when positioning the patient for transport. Normally, a patient with dyspnea in the absence of trauma will benefit from a head-uphill position in the toboggan or sitting position on a stretcher. Patients who have a serious chest injury may also benefit from being placed in a head-uphill position, which can reduce pressure on the diaphragm and thoracic organs and make breathing easier. However, many cases of thoracic trauma are accompanied by suspected spinal injury, which precludes transporting the patient in a seated position. In this case, consider elevating the head of the spine board to ease breathing efforts.

When the patient is in shock and breathing is the primary concern, keep the patient warm, oxygenated and in a head-uphill position. However, if profound hypovolemic shock is present, elevating the feet 8–12 inches above the level of the heart may be necessary and may be accomplished by placing the patient head-downhill during transport. The ultimate goal, of course, is to ensure that blood and oxygen reach the brain. Use common sense: for patients who are having difficulty breathing but have adequate perfusion, give oxygen, and transport head uphill; for patients in profound shock and poor perfusion, give oxygen and elevate the feet by transporting head downhill.

Table 23-2■ summarizes the actions to take in managing serious chest injuries.

**Table 23-2   Simple Management of Serious Chest Injury**

- Rapid care for ABCDs
- Support ventilation with bag-valve mask if needed
- Oxygen: 15 LPM via nonrebreather mask
- Immobilize spine if spinal injury suspected
- Use occlusive dressing on chest wounds, especially sucking wounds
- Rapid transport to definitive care at hospital
- Advanced Life Support en route if available
- Consider air medical transport

# STOP, THINK, UNDERSTAND

## Multiple Choice

Choose the correct answer.

1. L.A.P. is best described as_____
   a. last normal appearance, assessment, and palpation.
   b. laceration, avulsion, and penetration.
   c. look, auscultate, palpate.
   d. limited anterior pulses.

2. Which of the following actions do you take *first* for a patient who has been partially dug out of an avalanche but is apparently not breathing and has a thready pulse of 100? _____
   a. immediately begin ventilations with a bag-valve mask and high-flow $O_2$
   b. clear his chest, mouth, and nostrils of snow
   c. begin CPR
   d. quickly dig him out completely

3. What is the correct method for splinting a flail chest? _____
   a. Splint the flail segments above and below the fractured section using a soft, bulky dressing, a pillow, or clothing.
   b. Splint the flail segment by taping it to the surrounding ribs.

   c. Do not attempt to secure a flail segment, because doing so can cause serious injury to underlying organs.
   d. OEC Techicians should only allow self-splinting by the patient in a position of comfort.

4. Which of the following statements about an object impaled in the chest is true? _____
   a. Remove it *quickly*, then staunch any bleeding, administer $O_2$, and assist ventilations as needed.
   b. Remove it *slowly* to minimize damage, staunch any bleeding, and administer $O_2$ or assist breathing as needed.
   c. Leave and secure the object in place unless it must be removed to facilitate extrication or transportation.
   d. Never remove an impaled object because doing so may cause fatal bleeding.

5. The best treatment for a sucking chest wound is_____
   a. an occlusive dressing.
   b. load and go transport.
   c. ventilating the patient with a bag-valve mask.
   d. stabilizing the patient's chest wall with a pillow.

## Short Answer

When assessing a patient with chest injuries, you look, auscultate, and palpate. For each of these three actions, describe the clinical signs that you are looking to observe.

_____

_____

_____

_____

_____

 # CASE DISPOSITION

With the assistance of the other patrollers, you quickly immobilize the patient's spine on a long spine board, load him into a toboggan in a head-uphill position, and transport him to the first-aid room at the base lodge. Once inside, you take a full set of vital signs; the pulse has increased to 114, the blood pressure is 100/70, and the respiratory rate is 28 on high-flow oxygen. As you deliver your hand-off report to the paramedics, you show them a large bruise on the upper chest wall that extends beneath the patient's armpit. The paramedics agree with your assessment that the patient needs air transport.

Several days later during a patrol meeting, your medical advisor informs you that the patient was admitted to the hospital with a displaced posterior rib fracture that had punctured the lung. The patient had a significant pneumothorax that required installing a chest tube for several days. He compliments you on the care you and your team provided and states that the patient is expected to recover fully.

## Skill Guide

Date: _____

(CPI) = Critical Performance Indicator

Candidate: _____

Start Tme: _____

End Time: _____

## Managing an Open Chest Wound

**Objective:** To demonstrate the proper management of an open chest wound.

| Skill | Max Points | Skill Demo | |
|---|---|---|---|
| Determines the scene is safe. | 1 | | (CPI) |
| Introduces self and obtains permission to help/treat. | 1 | | |
| Initiates Standard Precautions. | 1 | | (CPI) |
| Assesses the ABCDs, controls any bleeding. | 1 | | |
| Stabilizes the cervical spine if injury is trauma induced. | 1 | | |
| Exposes the chest. | 1 | | (CPI) |
| Palpates entire chest checking for tenderness/deformities. | 1 | | |
| Applies an occlusive dressing and tape according to local protocol if sucking chest wound is present. | 1 | | (CPI) |
| Applies high flow oxygen via nonbreather. | 1 | | (CPI) |
| Treats for shock and maintains body temperature. | 1 | | (CPI) |
| Loads patient onto long spine board. | 1 | | |
| Readjusts occlusive dressing tape according to local protocol. | 1 | | |
| Transports patient and transfers to EMS personnel. | 1 | | |

Must receive 11 out of 13 points.

Comments: _____

Failure of any of the CPIs is an automatic failure.

Evaluator: _____  NSP ID: _____

PASS    FAIL

# Chapter Review

## Chapter Summary

Thoracic trauma is an inherent risk in many activities that take place in outdoor environments. The thoracic organs carry out some of the body's most vital functions and generally are well protected by the rib cage. Although resilient by nature, this protective structure is susceptible to damage when exposed to blunt or penetrating trauma and other mechanisms of injury. Should the integrity of the thoracic cavity be breached, damage to the organs within may quickly lead to a life-threatening condition. Even if the chest cavity is not penetrated, blunt force can damage organs in the chest. Because of the interrelated nature of these structures, thoracic injuries can involve more than one body system.

Serious chest injuries that occur in outdoor settings present OEC Technicians with several challenges, especially given that many of these injuries require prompt surgical intervention. Even minor chest trauma can compromise breathing. Recognizing the potential for serious injury is an essential step in reducing morbidity and mortality associated with thoracic trauma. Chest injuries are often considered load and go situations.

Chest trauma must be quickly identified, threats to life mitigated, and transport arranged to prevent shock or a potentially lethal outcome. As vital members of the emergency care system, OEC Technicians are uniquely qualified to render emergency care to injured patients, including those with a serious chest injury in backcountry environments. By using a standardized, systematic approach, OEC Technicians can quickly and accurately assess patients for external and internal chest trauma, determine its severity, and render appropriate care.

## Remember...

1. Both blunt and penetrating chest injuries can be life threatening.
2. Maintain a high index of suspicion for chest injury based on the mechanism of injury.
3. Assess the entire chest, including the upper back and armpits.
4. Provide oxygen to any patient with a suspected chest injury.
5. Treat sucking chest wounds with an occlusive dressing.
6. If the condition of a hypoxic patient with chest trauma worsens, consider a tension pneumothorax.

## Chapter Questions

### Multiple Choice

Choose the correct answer.

1. A $C_3$ spinal cord injury is more serious than a mid-thoracic injury because _____
   a. a vertebral injury at this level almost always severs the carotid artery.
   b. such a spinal cord injury is immediately fatal.
   c. a vertebral injury at this level affects the phrenic nerves, which controls the diaphragm and thus breathing.
   d. Actually, a mid-thoracic vertebral injury is more serious than a cervical one.

2. A contusion is best defined as _____
   a. a jagged cut.
   b. a bruise.
   c. a rib fracture.
   d. an external arterial bleed.

3. Which of the following assumptions should an OEC Technician make when assessing a patient with a chest injury? _____
   a. The injury is probably serious even if there is little obvious evidence of trauma.
   b. The patient is probably not seriously injured because the ribs can absorb a great deal of energy while protecting underlying organs.
   c. A patient with a chest injury should be transported slowly to minimize further injury.
   d. Low-flow $O_2$ should be administered through a nasal cannula to minimize further lung damage.

4. Which of the following statements defines and explains the implications of a posterior dislocation of the proximal clavicle? _____
   a. The clavicle has dislocated outward and can rupture the spleen.
   b. The clavicle has dislocated inward and places pressure on the great vessels and other surrounding structures.
   c. The clavicle has dislocated upward and can slice the jugular vein or carotid artery.
   d. This is a simple clavicular dislocation, which is not a dangerous injury.

5. Which of the following sets of injuries would you most suspect in a climber who has slowly tumbled down a soft snow chute, landed on the point of his ice ax, and has a thumb-sized hole in his chest just above his right nipple? _____
   a. flail chest, aortic rupture
   b. sternal fracture, myocardial contusion, sternoclavicular joint injury
   c. hemothorax, pneumothorax, hemopneumothroax, tension pneumothorax
   d. pericardial tamponade, commotio cordis

6. The most likely injury to a 14-year-old male who was hit in the chest by a hard line drive in a baseball game is_____
   a. a sucking chest wound.
   b. a myocardial contusion.
   c. commotio cordis.
   d. traumatic asphyxia.

7. What is your best immediate course of action when a woman in your climbing team develops the signs and symptoms of a spontaneous pneumothorax?_____
   a. descend rapidly
   b. call for a helicopter to evacuate her to the nearest trauma center
   c. administer high-flow $O_2$ with a nonrebreather mask; her condition will improve rapidly once she acclimatizes
   d. have patient sit and breathe slowly

8. Which of the following statements about chest injuries is true? _____
   a. When a moving body rapidly slows down or stops, the structures within the chest remain in motion for a short period of time longer, causing shearing injuries.
   b. It takes tremendous force to cause an internal chest injury because of the protection provided by the ribs, scapula, and sternum.
   c. Chest injuries can be caused only by direct blunt or penetrating trauma.
   d. A change in elevation must occur for a mild pneumothorax to worsen into a severe or life-threatening pneumothorax.

9. Which is the correct *question* for the following answer: "a constellation of three findings: distended neck veins, muffled heart sounds, and pulsus paradoxus" _____
   a. What is a tension pneumothorax?
   b. What is commotio cordis?
   c. What is a Beck's Triad?
   d. What is a coup-contrecoup injury?

# Matching

1. Match each of the following terms to its description.

_____ 1. aneurysm

_____ 2. closed chest trauma

_____ 3. commotio cordis

_____ 4. flail chest

_____ 5. blood in sac around heart

_____ 6. hemoptysis

_____ 7. hemothorax

_____ 8. myocardial contusion

_____ 9. occlusive dressing

_____ 10. open chest trauma

_____ 11. paradoxical motion

_____ 12. pleura

_____ 13. pneumothorax

_____ 14. pulmonary contusion

_____ 15. ruptured aorta

_____ 16. sucking chest wound

_____ 17. tension pneumothorax

_____ 18. traumatic asphyxia

**a.** the layers of tissue that forms a sac around the lungs

**b.** cardiac tamponade

**c.** used primarily for treating a sucking chest wound or a pneumothorax

**d.** a chest injury that involves penetration of the chest cavity

**e.** a bruise of the heart muscle

**f.** a bruise of the lung tissue

**g.** the accumulation of pressurized air within the pleural space that causes the displacement of the great vessels, tracheal deviation, jugular venous distention, and compression of the other lung

**h.** air in the pleural space

**i.** ballooning; weakening of an artery that predisposes it to rupture

**j.** two or more adjacent ribs that are fractured in two or more places, causing a free-floating segment

**k.** when one inhales a section of the chest goes inward

**l.** coughing up blood

**m.** an accumulation of blood in the pleural space

**n.** the inability of the chest wall to expand due to external pressure or massive crushing trauma, resulting in difficulty in breathing and hypoxia

**o.** sudden cardiac death due to blunt thoracic trauma without any observable thoracic or cardiac damage

**p.** chest injury that does not penetrate the thoracic cavity

**q.** development of a leak in the largest arterial blood vessel resulting in massive bleeding that is usually fatal

**r.** a chest wound that penetrates the pleura or lung, allowing air to be "sucked" into the pleural space upon each inspiration

2. Match each of the following conditions to the correct set of signs and symptoms.

_____ 1. aortic rupture and dissection

_____ 2. commotio cordis

_____ 3. pericardial tamponade

_____ 4. tension pneumothorax

_____ 5. sucking chest wound

_____ 6. traumatic asphyxia

**a.** a collapsed lung; the heart, great vessels, and trachea deviate to the opposite side

**b.** pain, shortness of breath, distended neck veins, muffled heart sounds

**c.** BP that changes with inhalation or exhalation

**d.** trauma in children that presents as Vtach or Vfib

**e.** acute chest or back pain, stabbing pain radiating between the shoulder blades, blood pressure that varies in each arm, rapid shock

**f.** profound hypoxia or anoxia, bulging eyes, purple color to face

# Scenario

*You are dispatched to a busy intersection on the mountain where two skiers have collided. You secure the scene and put on PPE. No witnesses are present. A quick assessment reveals that Skier 1 has a forearm injury, and that Skier 2 is self-guarding the left chest, has minor difficulty breathing, and reports chest pain of 6 out of 10 upon inhalation. Both patients are responsive and deny any neck, head, or back pain. You call for two toboggans, help, O$_2$, a trauma pack, and an ALS ambulance.*

*Skier 2 tells you that he was blindsided in the left rib area by Skier 1*

1. As you wait for help to arrive, the most important issue you should address is_____
   **a.** obtaining the name of Skier 2.
   **b.** obtaining the name of Skier 1.
   **c.** completing a SAMPLE interview.
   **d.** evaluating Skier 2 for serious chest injuries.

*You conduct a primary assessment on Skier 2. During secondary assessment, you note that a section of the patient's chest wall moves inward when he inhales. Palpation of the left side elicits pain. The patient experiences more pain with each inhalation and increasing difficulty breathing.*

2. These findings may indicate_____
   a. a pneumothorax.
   b. a hemothorax.
   c. a pericardial tamponade.
   d. flail chest.

*The toboggans and help arrive. You auscultate Skier 2's five lung lobes using a stethoscope.*

3. Which of the following findings could indicate a respiratory problem resulting from the impact?_____
   a. lung sounds clear
   b. right lower wheeze
   c. crepitus from a broken rib
   d. diminished lung sounds

4. On this load and go transport, the best position for the patient in the toboggan is_____
   a. head uphill.
   b. head downhill.
   c. on his left side with head downhill.
   d. sitting up.

# **S**uggested Reading

*Advanced Trauma Life Support for Doctors.* 2008. Chicago: American College of Surgeons.

Butler, F., J. Holcomb, S. Giebner, N. McSwain, and J. Bagian. 2007. "Tactical Combat Casualty Care 2007: Evolving Concepts and Battlefield Experience." *Military Medicine* 172(11): 1–19 (supplement).

Collier, B., R. Riordan, Jr., R. Nag, and J. Morris, Jr. 2007. *Wilderness Trauma and Surgical Emergencies,* Fifth Edition, edited by P. Auerbach. St. Louis: Mosby.

http://www.jems.com/news_and_articles/articles/jems/3308/cardiac_injury.html

http://www.sciencedirect.com/science/article/B6T35-4C1NHDP-1/2/b92477ac3a70b4c0ce3b008eaaa64765

http://www.trauma.org/archive/thoracic/CHESTflail.html

McGillicuddy, D., and P. Rosen. 2007. "Diagnostic Dilemmas and Current Controversies in Blunt Chest Trauma." *Emerg. Med. Clin. N. Am.* 25: 695–711.

Meredith, J., and J. Hoth. 2007. "Thoracic Trauma: When and How to Intervene." *Surg. Clin. N. Am.* 87: 95–118.

Misthos, P., S. Kakaris, E. Sepsas, K. Athanassiadi, and I. Skottis. 2004. "A Prospective Analysis of Occult Pneumothorax, Delayed Pneumothorax and Delayed Hemothorax after Minor Blunt Thoracic Trauma." *European Journal of Cardio-Thoracic Surgery* 25(5): 859–864.

*Prehospital Trauma Life Support.* 2006. National Association of Emergency Medical Technicians. St. Louis: Mosby.

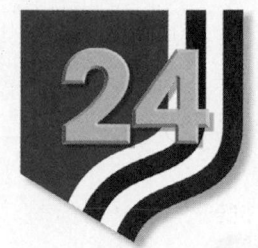

# Abdominal and Pelvic Trauma

Eric M. Lamberts, MD, FAAFP, ASAM

## ⊕ OBJECTIVES

**Upon completion of this chapter, the OEC Technician will be able to:**

**24-1** Identify and locate the major anatomical structures within the abdominopelvic cavity.

**24-2** List the functions of the major anatomical structures within the abdominopelvic cavity.

**24-3** List and describe at least six abdominopelvic injuries.

**24-4** Describe and demonstrate how to assess a patient with abdominopelvic trauma.

**24-5** Describe and demonstrate how to manage a patient with abdominopelvic trauma.

**24-6** Describe and demonstrate how to manage an evisceration.

**24-7** Describe and demonstrate how to manage an impaled object in the abdomen or pelvis.

**24-8** Describe and demonstrate how to manage a pelvic fracture.

## ⊕ KEY TERMS

evisceration, *p. 798*
femoral neck, *p. 806*

Kehr's sign, *p. 802*
pelvic binder, *p. 806*

straddle injury, *p. 798*
symphysis pubis, *p. 801*

## Chapter Overview

You have learned the anatomy and physiology of the abdominal and pelvic cavities, and also how to manage basic various gastrointestinal medical emergencies. Assessing and managing trauma adds another dimension to your skills. As you learn to assess and manage abdominopelvic trauma, the goal is not to determine the exact cause of the problem, but rather to identify a potentially serious emergency, render emergent care, and quickly move the patient toward definitive treatment.

*continued*

## HISTORICAL TIMELINE

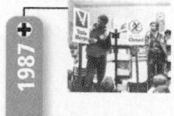

**1987** *Winter Emergency Care* is adopted by NSP.

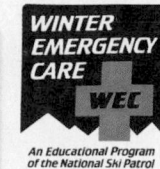

**1988** *Winter Emergency Care* is published by Warren Bowman, M.D.

# ✚ CASE PRESENTATION ✚

It is a mild day on the slopes, and on an intermediate trail you see a teenage girl skiing slowly in a wedge. You note that she is trying to control her speed by sticking her poles into the snow ahead of her. Suddenly, the tip of a pole catches in the snow and the handle jams into her abdomen. She immediately falls to the ground. When you reach her, she is lying on the snow, gasping for air, and clutching her abdomen. Her mother is nearby.

**What is your first step in assessment?**

Unlike other internal organs, the structures within the abdomen are poorly protected. Though better protected, the structures within the pelvis are not immune to damage. Both cavities are served by a vast network of blood vessels that, when injured, can lead to life-threatening bleeding. Blunt and penetrating injuries can harm the organs in the abdomen or the pelvis. When such injuries occur, solid organs bleed internally, or they leak enzymes that cause internal abdominal inflammation. When the bowel ruptures, bacteria enter these cavities, causing infection that can proceed to sepsis and death. If the abdominal aorta is damaged, massive bleeding can be rapidly fatal.

OEC Technicians must be ever vigilant whenever abdominal trauma is suspected. This chapter will give you the skills to adequately evaluate these injuries and provide field care as needed. Understanding which patients need prompt transport is one of the skills you will learn. The absence of signs or symptoms does not necessarily mean that a patient does not have an internal abdominal injury. A heightened index of suspicion and repeated assessments of patients are essential to reducing disability and death from abdominopelvic trauma.

⊕ 24-1  Identify and locate the major anatomical structures within the abdominopelvic cavity.

## Anatomy and Physiology

The anatomy and physiology of the abdominopelvic cavity have been described in detail in Chapter 16, Gastrointestinal and Genitourinary Emergencies. This section reviews anatomy and physiology with particular attention to trauma (Figure 24-1■).

**Figure 24-1** The organs in the abdominopelvic cavity.

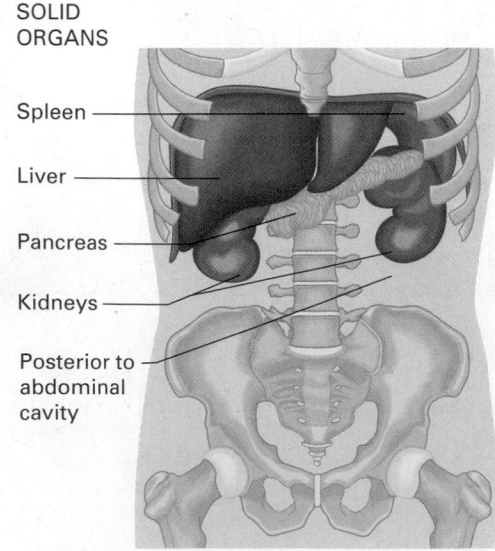

SOLID ORGANS

Spleen
Liver
Pancreas
Kidneys
Posterior to abdominal cavity

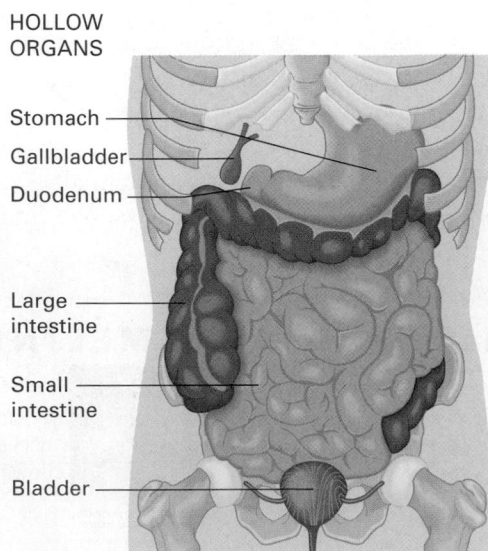

HOLLOW ORGANS

Stomach
Gallbladder
Duodenum
Large intestine
Small intestine
Bladder

The abdominal cavity is separated from the thoracic cavity by the diaphragm, the muscle that contracts to expand the lungs. The inferior margin of the abdomen is the pelvic brim, which is an imaginary plane formed by the top of the pelvic bones. The pelvic cavity is encased by the pelvic bones. Together, the abdomen and pelvis constitute the largest cavity in the human body.

Organs in the pelvic cavity are relatively protected from trauma by the bones of the pelvis—the ilium, the ischium, and the pubis. This is not the case with the abdominal organs, which are protected posteriorly by the spine and anteriorly and laterally only by the abdominal muscles and a layer of fat.

Some of the organs in or just behind the abdominal cavity are involved with processing blood: the kidneys remove toxins from the blood, the liver processes nutrients and chemicals in the blood, and the spleen helps to fight overwhelming infections and removes old red blood cells.

The aorta, the largest blood vessel in the body, and the companion inferior vena cava lie just in front of the vertebral column in the upper abdomen. In abdominal trauma, injury to blood-filled organs can cause life-threatening bleeding. The potential space inside the abdominopelvic cavity can fill rapidly with several liters of blood, producing life-threatening intra-abdominal blood loss before the abdomen starts to swell. Hypovolemic shock secondary to hemorrhage should *always* be of concern with abdominopelvic trauma.

During the assessment of patients, knowledge of abdominal and pelvic anatomy and physiology will provide OEC Technicians important clues. Localizing the site of injury can be very helpful in the management of abdominal injuries.

The abdomen is divided into four quadrants (Figure 24-2■). Injuries in each involve different organs, can have markedly different outcomes, and call for different

⊕ **24-2** List the functions of the major anatomical structures within the abdominopelvic cavity.

**Figure 24-2** The four quadrants of the abdomen.

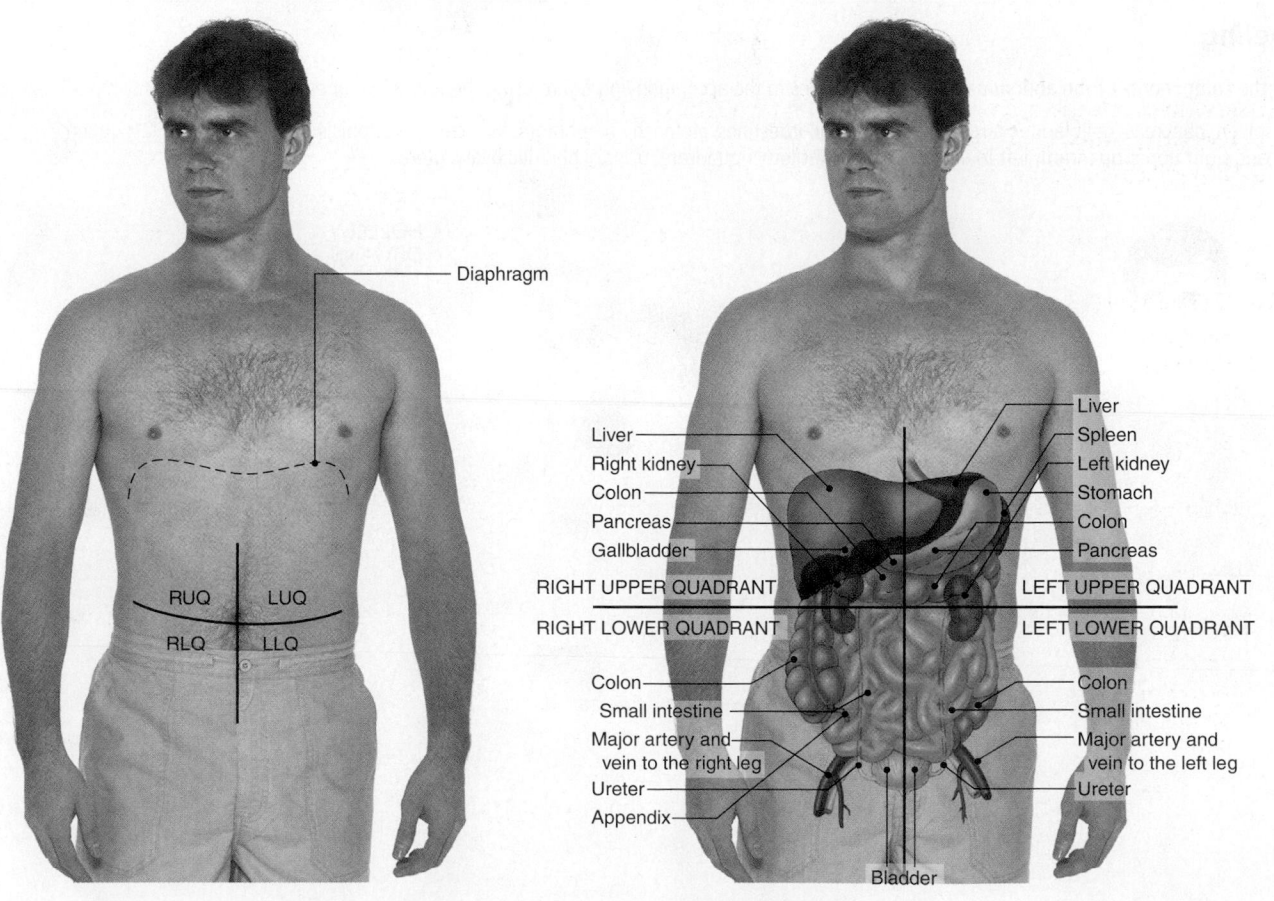

management strategies. Right upper quadrant (RUQ) trauma should make you consider liver injury, whereas left upper quadrant (LUQ) trauma should heighten your suspicion for spleen injury. Trauma to the midline of the upper abdomen should cause concerns for injury to the aorta, bowel, pancreas, spleen, or liver.

In some medical emergencies such as appendicitis, the location of presenting pain can confuse OEC Technicians because the visceral nerves involved do not enable precise localization of sensation. Fortunately in trauma, the location of the pain and tenderness can provide important clues to what structure or structures have been injured.

# STOP, THINK, UNDERSTAND

## Multiple Choice

Choose the correct answer.

1. Which of the following statements regarding the abdomen is false?_____
   a. The superior boundary of the abdomen is the diaphragm.
   b. The internal organs of the abdomen are well protected and thus at low risk of damage due to trauma.
   c. The structures within the pelvis are better protected than those of the abdomen.
   d. Both the abdominal and pelvic cavities are highly vascular and thus subject to life-threatening bleeding when injured.

2. Which of the following statements about abdominal injuries is true?_____
   a. Because the abdomen is a highly vascular area, abdominal injuries are easy for OEC Technicians to identify or diagnose.
   b. Because the abdominal cavity is so well protected, hemorrhage in this area is very rare.
   c. A patient with an abdominal injury and subsequent major internal bleeding may initially be asymptomatic (show no signs or symptoms).
   d. An OEC Technician can do little to minimize the risk of death due to abdominal trauma.

## Labeling

Label the components of the abdominal and pelvic cavities in the accompanying figure using the following labels:

liver, spleen, pancreas, gallbladder, large intestines, small intestines, stomach,  diaphragm, iliac crests, symphisis pubis, umbilicus, left upper quadrant, right upper quadrant, left lower quadrant, right lower quadrant, urinary bladder, ovary, uterus

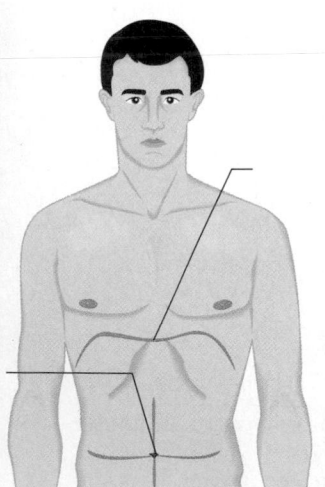

SOLID ORGANS

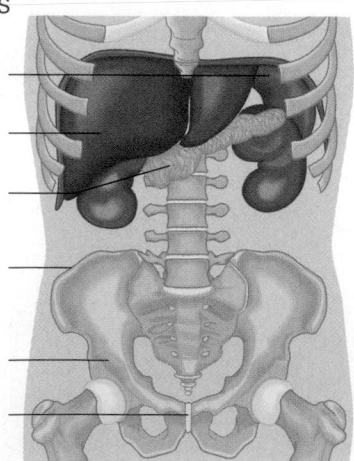

HOLLOW ORGANS

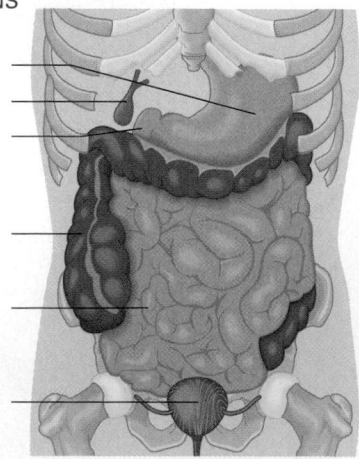

*continued*

**Female Reproductive System Illustrated**

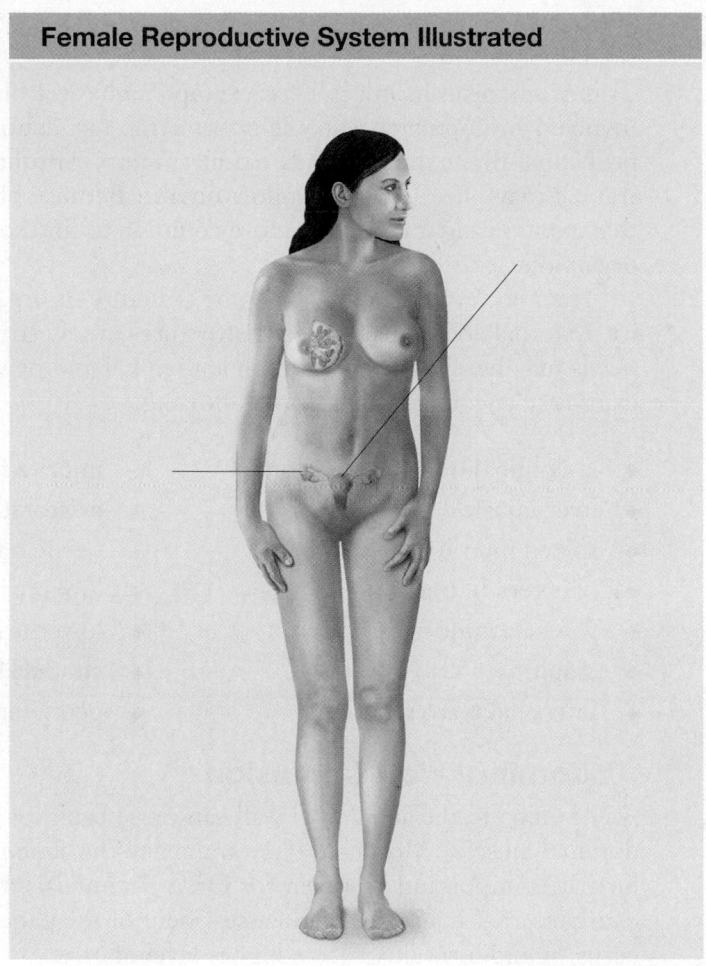

## Matching

1. Match each of the following organs with its primary function.

| | |
|---|---|
| _____ **1.** kidney | **a.** grinds and digests food |
| _____ **2.** liver | **b.** fights infection and removes old red blood cells |
| _____ **3.** spleen | **c.** processes chemicals in the blood |
| _____ **4.** aorta | **d.** removes waste |
| _____ **5.** stomach | **e.** stores urine until it can be excreted from the body |
| _____ **6.** bladder | **f.** largest blood vessel in the body |

2. For each of the following abdominal locations, indicate the underlying organ or organs that are most likely damaged. More than one organ may apply to each finding.

| | |
|---|---|
| _____ **1.** midline upper abdominal pain | **a.** liver |
| _____ **2.** left upper quadrant pain | **b.** spleen |
| | **c.** aorta |
| _____ **3.** right upper quadrant pain | **d.** pancreas |

⊕ **24-3** List and describe at least six abdominopelvic injuries.

# Common Abdominal and Pelvic Injuries

The mechanism of injury—for example, whether blunt or penetrating trauma is involved—can provide valuable information for identifying the nature of a patient's problems. Blunt trauma tends to cause injury to solid organs whereas penetrating trauma may affect solid or hollow organs. Because blunt trauma is more common than penetrating trauma, it is more common to find solid organ injuries than hollow organ injuries.

Trauma can injure more than one structure or organ in the abdominopelvic cavity. External abdominal or pelvic structures or any structure within the abdomen or pelvis may be damaged. Common abdominal and pelvic injuries that OEC Technicians may encounter include the following:

**eviscertion**   the protrusion of organs through an open abdominal wound.

- abdominal wall contusion
- liver injuries
- spleen injuries
- pancreas injuries
- vascular injuries
- diaphragm tear/rupture
- intestinal tear/rupture

- injuries from impaled objects
- **evisceration**
- pelvic fractures
- hip injuries
- lower urinary tract injuries
- **straddle injuries**
- genital injuries

**straddle injury**   an injury to the pelvis and the internal organs between the genitals and anus that results when a patient forcefully straddles a fixed object.

## Abdominal Wall Contusion

Any trauma to the abdominal wall can cause bruising of the skin and superficial abdominal muscles. Most mild blunt trauma to the abdomen does not cause internal injury. It is important, however, for OEC Technicians to realize that any trauma can cause internal injuries. Careful assessment of the patient is important, and any concerns should be evaluated at a higher level of care.

## Liver Injuries

Because the liver is the largest solid organ in the abdomen, injuries to it are common. Even though most of the liver is protected by the rib cage, it is vulnerable to both blunt and penetrating trauma. The liver's fibrous tissue and tough surrounding capsule enable it to withstand some trauma. However, because it is a highly vascular organ, injuries to it frequently cause internal bleeding (Figure 24-3■).

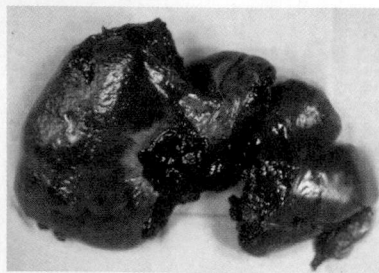

**Figure 24-3** A rupture of the liver may be caused by blunt trauma or penetrating trauma.

## Spleen Injuries

Like the liver, the spleen is partially protected by the lower rib cage and is a highly vascular organ. Because it is surrounded by only a thin membranous capsule and has relatively little fibrous material holding it together, it is one of the more fragile organs in the human body. Most injuries to it occur from blunt trauma. However, the spleen can also be injured from penetrating trauma or by a fractured rib. Even relatively minor trauma can cause splenic injury. If the delicate capsule ruptures, internal bleeding can be severe and can result in hypovolemic shock from hemorrhage (Figure 24-4■).

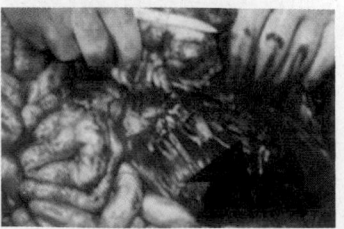

**Figure 24-4** Penetrating trauma to the spleen.

## Pancreas Injuries

The pancreas, a solid organ, can rupture or tear. Such injuries can cause digestive enzymes to leak into the abdominal cavity, which can destroy the pancreas and other surrounding structures and cause peritonitis. Abdomen impaction on the handlebars in a bicycle accident is the most common cause of pancreas injury. Pancreas injuries are becoming more common as a result of collisions in other outdoor sports, including snowmobiling and snowbiking (striking the handlebars), snowboarding (striking a terrain park rail), and kayaking (striking the front deck). Any injury to the middle of the abdomen above the naval can damage the pancreas.

## Vascular Injuries

The abdomen and pelvis contain numerous arteries and veins, both large and small. Among the larger vessels are the abdominal aorta, inferior vena cava, hepatic vessels, renal vessels, and the iliac arteries and veins. Rapid deceleration that results when the body hits a fixed object is the most common cause of vascular injury, although penetrating trauma also can damage blood vessels. Bleeding can be severe and may be immediately life threatening, depending on the size of the vessel, whether it is an artery or a vein, and the extent of vessel damage.

## Diaphragm Tear/Rupture

The diaphragm is vulnerable to both blunt and penetrating trauma. Severe blunt abdominal trauma can cause increased intra-abdominal pressure, causing the diaphragm to tear away from its attachments or causing holes in the diaphragm. The most common diaphragmatic injury is a diaphragmatic hernia, which occurs when one or more abdominal organs pass through (herniate) the diaphragm at the site at which the esophagus penetrates the diaphragm from the left side of the chest cavity. Penetrating objects can directly cause holes in the diaphragm. Regardless of the mechanism of injury, tears or holes in the diaphragm allow structures within the abdominal cavity, mainly the intestines, to migrate into the thoracic cavity. An injury to the diaphragm or the presence of abdominal organs in the chest cavity can compromise the patient's breathing.

## Intestinal Tear/Rupture

Some portion of the large intestine or the small intestine is located in every quadrant of the abdomen. Most intestinal injuries are due to penetrating trauma, which can cause undigested food and fecal matter to leak into the abdominal cavity, resulting in severe pain, infection, and peritonitis. Significant bleeding can also occur if a vessel in the intestinal wall is damaged.

## Impaled Objects

An impaled object that enters the abdominopelvic cavity can result in a variety of life-threatening injuries, depending on the structures that are damaged. Objects such as ski poles, tree branches, fence posts, knives, or pipes are common impaled objects (Figure 24-5■). They may enter the body on one side and protrude from the other side, or they may lodge within the abdomen or pelvis without exiting. Interestingly, most impaled objects in the abdomen or pelvis miss important organs or blood vessels, allowing the patient to do quite well with timely definitive care. Major complications are bleeding (initially) and infection (later).

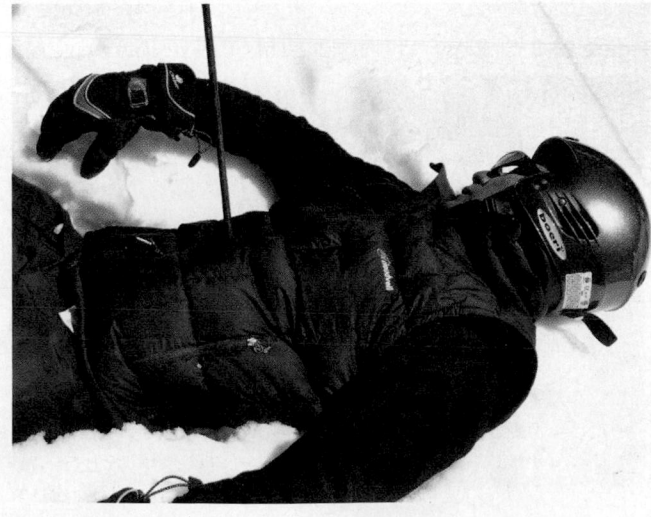

**Figure 24-5** An impaled object.
Copyright Candace Horgan

## Evisceration

Evisceration occurs when a tear in the abdominal wall exposes the intestines and/or other organs to the external environment (Figure 24-6■). Most often, evisceration is caused by a penetrating injury that tears an opening through the abdominal wall and peritoneum. It presents many problems, including severe bleeding, rapid heat loss, and the risk of infection. Evisceration is an uncommon (but certainly upsetting and challenging) injury for the patient, rescuers, and bystanders.

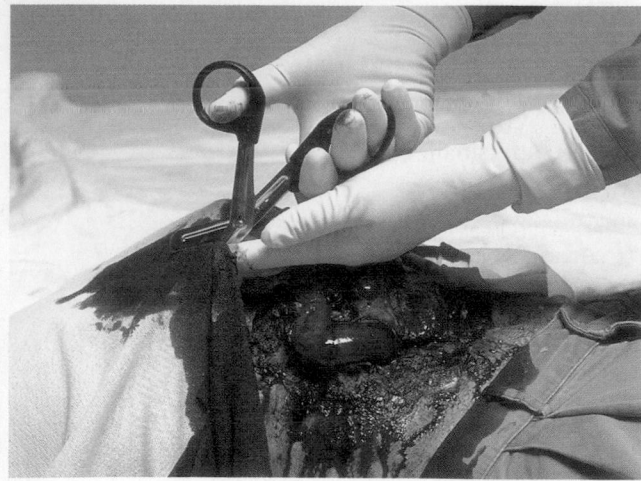

**Figure 24-6** Cutting away clothing at the site of an evisceration.

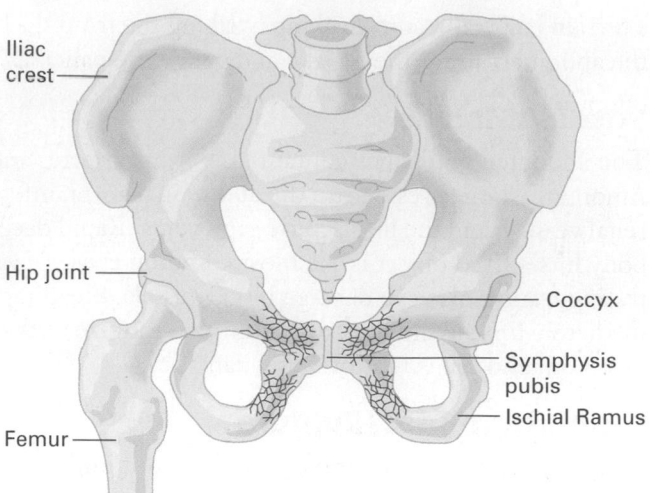

Iliac
crest

Hip joint

Coccyx

Symphysis
pubis

Ischial Ramus

Femur

**Figure 24-7** Fractures to the pelvis typically occur in these sites and
may result in injuries to internal organs.

## Pelvic Fractures

Even though the pelvic bones are among the sturdiest bones in the body, the pelvis
and the structures within the pelvic cavity are not immune to blunt or penetrating injury. Fractures involving the pelvic bones usually require great force and should be
suspected in high-speed collisions, falls from 20 feet or higher for adults and from
10 feet or higher for children, motor vehicle crashes, pedestrian-vehicle collisions,
pelvic gunshot wounds, or any other type of direct blunt trauma. Because the pelvis
is such a sturdy protector of the organs within it, forces sufficient to fracture the
pelvic bones may result in injuries to internal structures such as the urinary bladder
and blood vessels. The most significant complication of a pelvic fracture is acute internal bleeding. Because the pelvis forms a ring, it is likely to fracture in more than
one location (Figure 24-7■).

## Hip Injuries

Injuries involving the hip occur frequently in outdoor activities. Among the most common hip injuries encountered are hip fractures and hip dislocations (Figure 24-8■).
These injuries often are quite painful and require special care to prevent additional injury. Both injuries are covered in detail in Chapter 20, Musculoskeletal Injuries.

**Figure 24-8** Classic signs of hip dislocations: the left photo is anterior dislocation; the right photo is posterior dislocation.

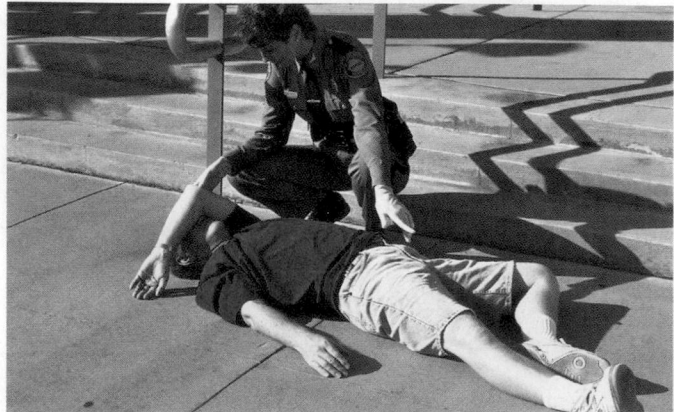

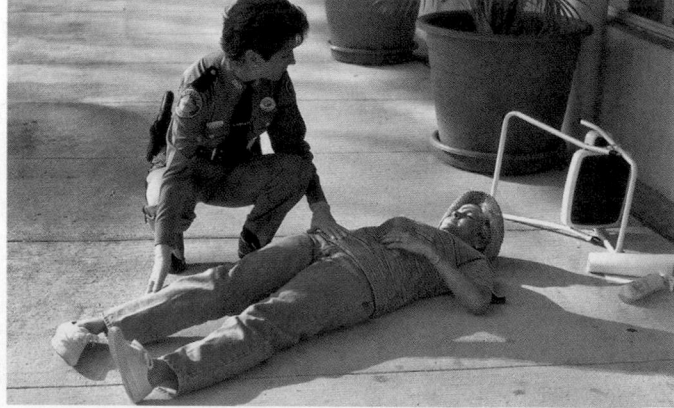

## Lower Urinary Tract Injuries

The urinary bladder is located behind and is protected by the **symphysis pubis**. If the symphysis fractures, bone fragments can lacerate the bladder. Most commonly this occurs from direct blunt trauma to the symphysis. Falls and straddle injuries are common sources of this type of trauma. In addition, blunt trauma can cause the bladder to rupture, which is much more likely to occur when the bladder is full. The pressure of a seat belt at the end of a rapid deceleration also can also rupture a full or distended bladder. If the forces are large enough, the urethra can be torn from the bladder. Injuries to the bladder or urethra can result in internal bleeding or in urine leaking into the pelvic cavity.

## Straddle Injuries

Genital trauma is generally not life threatening, but can be a challenge for both the patient and the rescuer. In outdoor settings, most genital injuries are caused by a straddle injury, which occurs when the patient's groin strikes an object such as a ski pole, a rail, or the top bar of a bicycle. In general, genital injuries in females are limited to external structures because the uterus and ovaries are well protected within the bony pelvis. The labia, however, are very vascular, and external injuries to them can cause profuse bleeding. Injuries to the male genitalia are often more serious, can be very painful, and can result in long-term complications.

## Genital Injuries

The external genitals can receive blunt or sharp trauma. In males, blunt trauma to the testicles can result in a hematoma in the scrotum. Lacerations can occur to the penis or scrotum and are seen most commonly when the genitals are caught in a zipper. In women, genital trauma causing a hematoma to the external labia or lips can be quite painful and can cause a lot of mental anguish for the patient. When evaluating genital injuries, always consider the patient's modesty.

# Assessment

Abdominal and pelvic injuries are often difficult to assess because the initial presentation can be relatively benign and then change for the worse. The assessment process follows the same guidelines already described in previous chapters. Emphasis is on recognizing that an abdominal or pelvic injury exists rather than identifying what organs have been affected. However, if OEC Technicians are aware of the locations of the abdominal organs, a higher degree of suspicion can be maintained for such injuries as a splenic rupture.

As with any incident, begin by ensuring that the scene is safe. Next, assess the patient's ABCDs and provide immediate treatment if needed.

A SAMPLE history with mechanism of injury is important, as is a good secondary assessment. As part of the history, be sure to ask the patient about any falls or collisions over the past few days because those injuries may have gone unrecognized until now. Remember, the most obvious injury is not always the most dangerous one.

As you perform the physical exam, note the presence of the following signs and symptoms that are consistent with an abdominopelvic injury:

- pain
- tenderness
- visible external wounds
- abdominal distention
- abdominal rigidity
- unexplained shock

**symphysis pubis** the site on the anterior pelvis at which the two pubic bones are joined together.

**24-4** Describe and demonstrate how to assess a patient with abdominopelvic trauma.

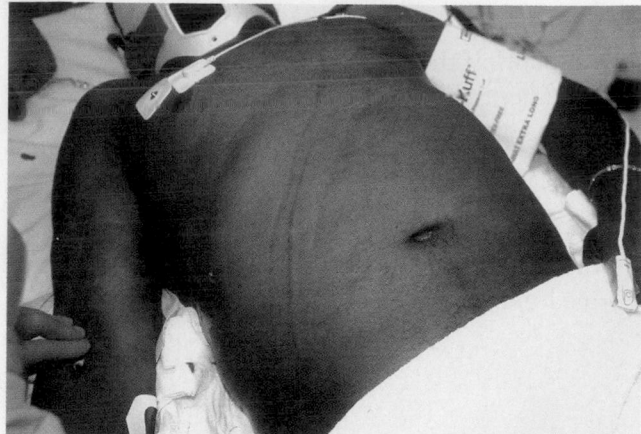

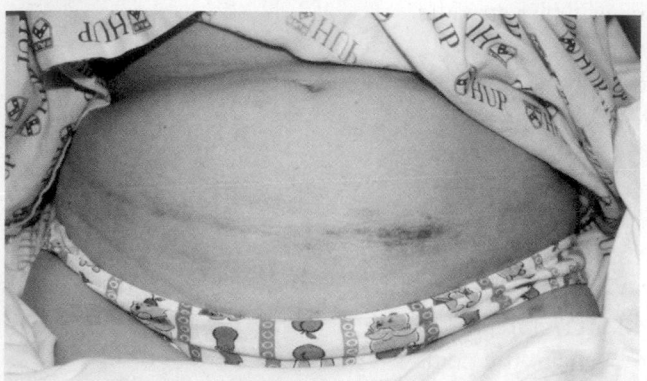

**Figure 24-9** A "seat belt" sign often indicates hidden injuries to internal organs. Copyright Edward T. Dickenson, M.D.

**Kehr's sign**   pain in an uninjured shoulder caused by the accumulation of blood beneath the diaphragm; a painful right shoulder indicates a lacerated liver, whereas a painful left shoulder indicates a lacerated spleen.

**Figure 24-10** The finding of pain or tenderness upon gentle palpation of the pelvic bones suggests a pelvic injury.

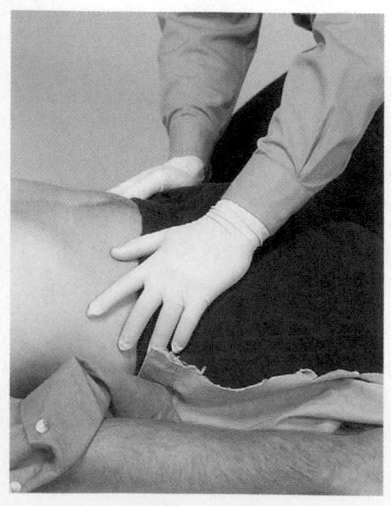

If the patient is in pain, ask where the pain is located and assess its nature using the OPQRST mnemonic described in Chapter 7, Patient Assessment. The location of pain, especially early on, is helpful in ascertaining which organs might have incurred injury. Early pain is often experienced where the initial impact occurred. Serious internal bleeding is not always obvious because most of the abdomimopelvic organs are supplied by visceral nerves, which provide the CNS vague or no pain messages in response to injury. In medical emergencies such as appendicitis, pain is often vaguely located initially and then becomes more localized as time goes on. In contrast, pain resulting from abdominal trauma pain is often initially localized in the place where the patient got hit and later becomes more generalized if blood, bile, or intestinal contents have leaked into the abdominal cavity and caused peritonitis.

Ask patients whether they have consumed alcohol or ingested any drugs. This is important because the symptoms of abdominopelvic trauma may be masked by these substances.

Inspect the abdomen for distension and overall symmetry. Abdominal distention, particularly if it is increasing over time, can be an indication of severe intra-abdominal bleeding. Note any discoloration of the abdominal wall. You may detect a large band of bruising across the lower abdomen, an area of discoloration known as the "seat belt sign" (Figure 24-9■). Although more commonly associated with rapid deceleration during vehicular crashes in which the abdomen slams against a seat belt, the seat belt sign also may be encountered if the abdomen strikes a fixed object such as a terrain park rail or a metal fencing cross bar. Also be sure to inspect the flank areas as well for discoloration.

Use the standard DCAP-BTLS assessment and palpate all four quadrants of the abdomen and the lower rib cage. Rib tenderness and crepitus are signs of rib fracture. Remember, the organs beneath a broken rib may be injured as well. Carefully palpate the abdomen, beginning in the quadrant farthest away from the site of pain.

When the spleen or liver is injured and bleeding from the organ irritates the underside of the diaphragm, pain can be referred to the shoulder on the same side as the injured organ, a finding known as **Kehr's sign**. Patients who complain of shoulder pain in the absence of an actual shoulder injury may have a ruptured spleen (in the case of left shoulder pain) or a lacerated liver (right shoulder pain).

Assess the integrity of the pelvis by placing your palms on the iliac crest on each side and applying *gentle* but firm inward (medial) pressure (Figure 24-10■). Bone crepitus, increased pain, or tenderness suggests a potential pelvic fracture. Palpate the pubic bones *gently*, but do not press downward or outward on any pelvic bone because doing so can worsen the fracture and/or cause more bleeding from ruptured pelvic blood vessels. In addition, only one rescuer should examine a patient for pelvic fracture. In the event that the pelvis is fractured, multiple examinations may lead to potentially life-threatening bleeding by disturbing the blood clot that has formed at the fracture site.

Genital injuries can be very painful and may be associated with pelvic fracture. The examination of potential genital injuries requires discretion on the part of rescuers. If injury is suspected, a brief exam is warranted. However, unless active bleeding is suspected, you may wish to wait to perform this exam in a more controlled environment such as the aid room. Preferably this exam should be performed by one OEC Technician with a second in attendance who are the same gender as the patient. If the patient is a child, ideally a parent or guardian should be present throughout the examination. However, while it is important to approach examinations of the pelvic region with care, do not delay an examination of a potentially life-threatening injury. If an examination is indicated, inspect the area for bleeding, discoloration, or soft-tissue injury.

Because the abdomen and pelvis are filled with numerous blood vessels, monitoring for shock is very important (Figure 24-11■). Several liters of blood can accumulate in these cavities. A rising pulse, a falling systolic blood pressure, and a decreasing level of responsiveness are ominous signs that must not be overlooked. Left upper quadrant injuries are especially worrisome because splenic injuries are especially prone to bleeding. So, too, are pelvic fractures, although any injuries in the abdominopelvic cavity have the potential for serious blood loss.

The importance of follow up exams and serial sets of vital signs cannot be overemphasized. If a patient with minimal symptoms develops abdominal distention, pain upon examination, an elevated pulse, or decreasing blood pressure, initiate management for shock and transfer to definitive care.

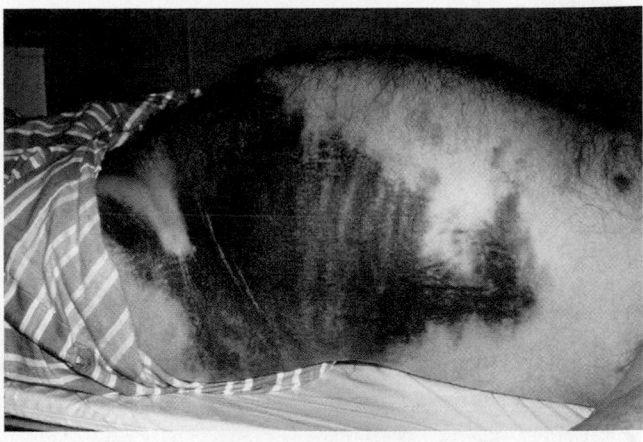

**Figure 24-11** Bruising of the abdomen is a sign of blunt trauma and possibly internal bleeding, which can be a life-threatening condition.

## STOP, THINK, UNDERSTAND

### Multiple Choice
Choose the correct answer.

1. Which of the following statements best describes the assessment of patients with traumatic abdominopelvic injuries?_____
   a. Pelvic and abdominal injuries are usually easy to assess because abdominopelvic structures are highly vascular and present with definitive signs and symptoms early on.
   b. Pelvic and abdominal injuries are often difficult to assess because the initial presentation can be relatively benign and then change for the worse.
   c. It is most important that the OEC Technicians determine which organ has been damaged because this provides important information to definitive caregivers on how best to treat the patient.
   d. It is not within the scope of OEC Technicians to determine whether or not an internal injury exists.

2. Which of the following statements regarding abdominal injuries is false?_____
   a. Sensations of pain may be vague or nonexistent.
   b. Early pain is often noted where the initial impact occurred.
   c. Pain often begins localized and then diffuses.
   d. Pain is usually local, specific, and easy to pinpoint.

3. Increasing abdominal distension following blunt trauma to the abdomen is most likely indicative of_____
   a. severe abdominal bleeding.
   b. swelling of an internal organ due to direct blunt trauma.
   c. the accumulation of fecal matter within the abdominal cavity.
   d. the accumulation of urine due to a ruptured bladder.

4. Kehr's sign is best defined as_____
   a. sudden, increasing abdominal swelling.
   b. absence of one of the two femoral pulses.
   c. a type of referred shoulder pain indicative of bleeding from the liver or spleen.
   d. a position that a patient with suspected internal injuries assumes to minimize pain.

5. Which of the following statements about assessing the integrity of the pelvis is true?_____
   a. Multiple examinations can lead to a worsening of bleeding.
   b. Multiple examinations are important to identify a worsening condition.
   c. OEC Technicians should not examine the bony pelvis to avoid doing damage to underlying organs or vessels.
   d. The best method for assessing the integrity of the pelvis is to have the patient attempt to stand.

6. Which of the following statements regarding examinations of genital injuries is true?_____
   a. Regardless of the severity of trauma, genital injury examination should wait until the patient reaches the privacy of an aid room or emergency department.
   b. If possible, genital injuries should be checked by two OEC Technicians who are the same gender as the patient.
   c. It is beyond the scope of an OEC Technician to examine the genitals in the field.
   d. A genital injury should be examined only if there is visible bleeding.

*continued*

## STOP, THINK, UNDERSTAND *continued*

7. Which of the following findings are serious indicators of internal injury? (check all that apply)

_____ **a.** Pulse rates, checked at five-minute intervals, that are (sequentially) 92, 108, 112, and 120

_____ **b.** Blood pressure readings, checked at five-minute interval, that are (sequentially) 120/86, 114/90, 106/86, and 96/76

_____ **c.** A marked increase in blood pressure

_____ **d.** A patient with a decreasing level of responsiveness

_____ **e.** Decreasing abdominal distension

_____ **f.** Left upper quadrant pain that radiates into the left shoulder

## True or False

Indicate which of the following statements are true (T) and which are false (F).

_____ **a.** Injury patterns in the abdomen are often determined by the MOI.

_____ **b.** Penetrating trauma may cause injury to hollow organs or to solid organs.

_____ **c.** Blunt trauma is more likely to cause injury to hollow organs than to solid organs.

_____ **d.** Blunt trauma is more likely to cause injury to solid organs than to hollow organs.

_____ **e.** Evisceration is usually caused by penetrating trauma.

_____ **f.** Because of their distance from one another, only one internal abdominopelvic organ at a time is typically injured by a traumatic force.

## List

List the six predominant signs and symptoms consistent with abdominopelvic injuries.

1. _____
2. _____
3. _____
4. _____
5. _____
6. _____

## Matching

Match each of the following injuries or organs to its description.

_____ **1.** impaled object

_____ **2.** pancreas

_____ **3.** intestinal rupture

_____ **4.** vascular injury

_____ **5.** pelvic fracture

_____ **6.** hip

_____ **7.** diaphragm

_____ **8.** evisceration

_____ **9.** liver

_____ **10.** spleen

_____ **11.** straddle injury

_____ **12.** bladder

**a.** This injury is caused by objects such as ski poles, tree branches, or knives and is characterized by initial bleeding and subsequent infection.

**b.** This may result in undigested food and fecal matter leaking into the abdominal cavity, resulting in severe pain and inflammation.

**c.** Rupture of this solid organ can cause digestive enzymes to leak into the abdominal cavity.

**d.** Rapid deceleration when the body hits a fixed object is the most common cause of this injury, which can result in severe bleeding.

**e.** This large organ is mostly protected by the rib cage; it is vulnerable to both blunt and penetrating trauma.

**f.** This highly vascular, fragile organ can be damaged by even minor trauma.

**g.** An injury to this structure can compromise breathing or cause the intestines to migrate into the thoracic cavity.

**h.** This relatively uncommon injury results from a tear in the abdominal wall.

**i.** This injury is most commonly caused by falls from 20 feet or higher, motor vehicle crashes, high-speed collisions, direct blunt trauma, or gunshot wounds.

**j.** This structure is frequently fractured or dislocated due to trauma associated with outdoor activities; additional injury can occur if it is not handled properly.

**k.** This can be lacerated by bone fragments from the symphisis pubis or ruptured by blunt trauma.

**l.** Is not usually a life-threatening injury but can bleed profusely and is generally more serious in males than females.

## CASE UPDATE

The patient's mother permits you to evaluate her daughter. You confirm that the patient's ABCDs are intact and that she does not have any spine pain. During your secondary assessment, the patient complains of severe pain in her "stomach." Examination of the abdomen reveals tenderness to palpation in the left upper quadrant. The patient's radial pulse is 124 and her respirations are 16. She says that she has no medical problems, is not taking any medications, has no allergies to medications, and last ate at breakfast approximately three hours ago. She appears to be breathing more easily but states that her "stomach really hurts."

**What will be your care and transport plan?**

## Management

As in any rescue situation, management of abdominopelvic trauma must center on keeping both patients and rescuers safe. If needed, move patients to a place where they can be safely managed, remembering that the spine may be injured. Because the potential for serious internal injury is great, activate EMS for transportation to definitive care as soon as a serious injury or threat to life is identified.

Following assuring that the scene is safe, focus initial treatment on correcting ABCD-related problems. Once these matters have been addressed, place patients into a position of comfort, which typically is supine with the knees slightly flexed, which reduces strain on the abdominal muscles. Place a small amount of padding under the patient's knees while maintaining spinal alignment and protecting the cervical spine as indicated. For cases involving a significant mechanism of injury with serious abdominal pain from trauma, OEC Technicians should carefully consider cervical and spinal immobilization. Next, place the patient on high-flow oxygen by nonrebreather mask. Open wounds should be dressed and bandaged according to the principles described in Chapter 18, Soft-Tissue Injuries.

Impaled objects should be secured in place. First, expose the wound, manually stabilize the object, and control bleeding. Then further stabilize the object with a bulky dressing. If the length of an impaled object compromises transport or rescue operations, you may need to cut the object to allow for transport. However, do not remove the object because doing so could lead to life-threatening hemorrhage. Keep the impaled object stationary when shortening it, as movement could cause additional internal injury.

Do not attempt to put eviscerated structures back into the abdomen. Instead, cover the area with a sterile dressing moistened with sterile water or saline solution, if available. If you do not have access to sterile fluids, then keep the area moist with water that is clean enough to drink. Do not use pond or stream water, which could have bacterial contamination. Do not allow the eviscerated abdominal contents to dry out. Keep the patient warm because evisceration can cause rapid, significant heat loss.

If during your assessment of the ABCDs the patient is having respiratory difficulty, you may need to assist the patient with ventilations. The patient may have a primary pulmonary problem, or if there is an abdominal injury, could have abdominal contents in the chest cavity from a torn diaphragm.

⊕ **24-5** Describe and demonstrate how to manage a patient with abdominopelvic trauma.

⊕ **24-6** Describe and demonstrate how to manage an evisceration.

⊕ **24-7** Describe and demonstrate how to manage an impaled object in the abdomen or pelvis.

**24-8** Describe and demonstrate
how to manage a pelvic
fracture.

**pelvic binder**   a device that is either
purchased commercially or made from a
folded sheet and is used to compress the
pelvis and control bleeding in a
traumatic injury.

In a suspected pelvic fracture, keep the patient supine and as comfortable as possible. A mechanism of injury that can cause a pelvic fracture warrants full spinal immobilization. Start with a cervical collar. To prevent further injury or disruption of the pelvic blood vessels, which is especially important if the patient must be transported a long distance or over uneven or rough terrain, consider stabilizing the pelvis using a **pelvic binder**. A pelvic binder may be purchased commercially, or it may be fabricated from a sheet or a table cloth. If you suspect a pelvic fracture, consider radioing for a sheet. A blanket is difficult to use because it is difficult to tie a knot in two ends of a blanket.

To stabilize the pelvic bones using a sheet binder, perform the following procedure (OEC Skill 24-1■):

1. Fold a sheet, lengthwise until it is approximately 10–18 inches wide, and place it crosswise on a long spine board where the patient's pelvis will be.
2. Maintaining spinal alignment, log roll the patient so that the buttocks are positioned on the sheet, with the sheet 1–2 inches above the top of the iliac crest (which is what a belt rides on).
3. Draw the two ends of the sheet together over the symphysis pubis and compress the greater trochanters of the femur.
4. Gently pull the ends of the sheet tight.
5. Tie the two ends of the sheet using an overhand knot, or wrap the two sheet ends around each other and secure in place using one or two nylon cable ties.

Keep the patient's knees slightly flexed by placing a rolled-up blanket under the knees. To further prevent movement, bind the patient's knees and ankles together using one or two cravats, and pad any voids. Complete the packaging by strapping the patient to the backboard.

**femoral neck**   the portion of the
femur that joins the femoral shaft to the
ball of the femur.

Patients with suspected hip dislocations should be transported in the most comfortable position, with the thigh immobilized. Suspected **femoral neck** fractures should be transported on a backboard. See Chapter 20, Musculoskeletal Injuries, for the details of how to care for hip injuries. If a co-existing spinal injury is suspected, immobilize the spine using Standard Procedures.

Shock is fairly common in abdominal and pelvic trauma and is treated in the usual manner. Patients who are in shock should not be given anything by mouth. As with other forms of serious trauma, ALS should be requested if available, and patients should be rapidly transported to a definitive-care facility (ideally a trauma center).

## STOP, THINK, UNDERSTAND

### Multiple Choice

Choose the correct answer.

1. In most cases of internal injury without suspected spinal injury, the patient is best placed in which position?_____
   a. Semi-Fowler position
   b. Trendelenburg position
   c. Recovery position
   d. Supine with the knees flexed

2. The best course of treatment for an impaled object that does not interfere with extrication or transport is to_____
   a. remove the object slowly to minimize bleeding or further damage, and then bandage with an occlusive dressing.
   b. remove the object quickly to minimize bleeding or further damage, and then bandage with an occlusive dressing.
   c. cut the object off at skin level, and then bandage with a bulky dressing.
   d. stabilize the object in place with bulky dressings.

3. Which of the following statements describes the best course of treatment for an evisceration?_____
   a. Gently attempt to put the eviscerated structures back into the abdomen, and then cover the wound with a moist, sterile dressing.
   b. Gently attempt to put the eviscerated structures back into the abdomen, and then cover the wound with a dry, sterile dressing.
   c. Do not attempt to put the eviscerated structures back into the abdomen; cover them with a moist, sterile dressing.
   d. Cut off the protruding part, bandage the remaining wound, and deliver the severed part to the emergency department wrapped in a wet dressing and placed in a bag of ice or cold water.

4. A patient suffering from a suspected pelvic fracture should be placed in which position?_____
   a. Supine position
   b. Recovery position
   c. Trendelenburg position
   d. Supported in a sitting position, with knees apart and flexed

##  CASE DISPOSITION

You administer oxygen to the patient on scene using a high-flow nonrebreather mask. Because she has significant abdominal pain, you radio for ALS transport. The girl is transported in a toboggan in a head-downhill position because you suspect shock. In the first-aid hut, the patient says, "I don't feel good." Further assessment reveals more generalized abdominal tenderness, and she tenses when you palpate her abdomen. There is no abdominal distention. Her pulse is now 132, and blood pressure is 98/50. Keeping the patient supine, you add blankets, raise her feet, and help load her into an ambulance. You later find out the patient had been admitted for an injury to her spleen.

# OEC SKILL 24-1 | Pelvic Stabilization

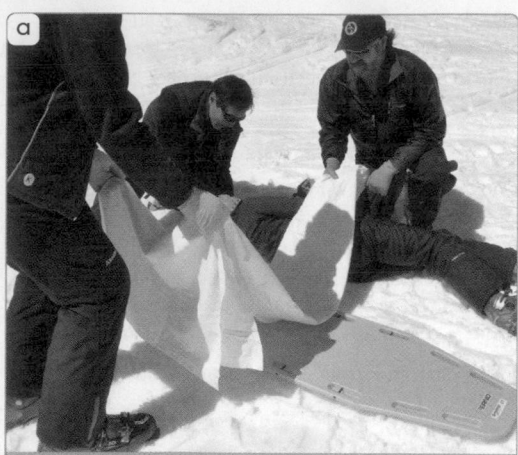

Prepare the sheet, and if you are using a backboard, wrap the sheet around the board.
Copyright Candace Horgan

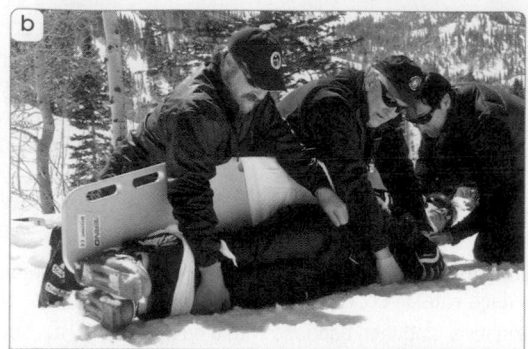

Log roll the patient, and place the patient such that the top of the sheet is 1–2 inches above the hip.
Copyright Candace Horgan

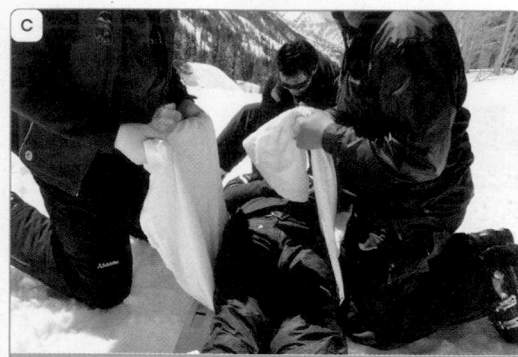

Draw the two ends of the sheet together over the symphysis pubis, and compress the greater trochanters of the hips.
Copyright Candace Horgan

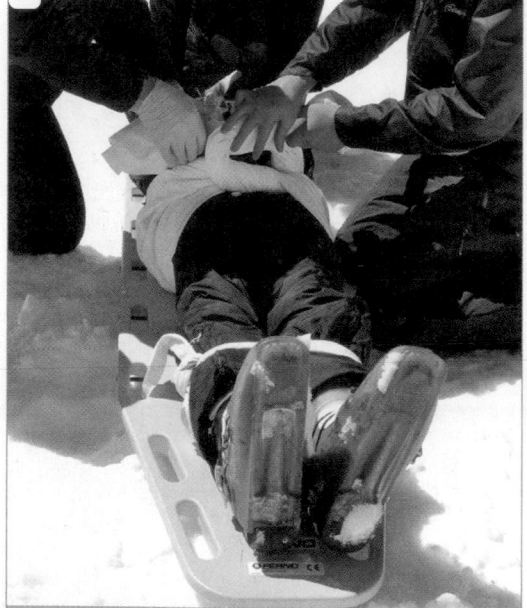

Tie the two ends using an overhand knot; finish immobilizing the patient and prepare for transport.
Copyright Candace Horgan

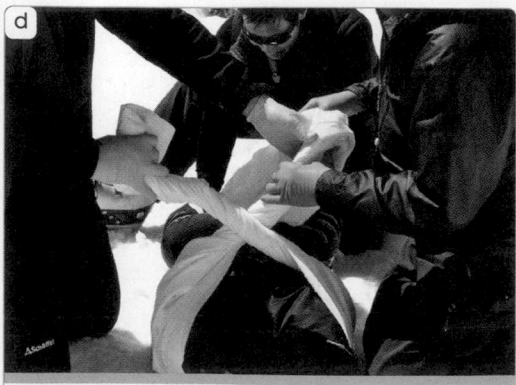

Gently pull the ends of the sheet tight.
Copyright Candace Horgan

## Skill Guide

Date: _____

(CPI) = Critical Performance Indicator

Candidate: _____

Start Time: _____

End Time: _____

## Pelvic Stabilization

**Objective:** To demonstrate ability to apply a pelvic/sheet binding to stabilize a suspected pelvic fracture.

| Skill | Max Points | Skill Demo | |
|---|---|---|---|
| Determines that the scene is safe. | 1 | | (CPI) |
| Introduces self, obtains permission to treat/help. | 1 | | |
| Initiates Standard Precautions. | 1 | | (CPI) |
| Maintains spinal alignment. | 1 | | (CPI) |
| Measures and applies a C-collar per local protocol. | 1 | | (CPI) |
| Folds a sheet lengthwise 12–18" wide and places it on a backboard where the pelvis will be positioned. | 1 | | |
| Log rolls patient onto backboard maintaining spinal alignment; positions patient so that the buttocks are positioned on the sheet 1–2" above the top of the iliac crest. | 1 | | (CPI) |
| Draws the two ends together over the symphysis pubis, compressing the greater trochanters of the femur. | 1 | | |
| Gently pulls the ends of the sheet tight. | 1 | | |
| Ties the two ends using an overhand knot, or wraps the two sheet ends around each other before securing the ends with one or two nylon cable ties. | 1 | | |
| Keeps the patient's knees slightly flexed, and pads under the legs/knees with a rolled-up blanket. | 1 | | |
| Secures the patient's knees and ankles with cravats, padding any voids. | 1 | | (CPI) |
| Secures the patient to the backboard, ensuring that the backboard straps do not go over or put stress on the injured area. | 1 | | (CPI) |

| Must receive 11 out of 13 points. |
|---|

Comments: _____

Failure of any of the CPIs is an automatic failure.

Evaluator: _____ NSP ID: _____

PASS    FAIL

# ✚ Chapter Review

## Chapter Summary

As the largest cavity in the body, the abdominopelvic cavity contains numerous solid and hollow structures and a vast network of blood vessels. Because injuries to these structures are not always obvious, OEC Technicians must carefully assess both the patient and the mechanism of injury. Frequent reassessment is needed because an initially stable patient can rapidly develop shock. Abdominopelvic injuries can be life-threatening. Overall management includes early recognition, treatment for shock, and rapid transportation to a trauma center.

## Remember...

1. The most obvious injury is not always the most serious one.
2. The initial presentation may be relatively benign; shock may develop over time.
3. Assessment of abdominal trauma includes examining all four quadrants and taking serial sets of vital signs.
4. Do not give a patient with abdominal trauma anything by mouth.

## Chapter Questions

### Multiple Choice

Choose the correct answer.

1. Which of the following statements regarding assessment of a patient who fell 6 feet from a rock face and landed straddling a boulder is true?_____
   a. OEC Technicians should refrain from examining possible genital injuries in the field.
   b. *Only* a same-sex OEC Technician should check for potential pelvic injuries; if a same-sex OEC Technician is not available, examination of the injury should wait until the patient is seen in the emergency department.
   c. If an injury is suspected, an exam is warranted.
   d. Because of the strength of the pelvic girdle, genital injuries are rare and rarely serious, so examining a potential genital injury is rarely warranted.

2. If you do not have any sterile saline with which to moisten a dressing to place on an open abdominal injury from which several inches of intestines are protruding, which of the following treatments is appropriate? _____
   a. water that is clean enough to drink
   b. milk warmed to room temperature
   c. a high-tannin green or black tea cooled to room temperature
   d. a dry dressing

3. Which of the following statements regarding abdominal or pelvic trauma are true? (check all that apply)
   _____a. The most obvious injury is not always the most dangerous injury.
   _____b. Assessment of abdominal trauma includes assessing all four abdominal quadrants.
   _____c. Assessing abdominal trauma includes serial sets of vital signs.
   _____d. It is acceptable to give a patient small amounts of food or water.

_____**e.** Unless signs and symptoms are obvious, patients with suspected abdominal trauma need not follow up with definitive medical care until signs or symptoms develop.

_____**f.** An initial presentation may be benign in spite of serious underlying damage.

_____**g.** Signs and symptoms of shock may develop slowly.

4. Which of the following sets of vital signs, taken at five-minute intervals, could be indicative of a serious internal injury?_____

   **a.** Pulse: 80, 92, 80, and 78; BP: 110/70, 112/70, 110/72, and 112/72

   **b.** Pulse: 78, 84, 92, and 99; BP: 128/78, 118/80, 112/84, and 100/70

   **c.** Pulse: 92, 88, 96, and 88; BP: 148/98, 148/96, 146/96, and 144/96

   **d.** Pulse: 96, 69, 98, and 102; BP: 120/84, 116/80, 110/76, and 120/70

5. Which of the following things could be assumed regarding potential abdominal injuries in a skier who has suffered a high-speed, blunt-trauma impact to the chest?_____

   **a.** Forceful exhalation at the time of impact could cause the diaphragm to rise and expose the upper abdominal quadrants to trauma.

   **b.** There is little or no concern about possible injury to the diaphragm because of the protection the rib cage provides.

   **c.** Thoracic and abdominal trauma do not occur concurrently because the diaphragm separates these two cavities.

   **d.** OEC Technicians should never assume anything.

6. What are the most important things to provide a teenager who has suffered an evisceration injury without accompanying spinal injury? _____

   **a.** Small sips of water at regular intervals, a dry dressing placed over the injury, ice packs applied indirectly over the injury, and rapid transport to the nearest emergency department.

   **b.** Oxygen applied at 4 LPM with a nasal cannula, a bulky pressure dressing secured to the wound, and rapid transport on a backboard with the patient prone and the knees bent.

   **c.** High-flow oxygen through a nonrebreather mask, a moist, sterile dressing covered with dry bandaging, blankets and other methods of keeping the patient warm, and rapid transport on a backboard (with the patient supine with the knees bent, or in a position of comfort).

## List

List five medical devices or other pieces of equipment that you could use to help a patient who has suffered a pelvic fracture and possible internal injuries in the field.

_____

_____

_____

_____

_____

## Scenario

*While you are on base duty in the treatment room, a 68-year-old male skier walks in and explains that he fell up on the mountain and has some minor discomfort in his lower midsection. After skiing down, the patient walked to his car and put his skis away before walking to the treatment room.*

*You assist the man into the treatment area and seat him on a chair. A primary assessment does not reveal any issues or external bleeding. As you start a secondary assessment, you take a SAMPLE history. The patient has no significant history and takes no prescription drugs. He explains that he lost control and then fell on his pole handle, which struck his groin.*

*Using the OPQRST mnemonic, you attempt to locate the source of pain, and the patient responds that he does not have any noticeable pain but that something does not feel right in his groin area.*

*Palpation does not identify any specific pain. While still in a seated position you lift each of the patient's legs while keeping the knee bent. When you lift his right leg, the patient reports pain in the groin area.*

**1.** Based on the MOI and the pain in the groin area, you suspect that the patient is experiencing a_____
   **a.** hip fracture.
   **b.** lower hernia.
   **c.** UTI.
   **d.** right-sided pelvic fracture.

*The patient denies any neck, head, or back pain.*

**2.** To treat this injury, you place the patient on a_____
   **a.** long board in a supine position with the knees flexed.
   **b.** long board in the right recumbent position.
   **c.** scope stretcher in the left recumbent position.
   **d.** long board in a supine position.

*With the help of additional patrollers, you lift and move the patient from a seated position to the stabilizing device. Because the likelihood of internal bleeding with this injury is high, you call an ALS ambulance for transport.*

*Commercially available girdles are available for stabilizing the injury.*

**3.** OEC Technicians can create a girdle by_____
   **a.** folding a sheet so that it is 8 inches wide and wrapping it around the patient's hip area.
   **b.** folding a sheet so that it is 12–18 inches wide, wrapping it around the patient's hips, and tying it off.
   **c.** placing a backboard strap around the patient's hip and drawing it tight.
   **d.** placing two straps over the patient's hip after placing the patient on the stabilizing device.

**4.** To better stabilize the patient on the transporting device, OEC Technicians should_____
   **a.** place a padded board from the hip to the foot along the lateral aspect of the patient's injured side.
   **b.** tie the patient's knees together with cravats.
   **c.** place a strap above and below the patient's flattened knees.
   **d.** tie the patient's knees together with cravats and pad under the bent knees.

# Suggested Reading

Abdominal Trauma, Blunt. http://www.emedicine.com/emerg/topic1.htm

Bernard, R. B., and B. A. McLellan. 1996. "Blunt Abdominal Trauma." *Emer. Med. Clinics of North America* 14(1): 151–169.

Lee, C., and K. Porter. 2007. "The Prehospital Management of Pelvic Fractures." *Emer. Med. J.* 24(2): 130–133.

# Cold-Related Emergencies

Marion C. McDevitt, DO
Colin K. Grissom, MD
Gregory A. Bala, MS

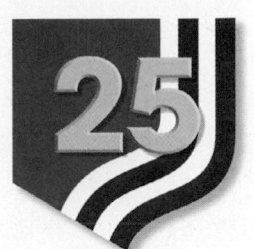

## ⊕ OBJECTIVES

**Upon completion of this chapter, the OEC Technician will be able to:**

**25-1** List and define the four mechanisms of heat loss.

**25-2** List the signs and symptoms of cold exposure.

**25-3** List the signs and symptoms of frostbite.

**25-4** List and explain the two classifications of hypothermia.

**25-5** List and explain the three categories of hypothermia related to severity.

**25-6** Define afterdrop and explain how to prevent it.

**25-7** Describe and demonstrate the assessment and emergency care of a patient with a cold injury.

**25-8** Describe and demonstrate the assessment and emergency care of a patient with frostbite.

**25-9** Describe and demonstrate the assessment and emergency care of an avalanche victim.

## ⊕ KEY TERMS

**afterdrop,** *p. 820*
**convection,** *p. 817*

**frostbite,** *p. 818*
**hypothermia,** *p. 819*

**thermoregulation,** *p. 815*
**wind chill,** *p. 817*

## Chapter Overview

The natural beauty of the great outdoors can be found almost anywhere. Whether you are high in the mountains, deep in the forest, or out in the desert, one thing is certain: you need to be prepared (Figure 25-1■). Weather is often the biggest challenge in any outing. It can be unpredictable, changing suddenly. As described in Chapter 2, a little preparation before traveling into the wilderness can save lives.

*continued*

## HISTORICAL TIMELINE

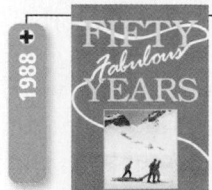

**1988** — 50th Anniversary of NSP held in Boston.

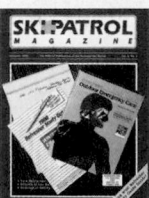

**1989** — Ski Patrol Magazine depicting the first OEC Refresher Guide.

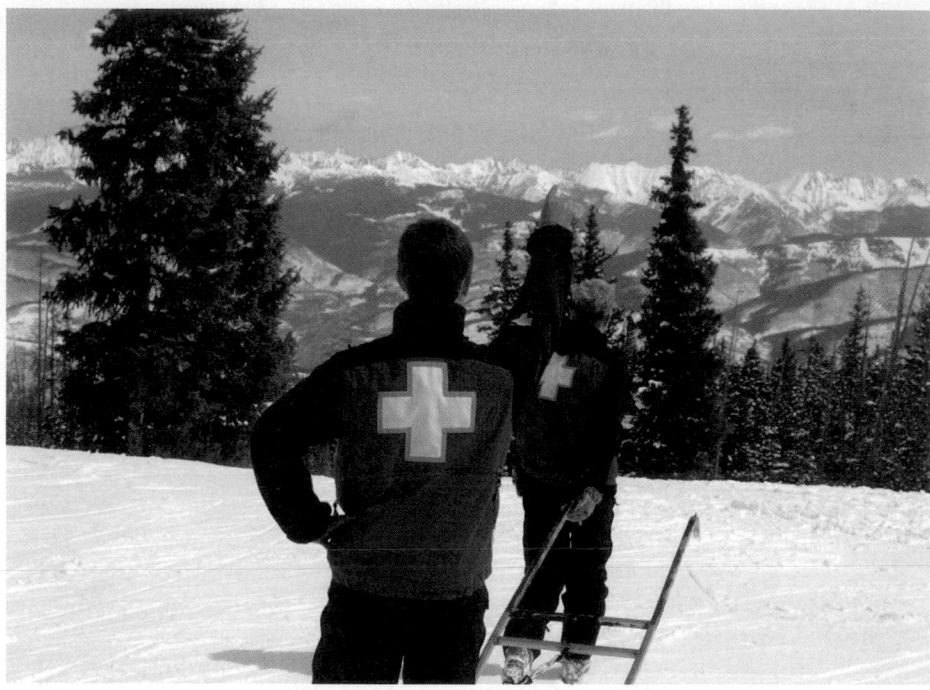

**Figure 25-1** The natural beauty of the outdoors can be found anywhere!
Copyright Scott Smith

Cold temperatures, in combination with inadequate preparation (i.e., necessary clothing, food, and shelter) and insufficient physiologic response, can overwhelm the body's mechanisms for regulating temperature. A variety of medical emergencies can result from exposure to cold, particularly during recreational activities in wilderness and high-altitude environments (Figure 25-2■). These emergencies include localized injuries (e.g., frostbite) and systemic illnesses (e.g., hypothermia and related problems). As an OEC Technician, you can save lives by recognizing and responding properly to these emergencies.

This chapter describes how the body regulates its core temperature and the ways in which body heat is lost to the environment. Also discussed are various forms of cold emergencies and how to assess and treat victims of frostbite, hypothermia, and avalanche.

**STAGES OF LOCAL COLD INJURY**

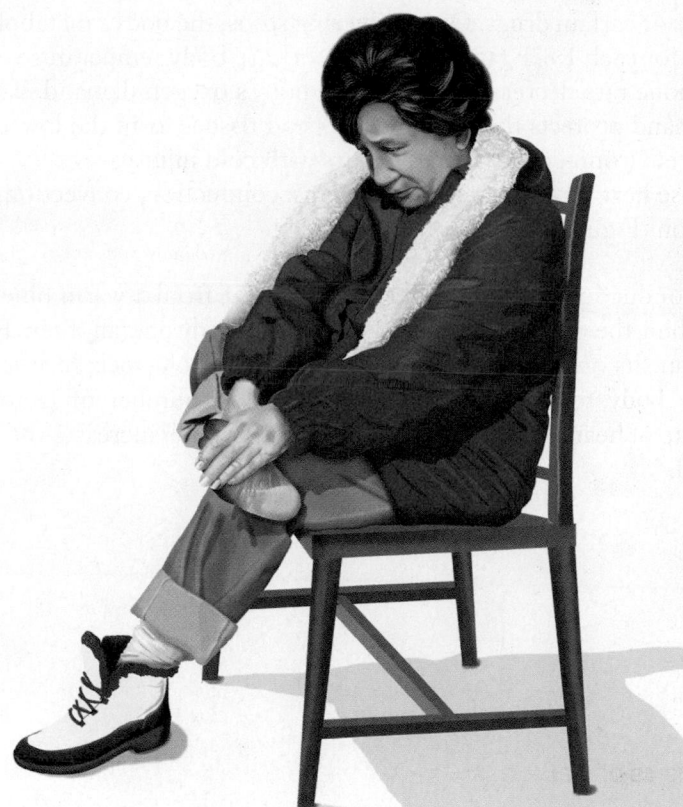

EARLY OR SUPERFICIAL COLD INJURY
usually involves the tips of the ears, the nose, the
cheek bones, the tips of the toes or fingers, and the
chin. The patient is usually unaware of the injury. As
exposure time lengthens or temperature drops, the
patient will lose feeling and sensation in the affected
area. The skin remains soft but cold to the touch,
and normal skin color does not return after palpation.
As the area rewarms, the patient may report a
tingling sensation.

LATE OR DEEP COLD INJURY
involves both the skin and tissue beneath it. The skin
itself is white and waxy with a firm to completely
solid, frozen feeling. Swelling and blisters filled with
clear or straw-colored fluid may be present. As the
area thaws, it may become blotchy or mottled, with
colors from white to purple to grayish-blue. Deep
cold injury is an extreme emergency and can result in
permanent tissue loss.

**Figure 25-2** Local cold injuries may progress from early or superficial to late or deep.

# Anatomy and Physiology

Humans evolved in tropical climates, making them much more adept at cooling (losing heat) than warming (reducing heat loss). As indicated in Chapter 7, normal body temperature is 95°–100.4°F (35°–38°C), with a median of 98.6°F (37°C). When the body's core (internal) temperature decreases, sensors located throughout the body send signals to the brain. In response, the brain sends messages to various body systems that reduce heat loss, generate heat (energy) production, or both. The process of maintaining normal body temperature is called **thermoregulation**. Body temperature is controlled by the hypothalamus, a small area of the brain located just above the brain stem. This area of the brain, in combination with the skin, blood vessels, muscles, and other organs such as the heart, lungs, and kidneys, work together to maintain homeostasis. The exact effects depend on how much core temperature changes.

When core temperature decreases, the body initially responds by constricting peripheral blood vessels. By reducing blood flow in the extremities, the body reduces heat loss through the skin. In addition, the body may divert, or shunt, blood away from colder areas. These two mechanisms are protective and ensure that the brain, heart, and other vital organs continuously receive warm blood. These mechanisms also decrease the surface temperature of the skin, so the body halts sweat production, allowing the skin to dry. In addition, body hairs stand on end to form a thin layer of trapped, warm air. If the core temperature continues to decrease, shivering begins.

**thermoregulation** the process of maintaining normal body temperature.

**25-1** List and define the four mechanisms of heat loss.

Shivering is an involuntary response that generates heat through repeated muscular contractions. Shivering is an effective means of heat production, but it ceases when core body temperature drops to below 90°F (32°C). Shivering also may be inhibited by traumatic injuries or certain drugs. Once shivering stops, the body's metabolic rate decreases 8 percent for each 1.8°F (1°C) reduction in core body temperature. Fortunately, as the metabolic rate decreases, so does the body's oxygen demand. This decline in oxygen demand protects the body's organs and tissues from the low-oxygen (or poor-perfusion) environment that often occurs with cold injuries.

The body can lose heat through four mechanisms: conduction, convection, evaporation, and radiation (Figure 25-3■).

+ **Conduction.** Conduction is the direct transfer of heat from a warm object to a colder object when the objects are in direct contact with one another. For instance, if a person sits on a snow-packed surface or on a cold rock, heat is transferred from the body to the snow or to the rock. A number of factors can accelerate the rate of heat loss, including wet clothing, which increases the rate of heat loss fivefold.

**Figure 25-3** The mechanisms of heat loss are:

a. Conduction
b. Convection
c. Evaporation
d. Radiation

**MECHANISMS OF HEAT LOSS**

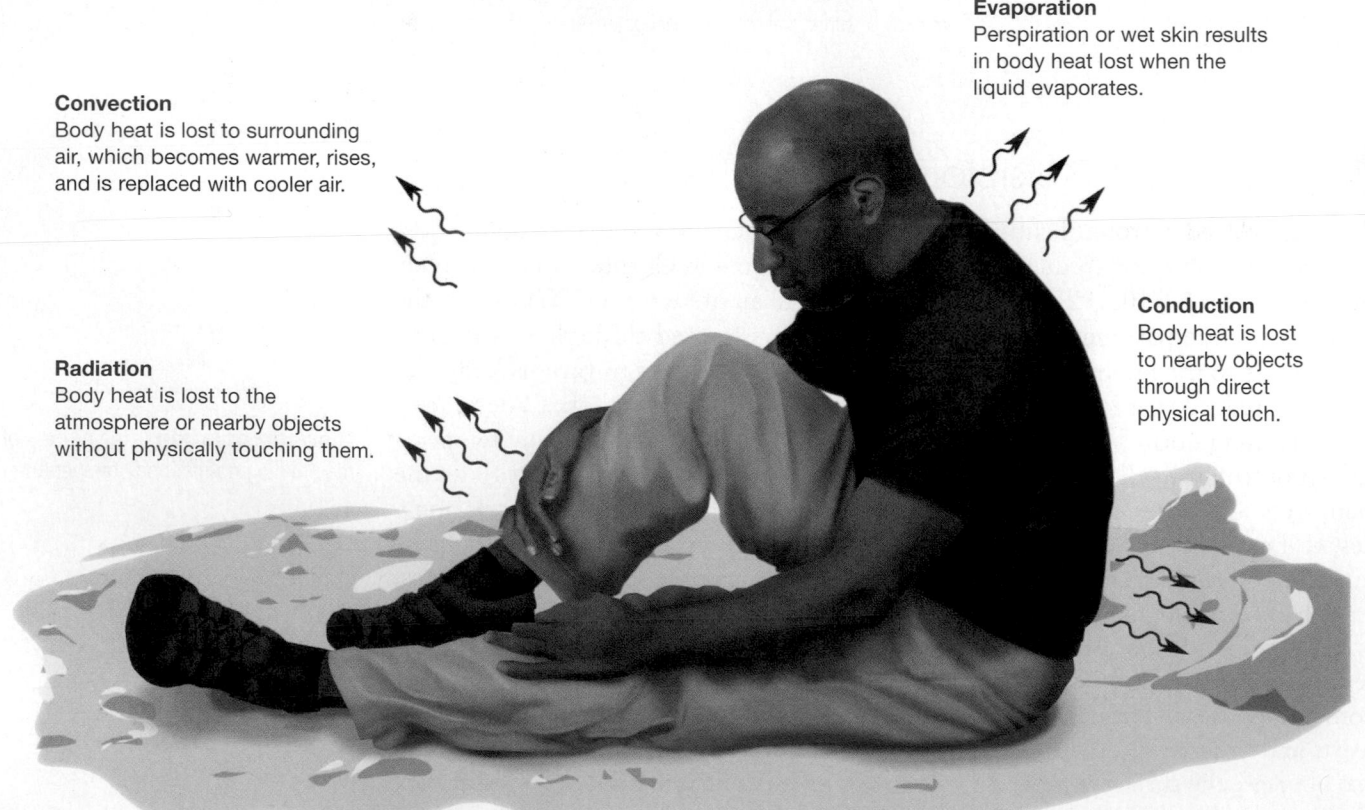

**Evaporation**
Perspiration or wet skin results in body heat lost when the liquid evaporates.

**Convection**
Body heat is lost to surrounding air, which becomes warmer, rises, and is replaced with cooler air.

**Conduction**
Body heat is lost to nearby objects through direct physical touch.

**Radiation**
Body heat is lost to the atmosphere or nearby objects without physically touching them.

WIND-CHILL INDEX

| WIND SPEED (MPH) | WHAT THE THERMOMETER READS (degrees °F) | | | | | | | | | | | |
|---|---|---|---|---|---|---|---|---|---|---|---|---|
| | 50 | 40 | 30 | 20 | 10 | 0 | −10 | −20 | −30 | −40 | −50 | −60 |
| | WHAT IT EQUALS IN ITS EFFECT ON EXPOSED FLESH | | | | | | | | | | | |
| CALM | 50 | 40 | 30 | 20 | 10 | 0 | −10 | −20 | −30 | −40 | −50 | −60 |
| 5 | 48 | 37 | 27 | 16 | 6 | −5 | −15 | −26 | −36 | −47 | −57 | −68 |
| 10 | 40 | 28 | 16 | 4 | −9 | −21 | −33 | −46 | −58 | −70 | −83 | −95 |
| 15 | 36 | 22 | 9 | −5 | −18 | −36 | −45 | −58 | −72 | −85 | −99 | −112 |
| 20 | 32 | 18 | 4 | −10 | −25 | −39 | −53 | −67 | −82 | −96 | −110 | −121 |
| 25 | 30 | 16 | 0 | −15 | −29 | −44 | −59 | −74 | −88 | −104 | −118 | −133 |
| 30 | 28 | 13 | −2 | −18 | −33 | −48 | −63 | −79 | −94 | −109 | −125 | −140 |
| 35 | 27 | 11 | −4 | −20 | −35 | −49 | −67 | −82 | −98 | −113 | −129 | −145 |
| 40 | 26 | 10 | −6 | −21 | −37 | −53 | −69 | −85 | −100 | 116 | −132 | −148 |

| Little danger if properly clothed | Danger of freezing exposed flesh | Great danger of freezing exposed flesh |
|---|---|---|

Source: U.S. Army

**Figure 25-4** Wind-Chill Index.

+ **Convection**. Convection is the direct transfer of heat through circulating air or fluid. The rate of heat loss is increased significantly when the skin is exposed directly to wind or cold water. Because of this, wind chill plays an important role in heat loss by displacing warm air next to the body. **Wind chill** is the apparent temperature felt on exposed skin and is a function of air temperature and wind speed. As air temperature falls, the chilling effect of air movement increases (Figure 25-4■). For example, a 10-mph wind lowers the apparent temperature to a greater degree at an air temperature of −4°F (−20°C) than a wind of the same speed would if the air temperature were 14°F (−10°C). Cold water accelerates heat loss by 25-fold.

+ **Evaporation**. Evaporation is the process where a liquid becomes a vapor. In humans, evaporation occurs primarily through sweating. When the body is overheated, sweat forms on the skin. The fluid absorbs body heat, which is transferred to the environment as the liquid sweat evaporates into a vapor.

+ **Radiation**. Radiation is the emission of infrared heat. Radiation may account for as much as 60 percent of heat loss, depending on the amount of the body directly exposed and the temperature difference between the body and the environment.

Chief among the factors that can predispose a person to a cold injury are alcohol and age (Figure 25-5■). Alcohol, one of the most common predisposing factors, causes peripheral vasodilatation in the skin, which leads to increased heat loss via convection. The smooth muscle in the veins in superficial soft tissues relaxes, causing the veins to widen or dilate, allowing more warm blood to reach the skin surface. The heat in the blood is then transferred to the environment. Alcohol also depresses the central nervous system, which can impair both the shivering response and judgment. Impaired judgment can lead to such irrational behaviors as not seeking appropriate shelter or not wearing appropriate clothing in a cold environment. The body's ability to self-regulate temperature adequately decreases

**convection** direct transfer of heat through circulating air; is increased when skin is exposed to wind.

**wind chill** the apparent temperature felt on exposed skin; is a function of the air temperature and wind speed.

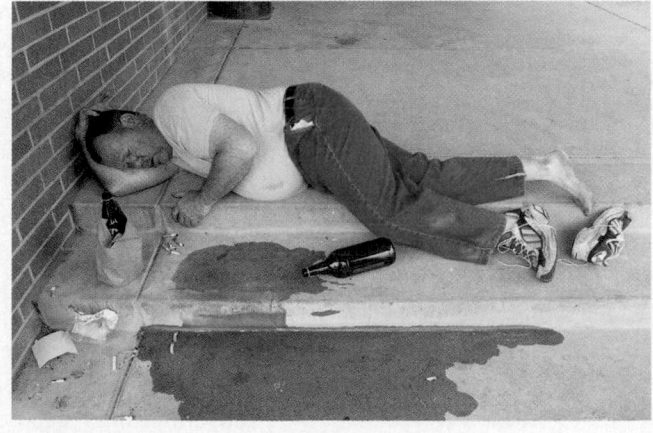

**Figure 25-5** Many factors may predispose a person to cold injury.

with advanced age. In older individuals, both body fat (needed for proper thermal insulation) and peripheral blood flow decrease. These factors, plus any chronic or underlying illnesses, put the elderly at high risk for cold injury.

Other factors that predispose a person to cold injury include:

+ Freezing temperatures
+ High winds
+ High altitude
+ Drug use
+ Previous frostbite injury
+ Overexertion, which produces fatigue and sweat
+ Poor fitting, inadequate, or wet clothing
+ Dehydration
+ Impaired circulation from chronic disease (such as heart disease or diabetes)
+ Poor nutrition

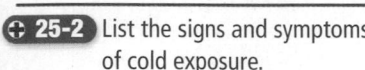

**25-2** List the signs and symptoms of cold exposure.

# Common Cold-Related Emergencies

Injury to the body from exposure to cold can be localized or involve the entire body. Directly exposing skin to a cold environment can cause frostnip or the more severe frostbite. As the entire body chills, hypothermia can occur (Figure 25-6■). If not reversed through internal or external mechanisms, it can become life threatening. The effects of cold weather illness can worsen if the affected individual does not seek warmth and shelter. Wind can exacerbate cold weather injury.

### Frostnip and Frostbite

**frostbite**  damage to tissues from freezing due to the formation of ice crystals between and within cells, rupturing the cells and leading to cell death.

**Figure 25-6** Directly exposing skin to a cold environment can cause frostnip or the more severe frostbite. As the entire body chills, hypothermia may occur.
Copyright Tristan Roberson

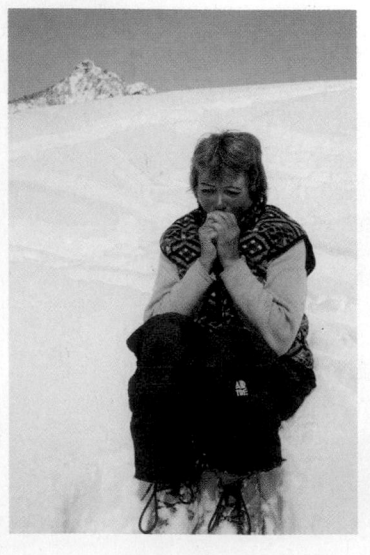

Frostnip, or chilblains, is a relatively minor, local cold injury that results from local vasoconstriction of blood vessels in response to cold. It does not involve freezing or permanent damage of the tissues. The ears, tip of the nose, fingers, and toes are prone to local cold injury such as frostnip. Affected areas are small, may appear yellowish to gray, may tingle at first, and then can be painful. Exposed body parts must be removed from exposure to the cold, and placing a warm hand over but not rubbing a frostnipped area is often enough to warm the affected area. Once the skin is warmed, no blisters appear, and the tissue is a normal color but may be slightly shiny.

**Frostbite** is the actual freezing of body tissue (Figure 25-7■). The same parts of the body that are affected by frostnip are most susceptible to frostbite. It may involve only superficial tissues, or it may extend to deep tissues and even bones in severe cases. Although frostbite generally occurs at temperatures below freezing, severity is not always related to absolute temperature, but instead is determined by the extent and duration of the freezing of the tissues.

Tissue injury from frostbite is produced in two ways. First, the actual freezing of the tissue forms ice crystals from within and between cells, extracting water from them. This leads to dehydration and chemical imbalances in the cells and damages proteins. The second and more significant mechanism of tissue injury is loss of blood supply to cells as capillaries and other small blood vessels are damaged. Additionally, damage to surviving capillaries and veins results in leakage of the liquid part of the blood (serum) out into the tissue. This causes sludging or thickening of the blood, making it semisolid. The blood eventually clots and forms blockages, further restricting blood flow. The lack of blood supply causes tissue death.

Obviously, the earlier the freezing is discovered and reversed, the less severe the overall injury will be. As with burns, the extent of damage caused by frostnip or frostbite is determined by how deeply the cold injury penetrates the skin and underlying structures. The conditions are categorized as follows:

+ *Superficial (frostnip).* Affects the first or top layer of skin; no permanent damage to the tissues results.
+ *Partial thickness (frostbite).* Affects the upper layers of skin; minor damage to the tissues results.
+ *Full thickness (frostbite).* Affects all the layers of skin plus muscle, and may even affect bone; severe damage to the tissues, including death, results.

Frostbite injury most commonly affects the distal parts of the extremities. The fingers and toes are affected most because they are farthest from the body core and large muscles that generate heat. Additionally, in cold conditions the blood supply to the extremities is greatly reduced by peripheral vasoconstriction, which shunts blood to the body core to preserve heat. Finally, during cold activities the extremities are subject to conductive cooling in addition to radiation and evaporative losses that the rest of the body endures. Hypothermia increases these physiologic responses, so all hypothermic patients must be closely evaluated for secondary frostbite injury.

The second most common sites for frostbite are the cheeks, nose, and ears. Wearing a protective mask, gator, or scarf can help prevent facial frostbite. Note, however, that constrictive clothing contributes to reduced blood flow and therefore reduced heat delivery to the area. The male genitalia are also common sites for frostbite.

## Hypothermia

**Hypothermia** is an abnormally low body temperature. Clinically, it is defined as a body temperature below 95°F (35°C) according to the American Heart Assocation (AHA). Hypothermia occurs when heat loss exceeds metabolic heat production and heat conservation. The condition can occur at temperatures well above freezing, especially when a person is in contact with flowing cold water or wind. As body temperature first drops (mild hypothermia), metabolism initially increases, causing shivering, which serves to warm the body. As core temperature drops further (moderate to severe hypothermia), body systems slow, causing clumsiness, stumbling, mental confusion, and eventually unresponsiveness. The patient is often unaware of what is happening, further exacerbating the seriousness of the condition.

Factors that predispose an individual to hypothermia include decreased heat production (due to insufficient food and decreased metabolism), impaired thermoregulation (causes include reduced shivering due to exhaustion, plus alcohol, drugs, critical illness, and trauma), and increased heat loss due to environmental exposure (resulting from inadequate insulation in cold temperatures or immersion in cold water).

Hypothermia is commonly divided into two types: primary hypothermia and secondary hypothermia.

### Primary Hypothermia

Primary hypothermia results from environmental exposure and is of two kinds: immersion hypothermia and non-immersion hypothermia.

Immersion hypothermia occurs when the entire body is underwater, or when only the head is above the water (Figure 25-8■). In cold water immersion, body core cooling rates are fast, but hypothermia does not occur as quickly as might be thought. A common misconception is that immersion in very cold water, even with protective

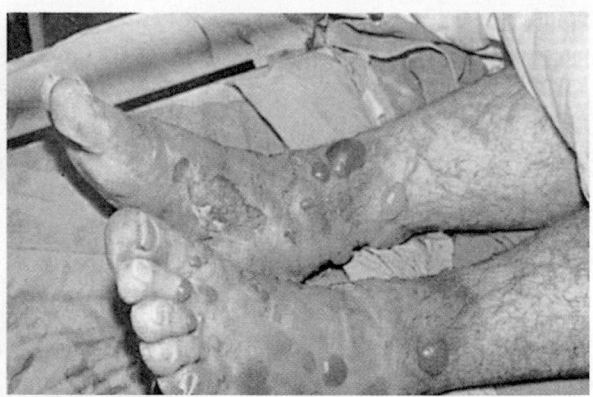

**Figure 25-7** Frostbite. In late or deep cold injury, the skin may appear white, waxy, and feel firm to frozen solid.

⊕ **25-3** List the signs and symptoms of frostbite.

---

### The Right Boot Fit

Tight fitting ski or hiking boots apply pressure to the top of the foot, constricting the dorsalis pedis artery on the top of the foot. This decreases blood flow to the toes and can exacerbate cold injury. If your feet get cold, loosen the buckle on the top of your ski boots or loosen the laces of your hiking boots to allow better blood flow to the toes.

NOTE

**hypothermia** an abnormally low body temperature; below 95°F (35°C).

---

⊕ **25-4** List and explain the two classifications of hypothermia.

**Figure 25-8** In cold water, even protective clothing may not be enough to protect against hypothermia.
Copyright Scott Smith

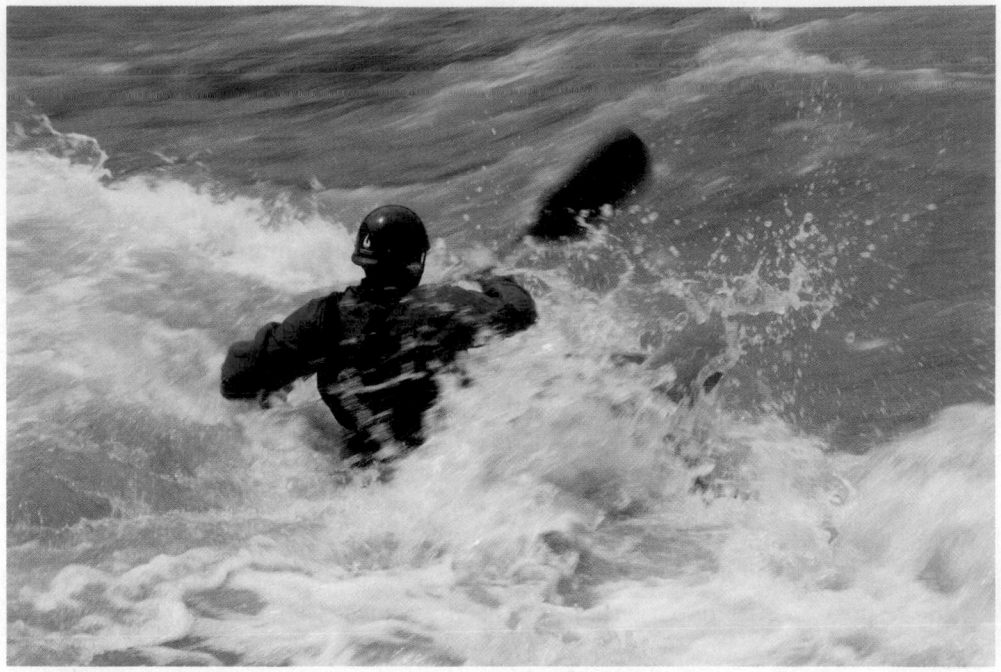

clothing, results in death from hypothermia within a few minutes. It actually takes more than 30 minutes for individuals to become hypothermic after falling into very cold water while wearing winter clothing, if the person is wearing a personal flotation device or can somehow hold his head above the water. The problem is that without a life jacket, the person must tread water, but muscle function in the arms and legs will be lost after 10 to 15 minutes, and drowning can occur.

Non-immersion hypothermia, or accidental hypothermia, occurs more slowly but may be accelerated by wind, rain, or snow if the person lacks adequate insulation (Figure 25-9■).

## Secondary Hypothermia

Secondary hypothermia occurs with systemic disorders and is frequently associated with traumatized or critically ill patients. In this situation, an injury or illness is the primary problem, and hypothermia is an associated secondary problem. Secondary hypothermia still can be severe and even life threatening.

## Classification of Hypothermia

**25-5** List and explain the three categories of hypothermia related to severity.

Hypothermia is categorized according to the patient's core temperature. The three categories of hypothermia are:

+ Mild hypothermia: core temperature of below 95°F (35°C)
+ Moderate hypothermia: core temperature of 86°–93.2°F (30°–34°C)
+ Severe hypothermia: core temperature below 86°F (30°C)

**afterdrop** a continued drop in core temperature after removal from cold exposure.

**25-6** Define afterdrop and explain how to prevent it.

## Afterdrop

**Afterdrop** is defined as a continued drop in core body temperature after removal from exposure to the cold. Typically, afterdrop occurs for a limited time, even *after* warming measures are initiated. It is thought to be caused by the return of cold blood from the extremities to the heart, resulting in a further drop in core body temperature. In severe cases, afterdrop can result in shock and cardiac arrest.

**STAGES OF HYPOTHERMIA**

**Mild:** Shivering is a response by the body to generate heat. It begins at a body temperature of 96.8°F (36°C) and ceases at 90°F (32°C).

**Moderate:**

**Apathy and decreased muscle function.** First fine motor function is affected, then gross motor functions.

**Decreased level of responsiveness** is accompanied by a glassy stare and possible freezing of extremities.

**Severe:**

**Decreased vital signs**, including slow pulse and slow respiration rate.

**Death.**

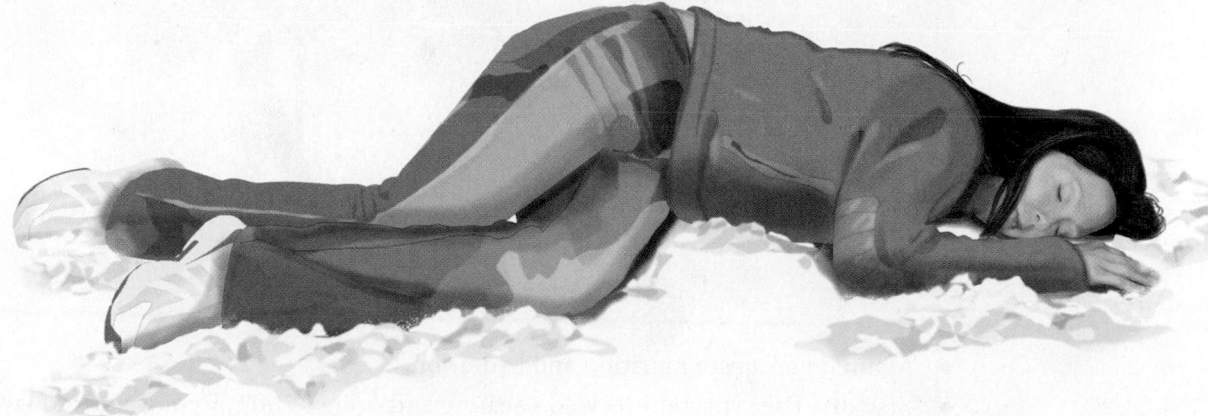

**Figure 25-9** Stages of hypothermia.

## Windburn

Windburn is an irritation of the skin that resembles superficial sunburn. It is partly due to the drying effect of the low humidity at high altitudes. It can be prevented to some extent by wearing a facemask or by applying a greasy sunscreen. Although windburn is not a cold injury, it can compound cold-related injuries, especially frostbite.

## Rescuer Preparation for Cold Weather Rescue

Do not become the victim! Prevention of a cold-related injury centers on protecting oneself from the mechanisms of heat loss. Convection, conduction, radiation, and evaporation all play important roles in frostbite. Because the nose and ears are frequently exposed to cold weather, wet conditions, and wind, they are especially vulnerable to convective and radiant heat losses. These areas are easily chilled and therefore susceptible to freezing if not adequately protected. Because OEC Technicians spend considerable time outdoors, they are at increased risk for cold injury (Figure 25-10■).

To reduce your risk:

✦ Know your environment and be prepared.

✦ Bring adequate appropriate clothing for the environment and use a strategy of layering insulation, with inner synthetic "wicking" insulating layers and an outer shell layer (Figures 25-11a–c■).

✦ Be attentive to yourself and your companions.

**Figure 25-10** Rescuers that work outside are at high risk for cold injury.
Copyright Studio 404

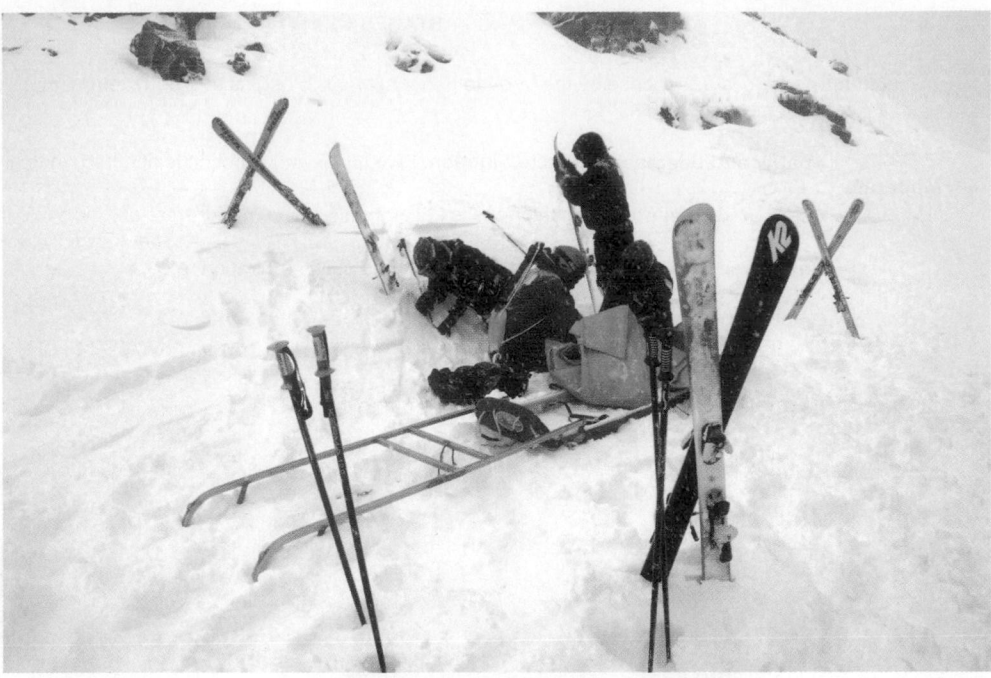

- ✦ Maintain adequate nutrition and hydration.
- ✦ Stay dry. Pace yourself to avoid sweating and overexertion. Remove or add layers of clothing as appropriate. Keep your feet dry.
- ✦ Avoid tight and restrictive clothing and boots.
- ✦ Change your socks often (at least daily, and never sleep wearing wet socks).
- ✦ Avoid alcohol, caffeine, and drugs, because they predispose you to cold injury.
- ✦ Do not tolerate numbness in your hands or feet.

For more information about how to prepare yourself adequately for outdoor rescue operations, refer to Chapter 3, Rescue Basics.

**Figure 25-11a** A rescuer needs to layer his clothing for the sometimes rapidly changing environment. The first layer should be light and breathable fabric.
Copyright Scott Smith

**Figure 25-11b** This rescuer has dressed for greater warmth by adding a jacket with wind-blocking protection.
Copyright Scott Smith

**Figure 25-11c** He has now covered both hands and head. His core will be warmed by the addition of the zipped up insulated vest with the standing collar.
Copyright Scott Smith

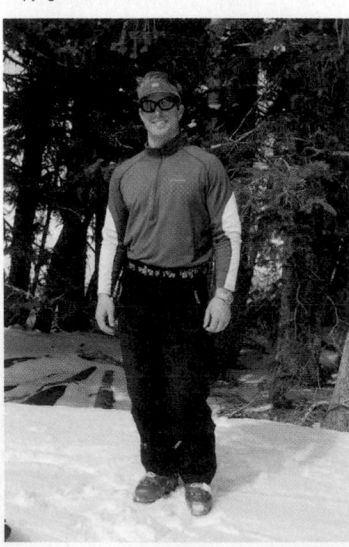

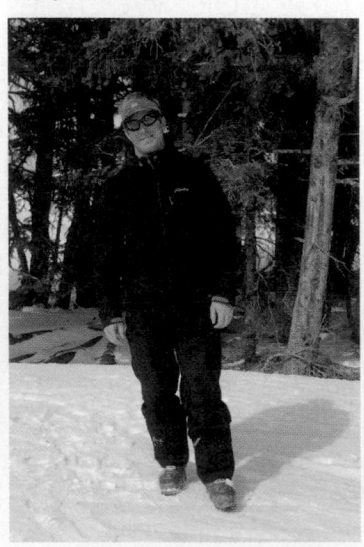

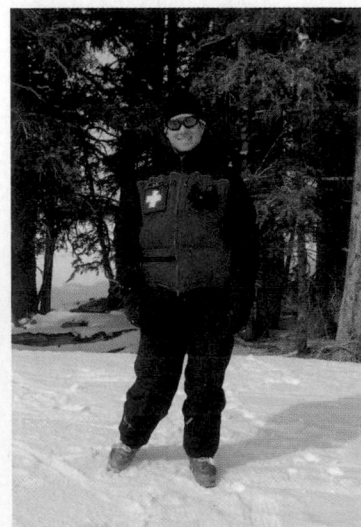

## STOP, THINK, UNDERSTAND

### Multiple Choice

Choose the correct answer.

1. When core body temperature decreases, the body initially responds by _____
   a. dilating peripheral blood vessels.
   b. shunting blood toward colder areas.
   c. maintaining even blood flow to all body parts.
   d. constricting peripheral blood vessels.

2. All of the following are protective mechanisms to ensure the brain, heart, and other vital organs receive warm blood, except _____
   a. shivering begins.
   b. body hairs stand on end.
   c. blood is shunted toward colder areas.
   d. sweat production ceases.

3. All of the following are true concerning frostnip, except _____
   a. it is a minor injury.
   b. upon rewarming, blisters occur.
   c. there is no permanent tissue damage.
   d. chilblains is another term for this cold injury.

4. Signs and symptoms of moderate to severe hypothermia include all of the following, except _____
   a. a core body temperature below 86°F (30°C).
   b. mental confusion.
   c. the onset of shivering.
   d. clumsiness and stumbling.

### List

1. List ten factors that may predispose a person to a cold injury.

   1. _____
   2. _____
   3. _____
   4. _____
   5. _____
   6. _____
   7. _____
   8. _____
   9. _____
   10. _____

2. List seven things that you can do to reduce your risk of cold-related injuries.

   1. _____
   2. _____
   3. _____
   4. _____
   5. _____
   6. _____
   7. _____

 # CASE UPDATE

You move the patient from the gondola and into the gondola base building, where you have room to work on her. Her clothes are wet and she appears to be dead. Her skin is pale and cold to the touch, and she is unresponsive. You immediately check her carotid pulse for 10 seconds, and you identify that it is very slow. There are no signs of trauma.

**What should you do now?**

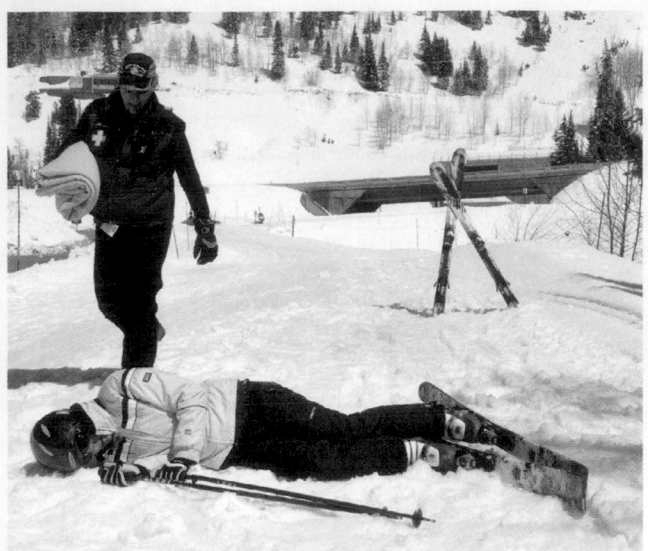

**Figure 25-12** OEC Technicians should have a blanket available to provide warmth and to treat the patient for shock.
Copyright Candace Horgan

**⊕ 25-7** Describe and demonstrate the assessment and emergency care of a patient with a cold injury.

**⊕ 25-8** Describe and demonstrate the assessment and emergency care of a patient with frostbite.

**Figure 25-13** As a late or deep cold injury begins to thaw, the injured area may change color from white to purple and become blotchy or mottled.

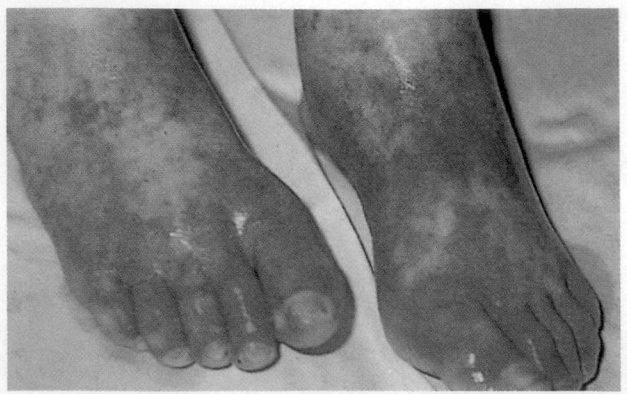

# Assessment of Cold Injuries

Overall assessment of cold injuries begins with scene safety. First and foremost, rescuers must not become patients because this can jeopardize the safety of everyone on scene. In the past some OEC Technicians have placed their jackets or clothing on a cold patient. If this will jeopardize the rescuer, it should not be done. It is better to rapidly transfer the patient to a warm environment. The OEC Technician should be prepared by having a blanket available for the patient (Figure 25-12■). "Space blankets" made of thin metallic material are lightweight and fit easily in a rescue pack.

Once the scene is considered safe, assess the patient's ABCDs just as you would any patient. However, some adjustments may be needed because heart rate and respirations can be very difficult to detect in a patient who is cold. For a patient with generalized hypothermia, the most recent 2010 AHA BLS guidelines recommend starting CPR if no pulse is detected after 10 seconds in an unresponsive patient. Performing inappropriate chest compressions because you failed to realize the patient had a very slow pulse can worsen the patient's condition by inducing cardiac arrhythmias such as ventricular fibrillation.

Once the primary assessment is complete, perform a quick secondary assessment as you remove the patient's cold or wet clothing and place him in warm blankets or wraps. Exercise caution, though, as excessive exposure of the body surface while performing a physical examination promotes further heat loss. Make every effort to limit the surface area exposed.

As part of the physical exam, look for signs of cold injury, such as frostbite, and carefully assess the patient for signs of hypothermia. Because cold injury patients may have coexisting injuries and/or illnesses, be sure to examine the patient fully using the DCAP-BTLS mnemonic, and obtain a complete SAMPLE history. Because the signs and symptoms of hypothermia may be exacerbated by alcohol, diabetes, altitude sickness, overdose, exhaustion, and other conditions, a thorough assessment of the patient is warranted.

## Frostbite

The earliest symptom of frostbite is pain at the involved site, although this is variable. This symptom is followed by numbness without pain, because as the tissue freezes, sensation and pain stop. The easing of pain is often mistaken for improvement of the condition.

Frostbite should be suspected if a painfully cold body part suddenly stops hurting but is not getting warmer. The affected part may initially feel soft but over time may become firm or woody to the touch. The affected area is initially white or waxy and then turns pale or red, depending on severity (Figure 25-13■). If the area involved is the head or face, someone other than the patient may be the first to notice it. Color changes in the hands and feet generally go unnoticed until these areas are uncovered.

Following warming, redness may persist over several days, followed by the appearance of clear or blood filled blisters. In severe cases, death of the affected tissue occurs. The affected area appears black, shriveled, and dry, a condition known as dry gangrene. Table 25-1■ lists the signs and symptoms of frostbite.

| Table 25-1 | Signs and Symptoms of Frostnip and Frostbite |
|---|---|
| Superficial (frostnip) | Skin appears cool and pale and may be painful; tissues remain intact |
| Partial thickness (frostbite) | Skin has white or gray colored patches that are not painful; tissue may indent if pressed; tissue loss, if present, is minimal |
| Full thickness (frostbite) | Skin is cold and feels hard or woody; tissue is white or gray and will not rebound when pressed; the area is numb (no pain); no pulse can be detected |

**Table 25-2** Severity of Hypothermia

| Severity of Hypothermia | Patient Presentation | Core Body Temperature |
|---|---|---|
| Mild | Alert but may be confused, shivering | below 95°F (35°C) |
| Moderate | Drowsy, decreased level of responsiveness, not shivering | 86°–93.2°F (30°–34°C) |
| Severe | Unresponsive, may not be breathing | < 86°F (< 30°C) |

## Hypothermia

As previously noted, hypothermia is divided into three categories that are defined by core body temperature ranges. In the field, measurement of core temperature can be difficult or impossible. Table 25-2■ presents a system for estimating core body temperature and the severity of hypothermia based on the patient's presentation.

### Mild Hypothermia

Generally, mild hypothermia (below 95°F or 35°C) first manifests as shivering, which can be vigorous. Shivering is an important mechanism that significantly increases muscle activity and heat production. It initially starts when the body's core temperature falls below 96.8°F (36°C). Unless other factors are present, shivering should enable the patient to overcome heat loss and elevate core temperature. In fact, most patients with mild hypothermia are able to warm themselves through shivering alone, although they still require protection from further heat loss in the form of warm, dry insulation for the body.

If core temperature continues to fall, uncontrollable shivering is observed until the core temperature reaches approximately 90°F (32°C). The exceptions to this are exhausted patients who are unable to shiver, and some cases of chronic exposure (greater than 6–8 hours) in which exhaustion occurs and shivering stops. Such patients generally remain responsive, although they may be confused and exhibit both a loss of judgment and decreased fine motor coordination (Figure 25-14■).

### Moderate Hypothermia

The transition to moderate hypothermia (86°–93.2°F or 30°–34°C) is characterized by cessation of shivering (usually at a core temperature of about 90°F or –32°C). A progressive slowing of metabolism also occurs, as evidenced by a slow pulse

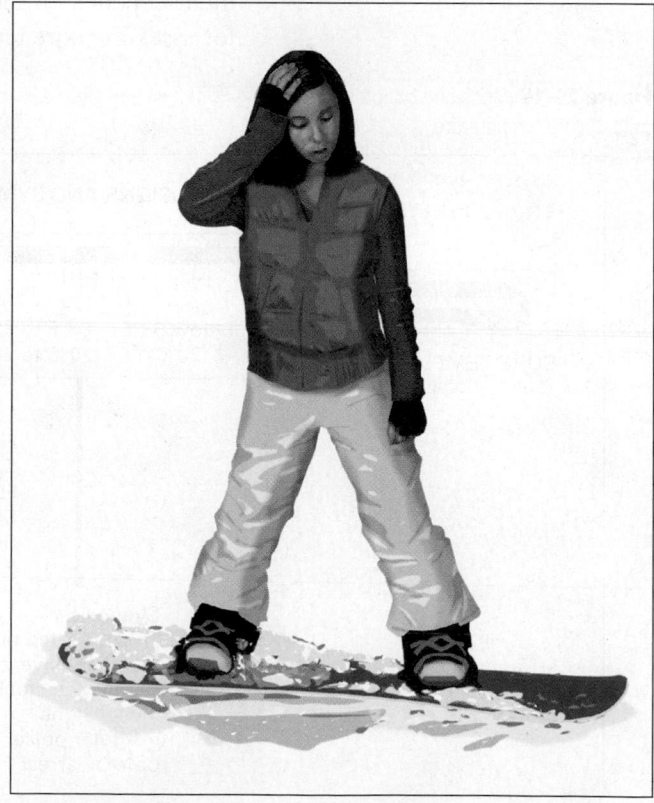

**Figure 25-14** Confusion is one of the first stages of hypothermia.

and/or slow respirations. As the heart rate falls and peripheral vasoconstriction relaxes, hypotension results. In other words, the heart beats more slowly and the blood vessels in the arms and legs relax, allowing more blood into the extremities and causing blood pressure to fall. The level of responsiveness continues to decrease from slurred speech and a staggering gait to unresponsiveness. The surface temperature of the skin gets much colder.

### Severe Hypothermia

As core temperature falls below 86°F (30°C), the heart is at risk of ventricular fibrillation, either spontaneously or in response to mechanical stimulation. For this reason, it is imperative to handle hypothermic patients gently and with great care. In severe hypothermia, mental status is severely depressed, resulting in coma. At core body temperatures nearing 77°F (25°C), the patient may appear clinically dead. Examination may reveal an unresponsive and comatose patient. The patient may be rigid, without palpable pulses or discernable respirations. The torso is cold to the touch. Pupillary eye reflexes and deep tendon reflexes are diminished or absent. Although apparently dead, the patient cannot be presumed dead unless those conditions persist after warming or obvious signs of fatal trauma are present. Suppression of energy-dependent processes markedly diminishes oxygen and metabolic demands. As cells become cold, they do not require as much oxygen and glucose. These decreased requirements explain the successful resuscitation of some hypothermic victims despite the appearance of death.

### Measuring Core Body Temperature

Important in the diagnosis of hypothermia is knowledge of the body's core temperature (Figure 25-15■), defined as the temperature of the vital organs in the *chest cavity*, including the heart, lungs, and large blood vessels. Knowing the core temperature enables you to classify hypothermia as mild, moderate, or severe. The aggressiveness of the treatment depends on the severity of hypothermia. Although multiple routes are available for assessing core temperature, the most effective procedure for the OEC Technician

**Figure 25-15** Signs and symptoms of a sinking core temperature.

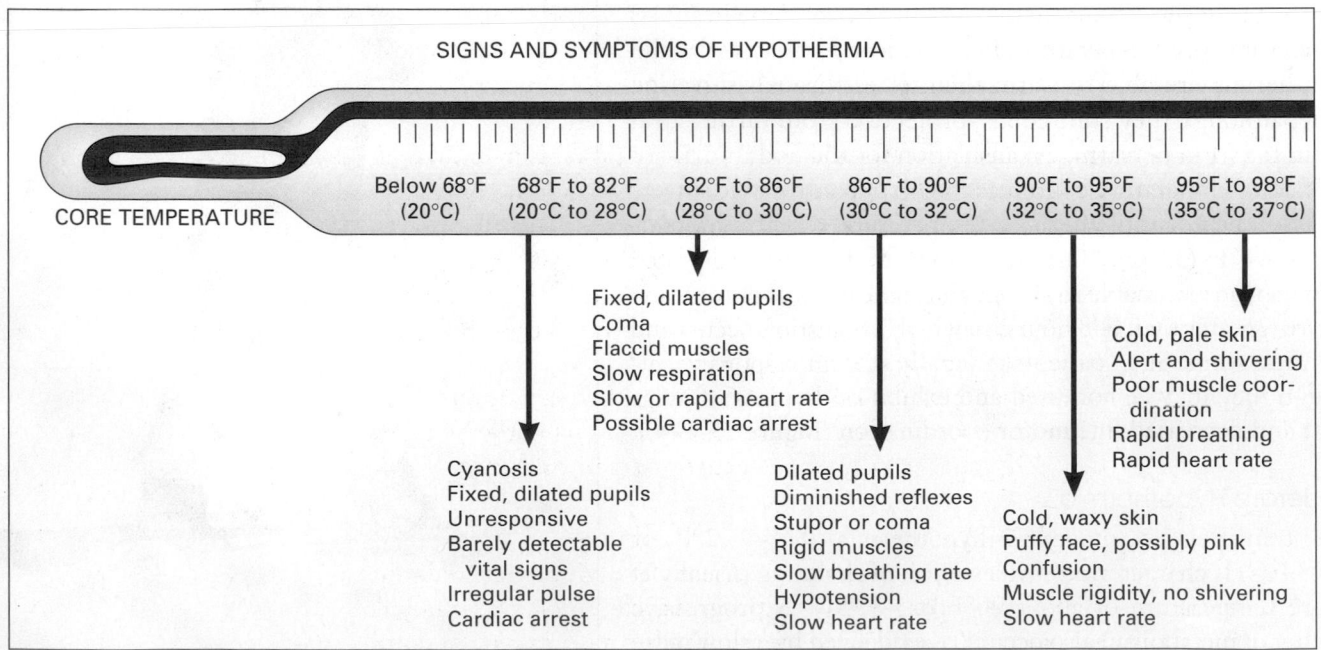

is the use of a low-temperature rectal thermometer. This instrument provides the best approximation of core temperature obtainable without the more-invasive temperature probes used in a hospital. An oral thermometer, however, used with the mouth closed gives a fairly accurate core body temperature. Other methods such as axillary or infrared tympanic thermometers are not advised. Additionally, it is important to recognize that in non-steady state conditions of cooling or warming, temperature gradients exist in the body, and differences may be observed between core and peripheral temperatures.

OEC Technicians should recognize the severity of hypothermia *clinically*. Using a rectal thermometer in the field (or, for that matter, in the aid room) is much less important than observing patients and placing them in a "category" of severity. This will give a close enough approximation of how cold a patient is, allowing you to begin your care.

# Management

The general principles of OEC treatment apply to all cases of cold injury, regardless of cause or severity. As with any situation, rescuer safety is the top priority and is ensured by mitigating any hazards that may be present. Always correct any ABCD-related problems first.

## Frostnip

Frostnip is usually easily treated by seeking shelter and warming the affected area by simply placing a warm hand or applying a warm chemical heat pack covered in cloth (so that it's not too hot). Do not rub the affected body part.

## Frostbite

The treatment for frostbite is rapid warming. Slow, gradual warming should be avoided because it is associated with greater tissue injury. Warming causes pain, sometimes severe pain, and this should be explained to the patient. Among the many factors to consider when re-warming frostbitten tissues are when, where, and how warming efforts should be performed.

### When to Warm Frostbitten Tissue

Ideally, tissues should be warmed as soon as possible following initial discovery, and in some instances prior to transport to a medical facility. Doing so may avoid further injury. However, circumstances or the lack of proper resources may prevent prompt warming. As a rule, warmed tissues must not be allowed to refreeze because in that case frostbitten tissue will become gangrenous, resulting in tissue death.

Judgment is required when deciding when to warm frozen tissue. If medical care is available in less than 2 hours, if the body part has spontaneously thawed, or if shelter and equipment are not available for thawing the part, then do not attempt to warm the tissue. If you are in the backcountry and shelter and proper equipment are available, and if rapid warming is possible and there is no possibility of refreezing, then thaw the body part. If the decision is made not to warm frozen tissue in the field, great care must be taken to protect the area from additional injury.

For patients who must self-evacuate, it is best to leave a foot frozen, because after it has thawed it will be too painful for walking. Because rapid warming in the field can be difficult, often the best field care is expeditious evacuation to medical care.

### Where to Warm a Frostbitten Body Part

Warming should be performed in a sheltered area where the patient's entire body can be kept warm. Additionally, proper equipment and sufficient resources should be available to warm the patient adequately and prevent refreezing. This is best done

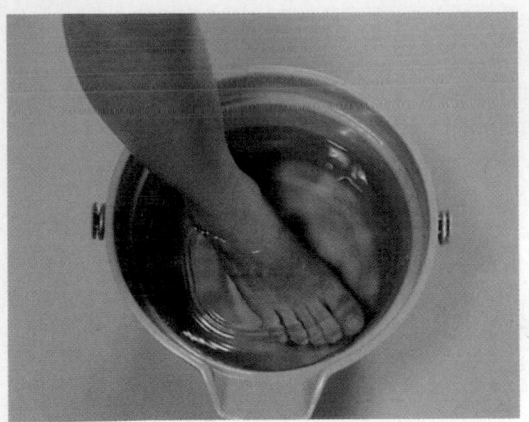

**Figure 25-16** If medical direction allows, warm the affected part by immersing it in warm water.

in a medical facility. If you are in the backcountry and a shelter such as a cabin is available, you can build a fire to heat water, and if refreezing will not occur, a frostbitten body part may be thawed.

### How to Warm a Frostbitten Body Part

Remove constrictive clothes, rings, watches, and so on. Using a vessel large enough to accommodate the limb, prepare a warm water bath that is heated to 102°–104°F (38.9°–40°C). Ideally, use a thermometer to check the water temperature. If one is not available, you should be able to comfortably place your hand in the water. Suspend the frostbitten part in the center of the warm water bath, using caution to not contact the sides or bottom. Keep the affected area in the bath for 20–30 minutes. Stir the water to keep it at a constant temperature, adding warm/hot water as needed. Allow the affected part to air dry if further heat loss is preventable (Figure 25-16■). DO NOT rub the tissues because this can cause sloughing and additional tissue damage.

Once the area is warmed, *aloe vera* ointment and dry dressings may be applied. If available, the patient may self-administer ibuprofen, but not acetaminophen or aspirin. Warming a frostbitten body part can cause severe pain that requires ALS for narcotic pain management. Be sure to place dressings between the digits. Elevate the affected area above the level of the heart to reduce swelling. In extended transport settings, such as during an expedition, daily wound care exams must be performed.

Initially it is difficult to determine the full extent of the injury. In fact, it may take several days to weeks for the final demarcation of tissue damage. The damaged or dead tissue will eventually become gangrenous and mummify, and it may even auto-amputate. This explains why amputation is not emergent and should be delayed. Extensive post-injury follow-up care is needed. Patients who have frostbitten areas with isolated, small (less than 1.5 cm), clear blisters may remain in the field if infection and subsequent refreezing can be prevented. Patients who are unable to walk, have large or blood-filled blisters, or have partial- or full-thickness cold injuries should be evacuated. Remember that people who have frostbite usually are hypothermic to some degree.

## Hypothermia: Prevent Heat Loss

Prevention of heat loss is key to the care of all cold injury patients. Move the patient gently to a shelter, and out of the wind. Relocation is best done on a litter, as self-evacuation of a patient with more than mild hypothermia can cause afterdrop. A heated building is best. If the only heat available is from a fire, make sure adequate ventilation of the smoke and carbon monoxide occurs. Replace the patient's wet or cold clothing with dry insulating clothing.

If shelter is not immediately available, protect the patient from the chilling effects of wind exposure and insulate him from the ground or other cold-conducting surfaces. Use insulating pads *beneath* the patient as a base; then add blankets or sleeping bags while maintaining adequate exposure of the patient's airway. This procedure will minimize convective and conductive heat loss while allowing for airway-related interventions, as needed. Place a wool hat on the patient's head to decrease radiant heat losses. A vapor barrier (i.e., a plastic sheet, space blanket, or large trash bag,) can be added to eliminate evaporative heat loss and to protect the insulation from getting wet. If wet clothing cannot be removed safely, place the vapor barrier between the clothing and the insulation. If the patient is dry, the barrier should be placed outside the insulation to further protect both patient and insulation from the elements. This method of insulating a hypothermic patient is referred to as a "hypothermia wrap" and is a highly effective method for conserving body heat.

## Warming Methods

Once heat loss has been minimized, attention may be turned toward warming the patient. The goal of warming efforts in the prehospital setting is to prevent afterdrop, a serious concern that must not be overlooked. In general, it is best to keep the patient lying down and still, both during and immediately following warming. A hypothermic patient who stands and walks after removal from the hypothermic environment will undergo more afterdrop than a patient who remains supine.

Warming methods are of two types: passive and active. Passive warming relies on retention of the patient's internal body heat (Figure 25-17■). In addition to the methods described in the section on preventing heat loss, shivering is the primary passive warming mechanism for patients in the field and is often all that is needed to warm patients who are mildly hypothermic.

Active warming, which involves the application of heat, may be separated into external and internal modalities. A common active external warming method is the application of hot packs or hot water bottles to major superficial arterial sites (e.g., neck, armpits, groin), the periphery (e.g., hands, feet), and the trunk (e.g., chest, abdomen). This technique does not provide enough heat to warm moderately or severely hypothermic patients who are not shivering. Thus, the use of hot packs for these patients provides limited benefit (Figure 25-18■).

Flexible plastic bladder-type systems containing warm water also may be used and have the advantage of contouring to the torso, which increases the surface area in contact and available for heat transfer. Chemical heat packs are not useful for warming the torso because the heat delivered is not sufficient. Do not apply heat sources directly to the patient's skin. Instead, insulate hot packs or hot water bottles in stockings, mittens, or between thin layers of clothing or blankets.

Other active external warming systems that are used in the field care of moderate to severe hypothermia include forced air warming systems and charcoal fuel heater systems. A forced air warming system utilizes hot air that flows through baffles or channels across the patient's body, warming it by convection. This system has been studied in both the prehospital and hospital settings and is a very effective active warming modality. Another effective backcountry system that has been well studied

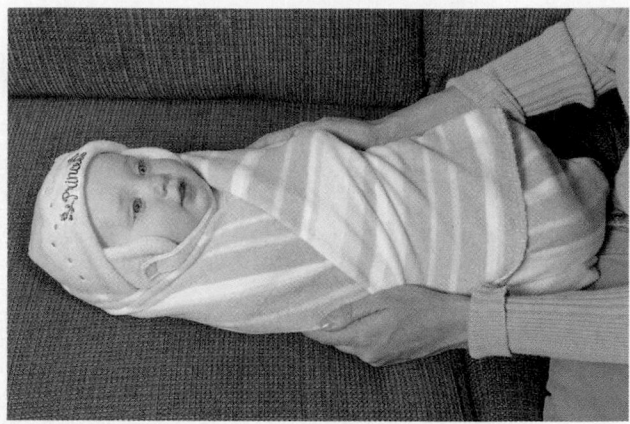

**Figure 25-17** It is important to keep pediatric patients warm to prevent hypothermia.

**Figure 25-18** One way to actively warm a mildly hypothermic patient is by placing heat packs in the groin, armpits, and on the chest. Remember to insulate the packs to prevent burns.

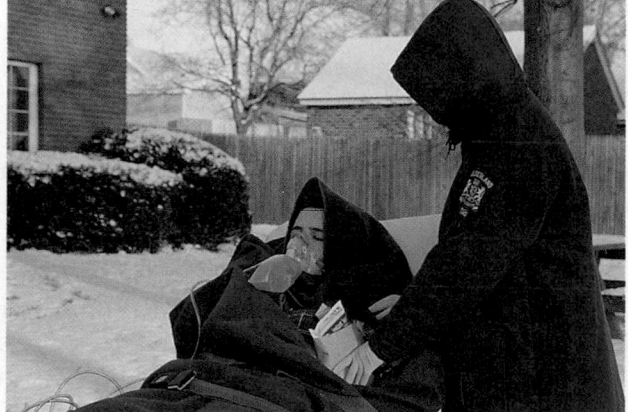

but is neither commonly used nor available is the charcoal fuel heater system. In this system, charcoal fuel is burned in a metal canister in a harness placed on the patient's chest. Heated air is blown through impermeable flexible tubing wrapped around the patient's torso. Ventilation of the burning charcoal is important to prevent carbon monoxide poisoning.

Active internal warming modalities that are available to OEC Technicians are limited to the application of heated, humidified oxygen at 40°C (if available) and to the consumption of warm beverages by patients who are responsive.

## Mild Hypothermia

If the patient is shivering vigorously, warming efforts should be augmented by applying active external warming modalities. This action, of course, is taken only after preventing further heat loss. Body-to-body contact is not necessary and may delay warming, especially if it extinguishes shivering by warming the skin but not the body core. Warm, high-energy, non-alcoholic drinks and high-energy foods containing sugar are helpful, providing that the patient is responsive, can hold an object in the hand, and can swallow without choking. This provides fuel to the body, which enables the muscles to continue to shiver, thereby generating additional heat.

Exercise will generate heat, but it may also precipitate afterdrop. If the patient is otherwise healthy and shivering vigorously, mild exercise may be initiated after 45–60 minutes of warming by shivering in an insulated environment. At this point, any afterdrop should be reversed. However, if any deterioration in physical or mental condition occurs during exercise, discontinue it immediately. Sometimes it is necessary for hypothermic patients to ambulate to leave an unsafe environment, but once in a safe location they should be placed in a supine position and treated for hypothermia.

## Moderate-to-Severe Hypothermia

Care for patients with either moderate or severe hypothermia is the same as that for those with mild hypothermia. However, patients who are moderately to severely hypothermic are extremely difficult to warm in the field, and these patients should be transported to an appropriate definitive care facility as quickly as possible for treatment with active external and/or internal warming techniques.

As a rule, the patient must be handled very gently and kept in a supine position. Because of the risk of inducing ventricular fibrillation, minimize patient movement while performing other life-sustaining measures. This is especially important when you remove the patient from the cold, and when you remove wet clothing and provide dry insulation.

Because the patient will not warm spontaneously, use of a hypothermia wrap is essential. Heat packs or warm water bottles may be applied as previously described. If medical care is remote and equipment is available, forced air or charcoal fuel systems should be considered. Body-to-body contact may be used if no other resources are available. These warming measures should not be performed in the field, however, if they delay transport to a hospital. If available and approved by your Medical Director and mountain management, deliver heated, humidified oxygen by nonrebreather mask at 12–15 LPM. Do not give a patient with altered mental status any warm drinks or food, as they may cause burns and/or choking.

Aggressive warming, such as whole-body warm-water immersion, should never be attempted because it may cause severe drops in blood pressure or ventricular fibrillation. Do not rub the extremities under any circumstances, as rubbing produces little frictional heat and may damage the skin and underlying tissue (especially if it is frozen). Rapidly transport the patient to a definitive care facility as soon as possible.

If the patient is severely hypothermic and presents without any signs of life, begin treatment immediately. A cold, rigid, apparently lifeless patient who is hypothermic may not actually be dead (Figure 25-19■). The apparent lack of pulse and apnea may be due to a very slow, faint heart rate and tissue rigidity. The time-honored tenet for caring for this type of patient is, "They are not dead until they are warm and dead!" Open the airway. Check for breathing and assess for a pulse for ten seconds. If cardiac activity is not detected, initiate CPR in the usual manner. Although the cold slows metabolism, the patient still needs oxygen, and rescue breathing or using a bag-valve-mask device (with ambient air or compressed oxygen) poses no danger to the patient. Improved ventilation and oxygenation may strengthen cardiac activity and make the pulse detectable.

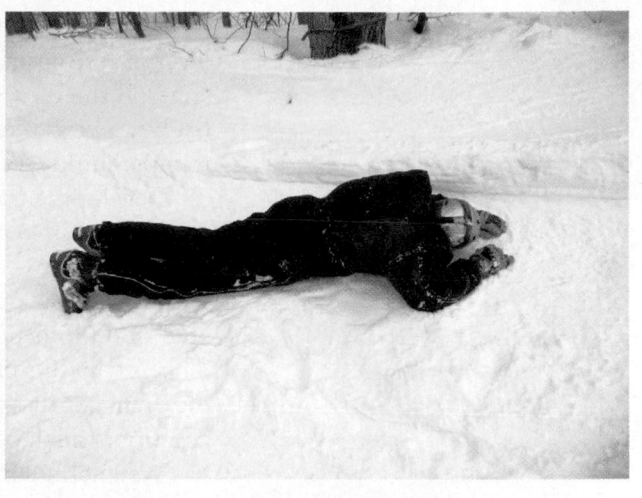

**Figure 25-19** A cold, unresponsive patient who is hypothermic may not be dead.
Copyright Edward McNamara

CPR may be indicated. However, the recommendations for CPR in a severely hypothermic patient periodically change. The specific procedure for providing CPR to a severely hypothermic patient should be confirmed with local medical advisors. Chest compressions should not be initiated on any hypothermic patient with signs of life (slow pulse or any respiratory effort) because this action may cause ventricular fibrillation. Additional treatment efforts should focus on heat loss prevention, warming, treatment of other injuries, and rapid evacuation and transport. Do not initiate chest compressions on a patient who has been submerged (drowning) in cold water for more than 1 hour, has a core temperature of less than 50°F (10°C), has obvious fatal injuries, is frozen (e.g., has ice in the airway), has a chest wall that is so stiff that compressions are impossible, or if the rescuers are exhausted or are in danger.

Use of an AED may be beneficial, although the protocols concerning its use in this situation may vary. If an AED is available to be used, the 2010 AHA BLS guidelines recommend continuing intermittent defibrillation attempts (if the AED advises) in a patient with severe hypothermia and core temperature less than 30°C as transport or rewarming is ongoing. Continue chest compressions in accordance with BLS protocol. The local Medical Director should provide input to this procedure.

### Hypothermia in an Extricated Avalanche Burial Victim

Rescue of an avalanche burial victim is a race against time. Asphyxiation is the major cause of death during avalanche burial, but hypothermia is the primary medical concern following extrication. The potential for serious trauma also is present in avalanche burial survivors, and such trauma may impair thermoregulation and accelerate the development of hypothermia.

Death from asphyxiation is time dependent. Avalanche burial victims who are extricated within 15 minutes have a greater than 90 percent chance of survival. The potential for survival is minimal when avalanche victims are buried for more than 35 minutes and have an obstructed airway and are in cardiac arrest on extrication. Survival beyond 35 minutes is usually dependent on whether the patient had an air pocket for breathing.

The initial priorities in the emergency management of an extricated avalanche burial victim are the same as for other patients: open the airway, ensure adequate ventilation (by digging the chest out of the snow so it can expand), and control external bleeding. Provide supplemental oxygen while maintaining spinal column immobilization.

⊕ **25-9** Describe and demonstrate the assessment and emergency care of an avalanche victim.

The severity of hypothermia in an avalanche burial victim may be assessed by the level of responsiveness and the duration of burial. If the avalanche victim is responsive and the duration of burial is less than one hour, then mild hypothermia is most likely, and treatment consists of providing warm dry insulation and warm sugar-containing liquids. Warming will occur through shivering.

Development of hypothermia during avalanche burial does not occur as quickly as during cold-water immersion. It generally takes more than 35 minutes of burial in an avalanche to cause moderate to severe hypothermia, but moderate or severe hypothermia may occur in avalanche burial victims *after extrication* because of accelerated development of hypothermia during exposure to a cold, windy environment. This is why it is important in the emergency care of avalanche burial victims to handle them gently and package them quickly using warming wraps in order to minimize additional heat loss.

Avalanche burial victims who have a depressed level of responsiveness and are not shivering because they have progressed to moderate or severe hypothermia will require medical transport to a hospital for definitive warming. Unresponsive avalanche burial victims who are breathing are likely moderately to severely hypothermic. Avalanche burial victims extricated after burials of 35 minutes or less who are pulseless have most likely died from asphyxiation, and although it is unlikely that resuscitation efforts will be successful, begin CPR. If CPR is unsuccessful after 30 minutes, usually the patient was already dead. However, you should continue CPR until higher-level medical personnel assume care. If burial time is greater than 35 minutes and core body temperature is less than 32°C, the victim may be severely hypothermic, and resuscitation efforts may be continued during transport to a medical facility.

## Treat Other Injuries/Illnesses

Cold injuries can occur in combination (e.g., frostbite and hypothermia) or be accompanied by other injuries, illnesses, or life-threatening conditions. Expeditiously treat all injuries and illnesses, whether associated with the cold injury or not, using appropriate methods described in other chapters. Immobilize the spine if indicated. Place fractures in the correct anatomic position, stabilizing them in the usual manner. Open wounds should be dressed before packaging the patient.

## Windburn

Treat windburn by applying soothing, greasy ointments or lotions. (Greasy sunscreens are useful for both preventing sunburn and treating windburn.)

# Evacuation and Transportation

A patient with mild hypothermia who has been adequately warmed and has returned to normal mental status need not be emergently evacuated. Take care to prevent a recurrence of cold injury, and monitor the patient to ensure resolution.

Any patient who does not respond to warming, who has moderate to severe hypothermia, or has severe frostbite must be evacuated as soon as possible and transported to a definitive care facility. Evacuation must be as gentle as possible to prevent ventricular fibrillation or additional tissue damage/injury. During transport, continue to monitor the patient's vital signs, the skin underneath any applied heat sources (for potential burns), and distal circulation (e.g., hands and feet). Reexamine the patient frequently unless doing so could increase heat loss or cause tissues to refreeze. If this potential exists, limit the patient's exposure to the best of your ability.

# STOP, THINK, UNDERSTAND

## Multiple Choice
Choose the correct answer.

1. All of the following are signs and symptoms of frostbite, except the _____
   a. core body temperature drops below 95°F (35°C).
   b. affected area is initially white or waxy.
   c. affected area appears black, shriveled, and dry.
   d. presence of clear or blood filled blisters.

2. All of the following are times in which you should not rewarm a frostbitten body part, except when _____
   a. medical care is available within two hours.
   b. there is a possibility of refreezing the body part.
   c. the body part has spontaneously thawed.
   d. the patient complains of pain while the body part is rewarming.

3. An avalanche victim extricated within _____ minutes has greater than a 90 percent chance of survival.
   a. 15
   b. 20
   c. 25
   d. 30

4. If a patient is extricated within 15 minutes, what is the percent chance of survival?
   a. 90%
   b. 20%
   c. 30%
   d. 45%

## List
List five steps you can take to minimize heat loss in the field.

1. _____
2. _____
3. _____
4. _____
5. _____

## Matching

1. Match each of the following descriptions to the correct category of hypothermia.

   _____ 1. mild hypothermia
   _____ 2. moderate hypothermia
   _____ 3. severe hypothermia

   a. the heart is at risk of ventricular fibrillation
   b. vigorous shivering occurs
   c. core body temperature is at 86°–93.2°F (30°–34°C)
   d. shivering stops
   e. core body temperature is below 86°F (30°C)
   f. core body temperature is at below 95°F (35°C)
   g. the patient appears to be clinically dead

2. Write "**yes**" in the line if the procedure should be tried to rewarm a hypothermic patient or "**no**" if the procedure should not be attempted.

   _____ a. Place the patient in a supine position.
   _____ b. Provide warm nonalcoholic high-energy drinks if the patient is responsive.
   _____ c. Apply heat packs/warm water bottles to patients with moderate to severe hypothermia.
   _____ d. Have mildly hypothermic patients exercise immediately.
   _____ e. Rapidly transport a patient with moderate to severe hypothermia to the hospital.
   _____ f. Attempt to immerse the whole body of patients with mild to severe hypothermia in warm water (if available).
   _____ g. Use body-to-body contact for patients with moderate to severe hypothermia, if no other resources are available.
   _____ h. Aggressively rub the patient's extremities to produce frictional heat.
   _____ i. Handle patients with moderate to severe hypothermia very gently to minimize the risk of ventricular fibrillation.
   _____ j. Begin CPR on patients with severe hypothermia even if they have minimum respirations and pulse.

# CASE DISPOSITION

You decide from her clinical picture that the patient is severely hypothermic. You direct someone to call 911. You ensure an open airway and use a bag-valve-mask device for rescue breathing. Others help the patient gently remove her wet clothes. You then place her in a hypothermia wrap with warm blankets and place warm water bottles in her axillae and groin.

The paramedics arrive, intubate the patient, and place her on a cardiac monitor, which shows that her heart has an organized rhythm with a very slow pulse. Additionally, the paramedics start intravenous lines and administer warm saline. They gently transfer her to the ambulance and take her to the hospital.

At the hospital her core body temperature initially is 79°F (26°C). The patient goes into ventricular fibrillation, an AED is used, and CPR is started. The patient has no response to initial defibrillation or the ACLS drugs given. In the ED, the patient is aggressively warmed, and eventually her heart regains a normal rhythm. The patient remains in the intensive care unit for a few days and later is discharged from the hospital.

# Chapter Review

## Chapter Summary

The outdoor environment presents many challenges. Weather changes, accidents, and poor planning can all be deadly. Cold weather injuries can be devastating, even fatal; the most important step in preventing cold injuries is preparation.

Frostbite can cause severe disability, but with quick identification and proper treatment, the severity can be minimized. The earliest symptom—pain at the involved site—is variable and is followed by numbness without pain as the tissue freezes. Commonly this stage is mistaken for improvement of the condition. Frostbite can occur on its own or as a result of avalanche burial or hypothermia. Poor judgment often plays a role in early stages of hypothermia, and hypoglycemia commonly accompanies frostbite. Responders should maintain a high level of suspicion because patients are not always aware of the severity of their condition. Once frostbitten tissue has thawed, refreezing must be avoided.

As OEC Technicians, we should always remember to avoid tight clothing and tight shoes. Do not tolerate numbness. Stay dry, hydrated, and well nourished. Avoid alcohol, caffeine, and drugs, as they predispose a person to cold injury.

Hypothermia is a common cold injury that can affect anyone almost anywhere and can occur at temperatures well above freezing, especially when water and wind are factors. As core body temperature drops (mild hypothermia), the body attempts to generate heat through shivering to warm the body. As core temperature drops further (moderate to severe hypothermia), body systems slow, causing clumsiness, stumbling, mental confusion, and eventually unresponsiveness and even death. Knowing the risk factors, signs and symptoms, and effective treatments can be lifesaving. Provide the patient with gentle care, and prevent afterdrop by keeping patients with moderate to severe hypothermia *supine* and warm.

Avalanche victims can have a multitude of problems, asphyxiation being foremost. Once the patient is extricated, hypothermia and traumatic injuries must be addressed.

## Remember...

1. "They're not dead until they're warm and dead."
2. Shivering ceases when body temperature is 90°F (32°C).
3. Handle suspected hypothermia patients gently.
4. Mild hypothermia can be treated with passive warming.
5. Moderate to severe hypothermia must be treated with active warming.
6. A slow, perfusing pulse is enough to sustain a severely hypothermic patient.
7. Do not warm a frostbitten area if it will be reexposed to freezing.
8. Frostbite requires rapid warming.

## Chapter Questions

### Multiple Choice

Choose the correct answer.

1. What is the process of maintaining normal body temperature called? _____
   a. thermoregulation
   b. homeostasis
   c. shunting
   d. adapting

2. All of the following are true concerning frostbite except _____
   a. ice crystals form between cells, extracting water from them.
   b. frostbite may affect only the upper layer of skin.
   c. frostbite may affect all the layers of skin, muscle, and bone.
   d. the most common sites for frostbite are the cheeks, nose, and ears.

3. What is the proper treatment for frostbite? _____
   a. slow, gradual rewarming
   b. placing a warm hand or warm chemical pack on the affected area
   c. rapid rewarming in water at 102°–104°F (38°–40°C)
   d. bringing the patient in from the cold and having them warm up the frozen body part at room temperature

4. What is the major cause of death in avalanche victims? _____
   a. starvation
   b. asphyxiation
   c. blunt trauma
   d. blunt trauma and starvation

5. At what temperature does shivering stop in hypothermic patients? _____
   a. 90°F (32°C)
   b. 82°–90°F (28°–32°C)
   c. 90°–95°F (32°–35°C)
   d. 95°F (35°C)

### Matching

Match each of the following descriptions to the type of heat loss that is occurring.

_____ **1.** conduction
_____ **2.** convection
_____ **3.** evaporation
_____ **4.** radiation

a. A hiker is emitting infrared heat.
b. A skier is sitting on the snow in his wet blue jeans.
c. A profusely sweating individual is running a marathon.
d. A snowmobiler falls into water through an open area in the ice.
e. A hiker lies down on a cold rock slab in a canyon.
f. An individual is skiing without a hat on a windy, 14°F (−10°C) day.

## Short Answer

**1.** Describe the difference between passive warming and active warming. Give examples of each type.

_____

_____

_____

_____

_____

_____

**2.** What is the key to the care of all cold injury patients?

_____

_____

**3.** Explain the meaning of "they're not dead until they're warm and dead."

_____

_____

_____

# Scenario

You are working the first aid station at the local state park. It is the last week of deer hunting season in December on a cold and damp day. A small group of hunters has parked its camper on the property and is hunting the backside of the 700-acre park.

One of the hunters on an ATV drives into the first aid area and advises you that another hunter is acting strange, shivering, and has slurred speech.

You jump on the area ATV with the portable trailer attached and follow to the scene. The ill hunter is found sitting next to a tree with wet hunting coveralls, and his rifle over his lap. As you shout to the hunter, he simply stares but doesn't respond.

**1.** The first action you take is to _____
   **a.** request one of the hunters remove the gun and empty the chamber.
   **b.** apply $O_2$.
   **c.** interview the bystanders.
   **d.** throw a blanket on the ill hunter.

Attempts to interview the patient provide very little information. During the primary assessment, the patient has a pulse of 60, a patent airway, and is breathing at 16 breaths per minute. A search of the neck reveals a Med Alert tag that indicates the hunter has diabetes. Questioning of the other hunters reveals that the group drank heavily last night but consumed no alcohol today. One of the buddies informs you that in one of the ill person's pocket is a glucose meter, and he knows how to use it. The glucometer returns a value of 110.

**2.** Based on the glucometer reading you would treat this patient _____
   **a.** for stroke because of the slurred speech.
   **b.** by giving glucose because of low sugar.
   **c.** for alcohol abuse.
   **d.** for hypothermia.

*A blanket is placed over the patient and oxygen applied with a nonrebreather at 10 liters to compensate for the altered mental status. The patient is placed in a left recumbent position in the trailer and transported to the first aid station at the park headquarters. All of the wet clothing is removed and the patient placed under an electric blanket. The core temperature is taken at 89°F.*

3. The primary hypothermia is classified as _____
   a. mild hypothermia.
   b. mild hyperthermia.
   c. moderate hypothermia.
   d. severe hypothermia.

*After 20 minutes, the core temperature rises to 90°F. The blood pressure is measured as 90/60 and the pulse rate is 70. The slurred speech is improving, but still not normal. Shivering has continued.*

4. The OEC Technician should _____
   a. continue to warm the patient and wait another 20 minutes to measure the results.
   b. call an ambulance and transport to hospital.
   c. release the patient to his buddies and return to hunting.
   d. release the patient to return to his camping trailer.

## Suggested Reading

McDevitt M. C., C. K. Grissom, and G. Bala. "Hypothermia: A review." *Ski Patrol Magazine*, Summer 2009.

State of Alaska Cold Injury Guidelines, http://www.chems.alaska.gov/EMS/Downloads_Rx.htm

Wilderness Medical Society. 2006. *Practice Guidelines for Wilderness Emergency Care*, 5th ed. W. W. Forgey, Ed. Globe Pequot Press, Guildford, Connecticut.

Auerback, Paul S., MD, MS. 2007. Wilderness Medicine, 5th ed., St Louis, Missouri: Elsevier.

EXPLORE PEARSON **myNSPkit**™

Please go to www.myNSPkit.com. Under Student Resources, you will find animations, videos, web links, and games related to this chapter—and much more. Look for information on **hypothermia physiology, cold weather adaptation techniques,** and other topics.

Register your access code from the front of your book by going to www.myNSPkit.com and selecting the appropriate links. If the in-cover access code has been redeemed, go to www.myNSPkit.com and follow links to **Buy Access.**

# Heat-Related Emergencies

Colin K. Grissom, MD
Marion C. McDevitt, DO
Gregory A. Bala, MS

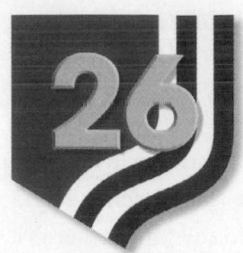

## ⊕ OBJECTIVES

**Upon completion of this chapter, the OEC Technician will be able to:**

**26-1** Explain the way the body normally adjusts to a hot environment.

**26-2** List the signs and symptoms of a patient with each of the four types of heat-related illness.

**26-3** Describe and demonstrate the assessment and emergency care of a patient suffering from each of the four types of heat-related illness.

**26-4** List the signs and symptoms of a patient who is a victim of a lightning strike.

**26-5** Describe and demonstrate the assessment and emergency care for a patient who has been struck by lightning.

**26-6** Explain what one can do to prevent heat-related illness.

## ⊕ KEY TERMS

**ambient temperature,** *p. 839*
**core body temperature,** *p. 839*
**heat acclimatization,** *p. 845*
**heat cramps,** *p. 843*

**heat exhaustion,** *p. 843*
**heat index,** *p. 840*
**heat-related syncope,** *p. 843*
**heat stroke,** *p. 843*

**humidity,** *p. 839*
**hyperthermia,** *p. 842*
**hyponatremia,** *p. 841*

## Chapter Overview

Exercising or traveling in a hot environment may be part of everyday life for some people, and for others it may be part of a planned outdoor adventure. Regardless, being active in hot environments requires daily precautions and advance preparation to prevent heat-related illnesses. Sometimes the need for precautions is obvious, as during a backpacking trip in a desert. At other times precautions one needs to take to prevent heat illness may be less obvious, as for athletes focusing on a sport during practice or a competition in a hot environment.

*continued*

## HISTORICAL TIMELINE

**1989**

NSP adopts the concept of a Senior Program.

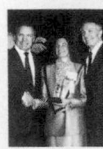

**1989**

Judy Bunce accepts the American Society of Association Executives for national recognition of WEC.

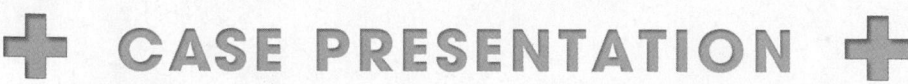

# CASE PRESENTATION

The summertime is a beautiful time to be in the desert, with morning temperatures that are tolerable but mid-day temperatures reaching 105°F. Because of the low humidity in the desert, higher temperatures can be tolerated, and the heat index is acceptable in the morning and evening, but even with 5 percent humidity, the heat index in the middle of the day is high enough to markedly increase the risk of heat illness during exercise.

Today you are with a group of backpackers who understand the importance of moving in the morning and evening hours to avoid the mid-day heat. You have found a sandstone overhang that provides some shade, where you will rest during the middle of the day, and you have ample water.

As you are resting, you see another group of backpackers who are still hiking in the middle of the day. One of the members, a young woman who looks about 20 years old, is clearly slower than are the others, is staggering, and bends over panting, and asks for rest and water. Her face is flushed.

**What should you do?**

**⊕ 26-1** Explain the way the body normally adjusts to a hot environment.

**core body temperature** the temperature in the part of the body that contains the vital organs.

**Figure 26-1** Your best defense against the dangers of hot environments is preparation and prevention.
Copyright Craig Brown

Insufficient preparation under hot conditions can lead to heat-related illness (Figure 26-1■). Whereas the mechanisms for adapting to cold are primarily behavioral, the body can, given enough time, physiologically adapt to heat. However, such an adjustment may take a week. The medical conditions that can result from exposure to heat vary from mild to severe to life threatening. OEC Technicians can care for people by recognizing and responding properly to these heat-related conditions.

This chapter describes how the body regulates its core temperature in hot environments. It then discusses the various forms of heat emergencies, including heat cramps, heat exhaustion, heat stroke, sunburn, and lightning injuries, and how to assess and treat those emergencies.

## Anatomy and Physiology

Normal **core body temperature** is 98.6°F (37°C). Regulatory mechanisms keep this internal temperature relatively constant, regardless of the **ambient temperature**, the temperature of the surrounding environment. When these regulatory systems are no longer able to cool the body, heat-related illness occurs.

In hot environments or during vigorous physical activity (which causes excess heat production), the body discharges excess heat through several mechanisms, including sweating (evaporative heat loss) and dilation of the blood vessels in the skin (radiant heat loss) (Figure 26-2■). This process, known as thermoregulation, is an important part of maintaining homeostasis.

Sweating is the body's most important cooling mechanism. When sweat on the skin evaporates, heat is lost. In environments with high **humidity**, such as tropical jungles, sweating is less effective for losing heat because evaporation occurs more slowly. In low-humidity environments, such as deserts, sweating is a more effective mechanism of heat loss. Dilation of blood vessels in the

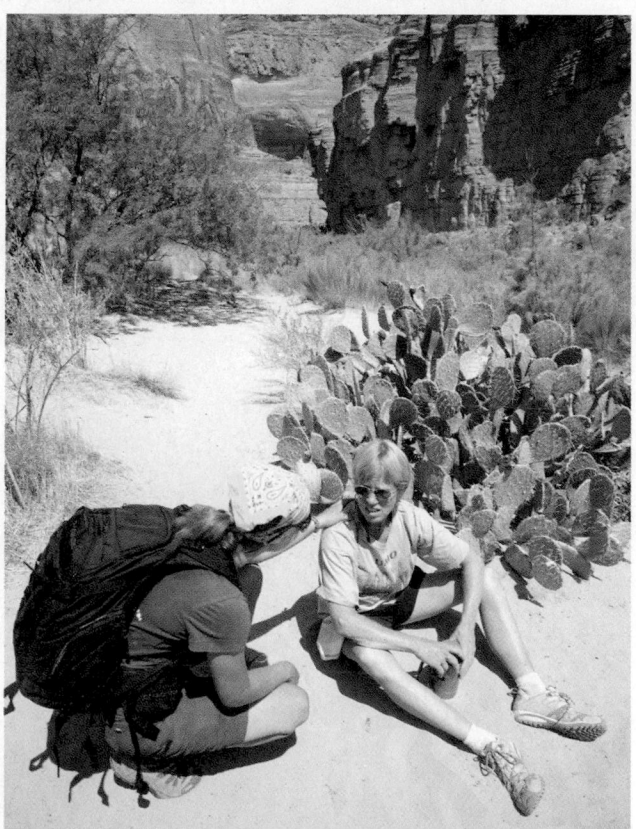

MECHANISMS OF HEAT LOSS

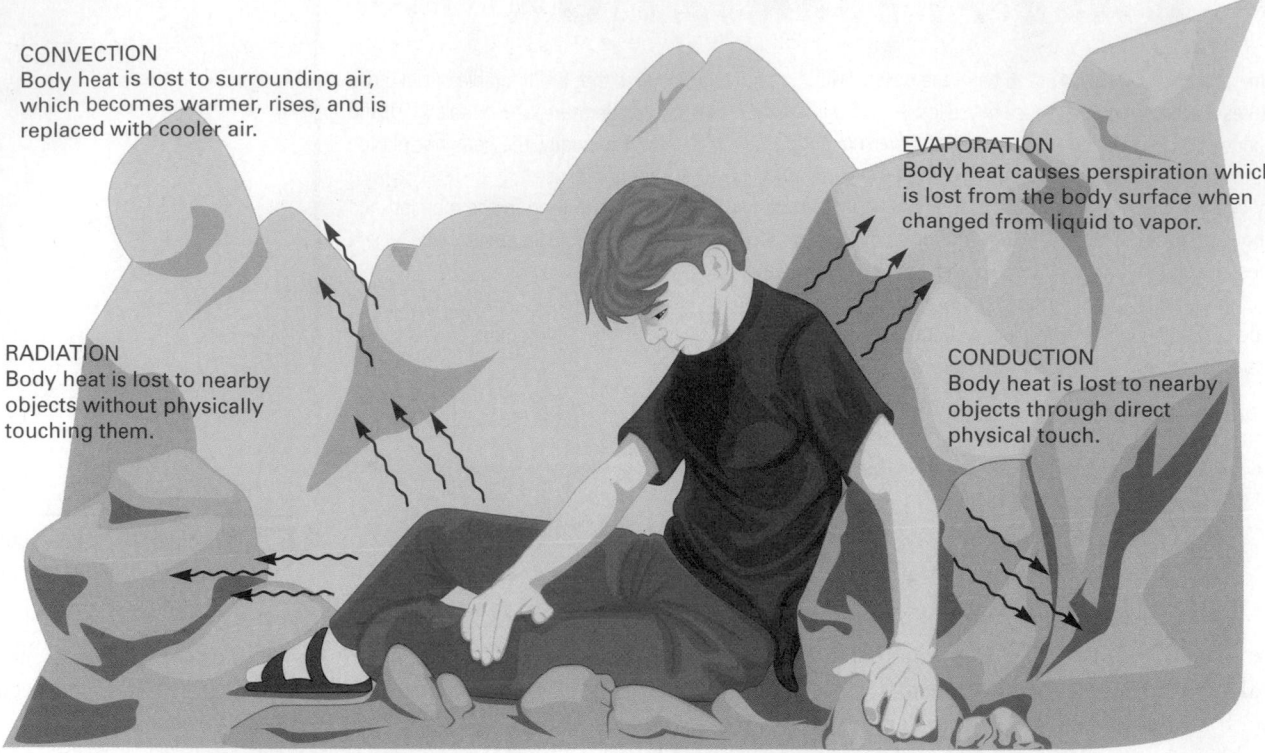

CONVECTION
Body heat is lost to surrounding air, which becomes warmer, rises, and is replaced with cooler air.

EVAPORATION
Body heat causes perspiration which is lost from the body surface when changed from liquid to vapor.

RADIATION
Body heat is lost to nearby objects without physically touching them.

CONDUCTION
Body heat is lost to nearby objects through direct physical touch.

**Figure 26-2** Mechanisms of heat loss.

**ambient temperature** the temperature in the immediate environment.

**humidity** the amount of water vapor in the air.

**heat index** a measure of the risk for heat illness; combines the effects of increasing ambient temperature and increasing humidity.

skin brings warm blood to the skin surface, allowing heat to radiate directly into the environment. When ambient temperature exceeds body temperature, loss of body heat by radiation from the skin is not effective for cooling, and sweating becomes the major mechanism for heat loss. This is the basis for the **heat index**, in which at higher humidities a given ambient air temperature translates into a higher heat index temperature, which in turn translates into a greater risk of heat illness (Figure 26-3■).

**Figure 26-3** The heat and humidity risk scale.

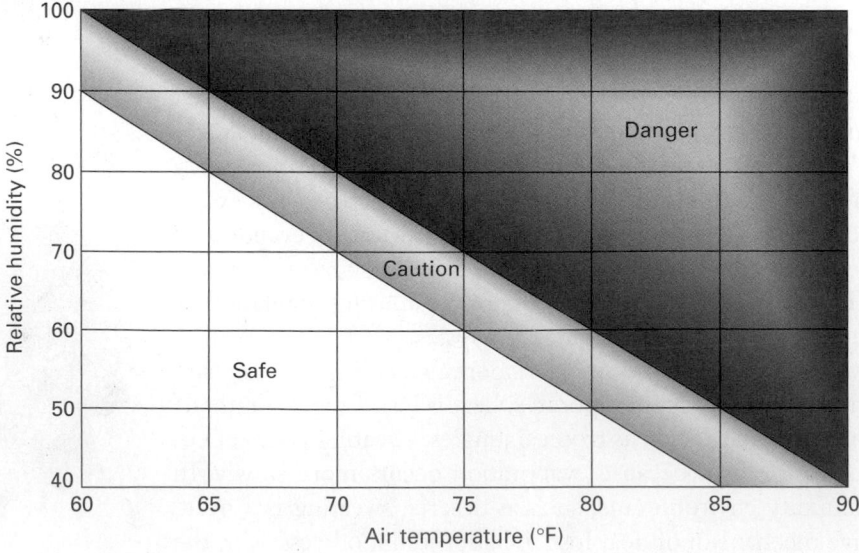

Adequate hydration is required for adequate heat loss from sweating. During exercise in hot environments, up to a liter of sweat can be lost each hour. Maintaining adequate hydration is essential to preventing heat illness, but overhydration also can be detrimental by diluting the sodium level in the blood (**hyponatremia**), which causes the swelling of brain cells. The key is to match hydration needs to the level of activity and the temperature of the environment, taking care to allow for adequate adjustment to the heat (heat acclimatization, discussed below), to avoid exercise during the hot part of the day, to take frequent rests, and to use thirst as an indication that additional hydration is necessary.

Unlike adaptation to cold, adaptation to heat depends on physiologic acclimatization (changes in the body to adapt to heat) rather than modifications in behavior alone. Prior heat exposure lowers the skin temperature at which sweating occurs, which initiates cooling of the body by the evaporation of sweat at a lower skin temperature. Physical training improves heat tolerance through the same mechanisms, and it also improves the efficiency of the cardiovascular system. Poor physical fitness, obesity, lack of heat acclimatization, and dehydration decrease an individual's heat tolerance. Chronic medical conditions increase the risk of heat illness, and heat may exacerbate chronic medical conditions.

**hyponatremia** dilution of the sodium level in the blood.

## STOP, THINK, UNDERSTAND

### Multiple Choice

Choose the correct answer.

1. The body's ability to cool itself through sweating and dilation of the blood vessels in the skin is known as_____
   a. hypertropic regulation.
   c. thermoregulation.
   b. hypotropic regulation.
   d. perspiration.

2. In environments in which the ambient temperature is greater than body temperature, the body cools itself through _____
   a. blood vessel dilation and radiation.
   b. sweating.
   c. conduction.
   d. syncope.

3. Which of the following statements about heat adaptation is true? _____
   a. It is largely based on modifications of behavior.
   b. The human body is largely incapable of adapting to hot environments.
   c. Prior heat exposure lowers the skin temperature at which sweating occurs.
   d. Cardiovascular conditioning has little or no affect on the body's ability to adapt to hot environments.

4. How much sweat can be lost during one hour of exercise in a hot environment? _____
   a. 1 ounce (30 cc)
   c. 1 pint (480 cc)
   b. 1 cup (240 cc)
   d. 1 liter (1,000 cc)

5. Which of the following are appropriate steps to take when hiking through the desert on a 105°F degree day? (check all that apply)
   _____a. Allow the body to adjust by exercising at a steady level and take frequent short breaks throughout the day.
   _____b. Find shelter and rest during the hottest part of the day.
   _____c. Match your level of hydration to the level of activity and the temperature of the environment.
   _____d. Force yourself to drink as much water as possible.
   _____e. Be well-conditioned and fit before undertaking such a trek.
   _____f. Avoid snacking.

**⊕ 26-2** List the signs and symptoms of a patient with each of the four types of heat-related illness.

**hyperthermia**    elevated core body temperature.

# Common Heat-Related Emergencies

## Heat Illness

Heat illness includes a group of disorders caused by exposure to a hot environment and failure of the body's normal mechanisms for regulating body temperature, electrolyte levels, and body fluid status. An abnormally high body temperature, known as **hyperthermia**, is characterized by a high core temperature, usually 101°F (38.3°C) or more (Figure 26-4■). Extreme or untreated hyperthermia can rapidly become life threatening.

Heat illness can occur in anyone exposed to hot environmental temperatures who does not maintain adequate hydration, especially while exercising.

Newborns, infants, the elderly, and the obese exhibit poor thermoregulation and are at greatest risk for heat illness. Newborns and infants are especially vulnerable if overdressed. Patients with such chronic medical conditions as heart disease, lung disease, and diabetes are at increased risk of heat illness. Alcohol and such drugs as amphetamines, cocaine, and medications, which dehydrate the body or decrease the body's ability to sweat, also make a person more susceptible to heat illnesses.

**Figure 26-4** Core body temperatures for heat illnesses and the corresponding efficiencies of hypothalamic regulation.

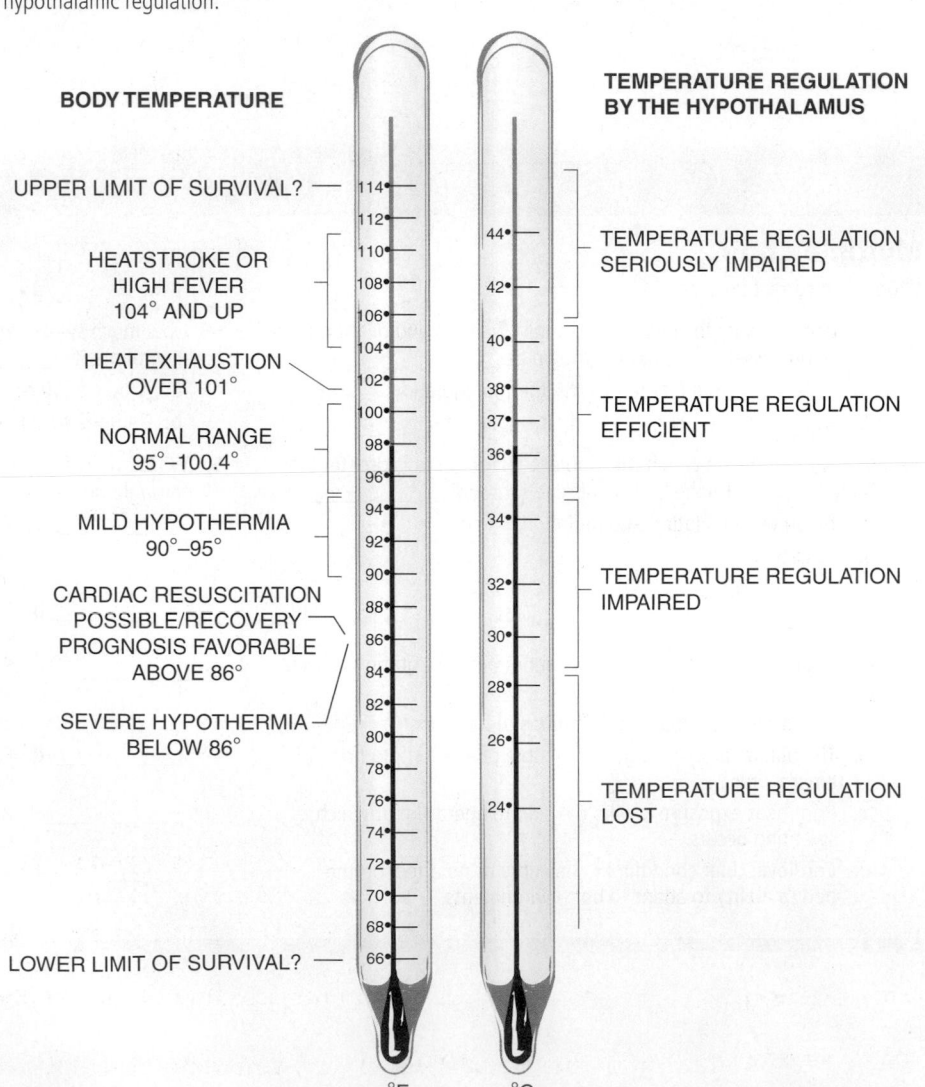

When the body's mechanisms for transferring heat to the environment are overwhelmed and the body is unable to tolerate the excessive heat, illness from heat exposure can take the following four forms:

- Heat-related syncope
- Heat cramps
- Heat exhaustion
- Heat stroke

## Heat-Related Syncope

Heat-related syncope is a condition that originates primarily in the cardiovascular system. Clinically, it is defined as a temporary loss of responsiveness or fainting due to a temporary loss of effective blood flow. Heat-related syncope occurs when the body is heat stressed and blood is diverted into the peripheral circulation (arms and legs) to allow heat to be lost at the body's surface. The blood does not return from the surface to the heart rapidly enough, which decreases brain perfusion and results in fainting. Although this condition may occur without warning while the patient is standing, it is often preceded by feelings of nausea or lightheadedness.

**heat-related syncope** fainting secondary to pooling of the blood in the extremities due to increased core body temperature.

## Heat Cramps

Heat cramps occur in large muscle groups after exercise in a hot environment and are caused by electrolyte disturbances and dehydration. Such cramps can be quite painful during the contraction (spasm) of the muscles. Stretching the muscles can alleviate the cramp, and rest, rehydration, and electrolyte replacement will prevent recurrence.

**heat cramps** painful muscle cramps that result from dehydration and electrolyte imbalances.

## Heat Exhaustion

Heat exhaustion is characterized by exhaustion, dizziness, nausea, headache, leg cramps, excessive sweating, and decreased urine output, with a core body temperature that is less than 104°F and a level of responsiveness that is normal or only mildly confused. Heat exhaustion is a common disorder resulting from dehydration to the point at which low body fluid volume (hypovolemia) causes signs and symptoms. When the body loses too much water and too many electrolytes through heavy sweating, the result is hypovolemia. The body responds rapidly to treatment, and changes in mental status do not persist or worsen.

**heat exhaustion** a condition characterized by fatigue, dizziness, nausea, and headache caused by dehydration and elevated core body temperature.

## Heat Stroke

Heat stroke is a life-threatening emergency identified by a decreased level of responsiveness and a core body temperature greater than 104°F (40°C). It is associated with an elevated heart rate, a high respiratory rate, and decreased sweating. The defining characteristic of heat stroke that differentiates it from heat exhaustion is a decreased level of responsiveness that persists or worsens, which should prompt immediate treatment and evacuation.

Heat stroke is the most serious heat illness and can occur from either exposure to heat without exertion (classical heat stroke) or exertion in a hot environment (exertional heat stroke). In heat stroke, the body's normal mechanisms for shedding excess heat are overwhelmed. Core body temperature rises (above 104°F or 40°C), and shock follows, which causes dysfunction of such organ as the brain, the heart and blood vessels, the liver, and the kidneys. Left untreated, heat stroke results in death.

Figure 26-5■ illustrates the various signs and symptoms of serious heat emergencies.

**heat stroke** a life-threatening elevation of core body temperature associated with shock and a deteriorating level of responsiveness.

**Figure 26-5** Signs and symptoms of serious heat emergencies.

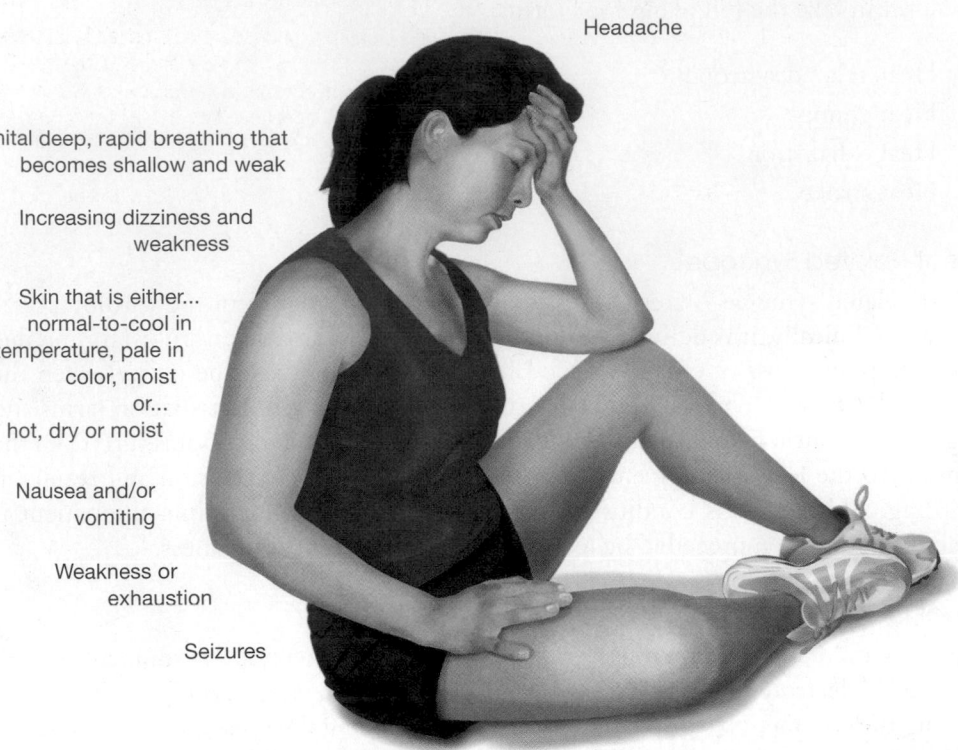

SIGNS AND SYMPTOMS OF HEAT EMERGENCY

Headache

Inital deep, rapid breathing that becomes shallow and weak

Increasing dizziness and weakness

Skin that is either...
normal-to-cool in temperature, pale in color, moist
or...
hot, dry or moist

Nausea and/or vomiting

Weakness or exhaustion

Seizures

Muscle cramps

# STOP, THINK, UNDERSTAND

## Multiple Choice
Choose the correct answer.

1. Hyperthermia is characterized by a core body temperature greater than approximately _____
   a. 99°F.
   b. 101°F.
   c. 104°F.
   d. 105°F.

2. What is the difference between classical heat stroke and exertional heat stroke? _____
   a. One is seen in the elderly, and the other is seen in pediatric patients.
   b. Exertional heat stroke is more severe than classical heat stroke.

   c. One is caused by heat exposure without exercise, and one is caused by exercising in a hot environment.
   d. Classical heat stroke is more severe than exertional heat stroke.

3. An elderly man who was found unresponsive inside a sweltering mobile home on a hot, humid day, has a body temperature of 103°F, and has flushed but dry skin is most likely suffering from_____
   a. carbon monoxide poisoning.
   b. heat exhaustion.
   c. carbon monoxide exhaustion.
   d. heat-induced syncope.

## Fill in the Blank

Heat illness is caused by exposure to hot environments and the body's failure to regulate _____, _____ and _____.

*continued*

## Matching

1. Match each of the following heat-related conditions to its description. The terms may be used more than once.

_____ 1. heat-induced syncope

_____ 2. heat stroke

_____ 3. heat exhaustion

_____ 4. heat cramps

a. a life-threatening condition characterized by a decreased level of responsiveness, a core body temperature of 104°F or higher, and elevated heart and respiratory rates

b. a temporary loss of responsiveness caused when blood is temporarily shunted to the peripheral circulation to support heat loss at the body's surface

c. a condition characterized by painful thigh or calf muscles caused by electrolyte imbalances and dehydration

d. usually occurs when an individual is standing and is preceded by nausea, lightheadedness, sighing, and yawning

e. characterized by decreased sweating or no sweating

f. a common condition among the elderly living in unventilated buildings or among young children left alone in cars

g. characterized by nausea, fatigue, dizziness, headache, excessive sweating, decreased urinary output, and elevated core body temperature below 104°F

2. Place the following signs and symptoms of hyperthermia in order from least severe (1) to life threatening (5).

_____ a. sweating
_____ b. heat exhaustion
_____ c. heat stroke
_____ d. syncope
_____ e. heat cramps

## Heat-Related Illness Prevention

To maximize tolerance to hot environments, a program for **heat acclimatization** is important. Individuals can improve their heat acclimatization before taking a wilderness trip to a hot environment by exercising daily in the heat for limited periods of at least one hour for at least several days (and preferably for one week). If this is not possible before a trip, then individuals should limit periods of exercise during the warmest parts of the day for the first week of the trip. Ensuring adequate hydration by consuming water or electrolyte drinks to maintain adequate fluid volume is also important before and during a trip into a hot environment.

During periods of exercise lasting several hours or more, salty snacks and adequate water intake are necessary to maintain adequate salt balance and prevent hyponatremia from salt and water losses in sweat. Urine that is a light yellow color is a good indicator of adequate hydration status, whereas darker urine indicates dehydration.

In addition to the physiological mechanisms of heat loss—sweating and blood vessel dilation—behavior is important for maintaining normal body temperature in hot environments. Wearing loose-fitting, lightweight, light-colored clothing and a wide-brimmed hat, avoiding exercise during the hottest part of the day, and resting frequently in the shade are all important measures for preventing heat illness (Figure 26-6■).

Adequate preparation is required to ensure that the body's heat-regulating mechanisms maintain normal body temperature in hot environments, especially during increased physical activity.

## Sunburn

Sunburn is a superficial burn of the skin caused by medium-wavelength ultraviolet (UV) light in sunlight. Repeated excessive sun exposure over many years may lead to chronic degenerative skin changes, such as excessive wrinkling, darkening, and thickening. Localized benign growths are common. Repeated sunburns are associated with an increased incidence of cancerous

**⊕26-6** Explain what one can do to prevent heat-related illness.

**heat acclimatization** adaptation of the body over time to a hot environment.

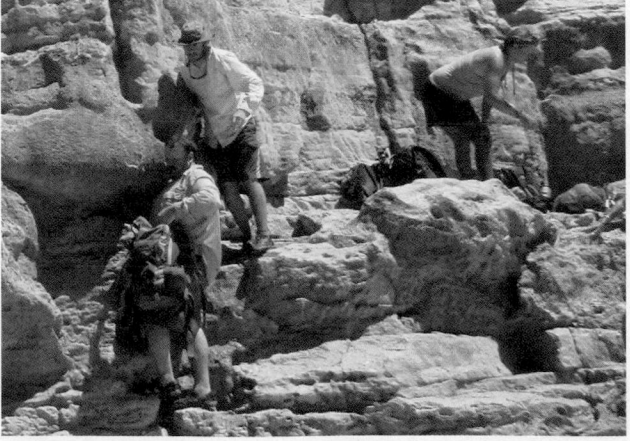

**Figure 26-6** To prevent hyperthermia in outdoor environments, wear loose-fitting, lightweight clothing.
Copyright Craig Brown

Table 26-1 Degrees of Sun Sensitivity as Classified by the Fitzpatrick Skin Phototypes System*

| Phototype (Class of Sun Sensitivity) | Unexposed Natural Skin Color and Hair Color | Sunburn and Tanning History After 45 Minutes of Exposure to Sun |
|---|---|---|
| Type I | Blond or red hair, ivory white skin, freckles | Burns easily, never tans |
| Type II | Blond hair, white skin | Burns easily, tans minimally |
| Type III | Brunette, white skin | Burns minimally, tans gradually |
| Type IV | Dark hair, olive, lightly tanned skin | Burns minimally, tans easily |
| Type V | Dark hair, moderate brown or tanned skin | Rarely burns, tans easily |
| Type VI | Black | Never burns, tans deeply |

* Adapted from *Fitzpatrick's Dermatology in General Medicine,* Fifth Edition. 1999. Burr Ridge, IL: McGraw-Hill Professional.

lesions. All of these changes can be delayed by avoiding excessive sun exposure and using proper skin protection.

Environments in which sunlight is more intense, such as at high altitude, or where sun is reflected, such as on snow or water, increase the risk of sunburn. At high altitude, atmospheric pressure decreases and the air is less dense, allowing more UV light to reach the skin in a given amount of time. Even on cloudy days, significant sunburn can occur to the skin or eyes in these environments. In general, individuals with fair skin, light-colored hair, or a prior history of sunburning easily should be more careful when at high altitude, on snow, or on water (Table 26-1■).

### Sunburn Prevention

Sunscreen can protect the skin by providing a mechanical or chemical barrier to sunlight. Zinc oxide and titanium dioxide are examples of mechanical (or physical) barriers that reflect the UV light in sunlight when applied to the lips and nose. More recently, sunscreens intended for application to large areas of skin contain zinc oxide or slightly less effective titanium dioxide for sun protection. These protect against UV rays. Chemical components of sunscreen absorb, rather than reflect, harmful UV rays (mostly UV-A) and are combined with zinc oxide or titanium dioxide for application to large areas of skin.

Most manufacturers of sunscreen creams, lotions, and lip salves now specify the sun protection factor (SPF) on the label. This number, which usually ranges from 4 to 50, refers to how long the skin is protected before becoming red from exposure to the sun. For example, the skin of an individual who wears an adequate amount of uniformly applied sunscreen with an SPF 20 will not burn until the skin has been exposed to 20 times the amount of solar energy that would normally cause it to burn. Unfortunately, this number can be misleading because other factors—including type of skin, time of day, altitude, amount of sweating, and frequency and adequacy of application of sun protection—influence how fast an individual will burn. UV radiation is greatest when the sun is directly overhead. Thin layers of clothing do not necessarily protect against exposure to sunlight. It should be emphasized that a thick hat with a brim and layers of clothing are effective measures to protect against sun exposure and may be more important than the use of sunscreen.

Sunscreen with an SPF of 30 or greater should be used in outdoor environments, especially at high altitude and on snow. There is probably no additional benefit to sunscreens with an SPF that is higher than 30. The key is to apply a thick coat of sunscreen on the skin before exposure to sunlight, and then to reapply it every few hours. Most individuals do not apply enough sunscreen and do not apply it frequently enough. The safety of sunscreen for children younger than 6 months old has not been established. The American Academy of Pediatrics recommends that infants be protected by clothing and shade. When adequate clothing and shade are not available, parents can apply a minimal amount of sunscreen with an SPF of at least 15 to small areas, such as the infant's face and the backs of the hands.

# STOP, THINK, UNDERSTAND

## Multiple Choice
Choose the correct answer.

1. Which of the following statements about acclimatization is true? _____
   a. It is dangerous to switch your daily jog from 40 minutes to 20 minutes and from early morning to mid-day before a desert hike to help you acclimatize.
   b. About a week before going to a hot climate, acclimatize by increasing your water intake by an additional 4–6 liters above your normal intake.
   c. When in a hot environment, avoid salty foods such as pretzels or crackers because they can cause fluid retention and dehydration.
   d. Drink enough water to keep your urine light yellow.

2. Sunburn is best described as_____
   a. a partial-thickness burn of the skin caused by medium-wavelength UV light in sunlight.
   b. a superficial burn of the skin caused by an exposure to medium wavelength UV light in sunlight.
   c. the absorption of too much heat into the dermal and epidermal layers of skin.
   d. destruction of the melatonin in the skin.

3. Which of the following statements about solar radiation is true? _____
   a. It can cause skin damage or eye damage even on cloudy days.
   b. It is more dangerous at sea-level than at 10,000 feet due to atmospheric reflection.
   c. It is less dangerous on a body of water than on sand because water absorbs medium-wavelength UV rays.
   d. It only affects blond-haired people, redheads, and people with light skin.

4. Which of the following statements about sunscreen is true? _____
   a. You do not need to apply sunscreen on cloudy days.
   b. The best type of sunscreen for your trunk, arms, and legs is a chemical with an SPF of 15 that absorbs UV radiation.
   c. The best type of sunscreen for your trunk, arms, and legs is a mixture of a chemical with an SPF of 30 that absorbs UV radiation and titanium dioxide or zinc oxide.
   d. Repeated use of chemical sunscreens is dangerous because they are toxic to the body.

5. UV radiation is greatest when the_____
   a. sun is directly overhead.
   b. sun is at a 45-degree angle to the body.
   c. sun is just above the horizon.
   d. sunlight is reflected and refracted such as when it passes through a canopy of leaves.

6. Which of the following statements concerning sunscreens is correct? _____
   a. Use a sunscreen with an SPF greater than 50 because the higher the SPF, the greater the protection provided.
   b. The right strength of sunscreen for any given individual should be determined by a dermatologist.
   c. Individuals with light skin should use a sunscreen with a lower SPF than individuals with dark skin.
   d. Sunscreen with an SPF of 30 is the best to use during regular sun exposure.

## Short Answer

Explain the difference between a physical sunscreen and a chemical sunscreen.

_____

_____

_____

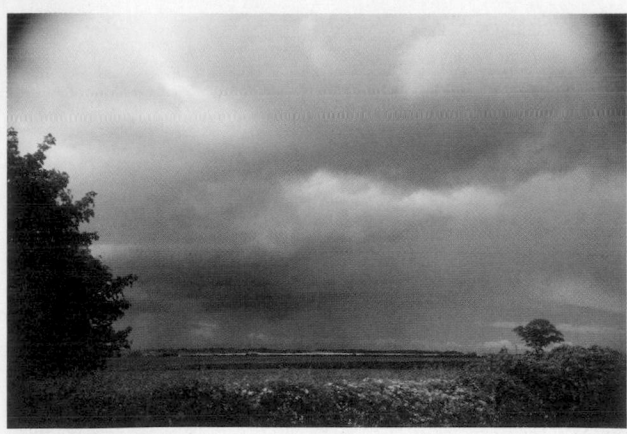

**Figure 26-7** These cumulonimbus clouds ("thunderheads") could well generate lightning.
Copyright Brian Cosgrove/Dorling Kindersley Media Library

## Lightning

Lightning is an atmospheric discharge of electricity that is capable of generating 300,000 amps and 2 billion volts. Although it depends on the resistance of the human body, which varies greatly among individuals, under the right conditions, it takes only 500 mAmps of direct current to kill someone. Most industrial applications using 30 or more volts are considered dangerous. Although typically associated with severe thunderstorms, the exact mechanism(s) responsible for the formation of lightning is still the subject of debate. Lightning is commonly thought to be caused by cumulonimbus clouds ("thunderheads") (Figure 26-7■) in which differential air currents create a difference in the electrical potential between clouds, or between clouds and the earth. In mountainous environments, cumulonimbus clouds that produce lightning tend to develop during the afternoon or evening. Lightning can occur during rainstorms, hailstorms, or snowstorms.

According to the National Weather Service, the odds of being struck by lightning during a lifetime of 80 years are 1 in 5,000. Between 1996 and 2005, an average of over 22 million lightning strikes occurred each year, and the average for lightning deaths during the 30 years from 1977 to 2006 was 62 deaths per year. (This figure may be as high as 70 deaths per year due to underreporting.) It is impossible to predict where lightning will strike.

⊕ **26-4** List the signs and symptoms of a patient who is a victim of a lightning strike.

### Facts About Lightning-Caused Injuries

+ Lightning injury is caused by direct electrical current at high voltage that lasts only 0.1 to 0.001 seconds in duration.

+ Respiratory arrest can result from injury to the respiratory control center of the brainstem.

+ Cardiac arrest can occur if the electrical current passes through the heart and disrupts its organized electrical activity.

+ Severe tissue damage by an electrical current may lead to the breakdown of muscle and the release into the circulation of chemicals that injure the kidney.

+ Lightning can cause unpredictable neurologic effects such as pain, paralysis, blindness, numbness, weakness, loss of hearing or speech, and unresponsiveness.

+ Significant internal tissue damage may not be obvious from the external burns at the sites at which electricity entered or exited the body.

+ Electrical current from lightning can cause muscular contractions that throw the patient off balance and cause injurious falls.

   + The fatality rate from a direct lightning strike is 30 percent; cardiac arrest is the most common cause of death.

   + The characteristic lightning-induced skin injury is known as "feathering" or "ferning" (Figure 26-8■).

### Reducing the Risk of Lightning Strikes

Although lightning is unpredictable, several commonly accepted techniques can reduce the chances of injury or death associated with lightning strikes. When lightning is in the area, or during a storm:

+ Seek shelter away from high points, exposed ridges, solitary trees, and trees taller than surrounding trees.

**Figure 26-8** A "feathering" or "ferning" pattern of a burn caused by a lightning strike.© David Effron, MD.

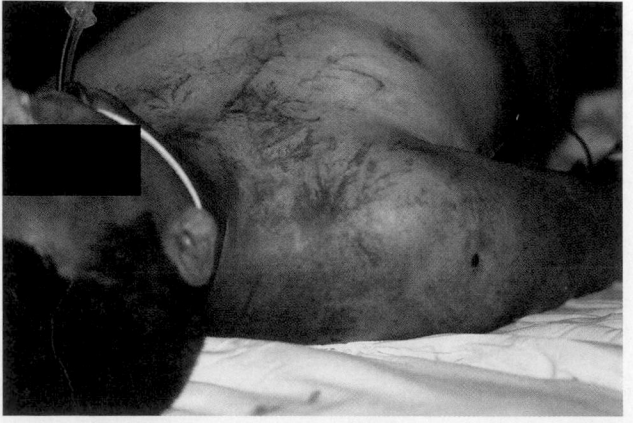

- Seek shelter in a forested area among trees or bushes, or in an area containing rocks of uniform size.
- Avoid open areas where you are one of the tallest objects.
- Avoid extremes of high ground or low ground.
- Do not stand in or near bodies of water.
- Avoid contact with metal objects.
- Put your feet together, squat low, tuck your head, and cover your ears. If possible, place your feet on a nonconductive material. Soil, non-metallic substances, and plastics may be used. Avoid being close to others; stay about 15 feet apart.
- Seek shelter deep in a dry cave, and stay away from the sides and the ceiling. Avoid small caves in which you must remain close to the walls or ceiling, because ground currents may flow through your body instead of taking a longer path through the cave wall.
- If you are boating, attempt to get to shore, waves and distance to the shoreline permitting.
- If you are on a chair lift or other elevated structure, get off as soon as possible.
- If available, large buildings and enclosed vehicles are usually safe.

The National Weather Service supports the use of the "30/30" rule: If you see lightning, count the time until you hear thunder. If this time is 30 seconds or less, immediately seek safe shelter, and wait 30 minutes or more after hearing the last clap of thunder before leaving your shelter. Even if you cannot see lightning, hearing thunder indicates that lightning is likely within striking range. The "30/30" rule cannot protect against the first lightning strike, so it is important to know the local weather forecast, and to seek appropriate shelter at the first sign of an impending storm.

If lightning overtakes you, the first precaution should be to descend as far as possible off exposed ridges or move out of clearings to lower, more-sheltered areas. Keep away from metal objects; remove your crampons, and place ski poles and ice axes a distance from your location. If there is no possibility of descending out of open areas to lower terrain, then you and all the members of your group should spread out and squat down, preferably while standing on insulated material, if possible. Stay away from exposed rock overhangs, where a ground current may pass through individuals seeking shelter. Within a ski area, clear all lifts of people when the danger of a lightning strike exists.

## STOP, THINK, UNDERSTAND

### Multiple Choice
Choose the correct answer.

1. Which of the following statements about lightning is false? _____
   a. It is impossible to predict where lightning will strike.
   b. Ski areas that operate in winter are at little or no risk of lightning strike.
   c. Lightning can be part of an advancing cold front.
   d. Clothing can explode off a lightning victim's body.

2. Your proper course of action when you see a flash of lightning and count 30 seconds before you hear thunder is to _____
   a. not worry about lightning strike because the storm is still far away.
   b. lie flat on the ground with your arms extended to minimize your height.
   c. seek shelter immediately.
   d. wait for three more cycles of lightning and thunder to determine if the storm is coming closer; if it is, seek shelter as soon as possible.

*continued*

**STOP, THINK, UNDERSTAND** *continued*

3. Which of the following are safe shelters in a thunderstorm? (check all that apply)

_____a. a lift operator's shack at the top of a chairlift

_____b. a shallow cave or overhanging cliff

_____c. in a forested area among trees or bushes, or among rocks of uniform size

_____d. in an open area in which you are the tallest object

_____e. in a large dip in the ground, such as a deep ditch or an empty swimming pool

_____f. off of a high point or a ridge line

_____g. crouched beside the members of your hiking group, at least 3 feet apart

4. While golfing in a foursome in a remote part of the course, you see lightning and hear thunder ten seconds later. What should you do?_____

   a. Grab your clubs and run like mad for the clubhouse.

   b. Leave your clubs, get in the cart, and drive quickly to the clubhouse.

   c. Separate from your clubs and friends, kick off your cleated shoes, and crouch down.

   d. Take shelter under a small stand of trees.

   e. Tuck your head between your legs.

## Fill in the Blank

1. Injury to the _____ control center in the brain can cause a lightning-strike victim to stop breathing.

2. Severe _____ damage can occur at the point of electrical current.

3. The _____(organs) may be secondarily injured due to an overload of breakdown products of injured muscle.

4. Lightning can cause a characteristic skin burn with a pattern resembling a_____ _____.

5. Cessation of electrical activity in the body after a lightning strike can cause_____ _____.

6. A direct effect on the nervous system can cause _____ in a victim.

---

 **CASE UPDATE**

You leave the shade of the rock overhang and walk out into the hot sun of a 105°F day to find a young woman who is sweating, asking for water, and complaining of fatigue, nausea, dizziness, and a headache. You offer to help and suggest that the young woman sit under the rock overhang, rest, and have some water and electrolyte drinks.

***What steps do you take to monitor her?***

---

⊕ **26-3** Describe and demonstrate the assessment and emergency care of a patient suffering from each of the four types of heat-related illness.

# Assessment

The assessment of heat-related injuries is fairly straightforward. OEC Technicians should perform a scene size-up, address safety issues, perform a primary assessment, address life-threatening issues, obtain a SAMPLE history, and perform a secondary assessment, which should include assessing for injuries using DCAP-BTLS and obtaining a complete set of vital signs. For any heat emergency, address any threats to life and provide adequate protection from direct exposure to the sun for both patients and rescuers (Figures 26-9a■ and 26-9b■). The sections that follow describe assessment findings for several heat-related injuries.

## Heat-Induced Syncope

Patients who suffer from heat-induced syncope are warm to the touch, may be lightheaded and have tachycardia, and may be hypotensive initially. Look for traumatic

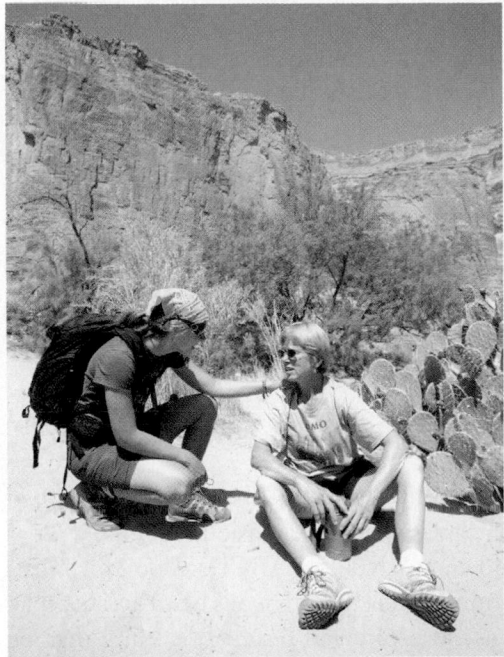

**Figure 26-9a** If you suspect hyperthermia, perform a primary assessment.
Copyright Craig Brown

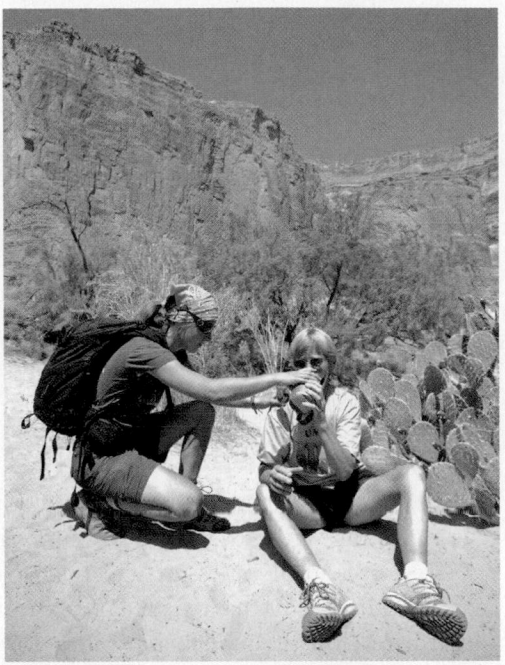

**Figure 26-9b** Address any life-threatening issues then move patient to shade as quickly as possible.
Copyright Craig Brown

injuries resulting from falling after fainting. As with all unresponsive patients, ensure that you open their airway and simultaneously check for breathing while checking for a carotid pulse. If there is no pulse or breathing, follow current CPR standards. If the patient has a pulse and is breathing, maintain the airway while conducting the secondary assessment. Patients receiving prompt care may rapidly regain responsiveness.

## Heat Cramps

The hallmarks of heat cramps are intense, painful muscle spasm and painful cramping in affected extremities. The cramping is often unrelenting. Abdominal cramping also may occur and can be quite severe. Hyperventilation is common.

## Heat Exhaustion

Depending on the severity of their condition, patients experiencing heat exhaustion exhibit a variety of signs and symptoms that include the following:

+ Weakness
+ Inability to work or participate in an activity
+ Headache
+ Mild confusion
+ Nausea
+ Faintness, lightheadedness
+ Decreased appetite
+ Tachycardia
+ Normal or slightly elevated body temperature
+ Warm skin
+ Sweating (moderate to heavy)

## Heat Stroke

Heat stroke is a life-threatening emergency characterized by an altered level of consciousness and organ dysfunction. Without prompt emergency treatment, heat stroke can be fatal. Classically, patients have hot, dry, flushed skin because the body's sweating mechanisms have been exhausted. However, heat stroke should be suspected in any patient that has an altered level of consciousness and does not respond quickly to treatment for heat exhaustion, even if the person is still sweating.

## Sunburn

The assessment of sunburn is the same as the assessment for other burns (Chapter 19, Burns). Depending on the amount of UV radiation exposure, sunburns can blister and result in second-degree burns.

## Lightning Strikes

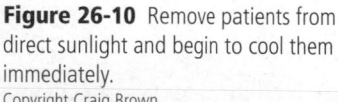
**26-5** Describe and demonstrate the assessment and emergency care for a patient who has been struck by lightning.

Because of the high incidence of cardiopulmonary arrest in patients who have sustained a lightning strike, the scene size-up, primary assessment, and basic life-support measures are critical. Assessment should be rapid and include the ABCDs. Look for burns and other trauma that resulted from the lightning strike. Spontaneous heart activity may return before spontaneous breathing returns, so prolonged rescue breathing may be necessary. Unlike patients who are still in contact with the source of an electrical shock, patients struck by lightning are not electrically charged and pose no threat to rescuers.

# Management

Ensure scene safety. In most cases of heat illness, move patients to a cooler location as soon as possible and/or shade patients from direct exposure to the sun (Figure 26-10■). The nature of further care is based on the cause of the suspected heat-related illness. If you suspect heat stroke, attend to any threats to life identified in your primary assessment. Provide appropriate hydration and any needed supportive measures such as oxygen therapy.

## Heat-Induced Syncope

For heat-induced syncope, place the patient into a supine position, which allows blood to flow to vital organs such as the brain. Remove the person from the heat source and elevate the patient's legs 10–12 inches, if needed. Provide supportive measures, including oxygen. For patients who are able to speak and swallow, give cool non-alcoholic liquids.

## Heat Cramps

Heat cramps generally respond favorably to oral electrolyte solutions such as commercial sports beverages. If one is not available, mix 1/4 to 1/2 teaspoon of table salt into a quart of cool water and add some pleasant flavoring. Gentle stretching or massage of the cramped muscles is usually beneficial and can provide some relief. After recovery, activity may be resumed. However, if the cramps return, a 24-hour rest period is recommended.

## Heat Exhaustion

Treat heat exhaustion promptly to prevent it from developing into heat stroke by taking the following actions (Figure 26-11■):

+ Immediately move the patient to a location that provides shade and a cooler temperature.

**Figure 26-10** Remove patients from direct sunlight and begin to cool them immediately.
Copyright Craig Brown

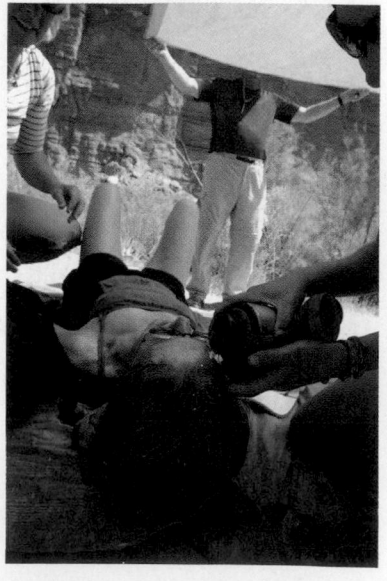

- Place the patient in a supine position with the legs elevated by available materials.
- Remove clothing (or at least loosen it) and cool the patient by fanning (either manually or electrically).
- Provide the patient high-flow oxygen.
- Rehydrate the patient with cool water, a cool electrolyte-containing solution, or 1/4 to 1/2 teaspoon of table salt added to a quart of cool water. Never force oral fluids for patients who are not fully responsive because they could aspirate the liquid into the lungs.

In most cases, these measures will improve the patient's condition. Lack of improvement or a worsening of symptoms may be indications of heat stroke. Because the distinction between heat exhaustion and heat stroke is not always clear, transport to a hospital for further evaluation and treatment any patient for whom any of the following conditions applies:

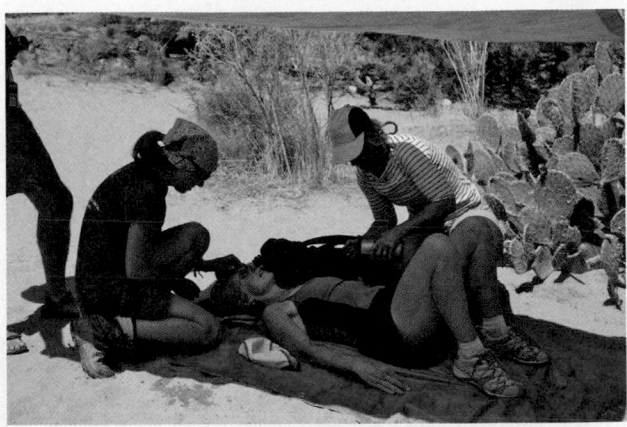

**Figure 26-11** Treat heat exhaustion promptly to prevent it from developing into heat stroke.
Copyright Craig Brown

- Symptoms that do not clear up promptly
- A decreasing level of responsiveness
- Body temperature that remains elevated
- The patient is very young, elderly, or has an underlying medical condition such as diabetes or cardiovascular disease

## Heat Stroke

As previously indicated, heat stroke is a true emergency that requires immediate attention. Recovery from heat stroke depends on the duration of the hyperthermia and the speed with which treatment is administered. Emergency treatment should begin immediately in the field and has one objective: *Lower the patient's body temperature by any means available.* Take the following steps when treating a patient with heat stroke:

- Notify EMS as quickly as possible for ALS transport to a hospital.
- Move the patient promptly from the hot environment to a cool, shaded environment.
- Shade the patient from direct sunlight.
- Remove the patient's clothing.
- Provide supplemental oxygen.
- The most effective cooling mechanisms are convection and evaporation, which are accomplished by keeping exposed skin wet and having a continuous flow of air across the skin. Naked patients may be sprayed with cool or lukewarm water while a fan blows air across the skin, or if necessary while a bystander manually fans the patient with a towel or a jacket.
- Conductive cooling can also be effective, particularly if ice packs are applied to areas of high blood flow, such as the armpits and groin.
- The immersion of patients in cold water is the most effective treatment but is best done under medical supervision.

If possible, check the patient's temperature frequently to determine if core body temperature is cooling. When the core body temperature reaches approximately 101°F (38.3°C), taper off the cooling efforts; rapid cooling below this point may lead to shivering (which will generate unwanted heat). If the patient returns to a

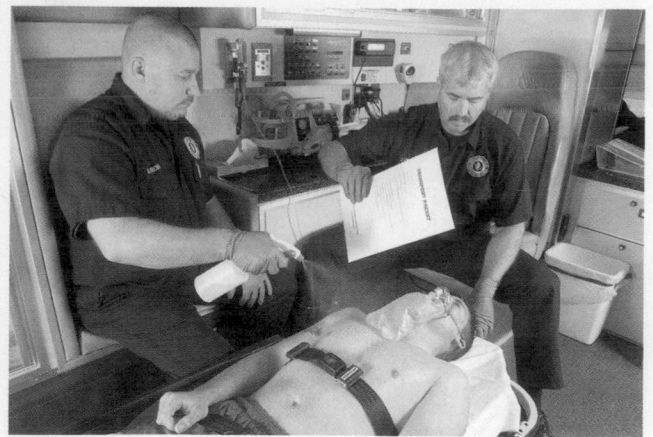

**Figure 26-12** If in doubt about the severity of a heat emergency, treat for heat stroke and transport to medical care as soon as possible.

level of responsiveness appropriate for oral hydration, give fluids. Anti-pyretic (anti-fever) medications such as aspirin or acetaminophen are not helpful. Rapid evacuation is indicated. Monitor patients carefully for a rebound increase in body temperature.

### Differentiating Between Heat Exhaustion and Heat Stroke

Heat stroke is differentiated from heat exhaustion by persistent profound mental status changes, hypotension/shock, and profound elevations in temperature. In heat exhaustion, mental status and blood pressure normalize rapidly upon rest in a supine position in the shade and oral rehydration. When there is doubt about whether a patient has heat exhaustion or heat stroke, treat as heat stroke and transport the patient to medical care as quickly as possible (Figure 26-12■). Table 26-2■ lists the criteria that help differentiate between heat exhaustion and heat stroke.

### Sunburn

Treatment for sunburn includes cool compresses and skin lotions containing aloe vera. Until the sunburn has resolved, prevent re-exposure to sunlight by wearing clothing that covers the affected areas.

**Table 26-2**    Differentiating Between Heat Exhaustion and Heat Stroke

| Finding | Heat Exhaustion | Heat Stroke |
|---|---|---|
| Occurs in high environmental temperatures? | Yes | Yes |
| May be associated with exercise? | Yes | Yes |
| Patient collapses? | Possible | Yes |
| Level of responsiveness | Mildly altered, improves quickly with treatment | Worsens over time, progresses to coma |
| Elevated core body temperature? | Yes, usually below 104°F | Yes, may be higher than 104°F |
| Pulse rapid? | Yes | Yes |
| Breathing rapid? | Yes | Yes |
| Responds to treatment in field? | Yes, rapidly | Sometimes; condition may worsen despite treatment |
| Shock, hypotension present? | No | Yes |
| Action to take in the field | Treat in the field | Evacuate and initiate treatment |
| Treatment | Cooling, rehydration | Rapid cooling |

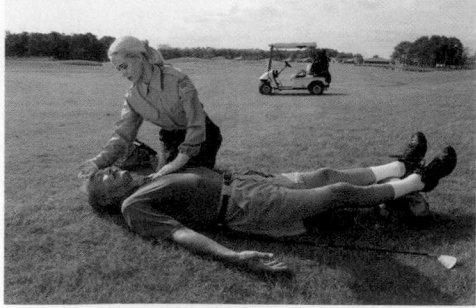

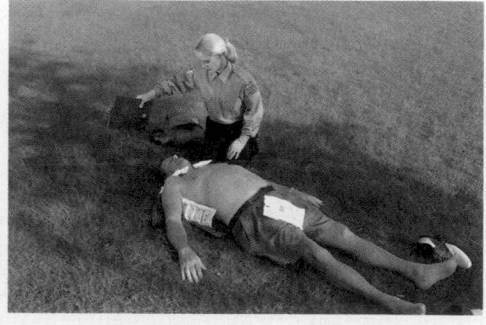

## Lightning Strikes

Care for patients who have sustained a lightning-strike injury in the same way as you would for any unresponsive patient: perform an appropriate primary assessment. Open the airway using the jaw-thrust maneuver and simultaneously check for breathing and a carotid pulse. Protect the spinal column because the patient could have a spinal injury from a fall. If breathing and a pulse are not present, begin CPR. If there is no pulse, early defibrillation with an AED is best. Because damage to the circulatory and respiratory systems is usually temporary and patients may be capable of full recovery, continue CPR. If a pulse returns but the patient is not breathing, continue rescue breathing as long as possible. Use a bag-valve mask and high-flow oxygen, if available.

For lightning-strike incidents involving multiple victims, care first for those in cardiac or respiratory arrest. This approach, called "reverse triage," is based on the assumption that patients who show signs of life (pulse and respirations, and perhaps movement, moaning, or talking) are likely to survive and thus should be treated *after* CPR is attempted on patients who appear dead. Quick treatment is crucial for increasing the chances that lightning-strike victims who are in cardiac or respiratory arrest can be successfully resuscitated. Remember, lightning-strike victims do not carry any residual electrical charge and are safe to touch.

## STOP, THINK, UNDERSTAND

### Multiple Choice

Choose the correct answer.

1. A significant change in behavior, hot flushed skin that is either dry or sweaty, and a strong rapid pulse can be indicative of which condition?_____
   a. heat-induced syncope
   b. heat stroke
   c. dehydration
   d. sunburn

2. Which of the following statements regarding patients with lightning-induced injuries are true? (check all that apply)
   _____a. The patient may still be electrically charged and thus can pose a threat to rescuers.
   _____b. CPR is rarely effective in lightning-strike victims due to the severe disruption of the heart's electrical system.
   _____c. Spontaneous heart action may return well before spontaneous respirations.
   _____d. The incidence of cardiac arrest in lightning-strike victims is low.
   _____e. Burns that appear to be superficial may actually be quite severe.
   _____f. Even if a patient appears to have made a full recovery, follow-up at a definitive-care facility is important because of the possibility of subsequent kidney failure.

3. You come across a family hiking on a hot, sunny day. The family's 4-year-old is lying on the ground, whimpering. Her skin is hot, dry, and flushed, and her mother tells you that her daughter "is refusing to talk to us." The best course of action is _____
   a. to explain to the parents that the child may be suffering from heat exhaustion or heat stroke and to obtain permission to assess and care for the child.
   b. to reassure the parents that children become crabby when it is hot, and that she should be all right after getting a drink of water.

   c. to commiserate with the parents that hiking with a tantruming child can be miserable, cluck sympathetically, and leave.
   d. to try to get the child to eat some saltine crackers or other salty food.

4. When a hiking companion begins to show signs and symptoms of heat exhaustion or heat stroke, another member of your party tells him to take acetaminophen or ibuprofen to lower his temperature. This course of action would be_____
   a. acceptable if the patient is 18 years of age or older and can tolerate these medicines.
   b. acceptable if the patient is 18 years of age or older, can tolerate these medicines, and if other cooling methods are employed at the same time.
   c. unacceptable because anti-pyretics are not effective for treating an elevated temperature resulting from heat exhaustion or heat stroke.
   d. acceptable only if other cooling methods fail to work.

5. After a patient suffering from heat stroke shows some improvement from being moved to a cooler environment, from having ice packs applied to the neck, groin and armpits, and from being sprayed with water and fanned, the next course of action *must* be to_____
   a. continue these measures and observe the patient until he recovers.
   b. gradually discontinue the cooling measures.
   c. offer the patient sips of a sports drink or lightly salted water and food.
   d. transport the patient immediately to definitive medical care by the fastest route possible, and alert the staff that you are enroute.

*continued*

STOP, THINK, UNDERSTAND *continued*

## Matching

Match each of the following heat-related illnesses to its description. Conditions may be used more than once.

_____ 1. heat cramps

_____ 2. heat exhaustion

_____ 3. heat stroke

_____ 4. heat syncope

a. unrelenting extremity cramping, hyperventilation
b. skin warm to the touch and lightheadedness after fainting
c. weakness, inability to keep hiking, nausea, tachycardia, warm sweaty skin
d. very hot sweaty, flushed skin, irrational behavior
e. unresponsiveness, weak pulse, decreased blood pressure

## Short Answer

1. Describe the field care provided to patients with heat-induced syncope or heat cramps.

   _____

   _____

   _____

2. Describe the field care provided to patients suffering from heat exhaustion.

   _____

   _____

   _____

3. Recovery from heat stroke depends on

   _____

   _____

4. The most important field treatment for a patient suffering from potential heat stroke is to

   _____

   _____

5. Why should the initial assessment and care of a lightning-strike victim be the same as that for an unconscious, unresponsive patient?

   _____

   _____

 **CASE DISPOSITION**

The exhausted, flushed, and sweating young woman sits in the cool shade of the overhang. Her respiration is 20/minute and her pulse is 100 beats/minute. She is responding appropriately to questions. She is able to drink a sports drink containing electrolytes, and once she lies down, she begins to look more comfortable. As you fan her with a piece of cardboard and she continues to rest and sip liquids over the next 30 minutes, her breathing slows and she becomes more talkative. Her pulse is now 80 beats/minute. Your findings suggest that she was suffering from heat exhaustion. Once the ambient temperature is cooler, you and your friends assist her on her walk out of the desert.

# ✚🛡 Chapter Review

## Chapter Summary

Heat illnesses include a group of disorders caused by exposure to a hot environment: heat syncope, cramps, heat exhaustion, and heat stroke. Unlike adaptation to cold, which involves only modifications in behavior, adaptation to heat depends on behavioral and internal mechanisms (physiologic acclimatization).

Patients with heat syncope (fainting) usually respond to supportive care. Heat cramps are painful muscle spasms that occur in large, heavily exercised muscle groups, such as the thigh or calf muscles, after vigorous exercise. Heat exhaustion occurs after exposure to a hot environment, especially during exercise; it is characterized by exhaustion, dizziness, nausea, excessive sweating, and decreased urine output; core body temperature is less than 104°F (40°C), and level of responsiveness is normal or mildly confused.

Heat stroke is a life-threatening emergency characterized by a decreased level of responsiveness, a core body temperature that is generally greater than 104°F (40°C), and increased pulse and respiratory rates. In heat stroke, the body's normal mechanisms for regulating body temperature and electrolyte and fluid balance fail. The most important defining characteristic of heat stroke is a decreased level of responsiveness that persists or progresses from confusion to coma, which should prompt immediate treatment and evacuation. In contrast, an altered level of responsiveness in heat exhaustion responds quickly to appropriate treatment.

Emergency management of heat cramps and heat exhaustion includes moving the patient from the hot environment to a cool shaded area, allowing the patient to rest, and providing oral hydration with cool, lightly salted water or an electrolyte solution. Heat stroke is a life-threatening emergency, and treatment should be started immediately while making plans for evacuation. Place patients in a cool shaded area, remove their clothing, wet their skin with cool water, and fan them aggressively to promote convective heat loss. Place ice packs at the neck, armpits and groin. The best care is to immerse patients in cold water with medical supervision.

Heat-related illness may be prevented by planning in advance and altering behavior. In hot environments, exercise outdoors during the early morning or late evening, have plenty of liquids available and stay well hydrated, wear a hat and light-colored, loose-fitting clothing, and gradually increase activity in the heat over days and weeks in order to allow physiologic acclimatization.

## Remember...

1. Allow the body to physiologically adapt to heat gradually, over several days (heat acclimatization).
2. Exercise in the early-morning or late-evening hours during hot weather.
3. Evaluate the risk of heat illness using the heat index.
4. The higher the heat and humidity, the greater the risk for heat illness.
5. Wear loose-fitting, light-colored clothing.
6. Drink plenty of water or electrolyte drinks.
7. Heat exhaustion responds rapidly to treatment.
8. Heat stroke is characterized by an elevated body temperature and an altered mental status.
9. Heat stroke is life threatening and does not respond quickly to treatment.
10. Patients struck by lightning are not electrically charged and (unlike victims of electrical injury) pose no threat to rescuers.
11. In a triage situation, care first for lightning-strike victims who appear dead.

# Chapter Questions

## Multiple Choice

Choose the correct answer.

1. The cooling mechanism that takes over when peripheral blood vessel dilation and radiation fail to cool the body adequately is_____

   a. syncope.
   b. shunting.
   c. an increased respiratory rate.
   d. sweating.

2. A 3-year-old child found unresponsive in a parked car with the windows closed during the summer is most likely suffering from_____

   a. heat cramps.
   b. heat-induced syncope.
   c. heat exhaustion.
   d. heat stroke.

3. Which of the following patients are at high risk for heat illnesses? (check all that apply)

   _____a. an infant dressed in a cap and a long-sleeved outfit/sweater
   _____b. an elderly person
   _____c. an obese person
   _____d. an athlete sitting and drinking from a personal water bottle
   _____e. a person snorting a line of cocaine
   _____f. an athlete out for a run
   _____g. a middle-aged person wearing a nasal cannula connected to a portable oxygen bottle
   _____h. a toddler with no hat, no sleeves, and no sunglasses sitting in a backpack carrier
   _____i. a healthy 7-year-old dressed in hiking shorts, boots, and a T-shirt and carrying a backpack with a water bottle in a side pocket

4. Which of the following actions would help you before and during a hike on the Bright Angel Trail from the south rim of the Grand Canyon to the Colorado River in mid-August? (check all that apply)

   _____a. Change your usual 40-minute daily jog from 7 a.m. to mid-day a week or more before leaving on your trip.
   _____b. A week before your trip, begin drinking increasing amounts of water each day, until you can tolerate drinking a full liter every 20 minutes.
   _____c. Eat salty snacks such as peanuts or crackers during the hike.
   _____d. Plan on stopping for only 5–10 minutes during each hour of the hike.
   _____e. Drink enough water to keep your urine completely clear (not yellow).
   _____f. Begin hiking before dawn, and sit out during the hottest part of the day.

5. The presence of dark-colored urine during a desert hike is indicative of _____

   a. thyroid disease.
   b. hyponatremia.
   c. dehydration.
   d. hyperthermia.

6. The heat index is _____

   a. a measure of discomfort urban dwellers can expect on a hot summer day.
   b. something outdoor enthusiasts should consider before choosing to exercise on a hot day.
   c. a measure of the risk for heat illness; it combines the effects of increasing ambient temperature and increasing humidity.
   d. a weather phenomenon that precedes thunderstorm activity.

7. Which of the following statements about sun protection is false? _____

   a. Cotton T-shirts provide adequate protection from the sun.
   b. Sunscreen with an SPF of 30 or greater should be applied before exposure to sunlight and reapplied several times during the day.
   c. Limit sunscreen use on children younger than 6 months of age to small areas such as the face or the backs of the hands.
   d. Cream- or oil-based sunscreens are best for use by snowboarders, skiers, and high-altitude hikers.

**8.** Which of the following locations provides a safe shelter during a thunderstorm? (check all that apply)

_____**a.** a shallow cave

_____**b.** an overhanging cliff

_____**c.** a field of uniform-sized boulders

_____**d.** a grove consisting of uniform-sized trees

_____**e.** a grove beneath the tallest, sturdiest tree

_____ **f.** just beneath a ridge line, crouching low

_____**g.** crouched in a wide drainage ditch

_____**h.** in a Quonset hut on the top of a mountain

_____ **i.** beneath a small grove of poplar trees in an open field

_____ **j.** in a large combine in an eastern-Washington wheat field

**9.** What is your next course of action for a patient suffering from apparent heat exhaustion whose temperature remains elevated and whose level of responsiveness has not improved despite appropriate care?_____

**a.** Continue what you are doing; it just takes some patients longer to improve.

**b.** Arrange to transport this patient to definitive medical care because this is most likely a case of heat stroke, and not a case of heat exhaustion.

**c.** Have the patient drink an additional bottle of sports drink or salt water and eat some salty food.

**d.** Stop what you are doing and immediately place the patient in the recovery position.

**10.** You are making camp in a campsite at Zion Park when your neighbors ask you for a sport drink. They explain that their 2-year-old, whom they carried in a backpack on a hike up the Angel's Landing trail this afternoon, has vomited and is now hot, flushed, sleepy, and confused. This child is most likely suffering from _____

**a.** fatigue and dehydration.

**b.** heat-induced syncope.

**c.** heat exhaustion.

**d.** heat stroke.

**11.** The care that this child needs is _____

**a.** emergent; this situation could be life threatening.

**b.** urgent, but she should respond to cooling and drinking a sports drink.

**c.** minor; she just needs a cool drink and a nap.

**d.** none of your business.

## List

List four ways to differentiate between heat exhaustion and heat stroke.

**1.** _____

**2.** _____

**3.** _____

**4.** _____

# Scenario

*An annual 10K foot race is being held today, and you have been asked to be at the halfway station because of your OEC skills. The ambient temperature is 98°F; the relative humidity is 92 percent.*

*About two hours into the race you notice a runner who appears to be staggering along the course. As he approaches your station, he collapses. You reach the patient and have two other volunteers stand on the course to divert runners away from you and the collapsed runner. During a primary assessment you find that the patient is unresponsive, has a pulse of 120, and has shallow, breaths at 28 per minute.*

*You call for help and carry the patient from the course to the covered treatment area a few feet away. The patient is very hot to the touch and has stopped sweating.*

1. Given these findings, you suspect that the patient is experiencing_____
   a. heat exhaustion.
   b. heat cramps.
   c. heat stroke.
   d. septic stroke.

*In the shade of the tent, you and your partners start fanning the patient and placing ice packs behind his neck, under his armpits, and in his groin area. During a secondary assessment, you notice a Med Alert bracelet that indicates that the patient is diabetic.*

2. Suspecting that hypoglycemia, and not heat illness, is the root cause for the patient's condition, you should_____
   a. start inserting glucose on a tongue depressor between the patient's cheek and gum.
   b. attempt to have the patient drink some cold orange juice.
   c. insert an OPA and continue to cool the patient.
   d. call for an ALS ambulance to administer IV therapy.

*While the ambulance is en route, you have the Registered Nurse on duty at your station use a glucose meter to measure the patient's blood sugar level. The glucose meter registers 40. A second set of vitals reads pulse at 110, blood pressure at 90/60, and respirations at 32 and shallow.*

3. Your prehospital treatment should be to_____
   a. monitor the airway and assist respirations with a bag-valve mask and high-flow oxygen.
   b. place the patient in the recovery position and monitor the airway.
   c. leave the patient in a supine position with his legs elevated.
   d. start CPR.

*The ALS ambulance arrives and immediately obtains an IV access. A recheck of blood sugar shows a level of 30. A member of the ambulance crew administers a bolus of dextrose, and the patient starts to regain consciousness, but he still has an altered mental status due to heat stroke. You assist the paramedics in preparing the IV drip set and normal saline bag to replace the lost fluid that contributed to the episode of heat exhaustion.*

## Suggested Reading

Auerbach, P. S. (Editor.) 2007. *Wilderness Medicine*, Fifth Edition. Philadelphia: Mosby.Forgey, W. W. (Editor.) 2006. *Wilderness Medical Society: Practice Guidelines for Wilderness Emergency Care*, Fifth Edition. Guilford, CT: Globe Pequot Press.

Forgey, W. W. (Editor.) 2006. *Wilderness Medical Society: Practice Guidelines for Wilderness Emergency Care*, Fifth Edition. Guilford, CT: Globe Pequot Press.

Tilton, B. 2004. *Wilderness First Responder: How to Recognize, Treat, and Prevent Emergencies in the Backcountry*, Second Edition. Guilford, CT: Globe Pequot Press.

 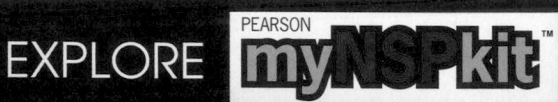

# Plant and Animal Emergencies

Joshua Kucker, MD

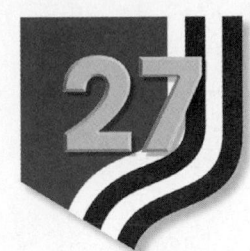

## ⊕ OBJECTIVES

**Upon completion of this chapter, the OEC Technician will be able to:**

**27-1** Compare and contrast poison, toxin, and venom.

**27-2** List and describe common toxic plants encountered in wilderness settings.

**27-3** Describe how plants can be harmful to humans.

**27-4** List and describe various land and marine creatures that may be harmful to humans.

**27-5** Describe and demonstrate how to assess a patient that has been injured following an encounter with a toxic plant, an animal, or some marine life.

**27-6** Describe and demonstrate how to manage an exposure to topical toxins.

**27-7** Describe and demonstrate the proper management of wounds caused by animals, including reptiles, insects, and spiders.

## ⊕ KEY TERMS

**antivenom,** *p. 873*
**bullae,** *p. 864*

**envenomation,** *p. 875*
**necrosis,** *p. 862*

**rash,** *p. 864*

## Chapter Overview

Anyone who has spent time in the outdoors should be aware of the risks posed by avalanches, lightning, or flash flooding. Injuries stemming from these events, although dramatic, are rare. Much more common are injuries and problems resulting from exposure to the many living wonders of the natural world—specifically, plants and animals, including insects.

This chapter discusses some common injuries resulting from exposure to plants and animals. Basic assessment considerations and treatment guidelines are also covered, as are recommendations for prevention.

As for any potential threats to life, plans for an emergency evacuation should always be in place. Although thousands of plant species and many thousands of insects

*continued*

## HISTORICAL TIMELINE

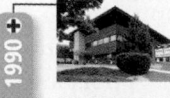

**1990** Office is consolidated with PSIA under management of the same Executive Director.

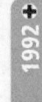

**1992** New Senior Program is implemented and the manual is published.

**1992**

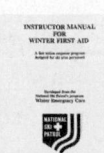

Instructor Manual for Winter First Aid published.

**CASE PRESENTATION**

It's a typical summer morning at the wilderness aid station. Blue skies radiate sunshine, the scenery captivates, and throngs of eager hikers and tourists abound. As you unlock the front door to begin your day, you see several people walking up the trail toward the building. You notice that whereas all of them are ambulatory, one person in the group is limping a bit as he walks. When he gets to the aid station, you learn that he is a 22-year-old male who is complaining of pain in his leg. He says that he was walking in the woods when he felt a sharp pain in his leg. When he looked down, he noticed two puncture holes in his calf above his boot. He thinks he may have seen a dark brown snake slithering away, but it "all happened so fast."

*What should you do?*

and other animals are potentially dangerous, this chapter is limited to those that are most frequently encountered. For plants, the focus is on skin-related injuries and toxicities from ingestions.

Even though the majority of encounters with plants and animals are benign, certain plants are highly toxic. Similarly, whereas most animal sightings are enjoyable events, species both large and small can inflict great injury. Maintaining the priorities of airway, breathing, circulation, and disability will help you assess and manage patients that have been injured by plants and animals. During the history and physical exam, OEC Technicians should focus on determining what the patient's plant or animal exposure has been, and whether any other patients have similar complaints.

## Anatomy and Physiology

⊕ **27-1** Compare and contrast poison, toxin, and venom.

The skin is composed of two major layers (Figure 27-1■). The outer layer, the *epidermis*, acts as a waterproof, protective barrier to invading organisms. Beneath it is the *dermis*, which contains hair follicles, blood capillaries, sweat glands, and nerve endings. The main functions of the dermis are sensation, temperature regulation, and fluid balance. Below the dermis is the *subcutaneous tissue* that contains many small blood vessels.

Injuries and topical exposures sustained from plants and animals nearly always affect the epidermis and dermis. Additionally, a forceful bite from a large animal can injure the underlying connective tissue, muscle, blood vessels, nerves, and bones. Not only can toxins from plants or animals cause local damage, but these poisons can enter the many blood vessels of the skin and be transported through the bloodstream to affect the cardiac, respiratory, and neurologic systems. In severe cases, respiratory or cardiac arrest can occur. The absorbed substances can act rapidly or slowly (sometimes over many hours) before system failure results.

**necrosis**   death of tissue.

When a toxin enters the vascular system, the rates at which it is absorbed by and distributed to a particular organ is dependent on the blood supply at each location. Some organs have a greater vascular supply and are affected rapidly. Because the blood supply to the extremities is not as great, the extremities are more prone to infection from an animal bite, and local **necrosis** at the bite site is common.

**Figure 27-1** A cross section of skin showing its layers.

It is important to understand the differences among a toxin, a poison, and venom. A toxin is a poison made by a living creature, whether plant or animal. A poison can come from a living creature or from chemicals or substances that do not come from living creatures. A venom is a specific toxin or poisonous secretion of an animal, most commonly from a snake, spider, or scorpion, usually transmitted by a bite or sting.

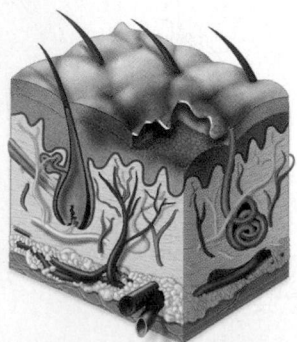

Skin reddened

# Adverse Effects and Emergencies from Common Plants and Fungi

The world is filled with a variety of plant life. Although most plants are benign or even beneficial to humans, some can cause harm, either through exposure to the skin (topical exposure) or through ingestion.

## Plants Toxic to the Skin

Localized skin reactions due to contact with plant material are a common occurrence in the outdoors. These reactions are typically a localized inflammatory response commonly called an allergic reaction (Figure 27-2a■). Chapter 14, Allergies and Anaphylaxis, contains details on allergic reactions. Plant toxins may cause itching only, or pain that can be severe enough to require evaluation by a physician and treatment with medications. Systemic effects may also be seen.

Poison Ivy, Poison Oak, and Poison Sumac

+ Description: These plants can be found in many forms, from low-lying vines to tall shrubs. The vines may often be found growing on tall trees with no leaves visible on the vines. Poison ivy and poison oak characteristically have three leaves grouped together, whereas poison sumac has seven leaves grouped together (Figure 27-2b–d■).

⊕ **27-2** List and describe common toxic plants encountered in wilderness settings.

⊕ **27-3** Describe how plants can be harmful to humans.

**Figure 27-2a** Blisters from contact with a poisonous plant.

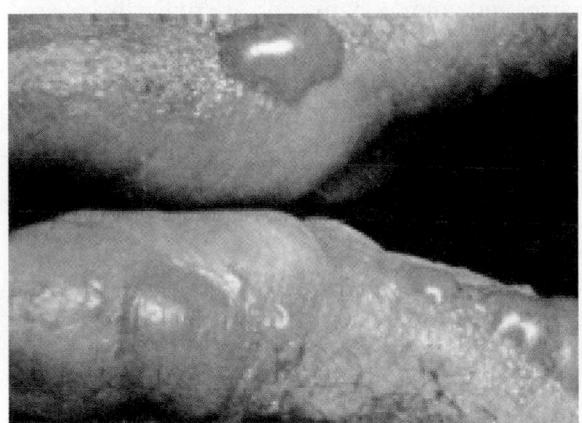

**Figure 27-2b** Poison ivy.

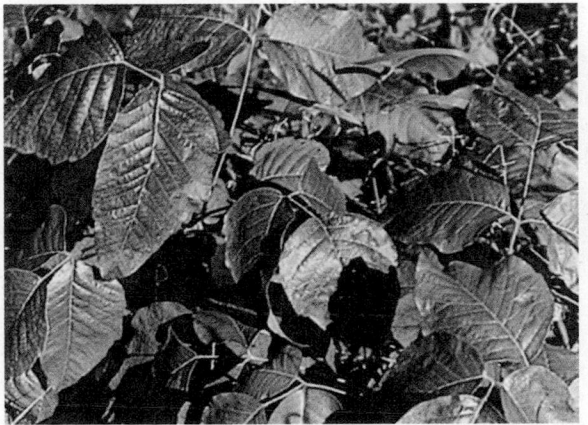

**Figure 27-2c** Poison sumac.

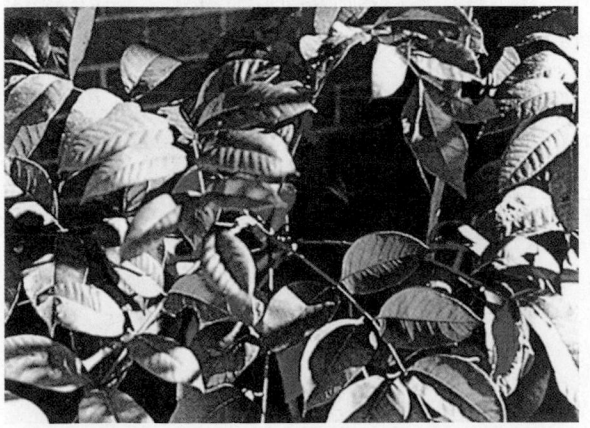

**Figure 27-2d** Poison oak.

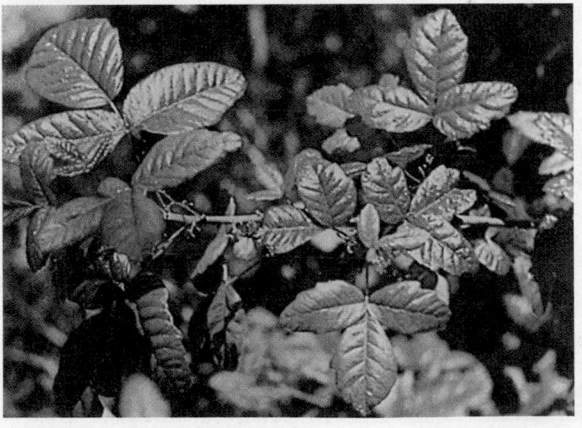

- Habitat: These plants typically grow in cool, wet environments that have plenty of shade.
- Toxic part: All parts of the plant are considered toxic. The plants secrete a toxic oil, known as urushiol oil, that may remain active even after the plant has been dead for up to 5 years. The oil can also be released into the air if the plant is burned.
- Toxic effects: Urushiol oil acts primarily on the skin. When the oil contacts the skin, it binds with skin proteins and forms an antigen. The resulting antigen-antibody reaction leads to a red, itchy, irritating **rash**. The more oil and the longer it is in contact with the skin, the more severe the rash. In severe cases, blisters or **bullae** may form. In addition to skin contact, the oil can also be inhaled, causing inflammation of the airways, difficulty breathing, and respiratory distress.

**rash** a temporary eruption on the skin.

**bullae** large blisters containing clear or bloody fluid.

### Stinging Nettle

- Description: Stinging nettles have soft green leaves on a wiry stem that can be from 3 feet to 7 feet tall (Figure 27-3■).
- Habitat: Stinging nettles grow in moist soil in forests with plenty of shade.
- Toxic part: The leaves and stem of this plant are covered with tiny hairs that can break off and become lodged in the skin.
- Toxic effects: Nettles that are stuck in the skin inject a chemical that causes a localized burning or stinging sensation. This burning may last from a few hours to up to a week.

### Cactus

- Description: Cacti grow in many sizes and unique shapes and are typically covered in spines (Figure 27-4■).
- Habitat: Cacti grow in hot, arid environments characterized by plenty of sun and limited water.
- Toxic part: The cactus plant is covered by spines that can break off and become stuck in the skin.
- Toxic effects: The spines do not contain a specific toxin. However, when one gets stuck in the skin, a localized inflammatory response causes pain and redness in the affected area.

**Figure 27-3** Stinging nettle.
Copyright Dorling Kindersley Media Library

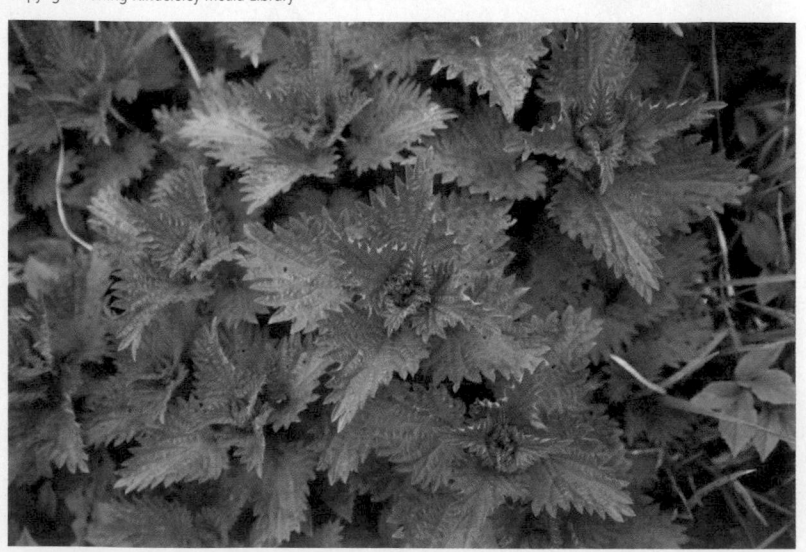

**Figure 27-4** Cactus.
Copyright Dorling Kindersley Media Library

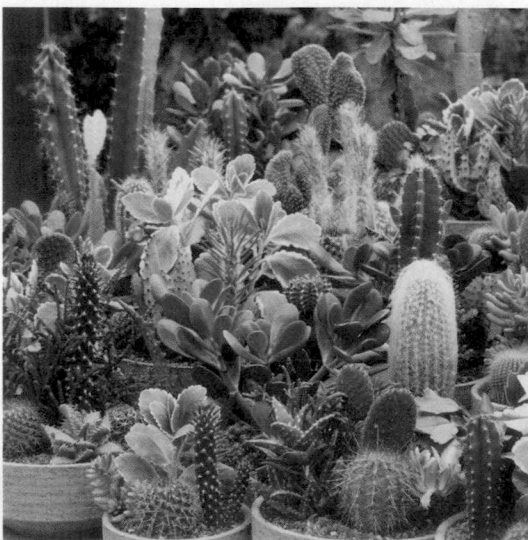

## Plants Toxic upon Ingestion

While the majority of toxic encounters from plants are topical in nature, outdoor enthusiasts may at times ingest vegetation or fruit that is harmful. Most common fruits and berries are rarely toxic. However, the ingestion of many other plants can lead to illnesses ranging from mild nausea to death.

The vast majority of toxic plant ingestions cause nausea and vomiting. Some toxic plants may produce cardiac effects, resulting in rhythm disturbances, whereas others may have neurological effects that produce hallucinations, confusion, or seizures. The onset of effects may occur within 15–30 minutes or over several hours. It is best not to ingest any plant material unless you are absolutely sure what it is.

Some toxic plants have medicinal purposes when the dose that is administered is small. Two of the more common of these plants are foxglove and the castor oil plant, which give us digitalis and castor oil laxative, respectively. Another is belladonna, which is used to treat diarrhea.

### Monkshood

- Description: Monkshood is a tall plant with a slim stem and blue blossoms (Figure 27-5■).
- Habitat: Monkshood typically grows in high montane environments near forest streams or on rocky slopes.
- Toxic part: While all parts of the monkshood plant are toxic, the toxic chemical is highly concentrated within the root of the plant.
- Toxic effects: When ingested, the poison causes nausea and digestive upset. Neurological effects, including nervous excitement, weakness, and paralysis, may also occur.

### Autumn Crocus

- Description: The autumn crocus is a low-lying plant with blossoms that bloom in the fall (Figure 27-6■).
- Habitat: The autumn crocus grows in meadows and grasslands.
- Toxic part: All parts of the autumn crocus plant are toxic when ingested.
- Toxic effects: Toxic effects initially begin with nausea, vomiting, and digestive upset and are followed by cardiovascular effects (e.g., arrhythmia) and shortness of breath. More severe effects include kidney failure, multisystem organ failure, and death.

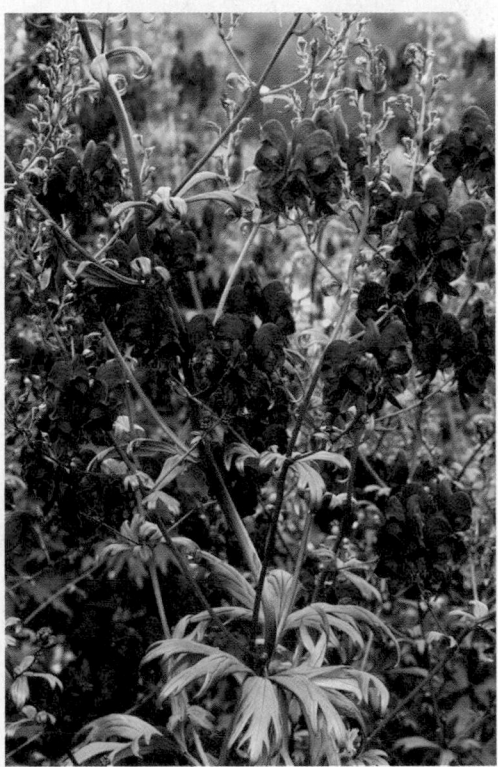

**Figure 27-5** Monkshood.
Copyright Clive Boursnell/Dorling Kindersley Media Library

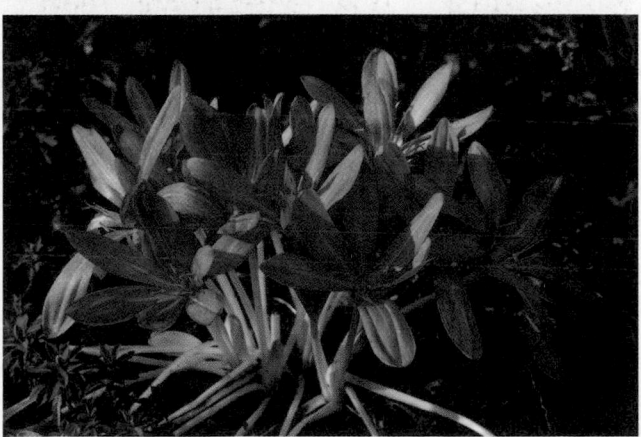

**Figure 27-6** Autumn crocus.
Copyright Roger Smith/Dorling Kindersley Media Library

### Lily of the Valley

+ Description: The lily of the valley grows to about 12 inches high and has bright green leaves that appear to grow directly out of the ground. The leaves are approximately 4 inches long by 1 1/2 inches wide. The plant is also characterized by small white flowers that are quite fragrant (Figure 27-7■).
+ Habitat: The plant is found within forested environments in partial shade.
+ Toxic part: All parts of the plant are toxic when ingested.
+ Toxic effect: When ingested, the plant causes nausea, vomiting, and headaches. Toxic effects on the heart can cause fatal arrhythmias.

### Foxglove

+ Description: The foxglove plant grows to about 4 feet high and has many small thimble-shaped flowers (Figure 27-8■).
+ Habitat: The plant is commonly found in wooded areas, both in sun and in partial shade.
+ Toxic part: All parts of the plant are toxic when ingested.
+ Toxic effect: The primary effects of ingestion of the foxglove plant are cardiovascular, resulting in arrhythmias that may be fatal. However, when used in small amounts medicinally, this plant's toxin can be beneficial to the heart and is called digitalis.

### Castor Oil Plant

+ Description: The castor oil plant can grow to the height of a small tree up to 10 feet tall. Its large leaves are palm shaped and have 7–9 lobes. The fruit of the tree is prickly and contains seeds of a shape that resembles that of coffee beans (Figure 27-9■).

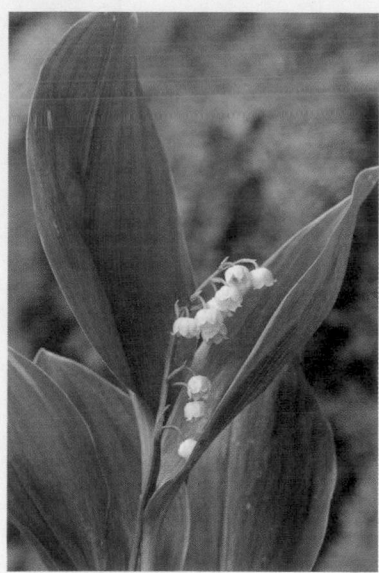

**Figure 27-7** Lily of the valley.
Copyright Deni Brown/Dorling Kindersley Media Library

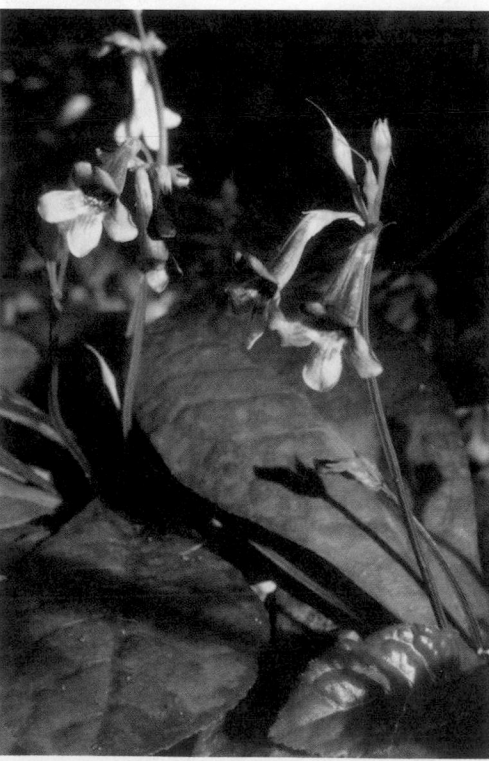

**Figure 27-8** Foxglove.
Copyright Dorling Kindersley Media Library

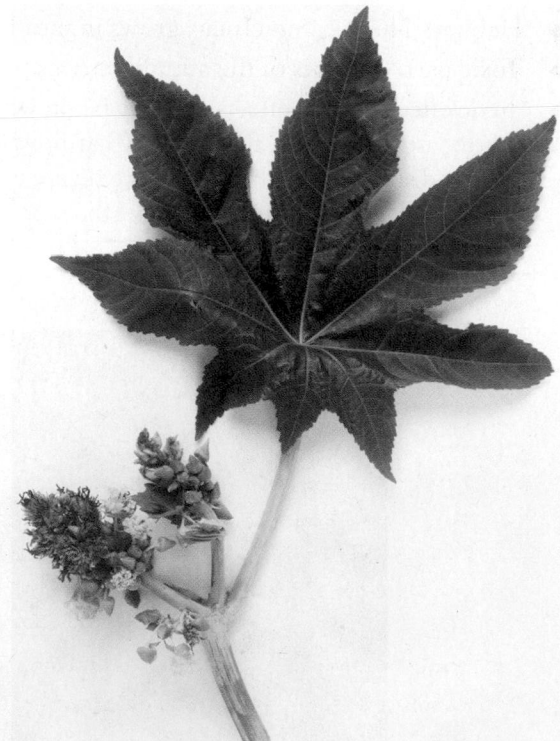

**Figure 27-9** Castor oil plant.
Copyright Steve Gorton/Dorling Kindersley Media Library

+ Habitat: The castor oil plant generally prefers warmer climates and is not cold hardy.
+ Toxic part: All parts of the plant are toxic. The toxin, known as ricin, is especially concentrated within the seeds and is highly toxic, even in small doses.
+ Toxic effect: Toxic effects include nausea, vomiting, digestive disturbance, and dehydration. The toxin can affect the entire body, leading to multisystem organ failure and death. In very small doses, it is used medicinally as a laxative called castor oil.

### Yew

+ Description: The yew plant is an evergreen growing up to 100 feet high. The berries are a characteristic bright red and resemble hollowed-out grapes (Figure 27-10■).
+ Habitat: The yew grows in dense forests on mountainsides.
+ Toxic part: All parts of the plant are toxic when ingested. The toxin is especially concentrated in seeds within the berries.
+ Toxic effect: Toxic effects include nausea, vomiting, diarrhea, and increased salivation. The effects can progress to shortness of breath, muscle spasms, and cardiovascular collapse.

### Water Hemlock

+ Description: The water hemlock grows to 8 feet high and has distinctive small green leaves and/or white flowers arranged in an umbrella-like shape at the very top.
+ Habitat: The water hemlock grows in wet meadows that have plenty of shade.
+ Toxic part: All parts of the plant are toxic.
+ Toxic effect: Toxicity begins with nausea and vomiting, followed by neurological effects of slowed speech, poor coordination, paralysis, and eventually death.

### Belladonna

+ Description: The belladonna plant grows as a branching shrub up to 5 feet in height. The bell-shaped flowers are typically a dark purple, and the berries are round and black.
+ Habitat: The plant grows in moist soil in shaded areas.
+ Toxic part: All parts of the plant are toxic when ingested.
+ Toxic effect: Toxic effects are quick in onset and include nausea, dry mouth, dizziness, visual disturbance, and agitation. The toxin also has cardiovascular effects that begin with a slowing of the heart rate and eventually lead to death. Medicinally, belladonna has been used in sedatives, stimulants, and antispasmodics (for the GI system), but in recent years it has fallen out of favor.

### Pokeweed

+ Description: The pokeweed plant grows up to 10 feet with large green alternating leaves and a reddish stalk or stem. Berries grow in large clusters and are typically a dark purple or black (Figure 27-11■).
+ Habitat: The plant grows in warm, moist, tropical environments.
+ Toxic part: All parts of the plant can be toxic to various degrees. The most toxic parts of the plant are the root and stem.
+ Toxic effect: Effects include nausea and vomiting, shortness of breath, spasms, and bloody diarrhea.

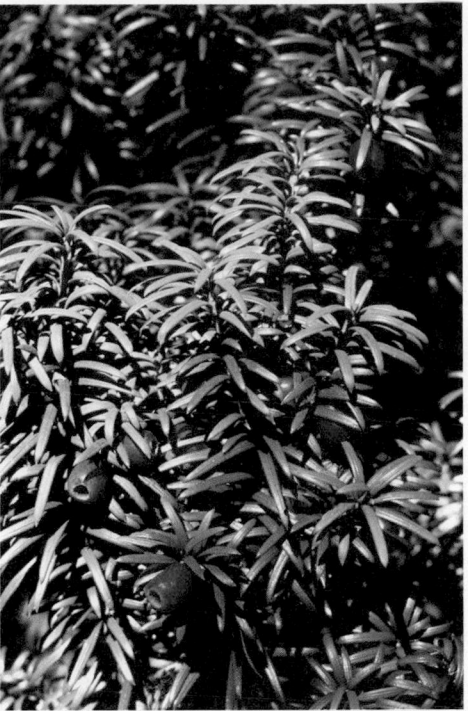

**Figure 27-10** Yew.
Copyright Roger Smith/Dorling Kindersley Media Library

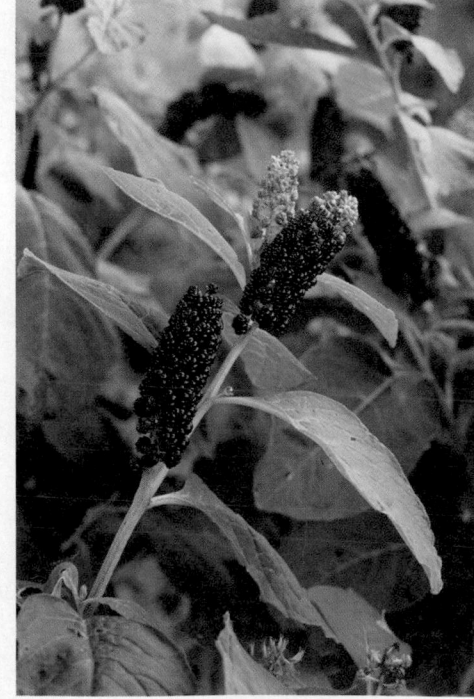

**Figure 27-11** Pokeweed.
Copyright Andrew Lawson/Dorling Kindersley Media Library

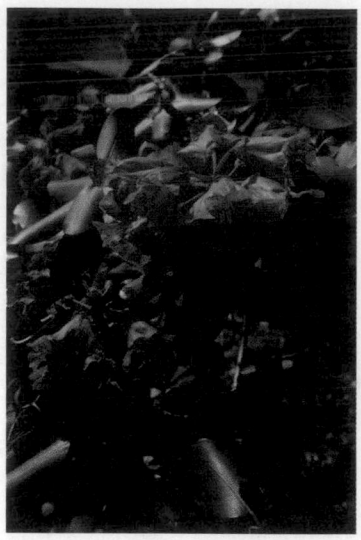

**Figure 27-12** Rhododendron.
Copyright John Glover/Dorling Kindersley Media Library

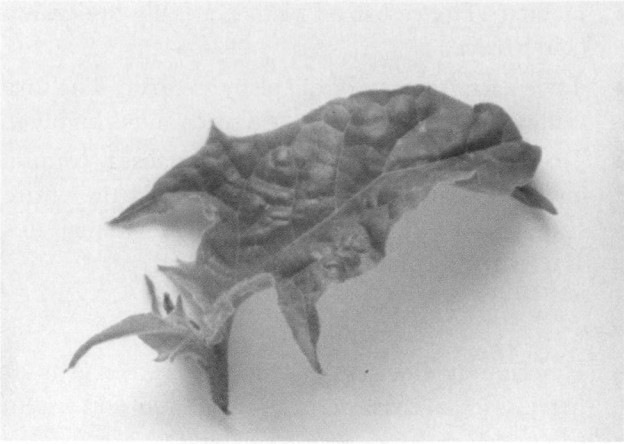

**Figure 27-13** Jimson weed.
Copyright Steve Gorton/Dorling Kindersley Media Library

## Rhododendron, Azalea

+ Description: The plants are evergreens that grow as rounded shrubs that are typically up to 10 feet tall. The leaves are dark green and are arranged in a spiral pattern. Flowers are arranged in the center of a grouping of leaves (Figure 27-12■).

+ Habitat: These plants grow in warm, wooded environments that have plenty of shade and water.

+ Toxic part: All parts of the plant are toxic when ingested.

+ Toxic effect: Toxic effects begin with nausea and vomiting, followed by bloody diarrhea, seizures, unresponsiveness, and death.

## Jimson Weed

+ Description: Jimson weed grows as a low shrub 3–5 feet tall. The leaves are a dark green and toothed, resembling the leaves of an oak tree (Figure 27-13■). Berries are spiny and grow off of the stem of the shrub.

+ Habitat: Jimson weed grows in moderate climates in partial sun.

+ Toxic part: All parts of the plant are toxic when ingested.

+ Toxic effect: Toxicity is marked by confusion and delirium.

## STOP, THINK, UNDERSTAND

### Multiple Choice

Choose the correct answer.

1. The initial focus on caring for a patient who is the victim of a plant or animal emergency is _____
   a. removing the source of the toxin.
   b. determining the MOI.
   c. maintaining scene safety.
   d. caring for the ABCDs.

2. Which of the following statements about poison ivy, poison oak, and poison sumac is true? _____
   a. The leaves are the most toxic part of the plant.
   b. Burning a poison ivy vine that has been dead for 5 years and inhaling the smoke can cause a respiratory reaction.
   c. A small or large exposure to urushiol oil can cause a severe reaction.
   d. Urushiol oil is a neurotoxin.

*continued*

3. Which of the following plants cause a mild, localized reaction that can last just a few hours? _____
   a. Poison ivy and poison sumac
   b. Cactus and stinging nettle
   c. Lily of the valley and yew
   d. Belladonna and pokeweed

4. A child who presents with nausea, vomiting, bloody diarrhea, and seizure and then loses responsiveness probably ingested_____
   a. belladonna.
   b. jimson weed.
   c. water hemlock.
   d. azalea.

5. Which of the following effects can result from ingesting toxic plants? (check all that apply)
   _____ a. Visual disturbances
   _____ b. Spasms or seizures
   _____ c. Unresponsiveness
   _____ d. Rashes
   _____ e. Death
   _____ f. Nausea and vomiting
   _____ g. Necrosis of the skin/underlying tissue
   _____ h. Cardiogenic effects
   _____ i. Salivation
   _____ j. Headache
   _____ k. Dehydration
   _____ l. Paralysis
   _____ m. Kidney failure

## Matching

Match each of the following to its description. Each term may be used more than once.

_____ 1. epidermis

_____ 2. dermis

_____ 3. subcutaneous tissue

   a. outermost layer of skin
   b. controls temperature and fluid/volume
   c. contains hair follicles, capillaries, sweat glands, and nerve endings
   d. a waterproof, protective barrier
   e. a transitional layer to muscles, tendons, and bones
   f. sensations occur in this layer
   g. topical exposure is less likely to reach this level

## Fill in the Blank

1. Localized tissue death at an animal bite site is called _____.

2. Large blisters filled with clear or bloody fluid are called _____.

3. Poison in the wound from a spider bite, snake bite, or wasp sting is known as_____.

4. A _____ is something you may ingest, inhale, absorb, or develop in the body that can disrupt bodily functions or damage structures.

5. A _____is a poison produced by a plant, an animal, or bacteria.

6. An individual who exhibits confusion and delirium after eating some spicy berries could have ingested _____.

## List

List three plants that can have cardiogenic effects.

_____

_____

_____

_____

## Short Answer

Explain the differences between a toxin and a poison.

_____

_____

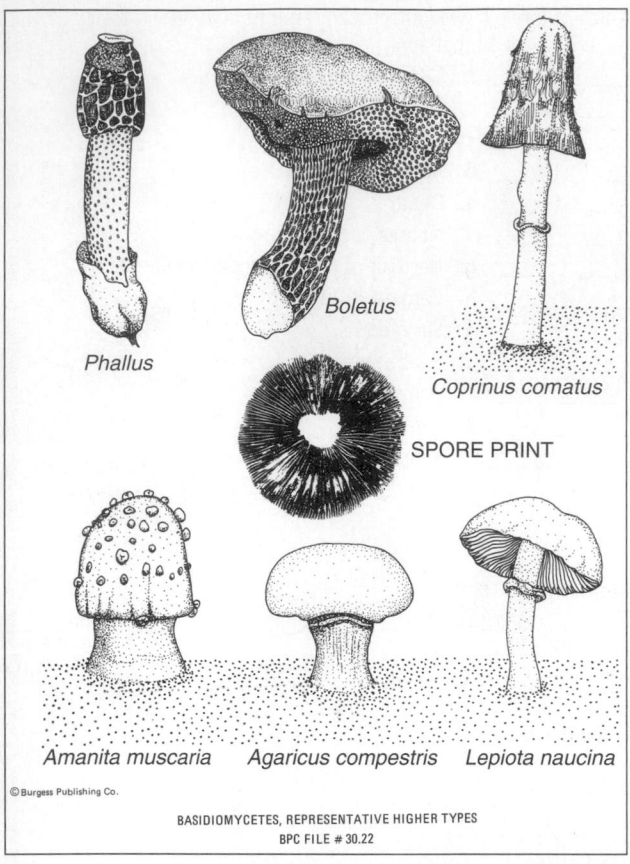

Phallus

Boletus

Coprinus comatus

SPORE PRINT

Amanita muscaria    Agaricus compestris    Lepiota naucina

© Burgess Publishing Co.

BASIDIOMYCETES, REPRESENTATIVE HIGHER TYPES
BPC FILE # 30.22

**Figure 27-14** Some examples of poisonous mushrooms.

## Poisonous Mushrooms

There are three main groups of mushrooms (which are fungi) that are dangerous to humans: the amanitas, the false morels, and a catch-all category known as little brown mushrooms, or LBMs (Figure 27-14■). Mushrooms in these groups cause virtually all of the fatal mushroom poisonings in the United States, with amanitas alone accounting for 90 percent of mushroom-related deaths.

Hundreds of other mushrooms also cause problems ranging from a mild stomach ache to severe physical distress, including vomiting, diarrhea, cramps, and loss of coordination. Two common poisonous mushrooms of this type are the jack-o-lantern and the green-spored lepiota. Although the effects of poisoning from these mushrooms may be alarming, they usually pass in 24 hours or less with no lasting effects. Some mushrooms, known as psilocybin mushrooms, contain chemicals that can produce hallucinogenic effects in humans and animals. The effects vary considerably among individuals.

### Amanita

- Description: The amanita mushroom is a large mushroom with a brightly colored top that is typically speckled with a white warty material (Figure 27-15■).
- Habitat: These mushrooms grow in large clumps in moist, shaded soil in woodlands.
- Toxic part: All parts of the mushroom are toxic.
- Toxic effect: Toxic effects are primarily neurologic and produce auditory and visual disturbances, sweating, salivation, and loss of equilibrium.

### False Morels

- Description: False morels have a wrinkled, irregular cap that is either saddle shaped or resembles a brain (Figure 27-16■). They may be black, gray, white, brown, or reddish.
- Habitat: False morels typically grow in moist soil around dead or dying trees.
- Toxic part: All parts of the mushroom can be toxic when ingested.

**Figure 27-15** An amanita mushroom.
Copyright Neil Fletcher/Dorling Kindersley Media Library

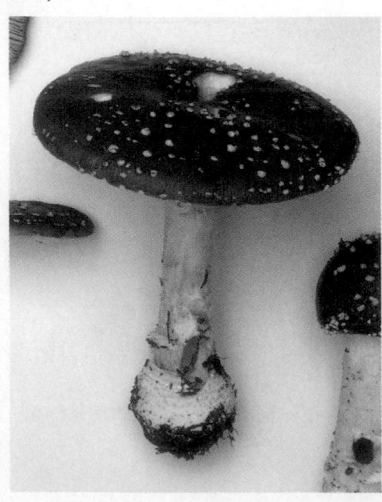

**Figure 27-16** A false morel mushroom.
Copyright Leighton Moses/Dorling Kindersley Media Library

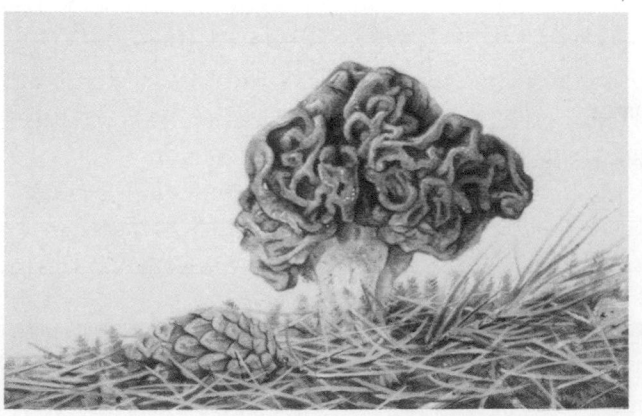

+ Toxic effect: Toxic effects include nausea, vomiting, diarrhea, and severe headaches. Ingestion can occasionally be fatal.

### Little Brown Mushrooms

+ Description: Literally hundreds of mushrooms belong in this category. All of these mushrooms are small brown mushrooms that are difficult to identify (Figure 27-17■).
+ Habitat: These mushrooms live in varied habitats; most grow in moist soil.
+ Toxic part: All parts of these mushrooms can be toxic when ingested.
+ Toxic effect: Toxic effects vary from mild nausea to hallucinations.

### Jack-o-Lantern

+ Description: The jack-o-lantern mushroom is a bright orange mushroom resembling a pumpkin. It is typically found in the fall.
+ Habitat: These mushrooms generally grow in shaded habitats east of the Rocky Mountains.
+ Toxic part: All parts of the mushroom are toxic when ingested.
+ Toxic effect: Toxicity ranges from mild to severe abdominal upset. Ingestion of these mushrooms is generally not fatal.

### Green-Spored Lepiota

+ Description: The green-spored lepiota is a large mushroom with a tan parasol-shaped cap and a large ring on the stem (Figure 27-18■). This mushroom has a greenish spore print (pattern and color produced after the cap of a mushroom is pressed against a white piece of paper).
+ Habitat: These mushrooms generally grow in open fields.
+ Toxic part: All parts of the mushroom are toxic when ingested.
+ Toxic effect: Ingestion of these mushrooms causes violent gastrointestinal upset.

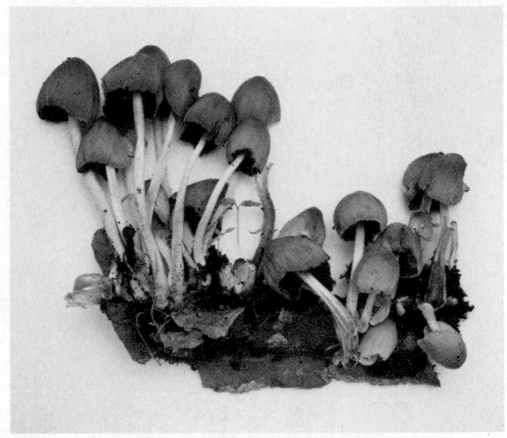

**Figure 27-17** Little brown mushrooms.
Copyright Neil Fletcher/Dorling Kindersley Media Library

**Figure 27-18** A lepiota mushroom.
Copyright Neil Fletcher/Dorling Kindersley Media Library

# Adverse Effects from Various Animals

## Spiders

While the vast majority of lesions attributed to spider bites are actually skin infections that developed from an insect bite, OEC Technicians must be aware that spider bites do occur and can result in significant morbidity. The spiders that bite and are of concern are the black widow, brown recluse, hobo, wolf, and funnel web.

### Black Widow Spider

+ Description: The black widow spider measures about 3/4-1 1/4 inches long. It has a jet black body and a characteristic red hourglass on its abdomen (Figure 27-19■).
+ Habitat: The black widow spider lives in trees and shrubs above ground but may also be found under logs and stones in woods and fields.
+ Characteristics of bite: Bites occur primarily between April and October and usually occur on the patient's hands and forearms. Most bites occur when the female spider is guarding her eggs. The bite site can resemble a "bull's-eye" or target and may sometimes become secondarily infected.
+ Toxic effect: The bite is initially painful and is followed by swelling and redness that can spread over the entire limb. Systemic signs and symptoms may develop, including nausea, abdominal pain, fever, sweating, and (in some cases) paralysis.

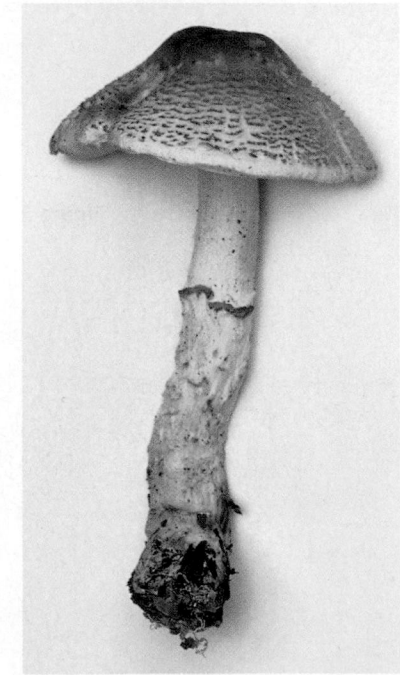

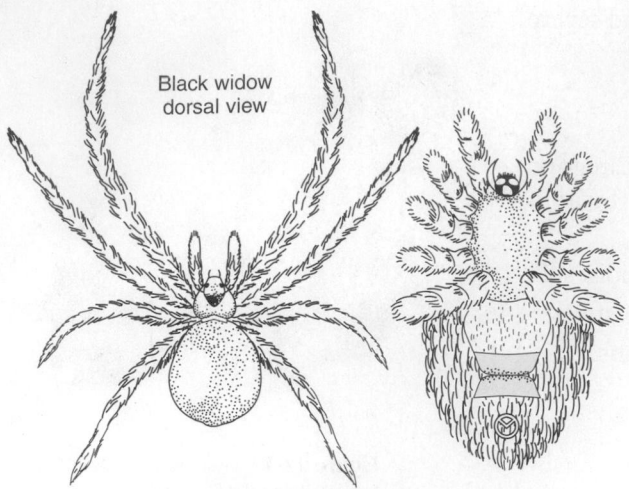

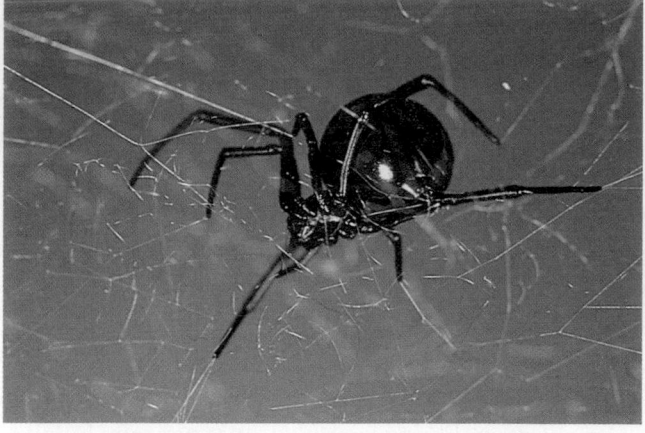

**Figure 27-19** A black widow spider.

## Brown Recluse Spider

+ Description: The brown recluse spider is light brown or dark brown and has a leg span up to 1 inch. It is identified by a characteristic violin or "fiddle" shape on its back, near the head (Figure 27-20■).

+ Habitat: The brown recluse spider typically is found under stones and in dark corners inside buildings. In the United States, the spider is found primarily in the Midwest and the Southwest.

+ Characteristics of bite: Local symptoms usually begin at the moment of the bite. A sharp stinging sensation is possible, although a victim may be unaware of having been bitten. If there is stinging, it usually subsides in 6–8 hours.

+ Toxic effect: The venom can destroy the walls of blood vessels, resulting in localized tissue death and skin ulcerations that can take a long time to heal. Although rare, death can occur due to renal failure.

## Hobo Spider

+ Description: The hobo spider is a small brown spider measuring about 1/2-3/4 inches in length. This spider has several chevron-shaped markings on the abdomen.

**Figure 27-20** A brown recluse spider.

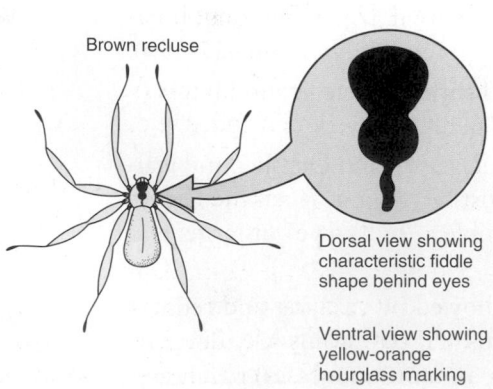

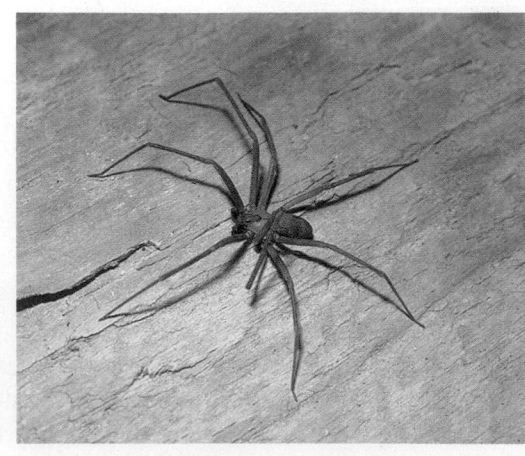

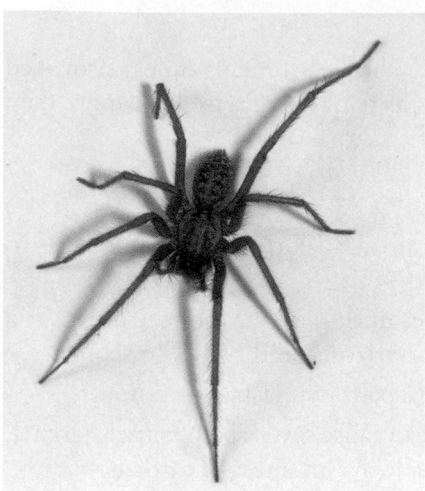

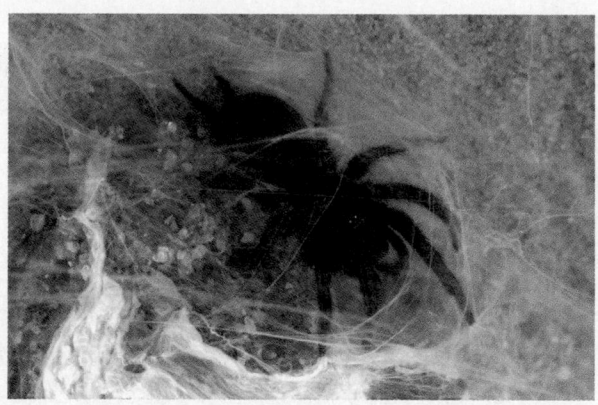

**Figure 27-22** A funnel web spider.
Copyright Jerry Young/Dorling Kindersley Media Library

**Figure 27-21** A wolf spider.
Copyright Frank Greenaway/Dorling Kindersley Media Library

+ Habitat: The hobo spider lives in damp locations such as wood piles and is found primarily in the Pacific Northwest.
+ Characteristics of bite: This spider may or may not inject venom into its bite, which is often painless. The bite site initially appears red and then disappears over several hours. Over the next 24 hours, a blister may form that later breaks open, becoming an open lesion.
+ Toxic effect: When venom is injected, an area of localized tissue death and skin ulceration often results.

## Wolf Spider

+ Description: The wolf spider ranges in size from very small to 1.5 inches. This spider characteristically carries its eggs and its young on its back (Figure 27-21■).
+ Habitat: The habitat of the wolf spider varies from coastal areas to woodlands.
+ Characteristic of bite: The bite is initially painful.
+ Toxic effect: Localized pain and swelling are typical. In fewer than 10 percent of cases, patients may also have systemic symptoms of nausea and/or headache.

## Funnel Web Spider

+ Description: Funnel web spiders are medium-sized to large spiders, with bodies that range from 2/8-2 inches in length. They are darkly colored, ranging from black to blue-black to plum to brown, with a glossy, hairless carapace covering the front part of the body (Figure 27-22■).
+ Habitat: Indigenous to Australia, funnel web spiders make their burrows in moist, cool, sheltered habitats—under rocks, in and under rotting logs, and sometimes in rough-barked trees.
+ Characteristic of bite: Some bites may be "dry," and if venom is injected, pain results.
+ Toxic effect: Bites cause mouth numbness, vomiting, abdominal pain, sweating, and salivation. It has been claimed that only approximately 10–25 percent of bites produce significant toxicity, but all bites should be treated as potentially life threatening. **Antivenom** to the bites of this spider was introduced in 1984 and is very effective.

**antivenom** a biological material (antibodies) administered to a patient to counteract exposure to a specific kind of venom; is produced by injecting the venom into an animal and then harvesting the antibodies that the animal makes against the venom.

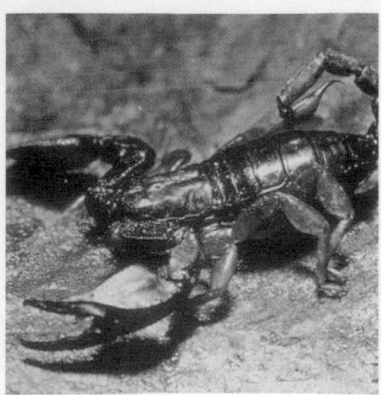

**Figure 27-23** A scorpion.

## Scorpions

Though fearsome in appearance, scorpions rarely bother humans unless provoked (Figure 27-23■). When they do sting, the vast majority of cases cause little more than local pain and discomfort.

### Bark Scorpion

+ Description: The bark scorpion is a small brown scorpion measuring up to 3 inches (Figure 27-24■).
+ Habitat: The bark scorpion lives in dark places during the heat of the day in arid environments. It is found in Texas, California, Arizona, and New Mexico.
+ Characteristic of sting: The sting causes severe pain that lasts 24–72 hours.
+ Toxic effect: The venom from a bark scorpion can cause severe pain, muscle jerking, nausea, vomiting, blurred vision, and occasionally disturbances of cardiac rhythm.

## Ticks

Located throughout the United States, ticks can transmit a wide variety of diseases from animals to humans. Transmission of tick-borne diseases occurs through the saliva of the tick while the tick is feeding on the blood of an animal host. Tick bites are typically painless, so the tick may stay attached to its host for 24 hours or more without the individual's knowledge. The best defense against tick bites is to prevent them by wearing appropriate clothing with long pants and sleeves and shoes with socks in areas known for ticks. Even proper clothing does not guarantee protection so it is still important to check your skin for them regularly, especially in the evening before going to sleep.

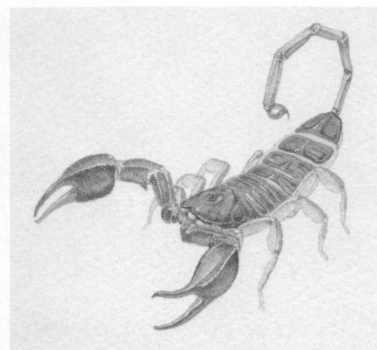

**Figure 27-24** A bark scorpion.
Copyright Dorling Kindersley Media Library

### Deer Tick

+ Description: The deer tick is a small tick (Figure 27-25■). Nymphs measure about 0.04 inches, whereas engorged (recently fed) adults measure about 0.16 inches.
+ Habitat: The tick lives in wood piles and tall grasses, and on deer.
+ Characteristic of bite: The bite is typically painless (Figure 27-26■). When the tick leaves, a characteristic rash that is described as a red circle surrounding a blanched white center (a target lesion) may be visible at the bite site.

**Figure 27-26** A tick embedded in the scalp.
Copyright Charles Stewart & Associates

**Figure 27-25** A deer tick.
Copyright Pfizer Central Research

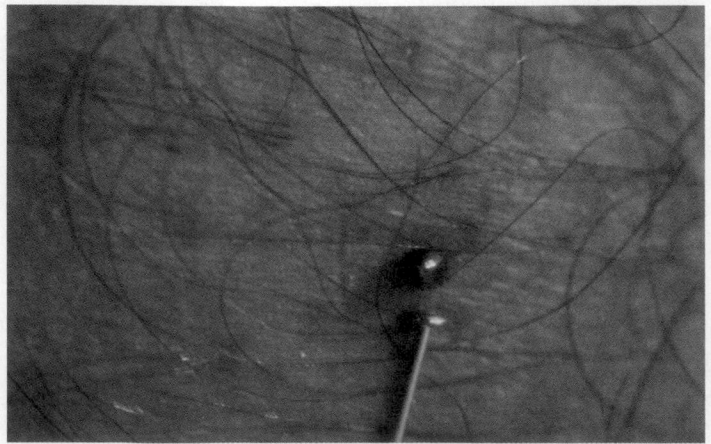

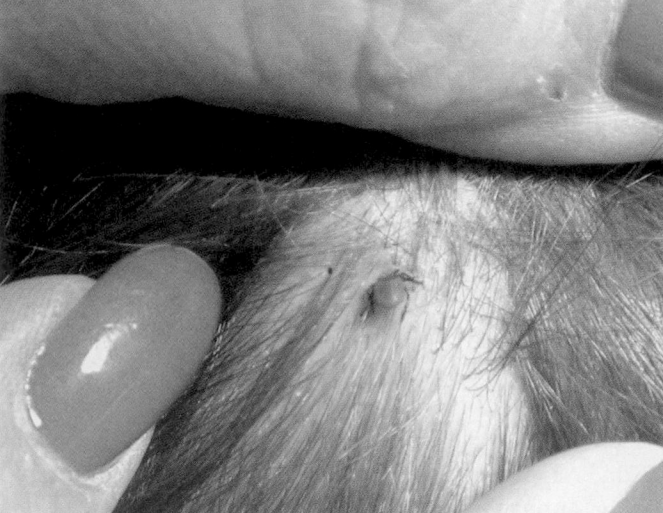

+ Disease transmitted: The primary disease transmitted by deer ticks is Lyme disease. Lyme disease characteristically begins with a rash that is followed by flu-like symptoms, including fever, nausea, and vomiting. As the disease progresses, patients develop generalized joint pain and may develop a facial droop. Sometime after the bite, people may develop both septic joints and meningitis.

### Wood Tick and Dog Tick

+ Description: These ticks are large ticks measuring up to 1/2 inch when engorged (Figure 27-27■).
+ Habitat: Dog and wood ticks typically live in woods and open fields.
+ Characteristic of bite: The bites of wood ticks and dog ticks are typically painless.
+ Disease transmitted: These ticks can transmit Rocky Mountain Spotted Fever; wood ticks are the vectors (transmitters) of this disease in the western United States, and dog ticks are the vectors in the eastern part of the country. Despite the disease's name, more recent cases have involved ticks from forested areas on the East Coast. The disease is characterized by fever, nausea, vomiting, and a full body rash consisting of small, red, raised areas.

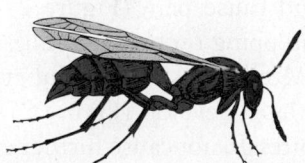

**Figure 27-27** A dog tick.
Copyright Dorling Kindersley Media Library

## Bees, Wasps, and Hornets

Bees, wasps, and hornets cause the most **envenomations** per year of any stinging creature (Figure 27-28■). The majority of stings cause pain and swelling in a localized

**envenomation** poisonous effects caused by bites or stings.

**Figure 27-28** Wasps, bees, and hornets commonly sting humans, causing local pain, redness, swelling, and subsequent itching. Always consider the possibility of an allergic reaction.

### WASPS, BEES, AND FIRE ANTS
The following members of this group commonly attack humans, causing local pain, redness, swelling, and subsequent itching. Always consider the possibility of an allergic reaction.

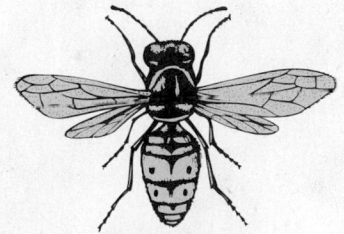

**HONEYBEE:** Found throughout the United States at any time of year, except in colder temperatures when they remain in their hives. In the Northeast and Midwest, they are major insects causing sting reactions. Hives are usually found in hollowed out areas such as dead tree trunks. Honeybees principally ingest nectar of plants, so they are often seen in the vicinity of flowers. The honeybee with its barbed stinger will self-eviscerate after a sting, leaving the venom sac and stinger in place.

**WASPS:** The most likely insect to cause sting reactions in the Southeast and Southwest. Wasps tend to nest in small numbers under the eaves of houses and buildings. Carnivores that are found in picnic areas, garbage cans, and food stands, they can deliver multiple stings at one time.

**YELLOW JACKET:** A principal insect causing sting reactions in the Northeast and Midwest. Yellow jackets tend to dominate in late summer and fall. Nests are located in the ground. Often seen in picnic areas and garbage cans, yellow jackets are ill-tempered and aggressive and can deliver multiple stings at one time. They will often sting without being provoked.

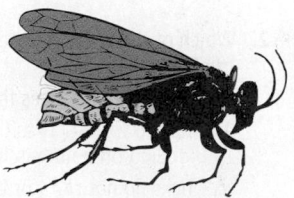 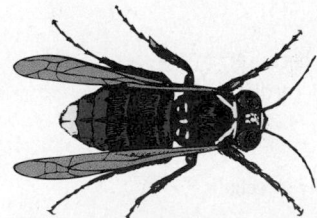

**YELLOW HORNET AND WHITE-FACED OR BALD-FACED HORNET:**
Seen mainly in the spring and early summer. Nests usually found in branches and bushes above ground. Carnivores that are seen in picnic areas, garbage cans, and food stands, they can deliver multiple stings at one time.

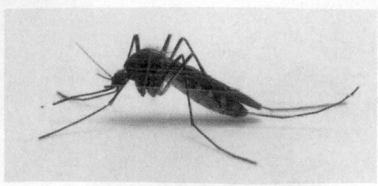

**Figure 27-29** A mosquito.
Copyright Frank Greenaway/Dorling Kindersley Media Library

area of the skin and in the nearby joint. In severe cases, anaphylaxis and death can occur (Chapter 14, Allergies and Anaphylaxis). The Africanized honey bee or so-called "killer bee" has recently extended its range into the southwestern United States and now exists as far north as southern Utah. A swarm of these bees can attack humans with deadly results.

## Mosquitoes, Fleas, and Biting Flies

Although bites from mosquitoes, fleas, and biting flies typically do not cause serious illness in the United States, they do cause localized redness, itching, and swelling (Figure 27-29■). Occasionally, a delayed reaction can lead to worsening edema and severe itching. Insect repellents containing DEET (N, N-Diethyl-meta-toluamide) are often quite effective in the prevention of bites.

For travelers outside of the United States, the greatest concern from mosquitoes is the transmission of diseases, primarily malaria, dengue fever, yellow fever, and encephalitis. Like ticks, mosquitoes transmit disease organisms while feeding on a host. Mosquitoes pick up the organisms while feeding on the blood of one host and transmit them to another host during a subsequent blood meal. Anyone planning to visit areas in which these diseases are endemic should consult with a tropical medicine specialist concerning the advisability of prophylactic medication or a vaccination.

**Figure 27-30a** A fire ant.

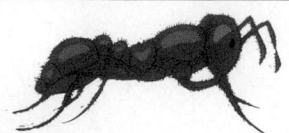

**FIRE ANT:** Can range from red to black and lives in loose dirt mounds. It is found throughout the southern states as far west as New Mexico. Fire ants may cause serious illness and/or allergic reactions. The ant attaches itself to the skin by its strong jaws and swivels.

**Figure 27-30b** Fire ant bites. An allergic reaction may ensue.

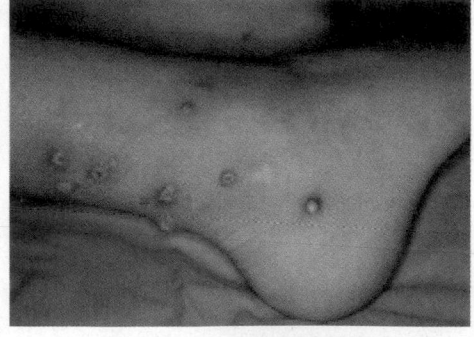

West Nile virus (WNV), first seen in the United States in 1999, is transmitted by mosquitoes. People who contract WNV usually have mild symptoms or no symptoms. Those with symptoms may have fever, headache, body aches, a skin rash, or swollen lymph glands. If West Nile virus enters the brain, the resulting encephalitis (inflammation of the brain) or meningitis (inflammation of the coverings of the brain) can be deadly. Eradication of mosquitoes from swamps and from standing water around homes is the best prevention strategy for WNV.

## Ants

Fire ants, a grouping of ants that includes five different species, are known to bite and cause pain (Figure 27-30a■). If threatened by direct provocation (e.g., stepping on their anthill), the ants will swarm and sting all at the same time. Most stings are painful at the injection site; in some cases, blisters, or bullae later develop (Figure 27-30b■). Aside from severe itching and pain, most bites do not cause further complications. Some sensitive individuals may have an allergic reaction much like that to a bee sting or a wasp sting. In addition, ant bites can become secondarily infected by excessive scratching.

# STOP, THINK, UNDERSTAND

## Multiple Choice
Choose the correct answer.

1. A scorpion sting can be serious because_____
   a. it can cause disturbances of cardiac rhythm.
   b. it can be fatal.
   c. it can cause paralysis.
   d. it is susceptible to secondary infections.

2. Which of the following statements about tick-borne diseases is true? _____
   a. Ticks carry diseases that they transmit directly to humans.
   b. Ticks transmit parasitic organisms through their saliva while feeding on a human host.
   c. Ticks do not carry or transmit diseases; the host becomes ill when tick bites become infected due to scratching.
   d. A tick must remain attached to a host for 24 hours or more in order for transmission of bacteria to occur.

*continued*

**3.** The greatest danger from a bee sting or a wasp sting is_____

   **a.** infection.
   **c.** paralysis.
   **b.** tissue necrosis.
   **d.** anaphylaxis.

**4.** Bullae are_____

   **a.** small male bovines.
   **b.** necrosed tissues caused by an ant bite.
   **c.** systemic rashes due to an allergic reaction to a bee sting.
   **d.** blisters that can be caused by an insect bite.

**5.** A unique feature of ants is _____

   **a.** that they contain a toxin that destroys epidermal and dermal tissue.
   **b.** that a large number of people develop a serious allergic reaction to their venom.
   **c.** that when disturbed, a swarm of ants bite all at the same time.
   **d.** that ants are incapable of stinging or biting.

**6.** Which of the following types of mushroom can produce hallucinogenic effects in humans and animals?_____

   **a.** Jack-o-lantern mushrooms
   **c.** Amanita mushrooms
   **b.** Psilocybin mushrooms
   **d.** False morel mushrooms

## Fill in the Blank

The most common mushroom-related deaths are caused by_____.

## List

**1.** List the three main groups of mushrooms that are fatal to humans.

   1. _____
   2. _____
   3. _____

**2.** List two types of mushrooms that can cause violent GI effects but are rarely fatal.

   1. _____
   2. _____

**3.** List four diseases transmitted by mosquitoes.

_____

_____

_____

## Matching

Match each of the following spiders to their description. Answers can be used more than once.

_____ **1.** black widow spider

_____ **2.** brown recluse spider

_____ **3.** hobo spider

_____ **4.** wolf spider

_____ **5.** funnel web spider

   **a.** a small brown Pacific Northwest spider that lives in wood piles and has chevron-shaped abdominal markings
   **b.** aas a jet-black body with a red hourglass on the abdomen; lives in trees, shrubs, and under logs and stones
   **c.** bite is painful and causes localized pain, swelling, nausea, vomiting, and increased heart rate.
   **d.** "Bull's-eye" bites, typically on the hands and forearms, with redness that can spread over limb; signs and symptoms include nausea, vomiting, abdominal pain, fever, sweating, and paralysis
   **e.** a spider that is endemic to the Midwest and the Southwest, has a fiddle shape on its back, and has a painless bite; venom destroys blood vessel walls, frequently causes ulcerations, and can cause fatal renal failure
   **f.** has a painless and often venomless bite; if envenomates, local tissue death can occur
   **g.** indigenous to Australia and can be deadly; however, antivenom is now available

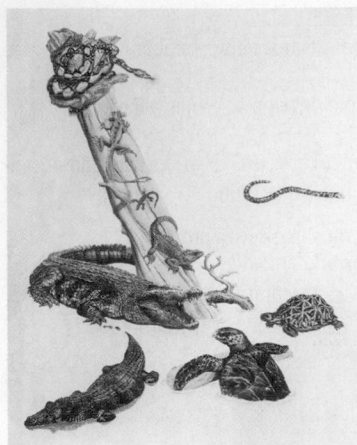

**Figure 27-31** Different types of reptiles.
Copyright Stephen Kirk/Dorling Kindersley Media Library

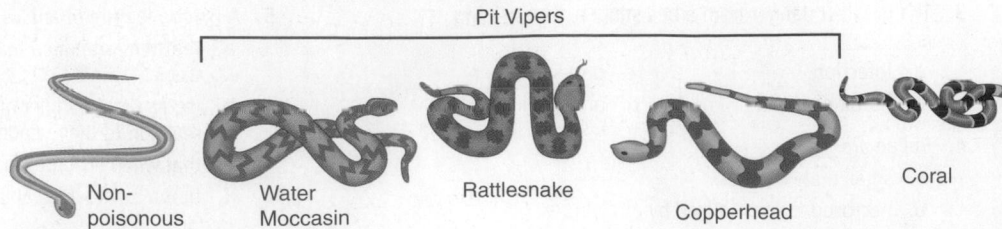

**Figure 27-32** Venomous snakes include pit vipers and the coral snake.

Pit Vipers

Non-poisonous · Water Moccasin · Rattlesnake · Copperhead · Coral

# Reptiles

Reptiles are cold-blooded animals that regulate their body temperature by moving into or out of the sun. These animals are also characterized by scales covering their skin (Figure 27-31■). Some reptiles produce venom for defense and to subdue prey.

Depending on the animal, venom may be secreted through its skin or saliva, or through a bite. Most reptile-related injuries are caused by snakes, both venomous and non-venomous. There are two families of venomous snakes in the United States: the pit vipers and the coral snakes (Figure 27-32■). Pit vipers have small depressions ("pits") between their nostrils and eyes that are used for detecting heat. In addition, they have movable fangs through which venom can be injected. Within the United States, the most common pit vipers of concern are rattlesnakes, copperheads, water moccasins, and massasaugas. Although not a pit viper, coral snakes are also venomous.

### Rattlesnake

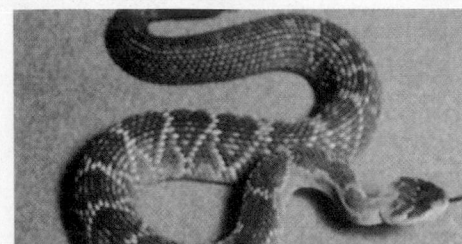

**Figure 27-33** A rattlesnake.

+ Description: There are approximately 30 species of rattlesnakes (Figure 27-33■). Often brown with a checkered or diamond skin pattern, they have a rattle at the end of the tail that is composed of modified scales. Rattlesnakes use their rattles as warnings and usually do not attack humans unless provoked.

MOTION OF STRIKE:
Shallow, slanting penetration is typical of snakebite, since snakes tend to hold the head level when striking. Wound depth and venom deposit vary with the species, the length of the fangs, and the snake's excitement. Even if the 1 1/4 inch fangs of the Eastern diamondback rattlesnake penetrate almost their full length, the slanting wound may be no more than 1/4 inch from the skin surface.

Bite pattern:

Fang · Pit · Elliptical pupil · Poison gland

• Immediate burning pain
• Swelling, discoloration
• Distinct puncture wound
• Blood oozing from wound

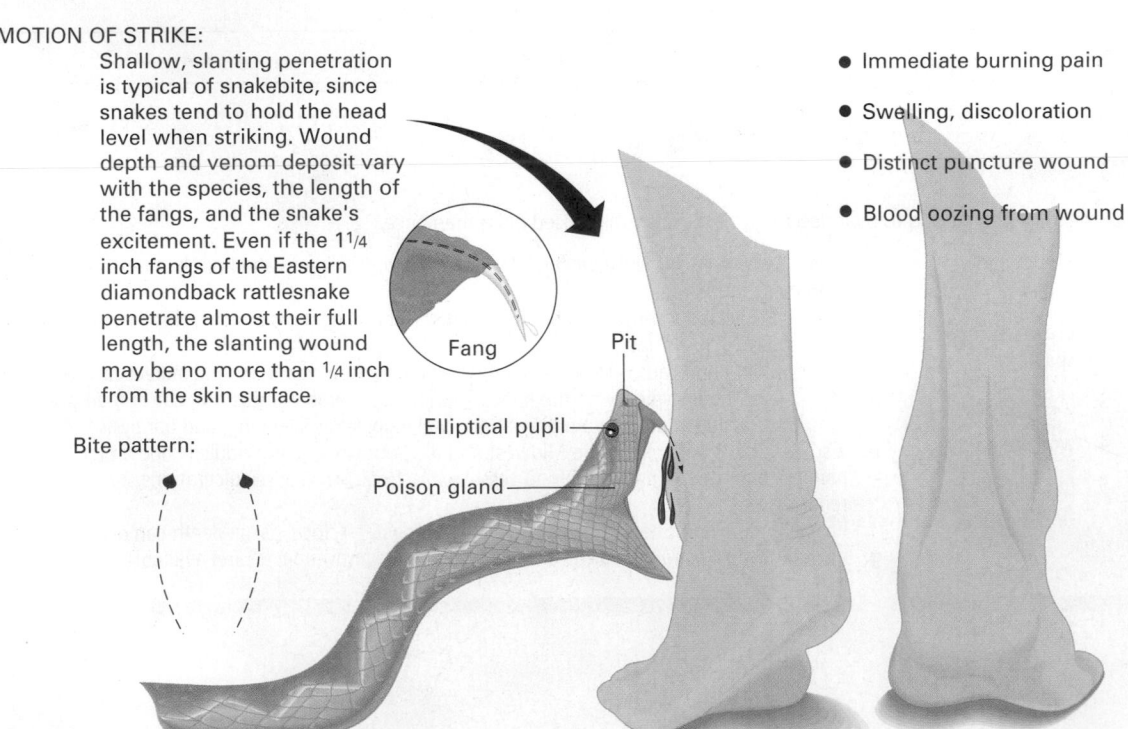

**Figure 27-34** A rattlesnake bite.

- ✦ Habitat: Rattlesnakes live in varied habitats, from arid environments to rocky outcroppings in forests.
- ✦ Characteristic of bite: Rattlesnake bites are typically very painful. There may be one or two puncture wounds or only a simple abrasion (Figure 27-34■).
- ✦ Toxic effects: Rattlesnake venom destroys tissue near the bite wound and can lead to the inability of blood clotting throughout the body, which can allow spontaneous internal bleeding. Without treatment, these bites are potentially fatal.

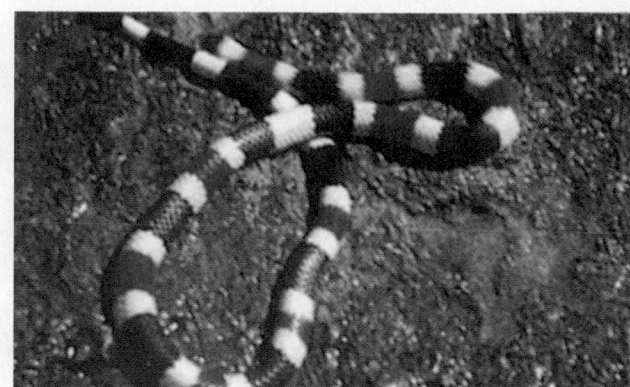

**Figure 27-35** A coral snake.

## Coral Snake

- ✦ Description: These snakes are covered with brightly colored bands. The phrase "red on yellow, kill a fellow; red on black, venom lack" is often remembered to help distinguish between harmful coral snakes and other similar-appearing but harmless snakes (Figure 27-35■). However, it is best to avoid contact with any potentially dangerous snake.
- ✦ Habitat: The coral snake lives in grasslands and dry desert regions.
- ✦ Characteristic of bite: Coral snakes tend to chew more than strike at their prey.
- ✦ Toxic effects: The venom of the coral snake is a potent neurotoxin that can lead to paralysis and respiratory failure.

⊕ **27-4** List and describe various land and marine creatures that may be harmful to humans.

## Alligator and Crocodile

- ✦ Description: These animals are large lizards with strong jaws that can open wide and easily crush bones. Ranging in size from 8–15 feet, these animals can weigh up to 1,000 pounds or more and are covered with thick scales (Figure 27-36■).
- ✦ Habitat: These animals live in warm environments in swamps and shallow water but will also climb onto land. Crocodiles live in fresh, brackish, or salt water, whereas alligators live in fresh water.
- ✦ Characteristic of bite: The bite typically results in massive soft-tissue damage, amputations, fractures, and severe internal bleeding.

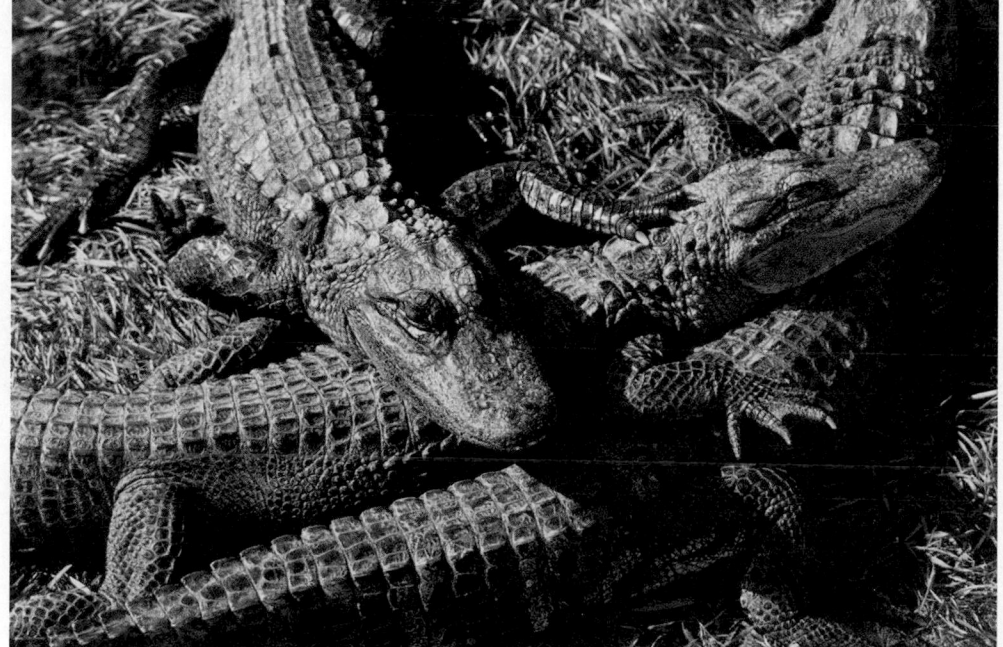

**Figure 27-36** Alligators.
Copyright Andy Holligan/Dorling Kindersley Media Library

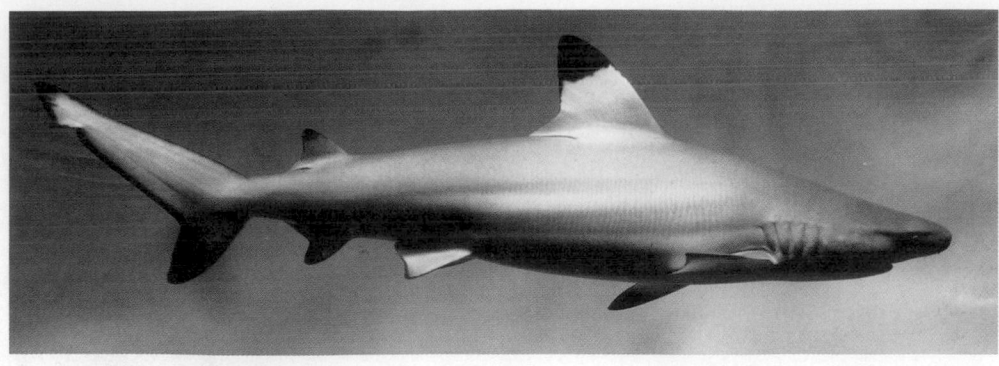

**Figure 27-37** A shark.
Copyright Frank Greenaway/Dorling Kindersley Media Library

## Marine Creatures

Many species of marine creatures can cause injuries in humans, either through localized soft-tissue injuries or via the injection of venom.

### Sharks

+ Method of injury: Sharks generally cause injury through their bite. Fortunately, shark attacks are rare, with fewer than 75 reported worldwide each year. Common shark species known to have attacked humans are great white, tiger, mako, bull, white tip reef, and black tip reef (Figure 27-37■).
+ Injuries: Shark bites cause soft-tissue injuries, fractures, and amputations. Death usually results from hemorrhage.

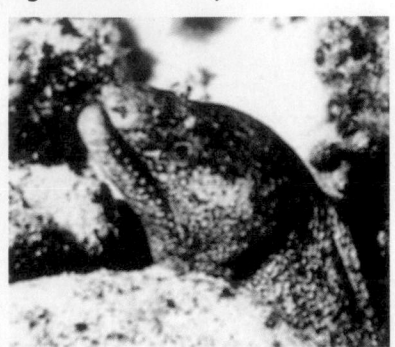

**Figure 27-38** A moray eel.

### Moray Eel

+ Method of injury: Injuries occur from the bite, which typically occurs when humans stick their hands into the eel's hole or when fishermen remove eels from a net.
+ Habitat: Moray eels live in hollow openings in coral and rock formations (Figure 27-38■).
+ Injuries: Moray eel bites are rarely fatal, but local tissue damage can be extensive. Partial arm amputations have been reported, and severe tendon injuries to the hands are common.

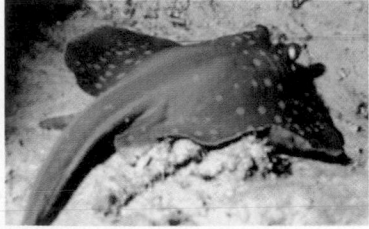

**Figure 27-39a** A stingray.

### Stingray

+ Method of injury: Stingrays are not typically aggressive (Figure 27-39a■). However, threatened stingrays can cause injury by striking with their barb-tipped tails.
+ Injuries: Injuries are generally local soft-tissue wounds (Figure 27-39b■). If the barb hits the chest or abdomen, internal injuries can occur.

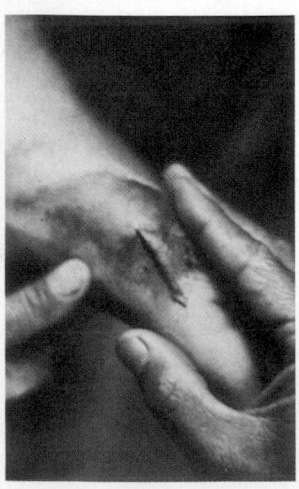

**Figure 27-39b** A stingray wound.

### Jellyfish

+ Method of injury: The tentacles of the jellyfish are covered with cells (nematocysts) that contain stinging chemicals used to kill their prey (Figure 27-40■). When a jellyfish's tentacles come in contact with a human, these chemicals are injected onto the skin.
+ Injuries: Jellyfish stings cause localized skin reactions. In addition, if the chemical is absorbed into the circulation, the results can be neurological and cardiovascular effects that lead to paralysis, respiratory failure, and cardiovascular collapse.

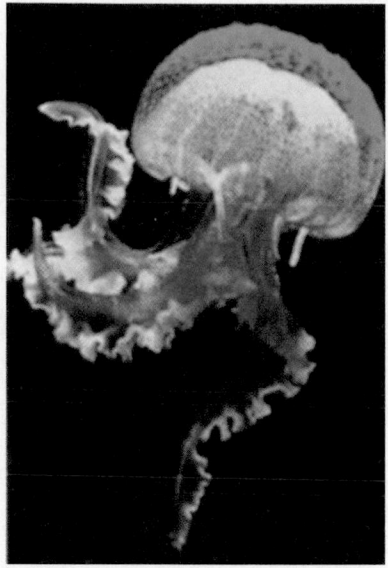

**Figure 27-40** A jellyfish.

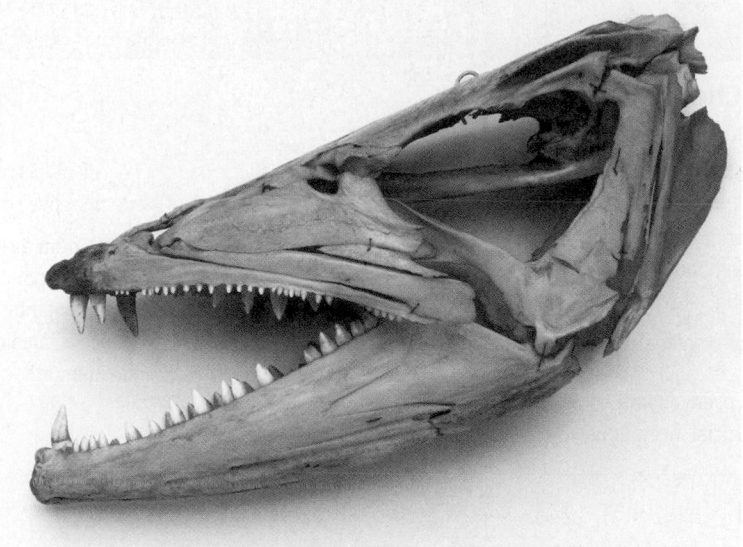

**Figure 27-41** The skull of a barracuda, a biting fish.
Copyright Colin Keates/Dorling Kindersley, Courtesy of the Natural History Museum, London

## Biting Fish

- Method of injury: A number of fish have been known to bite humans, including piranha, catfish, northern pike, muskellunge, and barracuda (Figure 27-41■).
- Injuries: Injuries are generally local soft-tissue wounds that range from minor to severe. Fish may occasionally cause fractures of the fingers or enough soft-tissue injury to result in massive hemorrhage.

## Spiny Aquatic Animals

- Method of injury: Numerous freshwater and saltwater fish and marine creatures have spines that can easily puncture or become imbedded in human skin. Sunfish, blue gill, bass, walleye, swordfish, and sea urchins are examples (Figure 27-42■).
- Injuries: Injuries are generally local soft-tissue wounds that range from minor to severe. Occasionally, spines may break off in a wound and result in a local infection.

**Figure 27-42** A spined fish.
Copyright Steve Gorton/Dorling Kindersley Media Library

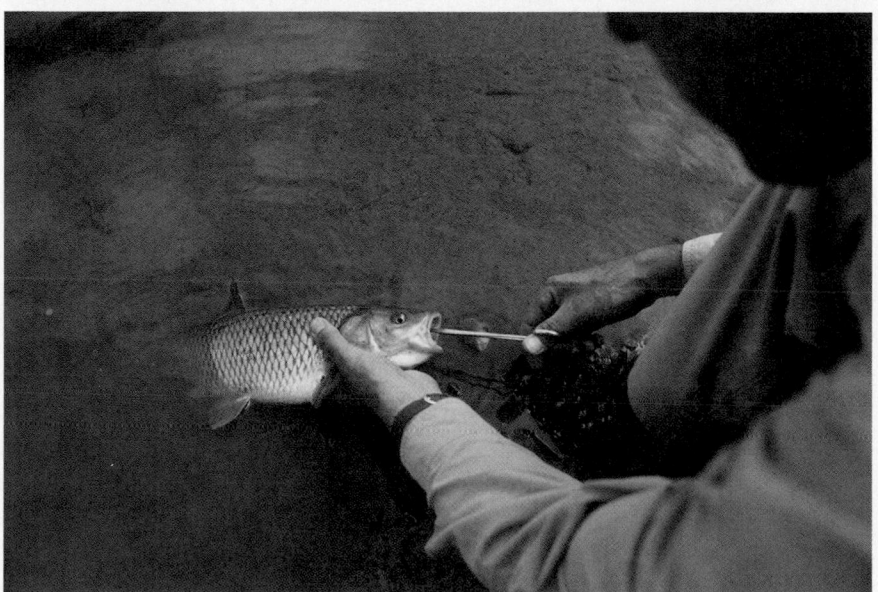

# STOP, THINK, UNDERSTAND

## Multiple Choice

Choose the correct answer.

1. The bite of a rattlesnake can be fatal by_____
   a. causing cardiac arrhythmia.
   b. preventing blood from clotting.
   c. causing paralysis of the respiratory muscles.
   d. causing sepsis.

2. The bite of an alligator or a crocodile is characterized by_____
   a. a deep, envenomated puncture.
   b. superficial lacerations.

   c. deep lacerations.
   d. massive soft-tissue damage, fractures, and amputations.

3. Death from a shark bite usually occurs from_____
   a. envenomation.
   b. drowning.
   c. cardiogenic shock.
   d. hemorrhagic shock.

## Matching

1. Match each of the following terms to its description.

   _____ 1. venom
   _____ 2. rattlesnake
   _____ 3. alligator
   _____ 4. cold-blooded animals
   _____ 5. pit viper
   _____ 6. coral snake

   a. regulates body temperature by moving into or out of the sun
   b. gives a warning by shaking its tail before it strikes
   c. a venomous snake in the United States that is not a pit viper
   d. a poison produced by some reptiles
   e. a type of snake in which the ability to sense heat guides their strikes
   f. a very large lizard that is capable of crushing bones

2. Match each of the following marine creatures to the type of injury it can inflict.

   _____ 1. spined fish
   _____ 2. moray eel
   _____ 3. shark
   _____ 4. stingray
   _____ 5. jellyfish
   _____ 6. biting fish

   a. injury resulting from the absorption of chemicals that can produce neurologic or cardiovascular effects
   b. bites that can range from superficial to fatal
   c. injured fingers or hands from reaching into this creature's home
   d. bites that can cause amputation, massive hemorrhage, and death
   e. has a barb which can cause a localized soft-tissue wound or internal injuries
   f. may leave an impaled object in the wound that can cause infection

## Mammals

Mammals are warm-blooded, vertebrate animals whose females have mammary glands for feeding the young. These animals are covered with hair and have bones in the inner ear that are used for hearing. Most injuries caused by mammals result from bites or the animal's claws. Because many mammals have powerful jaws, bites can cause soft-tissue damage, broken bones, and localized soft-tissue infections (Figures 27-43a■ and 27-43b■). They can also transmit diseases.

### Domestic and Wild Dogs, Wolves, Coyotes, and Foxes

+ Method of injury: Most members of the dog family (canids) cause puncture or tearing-type soft-tissue injuries. The extent of injury is largely dependent on the size of the animal, the strength of its jaws, and the disposition of the animal (Figure 27-44■). Occasionally, a tooth may break off and become lodged within the wound. Wild dogs, wolves, coyotes, and foxes rarely attack humans unless they are sick or are protecting their young.

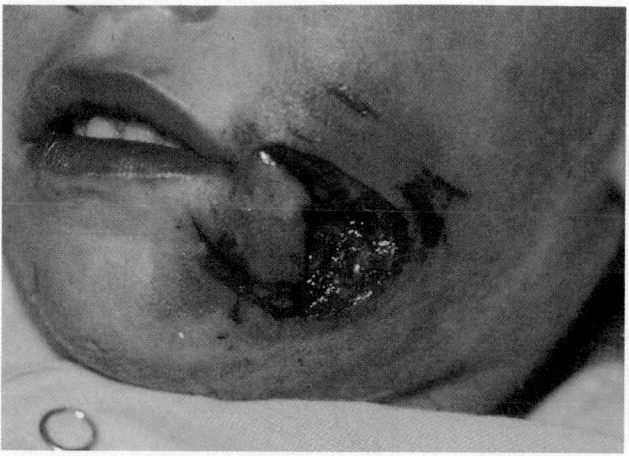

**Figure 27-43a** A horse bite.

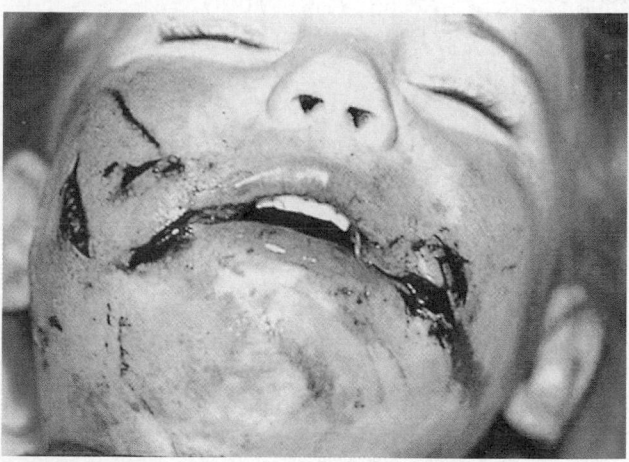

**Figure 27-43b** Dog bites.

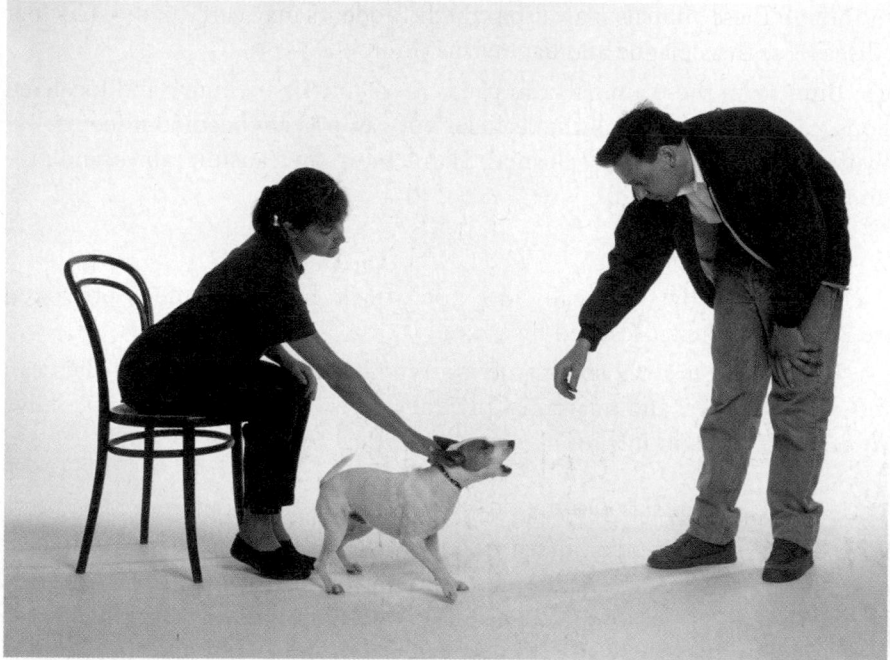

**Figure 27-44** Beware of a dog that is ready to bite.
Copyright Dorling Kindersley Media Library

- Injuries: Canid bites cause localized soft-tissue wounds, bleeding, occasional retained foreign bodies, fractures, and infections. Whenever a wild animal has bitten a human, assume that the animal is sick until proven otherwise, which raises the index of suspicion for diseases such as rabies.

## Domestic and Wild Cats

- Method of injury: Cat bites can cause deep puncture wounds. Domestic cats may also inflict scratches that inoculate bacteria into the skin. Cats generally pounce to sink their teeth into the neck of their prey (Figure 27-45■).
- Habitat: Most wild cats (e.g., mountain lion, bobcat, and lynx) are solitary creatures that live in forested areas and avoid human contact. However, with habitat encroachment and diminishing food supplies, wild cat attacks do occur.

**Figure 27-45** A cat.
Copyright Jerry Young/Dorling Kindersley Media Library

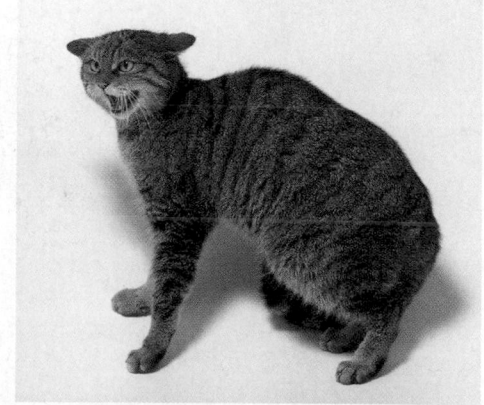

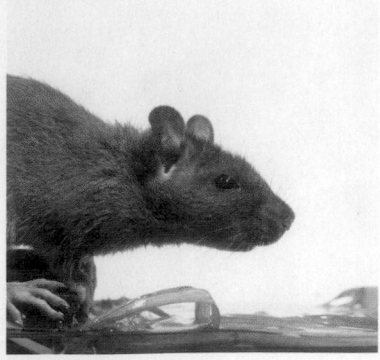

**Figure 27-46** A mouse.
Copyright Frank Greenaway/Dorling Kindersley,
Courtesy of the Natural Museum, London

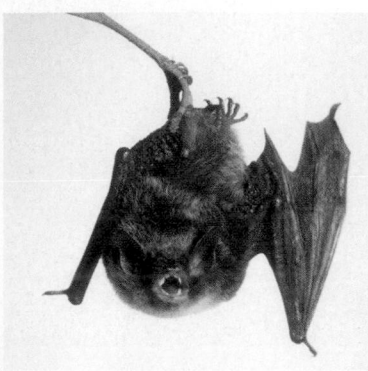

**Figure 27-47** A bat.
Copyright Frank Greenaway/Dorling Kindersley Media
Library

**Figure 27-48** Deer.
Copyright Frank Greenaway/Dorling Kindersley Media
Library

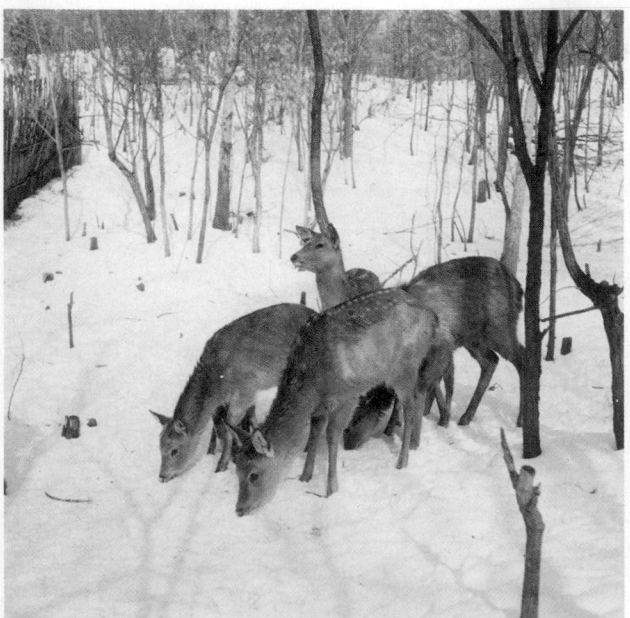

+ Injuries: Domestic cat bites are prone to becoming infected because the depth of the puncture wound prevents the wound from draining. Local tissues may become reddened and swollen; pain and fever may also occur. Bites on the neck and arms are common. Bites from wild cats can cause serious soft-tissue injuries and massive bleeding. Scratches from cats can result in bacterial infection.

### Pack Animals

+ Method of injury: Pack animals (e.g., horses, mules, llamas, and alpacas) used on wilderness adventures are typically tame and harmless to humans, but they may occasionally bite or kick.
+ Injuries: Bites or kicks can be severe and can result in soft-tissue injuries and fractures. Internal bleeding and head injuries are rare but do occur.

### Rodents and Other Small Mammals

+ Method of injury: Animals such as skunks, rabbits, rats, pika, squirrels, raccoons, and marmots generally only attack when provoked. Injury is typically caused by bites, although these animals may also scratch. Rodents may carry pathogens that cause diseases such as plague and hantavirus (Figure 27-46■).
+ Injuries: Bites from these animals can cause local soft-tissue injury and localized infections. Scratches are usually superficial but can quickly become infected, especially if they are not promptly cleaned. Skunk bites can transmit rabies, and rabbits can transmit tularemia.

### Bats

+ Method of injury: Bats typically do not attack humans unless provoked (Figure 27-47■). Injury is caused by a bite.
+ Injuries: Bites result in local soft-tissue injury and localized infections. Bats can transmit rabies, plague, and tularemia. In addition, even without a bite, the saliva of a bat can also transmit infections, usually rabies.

### Moose, Elk, Deer, and Bison

+ Method of injury: Most injuries occur when an inexperienced or unsuspecting hiker stumbles into the path of or foolishly attempts to touch one of these animals. Many injuries are caused by the animal charging the hiker and the hiker becoming knocked down or impaled on the animal's antlers (for moose, elk, and deer) or gored by the animal's horns (bison). Additionally, injuries may be caused by the animal's hooves or their sheer weight (Figure 27-48■). Most injuries and deaths to humans occur from collisions that result when the animal walks into the path of an oncoming vehicle.
+ Injuries: Incidents involving these animals cause soft-tissue injuries that range from minor to severe. Puncture wounds from antlers and horns are common. Internal injuries can also occur, as can head and spine injuries.

### Bear

+ Method of injury: Most bears do not attack humans unless provoked or defending their young. The exception to this involves grizzly bears, which have been known to attack unsuspecting hikers, fishermen, and other outdoor sports

# CASE UPDATE

Your patient, a 22-year-old male in moderate distress, is quite anxious about the bite marks on his leg. The affected leg is red and swollen. His pulse is 120, respirations are 18, and blood pressure is 110/90. No other signs of trauma are evident. He reports no medical problems, no medications, and no allergies.

*What do you do now?*

enthusiasts. Bears are great foragers and may wander into human camps looking for food. The best defense against bear incidents is to keep food away from tents and to store food in bear-proof containers. Most injuries are caused by the bear's powerful jaws and claws (Figure 27-49■).

- Injuries: Most encounters with bears produce soft-tissue injuries, but large wounds, hemorrhage, broken bones, internal injuries, and head or facial injuries can also occur.

## Assessment

In any harmful exposure to a plant or animal, OEC Technicians must first determine whether the situation is or could be life threatening. Once the scene is deemed safe, check to see if the patient is responsive. If the patient is not responsive, simultaneously open the airway and check for effective breathing while feeling for a carotid pulse. If the patient has a pulse but is not breathing begin rescue breathing. If the patient is not breathing and either there is no pulse or you are unsure if there is a pulse immediately begin chest compressions and follow the guidelines for CPR. During your initial assessment, when assessing for signs of shock, look for a neurologic emergency, life-threatening external hemorrhage, and other serious trauma.

Once life threats have been managed, perform a secondary assessment using the SAMPLE acronym and the DCAP-BTLS mnemonic, paying close attention to any known allergies. Begin by attempting to determine if the problem was a bite or sting, exposure to a plant (either contact or ingestion), or trauma from a large animal. Trying to identify the source of a plant or animal-related problem can be very challenging. A person walking in the woods, for example, could come in contact with poison ivy without knowing it. If the patient has a known environmental allergy (e.g., an allergy to yellow jacket stings), find out whether the patient has an epinephrine auto-injector (e.g., an "Epi-pen").

For animal or insect injuries, assess the affected area for signs such as a rash, pale or discolored skin, and general swelling. Closely examine the mouth and nose for evidence of swelling. Look for bite or fang marks (Figure 27-50■). Note the temperature of the patient's skin, because fever or chills may be present. Cool skin may also indicate that the patient is going into shock. Assess the patient for gastrointestinal signs and symptoms such as nausea and vomiting. Carefully assess the cardiovascular, respiratory, and neurologic systems for signs and symptoms because problems can develop within minutes. Reevaluate the patient frequently, because vital signs may deteriorate over time depending on the source of the problem.

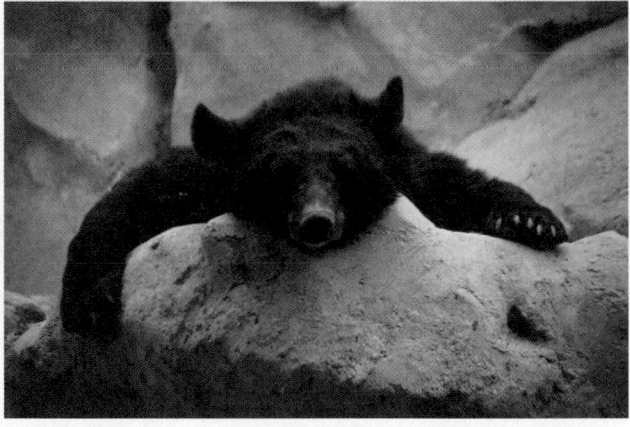

**Figure 27-49** A bear.
Copyright Christopher and Sally Gable/Dorling Kindersley Media Library

⊕ **27-5** Describe and demonstrate how to assess a patient that has been injured following an encounter with a toxic plant, an animal, or some marine life.

**Figure 27-50** After completing a primary assessment, begin the secondary assessment, including both SAMPLE and DCAP-BTLS. As part of assessing the incident, look for bite or fang marks.
Copyright Scott Smith

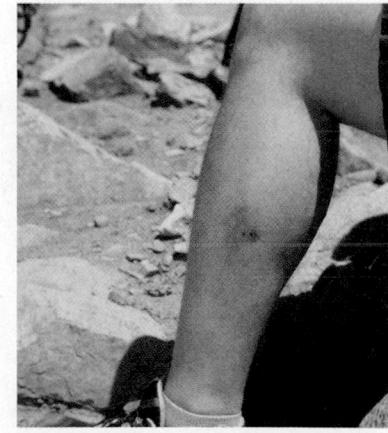

## Plants and Mushrooms

Skin contact with certain toxic plants can cause serious skin-related problems, allergic reactions, localized inflammation, or trauma from spines and needles. Evaluate the skin for signs of rash or trauma. Assess the extent of the rash or trauma and monitor them over time.

Gastrointestinal upset, abdominal pain (sometimes severe), muscle aches, and generalized weakness are common with the ingestion of toxic plants and mushrooms. Monitor the patient's vital signs frequently, carefully evaluating changes that may indicate that the patient is going into shock. Certain plants (e.g., deadly nightshade and cannabis) and certain mushrooms (e.g., peyote, psilocybin mushrooms) can produce hallucinogenic effects, including auditory and visual hallucinations.

## Spiders and Scorpions

Assess the site of spider or scorpion bites for localized soft-tissue injury and tissue necrosis. Assess skin color and temperature. Carefully monitor the site for signs that either a serious infection or tissue necrosis is developing (Figure 27-51■).

## Tick Bites

Generally it takes several days to a few weeks for systemic illness to result from a tick bite, although like any bite one can have an infection at the site. Monitor the attachment site for signs of a developing rash. Given that ticks can transmit serious diseases, also monitor the patient's vital signs. Assess for evidence of a fever, which could indicate that a serious infection is developing. Ticks usually remain on a host's body for an hour or two before attaching, so it is important to look for them and remove them as soon as they are discovered. To properly remove an attached tick, perform the following steps:

1. Grasp the tick as close to the surface of the patient's skin as possible, preferably with tweezers or gloved fingers (Figure 27-52■). Do not apply fingernail polish, isopropyl alcohol, or a hot match head to the tick because doing so can cause the release of toxins into the bite wound.
2. Pull the tick out with gentle, steady pressure, *taking care not to crush the tick's body* because this, too, can contaminate the wound with infectious fluids. Insure that all parts of the tick are removed.
3. After the tick is removed, disinfect the skin with isopropyl alcohol or another disinfectant.

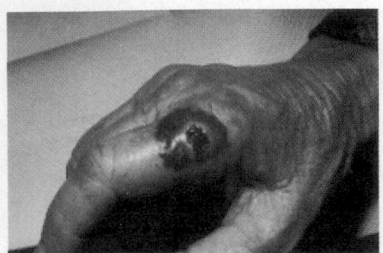

**Figure 27-51** A brown recluse spider bite wound several days after the bite.

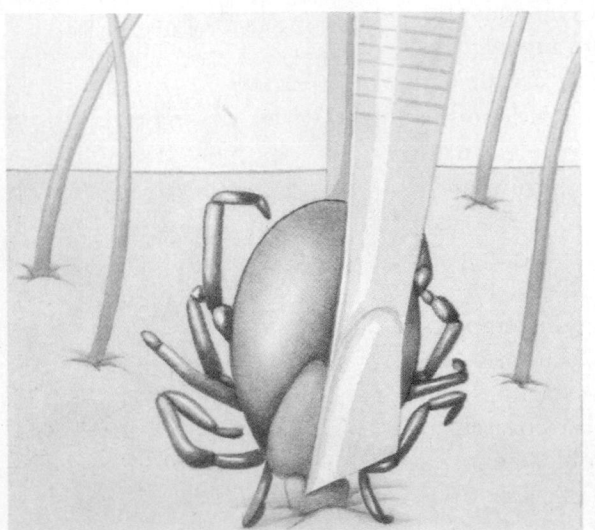

**Figure 27-52** When removing a tick, grasp the tick with tweezers as close as possible to the surface of the patient's skin.
Copyright Joanna Cameron/Dorling Kindersley Media Library

## Bee Stings

Monitor the site for localized inflammation and generalized signs of an allergic reaction. Since an allergic reaction can be severe, closely monitor the patient's vital signs, paying particular attention to swelling in and around the airway, change in voice, difficulty breathing, and instability of the patient's blood pressure (Figure 27-53■). Multiple stings are especially concerning and increase one's chances for serious reactions such as airway swelling, difficulty breathing, and anaphylactic shock.

## Mosquito, Insect, and Ant Bites

Assess the affected area(s) for localized inflammation, which, in most cases, should be minor. Given that mosquitoes can transmit serious diseases, closely monitor the patient for signs of fever as well as cardiovascular and neurological instability. Insect-transmitted diseases typically take several days to weeks to manifest themselves.

### Reptile Bites

Snake bites can be life threatening. Monitor the amount of inflammation around the bite wound, and look for signs of abnormal bleeding (i.e., bleeding from the gums or the nose). Monitor the patient's vital signs, paying close attention to any signs of shock.

Large reptiles such as alligators and crocodiles generally cause major tissue damage, fractures, and amputations. In these cases, most assessment is directly related to the ABCDs. Because an attack from these animals can result in massive injuries, monitor the vital signs carefully for signs of shock. Treat massive bleeding with compressive dressings using Standard Precautions. If hemorrhage from an extremity is uncontrollable, you may need to use a tourniquet.

### Injuries Caused by Marine Animals

Most injuries from marine animals cause local soft-tissue damage, but some injuries can cause cardiovascular or neurological instability. Evaluate the severity of any soft-tissue injuries and monitor the vital signs.

### Injuries Caused by Mammals

For injuries caused by large animals, pay close attention to the ABCDs and perform a complete secondary assessment. Assess all soft-tissue injuries for the degree of external bleeding (Figure 27-54■). Carefully evaluate the patient for evidence of internal injuries and head or spine injuries. Later, evaluate each soft-tissue injury for redness and swelling that may indicate a developing infection. Since small animals can transmit serious diseases which appear later, monitor the patient's vital signs and assess for cardiovascular and neurological instability.

# Management

As for any incident, ensure that the scene is safe to enter and free of any plant or animal life that could further harm patients or rescuers. Observe Standard Precautions to prevent contact with plant toxins or animal-transmitted diseases. Then, manage any ABCD-related problems, if present. If the patient is unresponsive, immediately open the airway and simultaneously check for breathing and for a carotid pulse. If there is no pulse, immediately begin chest compression in accordance with CPR guidelines. Request ALS assistance as needed. If an encounter with a large animal has resulted in trauma, assume a spine injury and manage accordingly. In the absence of significant trauma, place the patient in a position of comfort. Place patients who are in shock in a supine position and keep them warm. If indicated, apply high-flow oxygen by nonbreather mask at 15 LPM.

Further management of almost any serious animal-related injury, envenomations, or cases involving the ingestion of toxic plants or fungi should include urgent evacuation and transport to a definitive-care facility. Base your choice of transport (i.e., by ground or by air) on the length of transport, the severity of the injury or of the signs and symptoms, and local protocols. Given that the effects of many toxins take time to become evident, assume

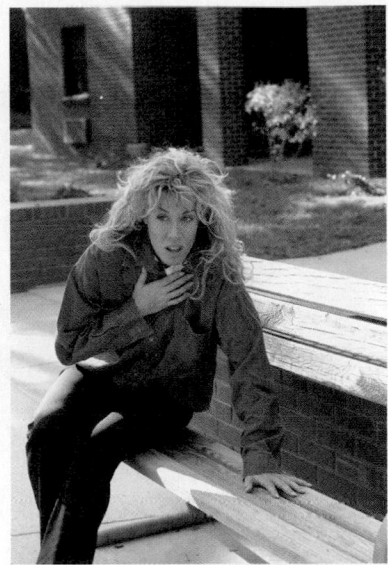

**Figure 27-53** In cases involving bee stings, closely monitor the patient's vital signs; pay special attention to indications of respiratory distress or anaphylactic shock.

⊕ 27-6 Describe and demonstrate how to manage an exposure to topical toxins.

**Figure 27-54** Examine patients for external bleeding and for other potential injuries.

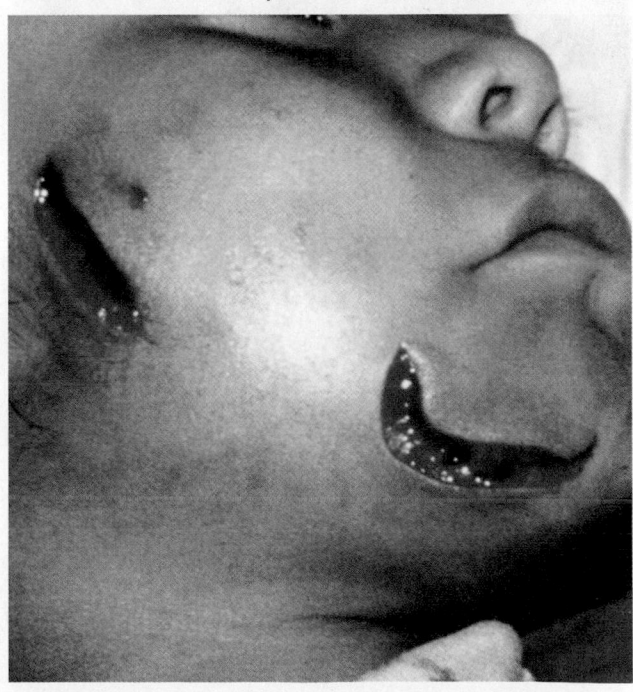

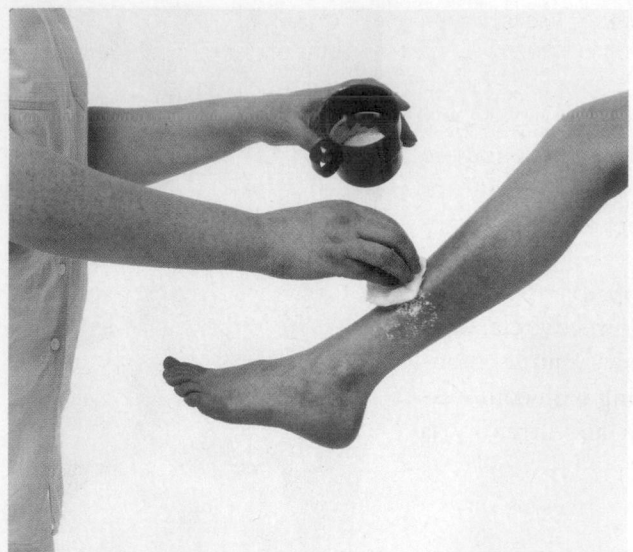

**Figure 27-55** *Tecnu* or *Oak-N-Ivy* commercial cleaners may be helpful for removing plant toxins from the skin.
Copyright Andy Crawford and Steve Gorton/Dorling Kindersley Media Library

⊕ **27-7** Describe and demonstrate the proper management of wounds caused by animals, including reptiles, insects, and spiders.

**Figure 27-56** If an intact stinger is still in place, remove it by scraping it off with the edge of a credit card.

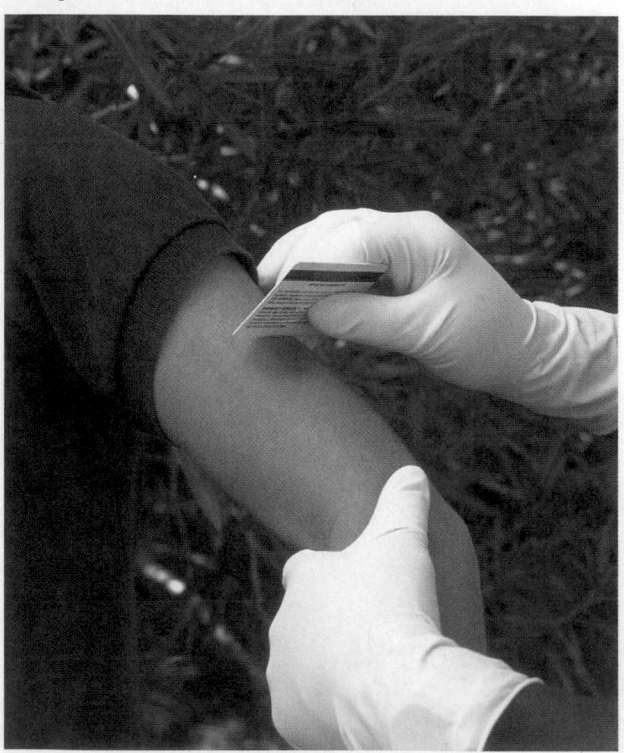

that patients have a life-threatening condition and plan accordingly. Descriptions of care for specific plant-related and animal-related problems follow.

## Care of Cases Involving Plant Toxins

The care for cases in which plant toxins have come into contact with the skin starts with skin decontamination. Protect yourself from contamination and remove any obvious resin or plant material that may be present. Next, vigorously wash the affected area with hot water and soap. Include cleaning under the patient's fingernails because toxins picked up from scratching may be present. If available, use commercial cleansers such as *Tecnu* or *Oak-N-Ivy*, which may help decontaminate the skin and medical equipment (Figure 27-55■). Depending on the severity of the rash, the patient may need to be evaluated and treated by a physician. Rashes typically respond well to oral steroids, which require a physician prescription. Itching and rash-related symptoms may be treated with diphenhydramine (Benadryl), which also requires the supervision of a physician. Clean all exposed clothing, equipment, and supplies by washing with hot water and soap.

If the injury is caused by a spine-bearing plant, remove large spines with tweezers as soon as possible. Smaller needles may be more challenging to fully remove and may require more specialized equipment. A physician should evaluate any area that continues to swell or becomes red, hot, and/or tender to the touch.

Patients that have inhaled smoke from a fire involving a poisonous or toxic plant such as poison ivy, poison oak, or poison sumac should be transported immediately to medical care because such smoke can cause significant respiratory problems.

## Care of Cases Involving Ingested Plant and Mushroom Toxins

For most cases involving the ingestion of plant or mushroom toxins, management by OEC Technicians involves supportive care. If you are able to identify the plant or mushroom and have access to a telephone, call 911 and ask for a poison control center. Personnel will be able to help you determine if the plant or mushroom is toxic, whether to induce vomiting, and whether emergent transport is indicated. They can also provide other valuable care-related information.

## Care for Cases Involving Biting and Stinging Creatures

If a stinger is present, scrape the stinger off the skin using the edge of a firm flat object such as a credit card (Figure 27-56■). Clean the bite area using soap and water. Apply ice, if available, to help reduce localized swelling and pain. For spider bites or scorpion stings, immobilize the area to prevent the venom from spreading. Continue to provide supportive care and arrange for transport. If the patient has a known allergy to certain insects, such as bees, they may have an epinephrine auto-injector. If indicated and authorized by your medical director and local protocols, you may need to assist the patient in administering an injection of epinephrine, following the procedure described in

Chapter 14, Allergies and Anaphylaxis. *Use the patient's own medication only.*

## Care of Snake Bites

Prompt evacuation and evaluation in a definitive-care facility are the primary focuses for a snake bite (Figure 27-57). "Wrap" the leg, proximal to distal (to the fang mark), snuggly with elastic bandages and apply a splint to avoid motion. Place the limb at the level of the heart to slow the spread of the venom and prevent swelling. Because physical exertion should be avoided, do not allow the patient to run or hike over a great distance because doing so will enhance the spread of the poison. *Never* follow the outdated recommendation to "suck the poison out"; not only does it not work, it can make the envenomation worse. Similarly, tourniquets are not recommended for snake bites. Also, do not apply ice to a snake bite, even if swelling is present, because doing so can slow the body's defensives against the toxin. The antivenom called *CroFab* may be indicated but should be administered by a physician only.

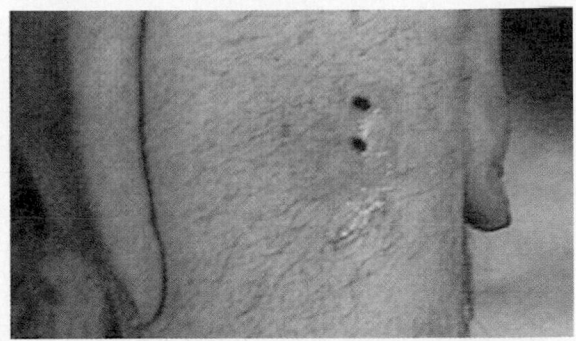

**Figure 27-57** A typical rattlesnake bite.

## Care of Injuries by Marine Creatures

For marine animal bites, control bleeding and transport the patient. If life-threatening hemorrhage is present, a tourniquet is recommended. Once safely out of the ocean, irrigate all wounds with fresh water and apply appropriate dressings as necessary. The treatment for any injury involving spines begins with removing the spines and decontaminating the affected area. For jellyfish stings, there are two important actions; preventing further nematocyst discharge and pain relief. To inactivate the nematocyst venom, liberally wash off the nematocysts from the affected area of skin with vinegar (4–6 percent acetic acid solution) as soon as possible for at least 30 seconds. Check with local authorities concerning frequently encountered species as this has been shown to work for only certain types of jellyfish (Figure 27-58). After the nematocysts are removed or inactivated with vinegar, the pain is treated by immersing the affected part in hot water (45 degrees C) for at least 20 minutes or longer if the pain persists. Additional care information may be obtained by contacting the Diver's Alert Network as found in Chapter 29, Water Emergencies. Any patient with a more systemic reaction should be emergently transported to a hospital. Even though some authors recommend giving patients antibiotics if transport is delayed, such an action is beyond the scope of OEC Technicians and is not recommended. X-rays are usually taken to look for retained foreign bodies and antibiotics are routinely administered in the hospital.

**Figure 27-58** Check with local authorities concerning marine species that may inflict injuries.
Copyright Nigel Hicks/Dorling Kindersley Media Library

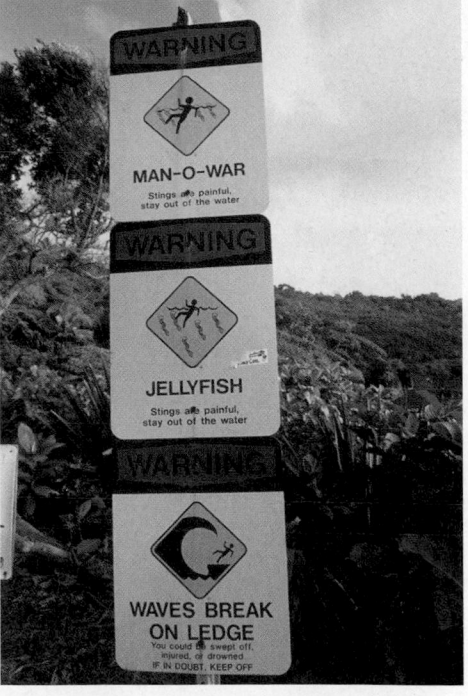

## Care for Animal Bites

Care for animal bites includes bleeding control and standard wound care. The mouths of all animals contain multiple types of bacteria that can enter a victim's tissues through a bite. Wash bites with sterile or clean water or a saline solution. Although larger wounds often require thorough cleaning and closure with sutures by a physician, smaller wounds (less than 2 cm) and punctures are typically left open to allow drainage. Immobilize suspected fractures in the usual manner. Any wound debridement and repair, which may be extensive, should be performed at the hospital by a physician. Because many rodents carry infectious diseases, a patient with a bite from these animals should be promptly transported to the hospital for treatment. Dog and cat bites pose a high risk of infection, and prophylactic antibiotics are sometimes recommended (Figure 27-59). If indicated, a tetanus booster will be given at the medical facility.

### Rabies

Even though rabies can be lethal, only two or three people die of rabies each year. The rabies virus is transmitted when the saliva of an infected animal is introduced through a bite. The most common carriers of the rabies virus are bats, raccoons, foxes, and skunks, though the total number of infected animals is extremely low. Many regions of the country have not had a documented case of a rabies infected animal in years. If not treated, the virus causes neurologic disease and ultimately death. Signs and symptoms include a flu-like illness that is followed by hallucinations, confusion, severe neurologic pain, agitation, swallowing difficulties, partial paralysis, and death.

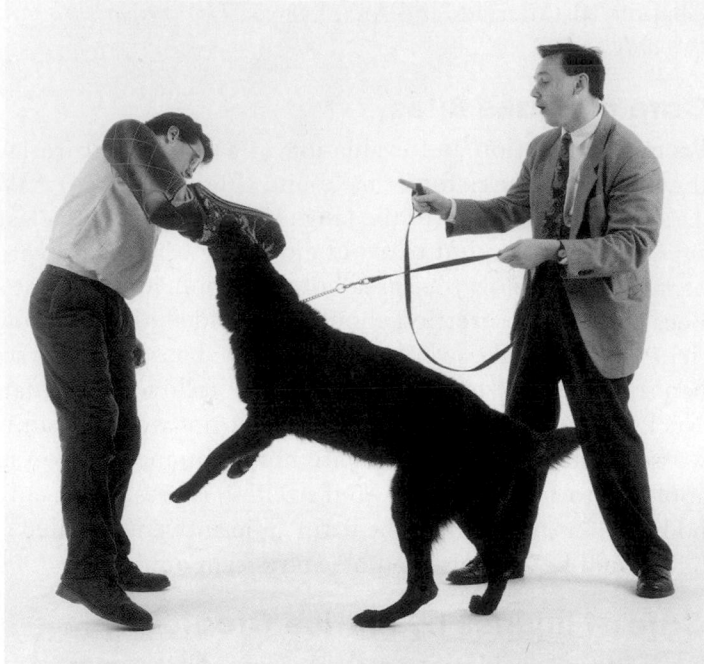

**Figure 27-59** Dog bites (and cat bites) often become infected.
Copyright David Ward/Dorling Kindersley Media Library

### Have Questions or Need Information?

The National Poison Center can provide valuable information regarding toxic plants and animals. This service is available 24 hours a day, 7 days a week by calling 1-800-222-1222 toll free.

## Large Animal-Related Trauma

Injuries caused by large animals are treated according to the signs and symptoms present. For instance, a large bite or kick requires the same type of care as that indicated by similar trauma caused by any other mechanism. Control external bleeding, splint possible fractures, and assume that a spine injury is present. Bandage wounds as indicated to prevent further contamination.

 **CASE DISPOSITION**

Your patient asks you about snakes in the area. You tell him that rattlesnakes are known to live in the park and that you are concerned that he may have been bitten by one. You splint his leg while keeping him supine, warm, and calm. You ask his friends to help you carry him to the trailhead a half-mile away so that he can avoid exertion. You arrange transport from the trailhead to the closest hospital so that he can be treated with antivenom. A week later you hear that except for local tissue necrosis, the patient is doing well and was just released from the hospital.

# STOP, THINK, UNDERSTAND

## Multiple Choice

Choose the correct answer.

1. Which of the following statements regarding assessment of a patient suffering from a plant-related or animal-related injury is false? _____
   a. It is necessary to determine the type of injury (i.e., whether it is from a bite or sting, from contact, or from ingestion).
   b. Consider the need for possible evacuation and transportation of the patient.
   c. Signs or symptoms may take minutes or hours to appear.
   d. If initially stable, it is highly unlikely that the patient's condition will later deteriorate.

2. Which of the following statements about the assessment of a patient who has ingested a toxic plant or mushroom is not true? _____
   a. Ingestion can cause gastrointestinal upset, a stroke, or a seizure disorder.
   b. Any neurological signs or symptoms are indicative of another problem such as a stroke or a seizure disorder.
   c. Skin contact can cause as severe a reaction as ingestion.
   d. A hallucinogenic effect may be attributed to the ingestion of mushrooms.

3. The development of hives, airway swelling, and breathing difficulty after a wasp sting in a patient with no known history of allergic reactions is most likely caused by_____
   a. anxiety.
   b. an exposure to some other toxin.
   c. anaphylaxis.
   d. neuropsychosis.

4. Which of the following statements about mosquito bites is false? _____
   a. They can cause an allergic reaction.
   b. They can transmit serious diseases.
   c. They can cause immediate gastrointestinal symptoms.
   d. They can cause neurologic problems that can result in death.

5. The most common result of an injury by a marine animal is _____
   a. local soft-tissue damage.
   b. anaphylaxis.
   c. systemic infection.
   d. gastrointestinal upset.

6. Which of the following assumptions should an OEC Technician make about an unresponsive patient who has been charged by a moose? _____
   a. It is unlikely that serious injury has occurred unless the patient was impaled by antlers.
   b. Blunt force abdominal trauma is rarely caused by a moose.
   c. There is high risk for spinal trauma.
   d. Diabetes is the most likely cause of the unresponsiveness.

7. Which of the following statements about poison ivy is true? _____
   a. Good commercial products are available for decontaminating exposed skin or contaminated medical equipment.
   b. Inhaling the smoke when this plant is burned is never injurious.
   c. Washing the skin with soap and water may be all that is necessary.
   d. If there is a severe rash, it is usually self-limiting and does not require treatment.

8. For a patient who has a large cactus spine imbedded in his thigh, the proper course of action is to_____
   a. bandage the wound but leave the spine in place.
   b. remove the spine, and then clean and bandage the wound.
   c. apply a constrictive band (not tourniquet) above and below the spine to prevent possible toxic envenomation by the plant, and then remove the spine.
   d. do nothing besides observing the site for signs of infection.

9. Proper care for a spider or scorpion bite includes_____
   a. scraping off the stinger, applying ice, and immobilizing the area.
   b. removing the stinger (if applicable), cleaning the area with soap and water, and then applying warm compresses to deactivate the toxin.
   c. applying a lightly constricting band above the wound, icing it, and immobilizing it.
   d. doing nothing unless signs or symptoms appear.

10. Your first course of action in helping someone who has been bitten on the ankle by a rattlesnake is to_____
    a. do nothing unless signs or symptoms appear, because most snakes do not envenomate humans.
    b. place a light constricting band above the bite, cut a small "X" over the puncture site or sites, and carefully suck out the venom with a venom extractor.
    c. place the patient supine with the leg lower than the heart, ice the wound, and arrange for rapid transport.
    d. wrap and immobilize the limb, place it at heart level, and arrange for rapid transport.

11. Your best course of action for helping a friend who has been bitten on the hand by a rattlesnake about two hours from the trailhead is to_____
    a. immediately help him hike out as quickly as possible.
    b. treat the wound, splint it at heart level, and then help him hike out as quickly as possible while being careful not to elevate his heart rate.
    c. treat the wound, splint it below heart level, and then have him remain absolutely still until help arrives.
    d. treat the wound, wrap the arm appropriately, place him in a supine position with the wound at heart level, and either carry him out or await an evacuation team.

*continued*

STOP, THINK, UNDERSTAND *continued*

## Short Answer

1. What should you do if you have questions regarding a toxin or poison?

_____

_____

_____

_____

2. How do you treat a jellyfish injury?

_____

_____

_____

_____

## Matching

Match each of the following animals with the injuries each is most likely to cause.

_____ 1. bear

_____ 2. dog

_____ 3. pack animal

_____ 4. rodent or bat

_____ 5. moose/ elk/deer/bison

_____ 6. cat

a. soft-tissue injury, localized infection, disease transmission
b. punctures and scratches, often on neck/arms; prone to infection
c. tearing injury, localized soft-tissue injury, retained foreign body, fractures
d. large wounds, hemorrhage, broken bones, internal injuries, and head and facial injuries
e. soft-tissue injury secondary to kick
f. blunt trauma, impalement, large puncture wounds

# Chapter Review

## Chapter Summary

The results of encounters with plants and animals in outdoor environments can range from minor annoyances to life-threatening injuries or diseases. Begin by assessing and stabilizing abnormalities of airway, breathing, circulation, and disability. If possible, try to identify the causative agent of injury and make sure that this agent will not also injure you. Treat soft-tissue injuries according to principles that have already been described in this textbook. When in doubt, transport out.

## Remember...

1. Most skin rashes from contact with toxic plants are not life threatening.
2. Skin rashes can become infected and should be evaluated by a physician.
3. Minor bites from wild animals are not usually life threatening.
4. Bites and scratches by certain small wild animals warrant evaluation for rabies.
5. Unexplained altered mental status or severe nausea/vomiting may be associated with ingestion of a plant or mushroom toxin.
6. When ingestion of a poisonous plant is suspected, obtain a history of what the individual ate.
7. Manage large bites and injuries as you would any traumatic wound.
8. Many stings, whether by insects or marine animals, can be managed with localized treatment.
9. Observation of signs of systemic involvement requires transport to a medical-care facility.
10. Taking preventative measures to avoid animal bites is the best course of action.

## Chapter Questions

### Multiple Choice

Choose the correct answer.

1. Which of the following is most likely to cause a localized skin reaction (rash)?_____
   a. envenomation
   b. inhalation
   c. contact with plant material
   d. punctures from fangs

2. Poison ivy, poison oak, and poison sumac typically grow in _____
   a. arid desert environments.
   b. hot and humid jungle environments.
   c. cold and barren tundra environments.
   d. shady, wet, and cool forest environments.

3. Hallucinations and mild nausea in a man who is staying in a remote campsite and ate some wild mushrooms are most likely caused by _____
   a. white mushrooms.
   b. jack-o-lantern mushrooms.
   c. little brown mushrooms.
   d. green-spored lepiota mushrooms.

4. Your best course of action to help a patient who is nauseated and vomiting and has a violent headache after eating a bunch of morels for dinner is to _____
   a. reassure her that although she is currently miserable, the signs and symptoms will pass.
   b. arrange for immediate transportation to a medical facility for treatment of false morel poisoning.
   c. have her drink syrup of ipecac or 1 tsp of salt in water to keep her vomiting; once the mushrooms are out of her system, she will recover without further intervention.
   d. observe her for 2–3 hours and then arrange for transportation if the situation has not resolved.

5. An individual who develops a target rash on the ankle followed by fever, nausea, and vomiting that progresses to joint pain and a facial droop is most likely suffering from_____
   a. tick-borne Lyme disease.
   b. a bite from a wolf spider.
   c. envenomation by a hobo spider.
   d. an HIV infection from a mosquito bite.

6. Your best course of action to care for a fellow hiker who has developed abdominal pain after eating a plant that no one can definitively identify is to _____
   a. ignore the situation unless signs or symptoms develop.
   b. plan for immediate evacuation of the patient because this situation can rapidly become life threatening.
   c. observe the patient and monitor his vital signs for the next several hours.
   d. have someone else eat the plant and see whether or not it makes him sick.

7. The proper technique for removing a tick imbedded in the skin is to_____
   a. apply nail polish, isopropyl alcohol, or a hot match to the tick's body to force it to back out so that its mouthparts are not left in the bite wound.
   b. grasp the tick firmly between your thumb and index finger, then gently crush its head while pulling it away from the skin.
   c. using a gloved hand or tweezers, pull the tick out with a gentle, steady pressure, without crushing it.
   d. do nothing and allow the tick to loosen itself because doing so minimizes the risk of separating its head from its body.

8. Which of the following statements about plant or animal injuries is true? _____
   a. Rub off poison oak contamination with a dry cloth.
   b. One should always be concerned about a delayed reaction to plant or animal toxins.
   c. Because vigorous washing of plant toxins can spread them, affected areas should be rinsed gently with water.
   d. Scraping the stinger off of a patient who has been stung by a hornet can cause the venom to transfer to the rescuer.

9. The best position to place a patient who has been struck on the foot by a venomous snake is_____
   a. flat, with the feet elevated above the heart.
   b. flat, with the feet at heart level.
   c. sitting so that breathing is easier, and with the feet above heart level.
   d. sitting so that breathing is easier, and with the feet below heart level.

10. A jellyfish sting can be treated with which of the following substances? (check all that apply)
   _____ a. hot water
   _____ b. isopropyl alcohol
   _____ c. aloe vera cream
   _____ d. milk
   _____ e. vinegar

## Short Answer

When monitoring a fellow camper who ingested a potentially toxic plant, what are you looking for?

_____

_____

_____

_____

## List

List the three types of poisonous snakes in North America.

_____

## Scenario

On a warm fall day, you and some friends hiking in the state park encounter another hiker lying on the side of the trail. Having only your OEC Technician's skills and the contents of a small fanny pack, you offer to assist, and he accepts. During the primary assessment, the patient tells you (between episodes of vomiting) that he feels hot, is nauseated, and has been vomiting. As he talks you notice a facial droop. You take Standard Precautions by putting on some gloves.

1. Based on the facial droop, your first impression and your course of action is_____
   a. that the patient has the flu and you will assist him out of the woods.
   b. that the patient has Bell's palsy and needs no assistance.
   c. that the patient may have eaten some mushrooms and needs assistance out of the woods.
   d. that the patient could be having a stroke and you will perform neurologic testing.

*Your evaluation identifies only the facial droop and no other neurologic signs. Applying the SAMPLE acronym to the interview in a secondary assessment, you learn that the patient is an avid hiker and hunter. Two weeks ago he bagged a trophy buck with a bow and arrow here in this park. He has no medical issues and does not take any medicines.*

2. Based on the patient's presentation and the information you now have, what would you do next during the secondary assessment?_____
   a. Listen to see if the patient is wheezing.
   b. Check for fruity breath, which suggests a diabetic emergency.
   c. Look for a red circle within a blanched white circle on the patient's skin.
   d. Ask the patient if he has consumed any wild plants.

*On the patient's lower back you find a red rash that resembles a bull's-eye.*

3. This finding leads you to believe that the patient has had_____
   a. a tick bite.
   b. a scorpion bite.
   c. a wolf spider bite.
   d. a brown recluse spider bite.

## **S**uggested Reading ○○○○○○○○○○○○○○○○○○○○○○○○○○○○○○○○○○○○○○○○○○○○○○○

American College of Emergency Physicians: www.acep.org

Auerbach, P. S. 1991. "Marine Envenomations." *New England Journal of Medicine* 325(7): 486–493.

Centers for Disease Control: www.cdc.gov

Gladman, A. C. 2006. "Toxicodendron Dermatitis: Poison Ivy, Oak, and Sumac." *Wilderness and Environmental Medicine* 17(2): 120–128.

Kunkel, D. B. 1984. "Bites of Venomous Reptiles." *Emergency Medical Clinics of North America* 2(3): 563–577.

Taplitz, R. A. 2004. "Managing Bite Wounds. Currently Recommended Antibiotics for Treatment and Prophylaxis." *Postgraduate Medicine* 116(2): 49–52, 55–56, 59.

wereyouwondering.com/poisonous Copyright 1983 by the Conservation Commission of the State of Missouri reprinted from the **Missouri Conservationist (mushrooms)**.

Wilderness Medical Society: www.wms.org

EXPLORE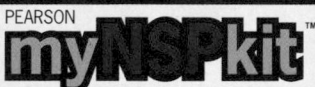

Please go to **www.myNSPkit.com**. Under Student Resources, you will find animations, videos, web links, and games related to this chapter—and much more. Look for information on poisonous plants, rabies prevention, and other topics.

Register your access code from the front of your book by going to **www.myNSPkit.com** and selecting the appropriate links. If the in-cover access code has been redeemed, go to **www.myNSPkit.com** and follow links to Buy Access.

# Altitude-Related Emergencies

Luanne Freer, MD, FACEP, FAWM

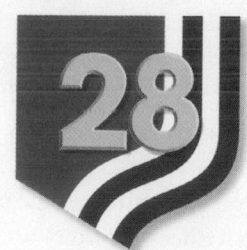

28

## ⊕ OBJECTIVES

Upon completion of this chapter, the OEC Technician will be able to:

**28-1** Define altitude.

**28-2** Describe the principles of altitude physiology.

**28-3** List risk factors for the development of altitude illnesses.

**28-4** Describe strategies to prevent altitude illness.

**28-5** List the signs and symptoms of the following altitude illnesses:
- acute mountain sickness
- high-altitude pulmonary edema
- high-altitude cerebral edema

**28-6** Describe how to assess a patient with altitude illness.

**28-7** Describe the treatment of a patient with altitude illness.

## ⊕ KEY TERMS

acclimatization, *p. 902*
acute mountain sickness (AMS), *p. 903*
altitude illness, *p. 898*
ataxia, *p. 905*

chilblains, *p. 907*
Gamow bag, *p. 913*
high-altitude cerebral edema (HACE), *p. 905*

high-altitude pulmonary edema (HAPE), *p. 904*
hypoxemia, *p. 900*
khumbu cough, *p. 906*
sleeping altitude *p. 903*

## Chapter Overview

Each year millions of people flock to the mountains and ski slopes for fresh air, spectacular views, and a nearly endless variety of outdoor activities (Figure 28-1■). Although beautiful and seemingly serene, the mountains hold many dangers that can quickly turn the adventure of a lifetime into a miserable or even life-threatening event. For the unsuspecting or unprepared, this means much more than simply suffering from burning thighs, sore muscles, or parched lips; it can mean intense headaches, rib-shattering coughing spells, pulmonary edema, coma-inducing brain

*continued*

## HISTORICAL TIMELINE

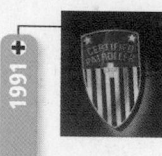

**1991** Code of ethics for patrollers is set by the Board.

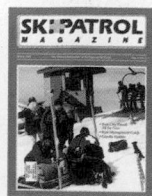

**1992** Junior classification is dropped for the new Student patroller classification.

# ✚ CASE PRESENTATION ✚

You are working first-aid duty in the patrol room at a resort that is at 9,000 feet above sea level when a 45-year-old man slowly walks in complaining of shortness of breath. Noticing that he looks unwell and is slightly cyanotic around his lips, you help him to the nearest gurney and begin to assess him. He tells you that he hasn't felt great since arriving on his flight from sea level two days ago. He denies any chest pain but says that he is extraordinarily tired, becomes short of breath "just walking to the bathroom," and has had a little dry cough. He has no significant past medical history, has not suffered any recent trauma, and is not currently taking any prescribed medications. He appears very concerned when he says, "I have never experienced anything like this in my life."

*What should you do?*

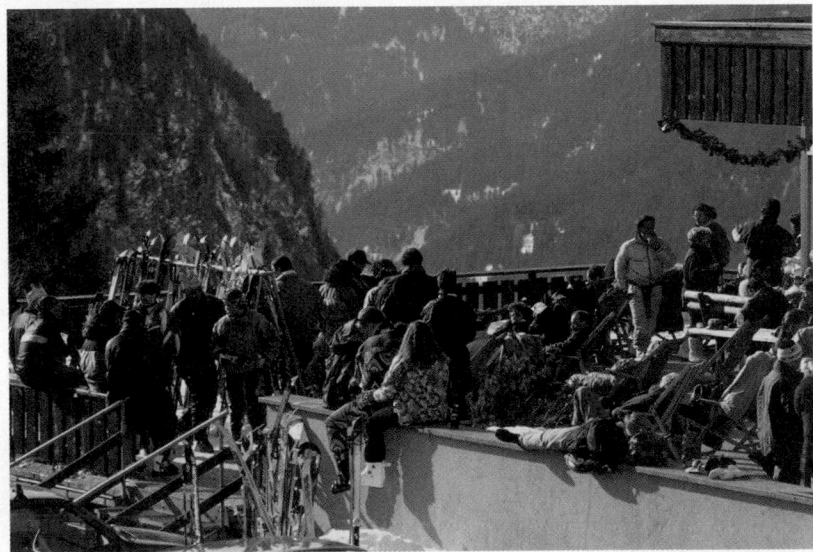

**Figure 28-1** The mountains hold beauty, exercise opportunities and adventure; however trouble can occur, potentially resulting into a life-threatening.
Copyright John Heseltine/Dorling Kindersley Media Library

**Figure 28-2** Altitude illness may affect up to 30 percent of visitors to the high-mountain resorts of the Rocky Mountains.
Copyright Wilderness Medical Society

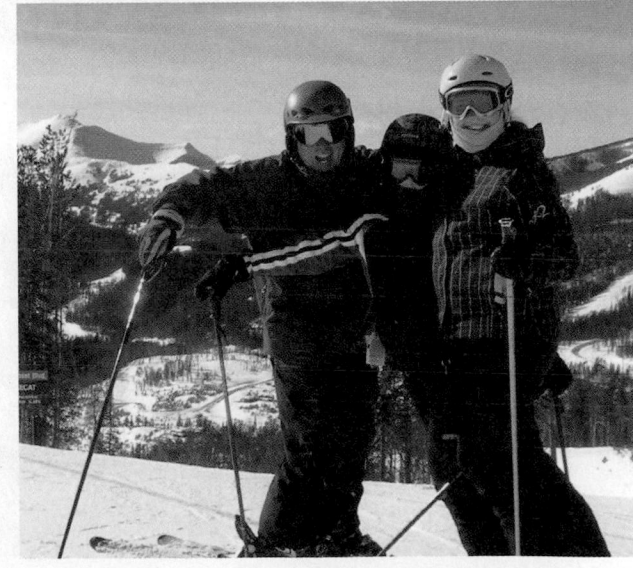

swelling, or even death. These illnesses are not caused by overexertion, heat, or the lack of proper equipment, but are due instead to high altitude, which can punish anyone who is not acclimatized to the thin air. Even hardy recreationalists are at risk. Altitude illness can affect up to 30 percent of visitors to the high-altitude resorts of the Rocky Mountains (Figure 28-2■).

Seasoned adventurers are not immune either; 50 percent of all hikers and climbers in the Himalayas suffer from some form of altitude illness. Fortunately, altitude sickness is preventable. The keys are knowing when to expect it, how to avoid it, how to identify it, and what to do if symptoms arise.

The human body is a remarkable organism that constantly makes internal adjustments in response to changes in the external environment. This ability to adapt has allowed humans to travel to and inhabit some of the most inhospitable places on earth, including high elevations. As altitude increases, though, air density decreases, so less oxygen is available. In response, the body's compensatory mechanisms make changes to improve the delivery of oxygen to the tissues and cells. Altitude illness occurs when the compensatory mechanisms are unable to keep up with the body's oxygen demand, resulting in problems that can range from mild annoyance to life-threatening conditions.

OEC Technicians, especially those who work in high-altitude mountain resorts, often encounter patients who are suffering from an altitude-related illness. As with all medical emergencies, the key to effective management is learning to recognize the signs and symptoms of acute altitude illnesses and promptly implementing appropriate treatment. This chapter will prepare you by providing a fundamental understanding of altitude illness, including its causes and its overall management.

This chapter discusses high altitude, how it affects the human body, and how the body attempts to adapt to it. It also describes how to distinguish among the different types of altitude illnesses, the signs and symptoms associated with each type, and techniques for managing specific altitude-related disorders. Because prevention is an essential component for reducing morbidity and mortality for any medical problem, the chapter also presents strategies for preventing altitude illness. By adopting and disseminating these strategies, OEC Technicians can help their patients avoid serious consequences from an altitude illness.

## Altitude Physiology

The body's ability to preserve homeostasis includes the ability to adapt to changes in altitude. Here we define altitude as the height or vertical elevation above sea level, which by convention is set at 0 feet (Figure 28-3■).

Although most **altitude illness** occurs at elevations higher than 8,000 feet above sea level, it can also occur at altitudes as low as 6,500 feet, because each individual's physiologic response to changes in altitude is different. The *rate of ascent* is very important in determining the probability of developing altitude illness; a rapid ascent is more likely to cause problems than a slower ascent (Figure 28-4■). Even though the deadliest forms of altitude sickness occur more frequently at extreme elevations, it can occur at intermediate altitudes as well.

---

⊕ **28-1** Define altitude.

---

⊕ **28-2** Describe the principles of altitude physiology.

**altitude illness** encompasses all types of illness due to altitude (AMS, HAPE, and HACE).

---

**Figure 28-3** Altitude is defined as the height or vertical elevation above sea level.
Copyright Gerald Lopez/Dorling Kindersley Media Library

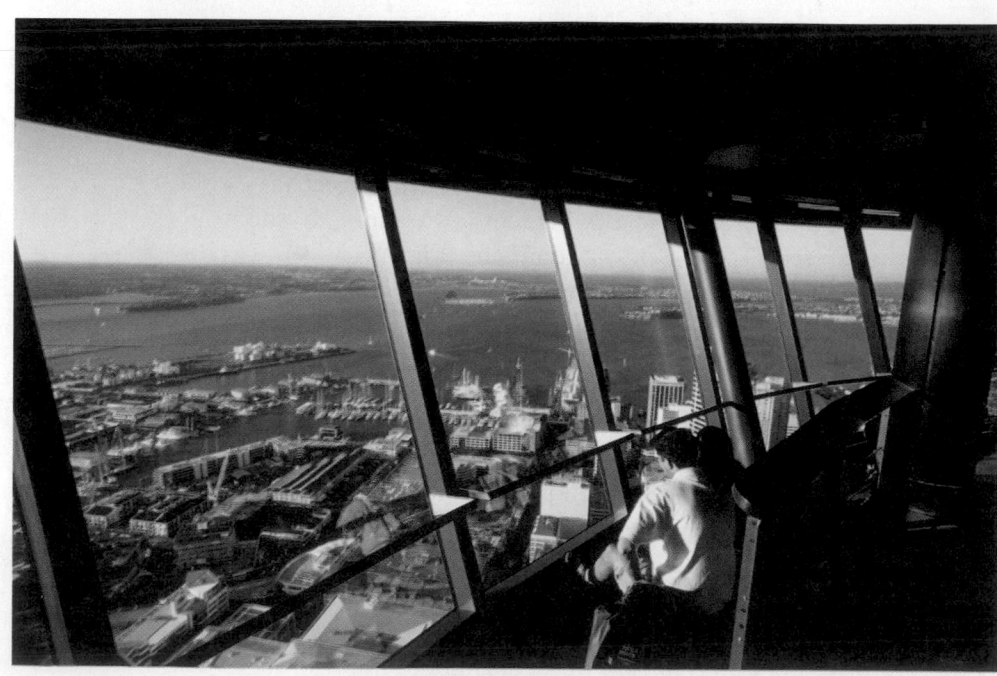

Interestingly, scientific evidence now suggests that the genetic makeup of some individuals helps them avoid altitude illness and acclimate to high altitudes more easily than other individuals.

## Altitude Classifications

Altitude is divided into five classifications: low altitude, intermediate altitude, high altitude, very high altitude, and extreme altitude (Figure 28-5■).

+ *Low altitude* is defined as elevations that are less than 5,000 feet (1,500 m). Thus low altitude extends from sea level to nearly one mile in elevation (Figure 28-6■). In most instances, the body's compensatory mechanisms can adapt to any altitude change within this elevation range. When symptoms do appear, they are usually minor and typically resolve within 24–48 hours, although patients with chronic medical conditions may suffer more serious or longer-lasting effects.

+ *Intermediate altitude* extends from 5,000 feet to 8,000 feet (1,500 m to 2,400 m). Depending on a person's genetic makeup, underlying health status, the altitude at which one starts, and the rate of ascent, the body's compensatory mechanisms typically adjust to altitude changes in this range within 72–96 hours. Preventative measures, when implemented early, can greatly minimize the problems that can occur at intermediate altitudes. Accordingly, physicians often recommend that travelers who plan to visit a higher elevation spend at least a few days at an intermediate altitude to allow their bodies to adjust.

+ *High altitude* is defined as elevations between 8,000 feet and 12,000 feet (2,400 m to 3,500 m). At high altitude, the physiologic effects of lower atmospheric oxygen pressure are generally first felt, resulting in decreased exercise performance and increased rate of respiration as the body attempts to increase its intake of oxygen. Because many mountain resorts are located at high altitude, large numbers of people

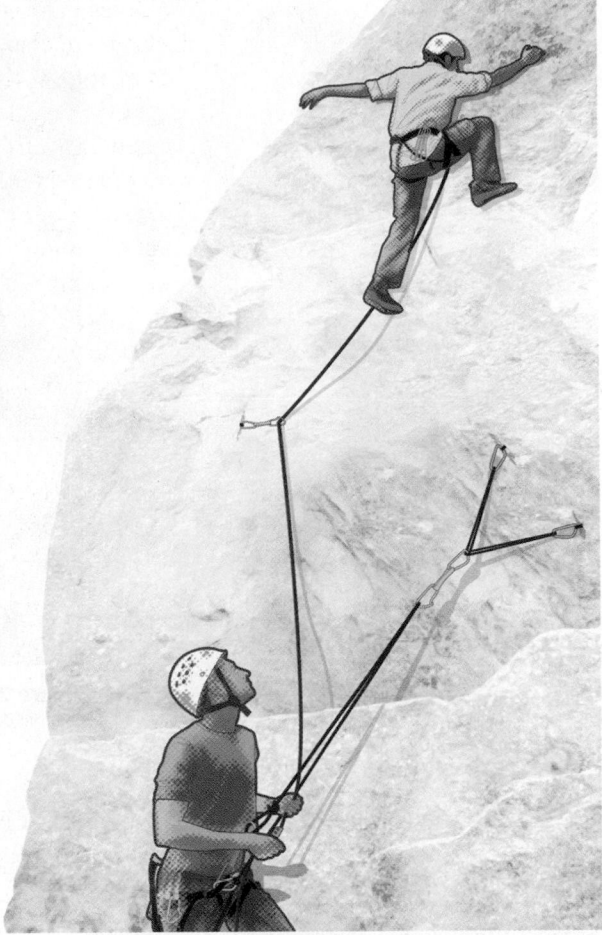

**Figure 28-4** The more rapid the ascent, the more likely it is that individuals will develop altitude illness.
Copyright Dorling Kindersley Media Library

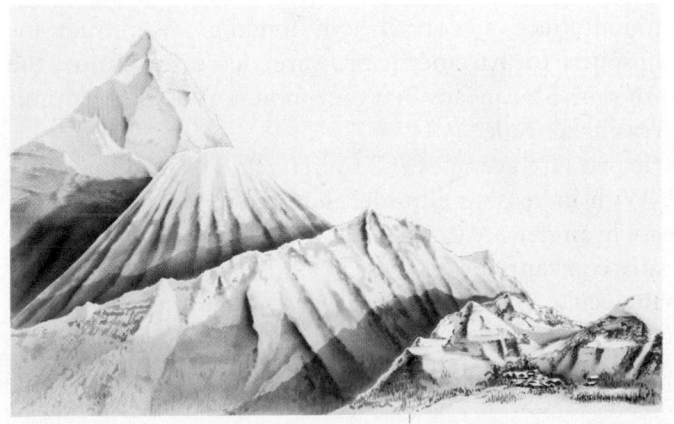

**Figure 28-5** Altitude is divided into five classifications.
Copyright Dorling Kindersley Media Library

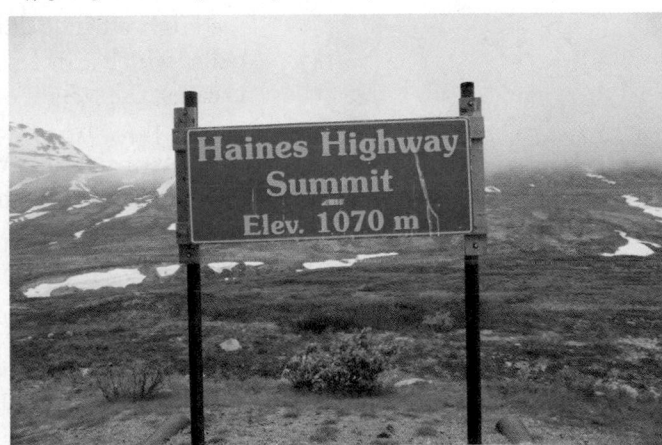

**Figure 28-6** Low altitude is defined as below 5,000 feet.
Copyright Nigel Hicks/Dorling Kindersley Media Library

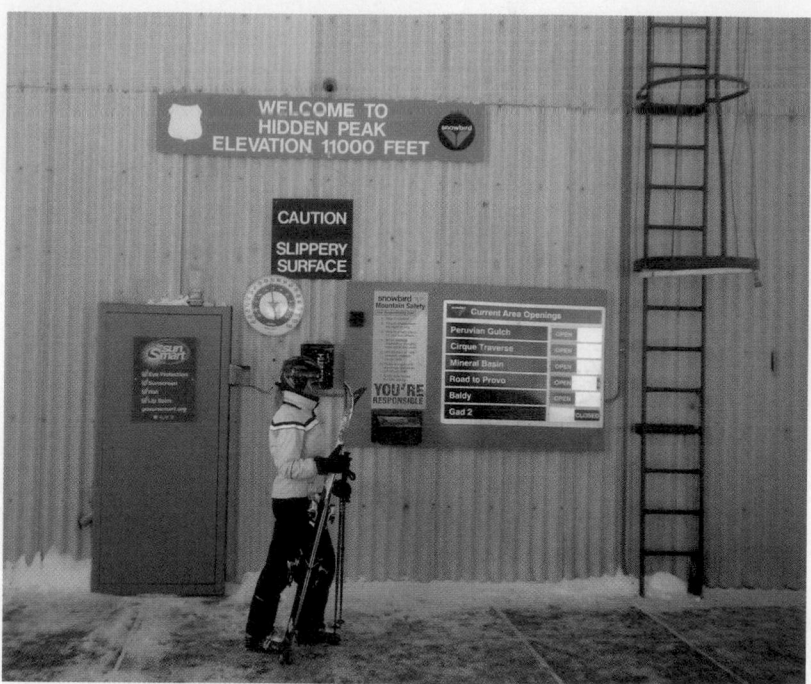

**Figure 28-7** High altitude is defined as 8,000–12,000 feet.
Copyright David Johe, MD

**hypoxemia**　insufficient oxygenation of the blood.

are vulnerable to high-altitude illness due to rapid ascent. In fact, altitude illness most commonly occurs within this altitude range (Figure 28-7■).

+ *Very high altitude* is defined as elevations of 12,000 feet to 18,000 feet (3,500 m to 5,500 m). At very high altitude, low blood oxygen content (**hypoxemia**) may occur during exercise and even during sleep. Visitors to very high altitude who have underlying lung disorders can be severely affected. Serious and deadly altitude illness occurs most commonly at very high altitude (Figure 28-8■).

+ *Extreme altitude* is defined as elevations greater than 18,000 feet (5,500 m). At these elevations, atmospheric oxygen levels are so low that work becomes difficult, and progressive deterioration of physiological function eventually outstrips the ability of the human body to acclimatize. For this reason, no permanent human habitation exists above 5,500 m. When ascending to extreme altitude, a period of acclimatization is critical because, without supplemental oxygen, visits that last more than a few moments can result in severe altitude illness and death (Figure 28-9■).

High altitude dramatically affects the amount of oxygen available to the body's cells, which can have a profound effect on normal body function. As altitude increases, the weight of the atmosphere (or barometric pressure) decreases, as does the partial pressure of oxygen in the air. This means that the amount of oxygen per unit volume of air is less with increasing altitude.

At sea level, the barometric pressure averages 760 mmHg, and oxygen makes up about 21 percent of the air. With increasing altitude, the barometric pressure decreases, which causes a decrease in air density (makes the air "thinner"). Although the concentration of oxygen remains constant, the decrease in air density means that each breath takes in fewer oxygen molecules. Thus, at 12,000 feet, the barometric pressure is only 483 mmHg, which means that roughly 40 percent fewer oxygen molecules are taken in per breath (Figure 28-10■). The result is hypoxia, which can lead to altitude illness.

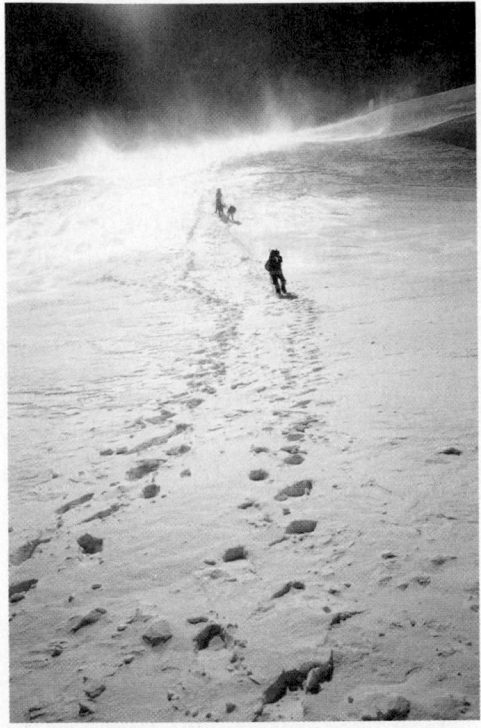

**Figure 28-8** Very high altitude is defined as 12,000–18,000 feet. Altitude illness is most likely to occur within this range of elevation.
Copyright Jamie Marshall/Dorling Kindersley Media Library

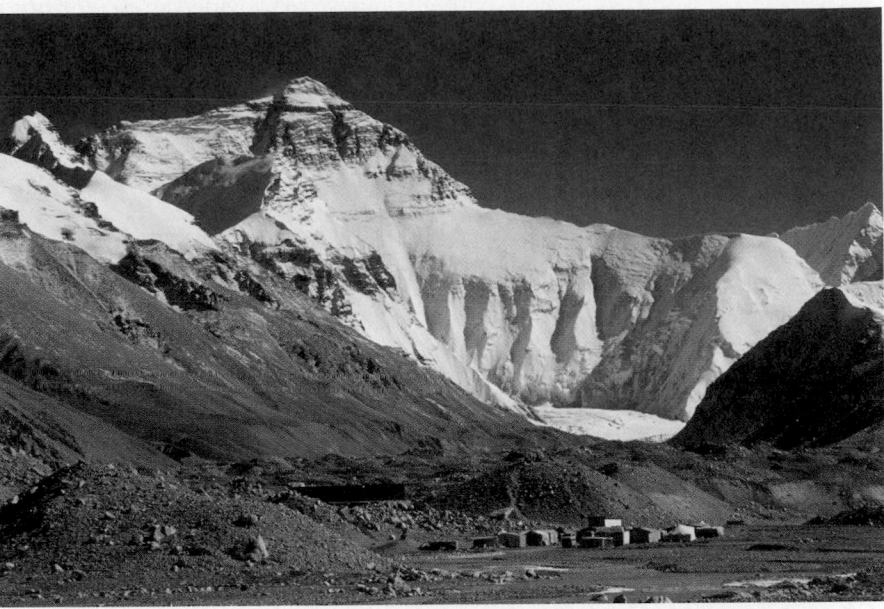

**Figure 28-9** Extreme altitude is greater than 18,000 feet. (This photo shows Mt. Everest.)
Copyright Ian Cumming/Dorling Kindersley Media Library

**Figure 28-10** As elevation rises, the oxygen concentration in the air is reduced, resulting in a lower oxygen intake per breath.
Copyright Wilderness Medical Society educational powerpoint series, 2008

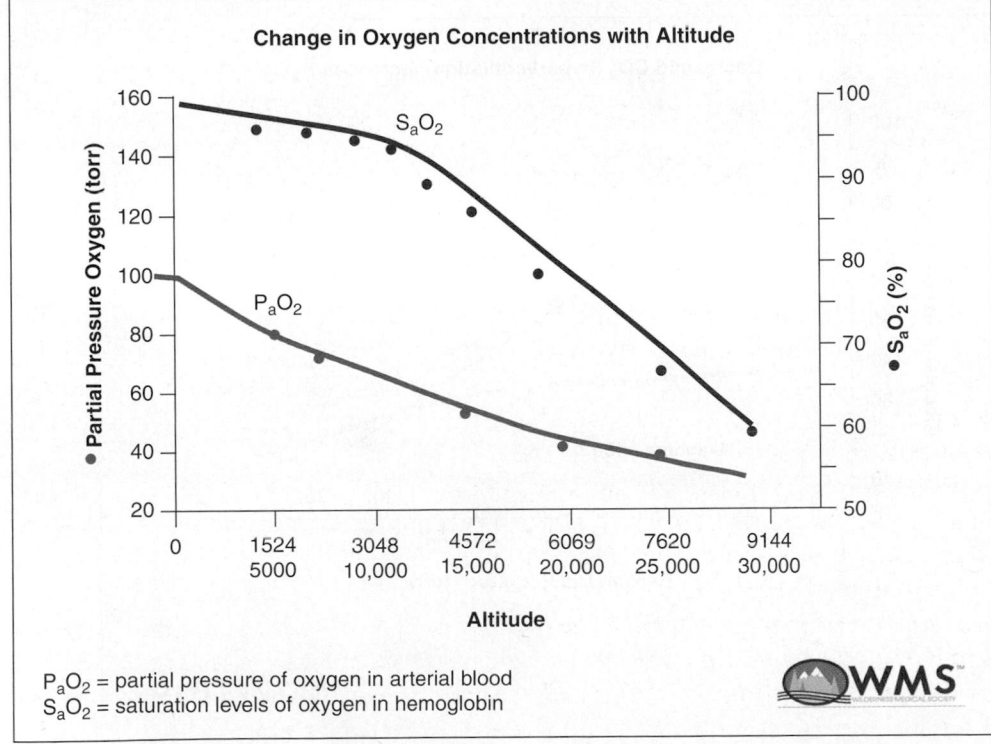

$P_aO_2$ = partial pressure of oxygen in arterial blood
$S_aO_2$ = saturation levels of oxygen in hemoglobin

The relationship of barometric pressure to altitude also changes with the distance from the equator: the air at higher altitudes is less dense in regions closer to the poles than in regions closer to the equator. Humans can survive these changes, however, if their bodies are provided sufficient time to adapt. If, for instance, a person who lives at sea level were to fly directly to the top of Mt. Everest (29,035 ft/8,848 m), they would quickly lose consciousness and die. However, some climbers who ascend gradually over many days are able to summit extreme-altitude peaks such as Everest without supplemental oxygen with only minor symptoms. This stark contrast is due to a physiological process known as altitude acclimatization.

## Altitude Acclimatization

**Acclimatization** to altitude is a process in which the body makes a series of physiological adjustments that increase the delivery of oxygen to the body's cells. This gradual adjustment to hypoxia allows a person to temporarily endure extreme altitudes. These physiological changes that help preserve homeostasis include the following adaptations:

+ *Increased rate and depth of respiration.* This change helps bring more oxygen into the body and is the result of a mechanism called the hypoxic ventilatory response (Figure 28-11■). The degree of this response is dependent on the individual's genetic makeup.

+ *Increased heart rate.* This adaptation allows more blood and oxygen to be pumped throughout the body and results in a mild elevation in systolic blood pressure.

+ *Increased red blood cell production.* This mechanism increases the amount of oxygen that can be carried to the tissues.

+ *Constriction of pulmonary blood vessels.* The blood vessels that go to and from the lungs constrict, increasing resistance to blood flow through the lungs. This resistance raises pulmonary blood pressure, helping "push" oxygen from the air sacs into the blood stream.

+ *Increased enzyme production (2, 3 DPG).* This mechanism facilitates the release of oxygen from hemoglobin, making oxygen available to body tissues.

⊕ **28-3** List risk factors for the development of altitude illnesses.

**acclimatization**    the body's physiologic process of gradual adjustment to changes in such factors as light, temperature, or altitude.

**Figure 28-11** The body compensates to the lower oxygen concentration at higher elevations by increasing the depth and rate of respiration. The trigger for this adjustment is the hypoxic ventilatory response.
Copyright Wilderness Medical Society educational powerpoint series, 2008

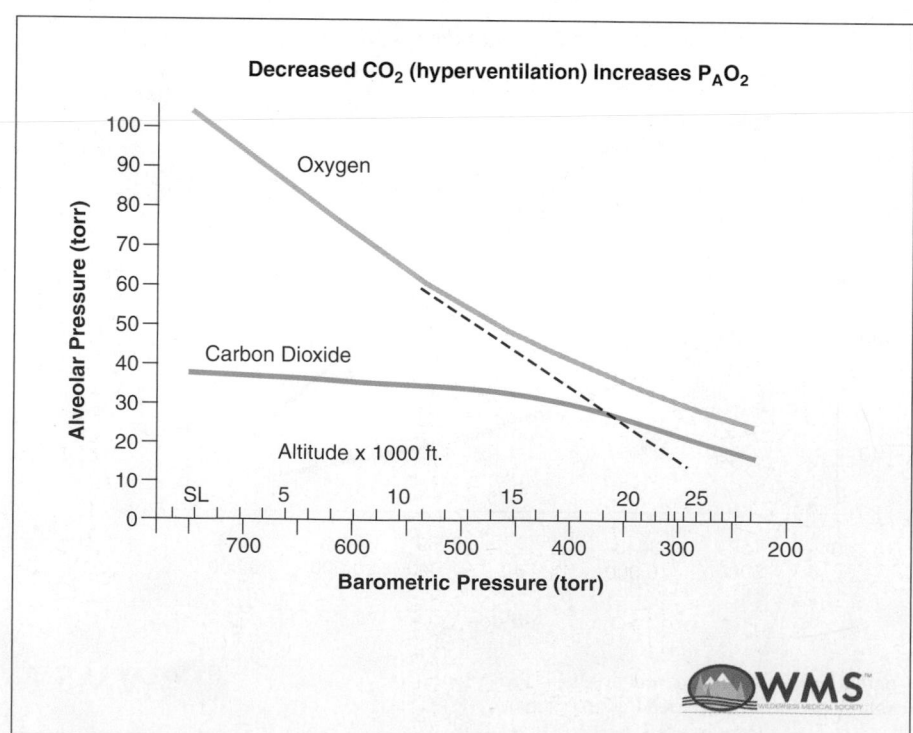

The ability to acclimatize varies from person to person, and even the most physically fit are susceptible to altitude-related illnesses (Figure 28-12■). Some people are able to adapt quickly to altitude changes without any apparent discomfort, whereas others develop varying degrees of altitude illness. A few individuals fail to acclimatize, even with gradual ascent, and they develop a life-threatening condition. The degree of hypoxia, the rate of ascent, and the individual's physiological makeup are the primary factors that determine whether the body successfully acclimatizes or becomes ill.

# Altitude-Related Problems

Among the altitude-related problems with which OEC Technicians should be familiar are acute mountain sickness, high-altitude pulmonary edema, high-altitude cerebral edema, and some other altitude-related problems.

## Acute Mountain Sickness

**Acute mountain sickness (AMS)** is a common condition that affects thousands of outdoor enthusiasts each year. AMS is defined as a usually mild medical condition that is caused by exposure to high altitude and includes the presence of a headache and feelings of generalized sickness in an otherwise healthy individual. (Figure 28-13■). It occurs when the rate of ascent outpaces the body's ability to adjust to the change in altitude. AMS rarely occurs at altitudes below 6,500 feet (2,000 m) and is more often encountered at altitudes greater than 8,000 feet (2,400 m). It is especially prevalent among individuals who rapidly ascend to high altitude from elevations below 2,000 feet.

The development and severity of AMS depend on several factors, including the rate of altitude ascent, the ultimate elevation attained (more importantly, the **sleeping altitude**), the time spent at altitude, the level of exertion, and genetic susceptibility.

AMS is characterized by mild to moderate headache accompanied by one or more of the following symptoms: dizziness, fatigue, shortness of breath, loss of appetite, nausea, sleep disturbances, and a general feeling of malaise (Figure 28-14■). These

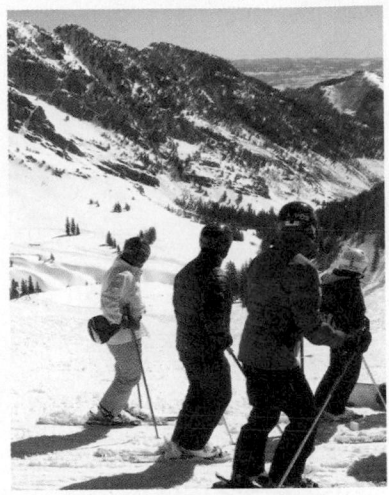

**Figure 28-12** Some individuals acclimatize more quickly than others. The rate of acclimatization is not based on their physical conditioning alone.
Copyright Denise Cheney

**acute mountain sickness (AMS)**   a usually mild medical condition that is caused by exposure to high altitude.

**sleeping altitude**   the altitude to which a climber descends to sleep to prevent AMS; is typically 500–1,000 feet below the highest elevation of that day's ascent.

**Figure 28-14** Signs and symptoms of acute mountain sickness (AMS).
Copyright Wilderness Medical Society educational powerpoint series, 2008

**Figure 28-13** Acute mountain sickness is defined as headache and feelings of sickness at high altitudes.

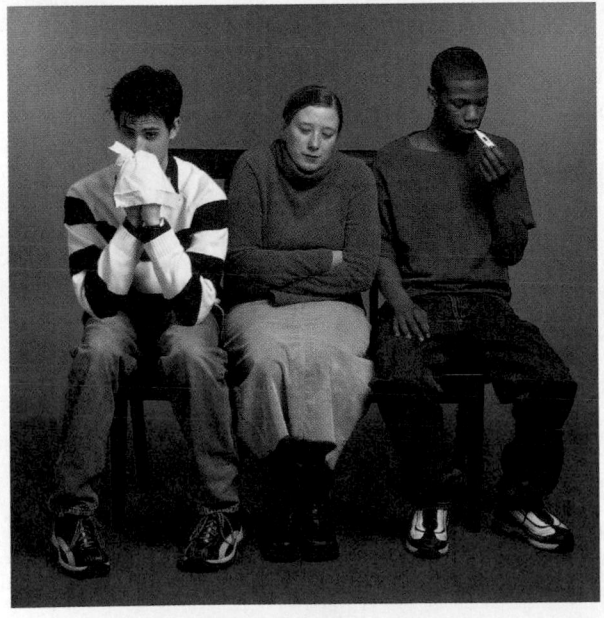

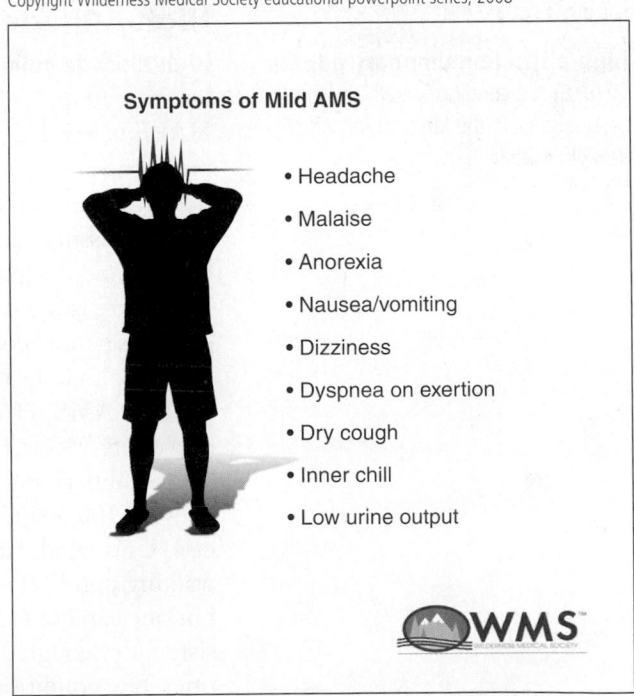

**Symptoms of Mild AMS**

- Headache
- Malaise
- Anorexia
- Nausea/vomiting
- Dizziness
- Dyspnea on exertion
- Dry cough
- Inner chill
- Low urine output

WMS

| Table 28-1 | Acute Mountain Sickness Self Assessment* |
|---|---|

If after recent ascent to altitude you have any degree of headache and score even one point in any of the other categories, you may have acute mountain sickness.

**Headache:**
0 None at all
1 Mild headache
2 Moderate headache
3 Severe (incapacitating) headache

**Gastrointestinal symptoms:**
0 Good appetite
1 Poor appetite or nausea
2 Moderate nausea or vomiting
3 Severe (incapacitating) nausea and vomiting

**Fatigue and/or weakness:**
0 Not tired or weak
1 Mild fatigue/weakness
2 Moderate fatigue/weakness
3 Severe (incapacitating) fatigue/weakness

**Dizziness/lightheadedness:**
0 None
1 Mild
2 Moderate
3 Severe (incapacitating)

**Difficulty sleeping:**
0 Slept as well as usual
1 Did not sleep as well as usual
2 Awoke many times, poor night's sleep
3 Could not sleep at all

*Source: Adapted from http://www.ismmed.org/ams_worksheet.htm

---

**28-5** List the signs and symptoms of the following altitude illnesses:

- acute mountain sickness
- high-altitude pulmonary edema
- high-altitude cerebral edema

**high-altitude pulmonary edema (HAPE)** a condition in which fluid accumulates in the lungs of individuals at high altitude.

---

symptoms, which many patients compare to the feeling of an alcoholic hangover, commonly develop within 12–24 hours after arrival at a higher altitude but can appear in as few as 4–6 hours in susceptible individuals. If the person is able to acclimatize successfully, the symptoms decrease in severity by about the third day. Because there are no specific diagnostic signs for AMS, it is often misdiagnosed as a viral flu-like illness, a hangover, exhaustion, dehydration, or a drug-related effect. Table 28-1■ provides a means of assessing whether an individual might be suffering from AMS.

## High-Altitude Pulmonary Edema

**High-altitude pulmonary edema (HAPE)** is a condition in which fluid accumulates in the lungs of an individual at high altitude. Unlike some other forms of pulmonary edema, HAPE is not due to a preexisting cardiac disorder. In cardiac pulmonary edema, fluid builds up in the lungs because the heart is not pumping correctly. In HAPE, fluid buildup is caused by excessive blood pressure in the pulmonary artery. The elevated blood pressure causes extracellular fluid to leak into the alveoli, which reduces gas exchange and oxygenation and results in cellular hypoxia.

HAPE is the most common cause of altitude-related death and rarely occurs at elevations below 8,000 feet. The incidence of HAPE among intermediate-altitude skiers is approximately 1 in 10,000 and most commonly affects young, healthy individuals.

Like AMS, HAPE develops as a result of several factors, including individual susceptibility, ascent rate, altitude reached, physical exertion, and certain underlying medical conditions. HAPE usually occurs within the first 2–4 days of ascent to altitudes above 8,200 feet (2,500 m) and is heralded by the onset of marked fatigue during exercise. Untreated, fatigue is soon accompanied by severe dyspnea upon exertion, such as walking uphill or up stairs. About half of HAPE patients have symptoms of AMS first, but one can get HAPE without having AMS first. Patients may also complain of a persistent dry cough during the early stages, and their nail beds and lips may become cyanotic. The condition typically worsens at night. Labored breathing at rest and audible chest congestion herald the development of a serious, potentially life-threatening condition (Figure 28-15■). HAPE may strike abruptly, especially in a sedentary person who may not notice the early stages. Pink (blood-tinged) frothy sputum is a very late finding and is accompanied by profound hypoxia.

Untreated, HAPE can be fatal within a few hours. Fortunately, it can be completely and easily reversed if recognized early and treated properly.

## High-Altitude Cerebral Edema

**High-altitude cerebral edema (HACE)** is a potentially deadly condition in which the brain swells. HACE is the most severe form of altitude illness and is most commonly encountered at elevations over 9,600 feet (3,000 m). HACE is preceded by AMS, and HAPE also may be present. About 3 percent of patients who develop acute mountain sickness go on to develop HACE.

HACE is a true medical emergency that can rapidly lead to death if not recognized and quickly treated (Figure 28-16■). It is characterized by a progression of symptoms that usually begins with headache and nausea and progresses to **ataxia** plus any of the following signs and symptoms: altered mental status, fatigue, drowsiness, difficulty speaking, paralysis, and coma. Hallucinations and psychotic behavior also are commonly observed. Although uncommon, seizures can occur. Death is due to brain herniation from increased intracranial pressure. The progression from AMS to HACE-induced coma may be as fast as 12 hours but usually requires 1–3 days. Recovery can be very quick, especially if treated early, but recovery can also be very slow and result in long-term complications, including decreased cerebral or neurologic function.

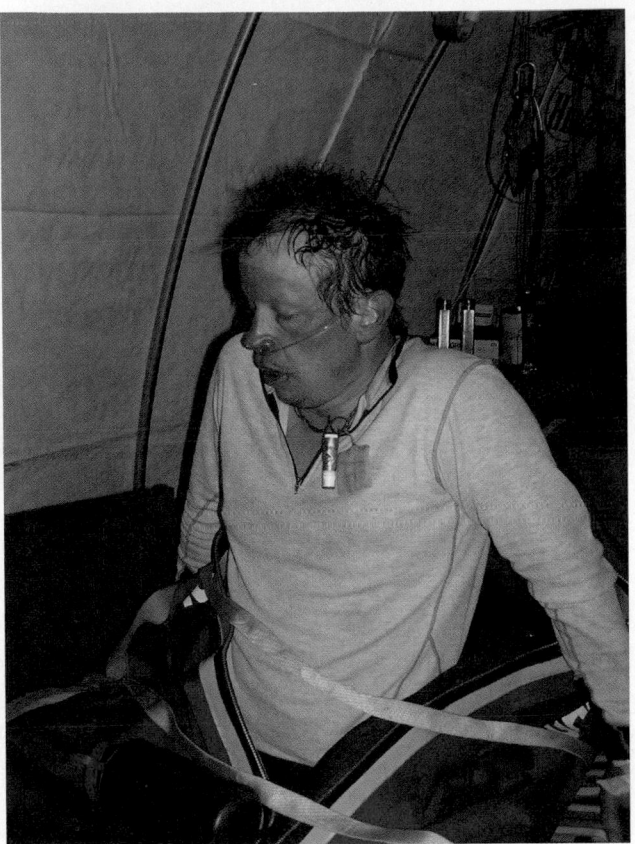

**Figure 28-15** High-altitude pulmonary edema (HAPE), a condition in which fluid accumulates in the lungs of individuals at high altitudes.
Copyright Luanne Freer, MD

**high-altitude cerebral edema (HACE)** a potentially deadly condition in which the brain swells in individuals at high altitude.

**ataxia** uncoordinated muscle movements; at high altitudes, it is associated with HACE.

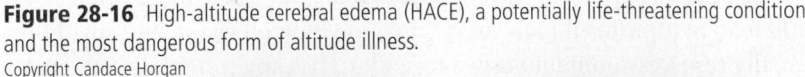

**Figure 28-16** High-altitude cerebral edema (HACE), a potentially life-threatening condition and the most dangerous form of altitude illness.
Copyright Candace Horgan

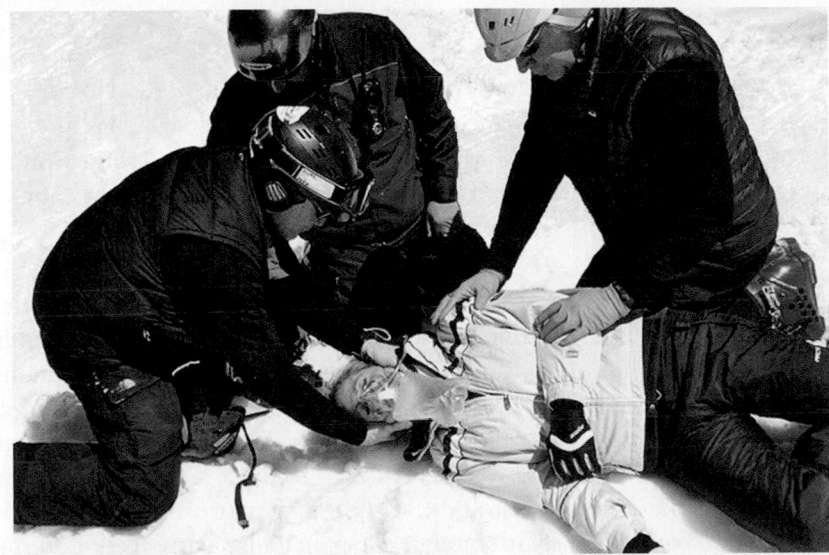

## Other Altitude-Related Problems

A decrease in available oxygen at altitude can complicate preexisting conditions, especially those involving the cardiovascular or respiratory systems, such as angina, congestive heart failure, and chronic respiratory conditions. Reduced oxygen availability can complicate pregnancy because of a reduction of oxygen delivered to the fetus.

In addition, altitude can adversely affect some medical equipment, most notably inflatable air splints, vacuum splints, and other pneumatic-based devices. The use of air splints at high altitude must be closely monitored, and because barometric pressure increases with decreasing elevation, air must be released from time to time as one descends to prevent overinflation. Failure to release pressure from these devices can result in compression on the involved extremity and neurovascular compromise.

Other medical conditions associated with altitude include khumbu cough, peripheral edema, high-altitude retinal hemorrhage (HARH), radial keratotomy (RK) blindness, solar keratitis, chilblains, and sunburn.

### Khumbu Cough

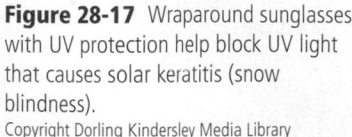

**khumbu cough**   a dry, persistent cough caused by inhaling excessively cold dry air that is typical at high altitude; also known as high-altitude bronchitis.

**Khumbu cough**, also known as high-altitude bronchitis, is a dry, persistent cough that affects nearly all people who spend time at altitudes above 14,000 feet (4,000 m). The condition is named after the Khumbu region in Nepal, near Mt. Everest, where it was first observed. Khumbu cough is caused by prolonged exposure to cold, dry air, which dries out the lower respiratory passages. The resulting severe bronchial irritation and constriction cause a cough that can become so severe that it can break ribs.

### Peripheral Edema

Mild to moderate edema of the face, hands, or feet is common among travelers at altitudes above 8,000 feet and is often seen without signs of acute mountain sickness. Altitude-related peripheral edema is noncardiac in origin and results from fluid leakage into the surrounding tissues. The condition is usually self-limiting and is not a sign of illness.

### High-Altitude Retinal Hemorrhage

High-altitude retinal hemorrhage (HARH) is a condition in which small blood vessels in the back of the eye rupture. The condition is encountered most often at elevations above 8,000 feet. Symptoms if present, can include blurred vision and small blind spots. HARH usually resolves spontaneously and seldom has any long-term effects.

### Radial Keratotomy Blindness

People who have had radial keratotomy (RK), an older surgical method to correct nearsightedness, may become blind at high altitude. This condition, which is not generally seen below 9,000 feet, begins with blurring of vision due to reduced refraction of light. Lasik, a newer procedure for vision correction, does not seem to cause the same effect.

**Figure 28-17** Wraparound sunglasses with UV protection help block UV light that causes solar keratitis (snow blindness).
Copyright Dorling Kindersley Media Library

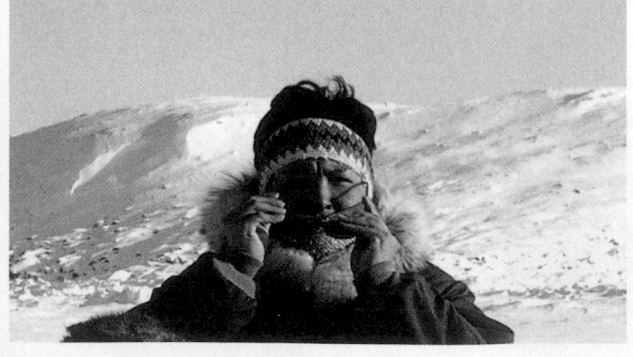

### Solar Keratitis

Exposure to the increased amount of UV radiation in sunlight at higher altitudes can cause solar keratitis, or snow blindness, in individuals who wear inadequate or no protective eyewear. UV light may be reflected off snow-covered terrain or water surfaces and can cause eye burns similar to those suffered by welders. Solar keratitis starts several hours after overexposure to UV light and begins with intense eye pain and a gritty feeling in the eyes.

Ideally, protective eyewear should be a "wraparound" type of sunglasses or glacier goggles to prevent light reaching the eyes from the side, and the addition of a visor helps deflect light entering from above (Figure 28-17■).

## Chilblains

**Chilblains** is an inflammatory response to exposure to cold, wet conditions that most commonly affects the skin of the ears, the tip of the nose, the fingers, and the toes (and rarely that of the legs and lower arms). Chilblains is characterized by blue or red edematous nodules that are painful to the touch. Although chilblains can occur at any altitude, it more commonly occurs at high altitudes. Chilblains is often misdiagnosed as frost nip or frostbite because it can have a similar appearance. The condition is usually self-limiting and generally has no long-lasting effects.

**chilblains**   a skin condition resembling frost nip that results from prolonged exposure to cold, wet conditions.

## Sunburn

Sunburn is more prevalent at higher altitudes because the decreased air density there increases one's exposure to the penetrating effects of the ultraviolet rays in sunlight (Figure 28-18■).

**Figure 28-18** The lower density of air at higher elevations increases the likelihood of sunburn from UV light. Remember to use protection on areas of exposed skin!
Copyright Andy Crawford and Steve Gorton/Dorling Kindersley Media Library

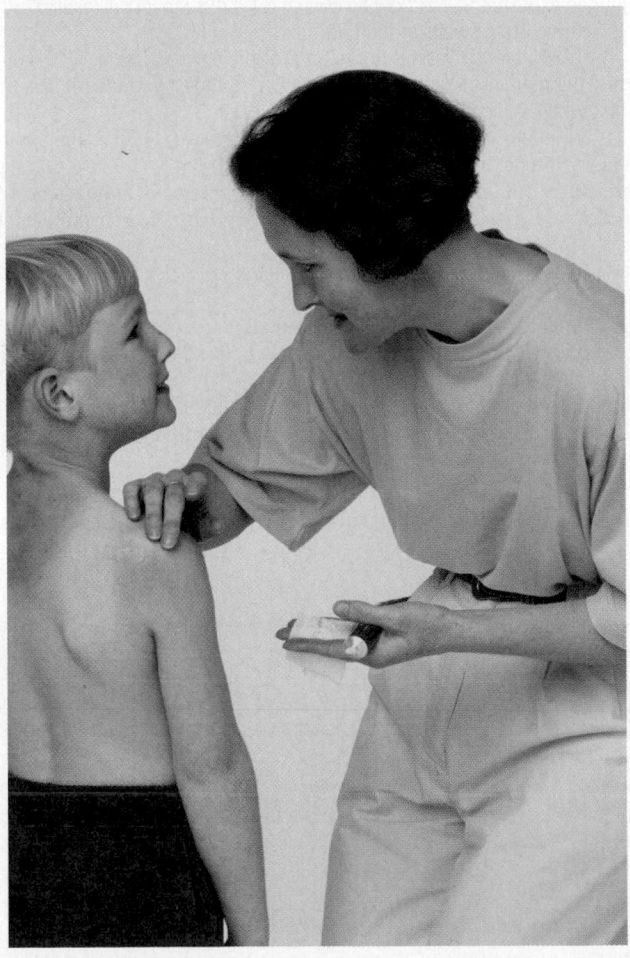

# STOP, THINK, UNDERSTAND

## Multiple Choice

Choose the correct answer.

1. How many altitude classifications are there?_____
   a. 5
   b. 4
   c. 3
   d. 2

2. How long does it take the body's compensatory mechanisms to adjust to conditions at intermediate altitudes (5,000–8,000 feet)?_____
   a. 12–24 hours
   b. 24–48 hours
   c. 48–60 hours
   d. 72–96 hours

3. Low altitude is defined as_____
   a. less than 4,000 feet.
   b. less than 5,000 feet.
   c. less than 5,500 feet.
   d. less than 6,000 feet.

4. When is altitude sickness likely to occur?_____
   a. Anytime an individual travels above 8,000 feet.
   b. When the body's compensatory mechanisms are unable to keep up with the body's oxygen demands.
   c. When the body's compensatory mechanisms keep up with the body's oxygen demands.
   d. Whenever an individual travels above 9,000 feet.

5. At which altitude classification may hypoxemia occur during exercise or sleep? _____
   a. intermediate altitude
   b. high altitude
   c. very high altitude
   d. extreme altitude

6. Serious and deadly altitude illness occurs most commonly in which of the following altitude classifications? _____
   a. intermediate altitude
   b. high altitude
   c. very high altitude
   d. extreme altitude

## Matching

Match each of the following altitude-related conditions with its best description. Conditions may be used more than once.

_____ 1. acute mountain sickness (AMS)

_____ 2. high-altitude pulmonary edema (HAPE)

_____ 3. high-altitude cerebral edema (HACE)

_____ 4. khumbu cough

_____ 5. high-altitude retinal hemorrhage (HARH)

_____ 6. solar keratitis

_____ 7. chilblains

_____ 8. sunburn

a. caused by prolonged exposure to cold, dry air, which dries out the lower respiratory passages
b. a condition in which the brain swells at high altitudes
c. a condition in which small blood vessels in the back of the eye rupture
d. symptoms of this condition include headache, dizziness, fatigue, shortness of breath, loss of appetite, nausea, sleep disturbances, and a general feeling of malaise
e. this condition results in blue or red edematous nodules that are painful to the touch
f. also known as high-altitude bronchitis
g. the most severe form of altitude illness; is commonly encountered at altitudes over 9,600 feet
h. often misdiagnosed as a viral flu-like illness, a hangover, exhaustion, dehydration, or a drug-related effect
i. the most common cause of death related to high altitude
j. snow blindness
k. this condition is often misdiagnosed as frost nip or frostbite
l. this condition is more prevalent at higher altitudes due to decreased air density and increased exposure to ultraviolet rays in sunlight
m. a condition in which fluid accumulates in the lungs of individuals at high altitude
n. this condition rarely occurs at altitudes below 8,000 feet; blood-tinged sputum accompanied by profound hypoxia are very late findings

 # CASE UPDATE

Upon examination of the patient, you notice that his breathing is labored, even at rest. The patient appears physically fit, which he confirms by saying, "I run and cycle more than 50 miles a week." His heart rate is 116, his blood pressure is 132/80, and his respirations are 36. A pulse oximeter measures the patient's oxygen saturation at 84 percent. The rest of the physical assessment is negative for any abnormal signs or signs of trauma.

**What do think is wrong with the patient? What should you do?**

# Prevention of Altitude Illnesses

With proper precautions, the incidence of altitude illnesses can be significantly reduced. However, as indicated previously, exceptional health or physical fitness does *not* render one immune to altitude illness. Thus, the prevention of altitude illness depends on proper acclimatization. Follow these guidelines to achieve proper altitude acclimatization:

+ Gradual ascent is the most effective way to prevent altitude illness.
+ Avoid rapid ascent to above 10,000 feet (3,000 m), especially if beginning the ascent at sea level.
+ Incorporate a layover of 2–3 days at an intermediate altitude—that is, between 8,000 feet and 10,000 feet (2,500–3,000 m). For individuals traveling from sea level, a 1-day layover at 6,000 feet (1,800 m) can dramatically decrease the chances of becoming ill (Figure 28-19■).
+ Once above 10,000 feet (3,000 m), limit increases in altitude to 1,000 feet (~300 m) per day. Then, for every 2,000 feet (~600 m) of elevation gained, take one or two extra rest days.
+ As you reach higher altitudes, more rest and a smaller altitude gain per day may be necessary.
+ Avoid heavy physical exertion for the first 24–48 hours at altitude.
+ Stay hydrated. Altitude acclimatization is often accompanied by fluid loss, so drink lots of liquids (sometimes 3–4 quarts per day) to remain properly hydrated (Figure 28-20■). As the respiratory rate increases at higher elevations, the amount of fluid lost during exhalations increases. Urine output should be copious and straw colored.
+ Avoid alcohol and other depressant drugs (including most sleeping pills) because they decrease the respiratory drive during sleep, which can worsen symptoms and cause AMS. Additionally, alcohol promotes diuresis and can lead to excessive fluid loss. Also avoid tobacco, which reduces peripheral circulation by constricting peripheral blood vessels.

**28-4** Describe strategies to prevent altitude illness.

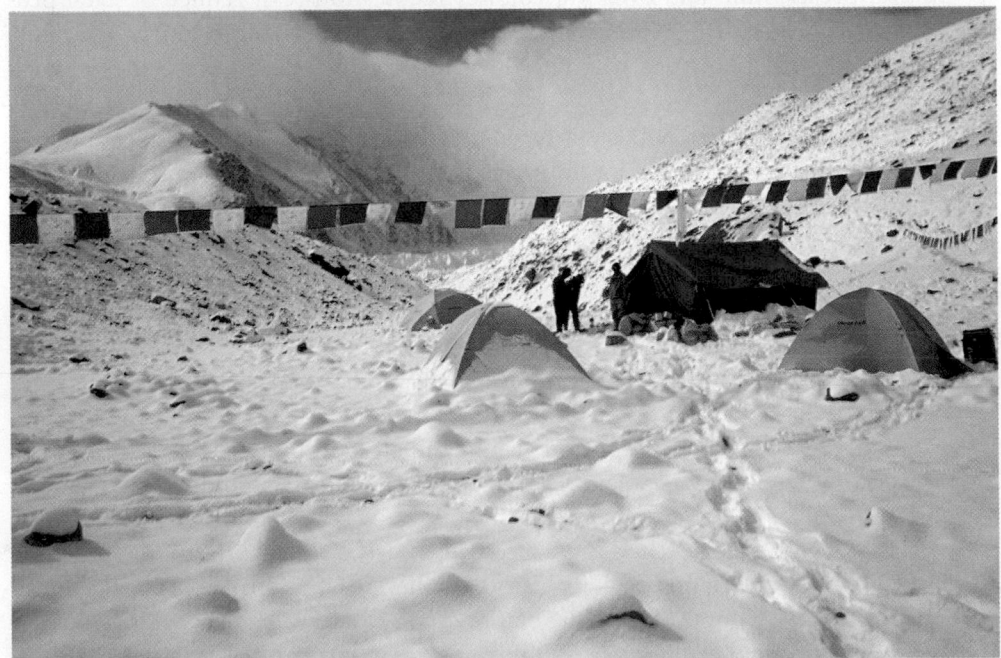

**Figure 28-19** Proper acclimatization, such as a 2- to 3-day rest period at high altitude (8,000–12,000 feet), can reduce the likelihood of altitude illness.
Copyright Jamie Marshall/Dorling Kindersley Media Library

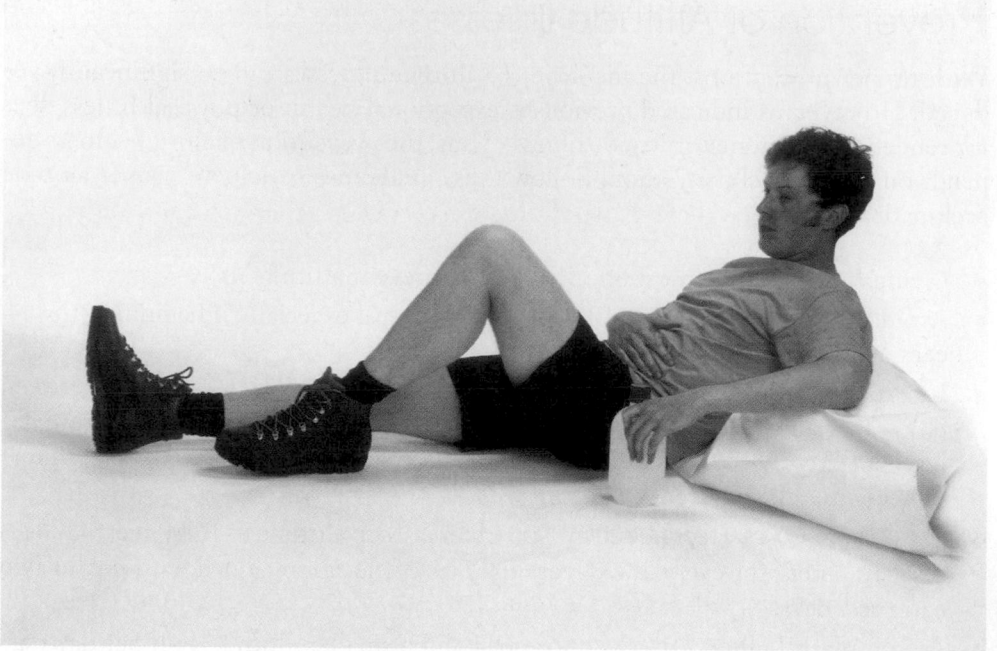

+ While at altitude, eat a high-carbohydrate diet (one that is approximately 70 percent carbohydrates).

+ If you begin to show symptoms of altitude illness, do not go higher until the symptoms resolve.

+ People acclimatize at different rates, so if you are traveling in a group, make sure everyone is properly acclimatized before going higher.

+ *"Climb high and sleep low."* This common mantra among climbers helps to reduce the adverse effects of climbing at high altitudes. If you are feeling well, climb during the day and then descend to a lower altitude to sleep at night.

Several prescription and over-the-counter medications can reduce or even prevent altitude illness. OEC Technicians should specifically ask high-altitude patients during the SAMPLE history whether they have taken one of these medications (Figure 28-21■).

*Acetazolamide* (Diamox) is a prescription medication that often is taken prophylactically to prevent AMS. The drug improves the bodies ability to acclimatize to altitude by forcing the kidneys to excrete bicarbonate. The resulting drop in blood pH stimulates hyperventilation and increased oxygen absorption. If taken early after the onset of AMS, acetazolamide can terminate AMS. Its effects may be delayed, so it is advisable to begin use 24 hours before ascent to altitude and to continue use for 48–72 hours at the maximum altitude attained. The prophylactic dose is 125 mg twice each day. Temporary side effects may include tingling of the lips and fingertips, blurred vision, and alteration of taste sensation.

Acetazolamide is a sulfonamide drug, so individuals who are allergic to sulfa drugs should not take it without prior testing. Because it is known to cause severe allergic reactions in people with no previous history of allergies, it is advisable to take a trial course of the drug before going to a remote location, where a severe allergic reaction could prove difficult to treat.

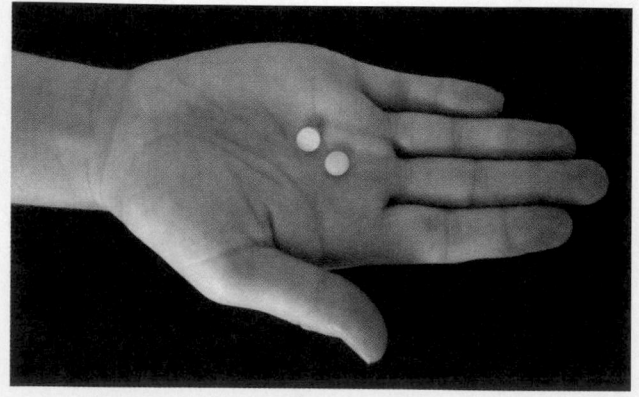

*Dexamethasone* is a prescription steroid that decreases swelling in the brain and in other structures and may reverse the symptoms of AMS. Dosage is typically 4 mg twice each day for a few days starting at the beginning of the ascent. Dexamethasone should be used with caution because it can mask signs of progressing disease. For this reason, it is recommended for prophylaxis in rare circumstances only.

*Gingko biloba* is an over-the-counter herbal supplement that has produced conflicting results in several studies. Accordingly, its use cannot be reliably recommended for AMS prophylaxis.

# Patient Assessment

⊕ **28-6** Describe how to assess a patient with altitude illness.

As has been stated throughout this text, the role of OEC Technicians is not to diagnose the underlying cause of a given problem, but instead to recognize patients who have signs and symptoms of an emergent condition and to quickly initiate life-saving treatment, if needed (Figure 28-22■).

As with any patient, the assessment process begins with a careful examination of the ABCDs. If a potentially emergent condition exists, initiate life-saving treatment in lieu of performing a complete physical examination, and refer the patient to a higher level of care. The primary assessment is followed by a secondary assessment, which includes a thorough history, a physical exam, and an assessment of the patient's vital signs.

OEC Technicians should ask patients about their medical history and symptoms using the SAMPLE acronym and the OPQRST mnemonic, respectively. Note whether patients have any underlying cardiac or respiratory conditions that could be worsened by altitude. For patients who are experiencing shortness of breath, ask if it is associated with any pain or persists during rest. Ask patients if they have ever had problems like this on previous visits to high altitude. Also ask patients if they have any AMS-related symptoms such as a headache, difficulty sleeping, nausea, vomiting, or excessive fatigue.

Physical examination of patients in outdoor settings is best accomplished using the L.A.P. exam, which involves looking, auscultating, and palpating (Figure 28-23■). Parts of the exam may need to be deferred until patients have been moved inside because environmental conditions can make examining patients especially challenging.

Begin the physical exam by allaying the patient's fears by explaining what you will do. Then place the patient into a position of comfort, which may well be an upright position that allows the person to breathe more easily. Note whether or not the patient appears short of breath at rest. Inspect the conjunctivae, lips, and nail beds for

**Figure 28-22** Ask the "SAMPLE" and "OPQRST" questions as an integral component of your assessment to fully understand what may be happening to a patient.
Copyright Studio 404

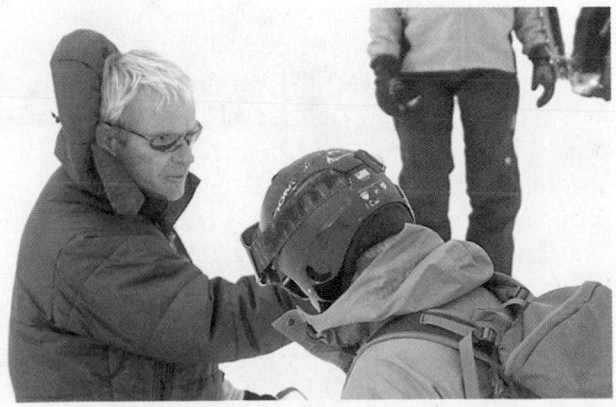

**Figure 28-23** Sometimes it is best to defer some aspects of the assessment until patients have been moved indoors.
Copyright Candace Horgan

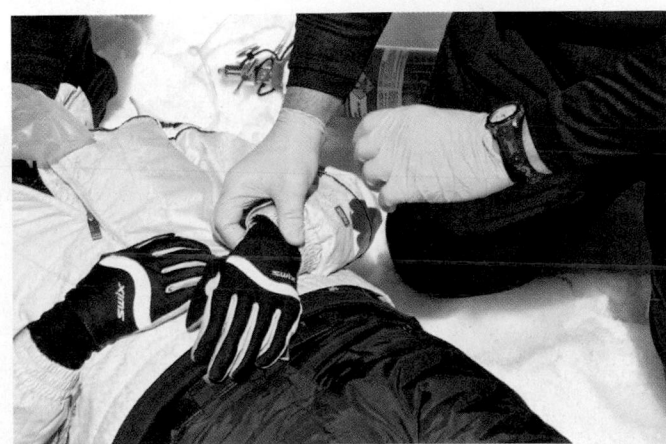

discoloration or cyanosis, and the face, hands, ankles, and feet for edema. Examine the inside of the mouth for any pink (blood-tinged) saliva or sputum. If a stethoscope is available and you have been trained to do so, auscultate the lungs for any abnormal sounds that could indicate the presence of pulmonary edema. See if there are any visual problems, especially a decrease in acuity.

Complete the physical exam by thoroughly palpating the body for areas of tenderness or swelling, and by assessing distal skin temperature, circulation, movement, and sensation. For patients who are complaining of symptoms that suggest AMS or HACE, attempt to assess them for ataxia by asking them to walk a straight line, heel to toe. Evidence of unsteadiness or an inability to maintain balance at altitude suggests HACE, which requires immediate treatment. Perform reassessments, including serial sets of vital signs, as needed.

---

⊕ 28-7 Describe the treatment of a patient with altitude illness.

# Patient Management

The treatment of patients who present with a suspected altitude-related disorder is generally supportive in nature, and early recognition is the key to a successful outcome. *The fundamental treatment for all cases of altitude illness is to descend to a lower elevation* (Figure 28-24■). Depending on the severity of symptoms, descent may need to be done urgently. Serious illnesses such as HAPE and HACE require more aggressive therapies, but OEC Technicians can begin effective early treatment. As with any emergency situation, scene and rescuer safety takes precedence over everything else. Do not risk yourself or others in a rescue. Be sure to remove potential hazards or move patients to a location where their conditions can be safely managed.

## General Management

Initial treatment for all altitude-related illnesses includes correcting any problems involving the ABCDs and placing patients into a position of comfort, unless spine immobilization is indicated. Immediate administration of high-flow oxygen via nonrebreather mask, especially when combined with rapid descent to a lower elevation, can be life saving. Keep patients warm by using jackets, blankets, reflective blankets, or sleeping bags as necessary, because cold stress elevates pulmonary pressures, decreases peripheral blood flow, and can worsen shock (Figure 28-25■). Anticipate

**Figure 28-25** Besides descent, treatment of altitude illness includes keeping patients warm and administering oxygen to treat for shock and decrease pulmonary edema.
Copyright Dorling Kindersley Media Library

**Figure 28-24** The fundamental treatment for all types of altitude illness is descent to a lower altitude.
Copyright Nigel Hicks/Dorling Kindersley Media Library

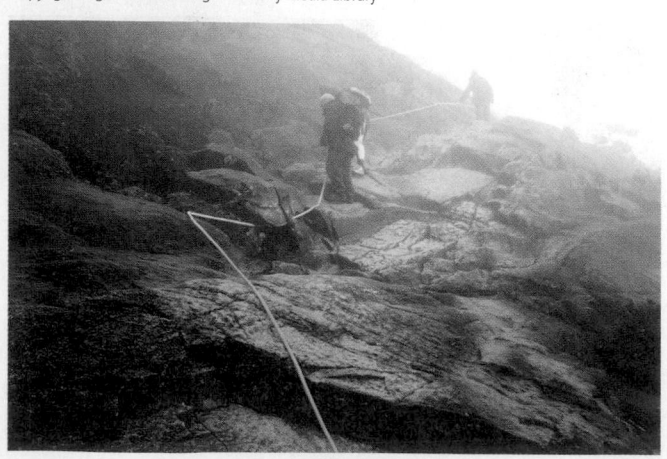

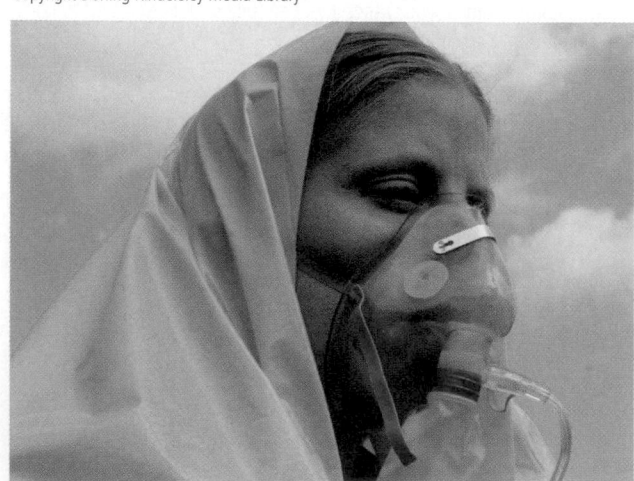

vomiting and be ready to clear the airway by removing the oxygen mask and turning patients onto their sides. Suction the airway as needed.

Continue to monitor vital signs and make preparations for transport because all patients with serious altitude illness require further evaluation and treatment at a definitive-care facility. Treatment of specific altitude-related disorders varies according to the underlying cause and the severity of symptoms.

## AMS Treatment

Treatment of AMS centers on treating symptoms, halting ascent, and waiting for altitude acclimatization to improve, which can take 12 hours to several days. In all cases, minimize exertion to prevent the worsening of symptoms. High-flow oxygen is particularly effective and can ease other symptoms such as headache and nausea. All other treatment is symptom based. For headache, which is a tell-tale sign of AMS, patients may self-administer conventional analgesics such as acetaminophen or ibuprofen. If symptoms do not resolve, descent is indicated.

## HAPE Treatment

The treatment of HAPE depends on equipment availability and other logistics. If oxygen is scarce or unavailable, the emergent treatment for HAPE is rapid descent to an elevation that is at least 1,500–3,000 feet (500–1,000 m) lower than the elevation at which symptoms were first observed. Unless there is no other way, avoid self-evacuation because it increases respiratory demands. Rescue groups should make delivery of oxygen to the patient a top priority.

If unlimited oxygen is available, descent may be delayed, at least for a while, because oxygen immediately reduces pulmonary arterial blood pressure. In severe cases, the use of specialized devices such as a **Gamow bag** can be life saving.

Following evacuation to a lower altitude, patients should be transported to a hospital for further evaluation and treatment, which typically consists of bed rest and supplemental oxygen. In severe cases, medications that reduce pulmonary blood pressure may be administered. Most patients recover rapidly. Upon release from the hospital, patients are advised to resume normal activities gradually and are warned that it can take up to 2 weeks to recover their strength completely.

## HACE Treatment

At the first sign of ataxia or a change in responsiveness, patients should be transported to a lower altitude, at least 1,500–3,000 feet (500–1,000 m) below the elevation at which the symptoms were first noticed. High-flow oxygen should be administered immediately, if available. If descent is not logistically possible, devices such as a Gamow bag can "buy time" until descent is possible and can significantly decrease morbidity and mortality. All other care is supportive in nature. Patients should be transported immediately to a hospital for definitive evaluation and treatment, which often includes the administration of steroids to reduce cerebral swelling (Figure 28-27■).

## Khumbu Cough Treatment

Khumbu cough is treated by placing a mask, a balaclava, or other cloth material over the mouth and nose to warm and humidify the air before it is inhaled into the lungs (Figure 28-28■). Warm beverages also can help keep the airway passages warm and moist. If available, inhaled steam can be both soothing and preventative. Prescription medications to suppress cough and to decrease airway inflammation may be curative.

### Gamow Bag

**NOTE**

A Gamow bag functions as a mini-hyperbaric chamber (Figure 28-26■). The patient is placed into the bag, which is then inflated to a pressure that simulates a temporary descent to a lower altitude.

**Gamow bag** a portable hyperbaric chamber that is used to treat high-altitude sickness.

**Figure 28-26** Use a Gamow bag if unlimited oxygen is available and descent must be delayed.
Copyright Leanne Freer, MD

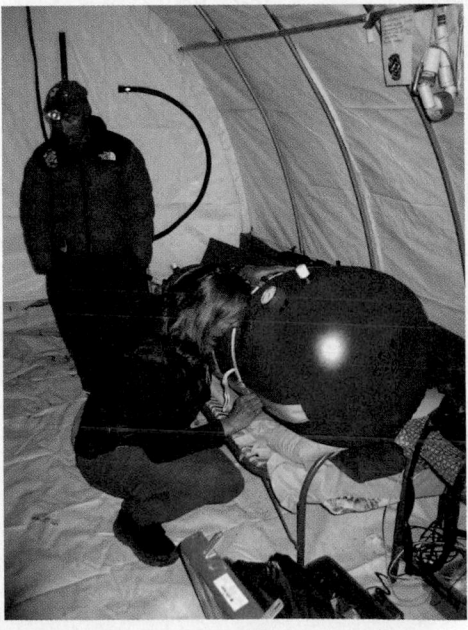

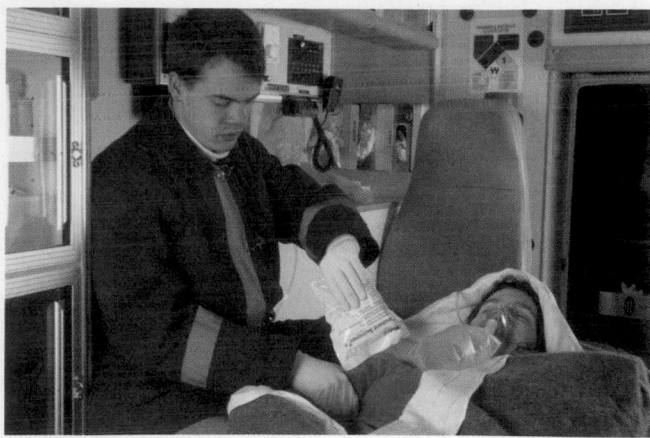

**Figure 28-27** Immediately after descent, patients with HACE must be transported to definitive care for further stabilization and treatment.
Copyright Dorling Kindersley Media Library

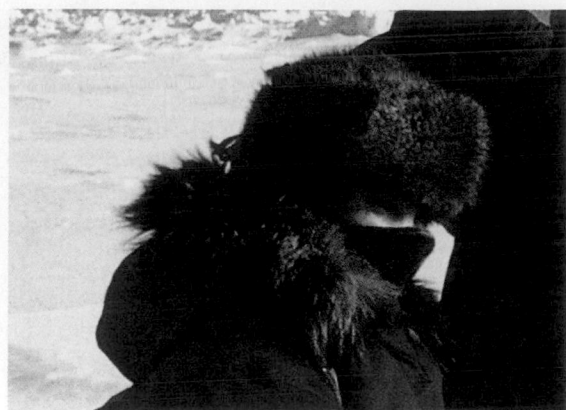

**Figure 28-28** Treatment of khumbu cough includes using a balaclava, a mask, and/or warm drinks to warm and moisten the air before it enters the mouth and nose.
Copyright Dorling Kindersley Media Library

## Treatment of Other Problems

Other medical problems that may be aggravated by high altitude are treated in the usual manner but may not resolve with conventional therapies until the patient is transported to a lower altitude. Altitude illness can be avoided by educating patients about proper preventative measures. Learning to recognize early symptoms of altitude illness is critical. Individuals with sleep apnea and related conditions may become severely hypoxic at high altitudes. Ask patients about this condition during your evaluation.

Patients experiencing visual problems need to descend with the help of "a guide." They should seek care from a physician, preferably one trained in pathological conditions of the eye.

# STOP, THINK, UNDERSTAND

## Multiple Choice

Choose the correct answer.

1. With what step should you begin the assessment of a patient with suspected altitude illness? _____
   a. a primary assessment
   b. a secondary assessment
   c. a medical history using the SAMPLE acronym and the OPQRST mnemonic
   d. a careful examination of the ABCDs

2. Which of the following statements is not a basic guideline for proper altitude acclimatization?_____
   a. be physically active for the first 24–48 hours at high altitude
   b. ascend gradually
   c. stay hydrated
   d. avoid alcohol and other depressant drugs

3. What are the three steps in the L.A.P. exam?_____
   a. listening, abnormalities, palpating
   b. looking, auscultating, palpating
   c. looking, auscultating, preventing
   d. listening, abnormalities, preventing

4. The fundamental goal of management for any patients experiencing altitude illness is to_____
   a. keep them at the same elevation until their bodies adjust.
   b. "climb high, sleep low" to help their bodies adjust.
   c. keep them hydrated.
   d. have them descend to a lower elevation.

5. Which of the following treatments is not an initial treatment for all altitude-related illnesses?_____
   a. Correct any problems with the ABCDs.
   b. Place patients in a position of comfort (unless spinal immobilization is necessary).
   c. Administer high-flow oxygen via a nonrebreather mask.
   d. Ascend slower to give the body a chance to acclimate.

6. Which of the following statements is not a basic guideline for proper altitude acclimatization?_____
   a. Climb high, sleep low.
   b. Avoid rapid ascent above 10,000 feet.
   c. Stay hydrated.
   d. Eat a high-protein diet (70 percent of calories from protein) while at high altitudes.

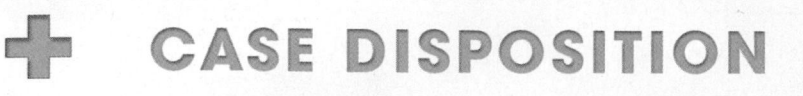

## CASE DISPOSITION

You are concerned that the patient has early signs of HAPE. You place him on high-flow oxygen, keep him comfortable, and mobilize resources to transport him to a hospital that is approximately 1,500 feet lower than your present location. Two days later, the patient's wife stops by the patrol room and thanks you "for taking such great care of my husband." She reports that his symptoms completely resolved within a day after descent and administration of supplementary oxygen. She further states that her husband was advised to either avoid going to a high altitude or to ascend more slowly on his next trip to a high elevation. He also was encouraged to speak with his private physician about using a prophylactic medication that can help prevent future episodes of HAPE.

# ⛨ Chapter Review

## Chapter Summary

Altitude illness is a common disorder that affects outdoor enthusiasts around the world. It is caused by reduced oxygen availability and can afflict even those who are extremely fit. Although the human body is capable of adapting rapidly to a variety of environmental conditions, it requires time to adjust to the internal and external changes that occur at high altitudes.

The body's compensatory mechanisms increase cardiopulmonary function whenever oxygen delivery to the cells must be increased. However, because the amount of oxygen available per breath is markedly reduced at high altitude when compared to low altitude, the body must work harder to keep up with oxygen demands. Problems arise when the body's need for oxygen outpaces oxygen availability, which results in hypoxia and a host of other problems ranging from merely inconvenient symptoms to life-threatening illness. Patients who have an underlying medical condition, especially those with cardiac or pulmonary disorders,

are most vulnerable to altitude-related illness and should proceed with caution and only after they have completely acclimatized.

The likelihood that OEC Technicians will encounter an altitude-related illness is high if they live and work in a high-altitude setting. This potential is compounded by guests who arrive after a quick ascent from a low altitude. In such individuals, symptoms can manifest quickly. Preventative measures, such as slow ascent and the use of prophylactic (prescribed) medications, may provide some protection but are no guarantee of immunity. It is therefore essential that OEC Technicians are able to recognize the signs and symptoms of altitude-induced conditions, including acute mountain sickness, HAPE, and HACE. Additionally, they must be prepared to act quickly to treat an altitude-related illness in order to halt the progression of symptoms and to reduce the chances of a potentially lethal outcome.

## Remember...

1. Altitude illness can become life threatening.
2. Once symptoms of AMS develop, do not ascend further until symptoms completely resolve.
3. Suspect HACE in the presence of headache and ataxia when at high altitude.
4. Descent with supplemental oxygen almost always improves the symptoms of altitude illness.

# Chapter Questions

## Multiple Choice

Choose the correct answer.

1. At what altitude classification do most people experience the physiological effects of lower atmospheric oxygen pressure?_____
   - **a.** low altitude
   - **b.** intermediate altitude
   - **c.** high altitude
   - **d.** very high altitude

2. Which of the following factors is not a primary determinant for whether the body successfully acclimates or becomes ill?_____
   - **a.** individual physiology
   - **b.** rate and depth of respirations
   - **c.** degree of hypoxia
   - **d.** rate of ascent

3. Which of the following physiological adjustments does not help preserve homeostasis during altitude acclimatization?_____
   - **a.** increased heart rate
   - **b.** silation of pulmonary blood vessels
   - **c.** increased rate and depth of respirations
   - **d.** decreased enzyme production

4. How far should a patient be brought down the mountain at the first sign of ataxia or a change in responsiveness (HACE)?_____
   - **a.** at least 500–1,000 feet
   - **b.** at least 1,000–1,500 feet
   - **c.** at least 1,500–3,000 feet
   - **d.** at least 3,000–4,000 feet

5. To treat HAPE, patients should be brought down_____
   - **a.** at least 500–1,000 feet.
   - **b.** at least 1,000–1,500 feet.
   - **c.** at least 1,500–3,000 feet.
   - **d.** at least 3,000–4,000 feet.

6. In treating AMS, waiting for the body to acclimate can take_____
   - **a.** 5–10 hours.
   - **b.** 7–12 hours.
   - **c.** 12–20 hours.
   - **d.** 12 hours to several days.

7. Two conditions that are characteristic of HACE are_____
   - **a.** ataxia and hallucinations.
   - **b.** loss of memory and unsteadiness.
   - **c.** loss of memory and inability to maintain one's balance.
   - **d.** inability to maintain one's balance and dilated pupils.

8. Which group of individuals is most vulnerable to altitude sickness?_____
   - **a.** All individuals are equally vulnerable.
   - **b.** Individuals who are 30 years old or older and have underlying medical conditions.
   - **c.** Individuals who arc 40 years old or older and have cardiac or pulmonary disorders.
   - **d.** All individuals who have underlying medical conditions, particularly cardiac or pulmonary disorders.

## List

1. List the signs and symptoms of acute mountain sickness.

   _____

   _____

   _____

   _____

**2.** List ten of the basic guidelines for preventing altitude sickness.

1. _____

2. _____

3. _____

4. _____

5. _____

6. _____

7. _____

8. _____

9. _____

10. _____

## Scenario

*Two 24-year-old male skiers walk into your patrol treatment room. Both arrived at the resort yesterday morning, and after a little "partying" last evening they put on their skis and hit the slopes, which are at about 7,900 feet of elevation. It is now noon, and the two men are complaining of flu-like symptoms and headaches.*

**1.** As an experienced OEC Technician, you know that _____

   **a.** as the altitude decreases, the percentage of $O_2$ in the air decreases.

   **b.** as the altitude decreases, the density of $O_2$ in the air decreases.

   **c.** as the altitude increases, the $O_2$ level increases.

   **d.** as the altitude increases, the air density and the available $O_2$ decrease.

**2.** When traveling to an intermediate altitude (5,000–8,000 feet), the average person can adjust in_____

   **a.** 12 hours.

   **b.** 72–96 hours.

   **c.** 5 days.

   **d.** 6 days.

**3.** After you perform a complete assessment using SAMPLE and OPQRST, you suspect that the patients are experiencing _____

   **a.** acute mountain sickness.

   **b.** high-altitude pulmonary edema.

   **c.** high-altitude cerebral edema.

   **d.** a seasonal flu attack.

*The two patients ask what can be done. You suggest that they could either drive down the mountain to the next town, where there is a community clinic and a doctor, or they could rest and acclimate to the elevation.*

**4.** You suggest they hydrate with non-alcoholic beverages and eat a diet that is _____

   **a.** low in carbohydrates.

   **b.** high in carbohydrates.

   **c.** high in protein.

   **d.** low in protein.

# Suggested Reading

Everest ER website: www.EverestER.org

Freer, L., and P. Hackett. 2008. "High Altitude Medicine" in *Expedition and Wilderness Medicine*, edited by B. Bledsoe, et al. Cambridge, MA: Cambridge University Press.

Hackett, P., and K. Zafren. 2007. High Altitude Medicine Slides (PowerPoint), available at www.wms.org

International Society Mountain Medicine website: www.ismmed.org

EXPLORE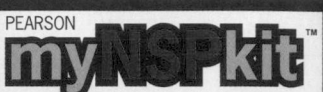

Please go to www.myNSPkit.com. Under Student Resources, you will find animations, videos, web links, and games related to this chapter—and much more. Look for more information on high-altitude sickness from the Wilderness Medical Society and other sources.

Register your access code from the front of your book by going to www.myNSPkit.com and selecting the appropriate links. If the in-cover access code has been redeemed, go to www.myNSPkit.com and follow links to Buy Access.

# Water Emergencies

Jeffrey Druck, MD

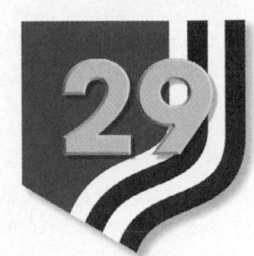

**29**

## ⊕ OBJECTIVES

**Upon completion of this chapter, the OEC Technician will be able to:**

**29-1** Compare and contrast dry drowning and wet drowning.

**29-2** Describe the physiologic response of the mammalian diving reflex.

**29-3** Define the following terms:

- submersion injury
- drowning
- near-drowning
- arterial gas embolism
- decompression sickness

**29-4** Describe the following gas laws:

- Boyle's law
- Henry's law
- Dalton's law

**29-5** List three types of barotrauma and indicate their causes.

**29-6** List nine ways in which a water-based emergency may be prevented.

**29-7** List the signs and symptoms of the following water-related emergencies:

- arterial gas embolism
- decompression sickness

**29-8** Describe how to manage a patient who has suffered a water-related emergency.

## ⊕ KEY TERMS

**arterial gas embolism (AGE),** *p. 928*
**barotrauma,** *p. 927*
**decompression sickness,** *p. 927*

**drowning,** *p. 925*
**laryngospasm,** *p. 922*
**mammalian diving reflex,** *p. 922*

**near-drowning,** *p. 926*
**partial pressure,** *p. 923*
**tonicity,** *p. 927*

## Chapter Overview

Water is earth's most abundant resource and covers approximately 70 percent of the planet's surface. Humans seem naturally attracted to water in every season and use it to engage in a variety of outdoor activities, including canoeing, rafting, kayaking, tubing, swimming, surfing, snorkeling, scuba diving, and fishing (Figure 29-1■). Even when frozen, water continues to serve as a popular source of recreation in such activities as

*continued*

## HISTORICAL TIMELINE

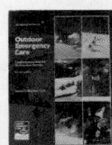

**1992** Interagency Liaison John Clair assists patrollers and ski areas in obtaining hepatitis B vaccine thru an arrangement with a pharmaceutical company.

**1993** (WEC) OEC Second Edition is published.

## ✚ CASE PRESENTATION ✚

You and several friends are hiking near a local lake on a beautiful spring day when you hear shouts for help. As you near the scene, you come upon bystanders who tell you they did not see what happened. When you and your companions reach the water's edge, you see a 14-year-old male floating in the water, approximately four feet from shore. You can clearly see the bottom of the lake, which is littered with rocks of various sizes. Looking up, you see a rock ledge extending approximately ten feet above the water's edge. You identify yourself as an OEC Technician and quickly assess the patient. He is unresponsive and cyanotic. He is not breathing, has a weak carotid pulse, and his skin is cool to the touch. You notice that he has a large gash on the top of his head.

*What should you do?*

---

ice skating, ice hockey, ice fishing, ice climbing, and snow machine racing. Given our attraction to water, it stands to reason that injuries often occur in and around this medium.

Water-related injuries are among the most prevalent types of injury encountered in outdoor recreation. Water-related emergencies can occur any time and nearly anywhere. When people think of a water emergency, the image that usually comes to mind is of someone drowning in a recreational body of water, such as a swimming pool, a lake, or the ocean. But drowning can also occur in a bathtub, a well, or a creek (Figure 29-2■). In fact, a person can drown in as little as 2 inches of standing water, in a bucket, or in a puddle like those found in any ski resort's parking lot.

OEC Technicians will likely face a water-related emergency at some point in their career, so you must be prepared to respond to this type of incident and initiate emergency care in a timely fashion. In general, the assessment and initial stabilization of a patient with a water emergency are similar to those performed for other seriously injured patients. Understanding the subtleties and complications inherent to water-related emergencies will enable OEC Technicians to more rapidly identify the problem and to render appropriate treatment in preparing patients for definitive care.

**Figure 29-1** People gravitate to water activities throughout the year. A water-related emergency may happen at any time.
Copyright Scott Smith

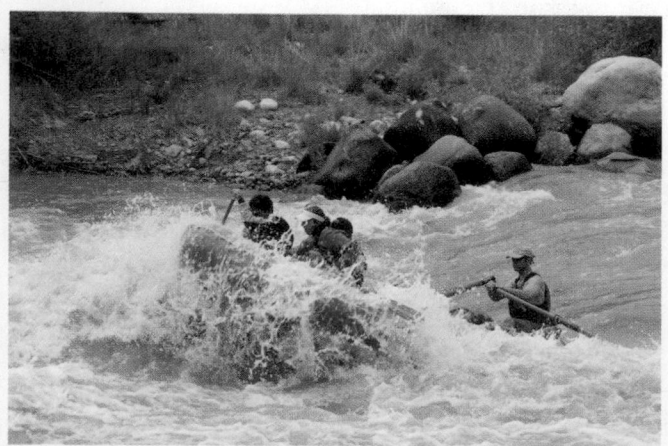

**Figure 29-2** Drowning can occur in as little as 2 inches of water. This child is in more than 2 inches of water.
Copyright Paul Wilkinson/Dorling Kindersley Media Library

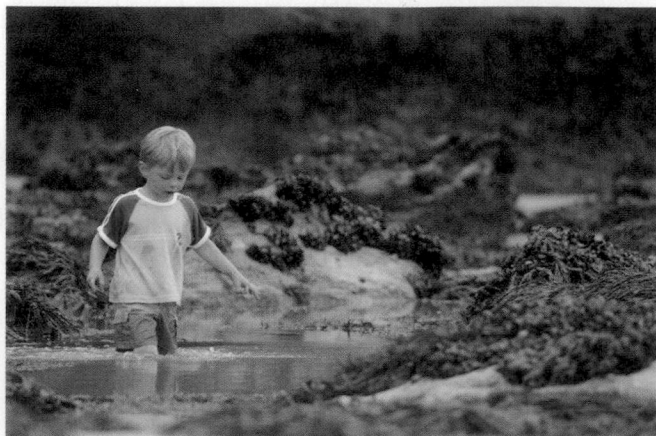

# Anatomy and Physiology

Under normal conditions, the process of breathing is automatic. Air enters the oro- or nasopharynx, passes through the vocal cords and the larynx, then into the trachea and bronchioles, and down into the alveoli. From there, oxygen molecules diffuse into the blood and are transported by red blood cells throughout the body (Figure 29-3■). When a person's airway is submerged under water or another liquid for more than a few seconds, this vital process is interrupted, which sets into motion a series of events that immediately affects homeostasis. Unless corrected, this situation can quickly lead to death by drowning.

The pathophysiology of drowning is complex and involves several body systems, chief of which are the respiratory and cardiovascular systems. A person submerged under water reflexively holds his breath. Depending on a person's overall health and conditioning, the person can hold off breathing for only a few seconds or up to several minutes, after which the body's need for oxygen overrides any further attempts at breath holding. Panic quickly sets in as oxygen levels in the brain begin to drop. In an attempt to bring more oxygen into the body, the person begins to gasp and may aspirate small amounts of water (Figure 29-4■). As a result, the larynx may spasm, completely closing the airway. The resulting anoxia causes the person to lose consciousness and induces electrical disturbances within the heart, leading to cardiac arrest. The airway muscles then relax, which allows water to rush into the lungs. Table 29-1■ lists the pathophysiological events that occur in drowning.

**29-1** Compare and contrast dry drowning and wet drowning.

**29-2** Describe the physiologic response of the mammalian diving reflex.

**Figure 29-3** An overview of ventilation and perfusion.

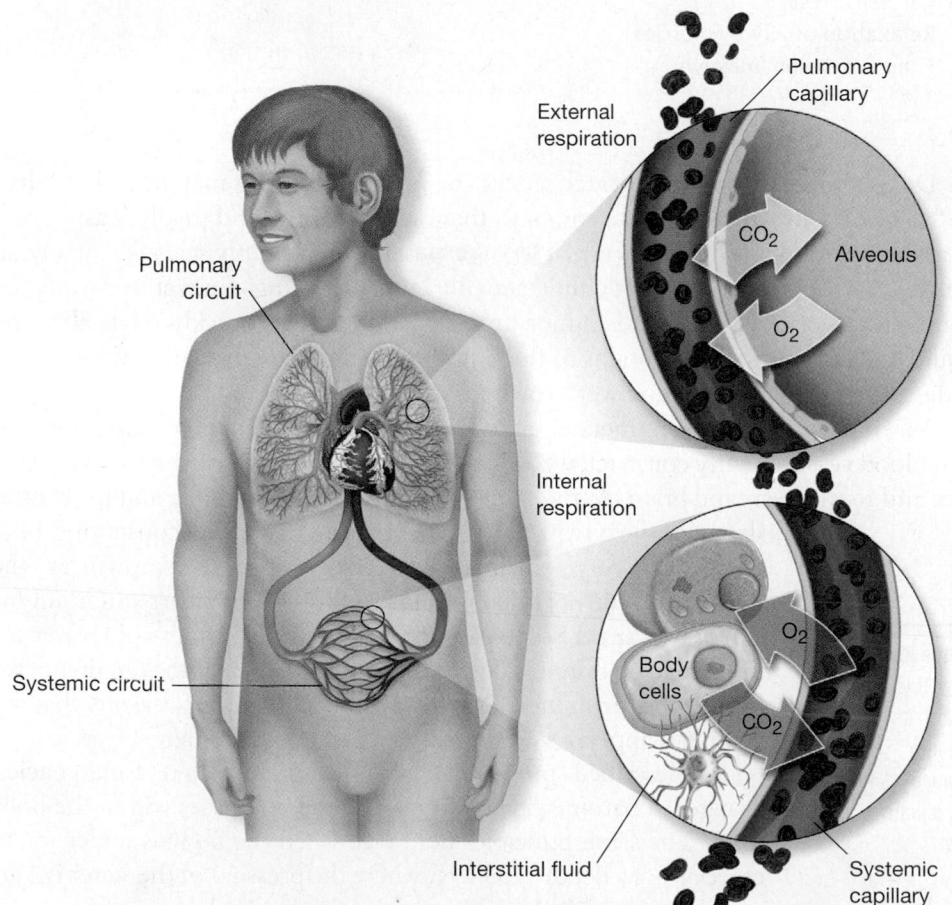

**Figure 29-4** The aspiration of water and other events can lead to dire, even fatal outcomes.
Copyright Dorling Kindersley Media Library

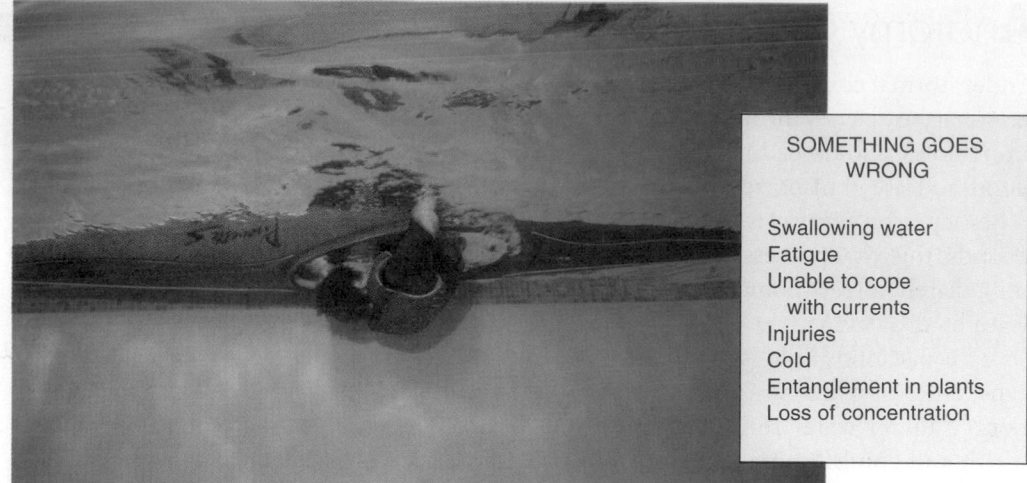

SOMETHING GOES WRONG

Swallowing water
Fatigue
Unable to cope
  with currents
Injuries
Cold
Entanglement in plants
Loss of concentration

| Table 29-1 | Events in the Pathophysiology of Drowning |
|---|---|

- Panic
- Gasping
- Possible aspiration of liquid (minor)
- Laryngospasm
- Hypoxia
- Loss of consciousness
- Myocardial irritability (electrical disturbances)
- Cardiac arrest
- Relaxation of airway muscles
- Fluid aspiration (massive)

**laryngospasm**   spasm of the vocal cords that prevents air movement through the respiratory tract.

**mammalian diving reflex**   a reflexive response to diving in many mammals that is characterized by physiological changes that decrease oxygen consumption (including slowed heart rate and decreased blood flow to the abdominal organs and muscles) until breathing resumes.

### What Is an Atmosphere?

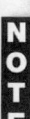

One atmosphere equals the pressure of air at sea level (14.7 pounds per square inch). Put another way, if you took all the air above one square inch of the earth's surface at sea level and weighed it all the way into space, that air would weigh 14.7 pounds. Because water is more dense than air, it takes one inch square column of water only 33 feet high to equal one atmosphere.

Depending on how much water enters the lungs, drowning may be either "dry" or "wet." Dry drowning is more common than wet drowning and involves aspiration of a small amount of fluid and violent **laryngospasm**, which tightly seals the airway. In this form of drowning, very little fluid actually enters the lungs. In wet drowning, by contrast, either laryngospasm is minor or the airway muscles quickly relax, allowing liquid and any material it contains to flood into the lungs. Dry drowning usually precedes wet drowning, although wet drowning may occur alone.

As soon as the body is immersed or submerged in extremely cold water, peripheral blood vessels tightly constrict, which shunts warm blood away from the body surface and to the heart and brain. At the same time, the body's metabolic and heart rates slow significantly, reducing oxygen demand and conserving oxygen. This very effective protective response, known as the **"mammalian diving reflex,"** helps to protect the heart and brain for a period of time. Some patients have survived under cold water for more than 60 minutes due to this reflex. The mammalian diving reflex is most prominent in young children and, for reasons that are not clear, appears to diminish as a person gets older.

As described in Chapter 28, Altitude-Related Emergencies, changes in barometric pressure affect the way gases within the body react. The same principles hold true when the body is under water, especially at a depth of 33 feet, where the pressure of the water is 2 atmospheres (ATM): 1 ATM from the air plus 1 ATM from the water.

Fully understanding how diving injuries occur requires a basic understanding of three laws that affect gases: Boyle's law, Henry's law, and Dalton's law.

## Boyle's Law

Briefly, Boyle's law states that at a constant temperature, the volume of a gas is inversely proportional to the pressure exerted by that gas. In other words, as one descends in a body of water and the water pressure increases, the pressure inside the chest cavity and the lungs increases, which causes the volume of gas within the lungs to decrease. Thus, if you have 6 liters of air in your lungs and you dive to 33 feet (2 atmospheres of water pressure and 1 atmosphere of air pressure for a total of 3 atmospheres), the volume of air in your lungs is reduced (compressed) by half, to 3 liters. Conversely, when pressure decreases, the volume of a gas increases (expands).

When you ascend from a depth of 33 feet to the surface, the volume of gas within your lungs will attempt to increase. Because the total volume of the lungs is limited by the size of the chest, the resulting increase in pressure (as the gas tries to expand) within the lungs can rupture them. The same is true for any other air-filled body cavity or body structure.

## Henry's Law

Henry's law states that at a given temperature, the amount of gas that will dissolve in a liquid is directly proportional to the **partial pressure** of the gas.

This means that a gas such as nitrogen will remain dissolved in the blood so long as the partial pressure remains constant. If the external pressure suddenly decreases, bubbles may form. Should bubbles form within the bloodstream, they can lodge in a vessel and obstruct blood flow, resulting in a variety of problems.

## Dalton's Law

Dalton's law states that the pressure of a mixture of gases is the sum of the partial pressures of all the gases in that mixture. At sea level, air pressure is one atmosphere or 14.7 pounds per square inch (psi). If the gas at the water's surface is a mixture containing just two gases, 20 percent oxygen and 80 percent nitrogen (which is close to what is in air), then the pressure exerted by the oxygen is $0.20 \times 14.7$ psi or 2.94 psi, and the pressure exerted by the nitrogen is $0.80 \times 14.7$ or 11.76 psi. The pressure at a depth of 66 feet is 3 atmospheres, or 44.1 psi. In the same mixture of gases, the pressure from oxygen is $0.20 \times 44.1$, or 8.82 psi, whereas the pressure from nitrogen is $0.80 \times 44.1$, or 35.28 psi. So as one goes deeper under water, the pressure from nitrogen is greatly increased.

⊕ **29-4** Describe the following gas laws:

- Boyle's law
- Henry's law
- Dalton's law

### Boyle's Law

NOTE

At a constant temperature, the volume of a gas is inversely proportional to the absolute pressure of the gas. Translation: when pressure decreases, the volume of a gas increases, and vice versa.

**partial pressure**   the pressure of a single gas within a mixture of gases; the partial pressure of each gas in a mixture of gases is equal to the pressure that gas would exert if it occupied the same volume alone at the same temperature.

### What Is Partial Pressure?

NOTE

In a mixture of gases, each gas is responsible for part of the total pressure of the mixture. Put another way, the partial pressure of each gas in a mixture of gases is equal to the pressure that gas would exert if it alone occupied the same volume at the same temperature.

### Why Do Carbonated Beverages Bubble?

NOTE

When you open a bottle of carbonated beverage, you reduce the pressure over the surface of the liquid, so bubbles come out of the liquid and go into the air above the liquid.

### Henry's Law

NOTE

At a given temperature, the amount of gas that will dissolve in a liquid is directly proportional to the partial pressure of that gas. Translation: at higher pressures, more gas will dissolve in a liquid; when the pressure decreases, the gas will come out of the liquid and form bubbles.

### Dalton's Law

NOTE

The pressure of a gas mixture is the sum of the partial pressures of all the gases in the mixture. Translation: the overall pressure of a gas is made up of the pressure of each individual gas, added together.

# STOP, THINK, UNDERSTAND

## Multiple Choice

Choose the correct answer.

1. Which of the following statements best describes the "mammalian diving reflex"? _____
   a. The heart rate increases, forcing blood to the heart and brain.
   b. The heart rate increases while body metabolism slows, reducing oxygen demand.
   c. Blood vessels constrict, and the heart rate and body metabolism slow, reducing oxygen demand.
   d. Blood vessels dilate, and the heart rate and body metabolism increase, supplying the brain with needed nutrients.

2. When individuals are submerged in water, they may begin to gasp, causing the _____ to spasm and completely closing the airway.
   a. mouth
   b. trachea
   c. esophagus
   d. larynx

3. How deep must water be for a human to drown in it? _____
   a. 2 inches
   b. 12 inches
   c. 1.5 feet
   d. 2 feet

4. Which law states that at a given temperature, the amount of gas that will dissolve in a liquid is directly proportional to the partial pressure of the gas? _____
   a. Dalton's law
   b. Henry's law
   c. Boyle's law
   d. Newton's law

5. In what age group is the "mammalian diving reflex" most prominent? _____
   a. young children
   b. teenagers
   c. adults
   d. senior citizens

## Fill in the Blank

1. _____ drowning involves aspiration of a small amount of fluid and violent laryngospasm.

2. In _____ drowning, laryngospasm is minor and allows liquid and materials it contains to flow into the lungs.

# Common Water Emergencies

⊕ 29-3 Define the following terms:
- submersion injury
- drowning
- near-drowning
- arterial gas embolism
- decompression sickness

**Figure 29-5** Water-related emergencies often involve a variety of physical injuries. Copyright Scott Smith

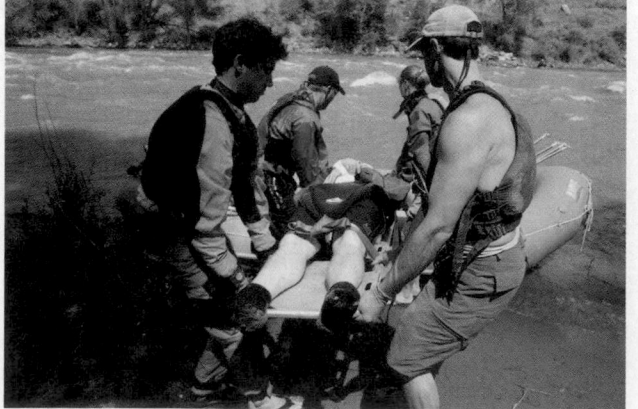

The types of emergencies encountered in and around water are virtually limitless and include many of the medical and traumatic disorders previously described in this textbook. In addition, several emergencies are unique to water environments or are encountered only when an individual is exposed to changes in atmospheric pressure. Among the water-related emergencies that OEC Technicians may encounter are submersion injuries, barotrauma, nitrogen narcosis, swimmer's ear, breath holding, trauma, injuries by aquatic animals, and aggravation of existing medical conditions.

OEC Technicians will no doubt face other forms of trauma in aquatic environments, including soft-tissue, orthopedic, and neurologic injuries (Figure 29-5■). Such injuries may be caused by the environment, by the equipment used, or from an unexpected or violent encounter with an aquatic animal. Emergencies are not always traumatic, though, and many emergencies may be brought on by the physical exertion associated with various water sports, especially in individuals with a preexisting medical condition. Hypothermia may also occur in aquatic environments and is discussed in detail in Chapter 25, Cold-Related Emergencies.

## Submersion Injuries

A submersion injury is any injury that occurs while a person is under water. Remember, only the airway need be submerged. Submersion injuries are the fifth-leading cause of traumatic injury in the United States and can occur nearly anywhere. OEC Technicians should be familiar with two types of submersion injuries: drownings and near-drownings.

## Drowning

**Drowning** is defined as suffocation by submersion that results in death within 24 hours following removal from the water. Each year, approximately 400,000 drowning deaths occur worldwide, of which approximately 3600 deaths occur in the United States. Drowning is the second-leading cause (after motor vehicle trauma) of accidental death in children ages 1 month to 14 years old, and is the leading cause of accidental death in children ages five years and younger (Figure 29-6■). In the United States, 90 percent of all drowning deaths occur in fresh water, and 50 percent occur in swimming pools. Children less than one year of age tend to drown in bathtubs and buckets because they cannot get out by themselves when they fall into the water. Older children aged 1–4 drown in swimming pools while those aged 5–14 years tend to drown in lakes, ponds, rivers, and oceans. Nearly one-third of all drownings occur in non-summer months.

Among the many factors that contribute to drowning are panic, poor judgment, fatigue, muscle or stomach cramps, inability to swim, trauma, spinal cord injuries, disorientation, and physical immobility from cold or some kind of physical restraint (e.g., another person holding on or entanglement in seaweed) (Figure 29-7■). Alcohol is

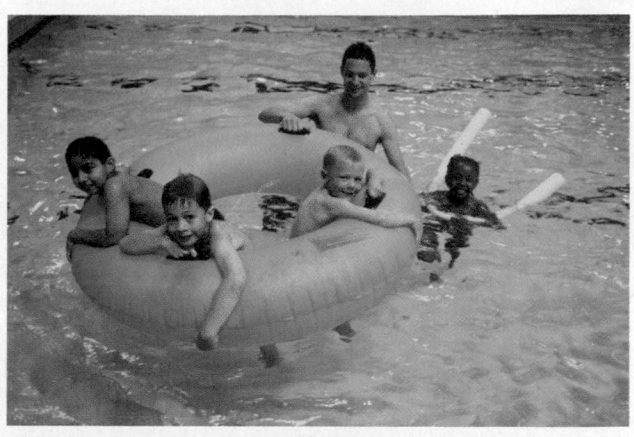

**Figure 29-6** Drowning is a leading cause of accidental deaths among children. Copyright Zena Holloway/Dorling Kindersley Media Library

**drowning**   suffocation by submersion in water.

**Figure 29-7** Factors that contribute to drowning.

SOMETHING GOES WRONG

Swallowing water
Fatigue
Unable to cope
  with currents
Injuries
Cold
Entanglement in plants
Loss of concentration

PANIC

INEFFICIENT BREATHING

DECREASED BUOYANCY

EXHAUSTION

DROWNING

CARDIAC ARREST

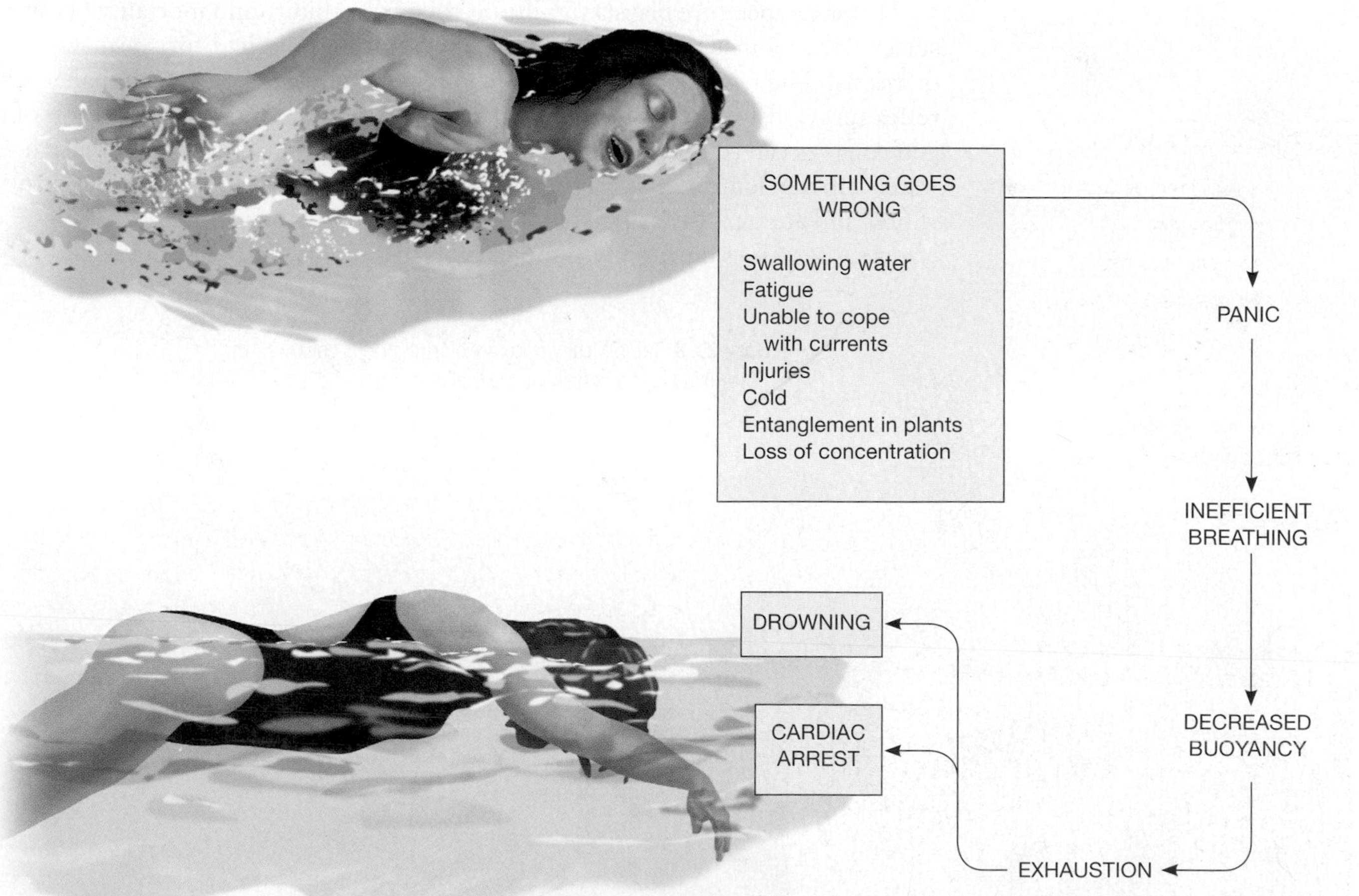

another contributing factor and is implicated in more than half of all drowning deaths in adolescents and adults. Males are four times more likely to drown than are females, probably because of their greater likelihood of engaging in dangerous behaviors.

A preexisting illness also can increase the risk of drowning. For instance, drowning is the leading cause of accidental death among patients with a history of seizure activity, and the bathtub is the most common site in which such drownings occur.

Certain activities are associated with an increased risk for drowning. Boating, for example, including rafting, kayaking, and tubing, accounts for more than half of all drowning deaths. Sadly, many of these deaths are preventable; studies indicate that personal flotation devices (PFDs) were not worn in 90 percent of all boating-related deaths.

Additionally, drowning can occur after diving into shallow or obstacle-filled water. A head or spine injury from striking the bottom or striking an unseen object can render injured individuals unable to save themselves.

## Near-Drowning/Secondary Drowning

**near-drowning** survival for at least 24 hours after being suffocated by submersion in water.

**Near-drowning** is defined as survival for more than 24 hours after being suffocated by submersion. In this case, the patient may initially present in respiratory or cardiac arrest but is resuscitated. Patients who die within 24–72 hours are said to die from secondary drowning. Of the estimated 15,000–70,000 near-drownings that occur each year in the United States, approximately 15 percent die from secondary drowning.

A variety of water conditions can complicate drowning and near-drowning. Among the conditions of greatest concern are water temperature (cold or warm) and the water's salinity (whether it is fresh water or salt water). In addition, debris (sand or other small particles) and algae and other microorganisms may be suspended in the water and can be aspirated.

Water temperature plays a significant role in morbidity and mortality because the survival rate is much higher for cold-water submersions than for warm-water submersions. The reason is that cold-water submersion triggers the mammalian diving reflex (previously described), and the resulting bradycardia and preservation of oxygen reserves can increase the survival rate of submersion victims. Even though cold-water submersion can occur at any time of year, most incidents occur during the winter and are typically associated with falling through the ice (Figure 29-8■). Cold-water submersions during the summer typically involve high mountain lakes, rivers,

**Figure 29-8** The difficulty of cold-water rescues is enhanced by hypothermia and potentially by the breaking apart of the ice.

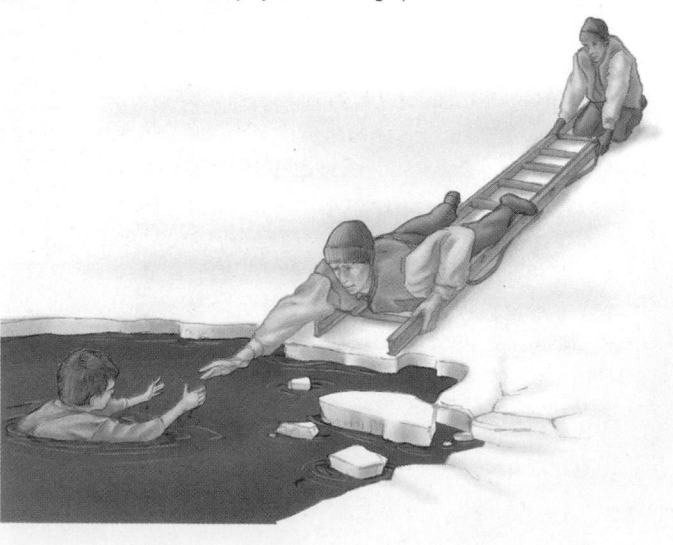

and streams. Submersion in warm or hot water (in bath tubs or hot tubs) can cause vasodilation and quickly lead to distributive shock.

Water salinity affects the movement of water within the body. Because fresh water has a lower **tonicity** (a lower salt concentration) than alveolar fluid, aspirated water moves into the lung tissue and then into the bloodstream, causing low blood sodium (hyponatremia) and increased blood volume (hypervolemia). Note, however, that an adult male would have to aspirate more than 7 liters of water for these effects to occur. Wet drowning will normally occur first with the aspiration of 7 liters of water.

Conversely, salt water has a higher tonicity than the water in body tissues. Thus, aspiration of salt water causes fluid to leave the bloodstream and enter the lungs, causing hypovolemia and hypernatremia. Again, large volumes of salt water must be aspirated for significant fluid shifts to occur. The finding that only 15 percent of drowning victims have electrolyte abnormalities suggests that massive fluid shifts are uncommon. Because few people drown from large volumes of aspirated water, the salinity of the water is less important than the temperature of it.

Water, especially moving water, contains millions of suspended particles per liter that may be aspirated, causing a host of problems depending on the particles' sizes and composition. Dirt, rocks, and other inorganic debris may become lodged anywhere along the air passageways, reducing airflow and oxygenation. Pathogens such as bacteria or parasites such as *Giardia* may be aspirated deep into the delicate pulmonary tissues, resulting in local or systemic infections. Organic matter such as algae, seaweed, and other aquatic life can also block or damage the lower airways.

## Barotrauma

**Barotrauma** is a form of trauma that is caused by the difference in the pressure within air-filled structures of the body (e.g., the lungs, intestines, and the middle ear) and the pressure of the external environment. Such pressure differences result from the expansion or compression of the gas within those body structures. If the pressure within the structure becomes too great, the structure can rupture; a reduction in pressure can create a vacuum, which also causes medical problems.

Barotrauma is a common disorder among divers and can occur during rapid descent or ascent. According to the Divers Alert Network (DAN), an international organization that provides information to divers and rescuers, approximately 1,000 cases of DCI (decompression illness) occur each year.

There are three basic types of dive injuries with which OEC Technicians should be familiar: decompression sickness, arterial gas embolism, and squeeze.

### Decompression Sickness

**Decompression sickness**, also known as DCS or more commonly as "the bends," is a buildup of nitrogen bubbles within the body (Figure 29-9■). It occurs primarily in scuba divers who ascend too rapidly, but it may also occur if a diver travels to high altitude (by either plane or car) too quickly after diving. DCS results when dissolved nitrogen within the blood forms bubbles.

To illustrate this process, consider a bottle of carbonated soda. Dissolved within the liquid soda is carbon dioxide ($CO_2$), a gas that gives the liquid its characteristic "fizz." The $CO_2$ cannot be seen because it is under pressure. Once the bottle is opened, however, the pressure within the bottle is rapidly released, causing $CO_2$ bubbles to form. In a diver who has ascended from a depth, dissolved nitrogen in the blood forms bubbles as the pressure of

**tonicity** a property of solutions that relates to the concentration of solutes (such as salt) it contains, and how the water in a solution moves across a cell membrane; water in a solution crosses a cell membrane from the side that has the lower tonicity (a hypotonic solution) to the side that has the higher tonicity (a hypertonic solution); pure water is hypotonic to the solution within cells because that solution contains salts.

⊕ **29-5** List three types of barotrauma and indicate their causes.

**barotrauma** trauma that is caused by differences in pressure between the body and the environment.

**decompression sickness** formation of nitrogen bubbles in tissues from a too-rapid ascent.

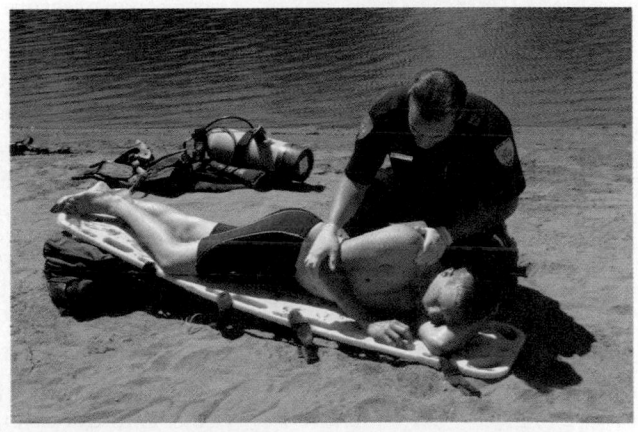

**Figure 29-9** This patient has decompression sickness ("the bends") and has been placed in the recovery position while awaiting ambulance transport to a medical facility.

| Table 29-2 | Signs and Symptoms of Decompression Sickness (DCS) |
|---|---|
| **Body System** | **Signs and Symptoms** |
| Integumentary | Itching, rash, swelling, discoloration |
| Musculoskeletal | Mild to severe joint pain (e.g., shoulder, elbows, knees); pain may radiate down arms/legs; low back pain |
| Audiovestibular | Nausea/vomiting, ringing in the ears, hearing loss, dizziness, lack of balance (including difficulty walking) |
| Nervous | Headache, numbness, difficulty speaking or swallowing, extreme fatigue, visual disturbances, difficulty urinating |
| Respiratory | Shortness of breath, severe cough |
| Cardiovascular | Chest pain, irregular pulse, shock, cardiac arrest |

the water is reduced by ascent. These bubbles then migrate from the bloodstream and into the tissues, causing severe muscle and joint pain. Sometimes, large nitrogen bubbles can become emboli and block blood flow to critical organs.

DCS is further divided into two subcategories, based on the severity of symptoms. Type I DCS is the less serious form of decompression sickness and typically resolves within a few minutes (Table 29-2■). Type II DCS can be immediately life threatening and affects multiple body systems, including the pulmonary, cardiovascular, vestibular, and nervous systems.

### Arterial Gas Embolism

**arterial gas embolism (AGE)** a condition that occurs immediately after rapid ascent in which air bubbles enter the bloodstream from a ruptured alveolus and lodge in an artery.

**Arterial gas embolism (AGE)** is a serious medical problem caused by a rapid ascent during which a diver does not exhale properly. When this occurs, the gas within the lungs expands and the alveoli rupture. The air from the ruptured portions of the lung then enters the pleural space, mediastinum, or bloodstream, resulting in a pneumothorax, pneumomediastinum, or air emboli, respectively (Figure 29-10■). According to DAN, approximately 6 percent of all diving problems reported to DAN involve AGE.

### Squeeze and Reverse Squeeze

*Squeeze* is a generic term used to describe the effects of too much external pressure on various parts of the body. Reverse squeeze occurs when there is too much pressure within a body compartment or organ. Squeeze can affect the external ear if the canal between the middle ear and the nasopharynx (the Eustachian tube) is obstructed when descending to depth. The obstruction prevents the pressure in the middle ear from increasing to equilibrate with the pressure outside the eardrum. The resulting excessive pressure on the outside of the eardrum causes it to rupture. In reverse squeeze, the opposite occurs. During ascent, the eardrum can rupture from too much pressure in the middle ear pushing outward. Both situations result in severe ear pain. You may have experienced the sensation of pressure buildup or release (without the eardrum rupturing) during ascent or descent in an airline flight. This is what makes some small children cry while flying as they cannot equilibrate the pressure as well as adults can. Inner ear barotrauma is generally caused by severe pressure changes between the middle and inner ear and most commonly occurs during rapid ascent.

Other forms of squeeze include sinus squeeze, in which trapped air within the sinus cavity expands, and tooth squeeze, in which air trapped in a cavity or a filling expands. Both can occur during ascent or descent. "Mask" reverse squeeze occurs inside a diver's face mask upon descent, causing a suction-like effect that can cause the blood vessels in the eyes to rupture.

**Figure 29-10** A diagram of an air embolus within an artery.

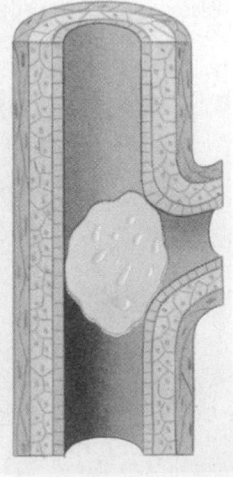

Air Embolus

## Nitrogen Narcosis

Nitrogen narcosis, or "rapture of the deep," is a condition that generally affects divers who descend to depths greater than 100 feet (30 m), but it has been reported to occur at depths as shallow as 33 feet. This condition is characterized by altered responsiveness and impaired judgment, resulting in effects that are similar to alcohol intoxication. The effects increase in severity the deeper the diver descends. Unless it is recognized and steps are taken to reverse the effects, nitrogen narcosis can result in irrational behavior, such as taking off one's oxygen regulator, which can rapidly lead to death. The exact cause of nitrogen narcosis is not fully understood, but is thought to be related to the effects of nitrogen on nerve transmission. The condition is easily reversed by ascending, sometimes as little as 10 feet.

## Swimmer's Ear

Swimmer's ear is an acute bacterial infection of the external auditory (ear) canal that occurs when the skin barrier within the canal is disrupted, often by remaining wet for a prolonged period of time (Figure 29-11■). Other causes of swimmer's ear include sticking an object such as a finger or cotton-tipped swab into the ear, the repeated use of ear plugs, and dry, cracked skin. Patients usually present with severe ear pain, a yellowish discharge from the ear, and tenderness upon pushing on the tragus (the anatomical bump in front of the ear canal). Children and teenagers are more prone to this disorder, as are individuals with diabetes and immune system disorders. Most of the many preventative treatments available are mildly acidic or alcohol-based solutions that make the ear canal inhospitable to bacteria.

## Breath Holding

In an effort to travel farther or deeper under water, swimmers will sometimes intentionally hyperventilate to dramatically increase the amount of oxygen in their lungs and allow them to hold their breath longer (Figure 29-12■). Unfortunately, hyperventilating also decreases the amount of carbon dioxide in the lungs, which removes the body's stimulus to breathe. As a result, the person may pass out and drown. This condition most commonly affects children and young adults, and swimming pools are the most frequent setting.

**Figure 29-12** Hyperventilation and then breath holding entail the risk of losing consciousness and drowning.
Copyright David Peart/Dorling Kindersley Media Library

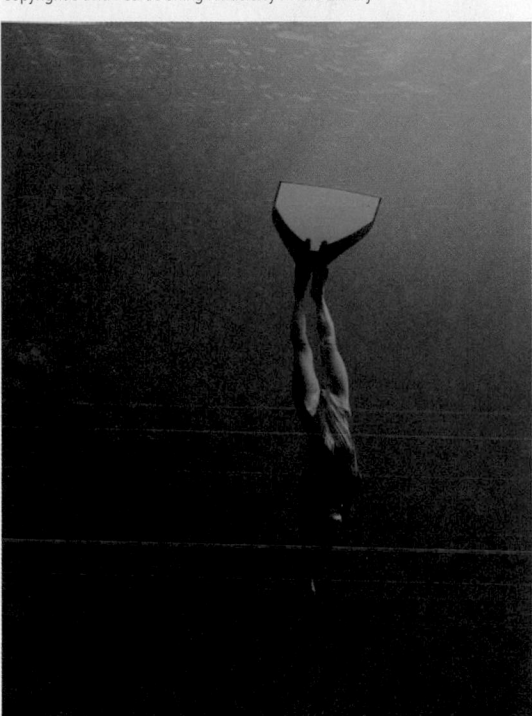

**Figure 29-11** The external ear (auditory) canal, the site at which swimmer's ear occurs.

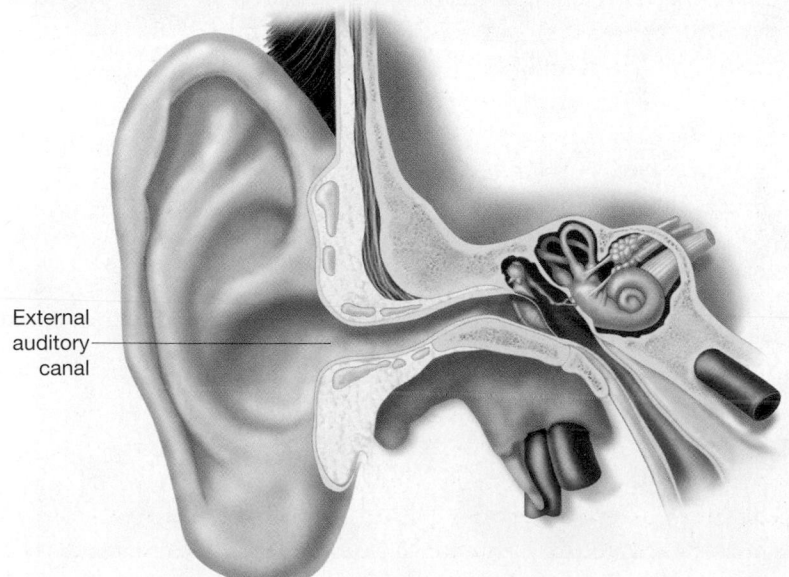

External auditory canal

## Trauma

Accidental injury in and around the water is common and results in a variety of injury patterns well known to OEC Technicians. Soft-tissue injuries are the most common type of water-related injury encountered, followed by neurological injuries involving the cervical spine or the upper thoracic spine. Injury sources include sharp rocks, sticks, abrasive surfaces, and fish hooks. Spine injuries are usually caused by diving into shallow water.

Each year, approximately 6,500 diving-related injuries are treated in the United States, of which 5 percent require hospitalization. Orthopedic injuries, including fractures and joint dislocations, are frequently encountered and often result from falling onto a hard or uneven surface or from being violently twisted while in swiftly moving water (Figure 29-13■). Boating accidents, especially those involving powered watercraft, can produce many of the same injury patterns observed with other high-speed, deceleration-type injuries, such as those associated with snow machine, ATV, and automobile collisions.

## Injuries by Aquatic Animals

The waters of the world contain a great variety of aquatic life that can inflict serious traumatic or toxicological injuries to humans. Fresh water fish such as northern pike, walleye, or muskellunge have many sharp teeth, whereas species such as bass, sunfish, and crappie have sharp dorsal spines, all of which can cause a variety of soft-tissue injuries. Saltwater animals such as sharks, barracuda, and moray eels have powerful jaws and razor-sharp teeth and can inflict serious, even life-threatening wounds (Figure 29-14■). Turtles have powerful jaws and some species, such as snapping turtles

**Figure 29-13** In rapidly flowing water, injuries can result from striking objects below the surface and from twisting caused by the current.

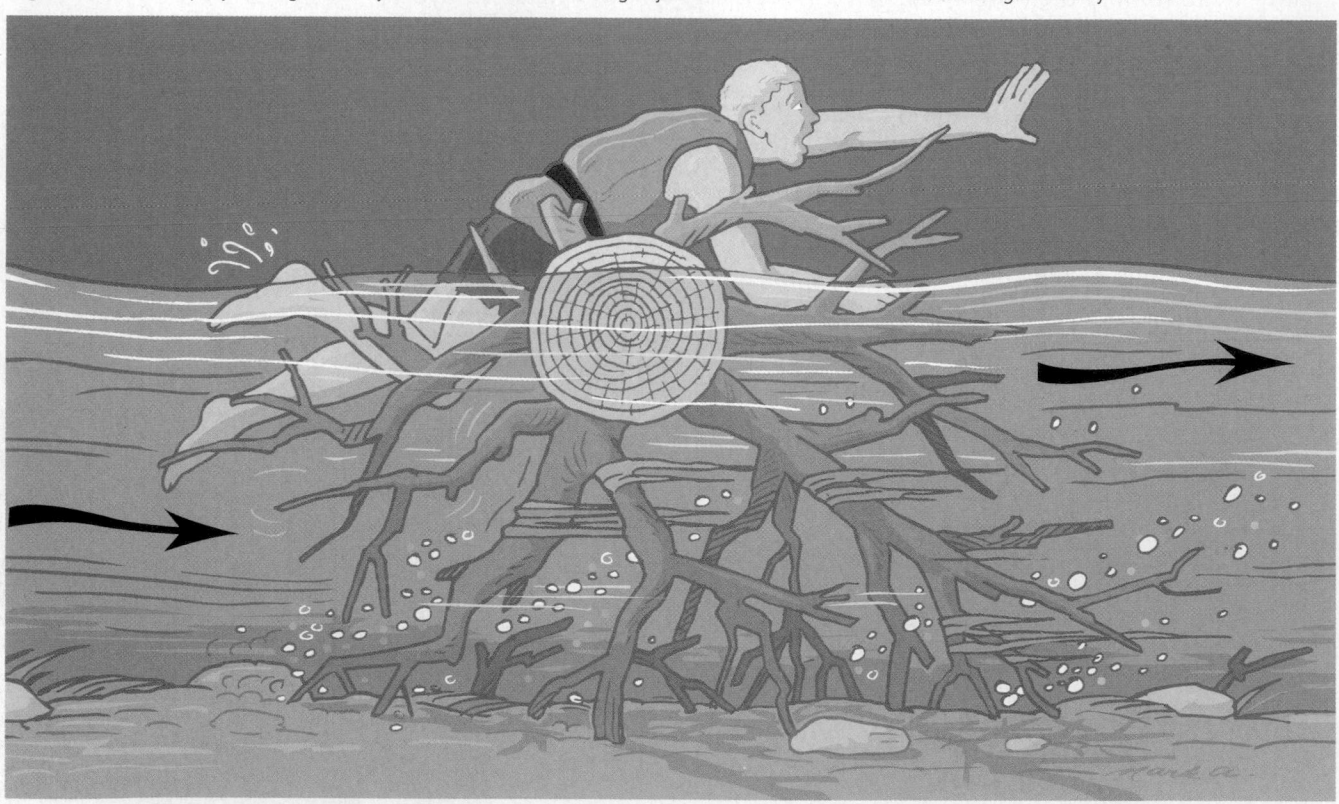

and sea turtles, can deliver bone-crushing bites. Even relatively small marine animals such as sea urchins or jellyfish can inflict neurologic, cardiovascular, or dermatologic injuries from toxins, stings, or spines. For more information about marine animals, see Chapter 27, Plant and Animal Emergencies.

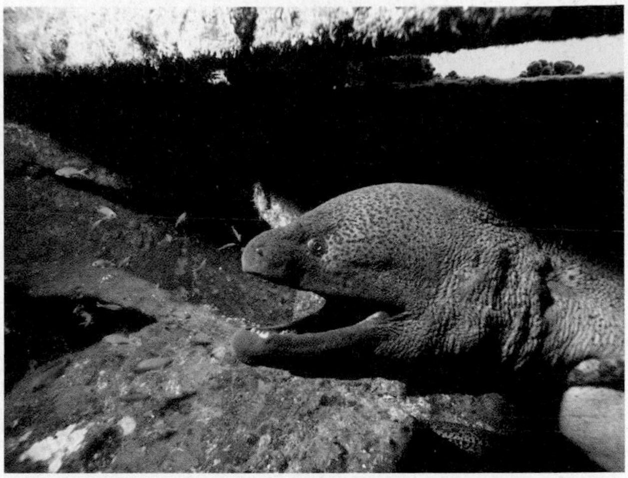

## Aggravation of Existing Conditions

Water-based sports such as swimming, white-water rafting, and scuba diving are physically demanding activities that increase the body's metabolic needs. As a result, they can worsen underlying medical disorders, especially cardiac, pulmonary, and diabetic conditions. Water-related problems in people with existing conditions can be more severe because of the medical disorder.

# Preventing Water Emergencies

As with other sports, water-based activities carry certain inherent risks of injury. Fortunately, many of these risks can be mitigated or prevented altogether by heeding the following recommendations:

+ Avoid alcohol when around water.
+ Use proper safety equipment, including approved personal floatation devices (PFDs) (Figure 29-15■).
+ Never swim alone.
+ Monitor the activities of anyone who is in the water (Figure 29-16■).
+ Never enter swiftly moving water.
+ Confirm water depth before diving; never dive into water that is not deep enough.
+ Check the thickness of the ice before traversing it.
+ Scuba dive conservatively; ascend slowly while breathing normally.
+ Watch for rip currents.

**Figure 29-14** Many varieties of aquatic life, including this moray eel, may inflict serious, even life-threatening injuries.
Copyright David Peart/Dorling Kindersley Media Library

**⊕ 29-6** List nine ways in which a water-based emergency may be prevented.

**Figure 29-15** These arm flotation devices are *not* approved personal floatation devices (PFD).
Copyright Zena Holloway/Dorling Kindersley Media Library

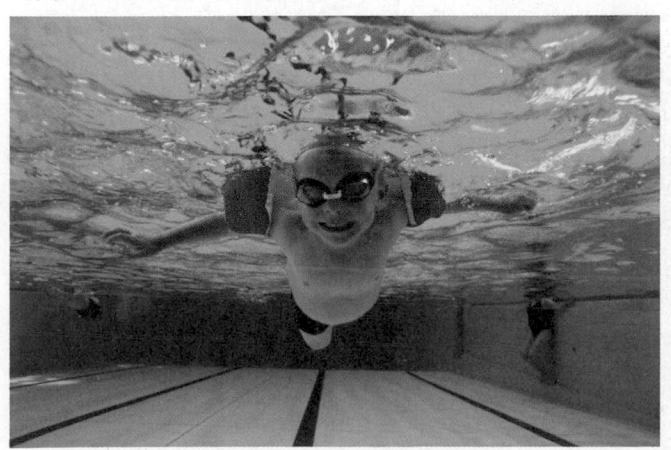

**Figure 29-16** Continually monitor the activities of anyone who is in the water.
Copyright Linda Whitwam/Dorling Kindersley Media Library

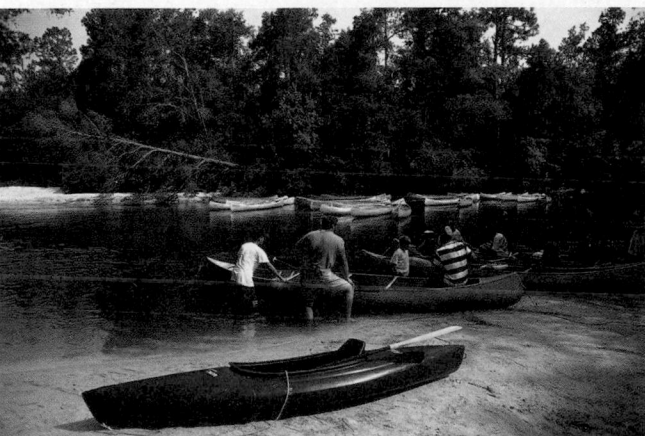

# STOP, THINK, UNDERSTAND

## Multiple Choice

Choose the correct answer.

1. Which of the following statements correctly describes what may happen in "mask" reverse squeeze? _____
   a. The mask may work loose while descending, and pressure may cause blood vessels in the eyes to rupture.
   b. The mask may cause a suction-like effect upon descent, which can cause the blood vessels in the eyes to rupture.
   c. The mask may cause a suction-like effect upon ascent, which can cause the blood vessels in the eyes to rupture.
   d. The mask may work loose while ascending, and pressure may cause blood vessels in the eyes to rupture.

2. Which of the following phenomena explains why the rate of survival in cold-water drowning is much higher than that in warm-water drowning? _____
   a. nitrogen narcosis
   b. Boyle's law
   c. barotrauma
   d. the mammalian diving reflex

3. For a submersion injury to occur, which of the following anatomical parts must be submerged? _____
   a. legs
   b. airway
   c. upper torso
   d. neck

4. Males are _____ times more likely to drown than are females.
   a. 2
   b. 3
   c. 4
   d. 5

5. Which of the following conditions is *not* one of the three basic types of barotrauma? _____
   a. reverse rush
   b. squeeze
   c. arterial gas embolism
   d. decompression sickness

6. Which of the following statements describes the easiest way to reverse nitrogen narcosis? _____
   a. Rapidly descend 10 feet.
   b. Ascend, sometimes as little as 10 feet.
   c. Stay at the same depth until your body adjusts.
   d. None of the above.

7. In the United States, _____ percent of all drowning deaths occurs in fresh water and, _____ percent occur in swimming pools.
   a. 50, 25
   b. 50, 20
   c. 90, 75
   d. 90, 50

8. Which of the following recommendations does *not* help mitigate or prevent water emergencies? _____
   a. Check the thickness of the ice before traversing it.
   b. Never enter swiftly moving water.
   c. Swim alone only if you are familiar with this body of water.
   d. Avoid alcohol when around water.

## Fill in the Blank

If you have a membrane that is permeable to water with salt water on one side and fresh water on the side, water will cross the membrane from the _____ solution to the _____ solution.

 **CASE UPDATE**

You assist in removing the patient from the water while maintaining C-spine precautions. You direct some of your companions to summon help and then immediately begin rescue breathing using a pocket mask.

*What should you do now?*

# Patient Assessment

The assessment of patients with a water-related emergency is not substantially different from the assessment of patients with any other emergency. First and foremost is ensuring the safety of yourself and others. Safety measures may include donning a personal floatation device, a helmet, and other safety equipment as directed by your area management or as the situation requires—and, as always, Standard Precautions. If you are not trained in water rescue techniques or do not have the proper equipment, wait for the arrival of specialized water rescuers (Figure 29-18■).

Once the scene is safe, quickly assess the patient's ABCDs and correct all potential threats to life before proceeding to a secondary assessment. In any submersion injury, carefully assess and protect the spine to prevent additional neurologic injury. Whenever possible, this should be initiated before the person is removed from the water. It may be easier to apply a cervical collar and place the patient onto a backboard in shallow water than to perform these procedures after you have removed the person from the water.

**29-7** List the signs and symptoms of the following water-related emergencies:

- arterial gas embolism
- decompression sickness

**Figure 29-17** Ensuring the safety of the rescuer(s) is an essential part of any water-related emergency.

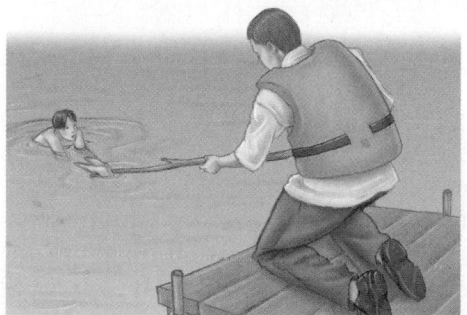

Reach

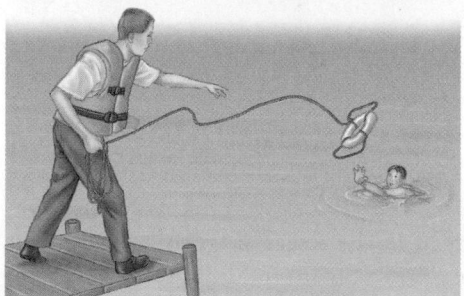

Throw

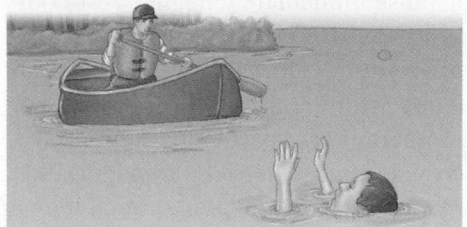

Then go

**Figure 29-18** If you are not trained in water rescue, wait for professional rescuers.

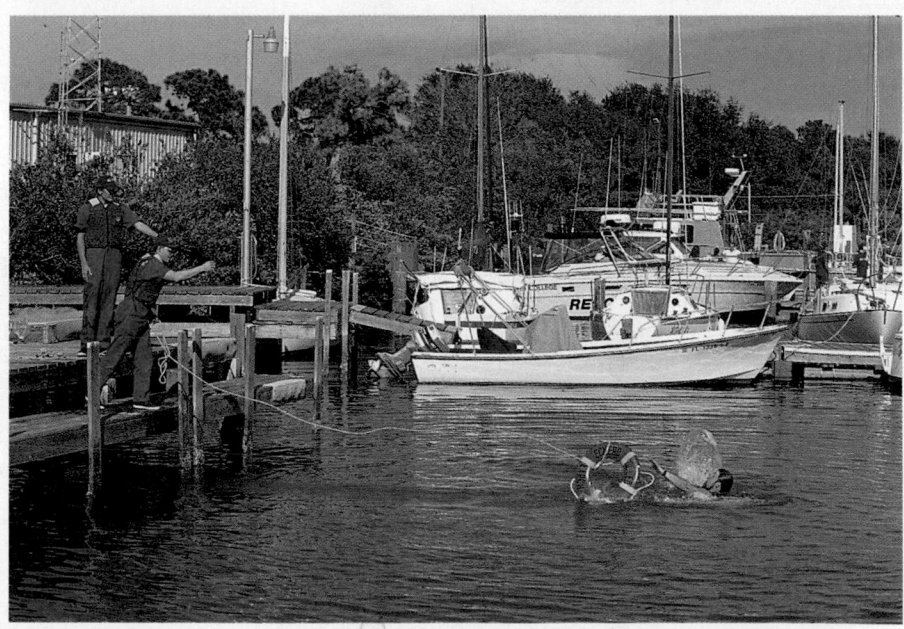

Unless the patient has serious or life-threatening injuries, perform a complete secondary assessment using the DCAP-BTLS mnemonic. Additionally, perform a complete neurologic exam on all non-critical patients. Assess the vital signs, level of responsiveness, skin condition, and capillary refill frequently because each may provide early indications of the presence of a serious underlying injury. As part of the history, attempt to obtain as much information as possible about what has occurred, including how long the person was submerged, water temperature and salinity, and the person's appearance immediately after being removed from the water. If possible, determine if the patient has a pre-existing medical condition or is taking any medications.

Carefully assess any patient who appears fine after a near-drowning event because the onset of symptoms may be delayed. Listen to the patient's breathing for any unusual noises. Patients with a history of recent scuba diving or deep-water snorkeling should be further assessed for possible AGE or DCS.

Arterial gas embolism may present with the following signs and symptoms:

+ Itchy, mottled skin
+ Bloody frothy sputum
+ Altered LOC, confusion
+ Dyspnea
+ Chest pain
+ Muscle and joint pain
+ Blurred vision
+ Nausea, vomiting
+ Numbness, paralysis
+ Decreased coordination
+ Staggering gait

The signs and symptoms of decompression sickness ("the bends") depend on the severity of the injury. Type I DCS is characterized by joint pain, itchy or burning skin, and a skin rash that is blotchy in nature. The pain can be mild to intense and usually resolves within a short period of time, often within 10 minutes of onset. Type II DCS can be immediately life threatening and present with severe dyspnea, hypovolemic shock, spinal paralysis, or coma.

**⊕ 29-8** Describe how to manage a patient who has suffered a water-related emergency.

## Patient Management

The treatment of a patient who has suffered a water-related injury depends on the nature of the injury and the severity of the patient's symptoms. Remove all patients from the water as quickly as possible. Rescue breaths may be given in the water; however chest compressions are usually not practical in the water (Figure 29-19■). For any patient who has a submersion injury, after removal from the water, open the airway and simultaneously check for breathing and a carotid pulse. If there is no breathing or pulse immediately begin chest compressions in accordance with the 2010 CPR standards. If the patient has a pulse but is not breathing, immediately begin rescue breathing. There is no evidence that water in the respiratory system acts as an obstructive foreign body, so do not attempt to remove it. Call for advanced medical providers and transportation as soon as possible. For any patient with a possible spinal injury, initiate spinal precautions, preferably while the patient is still in the water (Figure 29-20■).

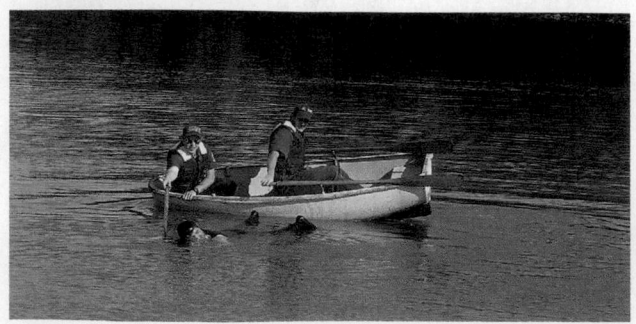

**Figure 29-19** Remove submersion patients from the water as quickly as possible; rescue breathing may be performed in the water, but chest compressions are not effective in the water.

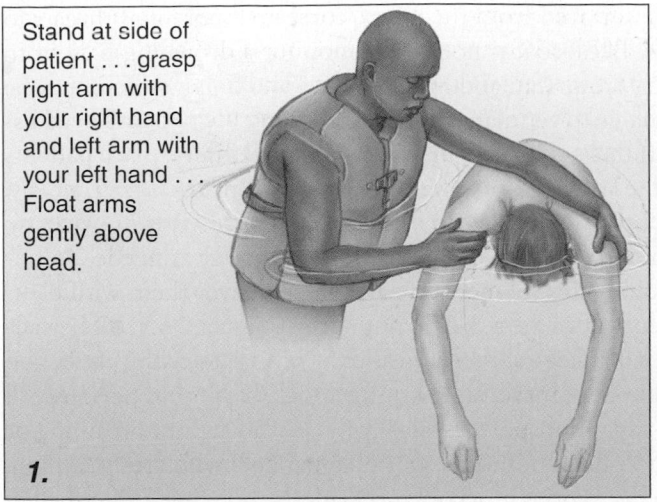

1. Stand at side of patient . . . grasp right arm with your right hand and left arm with your left hand . . . Float arms gently above head.

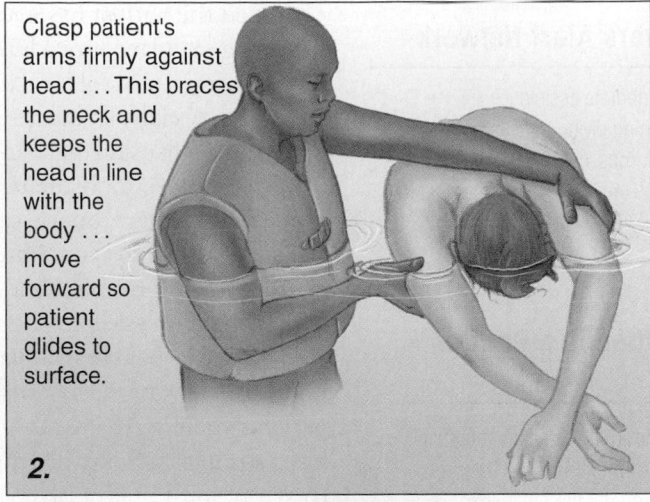

2. Clasp patient's arms firmly against head . . . This braces the neck and keeps the head in line with the body . . . move forward so patient glides to surface.

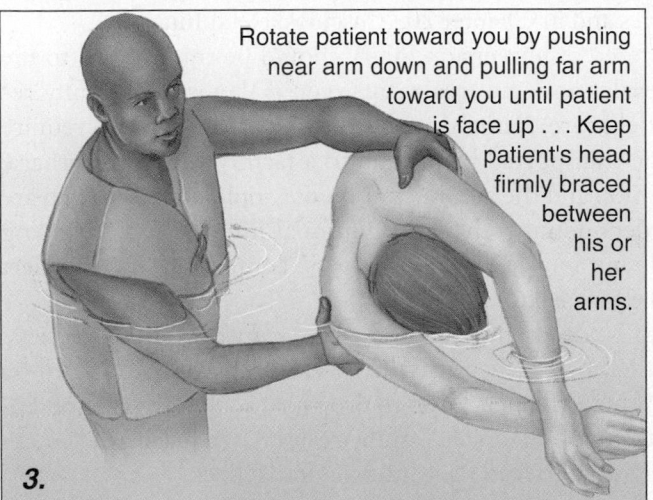

3. Rotate patient toward you by pushing near arm down and pulling far arm toward you until patient is face up . . . Keep patient's head firmly braced between his or her arms.

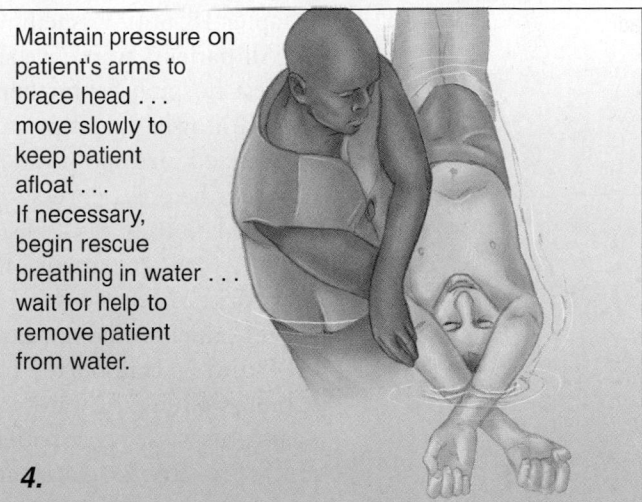

4. Maintain pressure on patient's arms to brace head . . . move slowly to keep patient afloat . . . If necessary, begin rescue breathing in water . . . wait for help to remove patient from water.

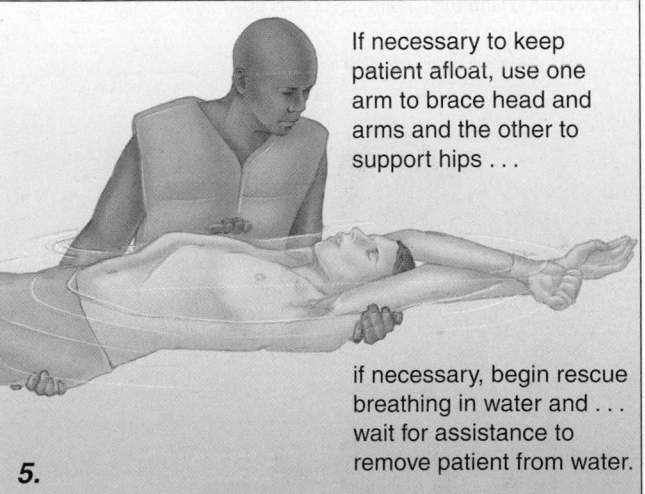

5. If necessary to keep patient afloat, use one arm to brace head and arms and the other to support hips . . . if necessary, begin rescue breathing in water and . . . wait for assistance to remove patient from water.

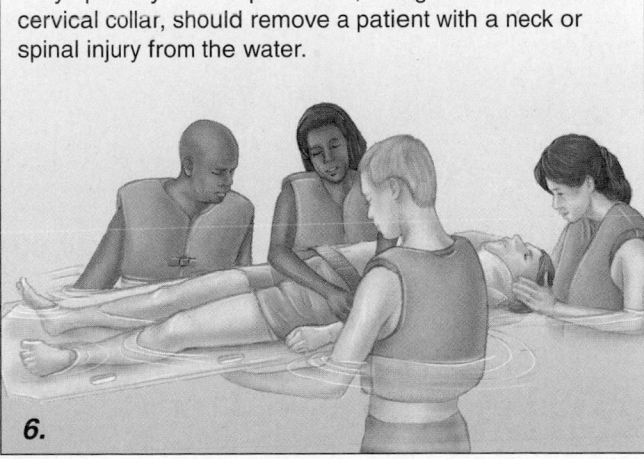

6. Only specially trained personnel, using a backboard and cervical collar, should remove a patient with a neck or spinal injury from the water.

**Figure 29-20** Water rescue technique; note the precautions for a spinal injury.

**Divers Alert Network**

NOTE

For immediate assistance concerning diving injuries or barotraumas, call 1-919-684-4326 or 1-800-446-2671.

**When Is a Patient Dead?**

NOTE

Even though death is no laughing matter, remember that: They're not dead until they're warm and dead!

Once the patient has been removed from the water, correct all potential threats to life using standard procedures. Because it is not uncommon for a drowning patient to have a foreign body obstructing the airway, abdominal thrusts and finger sweeps may be needed, especially if you are unable to ventilate after repositioning the patient's head using the jaw-thrust maneuver. If there is no concern for spinal cord injury, place patients onto their sides to facilitate the drainage of water and debris from the upper airway. Once a patient is properly secured to a spine board and a cervical collar is in place, tip the spine board to allow water and debris to drain. Suction the airway as needed.

As soon as possible, thoroughly dry submersion patients and cover them with blankets, jackets, or a sleeping bag to reduce the risk of hypothermia (Figure 29-21■). If available, wrap the patient in a space blanket to prevent further heat loss. Place the patient on high-flow oxygen via a nonrebreather mask, and treat for shock, if present. Seriously ill patients require ALS care and rapid transport, especially those who are not breathing or have a pneumothorax or tension pneumothorax. In stable patients who are breathing, treat any soft-tissue or orthopedic injuries in accordance with the principles described in Chapter 18, Soft-Tissue Injuries and in Chapter 20, Musculoskeletal Injuries.

All patients who have suffered a submersion injury should be transported to the nearest hospital for further evaluation and treatment, even if they seem to fully recover following appropriate field care. Patients with suspected AGE or DCS require specialized care and should be transported by ground to a facility with a hyperbaric chamber because repressurization and the administration of supplemental oxygen are required to treat these disorders definitively. For additional information regarding the emergent treatment of diving injuries or barotraumas, contact the Divers Alert Network, 24 hours a day, 7 days a week.

All patients who appear to be dead after removal from *cold* water should receive CPR and be transported to the hospital because the severe bradycardia induced by submersion in cold water can cause the heart rate to drop so low that the person appears pulseless. These patients can often be successfully resuscitated, even after an extended time under water, and go on to lead healthy, productive lives.

**Figure 29-21** Dry off and warm the patient as soon as possible to reduce the risk of hypothermia and shock.
Copyright Andy Crawford and Steve Gorton/Dorling Kindersley Media Library

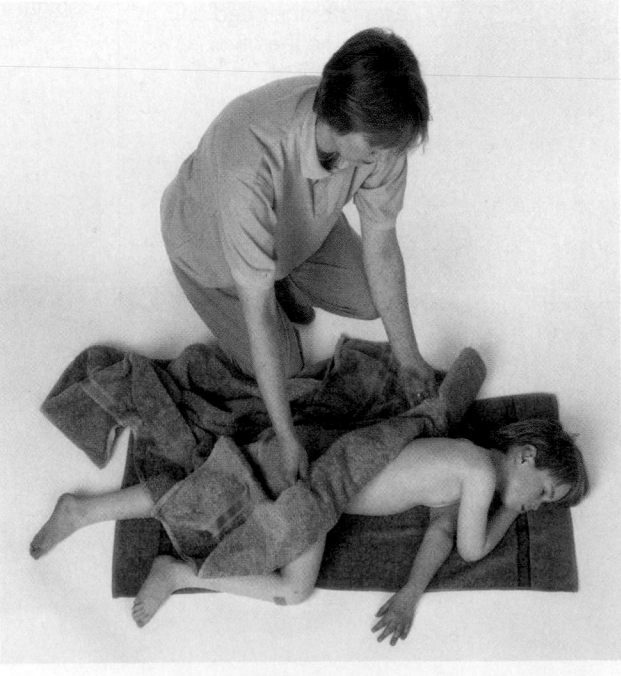

# STOP, THINK, UNDERSTAND

## Multiple Choice
Choose the correct answer.

1. Which of the following findings is *not* a sign or a symptom of arterial gas embolism? _____
   a. blurred vision
   c. muscle/joint pain
   b. paralysis
   d. bleeding from the ears

2. When gathering the history for a submersion patient, which of the following pieces of information is *not* relevant? _____
   a. how long the patient was submerged
   b. the salinity of the water
   c. how long the patient waited to go swimming after eating
   d. the water temperature

3. What is your first priority when assessing a victim during a water rescue? _____
   a. making sure the patient is breathing
   b. making sure the patient has a pulse
   c. making sure the patient has an airway
   d. ensuring your own safety

4. In Type I decompressions sickness (DCS), the pain usually resolves within _____ minutes.
   a. 25
   c. 10
   b. 15
   d. 5

5. Which of the following terms is another name for decompression sickness? _____
   a. "The bubbles"
   c. "The gases"
   b. "The bends"
   d. "The folds"

6. Which of the following findings is *not* a sign or a symptom of Type II decompression sickness? _____
   a. spinal paralysis
   c. shivering
   b. hypovolemic shock
   d. severe dyspnea

7. Cold-water drowning may cause severe _____, which can cause the heart rate to drop so low that the person appears pulseless.
   a. bradycardia
   c. ventricular fibrillation
   b. tachycardia
   d. atrial fibrillation

## List

List three precautions that should be considered during water rescues.

1. _____
2. _____
3. _____

 **CASE DISPOSITION**

You continue rescue breathing while others dry the patient off and cover him with towels, all the while ensuring that full spinal immobilization is maintained. Within a few minutes, he starts to breathe on his own. Other rescuers who have arrived transport the patient to a trauma center, where he is diagnosed with a cervical spine fracture. Although his road to recovery will be long, he is expected to regain full neurologic function after spinal surgery.

# ⛨ Chapter Review

## Chapter Summary

OEC Technicians may see a wide range of medical and traumatic emergencies as a result of water-related outdoor recreation activities. Water emergencies can occur any time and anywhere and may be life threatening. Additionally, OEC Technicians must be prepared to manage a water-related emergency even in settings that lack a body of water because drowning can occur in a bathtub, a toilet, a bucket of water, or a shallow puddle.

The treatment of a water-related emergency is generally no different than that provided to any other trauma patient. It centers on correcting any deficiencies involving the ABCDs and treating the patient for hypothermia and shock, if present. Drowning is among the most common forms of water emergency and must be quickly managed to prevent a lethal outcome. Due to the body's innate physiological functions, a person may be successfully resuscitated, even after being submerged in cold water for a long period of time.

Conditions such as barotraumas are especially dangerous and present unique challenges in that they generally require urgent transport to a hospital, preferably to a hospital that is capable of definitively managing diving injuries. All patients who suffer a submersion injury should be transported to the hospital for follow-up, even if they appear normal, because complications can arise several hours or even days after the incident and may be mitigated by prompt treatment.

## Remember...

1. Spinal cord injury should be suspected in any patient with a submersion injury to which there was no witness.
2. All near-drowning patients should be transported to a hospital.
3. Consider DCS and AGE in all patients with a history of diving.
4. Provide high-flow oxygen to all patients who have suffered a submersion injury.
5. The mammalian diving reflex may enable a person to survive prolonged submersion.
6. They're not dead until they're warm and dead!

## Chapter Questions

### Multiple Choice

Choose the correct answer.

1. Which of the following statements explains the phrase "They're not dead until they're warm and dead"?_____
   a. Warm-water drowning victims have a better chance of survival.
   b. Patients who appear dead at the scene probably are.
   c. Cold water causes the heart rate to drop so low that the victim appears pulseless.
   d. Cold water causes the heart rate to drop so low that the victim must be warmed up rapidly.

2. Which of the following conditions is *not* among the water emergencies an OEC Technician may encounter? _____
   a. swimmer's ear
   b. nitrogen narcosis
   c. barotraumas
   d. inverse "bends"

3. Which gas law explains that as a diver goes deeper under water, the partial pressure from nitrogen in comparison to oxygen in the volume of air in the lungs greatly increases?_____
   a. Boyle's law
   b. Henry's law
   c. Dalton's law
   d. Newton's law

**4.** Which gas law means that as a diver goes deeper under water, the pressure from nitrogen greatly increases? _____

    **a.** Boyle's law                        **c.** Dalton's law

    **b.** Henry's law                        **d.** Newton's law

**5.** Individuals who die within _____ hours after removal from the water are said to have died from secondary drowning.

    **a.** 12–24                            **c.** 24–72

    **b.** 24–36                            **d.** 36–72

**6.** Divers encounter another atmosphere of pressure for every _____ feet they descend.

    **a.** 23                               **c.** 33

    **b.** 28                               **d.** 41

**7.** Alcohol intoxication is involved in more than _____ percent of all drowning deaths in adolescents and adults.

    **a.** 40                               **c.** 55

    **b.** 50                               **d.** 65

**8.** In breath holding, swimmers sometimes intentionally hyperventilate, which _____ and may remove the body's stimulus to breathe.

    **a.** decreases the oxygen and increases the carbon dioxide in their lungs

    **b.** increases the oxygen and increases the carbon dioxide in their lungs

    **c.** decreases the oxygen and decreases the carbon dioxide in their lungs

    **d.** increases the oxygen and decreases the carbon dioxide in their lungs

**9.** When dealing with a submersion injury, when is the best time to apply a C-collar and place the patient on a backboard? _____

    **a.** After the patient has been brought out of the water.

    **b.** In shallow water, before the patient is on the shore.

    **c.** In deeper water, so the patient can be moved safely.

    **d.** Water depth is irrelevant; use the C-collar and the backboard wherever they are located.

## Short Answer

List in order and explain the four water rescue methods.

_____

_____

_____

_____

## List

**1.** Excluding drowning, list seven different types of water emergencies.

    **1.** _____

    **2.** _____

    **3.** _____

    **4.** _____

    **5.** _____

    **6.** _____

    **7.** _____

2. List the ten events in the pathophysiology of dry drowning.

1. _____

2. _____

3. _____

4. _____

5. _____

6. _____

7. _____

8. _____

9. _____

10. _____

## Matching

Match each of the following terms with its description.

_____ **1.** arterial gas embolism (AGE)

_____ **2.** barotraumas

_____ **3.** Boyle's law

_____ **4.** Dalton's law

_____ **5.** decompression sickness (DCS)

_____ **6.** drowning

_____ **7.** Henry's law

_____ **8.** laryngospasm

_____ **9.** near-drowning

_____ **10.** secondary drowning

**a.** states that the amount of a gas that will be absorbed by water increases as the gas pressure increases

**b.** the formation of nitrogen bubbles in tissues from too rapid of an ascent; usually occurs hours after ascent

**c.** suffocation by submersion in water

**d.** states that when pressure decreases, the volume of gas will increase, and vice versa

**e.** survival for at least 24 hours after being suffocated by submersion in water

**f.** spasm of the vocal cords that prevents air movement through the respiratory tract

**g.** refers to patients who die within 24–72 hours after being suffocated by submersion in water

**h.** a condition following a rapid ascent in which air bubbles from a ruptured alveolus get lodged in the bloodstream

**i.** trauma that results from pressure differences between the body and the external environment

**j.** states that the total pressure exerted by a gas mixture equals the sum of the partial pressure of each gas in the mixture

## Scenario

*You just started the day shift when you get a call that a snowmaker driving a snowmobile fell through the ice at the pond. You arrive to find the patient head down in about 5 feet of icy water. Additional OEC Technicians are responding with the AED, $O_2$, a backboard, and a trauma sled. You make a request for an ALS ambulance.*

*Two other snowmakers have tied ropes around their waists, secured the other ends of the ropes to a tree, and crawled to the opening in the ice. They grab the victim by the feet, pull him out of the water, and then drag him by the collar of his jacket to a safe position on the shore. The two rescuers estimate the time the patient spent in the frigid water to be no more than 15 minutes.*

*You and another OEC Technician remove the patient's snowmobile helmet and open the airway with a modified jaw-thrust maneuver. The patient is not breathing and is pulseless.*

**1.** After ensuring scene safety for a drowning victim with possible trauma, OEC Technicians should first_____
   **a.** apply the AED and shock the patient immediately.
   **b.** protect the patient's neck and spine and initiate CPR.
   **c.** apply a cervical collar and place the patient on a backboard.
   **d.** prepare to "load and go."

**2.** If after 2 minutes of CPR the patient is reassessed and neither breathing nor a pulse is detected, OEC Technicians should_____
   **a.** continue CPR, place the patient on a backboard, and transport to the nearest hospital.
   **b.** attempt to warm the patient up and remove all wet clothing.
   **c.** discontinue CPR because the patient was under cold water for up to 15 minutes.
   **d.** continue CPR, initiate the use of the AED, and transport after three unsuccessful shocks.

*The patient is transported by the ALS unit while CPR is continued. At the hospital, the patient's core temperature was raised, and the patient was revived by CPR and cardiac drugs.*

## Suggested Reading

Aish, M. A., and N. Kissoon. 2008. "Submersion Injuries." In *Emergency Medicine*, edited by J. C. Adams. Philadelphia: Saunders.

Auerbach, P. *The DAN Guide to Dive Medical Frequently Asked Questions (FAQ)*. Divers Alert Network, North Carolina, 2003.

Burford, A. E., et al. 2005. "Drowning and Near Drowning in Children and Adolescents." *Pediatric Emergency Care* 21(9): 610–616.

Centers for Disease Control and Prevention, National Center for Injury Prevention and Control. Web-based Injury Statistics Query and Reporting System (WISQARS). Available at: http://www.cdc.gov/ncipc/wisqars

Druck, J. 2006. "Altitude Illness and Dysbarisms." In *Emergency Medicine Secrets*, edited by V. J. Markovchick and P. T. Pons. St. Louis, MO: Mosby.

Salomez, F., and J. L. Vincent. 2004. "Drowning: A Review of Epidemiology, Pathophysiology, Treatment and Prevention." *Resuscitation* 63(3): 261–268.

Shepherd, S. M., J. Martin, and W. H. Shoff. "Drowning." emedicine.medscape.com/article/772753-overview

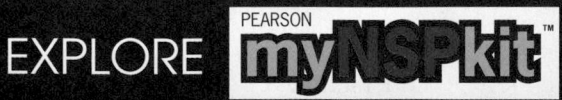

EXPLORE **PEARSON myNSPkit™**

Please go to www.myNSPkit.com. Under Student Resources, you will find animations, videos, web links, and games related to this chapter—and much more. Look for information on drowning prevention and the Centers for Disease Control and Prevention information on drowning.

Register your access code from the front of your book by going to www.myNSPkit.com and selecting the appropriate links. If the in-cover access code has been redeemed, go to www.myNSPkit.com and follow links to **Buy Access**.

# Pediatric Emergencies

David Walker, MD
Brigitte Schran Brown, M.Ed, MA, EMT

## ⊕ OBJECTIVES

**Upon completion of this chapter, the OEC Technician will be able to:**

**30-1** List and describe the anatomical and physiological differences between children and adults.

**30-2** List and describe the six stages of child growth and development.

**30-3** List the normal range of vital signs for each pediatric age group.

**30-4** Understand and be able to incorporate communication tips and techniques for assessing and interacting with a pediatric patient.

**30-5** Describe the signs and symptoms of respiratory distress and failure in a child.

**30-6** List and describe the signs and symptoms of various pediatric disorders.

**30-7** List the most common cause of cardiac arrest in pediatric patients.

**30-8** List common causes of seizures in pediatric patients.

**30-9** List five indicators of potential child abuse and neglect.

**30-10** Define sudden infant death syndrome.

**30-11** Describe and demonstrate how to assess a pediatric patient, using the pediatric assessment triangle.

**30-12** Describe and demonstrate how to manage common pediatric illnesses and injuries.

## Chapter Overview

Helping a pediatric patient can be one of the most rewarding experiences an OEC Technician can have. It also can be one of the most stressful.

This chapter describes strategies to help OEC Technicians communicate with pediatric patients and their caregivers and will provide you a greater level of understanding and confidence when dealing with the remarkable and complex world of children.

It is essential that you are able to recognize the often-subtle clues that children may exhibit when they are ill or injured. Children can present with very different illnesses,

*continued*

## HISTORICAL TIMELINE

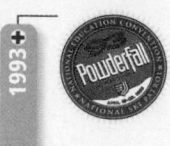

1993 — First "Powderfall" is held at Snowbird, Utah.

1993 — 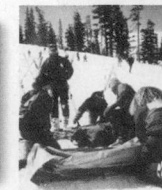 The National Senior Auxiliary program is adopted.

## ⊕ KEY TERMS

adolescent, *p. 949*

child abuse, *p. 960*

child neglect, *p. 960*

decompensated shock, *p. 943*

epiglottitis, *p. 951*

fontanel, *p. 945*

infant, *p. 947*

meningitis, *p. 954*

newborn, *p. 947*

pediatric assessment triangle, *p. 963*

preschool period, *p. 947*

retraction, *p. 945*

school-aged child, *p. 948*

shaken baby syndrome, *p. 961*

sudden infant death syndrome (SIDS),
*p. 957*

toddler, *p. 947*

tripod position, *p. 964*

problems, and patterns of trauma than adults (Figure 30-1■). A child's unique physiology changes continually from birth to adulthood, which can make assessment and care difficult for OEC Technicians. Problems such as respiratory distress, temperature regulation, or trauma can be more difficult to manage in young patients. Additionally, a child's ability to compensate for shock can cause a seemingly stable patient to spiral suddenly into **decompensated shock**.

## Anatomy and Physiology

Children are not miniature adults. Although they and adults share the same basic anatomy and physiology, inherent differences in intellectual capacity, size, proportion, and metabolism make pediatric patients unique. These differences change throughout childhood, resulting in large variations in behavior, vital signs, and the physical and emotional ability to cope with the stresses of injury and illness.

Two of the most important anatomic differences between children and adults are the size of the airway and the mechanism of breathing. These differences are especially relevant in infants and younger children. As a group, children have relatively small mouths and airways. Until approximately eight years old, a child's tongue is proportionally larger and more bulbous in relation to the oral cavity, which increases the risk of airway obstruction by the tongue. Something as simple as swollen tonsils and adenoids can cause serious respiratory distress in children (Figure 30-2■).

As children age, the oral cavity enlarges, the jaw elongates, and the tongue becomes proportionately flatter and smaller, allowing a relatively larger airway. The larynx sits higher and more anteriorly in the neck and is funnel shaped. Unlike an adult, the narrowest part of the child's airway is at the opening of the glottis. Thus because airway obstructions occur inferior to or below the vocal cords, the risk and severity of foreign-body airway obstruction are increased in children.

A child's trachea is shorter and smaller in diameter, and it is more flexible because the tracheal cartilages have not yet fully developed. For this reason, OEC Technicians must be careful when opening the airway of an unresponsive child because hyperextension of the neck can cause the trachea to become compressed or even collapsed.

Anatomically, a child's head is proportionally *larger* and heavier in relation to the body than is an adult's head (Figure 30-3■). The younger the child, the more pronounced this proportional difference is. Because of their proportions, young children are more susceptible to heat loss from the head, and during rapid deceleration the head is propelled forward first, before the body. A child's larger head also causes neck

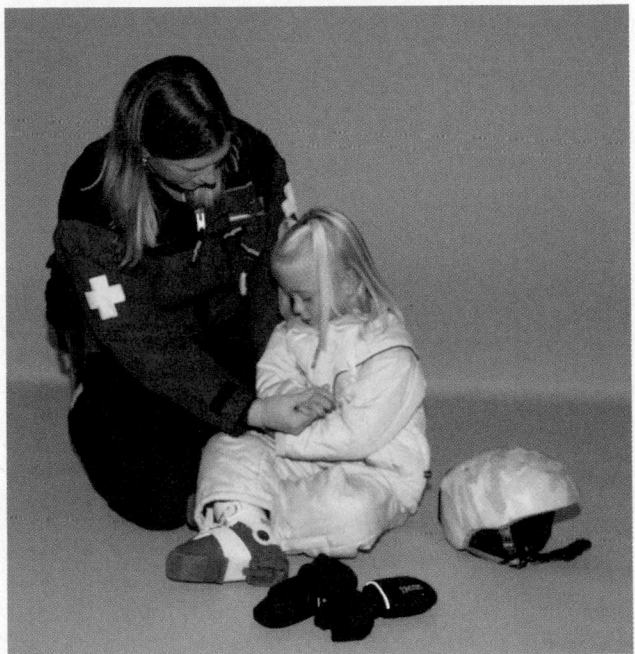

**Figure 30-1** Children can present special challenges for emergency care providers because their medical needs differ from those of adults.
Copyright Mike Halloran

**decompensated shock** shock that results from the body's inability to compensate for low blood volume or inadequate tissue perfusion.

⊕ 30-1 List and describe the anatomical and physiological differences between children and adults.

## CASE PRESENTATION

You are paddling on the day-stretch of a popular whitewater river when you notice a woman on shore frantically waving you down. As you paddle up to her, she tells you that her eight-year-old granddaughter slipped getting out of her kayak and landed on a rock with her arm outstretched. You find the girl sitting with her legs in the water, cradling her arm against her life-jacket. She is shivering violently and her lips are blue. Her grandmother tells you that her upper arm and shoulder hurt. The girl is whimpering but screams and begins to cry when you approach.

**What should you do?**

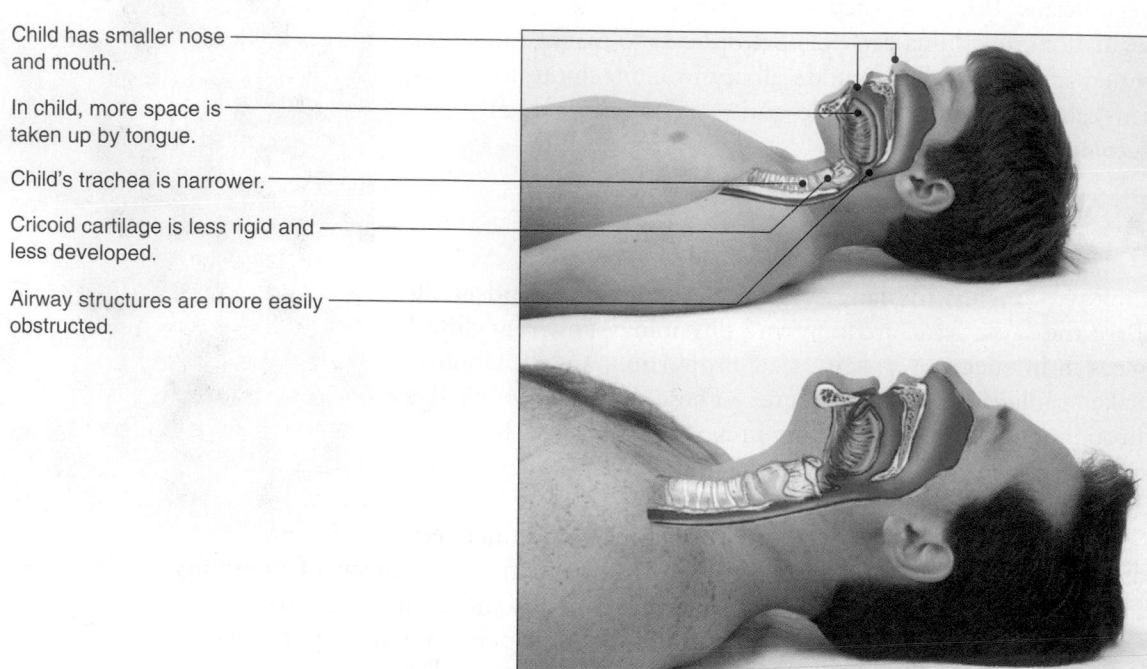

Child has smaller nose and mouth.

In child, more space is taken up by tongue.

Child's trachea is narrower.

Cricoid cartilage is less rigid and less developed.

Airway structures are more easily obstructed.

**Figure 30-2** The respiratory anatomy of children compared to that of adults.

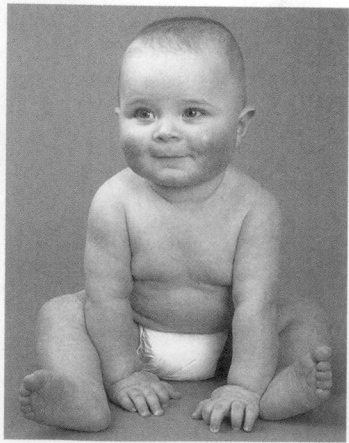

**Figure 30-3** Compared to adults, a child's head is larger in proportion to the body.

flexion when a spine board is used, which has implications for airway management and for maintaining a neutral C-spine alignment when a child's neck is immobilized.

A child's brain is proportionally *smaller* than an adult's brain, and it does not completely fill the cranial cavity. The extra space between the skull and the brain allows the child's brain to move more within the skull when the head is moved quickly. The combination of a large, heavy head and room for the brain to move within the skull puts infants, toddlers, and preschoolers at greater risk for both head injury and traumatic brain injury. Interestingly, even though the heads and brains of adolescents are proportionally smaller than those of adults, adolescents have the highest rate of traumatic brain injuries, a finding that is attributed less to anatomy than to adolescents' greater risk-taking and inability to fully comprehend the consequences of their actions.

Children also have a greater body surface area than adults, thinner skin, and less muscle mass and body fat. Thus, children are at greater risk for heat loss, faster absorption of toxins through the skin, morbidity from burns, and multiple organ injuries.

A child's musculoskeletal system is immature and grows rapidly, especially during the first year of life. The brain of an infant can grow because the cranial bones are not fused but instead are separated by gaps called **fontanels**. The larger of a newborn's two fontanels, the anterior fontanel, is located superior to the frontal bone; the posterior fontanel is superior to the occipital bone. By 18–20 months of age, both fontanels close, making the skull one continuous bony structure.

A child's bones, joints, and ligaments are softer and more flexible than those of an adult. The thoracic cage also is more pliable. As a result, a child's musculoskeletal system generally can absorb more force without breaking. This is not entirely advantageous, however, because the energy is transferred through the bones and muscles to the underlying structures, resulting in a higher rate of internal organ injury. This ability of a child's bones to bend explains why greenstick fractures are common in children.

Growth plates, known as epiphyses, are found at the ends of long bones as well as within the bones, the pelvis, and skull (Figure 30-4■). With proper nutrition (especially an adequate supply of calcium), the epiphyses produce cartilage, which later calcifies into bone. The area of the growth plate between the uncalcified cartilage cells and the calcified bone cells is weak, and fractures at this site are common. Growth plates begin closing around age 12 and usually disappear by age 16.

Compared to adults, children have a higher rate of metabolism (burn energy more quickly) and have fewer energy reserves. This explains why children exhibit great bursts of energy followed by sudden, profound fatigue. It also explains why children need regular meals and can consume enormous amounts of carbohydrates with few, if any, ill effects. The younger the child, the more frequently meals are needed.

Children and adults also differ in how they breathe. With few exceptions, newborns breathe through their nose. If a newborn's nose becomes obstructed by mucus or a foreign body, breathing difficulty will occur quickly. Also infants and small children rely on diaphragmatic breathing because their intercostal muscles are not yet fully developed. As a group, children of all ages breathe at a faster rate and have a greater minute volume than do adults. The body's primary response to respiratory distress is to increase the rate and effort of breathing. Because children start with a faster rate and effort of breathing, they tire easily and have a higher incidence of respiratory failure. This is the reason why *many* pediatric emergencies begin with respiratory distress. Because a child's chest wall is less muscular, intercostal **retractions** are more pronounced.

Unless born with a birth defect, most children have very healthy cardiovascular and nervous systems. Despite this, they are vulnerable to a variety of toxins, both natural and man-made. Children have a proportionally smaller blood volume than adults yet bleed at the same rate. They also have a higher heart rate and lower blood pressure. Additionally, a child's arteries are able to constrict more quickly than an adult's arteries. This combination enables a child to compensate better *initially* to shock. However, the compensatory mechanisms can fail quickly, which can cause an apparently healthy child to suddenly go into life-threatening shock, often with little or no warning. Hypovolemia, whether due to blood loss, vomiting, or diarrhea, can quickly lead to decompensated shock.

Due to an underdeveloped hypothalamus, children have difficulty regulating body temperature, which places them at high risk for both hyperthermia and hypothermia. A child's temperature can rapidly rise to 105°F (40.5°C), creating an emergent condition. Equally important, the larger ratio of skin surface area to body mass in children (infants through school age) can cause rapid cooling, which when combined with a slow central nervous system response, can result in hypothermia.

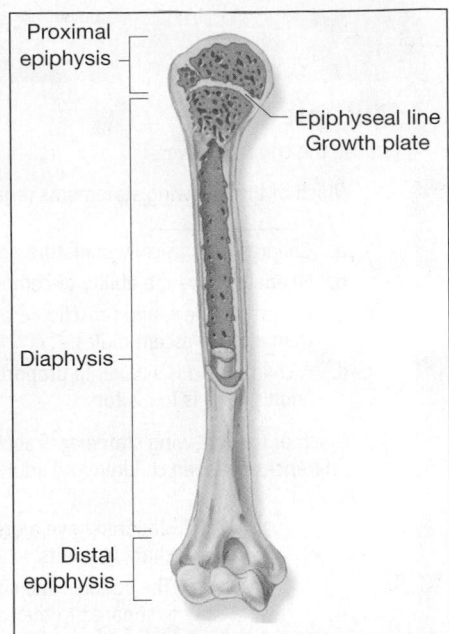

**Figure 30-4** The anatomy of a long bone.

**fontanel** an unfused suture between the bones of the skull of a newborn that allows expansion of the growing brain; the fontanels close at approximately 18–20 months of age.

**retraction** the condition in which muscles pull in between the ribs and above the sternum upon inhalation.

# STOP, THINK, UNDERSTAND

## Multiple Choice
Choose the correct answer.

1. Which of the following statements regarding pediatric patients is true? _____
   a. Children are basically miniature adults.
   b. Neonates have the ability to comprehend abstract concepts.
   c. Infants, toddlers, and preschoolers are at less of a risk of TBI than are adolescent males.
   d. A child's head is smaller in proportion to his torso than an adult's head is to his torso.

2. Which of the following statements about size and proportion differences between children and adults are true? (check all that apply)
   _____ a. Children have a greater body surface area than do adults.
   _____ b. The younger the child, the thicker is the skin compared to that of an adult.
   _____ c. Children proportionately have less muscle mass but more fat than do adults.
   _____ d. Compared to an adult, a child's head is proportionately larger and heavier in relation to its body.
   _____ e. A young child's airway and mouth are proportionately larger than those in adults.
   _____ f. Compared to an adult, a child's tongue is proportionately larger and more bulbous in relation to the oral cavity.
   _____ g. A child's trachea is shorter and smaller in diameter than is an adult's.
   _____ h. A child's trachea is firmer and more rigid than is an adult's.

3. A purpose of the fontanelles in an infant's skull is to_____
   a. allow for greater perfusion of the dura mater and pia mater.
   b. regulate the amount of cerebrospinal fluid.
   c. allow the infants brain to hold more blood.
   d. give the brain room to grow.

4. Which of the following statements about a child's bones, joints, and ligaments are true? (check all that apply)
   _____ a. They are harder than an adult's.
   _____ b. They are more flexible than an adult's.
   _____ c. A child's thoracic cage is more pliable than an adult's.
   _____ d. Energy from blunt trauma is better absorbed by a child's skeleton than by an adult's skeleton.
   _____ e. The growth plate in a child's long bone can fracture easily.

5. Which of the following statements regarding a child's physiology is not true? _____
   a. Children can compensate well for shock for a relatively long length of time.
   b. A child's arteries are able to constrict more quickly than are those of an adult.
   c. Children have difficulty regulating their body temperature.
   d. Children generally have very healthy nervous and cardiovascular systems.

6. The ratio of skin surface area to body mass in children is_____
   a. 10 percent smaller than in adults.
   b. 20 percent smaller than in adults.
   c. equal to that in adults.
   d. greater than that in adults.

7. The underdeveloped hypothalamus in children places them at high risk for_____
   a. hyperthermia.
   b. hypothermia.
   c. hyperglycemia.
   d. hyperthermia and hypothermia.

## Short Answer
Proportionally for their size, the blood volume of children is (circle one) less than / equal to / greater than that of adults. Discuss what this has to do with shock in children.

_____

_____

_____

⊕ 30-2  List and describe the six stages of child growth and development.

⊕ 30-3  List the normal range of vital signs for each pediatric age group.

# Human Growth and Development

Between birth and the age of 18, humans undergo a great variety of physical, intellectual, emotional, and social changes. Language evolves from crying and grunts to organized spoken words and written communication. The rate of change varies from child to child, but the pattern of development leading to adulthood moves through six identifiable but overlapping stages (Table 30-1■):

1. The newborn (neonatal) stage
2. Infancy
3. The toddler stage
4. The preschool period
5. The school-age period
6. Adolescence

## The Newborn Stage

The **newborn** period (also called the neonatal period) begins at birth and spans the first 28 days of life (Figure 30-5■). Immediately after emerging from the womb, newborns have the same basic biological needs as adults. To begin breathing, a neonate must have a patent airway, the urge to breathe, and lungs that are mature enough to be able to absorb oxygen. The lungs of newborns continue to produce surfactant, a chemical first produced at 32 weeks of pregnancy that enables the alveoli to inflate properly. Without this chemical, a newborn's chances of survival are markedly decreased.

Newborns chill rapidly, so a warm environment and protection with a blanket and a cap are essential. During this early part of life, infants express needs and displeasure by crying and respond to various stimuli, including light, sounds, normal or cold temperatures, and hunger.

## Infancy

Infancy encompasses months 2 through 12 (Figure 30-6■). **Infants** are completely dependent on their caregivers. Infants are able to recognize faces and can exhibit facial expressions, and they can switch from crying to cooing when their needs are met. Gross motor skills develop rapidly. By the end of infancy (1 year of age), infants typically progress from rolling over to pulling themselves up to a standing position. Some even begin walking.

## The Toddler Stage

The **toddler** stage of development encompasses the period from 12 months to 36 months (Figure 30-7■). The average age for children to start walking is between 8 months and 14 months of age. Infinitely curious, toddlers begin exploring, climbing, and opening drawers. In conjunction with this natural curiosity comes a lack of comprehension about the consequences of actions. Thus, toddlers are at high risk of serious injury from falls, electrocution, burns, poisoning, and being struck by automobiles.

At one year, toddlers can use several key words such as their names, "mama," "papa," "no," "cup," and "ball." By the time they are 18–24 months, children can typically speak up to 20 words. By age 2, children can follow simple requests. Fine motor skills are developing and toddlers can use a spoon, even though most prefer to eat with their fingers. With a developing vocabulary of about 50 words, 3-year-olds can speak in short three- or four-word sentences.

Toddlers grow anxious when approached or held by a stranger, and although they engage in independent play, they want a caregiver to be nearby. Although they begin to socialize with peers, they are generally incapable of sharing toys with another child.

## The Preschool Period

The **preschool period** spans the ages of 3–5 years (Figure 30-8■). Preschoolers can communicate quite clearly and begin to answer simple questions. "Why" is a favorite word, as is "no." Developing sentence structure enables preschoolers to engage in simple conversations. Thinking is still concrete and focuses largely on the here and now.

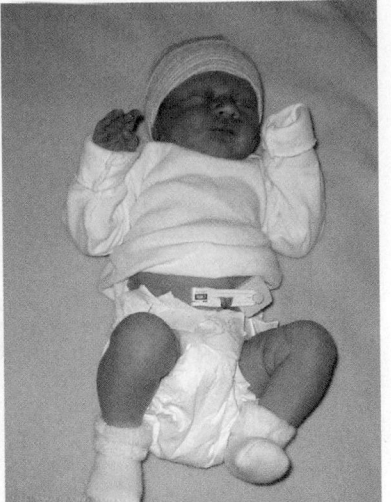

**Figure 30-5** A newborn: birth to 28 days.

---

**⊕ 30-4** Understand and be able to incorporate communication tips and techniques for assessing and interacting with a pediatric patient.

**newborn** a child in the first month of life; children in this stage are also said to be in the neonatal period.

**infant** a child ages 2–12 months.

**toddler** a child ages 12–36 months; the stage at which a child begins to explore, climb, and speak simple words or phrases.

**preschool period** the period of childhood during ages 3–5 years; a time in which a child gains fine motor skills and greater independence.

**Figure 30-6** An infant: 2–12 months.

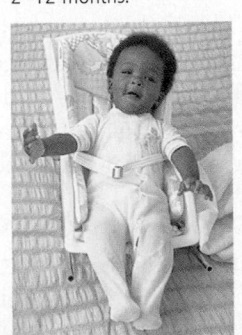

**Figure 30-7** A toddler: 12–36 months.

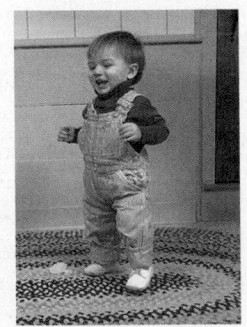

**Figure 30-8** A preschool child: 3–5 years.

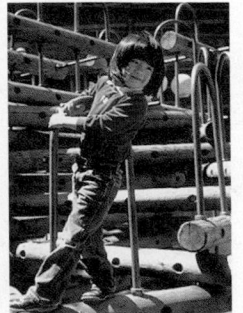

| Table 30-1 | Human Growth and Development | |
| --- | --- | --- |
| **AGE** | **PHYSICAL DEVELOPMENT** | **INTELLECTUAL DEVELOPMENT** |
| **NEWBORN** 0–1 Month | Responds to light, temperature (cold or hot), hunger (taste), and sound | Minimum development |
| **INFANT** 1–12 Months | Rolls over at first, then crawls, pulls up; walks at about 1 year | Visually alert, plays with hands; at six months plays briefly with toys; learns names (mom, dad); learns to pinch; puts toys in mouth and laughs; laughs when a Jack in the Box pops up |
| **TODDLER** 12–36 Months | Learns to walk up to 14 months, then kneels; at 18 months to 3 years, learns to sit unaided, goes up and down stairs sitting and runs, and tries to throw a ball; spatial awareness increases; can play pat-a-cake | Opens and closes containers; learns to scribble; shows handedness; holds a spoon to eat; can stack up 3–6 blocks; identifies people in photos |
| **PRESCHOOL CHILD** 3–5 Years | Develops balance; learns to climb stairs at age 3; can skip; can pedal a tricycle | Very developed imagination; can understand directions; fantasies seem real; says "I'm hurt 'cause I was bad"; learns alphabet, numbers, and colors; understands concepts of past, present, and future |
| **SCHOOL-AGE CHILD** 6–12 Years | Learns to ride a bike around age 6; learns specific skills for sports; muscles begin to develop | Learns to read; develops math skills; learns about more than their immediate surroundings and about their impact on others |
| **ADOLESCENT** 13–18 Years | Can lack coordination during growth spurt but later becomes efficient and very skilled at sports | Learns life skills; easily comprehends complex problems; understands government |

Gross motor skills continue to develop, and between ages 3 years and 4 years many preschoolers enjoy riding a tricycle and can walk on tip-toes with ease. They know the primary colors, can hold a crayon correctly, and can reproduce a circle on paper. They can draw stick figures and can stack and create more complex structures with building blocks.

Socially, preschoolers seek greater independence, can use the toilet by themselves, and use eating utensils properly. By 4 years of age, preschool children can hop, sit cross-legged, and throw, catch, bounce, and kick a ball. Imagination and inquisitiveness develop, as do fine motor skills and eye-hand coordination. To developing preschoolers, play enables them to explore their world and further develop physical and social skills. By now children understand humor and can comprehend abstract concepts such as the past, the present, and the future.

Five-year-olds can skip and have developed balance. (This age is generally the earliest age to begin skiing or snowboarding.) They can count, can draw people more accurately (with correct facial features), and have expanded their knowledge of colors. Dressing and undressing is done independently, as is hand washing. Awareness of gender differences emerges, as does the enjoyment of simple riddles, jokes, and potty humor. These children can understand the time of day as it relates to their activities and routines, and they are less stressed if routines are broken.

Language continues to develop, as the complexity of grammar increases and the progression of thoughts advances. By age six, children have usually developed the intellectual and social skills needed to begin school.

## The School-Age Period

**school-aged child** a child, ages 6–12 years.

By the time they reach 6 years of age, children can take care of most of their basic physical needs, with some help (Figure 30-9■). They answer questions directly and are much less dependent on their caregivers, but in the United States at least they still

| EMOTIONAL DEVELOPMENT | SOCIAL DEVELOPMENT | LANGUAGE DEVELOPMENT |
|---|---|---|
| Cries if unhappy | Dependent on caregiver | Occasional unintelligible noise |
| Still cries when unhappy, coos and smiles when happy | Recognizes parents; is unafraid of strangers until 6 months | Makes baby sounds, utters syllables |
| Early shows of affection; likes to look at books; explores more with no sense of danger; later role plays; does not understand sharing; becomes clingy when upset; wants instant gratification, has tantrums, and can be stubborn; does not like to be restrained | Feeds self with fingers; drinks from a cup with a lid; helps caregiver with getting dressed; is mischievous; is selfish, saying "mine"; begins toilet training | Understands simple words, including name but also screams if wants something; by age 3, can speak 50 words and understands many more; starts simple three-word sentences |
| Understands humor; becomes very inquisitive; develops fantasies and a vivid imagination | Begins to share; can use the toilet; eats with utensils; can dress independently; can wash hands | Can answer simple questions; can have a conversation; starts vocabulary and grammar develop |
| Emotional and physical pain becomes differentiated; can make own decisions | Develops understanding of right from wrong; begins to develop team skills | Can answer more complex questions directly; becomes more efficient with communication skills |
| Has first loving and emotional experience with individuals of the opposite sex; understands authority and laws | Joins clubs and sports teams; understands society | Develops vocabulary of words; develops the ability to write a story with correct grammar |

depend on others for food, water, and shelter. They can differentiate emotional and physical pain but still find it difficult to control their emotions. They begin to participate in sports and school activities, and they understand the concept of being part of a team. Although they can generally be addressed in the same manner as an adult, they still require simple language. Six-year-olds can usually make their own decisions and have begun to develop a good understanding of which things can hurt them physically.

The difference between right and wrong becomes established in school-aged children, and they begin to understand the consequences of their actions. If these concepts are not learned at this age, it becomes increasingly difficult for children to develop the concept of acceptable moral behavior. Parents and teachers influence a child's notions of good and bad societal behavior the most during this age, although adolescents continue to form values well into adulthood. At around age 10, children begin to be concerned about being accepted by others and living up to others' expectations, and generally these values remain throughout their lives.

**adolescent** an individual, ages 13–18 years; focus shifts from parents to peers; decision making, abstract thinking, and complex memorization skills develop.

## Adolescence

An **adolescent** encompasses the ages of 13 years to 18 years of age (Figure 30-10■). During this period, children become increasingly independent and mature rapidly. Their focus shifts from their parents or caregivers to their peers. Decision making, abstract thinking, and complex memorization skills are developed. At this age, many teens (especially males) feel invincible, which leads to a higher incidence of accidents and injuries. Many of these mishaps stem from their demand for greater independence, hormonal fluctuations, and an incomplete (often immature) understanding of the consequences of their actions.

During adolescence, teenagers often become very sensitive to their own appearance. Independence and privacy become increasingly important.

**Figure 30-9** School-age children: 6–12 years.

**Figure 30-10** Adolescents: 13–18 years.

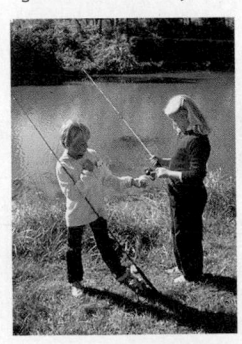

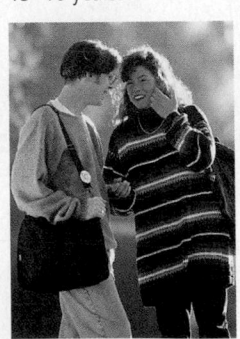

Sexuality develops and sexual behavior may begin, although the maturity to handle difficult choices or peer pressure may be lacking, which can lead to substance abuse or pregnancy.

Adolescents communicate much like adults, and most can understand very complex, abstract problems. They understand the principles of law and government and develop opinions on social, political, and moral issues. Their opinions can easily be influenced by peers, and they may choose older peers or adults (parent, teacher, coach) whom they wish to emulate.

# Common Pediatric Illnesses and Injuries

Children suffer a variety of medical disorders and traumatic injuries. Although most of these conditions are similar in nature and frequency to those seen in adults, some are unique to the pediatric population. Moreover, some disorders occur more frequently in certain pediatric age groups than in others. Because children have small airways and immature immune systems, respiratory emergencies are common.

## Airway Problems

**30-5** Describe the signs and symptoms of respiratory distress and failure in a child.

The most common upper airway conditions that cause respiratory emergencies in children are croup, tonsillitis, and foreign-body airway obstruction. Lower airway problems such as bronchiolitis, pneumonia, and asthma also occur.

### Croup

**30-6** List and describe the signs and symptoms of various pediatric disorders.

Croup is an inflammation of the larynx, trachea, and bronchi that typically results from an airborne viral (and sometimes bacterial) infection that primarily affects children between the ages of 6 months and 3 years (Figure 30-11■). Croup is characterized by sudden onset of a sharp, seal-like barking cough. Most cases of croup occur in the late fall and winter and are preceded by 2–3 days of "cold-like" symptoms (runny nose, increased mucus production, and fever). Although most cases are mild and resolve without complications, croup can produce severe respiratory distress.

### Tonsillitis

Tonsillitis, an inflammation of the tonsils, is a common childhood disease that primarily affects children ages 5–15 years. It may result from a viral infection or from "strep throat," a bacterial infection. Tonsillitis is characterized by severe sore throat and difficulty swallowing. While painful, it rarely results in respiratory distress.

**Figure 30-11** Croup, an inflammation of the larynx, can cause airway obstruction.

### Foreign-Body Airway Obstruction

Because young children often explore their world by placing objects in their mouths, small objects such as food, toy parts, or coins can become lodged in a child's airway, resulting in partial or complete obstruction. Food is the primary cause of foreign-body airway obstruction in older children and is primarily due to either putting too much food in the mouth or not completely chewing food. Dislodged teeth or vomitus can also cause partial or complete airway obstruction.

### Bronchiolitis

Bronchiolitis is inflammation of the bronchioles caused by a viral infection. Although it can affect children of all ages, most cases occur in children under 2 years old. Bronchiolitis, which most commonly occurs in the fall and winter, develops over a period of 2–3 days and is characterized by fever, cough, and difficulty breathing, which in some cases can be severe.

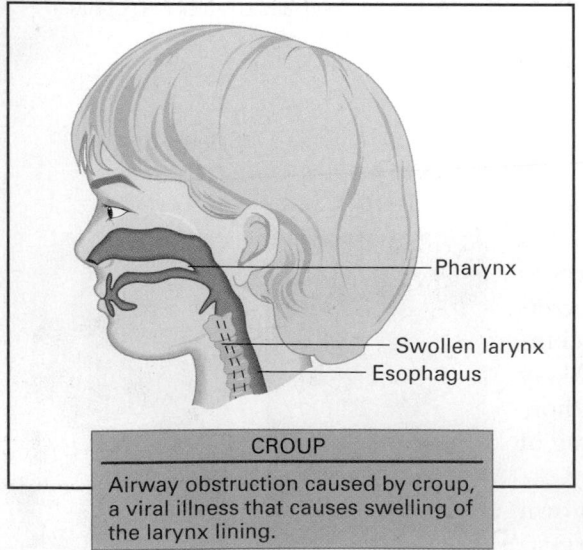

Pharynx

Swollen larynx
Esophagus

**CROUP**
Airway obstruction caused by croup, a viral illness that causes swelling of the larynx lining.

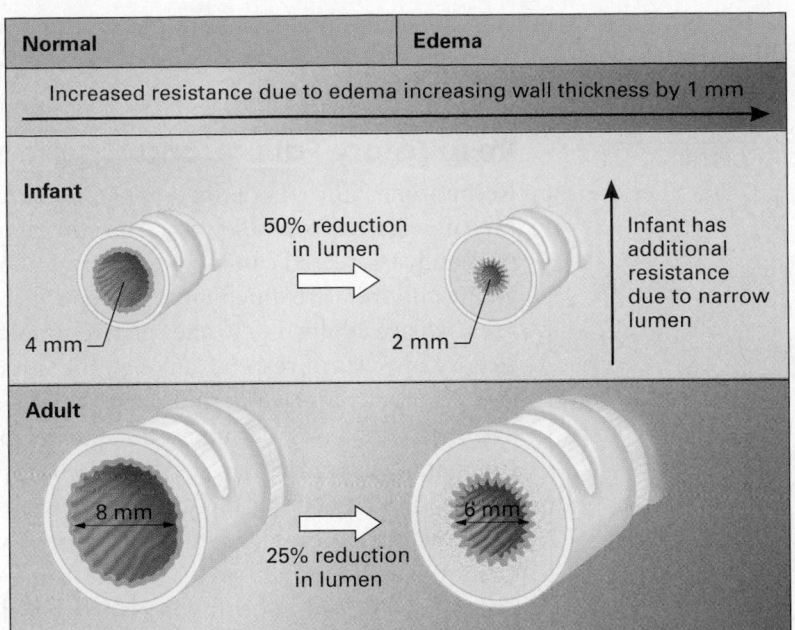

| Normal | Edema |
|---|---|

Increased resistance due to edema increasing wall thickness by 1 mm

**Infant**

4 mm — 50% reduction in lumen — 2 mm

Infant has additional resistance due to narrow lumen

**Adult**

8 mm — 25% reduction in lumen — 6 mm

**Figure 30-12** In asthma, inflammation of the airways reduces their diameter, causing respiratory difficulty.

## Pneumonia

Pneumonia is a viral or bacterial infection of the lung that is often preceded by an upper respiratory infection, a fever, and a cough. It can occur any time of year but is most commonly encountered during the winter and spring. Although pneumonia can occur at any age, children who have aspirated a foreign body or have a history of either recurring respiratory infections (e.g., bronchiolitis) or chronic illnesses are at greater risk for contracting pneumonia. Untreated, pneumonia can lead to respiratory distress, respiratory failure, and even respiratory arrest. A similar condition can occur when the lungs are exposed to certain chemicals.

## Asthma

Asthma is a reactive disease of the small airways that is characterized by marked constriction of the bronchioles and wheezing (Figure 30-12■). Its pathophysiology was described in Chapter 13, Respiratory Emergencies. Among the most common causes of asthma are viral illnesses, pollen, exercise, and exposure to cold air. Although asthma is the most common chronic childhood illness in the United States, affecting an estimated 10–12 percent of children, the disease can affect individuals of any age. Children who suffer from childhood asthma usually have the condition by the time they reach 5 years of age.

## Epiglottitis

**Epiglottitis**, a true medical emergency that can produce life-threatening respiratory distress, is severe inflammation of the epiglottis that can completely block the upper airway (Figure 30-13■). Epiglottitis results from a bacterial infection and is characterized by high fever, sore throat, and an inability to swallow. The hallmark of epiglottitis is a patient who is sitting forward, is very still, and is drooling. If not treated quickly, epiglottitis can result in death.

**epiglottitis**   an inflammation and swelling of the epiglottis, the small, leaf-shaped structure that covers the larynx when a person swallows and prevents food from entering the trachea.

**Figure 30-13** Epiglottitis can obstruct or completely block the airway.

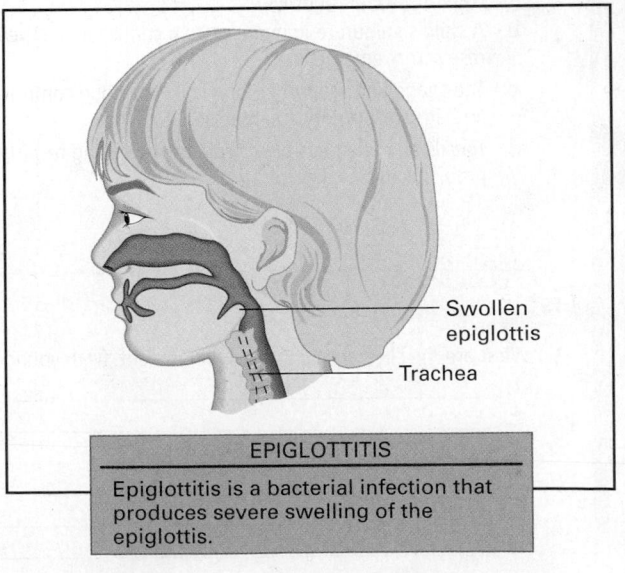

Swollen epiglottis

Trachea

**EPIGLOTTITIS**

Epiglottitis is a bacterial infection that produces severe swelling of the epiglottis.

⊕ **30-7** List the most common cause of cardiac arrest in pediatric patients.

Although now a rare disease in children thanks to vaccination for *H. influenza*, the disease most commonly affects children ages 1.5–7 years. It is still seen in immigrant and nonvaccinated populations.

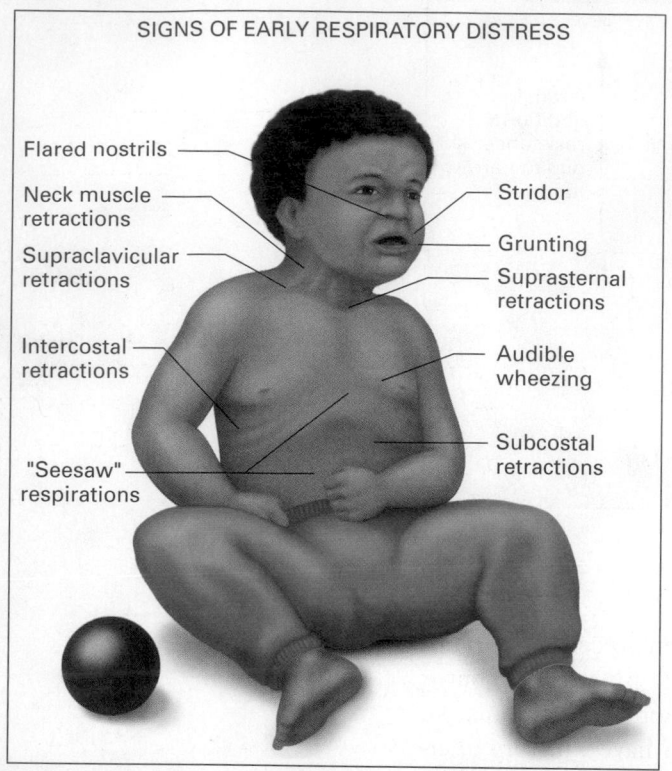

SIGNS OF EARLY RESPIRATORY DISTRESS

Flared nostrils
Neck muscle retractions
Supraclavicular retractions
Intercostal retractions
"Seesaw" respirations
Stridor
Grunting
Suprasternal retractions
Audible wheezing
Subcostal retractions

**Figure 30-14** Some signs of respiratory distress.

## Respiratory Failure and Cardiac Arrest

Respiratory failure is defined as the inability of the lungs to exchange gases properly. It is a true emergency that if not immediately corrected can be quickly fatal. Children, especially young children, are much more susceptible to respiratory failure than are adults due to the relative immaturity of their accessory muscles of respiration (e.g., the intercostal, trapezius, and sternocleidomastoid muscles). When a child becomes dyspneic, the body compensates quickly by increasing the heart and respiratory rates. Although temporarily effective, this process has a potentially fatal drawback: as the heart rate dramatically increases, so does the heart's oxygen needs. The resulting increased effort to breathe can easily exhaust and overwhelm a child, resulting in respiratory distress and possibly respiratory failure (Figure 30-14■).

As exhaustion occurs, the respiratory rate slows and the child becomes hypoxic. Cardiac arrest subsequently occurs due to anoxia. For this reason, most cases of cardiac arrest in children are preceded by respiratory failure. The development of relative bradycardia in a child with respiratory distress is an ominous sign of impending cardiac arrest. Other causes of pediatric cardiac arrest include trauma, drowning, poisoning, and an underlying congenital defect.

# STOP, THINK, UNDERSTAND

## Multiple Choice

Choose the correct answer.

1. Which of the following statements regarding pediatric respiratory emergencies is not true? _____
   a. The small size of the pediatric airway contributes to pediatric respiratory emergencies.
   b. A child's immature immune system contributes to pediatric respiratory emergencies.
   c. The shape and proportion of a child's tongue contributes to pediatric respiratory emergencies.
   d. Tonsils and adenoids play a role in preventing respiratory problems in children.

2. Which of the following statements about respiratory failure in children is not true? _____
   a. It can quickly become fatal if not treated.
   b. Children are less susceptible to respiratory failure than are adults.
   c. In children, the body compensates for dyspnea by increasing the heart and respiratory rates.
   d. Respiratory failure is almost always preceded by exhaustion.

3. Cardiac arrest that quickly follows respiratory failure in children results from _____
   a. exhaustion.          c. airway obstruction.
   b. hypoglycemia.        d. anoxia.

## List

1. What are the six stages of child development, from youngest to oldest?
   1. _____
   2. _____
   3. _____
   4. _____
   5. _____
   6. _____

*continued*

**2.** What are four common causes of upper airway emergencies in children?

1. _____
2. _____
3. _____
4. _____

**3.** What are three common causes of lower airway emergencies in children?

1. _____
2. _____
3. _____

## Short Answer

Why is it important for an OEC Technician to understand the various developmental stages of childhood?

_____
_____
_____
_____
_____

## Abdominal Pain

Abdominal pain is a common childhood disorder. Of the many causes of pediatric abdominal pain, the most common is constipation or stool holding. This condition can occur due to changes in dietary or sleep patterns and dehydration. When in outdoor settings or when simply confronted with an unfamiliar restroom, shyness about defecation may cause some children to intentionally withhold a bowel movement, sometimes for up to a week. The resulting accumulation of feces in the bowel causes constipation and pain.

Gastroenteritis and appendicitis are two other medical sources of pediatric abdominal pain that OEC Technicians may encounter. Gastroenteritis can occur at any age, has numerous causes, and may mimic several very serious conditions. Appendicitis occurs much less commonly in children than in adults, but if unrecognized it can lead to peritonitis, shock, and death. Of the other conditions that cause abdominal pain in children, most are rare and beyond the scope of this text. As a rule, any child who presents with severe abdominal pain and appears ill should be evaluated by a physician.

## Nausea, Vomiting, and Diarrhea

Nausea, vomiting, and diarrhea, collectively referred to as "NVD," are among the most common complaints OEC Technicians encounter in children and are associated with a variety of pediatric illnesses and injuries. This triad of complaints has many causes, including gastroenteritis, viruses, bacteria, parasites, tainted or unfamiliar food, lack of sleep, and overstimulation. Depending on the underlying cause, NVD can range in severity from mild to life threatening. Severe vomiting and diarrhea can lead to marked dehydration, hypovolemia, and shock.

## Seizures

As described in Chapter 11, Altered Mental Status, a seizure is an electrical disturbance within the brain that results in alterations in awareness, attentiveness, responsiveness, behavior, and/or body movement. Seizures may be classified as either partial (affecting one part or side of the body) or generalized (affecting both sides simultaneously). The many causes of seizure include fever, hypoxia, diabetes, epilepsy, toxins, and head injury.

⊕ **30-8** List common causes of seizures in pediatric patients.

Febrile seizures are the most common type of pediatric seizure, accounting for approximately half of all cases. Most febrile seizures occur in children between the ages of 6 months and 5 years and typically affect otherwise healthy children who have the combination of an infectious illness and an elevated temperature. Febrile seizures are generalized in nature, usually last less than 5 minutes, and have a post-ictal phase lasting several minutes. Most febrile seizures are harmless; there is no evidence that febrile seizures, *by themselves*, cause death, brain damage, epilepsy, mental retardation, a decrease in IQ, or learning difficulties.

Children are susceptible to status epilepticus, a condition that is characterized by a seizure lasting more than 10 minutes, a prolonged post-ictal state, or three or more seizures in a row between which the patient does not return to normal mental status. Status epilepticus is a true emergency that requires immediate medical care.

A less serious type of seizure that may be seen in children is the "absence seizure," which lasts from a few seconds to a minute or more and is characterized by a period in which the child remains awake but is momentarily unresponsive to external stimuli. Typically benign, a child may experience multiple absence seizures in a single day. The cause of this type of seizure is unknown, and most children outgrow this condition by the age of 18–22 years.

## Meningitis

**meningitis** an inflammation of the membranes covering the spinal cord and brain; may be caused by viruses or bacteria.

**Meningitis**, inflammation of the meninges, is a potentially life-threatening condition that is considered a true medical emergency and requires prompt medical care. Meningitis due to a bacterial or viral infection usually develops over 1–4 days and may be highly contagious. It is characterized by lethargy, high fever, severe headache, and a stiff, sore neck. In infants, the fontanels may bulge outward. Young children are especially vulnerable to meningitis, especially from birth to 5 years of age.

## Poisoning

Toddlers and preschool children are at high risk of accidental poisoning due to their inexperience in distinguishing candy from medications or harmless plants from those that are toxic (Figure 30-15■). Infants are at greatest risk because they constantly put things in their mouth. Unfortunately, many toxic substances smell good or taste good, and even small amounts of some toxins can make a child very ill.

Children can be poisoned by medications, both prescription drugs and over-the-counter drugs such as aspirin or acetaminophen (Tylenol). Some medications, especially those formulated for pediatric patients (e.g., cough syrups, pain relievers, children's vitamins) taste like candy. If ingested in large amounts, overdose and toxicity can quickly occur.

Pediatric poisonings can also occur from petroleum-based solvents, rodent poison, antifreeze, or just about anything that is kept unlocked within a curious child's reach such as under the kitchen sink. Long-term lead poisoning can occur from eating lead-based paint on toys or on the railings of a staircase. Some items from China have been shown to have cadmium in the paint, which is also very poisonous. Also the ingestion of too many vitamin tablets can result in iron toxicity.

Adolescents also can be poisoned either accidentally or intentionally. Excessive alcohol consumption is the most common type of poisoning encountered among individuals in this age group. The liver in teenagers cannot process alcohol as efficiently as can the liver in adults, so excessive alcohol intake can lead to alcohol toxicity, respiratory depression, or respiratory arrest. Intentional overdose may be related to underlying depression and may constitute a suicide attempt (Figure 30-16■).

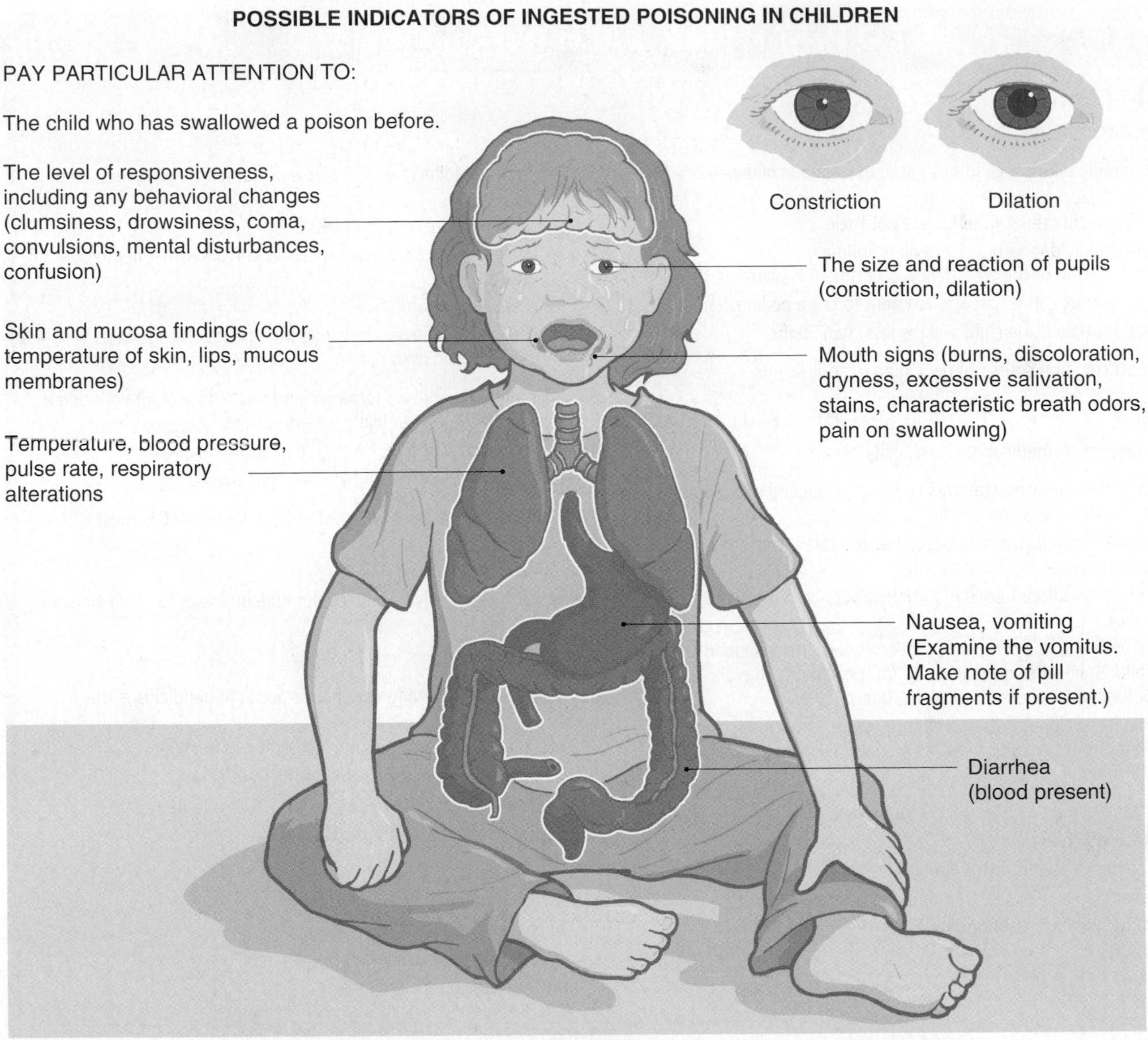

## POSSIBLE INDICATORS OF INGESTED POISONING IN CHILDREN

PAY PARTICULAR ATTENTION TO:

The child who has swallowed a poison before.

The level of responsiveness, including any behavioral changes (clumsiness, drowsiness, coma, convulsions, mental disturbances, confusion)

Skin and mucosa findings (color, temperature of skin, lips, mucous membranes)

Temperature, blood pressure, pulse rate, respiratory alterations

Constriction          Dilation

The size and reaction of pupils (constriction, dilation)

Mouth signs (burns, discoloration, dryness, excessive salivation, stains, characteristic breath odors, pain on swallowing)

Nausea, vomiting (Examine the vomitus. Make note of pill fragments if present.)

Diarrhea (blood present)

**Figure 30-15** Possible signs and symptoms of ingested poisoning in children.

**Figure 30-16** Adolescents can overdose on prescription drugs either accidentally or intentionally.
Copyright Edward McNamara

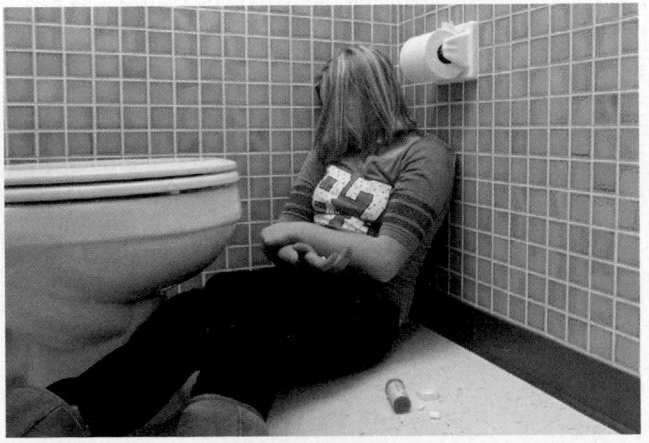

# STOP, THINK, UNDERSTAND

## Multiple Choice

Choose the correct answer.

1. A situation in which a child has eaten at least 50 children's vitamins is_____
   a. benign; children's vitamins are not toxic.
   b. potentially dangerous; immediate follow up with a pediatrician or the emergency department is warranted.
   c. worrisome; call for an appointment to see a pediatrician.
   d. serious only if the child weighs less than 50 lbs.

2. The most common source of poisoning in adolescents is_____
   a. food.
   b. prescription medications.
   c. alcohol.
   d. vitamins.

3. Which of the following statements about prolonged vomiting or severe diarrhea in young children is true? _____
   a. While uncomfortable, these conditions rarely cause severe consequences for children.
   b. These conditions can lead to dehydration and hypovolemic shock.
   c. Nausea and vomiting are of little concern in very young children because neonates and infants typically have unformed stools and spit up routinely.
   d. In older children these conditions are psychosomatic and result from such situations as having to use an unfamiliar restroom.

4. The most common cause of pediatric seizures is_____
   a. traumatic brain injury.
   b. cerebral palsy or birth trauma.
   c. fever.
   d. congenital brain abnormality.

5. Which of the following statements about febrile seizures is true? _____
   a. They are generally harmless.
   b. They can quickly cause brain damage and other neurologic disorders.
   c. They can be fatal.
   d. They have a proven link to learning difficulties such as dyslexia and dysgraphia.

6. An infant who appears lethargic and has bulging fontanels and a fever of 104°F is most likely suffering from_____
   a. influenza A or B.
   b. NVD.
   c. febrile seizure disorder.
   d. meningitis.

7. The condition of the infant described in Question 6 is most likely_____
   a. not dangerous.
   b. dangerous only if body temperature increases to 105°F or higher.
   c. urgent.
   d. life threatening.

8. Which of the following statements about appendicitis is true? _____
   a. It is the second leading cause of death in children.
   b. It is more common in children than in adults.
   c. It is characterized by severe left lower quadrant pain.
   d. It can lead to peritonitis and shock.

9. NVD stands for_____
   a. neurovascular deformity.
   b. nausea, vasculitis, diarrhea.
   c. neurologic vascular deformity.
   d. nausea, vomiting, diarrhea.

## Short Answer

1. Name and describe three common causes of abdominal pain in children.

   _____

   _____

   _____

   _____

2. What are the primary causes of NVD?

   _____

   _____

   _____

   _____

*continued*

**3.** What are some of the reasons why infants, toddlers, and preschoolers are at high risk of accidental poisoning? _____

_____

_____

_____

_____

## Sudden Infant Death Syndrome

The unexpected death of an infant due to undetermined causes is classified as a case of **sudden infant death syndrome (SIDS)**. Each year approximately 2,500 infants in the United States die from SIDS.

The exact cause of SIDS is unknown; there is still no universally accepted reason why apparently healthy children die unexpectedly. It does not appear that SIDS is caused from suffocation, and research has shown that there may be a tendency for SIDS to run in families. Some researchers speculate that SIDS is preceded by sleep apnea (periods of not breathing while at rest) and anoxia (lack of oxygen). Many believe that there are several different causes of SIDS. A reduction in the incidence of SIDS over the past 15 years is likely due to the recommendation of several practices, including avoiding redundant soft bedding and soft objects in the infant's sleeping environment, avoiding having adults sleeping with an infant in the same bed, and (first and foremost) placing babies on their backs for sleep times (Figure 30-17■).

In a typical SIDS case, parents will attempt to awaken the infant in the morning, only to find that their baby is dead. In addition to profound grief, many parents suffer severe guilt following the death of a child from SIDS.

## Trauma

Children of all ages are inherent risk takers and frequently engage in activities that can result in serious bodily injury. Accidental trauma is the leading cause of death in children older than 1 year, accounting for more childhood deaths annually than all other sources combined. The leading cause of death from accidental trauma is vehicle crashes, followed by firearm-related injuries and drownings (Figure 30-18■). Blunt trauma is the leading mechanism of injury.

⊕ **30-10** Define sudden infant death syndrome.

**sudden infant death syndrome (SIDS)** the sudden, unexplained death of an infant in which a postmortem examination fails to determine the cause of death.

**Figure 30-17** Putting infants on their backs while they sleep reduces the likelihood of death from SIDS.

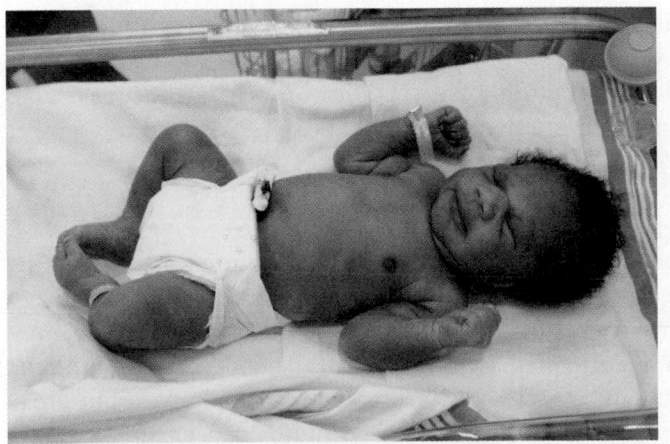

**Figure 30-18** Accidental trauma is the leading cause of death in children over 1 year of age.

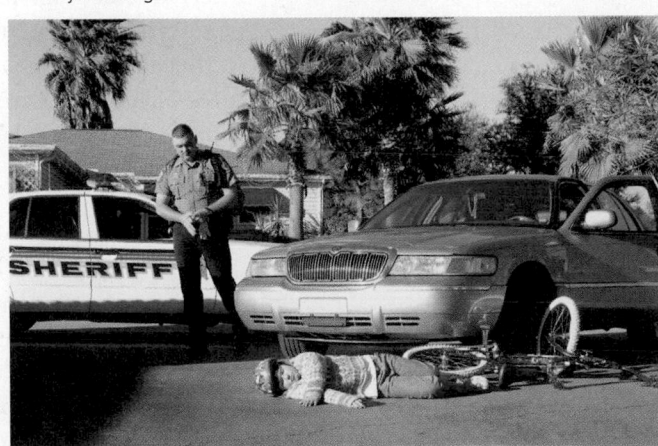

## Head and Neck Injuries

Head injury is a common pediatric injury, and among infants and toddlers the primary source of head injury is falls. Because infants and toddlers have a relatively large head, weak neck muscles, and flexible bones and ligaments, they have difficulty controlling head movement. As a result, the head tends to lead the way in a fall. Injuries occur to the surface of the head and face, the skull and within the skull. Due to the highly vascular nature of a child's head and the thinness of the skin, head injuries can result in significant bleeding.

In general, head injuries tend to be more severe in children. Small children with severe traumatic brain injuries can rapidly develop elevated intracranial pressure. The relatively small size of the brain compared to the skull allows blood to fill the inside of the skull, causing a cerebral hematoma that results in brain herniation, often before significant symptoms are noticed. Among adolescents, motor vehicle collisions are the leading cause of head injuries, followed by trauma resulting from acts of violence.

Compared to adults, toddlers and preschoolers have a lower incidence of spine injury. However, spine injuries in children tend to be high cervical injuries and therefore are more lethal. During adolescence, the adult pattern of neck injuries is seen. Among adolescent males, diving injuries are a common source of cervical-spine injury.

## Chest and Abdomen Injuries

Because the chest wall in young children contains more cartilage, less bone, and less muscle than that of an adult, the transmission of the energy of blunt trauma to the underlying organs is increased. As a result, flail chest and displaced broken ribs due to blunt trauma are rare in younger children, but contusions of the lungs or heart, hemothorax, and pneumothorax can occur.

A potentially life-threatening pediatric chest injury is commotio cordis, the sudden death of a healthy preadolescent (most often a male) who is struck in the chest by a hard object such as a baseball, or strikes a hard surface with the chest, such as might occur during snowboarding, skiing, or mountain biking. The transmission of the blunt force through the child's chest wall to the heart interrupts the normal electrical pattern of the heart, resulting in ventricular fibrillation and, if not immediately treated by defibrillation, sudden cardiac death.

Because of the small size of a child's thorax, injuries that appear to involve the chest only also may cause injuries to abdominal organs (Figure 30-19■). Immature muscle provides less anterior and posterior protection to the abdominal organs. In blunt force trauma, more energy is transmitted to the intra-abdominal solid organs (liver and spleen) and to the kidneys. Injuries to these organs can result in significant internal bleeding, leading to hypovolemic shock. Hollow organ trauma in nonpenetrating injuries to the abdomen is less common in children than in adults.

Because the pelvic bones in younger children are softer and more flexible, fractures of the pelvis are less likely in children than in adults. Because a teenager's pelvis is more like an adult's, they are at increased risk of fracture as compared to younger children.

## Extremity Injuries

As explained in the anatomy section of this chapter, the ends of the long bones of children (and the bones of the skull and pelvis as well) contain growth plates. The sites of the growth plates are more prone to a fracture than are the shafts of the bones. In children, the more elastic and pliable bone shafts tend to bend instead of break into pieces, and when they bend, the result is a greenstick fracture.

### Pediatric Trauma

NOTE

For any given mechanism of injury, children are more likely than adults to have more severe injuries and injuries that affect more than one body system.

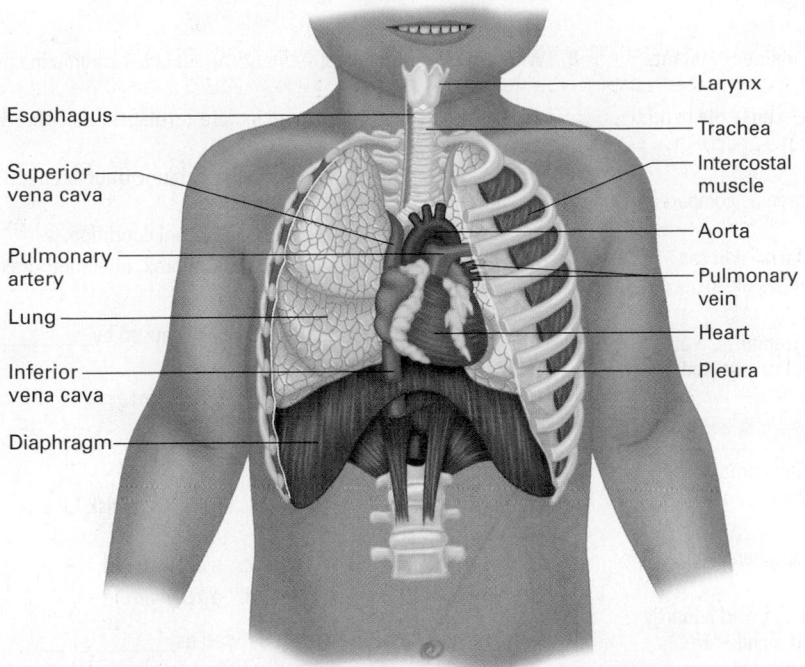

**Figure 30-19** Due to a child's size, injuries to the chest can also involve injuries to the abdomen.

## Burns and Electrocutions

Burns are among the most common childhood injuries, affecting approximately 88,000 children under 14 years of age in the United States each year. Scald-related burns are the most common type of burn, especially among toddlers and preschool children who pull hot fluids down onto themselves. Injuries involving open flames most commonly affect school-age children and adolescents. Chemical burns occur less frequently and affect older children more often than younger children. Infants and toddlers are more susceptible to electrical burns than are older children due to their curiosity and lack of understanding of electricity. Electrical injuries most commonly occur when a toddler or preschooler sticks a metal object into a wall outlet or when an infant chews on a live electrical cord. Most burn and electrocution injuries occur within the home.

## STOP, THINK, UNDERSTAND

### Multiple Choice

Choose the correct answer.

1. SIDS stands for_____
   a. sudden infant death syndrome.
   b. systematic infant disease spectrum.
   c. a system for assessing pediatric patients using skin (color and tone), irritability, disability, and sensory response.
   d. standard infant disability scale.

2. The leading cause of death in children is_____
   a. SIDS.
   b. poisoning.
   c. cardiac arrest.
   d. trauma.

3. The most common cause of traumatic brain injury in children is_____
   a. a fall.
   b. motor vehicle collisions.
   c. shaken child syndrome.
   d. prolonged febrile seizures.

*continued*

STOP, THINK, UNDERSTAND *continued*

4. Which of the following statements about head injuries in infants and toddlers is true? _____
   a. A child's large head and weak neck muscles cause the head to lead the way in a fall, subjecting it to a greater chance of injury.
   b. Head injuries tend to be less severe in children as compared to adults.
   c. A young child's facial fat pads and thicker facial skin can result in a severe head injury with few or no visible signs of external injury.
   d. An increase in intracranial pressure due to traumatic brain injury is common in adolescents and adults but less common in younger children.

5. Which of the following statements is true? _____
   a. Brain swelling and herniation in a child usually progresses slowly and is almost always characterized by increasing nausea, vomiting, and lethargy.
   b. The signs and symptoms of brain swelling and herniation can progress rapidly.
   c. The severity of the nausea, vomiting, headache, and lethargy that develop with a traumatic head injury in a child are directly proportional to the amount and severity of brain swelling.
   d. Children never show signs of head trauma until it is too late.

6. The most common cause of head trauma in adolescents is_____
   a. falls.
   b. sports injuries.
   c. motor vehicular accidents.
   d. acts of violence.

7. Which of the following statements about spinal injury in children are true? (check all that apply)
   _____ a. Toddlers and preschoolers have a lower incidence of spinal trauma than do adults.
   _____ b. Spinal injuries in children tend to be higher on the spinal column than those in adults and are therefore more lethal.
   _____ c. Spinal injuries in adolescents are typically less severe than those in adults.
   _____ d. Spinal injuries in young children tend to be lower on the spinal column and are therefore less severe than those in adults.

8. Which of the following statements about chest trauma in children is not true? _____
   a. A child's chest wall contains more cartilage, less bone, and less muscle than that of an adult.
   b. Children suffer less transmission of blunt-trauma energy to underlying organs than do adults.
   c. Commotio cordis is a potentially lethal condition.
   d. Children are not immune to hemothorax, pneumothorax, or pericardial tamponade.

9. With commotio cordis, death is typically caused by_____
   a. a long fall.
   b. a blow to the chest directly over the heart.
   c. overexertion.
   d. blunt force trauma to the abdomen.

10. Which of the following individuals is at greater risk for a pelvic fracture? _____
    a. a 1-year-old        c. a 10-year-old
    b. a 5-year-old        d. a 16-year-old

11. A "greenstick" fracture is best defined as_____
    a. an incomplete break through the epiphyseal plate of a long bone.
    b. a comminuted mid-shaft fracture of a long bone.
    c. the result of excessive bending of the shaft of a long bone.
    d. occurring when a piece of a long bone is sheared off entirely.

12. When compared to trauma injuries in adults, trauma injuries in children are likely to be_____
    a. less severe.
    b. more severe and affect a single body system.
    c. more severe, cause more injuries, and affect multiple body systems.
    d. less severe to bones of the extremities, muscles, and ligaments, but more severe to the hips, pelvis, and internal organs.

13. Of the following, the most common injury in children under age 14 is_____
    a. blunt chest trauma.
    b. penetrating abdominal injury.
    c. a broken pelvis.
    d. burns.

---

**⊕ 30-9** List five indicators of potential child abuse and neglect.

**child abuse**   any act or failure to act on the part of a parent, a caregiver, or any adult that results in serious physical or emotional harm or imminent risk of harm to a child.

## Child Abuse and Neglect

Child abuse is a legal term, not a medical diagnosis, and its definition can vary according to state or provincial law. **Child abuse** is defined as any act, or the failure to act on the part of a parent, a caregiver, or any adult that results in serious physical or emotional harm or imminent risk of harm to any child. As with adults, abuse can be physical, emotional, psychological, or sexual. **Child neglect** is more common than physical abuse and is defined as the failure to provide for the shelter, safety, supervision, and nutritional needs of a child (Figure 30-20a–c■).

Sadly, many children in the United States are abused or neglected. Child abuse transcends all cultures, socioeconomic classes, races, and religions. Most abusers are a parent or someone who is close to the child (e.g., a step-parent, a divorced parent's

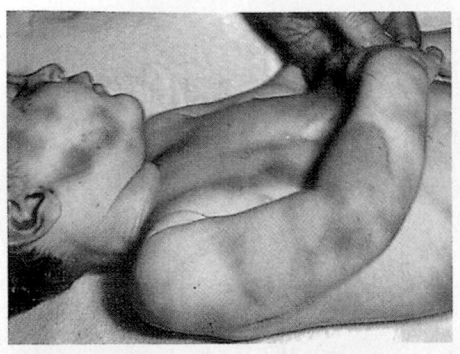

**Figure 30-20a** Physical abuse in a child: multiple fatal injuries.

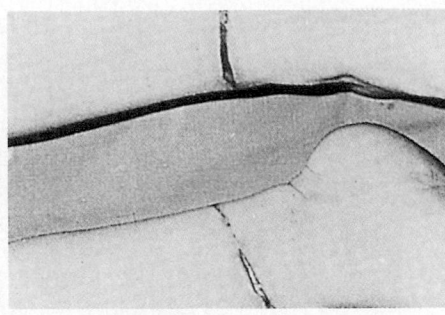

**Figure 30-20b** Physical abuse in a child: cuts from restraints.

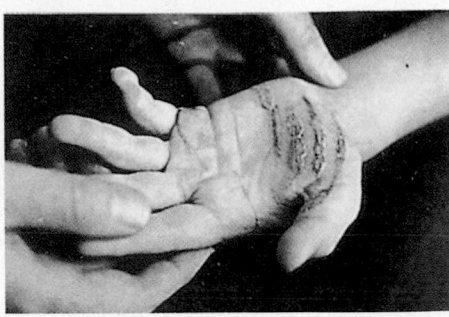

**Figure 30-20c** Physical abuse in a child: burns from a stove.

significant other, a caregiver, a sibling, a relative, or a family friend). Each year nearly 2,000 children die from abuse or neglect; 75 percent of them are under 4 years old.

Cultural norms concerning the treatment of children vary widely. What one culture may view as appropriate care and discipline of a child may be viewed in another culture as abusive. Child abuse is not a new phenomenon, but instead a painful part of human culture for millennia.

One form of physical abuse of which OEC Technicians should be acutely aware is **shaken baby syndrome**. Also known as abusive head trauma, shaken baby syndrome is a condition that results when a person picks up and intentionally shakes a newborn, an infant, or a young toddler. The ensuing "whiplash" effect causes the child's brain to forcefully contact the bones within the skull. Traumatic brain injury can result, often with fatal consequences. Studies show that most cases of shaken baby syndrome are perpetrated by the child's caregiver or someone close to the child. Shaken baby syndrome should be suspected in cases of head injury in a child that is less than 1 year old and for which the caregiver cannot give a plausible explanation of what happened to the child.

Even though child abuse is a crime in all states and provinces, the laws regarding the reporting of possible abuse vary. Most states and provinces allow anonymous reporting to prevent retaliation against the person who reported the suspected abuse. Generally, individuals who report suspected abuse are legally shielded from lawsuits, but only if they report suspected abuse to the proper agency. In some jurisdictions, medical personnel are required by law to report any suspicion of abuse and are subject to penalties if they do not. OEC Technicians should determine the legal requirements regarding the reporting of suspected abuse in their locations.

The report of abuse activates an investigation by specially trained social workers, nurses, and physicians, who look for the signs and symptoms of abuse. In most cases, the investigation is stopped if corroborating evidence is not found. If abuse is substantiated, intervention services are implemented.

## Shock

Shock is a state of inadequate tissue perfusion that can have medical or traumatic origins. In children, hypovolemic and distributive shock occur more frequently than cardiogenic or obstructive shock. The signs of shock in children are illustrated in Figure 30-21■.

Hypovolemia is the most common cause of shock in children. It can occur from dehydration due to vomiting and/or diarrhea, from acute external blood loss, or from internal bleeding. Whereas most adults can easily tolerate the loss of a pint of blood (the amount typically removed during blood donation), a pint can equal 30 percent of the total blood volume of an infant or small child.

**child neglect** a failure to act on the part of a parent, a caregiver, or other responsible adult to provide for the physical, emotional, educational, safety, or social needs of a child to the extent that emotional, developmental, or physical harm may occur.

**shaken baby syndrome** a condition in which an infant or toddler is picked up and violently shaken, causing a traumatic brain injury.

**Figure 30-21** Signs of shock in a child.

**SIGNS OF SHOCK (HYPOPERFUSION) IN A CHILD**

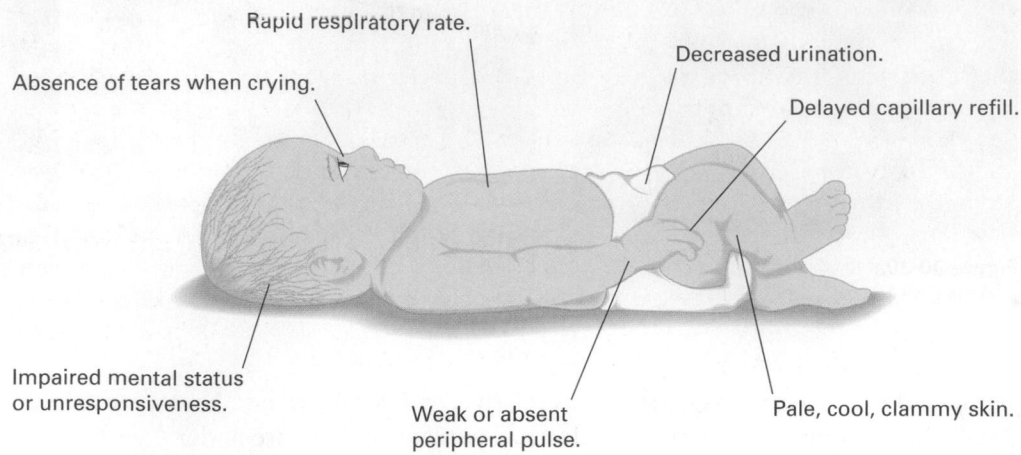

- Rapid respiratory rate.
- Absence of tears when crying.
- Decreased urination.
- Delayed capillary refill.
- Impaired mental status or unresponsiveness.
- Weak or absent peripheral pulse.
- Pale, cool, clammy skin.

The second most likely cause of shock in a child is sepsis. Additionally, anaphylaxis resulting from an insect bite, a food allergy, or exposure to a poison also can cause shock. Cardiogenic shock is rare except in children who have a congenital heart condition. Obstructive shock can occur and is usually due to blunt chest trauma that results in pericardial tamponade or a tension pneumothorax.

## STOP, THINK, UNDERSTAND

### Multiple Choice
Choose the correct answer.

1. Which of the following statements about child abuse are true? (check all that apply)
   - _____ a. Child abuse includes exposing a child to the risk of imminent harm.
   - _____ b. Child abuse is a fairly recent social phenomenon.
   - _____ c. Child abuse is a legal term, not a medical diagnosis.
   - _____ d. Child abuse primarily occurs among the poor.
   - _____ e. Most perpetrators of abuse are strangers to the child.
   - _____ f. A person required to report child abuse must have absolute proof prior to reporting.

2. Which of the following statements regarding the reporting of child abuse or neglect by OEC Technicians is not true? _____
   a. OEC Technicians should be familiar with local laws governing mandatory reporting of suspicion of abuse or neglect by EMS or health care providers.
   b. Individuals required to report child abuse should not report child abuse unless they are quite certain that an injury resulted from abuse.
   c. Doctors need not report abuse since the law protects them from prosecution.
   d. Generally, individuals reporting suspected abuse are legally shielded from lawsuits, but only if they report suspected abuse to the proper agency.

3. The two most common forms of shock in children are_____
   a. hypovolemic and distributive.
   b. hypovolemic and cardiogenic.
   c. obstructive and anaphylactic.
   d. obstructive and distributive.

4. A pint of blood, the amount taken from an adult during blood donation, is equivalent to approximately what percentage of a small child's blood volume? _____
   a. 10 percent
   c. 50 percent
   b. 30 percent
   d. 75 percent

5. Abusive head trauma is one name for abuse that occurs when a caregiver_____
   a. picks up and violently shakes a child or infant.
   b. strikes a child over the head with an object.
   c. slaps or punches a child in the face or on the head.
   d. fails to restrain a child in a child safety seat and the child's head strikes the windshield during a collision.

6. When cardiac arrest occurs in children, it usually results from_____
   a. respiratory failure.
   c. blunt trauma to the chest.
   b. exsanguination.
   d. blunt trauma to the head.

# CASE UPDATE

Smiling, you approach the young patient and crouch down beside her. You introduce yourself to her and to her grandmother and reassure both of them that you are there to help. You ask and receive the grandmother's permission to examine the child. Sensing her fear and pain, you ask the child her name. Although the grandmother already told you what happened, you ask the girl, "What happened?" and "Where does it hurt?" In response to your calm, caring approach, she stops crying and points with her left index finger at her right upper arm and shoulder.

With the grandmother's assistance, you carefully lift the child out of the water and onto more stable ground, being careful to protect her injured arm and shoulder.

Recognizing that an 8-year-old has trouble regulating her internal temperature, you gently wrap the girl's legs in a space blanket. With the help of other OEC Technicians, you carefully remove the child's life-jacket, compliment her for wearing a helmet, and continue to wrap her torso in the space blanket.

**What should you do now?**

# Assessment

Assessment of a pediatric patient follows the same steps as that of an adult. However, you may need to modify the assessment based on the child's age and level of development.

When assessing a child, remember that the heart rate and respiration rate can change very rapidly because of the child's emotional response to injury or fear of being approached by a stranger. The child's crying can make assessment very difficult. More importantly, the metabolic compensation mechanisms in a child's body can make the condition appear stable when, in fact, the patient is in shock. For these reasons and others, OEC Technicians must not assume that all is well with a child who does not exhibit signs of serious illness or injury. Instead, it is very important that OEC Technicians carefully evaluate both the child and the mechanism of injury or nature of illness, and place this information in context with the assessment findings, the child's history, age, and developmental stage, and the parent's knowledge of what is normal and abnormal for the child.

## Scene Size-Up, MOI, and Consent

As with any incident, the assessment process begins with a scene size-up. Remove all potential hazards that are present. Especially for young patients, do not overlook seemingly innocuous objects such as a pencil, keys, or small objects that could become a hazard in the hands of a curious child. If numerous potential hazards are present, consider moving patients who do not have a spinal injury and their caregivers to a safer, more secure location. If trauma is suspected, attempt to determine the mechanism of injury, and be sure to assess it carefully and in context with the child's anatomy and developmental stage. As with any patient, observe proper Standard Precautions.

As you approach the patient, begin to formulate a general impression of the patient's overall condition. To facilitate this process, the American Academy of Pediatrics recommends the use of the **pediatric assessment triangle** (Figure 30-22■), which enables rescuers to quickly assess a child's appearance, work of breathing, and circulation to skin.

By evaluating these criteria, OEC Technicians can quickly determine whether a child is "sick" or "not sick." In most instances, this exam can be performed in just a few seconds by simply looking and listening as you approach the patient.

⊕ **30-11** Describe and demonstrate how to assess a pediatric patient, using the pediatric assessment triangle.

**pediatric assessment triangle** an assessment tool that utilizes a pediatric patient's appearance (mental status, body position, and muscle tone), work of breathing (visible movement, effort, and audible sounds), and circulation (skin color) to assess the patient's well-being.

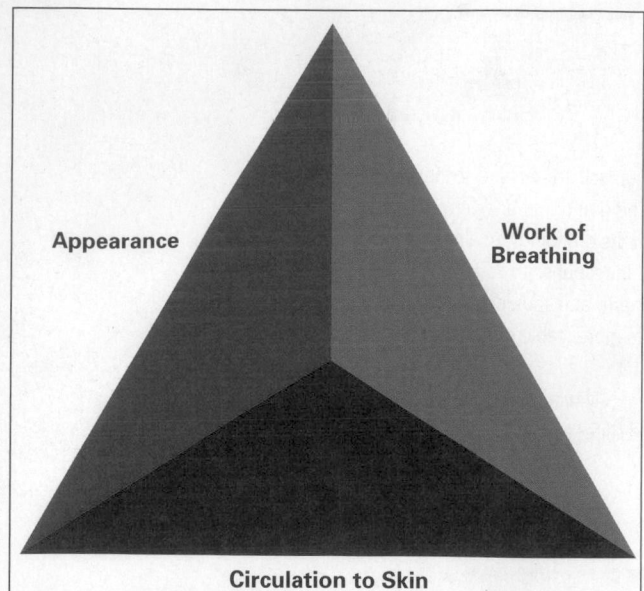

**Figure 30-22** The pediatric assessment triangle.
Used with permission of the American Academy of Pediatrics

**tripod position**    a position in which a patient sits upright and leans forward onto outstretched arms; the head and chin are thrust forward in an attempt to keep the airway open.

**Figure 30-23** As you approach the child, observe the patient's appearance.
Copyright Craig Brown

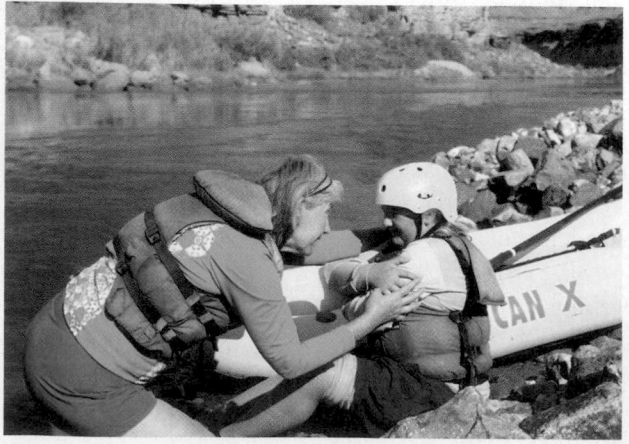

If a parent is present, be sure to ask for permission (consent) to assess and care for children under 18 years of age (or under the age of majority in your state or province). Emancipated minors may provide their own consent for care. If there are no contraindications (e.g., a suspected spinal injury), leave a young child in the caregiver's arms because this will help both of them to feel more secure and in control. Remember, to a young child, you are a stranger. Many children obtain cues from their parent or caregiver that may dictate their response. If the parent is comfortable with your approach and assessment, the child will likely be less afraid and more cooperative. If a parent or caregiver is not present, and the child needs care, implied consent takes effect (see Chapter 1, Introduction to Outdoor Emergency Care).

### The Child's Appearance

As you approach the child, observe the patient's appearance (Figure 30-23■). Is the child obviously injured or ill? A child who is unresponsive, has labored breathing, is pale, and/or has major bleeding should alert you to a possible life-threatening problem. Obvious limb deformities, "painful" crying, or an apparent decreased level of responsiveness are also signs of a serious condition. If there are no obvious findings of major illness or injury, continue to observe the patient for other clues, and ask yourself the following questions:

+ *Is the child active and moving about, or instead sits still and is quiet?* Children who are laughing or playful are not seriously ill. A child who sits still or is sitting forward and drooling is in a condition that warrants rapid transport.

+ *Does the child make eye contact?* It is generally a good sign if a child immediately focuses on your face and can follow your movements. Likewise, toddlers or preschoolers who make eye contact with you, start crying, and then immediately seek their parent are probably not seriously ill. Such children are responding in an age-appropriate manner to a stranger. Children who do not engage you or look at you and then refocus on themselves, have a weak cry, or are not moving should alert you to a possible serious medical condition.

+ *Does the child appear irritable or agitated?* Under normal conditions, a parent or caregiver should be able to console and quiet a child. Children who are ill often cry or whine upon even small movements or changes in position and often cannot be comforted. An infant who is paradoxically irritable—that is, one who becomes quiet when left alone but is irritable when in the caregiver's arms—should be considered very ill.

+ *Does the child respond to his caregiver's voice?* A child who quiets, smiles, or appropriately responds to a caregiver's voice is generally less ill than one who does not.

### Respiratory Effort

Observe children for signs of increased respiratory effort (Figure 30-24■). In most cases, the appearance of a child in respiratory failure is striking. A child who is in respiratory distress is typically found sitting upright and may assume the **tripod position**. Infants may also extend the head and neck into the "sniffing" position, with the nose in the air, which straightens the airway as much as possible to allow as much air as possible to reach the lungs. Children with epiglottitis may be drooling because swallowing is extremely painful.

Look for the use of accessory muscles and for nasal flaring. The child's head may bob up and down as the sternocleidomastoid muscles contract during inhalation and relax during exhalation. Paradoxical breathing, also known as see-saw breathing, may be present; the abdomen extends outward and the chest collapses inward upon inhalation. During exhalation, the opposite occurs: the abdomen sinks inward and the chest protrudes outward. If the patient is shirtless, look for retractions, in which the soft tissues above the sternum and clavicles and between and below the ribs sink inward upon inhalation. Be aware that in older children, retraction becomes less obvious.

Listen to how the child is breathing. Respiratory sounds can vary greatly with the severity of distress, ranging from an almost inaudible sigh to wheezing or grunting. Sounds can be heard during inhalation, exhalation, or both. Wheezing may be heard during inhalation or exhalation, whereas grunting is heard only during exhalation. In children, wheezing is a high-pitched whistling sound. Grunting is a low-pitched sound that may sometimes resemble a whimper. It is usually constant but can be intermittent. Grunting opens the smallest passages to the alveoli, maximizing gas exchange. Both wheezing and grunting indicate lower airway problems and severe respiratory distress. A high-pitched barking cough suggests croup.

Observe how fast the child is breathing, realizing that pain, anxiety, fear, excitement, and other factors can increase the breathing rate, and that the normal rate of respiration depends on the age of the child. Even though crying can make it difficult to assess the rate of breathing, it generally indicates that air is moving in and out of the lungs well. When assessing breathing effort, ask yourself not only "Is air moving?" but also "Is air moving *well*?"

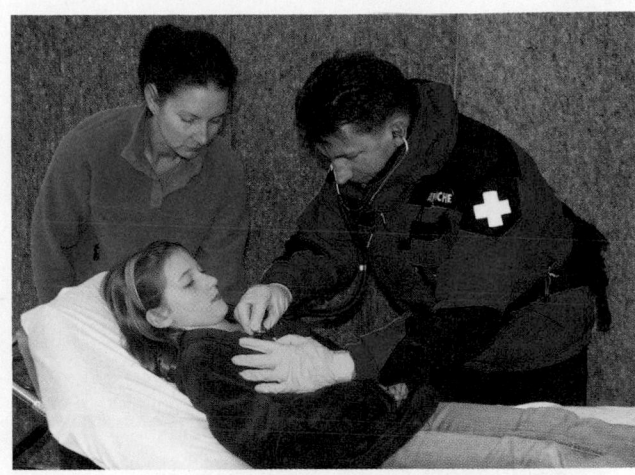

**Figure 30-24** Observe children for signs of increased respiratory effort.
Copyright Mike Halloran

### Circulation

Assess the child's skin color for clues regarding the perfusion of the patient's tissues. If low-light levels, cold environments, or dark skin make assessment more difficult, assess the sclera of the eyes, the lips, or the palms of the hands. The skin should appear pink, not pale, mottled, or gray or blue. If the skin is pink, the child is generally well oxygenated and has good tissue perfusion. An exception to this is carbon monoxide (CO) poisoning, in which the skin may appear pink or red but blood oxygen levels are very low.

Paleness suggests that either the blood is either poorly saturated with oxygen or that circulation is poor, as is seen with excessive blood loss, respiratory distress, or heart failure. Mottled skin (areas of red, purple, and white patches) or gray skin also indicates poor tissue perfusion. Cyanosis, a bluish tint to the skin and mucous membranes, is an ominous sign that indicates a serious respiratory problem or hypoxia.

### Questions to Be Asked Following a General Impression

*Is the child sick or not sick?*

*Is the child having a problem breathing?*

*What is the likely cause of the illness or injury?*

*Are urgent interventions needed?*

*Should rapid transport and EMS help be initiated?*

NOTE

## Primary Assessment

Upon making physical contact with the patient, perform a primary assessment in the usual manner (Figure 30-25 ■). Pay close attention to potential threats to life and correct any that may be present. Much of the primary assessment may already have been performed as part of the pediatric assessment triangle. Because cardiac arrest

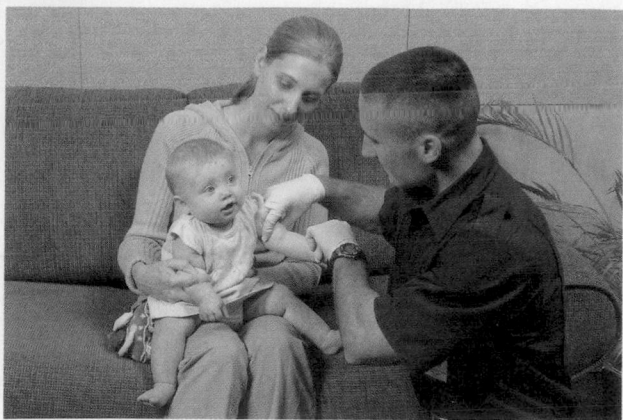

**Figure 30-25** Perform a primary assessment.

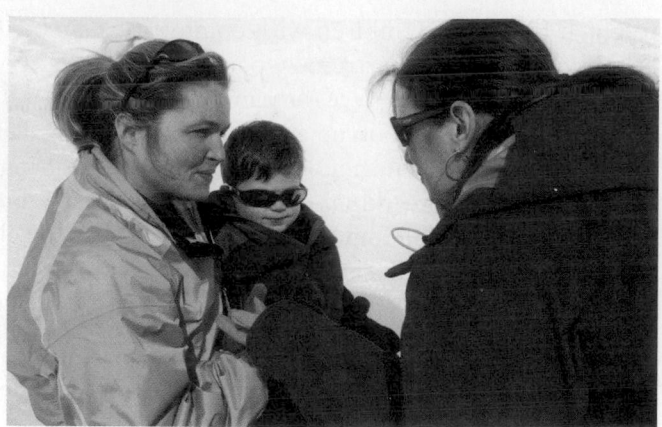

**Figure 30-26** Get down to the child's eye level and introduce yourself to the child and the caregiver.
Copyright Tristan Roberson

> **NOTE**
>
> ### Signs of Complete Airway Obstruction
>
> *Inability to cough*
>
> *Inability to speak or cry*
>
> *Respiratory arrest*

in pediatric patients is generally preceded by respiratory failure, assess the airway and respirations very carefully. Also, because a child's condition can change quickly, reassess the ABCDs frequently. If there is any evidence of ABCD-related compromise, request ALS assistance immediately and rapidly transport the patient to a definitive-care facility.

## Secondary Assessment

Next, perform a secondary assessment. Depending on the child's age and stage of development, you may need to use a somewhat different strategy. The success of the secondary assessment often is directly related to an OEC Technician's *ability to effectively communicate and interact* with patients and their caregivers.

### The History

For toddlers or preschoolers, most (if not all) of the SAMPLE history will come from the caregiver, who thus becomes an integral part of both the assessment process and the child's care-giving team. Establishing trust with both patients and caregivers early on is critical.

Approach children slowly and gently, crouching beside them so that you are at their eye level. Smile. Introduce yourself to both caregiver and child (Figure 30-26■). Ask for both of their names, and ask children directly what they like to be called. Speak in a normal, calm, and unhurried tone of voice, using words a child can understand. If the adult begins by telling you what happened, actively listen. Then, turn your attention to the child and paraphrase this information to the patient. For example, you might say, "It sounds like you took a pretty hard tumble on your arm! Can you show me where it hurts?" This acknowledges the information given by the caregiver and incorporates the child into the SAMPLE process. Alternate speaking and looking at the child and the caregiver, posing questions to both. Modify the words you use for body parts as appropriate. Use words such as "tummy" for preschoolers or younger school-aged children, and "belly" or "abdomen" for teens.

School-aged children and adolescents should be treated as adults with respect to their need for respect and privacy. If you suspect possible substance abuse, pregnancy, or other privacy issues, have your partner interview the caregiver separately while you interact with the patient.

# STOP, THINK, UNDERSTAND

## Multiple Choice

Choose the correct answer.

1. The most likely reason a weak, crying infant would crane the head and neck with the nose in the air is_____
   a. an attempt to straighten the airway to allow more air into the lungs.
   b. crankiness.
   c. a stomachache.
   d. an attempt to defecate.

2. What can you learn about the condition of a 2-year-old who stops whining and reaches for her mother when she comes into the room?_____
   a. The child is probably very ill.
   b. While ill, the child's condition is probably not critical.
   c. The child is probably fine and just wanted her mother.
   d. There is little or nothing in this information to help you evaluate the seriousness of this child's condition.

3. The grunting sounds of a resting 4-year-old who is running a low-grade fever and is pale could indicate_____
   a. respiratory distress.
   b. stool holding or constipation.
   c. irritation with his mother for not picking him up.
   d. a mental or psychological disorder.

4. Which of these is not in the pediatric triangle?_____
   a. response to pain
   b. appearance
   c. circulation to skin
   d. work of breathing

5. One of the most important questions to ask yourself about a sick child is whether _____
   a. the child can speak in full sentences.
   b. the child has a fever.
   c. air is moving well in and out of the lungs.
   d. the child can cough.

6. The best way to assess circulation in a dark-skinned 7-month-old patient is to_____
   a. gently pinch the skin on the back of the hand and see how quickly it returns to its original color.
   b. look at the child's sclera, palms, or lips.
   c. check capillary refill in the child's nail beds.
   d. ask a caregiver to tell you if the child looks normal.

7. If no spinal injury is suspected, the best place to examine a toddler is_____
   a. on an examination table.
   b. on a bed or gurney.

   c. in a parent's or caregiver's arms.
   d. sitting on the floor with the child in your lap.

8. The pediatric assessment triangle includes a rapid assessment of the_____
   a. child's appearance, work of breathing, and circulation to the skin.
   b. mechanism of injury, skin color, and respiratory rate.
   c. respiratory rate and effort, pulse, and level of responsiveness.
   d. child's level of responsiveness, ability to cry, and pulse.

9. In which of the following cases would you suspect a potentially life-threatening illness or injury? (check all that apply)
   _____ a. A child who is sitting forward, is quiet, and is drooling.
   _____ b. A child who is pale and bleeding heavily from an arm laceration.
   _____ c. A child who took a hard fall skiing and is sitting in the snow giggling.
   _____ d. A quiet child of any age who will not make eye contact with you, turn toward your voice, or acknowledge your presence in any way.
   _____ e. A child who is using accessory muscles to breathe.
   _____ f. A infant who exhibits "see-saw" respirations.
   _____ g. A child who refuses to move.
   _____ h. A child who is whimpering but not crying after a fall.

10. Which of the following statements regarding the assessment of a pediatric patient are correct? (check all that apply)
   _____ a. Assessing a child is the same as assessing an adult.
   _____ b. Pediatric assessments should be modified according to the child's age and developmental level.
   _____ c. Changes in a child's heart and respiratory rate are almost always indicative of decompensating shock.
   _____ d. A crying child generally means a seriously injured child.
   _____ e. OEC Technicians should make every effort possible to quiet a crying child before beginning an exam.
   _____ f. OEC Technicians should ensure that innocuous but potentially hazardous items such as keys, pens or pencils, or other small objects are not within reach of a small patient.

## Short Answer

1. When approaching a child, what are some of the techniques you should use?

   _____
   _____
   _____
   _____

*continued*

**STOP, THINK, UNDERSTAND** *continued*

2. Describe the appearance of a child who is in respiratory failure.

_____

_____

_____

_____

3. Describe the best physical position for a rescuer to take when approaching a child.

_____

_____

_____

_____

## Honesty, Trust, and Communication

When caring for a child, always be honest. If something you will do will cause the child pain, say so in a kind way. Trust is essential when interacting with a pediatric patient. Once lost, it may be impossible to regain, and lost trust can affect other OEC Technicians who may become involved in a patient's treatment. How you interact with children and caregivers can truly "make or break" events at the scene.

Explain to children (if old enough to understand) and to caregivers what you are doing, step by step, *before* you do it. Children under 6 years of age might not be able to explain what is wrong or localize pain. For example, a child with a fractured humerus might scream when touched anywhere on the body. Screaming or crying due to pain, fear, or the desire to block out the situation can make communication difficult or impossible. Although it may be difficult, understand that crying is a normal way for children to cope with a frightening or stressful situation. At all times, refrain from showing irritation or anger, even if it is difficult to do so.

Try gently placing a hand on the child's (uninjured) arm, and make eye contact. Quietly ask children if they are afraid or in pain, and acknowledge and accept what they tell you. Show understanding, such as nodding and saying calmly, "I'd be feeling scared too, if I fell and hurt myself." Offer honest reassurance such as, "We are going to do everything we can to make you better." Be careful not to promise something you cannot provide, such as a guarantee that nothing you do will cause pain. Never belittle or admonish the feelings of either a child or a caregiver; instead, show acceptance, respect, and provide reassurance that you are there to help.

Also, be careful how you phrase questions to avoid placing yourself in a no-win situation. For example, asking a child, "Is it okay if we splint your arm now?" might land you in a trust-breaking impasse if the child answers "No." Instead, offer the patient or caregiver a choice, such as "Would you like me or (OEC Technician) Emily to put the splint on your arm?" or, "Can I help your mother (or father) put this splint on you?" while *you* apply the splint (with the parent's help). This empowers the child through choices and ensures the needed outcome (in this case, splinting the arm).

Nearly all children settle down and communicate with an OEC Technician if they are made as comfortable as possible (Figure 30-27■). Providing warmth—or better yet, moving an injured child indoors as

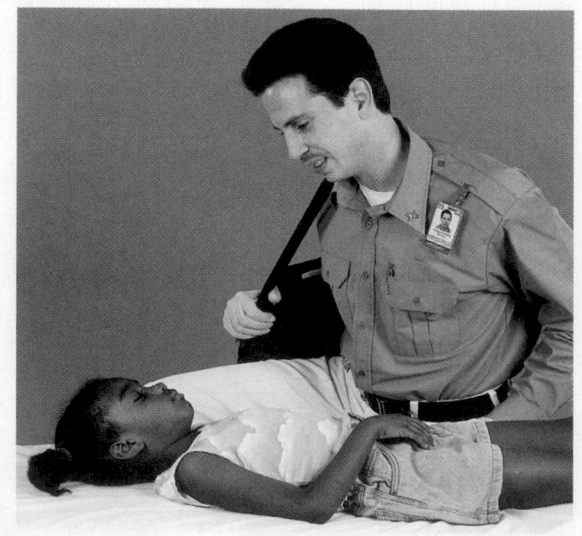

**Figure 30-27** Make the child as comfortable as possible.

quickly as the situation will allow—is a good first step in providing for the child's safety, comfort, and well-being.

When obtaining the SAMPLE history, be sure to ask when the child was last well. Parents will often state that the child was well when put to bed but awoke during the night complaining of symptoms. Ask about the child's normal appearance and behaviors, including eating habits; this information is essential, especially when assessing young children who may not understand questions or be able to answer them. Have the caregiver describe any abnormal behaviors and explain what the corresponding normal behaviors are. If, for example, a parent reports that a child "spaced out for a while" or that an infant was grunting rhythmically while lying unresponsive in his crib, the problem could be related to seizure activity.

If the initial complaint is pain, assess the symptoms using the standard OPQRST mnemonic, using age-appropriate words and terms. Be sure to ask where the pain is located, because ear or throat pain may indicate the presence of an infectious disease such as tonsillitis or epiglottitis. Also ask if the pain is associated with nausea, vomiting, or diarrhea; if it is, ask how long NVD has been present, and how many known episodes of NVD the patient has had.

Gastroenteritis usually presents with repeated episodes of vomiting and is frequently accompanied by five or more explosive watery stools per day. Although vomiting usually lasts approximately 12 hours, diarrhea may persist several days to a week. If the patient is very young, ask if the child has had episodes of crying, and if so, how many hours or days it has been occurring.

Ask the parents of young children about fluid intake and output. For newborns and infants, ask how many bottles or feedings the child has had in the past 24 hours. Ask if the feedings have been of a normal frequency and amount, and if the child has experienced excessive urination or has had diarrhea.

Be sure to ask about any medications, vitamins, and nutritional supplements a pediatric patient may be taking, including over-the-counter medicines and herbal supplements.

Also ask if anything was done to help relieve the child's symptoms before your arrival on scene. For cases of croup, the parents may state that they placed the child next to a humidifier or took the child into the cool night air, whereupon the symptoms lessened or disappeared. They also may have given the child acetaminophen to control a fever.

## The Physical Exam

The physical exam of a pediatric patient can be challenging. The order in which the exam is performed may need to be modified according to the child's age and the suspected severity of the problem. For instance, it is often more productive to assess newborns and infants using a toes-to-head approach, instead of the traditional head-to-toes approach. The exam for these patients can often be made easier using a "peek-a-boo" approach. For preschool children, the exam may be facilitated by distracting the child with a toy or a tongue blade. Many emergency-care providers have toys that are used specifically for this purpose. Let the child play with the toy as you perform your exam. Additionally, involve the child in the exam process by allowing him to assist. If appropriate (based on the medical problem), infants or small children will usually feel more secure if you allow them to remain in their parent's arms.

Children are naturally curious, and young children may be far more willing to allow you to listen to their lungs if you let them listen to their own lungs first. Some children may become frightened if you examine their head first. In this case, examine the trunk and extremities first, and the head and neck last. Be aware when performing a physical exam that many children are ticklish and may flinch when their bodies are touched.

Most school-age children have been examined by a pediatrician and understand the process of a physical exam. Some may be fearful you are going to give them a "shot." Acknowledge their fear and be honest and reassuring about what you will and will not do. For example, you might say something like, "I don't like shots, either! But don't worry, I don't give shots." Be careful not to make statements such as this if you know that other members of the care team or ambulance crew may later need to give them a shot.

The physical exam of pediatric patients can be challenging. The order in which the exam is performed may need to be modified according to a child's age and the suspected severity of the problem. For instance, it is often more productive to assess newborns and infants using a toes-to-head approach, instead of the traditional head-to-toes approach.

Before the text discusses the details of a physical examination for pediatric patients, consider the following tips that can make examining children easier:

1. Identify yourself to caregivers (if present) and to pediatric patients who are old enough to understand. Talk to the child but include the parent or caregiver in the conversation. Use your first name, saying, "Hi, I'm David. What's your name?" Ask permission to care for the child if a parent or caregiver is present. In most states implied consent takes effect when an injured or sick child is alone and you are giving appropriate aid.

2. If the parents are not present, tell the child in simple language that someone will find them as soon as possible. Assigning the task of finding the parents to another OEC Technician in the presence of the child can reassure the child that the parents will be on the way as soon as possible.

3. If the patient is unresponsive or is severely injured or ill, correct problems relating to the ABCDs. Call for help and transport rapidly. Move as quickly as possible without creating more anxiety for the child or caregivers.

4. If the child does not have life-threatening injuries, proceed in a calm, reassuring, relaxed pace. Include pediatric patients in the care by giving them a toy or an inflated glove, or by letting them listen to their own heart/lungs first.

5. Sit, kneel, or squat so that you are down at a child's level. Standing over small children can make them feel fearful or threatened. Try to avoid loud or distracting noises, including transmissions from your radio. Try to keep bright light out of a patient's eyes, and keep the number of rescuers who are interacting with the patient to a minimum.

6. Be friendly and include both the patient and caregivers when speaking. Try to alleviate any fears any of them might have. Acknowledge and accept each patient's feelings. Smile sincerely.

7. Allow smaller children to remain in their parent's arms, if possible. Doing so can be comforting and reassuring to both.

8. Always be honest with pediatric patients. Some may be fearful, for instance, that you are going to give them a "shot." Avoid telling them "this won't hurt" when you know it might. Acknowledge their fear and be honest and reassuring about what you will and will not do. Helping a patient breathe through pain can also facilitate getting a painful procedure done. When applying a splint to a child's broken arm, for example, try acknowledging that it might hurt and then suggesting that the child take a deep breath in through the nose and then blow it out hard through the mouth ("smell the roses, blow out the candle") while you manipulate the arm.

9. Ask pediatric patients where it hurts, or ask caregivers where they suspect it hurts, and examine that area *last*. Obviously, if a body part requires a life-supporting measure, do this first. If a child points to a wrist, for example, examine the rest of the child's body, then examine the rest of the injured arm, and only then gently palpate the wrist. If you touch the painful wrist first, you might have a difficult time examining the rest of the patient.

10. If you need to use any equipment for the exam or for care, explain what you are doing in language your patient can understand. Whenever possible, allow a child to touch or examine the equipment first. Ask patients if they have any questions, and then answer them honestly and simply.

11. Although most school-age children have been examined by a pediatrician and understand the process of a physical exam, young children might not understand what you mean by, "I'm going to examine you." Accordingly, explain each step of the examination as you do it. Be willing to stop to answer questions or to reassure the child.

12. Maintain good eye contact with patients, both to maintain their confidence and to pick up subtle clues, such as a small grimace that indicates that something hurts. Speak directly to pediatric patients in simple language and reassure them that you are there to help them.

13. Make sure pediatric patients understand what you are saying. Ask questions such as, "Do you know how to take a deep breath? Can you do it for me?" Or better yet, show them how to do it. Simple praise, such as, "Oh, that was a great deep breath!" can work wonders in gaining the cooperation of preschoolers.

14. Continually reassure anxious caregivers. Never lose your cool, and never get excited.

**Figure 30-28** The respiratory rate is the most important vital sign in a child.

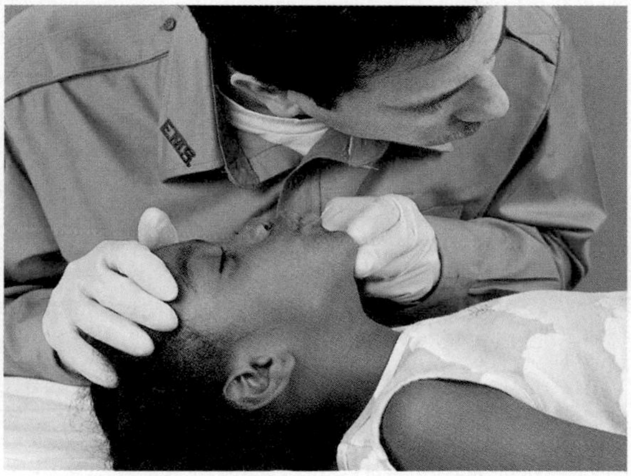

Begin each physical exam by obtaining an initial set of vital signs. See Table 30-2■. At a minimum, include the pulse rate and the respiration rate, the latter of which is the most important vital sign in young children (Figure 30-28■). Because children have a more variable breathing rate than that of adults, count breaths for 30 seconds and then multiply the count by 2. In general, a respiratory rate greater than 60 per minute or less than 15 per minute is cause for concern.

Assess circulation by measuring the peripheral pulse and blood pressure. Among the places to check the pulse are the brachial or femoral pulse in infants, the brachial pulse in small children, and the radial or carotid pulse in older children (Figures 30-29a–c■).

**Table 30-2** Normal Values for Pediatric Vital Signs

| | Infants (Birth–1 year) | Children (1–8 years) |
|---|---|---|
| Pulse | 100–120 beats per minute | 80–100 beats per minute |
| Respirations | 25–50 respirations per minute | 15–30 respirations per minute |
| Blood pressure | | |
|   Systolic | 75–95 mmHg | 80–100 mmHg |
|   Diastolic | 75–95 mmHg | 70–110 mmHg |
| Temperature | 36.1–38.0° C | 36.1–38.0° C |
| | (97.0–100.4° F) | (97.0–100.4° F) |
| Pulse oximetry | > 95% | > 95% |
| Mental status | GCS = 15 | GCS = 15 |

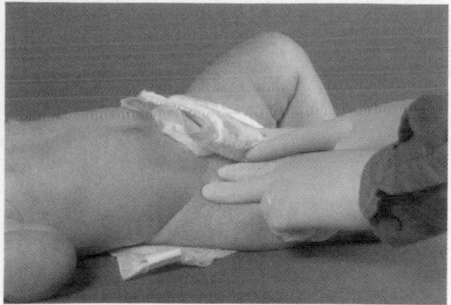

**Figure 30-29a** Assessing the femoral pulse in an infant.

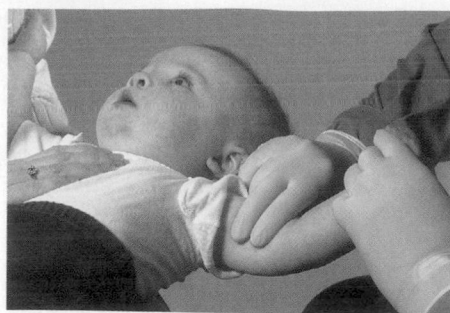

**Figure 30-29b** Checking the brachial pulse in an infant.

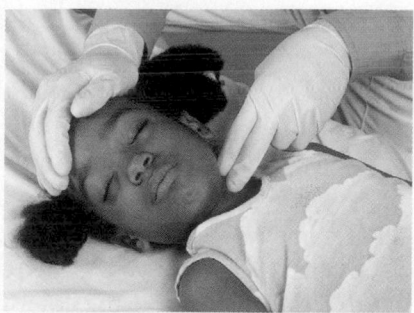

**Figure 30-29c** Assessing the carotid pulse in an older child.

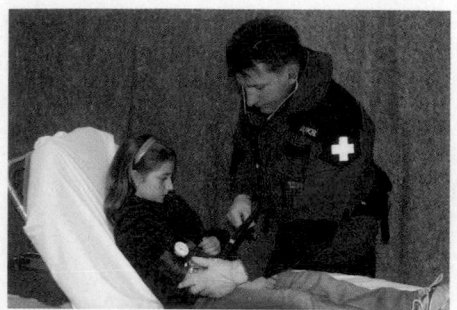

**Figure 30-30** Take a child's blood pressure using a pediatric blood pressure cuff.
Copyright Mike Halloran

Measure blood pressure using a properly sized pediatric cuff (Figure 30-30■). A standard adult-sized BP cuff usually can be used for teenagers. Note that blood pressure can be very difficult to measure in children under 3 years. Remember that because children can compensate well for shock initially, blood pressure is not a reliable indicator of shock.

For school-age children and adolescents, perform a head-to-toe examination in the usual fashion. For preschoolers and younger children, after completing the primary assessment, begin the physical exam by gently palpating the extremities, leaving out any part that could hurt *until the end of the entire exam* (Figure 30-31■).

Assess capillary refill and distal pulses (Figure 30-32■). Check distal sensation by gently scratching a child's hand or foot. Small children will withdraw the extremity if they have sensation, whereas older children can tell you they can feel you. Assess skin color and note any skin tenting, if present. Examine the pelvis gently, in the same way you would for an adult (Figure 30-33■).

Expose and inspect the abdomen, looking for any signs of injury using the DCAP-BTLS mnemonic (Figure 30-34■). Gently palpate each abdominal quadrant leaving until last the quadrant the child has identified as being painful (Figure 30-35■). Watch each child's response carefully, because even minor trauma can cause splenic or liver injuries in children due to the poor protection their undeveloped abdominal muscles provide.

Expose the chest to look for evidence of trauma, again using DCAP-BTLS (Figure 30-36■). Due to thoracic flexibility, children can receive significant injuries within the chest cavity with only minor external chest wall findings. Whenever children will tolerate it, listen to the lungs, noting any abnormal sounds.

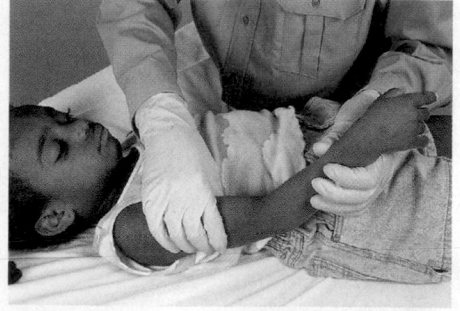

**Figure 30-31** For preschoolers and younger children, begin the physical exam by palpating the extremities.

**Figure 30-32** Assessing capillary refill in a child.
Copyright Mike Halloran

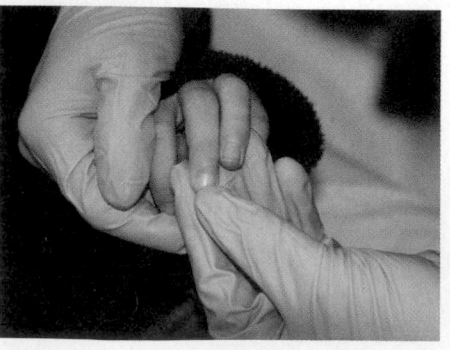

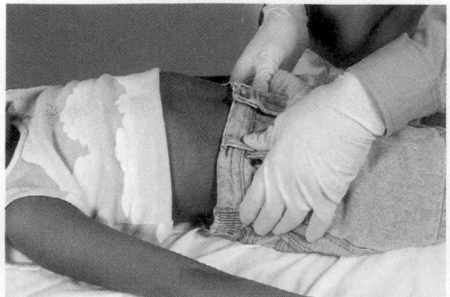

**Figure 30-33** Assess the pelvis in a child gently, in the same way you would use for an adult.

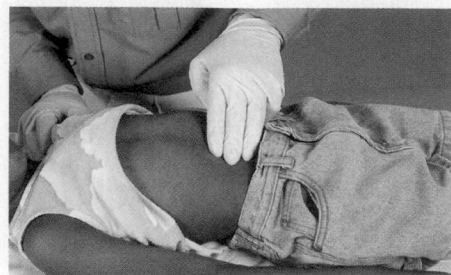

**Figure 30-34** Expose and inspect a child's abdomen using the DCAP-BTLS mnemonic.

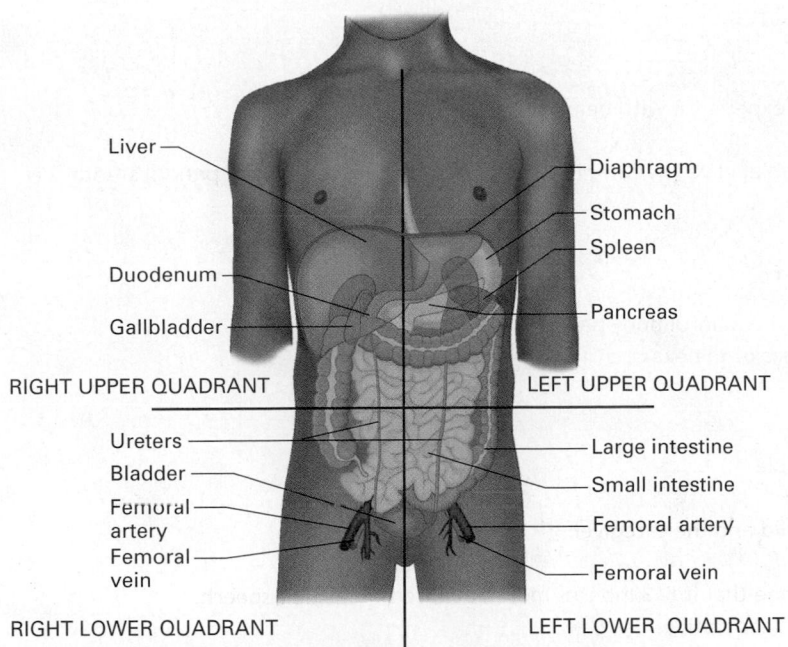

Liver
Diaphragm
Stomach
Spleen
Duodenum
Gallbladder
Pancreas

RIGHT UPPER QUADRANT    LEFT UPPER QUADRANT

Ureters
Bladder
Femoral artery
Femoral vein
Large intestine
Small intestine
Femoral artery
Femoral vein

RIGHT LOWER QUADRANT    LEFT LOWER QUADRANT

**Figure 30-35** The four abdominal quadrants.

Palpate the entire spine (Figure 30-37■). Be sure to watch the child's facial expressions for any indications of pain; such findings are an indication of the need for spinal immobilization.

Gently inspect and palpate the head and face of children as you would for an adult (Figure 30-38■). However, be careful when assessing a newborn or infant's head because the fontanels are delicate. Note whether the fontanels are level with the scalp (normal) or are either sunken or bulging (both abnormal). Look in the child's nose and ears for blood or fluid. Check the nose and mouth for excess mucus, swelling, or obstructions. Gently palpate the neck, again looking at the child's face for signs of discomfort (Figure 30-39■).

Finally, assess any other area(s) that appear to be injured. Be gentle, take time to explain what you will do before you do it, and warn patients about any part of the exam that might produce discomfort. Table 30-3■ summarizes the approaches to examining the different age groups of pediatric patients.

Continue to monitor pediatric patients and perform frequent reassessments, including respiratory and circulatory status, level of responsiveness, skin color, and vital signs, for valuable clues concerning whether or not patients are responding to care.

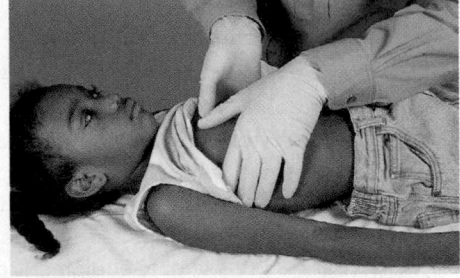

**Figure 30-36** Expose the chest to look for signs of trauma.

**Figure 30-38** Inspect and palpate the child's head and face.

**Figure 30-39** Examine the neck, watching the child's face for signs of discomfort.

**Figure 30-37** Palpate the child's entire spine.

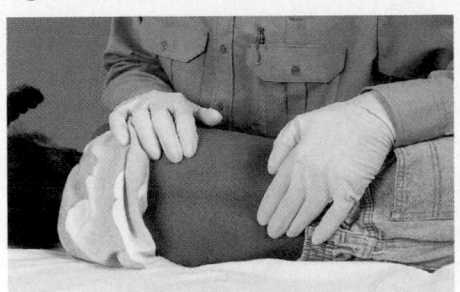

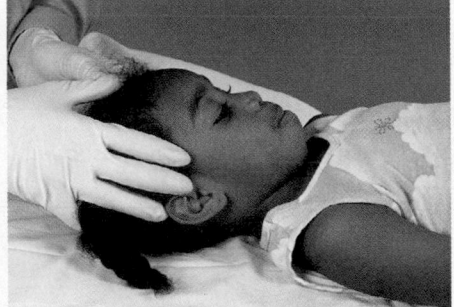

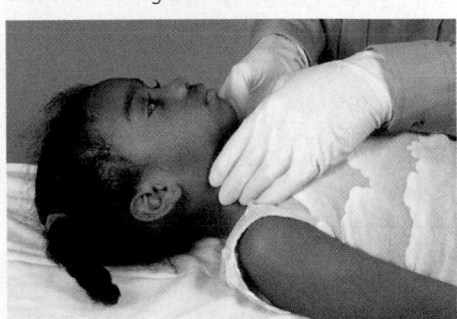

**Table 30-3**  Age-Based Assessment of Children

**Infants: ages 1 month to 1 year**

- Child is aware of surroundings but has limited experience with being examined.
- Examine the child in a caregiver's arms.
- Engage the caregiver in the evaluation; if possible, have the caregiver assist whenever removing the patient's clothes is necessary.
- Approach at the level of the child.
- Move slowly and calmly during the exam.
- Tell the caregiver what you are doing.
- Examine the least painful body parts first, and the painful body part last.
- Inform the caregiver about possibly painful parts of the exam.

**Toddlers: ages 12–36 months**

- May be fearful of strangers.
- Examine the child in a caregiver's arms, if possible.
- Approach at the level of the child.
- Move slowly and calmly, talking to both the child and the caregiver.
- Address the child first.
- Recognize that children can understand language that is 6–8 months more advanced than their speech.
- Toddlers may push your hands away and be uncooperative.
- Be gently persistent. The child's resistance will lessen.
- Avoid asking any question that a child can answer "no."
- Perform the most painful part of the exam last (if possible).
- Inform both the child and caregiver whenever pain could be associated with part of the exam.

**Preschool children: ages 3–5 years**

- They can move between fantasy and reality and are magical thinkers.
- They have good verbal skills and can be quite vocal.
- History taken from them is not always accurate; rely on the caregiver instead.
- If very sick, preschoolers can regress to the level of a toddler.
- Let patients decide whether or not they want to be examined in a caregiver's arms.
- Before you do something, use simple language to explain what you are going to do.
- Allow patients to examine equipment or listen to their own heart through a stethoscope first.
- Limit a patient's options to two choices.
- Praise good behavior in patients.
- Because a preschooler's temperament can change rapidly and unexpectedly, expect "meltdowns" or regressions in behavior.

**School-aged children: ages 6–12 years**

- These children understand cause and effect and recognize authority.
- Speak to children in simple terms and include caregivers.
- Perform the physical assessment in a head-to-toes fashion. (Touch the painful part last, if possible.)
- Respect each child's modesty and need for privacy.
- School-age children may respond better to a same-sex examiner.
- Inform school-age children what you are going to do before you do it.
- Inform patients if some part of the examination might hurt.
- If seriously injured children regress and become mute, involve caregivers in the examination.

**Adolescents: ages 13–18 years**

- They are rational and analytical.
- Decision making and control skills are not as advanced as analytic and verbal skills.
- Ask their permission to examine them.
- Respect their privacy.
- Evaluate and examine them apart from a parent's or caregiver's presence, especially if substance abuse or pregnancy may be involved.
- Respect their independence.
- Obtain the history directly from patients.
- Treat adolescents as you would an adult.
- Be direct and honest.

| Table 30-4 | When to Suspect Child Abuse |
|---|---|

- Multiple injuries (mix of new, old, and/or partially healed injuries)
- Bilateral injuries (injuries on both sides of the body)
- Circumferential bruising (bruise extends completely around an extremity)
- Bruises located in unusual places (especially the genitalia)
- Pattern bruises (e.g., an outline of an adult's hand, or a clear line of demarcation)
- Age-inappropriate injuries (e.g., a skull fracture in a child who is too young to walk)
- Inconsistent histories from the child and caregiver or from two caregivers
- History that is vague or changes over time
- Older children who cannot or will not provide an explanation for their injuries
- Any infant with an altered level of responsiveness

Because children can deteriorate quickly, never take your eyes off pediatric patients. Assess the vital signs every 3–5 minutes for children who are ill or injured, and every 10 minutes for pediatric patients with no apparent problems.

Even though some adults may express their fear and genuine worry for an injured child by acting angry, it is prudent to suspect child abuse whenever a parent or caregiver becomes verbally abusive to a child or berates the child for getting hurt. Calling a child names such as "stupid" or "idiot" also may be indicators of emotional or physical abuse. While it is common for a child to fear that a parent will be angry that the child got hurt ("Dad's going to be mad that we have to go home because I broke my leg"), children who completely withdraw from or cringe at the sight of a parent or caregiver should be considered at risk. Table 30-4■ lists additional signs of potential child abuse, which include bilateral injuries, bruises of various ages, histories that are inconsistent with the injury pattern, and suspected long bone fractures or head injuries in a child under 1 year of age.

# Management

⊕ 30-12 Describe and demonstrate how to manage common pediatric illnesses and injuries.

The basic principles for treating pediatric patients are the same as those for treating adults: mitigate any hazards and correct any ABCD-related problems. CPR for children, infants, and newborns is discussed in Chapter 15, Cardiovascular Emergencies. Because children have a smaller blood volume, control external bleeding aggressively; children easily can go into shock from a minor head laceration that is bleeding profusely. Even though children have vigorous compensatory physiologic mechanisms that allow them to respond to serious illness or trauma, compared to adults they have a smaller compensatory reserve and can go into shock quickly, often without exhibiting any external signs. Any child who looks sick and does not *appear* to be getting better with care is probably getting worse, even if the vital signs remain unchanged. For children who appear sick or injured, summon advanced life support personnel and/or arrange for rapid transportation to a definitive-care facility.

**Figure 30-40** In an infant that requires ventilation, do not hyperextend the neck.

You may need to modify how you deliver care based on a child's developmental stage. For instance, if ventilations are required, avoid hyperextending the necks of young children, or the airway may collapse (Figure 30-40■). For children under 1 year of age, open the airway by using the head-tilt, chin-lift maneuver to place the patient in a "sniffing" position (Figure 30-41■). Administer any needed ventilations at the respiratory rate that is normal for that child's age group.

If spine injury is suspected, apply a pediatric cervical collar and immobilize the child to a long spine board. If a pediatric collar is not

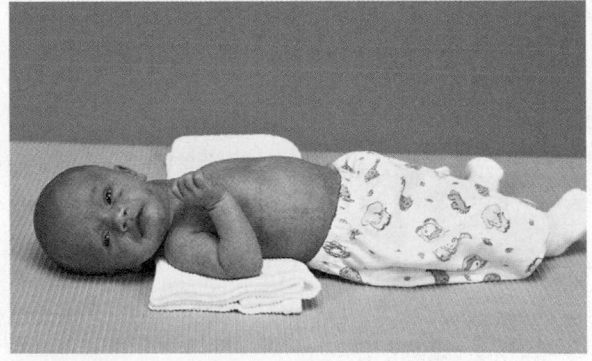

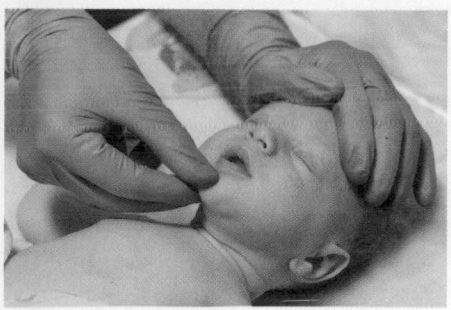

**Figure 30-41** Use the head-tilt, chin-lift for children under 1 year of age.

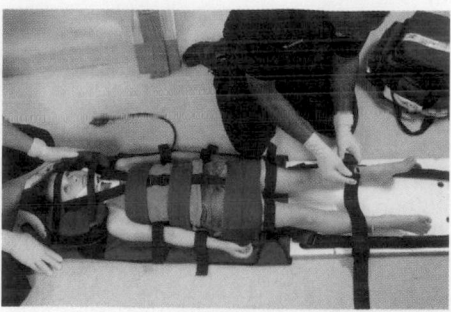

**Figure 30-42** Children, infants, and toddlers can be immobilized with a vest-style immobilization device.

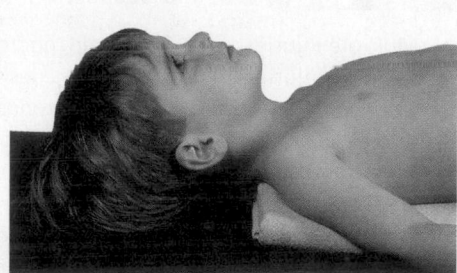

**Figure 30-43** Padding beneath the shoulders of a child on a backboard helps keep the airway open.

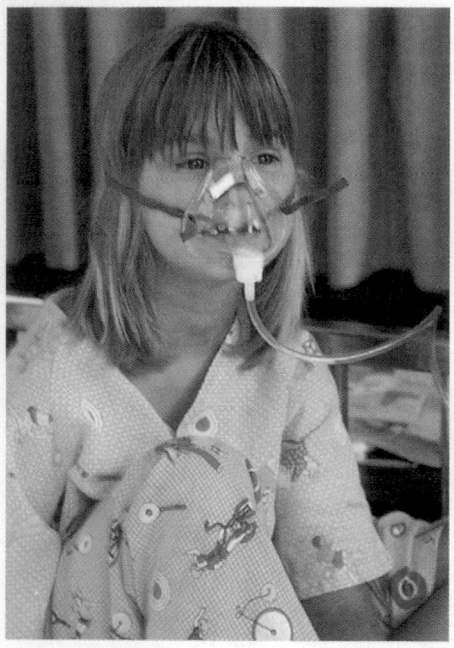

**Figure 30-44** Administer oxygen to a child using a pediatric mask.

available, one can often be fabricated using a covered malleable splint, such as a SAM™ splint. Often infants, toddlers, and children can be effectively immobilized using a vest-style immobilization device (Figure 30-42■). Padding may be needed beneath the thorax, when placing a young child on a long spine board, to bring a younger child's head into a neutral position. For infants, toddlers, and preschoolers, pad beneath the shoulders and torso to keep the airway open (Figure 30-43■).

Because respiratory-related problems are more common than cardiac disorders in children, administer high-flow oxygen using a pediatric mask if a child has an altered level of responsiveness, appears ill, or has obvious injuries (Figure 30-44■). Because some children (especially young children) can become frightened by an oxygen mask, lessen their anxiety by applying brightly colored stickers of popular cartoon characters, superheroes, or animals to the mask before putting the mask on their face. Parents or caregivers can often help a child accept the use of an oxygen mask. Alternatively, you or a caregiver may hold the oxygen mask near the patient's face, a process known as "blow-by oxygenation" (Figure 30-45■).

Fractures, if present, should be splinted in the usual fashion. Malleable splints are highly effective for splinting fractures in pediatric patients. If the fracture involves the clavicle, shoulder, or upper extremity, be sure to apply a

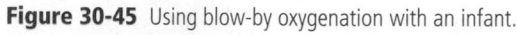

**Figure 30-45** Using blow-by oxygenation with an infant.

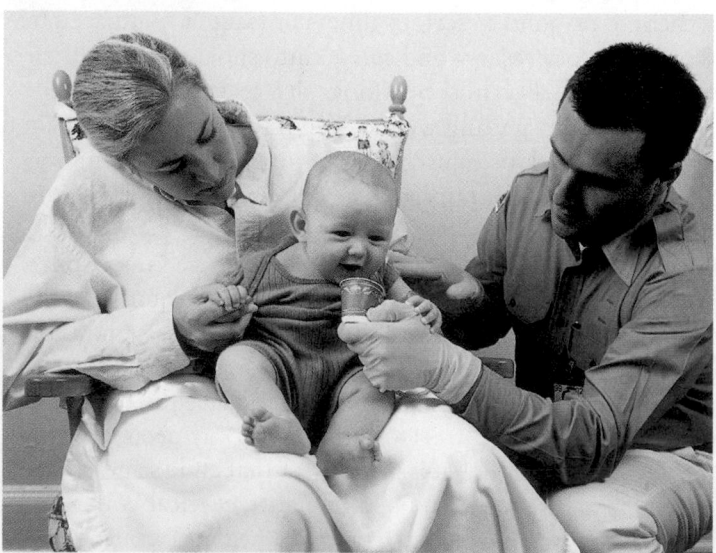

sling and swathe to decrease movement and to lessen pain. If available, use a pediatric traction splint for a mid-shaft femur fracture in a small child. For teenagers, an adult splint will usually work.

The symptoms of some pediatric airway-related disorders, such as croup, tonsillitis, and bronchiolitis, may be decreased with cool and/or humidified air such as might be obtained by taking the child outdoors. Other problems such as asthma and epigolittis are potentially life threatening and require more advanced care in a definitive-care setting. In these cases, rapid transportation with basic life support measures is the mainstay of field care. For a child with asthma, assist the older child or the caregiver in administering medicine from the child's own metered dose inhaler.

Manage foreign-body obstructions according to current American Heart Association guidelines and/or the techniques described in Chapter 13, Respiratory Emergencies. Because a foreign body can become lodged beyond a child's vocal cords, aggressive airway management may be required to relieve the obstruction. In this case, continue BLS maneuvers while rapidly transporting the patient toward ALS care.

Nausea, vomiting, and diarrhea are difficult to manage in the field. If severe, NVD could indicate the presence of an abdominal problem that might require surgery, so do not allow the patient to take anything by mouth and rapidly transport to definitive care.

Manage seizures as described in Chapter 11, Altered Mental Status. Do not attempt to physically restrain a child who is actively seizing, and do not allow anyone to place anything in the child's mouth. Once the seizure has stopped, open and clear the airway as necessary. If no spine injuries are suspected, place the child in the recovery position and continue to monitor the child's airway and vital signs (Figure 30-46■). Febrile seizures are managed by placing cool cloths in both axillae, in the groin, and on the forehead to reduce body temperature. An acetaminophen suppository can be inserted by a parent or a caregiver. Febrile seizures are benign, however it is important to protect the child from trauma during the event. Focus on reducing the fever and attempting to determine the cause of the elevated temperature and the seizure.

Sadly, there is little OEC Technicians can do to help a SIDS patient. By the time the infant is discovered, advanced signs of death (i.e., rigor mortis, livor mortis) are often apparent. In such circumstances, OEC Technicians should turn their attention to the parents or caregivers. Summon law enforcement if required in your state or province, and comfort the family as best as possible.

Manage other pediatric medical conditions as you would for an adult, following the recommendations described in previous chapters. Trauma-related pediatric problems also are managed as described in other chapters; pay special attention to controlling external bleeding (Figure 30-47■).

Pediatric shock, whether due to a medical or a trauma-related cause, can be extremely difficult to manage in the field due to the child's inability to compensate once initial compensatory mechanisms fail. If shock is suspected, immediately evacuate the patient by ALS transport to a definitive-care facility, preferably one that specializes in pediatric emergency care.

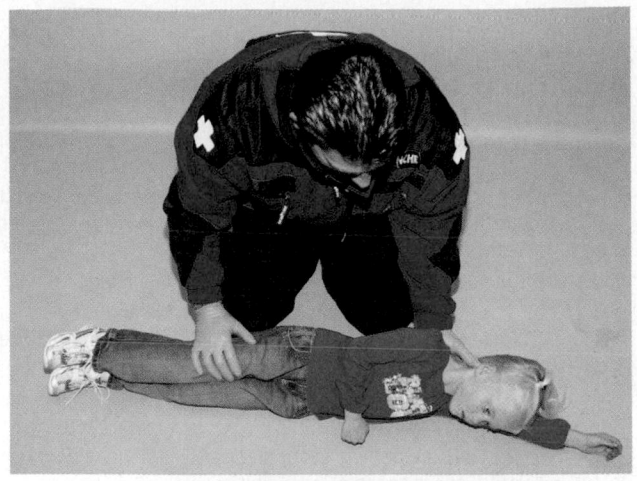

**Figure 30-46** If no spine injury is suspected, place a child who had a seizure in the recovery position.
Copyright Mike Halloran

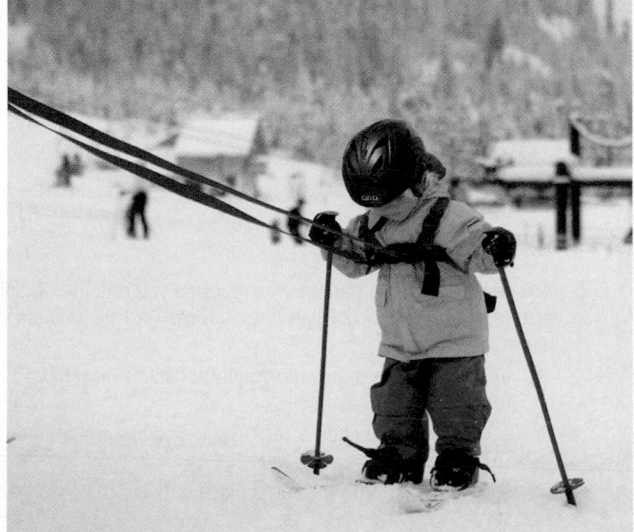

**Figure 30-47** Many children participate in outdoor recreational activities, so OEC Technicians need to know how to treat children. Remember: children are not "little adults."
Copyright Craig Brown

# STOP, THINK, UNDERSTAND

## Multiple Choice

Choose the correct answer.

1. When asking a 16-year-old patient with severe abdominal pains about the possibility of pregnancy or the date of her last normal menstrual period, you should _____

   a. include the mother because the child is a minor.

   b. have your partner take the mother aside and ask her questions while you privately ask the patient about issues such as pregnancy.

   c. not ask this type of question because it violates patient privacy laws.

   d. not ask the patient about pregnancy but should let her bring it up if she is concerned about it.

2. Before you attempt to realign a tib-fib fracture in a 7-year-old girl, you should say to her, _____

   a. "Don't worry; this won't hurt a bit."

   b. "This may hurt a lot, so go ahead and close your eyes."

   c. "Big girls don't cry."

   d. "It might hurt when I move your leg, but it should feel better as soon as it's in the splint."

3. Which of the following questions are important to ask the parent of an ill child? (check all that apply)

   _____ a. Whether or not there is a family history of child abuse or neglect.

   _____ b. Whether or not the child looks "normal" to the parent.

   _____ c. When the child last appeared normal or well.

   _____ d. Whether the child is toilet trained or not.

   _____ e. How often the child vomited during the night.

   _____ f. Whether or not the child has urinated recently.

   _____ g. How many bottles/glasses of water, juice, or formula the child has had in the past 24 hours.

   _____ h. Whether any fruit juice the child consumed was natural or made with corn syrup.

   _____ i. Whether the child takes any medications, vitamins, or supplements.

   _____ j. What the parent has done to relieve any symptoms.

4. When assessing a child, it is best to assess an injured arm_____

   a. first, to get it over with.

   b. after assessing the uninjured arm.

   c. in the usual order in which you are accustomed to doing your exam.

   d. last.

5. A 6-year-old trauma patient winces when you palpate his spine but denies that it hurts when you ask him. Your next course of action is to _____

   a. assume a spinal injury based on the child's nonverbal cue for pain.

   b. accept what the child is telling you and assume there is no spinal injury.

   c. repeatedly palpate the same place and ask the child, "Are you sure?" several times.

   d. tell the child "I think you're lying to me."

6. Why should rescuers never hyperextend the neck of a very young pediatric patient when administering rescue breathing? _____

   a. Because doing so could cause spinal damage.

   b. Because it is not necessary to do so.

   c. Because hyperextension could cause the airway to collapse.

   d. Because hyperextension could cause the tongue to occlude the airway.

7. Which of the following statements regarding administering oxygen to children is true? _____

   a. Oxygen administration can cause blindness in infants and thus should be avoided.

   b. An alert, oriented child with only a possible broken arm who is breathing at 24 breaths per minute needs oxygen therapy.

   c. Using "blow-by oxygenation" for a child who resists the application of an oxygen mask is an adequate method for administrating high-flow, high concentrations of oxygen in children.

   d. High-flow oxygen can damage a child's lungs and should thus be avoided.

8. After several attempts at removing a bottle cap that is firmly lodged in the throat of a 3-year-old and is blocking the airway have failed, your next course of action is to_____

   a. attempt to carefully remove the cap with long-handled tweezers or hemostats.

   b. stop attempts and administer high-flow oxygen until advanced life-support help can arrive.

   c. continue attempts while simultaneously moving as quickly as possible toward advanced help.

   d. stop attempts and tell the parents you are sorry; there is nothing else you can do.

9. The correct course of action for treating an 11-year-old boy in the post-ictal phase of a first-time seizure is to_____

   a. monitor the boy's airway, place him in the recovery position, and summon ALS.

   b. stabilize the boy's head so that he does not harm himself.

   c. tell the parent the boy should be alright now, to let him "sleep it off," and to suggest they follow up with the child's pediatrician as soon as is feasible.

   d. transport the boy only if the seizure was febrile or status epilepticus; otherwise, this is a benign condition that warrants nothing more than informing the child's pediatrician.

10. An angry 3-year-old boy hits you while you are examining him. Your best course of action is to _____

    a. hit him back lightly to show him how it feels.

    b. yell at him and tell him he is being bad.

    c. ask the parent to "control your child" or you won't be able to finish your assessment.

    d. understand that this is a normal response by a frustrated toddler, and ask the parent to help distract the child while you finish your assessment.

*continued*

11. A 5-year-old girl begins screaming whenever you attempt to examine her. Your best course of action is to _____
   a. firmly take her hands in yours, make eye contact with her, and gently but firmly tell her to calm down because you have to finish the examination.
   b. ask her what she is afraid of, acknowledge and accept what she tells you, be reassuring and try not to become irritated, and do your best to finish the exam in spite of her screaming.
   c. have her parent or caregiver hold her down while you finish your exam.
   d. walk away until the child can compose herself.

## Fill in the Blank

1. _____ is the developmental stage in which a child's focus shifts from parents to peers.

2. Any act, or failure to act, on the part of a parent, caregiver, or any adult, that results in serious physical or emotional harm or imminent risk of harm to a child will be identified as _____ _____.

3. A failure to act on the part of a parent, caregiver, or other responsible adult, to provide for the physical, emotional, educational, safety, or social needs of a child to the extent that emotional, developmental, or physical harm may occur will be identified as _____ _____.

4. A child may _____ rather suddenly, resulting in severe shock.

5. The _____ of newborns allow brain expansion.

6. Neonates generally breathe through their _____.

## Short Answer

Why should the vital signs of pediatric patients be reassessed frequently?

_____

_____

# CASE DISPOSITION

After confirming that there are no immediate threats to life, you perform a secondary assessment, which reveals an obvious deformity over the lateral third of the right clavicle. There is also considerable bruising and swelling over the girl's right upper arm. The girl begins to cry again, and you ask her why. She tells you she is afraid that you will hurt her, or worse, give her a shot. You reassure her that you don't give shots, and tell her that you'd like to splint her arm, which will help take away some of the pain. You explain, however, to both the girl and her grandmother, that it might hurt when you move the arm into the splint and sling. The girl looks at her grandmother, who gives her an encouraging smile and tells you, "We'll both be big girls."

The grandmother holds the child's uninjured hand while you and the other OEC Technicians prepare to carefully splint, sling, and swathe the girl's injury. You tell the girl that when you move her arm, she should take a deep breath in through her nose and blow it out hard through her mouth by instructing her to "smell the roses and blow out the candle!" You continue to talk to the girl quietly, telling her a story while you splint the arm. When you are done she tells you it feels better.

You accompany the child and her grandmother downriver in a large oar boat, keeping a close eye on the girl's respirations, appearance, and vital signs. Her vital signs remain stable. An ambulance takes her to the hospital.

The next day, the child's mother calls and tells you that her daughter did indeed suffer a broken clavicle. Fortunately, her humerus was not broken and her arm was only deeply bruised. She thanks you for your calm, caring approach in helping her child.

# Chapter Review

## Chapter Summary

Children are unique beings that can present OEC Technicians with a variety of challenges. Due to anatomical and developmental differences, pediatric patients can present with injury and illness patterns that differ markedly from those in adults. Additionally, immature body systems and poor compensation mechanisms can cause a child to decompensate quickly, often with little or no apparent warning. It is for this reason that children must not be considered "little adults."

Like adults, children engage in a wide variety of outdoor recreational activities. Thus OEC Technicians will likely encounter children who are ill or injured. By learning how to recognize common pediatric disorders and by approaching pediatric patients in a caring, friendly manner, OEC Technicians will be able to assist children throughout their growth and development.

## Remember...

1. Children are not miniature adults; they do not see, perceive, or respond to the world as adults do.
2. Children undergo six growth and development stages: the newborn stage, infancy, the toddler stage, the preschool period, the school-age period, and adolescence.
3. Whenever possible, incorporate caregivers or parents into the assessment process.
4. Be sensitive to an adolescent's need for independence, respect, and privacy.
5. A child can maintain a normal blood pressure and appearance during compensated shock.
6. Children can change rapidly from compensated shock to decompensated shock.

7. Assume that the condition of a child who looks sick and is not improving with care is worsening.
8. Report suspected child abuse to the proper authorities.
9. Approach children slowly and gently. Smile and be friendly.
10. A child who is crying or screaming has a patent airway.
11. A slow heart rate in a child with respiratory distress is an ominous sign of severe illness and impending cardiac arrest.
12. Cardiac arrest in children is usually preceded by respiratory failure.
13. Parents often demonstrate their fear by showing anger or irritation.

## Chapter Questions

### Multiple Choice

Choose the correct answer.

1. A 12-year-old child who presents with a headache, a fever, and a stiff neck is most likely suffering from _____
   a. measles or mumps.
   b. viral influenza.
   c. meningitis.
   d. pneumonia or bronchiolitis.

2. A 15-year-old boy who is struck in the chest with a baseball, collapses, and is apparently pulseless is most likely suffering from_____
   a. a high cervical injury affecting the respiratory and cardiac control centers.
   b. a hemothorax or a pneumothorax.
   c. cardiac tamponade.
   d. commotio cordis.

**3.** Which of the following injuries are more likely to occur in a 9-year-old boy who has suffered blunt chest trauma by striking his chest on the handlebars of his bicycle?_____

    **a.** commotio cordis, mediastinal injuries, clavicular fracture

    **b.** thoracic spine inury, shoulder separation, flail chest

    **c.** humeral fracture, ruptured spleen or liver, posterior clavicular dislocation

    **d.** pneumothorax, shoulder dislocation, C-spine fracture

**4.** You respond to a national park campground and find an unresponsive 7-month-old child that shows no physical evidence of trauma. The child's father tells you that the child fell over and struck his head on a rock the day before. What assumption should you make about this situation? _____

    **a.** The infant is suffering from a blunt-trauma closed head injury caused by the fall.

    **b.** This child is in the early stages of SIDS.

    **c.** The MOI does not match the child's level of development; you suspect possible child abuse.

    **d.** A birth defect or other illness may be causing the child's decreased level of responsiveness.

**5.** A 6-year-old girl is brought in to your ski area aid station, and while examining her you notice multiple injuries and scars in various stages of healing. You suspect that this child might be the victim of child abuse. Your best course of action is to _____

    **a.** observe how the parents interact with the child; if they appear concerned and caring, it is probably not child abuse.

    **b.** continue with your assessment and care of the child, but make a mental note to call a hospital social worker or a child protection agency to voice your concerns.

    **c.** question the parents about the injuries, and if their explanations seem plausible, assume it is not child abuse.

    **d.** do nothing; it is not your business to determine whether or not abuse has occurred.

**6.** Your *initial* response to an 11-year-old girl who is brought into your ski area aid station, begins to cry, and says that "Dad is going to be really mad at me for getting hurt" is to_____

    **a.** be reassuring; you realize that children of this age frequently express concerns of this nature when they are stressed.

    **b.** ignore the comment; what goes on in other people's families is not your concern.

    **c.** immediately contact law enforcement and ask them to take this child into emergency protective custody.

    **d.** tell the child that it is very likely that her father is going to respond in such a manner.

**7.** The most likely cause of lethargy and decreased responsiveness in a 3-year-old girl who has been vomiting and having multiple bouts of severe diarrhea throughout the night is _____.

    **a.** fatigue from being up and ill all night.

    **b.** crankiness because she is not feeling well.

    **c.** that she is afraid of you.

    **d.** that she may be going into hypovolemic shock.

**8.** Which of the following are factors that can help you determine the severity of a child's illness? (check all that apply)

    _____ **a.** Whether or not the child is active and moving or is still and quiet.

    _____ **b.** Whether or not the child makes eye contact with you, even briefly.

    _____ **c.** Whether or not the child cries or whines when moved or picked up.

    _____ **d.** The fact that the child learned to walk at 11 months of age.

    _____ **e.** The fact that the child turns toward its mother and begins crying "Up Mommy, up, up!"

    _____ **f.** The fact that a 3-year-old child pushes away the doll you offer her before you begin your assessment.

    _____ **g.** The presence of multiple bruises, cuts, and scrapes on the legs of a 3-year-old child.

    _____ **h.** The fact that a child is listless and pale.

9. You have established a rapport with a 10-year-old boy who has suffered a femur fracture. After the medic unit arrives, the medic tells you that she will need to start an IV on the child, who then begins to scream hysterically. Which of the following courses of action is your best option? _____

   **a.** Step back and let the medic handle this; it is her patient now.

   **b.** Get close to the patient, make eye contact with him, and gently ask him if he is afraid. Reassure him that it's normal to feel afraid, and that you will stay right there with him if he would like you to.

   **c.** Tell him that "it will only hurt for a moment" and to calm down.

   **d.** Tell him you understand that he's scared, then get it over with quickly by helping to hold him down while the medic starts the IV.

## Matching

1. Match each of the following developmental stages to its description. Each term may be used more than once.

   | _____ **1.** infancy | **a.** asks "why" a lot and can engage in simple conversations |
   | _____ **2.** toddler stage | **b.** can ride a tricycle and walk on tip-toes |
   | _____ **3.** preschool period | **c.** focus shifts from parents/caregivers to peers |
   | _____ **4.** school-age period | **d.** can hop, sit cross-legged, skip, and throw a ball |
   | _____ **5.** adolescence | **e.** likes to say "No!" |
   | | **f.** recognizes faces; can mimic facial expressions |
   | | **g.** begins exploring, climbing, and opening drawers |
   | | **h.** begins to participate in team sports |
   | | **i.** is very sensitive about one's appearance |
   | | **j.** If differentiating between right and wrong (acceptable behavior) is not learned at this age, it probably never will be learned. |
   | | **k.** develops stranger anxiety |

2. Match each of the following respiratory emergencies to its description. Each emergency may be used more than once.

   | _____ **1.** asthma | **a.** food is the most common cause of this problem in older children |
   | _____ **2.** bronchiolitis | **b.** pollen, exercise, or cold air can trigger this common respiratory disease |
   | _____ **3.** croup | **c.** a viral infection that causes inflammation of the larynx, trachea, and bronchi |
   | _____ **4.** foreign body airway obstruction | **d.** a viral or bacterial infection of the lungs, often preceded by fever and cough |
   | _____ **5.** pneumonia | **e.** individuals with a history of chemical exposure to the lungs are more prone to this illness |
   | _____ **6.** tonsillitis | **f.** primarily affects children between 6 months and 3 years of age; this condition has a sudden onset of a barking cough and is often preceded by a runny nose and a fever |
   | | **g.** inflammation of smaller airway passages of the lungs; is characterized by fever, cough, and respiratory distress |

## List

List the six causes of seizure in children.

1. _____

2. _____

3. _____

4. _____

5. _____

6. _____

## Short Answer

Define status epilepticus.

_____

_____

_____

_____

## Scenario

*You receive a call from the ski resort's day-care center about a 6-year-old girl that appears to be very sick. Upon arriving at the center, you take one of its workers aside to learn what you can about the situation. The scene is safe and you have received permission through the center to assess the situation, so you approach the child. You get down on one knee so that you are at the child's level, and you tell her that you are going to help her.*

1. Compared with adults, two of the most important anatomical differences in children are that children have_____
   a. a larger head and a smaller body surface.
   b. more muscle and less body fat.
   c. thicker skin and more muscle.
   d. a smaller airway and a reduced ability to sweat.

2. The most important thing to ascertain during the assessment is_____
   a. whether the child has any allergies.
   b. if there are any abnormalities with the child's ABCDs.
   c. where the child's mother is.
   d. if the day-care center worker knows anything about the family's history.

*You complete a primary assessment and start a secondary assessment. Your attempts to reach the parents are unsuccessful. Your secondary assessment indicates that this 6-year-old girl is lethargic and has a high fever, a severe headache, and a stiff sore neck.*

3. The girl's symptoms are consistent with _____
   a. meningitis.
   b. a febrile seizure.
   c. pneumonia.
   d. croup.

*Because the girl's condition is a true medical emergency, you call an ambulance for transport. You also request and receive from the day-care center a list of the names of all the other children at the day-care center and their parents' phone numbers.*

4. You give the list to the paramedics for delivery to the emergency department physician because _____
   a. the children could be eye witnesses.
   b. the other children could have been exposed to a substance that caused the girl's reaction.
   c. the girl's medical condition could be highly contagious.
   d. the doctor may need to make a call to the Department of Child Services.

## Suggested Reading

Markenson, D. S. 2001. *Pediatric Prehospital Care*. Upper Saddle River, NJ: Pearson. http://emedicine.medscape.com/emergency_medicine

Murphy, M. F., et al. 2008. "The Young Airway." *JEMS* (33)6: 58–71. http://www.peppsite.com

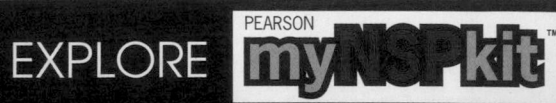

EXPLORE   PEARSON myNSPkit™

Please go to www.myNSPkit.com. Under Student Resources, you will find animations, videos, web links, and games related to this chapter—and much more. Look for information on epiglottitis, febrile seizures, the pediatric physical exam, and more.

Register your access code from the front of your book by going to www.myNSPkit.com and selecting the appropriate links. If the in-cover access code has been redeemed, go to www.myNSPkit.com and follow links to **Buy Access.**

# Geriatric Emergencies

Ricky C. Kue, MD, MPH

## ⊕ OBJECTIVES

**Upon completion of this chapter, the OEC Technician will be able to:**

**31-1** Describe six physiologic changes that occur with aging.

**31-2** Describe effective methods for communicating with geriatric patients.

**31-3** Describe the effects of the following illnesses and diseases on geriatric patients:

- cardiovascular and respiratory disease
- neurological diseases
- gastrointestinal (GI) diseases
- altered mental status

**31-4** Describe how the chronic use of medication can affect the results of an assessment of geriatric patients.

**31-5** List four trauma considerations that are unique to geriatric patients.

**31-6** Describe the general management of geriatric patients.

**31-7** Describe how to manage a geriatric patient with advanced directives.

## ⊕ KEY TERMS

**bronchodilator,** *p. 993*
**geriatric,** *p. 987*
**heart contractility,** *p. 994*
**kyphosis,** *p. 989*

**lordosis,** *p. 989*
**nephron,** *p. 989*
**osteoporosis,** *p. 989*
**polypharmacy,** *p. 993*

**scoliosis,** *p. 989*
**syncope,** *p. 992*
**vital capacity,** *p. 988*

## Chapter Overview

Seniors represent the fastest growing population segment in the United States, and this group is projected to grow exponentially as the Baby Boomer generation retires. A senior is defined as a person who is 65 years of age or older.

According to the U.S. Census Bureau, seniors currently constitute approximately 12 percent of the total U.S. population, and they are projected to represent 21 percent of the total population by 2050. Each year millions of people take to the

*continued*

## HISTORICAL TIMELINE

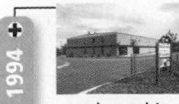

1994 — 10,000-sq.-ft. warehouse is purchased in Lakewood, Colorado with the Professional Ski Instructors Association (PSIA).

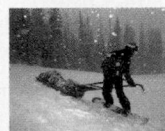

1994 — Snowboarders are allowed to join NSP.

# CASE PRESENTATION

You receive a call for a skier who was found down. Upon arrival you find an elderly man standing near the off-ramp of a lift. He is accompanied by several family members and appears to be well. The patient states that he was waiting for his family to unload from the lift when he turned and fell. "I just bumped my head." Upon questioning the patient, he tells you that he briefly "saw stars" after the incident and now complains of feeling "a little dizzy."

A small hematoma begins to form on his forehead. He denies any cervical spine tenderness and has no other complaints. Upon checking his pulse, you note that it is strong but slow and slightly irregular. The rest of the physical exam is unremarkable. The man's wife tells you that the patient is on medications for high blood pressure and "for a mechanical heart valve." The man says that he is embarrassed that his clumsiness has resulted in so much attention, insists that he will be fine despite the dizziness, and wants to continue skiing. Something about the situation makes you uneasy.

***What should you do?***

outdoors to engage in a wide variety of activities. Increasingly, this includes large numbers of seniors.

Many seniors are avid snow sports enthusiasts. A 2009 study by the National Ski Areas Association shows that the long-term aging pattern is due to the increase of snow riders aged 45 and over. Since 1998, the proportion of visitors aged 45–54 has increased from 14.0 percent to 19.3 percent; the proportion of visitors aged 55–64 has increased from 4.6 percent to 8.5 percent; and the proportion of visitors aged 65+ has risen from 2.4 percent to 3.5 percent. Despite improvements in their overall health and activity level, seniors cannot escape the inevitable changes that come with aging (Figure 31-1■).

The elderly have unique health care needs. As people age, they become physiologically different than when they were young. These differences make the health care needs of geriatric patients much different than those of younger patients. Fortunately, thanks to advances in medicine and technology, today's seniors are healthier, live longer, and are far more active than the elderly of the past. Seniors increasingly participate in activities that could bring them to the attention of ski patrollers and other OEC Technicians.

The effects of aging can affect your assessment findings and management approach. For example, a greater tolerance for pain in elderly patients may mask serious injury, and changes in the curvature of the cervical and thoracic spine can make it much more difficult to immobilize an elderly person's neck and back using standard practices and equipment. Elderly patients also may have more complex medical histories than younger patients. Additionally, seniors may take more medications, often for more than one chronic condition at a time. Some of these medications can reduce the efficiency of the body's compensatory mechanisms during stress, and some combinations of medications can cause drug interactions further confusing the clinical picture. Finally, aging can present communication challenges by reducing the ability of sen-

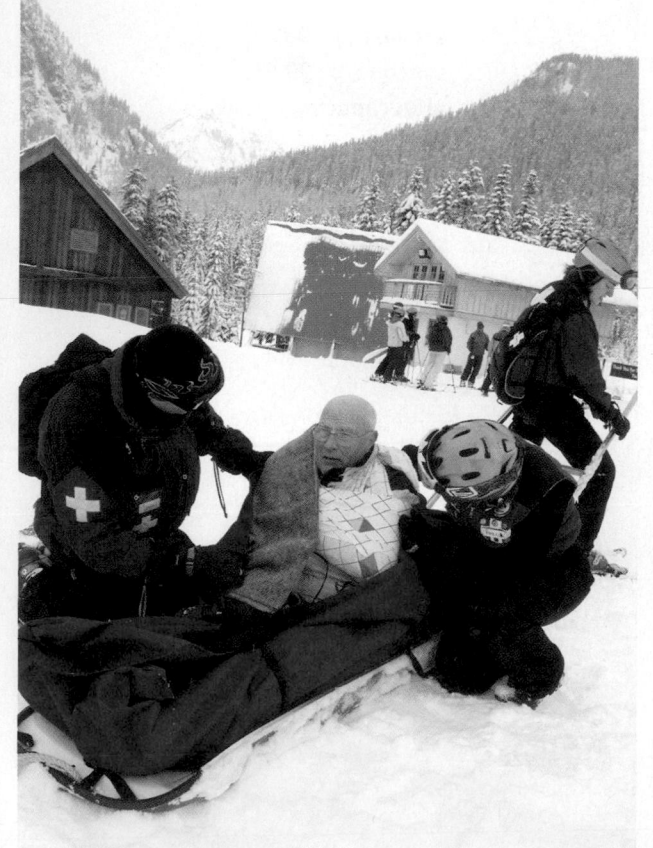

**Figure 31-1** More seniors now enjoy outdoor activities, but the effects of aging increase their risk of injury.
Copyright Craig Brown

iors to hear, see, and process information. Generational differences also can impede effective communication: seniors and younger people alike may harbor certain myths and generalizations regarding the attitudes and behaviors of the other generation.

As an OEC Technician, you will increasingly encounter geriatric patients as they venture into the outdoors in record numbers. A fundamental understanding of the aging process and geriatric physiology, knowledge of medications and their affects, combined with a strategy to promote effective communication, will prepare you to address the unique medical needs of our nation's elderly, enabling them to remain socially and physically active throughout their golden years.

## Physiologic Changes of Aging

The aging process is accompanied by numerous physiologic changes that make **geriatric** patients inherently different from younger patients. The changes that occur with aging can alter the body's response to various medical disorders and traumatic injuries (Figure 31-2■). However, age-related changes need not make the elderly frail

**⊕ 31-1** Describe six physiologic changes that occur with aging.

**geriatric** pertaining to elderly persons or to the aging process.

**Figure 31-2** Changes in the body systems of elderly individuals.

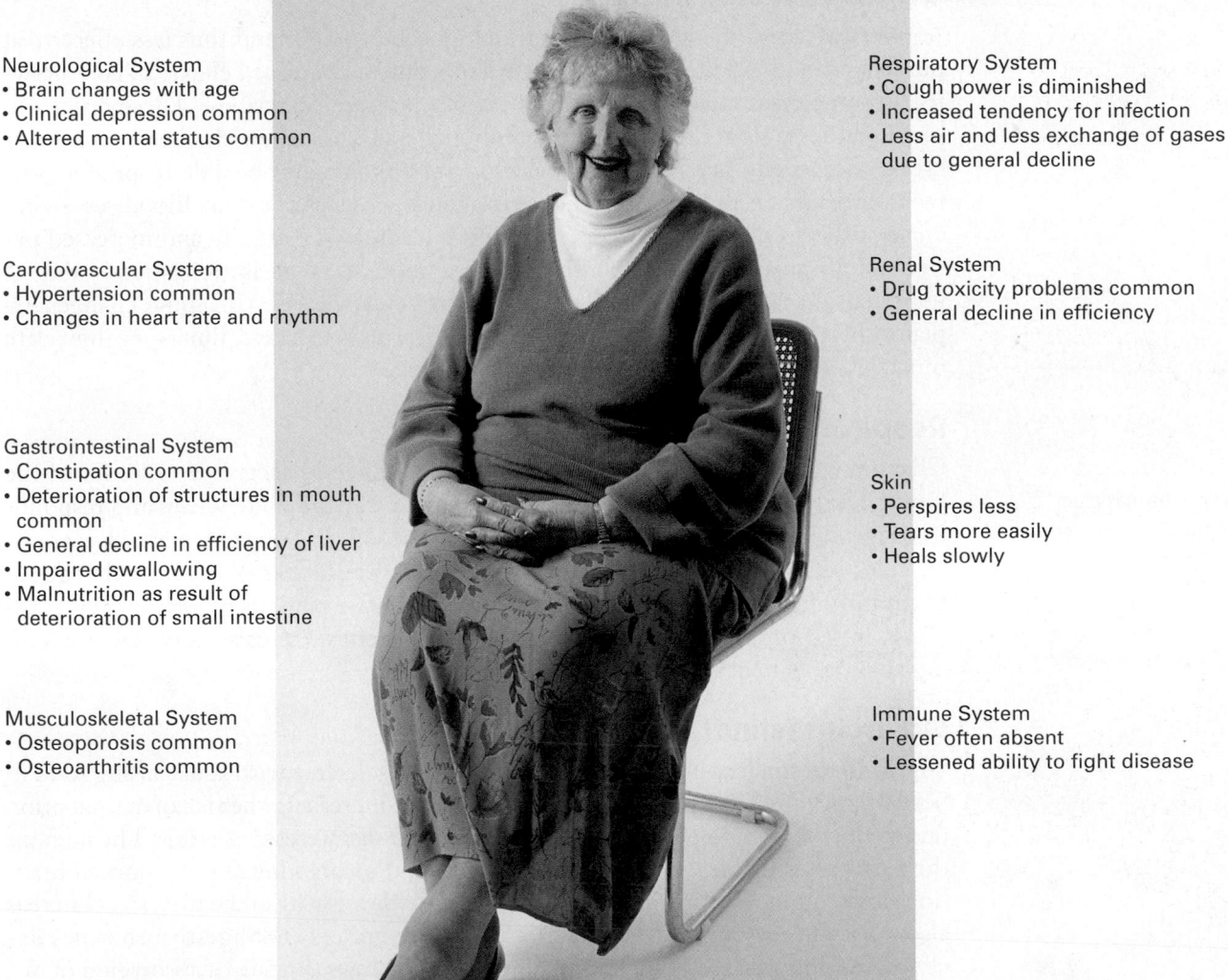

**Neurological System**
• Brain changes with age
• Clinical depression common
• Altered mental status common

**Cardiovascular System**
• Hypertension common
• Changes in heart rate and rhythm

**Gastrointestinal System**
• Constipation common
• Deterioration of structures in mouth common
• General decline in efficiency of liver
• Impaired swallowing
• Malnutrition as result of deterioration of small intestine

**Musculoskeletal System**
• Osteoporosis common
• Osteoarthritis common

**Respiratory System**
• Cough power is diminished
• Increased tendency for infection
• Less air and less exchange of gases due to general decline

**Renal System**
• Drug toxicity problems common
• General decline in efficiency

**Skin**
• Perspires less
• Tears more easily
• Heals slowly

**Immune System**
• Fever often absent
• Lessened ability to fight disease

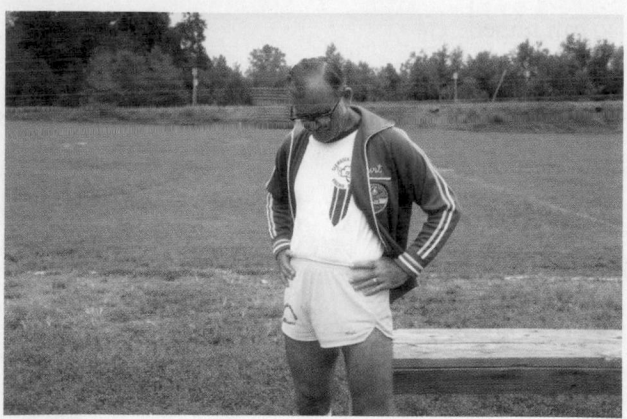

**Figure 31-3** These days seniors are pursuing active lifestyles more often than ever.

or helpless. Far from it, seniors increasingly maintain an active lifestyle that includes participating in and enjoying a variety of outdoor activities (Figure 31-3■).

## Neurological Changes

As the body ages, changes within the nervous system make the brain and peripheral nerves less effective at processing data and transmitting impulses between various parts of the body. Such changes can seriously affect the body's ability to respond to disease or trauma. The total number of brain cells decreases, causing the brain to shrink in size. By age 85, total brain weight can be reduced by as much as 10 percent. Cerebral blood flow is reduced, which can decrease the amount of glucose and oxygen that reaches brain cells. Nerve impulses are slowed, resulting in slowed reflexes, longer reactions times, and reduced perception of stimuli such as light, sound, and pain. As a result of reduced visual and auditory acuity, geriatric patients may not see hazards or hear warnings until it is too late. The inner ear balance organs may be less effective, allowing older people to fall down easier. Additionally, the reduction of pain perception with age may lead seniors to underestimate the seriousness of their injuries.

## Cardiovascular Changes

As the heart ages, the walls of the ventricles become stiffer and thus less effective at pumping blood. Additionally, heart rate slows due to decreased electrical conductivity. In some cases medications called beta-blockers are prescribed. These drugs can physiologically slow the heart rate intentionally and not allow the heart rate to increase as needed. As a result, the hearts of seniors may not be able to produce the tachycardia that is the normal response to acute blood loss or shock. Blood vessels become stiffer from atherosclerosis, resulting in decreased elasticity and increased peripheral vascular resistance, both of which increase a geriatric patient's risk of hypertension, cardiac disorders, and cerebrovascular disease. All these changes explain why a geriatric patient's cardiovascular responses to stress, illness, or injury are much less effective than those of younger patients.

## Respiratory Changes

**vital capacity**   the maximum amount of air that can be expired following a maximum inhalation.

Changes within the respiratory system of seniors include decreased elasticity of the lungs, decreased **vital capacity**, and changes in the way the body senses and responds to oxygen and carbon dioxide levels within the blood. In fact, a healthy 90-year-old has approximately half the lung capacity of a healthy 30-year-old. These changes in respiratory function ultimately affect the way geriatric patients maintain oxygen reserves in response to stress. Additionally, the gag reflex decreases with age, increasing an older patient's risk of aspiration.

## Gastrointestinal Changes

The sense of smell and the abundance of taste buds decline with age, causing food to be less appealing. The gums and teeth deteriorate, increasing the risk of malnutrition due to the inability to chew food and the resulting disinterest in eating. Throughout the gastrointestinal tract—from the esophagus to the large intestines—normal function slows, often resulting in constipation. Activity levels within the liver and pancreas also are reduced. Overall, the secretion of gastric buffers and digestive enzymes declines, causing a marked decrease in digestion that slows the rate of absorption of nutrients, water, and oral medications. Older patients are at higher risk for various GI disorders, including obstruction, ulcers and perforations (Figure 31-4■).

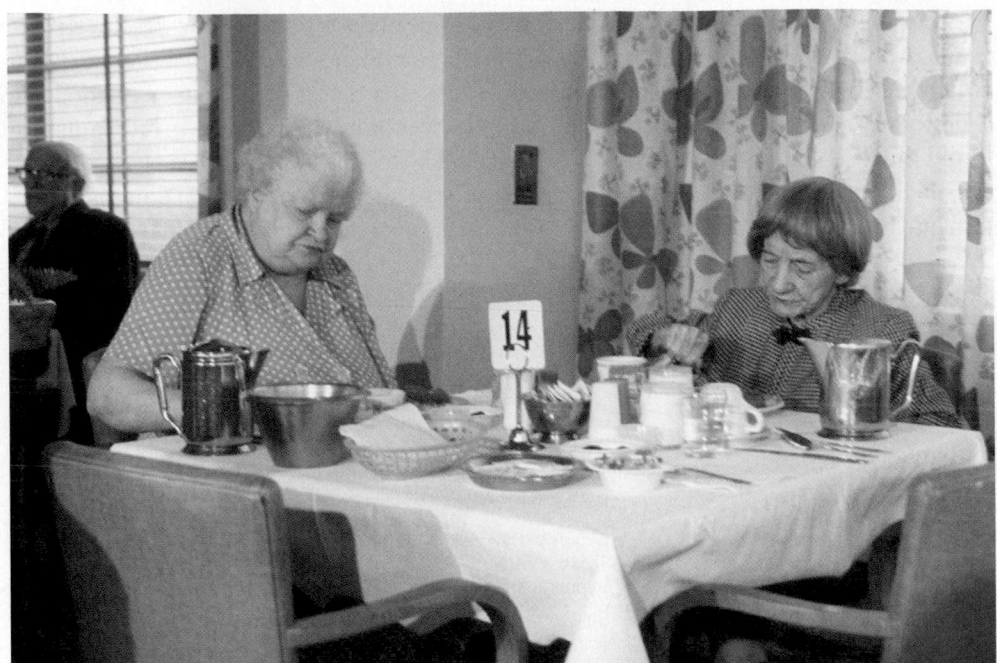

**Figure 31-4** Age-related changes throughout the gastrointestinal system impair the nutritional status and overall health of seniors.

## Changes in Renal Function and Electrolyte Balance

With advancing age, the kidneys become less effective at filtering drugs, toxins, and waste products out of the blood; one result is that the systemic effects of medications may be prolonged. **Nephron** function decreases by 30–40 percent, which can alter water balance and electrolyte levels within the body. Urine production and excretion are affected as well. By the time a person reaches 65, total body water can decrease by as much as 30 percent, making geriatric patients more susceptible to fluid loss and dehydration during physical activity and reducing their ability to respond to shock.

## Musculoskeletal Changes

Bones lose density and muscle mass declines as the body ages. **Osteoporosis**, a disease that results in decreased bone density due to excessive mineral loss, affects as many as 28 million Americans (Figure 31-5■). This condition predisposes seniors to fractures of the hips, spine, and wrists. The natural curvatures of the spine can become altered with increasing age, causing scoliosis, kyphosis, or lordosis. **Scoliosis** is an abnormal lateral curvature of the spine that causes the spine to curve in an "S" shape. **Kyphosis** is an abnormal curvature, usually in the upper thoracic spine, that produces a "humpback" appearance. Increased **lordosis** causes "swayback," or excessive inward curvature of the lumbar spine. Scoliosis and kyphosis can affect lung function, whereas lordosis causes lower back pain.

Aging also causes changes in collagen within musculoskeletal tissues, resulting in stiffer, less flexible ligaments and predisposing geriatric patients to torn ligaments from trauma. Cartilage begins to degenerate due to the loss of water, resulting in degenerative arthritis of the joints. Muscle tissue becomes more susceptible to injury, and muscle mass atrophies. The rib cage stiffens and the respiratory muscles lose strength, contributing to a decrease in lung vital capacity.

## Integumentary and Endocrine Changes

With aging, the skin thins by as much as 20 percent and loses both elasticity and underlying fat content, predisposing the skin to bruising and to increased heat loss and hypothermia. As the skin becomes less elastic, it is more susceptible to tearing and other

**nephron**  the smallest functional unit of the kidney.

**osteoporosis**  a disease process that leads to a reduction in bone mass.

**scoliosis**  abnormal lateral curvature of the spine.

**kyphosis**  abnormally increased dorsal curvature of the thoracic spine.

**lordosis**  abnormally increased anterior curvature of the spine (usually the lumbar spine).

**Figure 31-5** The loss of bone density in osteoporosis make bones less elastic and more brittle.

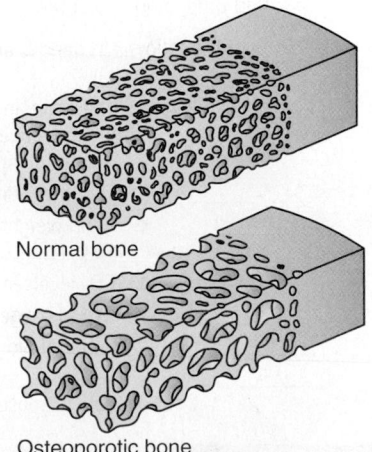

Normal bone

Osteoporotic bone

dermatologic injuries, an important consideration when lifting or moving elderly patients. Additionally, because the body has fewer sweat glands with age, a patient's risk of hyperthermia is increased because the body is less effective at cooling itself. Endocrine function also diminishes because the pancreas becomes less effective in regulating blood glucose. Half of all individuals over age 65 have or will develop Type 2 diabetes, especially if they are obese. Immunologic response also is decreased, making geriatric patients more susceptible to infections and increasing the time it takes them to heal.

# STOP, THINK, UNDERSTAND

## Multiple Choice

Choose the correct answer.

1. Which of the following statements regarding the geriatric population is true? _____
   a. Overall, geriatric health is on the decline due to physical inactivity and poor diet.
   b. Few changes in the overall health and well-being of the elderly population have occurred over the past several decades.
   c. Today's seniors are less active but healthier than previous generations due to improvements in health care.
   d. Overall, today's seniors are healthier and more active than ever before.

2. Which of the following statements is true? _____
   a. Atypical symptoms in the elderly are indicative of poor health.
   b. Norms in vital signs, symptoms, and overall physiology remain constant throughout adulthood in a healthy individual.
   c. An elderly patient may present with symptoms that are atypical for a young patient but normal for an older patient.
   d. Atypical symptoms in an elderly individual generally signify deteriorating health or impending shock.

3. Which of the following assumptions can you make regarding an elderly patient? _____
   a. Most physiological changes due to aging render the elderly frail or helpless.
   b. Elderly patients who maintain active lifestyles and participate in outdoor activities will not show the physiological changes typical of most seniors.
   c. The physiological changes caused by aging are due to inactive, unhealthy lifestyles.
   d. The physiological changes that occur with age do not necessarily make seniors frail or unable to participate in sports and other vigorous outdoor activities.

4. Which of the following changes are typical for seniors? (check all that apply)
   _____ a. The brain and peripheral nervous system are less effective at processing and transmitting data and impulses.
   _____ b. The total number of brain cells decreases.
   _____ c. Brain weight decreases by as much as 10 percent.
   _____ d. $CO_2$ levels in the blood increase.
   _____ e. Blood oxygen levels permanently decrease.
   _____ f. Cerebral blood flow decreases.
   _____ g. Sensitivity to stimuli such as light, sound, and pain increase.

5. Which of the following statements regarding a geriatric patient's cardiovascular response to hypovolemia resulting from trauma is true? _____
   a. There is little difference in cardiovascular response to hypovolemia between younger and older patients.
   b. Severe tachycardia can occur in an elderly patient secondary to trauma and blood loss.
   c. A generally slower heart rate in geriatric patients can prevent the normal increase in heart rate seen with hypovolemia.
   d. It is not uncommon for an elderly patient's pulse rate to decrease significantly during trauma.

6. Compared to the lung capacity of a 30-year-old, the lung capacity of a healthy 90-year-old is_____
   a. about the same.
   b. about 10 percent less.
   c. about 50 percent less.
   d. slightly greater due to decreased elasticity in lung tissue.

7. Seniors are at greater risk of hip, spine, and wrist fractures because of _____
   a. atherosclerosis.
   b. arteriosclerosis.
   c. hyperacidosis.
   d. osteoporosis.

8. Elderly patients have more risk of rupturing their Achilles tendon because _____
   a. they are less active, making the tendon subject to injury.
   b. the muscles in the calf are weaker.
   c. collagen within the tendon is stiffer and less flexible.
   d. the tendon is thinner due to age.

9. Compared to a younger patient, an elderly patient is considered to be at what risk of dehydration?_____
   a. greater
   b. lesser
   c. equal

10. Compared to a younger person, how susceptible to hypothermia or hyperthermia is a geriatric patient?_____
    a. more
    b. less
    c. equally

# Common Geriatric Illnesses and Conditions

## Altered Mental Status

Among the many causes of altered mental status in elderly individuals are infection, head injury, stroke and TIA, acute cardiovascular conditions, and endocrine disorders such as hypoglycemia (Figure 31-6■). OEC Technicians also should consider environmental factors that change mental status, such as hypoxia due to high altitude, hypothermia, and hyperthermia. Toxicological ingestions, medications, stings, and envenomations also can alter normal thought processes. Additionally, the aging process increases an elderly individual's risk for such conditions as dementia and Alzheimer's disease. Common causes of altered mental status in seniors, such as hypoxia and hypoglycemia, may be due to a variety of underlying conditions.

## Hypertension

Essential hypertension is clinically defined as a systolic blood pressure greater than 140 or a diastolic pressure greater than 90, as seen on more than one measurement and without an apparent cause. Blood pressure increases as we age. Physicians once believed that slight elevations in blood pressure were acceptable in elderly individuals. Today, however, most physicians urge older individuals to keep blood pressure below the recommended normal values, and yet only 25 percent achieve adequate blood pressure control. Untreated, hypertension is a serious medical disorder that can adversely affect other body systems, and it is a major risk factor for such diseases as myocardial infarction and stroke.

Because hypertension affects more than two-thirds of all seniors, it is important to recognize that any abnormally high blood pressure warrants further investigation. Patients with a systolic reading of 200 or more or a diastolic pressure of greater than 120 require *urgent* evaluation by a physician.

**31-3** Describe the effects of the following illnesses and diseases on geriatric patients:

- cardiovascular and respiratory disease
- neurological diseases
- gastrointestinal (GI) diseases
- altered mental status

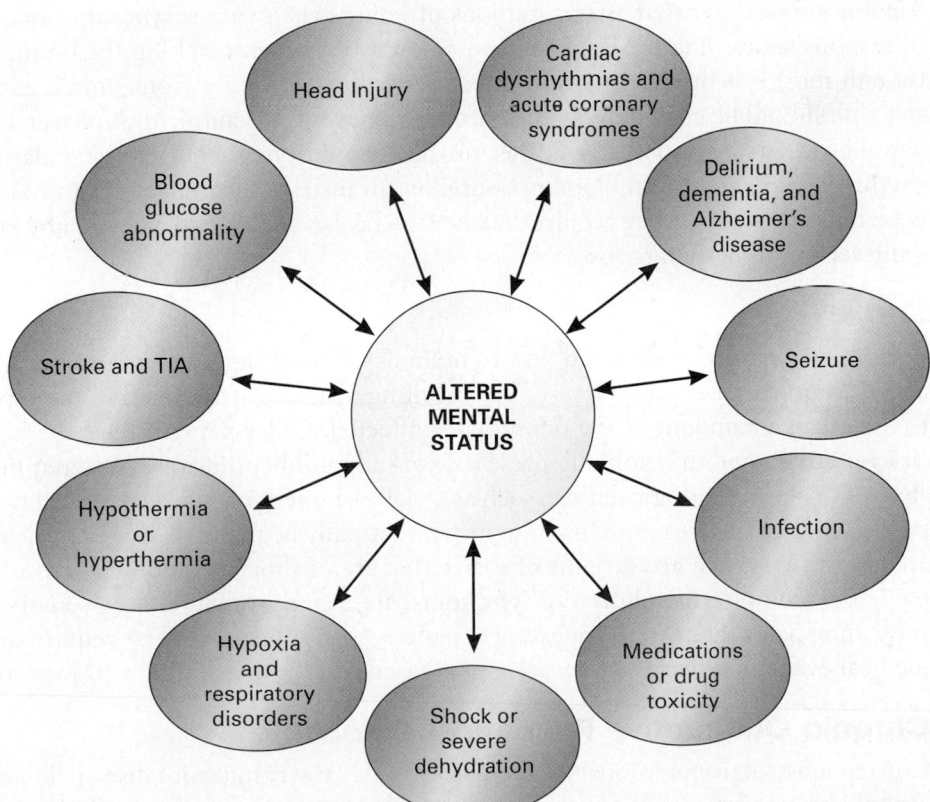

**Figure 31-6** Common causes of altered mental status in elderly patients.

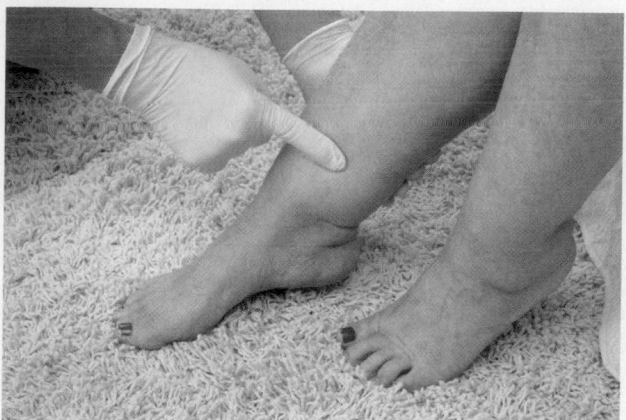

**Figure 31-7** Swelling (edema) of the ankles is a sign of CHF. Removal of the pressure exerted by the examiner's finger may leave an indentation in the swollen tissue, a sign called "pitting edema."

**syncope**   a transient loss of responsiveness resulting from inadequate cerebral blood flow.

## Myocardial Infarction

The incidence of myocardial infarction (MI) increases with age and is aggravated by risk factors such as uncontrolled hypertension, high blood cholesterol levels, diabetes, smoking, obesity, and a strong family history of coronary artery disease. MI can also be provoked by rigorous physical activity in susceptible individuals. Chest pain is the most common symptom of a heart attack and is often accompanied by pain or numbness in the jaw or left arm and by shortness of breath. In seniors, the signs and symptoms of an MI may not be straightforward. Geriatric patients may complain only of weakness or of a general feeling of unease. They also may complain of neck pain, back pain, or mild chest discomfort. Such presentations, which are considered "atypical" for younger cardiac patients, appear to be the norm for geriatric heart attack patients. Maintain a high index of suspicion for heart attack in older patients, and be vigilant for subtle symptoms of heart attack in seniors who have risk factors for coronary artery disease.

## Congestive Heart Failure

Congestive heart failure (CHF) is a condition in which the heart cannot pump enough blood to meet the needs of the body's other organs. As you learned in Chapter 15, Cardiovascular Emergencies, heart failure results from ineffective pumping by the right or left ventricle or both and is commonly caused by long-standing hypertension or by a previous heart attack that damaged the heart muscle. Seniors who have CHF typically take medications that improve the pumping strength of the heart, control blood pressure, or help reduce fluid levels and swelling in the body (Figure 31-7■). Physical exertion can aggravate the condition, as can ascending to high altitude.

## Syncope

A common disorder that affects millions of seniors each year is **syncope**, a brief loss of responsiveness due to an inadequate amount of oxygen reaching the brain. Even though most syncopal episodes in the general population are from simple fainting, syncope should be considered a life-threatening event in seniors until proven otherwise because it may stem from other medical conditions such as an irregular heart rhythm, a sudden drop in blood pressure, or a transient ischemic attack (TIA). Syncope in the elderly usually requires further medical evaluation to rule out any potentially serious underlying causes.

## Stroke

A stroke is a reduction of blood flow to brain tissue resulting from narrowing, blockage, or rupture of a cerebral artery. The resulting neurologic dysfunction corresponds to the area and amount of the brain that is affected. Older patients have the highest risk for stroke and may initially present with only mild confusion or altered mental status. Typical neurologic deficits such as facial asymmetry, slurred speech, abnormal behavior, or changes in limb function may not initially be present. Transient ischemic attacks (TIA), which are variants of stroke that are of short duration and are accompanied by complete resolution of symptoms, are also prevalent among seniors. Despite an apparently normal appearance, patients with presumed TIA require urgent medical evaluation because they are at increased risk for developing a serious stroke.

## Chronic Obstructive Pulmonary Disease

Chronic obstructive pulmonary disease (COPD) is any respiratory disease, including chronic bronchitis, emphysema, and asthma, that results in an increased obstruction

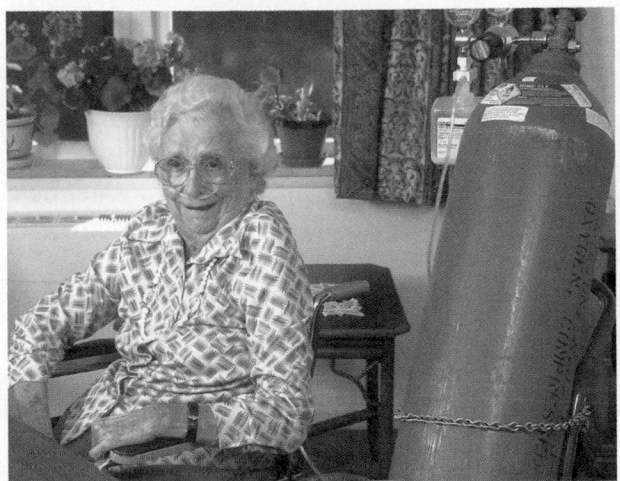

| Table | **31-1** | Causes of Abdominal Pain in Elderly Patients |
|---|---|---|

Appendicitis
Cholecystitis/biliary colic
Bowel obstruction
Bowel perforation
Mesenteric ischemia
Abdominal aortic aneurysm
Gastritis and GI bleeding
Pancreatitis
Diverticulitis
Hernias

**Figure 31-8** This COPD patient is using a nasal cannula to administer continuous low-flow oxygen at home.

to expiratory airflow. Seniors are at greater risk for COPD due to the effects of long-term smoking, which is the leading cause of COPD, and various occupational exposures. Additionally, COPD is markedly worsened by age-related changes that result in less-effective gas exchange. Older patients with COPD are very sensitive to sudden changes in exertion and typically require low-flow supplemental oxygen therapy as well as inhaled **bronchodilators** to maintain homeostasis (Figure 31-8■). This delicate balance in respiratory function can be compromised during even mild physical activity or as a result of a rapid ascent to a higher altitude.

**bronchodilator** an agent that causes expansion of the air passages within the lungs.

⊕ **31-4** Describe how the chronic use of medication can affect the results of an assessment of geriatric patients.

## Abdominal Emergencies

Elderly patients who present with an acute abdomen represent true emergencies because the underlying cause could be a life-threatening condition such as a ruptured abdominal aortic aneurysm, a bowel obstruction or rupture, GI bleeding, or peritonitis (Table 31-1■). In fact, over 60 percent of the causes of abdominal pain in elderly patients require surgical intervention, nearly double the rate for younger patients. Due to the age-related reduction in pain sensation, even serious causes of abdominal problems may present with few or no signs or symptoms in seniors. Thus because older individuals tend to have more serious conditions associated with abdominal pain, arranging rapid transport to a physician for evaluation is very important for geriatric patients.

**polypharmacy** the simultaneous use of several medications in combination.

**Figure 31-9** Seniors currently consume more than 30 percent of all prescription medications and are projected to consume 50 percent by 2020!
Copyright Beverly Henrickson

# Medication Use in the Elderly

Longevity and quality of life in the elderly has improved greatly in recent decades, thanks in part to the many new medications created each year. As a group, seniors consume more than 30 percent of all prescription drugs in the United States, and their consumption is projected to increase in proportion to 50 percent by the year 2020 (Figure 31-9■).

More than 40 percent of elderly patients take five or more medications weekly, whereas 12 percent take ten or more each week. The concurrent use of multiple medications, known as "**polypharmacy**," is common among older patients because they often have multiple, coexisting medical conditions. Taking

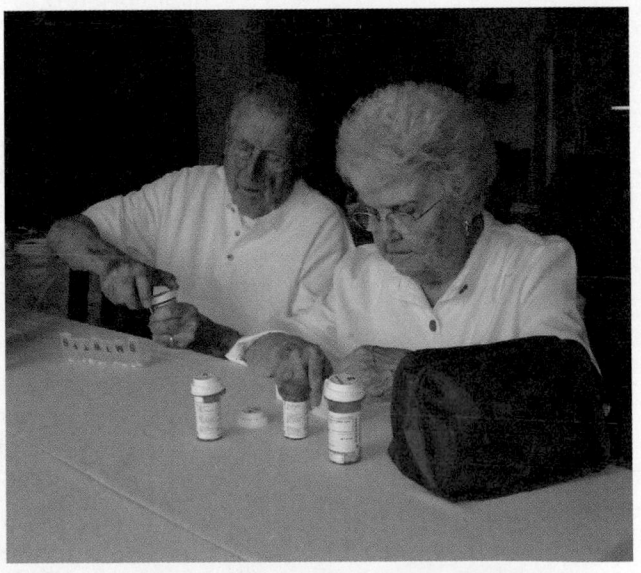

medications in combination can cause a host of adverse reactions and can significantly affect assessment findings. Ask geriatric patients about their use of herbal supplements and over-the-counter medications because some seniors may not consider them true "medications."

Ask elderly patients directly if they share medications with friends or family because they may not readily admit to this practice. Obtaining a complete accounting of senior patients' past medical history and medications during the SAMPLE history can help you and higher-level providers provide better care for geriatric patients.

Unfortunately, elderly patients may not know the names of all the medications they take. In such situations, OEC Technicians should ask what each medication is used for, because this information may well provide clues that may help identify the medication. For instance, a patient may say, "it makes me have to pee" or "it makes my heart beat slower."

Medications for treating hypertension are among the most commonly prescribed classes of medications among older patients. A few examples of these cardiovascular medications are beta-blockers, calcium-channel blockers, and diuretics. Beta-blockers make the heart contract more efficiently and are used to manage cardiac arrhythmias. These medications are highly effective in reducing the amount of stress placed on the heart and are commonly used to lower blood pressure. Unfortunately, they also can adversely affect the body's compensatory mechanisms when the body is stressed or in shock. For example, the expected increased heart rate in response to blood loss in a patient with traumatic internal bleeding may not occur if the patient's heart rate is being slowed by beta-blockers. Common beta-blockers include metoprolol (Lopressor), propranolol (Inderal), and atenolol (Tenormin).

**heart contractility** the capacity of cardiac muscle cells to shorten in response to a suitable stimulus.

Calcium-channel blockers reduce heart rate, blood pressure, and (to a lesser degree) **heart contractility**. Like beta-blockers, calcium-channel blockers can potentially counteract the normal compensating mechanisms during stress or trauma. Common calcium-channel blocking agents include diltiazem (Cardizem), nifedipine (Procardia), and verapamil (Isoptin).

Diuretics decrease the volume of circulating fluid within the cardiovascular system in order to reduce blood pressure. By causing the kidneys to excrete more urine, diuretics alter the body's fluid and electrolyte balance. Elderly patients who take these medications are more susceptible to hypotension, dizziness, syncope, and slower heart rates and may exhibit shock faster due to a lower blood volume. Common diuretics include hydrochlorothiazide (HCTZ), triamterene (Dyazide), and furosemide (Lasix).

Blood "thinners" are another class of medications that deserve special attention when encountered with a geriatric patient. Those medications are commonly prescribed to patients with a history of mechanical heart valve replacement, an irregular heartbeat, or blood clots in the legs (deep vein thrombosis) or lungs (pulmonary embolism). Blood thinners can increase or prolong trauma-related bleeding. Even a nosebleed or a "slight concussion" could have disastrous consequences due to uncontrollable bleeding. A patient with blunt abdominal trauma may harbor occult abdominal bleeding that is accelerated by a blood thinning medication. Head trauma may cause serious bleeding inside the skull. Thus, any trauma patient who is on a blood thinner should be carefully examined, no matter how trivial the injury. Common blood thinners include warfarin (Coumadin), clopidogrel (Plavix), and enoxaparin (Lovenox). Aspirin has blood thinning properties also. Because of the increased risk of bleeding, many trauma systems recommend that patients on blood thinners who have any *significant* mechanism of injury be transported not to a local ED, but instead to a trauma center, where the large quantities of blood products often needed by such patients are available.

# STOP, THINK, UNDERSTAND

## Multiple Choice
Choose the correct answer.

1. In elderly patients, hypertension is best defined as_____
   a. BP that increases gradually and continually with age.
   b. a sustained BP that is greater than 140/90.
   c. a normal part of aging.
   d. a 20-point increase in either systolic or diastolic pressure above the patient's normal BP at age 30.

2. CHF is best described as_____
   a. a condition in which the ventricles no longer pump blood effectively.
   b. hardening of the carotid arteries, which causes confusion and dementia.
   c. a stroke.
   d. hypertension.

3. Syncope is best defined as_____
   a. dizziness caused by either hypoglycemia or hyperglycemia.
   b. confusion due to dementia.
   c. a brief loss of responsiveness due to inadequate oxygen reaching the brain.
   d. a "mini-stroke" that warns of an impending larger stroke.

4. Which of the following statements about stroke is not true? _____
   a. A stroke is caused by a sudden narrowing, blockage, or rupture of an artery in the brain.
   b. Older individuals are at lower risk for stroke than are younger individuals because younger individuals have greater arterial elasticity.
   c. A stroke may initially present with only mild confusion or altered mental status.

   d. The resulting neurologic dysfunction from a stroke corresponds to the size and location of the brain tissue that is affected.

5. The primary cause of COPD is_____
   a. smoking.
   b. aging.
   c. stroke.
   d. congestive heart failure.

6. Which of the following statements about abdominal emergencies is true? _____
   a. An elderly patient suffering from a serious abdominal emergency will typically exhibit severe signs and symptoms such as pain, syncope, nausea, and vomiting.
   b. The majority of elderly patients suffering from abdominal emergencies will not require surgical intervention.
   c. Older patients tend to have more serious conditions associated with even mild abdominal pain than do their younger counterparts.
   d. Abdominal complaints in elderly patients are typically due to poor digestion or bad diet and can generally be ignored unless severe signs or symptoms develop.

7. Polypharmacy is best described as_____
   a. obtaining prescriptions from multiple doctors at multiple pharmacies.
   b. the concurrent taking of multiple medications by one individual.
   c. an illegal pharmaceutical practice that can result in fatal overdoses.
   d. an accidental overdose of a medication.

## Matching
Match each of the following medication types to the effects it may cause.

_____ 1. beta-blocker
_____ 2. calcium-channel blocker
_____ 3. blood thinner
_____ 4. diruetic

a. a nosebleed (epistaxis) that will not stop bleeding
b. a trauma patient suffering from severe hypovolemia whose pulse rate does not increase in spite of the blood loss
c. a patient who suffers from hypotension, dizziness, and syncope
d. a patient with severe internal bleeding whose blood pressure and pulse remain "normal"

## List
Typical signs or symptoms of a myocardial infarction include chest pain, shortness of breath, and pain radiating into the jaw or arms. List the *atypical* signs and symptoms that elderly patients may experience.

1. _____
2. _____
3. _____
4. _____
5. _____

# CASE UPDATE

Upon examination of the patient, you find that he has a BP of 180/92, a HR of 58, and normal respirations. Your partner reviews the patient's medications with a family member and reports that he is taking warfarin, lopressor, and aspirin. As you continue with your evaluation, the patient vomits and then says, "It must have been something I ate for lunch." His mental status is unchanged; he is alert, oriented, and cooperative. The rest of his neurological evaluation is normal. His only request is that someone help him back to the lodge so he can lie down and rest for the remainder of the day. You sense something is wrong with this patient.

**What should you do?**

---

**⊕ 31-5** List four trauma considerations that are unique to geriatric patients.

# Trauma Considerations in Elderly Patients

Seniors in the United States are engaging in far more outdoor activities than in years past, and as more seniors venture outdoors, their risk for trauma is increased. Geriatric trauma patients require special considerations, because for a given type of trauma, seniors have higher mortality rates compared with those of younger patients. The mortality rate of seniors from traumatic brain and spinal cord injuries, for example, is higher than that of patients younger than 65 and rises exponentially with age. As an independent risk factor, age presents the greatest increase in risk for a poor outcome of trauma cases. These statistics are important to OEC Technicians because they will be increasingly likely to encounter older patients with a traumatic injury, whether from skiing, hiking, mountain climbing, or other outdoor activities.

Assessment of seniors can be particularly tricky. What may appear to be a relatively minor complaint could be seen, after careful evaluation, to be a life-threatening injury. In older adults, a trivial mechanism of injury can lull OEC Technicians into thinking that nothing is wrong with the patient. Other factors besides age, including underlying disease and medication use (especially blood thinners), must be considered because they can alter the clinical picture or increase a patient's potential morbidity and mortality.

The geriatric population has a higher incidence of trauma from inadvertent falls than do other age groups. Among the most common serious traumatic injuries affecting the elderly population, whether from falls or other mechanisms of injury, are pelvic and hip fractures, traumatic brain injury, and cervical spine injury.

## Falls

Falls represent one of the most common mechanisms of injury in elderly adults and are a significant source of morbidity and mortality. Approximately 8 percent of adults 65 and older visit the emergency department each year due to a fall-related injury, and about 25 percent of these patients ultimately require in-patient medical care. More importantly, falls cause 12 percent of all deaths in the geriatric population, both directly and indirectly.

Many falls are caused by an underlying medical condition that may be unknown to the patient. Although the outdoors presents numerous trip-and-fall hazards, OEC Technicians should not automatically assume that a fall was due to clumsiness or inattentiveness. Instead, it is vital that OEC Technicians evaluate not only the traumatic injuries related to a fall but also the potential cause of the fall. Some falls result from

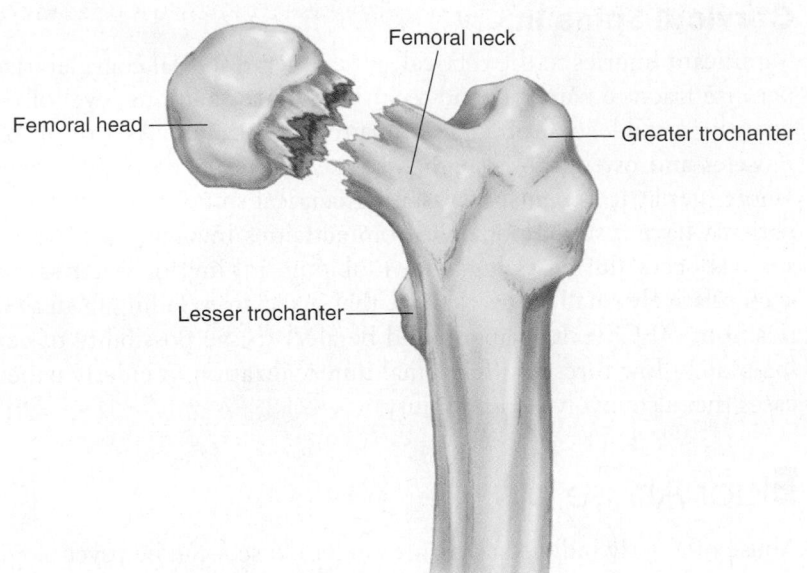

Femoral neck

Femoral head

Greater trochanter

Lesser trochanter

**Figure 31-10** A displaced femoral neck fracture—commonly known as a fractured hip—is a common result of a fall among seniors.

a medical cause, such as a syncopal episode. Red flags in the medical history that suggest this possibility include palpitations, chest pain, lightheadedness or dizziness before the fall, shortness of breath, diabetes and weakness. These symptoms, whether they occur before or immediately after a fall, should be considered indicators that some underlying medical problem may have caused the fall and that further evaluation by a physician is required. Falls can cause a host of other problems, including long-bone fractures, head injuries, and internal bleeding.

## Hip and Pelvic Fractures

Fractures of the hips and pelvis that result from osteoporosis are common among elderly patients and most often result from a fall (Figure 31-10■). Other common mechanisms of injury that can produce a hip or pelvic fracture are low-speed collisions, bicycle crashes, equestrian and snow sports mishaps, and other forms of blunt trauma. Older patients have more bleeding complications from hip and pelvic fractures and are more prone to multiple fractures, which increase morbidity and mortality. Hip or pelvic fracture must be considered when evaluating hypotensive geriatric patients who have an altered mental status in the absence of obvious evidence of external bleeding, chest or abdominal trauma, or long-bone fracture.

## Traumatic Brain Injury

Two major age-related changes put geriatric patients at greater risk of traumatic brain injury: the dura mater becomes more adherent to the skull, and the brain shrinks in size. The combination of these two changes increases the space between the outside of the brain and the inside of the skull, allowing for more brain movement within the skull. Deceleration head trauma, even with a relatively minor mechanism of injury, can cause brain injury. Additionally, the use of warfarin or other blood thinning medications and the presence of chronic medical conditions such as hypertension or diabetes dramatically increase the risk of bleeding within the skull. These factors explain why an older person who experiences apparently minor head trauma can have a severe traumatic brain injury. The typical symptoms associated with traumatic brain injuries (Chapter 21, Head and Spine Injuries) may not be readily apparent in geriatric patients. Maintain a high level of suspicion of brain injury in any geriatric patient who has suffered a head injury; pay especially close attention to any changes in the patient's level of responsiveness (Figure 31-11■).

**Figure 31-11** Suspect a traumatic brain injury in any older person with head trauma.
Copyright Eddie Sperling Photography

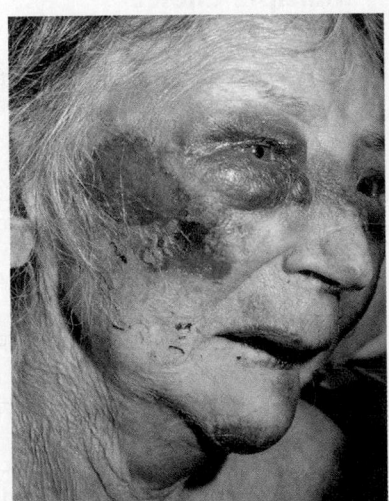

## Cervical Spine Injury

Significant injuries to the cervical spine deserve special consideration among seniors because fracture patterns tend to involve more than one level of the spine, are frequently unstable, and often accompany head trauma. As a result of weakened neck muscles and osteoporosis, high cervical injuries at the $C_1$–$C_2$ region are common among geriatric patients. Devastating cervical spine injury and paralysis in geriatric patients have resulted not only from activities involving jarring or shearing forces such as occur during skiing, snowmobiling, rafting, or water skiing, but also from such relatively small forces as those that occur from falling from a standing or seated position. OEC Technicians should be alert to the possibility of cervical injury and maintain a low threshold for spinal immobilization in elderly patients, especially in cases that also involve a head injury.

# Elder Abuse

Abuse of elderly individuals—called elder abuse—can be psychological, financial, or (most commonly) physical. Abuse of an elderly individual that results from acts of omission is known as elder neglect. Other non-physical forms of abuse exist.

When taking a history for an elderly patient for whom you suspect abuse, be simple, direct, nonthreatening, and nonjudgmental. Any history from an injured senior that is inconsistent with the observed pattern of injuries should raise suspicion for elder abuse.

The finding upon a physical exam of injuries at various stages of healing (e.g., older bruises, healing cuts, and fresh bruises) in elderly patients should raise suspicion of elder abuse. Intentional burns, cord or rope marks, or cigarette burns on the thin skin of elderly individuals can provide clues to identify potential elder abuse.

OEC Technicians should focus on recognizing possible elder abuse and ensuring appropriate intervention. In most states mandated reporters include physicians, nurses, emergency medical technicians, and law enforcement officers. It is impractical to address the issue of elder abuse at the scene; instead, treat all life-threatening injuries, arrange for transport to a hospital, and then immediately report your concerns about elder abuse to the appropriate authorities.

## STOP, THINK, UNDERSTAND

### Multiple Choice

Choose the correct answer.

1. Which of the following statements describes the best way to deal with an elderly trauma patient who has a minor complaint, no severe signs or symptoms, and a minor mechanism of injury?_____
   a. Have a "wait and see" attitude.
   b. Ignore such patients; they are usually lonely and are looking for some attention.
   c. Arrange immediate transport to a trauma center, regardless of the patient's wishes.
   d. Maintain a high index of suspicion and perform a careful assessment.

2. The most common mechanism of injury among geriatric patients is_____
   a. motor vehicle accidents.     c. asphyxiation.
   b. drowning.                     d. falling.

3. Which of the following actions should you next take for an elderly patient who has fallen while on a hike?_____
   a. Ask the patient about the events that led up to the fall.
   b. Respect the patient's privacy and avoid embarrassing the patient by focusing on the injury and not on preceding events.
   c. Assume that this elderly patient fell due to diminished vision and minor syncope.
   d. Assume that the patient fell due to some underlying medical condition and immediately take action to address a probable medical complaint.

*continued*

4. For a geriatric patient who has fallen, has hypotension and altered mental status, and has no obvious external bleeding and no obvious head, chest, or abdominal trauma, you should assume_____
   a. nothing; you should never make any assumption about any patient.
   b. that the patient may be suffering from a hip fracture.
   c. that the patient is suffering from dementia.
   d. that the patient may be suffering from a bleed in the head.

5. The two major physiologic factors that put seniors at higher risk for traumatic brain injury are_____
   a. a thinner, more brittle skull and weaker cervical vertebrae.
   b. a brain that enlarges while the dura mater thins, leaving less room in the skull and a brain that is more easily damaged.
   c. a brain that shrinks and dura mater that is more adherent to the skull, which increases the amount of movement the brain can have within the skull.
   d. weakened arteries and weakened veins, which can rupture more easily and cause hemorrhage.

6. Which of the following statements about cervical spine injuries in elderly patients are true? (check all that apply)
   _____ a. Fractures tend to involve more than one level of the spine and are frequently unstable.
   _____ b. It is rare to see cervical injuries at the $C_1$–$C_2$ level in elderly patients.
   _____ c. Paralysis can result from something as simple as falling out of a chair.
   _____ d. The correlation between head injuries and cervical spine injuries is high in elderly patients.
   _____ e. The likelihood of a cervical spine injury and the subsequent need to use a backboard generally diminish with the age of the patient.

7. The mortality (death) rate for elderly trauma patients is _____ the rate for younger trauma patients.
   a. less than
   b. approximately equal to
   c. greater than

# Additional Considerations

Several medical advancements have vastly improved the quality of life for seniors and have increased their ability to participate in various outdoor activities: joint replacement, implantable devices, and external ports and apparatus. OEC Technicians must be aware of these developments because they can influence treatment decisions.

## Artificial Joints

As a result of advances in orthopedic surgery techniques, geriatric patients can now undergo complete joint replacement, enabling them to continue their favorite outdoor activities, often at a higher performance level (Figure 31-12■). Commonly replaced joints include the shoulder, hip, and knee. Vertebral discs can also be replaced, and vertebrae can be fused. Artificial hip and shoulder joints dislocate more easily, and such patients may require novel ways of immobilization for transport. Additionally, patients who have had spinal surgery are more likely to have back or neck problems following a spinal insult. Because of these developments, OEC Technicians may need to alter their evaluation of these patients.

## Implantable Devices

The increased use of implantable devices—cardiac pacemakers, internal defibrillators, artificial heart valves, neurostimulators, cochlear devices, and internal drug pumps—has allowed seniors who could no longer participate in outdoor activities to again enjoy those activities.

Although each of these devices provides numerous therapeutic benefits, they also may cause or worsen many medical conditions. For instance, failure of a cardiac pacemaker can cause life-threatening arrhythmias or cardiac arrest and can override the heart's compensatory mechanisms in a patient in

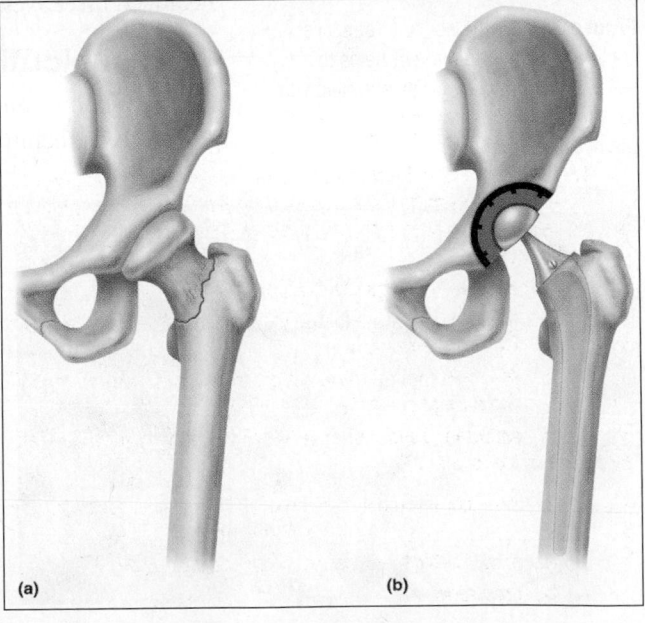

**Figure 31-12** A fractured hip (a) and the hardware used for a total hip replacement (b).

(a)    (b)

shock. Failure of an internal drug pain pump can lead either to life-threatening narcotic overdosing or to withdrawal when narcotic pain medicine is no longer being delivered properly. Failure of an implantable cochlear device affects hearing and can hinder communication.

Implantable devices also can be compromised by factors in the external environment. For instance, portable radios, microwaves, and magnetic objects may inactivate a cardiac pacemaker or an implantable defibrillator and can cause interference with cochlear devices.

## External Openings, Ports, and Apparatus

Many elderly patients with endocrine, GI, or GU disorders rely on an external port to assist with a normal body function or to facilitate a therapeutic intervention. A patient may have a urinary catheter to collect urine, or an abdominal colostomy bag that collects feces from the large intestine. Some patients may have a temporary or permanent shunt or catheter placed into one of the large veins of the arm or chest for kidney dialysis or for the administration of medications such as chemotherapeutic drugs. Problems can arise with any of these openings or ports, and the most frequent problems involve clogging or infection.

OEC Technicians also encounter portable drug infusion pumps and battery-operated oxygen devices. Portable infusion pumps are used to provide medications such as insulin in either a continuous dose or in timed increments. External diabetic pumps, which have a catheter that is inserted into the skin, usually in the abdomen, can be as small as a digital pager and often are found in a shirt pocket or attached to the patient's belt. Malfunction can cause hyperglycemia or hypoglycemia. Battery-operated oxygen tanks of various sizes are used to treat respiratory ailments. Even though most external medical apparatus units are hermetically sealed, problems can arise should dirt or other debris enter the system and interfere with the device's internal systems.

**⊕ 31-7** Describe how to manage a geriatric patient with advanced directives.

**⊕ 31-2** Describe effective methods for communicating with geriatric patients.

## Advanced Directives

The use of advanced directives—legal documents that provide guidance regarding a patient's wishes in the event the patient is unable to communicate during a life-threatening medical emergency—is increasing in the United States, especially among the elderly. Chapter 1, Introduction to Outdoor Emergency Care, provides more information about advanced directives.

## Communicating with Elderly Patients

Effective communication with an ill or injured patient is essential and is a hallmark of a good OEC Technician. Effective communication is especially important in gathering the history and assessing geriatric patients. Always show the utmost respect for elderly patients, and avoid being overly casual or too aggressive with them. Practicing the following recommendations can help you both reduce a geriatric patient's anxiety and more quickly identify the problem and implement a treatment strategy (Figure 31-13■).

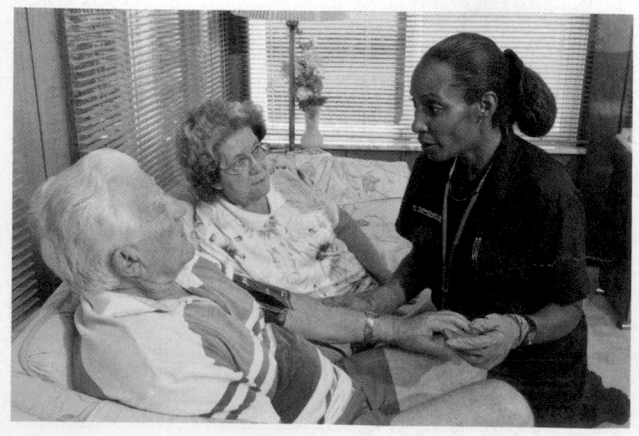

**Figure 31-13** The ability to effectively communicate with a patient helps to reduce the patient's anxiety and help you to more quickly identify the problem and the necessary treatment.

When making contact with an elderly patient at the scene, eliminate distractions such as music or other loud noises. Place yourself at the patient's level and maintain eye contact. Do not assume that all elderly patients are hard of hearing; use a normal speaking voice. If it becomes evident that the patient cannot hear you, increase the volume of your voice slightly until the patient can hear you. Speaking in a lower octave may help the patient hear you better.

OEC Technicians should be aware that autonomy is very important to seniors. Allow elderly patients to remain in control of their bodies, and obtain their consent before assessing or treating them. When addressing seniors, always use "Mr.," "Mrs.," or "Ms." followed by their last name. Avoid using a nickname or a first name unless the patient requests it. As you build rapport, the interaction may take on a more casual tone, but you should not be the one to initiate it. Also avoid terms such as "hon" or "sweetie" because seniors generally consider them offensive or demeaning.

Be clear and purposeful in your conversations with patients. Speak directly to patients at all times, even if they seem unable to understand you. To avoid confusion, have only one OEC Technician speak with a patient, and ask only one question at a time.

Do not direct your questions to a patient's family or friends as if the patient were not there. If a patient is unable to speak and family or friends are present, designate one person to speak on the patient's behalf. Having multiple people trying to answer for the patient is too confusing.

When obtaining a history, making more open-ended requests such as "Tell me about your pain" allows the patient to describe what occurred or is transpiring. Close-ended questions such as "Is the pain sharp or dull?" can be useful for clarifying specific points or obtaining specific information.

Use active listening skills to better understand a patient's complaints or symptoms. If, for example, a patient denies having "chest pain" and instead describes it as "discomfort," confirm your understanding by saying something like "So, you're experiencing discomfort in your chest. Is that correct?" As your exam progresses, continue to refer to the symptom as "discomfort." Whenever possible, use lay terms instead of complex medical terminology. Using these strategies will increase the effectiveness of your interview and will allow you to obtain a more complete medical history.

## Assessment

Assessment of geriatric patients is no different from assessment of any other patient (Figure 31-14■). It includes a scene size-up, a primary assessment, a secondary assessment, and ongoing reassessment.

The scene size-up includes an evaluation of the surroundings for any potential hazards that may endanger you or others. In cases involving trauma in an elderly person, take an extra moment to look for clues about what might have contributed to the patient's problem. For instance, loose rocks, slippery surfaces, uneven terrain, and exposed roots can all create trip-and-fall situations in outdoor environments, whereas loose rugs, torn carpeting, exposed power cords, benches, and other floor-level objects can cause indoor falls. Walking in rigid ski boots, hiking boots, or cycling shoes also can cause inadvertent stumbling, especially when combined with the less-acute senses and unstable balance of some elderly individuals. Sudden acceleration, deceleration, or descent, such as might be encountered while sledding, skiing, cycling, or rappelling, also may be a contributing factor by causing a precipitous but temporary drop in blood pressure. Even viewing a broad vista or a steep drop-off can induce dizziness and fainting in susceptible elderly individuals.

Begin the primary assessment by evaluating the ABCDs to identify any life-threatening problems that require immediate attention. Table 31-2■ lists some specific physiological effects of aging that can affect the assessment of elderly patients.

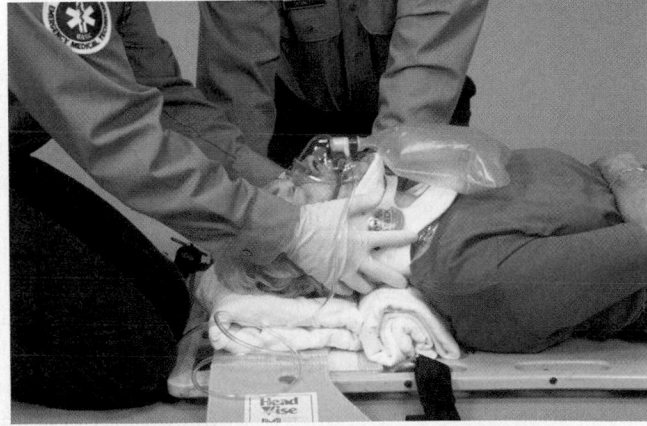

**Figure 31-14** Assessment of geriatric patients is the same as that for all other groups of patients.
Copyright Craig Brown

**Table 31-2** Some Physiological Effects of Aging and Their Implications for Assessment

| Effect | Result | Implications for Assessment |
|---|---|---|
| Deposition of cholesterol within thickened arterial walls | Increases risk of heart attack, stroke, and hypertension | Heart attack and stroke more likely |
| Decreased cardiac output | Diminished physical activity and reduced tolerance of physical stress | More prone to falls; more complaints of fatigue |
| Decreased elasticity of lungs and decreased activity of cilia | Decreased ability to clear foreign substances from lungs | Higher risk of pneumonia and other respiratory infections |
| Fewer taste buds, less saliva; reduced acid production and slower movement along the digestive tract | Less enjoyment of eating; difficulty chewing and swallowing; early feeling of fullness when eating; difficulty digesting and absorbing food; constipation | Weight loss; abdominal pain common |
| Diminished liver and kidney function | Increased toxicity from alcohol and medications; diminished ability of blood to clot | Need for reduced doses of medication; bleeding tendencies |
| Diminished thyroid function | Decreased energy and tolerance of heat and cold | Increased risk of hypothermia and hyperthermia |
| Decreased muscle mass, loss of minerals from bones | Decreased strength | Falls more likely; minor falls more likely to cause fractures |
| The presence of multiple medical conditions | Use of many different medications, sometimes prescribed by different physicians | Increased risk of medication error; potentially harmful medication interactions more common |
| Deaths of friends and family | Depression; loss of social support | Increased risk of suicide |
| Loss of skin elasticity, shrinking of sweat glands | Thin, dry, wrinkled skin | Increased risk of injury (requires gentle handling to avoid skin and subcutaneous tissue injuries) |

Evaluate each patient's neurological status because it may provide the only clue that a potential life-threatening emergency exists. The response you get when you first ask a patient what happened or what is wrong will give you important neurologic information. Be suspicious of any apparent change in mental status, however minor, and do not assume that any behavioral abnormalities are simply "due to old age." Consult a family member or caretaker, if present, to determine whether a patient's mental status is normal or abnormal. Any abnormal findings should be explored further in an effort to evaluate the extent of the deficit. Carefully document your findings on the patient care report because they will serve as the baseline for future mental status exams.

Next, obtain a baseline set of vital signs. Then begin a secondary assessment with a SAMPLE history. As you talk with the patient, use the communication strategies described earlier in the chapter, and demonstrate active listening skills. Be aware that because an elderly patient may have multiple concurrent medical conditions, signs and symptoms of one disorder can overlap or mask those of another disorder.

Obtain a full accounting of the patient's current or recent medications, including all over-the-counter medications and homeopathic remedies. Obtaining information about past surgeries and current medical conditions may help explain the patient's current condition. If elderly patients do not volunteer information during the history-gathering process, ask specific questions to get the information you need. Be sure to ask patients when they last ate, because an imbalance between the calories consumed and the calories expended during outdoor activity may help to explain altered mental status, fatigue, dizziness, or weakness. If pain is present, fully explore its extent and severity using the OPQRST mnemonic.

Perform a thorough head-to-toes physical exam using the DCAP-BTLS mnemonic. Some injuries may not readily be apparent to elderly patients. Ask any patient with artificial joints if those joints feel normal. Examine the patient's skin for tenting, which may indicate underlying dehydration or hypovolemia.

Obtain vital signs every 5 to 10 minutes to look for indications that the patient's condition is changing. Check the pulse for regularity and equality on both sides of the body. If, for example, the chief complaint is abdominal pain with dizziness or weakness, check both femoral pulses because unequal pulses can indicate a cardiovascular-related problem such as an aortic aneurysm. Remember that a patient's medications can alter the vital signs. Patients who take a beta-blocker, for example, often cannot generate a tachycardic response, even in response to hypovolemia or acute blood loss. If a patient has an implantable or external medical device, ask if it appears to be operating normally. Likewise, have the patient or a family member check any openings or ports for patency and proper functioning.

# Management

Geriatric patients are typically more complex to manage than are younger patients because of their complex medical histories, their use of multiple medications, and age-related physiological changes. Additionally, any delays in treatment may cause their condition to worsen more than would be expected for younger patients. As a result, geriatric patients often require more aggressive treatment to mitigate complications related to poor cardiac output, respiratory distress, blood loss, or shock. Therefore, maintain a high index of suspicion for injury and disease; if something does not seem right, refer or transport elderly patients to a higher level of care.

Should you identify a life-threatening problem while your transportation is on scene, interrupt the secondary assessment, provide immediate appropriate emergent care for the problem, and transport the patient to a higher level of care.

As for any patient, initial management of geriatric patients centers on correcting all life-threatening problems discovered during the primary assessment. Aggressively manage airway and breathing concerns as soon as they are identified. Control external bleeding using the techniques described in Chapter 18, Soft-Tissue Injuries. Even though blood thinners can make controlling hemorrhage more difficult in elderly patients, direct pressure (perhaps including a pressure bandage) is often all that is needed. The control of bleeding may take longer than normal. Treat suspected hypoxia with the appropriate airway adjunct and high-flow oxygen. Because even minor alterations in a patient's level of responsiveness may indicate underlying cerebral hypoxia, especially at higher altitudes or as a result of rigorous physical activity, the use of supplemental oxygen can be very beneficial. If hypoglycemia is suspected, treat as described in Chapter 11, Altered Mental Status.

If spinal injury is suspected, immobilize the spine as described in Chapter 21, Head and Spine Injuries, taking into consideration the fact that a spinal column abnormality, osteoporosis, or other degenerative spine disease can make cervical collar placement or long spine board immobilization difficult in elderly patients. Use towels, jackets, or other material to fill any voids (including the back of the head) and pad bony prominences to reduce overall movement, make the patient more comfortable, and reduce the incidence of pressure sores (Figure 31-15■).

Treat the specific medical disorders encountered in the order of severity, giving precedence to those that negatively affect the ABCDs. If the patient has a history of asthma, is exhibiting signs of respiratory distress that do not resolve with high-flow

**⊕ 31-6** Describe the general management of geriatric patients.

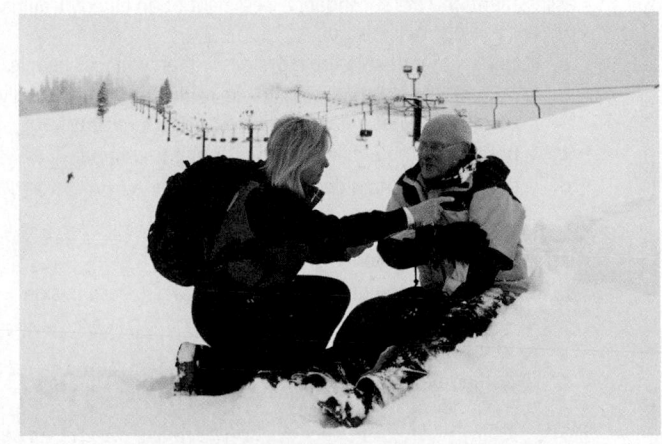

**Figure 31-15** Padding is especially important for elderly patients.

oxygen, and is in possession of a personal inhaler, consider assisting the patient in taking the medication if your state and local protocols allow it. Likewise, you may need to assist a patient who has severe chest pain and a history of heart attack in taking a nitroglycerin tablet or an aspirin, if permitted within your jurisdiction.

Dress and bandage all soft-tissue injuries in the usual manner. Splint and stabilize obvious fractures to minimize pain, swelling, blood loss, and potential emboli, being careful not to over-manipulate fragile joints or bones and possibly cause additional injury. Stabilize pelvic fractures by carefully binding the pelvic girdle as described in Chapter 20, Musculoskeletal Injuries. Treat a dislocated artificial joint in the same way you would treat any dislocated joint. Aggressively manage hypotension and shock —even if the classic signs of shock are not evident due to the physiologic changes of aging, medication use, and other factors—by placing the patient in a supine position with the feet elevated 8–12 inches. Keep patients warm by covering them with a blanket.

Transport patients who require further evaluation or additional treatment to an emergency care facility, preferably one that has a geriatric specialist on staff.

# STOP, THINK, UNDERSTAND

## Multiple Choice
Choose the correct answer.

1. An advanced directive is best defined as _____
   a. a mentally capable patient's legal refusal or acceptance of help during a life-threatening medical emergency.
   b. a patient's inability to give either informed consent or refusal for care during a life-threatening medical emergency due to a physical or mental handicap.
   c. consent for care by a patient's parent or spouse during a life-threatening medical emergency regardless of the patient's wishes.
   d. a legal document that provides guidance regarding a patient's wishes during a life-threatening medical emergency when the patient is unable to express those wishes.

2. A very slight change in mental acuity between the primary assessment and the secondary assessment of an elderly trauma patient is likely indicative of_____
   a. fatigue; older people tire more easily than younger people.
   b. a normal age-appropriate behavior; older patients normally have a somewhat diminished level of mental acuity.
   c. a possible neurologic deficit caused by the trauma.
   d. a sign of developing dementia.

3. "Tenting" of the skin could be indicative of_____
   a. dehydration or hypovolemia.
   b. tissue breakdown due to an age-related decrease in skin elasticity.
   c. extreme or rapid weight loss.
   d. hypothermia or hyperthermia.

4. Subtle changes in vital signs in an elderly patient are_____
   a. normal.
   b. possible indicators of an underlying disease process.
   c. a serious indicator of impending circulatory failure.
   d. a temporary phenomenon caused by an emotional response to trauma.

5. Your best course of action for an elderly patient who complains of dizziness, weakness, and associated abdominal pain is to_____
   a. urge the patient to go home and rest.
   b. suggest that the patient use the restroom because a full bladder or bowel could cause syncope.
   c. check the patient's femoral pulses bilaterally.
   d. immediately summon a higher level of medical care because these symptoms could be indicative of a very serious medical problem.

6. Your next course of action for a patient who says that a colostomy port may be blocked is to_____
   a. assist the patient or have a family member assist the patient in checking the port for patency.
   b. ignore the problem because the patient can fix it later.
   c. call for a higher level of medical care because this situation could quickly become life threatening.
   d. show the patient where the restroom is because colostomy ports can be contaminated with fecal matter.

*continued*

7. If a 72-year-old man tells you that he is feeling short of breath and anxious, you should_____
   a. reassure him and continue your exam.
   b. ignore the comment because focusing on anxiety can make it worse.
   c. give him a few moments to relax before resuming your exam.
   d. immediately place him on high-flow $O_2$, assess him, and arrange for transportation to a higher level of medical care while continuing to monitor his condition.

8. Which of the following statements about backboarding an elderly patient is correct? _____
   a. Backboard elderly patients just as you would younger adult patients.
   b. It is necessary to tighten the straps more securely in an elderly patient.
   c. Because hip fractures occur easily in elderly patients, cross the straps loosely over the lower abdomen instead of the usual placement over the bony pelvis.
   d. Use towels, jackets, and other padding material to fill any voids, and pad all bony prominences.

9. Which of the following statements is true? _____
   a. Elderly patients are more likely to develop early signs and symptoms of shock than are younger patients.
   b. Elderly patients may show few or no signs of shock even with severe blood loss.
   c. There is no difference in the development of the signs and symptoms of shock in elderly patients and younger adult patients.
   d. Elderly patients exhibit the same signs and symptoms of shock that younger patients exhibit, but those findings take longer to become evident.

 **CASE DISPOSITION**

You are concerned that the patient may have a head injury. You also are worried about the patient's high blood pressure. Accordingly, you place the patient on high-flow oxygen, keep him comfortable, and mobilize resources to transport him to the hospital. Although the patient initially refuses treatment, you tell him your concerns and gain his cooperation. Reluctantly, the patient goes by ambulance to the emergency department at a nearby trauma center.

That evening, the ambulance crew gives you an update on the patient. He became increasingly lethargic while en route. He was diagnosed with a subdural hematoma. The warfarin he was taking increased the intracranial bleeding from a relatively trivial head injury to a serious condition. Following aggressive treatment that included surgery, his prognosis is good because of your knowledge of the aging process and your insistence that he be evaluated at a hospital.

# Chapter Review

## Chapter Summary

Seniors are the fastest growing population segment in the United States and will continue to be so for many years as members of the "Baby Boomer" generation age. Thanks to advances in technology, nutrition, healthcare, outdoor apparel, and equipment, today's seniors are far more active than their counterparts from previous generations. They also are healthier and able to engage in a wide range of outdoor activities, and they place demands on their bodies that only a few decades earlier were considered ill-advised or altogether impossible. The many age-related changes the human body undergoes as it ages can affect the way it responds when stressed, ill, or injured. As a result, it is highly probable that OEC Technicians will encounter older patients in increasing numbers.

Geriatric patients pose unique challenges to OEC Technicians. Accordingly, OEC Technicians need to understand age-related physiologic changes, the illnesses and injuries to which seniors are most prone and the medications prescribed to manage those conditions, and the medical devices that geriatric patients may use to maintain health while engaging in outdoor activities.

Finally, OEC Technicians must maintain a high index of suspicion when assessing elderly patients for injury or disease be-

cause numerous factors can mask these patients' clinical signs and symptoms. By combining their knowledge of the aging process with a thorough assessment of the patient's condition, OEC Technicians can provide geriatric patients high-quality on-scene care and advocate for further evaluation and treatment. Their care can help seniors resume their participation in and enjoyment of outdoor activities for many years to come.

# Remember...

1. The elderly population is the fastest growing population in the country.
2. Aging causes physiologic changes that increase a geriatric patient's risk for disease and injury.
3. Geriatric patients should be considered high-risk patients because many have multiple medical conditions.
4. Polypharmacy can affect clinical findings.
5. Speak directly and clearly to geriatric patients.
6. Address seniors as "Mr.," "Mrs.," or "Ms." followed by their last names.
7. Never assume that geriatric patients cannot understand you simply because they are elderly.
8. "Atypical" complaints are normal for geriatric patients.
9. Have a low threshold for advising geriatric patients to undergo further evaluation.
10. Consider the underlying cause of a fall in geriatric patients.
11. Elderly patients are at greater risk for mortality due to traumatic injuries.
12. Elderly patients have low compensatory reserves and thus benefit from aggressive intervention.
13. Have a high index of suspicion for cervical spine injuries in elderly patients.
14. Never attribute altered mental status to old age alone.

# Chapter Questions

## Multiple Choice

Choose the correct answer.

1. Which of the following statements correctly reflects your primary concern about moving an elderly patient?_____
   a. The patient's bones are so brittle that they may break when you move him.
   b. The patient's skin is less elastic and thus more susceptible to tears and other dermatologic injuries.
   c. The patient is likely to become uncooperative or combative.
   d. Decreased central nervous system function may cause the patient to become dizzy and to vomit.

2. What assumptions should you make about a 75-year-old male hiker who appears confused on the trail?_____
   a. He is probably exhibiting signs and symptoms of typical age-related dementia.
   b. He may be showing signs of altered mental status (AMS) caused by trauma.
   c. He probably has Alzheimer's disease.
   d. His confusion is probably normal; respect this elderly patient's privacy and leave him alone.

3. Which of the following actions demonstrate good communication skills with seniors? (check all that apply)
   _____ a. Speak louder than usual.
   _____ b. If possible, eliminate distractions such as loud music or background noise.
   _____ c. Do not maintain eye contact, because it is rude for a younger person to do so with an elder.
   _____ d. Address elderly patients by their first names.
   _____ e. Use calming terms such as "sweetie" or "hon".
   _____ f. Minimize the patient's confusion or distractions by directing your questions to family members.
   _____ g. Communicate one-on-one with elderly patients as much as possible.
   _____ h. Use close-ended questions rather than open-ended questions.

4. When your assessment findings are "normal" but elderly patients do not seem "right" to you, you should_____
   a. transfer or transport such patients to a higher level of medical care.
   b. tell the patients to go home and rest and see how they feel later.
   c. repeat the assessment two or three more times.
   d. assume that nothing is wrong and suggest that such patients resume normal activities as they see fit.

5. Compared to an unresponsive younger patient, an unresponsive geriatric patient's risk for aspiration is_____
   a. lower.
   b. the same.
   c. higher.

## Matching

1. Match each of the following conditions to its description.

   _____ 1. kyphosis
   _____ 2. lordosis
   _____ 3. osteoporosis
   _____ 4. scoliosis

   a. a decrease in bone density due to mineral loss
   b. "humpback" curvature of the upper thoracic spine
   c. "swayback" appearance due to inward curvature of the lumbar spine
   d. a lateral curvature of the spine

2. Match each of the following medication types to its action.

   _____ 1. beta-blockers
   _____ 2. calcium-channel blockers
   _____ 3. diuretics
   _____ 4. blood thinners

   a. make the heart contract more efficiently, manage cardiac arrhythmias, and lower blood pressure
   b. help decrease the volume of circulating fluid within the cardiovascular system
   c. reduce heart rate, blood pressure, and heart contractility
   d. are typically prescribed to patients with a history of mechanical heart valve replacement, irregular heartbeat, deep vein thrombosis, or pulmonary embolism

3. Match each of the following devices or processes with its function.

   _____ 1. urinary catheter
   _____ 2. colostomy
   _____ 3. shunt catheter
   _____ 4. infusion pump

   a. drains feces
   b. provides access to a vein for kidney dialysis
   c. drains urine
   d. administers insulin

## Scenario

*You are called to the ski lodge off the main parking lot to see a woman who is not feeling well. When you arrive, you find a 78-year-old woman who has traveled with her family to watch her grandchildren ski. She is awake, alert, and oriented to person only (she knows her name); she seems confused about where she is and the day of the week. She is complaining of a headache and nausea, and while you are there she vomits. Her daughter tells you that her mother's mental status and slurred speech are not normal for her. The scene is secure, and you ask bystanders to move back.*

1. This woman may have any of the following except_____
   a. diabetes.
   b. stroke.
   c. dementia.
   d. head injury from previous fall.

*The daughter verifies that the patient does not have diabetes and has not consumed alcohol. Next you administer the Cincinnati Stroke Test and observe positive findings.*

**2.** Based on the findings, the patient's presentation, and statements by the daughter, you suspect that the patient is having _____

    **a.** an MCI.

    **b.** a TIA or CVA.

    **c.** an ABC.

    **d.** a UTI.

*Prompt action is critical for patients with suspected strokes. Administration of a drug called TPA must be made within 3 hours of the onset of clot formation and cannot be used for a hemorrhage.*

**3.** Which of the following questions should you ask the daughter next?_____

    **a.** Has your mother ever had an attack like this before?

    **b.** What time did your mother eat her last meal?

    **c.** What prescribed medicines is your mother taking?

    **d.** How long ago did your mother last have her normal mental status?

*You note some weakness to the left side of her face. She takes medications for her heart and for hypertension.*

*Her vital signs are pulse: 100 and irregular; respirations: 20; blood pressure: 170/110; and her skin is pale, cool, and dry.*

*You provide oxygen, place the patient in a position of comfort, and monitor the vital signs and airway while you wait for the ALS unit.*

## Suggested Reading

Birnbaumer, D. M. 2006. "The Elderly Patient." In *Rosen's Emergency Medicine*, Sixth Edition, edited by J. A. Marx. St. Louis, MO: Mosby Elsevier.

Forinash, K., and D. M. Meade. 2000. "Trauma in the Elderly." *EMS Magazine* (29)9: 79–88.

Hawks, T., 2008/09 NSAA National Demographic Study. August 2009. RRC Associates, pg. 7.

Kahn, J. H., and B. Magauran. 2006. "Trends in Geriatric Emergency Medicine." *Emergency Medicine Clinics of North America* 24(2): 243–260.

 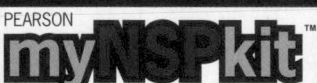

# Outdoor Adaptive Athletes

Bruce Evans, MD

## OBJECTIVES

**Upon completion of this chapter, the OEC Technician will be able to:**

**32-1** Define and contrast the following terms:
   a. disability
   b. handicap
   c. impairment

**32-2** List and describe two disorders that cause intellectual disabilities.

**32-3** List two disorders that cause progressive physical disabilities.

**32-4** Describe four elements of effective communication with a person who has an intellectual disability.

**32-5** Describe how to assess and care for physically disabled athletes.

**32-6** List the signs and symptoms of autonomic dysreflexia.

**32-7** Describe and demonstrate how to assess an adaptive athlete.

**32-8** Describe and demonstrate how to care for an adaptive athlete who is injured or ill.

**32-9** Describe and demonstrate how to manage an above-the-knee amputee with a femur fracture of the same leg.

## Chapter Overview

Many athletes today have some form of impairment but are able to participate in recreational sports and even compete in organized events. The physical and societal barriers these athletes face while participating in outdoor sports can be profound. Whether the athlete's impairment is physical or intellectual, just getting from the parking lot to the venue can mean facing challenges that most of us have never even had to consider, much less overcome.

*continued*

## HISTORICAL TIMELINE

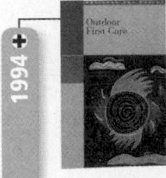

**1994** The NSP Board votes to change WEC to OEC. A new program, *Outdoor First Care*, is also introduced.

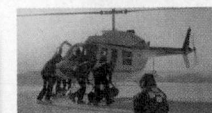

**1996** NSP home page debuts on the World Wide Web.

## ⊕ KEY TERMS

adaptive athlete, *p. 1011*

adaptive equipment, *p. 1019*

Americans with Disabilities Act (ADA), *p. 1010*

athetoid cerebral palsy, *p. 1016*

attention deficit disorder (ADD), *p. 1012*

autonomic dysreflexia (AD), *p. 1016*

autism spectrum disorders (ASDs), *p. 1013*

bi-ski, *p. 1023*

bucket, *p. 1023*

cerebral palsy (CP), *p. 1016*

cognitive disability, *p. 1013*

disability, *p. 1011*

Down syndrome (DS), *p. 1018*

dyslexia, *p. 1012*

dystonic cerebral palsy, *p. 1016*

expressive aphasia, *p. 1031*

four tracker, *p. 1024*

handicap, *p. 1011*

impairment, *p. 1011*

intellectual disability, *p. 1012*

mono-ski, *p. 1023*

multiple sclerosis (MS), *p. 1017*

muscular dystrophy (MD), *p. 1017*

ostomy bag, *p. 1016*

outriggers, *p. 1023*

paraplegic, *p. 1016*

prosthetic, *p. 1020*

quadriplegic, *p. 1016*

sit-board, *p. 1023*

sit-ski, *p. 1023*

ski bra, *p. 1024*

sliding board, *p. 1022*

spastic cerebral palsy, *p. 1016*

spina bifida (SB), *p. 1017*

spinal cord injury (SCI), *p. 1016*

stoma, *p. 1031*

tether, *p. 1023*

three tracker, *p. 1024*

two track skiing, *p. 1024*

visual impairment, *p. 1015*

---

**Americans with Disabilities Act (ADA)** legislation passed in 1990 designed to prevent discrimination against individuals with disabilities.

**disability** any condition that impairs normal function or daily activity.

**impairment** any loss or limitation of physical or intellectual function.

**handicap** any condition that impairs normal physical or intellectual function.

**adaptive athlete** a person with a physical or intellectual disability who participates in a sport.

Many factors determine whether an individual with a disability or impairment is capable of participating in a sport. Active participation usually requires a mental ability equivalent to performing activities of daily living (e.g., dressing oneself, brushing one's teeth); passive participation (e.g., sitting in a sit-ski) requires less mental capacity. Physical participation depends on the person's balance, muscle strength, coordination, and neurologic processes; impairment of one or more of these functions can make active participation difficult. Sometimes simply the desire to participate helps adaptive athletes perform at a higher level than expected.

Participation in outdoor sports has become more popular for adaptive athletes in recent years due to improved access and innovative equipment. In 1990, the U.S. Congress passed the **Americans with Disabilities Act (ADA)**, which prompted many ski resorts and other facilities to begin removing physical obstacles to wheelchair access. Nearly all governmental recreational facilities have also made outdoor activities accessible to individuals with handicaps. New facilities and structures must comply with ADA standards for access (Figure 32-1 ■). The resulting improved access for athletes

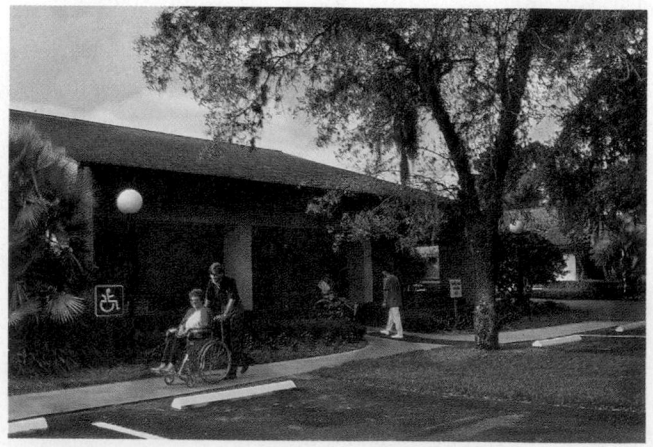

**Figure 32-1** Buildings, facilities, and vehicles must now comply with ADA standards for accessibility.

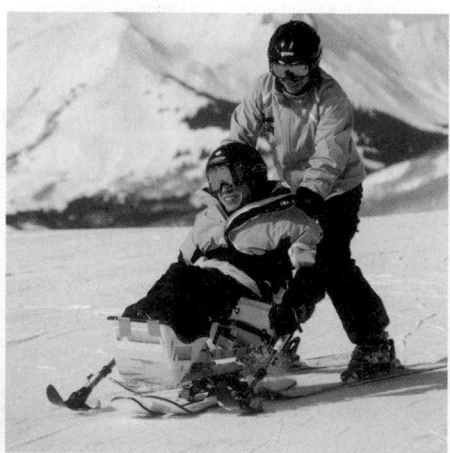

**Figure 32-2** Adaptive athletes of all abilities and ages are able to participate in a variety of outdoor sports today.
Copyright Pat Pielsticker Bittle

## + CASE PRESENTATION +

You are stationed at your ski resort's recreational race course during a special event for disabled athletes when an adult chaperone waves you over to her group. As you approach, you notice a competitor sitting on the snow wearing her race course bib and helmet. The chaperone explains that the girl, who is 14 years old, has not been acting normally since she finished her last race about 10 minutes ago. The chaperone explains that the athlete is usually much more interactive, and that even though the skier negotiated the race course without mishap, she had experienced "a few falls" during the day.

You continue to interact with the chaperone while calmly approaching the skier. Kneeling down so that you can begin your visual assessment and address her at eye level, you notice that she appears to be staring off in one direction and does not make eye contact with you. She does not respond to your questions and seems unable to follow verbal instructions. You become concerned that the patient's mental status may be different than her normal status, even in the absence of any reported trauma. You suspect that this encounter will require more than one rescuer, so you radio dispatch for equipment and assistance.

*What should you do while you are waiting for assistance?*

---

with impairments has added to the growing popularity of outdoor programs for a wide range of participants. At the same time, incorporating new materials that are less expensive, stronger, and lighter into adaptive equipment has meant more independence for more athletes with impairments (Figure 32-2■). Finally, outdated stereotypes about which recreational opportunities are appropriate for athletes with sensory, motor, or intellectual impairments have given way to more commonsense ideas about having fun in outdoor environments.

As a result of these changes, OEC Technicians now need to consider whether an injured or ill athlete may have some type of impairment. More importantly, such impairments may present unique challenges that rescuers must incorporate into their assessment and management plan. Disabled athletes, for example, may be at higher risk for certain injuries, and specialized equipment may be required to evacuate these atheletes from the scene. Guides, instructors, or other companions accompanying a disabled athlete may be able to offer invaluable insight and assistance. Being alert to these and other considerations can enable OEC Technicians to provide the best assistance to an injured or ill athlete with an impairment.

## Common Disabilities

The words you use when offering aid to an athlete with a disability are important, both to demonstrate proper respect to your patient and to ensure that proper care is provided. A **disability** is any physical or intellectual condition that impairs normal function or daily activity, whereas an **impairment** is a loss of a physical, physiological, or psychological ability or the inability to perform a task in daily life. An individual can have an impairment and not have a disability. Individuals with disabilities, whether genetically inherited or acquired through trauma or illness, prefer the term *disability* to the term **handicap**. The National Ski Patrol has adopted the term **adaptive athlete** to describe any individual with an impairment who participates in a sport or an outdoor activity (Figure 32-3■).

It is estimated that up to 20 percent of the U.S. population has some form of intellectual or physical impairment. A person can have an intellectual disability or a

⊕ **32-1** Define and contrast the following terms:

   **a.** disability

   **b.** handicap

   **c.** impairment

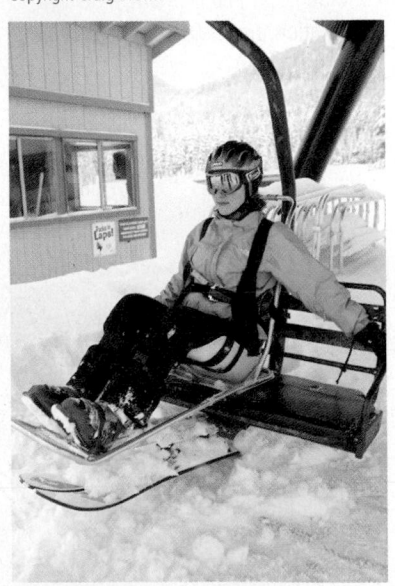

**Figure 32-3** The National Ski Patrol considers any individual with an impairment who participates in a sport as an adaptive athlete.
Copyright Craig Brown

## Disability or Impairment?

A person with one arm has a significant impairment in life but would have no disability with respect to reading a book, eating, or skiing down a slope. However, the same person may have a disability with respect to tying a shoelace.

physical disability, or both. Intellectual impairments can involve a learning disability, be cognitive, or be related to psychological or personality problems. Communication with intellectually impaired people during assessment may be difficult.

Many physically impaired people are able to participate in outdoor activities and sports. Neurologically impaired people, amputees, and people with a muscular disease make up the largest percentage of physically impaired athletes. Some individuals have both intellectual and physical impairments, some with severe disability. However, many of these individuals, such as those with Down syndrome, are able to participate in modified versions of a sport under the close supervision of aides.

---

# STOP, THINK, UNDERSTAND

## Multiple Choice

Choose the correct answer.

1. The inability to perform a task in daily life is_____
   a. a disability.
   c. an impairment.
   b. a handicap.
   d. a disillusion.

2. A person who has an impairment_____
   a. is crippled.
   b. is handicapped.
   c. may or may not be disabled.
   d. has both physical and mental problems.

3. The largest percentage of athletes with a physical impairment have what type of disability? _____
   a. cognitive
   b. learning, psychological, or personality
   c. neurologic impairment, amputation, or a muscle disease
   d. down syndrome

---

⊕ **32-2** List and describe two disorders that cause intellectual disabilities.

**intellectual disability** any condition that impairs normal information processing.

## Intellectual Disabilities

It is very likely that OEC Technicians will provide care to patients with **intellectual disabilities**. A rescue team's ability to meet the emergent medical and emotional needs of these athletes depends on understanding the unique features of those disabilities.

Intellectual disabilities include a wide range of conditions, including learning disorders, attention deficit disorders, dyslexia, autism, psychological impairment (psychotic and emotional), and other cognitive disorders. Additionally, not all athletes with a specific syndrome or category of disability have the same degree of impairment or the same types of behaviors. As a result, broad descriptive terms such as "mentally challenged" or "mentally retarded" are neither useful nor acceptable. Knowing the key features associated with specific disabilities can help OEC Technicians anticipate how to provide the best possible care for these athletes.

### Learning Disorders

**attention deficit disorder (ADD)** a behavioral syndrome that causes short attention span, impulsive behavior, and restlessness.

**dyslexia** an impairment of information processing that makes learning new information difficult.

People with learning disorders typically have one of two main disorders. **Attention deficit disorder (ADD)** is typically a genetically inherited disability characterized by a short attention span. Hyperactivity, impulsive behavior, and restlessness are also commonly seen in association with ADD (Figure 32-4■). **Dyslexia** is another learning disorder in which individuals have difficulty processing new information. This results in delays when learning a new skill or sport. Learning disorders are not necessarily associated with below-normal intelligence, but they may impair an athlete's ability to communicate with or respond to a rescuer.

### Autism Spectrum Disorders

**Autism spectrum disorders (ASDs)** are developmental disabilities with a wide variety of manifestations that affect communication and behavior. Individuals with ASDs, which include autism, Asperger's syndrome, and atypical autism, are challenged by participating in what most people consider normal, day-to-day interactions.

According to the U.S. Centers for Disease Control and Prevention (CDC), ASDs are the fastest growing developmental disabilities in the United States. People with an ASD are seven times more likely to come into contact with rescuers than are individuals from the general population. Individuals with an ASD often have both learning and language impairments that limit effective communication. Unfamiliar environments or strangers may cause repetitive movements, fear, or aggression. Moving away from a rescuer or appearing to ignore a stranger are two examples of ways in which an athlete with an ASD may respond to an OEC Technician. Many people with an ASD do not exhibit outwardly visible signs of this disability until they experience a problem. People with ASDs are prone to wander and are attracted to bodies of water (e.g., lakes, pools), a combination that explains why drowning is the leading cause of death for people with an ASD.

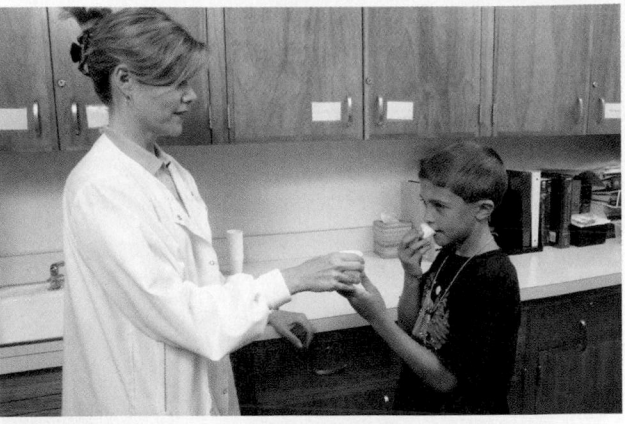

**Figure 32-4** Medicines can help control the impulsiveness and restlessness commonly seen with some ADD patients.

**autism spectrum disorders (ASDs)** developmental disabilities that impair communication with others.

## Cognitive Disabilities

**Cognitive disabilities** result from traumatic brain injuries (TBI) or any loss of brain function that limits the ability to process information. Sensory perception, coordination, movement, and communication can all be affected. Seizures and physical impairments can be associated with cognitive disabilities. Because these individuals usually have coordination problems, they must use equipment that does not require them to balance or use muscular control.

**cognitive disability** an impairment of brain function that limits the ability to process information.

### Autonomic Dysfunction

Autonomic dysfunction (AD) or dysautonomia is a disease that affects the autonomic nervous system. The effects of dysautonomia are numerous and vary widely from person to person from mild, with minimal impairment, to severe, leaving the affected person completely bedridden and disabled.

### Mental Illness

Mental illnesses also manifest as a wide variety of symptoms and behaviors. Schizophrenia and manic-depressive disorder are examples of impairments that can cause sudden personality changes or bizarre behaviors. OEC Technicians must be able to differentiate among the various types of mental illnesses. For more information about mental illness, refer to Chapter 33, Behavioral Emergencies and Crisis Response.

## Intellectual Difficulties

A multitude of genetic and environmental factors can cause life-long intellectual disabilities. "Mental retardation" is an outdated general label that implied a below-average intelligence quotient, or IQ. This term has been abandoned and is not helpful in assessing and treating patients in outdoor environments. OEC Technicians will encounter adaptive athletes who have below-average intellectual capacity due to difficulties in learning or socialization. Among the prenatal causes for impaired intellectual function are inherited genetic conditions (e.g., Down syndrome, fragile X syndrome), fetal alcohol syndrome, and syndromes that affect embryonic brain growth. Birth or infant asphyxia, brain trauma, lead or mercury poisoning, and meningitis can also affect mental development and ability.

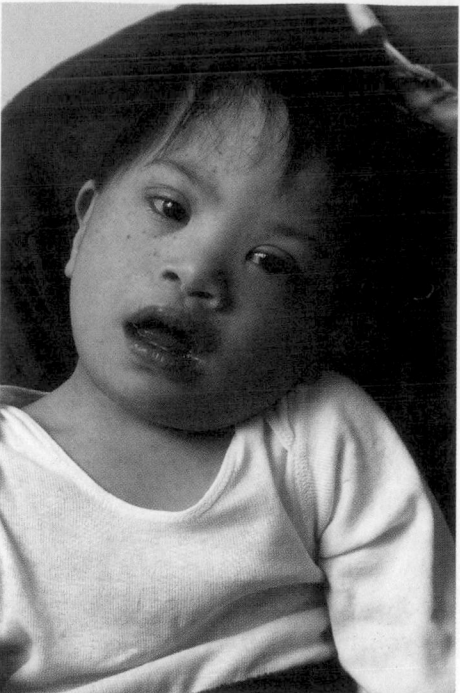

**Figure 32-5** Caring for individuals with some disabilities requires a lot of understanding, patience, and compassion.

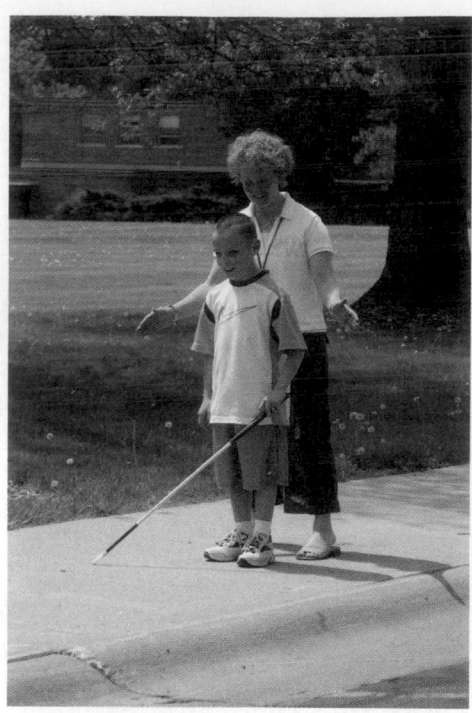

**Figure 32-6** A patient's caretaker can play a very important role in aiding OEC Technicians.

OEC Technicians must realize that people with life-long intellectual and social development deficits need tremendous understanding and kindness during the assessment and treatment processes in outdoor environments (Figure 32-5■). These patients are out of their usual surroundings and may be frightened or disoriented. Always try to communicate with these patients in the same manner as with other patients, even though this may not always be possible. Each patient's caretaker is *very* important in helping you to communicate with these patients (Figure 32-6■). Patients with intellectual impairments exhibit anxiety, hyperactivity or apathy, bad judgment, and impulsiveness. They are also easily distracted, which can hinder both assessment and management. It is essential that OEC Technicians remain patient and act with friendliness and understanding.

# STOP, THINK, UNDERSTAND

## Multiple Choice

Choose the correct answer.

1. The fastest growing developmental disability in the United States is_____
   a. dyslexia.
   b. attention-deficit disorder (ADD).
   c. autism spectrum disorders (ASDs).
   d. hyperactivity.

2. Moving away from or ignoring a rescuer can be due to which of the following disorders? _____
   a. ADD
   b. Autism
   c. Hyperactivity disorder
   d. Dysautonomia

3. The leading cause of death for individuals with an ASD is
   _____
   a. TBI.
   b. suicide.
   c. vehicular accidents.
   d. drowning.

4. Cognitive disabilities are primarily caused by _____
   a. a TBI.
   b. seizures.
   c. substance abuse.
   d. birth defects.

*continued*

5. Two disabilities that can cause sudden personality change or bizarre behavior are_____
   a. schizophrenia and manic-depressive disorder.
   b. dyslexia and dysgraphia.
   c. ASD and Asperger's syndrome.
   d. ADD and ADHD.

6. Which of the following statements about mental retardation is correct? _____
   a. It encompasses social dysfunctions such as ASDs.
   b. It encompasses cognitive impairments such as dyslexia or dysgraphia.
   c. It can manifest itself in behavioral disorders such as schizophrenia or manic depression.
   d. It is an incorrect and unacceptable label.

7. Which of the following actions are important components for assessing an individual with an intellectual or social disability? (check all that apply)
   _____ a. Respond with kindness.
   _____ b. Respond with patience.
   _____ c. Involve the patient's caretaker.
   _____ d. Speak louder than usual.
   _____ e. Try to communicate in the same manner as you would with any patient.
   _____ f. Do not speak until the patient makes eye contact with you.
   _____ g. Realize that if the patient grows frustrated it is because he does not understand you.
   _____ h. Realize that if the patient grows frustrated it is because you do not understand him.
   _____ i. Attempt to determine the exact type of disability this patient has.

## Fill in the Blank

The two primary inherited genetic conditions that cause below-average intellectual capacity are _____ and _____.

## List

List four things that can adversely affect mental development and ability.
1. _____
2. _____
3. _____
4. _____

## Physical Disabilities

Skiers with physical limitations resulting from spinal cord injuries, cerebral palsy, or amputation are often able to overcome their disability by using specialized equipment. Other physical limitations, such as **visual impairment**, can be overcome through assistance from a guide or a specially trained skiing partner (Figure 32-7■). Young war veterans with amputations are increasingly becoming active in many outdoor activities. As a result, it is highly likely that OEC Technicians will encounter athletes with physical disabilities.

⊕ **32-3** List two disorders that cause progressive physical disabilities.

**visual impairment** a range of visual disabilities that include legal blindness, partial sightedness, and complete blindness.

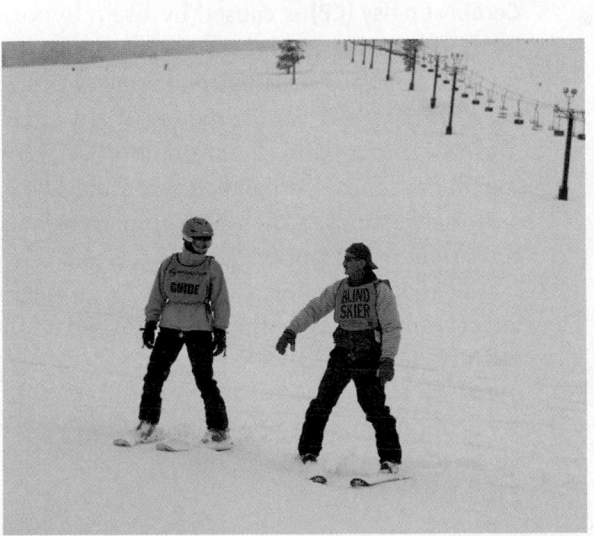

**Figure 32-7** The physical limitations imposed by visual impairment can be overcome through the use of a guide. Copyright Craig Brown

**⊕ 32-6** List the signs and symptoms of autonomic dysreflexia.

**spinal cord injury (SCI)** damage to the spinal cord due to trauma.

**paraplegic** people who do not have use of their legs.

**quadriplegic** people who have lost function in all four extremities are called quadriplegics.

**autonomic dysreflexia (AD)** abnormal function of the nervous system associated with spinal cord injuries; can lead to dangerously high blood pressure.

**ostomy bag** a bag for collecting urine or feces that attaches to the body with adhesive tape.

**cerebral palsy (CP)** a brain injury before, during, or shortly following birth that results in a non-progressive, non-contagious muscular motor disorder.

**spastic cerebral palsy** a form of CP that causes constant, involuntary muscle contractions.

**athetoid cerebral palsy** a form of CP that causes slow, writhing muscle contractions.

**dystonic cerebral palsy** a form of CP associated with extreme muscle rigidity.

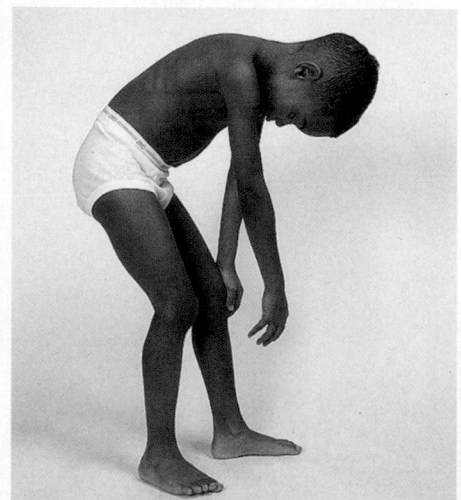

**Figure 32-8** A person with cerebral palsy is at increased risk of an extremity injury during a fall.

## Spinal Cord Injuries

**Spinal cord injuries (SCI)** can result from trauma, congenital malformations, tumors, or other progressive conditions. Nerve damage within the spinal cord typically affects sensory perception and motor control at a certain level of the spinal cord, above which the athlete may have normal sensation, coordination, and muscle strength. People who do not have use of their legs are called **paraplegics**, while people who have lost function in all four extremities are called **quadriplegics**. Because adaptive athletes may not be able to feel trauma or cold-related injuries below the level of their spinal cord injury, OEC Technicians should consider these possibilities when assessing and caring for a patient with a preexisting SCI.

Adaptive athletes with SCI are at risk for developing **autonomic dysreflexia (AD)**, which can occur as a result of new trauma above or below the level of a preexisting cord injury. AD may be triggered by a variety of other things, including very minor trauma, having an overfull bladder, hyperthermia, hypothermia, and physiologic stressors not apparent on physical exam. AD may initially present without symptoms but can quickly lead to feelings of panic or anxiety. It can cause a rapid increase in blood pressure to dangerously high levels, resulting in headache and/or blurry vision. Physical findings sometimes include altered mental status and skin changes such as sweating or flushing. OEC Technicians should be alert for potential mechanisms that could cause AD, during both assessment and management. Simply unblocking an obstructed catheter may prevent or relieve AD. AD is a true medical emergency, and OEC Technicians should make every effort to determine the source of the problem and to correct it. Often, SCI patients can assist you in determining the cause.

Even in the absence of emergent AD, adaptive athletes with SCIs have a loss of autonomic nervous system control of body function below the level of cord injury. A variety of adjunct devices can help overcome some of these disabilities. A bladder catheter that passes through the urethra to an external urine collection bag, for instance, may be used to collect urine. Another example is a urostomy, a surgically created port in the anterior abdomen or near the kidneys that drains the urinary system. Patients may have an **ostomy bag**, a clear plastic bag that enables the collection of feces through a surgically created port in the abdominal wall. If the port connects to the small bowel, the patient has an ileostomy bag; a port that connects to the large intestine has a colostomy bag.

## Cerebral Palsy

**Cerebral palsy (CP)** is caused by brain hypoxia just before, during, or following birth. The subsequent brain injury typically results in impaired voluntary motor function and coordination in one of three patterns. **Spastic CP**, the most common form of CP, is characterized by intermittent or repetitive involuntary muscle contractions in one or more extremities, causing jerking body movements and impaired balance. **Athetoid CP** causes slow, involuntary movements and contractions, which also impair balance. **Dystonic CP** is characterized by rigidity in one or more extremity.

All adaptive athletes with CP are at increased risk of extremity injury during falls (Figure 32-8■). They may not be able to protect or relax an extended extremity during an accident. Trauma may worsen spasticity, making field treatment of the injured extremity difficult. Stabilizing a suspected fracture or dislocation injury in a position of comfort is often better than attempting to apply traction or reposition the extremity. Among individuals with CP, those with athetoid or mild spastic CP are most likely to ski. Whereas many of them can walk, they may prefer to sit to ski. Individuals with dystonic CP have the most problems skiing because their rigid muscles make it difficult to accommodate them in a sit-ski.

## Multiple Sclerosis

**Multiple sclerosis (MS)** is an intermittently progressive disease that causes degeneration of both central and peripheral nerves. Each progression is often associated with exacerbations that can cause a rapid onset of motor and sensory deficits. Impairments vary widely but typically include paralysis, balance problems, reduced stamina, and visual deficits. Mood changes and slurred or slowed speech may also occur during exacerbations, making assessment more difficult. Individuals with milder MS may be able to stand to ski, but as the condition progresses it may become difficult for these individuals to ski while sitting. Although individuals with MS generally function at a high mental capability, their affect changes as the disease progresses.

**multiple sclerosis (MS)** a progressive neurologic syndrome that causes weakness, paralysis of the extremities, and visual deficits.

## Spina Bifida

**Spina bifida (SB)** results from a congenital malformation of the spine and spinal cord, often at the lumbar level. Adaptive athletes with SB frequently have sensory or motor deficits below the level at which the spinal cord is malformed. Allergies to natural latex rubber in SB patients can cause anaphylactic shock and death. Some SB patients also have abnormal cerebrospinal fluid (CSF) circulation, which can cause a damaging increase in pressure on the brain and spinal cord. A surgically implanted drainage tube known as a shunt allows excess CSF to flow into the abdomen. If this tube becomes kinked or blocked, the accumulation of CSF around the brain can cause life-threatening pressure to build up within the skull. Although infection is a leading cause of shunt malfunction, trauma may damage the drainage system. Therefore, any patient with a shunt who reports a worsening headache or has changes in mental status requires emergent physician evaluation.

**spina bifida (SB)** a congenital malformation that results in gaps within the bony spine that expose the spinal cord to injury.

**muscular dystrophy (MD)** a syndrome characterized by progressive muscle degeneration.

## Muscular Dystrophy (MD)

**Muscular dystrophies (MD)** affect the skeletal muscles such that the arms and/or legs become difficult to use (Figure 32-9■). Patients with MD have spinal curvature, lax joints, weak and wasted muscles, and are easily fatigued, but they have normal mental status. The most common form of childhood MD affects males more than females, and most of these children die following the teenage years. Most adaptive athletes with MD sit to ski.

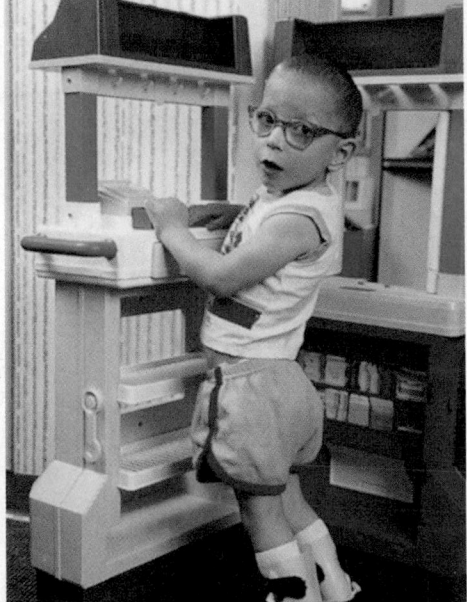

**Figure 32-9** Muscular dystrophy causes skeletal muscles to become very weak.

## Amputations

Individuals with amputations are the largest group of adaptive athletes, and they use a wide variety of adaptive equipment and prosthetics to overcome physical impairments. Amputations can be congenital, traumatic, or surgical in origin, and some people have more than one amputated extremity. The relative impairment resulting from amputation depends on whether the amputated extremity is an arm or a leg, and how much of the extremity was lost. Loss of an upper extremity affects the ability to participate in many activities but has little effect on participation in snow sports. An adaptive athlete with a single amputation below the knee can either use an artificial leg with a ski mounted to it, or ski on one ski. Most double lower amputees sit to ski, especially if the amputations are above the knee.

# STOP, THINK, UNDERSTAND

## Multiple Choice
Choose the correct answer.

1. Which of the following statements regarding the assessment of a paraplegic patient with a mid-lumbar SCI is false? _____
   a. The patient will be unable to feel that his lower leg is broken.
   b. The patient is at risk for developing AD.
   c. The patient will be able to wiggle the toes in the affected leg.
   d. The patient should have normal CMS of the upper extremity.

2. Sweating, flushing, altered mental status, or elevated BP in a paraplegic patient should alert an OEC Technician to what condition? _____
   a. Anxiety
   b. A TBI
   c. Shock
   d. AD

3. Which of the following statements about autonomic dysreflexia (AD) is false? _____
   a. AD can be caused by something as simple as an overly full bladder.
   b. AD is life threatening and a true medical emergency.
   c. Once the signs/symptoms of AD develop, there is no way for an OEC Technician to relieve or stop the development of this condition.
   d. An SCI patient can often help determine the cause of the dysreflexia.

4. A patient with CP is at greater risk for which of the following types of injury? _____
   a. a TBI
   b. an internal injury
   c. an SCI
   d. an extremity injury

5. A progressive disease in which a patient may initially be able to stand to ski but may ultimately end up in a sit-ski or a bucket ski is_____
   a. spina bifida.
   b. autonomic dysreflexia.
   c. muscular dystrophy.
   d. dystonic cerebral palsy.

6. Which of the following statements about amputee athletes is true? _____
   a. Patients with upper extremity amputations can rarely participate in snow sports due to significantly reduced balance.
   b. An individual with a single amputation below the knee can ski either standing or sitting.
   c. Amputation can impair cognitive function.
   d. An individual with congenital amputation has a harder time skiing than a person with a traumatic amputation.

## Fill in the Blank

1. A tubular device that collects urine in SCI patients is a _____. An external portal on the abdominal wall for the diversion of urine is a _____, while an external bag attaching to the abdominal wall for feces is called a _____. The abdominal wall portal from the small intestines is called a _____.
2. Hypoxia of a fetus/newborn before, during, or following birth can cause _____.
3. The most common form of CP, which causes involuntary muscle contractions in one or more extremity, is _____._____. CP that causes slow, involuntary movements and rigidity in one or more extremity is characteristic of _____ CP.

## Visually and Hearing Impaired Adaptive Athletes

Outdoor enthusiasts who are visually or hearing impaired represent a large percentage of adaptive athletes. Blind skiers are seen around the world, often on gentle slopes with guides acting as their "eyes." The pattern of injuries seen in blind participants in snow sports is similar to that of participants with normal vision, but the incidence of injury is higher. Because blind individuals may be more anxious after injury, explain in detail the steps you will take in providing care.

Individuals with hearing impairments can generally participate in any outdoor activity. Many hearing-impaired patients can read lips, but to do so they must be able to clearly see your mouth. Although some individuals with hearing impairments may have some speech problems, most communicate well, with or without the use of sign language. Interestingly most deaf people sound the same, using the same "tones" when speaking (Figure 32-10■).

## Combined Physical and Intellectual Disability

**Down syndrome (DS)** is a range of genetic disorders, caused by the presence of an extra chromosome, that results in physical and intellectual disabilities that vary widely from

**Down syndrome (DS)** a genetic disability that causes intellectual impairment and physical anomalies.

**adaptive equipment** modified sport gear that helps its user overcome a functional impairment.

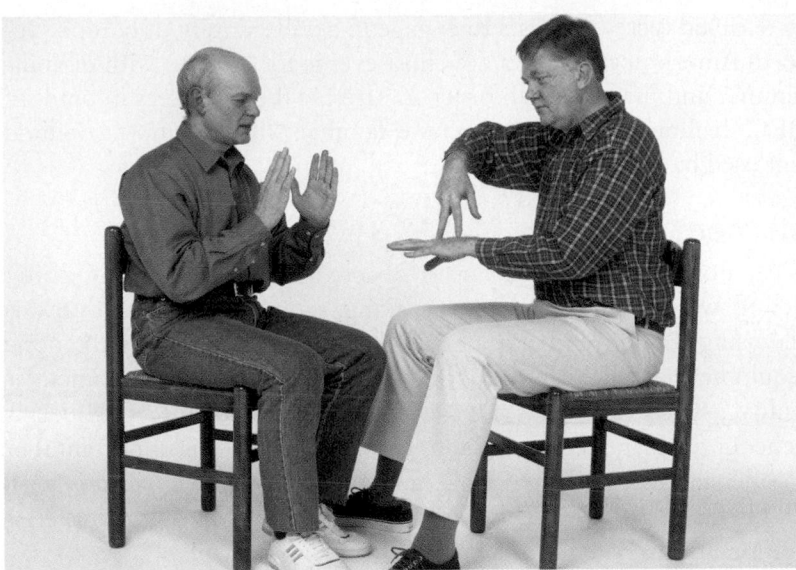

**Figure 32-10** Most individuals with a hearing impairment can communicate well, with or without the use of sign language.
Copyright Andy Crawford/Dorling Kindersley Media Library

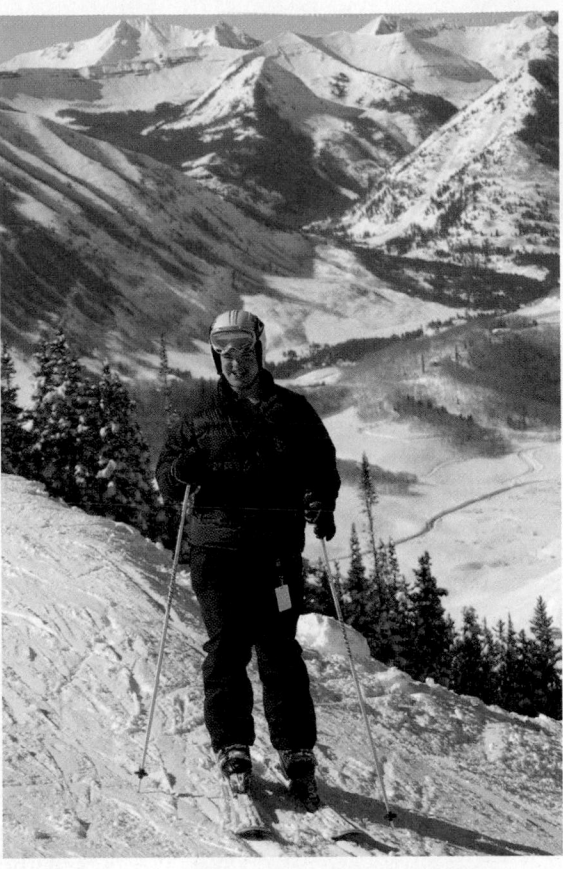

**Figure 32-11** The physical and intellectual abilities of adaptive athletes with Down syndrome vary widely among individuals.
Copyright Pat Pielsticker Bittle

**Figure 32-12** A medal from the Paralympic Games.
Copyright Andy Crawford/Dorling Kindersley Media Library

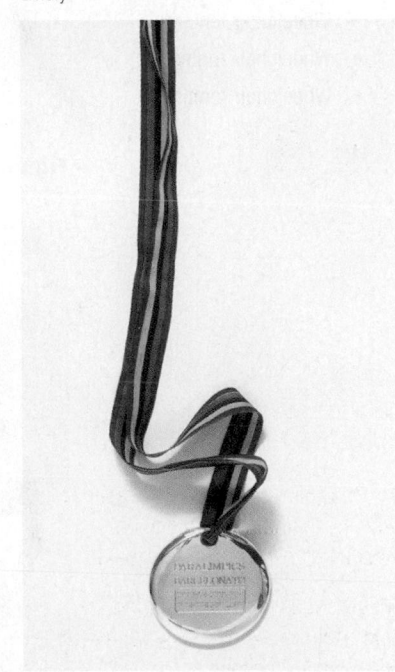

one individual to another (Figure 32-11■). The characteristic facial features, body appearance (including short stature), and pleasant nature of individuals with Down syndrome are typically associated with but not predictive of the degree of intellectual impairment. Because adaptive athletes with Down syndrome are often highly competitive and less likely to complain about an injury or illness, they should be carefully evaluated to avoid dismissing a potentially serious injury. These individuals are at increased risk of musculoskeletal injuries due to lax ligaments, especially the atlanto-axial ligament, which stabilizes $C_1$ relative to $C_2$ in the upper portion of the cervical spine.

# Adaptive Equipment

**Adaptive equipment** enables athletes with a wide range of physical disabilities to participate in outdoor sports. The use of adaptive equipment for winter sports began in Europe, where disabled combat veterans began skiing for rehabilitation and recreation. In 1942, Franz Wendel, a German veteran of World War II and an amputee, made the first outriggers from crutches and short skis. By the late 1940s, the Austrian Ski Association had a program for disabled skiers. In 1968, Arapahoe Basin ski resort in Colorado started a handicapped ski program, which was moved to nearby Winter Park resort in 1970. The U.S. Handicapped Ski Team, predecessor to the U.S. Disabled Ski Team, was organized in 1974.

Originally conceived by Eunice Kennedy Shriver, the first summer Special Olympics was held in Chicago in 1968 and was followed by the first winter Special Olympics in Steamboat Springs, Colorado, in 1977. In 2003, the Special Olympics went worldwide, and it now hosts many events for all disabled athletes.

The Para Olympic Games began in the summer in Rome in 1960, and it was followed by the first Para Olympic Winter Games in 1976 held in Sweden, which hosted athletes from 12 countries. Disabled athletes from all over the globe now participate every two years in various events following the regular Olympic Games. The Salt Lake Paralympic Games of 2002 hosted 416 athletes from 36 nations (Figure 32-12■). The successes of these athletes, combined with improvements in equipment, have made it possible for many disabled recreationalists to engage in a wide variety of outdoor activities. Many North American ski resorts now host events for athletes with disabilities during the summer and the winter. In order to care for these athletes in outdoor environments, OEC Technicians need to become familiar with the most common types of equipment used by adaptive athletes.

## General Equipment

Adaptive athletes can now participate in a variety of activities, including snow skiing and boarding, cycling, water skiing, canoeing/kayaking, sailing, rowing, and various wheelchair events, using specialized equipment (Figure 32-13■). Although generic adaptive sports equipment is available, sometimes the design of this equipment is based on an individual participant's needs (Figure 32-14■). Because OEC Technicians will increasingly encounter adaptive athletes and their equipment, it is important that they have a basic understanding of the types of equipment these individuals use, both for recreation and for the activities of daily living, as well as the types of prosthetics that people with amputations use daily.

An artificial body part that substitutes for a lost body part is a **prosthetic** (Figure 32-15■). Even though prosthetics can replace any body part, from a heart valve to a leg, only musculoskeletal parts are considered in this chapter. A below-the-knee amputation is known as B/K amputation, whereas an above-the-knee amputation is an A/K amputation. Artificial legs come in many designs (Figure 32-16■) and can have only an ankle joint or both a knee joint and an ankle joint, depending on where the leg was amputated. Some artificial legs are designed for a particular sport. For example, some track athletes use legs that function like springs to run quite fast in some sprinting events. Although arms can be amputated at any level, most artificial arms have a hook-shaped pinching device that enables objects to be grasped and manipulated. Newer artificial arms may have a hand controlled by computer chips that can open and close and look and function very much like a real hand (Figure 32-17■).

Many people use a cane while walking, either to help with balance or to partially unload one leg. By acting as an extension of one arm, a cane aids balance by giving its user a third point of contact with the ground. Although most people hold a cane in the hand on the side opposite the leg with a problem, a cane can be used on the same side

**Figure 32-14** Much of the equipment adaptive athletes use is custom made.
Copyright Andy Crawford/Dorling Kindersley Media Library

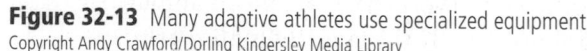

**Figure 32-13** Many adaptive athletes use specialized equipment.
Copyright Andy Crawford/Dorling Kindersley Media Library

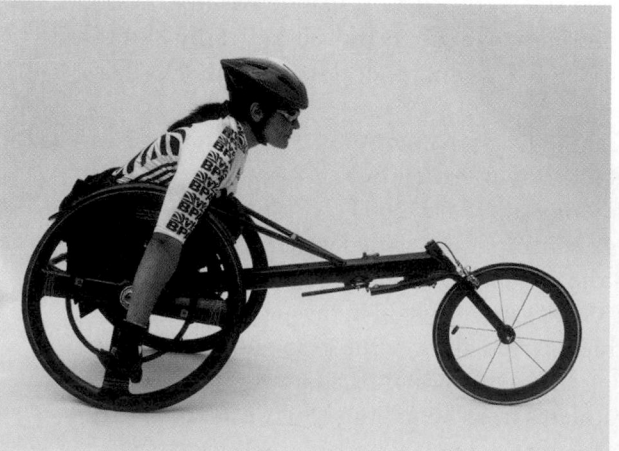

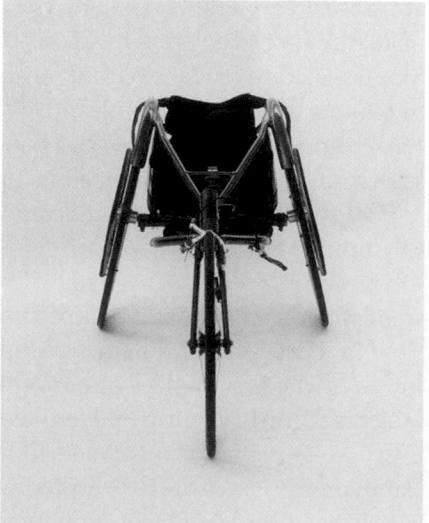

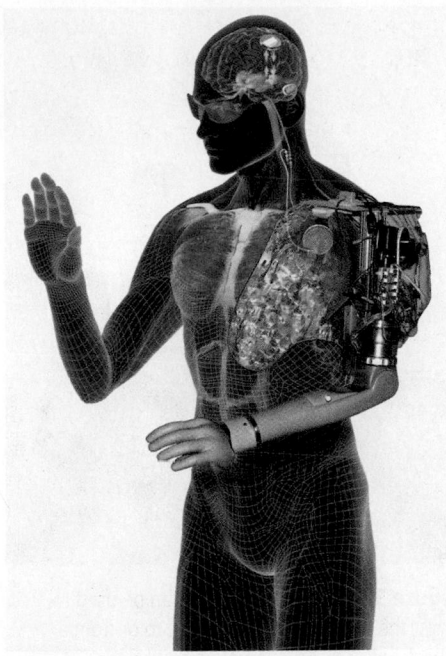

**Figure 32-15** A prosthetic is an artificial body part used as a substitute for a lost body part.
Copyright Dorling Kindersley Media Library

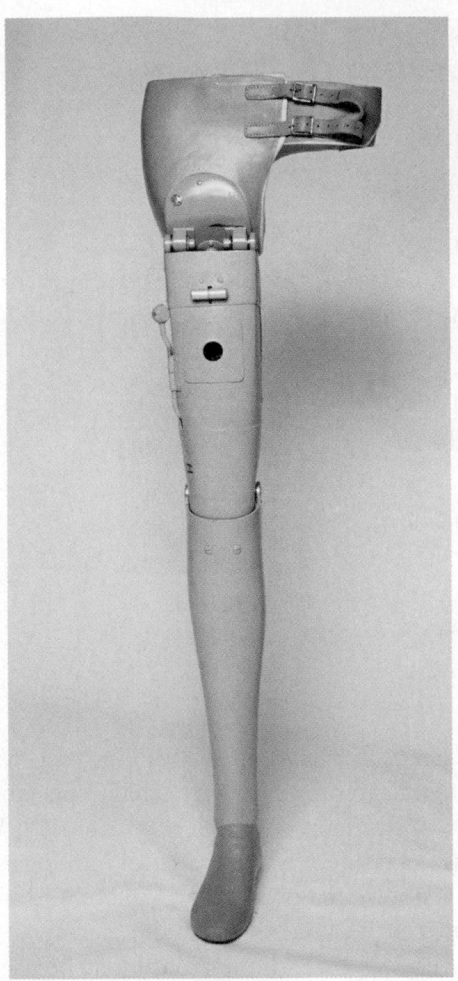

**Figure 32-16** Artificial legs come in many shapes, sizes, and designs.
Copyright Image Source/PunchStock

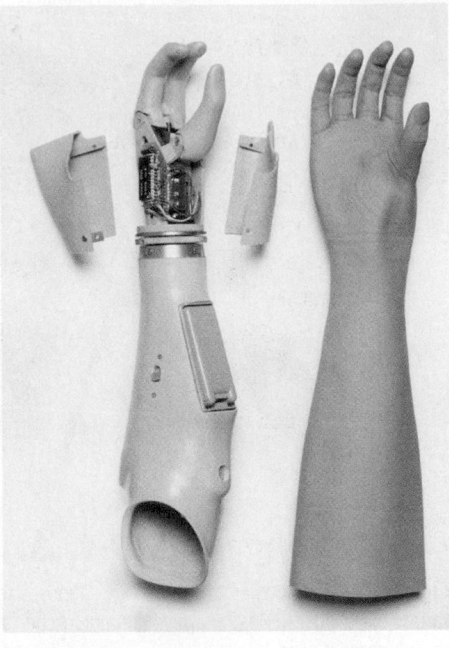

**Figure 32-17** Two types of artificial arms.
Copyright Jane Stockman/Dorling Kindersley Media Library

as the affected leg to allow some weight to be transferred from the leg to the cane. This task is better performed by a crutch, but some individuals prefer a cane over a crutch.

Crutches come in different sizes and designs and are made of different materials, primarily wood or lightweight aluminum. Standard crutches transfer some body weight to the armpits, but most of the body's weight is borne by the hands and wrists and transferred to the shoulders. Thus to use crutches effectively, a person must have sufficient upper body strength. The use of two standard crutches either takes all the body's weight off of one leg or enables a part of the body's weight to be applied to one or both legs. Use of a single crutch on the same side as an injured leg takes some of the body's weight off that leg.

Other types of crutches, including the Canadian and Lofstrand crutches, are made of aluminum or another lightweight metal and are designed to transfer body weight from the hands/wrists to the shoulders only (Figure 32-18■). There is no weight transferred to the armpits. The forearm part of the crutch aids balance. Most adaptive sport crutches are modifications of these crutches.

The primary modes of transportation for those who cannot walk are wheelchairs, which come in many designs and have countless features to meet a person's individual needs. They may be self-propelled, pushed by another person, or powered by an onboard battery system. Many come with removable sides or leg extensions that ease transfers to and from the chair. Some come with a padded seat, whereas others have

**prosthetic** an artificial body part that substitutes for a missing human body part.

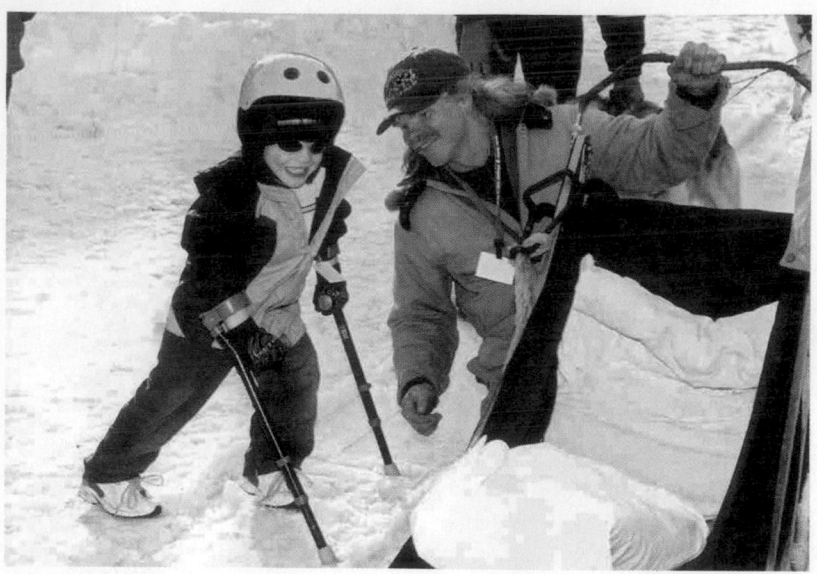

**Figure 32-18** Crutches come in many shapes, sizes, and materials and are used for a variety of purposes. Most adaptive sports crutches are modified versions of the crutches shown here.

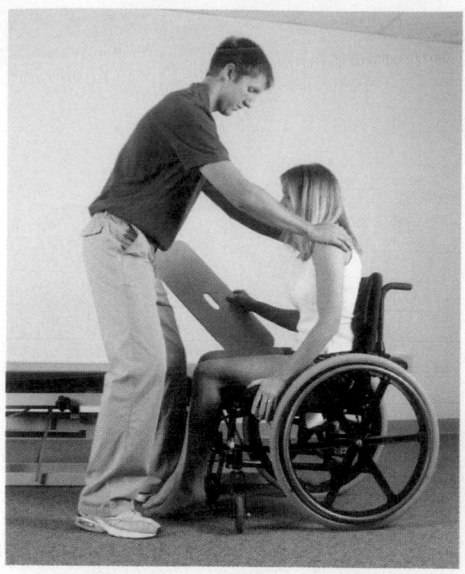

**Figure 32-19** A sliding board can be used to assist the transfer of an individual to or from a wheelchair.

a bucket seat to aid upper body posture. Wheelchairs designed especially for sports are smaller, more lightweight, have specialized wheels, and are built for the unique needs of the sport in which they are used. With the exception of motorized wheelchairs, all modern wheelchairs fold up for easy transport in a vehicle.

A smooth, flat board approximately 12 inches wide and 3 feet long called a **sliding board** may be used to assist the transfer of an individual from or to a wheelchair (Figure 32-19■). A sliding board may be used by the disabled person alone, or others may use one to slide the person after performing a "total lift" when the disabled person cannot assist in the transfer.

Individuals with little or no leg muscle function may opt to use a sling device to move their leg while sitting. With this device, the person places a loop around the foot and, keeping the leg straight, uses the arms to move the leg to the desired position.

**sliding board** a flat board, 12 inches by 36 inches, made of smooth wood or plastic, used to transfer someone to or from a wheelchair.

## Snow Sports Equipment

Technological improvements in many different types of equipment have made virtually any winter sport or activity accessible to adaptive athletes. The specific equipment used depends on each athlete's physical and mental capacities and specific needs. Some adaptive skiers can participate without an assistant, whereas others may need one or two helpers (Figure 32-20■). Some adaptive equipment requires little or no assistance to use, while other devices are completely controlled by helpers. OEC Technicians need to become familiar with the use of such equipment, including getting users into and out of the devices, and to know how to remove a person from a chairlift using specialized adaptive equipment.

Adaptive alpine skiers can be categorized into four major groups: sit-down skiers (who use a mono-ski, a bi-ski, or a sit-ski), three-track and four-track skiers, blind guided skiers, and two-track or stand-up skiers. Individuals of each group use unique equipment. Other adaptive snow sports riders may use snow bikes and sitting snow boards. Important aids used in conjunction with major snow sport equipment include tethers and outriggers.

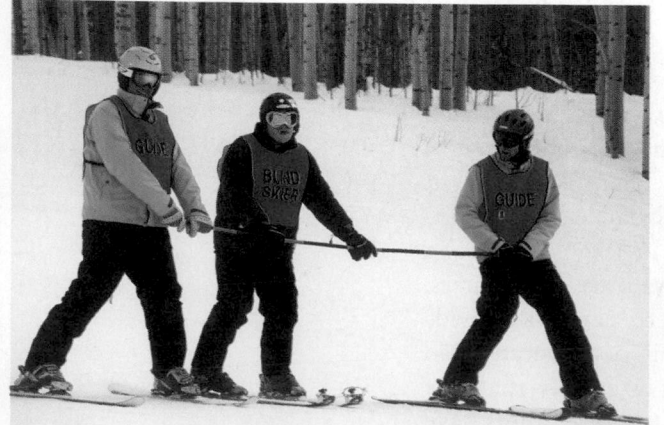

**Figure 32-20** This adaptive skier is being aided by two helpers.
Copyright Pat Pielsticker Bittle

A **tether** is a strap (or pair of straps) that is attached either to the sit-down device or to the skier's waist and is held by a helper skier, who both guides the adaptive skier and prevents the buildup of too much speed (Figure 32-21■). An **outrigger** is essentially a lightweight metal Lofstrand crutch that is attached to a small ski and used to aid a stand-up or sit-down skier in balancing and steering (Figure 32-22■). Currently available commercial outriggers come with hinged skis that can be folded upward to convert the outrigger into a crutch.

A **sit-ski**, which allows a person to ski in a seated position, consists of a **"bucket"** or seat on which the athlete sits plus one or two skis attached to the bucket (Figure 32-23■). The adaptive skier's feet are strapped into extensions of the frame to which the bucket is attached, and the skier turns the sit-ski by moving the head, the shoulders, or hand held outriggers. A sit-ski with two skis, called a **bi-ski**, can be skied independently or skied using stabilizing outriggers and/or a tether controlled by an assistant. The presence of two skis provides a relatively stable platform, so many beginning adaptive skiers use a bi-ski first. A **mono-ski**, which has only one ski under the bucket, is more difficult to use than a bi-ski but is easier to turn for expert adaptive skiers. Sit-skis include a mechanism to raise or lower the bucket for getting onto a chairlift. Since the advent of snowboards, some adaptive athletes are now attaching a "board" to their bucket, producing a **sit-board**.

Every time an adaptive athlete in a sit-ski gets onto a chairlift, someone must attach a safety strap to the back of the chair (Figures 32-24a–b■). The strap, which prevents the adaptive athlete from falling out of the chairlift, is necessary because the

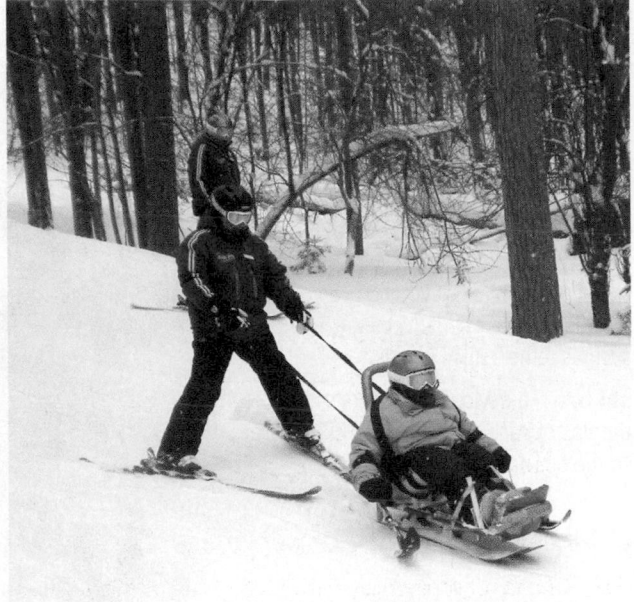

**Figure 32-21** A helper using a tether to aid an adaptive skier.
Copyright David Johe

**tether** a strap (or pair of straps) that is attached to an adaptive skier's waist or to a sit-ski to guide the skier and prevent excessive speed.

**outriggers** short skis mounted on crutch-type ski poles that provide better balance for a disabled skier.

**sit-ski** a device consisting of two basic components: a "bucket" or seat on which the adaptive athlete sits, and one or two skis attached to the bucket.

**bucket** the seat of a sit-ski, which may have one or two skis mounted to the base of the seat.

**bi-ski** a sit-ski with two skis attached to the bottom of the device.

**mono-ski** a sit-ski with one ski attached to the bottom of the device.

**sit-board** a device in which a bucket used for sitting is attached to a snowboard.

**Figure 32-23** A sit-ski.
Copyright Craig Brown

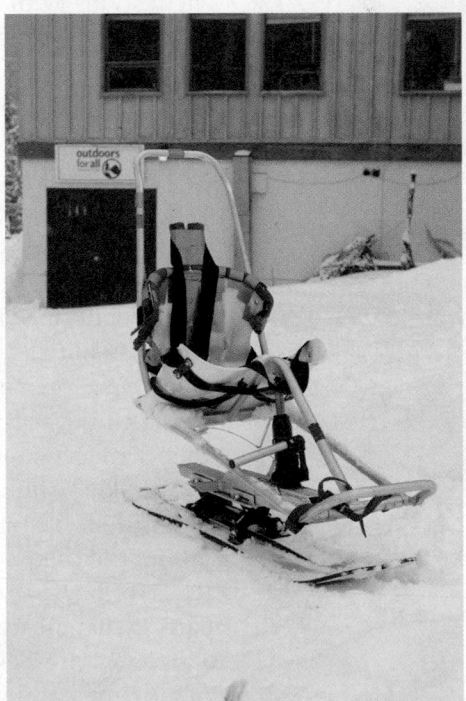

**Figure 32-22** An outrigger.
Copyright David Johe

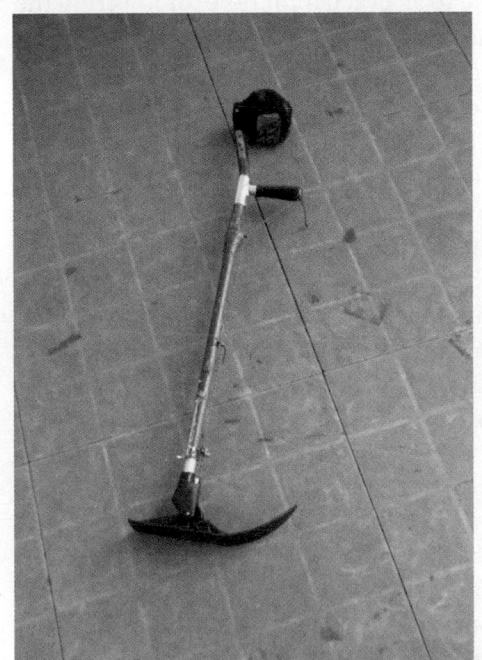

**three tracker** a skier with one leg who uses one ski and outriggers on both arms.

**four tracker** a skier with two legs (one or both of which may be a prosthetic) who also uses two outriggers.

**two track skiing** the use of two skis only by an adaptive skier; can include the use of adaptive equipment such as tethers and ski bras.

**ski bra** a device that attaches near the tips of each ski to hold the skis apart so the tips cannot cross.

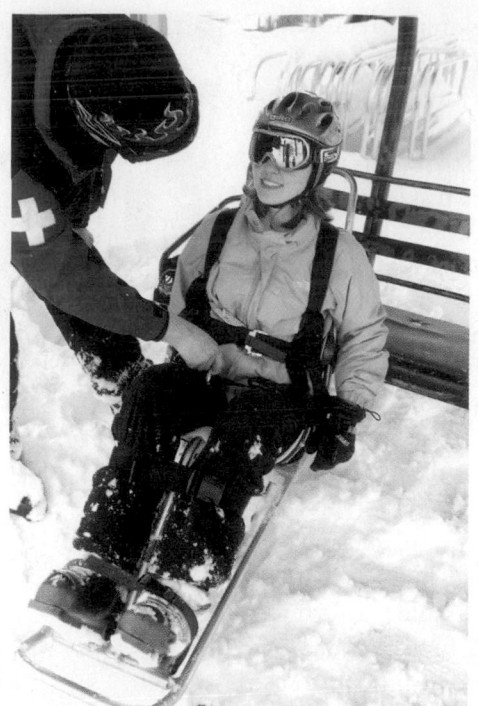

**Figure 32-24a** A safety strap must be attached to the back of the chair when loading a sit-ski. This OEC Technician is helping to load this woman using a sit-ski onto a chairlift.
Copyright Craig Brown

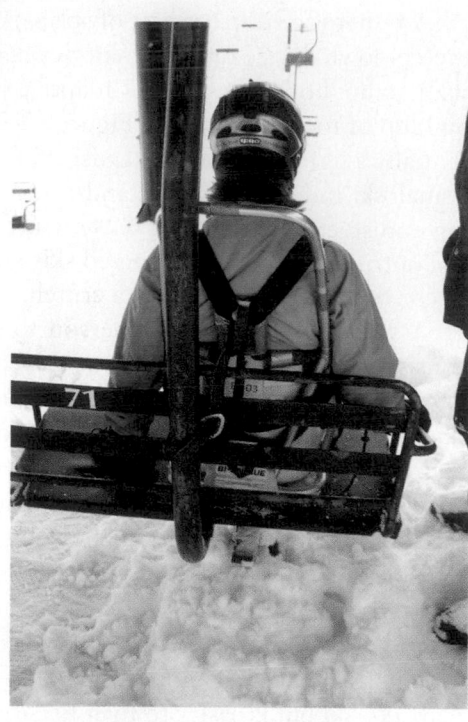

**Figure 32-24b** The OEC Technician has attached the safety strap to the back of the chair.
Copyright Craig Brown

**Figure 32-25** This adaptive athlete is enjoying three-track skiing.
Copyright Tom Stillo

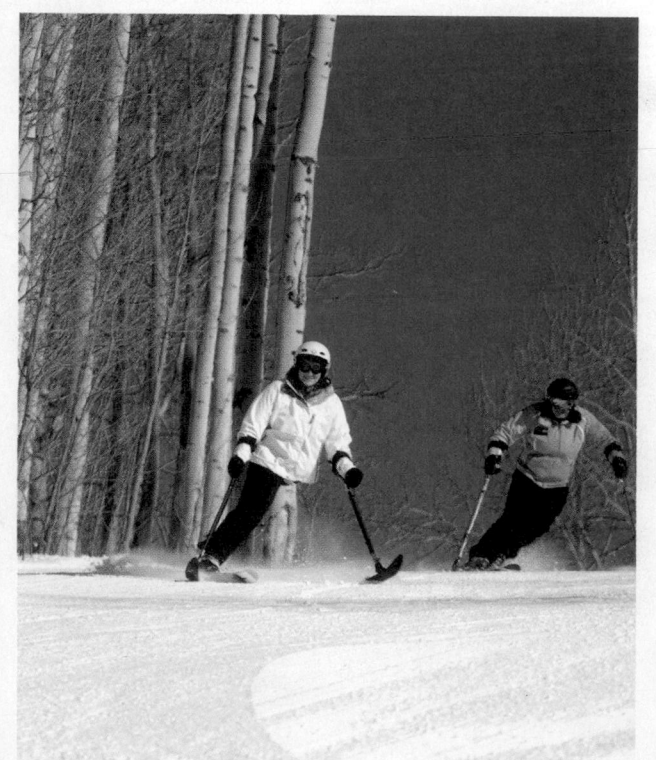

safety bar may not fully close due to the size of the seat or the sit-ski's bucket. Additionally, each sit-ski comes with evacuation straps, which generally are placed between the person's legs and one on either side of the bucket, plus "hooks" (specially placed for balance) where these straps attach. These straps form a mechanically advantageous triangular construct that can be attached to an evacuation rope for lowering the sit-ski from the lift to the ground, should evacuation be needed. OEC Technicians manage a sit-board in a similar way.

Adaptive athletes who can stand and balance themselves typically use either the two-track, three-track, or four-track method of skiing. **Three trackers** use two outriggers plus one ski, whereas **four trackers** use two outriggers plus two skis, one or both of which may be attached to artificial legs. These skiers are fairly independent once they have learned to use the equipment, but some may initially require a tether. A person with one leg may three-track, leaving the artificial leg off (Figure 32-25■), or four-track with the artificial leg in place. Athletes with leg problems other than an amputation may also four-track.

Any skier who can stand and maintain balance while in motion without outriggers can engage in **two track skiing**, with or without the aid of tethers or ski bras. A **ski bra** is a device that attaches to the front of each ski and holds the skis a fixed distance apart, so that the tips do not cross. Two-track skiing is best suited to athletes with developmental and cognitive disabilities, visual impairment, or hearing impairment.

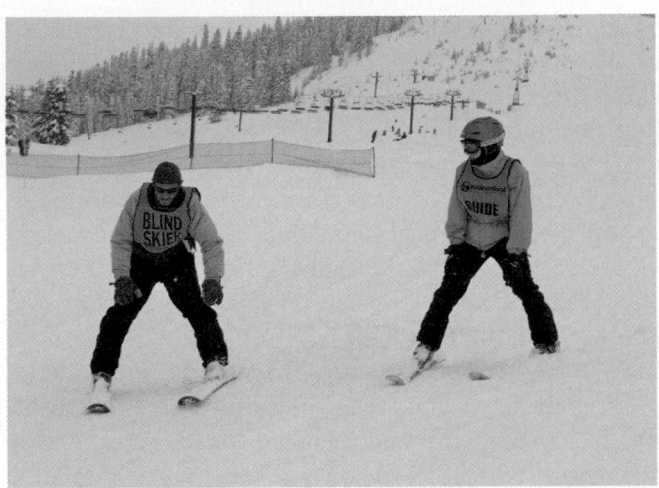

**Figure 32-26** This assistant to a blind skier is monitoring his movements and providing oral directions.
Copyright Craig Brown

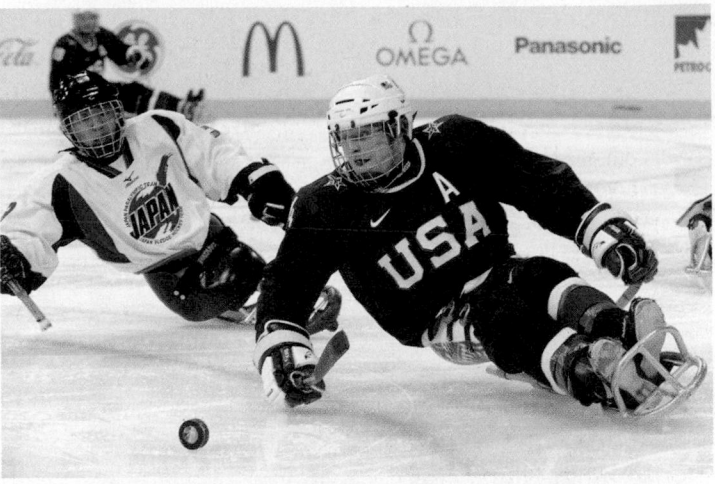

**Figure 32-27** Sled or sledge hockey enables adaptive athletes to play ice hockey.
Copyright Richard Lam Photography

Blind skiers always require an assistant who constantly monitors their movements and provides oral "directions" (Figure 32-26■). These skiers may be on a loose tether, especially when learning.

One of the simplest ways an adaptive athlete can participate in winter sports is to use a snow-slider. This device, similar to a walker, allows the athlete to stand on skis and to move forward on a flat surface by sliding one ski in front of the other, usually with the help of an assistant.

Some adaptive athletes use snow-bikes, which are tricycle-like devices that have skis instead of wheels. They are best used on relatively flat surfaces but may be used on slopes by experienced athletes.

Sledge hockey, or sled hockey as it is called in the United States, is a sport that enables adaptive athletes to play a slightly modified version of ice hockey while sitting in a sled that has two large parallel skate blades under it (Figure 32-27■). The athletes propel themselves around an ice rink using a pair of special hockey sticks, each of which has a standard blade on one end for handling the puck and small "picks" on the other end for propelling the sled. An inline skate version of this sport has recently been developed to allow the same game to be played off the ice, using two rows of inline wheels under the bucket seat.

Ski lifts are required to reasonably accommodate adaptive skiers (Figure 32-28■). Gondolas, trams, and chair lifts must be designed for this purpose. Gondolas and trams must have doors wide enough to accommodate disabled athletes. Chair lifts should be accompanied by a sign that indicates how high the lift's seat is, so adaptive athletes can adjust the heights of their buckets to get on the lift. These guidelines are set by the Americans with Disabilities Act.

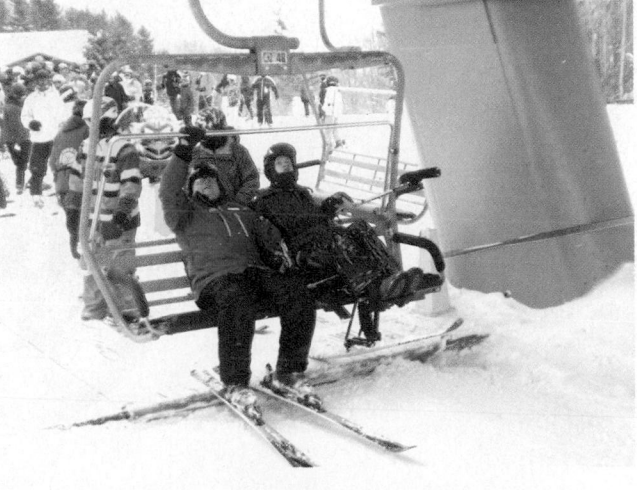

**Figure 32-28** Ski lifts are required to reasonably accommodate adaptive skiers.
Copyright David Johe

## Warm Weather Sports Equipment

Many different types of equipment are available to assist adaptive athletes who wish to participate in a variety of warm weather sports, including water sports, cycling, horseback riding, basketball, hiking, running, and climbing.

Every athlete who participates in any water sport should wear a properly fitting Coast Guard–approved buoyancy device

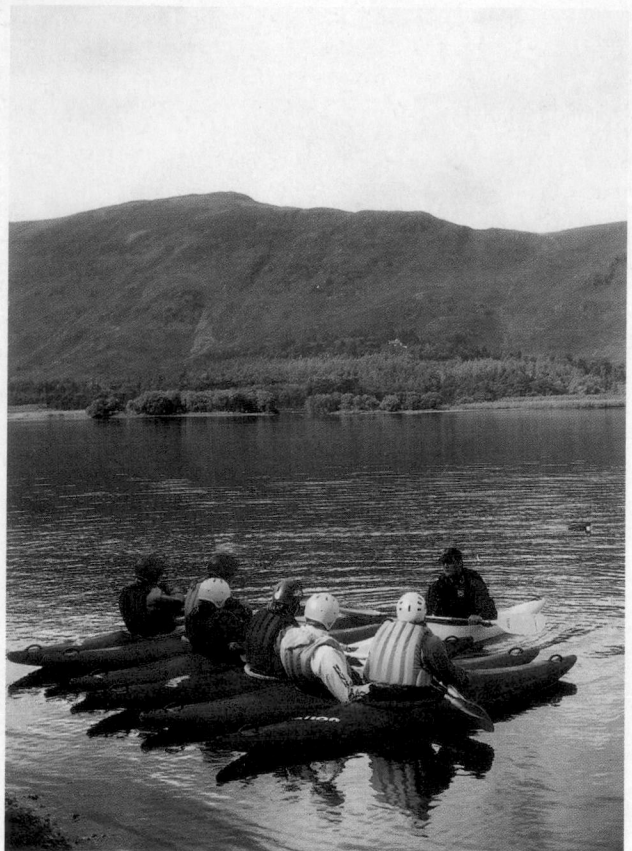

**Figure 32-29** Kayakers in safety gear listening to their guide.
Copyright Kim Sayer/Dorling Kindersley Media Library

(life jacket) (Figure 32-29■). Many paraplegics are accomplished swimmers who use only their arms for propulsion. Adaptive sailors who have little or no mobility can use specialized seats and rigging and "puff technology," which enables even quadriplegic sailors to use their mouths to "puff" or "suck" on tubes to activate computerized motors that control the rudder and sails. Canoeing and kayaking can be accomplished using specialized seats, paddles, backrests, and pontoons for stability. Water skiing, too, can be done with sit-down water skis, special booms and ropes, twin skis, and other devices.

Cycling is a highly popular sport among adaptive athletes, and many different types and styles of adaptive bikes are available. Tandem, recumbent, and hand-powered bikes enable nearly anyone with a disability to power a cycle. Special "trident" cycles enable many participants with balance problems to ride in comfort and with confidence. Other adaptive features include special seats, gearing, pedals, and controls (Figure 32-30■).

Adaptive horseback riders can choose among many different types of saddles, bridles, bits, and arena "toys" for use in specialized riding programs. Wheel-chair basketball is very popular today and features special competition chairs that are easy to maneuver. A variety of adaptive equipment is also available for adaptive hikers and climbers.

The equipment and prosthetic devices adaptive athletes use in all these activities are typically expensive, and they are so carefully custom fitted to each athlete that the athletes consider them extensions of their bodies. Accordingly, OEC Technicians should take special care in handling and transporting the equipment of ill or injured adaptive athletes. When caring for each of these patients, keep their equipment nearby and ensure that it is transported with the athlete.

**Figure 32-30** A cycle can be modified to provide a special seat, gearing, pedals, and controls suitable for adaptive athletes.
Copyright Andy Crawford/Dorling Kindersley Media Library

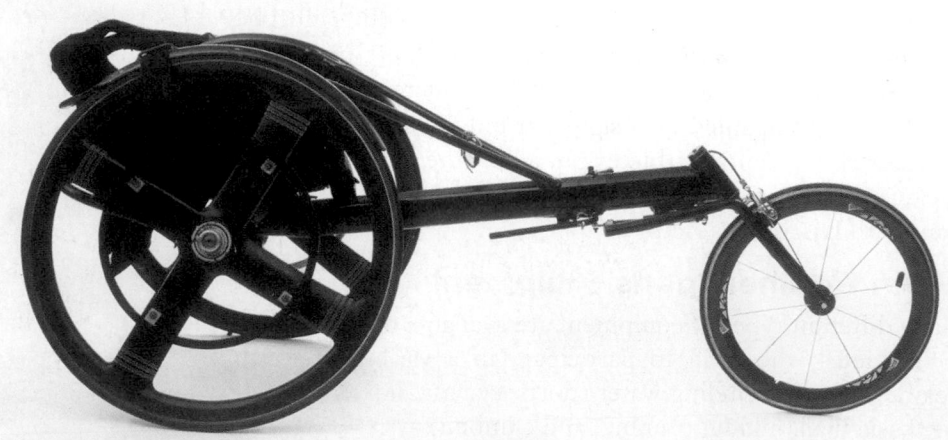

# STOP, THINK, UNDERSTAND

## Multiple Choice

Choose the correct answer.

1. Which of the following statements about adaptive equipment is false? _____
   a. Most adaptive equipment is very expensive.
   b. Many adaptive athletes consider their equipment an extension of themselves.
   c. By law, ski lifts must be able to accommodate adaptive athletes and their equipment.
   d. Adaptive equipment is generally very durable, so little or no harm will come to it if it must be tossed aside during a rescue operation.

2. The reason a patient with Down syndrome might become combative shortly after taking a fall while ice skating most likely relates to_____
   a. the nature of athletes with Down syndrome.
   b. a possible TBI.
   c. autonomic dysreflexia.
   d. the patient's frustration over not being able to communicate with rescuers.

3. Which of the following statements about individuals with Down syndrome are true? (check all that apply)
   _____ a. Individuals with Down syndrome typically exhibit anger and out-of-control behavior when stressed.
   _____ b. Athletes with Down syndrome are often highly competitive and less likely to complain about an injury.
   _____ c. A laxity of ligaments can increase the chances of musculoskeletal injury in athletes with Down syndrome.
   _____ d. An athlete with Down syndrome is less likely to suffer a cervical spine injury than are other athletes.
   _____ e. Patients with Down syndrome exhibit extremely obvious clinical signs when injured.

## Fill in the Blank

1. Individuals who have suffered a brain injury and can no longer live on their own or take care of themselves are said to have a/an_____.

2. An opening created surgically on the abdominal wall for excretion of urine is called a/an_____.

3. A progressive, neurological syndrome that causes weakness, paralysis of the extremities, and visual deficits is _____.

4. A sit-ski with two skis mounted to the base of the seat is a/an _____.

5. An impairment of information processing that makes learning new information difficult is_____.

6. A collection device that adheres to the abdominal wall and used to collect urine or feces is a/an _____.

7. Loss of all or part of an extremity from trauma or surgery is _____.

8. A condition occurring at or near the time of birth that results in loss of muscle control, making walking or balancing difficult, is _____.

9. A potentially deadly condition that is associated with spinal cord injury patients that starts with a dangerously high blood pressure is _____.

10. A genetic syndrome that causes progressive muscle degeneration is_____.

11. Any condition that impairs normal physical or intellectual function is a/an _____.

12. A congenital deformity that exposes the spinal cord because part of the posterior bony spine is absent is _____.

13. _____ CP causes slow, writhing muscle contractions.

## Short Answer

1. What is the ADA of 1990, and what is its purpose?

   _____
   _____
   _____
   _____

*continued*

STOP, THINK, UNDERSTAND *continued*

2. What is "puff technology?"

_____

_____

_____

_____

# CASE UPDATE

The adaptive athlete has remained sitting on the snow while you've established that her ABCDs appear to be intact. You've already introduced yourself to her and told her what you're doing. During your assessment of the patient the chaperone listed the patient's medications and described her known seizure disorder. As another patroller arrives with a fully loaded toboggan, the patient begins to have a tonic-clonic seizure.

You rapidly move behind the patient to stabilize her head and neck as you roll her into a recovery position to protect her airway should she vomit. Your partner immediately comes to the patient's side and provides oxygen via a nonrebreather mask. You consider a head injury or a new illness as possible causes for the current seizure. The patient's seizure activity stops spontaneously after about a minute.

**What should you do now?**

---

⊕ **32-7** Describe and demonstrate how to assess an adaptive athlete.

⊕ **32-8** Describe and demonstrate how to care for an adaptive athlete who is injured or ill.

**Figure 32-31** OEC Technicians can be presented with unique challenges when dealing with an injured adaptive athlete. Copyright Greg Bala

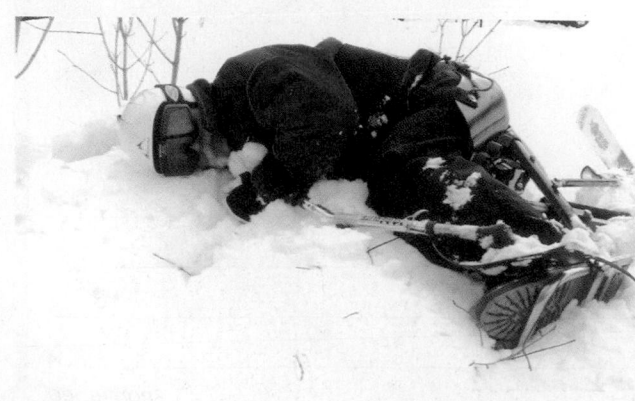

# Assessment

The evaluation of trauma or illness in adaptive athletes may present OEC Technicians with unique challenges (Figure 32-31■). Communicating with patients and understanding their needs may be difficult. The physical exam might require modification or special considerations for unique injuries. The principles of a good assessment, however, apply to all adaptive athletes, whether their disability is intellectual or physical. Respect for the patient and common sense are an OEC Technician's best guideposts for performing a useful and accurate evaluation.

The principles of assessing adaptive athletes are essentially the same as for any other patient: they begin with a scene size-up and are followed by a primary assessment and the correction of any ABCD-related problems. Because some patients are allergic to natural latex rubber, OEC Technicians should use latex-free disposable gloves and equipment, whenever possible.

As indicated in Chapter 8, Medical Communications and Documentation, good communication provides the basis for understanding and is one of the hallmarks of a highly trained rescuer. When interacting with an adaptive athlete, good communication is even more essential. Start every encounter with an adaptive athlete as you would any other assessment, using the following basics of effective communication:

- Introduce yourself as rescuer patroller or OEC Technician, using your first name and title. Do not assume that the patient knows your role or can read your name badge.

- Ask if you can offer assistance, and ask specifically how you can help. If the adaptive athlete is unable to provide this information, ask the athlete's guide or companion how you can best provide assistance.

- Consider the level of stress that injured or ill adaptive athletes are experiencing. Pain from an injury or anxiety caused by being separated from a skiing guide may reduce their ability to communicate with you.

- Speak directly to adaptive athletes, using a clear voice and calm demeanor.

- Use the responses of adaptive athletes and their companion to guide your assessment and management.

- Speak to the adaptive athlete, and not to the athlete's disability. Refer to the person by name, not by condition. Do not say, "I'm going to help the kid with Down's."

- Appreciate that you may not be familiar with the impairments of an adaptive athlete, and that the encounter may be stressful for you as a rescuer.

- Communicate with the patient's companion, relative, or caregiver because they may have important information that guides your care.

Effective communication includes addressing the patient at an appropriate level for eye contact, as when kneeling to speak with a wheelchair or sit-ski athlete. OEC Technicians can gain the confidence of injured or ill adaptive athletes if they ask how they can help, and how best to care for them and their equipment (Figure 32-32■).

Begin the secondary assessment by obtaining a medical history using SAMPLE and OPQRST (if applicable). If necessary, ask the patient's guide or companion for information such as the individual's "baseline" mental status. A new headache or a change in responsiveness should alert a rescuer to the possibilities of a closed head injury or the development of autonomic dysreflexia. Some adaptive athletes take multiple medications, and medical conditions such as seizure disorders are associated with certain physical disabilities.

Perform a physical exam using DCAP-BTLS. As you perform the physical exam, be sure to explain in detail what you are doing, to help reduce the patient's anxieties. Patients who lack sensation due to central or peripheral nerve damage may not be aware of traumatic or cold/heat-induced injuries. A thorough physical exam is a crucial part of the assessment, but it should not outweigh the risks of prolonging the patient's exposure to cold or hot temperatures. Obtain a complete set of vital signs, repeating at regular intervals as needed.

## Assessing Athletes with Intellectual Disabilities

Impairments caused by intellectual disabilities are likely to affect communication between an adaptive athlete and OEC Technicians to some degree. A severe disability, for example, may mean that an OEC Technician must rely on the athlete's guide to answer history-related questions and provide valuable information regarding assessment findings (e.g., what is normal, and what is abnormal). Intellectual disabilities may slow an adaptive athlete's ability to respond to questions or appreciate the importance of scene safety, including the need to move quickly to a safer location. Withdrawing from an OEC Technician or telling a family member the answer to your questions may be part of a patient's normal reaction to fear, pain, or an unfamiliar face.

**32-4** Describe four elements of effective communication with a person who has an intellectual disability.

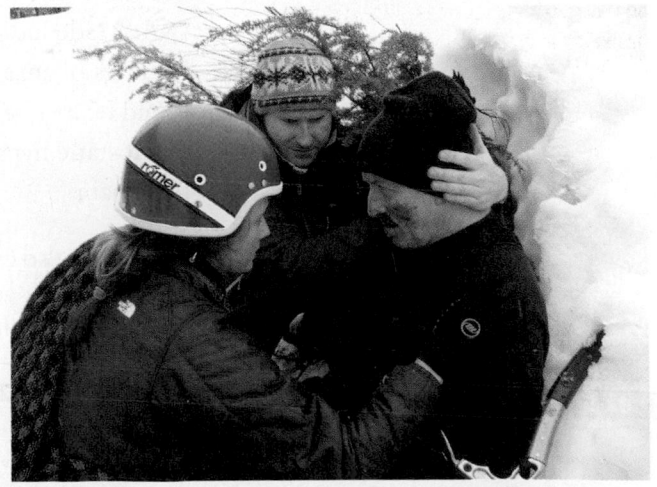

**Figure 32-32** Good communication when assessing adaptive patients includes making appropriate eye contact.
Copyright Brigitte Schran Brown

Avoid using phrases that have more than one meaning, such as "knock it off." Because open-ended questions may be too difficult for an intellectually impaired adaptive athlete to understand in a stressful situation, ask questions that can be answered yes or no. Avoid frightening patients by making sudden movements or by speaking in a loud voice. On-scene stimuli, such as noise from snowmaking equipment, may distract patients. Establishing personal space boundaries or understanding the need for a physical exam may be very difficult and stressful for adaptive athletes with an intellectual disability. Certain disabilities are associated with behaviors or clues that rescuers can use to perform the best possible assessment.

Adaptive athletes with learning disorders or cognitive disabilities may not be able to process questions normally, or understand what you are doing. Mental illness may cause a personality or behavior change that impairs an adaptive athlete's ability to follow instructions.

Remaining calm is essential in helping an adaptive athlete with an intellectual disability. Asking direct, clear questions is reassuring and helps you gain insight during your assessment. Using simple, one-step directions and visual examples of what you intend to do can make the encounter less stressful for the patient. Take full advantage of the skiing guide or relative to learn about your patient and how you can provide the best care.

Direct other rescue team members to manage any distractions in and around the scene. Once personal boundaries have been established, ask the patient if you can check for medical alert jewelry or ID as part of the physical exam. Assume that any impairment in mental status could be the result of a new injury or illness, or that an established intellectual disability may mask an emergent condition.

The calm, easy-going manner of adaptive athletes with Down syndrome can be deceiving; because they tend to minimize pain or complaints, they may have a serious injury that could be overlooked without a careful exam. Additionally, loose ligaments in the upper cervical spine or apparent joint instability should prompt rescuers to carefully reevaluate the mechanism of injury and related physical findings.

Adaptive athletes with autism spectrum disorder also tend to minimize complaints of pain. Because ASD is by definition a disability of communication, these patients may appear to ignore questions or repeat what you have said. They may avoid eye contact or attempt to move away from you. Using simple, concrete phrases can help direct the assessment.

Patients with autonomic dysfunction present with a wide range of signs and symptoms, including one or more of the following:

- Excessive fatigue
- Excessive thirst (polydipsia)
- Lightheadedness, dizziness, or vertigo
- Feelings of anxiety or panic (not mentally induced)
- Rapid heart rate or slow heart rate
- Orthostatic hypotension, sometimes resulting in syncope
- Joint pain

They may also experience headaches, pallor, malaise, facial flushing, constipation, diarrhea, nausea, acid reflux, visual disturbances, numbness, nerve pain, trouble breathing, chest pains, and (in some cases) loss of responsiveness and seizures.

## Assessing Adaptive Athletes with Physical Disabilities

⊕ **32-5** Describe how to assess and care for physically disabled athletes.

Communicating with adaptive athletes who have physical impairments may also challenge OEC Technicians, particularly if the athlete has a sensory disability. Blind or deaf athletes require rescuers to modify the type or style of communication used in assessment and treatment, but not the basic content. Courtesy and professionalism allow the rescuer to make the best assessment possible.

Hearing-impaired patients often rely on lip reading. Because of this, OEC Technicians should directly face patients and speak slowly. Remove face coverings to make lip reading easier. Written communication is preferred by some deaf athletes and is especially useful when asking for contact information. Visually impaired athletes require more assistance with orientation, especially in unfamiliar settings. Verbal cues from OEC Technicians can be used to reassure patients that the scene is safe or to establish the role and identity of rescuers. As always, ask the patient how you can help. Ask if you can touch the patient (and let them know how and where you will do that) before beginning your exam or treatment.

Adaptive athletes with amputations, spinal cord trauma or impairment, or peripheral neurological conditions generally communicate as any other individual would, but their level of anxiety may be higher.

Disabilities from stroke or traumatic brain injury (TBI) often cause specific motor and/or sensory deficits. Signs such as muscle wasting (the weakening, shrinking, or loss of muscle mass) or flexor tendon contractures (which can cause permanent contortion of a joint or limb) may be evident in patients with preexisting brain injuries. These conditions can make assessment more difficult but should alert OEC Technicians to extremities that are at a higher risk for injury. Another manifestation of TBI may be **expressive aphasia**, which is a limited ability to speak or respond to questions. It may be difficult to establish whether a patient with a TBI has a preexisting intellectual disability or altered mental status as a result of a new injury. A relative or caretaker may be able to help you determine if something new has happened in regard to the patient's mental status.

Occasionally, the mechanism of injury involves the patient's adaptive equipment (Figure 32-33■). Falls while using outriggers or bucket seats tend to cause more injuries to the upper extremities. Extremities can also be injured at the site of amputation by a prosthetic limb.

Ostomy bags and tubing should be examined for damage or associated bleeding from the **stoma** site. The adhesive tape securing the bag to the stoma site can be pulled loose. Tubing can become blocked during extrication or when packaging the patient for transport. Observe Standard Precautions at all times when inspecting or handling a collection bag or inspecting an ostomy site.

# Management

As for the management of any injury or illness, the need to evacuate a disabled patient must be weighed against the time required for reassessments during transport. A rescuer may need to prioritize transportation over serial evaluations, except as needed to ensure that a patient's ABCDs and mental status are stable.

Calling for additional assistance when starting an encounter with an adaptive athlete is often indicated. A rescuer may need additional help with crowd or traffic control, or a patient's equipment may necessitate more lifting in preparation for transport. Adaptive equipment may need to be transported alongside the patient. Finally, calling ahead alerts clinical staff that a patient with special needs is en route and may allow time for notification of group leaders or family members who can assist in caring for the adaptive athlete.

**expressive aphasia**   the inability to express speech normally.

**stoma**   a surgical port created in the body.

---

⊕ **32-9** Describe and demonstrate how to manage an above-the-knee amputee with a femur fracture of the same leg.

**Figure 32-33** The adaptive equipment in use at your ski area can be a part of the MOI.
Copyright Kari Taylor

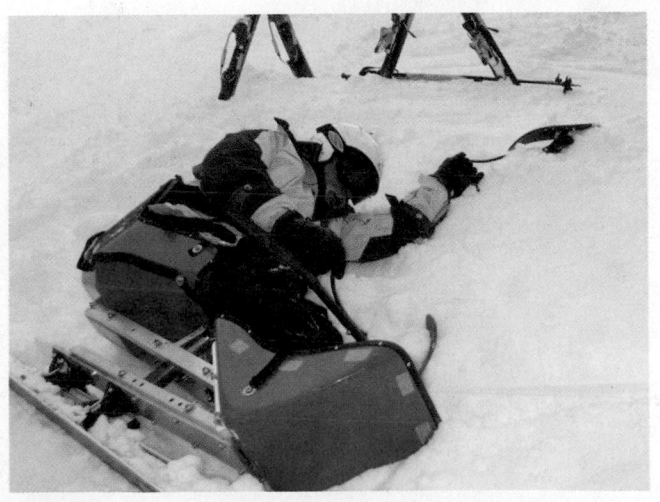

Using clear and concise communication when managing an adaptive athlete's injuries is an OEC Technician's greatest asset. Demonstrating what you need to do next is a powerful way to communicate your intentions and may relieve anxiety and build confidence in your care. Rescuers should expect that some athletes will have unpredictable reactions to treatment. A patient with an intellectual disability, for example, may panic when wrapped in the weather-proof tarp of a toboggan.

Stabilization of injuries in amputees often means splinting in a position of comfort. Using traction for a mid-shaft femur fracture in a below-the-knee amputee is not practical in outdoor environments. In general, immobilize above and below a fracture or dislocation, using a quick splint if possible. Use extra padding to avoid pressure on areas without sensation, whether those areas are close to the injury or not. Also, do not put pressure on an ostomy bag. Modify splints and strapping if needed, but never force an injured extremity into a rigid splint. Splints may aggravate muscle spasticity in such conditions as cerebral palsy. Offering the patient choices may further reduce anxiety. Providing simple options, such as riding in a toboggan with the head uphill or downhill, may reduce a patient's stress.

Getting a disabled athlete out of specialized equipment requires common sense and ingenuity. For example, if someone in a "bucket seat" with the legs attached to a frame has injured a lower leg, it may be better to leave the patient in the device (which immobilizes the leg) until more help is available (Figure 32-34■). Evaluate the situation and do what is easiest and safest for the patient.

Adaptive equipment and prosthetic limbs often cost thousands of dollars. These items should be transported with or alongside the patient whenever possible. Reassure adaptive athletes that their equipment has been cared for appropriately.

Adaptive athletes may be accompanied by service animals, especially at base areas (Figure 32-35■). Make every effort to maintain the normal relationship between injured adaptive athletes and their service animals, including proximity. Doing so will comfort both the patients and their service animals during an obviously stressful situation.

For injured adaptive athletes who depend on a wheelchair, inquire how to secure their equipment so that you can make it available to them when they are ready to leave an aid station or clinic. Be aware that wheelchairs are typically very expensive. Motorized chairs can be heavy and awkward to transport.

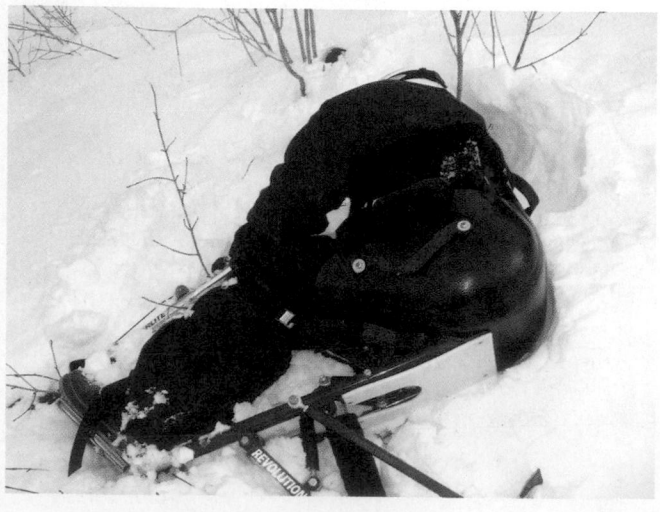

**Figure 32-34** It can be better to leave injured adaptive athletes in their adaptive devices until their arrival at an aid room.
Copyright Greg Bala

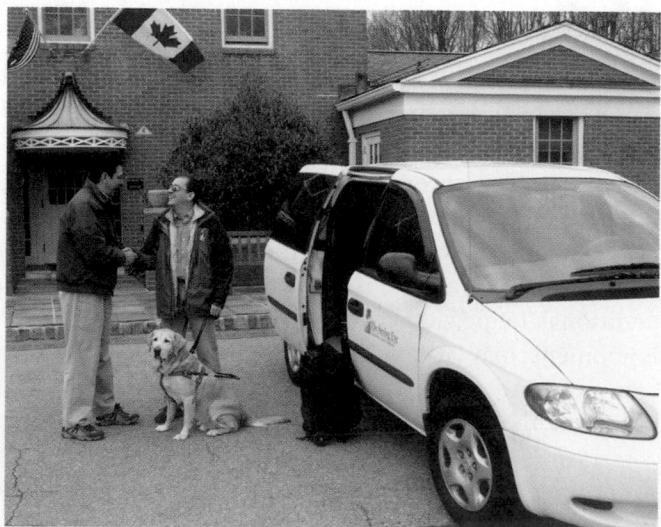

**Figure 32-35** Service animals often accompany adaptive athletes in the base area.

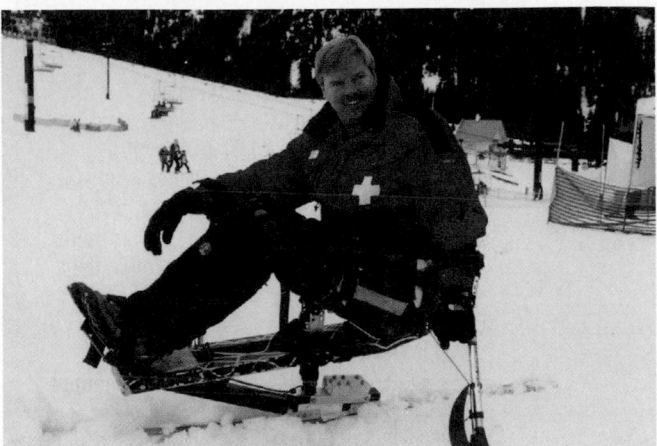

**Figure 32-36a** This adaptive skier has achieved certification as an OEC Technician.
Copyright Brigitte Schran Brown

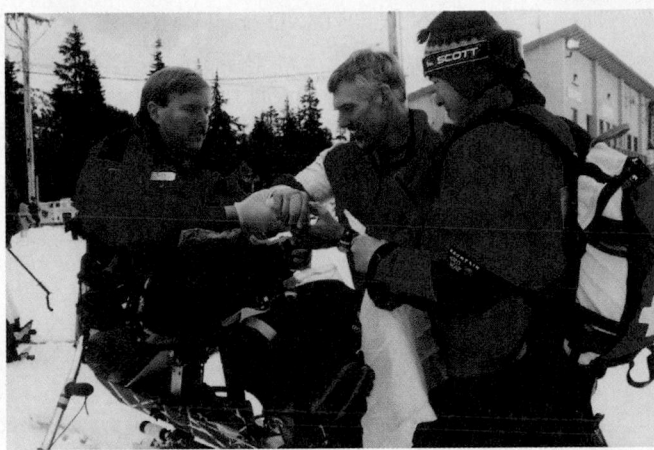

**Figure 32-36b** An adaptive patroller practicing outdoor emergency care on fellow patrollers.
Copyright Brigitte Schran Brown

## Lift Evacuation Considerations

Give adaptive athletes priority when evacuating chairlifts. Athletes with intellectual disabilities may have difficulty tolerating chairlift evacuation delays, whereas athletes with mobility problems have an increased risk of cold and other exposure injuries. Working with the lift evacuation team to ensure that adaptive athletes are evacuated first is standard practice in lift evacuations in most resorts.

Skiers with visual impairments may need additional oral coaching and reassurance during an evacuation, even if they have a guide with them in the same chair. During chair evacuation, OEC Technicians must communicate constantly with blind skiers, because evacuation is more difficult for individuals without sight. Always evacuate a blind skier first, and the blind skier's assistant second. Because blind skiers may be disoriented until their guide or skiing partner can join them on the hill, have someone remain with and talk to them so that they can feel safe. Once a blind skier's assistant is off the lift, that person can help with the skier's care.

The equipment of sit-skiers typically has leash devices and a minimum of three contact points for attachment to an evacuation line. Secure all of the contacts with locking carabiners, and inspect all webbing before the evacuation proceeds. Each ski area must develop its own plan for evacuating skiers from non-surface ski lifts.

## STOP, THINK, UNDERSTAND

### Multiple Choice
Choose the correct answer.

1. Which of the following statements regarding the assessment of an injured adaptive athlete is true? _____
   a. The principles of the exam must be modified to accommodate an adaptive athlete.
   b. OEC Technicians should use latex-free exam gloves because many patients, especially those with spina bifida, are allergic to them.
   c. When examining an adaptive athlete, an OEC Technician should speak more slowly and somewhat more loudly than usual.
   d. OEC Technicians should approach the exam with the assumption that the adaptive athlete will most likely not be able to understand them.

2. Which of the following assumptions should an OEC Technician make concerning a patient with Down syndrome who has a bad headache after a skiing fall, given that the patient's caregiver reports that the patient normally has headaches?_____
   a. This headache could be indicative of a closed head injury.
   b. Given that this adaptive athlete normally gets headaches, this finding is probably insignificant.
   c. Patients with Down syndrome tend to overdramatize their injuries.
   d. An OEC Technician should never assume anything.

*continued*

STOP, THINK, UNDERSTAND *continued*

3. Which of the following assumptions should OEC Technicians make concerning a patient with an intellectual disability who appears drowsy and seems to be ignoring them during the exam?_____

   a. This behavior is normal behavior for a patient with an intellectual or cognitive disability.

   b. The patient is ignoring the OEC Technician because she is growing frustrated over her inability to communicate with the rescuer.

   c. This behavior could be an indication of a serious head or internal injury.

   d. An OEC Technician should never assume anything.

4. Which of the following statements about patients with intellectual disabilities is true? _____

   a. The disability may slow the ability of these patients to respond to your questions.

   b. Many patients with an intellectual disability will not respond to a stranger, so questions should be directed to a caregiver.

   c. It is appropriate to use open-ended questions such as "Tell me where it hurts."

   d. The answers given by an athlete with intellectual disabilities are frequently inaccurate.

5. Which of the following actions are proper components of an assessment of an adaptive athlete? (check all that apply)

   _____ a. Introduce yourself as a ski patroller/OEC Technician using your first name and title.

   _____ b. Ask adaptive athletes to explain specifically how you can help them.

   _____ c. Examine adult adaptive athletes apart from their ski guide or caregiver to maintain their privacy.

   _____ d. Speak directly to the adaptive athlete using a clear voice and a calm demeanor.

   _____ e. Speak directly to the caregiver if the adaptive athlete has a cognitive disability.

   _____ f. Proceed with the exam as you normally would.

6. Which of the following findings are signs or symptoms of patients with autonomic dysfunction? (check all that apply)

   _____ a. excessive fatigue

   _____ b. polydipsia

   _____ c. severe agitation

   _____ d. tachycardia or bradycardia

   _____ e. orthostatic hypotension

   _____ f. joint pain

   _____ g. facial flushing

   _____ h. uncontrollable laughter

   _____ i. chest pain

 # CASE DISPOSITION

Because you suspect that trauma is a factor in this case, you apply a cervical collar while the patient is still on the ski slope. Because she has remained confused and unresponsive to questioning, you and your partner elect to transport her in the toboggan on a long spine board with the cervical collar in place. You maintain high-flow oxygen during transport to the clinic and check the patient's level of alertness several times while your partner steers the toboggan. You've radioed ahead to the clinic about the seizure, so the staff is waiting for your arrival and helps transport the patient into the treatment area. A family member and the chaperone meet the patient at the clinic and describe the patient's gradual return to baseline mental status. You advise hospital follow-up and arrange transport. X-rays of the patient's cervical spine show no evidence of injury, but a CAT scan of her brain shows a small subdural hematoma. Even though the patient had a history of seizures, you made the correct decision to have her evaluated for a new condition, which probably saved her life.

# Chapter Review

## Chapter Summary

Adaptive athletes who have overcome a disability are increasingly participating in outdoor recreational activities, including skiing and snowboarding and patrolling (Figures 32-36a■ and 32-36b■). OEC Technicians must learn and practice the best ways to meet the needs of these athletes when they become injured or ill. Rescuers should convey respect for adaptive athletes and for their disability by using the basics of good communication. Speaking to the athlete instead of speaking to the disability is another way to convey respect. Life-threatening emergencies are no more common among adaptive athletes than among any group of patients, and OEC Technicians must focus on the ABCDs and important clues to potentially critical conditions, including altered mental status and abnormal vital signs. Remaining calm, reassuring the patient, and using additional resources help OEC Technicians provide the best care for all adaptive patients, regardless of their disability.

## Remember...

1. Assume that altered mental status is the result of a new injury or illness.
2. Adaptive athletes with sensory and movement disorders are at higher risk for cold-weather injuries.
3. Ask adaptive athletes how you can assist them. Ask the athlete's skiing guide or chaperone for information and assistance.
4. Describe and demonstrate how you will help an adaptive athlete before doing a procedure.
5. Ask about medications and medical history. Look for medical alert jewelry or other alerts to help identify preexisting medical conditions.
6. Request additional rescuers when caring for athletes with disabilities.
7. Collect an adaptive athlete's equipment, and transport it with the athlete.
8. Paraplegics are at an increased risk for hypothermia and frostbite.
9. Patients with spina bifida are allergic to latex. Always use latex-free gloves when treating these patients to avoid an anaphylactic reaction.

## Chapter Questions

### Multiple Choice

Choose the correct answer.

1. While you are examining a paraplegic skier in a bucket ski who says he was not going very fast when he fell, he suddenly complains of a headache and anxiety. His blood pressure is 170/120. This patient is most likely suffering from _____
   a. autonomic dysreflexia.
   b. hypertension.
   c. a panic or anxiety attack.
   d. internal injuries.

2. The best care for a patient with spastic CP who has fallen and suffered a potential mid-shaft femur fracture is to _____
   a. apply a traction splint.
   b. make one attempt at realigning the fracture and then splint the injured limb in the anatomically correct position.
   c. secure the patient to a backboard without splinting the limb and then tie the lower extremities together.
   d. splint the injured leg in a position of comfort.

3. Which of the following actions describes the best way to communicate with a deaf patient who has become separated from his partner?_____
   a. Hold off on doing your assessment until the patient's partner can be located.
   b. Using a pen and paper, write down your questions and have the patient write down his answers.
   c. Make eye contact and assume the patient can probably read lips.
   d. Use gestures to communicate (such as grimace as if in pain), point to a body part, and cock your head questioningly to ask whether or not this area hurts.

4. Which of the following statements describes the correct course of action regarding the presence of an ostomy bag in a paraplegic athlete who has fallen from a rock face and complains of chest pain?_____
   a. Continue with your assessment and ignore the ostomy bag because OEC Technicians do not deal with ostomy ports.
   b. Expose the bag and port and check for bleeding from the stoma site.
   c. Ask the patient to check his own bag to be sure it is intact.
   d. Carefully remove and tie off the bag, then cover the site with sterile gauze.

5. Which of the following statements describes the best course of action concerning a patient with an intellectual disability who panics when you cover her with a waterproof tarp in a toboggan?_____
   a. Reassure her that the tarp will keep her dry and continue with the transport.
   b. Tell her to breathe deeply because she will soon be at the first-aid hut.
   c. Ask her caregiver to help calm her down.
   d. Tell her that you understand that the tarp is making her feel panicky and then offer to remove it.

6. Your best course of action when transporting an injured adaptive athlete who is being accompanied by a service dog even though your recreation area has a strict "no pets" policy is to_____
   a. ask the patient's caregiver or partner to take the dog to the car.
   b. explain that the dog may come with you to the aid station but must be leashed up outside.
   c. ask a fellow OEC Technician or the patient's caregiver or partner to play with the dog outside until the patient is ready to go.
   d. allow the dog to accompany the patient into the aid room.

7. Which of the following statements regarding applying a splint to a patient with cerebral palsy who has an obvious tib/fib fracture is incorrect? _____
   a. The splint can aggravate muscle spasticity.
   b. The splint can help reduce muscle spasticity.
   c. It is acceptable to forego a splint and position this patient in a position of comfort.
   d. It is acceptable to use a rigid splint on this patient as long as it does not appear to be causing the patient discomfort.

8. Which of the following statements best summarizes communication with an adaptive athlete?_____
   a. Speak to the athlete rather than to the disability.
   b. Most patients with cognitive disabilities will be unable to understand you.
   c. Most patients with intellectual disabilities will be able to understand you only if their IQ is at least 90.
   d. The likely reason that patients with cognitive disabilities grow increasingly agitated and shut down is that you are not communicating well with them.

9. Which of the following statements regarding lift evacuation considerations for adaptive athletes are correct? (check all that apply)
   _____a. Adaptive athletes should be given priority when evacuating a chairlift.
   _____b. Adaptive athletes and their caregivers should be evacuated last.
   _____c. A patient with cognitive or intellectual disabilities may become agitated and anxious while waiting for evacuation from a chairlift.
   _____d. Skiers or snowboarders with visual impairments may need additional oral coaching during an evacuation, even if they have a guide with them in the same chair.
   _____e. When evacuating blind skiers, evacuate their caregivers first and the blind skiers second.
   _____f. Chairlift evacuation of an adaptive athlete in a sit-ski is a requirement for all OEC Technicians taking an OEC course.

## Matching

Match each of the following physical impairments to its description.

_____ **1.** cerebral palsy

_____ **2.** multiple sclerosis

_____ **3.** muscular dystrophy

_____ **4.** spina bifida

**a.** a congenital malformation of the spine and spinal cord

**b.** a condition that makes use of the legs or arms difficult; patients may have spinal curvature and weak, wasted muscles

**c.** caused by brain hypoxia just before, during, or after birth; the subsequent brain injury impairs voluntary motor function and coordination

**d.** a progressive disease that causes degeneration of both the central and peripheral nervous systems

# Scenario

*You receive a call concerning an injured skier in the woods on Fiddler Slope. Upon arrival at the scene you find a male patient on a sit-ski down an embankment and against a tree. Two other skiers who saw the accident remained with him until your arrival.*

**1.** An adaptive athlete is a person who _____

   **a.** cannot participate in sports without full physical support.

   **b.** is mentally restricted.

   **c.** is physically or mentally challenged and participates in sports.

   **d.** needs specially designed equipment.

*After securing the scene and taking Standard Precautions, you approach the patient, who is responsive, alert, and oriented to person, place, and time. The patient has a double amputation just above the knees from a motorcycle accident. The witnesses tell you that the injured skier swerved and went off the trail to avoid colliding with two young out-of-control skiers.*

*The patient, who is still strapped in the sit-ski, has no visible evidence of bleeding but complains of severe pain in the right femur area. You call for additional patrollers to bring a trauma sled and request an ALS ambulance.*

**2.** To remove outriggers the injured skier was also using, you_____

   **a.** remove them from the rear bottom of the sit-ski.

   **b.** remove them from the front bottom of the sit-ski.

   **c.** remove the straps of the poles from the injured skier's wrists.

   **d.** remove them from the sit-ski seat.

*Help arrives with the requested equipment. You create an extrication plan after asking the injured man about any special information concerning this sit-ski. You employ the aid of the witnesses and the additional patrollers to secure the patient and remove him from the sit-ski. Based on the MOI you ensure cervical stabilization for this patient.*

**3.** You perform a secondary assessment by gathering a medical history using _____

   **a.** PEARRL.

   **b.** SAMPLE.

   **c.** DCAP-BTLS.

   **d.** AVPU.

**4.** You complete a physical exam using _____

   **a.** SAMPLE.

   **b.** OPQRST.

   **c.** AVPU.

   **d.** DCAP-BTLS.

*While many skiers using sit-skis experience upper extremity injuries, you found none during the assessment.*

5. To treat the suspected femur fracture, you should _____
   a. not apply any splint because no traction can be applied to a shortened extremity.
   b. use a Kendrick traction device in a shortened position.
   c. use a quick splint to stabilize the leg above and below the fracture site.
   d. use a ski pole to improvise a device to place traction on the end of the stump.

*With a cervical collar applied and the stump stabilized, you place the patient on a long board. You request that the receiving hospital be advised of the patient's injury. After the patient is secured in the toboggan, with the injury uphill, the additional patrollers and friends help transport the patient's customized ski equipment down to the base.*

## Suggested Reading

Autism Society of America: www.autism-society.org

"Emergency Managers, Responders, Service & Care Providers" at www.disabilitypreparedness.gov

"Overcoming Communication Barriers in Emergency Situations" at www.patientprovidercommunication.org

"Tips for First Responders!" at http://cdd.unm.edu/products/tipsforfirstresponders.htm

## EXPLORE PEARSON myNSPkit™

Please go to www.myNSPkit.com. Under Student Resources, you will find animations, videos, web links, and games related to this chapter—and much more. Look for information for responders to persons with disabilities, overcoming communication barriers, and more.

Register your access code from the front of your book by going to www.myNSPkit.com and selecting the appropriate links. If the in-cover access code has been redeemed, go to www.myNSPkit.com and follow links to **Buy Access**.

# Behavioral Emergencies and Crisis Response

Matthew J. Levy, D.O., M.S., NREMT-P

## ⊕ OBJECTIVES

**Upon completion of this chapter, the OEC Technician will be able to:**

**33-1** Define the following terms:
   a. behavior
   b. behavioral emergency

**33-2** Compare and contrast neurosis and psychosis.

**33-3** List and explain four factors that can cause stress or lead a person to behave strangely.

**33-4** List the signs and symptoms of common behavioral emergencies.

**33-5** Identify techniques to help maintain rescuer safety when responding to a behavioral emergency.

**33-6** Describe and demonstrate how to assess a patient with a behavioral emergency.

**33-7** Describe and demonstrate the treatment of a patient with a behavioral emergency.

**33-8** List the indications for restraining a patient.

**33-9** Describe and demonstrate how to properly restrain a patient.

**33-10** List the five phases of the Kübler-Ross grieving process.

## Chapter Overview

As an OEC Technician, you will encounter emergencies that vary in complexity and severity. You will also interact with a diverse population of people who are in **crisis**, and depending on the situation, you may encounter people who are behaving in an unexpected, unusual, or possibly dangerous manner (Figure 33-1■). This behavior may be caused by a variety of conditions ranging from relatively minor to immediately life

*continued*

## HISTORICAL TIMELINE

1996 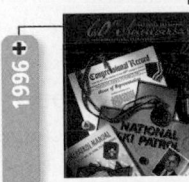 National Board recognizes a new "national education committee."

1998 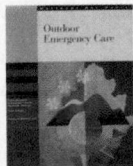 *OEC* Third Edition is published.

## ⊕ KEY TERMS

behavior, *p. 1040*
behavioral emergency, *p. 1040*
crisis, *p. 1039*
dependent lividity, *p. 1048*
depression, *p. 1044*

livor mortis, *p. 1048*
neurosis, *p. 1043*
positional asphyxia, *p. 1059*
psychosis, *p. 1043*
reasonable force, *p. 1058*

restraint, *p. 1058*
rigor mortis, *p. 1048*
schizophrenia, *p. 1045*
suicide, *p. 1045*

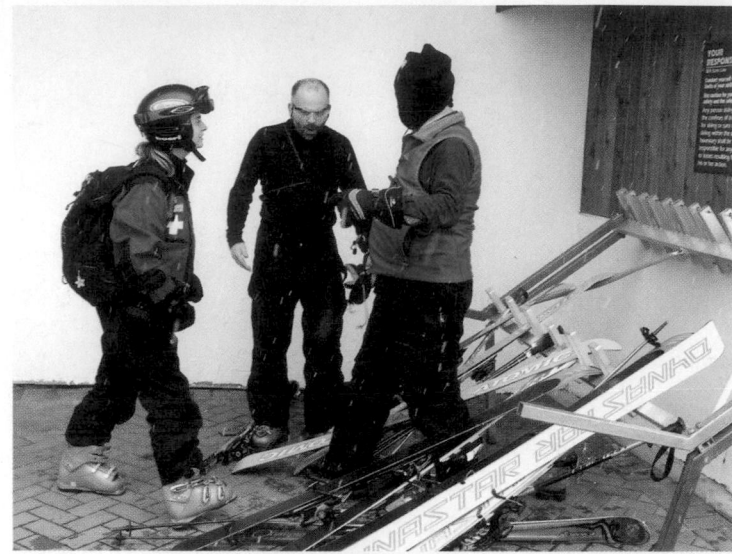

**Figure 33-1** For an OEC Technician who is interacting with an individual who is behaving abnormally, safety is a primary concern.
Copyright Craig Brown

⊕ **33-1** Define the following terms:

 a. behavior
 b. behavioral emergency

**crisis** a state of emotional turmoil within an individual in which the balance between thoughts and emotions is lost.

**behavior** an individual's actions or reactions in response to external or internal stimuli.

**behavioral emergency** a situation in which a person acts in a way that is unacceptable or intolerable to others and oftentimes poses a danger to themselves or others.

threatening. Regardless of the cause, safety remains your primary concern as an OEC Technician, and it must be ensured at all times. Failure to recognize abnormal behavior or an unsafe situation could result in serious injury to you, the patient, or others.

**Behavior** is an individual's actions or reactions in response to external or internal stimuli. Some behaviors are physical manifestations of underlying emotions, such as yelling, laughing, or crying. Whether one's behavior is considered normal or abnormal is subjective and largely depends on social norms, which vary from region to region and from culture to culture. Therefore, what is acceptable behavior in one community may not be acceptable in another. When a person's behavior differs from accepted norms, the person's actions are considered abnormal. If the shift in behavior is severe enough, the person is considered to be experiencing a behavioral emergency.

A **behavioral emergency** is a form of altered mental status. Behavioral emergencies exist when an individual exhibits abnormal thoughts or actions within a given set of circumstances that are considered to be dangerous to the patient or to others. The determination is usually made by others, not by the individual, with the noted exception of suicidal patients who call for help for themselves. A key concept in this definition is that the behavior must be taken into *context within the situation*. For example, the mother of a missing child might yell, scream, cry, or display other emotional outbursts. In the context of this situation, this behavior might not be considered unusual. However, if she were to become uncontrollable, her behavior might be considered abnormal. Likewise, if she behaved in the same way without any apparent cause, the situation might be considered a behavioral emergency.

As an OEC Technician, you must carefully approach patients who exhibit abnormal behavior to evaluate them and the circumstances involved. The underlying cause may be a medical, chemical, traumatic, or psychiatric disorder. Thus it is important that you quickly recognize the existence of a behavioral emergency and implement

**CASE PRESENTATION**

You receive a call to respond to a person "having an anxiety attack." Upon your arrival, you find a visibly upset male who appears to be in his 20s sitting on a bench along one of the area's popular trails. The man, who is wild-eyed and appears to be anxious, is yelling at a nearby female, who identifies herself as the man's sister. Upon identifying yourself, the man yells angrily at you to "Get away or someone will get hurt!" while repeatedly clenching and un-clenching his fists.

**What should you do?**

effective strategies for safeguarding the patient and others while addressing any threats to life. This chapter presents a basic introduction to behavioral emergencies, their causes, and general management principles. In addition, this chapter describes death and the grieving process as well as the potential effects of acute or cumulative stress on rescuers.

## Anatomy and Physiology

As described in previous chapters, the human body is a remarkable organism that performs millions of tasks simultaneously and is capable of adapting to various internal and external conditions while preserving homeostasis. This ability is controlled by the central nervous system—specifically the brain, a complex organ that constantly receives messages from the body's numerous sensory receptors. In response to various stimuli, whether social or physical, the brain initiates a variety of corrective actions to return the body to a state of equilibrium as quickly as possible.

*Stress* is defined as a person's total response to environmental demands or pressures. When exposed to stress, the body responds by making a physical, mental, or emotional adjustment. Stress is caused by a stimulus, a perceived threat or a stress-inducing factor known as a stressor.

In humans, stress results from interactions between individuals and their environment that are perceived as straining or exceeding their adaptive capacities and threatening their well-being. Stress is a normal part of life and may be caused by internal or external factors. When the body is stressed, its "fight or flight" system automatically triggers a series of responses throughout the body, including the release of the neurotransmitters epinephrine, norepinephrine, and dopamine. In addition to preparing the body for stress, these chemicals activate a part of the brain known as the amygdala, which triggers an emotional response to the stressor.

The fight-or-flight system is highly effectively for short periods of time. However, when the body receives too much stress at one time or suffers prolonged stress, serious imbalances can cause cerebral impairment, altering mental processes and causing abnormal behavior. How an individual responds to stress depends on a variety of factors, including age, overall health, genetics, individual physiology, personality, attitude, and self-image (Figure 33-2■).

Some medical researchers believe that structural abnormalities or chemical imbalances within the brain can impede normal brain function and alter one's perception of reality. When this occurs, sensory input may be falsely interpreted or misinterpreted, which can lead to bizarre, violent, and even homicidal or suicidal behavior.

**Figure 33-2** How each individual responds to stress depends on a variety of factors.

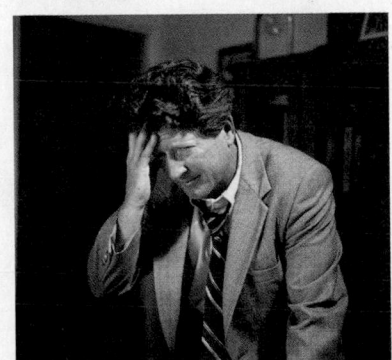

## STOP, THINK, UNDERSTAND

### Multiple Choice

Choose the correct answer.

1. What is the most important consideration in any situation you may encounter as an OEC Technician? _____
   a. identifying yourself as an OEC Technician
   b. maintaining a patient's airway
   c. ensuring safety
   d. determining the mechanism of injury

2. Abnormal behavior is largely_____
   a. a diagnosis.
   b. a response to the environment.
   c. subjective and dependent on varying social norms.
   d. not something an OEC Technician should determine.

3. A behavioral emergency is best described as_____
   a. a judgment call.
   b. an inappropriate response to a situation.
   c. a form of altered mental status.
   d. an emotional response from a patient that an OEC Technician feels unable to handle.

4. A behavioral emergency_____
   a. may be handled only by a person with a higher level of training than an OEC Technician.
   b. must be considered in the context of the situation in which it is occurring.
   c. must be considered to occur any time a person appears to be distraught.
   d. is almost always dangerous to an OEC Technician.

5. Stress is best defined as_____
   a. a person's total response to environmental demands or pressures.
   b. a physical or emotional response to a situation that can harm the body.
   c. a period of heightened anxiety.
   d. anything that elevates a person's pulse rate, respiratory rate, and blood pressure.

---

Often, medications are administered to patients with a diagnosed behavioral disorder to correct chemical imbalances.

⊕ **33-3** List and explain four factors that can cause stress or lead a person to behave strangely.

⊕ **33-4** List the signs and symptoms of common behavioral emergencies.

# Common Behavioral Emergencies

Among the many factors that can cause stress or lead a person to act strangely are the following conditions:

+ medical disorders
+ chemical exposures
+ trauma
+ behavioral conditions

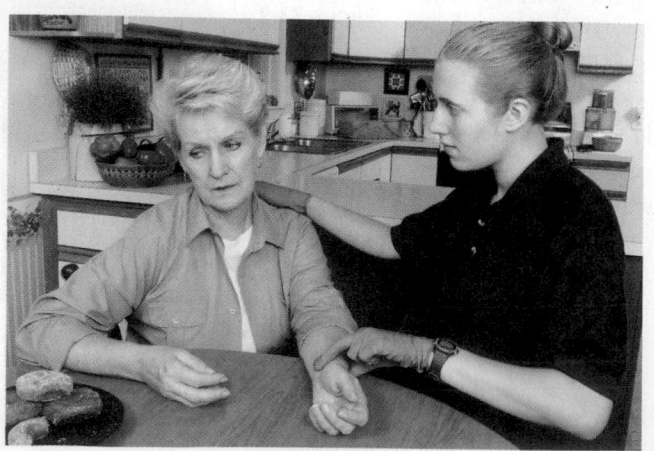

**Figure 33-3** Medical conditions such as diabetes can cause an altered mental status.

### Medical Disorders

In many instances, the source of a person's apparent behavioral emergency can be traced to an underlying medical condition. Whenever you detect an alteration in mental status, always consider potential medical conditions that can be easily treated, including hypoxia and hypoglycemia. As described in previous chapters, the brain requires a steady supply of oxygen and glucose and quickly malfunctions when levels of either of these crucial nutrients become too low. Possible medical causes of abnormal behavior include epilepsy, seizures, cardiopulmonary disorders, hypotension, dehydration, electrolyte imbalance, and diabetes (Figure 33-3■). Carbon monoxide poisoning, as from a malfunctioning or poorly ventilated heater or generator, can also cause hypoxia and should be considered as well.

## Chemical Exposures

The use of mind-altering substances such as alcohol or drugs often mimics the signs and symptoms of a behavioral emergency (Figure 33-4■). As indicated in Chapter 12, Substance Abuse and Poisoning, alcohol is the most commonly abused substance in the United States and is frequently associated with both altered mental status and bizarre behavior. Individuals who abuse alcohol or drugs can be depressed, agitated, or even violent. In addition, many wild plants, berries, and mushrooms can also produce adverse effects, resulting in a wide range of symptoms that may invoke bizarre behavior.

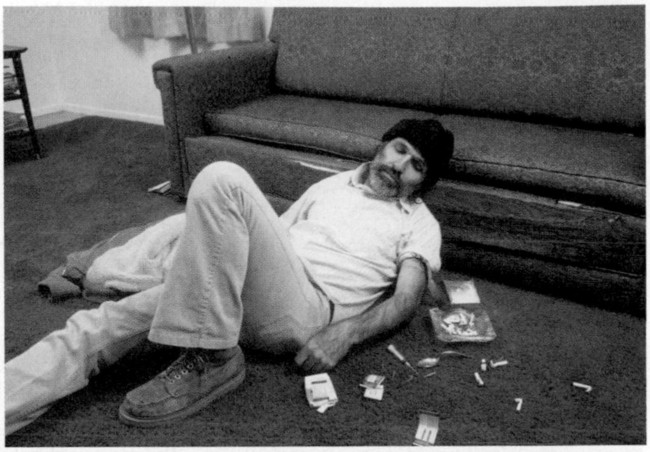

## Trauma

Brain injuries can cause altered responsiveness and behavioral disorders. A concussion or an intracranial hemorrhage especially in closed head injuries without external signs of trauma, may initially appear to be an underlying psychiatric disorder. Patients with a head injury can present with a wide range of signs and symptoms, including confusion, irritability, agitation, verbal outbursts, irrational behavior, and personality changes (Figure 33-5■). Acute blood loss at any site in the body is another potential cause of abnormal behavior and may produce many of these same signs and symptoms due to brain hypoxia. Environmental conditions, including hypothermia and hyperthermia, are also associated with bizarre behavioral changes.

## Behavioral Conditions

The human psyche is highly complex, and a full discussion of specific psychiatric disorders goes well beyond the scope of this text. The following brief description presents some of the most common behavior-related emergencies that OEC Technicians may encounter (Figure 33-6■). For ease of presentation, most behavioral conditions are categorized as either a neurosis or a psychosis. A **neurosis**, also known as a neurotic disorder, is characterized by abnormal behavior in a person who remains firmly in touch with reality. This sharply contrasts with a **psychosis**, or a psychotic disorder, which is characterized by abnormal behavior and altered perceptions of reality. These

**Figure 33-4** The ingestion of alcohol or drugs can alter mental status; at times the signs and symptoms mimic those of a behavioral emergency.

**⊕ 33-2** Compare and contrast neurosis and psychosis.

**neurosis** a condition in which a person exhibits abnormal behavior but remains able to understand the normal boundaries of reality.

**psychosis** a condition in which a person exhibits abnormal behavior and has altered perceptions of reality.

**Figure 33-6** Most common behavior-related emergencies that OEC Technicians encounter can be categorized as either a neurosis or a psychosis.

**Figure 33-5** Head trauma and cold injuries can cause altered responsiveness and behavioral disorders.
Copyright Scott Smith

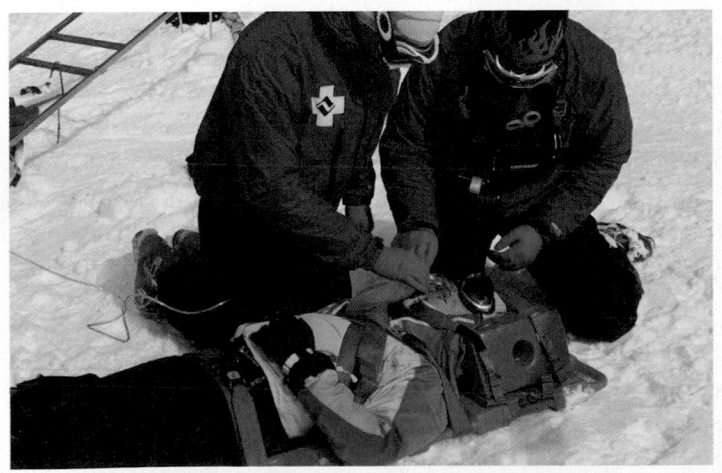

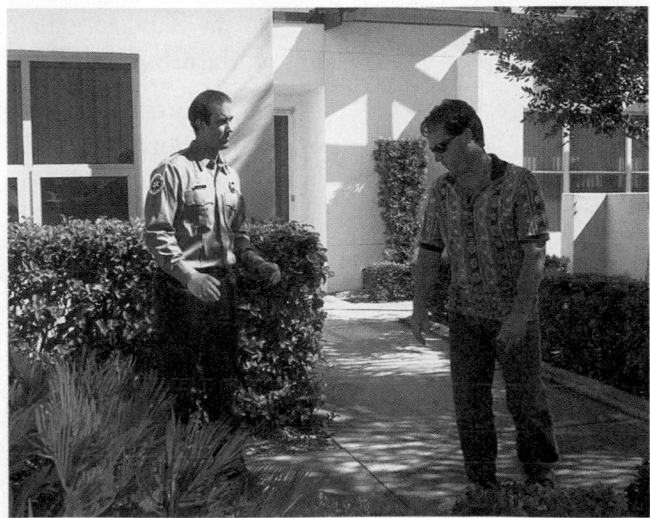

## Table 33-1    Causes of Behavioral Alterations

- Reduced oxygen to the brain (hypoxia)
- Very low blood pressure
- Low blood sugar (hypoglycemia)
- Illnesses such as a seizure disorder, Alzheimer's disease, or infections
- Dehydration
- Abnormal electrolyte levels
- Situational stress (e.g., witnessing the death of a loved one)
- Head injuries
- Environmental exposures (hypothermia or hyperthermia)
- Accidental ingestion of mind-altering substances such as wild herbs, berries, or mushrooms
- Ingestion of drugs or alcohol
- Psychiatric disorders

### NOTE

#### Hallucinations

Hallucinations are perceptions of things that are not present in the real world by a person who is awake and responsive. Hallucinations may involve any of the five senses (hearing, sight, smell, touch, or taste) and may be caused by any number of medical, chemical, traumatic, and psychotic conditions (especially schizophrenia). Auditory hallucinations are more common than visual hallucinations with psychiatric disorders, whereas visual hallucinations are more commonly associated with an underlying medical or traumatic condition.

altered perceptions may include believing that one possesses super-human powers or abilities, having delusions of grandeur, or having feelings of divine superiority. Table 33-1■ lists some causes of behavioral alterations. Psychotic individuals often have visual or auditory hallucinations, which can lead the person to engage in dangerous or homicidal behaviors. Patients with a psychosis-based emergency are generally considered more dangerous than those with a neurosis-based emergency due to their increased tendency to exhibit violent or homicidal behavior.

### Neurotic Disorders

The neurotic disorders listed here are those identified as more common. A person who is not in reality can also have these disorders as part of a psychotic disorder.

**Anxiety**    Anxiety is a generic term used to describe a vague feeling of apprehension, uneasiness, or dread that can build over time or come on suddenly. It is the most common emotional disorder in the United States, affecting more than 25 million people. Anxiety is a normal reaction that occurs when one is faced with a stressful situation, and not all anxiety is harmful. In fact, certain amounts of anxiety can make a person more alert or careful or prompt a person to take purposeful action. Excessive anxiety, however, can result in feelings of impending doom and an inability to function. Over time, anxiety can lead to clinical depression and other health problems.

**depression**    a clinical state marked by feelings of sadness and self-loathing.

**Depression**    Depression is also a common but serious mental disorder that affects millions of people worldwide. **Depression** is defined as having feelings of sadness, worthlessness, hopelessness, or despair and can become so severe that it interferes with normal living. Depression is characterized by low self-worth, guilt, loss of interest in once-pleasurable things, sleep or appetite disturbances, and poor concentration. Most episodes of depression are brief, lasting only a few days. Severe depression, however, can last for months or even years and can lead to self-destructive behaviors or suicide attempts.

**Paranoia**    Paranoia is a condition in which individuals believe that they are in imminent danger of being harmed (e.g., physically, emotionally, financially) by others who are plotting against them. The condition is characterized by feelings of deep suspicion, irrational fear, severe distrust of others, delusions, and eccentric behavior.

Paranoid individuals often believe that they are being unfairly persecuted. Paranoia is often associated with other behavioral conditions and can present by itself as part of a neurosis or as a symptom of a deep rooted psychosis such as schizophrenia.

**Agitation** *Agitation* is defined as excessive restlessness and increased mental or physical activity. It can occur suddenly or develop gradually over time and is characterized by irritability, tension, heightened sensitivity, and excessive motion. The causes of agitation are numerous and are beyond the scope of this chapter. When associated with a mental disorder, agitation often precedes more aggressive behavior and is considered a warning sign for impending violence (Figure 33-7■).

## Psychotic Disorders

Psychotic individuals can have anxiety, depression, paranoia, or agitation. However, psychotic people do not understand the difference between what is real and not real.

**Schizophrenia** The type of psychosis known as **schizophrenia** is a complex mental disorder in which a person cannot differentiate between what is real and what is not real. It is characterized by impaired reasoning, emotional instability, paranoia, auditory or visual hallucinations, delusions, and (in many cases) violent behavior. Schizophrenia is a serious, lifelong mental disorder that in many cases can be effectively managed with medication. People who have schizophrenia and discontinue their medications can pose a danger to themselves and others.

**Bipolar Disorder** Bipolar disorder, formerly known as manic-depressive illness, is a common psychiatric disease that has been likened to an emotional rollercoaster of highs and lows. It is characterized by alternating, intermittent periods of euphoria, known as mania, and periods of depression. During the manic phase, a person experiences an emotional high that may be exhibited as increased excitability, increased energy levels or activity, elevated mood, restlessness, or impulsive behavior (such as hypersexuality or compulsive spending). During this phase, the person can become physically violent or dangerous. The depression phase is characterized by increased irritability, frustration, feelings of worthlessness, and thoughts of suicide. Because people with bipolar disorder can develop psychosis, it is distinctly different from neurotic depression and other forms of mania.

## Suicide

**Suicide**, the intentional taking of one's life, is a problem that affects thousands of individuals each year and is growing in magnitude, particularly among the young and the elderly. It is the eighth leading cause of death in the United States and is the third leading cause of death among young people ages 15–24. Anyone, regardless of race, sex, or socioeconomic background, can become suicidal if the level of emotional distress is severe enough. Among the many reasons a person might attempt suicide are depression, a high-stress lifestyle, mental or physical pain, family trauma or abuse, and social, economic, or psychiatric problems. People who have tried suicide before, have a family history of suicide, are depressed, or take illegal drugs are at greater risk for suicide.

The ways in which individuals may take their own lives are limited only by their imaginations. Among the most common methods are hanging, drug overdose, jumping from heights, carbon monoxide poisoning, and the use of weapons—especially

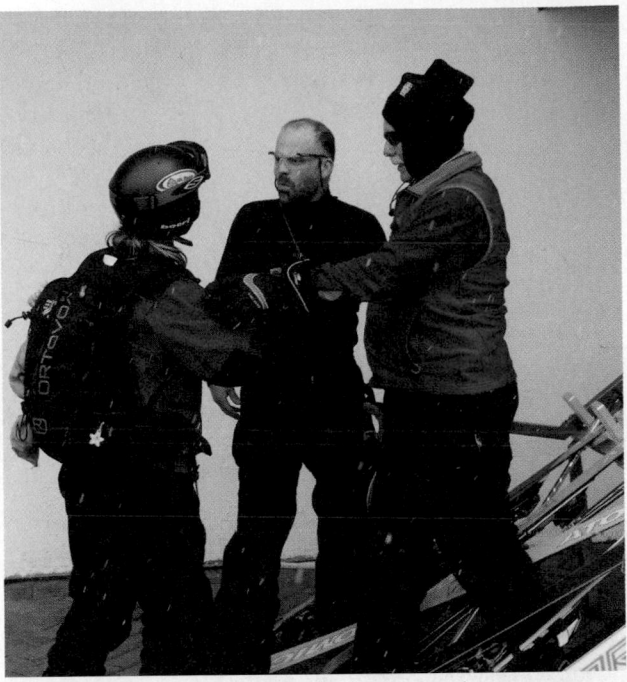

**Figure 33-7** Agitation that is associated with a history of mental disorder may be a warning that more aggressive or violent behavior is impending.
Copyright Craig Brown

**schizophrenia** a psychiatric disorder in which a person cannot distinguish what is real from what is not real.

**suicide** the intentional taking of one's own life.

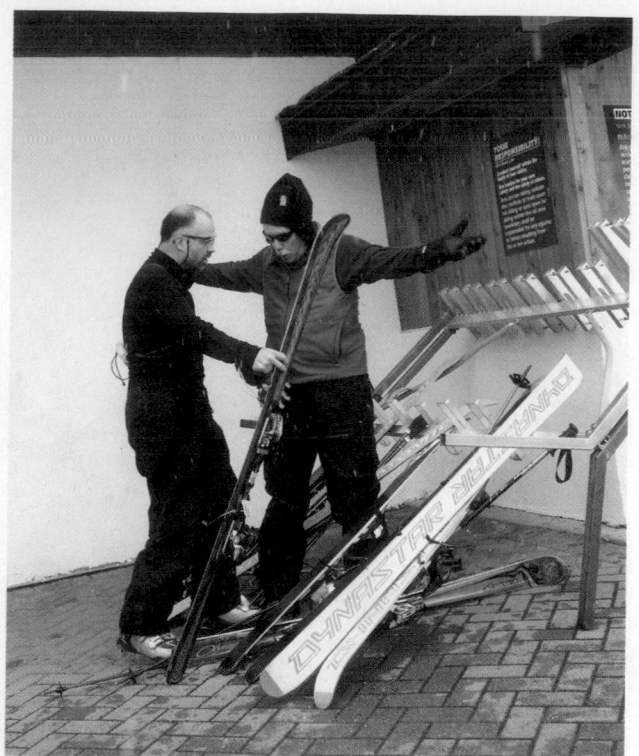

**Figure 33-8** Verbal abuse, the most common form of abuse, may lead to physical abuse.
Copyright Craig Brown

firearms, which account for more than half of all suicides. Many suicides and suicide attempts go unreported because they are masked by risky behaviors that can result in serious injury or death. OEC Technicians should be aware of this when assessing patients. Individuals who have made a very superficial wound on the body or have taken four pills and then immediately tell someone they did so have committed a suicidal gesture. Such gestures indicate a serious situation, and even if the results of the suicidal act are not life threatening, psychiatric care is urgently needed. A patient who has made a suicidal gesture cannot be left alone or allowed to refuse medical care. OEC Technicians do not need permission to care for individuals who are suicidal or homicidal.

## Violence

Violence, the use of force to abuse, damage, or injure, is an unfortunate by-product of numerous disorders, including mental illness. Violence may be directed inward (as in a suicidal individual), or it may be directed outward, toward others. It may be intentional, or it may be unintentional, as occurs in patients who are severely hypoxic or have suffered traumatic injury and become violent due to the body's fight-or-flight response. Violence is also associated with several forms of mental illnesses, especially depression, paranoia, and schizophrenia. It may also occur independent of a mental illness, most often in the form of physical assault. Patients who exhibit violent behavior may be neurotic (and fully aware of their surroundings) or psychotic and completely out of touch with reality.

## Abuse

Abuse is a criminal act that each day affects millions of people around the world. Abuse can take several forms. Verbal abuse, the most common form, involves the use of hurtful words and may include sarcasm, verbal humiliation, name calling, and personal attacks on a person's character or abilities (Figure 33-8■). Verbal abuse may lead to physical abuse, which involves force or violence that results in pain, physical humiliation, or bodily injury. Sexual abuse involves forcing a sex act on another person against their will. Rape is a particularly heinous form of sexual abuse that involves unlawful sexual intercourse or forcing another person to perform a sex-related activity.

# STOP, THINK, UNDERSTAND

## Multiple Choice
Choose the correct answer.

1. The general term for any disorder in which a person exhibits abnormal behavior but remains firmly in touch with reality is_____
   a. neurosis.
   b. psychosis.
   c. depression.
   d. agitation.

2. The general term for any disorder in which an individual exhibits abnormal behavior and has an altered perception of reality is_____
   a. neurosis.
   b. psychosis.
   c. depression.
   d. anxiety.

3. The third leading cause of death among individuals ages 15–24 is_____
   a. motor vehicle accidents.
   b. overdoses.
   c. suicide.
   d. trauma.

4. Which of the following is not a common method of suicide in the United States?_____
   a. a drug overdose
   b. carbon monoxide (CO) poisoning from a car exhaust
   c. hanging
   d. the use of a sharp instrument

*continued*

5. Paranoia is best described as a condition in which individuals_____
   a. believe that others are plotting to harm them.
   b. believe that if they don't exercise regularly they may develop coronary artery disease.
   c. fear that giving their child a measles vaccine may cause autism.
   d. fear that they will fail their OEC final if they don't read the text.

6. Which of the following statements regarding agitation is true?
   _____
   a. An agitated individual rarely poses a threat to rescuers.
   b. Agitation is a concern only if it is coupled with hypoglycemia.

c. Agitation precedes more aggressive behavior and should be considered a warning sign for possible violence.
d. Agitation is a form of psychosis.

7. A condition in which a person cannot differentiate between what is real and what is not, and that is characterized by hallucinations, delusions, and possible violence, is _____
   a. depression.
   b. schizophrenia.
   c. paranoia.
   d. agitation.

## Fill in the Blank

The two most common medical causes of abnormal behavior are _____ and _____.

## Matching

Match each of the following terms to its description.

_____ 1. abuse

_____ 2. agitation

_____ 3. anxiety

_____ 4. bipolar disorder

_____ 5. depression

_____ 6. hallucination

_____ 7. neurosis

_____ 8. paranoia

_____ 9. psychosis

_____ 10. schizophrenia

_____ 11. suicide

_____ 12. violence

a. A condition characterized by abnormal behavior in which the individual remains in touch with reality.
b. A feeling of despair or sadness characterized by low self-worth, guilt, and sleep or appetite disturbances.
c. The intentional taking of one's own life.
d. A condition characterized by abnormal behavior in which the individual has an altered perception of reality.
e. A feeling of apprehension, dread, or impending doom.
f. A belief that one is in imminent danger of being harmed by others who are plotting against you.
g. Excessive restlessness and heightened mental or physical activity.
h. A by-product of numerous disorders that is defined as the use of force to abuse, damage, or injure.
i. A type of psychosis in which a person cannot differentiate between what is real and what is not; is characterized by impaired reasoning, hallucinations, delusions, and possible violence.
j. Sensing things that are not present.
k. A condition characterized by roller-coaster highs and lows; also known as manic/depressive illness.
l. A criminal act against a person that includes verbal, physical, and sexual forms.

# Death and Grief

Death is the inevitable terminal phase of any organism's life cycle. Regardless of its cause—medical illness, traumatic injury, or suicide—the death of another human being evokes a variety of behavioral responses in survivors, including rescuers. Some of these responses may be considered abnormal, whether directed inwardly or outwardly.

Because OEC Technicians often work in remote settings and care for patients who may not be discovered for some time or cannot reach definitive care quickly, it is important that OEC Technicians be able to identify those patients whose illnesses or injuries are not survivable. Anyone who finds a deceased person may experience significant psychological effects, and counseling may be needed to help the finder cope with this stress.

## Obvious Signs of Death

Under most conditions, OEC Technicians initiate life-saving interventions on any patient who is pulseless and apneic and then immediately transport that patient to a

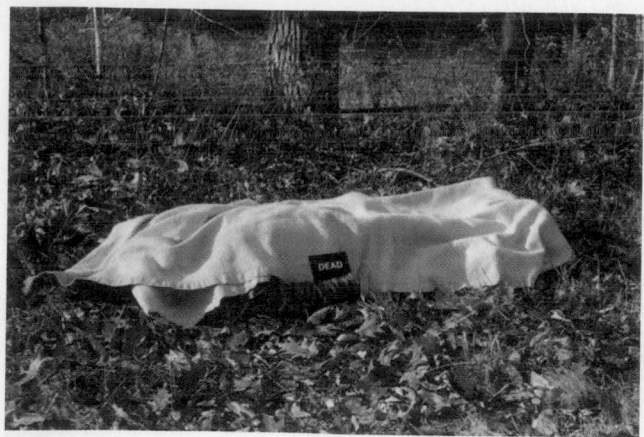

**Figure 33-9** Any rescuer who finds a deceased individual can experience a significant psychological reaction.
Copyright Mike Halloran

**livor mortis**   a purplish discoloration of the skin in the lowest parts of the body due to the settling of blood following death; also called dependent lividity.

**dependent lividity**   a purplish discoloration of the skin in the lowest parts of the body due to the settling of blood following death; also called livor mortis.

**rigor mortis**   stiffening of the body after death.

---

⊕ **33-10**  List the five phases of the Kübler-Ross grieving process.

**Figure 33-10** Listening to individuals who are experiencing grief can aid them in the grieving process.

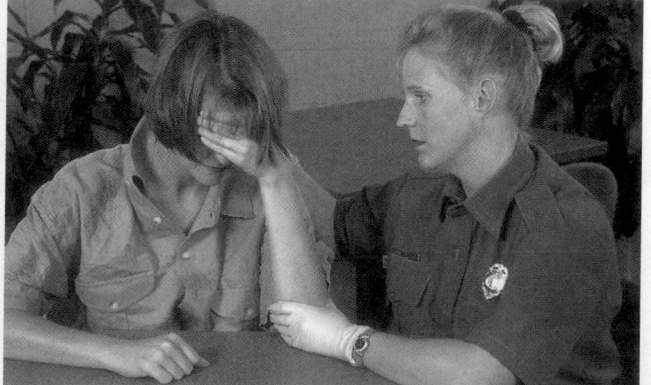

definitive-care facility. In some instances, however, these techniques will clearly be futile and should be withheld (Figure 33-9■).

The decision to withhold interventions should be made either with the direct collaboration of a physician or when the following obvious signs of death are apparent:

+ Prolonged cardiac arrest
+ Documented pulselessness and apnea for more than 30 minutes (the exception to this is any potentially hypothermic patient)
+ **Livor mortis**, a purplish discoloration of the skin due to the pooling of blood in the subcutaneous tissues that are closest to the ground; also called **dependent lividity**
+ **Rigor mortis**, the stiffening of the body after death
+ Decapitation, the traumatic separation of the head from the body
+ Obvious mortal injuries associated with cardiac arrest
+ Decomposition (putrefaction of body tissues)

Death may also be confirmed if the patient is both pulseless and apneic and has a valid Do Not Resuscitate order (DNR). As before, the decision to not initiate resuscitative measures should either be made in direct consultation with a physician or be based on local protocols. Even though only physicians and coroners pronounce people dead, starting CPR is of little value for individuals with any of the previously listed findings.

## Grief

Following a death, it is common for people who have known the deceased person to experience a period of grief—an emotional, often painful, reaction to the loss of a loved one (Figure 33-10■). Grief is a normal response to loss and can result in a wide range of reactions that were documented and categorized by Dr. Elisabeth Kübler-Ross in her book *On Death and Dying*. Individuals who are grieving a death or have learned of an impending death typically experience the following five phases of the grieving process:

+ denial
+ anger
+ bargaining
+ depression
+ acceptance

During the denial phase, a person refuses to believe that a loss has occurred or will occur, or to acknowledge the events leading up to the loss. This phase is followed by the anger phase, in which the person becomes enraged by the circumstances. Next, the person enters the bargaining phase, which involves attempts to negotiate with oneself or one's higher power in an effort to postpone or undo the loss. The fourth phase, depression, occurs when the person realizes that nothing can change the situation. This phase is followed by the acceptance phase, during which the person comes to terms with the loss and becomes ready to move forward.

The phases of grief occur in no specific timeframe, and not every grieving person goes through every stage or experiences the stages in the order listed. In fact, people may remain stuck

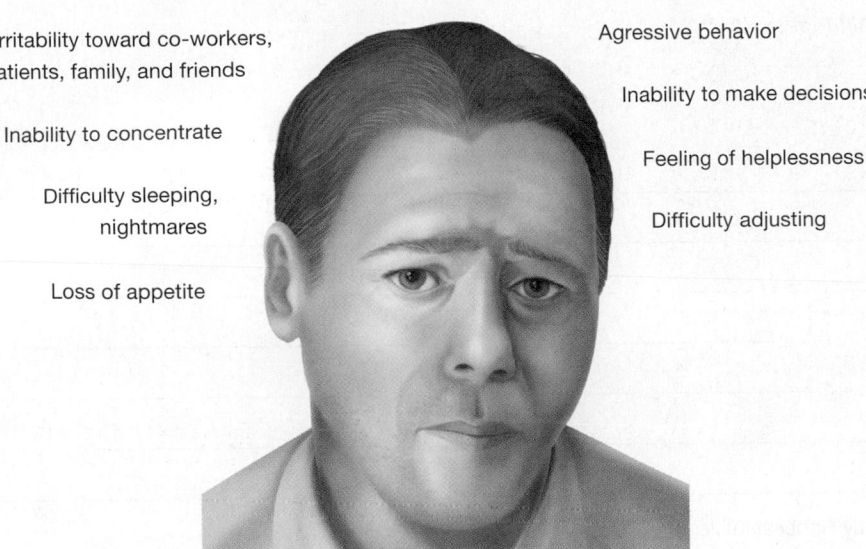

Irritability toward co-workers, patients, family, and friends

Inability to concentrate

Difficulty sleeping, nightmares

Loss of appetite

Agressive behavior

Inability to make decisions

Feeling of helplessness

Difficulty adjusting

**Figure 33-11** The warning signs of stress.

in one phase for months or even years. In addition, a person may revert to a previous phase during the healing process, as often occurs during evocative times such as holidays, birthdays, or anniversaries.

## Post-Traumatic Stress Disorder

Post-traumatic stress disorder, or PTSD, is an anxiety-related condition that may occur following exposure to a traumatic incident such as a critical injury, a violent event, or an unexpected death. The condition can affect the patient, family members, and rescuers. Symptoms are highly individualized and may either occur immediately following the incident or not become apparent for weeks, months, or even years afterward. The condition is characterized by feelings of helplessness, difficulty adjusting, sleep or eating disturbances, heightened awareness, aggressive behavior, interpersonal relationship challenges, and an inability to cope with normal, everyday situations (Figure 33-11■). Untreated, the condition can cause long-term health problems, including depression and suicidal thoughts. This condition is explained in more detail in Chapter 3, Rescue Basics.

## STOP, THINK, UNDERSTAND

### Multiple Choice
Choose the correct answer.

1. Which of the following patients does not exhibit an obvious sign of death? _____
   a. a patient with rigor mortis
   b. a patient with livor mortis
   c. a hypothermic patient who is pulseless and apneic for more than 30 minutes
   d. a decapitated patient

2. Three months after you and a colleague dug a body out of an avalanche, your colleague tells you that she is having recurrent nightmares, is unable to sleep soundly, is losing weight, and is yelling at her husband a lot. From what condition is your colleague most likely suffering? _____
   a. schizophrenia          c. anxiety
   b. depression             d. PTSD

3. Which of the following is not one of the four major common neuroses? _____
   a. manic depressive       c. depression
   b. anxiety                d. paranoia

*continued*

STOP, THINK, UNDERSTAND *continued*

## List

1. List the seven obvious signs of death.

   1. _____

   2. _____

   3. _____

   4. _____

   5. _____

   6. _____

   7. _____

2. List the five stages of grief as described by Elisabeth Kübler-Ross.

   1. _____

   2. _____

   3. _____

   4. _____

   5. _____

 # CASE UPDATE

Your immediate concern is for your own safety and for that of others near the irate man. As other OEC Technicians clear bystanders from the scene, you attempt to defuse the situation using a calm and caring tone. You assure the man that you are here to help him. Within a few minutes, he begins to settle down, and then he starts to cry.

After obtaining his permission, you carefully approach the man in a non-threatening manner. He agrees to let you take his vital signs. His heart rate is 105 bpm, his blood pressure is 126/72, and his respiratory rate is 32. His skin is somewhat sweaty and warm to the touch. As you begin to build trust, you learn that the patient's brother died one year ago today. The two siblings were hiking up to the top of their brother's favorite ridge, where they planned to release his ashes to the wind. Today is the patient's first time hiking in over 5 years. He is still upset and repeatedly says, "I can't believe that he's gone."

The patient is now breathing deep and hard and continues to cry intermittently, but he is alert and oriented to place, date, and time. During your assessment, you learn that the patient has not eaten since last night, and that he never eats breakfast. It is now mid-day. With prompting, you get the patient to agree to eat an energy bar while you continue your assessment. He complains that his lips and hands are tingling and that he feels like he may "pass out." The physical assessment is unremarkable for obvious trauma, although the patient's fingers are now tightly contorted. He begins to become agitated because he cannot open his hands. He denies that this has ever happened before or having used any mind-altering substances.

***What should you do now?***

# Assessment

## Scene Safety

As indicated in previous chapters, maintaining the safety of rescuers and others is of paramount importance. This is *especially* true in any situation involving people exhibiting abnormal behavior (Figure 33-12■). It is therefore essential that OEC Technicians rapidly identify potentially dangerous situations and remain mindful of the fact that individuals experiencing a behavioral emergency can become violent. Even though conventional thought holds that medical personnel should not initiate patient care until law enforcement personnel have secured the scene, given the sometimes remote nature of outdoor emergency care, it is not always possible to wait until someone arrives on scene. In these instances, always follow your "gut" instinct. If something doesn't feel right, it probably isn't right. Use your best judgment at all times.

When approaching a patient who may be having a behavioral emergency, make mental notes about the scene and look for at least two escape routes. Whenever possible, remain near an egress route, and never let the patient get between you and it. Approach patients from a direction that enables them to see you so that you do not surprise them. Announce that you are a patroller or an OEC Technician and are there to help. Always attempt to speak to the patient at eye level. Speak in a soft but firm voice. Avoid yelling or raising your voice even if the patient does not reciprocate. Maintain a comfortable distance from patients (ideally at least 3 feet away or out of arms length) until they have given you permission to approach them. Avoid sudden movements, which may startle patients and invoke an aggressive or violent response. Assume that patients could be dangerous, and act accordingly. If at any time the scene becomes unsafe, evacuate to a safer location and await additional assistance. Never approach a patient who has a weapon (Figure 33-13■).

If you have a portable communications device, use it to quickly summon any needed help. Many modern public safety two-way radios are equipped with a distress button that, when activated, alerts others on the same frequency that you are in trouble. Be aware that radio static and loud radio traffic can agitate an emotionally unstable individual. A high-powered flashlight can not only illuminate the scene but can also temporarily blind a person who is acting aggressively or charging toward you. Be prepared to quickly drop your equipment or pack and evacuate the scene if it suddenly becomes unsafe.

Situational stressors, such as witnessing the death or injury of a loved one, can cause a person to respond with fear, anger, or grief. Remember that these responses are typical under the circumstances. Often, as you take control of the situation, the patient will begin to calm down. It is important to keep your emotions under control while you give patients time to gain control of their emotions. Be honest with patients, explaining what you are going to do before you do it, and continue to observe them for any changes in their behavior.

## Patient Assessment

The assessment process begins with a rapid evaluation of the patient's ABCDs. If the patient has been speaking to you, the

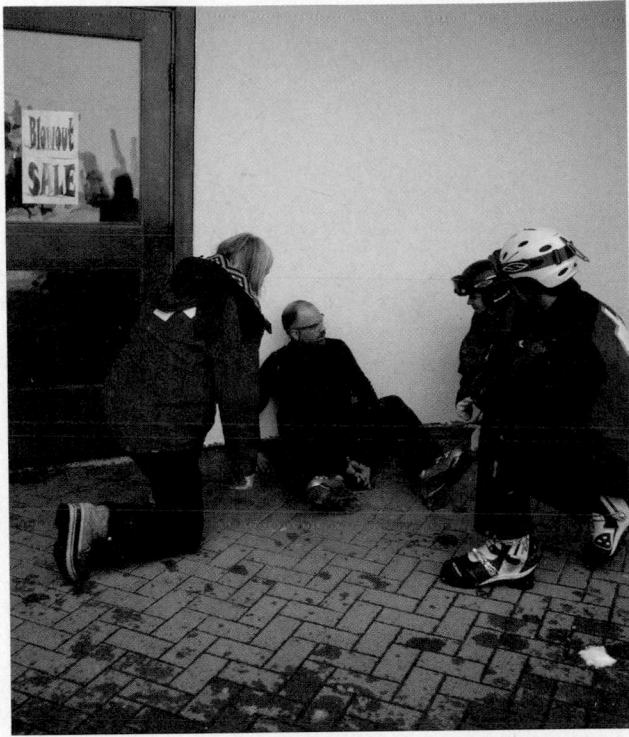

**Figure 33-12** Scene safety is especially important when someone exhibiting abnormal behavior is involved.
Copyright Craig Brown

⊕ **33-5** Identify techniques to help maintain rescuer safety when responding to a behavioral emergency.

⊕ **33-6** Describe and demonstrate how to assess a patient with a behavioral emergency.

**Figure 33-13** Never approach a patient who has a weapon.

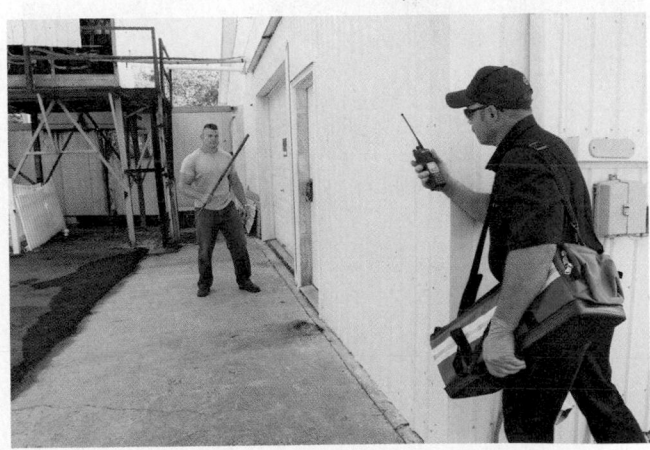

| **Table 33-2** Signs and Symptoms of a Behavioral Emergency |
| --- |
| • Agitation<br>• Paranoia<br>• Speech that appears stressful<br>• Bizarre thinking or actions<br>• Self-destructive behavior or attempted suicide<br>• Mental confusion<br>• Hostility/anger/uncontrolled rage<br>• Uncontrolled crying |

person's airway and breathing are not likely compromised. Correct any ABCD problem before proceeding to the physical assessment. Realize that some ABCD problems may not be immediately evident. For instance, the respirations of a patient who took an overdose of drugs in a suicide attempt may be normal at first but may then become compromised once the drugs take effect. For this reason, regularly monitor the ABCDs of any patient with documented altered mental status.

Patients with a behavior-related problem can range from withdrawn and quiet, to agitated and overly talkative, to hostile and threatening. In some cases the patient is simply "not acting right." A patient's behavior may change quickly or slowly, and some changes may not be immediately obvious. For this reason, patients with any behavior considered abnormal, bizarre, or unacceptable must be carefully evaluated by a physician. OEC Technicians are discouraged from attempting to diagnose the underlying cause of a patient's behavior and instead should protect the patient from harm. However, OEC Technicians should be able to determine if a patient is in touch with reality, and whether they are anxious, depressed, or dangerous. See Table 33-2■ for a list of the signs and symptoms of a behavioral emergency.

Once the scene is secured, approach the patient carefully, identifying yourself and then stating why you are there (Figure 33-14■). When evaluating a patient who appears to be having a behavioral emergency, it is important to determine if the patient is in touch with the real world. Observe the patient's appearance and overall demeanor. Does the person exhibit poor judgment? Is the person wearing clothing that is appropriate for the prevailing conditions? Does the person appear calm, or does the person instead exhibit signs of aggression such as tensing muscles (especially the jaw muscles), clenching the fists, pacing back and forth, or punching the air or inanimate objects? Does the person appear happy, sad, angry, or emotionless? Is the patient alert and oriented? Figure 33-15■ illustrates the continuum of responses of patients during a behavioral emergency.

Individuals who have certain chronic mental diseases, such as schizophrenia, do not function within the normal boundaries of reality. When in crisis, these individuals are often not oriented to the situation, place, or time and appear confused and disorganized. They may not even know who they are. People who have an underlying neurotic disorder can also exhibit bizarre behavior, but they generally function within reality and know who they are, what date it is, where they are, and what has happened, unless other factors such as alcohol or drug use are involved. In these situations, it is generally appropriate to immediately request additional help in managing both the surrounding area and the patient if the situation escalates.

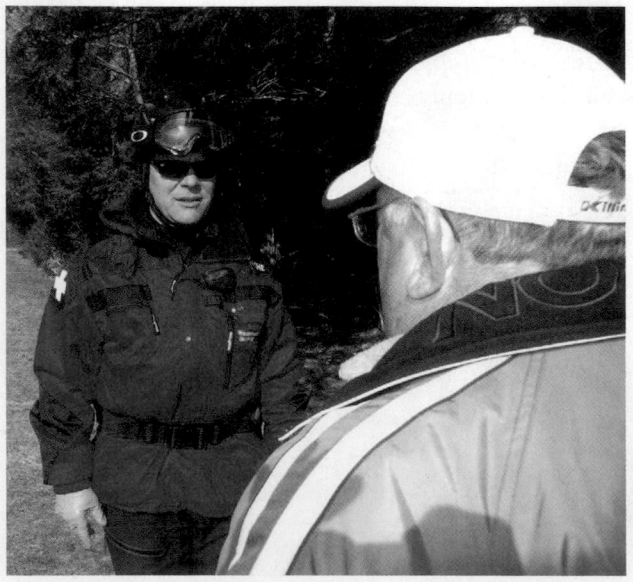

**Figure 33-14** Approach a person who may be having a behavioral emergency carefully; identify yourself and explain your purpose.
Copyright Edward McNamara

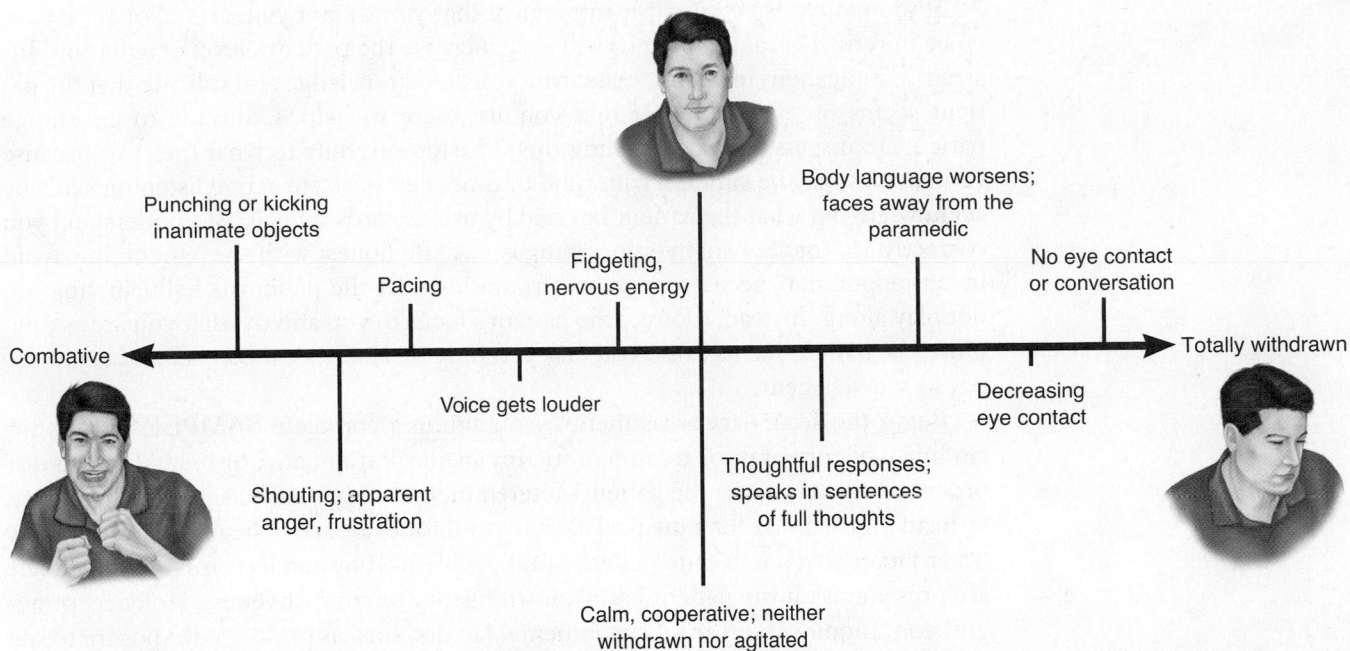

Combative ◄————————————————————————————————————► Totally withdrawn

Punching or kicking inanimate objects

Pacing

Fidgeting, nervous energy

Body language worsens; faces away from the paramedic

No eye contact or conversation

Voice gets louder

Shouting; apparent anger, frustration

Thoughtful responses; speaks in sentences of full thoughts

Decreasing eye contact

Calm, cooperative; neither withdrawn nor agitated

**Figure 33-15** OEC Technicians can use their interpersonal skills to bring a patient, whether combative or withdrawn, to the calm, cooperative state in the center of the continuum of responses to a behavioral emergency.

As the patient speaks, listen to both the words and the tone of voice. Is the patient yelling and using obscenities? Does the person express homicidal or suicidal thoughts? Is the patient's speech fast or slow? Are the words slurred, pressured (i.e., the speaker can't get them out fast enough), or threatening? Does the person raise or lower his voice by an octave? Does the person make sense? Is the patient oriented to time, situation, people, and place? Does the person appear to be functioning within the realm of reality?

Maintain a safe distance until the patient calms, and encourage the patient to talk. Do not make physical contact at this point because doing so could invoke an aggressive or violent response. Again, call for additional security personnel, including local police authorities should the patient require forcible restraint. Refer to Table 33-3■ for additional suggestions on how to approach behavioral emergency patients.

Calming a patient having a behavioral emergency is essential for performing an assessment. Explain to the patient, in simple terms, what you are doing before assessing them or rendering treatment. Unless the patient requires emergent treatment, proceed without hurrying to avoid upsetting the patient.

**Table 33-3** Approaching and Caring for the Behavioral Emergency Patient

- Maintain your safety at all times; always have an escape route.
- Approach patients in a way that they can see you.
- Avoid unnecessary physical contact with patients.
- Try to calm patients.
- Take time to talk to patients and to listen to their responses.
- Never lie to patients.
- Never play along with any auditory or visual hallucinations.
- Review the medical conditions that might resemble a behavioral emergency.
- Treat any life-threatening problems you encounter.
- Monitor patients for signs of agitation or worsening of their condition.

If the patient is yelling, it is imperative that you do not yell, argue, or raise your voice in return because doing so will only increase the patient's level of agitation. Instead, ask questions in a calm, reassuring voice. Acknowledge and validate that the patient seems upset, and repeat that you are there to help. Continue to encourage patients to discuss what is troubling them. Listen carefully to what they say, because verbal clues may be subtle. From time to time, demonstrate active listening skills by acknowledging what the patient has said by using words such as "If I understand you correctly . . ." or "So what you're saying is. . . ." Be honest with the patient, but avoid being judgmental, accusatory, or confrontational. If the patient is hallucinating, do not play along. Instead, redirect the patient's focus to you and to what you are asking. Once the patient seems calm, you may carefully make physical contact and begin the physical assessment.

Begin the secondary assessment by obtaining a complete SAMPLE history, including a history of prior treatment for any medical, traumatic, or mental health disorders that might cause the patient's altered mental status, such as diabetes, epilepsy, or head injury. Look for a medical alert tag and for evidence of head trauma or of any other factor that could cause a behavioral problem. If bystanders or family members are present, ask if the patient has a known history of combativeness, violence, or aggression. Inquire about any environmental factors, such as prolonged exposure to sun or cold, ingestion of wild plants, or dehydration, that might precipitate the observed behavior. It is essential that any patient who appears to be psychotic be carefully assessed for a treatable medical or traumatic condition.

If the patient has a history of a previous medical or traumatic condition, assess the condition in the usual fashion and treat accordingly. If the patient has a history of mental illness, ask whether the patient has been prescribed any medications for that illness, and whether the patient is taking those medications as directed. Refer to Table 33-4■ for a list of psychotropic agents. If the patient may have overdosed on a medication or some other substance, gather as much information as possible about the ingested product, including the name of the substance, the quantity ingested, and when the ingestion occurred. Try to learn why the patient took the substance by asking, "What did you want to happen?" Also, ask if the patient consumed any alcohol, including the type (e.g., beer, bourbon, vodka) and quantity ingested.

As you assess the patient, note the presence of any signs or symptoms that might suggest a behavioral emergency, including the following:

+ Agitation: repetitive motions, threatening actions
+ Paranoia: thoughts that someone or something is going to harm them; often accompanied by anxiety and fear
+ Pressured speech: a very rapid, difficult-to-understand speech pattern; can be also seen in patients on stimulants such as cocaine or methamphetamine
+ Bizarre thinking or actions: a frequent reason why someone calls for help or is concerned about a behavioral emergency

**Table 33-4** Psychotropic Agents

| | |
|---|---|
| • Amitriptyline (Elavil) | • Nortriptyline (Pamelor) |
| • Doxepin (Adapin) | • Paroxetine (Paxil) |
| • Fluoxetine (Prozac) | • Phenelzine (Nardil) |
| • Fluvoxamine (Luvox) | • Sertraline (Zoloft) |
| • Imipramine (Tofranil) | • Tranylcypromine (Parnate) |

- Self-destructive behavior or attempted suicide: physical actions or verbal statements indicating that the patient is trying or did try to hurt himself
- Mental confusion: disorganized words or thoughts that are difficult to follow during a conversation
- Hostility/anger/uncontrolled rage: can pose a danger to the patient, the rescuers, and those around them
- Uncontrolled crying: inconsolable despite the rescuer's attempts at calming
- Unusual appearance: withdrawn stance, clothing in disorder, poor personal hygiene, too many or not enough clothes for the ambient temperature

Patients with anxiety exhibit a wide range of signs and symptoms that may include fear, apprehension, agitation, crying, and hyperventilation. Patients may also present with dyspnea, which is usually benign. If the anxiety is severe, the patient may hyperventilate (exhibit tachypnea and breathe deeply). As carbon dioxide levels in the blood decrease, the patient begins to exhibit the hallmark signs and symptoms of hyperventilation: tingling around the mouth, hands, or feet, and tight spasms in their hands and feet (a condition known as carpal-pedal spasms). If these findings are not immediately corrected, the patient may faint. Fortunately, the condition is fairly benign.

Patients who are depressed are often withdrawn, introspective, and relatively quiet. Such patients may or may not admit to being depressed but may exhibit apathy toward their appearance, health, or general well-being. Patients who are willing to talk may express feelings of worthlessness, despair, or profound sadness. They may also reveal that they have experienced one or more life changes such as the loss of a loved one, the loss of a job, or some other personal tragedy. Such patients may also describe a host of symptoms, such as a loss of appetite, problems sleeping, or frequent somatic complaints such as headaches or "stomach aches."

Patients who are chronically depressed frequently take medication to control their depression. Patients who stop taking their medications or experience more severe depression may begin thinking about suicide. Even though the role of OEC Technicians does not include diagnosing suicidal intent, briefly assess the patient's suicide risk by noting whether the patient exhibits or articulates indications that might suggest a high risk for suicide. This is especially important in interacting with individuals who are refusing medical care. As part of the exam process, note the presence of current wounds or old scars, especially over arterial sites such as the wrist, inside the elbow, and neck. Be suspicious of any solo activities that have a high potential for death. Do not be afraid to ask the patient directly, "Are you trying to hurt yourself?" because many patients are relieved that someone has heard their cry for help.

Patients with paranoid tendencies can be difficult to assess because they are typically suspicious of anyone who attempts to help them. Some patients may accuse you of attempting to harm them; others may openly seek your protection. The irrational fears of paranoid patients often lead these patients to refuse a physical examination or the use of medical equipment such as a blood pressure cuff on them. paranoid patients who are psychotic may complain of hearing voices that feed their anxieties.

Patients who have a psychotic disorder such as schizophrenia are among the most difficult behavioral emergency patients to assess, especially if they are concurrently paranoid. These patients often have auditory hallucinations of voices that instruct them to harm themselves or others or to engage in bizarre or dangerous activities. It is important to ask schizophrenic patients if they have taken their medications as prescribed, because schizophrenic attacks are often precipitated by the patient's noncompliance with

**Table 33-5** Signs of Physical Abuse

- Bruises or injuries of various ages, especially in young children
- Injuries that are not age appropriate (e.g., a long bone fracture in a child under 1 year)
- Fear of physical contact
- Exaggerated startle reflex
- Obvious fear of a spouse, significant other, parent, guardian, or sibling
- Suspicious injuries that are "explained away" by the patient or a significant other

**Table 33-6** Signs and Symptoms of Sexual Abuse

- Frequent, unexplained somatic complaints (e.g., headaches, stomach aches)
- Description of inappropriate touching or physical contact of a sexual nature
- Self-mutilation
- Poor personal hygiene

their medications. Patients who appear to be psychotic do not think or act rationally, so reasoning with them can be extremely difficult, if not impossible. Beside being paranoid, psychotic patients can also describe symptoms of depression, anxiety, or mania.

Any patient who has been abused, whether only recently or over a long period of time, may exhibit numerous behavior-related signs and symptoms. Abuse is a crime that, if suspected, must usually be reported to those who will be caring for the patient and to law enforcement officials. Abuse should be suspected whenever any tell-tale signs or symptoms are present. Signs of physical abuse are listed in Table 33-5■, and signs and symptoms of sexual abuse are listed in Table 33-6■.

Complete the secondary assessment as you would for any patient, using the OPQRST and DCAP-BTLS mnemonics, noting all pertinent signs or symptoms and documenting them on the patient care report. Obtain a complete set of vital signs and monitor them frequently, especially if the patient has ingested any drugs or alcohol. Continue to treat patients in a dignified, caring manner, regardless of their appearance, attitude, or behavior, and document all assessment findings on the patient care report. Be ready to protect yourself if you detect even the possibility of aggressive or violent behavior.

⊕ **33-7** Describe and demonstrate the treatment of a patient with a behavioral emergency.

# **M**anagement

The treatment of patients having a behavioral emergency is both preventative and supportive. Prevention efforts center on keeping patients safe and away from hazards or potential weapons, and on preventing them from harming themselves or others. As with any patient, treatment begins by correcting any potential threats to life, including any external hemorrhage resulting from self-inflicted wounds.

Until proven otherwise, assume that the patient's abnormal behavior results from an underlying medical condition. Because many behavioral emergencies, including apparent psychosis, are due to hypoxia, place the patient on oxygen using a nonrebreather mask at 15 LPM. Likewise, if the symptoms of hypoglycemia are present, consider administering glucose as described in Chapter 11, Altered Mental Status, being careful to adhere to all state, provincial, or local protocols. Continue to calm and reassure the patient as you provide treatment. Be empathetic to the patient's feelings, and redirect the patient's attention as needed to reduce anxiety, paranoia, or suicidal thoughts. Finally, remember that special patient situations warrant additional help in the form of additional patrollers, area management, and (if appropriate) police authorities.

Consider restraining patients who exhibit violent behavior or present a danger to themselves or others, following all local protocols and procedures. This is especially important for any patient who presents with psychosis. Continue to provide supportive care as needed, and transport the patient to the nearest definitive-care facility for further evaluation and ongoing treatment. Be sure to carefully document the patient encounter on the patient care report, including the patient's behavior and response to treatment. Use direct quotes as appropriate to convey the patient's feelings.

# STOP, THINK, UNDERSTAND

## Multiple Choice

Choose the correct answer.

1. You are working to stabilize a critically injured patient at a scene involving multiple injured people and some fatalities. A woman approaches you screaming hysterically that she cannot find her daughter. What is your best course of action? _____
   a. Tell her you are sorry but you are too busy to help her right now.
   b. Acknowledge that she must be feeling very frightened and anxious, and ask a passer-by or a fellow rescuer to help her.
   c. Tell her to "get out of your face" and that "lots of other people can't find their kids, either."
   d. Stop what you are doing and help this woman find her daughter.

2. A pale, diaphoretic man who is suffering from chest pains and an irregular heartbeat tells you that "my mother is standing right next to you!" The patient's wife whispers to you that the man's mother passed away three years ago. What is your appropriate response?
   _____
   a. Tell the patient you are glad his mother is there for him.
   b. Firmly tell the patient that he is hallucinating, that his mother is not there.
   c. Pretend you didn't hear the patient and ignore his remark.
   d. Gently tell the patient, "I can't see her," and then redirect the patient to answering some SAMPLE questions.

3. A patient with a prior history of anxiety and panic attacks is sitting in the lodge cafeteria. His vital signs are a pulse rate of 110 bpm and a respiratory rate of 32 breaths per minute. He denies any accident or illness but says that his lips are tingling and he feels as if he is going to faint. What is your best course of action?
   _____
   a. Have him lie down, calm him, and have him breathe in a slow, controlled fashion.
   b. Call immediately for an ambulance with ALS.
   c. Tell him to start coughing so that he does not go into cardiac arrest.
   d. Slap him, because this will shock him enough to calm him down.

4. You are caring for a 20-year-old male snowboarder who suffered a fractured femur after he ducked under a "Danger, Cliff Ahead" sign and attempted to board off the cliff. Which of the following actions would be appropriate for you to take with this patient?
   _____
   a. Say, "That was a really dumb thing to do."
   b. Gently ask, "Are you trying to hurt yourself?"
   c. Shake your head and say, "What were you thinking?"
   d. Gently ask, "Have you tried to commit suicide before?"

5. Which of the following statements is true? _____
   a. Any patient exhibiting abnormal behavior should be assumed to have a psychiatric disorder until proven otherwise.
   b. Any patient exhibiting abnormal behavior should be assumed to be suffering from psychosis until proven otherwise.
   c. Any patient exhibiting abnormal behavior should be assumed to have an underlying medical condition until proven otherwise.
   d. An OEC Technician should not make any assumptions about a patient exhibiting abnormal behavior.

6. You are called to a scene in which a patient is behaving bizarrely, including yelling at you and others to "just leave me alone!" A friend of the patient tells you that the patient has diabetes and hasn't eaten in several hours. What is your best course of action?
   _____
   a. Reassure the patient, and then sit back and wait for him to recompose himself.
   b. Tell the friend to get the patient a hamburger and make him eat it.
   c. Speak calmly and reassuringly to the patient, and encourage him to allow you to administer oral glucose to him by mixing two packets of sugar into a glass of orange juice.
   d. Firmly tell the patient that his behavior is unacceptable, and that if he doesn't calm down you will have to notify law enforcement authorities.

*continued*

**STOP, THINK, UNDERSTAND** *continued*

7. Which of the following directives regarding approaching a patient with a potential behavioral emergency are appropriate or correct? (check all that apply)

_____ a. Listen to your gut instinct.

_____ b. Make mental notes about possible escape routes.

_____ c. Do not let the patient get between you and your escape route.

_____ d. Approach the patient quietly from behind.

_____ e. Tell the patient you are there to help.

_____ f. Do not identify yourself as an authority figure such as an OEC Technician because doing so could trigger a psychotic episode.

_____ g. Stand above the patient because being at the patient's eye level makes you vulnerable to attack.

_____ h. Speak loudly and firmly.

_____ i. Never approach the patient directly, even if you have received permission to do so.

_____ j. Avoid sudden movements.

_____ k. Speak loudly and firmly to assert your authority.

_____ l. Do not make any assumptions about the patient.

---

**⊕ 33-8** List the indications for restraining a patient.

**⊕ 33-9** Describe and demonstrate how to properly restrain a patient.

**restraint**   any method, physical or mechanical, that restricts the movement of a patient.

**reasonable force**   the minimum force needed to keep a patient from hurting himself or others.

**Figure 33-16a** Sometimes the use of physical restraint becomes necessary due to an individual's violent behavior.
Copyright Craig Brown

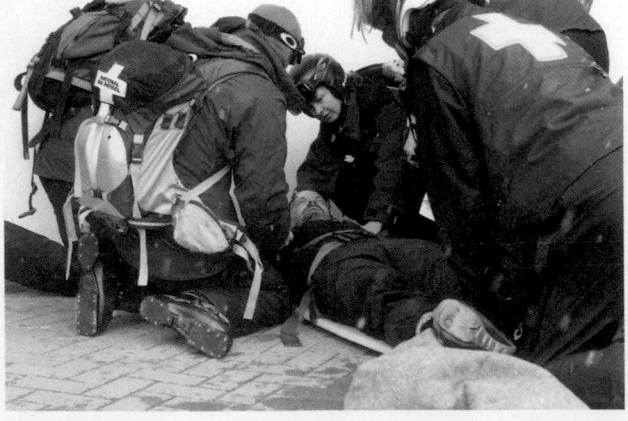

## Restraints

When a patient's behavioral emergency escalates to the point at which words are no longer calming and the patient poses an imminent threat of violence, physical restraint is needed (Figure 33-16a■). Under these circumstances, there is no alternative but to protect the safety of the patient, the rescuers, and bystanders. The most common indication for the use of restraints is a violent psychotic patient.

Before applying restraint, OEC Technicians should decide if the patient has the capacity (or ability) to refuse medical care. If the patient does and is not an imminent danger to himself or others, you should neither touch nor threaten to touch the individual. Assessing for the capacity to refuse medical care is a complex issue that is beyond the scope of this chapter, and it is ultimately dictated by local protocols with the guidance of medical direction. Ask for the assistance of area security or law enforcement personnel in isolating the individual, both for your safety and for the safety of others.

Restraint is a process that restricts a patient's normal movement; its ultimate goal is to prevent the patient from harming himself or others. OEC Technicians should be familiar with two forms of restraint: physical restraint, which involves directly holding onto a patient, and mechanical restraint, which involves the use of equipment such as a flexible band, strap, or cuff. Only patients who are clearly demonstrating an imminent danger to themselves or others should be restrained. It is best to seek the patient's cooperation to avoid the need for restraint. Unfortunately, this may not always be possible.

Restraining a patient, if necessary, is best done by law enforcement officials or a higher level of medical authority. Whereas law enforcement personnel can restrain anyone if they have probable cause, this is not true for medical personnel (Figure 33-16b■). Most states and provinces have specific laws governing the use of restraints by those outside of law enforcement. In fact, physicians have very limited abilities to order prehospital personnel to medically restrain a patient. When permitted, the prevailing tenet is to use only **reasonable force**, the minimum amount of force required to keep the patient from hurting himself or others. Many factors contribute to determining this level of force, including the patient's size, strength, mental attitude, and degree of agitation; the type of abnormal behavior; and the availability of restraint equipment and personnel. OEC Technicians must be familiar with their local protocols regarding the use of restraints and the procedures for restraining a combative patient. They should also be aware that use of excessive force can have both civil and criminal legal consequences.

If it becomes necessary to restrain a patient, all on-scene personnel must work together. Ideally, a minimum of five people are required to safely restrain a patient: one person to hold each extremity, and one person to hold the patient's head in neutral alignment. If the patient must be mechanically restrained, a sixth person is needed to apply the mechanical restraints. The patient and/or the rescuers are more likely to be injured when too few personnel are available to properly restrain a patient. A team leader should be designated, and that leader should brief all personnel involved on their respective roles.

Once a plan is established, the team should move into position upon a receiving a pre-established signal. A simple show of force will often prompt a patient to submit peacefully. The team leader should always attempt to seek the patient's cooperation and consent to treatment. If the patient remains noncompliant, then it becomes necessary to restrain the patient. Throughout the restraining process, continue to talk to the patient, providing instructions in a firm voice. Be polite at all times. Use statements such as, "Sir, please stop fighting us," "We are here to help you," and "Please lie down." Once the patient is physically restrained, use only enough force to keep the patient submissive; any additional force may be considered excessive. See OEC Skill 33-1■.

Under most circumstances, any patient that required physical restraint to be brought under control should be mechanically restrained until examined by a physician. Such patients should be placed face up on a backboard to facilitate safe transport and the monitoring of vital signs. The exact method by which you mechanically restrain a patient should be consistent with local protocol as approved by your medical director. In one widely accepted technique, one of the patient's arms is secured to the board above the patient's head to prevent the patient from sitting up. The patient's other arm should be extended alongside the torso and tied to the board. The legs, too, should be securely tied to the lower end of the board while remaining a neutral alignment. Additional straps may be secured across the patient's hips and chest to further increase restraint. Be ready to tip the board on its side should the patient vomit. Never stick your finger in a restrained patient's mouth. Additionally, never restrain a patient in a prone position, and never "hog-tie" a patient because in both cases death can result due to **positional asphyxia**.

Positional asphyxia is a lethal condition in which the patient's own body weight impairs the ability to breathe, resulting in suffocation and death. Continuously monitor a restrained patient, paying close attention to the patient's ABCDs, skin color, vital signs, and distal CMS. Ideally, the vital signs and distal CMS status should be reevaluated every 5–10 minutes.

Handcuffs may only be used by law enforcement personnel who should physically accompany the patient to the hospital. Restrained patients often try to persuade medical personnel to remove the restraints. However, once applied, restraints should remain in place until the patient is turned over to the definitive-care facility's personnel. Be sure to provide thorough documentation of both the patient's behavior before, during, and after the application of restraints and your reasons for using restraints. Documentation should also include what efforts were taken to avoid restraining the patient, the restraint method(s) used, the total time the patient was restrained, and all ongoing CMS exams.

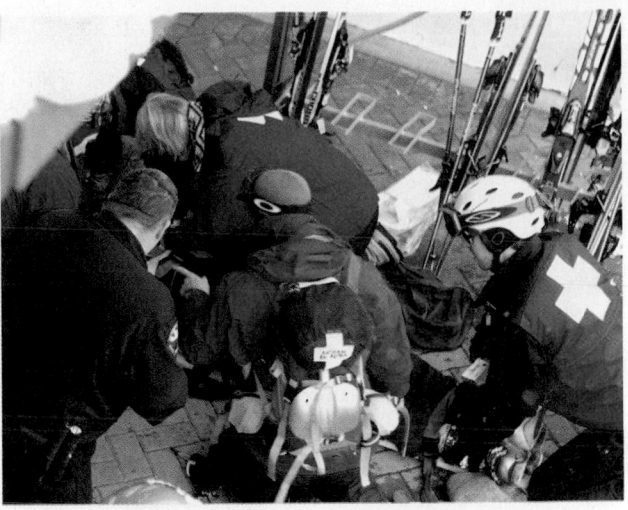

**Figure 33-16b** Even though law-enforcement personnel need only probable cause to restrain anyone, this is *not* the case for medical personnel.
Copyright Craig Brown

**Behavior and Injury**

One of the most difficult situations to deal with is how to handle the head injured patient who is aggressive, appears psychotic, will not listen to reason, and yet needs spinal immobilization due a traumatic injury. You will need help from another trained rescuer to provide careful handling for this person who is exhibiting behavioral issues. Aggressive restraint in order to immobilize this patient to a spine board may be necessary; however it is important to exercise care and not cause more harm to the patient.

**positional asphyxia** a fatal condition in which a patient's body weight impairs the ability to breathe, resulting in suffocation.

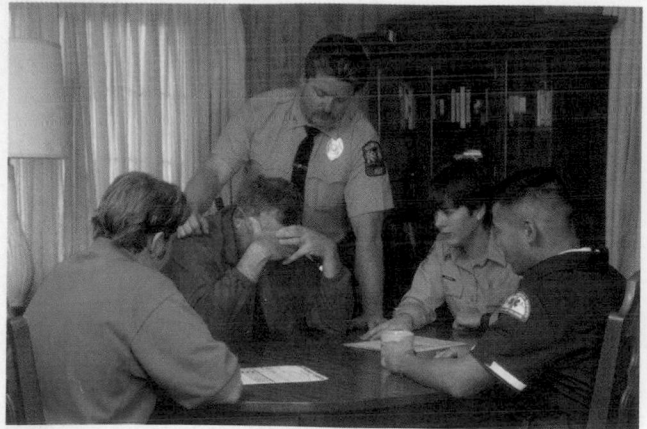

**Figure 33-17** Some communities have CISM organizations that can help rescuers process and work through a psychologically traumatic incident.

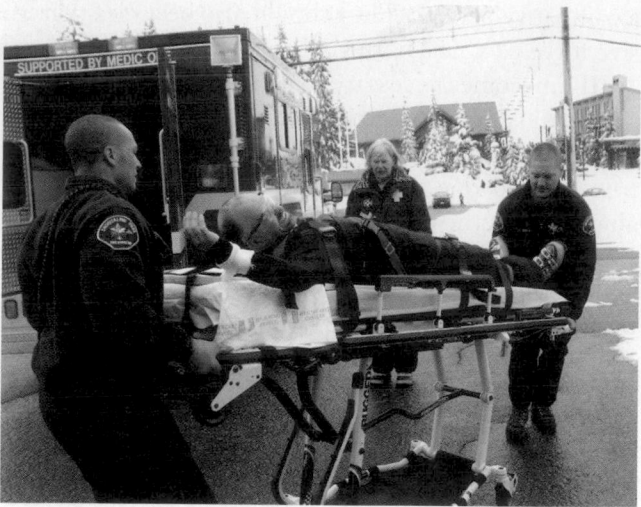

**Figure 33-18** Individuals who exhibit abnormal behavior should be considered to have a medical illness and transported to a medical facility for further evaluation.
Copyright Craig Brown

## Critical Incident Stress

As an OEC Technician, you are not immune to the emotional and psychological consequences of managing ill or injured patients and witnessing death. The consequences may be either short lived or long term. Rescuers and others involved in extraordinary circumstances can be adversely affected by such encounters and can suffer a variety of symptoms of post-traumatic stress disorder, including difficulty concentrating, inability to sleep, repeatedly replaying the incident, headache, gastrointestinal abnormalities, profound sadness, and depression. Fortunately, professional help is available to rescuers who may need assistance in working through the aftermath of a traumatic incident, and many agencies have formal agreements with a local critical incident stress management (CISM) team created for this very purpose (Figure 33-17■). If you find yourself disturbed by an incident, seek assistance (Figure 33-18■). You are not alone.

## STOP, THINK, UNDERSTAND

### Multiple Choice
Choose the correct answer.

1. Which of the following statements about the use of restraints is true? _____
   a. Law-enforcement personnel may restrain anyone if they have probable cause.
   b. OEC Technicians may restrain anyone if they have probable cause.
   c. An OEC Technician may restrain a combative patient who is a danger to others and is capable of refusing medical care.
   d. An OEC Technician may restrain an angry patron at a ski resort who is threatening to punch a snowboarder who collided with his son.

2. The goal of restraint is to _____
   a. enable you to administer medical care to a patient who is refusing care.
   b. prevent a patient from harming himself or others.
   c. force an out-of-control patient to calm down.
   d. prevent a mentally competent patient who has harmed someone from leaving the scene.

*continued*

3. If restraining a patient has become necessary, what is the ideal minimum number of people required to safely administer non-mechanical restraint? _____

   a. two
   b. three
   c. four
   d. five

4. How frequently should the ABCDs be assessed on a stable patient who has been restrained? _____

   a. Every 5 minutes.
   b. Every 15 minutes.
   c. Whenever some aspect of the patient's condition appears to change.
   d. Immediately after applying the restraints and again just before transferring the patient to a higher level of care.

5. What is the correct course of action when a restrained patient calms down and asks you to please remove the restraints? _____

   a. Tell the patient you will do so if they promise to remain calm.
   b. Remove the restraints immediately because not doing so constitutes assault on the patient.
   c. Leave the restraints on, because only a definitive medical care provider can remove them.
   d. Tell the patient you will loosen or remove only one of the arm restraints to reduce the feeling of claustrophobia.

6. The use of a critical incident stress management team is _____

   a. indicative of psychological weakness.
   b. a beneficial strategy for working through traumatic incidents.
   c. only necessary in the first week or so following a traumatic event.
   d. available to EMS, fire, and law-enforcement personnel, but not to OEC Technicians.

7. A behavioral emergency is _____

   a. a sign of psychological weakness on the part of the patient.
   b. something OEC Technicians will rarely, if ever, have to deal with.
   c. something to be dealt with firmly.
   d. a possible response to an injury or illness.

# ✚ CASE DISPOSITION ✚

You try to calm the patient by having him breathe in a slow, controlled fashion. After several minutes, he calms down and stops crying. Shortly thereafter, the tingling subsides, so he now has full use of his hands and no longer feels faint. He drinks some bottled sports drink from his backpack. Embarrassed, he tells you that he has been very stressed since his older brother died, and he thanks you for your kindness. You and another OEC Technician accompany the patient and his sister to the top of the ridge, which is only a quarter mile away. From a respectful distance, you watch as the pair opens an urn and throws ashes off the ridge. As the two hug each other, you smile, knowing that the healing process has begun.

This behavioral emergency was likely brought on by the combination of anxiety, grief, and low blood sugar. The techniques used to manage the patient and his behavior enabled the OEC Technician to de-escalate what could have been a potentially difficult situation.

## OEC SKILL 33-1 Physical/Mechanical Restraint of a Patient

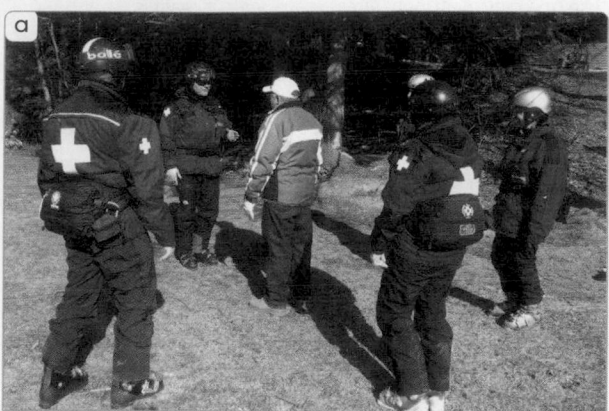

**a** Make a plan involving all the rescuers and then have one person speak calmly with the patient.
Copyright Edward McNamara

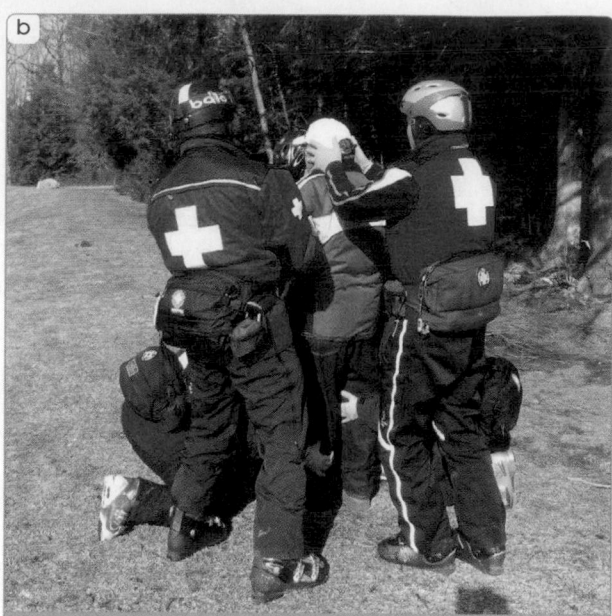

**b** The team moves into position upon receiving a preestablished signal. Each member of the team should restrain either a single limb or the head.
Copyright Edward McNamara

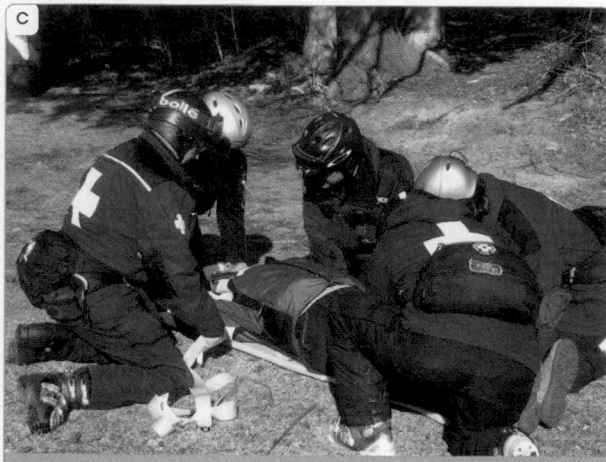

**c** Firmly support the patient as you lower him to the ground or onto a backboard.
Copyright Edward McNamara

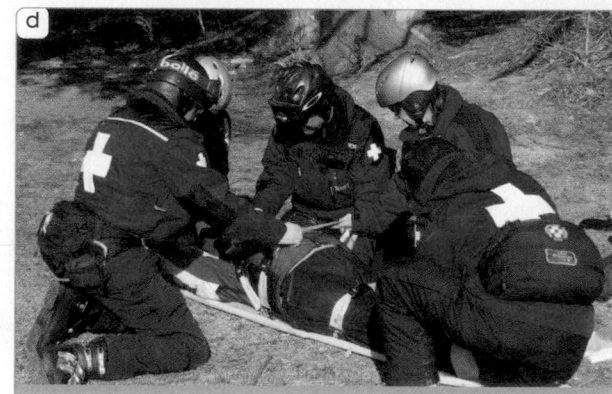

**d** Secure the patient with his right arm over his head and his left arm along his torso.
Copyright Edward McNamara

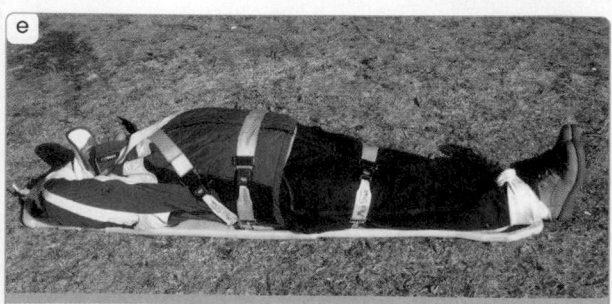

**e** Tie the patient down completely using as many straps as needed; be prepared to tilt the board if the patient should vomit.
Copyright Edward McNamara

## Skill Guide

Date: _____

(CPI) = Critical Performance Indicator

Candidate: _____

Start Time: _____

End Time: _____

## Patient Restraint

**Objective:** To demonstrate the ability to safely restrain a patient.

| Skill | Max Points | Skill Demo | |
|---|---|---|---|
| Determines scene is safe. | 1 | | (CPI) |
| Introduces self, obtains permission to treat/help. | 1 | | |
| Initiates Standard Precautions. | 1 | | (CPI) |
| Secures the scene. | 1 | | |
| Determines if patient can refuse care. | 1 | | |
| Calls for additional help or assistance per local protocol. | 1 | | (CPI) |
| Assembles 5 people for physical restrain, 6 people for mechanical restraint. | 1 | | |
| Uses appropriate language with patient to not escalate situation. | 1 | | (CPI) |
| Places patient on spine board. | 1 | | |
| Secures one of the patient's arms above the head. | 1 | | |
| Secures patient's other arm at side. | 1 | | |
| Prepares for patient vomiting (has suction equipment available for use if needed). | 1 | | (CPI) |
| Monitors vital signs every 5–10 minutes. | 1 | | (CPI) |
| Maintains patient restraint until care is transferred. | 1 | | |

Must receive 11 out of 14 points.

Comments: _____

Failure of any of the CPIs is an automatic failure.

Evaluator: _____ NSP ID: _____

PASS     FAIL

# ⛊ Chapter Review

## Chapter Summary

Abnormal or bizarre behavior is not an unusual occurrence in prehospital settings and is a sign that the central nervous system is in distress due to a variety of causes, not all of which are psychiatric in origin. Patients who exhibit inappropriate behavior are typically normal people who are confronting extraordinary circumstances and have become unable to control their emotions. Altered mental status can also be caused by a traumatic or medical condition that changes a patient's behavior. Accordingly, abnormal behavior with altered mental status is considered a medical condition until proven otherwise, an approach that ensures that an underlying medical or traumatic problem is not overlooked.

Mental illness is a complex collection of disorders that cannot be accurately diagnosed in the field and instead requires careful, thorough evaluation by a trained mental-health professional. The goals of treating a patient exhibiting abnormal behavior in a prehospital setting are to ensure the safety of everyone involved, correct potential threats to life, and treat symptoms as they become apparent. Given that many cases of abnormal behavior are medical in origin, provide supplemental oxygen and glucose whenever they are indicated. If the patient appears to be psychotic, usual reasoning methods on the part of the OEC Technician may not be effective.

OEC Technicians will encounter people in crisis. By being empathetic to the person's plight and demonstrating a caring demeanor, OEC Technicians may be able to de-escalate a potentially violent or hazardous situation. Like their patients, OEC Technicians are not immune to the stressors inherent to emergencies and may find themselves having difficulty handling their feelings. Should this occur, it is imperative that OEC Technicians recognize the signs of post-traumatic stress in themselves and their colleagues and seek follow-up care.

## Remember...

1. Personal safety is the top priority when managing a behavioral emergency.
2. A behavioral emergency exists when a person exhibits abnormal thoughts or actions.
3. The cause of a behavioral emergency may be medical, chemical, traumatic, or psychiatric.
4. Signs and symptoms of a behavioral emergency include panic, agitation, violence, and self-destructive behavior.
5. The five stages of grief are denial, anger, bargaining, depression, and acceptance.
6. Calming patients is one of the most important components of managing a behavioral emergency.
7. If appropriate, call for help, including area security personal and police authorities.
8. Always keep your cool.

## Chapter Questions

### Multiple Choice

Choose the correct answer.

1. You should consider a situation in which an individual swallows four aspirin tablets and then says he wants to die to be_____
   a. silly and insignificant.
   b. something you should ignore because focusing on it becomes attention getting.
   c. a serious suicide attempt.
   d. a suicidal gesture.

2. What is your best course of action regarding an obviously agitated patient who has a profusely bleeding gash on his head from a fallen rock and who threatens you if you come any closer?_____
   a. Leave the scene immediately because it is not safe, and remain as far from the man as you can.
   b. Try to reason with the individual.
   c. Ignore his request, speak reassuringly, and proceed with treating his wound.
   d. Call for assistance, and then continue to speak reassuringly to the patient from a distance so he does not feel threatened and then care for the patient since he may have a head injury.

3. Under which of the following circumstances may an OEC Technician restrain a patient? _____
   a. When a patient who is capable of refusing medical care poses a danger to himself or others.
   b. When a patient suffering from a gash on his thigh blocks a chairlift off-ramp and angrily tells rescuers, "Leave me alone; I'll move when I'm damn good and ready".
   c. When a moderately inebriated woman has bitten another woman in a bar for flirting with her boyfriend.
   d. When a patient with a head injury becomes combative and incapable of refusing medical care.

4. Which of the following positions is correct for placing a patient in mechanical restraints? _____
   a. Supine, with both arms secured above the patient's head and both legs straight.
   b. Supine, with the right arm secured above the patient's head, the left arm secured at the patient's side, and both legs straight.
   c. Prone, with both arms secured above the patient's head, and both legs secured to the backboard.
   d. Curled up on the left side with both hands and both feet tied together.

## Matching

1. For each of the following descriptions, indicate whether the individual is suffering from a neurosis or from a psychosis.

   _____ 1. neurosis
   _____ 2. psychosis

   a. an individual who is depressed
   b. an individual who tells you he is capable of surviving a snowboard jump off an 80-foot-high cliff
   c. an anxious individual who washes his hands 20–30 times a day out of fear of contracting AIDS
   d. an individual who tells you his deceased mother is telling him to jump off a cliff
   e. an individual who believes he is Jesus

2. For each of the following descriptions, indicate whether the individual is most likely suffering from a medical/traumatic condition or from a psychiatric disorder.

   _____ 1. psychiatric disorder
   _____ 2. medical/traumatic condition

   a. a skier who launched off of a 30-foot cliff and tells you he did so because God told him to do it
   b. an individual who wanders into your aid room and tells you he keeps hearing voices in his head
   c. an individual who wanders into your aid room and tells you that he sees flashing lights and swirls moving across his range of vision
   d. an individual suffering from chest pains who tells you his deceased mother is standing next to you
   e. an individual found sitting alongside a hiking trail who shrieks at you to "Shut up, shut up! Turn the voices off!"
   f. a pale and diaphoretic individual who is yelling that his chest hurts

## Scenario

*You receive a call for medical assistance for a teenager in the Main Lodge. Upon arrival you find a young male who is totally out of control; he is cursing and throwing objects at people.*

1. The first action you should take is to_____
   a. immediately leave the area.
   b. clear the area of any bystanders and ask if any of them knows the teenager.
   c. rush in and restrain the teenager.
   d. walk up and ask the teenager face to face what is wrong.

*A bystander tells you that the teenager has been diagnosed with bipolar disorder and has not been taking his prescribed lithium. The youth has also been depressed and is taking unprescribed tranquilizers.*

2. A patient who has bipolar disorder and is in a depressive phase_____
   a. may have episodes of spending sprees.
   b. experiences unusual highs.
   c. may talk faster than normal and cannot focus.
   d. may demonstrate suicidal tendencies.

*Realizing that the situation is serious, you call for additional help, including members of management, police personnel, an ambulance, and O₂. You announce that you are a medical responder and want to help, and then you occupy a safe position next to a nearby exit.*

3. Which of the following actions is not appropriate? _____
   a. Take extra time to listen to the patient.
   b. Diffuse the situation by restraining the patient.
   c. Ask the patient what is wrong.
   d. Keep at least 3 feet from the patient until the patient says coming closer is okay.

*While waiting for your requested assistance, you ask the patient if it is okay to take his pulse. After receiving permission, you reach out and wait for the patient to present his arm. His pulse is 100 bpm and strong and regular. The O₂ arrives with assisting personnel. When you ask the patient if he would sit down and let you administer nasal oxygen, he refuses.*

*When the ambulance crew and police officer arrive, you ask them to stay back. You take a few steps away from the patient to update the police officer and ambulance crew concerning the patient's history and pulse rate. With assistance from the police officer, you hand over care of the patient to the ambulance crew, who transport the patient to the hospital, where he is admitted and administered the proper medications for controlling his condition. You return to your base to create an incident report.*

## Suggested Reading

Auerbach, P. S. 2007. *Wilderness Medicine*, Fifth Edition, Chapter 30: Mental Health in the Wilderness. St. Louis: Mosby.

Mistovich, J. J., B. Q. Hafen, and K. J. Karren. 2010. *Prehospital Emergency Care*, Ninth Edition. Upper Saddle River, NJ: Pearson Education.

Mitchell, J.T., Resnik, H.L.P. *Emergency Response to Crisis: A Crisis Intervention Guidebook for Emergency Service Personnel*, Upper Saddle River: Pearson Education.

EXPLORE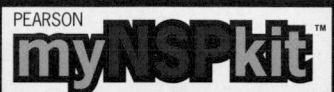

Please go to www.myNSPkit.com. Under Student Resources, you will find animations, videos, web links, and games related to this chapter—and much more. Look for information on application of soft restraints, schizophrenia, bipolar disorder, helping the combative patient, and more.

Register your access code from the front of your book by going to www.myNSPkit.com and selecting the appropriate links. If the in-cover access code has been redeemed, go to www.myNSPkit.com and follow links to **Buy Access**.

# Obstetric and Gynecologic Emergencies

Nici Singletary, MD, FACEP

## ⊕ OBJECTIVES

**Upon completion of this chapter, the OEC Technician will be able to:**

**34-1** Identify the major anatomical structures within the pelvic cavity.

**34-2** List the functions of the female genitourinary and reproductive system.

**34-3** List the functions of the major gynecologic structures.

**34-4** List three causes of abdominal pain of gynecologic or obstetrical origin.

**34-5** List four possible causes of vaginal bleeding.

**34-6** List the three stages of a normal pregnancy.

**34-7** List three possible consequences of abdominal trauma in a pregnant patient.

**34-8** Describe four possible complications of pregnancy.

**34-9** Demonstrate how to examine a female patient with abdominal or pelvic pain.

**34-10** Describe how to assess the abdomen of a pregnant patient.

**34-11** Describe the process of assisting an emergency delivery.

**34-12** Describe the management of a pregnant patient with abdominal trauma.

## Chapter Overview

The female anatomy is unique in that it enables reproduction and the continuation of the human species. The normal cycle of ovulation—the production of an egg—is typically followed either by menstruation (if the egg is not fertilized) or by pregnancy (if fertilization occurs).

Gynecological emergencies are emergent conditions unique to women and involve the genital or reproductive tract. Obstetric emergencies pertain to a woman

*continued*

*continued*

## HISTORICAL TIMELINE

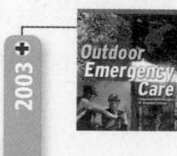

**2003** *OEC Fourth Edition* is published.

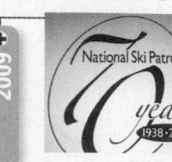 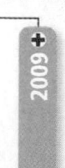

**2009** NSP celebrates its 70th anniversary during its annual board meeting in Denver, Colorado.

**2009** Editorial work is underway on OEC Fifth Edition.

## ⊕ KEY TERMS

| | | |
|---|---|---|
| **abruptio placentae**, *p. 1078* | **gestation**, *p. 1071* | **pelvic inflammatory disease (PID)**, *p. 1074* |
| **cystitis**, *p. 1074* | **gestational period**, *p. 1071* | **placenta previa**, *p. 1078* |
| **dysmenorrhea**, *p. 1073* | **hematuria**, *p. 1074* | **preeclampsia**, *p. 1078* |
| **eclampsia**, *p. 1078* | **miscarriage**, *p. 1078* | **reproductive age**, *p. 1073* |
| **ectopic pregnancy**, *p. 1074* | **ovarian cysts**, *p. 1074* | |

who is pregnant or is delivering an infant, or in the period immediately after delivery, even if the emergency is related to a nonreproductive medical condition such as asthma. During pregnancy a medical or traumatic emergency can potentially result in the injury or death of two patients; the mother and the fetus. The health and well-being of the mother affects the fetus, and vice versa. For OEC Technicians, this situation presents unique challenges because caring for a pregnant woman means you are in fact managing two patients (Figure 34-1■).

The organs that constitute the genitourinary and reproductive system lie primarily in the pelvis, although during pregnancy the expanding uterus rises out of the pelvic cavity and into the abdominal cavity. The relative proximity of the genitourinary, reproductive, and gastrointestinal systems and common nerve pathways explain why the signs and symptoms associated with gastrointestinal problems and obstetrical or gynecologic problems are often similar. When evaluating and caring for a female of reproductive age who has abdominal or pelvic pain, always consider the possibility of pregnancy, even if she denies that possibility. Bear in mind that such patients may have a problem related to the gastrointestinal, genitourinary, or reproductive systems. For a complete review of acute abdominal emergencies that are not related to the reproductive system, please refer to Chapter 16, Gastrointestinal and Genitourinary Emergencies.

Gynecologic emergencies are common, but fortunately they are not usually life threatening. Obstetrical emergencies, by contrast, often threaten the life of the fetus and/or the mother, even when the mother's appearance and vital signs are deceptively normal. Although OEC Technicians may not be likely to encounter women in advanced stages of pregnancy in outdoor environments, many athletic women continue to exercise and enjoy outdoor activities well into their pregnancies. It is likely that you will eventually be called upon to care for a pregnant woman who is in labor or has a medical or traumatic emergency. The goals for management of gynecologic—and particularly obstetrical—emergencies are the rapid identification of a potentially serious or life-threatening condition followed by immediate treatment and evacuation to a care center.

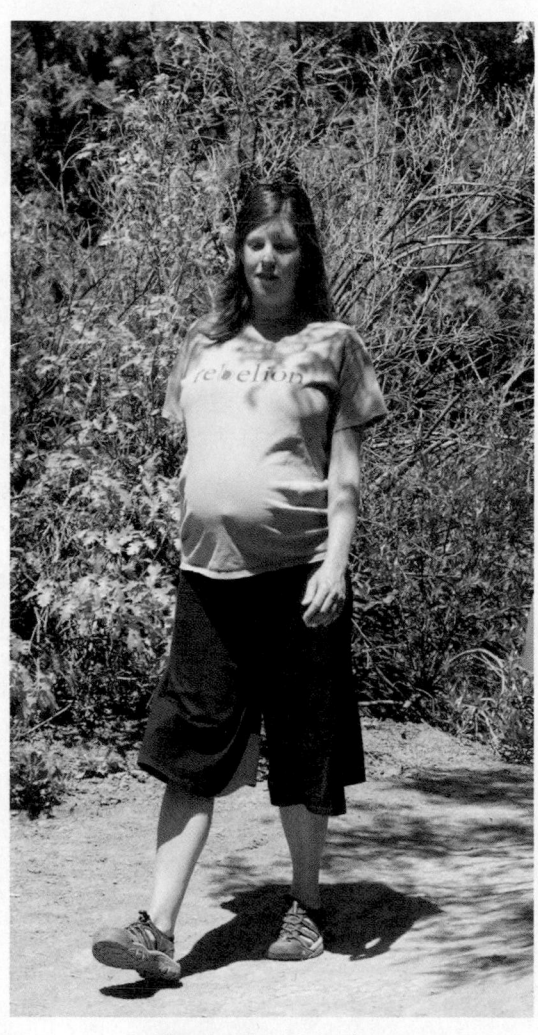

**Figure 34-1** Caring for a pregnant woman means that you are in fact caring for two patients.
Copyright Scott Smith

## Anatomy & Physiology

The woman's genitourinary, gastrointestinal, and reproductive systems are located within the abdominopelvic cavity. As previously described, the boundaries of the pelvic cavity include an imaginary line extending between the iliac crests (superior), the ischium (inferior), internal muscles (anterior), the ileum (lateral), and the sacrum (posterior). Thus, with the exception of the anterior wall, the pelvic organs are well protected by the pelvic bones. The major internal structures of the female

⊕ **34-1** Identify the major anatomical structures within the pelvic cavity.

⊕ **34-2** List the functions of the female genitourinary and reproductive system.

# CASE PRESENTATION

You are called to the ski school instruction area, where a 26-year-old woman who is observing her toddler in a class has slipped and fallen on hard packed snow. The woman is 34 weeks pregnant and is complaining of severe abdominal pain. Upon your arrival, the woman is lying supine on the snow with both knees flexed. She is awake and oriented, and very worried that her unborn child may have been injured. A ski school instructor witnessed the incident and reports that she fell onto her left side, striking her abdomen. The woman describes her abdominal pain as "sharp" and "all over," and unlike the labor contractions she had during her first delivery. She does not feel any leakage of fluid and denies feeling lightheaded. She reports that her second pregnancy has been uncomplicated to date, and that a recent ultrasound showed a single male fetus. She denies any injury other than that to her abdomen. As you assess the patient, you notice that her radial pulse is quite weak and seems faster than normal.

*What should you do?*

---

**⊕ 34-3** List the functions of the major gynecologic structures.

reproductive system are the ovaries, the fallopian tubes, the uterus, and the vagina (Figure 34-2■), as well as the perineum.

## Ovaries

An ovary is one of two solid reproductive organs located in the right and left lower quadrants. The ovaries contain the ova, or germ cells, and also produce the hormones progesterone and estrogen.

## Fallopian Tubes

The fallopian tubes are two hollow structures that begin in the right and left lower quadrants, near the ovaries, extend downward into the pelvic cavity, and connect to either side of the uterus. An ovum is typically fertilized here, and the tubes serve as a conduit for the mature egg as it travels from an ovary to the uterus.

**Figure 34-2** The female reproductive system.

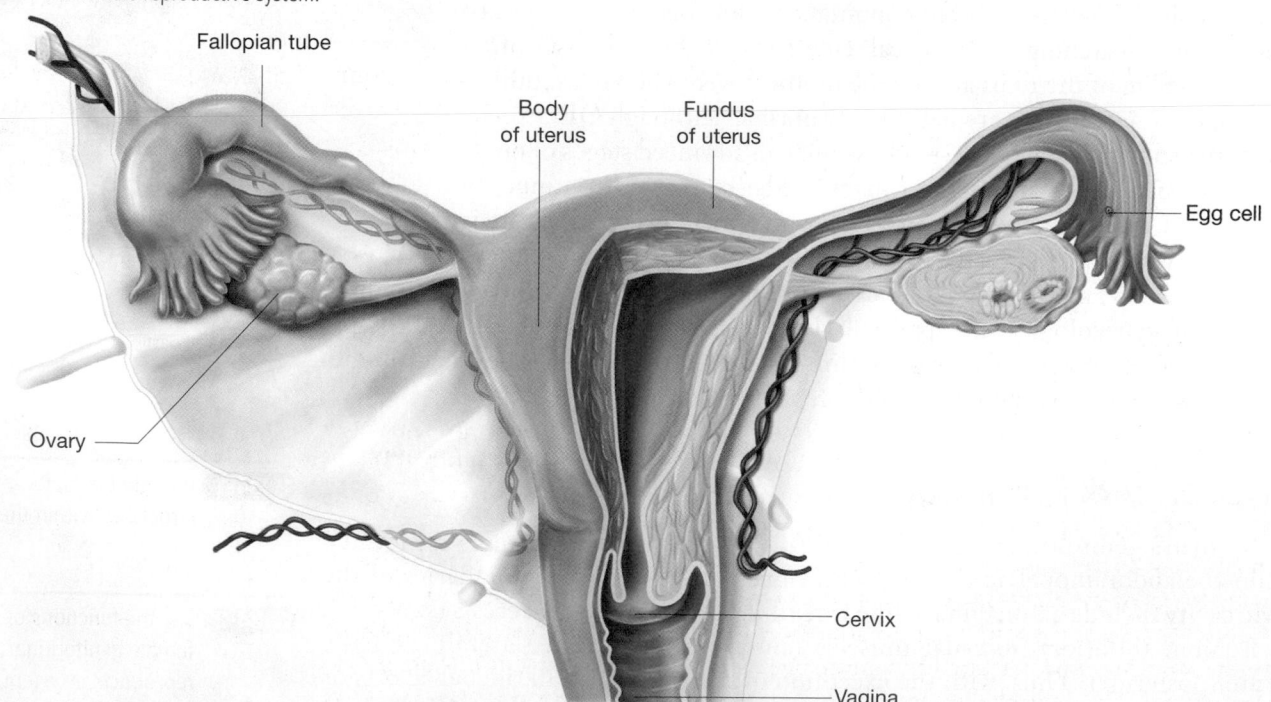

## Uterus

The uterus is a hollow muscular organ in which the fertilized ovum develops into a fetus. The uterus is about 3 inches in length in a non-pregnant female and is supported in the pelvic cavity (behind the urinary bladder and in front of the rectum) by various ligaments. The large, upper, rounded end of the roughly pear-shaped uterus is known as the *fundus*; the elongated lower portion, or *cervix*, ends in an opening known as the *os*. The uterus is normally palpable only during pregnancy.

## Vagina

The vagina is a hollow muscular tube extending from the uterus to an exterior opening, the *vulva*. It serves as an opening for menstrual flow, and is part of the birth canal. During heterosexual intercourse a man's penis is put into the vagina.

## Perineum

The perineum is the outer soft tissue that in a female extends from the vaginal opening to the anus. The perineal area may be torn during childbirth.

## The Reproductive Cycle

The female reproductive cycle begins with ovulation—that is, the release of an ovum or egg from an ovary. This cycle occurs about once every 28 days during a woman's reproductive years (approximately ages 15–50). The ovum travels through a fallopian tube to the uterus, the lining of which becomes thicker and richer in blood vessels in order to receive the ovum. If the ovum has been fertilized, it implants and grows in the lining of the uterus. If not, the ovum dies, and the lining of the uterus breaks down and is expelled through the vagina in the form of menstruation, or a menstrual period, which normally lasts for 5–7 days.

Following fertilization of an ovum by a sperm, an embryo is formed. The embryo is referred to as a fetus from the beginning of the 9th week of pregnancy until delivery. In humans, birth normally occurs from 37 to 42 weeks of pregnancy.

**Gestation** is the time between conception and delivery of a child (approximately 266 days in humans). The **gestational period** is considered to begin on the first day of a woman's last normal menstrual period before fertilization, which is about 2 weeks before fertilization occurs. The gestational period is divided into three trimesters of 12 weeks each. Delivery before 37 weeks is considered "preterm" or premature and can result in a wide spectrum of problems for the infant, most of which result from immature lungs that cannot exchange oxygen. In general, an infant born before the third trimester of pregnancy has a very low chance of survival.

A number of physiologic changes that are important for OEC Technicians to recognize occur during pregnancy. First, the fetus develops within the mother's uterus inside a bag-like amniotic sac that is filled with up to a liter of clear amniotic fluid. This fluid helps to insulate, cushion, and protect the developing baby. Nourishment is provided from the mother via a vascular placenta, which adheres to the uterine wall and is connected to the baby by the umbilical cord. Early in pregnancy, the uterus and developing fetus are protected by the pelvic bones and are not palpable. After 12 to 13 weeks, however, the uterus emerges from this protective bony enclosure, making it vulnerable to direct trauma. By 20 weeks, the uterus rises to the level of the umbilicus—a useful landmark when assessing a pregnant woman. Toward the end of pregnancy, the uterus can extend as high as the diaphragm (Figure 34-3■). Thus, the uterus may be found in all four quadrants of the abdomen as well as the pelvis at the end of a full-term pregnancy.

After 28 weeks of gestation, maternal blood volume (both red blood cell and plasma components) rises. The maternal heart rate increases by 15–20 beats per minute by the third trimester. The respiratory system is also subject to changes during pregnancy. As

**gestation** the period during which a female is pregnant; in humans it is about 266 days, from fertilization of the egg until birth.

**gestational period** the time from the first day of a woman's last normal menstrual period before fertilization, which is about 2 weeks before fertilization, until birth.

**Figure 34-3** The structures within a woman during a full-term pregnancy.

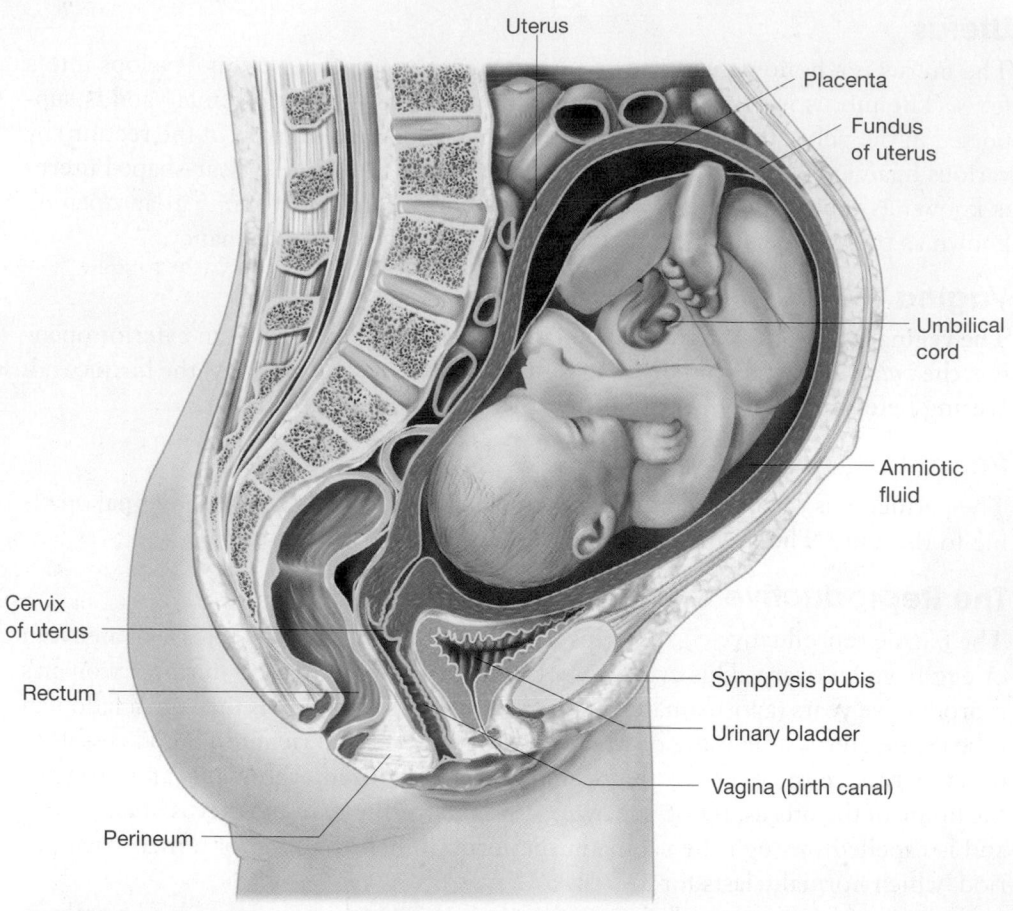

Uterus

Placenta

Fundus of uterus

Umbilical cord

Amniotic fluid

Cervix of uterus

Rectum

Symphysis pubis

Urinary bladder

Vagina (birth canal)

Perineum

the uterus expands, the diaphragm is pushed upward into the thorax, and the ribs compensate by flaring out. The mother's need for oxygen increases as the fetus and uterus grow and as blood volume increases. The respiratory system adapts to this need through a variety of mechanisms that result in a slight increase in respiratory rate.

Changes in maternal physiology also affect blood pressure. Systolic and diastolic blood pressures decrease by 4–6 mmHg and 8–15 mmHg, respectively, reaching their lowest point in mid-pregnancy before returning to normal levels by full term. What does this all mean for OEC Technicians who are assessing a pregnant woman? First, blood pressure, pulse rate, or respiratory rate may not change during the first trimester. However, from the mid-second trimester on, a healthy woman with a typical uncomplicated pregnancy may have a normal blood pressure of 96/60 and a pulse of 100—values that would potentially be considered indicative of shock in a non-pregnant female. Accurate blood pressure measurements are obtained with the patient lying on her left side, a position that prevents the pregnant uterus from placing pressure on the vena cava.

Because of the physiologic changes of pregnancy, a woman may lose 30–35 percent of her blood volume to hemorrhage before showing any signs of shock. However, even though a woman's vital signs may appear stable, her fetus will be in shock due to the combination of decreased blood flow from the uterus to the placenta and the shunting of blood away from the fetus. OEC Technicians should always anticipate the development of shock in a pregnant trauma patient—and in her fetus—even in light of normal vital signs.

## STOP, THINK, UNDERSTAND

### Multiple Choice

Choose the correct answer.

1. Which of the following statements concerning an obstetric emergency is true? _____
   a. It pertains only to complications with the fetus.
   b. It pertains to any medical or traumatic emergency involving a pregnant woman.
   c. An unborn baby is so well protected that trauma rarely affects it.
   d. Obstetric emergencies involve only emergency deliveries in prehospital settings.

2. What are the goals for the management of gynecologic and obstetric emergencies? _____
   a. To rapidly identify a life-threatening condition and thereby deliver a healthy baby in the field.
   b. To stop or delay imminent childbirth until the pregnant woman can reach a hospital.
   c. To rapidly identify potentially serious or life-threatening conditions and immediately care for and evacuate the patient to definitive medical care.

d. OEC Technicians are not authorized to handle this type of emergency.

3. A full-term pregnancy lasts about how long? _____
   a. 20–24 weeks          c. 37–42 weeks
   b. 32–36 weeks          d. 42–46 weeks

4. Pregnancy is divided into three trimesters of how many weeks each? _____
   a. 8                    c. 12
   b. 10                   d. 16

5. What is the function of amniotic fluid? _____
   a. to cushion and protect the baby
   b. to provide nourishment for the baby
   c. to allow the uterus to expand as the baby grows
   d. to prevent the implantation of another ovum during an existing pregnancy

### Short Answer

1. An ovum (or egg) is released from an ovary about every _____ days during a woman's reproductive years, which encompass approximately age _____ to _____.

2. A baby delivered before _____ weeks of gestation is considered to be premature.

# Common Obstetrical and Gynecological Emergencies

## Abdominal Pain

Abdominal pain is the most common presenting complaint for women of **reproductive age** undergoing an obstetrical or gynecological emergency. Among the myriad causes of gynecological abdominal pain are the following conditions:

+ dysmenorrhea
+ cystitis
+ ovarian cysts
+ pelvic inflammatory disease
+ ectopic pregnancy

### Dysmenorrhea

Also known as menstrual "cramps," **dysmenorrhea** is defined as painful menstruation during each menstrual cycle. It usually begins in adolescence, and may occur during each menstrual cycle. Dysmenorrhea usually begins with the onset of menstruation and causes lower abdominal and pelvic discomfort that may be described as dull throbbing, or crampy. The pain lasts for the first 2–3 days of menstruation and may radiate to the lower back or thighs. Dysmenorrhea can be associated with other signs

**34-4** List three causes of abdominal pain of gynecologic or obstetrical origin.

**reproductive age**   the portion of the life cycle in which individuals can produce offspring—typically, years 15–50 among women, although some women can become pregnant at a younger age or at an older age.

**dysmenorrhea**   painful menstruation including cramps in the lower abdomen.

and symptoms such as headache, nausea, vomiting, or diarrhea. The pain is often relieved with over-the-counter anti-inflammatory medications such as ibuprofen. Application of heat to the lower abdomen or back (as from a hot water bottle or a heating pad) and lying with the knees pulled up toward the abdomen may also be helpful.

### Cystitis

**cystitis** an inflammation of the bladder, usually caused by a bacterial infection.

**Cystitis** is an inflammation of the bladder, usually caused by a bacterial infection. Although this is a urinary condition, it is discussed in this chapter because the urinary tract is closely associated with the female reproductive anatomy. This condition is very common in women and may be related to the relatively short length of the urethra, which allows bacteria to ascend from the urethral opening to the bladder. Although dysuria (painful, stinging urination) is typically associated with cystitis, many women experience midline lower abdominal pain that worsens with urination and may be associated with either **hematuria** (blood in the urine) or increased urgency and frequency of urination.

**hematuria** blood in the urine.

### Ovarian Cysts

**ovarian cysts** sacs that develop on the surface of an ovary and contain either fluid or a semisolid material.

**Ovarian cysts** are sacs that develop on the surface of an ovary and contain fluid or a semisolid material. Cysts may be chronic and multiple, or they may be associated with ovulation or pregnancy. They can be quite large, up to 10 cm in diameter. Most are harmless, even painless, and resolve on their own, whereas others cause severe pain that is usually localized to the area overlying the affected ovary in the extreme right or left lower quadrants. Occasionally, an ovarian cyst may be complicated by hemorrhage within the cyst or by a twisting of the ovary. Both conditions result in severe abdominal pain that may become diffuse. Women with a history of painful ovarian cysts are usually treated successfully with an over-the-counter anti-inflammatory such as ibuprofen.

### Pelvic Inflammatory Disease (PID)

**pelvic inflammatory disease (PID)** an inflammatory condition of the female reproductive tract, particularly the fallopian tubes; is usually caused by sexually transmitted microorganisms.

**Pelvic inflammatory disease (PID)** is an inflammatory condition of the female reproductive tract, particularly the fallopian tubes, that is usually caused by sexually transmitted microorganisms such as chlamydia or gonorrhea. The signs and symptoms of PID include severe diffuse lower abdominal pain that is constant and may radiate to the lower back, and vaginal discharge. The hallmark of PID is a patient who presents bent over at the waist and walks in short, deliberate steps. Symptoms often begin just after a menstrual period and may result in adhesions in the fallopian tubes and subsequent risk of sterility or of an ectopic pregnancy (described next).

### Ectopic Pregnancy

**ectopic pregnancy** a pregnancy occurring in a site other than within the uterus.

Occasionally, a fertilized egg will implant outside the uterus, or an "ectopic" location. An **ectopic pregnancy** is a serious and potentially life-threatening condition. Up to 95 percent of ectopic pregnancies occur in a fallopian tube, which is too narrow for a developing embryo. As the embryo develops, the fallopian tube stretches, causing a dull pain over the affected lower quadrant. Occasionally light vaginal bleeding or "spotting" occurs during the first months of pregnancy because the fallopian tube bleeds as it stretches. The spotting may be misinterpreted as a menstrual period. Women with this condition may be unaware that they are pregnant or simply deny being pregnant. With time, the tube ruptures, resulting in major internal bleeding, severe pain, and hemorrhagic shock or even death. Blood within the abdomen may cause referred pain in the left shoulder. Up to 50 percent of women with ectopic pregnancies have a history of prior PID.

## Vaginal Bleeding

Vaginal bleeding may be physiologic (that is, "normal" vaginal bleeding during a menstrual period) or may result from hormonal or organic problems of the reproductive system. In a non-pregnant female, the most common cause of vaginal bleeding is menstruation, the cyclical discharge of about 25–65 mL blood and tissue that begins about 2 weeks after ovulation if fertilization does not occur. Bleeding usually lasts for 5–7 days and gradually decreases in flow. The amount of bleeding varies from female to female and is most easily quantified by the number of pads or tampons used per day (or per hour for heavier bleeding).

For most women, the amount of menstrual flow is relatively consistent from one period to the next. On occasion, however, an increase in flow—possibly related to hormonal fluctuations or stress—causes a woman to seek medical attention. In addition, some women will develop mid-cycle bleeding that simulates a period. These episodes, referred to as "abnormal vaginal bleeding," may have benign causes (such as stress) or may result from more serious diseases (such as uterine or cervical cancer). Fortunately, most abnormal vaginal bleeding does not cause significant hypovolemia, even when it occurs over several days. However, abnormal vaginal bleeding always requires further evaluation by a physician, especially if accompanied by signs or symptoms of shock, such as dizziness, diaphoresis, fainting, pallor, tachycardia, or hypotension, or if the bleeding is heavy enough to require a new pad or tampon every 15 minutes or is associated with the passage of large clots. If any of these findings are noted, transport the patient immediately to an emergency department.

## Gynecological Trauma

Blunt-force trauma to the external genitalia is an unusual injury, but one that OEC Technicians may encounter, especially in mountain biking, skiing, or snowboarding accidents. Blunt forces, such as straddle injuries from a bicycle, may result in painful vulvar hematomas, perineal lacerations, vaginal bleeding, or pelvic fractures. The urethra or bladder may be torn, causing either hematuria or the inability to urinate. Swelling associated with genital trauma may also cause an inability to urinate and urinary retention. Because the genital tissue is richly vascular, lacerations may bleed profusely but are usually controllable with direct pressure. Internal bleeding due to a vaginal or cervical laceration is much more difficult to control and requires immediate treatment by a physician.

## Sexual Assault

Sexual assault is a form of trauma defined as any physical contact of a sexual nature without voluntary consent. Forms of sexual assault include inappropriate touching, child molestation, and vaginal, anal, or oral penetration. The perpetrator may be of either sex but is typically male and someone known to the victim or a member of her family, rather than a total stranger. Many victims are adolescent females and children (Figure 34-4■). In the United States in the year 2000, one woman in six, and one man in 33, reported an attempted or completed rape.

Sexual assault may occur with enough force to cause physical trauma, both internal and external. Other health problems resulting from rape include sexually transmitted diseases, chronic abdominal pain, and headaches. The psychological trauma is often more severe than the physical trauma and is

⊕ **34-5** List four possible causes of vaginal bleeding.

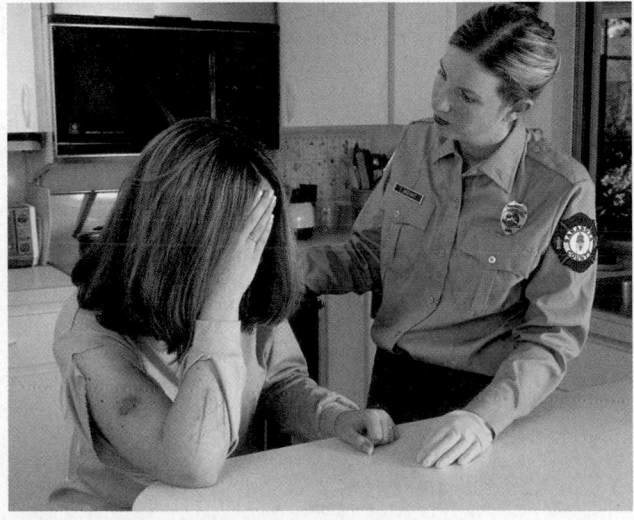

**Figure 34-4** Many sexual assault victims are adolescent females and children.

potentially long lasting. Victims of sexual assault often suffer from anxiety, fearfulness, eating disorders, and chronic depression that may even lead to suicide. In 2009, 89,000 women reported they were raped in the United States. There are estimates that another 75,000 rapes of women went unreported. In many states, OEC Technicians are mandated by law to report suspected sexual assault to law enforcement officials.

## STOP, THINK, UNDERSTAND

### Multiple Choice

Choose the correct answer.

1. Which of the following statements concerning the physiological changes in a pregnant woman is false?_____
   a. At 28 weeks, maternal blood volume increases.
   b. By the 3rd trimester, maternal heart rate increases by 15–20 beats/minute.
   c. Maternal BP increases by 10–20 mmHg and is highest just before delivery.
   d. Maternal BP decreases by 8–15 mmHg and is lowest at approximately 20 weeks.

2. In which position should you place a pregnant patient when taking her vital signs? _____
   a. lying on her left side
   b. lying on her right side
   c. sitting up
   d. lying supine with her knees bent

3. What percentage of her blood volume might a pregnant woman lose before she shows signs or symptoms of shock? _____
   a. 5–10 percent          c. 30–35 percent
   b. 15–25 percent        d. More than 40 percent

4. You are caring for a pregnant woman injured in a fall. Which of the following statements regarding the health and well-being of this mother and her unborn child is true? _____
   a. The mother may show no signs or symptoms of shock and have stable vital signs even though the fetus is already in shock.
   b. A fetus will go into shock only after the pregnant woman has.

   c. The woman's uterus and the developing fetus are so well protected by the bony pelvis and amniotic fluid that fetal shock is a very rare occurrence.
   d. Maternal or fetal shock is a rare occurrence due to the increased maternal blood volume, which serves as a compensatory mechanism.

5. Which of the following statements about a woman who does not know if she is pregnant, whose last normal menstrual period was 10 weeks ago, and who is complaining of severe abdominal pain that radiates into her left shoulder is true?_____
   a. This patient may be suffering from an ectopic pregnancy, which can quickly become life threatening.
   b. This patient may be suffering from an ovarian cyst, which although uncomfortable is not life threatening.
   c. This patient may be suffering from dysmenorrhea, which although uncomfortable is not life threatening.
   d. An OEC Technician is not authorized to make this type of determination.

6. Which of the following statements regarding sexual assault is false? _____
   a. Sexual assault may occur with enough force to cause physical trauma, both internal and external.
   b. The perpetrator in most cases of sexual assault is a stranger.
   c. The psychological trauma of sexual assault is often worse than the physical trauma.
   d. Victims of sexual assault often suffer from chronic depression, anxiety, fearfulness, or eating disorders.

### Short Answer

List and describe the signs and symptoms of abnormal vaginal bleeding.

_____

_____

_____

_____

*continued*

## Matching

**1.** Match each of the following structures to its description.

_____ 1. cervix
_____ 2. fallopian tube
_____ 3. fundus
_____ 4. ovary
_____ 5. perineum
_____ 6. uterus
_____ 7. vagina

a. a soft, outer tissue of the female reproductive anatomy; often tears during delivery
b. a hollow, muscular tube extending from the uterus to an exterior opening
c. produces progesterone and estrogen; contains ova
d. a hollow, muscular organ in which a fertilized ovum develops
e. serves as a conduit for a mature egg as it travels from an ovary to the uterus
f. the top of the uterus
g. the bottom of the uterus

**2.** Match each of the following terms to its description.

_____ 1. cystitis
_____ 2. dysmenorrhea
_____ 3. ectopic pregnancy
_____ 4. ovarian cyst
_____ 5. PID

a. a potentially life-threatening condition in which a fertilized egg develops outside of the uterus, usually in a fallopian tube; is characterized by severe lower abdominal pain, spotting or bleeding, and possible referred pain in the left shoulder
b. an inflammatory condition, usually secondary to an STD (sexually transmitted disease), in which the patient presents with diffuse low abdominal pain, sometimes fever, vaginal discharge, and a doubled-over gait
c. menstrual "cramps"
d. an inflammation of the bladder caused by a bacterial infection; is characterized by lower abdominal pain and pain or burning upon urination
e. a fluid-filled sac on an ovary; may rupture and can cause localized pain over the affected ovary

# Pregnancy: Normal Physiologic Changes

⊕ **34-6** List the three stages of a normal pregnancy.

The vast majority of pregnancies are considered normal and low-risk events. During the first trimester, a pregnant woman may notice swelling of her breasts, fatigue, nausea, and the need to urinate frequently. Vomiting is common, especially in the morning, and when severe or protracted it may prompt the woman to seek medical attention.

By the end of the 12th week, the baby's vital organs have developed, its bones start developing, and the limbs become more pronounced. At this point, the fetus is about 4 inches long. By the second trimester, nausea resolves. The mother's breasts continue to grow and the uterus begins to expand out of the pelvis. Women may find it more difficult to sleep on their backs during this stage, or they may experience backache, gas, or constipation. Prenatal care includes testing for diabetes, hypertension, and other conditions that may increase the risk for premature labor and delivery or fetal-maternal mortality. During the second trimester the fetus continues to grow, and facial features become more distinguishable. The brain and spinal cord continue to grow, and the kidneys and liver begin functioning. The woman will now feel the baby's movement. By the end of this trimester, hair, nails, and eyelids begin to form.

During the third trimester, the fetus maintains steady growth. The brain continues to develop, eyelashes form, and the eyes open. By week 30, the fetus weighs about 3 pounds. The additional weight gain can make a pregnant woman feel off balance, creating a risk for falls, especially during outdoor recreational activities. Some swelling of the feet and hands is common, as are indigestion, fatigue, difficulty breathing (due to the growing uterus expanding high into the abdomen), and difficulty sleeping. By the end of the third trimester, the fetus rotates within the uterus to a head-down position in preparation for delivery.

**(34-8)** Describe four possible complications of pregnancy.

**placenta previa**    low implantation of the placenta such that it partially or completely covers the internal opening of the uterus; upon the onset of any contractions and cervical dilation, or when the cervix begins to dilate at the onset of labor, the placenta is stretched and pulled from the uterine wall, producing painless bleeding that may be life threatening to both mother and fetus.

**abruptio placentae**    premature separation of a normally situated but improperly implanted placenta; it usually occurs late in pregnancy but may occur during labor.

**preeclampsia**    a toxemia during pregnancy characterized by high blood pressure and edema of the hands or face; also called pregnancy-induced hypertension (PIH).

**eclampsia**    a potentially life-threatening disorder in pregnant women that is characterized by hypertension, generalized edema, and proteinuria (protein in the urine); involves the seizures of the convulsive stage of preeclampsia-eclampsia syndrome, which are not attributable to another cerebral condition such as epilepsy.

**miscarriage**    a common term for a spontaneous abortion; the spontaneous termination of a pregnancy before about 20 weeks of gestation, at which time the fetus is not yet sufficiently developed to survive.

# Complications of Pregnancy

## Hemorrhage

Vaginal bleeding during the first trimester of pregnancy can occur and may signal an impending miscarriage or an ectopic pregnancy. After the first trimester, bleeding results from either a placenta that is implanted abnormally low over the cervix (**placenta previa**), or from premature separation of the placenta from the wall of the uterus (**abruptio placentae**). The former condition presents with painless, dark-red vaginal bleeding, whereas abruptio placentae is associated with severe abdominal pain, a firm, contracted uterus, and bright-red vaginal bleeding. Both conditions can result in fetal and/or maternal death, and either mandates immediate evaluation by an obstetrician. Another form of hemorrhage associated with pregnancy is postpartum hemorrhage, which is bleeding in excess of 500 mL following a vaginal delivery. Firm, downward massage of the woman's lower abdomen after delivery stimulates the uterus to contract and should promptly resolve this form of bleeding. Refer to Table 34-1■ for a complete list of causes of vaginal bleeding during pregnancy.

## Pregnancy-Induced Hypertension (PIH)

Pregnancy-induced hypertension, or "toxemia," is a form of high blood pressure that develops during pregnancy. Also known as **preeclampsia**, PIH develops after the 20th week of gestation and is more common in a first-time pregnancy (primagravida), in twin pregnancies, and in women with preexisting diabetes. OEC Technicians may observe the following two characteristics of this condition:

+ Blood pressure greater than 140/90 (or a significant rise in one or both pressures)
+ Edema of the face and/or hands

Pregnancy-induced hypertension may be complicated by seizures, a condition known as **eclampsia**. This severe form of PIH usually develops late in pregnancy, close to the time of delivery. Although a woman with eclampsia should be treated with supplemental oxygen, airway maintenance, and positioning on her left side, the definitive treatment is emergent delivery of the infant.

## Miscarriage

A **miscarriage**, or spontaneous abortion, is the loss of a pregnancy prior to 20 weeks of gestation, before the fetus is able to survive outside the uterus. Any fetus less than 24 weeks will have little chance of survival, and even at 24 weeks the chances of survival are slim. Spotting or bleeding is the primary sign, and it may be accompanied by lower abdominal cramping. About a fourth of all pregnant women experience some spotting or bleeding in the first two trimesters, representing a "threatened abortion." Up to half of these women eventually miscarry completely and pass blood, fetal tissue, and the placenta. At times, only a portion of the tissues are expelled, re-

| Table **34-1** Causes of Vaginal Bleeding During Pregnancy |
| --- |
| Ectopic pregnancy |
| Threatened abortion |
| Placenta previa |
| Abruptio placentae |
| Uterine rupture |
| Postpartum hemorrhage/uterine atony |

sulting in an incomplete abortion and heavy, continuous vaginal bleeding accompanied by cramping and the passage of clots.

## Supine Hypotensive Syndrome

After 20 weeks of gestation, the enlarged uterus can compress the vena cava when a pregnant woman is in a supine position. Such compression decreases blood return to the heart and subsequently cardiac output by 30–40 percent and can result in profound maternal hypotension. OEC Technicians can easily prevent this condition by simply placing the mother in the left lateral recumbent position or by elevating the right hip approximately 1–2 inches. If the mother is on a long spine board, the board can be tipped so that the patient is slightly tilted onto her left side. Additionally, the abdominal contents can be manually pushed to the left, moving the uterus off of the vena cava.

# Childbirth

Few emergencies cause more anxiety for an OEC Technician than an emergency delivery—and yet, only a century ago, almost all childbirth took place outside of a hospital, usually at home. Today, accidental delivery outside of a hospital is more common in women with little or no prenatal care and in women who have had multiple pregnancies. Babies of these women have a higher incidence of fetal mortality than in-hospital deliveries. As an OEC Technician, the most likely scenario you will encounter is a teenager at a ski area who denies being pregnant but complains of regular intermittent abdominal pain and has physical findings consistent with pregnancy (for example, an enlarged uterus, a lack of menstrual periods, stretch marks, and fetal movement).

Childbirth begins with labor, which can be gradual or abrupt in onset and is divided into three stages (Figures 34-5a–c■). The first stage begins with irregular lower abdominal uterine contractions and is often accompanied by lower back pain. As labor progresses, the contractions become more intense and painful, last longer, and become more regular. Toward the end of the first stage, contractions recur at 3- to 4-minute intervals and last about 50–60 seconds. The cervix generally dilates. Then, in the second stage, the fetus descends through the birth canal, and the baby is delivered. The third stage involves the delivery of the placenta.

Signs of imminent delivery include:

+ Bloody show (passage of the mucus plug that seals the cervix throughout pregnancy)
+ Rupture of the amniotic sac (the "bag of waters")
+ The urge to push or defecate

Leaked fluid is usually clear but may also appear tea-stained or be pea-colored from fetal stool (known as meconium). The urge to have a bowel movement is a normal sensation indicating that delivery is about to occur. Do not allow the patient to go to a bathroom, and reassure her that this is a normal sensation that means she is about to deliver the baby. If she feels the urge to push or to have a bowel movement, inspect the perineum for

**34-11** Describe the process of assisting an emergency delivery.

**Figure 34-5** (a) The first stage of labor extends from the beginning of contractions to full cervical dilation. (b) During the second stage of labor, the baby enters the birth canal and is born. (c) The third stage of labor involves the delivery of the placenta.

**First stage:**
beginning of contractions to full cervical dilation

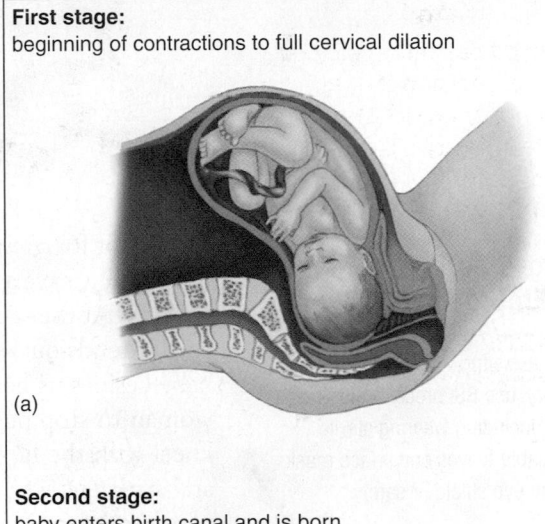

(a)

**Second stage:**
baby enters birth canal and is born

(b)

**Third stage:**
delivery of the placenta

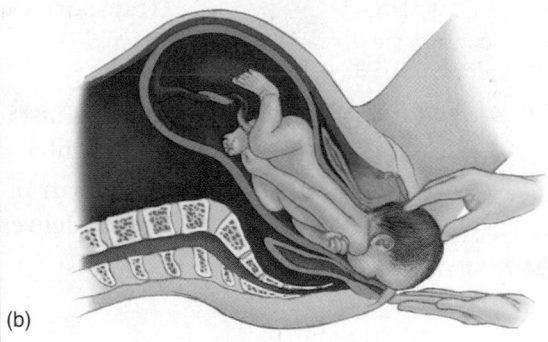

(c)

**Figure 34-6** A patient with a prolapsed umbilical cord being treated and who will then be transported to the hospital by a paramedic unit.

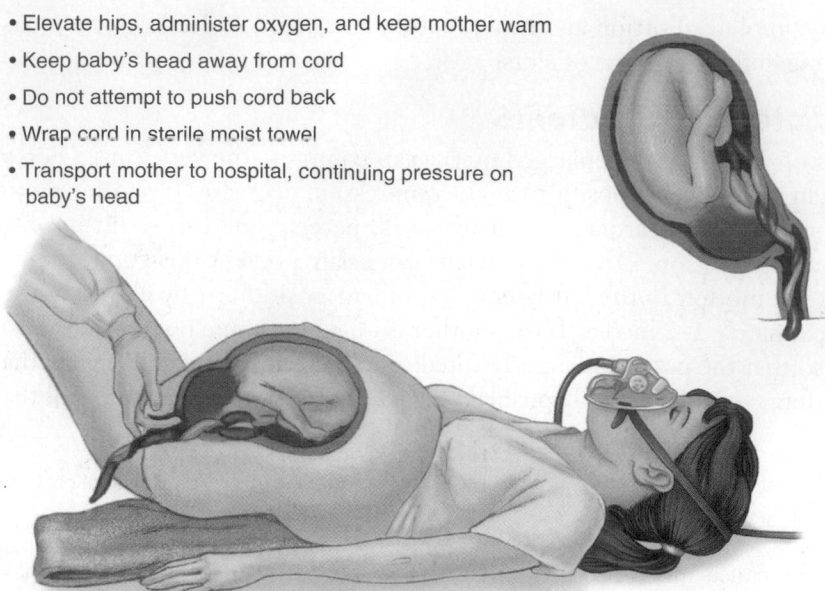

- Elevate hips, administer oxygen, and keep mother warm
- Keep baby's head away from cord
- Do not attempt to push cord back
- Wrap cord in sterile moist towel
- Transport mother to hospital, continuing pressure on baby's head

### Always be Prepared for an Emergency Delivery

**NOTE**

When assisting with an emergency delivery, use BSI precautions at all times, including wearing sterile disposable gloves and a face mask with an eye shield or safety glasses.

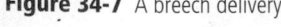

bulging or for *crowning*, which is the appearance of the infant's head at the vaginal opening. Ideally, have a second rescuer present for this examination and/or to assist with the delivery. At the same time, look for a prolapsed umbilical cord, in which the umbilical cord extends out of the vagina (Figure 34-6■). If the umbilical cord or any part of the baby besides its head (a foot, for example) is visible at the vaginal opening, instruct the woman to stop pushing, and assist her into a knees-to-the-chest position; having her kneel with the hips flexed slightly more than 90 degrees, and resting her upper chest and arms against a bed or the ground will create this position. Place the mother on supplemental oxygen while arranging emergent transfer to advanced medical care.

Transport a woman in labor to a higher level of care under the following circumstances:

+ If it takes less than 20 minutes to get there
+ If the umbilical cord is visible in the vagina (a prolapsed cord)
+ If any part of the baby other than the top of the head is visible in the vagina (a breech delivery) (Figure 34-7■)

**Figure 34-7** A breech delivery.

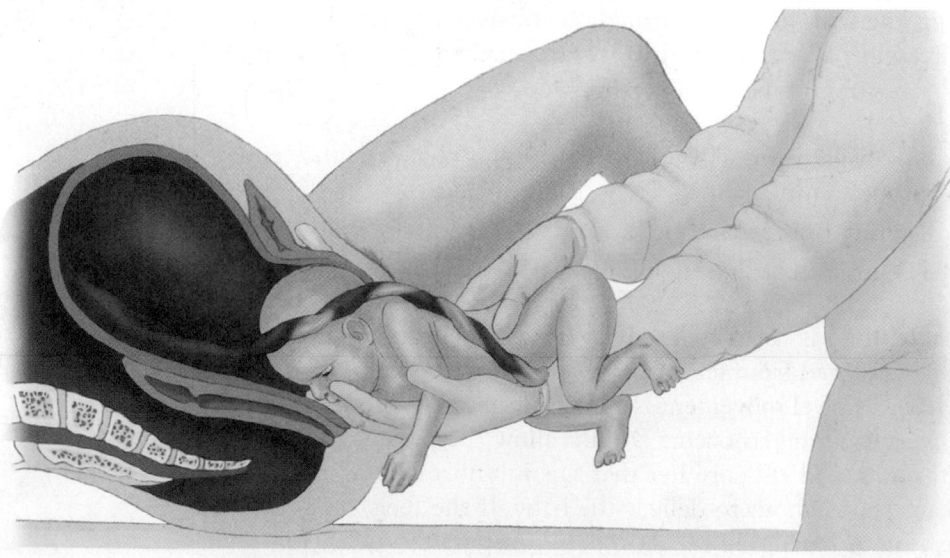

- If the woman says her doctor says she will need a C-section
- If this delivery is the woman's first, and the amount of the baby's head that is visible is smaller than 1 inch across

Any signs of imminent delivery require that OEC Technicians be prepared to assist with immediate delivery. If delivery is not imminent, place the patient in left lateral recumbency and provide supplemental oxygen while arranging transportation to a hospital (Figure 34-8■). If the baby is crowning, perform the following steps to assist the woman with an emergency delivery:

1. Use a sterile disposable obstetric (OB) delivery kit, if available (Figure 34-9■). If one is not available, improvise by obtaining clean towels and sheets, a blanket for the baby, 4-inch by 4-inch gauze sponges, scissors or a straight-edged razor, a soft rubber bulb syringe, white cloth tape, and two clean cotton shoelaces, all of which you should sterilize with boiling water if there is time to do so. Use BSI precautions at all times, including sterile disposable gloves and a face-mask with an eye shield or glasses. A gown may prevent splashing of body fluids on you during the delivery. Following delivery, place all supplies that were soiled with body fluids in a biohazard bag and dispose of them properly.

2. Remove the woman's clothes from the waist down, placing her in semi-Fowler's position on a firm, sturdy padded table if available (a bed may be too low or too soft) (Figure 34-10■). If such a table is not available, use any firm elevated flat surface. Use a folded blanket or large towel to elevate her buttocks 2–4 inches in relation to the middle of her back. Bend her hips and flex and spread her knees apart, always protecting her modesty. Place one end of a clean sheet or large towel under her buttocks and allow the other end to unfold to the floor, creating a clean delivery "field." Sit between the woman's legs and place other sheets

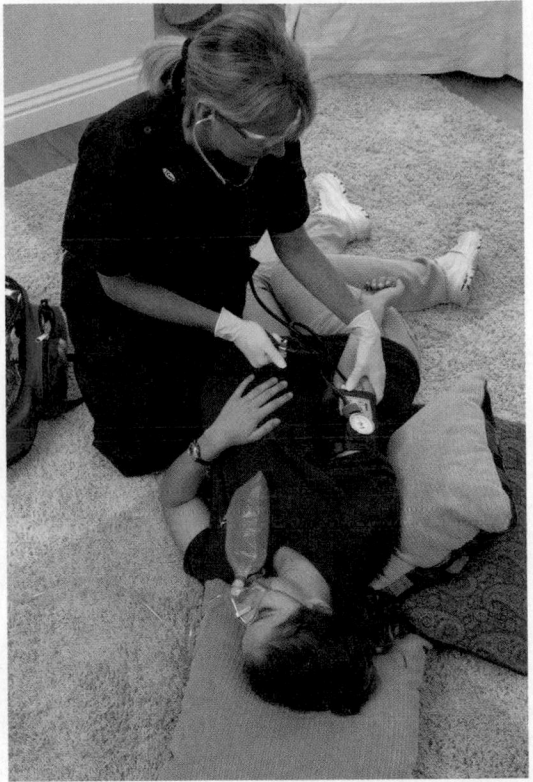

**Figure 34-8** If birth is not imminent, place the woman in left lateral recumbency to keep pressure off the inferior vena cava.

**Figure 34-10** For a women who is already unclothed, use padding, blankets, and sheets to position the woman for delivery.

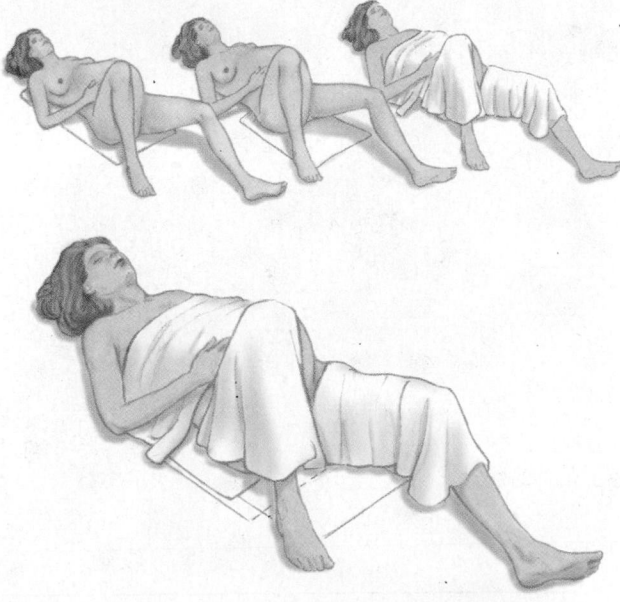

**Figure 34-9** Contents of an obstetric (OB) kit.

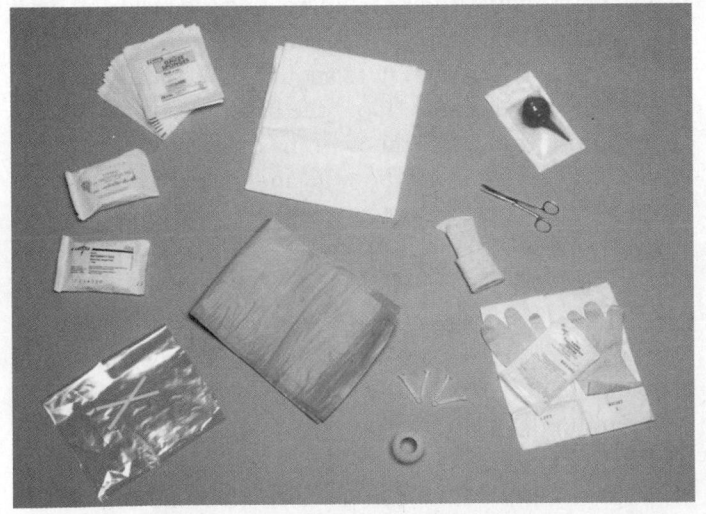

or towels in front of you to soak up blood or amniotic fluid during the delivery. Put your OB kit or other sterile supplies on a firm level surface beside you. Station another OEC Technician at the woman's head to provide reassurance.

3. Time the woman's contractions from the start of one contraction to the start of the next. Then, while feeling the abdomen, note the duration of a single contraction by recording the time between the onset of a contraction and its completion. Encourage the woman to rest between contractions. See OEC Skill 34-1■.

4. Once the baby is crowning, allow the woman to push the baby's head out; support its head with your gloved hand as it emerges. Applying gentle pressure with your hand will allow the head to come out in a controlled fashion and help prevent the baby's head and body from suddenly popping out. Applying this gentle pressure can markedly reduce the severity of the women's perineal tissues tearing. The head usually emerges face down. Once the head has emerged, it will rotate slightly, allowing you easier access to the baby's face and airway.

Instruct the woman to stop pushing, and only if there is obvious obstruction to spontaneous breathing, immediately suction the baby's mouth and then the nostrils, using a soft rubber bulb syringe. Suctioning the nostrils before the mouth may stimulate the baby to gasp and thereby aspirate any fluid in the nose or pharynx. Note if the fluid in the baby's mouth and nose does not appear clear, a sign of meconium (stool), in the amniotic fluid. This is a condition called meconium aspiration and causes inflammation in the baby's lungs after birth. Next, feel for the umbilical cord around the baby's neck. If present, gently lift the cord over the baby's head. Because the cord may wrap around the neck more than once, check again to ensure that the cord is not around the baby's neck. If you are unable to lift the cord over the baby's head, immediately place two clamps or umbilical ties around the cord about 2 inches apart and then cut the cord between the clamps.

5. After delivering the head, you should see the baby's upper shoulder. With one hand on either side of the baby's head, gently guide the head down slightly to help deliver the shoulders as the woman pushes. After this, you may need to guide the head up slightly to deliver the lower shoulder. Support the baby's head with one hand and its upper body with your other hand as the shoulders are delivered. Never pull the baby from the birth canal.

Once the head and shoulders are delivered, the rest of the baby slips out quickly because its body is covered with a white, cheesy substance (vermix caseosa). Once the baby emerges, rotate it 180 degrees so that the supine newborn is against your body with one hand holding the head and neck and the torso is resting on the same hand's forearm. Again if there is obvious obstruction to spontaneous breathing, suction the mouth and nose. Hold the baby's head and neck in a neutral position at all times to maintain an open airway. Have an assistant record the time and location of the birth for later entry on a birth certificate.

6. Should transportation to an EMS access point or medical facility be delayed more than 20 minutes, you will need to cut the umbilical cord (Figure 34-11■). Place two clamps or tie two cloth shoelaces about 7–10 cm (2.75–4 inches) from the baby and about 5–10 cm (2–4 inches) apart, then cut the cord between the clamps or laces.

7. The delivery of the placenta is the third stage of labor (Figure 34-12■). Allow the placenta to come out of the

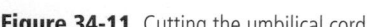
**Figure 34-11** Cutting the umbilical cord.

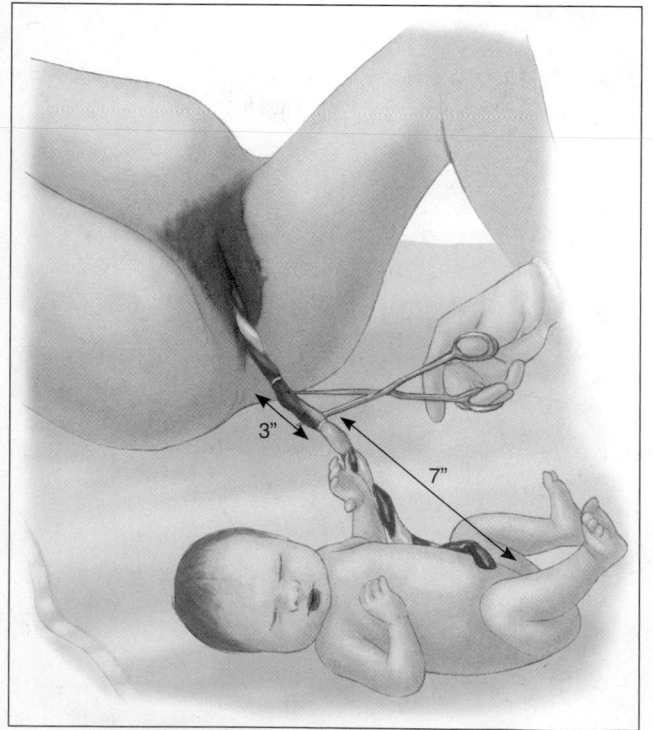

3"

7"

vagina by itself. Pulling on the umbilical cord that is still attached to the placenta can be harmful. The placenta should separate from the inside wall of the uterus about 20–30 minutes after the baby is delivered. If transport is available once the baby is born, do not wait on the delivery of the placenta. However, if the placenta does come out of the vagina, put it in a plastic bag and send it to the hospital with the mother and her baby.

Put a sanitary pad over the mother's vagina and have her lie on her back with her legs straight. Vaginal bleeding slows after the placenta is out and the uterus starts to shrink. Massage the mother's lower abdomen in a circular motion where the uterus is located to help her uterus shrink and to aid in the production of oxytocin, a hormone that makes the uterine muscles contract.

Always transport the mother, baby, and placenta to the hospital or to some other ALS access point. If there is excessive bleeding, place the mother in the Trendelenburg position, provide supplemental oxygen, and monitor her vital signs. Apply sanitary napkins to the perineum, as needed, an especially helpful practice when bleeding is the result of lacerations of the birth canal or perineum. Do not place a tampon or any dressings inside the vagina.

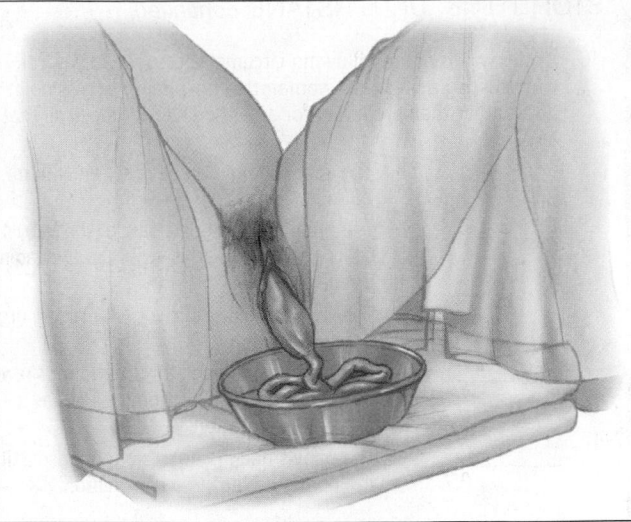

**Figure 34-12** Delivery of the placenta, the third stage of labor.

## STOP, THINK, UNDERSTAND

### Multiple Choice
Choose the correct answer.

1. From which of the following conditions is a pregnant woman with an elevated BP of 140/90 and edema of her face and hands most likely suffering? _____
   a. obesity due to a poor diet
   b. pregnancy-induced hypertension, toxemia, or preeclampsia
   c. dysmenorrhea, cystitis, or pelvic inflammatory disease
   d. a normal pregnancy, because a pregnant woman's blood pressure usually rises somewhat, and swelling of the face and hands is normal

2. From which of the following conditions is a woman who is 24 weeks pregnant and has a blood pressure of 80/52 most likely suffering? _____
   a. PID
   b. preeclampsia
   c. supine hypotensive syndrome
   d. a normal pregnancy, because a pregnant woman's blood pressure usually drops during the first and second trimesters

3. Which of the following statements correctly describes the way to treat the woman in Question 2? _____
   a. Place a sanitary pad between her legs, put her in a position of comfort, and transport her rapidly to the hospital.
   b. Place her in a supine position with her knees elevated, and transport her rapidly to the hospital.

   c. Place her on her left side and manually push and displace her uterus to the left.
   d. Do nothing; reassure her that what is happening is normal and suggest that she follow up with her obstetrician.

4. Which of the following statements about childbirth (delivery) is false? _____
   a. Deliveries outside of a hospital are more common in women who have had little or no prenatal care.
   b. The most likely field delivery situation an OEC Technician will encounter is a teenager who denies that she is pregnant.
   c. Field delivery is considered an immediately life-threatening emergency due to the remote location and the possibility of complications.
   d. There is a higher incidence of fetal mortality for field deliveries than for in-hospital deliveries.

5. Which of the following statements is false? _____
   a. If transport time to the hospital is longer than 20 minutes, an OEC Technician should clamp and cut the umbilical cord.
   b. Umbilical cord clamps should be placed 7–10 cm (2.75–4 inches) from the baby and 5–10 cm (2–4 inches) apart.
   c. If the placenta has not been delivered within 30 minutes, an OEC Technician should gently pull on the umbilical cord while simultaneously massaging the mother's abdomen.
   d. If the placenta has been delivered, it should be transported to the hospital with the mother and infant.

*continued*

## STOP, THINK, UNDERSTAND *continued*

6. Under which of the following circumstances should you consider transporting a pregnant woman to a hospital or access point for EMS rather than preparing for a field delivery? (check all that apply)

_____ **a.** The access point can be reached within 20 minutes.

_____ **b.** The umbilical cord or a part of the baby's body other than the head is visible in the vaginal opening.

_____ **c.** The woman tells you she has a strong urge to defecate.

_____ **d.** The woman has been informed that she will require a cesarean section, or she has a breech presentation.

_____ **e.** The baby's head is not visible on inspection of the perineum during a contraction.

_____ **f.** This is the woman's first delivery, and when the baby's head is visible during a contraction you can see only about an inch of the baby's head.

7. Which of the following signs and symptoms are common indications of an imminent delivery? (check all that apply)

_____ **a.** bloody show

_____ **b.** rupture of the amniotic sac (the "bag of waters")

_____ **c.** a burning sensation upon urination

_____ **d.** the urge to push or defecate

_____ **e.** irregular, lower abdominal contractions

_____ **f.** diarrhea

_____ **g.** perineal bulging/crowning

## Short Answer

1. Describe the position in which a pregnant woman who has received a traumatic injury should be transported.

_____

_____

_____

2. Why is it important to suction a newborn infant's mouth before suctioning the nose?

_____

_____

_____

3. Why is it important to note whether or not the amniotic fluid is clear?

_____

_____

_____

## Matching

Match each of the following conditions to its description.

_____ **1.** abruptio placentae

_____ **2.** placenta previa

_____ **3.** preeclampsia

_____ **4.** supine hypotensive syndrome

**a.** characterized by a significant rise in maternal blood pressure and edema of the hands and/or face

**b.** characterized by a severe drop in maternal blood pressure due to the weight of the fetus on the woman's vena cava

**c.** characterized by painless, dark-red vaginal bleeding

**d.** characterized by severe abdominal pain, a firm, contracted uterus, and bright-red vaginal bleeding

**Table 34-2** APGAR Scoring System

| Points | 2 | 1 | 0 |
| --- | --- | --- | --- |
| Appearance | Body completely pink | Body pink, limbs blue | Body completely blue or pale |
| Pulse | Greater than 100 | Less than 100 | Absent |
| Grimace or irritability | Crying | Feeble cry when stimulated | Does not cry or react to stimuli |
| Activity or muscle tone | Active | Some weak motion | Body limp, no tone |
| Respiration | Strong cry | Weak cry | None |

# Basic Care of Newborns

Once an infant is delivered, vigorously dry it off and wrap it in a blanket, towel, or space blanket, covering the entire baby except for its face. A baby's body temperature can drop very quickly, and neonatal hypothermia is reported in about half of all pre-hospital deliveries. While drying and stimulating the baby, assess its APGAR score, a scoring system used to evaluate a newborn's health status (Table 34-2). In determining an APGAR score, either 0, 1, or 2 points are assigned at 1, 5, and 10 minutes after birth, for each of the following five categories:

**A**ppearance
**P**ulse
**G**rimace or irritability
**A**ctivity or muscle tone
**R**espirations

The APGAR score is helpful in determining if the baby is doing well outside the uterus or if it needs resuscitation. If the infant is in need of resuscitation before the 1-minute score, do not wait; begin resuscitation efforts. Should the 5-minute score be less than 7, continue obtaining scores every 5 minutes up to 20 minutes.

Begin your evaluation of a newborn with the ABCDs. The airway was initially suctioned after the head was delivered and again after the baby was delivered only if there was obvious obstruction to spontaneous breathing. Usually an infant begins crying vigorously within 15–20 seconds after delivery, often while being dried. If not, use your fingers to either flick the soles of the infant's feet or rub the infant's back (Figure 34-13■). Should the infant not begin to breathe after 10–15 seconds, begin resuscitation.

If the infant appears to be breathing well, determine its pulse rate by palpating the brachial pulse or by palpating the umbilical cord. A newborn's pulse rate should be *at least* 100 beats/minute. If it is less, begin positive pressure ventilations with supplemental

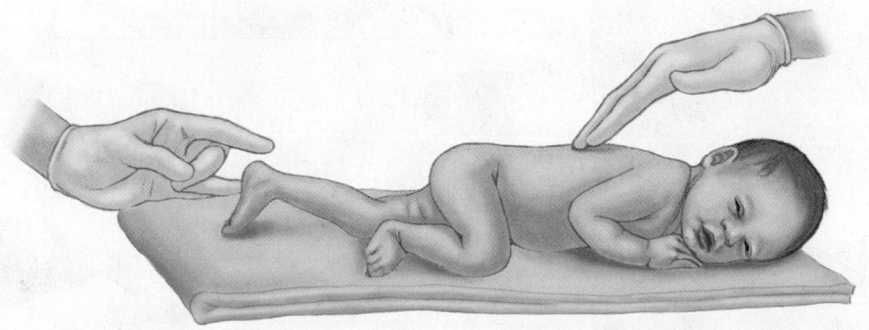

**Figure 34-13** To stimulate a newborn infant to breathe, flick the soles of the feet or rub the back.

oxygen using an *infant* bag-valve mask (BVM) placed over the baby's nose and mouth at a rate of 40–60 breaths per minute. Bag the baby using just enough pressure to observe the chest rising. Reassess the pulse rate after 90 seconds, and if less than 60 beats/minute, give oxygen at low concentrations, and increase it as needed until the heart rate is at least 100 beats/minute. Assisted ventilation is the most effective action in neonatal resuscitation and usually brings the heart rate up to 100 beats/min. Once the pulse rate reaches 100, gradually reduce the rate and pressure of the BVM ventilations until it is apparent that the infant is breathing well on its own and is maintaining good color.

An infant's skin color is another indicator of its well being using the APGAR scale. A lack of oxygen in the infant's bloodstream causes cyanosis of the face and trunk, *normally*, for up to several minutes after delivery as the hemoglobin becomes saturated with oxygen. Full oxygen saturation takes up to ten minutes. Therefore newer evidence has shown that clinical assessment of skin color is a very poor indicator of the newborn's oxygen saturation of hemoglobin during the period immediately after birth. For infants with strong, regular respirations and cyanosis, administer high-flow oxygen using "blow-by $O_2$," in which the end of the tubing is placed close to the infant's nostrils (Figure 34-14■). If the newborn is not breathing begin ventilation with room air first, and increase the oxygen percentage in the ventilations slowly. There is growing evidence that hypoxia and (even briefly) over oxygenation of the newborn can result in an adverse outcome.

Infants with a pulse rate lower than 60 beats/min, or a pulse rate remaining between 60 and 100 beats/min despite adequate ventilation with supplementary oxygen for 30 seconds, should be given chest compressions (CPR) (Figure 34-15■). In this situation, even though a pulse may be palpable, the heart rate and cardiac output are inadequate for supporting the infant's life. Perform the chest compression technique and compression rates specified by current standards for health professionals as published by approved NSP CPR certification program providers as discussed in Chapter 15, Cardiovascular Emergencies. CPR should be continued until the infant responds with adequate respirations and a heart rate greater than 60, or until pronounced dead by a physician. Although it can be distressing to perform CPR on an infant, remember that infants are quite resilient and can survive prolonged effective CPR without brain damage.

**Figure 34-15** Infants with an inadequate pulse rate require chest compressions.

**Figure 34-14** Provide "blow-by" $O_2$ by placing the oxygen tubing, a mask, or a paper cup near the infant's nostrils.

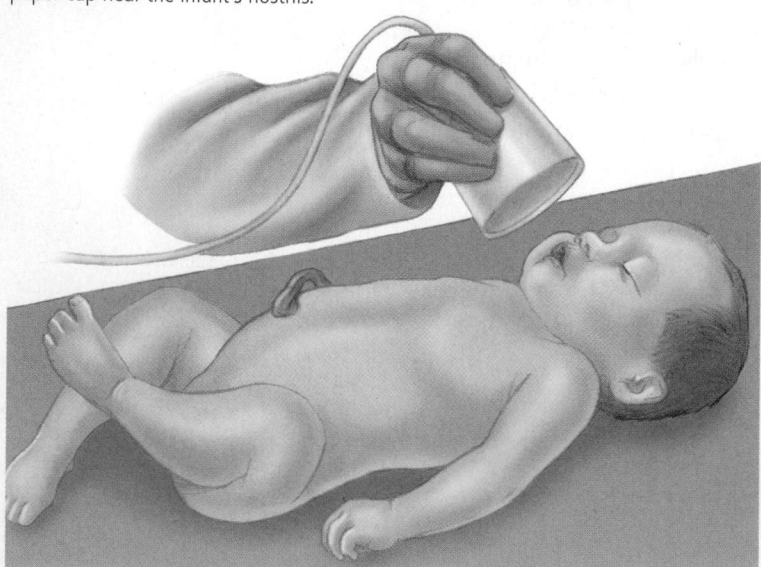

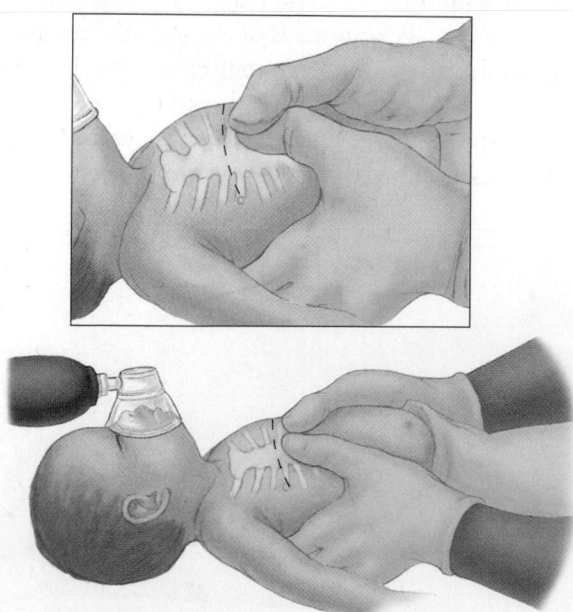

# STOP, THINK, UNDERSTAND

## Multiple Choice

Choose the correct answer.

1. APGAR stands for which of the following? _____
   a. appearance, pulse, gestation, airway, respirations
   b. airway, pulse, grimace, aptitude, respirations
   c. airway, presentation, grip, aptitude, rotation
   d. appearance, pulse, grimace, activity, respirations

2. A newborn's pulse rate should be at least_____
   a. 100 beats per minute.      c. 80 beats per minute.
   b. 90 beats per minute.       d. 70 beats per minute.

3. If a newborn does not begin crying 15–20 seconds after delivery, you should take all of the following actions except_____
   a. gently toweling off the infant.
   b. flicking the soles of the infant's feet.
   c. rubbing the infant's back.
   d. carefully holding the infant upside-down by gripping its ankles with one hand, and then gently smacking its bottom with the other.

4. How long should you wait before beginning resuscitation on a newborn that is not breathing? _____
   a. 10–15 seconds      c. 60 seconds
   b. 30 seconds         d. 5 minutes

5. To determine the pulse rate of a newborn, you should palpate the pulse at the_____
   a. carotid artery or listen to the chest with a stethoscope.
   b. femoral artery.

   c. radial artery.
   d. brachial artery or the umbilical cord.

6. If a newborn's pulse rate is less than 60 beats per minute, what should you do first? _____
   a. Immediately begin CPR.
   b. Immediately oxygenate the infant using a nonrebreather mask at 15 LPM.
   c. Begin rescue breathing with an infant bag-valve mask.
   d. Place the infant on the mother's abdomen and allow it to nurse.

7. At what rate should you resuscitate a newborn that is not breathing? _____
   a. 50–70 breaths per minute
   b. 40–60 breaths per minute
   c. 30–40 breaths per minute
   d. 12–20 breaths per minute

8. If a vigorous newborn you have just delivered is cyanotic around the trunk and face, what should do you first? _____
   a. Realize that this may be normal for a newborn.
   b. Begin resuscitation with a bag-valve mask.
   c. Massage the newborn's back.
   d. Place the newborn with the head slightly downhill to allow mucus to drain from its nose and mouth.

## Matching

Match each of the following actions with the condition for which it is proper. The actions can be used more than once.

_____ 1. Place the pregnant woman on her left side.
_____ 2. Administer high-flow $O_2$.
_____ 3. Firmly massage the uterus downward.
_____ 4. Rapidly transport the woman to the ED.

a. pregnancy-induced hypertension (preeclampsia)
b. supine hypotensive syndrome
c. placenta previa
d. abruptio placentae
e. post-partum hemorrhage

## Short Answer

Describe the process of taking an APGAR score, and indicate how often a score should be taken.

_____

_____

_____

### One Victim but Two Patients

When you are caring for a pregnant trauma victim, you are really caring for two patients. The expectant mother will understandably be very concerned, even distraught, about potential injury to her baby. A calm, reassuring manner will help ease her anxiety.

**⊕ 34-7** List three possible consequences of abdominal trauma in a pregnant patient.

**Figure 34-16** The two main risks for an active pregnant woman are falling and collisions.
Copyright Craig Brown

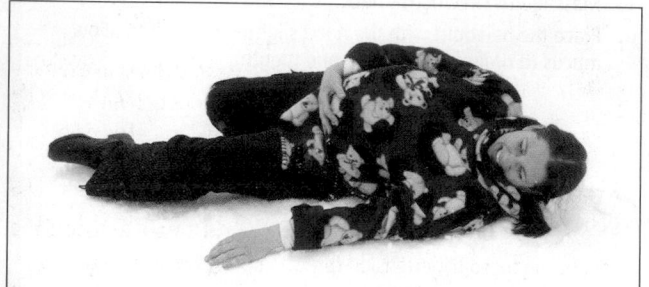

# Trauma During Pregnancy

According to the American Congress of Obstetricians and Gynecologists, "Most forms of exercise are safe during pregnancy. However, some types of exercise involve positions and movements that may be uncomfortable, tiring, or harmful for pregnant women." Because of the variety of demands in certain sports and of the health status and fitness of pregnant female athletes, there is no standard timeline for the permissibility of competition during pregnancy. As OEC Technicians, you are more likely to provide emergency care to a pregnant woman who is injured while participating in a sport such as skiing than you are to deliver a baby. Many women who are fit or athletic continue to ski through the second trimester, and occasionally into the third trimester. The two main risks for pregnant women who participate in sports are falling and collisions. An indirect blow to the abdomen can be just as dangerous as a direct blow and could potentially harm the developing fetus or the woman's enlarged uterus (Figure 34-16■).

Three potentially dangerous consequences of a fall or collision are a ruptured uterus, abruptio placentae and premature labor, and the rupture of membranes. Uterine penetration by a foreign body is also a possibility but is exceedingly rare. The most common cause of fetal death—after the death of the mother and trauma during pregnancy—is abruptio placentae (Figure 34-17■). This condition is typically the result of a shearing force produced when the body stops moving before the internal organs do. The amount of shearing force and the extent of the resultant indirect injury are determined by the rate of deceleration, and not necessarily by how fast the body was moving. When shearing forces cause the placenta to separate from the uterus, all blood flow and nutrient transfer to the fetus is interrupted, resulting in fetal death. Classic signs and symptoms include vaginal bleeding, abdominal pain, constant uterine contractions, and expanding uterine height.

Uterine rupture is less common and presents with sharp pain following direct trauma to the abdomen. The normally smooth contour of the abdomen of the pregnant woman may become irregular, and fetal parts become more easily palpated. Rupture may also present with minimal signs and symptoms. Sadly, fetal death is a common outcome of uterine rupture, and

**Figure 34-17** Abruptio placentae.

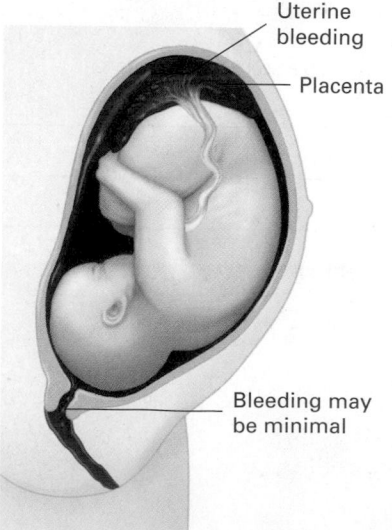

Uterine bleeding

Placenta

Bleeding may be minimal

**Figure 34-18** Amniotic sac rupture.

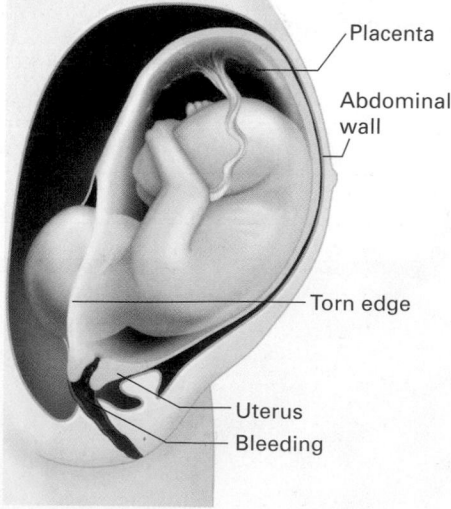

Placenta

Abdominal wall

Torn edge

Uterus

Bleeding

# CASE UPDATE

Recognizing that this woman, who is 34 weeks pregnant, has sustained blunt abdominal trauma, you assess her for additional trauma, including any obvious bleeding, tenderness in the neck, spine, or abdomen, and neurological deficits. You note that the patient's abdomen is diffusely tender. The uterus rises to about 5 finger widths above the umbilicus and is very firm to the touch. You get assistance in positioning the patient onto her left side and obtain her vital signs. Her blood pressure is 90/60, her pulse is 110, and her respirations are 20 and shallow.

***What are the potential consequences of blunt abdominal trauma during pregnancy? What should you do next?***

if the woman is unable to receive emergent medical care at a hospital, she may die as well.

Premature rupture of the amniotic sac (Figure 34-18■) often causes leakage of clear or blood-tinged fluid from the vagina. Early labor may ensue or be precipitated by trauma to the abdomen. It is unlikely that you will need to deliver a baby under these circumstances, but nonetheless you should be prepared to do so.

As stated previously, pregnant women may lose 30–35 percent of their blood volume *before* showing signs of shock. While the woman's vital signs may appear stable, the fetus will be in shock due to decreased blood flow from the uterus to the placenta and the shunting of blood. Thus, OEC Technicians should *always* anticipate the development of shock in a pregnant trauma patient—and in her fetus—even given normal vital signs, and should provide high-flow oxygen, rapid evacuation, and immediate transportation to ALS providers or a definitive-care facility, where intravenous fluids can be administered.

## Assessment

The assessment of a woman with a gynecologic or obstetrical complaint is unique in that the history must include information concerning her reproductive cycle. Fortunately, most gynecologic emergencies are not life threatening. Obstetrical emergencies, however, can threaten the life of both the woman and the fetus. In addition, because a woman may not be aware that she is pregnant, always consider the possibility that any female patient of reproductive age may be pregnant.

Begin your assessment, as always, with an evaluation of the ABCDs and vital signs. Use the SAMPLE acronym and the OPQRST mnemonic to guide you in obtaining both a general medical history and a history of the current illness or injury (Figure 34-19■).

Whether the patient is known to be pregnant or not, ask these questions:

- When was your last (normal) menstrual period, and when is the next period expected?
- If you are late for an expected menstrual period, could you be pregnant?
- Have you had a recent pregnancy test?

### First Steps in Treating a Pregnant Trauma Patient

**NOTE**

Early critical intervention for a pregnant woman with trauma includes placing her on high-flow oxygen and positioning her on her left side (perhaps by tipping the spine board to the left). Treat her for shock even in the presence of normal vital signs.

**34-9** Demonstrate how to examine a female patient with abdominal or pelvic pain.

**34-10** Describe how to assess the abdomen of a pregnant patient.

**Figure 34-19** Begin your assessment of a pregnant woman as you would any other assessment—with an evaluation of the ABCDs and her vital signs.
Copyright Craig Brown

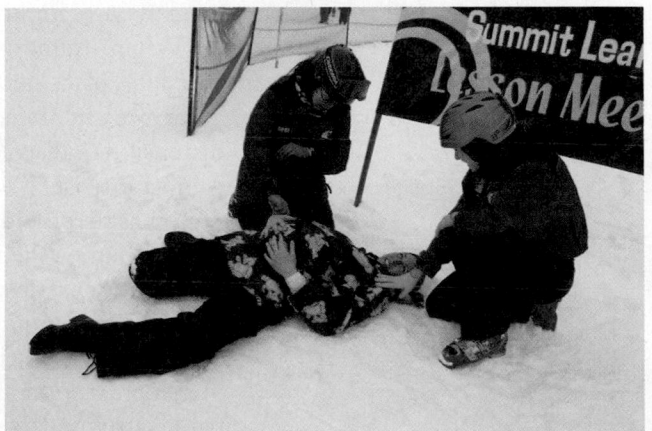

If her complaint is related to vaginal bleeding, ask the following questions:

+ How many pads or tampons have you used in the past 24 hours?
+ Have you passed any clots?
+ Have you noted any dizziness upon standing?
+ Have you received any trauma to your genital area?

If her complaint is related to abdominal pain, ask these questions:

+ Have you experienced this type of pain before (with menstruation, or between menses)?
+ Have you noted any recent vaginal bleeding or spotting?
+ Do you have any abnormal vaginal discharge, burning during urination, fever, or back pain?

If she is known to be pregnant, ask the following questions:

+ When is the expected due date?
+ Have you had any prenatal care?
+ Have you been pregnant before? If yes, did you have any deliveries, and were there any problems delivering?
+ Do you have any prenatal or preexisting medical conditions such as gestational diabetes, or a history of high blood pressure or twins?
+ Has your water broken (membranes ruptured)?
+ Have you noted any vaginal bleeding since the injury?
+ Have you felt the baby move since the injury?

Note that fetal movement can be detected by a pregnant woman after about 20 weeks of gestation and is a good sign of fetal well being. Also, if abdominal pain is present *in a pregnant woman*, determine the quality, location, and timing, and whether any back pain is present. Remember that conditions other than pregnancy may be the cause of the pain.

Be mindful at all times of a woman's need for privacy. Although a gynecologic or obstetrical history is crucial, try to ask the necessary questions in a way and in a place where others cannot overhear your conversation. In general, undressing a woman in an outdoor environment to perform an examination is not necessary; wait until she has reached a patrol facility or other first-aid facility where a female assistant can help with the inspection of the affected areas in privacy. If evacuation will take a long time and you feel that you need to, for example, inspect for crowning in a woman in labor who feels the need to push, improvise some screening using clothing, sheets, towels, or sleeping bags.

When examining a non-pregnant woman who has abdominal pain or vaginal bleeding, place her in a position of comfort—usually, supine with her knees flexed to allow the abdominal and pelvic muscles to relax. Look at the abdomen, noting any distension or discoloration. Have the patient use one finger to point to where her pain is most intense. Next, palpate the four quadrants of the abdomen and the suprapubic region as described in Chapter 16, Gastrointestinal and Genitourinary Emergencies. Note whether the woman reveals tenderness or shows guarding. OEC Technicians need not examine a non-pregnant woman's genital region unless she has a history of trauma and ongoing hemorrhage.

For a woman with a known pregnancy, note whether the uterus feels tight, as during a contraction, or if there is tenderness upon palpation. If the uterus is easily palpable, attempt to detect any fetal movement.

# Management

For non-pregnant women, begin by making sure the scene is safe, and care for any ABCD problems. For patients with heavy vaginal bleeding, severe abdominal pain, or signs and symptoms of shock, administer high-flow oxygen, and arrange for rapid transportation via ALS to a definitive-care medical facility. Monitor vital signs regularly while awaiting transport. Do not allow the patient to eat or drink while under your care as surgical intervention may be necessary. Abdominal pain may be associated with nausea or vomiting so anticipate the need to provide an emesis basin. Suction as needed to clear the airway.

The general management of a pregnant woman following trauma is similar to that of any other trauma victim, but with a few additional considerations. Following the scene survey and BSI precautions, begin—as always—with the ABCDs and a rapid assessment. Early critical interventions include application of high-flow oxygen—even without maternal signs of shock or respiratory difficulty. Suction as needed to clear the patient's airway. If possible, position the woman on her left side, or if her injuries prevent this, either elevate the right hip or manually displace the uterus until she is immobilized on a spine board to avoid possible supine hypotension from pressure on the vena cava (Figure 34-20■). When immobilizing a pregnant woman on a spine board, avoid placing any straps directly over her abdomen. Then tip the spine board to the patient's left by placing a patrol pack or a folded blanket under the right side of the board. Abdominal pain may be associated with nausea or vomiting, so anticipate the need to provide an emesis basin or to assist with removing an oxygen mask.

Transport rapidly but gently, reassessing the patient regularly (Figure 34-21■). In late stages of pregnancy, the uterus pushes up toward the diaphragm and makes it more difficult to take a deep breath. This can be compounded by transporting the woman in a toboggan with her head downhill, and should be avoided if possible. In the case of shock or suspected fetal shock for which transport in a head-downhill position is needed, an object such as a fanny pack can be placed under the head of the board to bring the board to a more neutral position, thus lessening respiratory difficulties while simultaneously treating shock.

⊕ **34-12** Describe the management of a pregnant patient with abdominal trauma.

**Figure 34-20** If possible, place the woman on her left side, or elevate her right hip or manually displace the uterus. Avoid placing straps over her abdomen.
Copyright Craig Brown

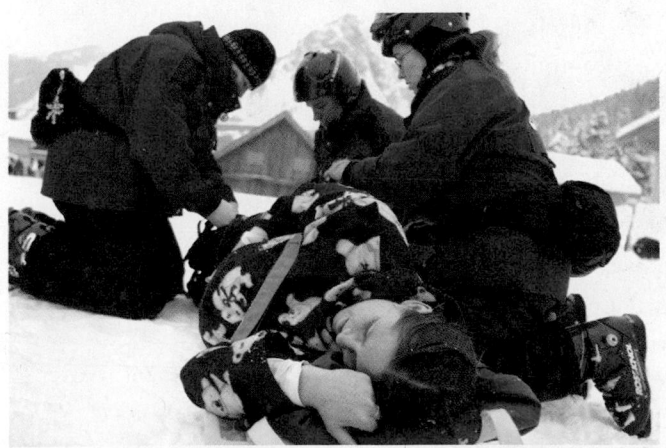

**Figure 34-21** Most women with any gynecologic or obstetrical complaint will require further evaluation by a physician at a medical facility.

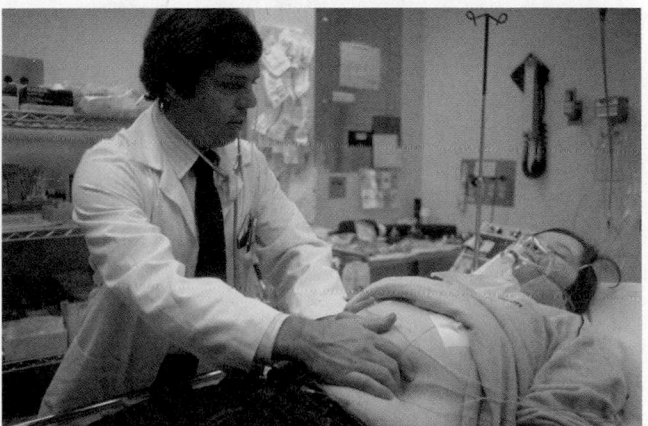

# CASE DISPOSITION

After placing your patient on her left side, her pulse rate remains at 110 but is much stronger, and a repeat blood pressure reading is now 105/70. She continues to complain of severe abdominal pain, and reassessment shows her uterus to be continuously firm. You place the patient on high-flow oxygen by nonrebreather mask while arranging emergency transportation to the hospital.

You transport the patient, lying on her left side, by toboggan to the patrol facility, where an ALS ambulance crew is awaiting her arrival. Two days later, the patient's husband stops by the patrol room to thank you and the other patrollers. He reports that his wife was diagnosed at the hospital with abruptio placentae. She underwent an emergency caesarian section to deliver a 3-pound baby boy who is on a ventilator in the neonatal intensive care unit but is doing well. He tearfully notes that without your prompt care and rapid evacuation, he could have lost not just his wife, but his newborn son as well!

## OEC SKILL 34-1 | Assisting with Childbirth

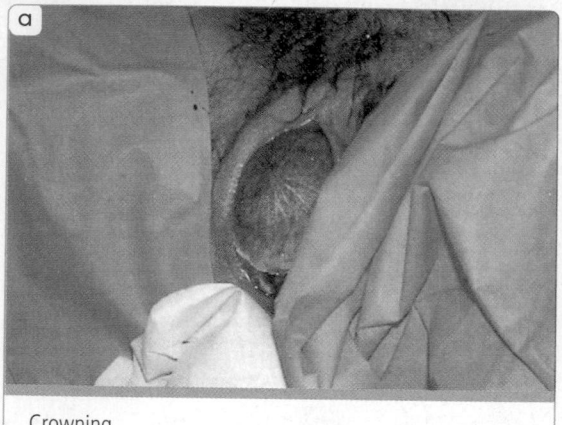

Crowning.

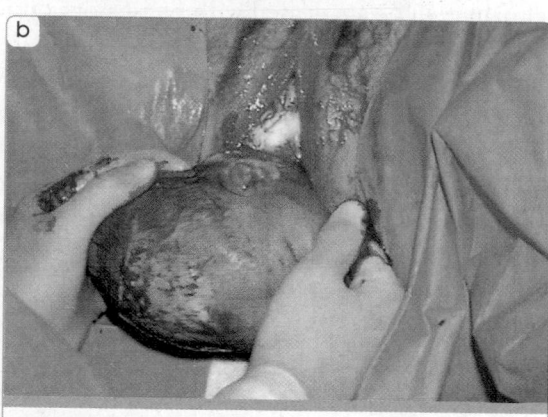

Head delivers and turns.

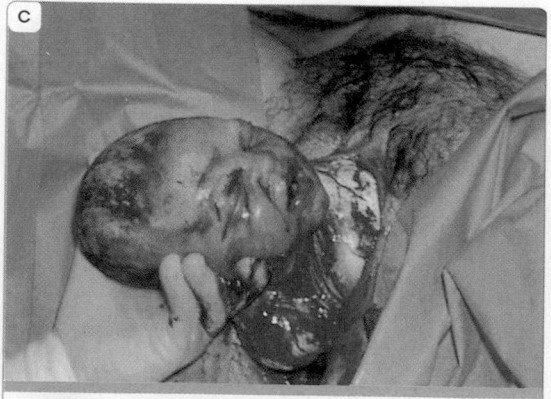

Shoulders deliver.

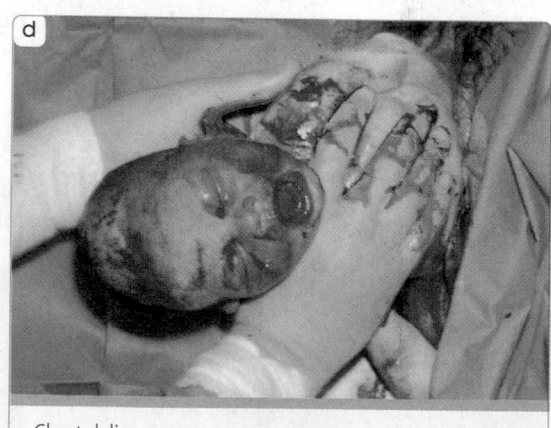

Chest delivers.

## OEC SKILL 34-1 | Assisting with Childbirth

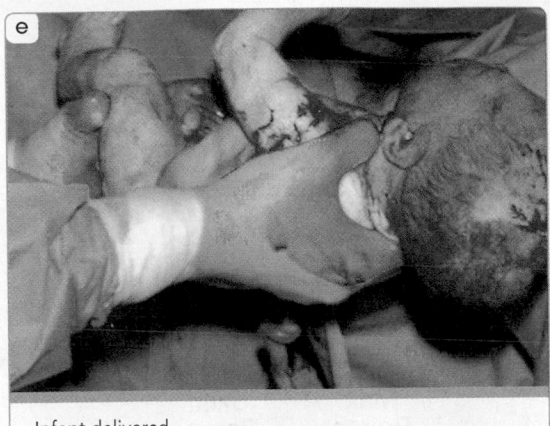

Infant delivered.

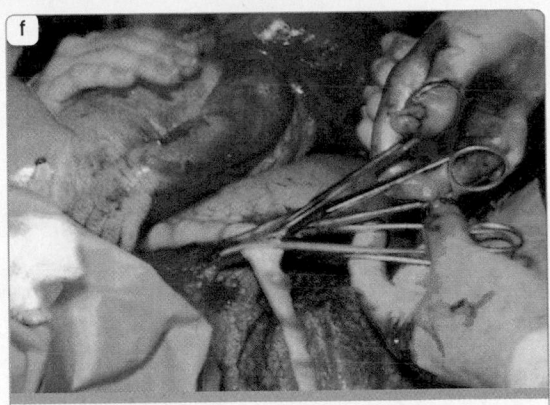

Cutting of the cord.

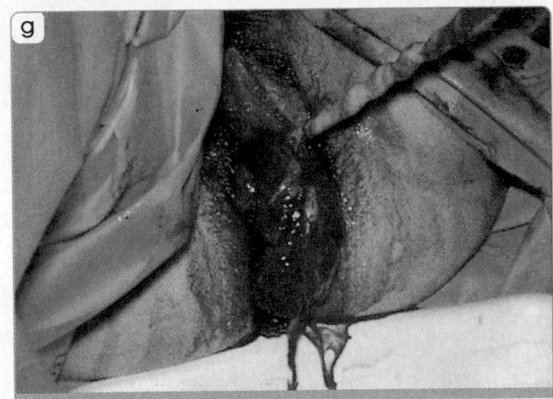

Placenta begins delivery.

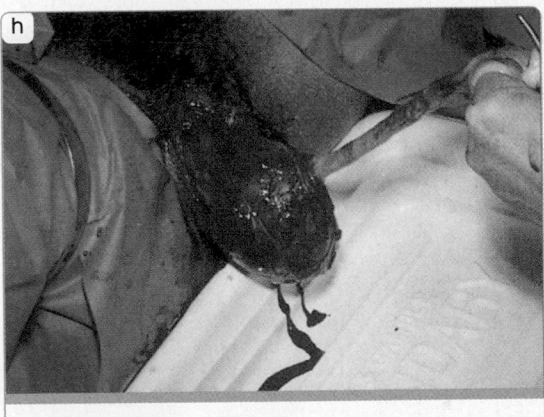

Placenta delivers.

## Skill Guide

Date: _____

(CPI) = Critical Performance Indicator

Candidate: _____

Start time: _____

End time: _____

## Assisting with Normal Childbirth

**Objective:** To demonstrate ability to assist in a live, uncomplicated delivery of a newborn.

| Skill | Max Points | Skill Demo | |
|---|---|---|---|
| Determines scene is safe. | 1 | | (CPI) |
| Introduces self, obtains permission to treat/help. | 1 | | |
| Initiates Standard Precautions. | 1 | | (CPI) |
| Obtains disposable sterile OB delivery kit or improvises with towels, sheets, blankets, etc. | 1 | | |
| Assists mother in removing clothing, positioning mother on firm padded surface and provides privacy. | 1 | | (CPI) |
| Positions mother in a semi-Fowler's position, elevates pelvis 2"–4" keeping knees flexed. | 1 | | |
| Times contractions from start of one contraction to the beginning of the next. Notes duration of contraction by feeling the abdomen. | 1 | | (CPI) |
| When the baby is crowning, encourages mother to push while supporting the head of the baby. Applies gentle pressure with his hand to allow head to come out in a controlled fashion. | 1 | | (CPI) |
| After head has emerged, instructs mother to stop pushing and immediately suction baby's mouth, nostrils with soft rubber bulb syringe. Notes if fluid is not clear (possible meconium in fluid). | 1 | | (CPI) |
| Checks position of umbilical cord. If around the baby's neck, gently lifts cord over the baby's head. If unable to lift over head, places 2 clamps 2" apart and cuts cord. | 1 | | (CPI) |
| Guides baby's head down to deliver the shoulder as mother pushes. Supports baby's head with non-dominant hand and slides dominant hand under the baby's body as it emerges. Suctions nose and mouth again. | 1 | | |
| Records time and location of the birth. | 1 | | (CPI) |
| If transport to hospital is >20 min, cuts umbilical cord. | 1 | | |
| Dries infant, wraps in blanket, assesses APGAR and record. | 1 | | (CPI) |
| Prepares for delivery of placenta approx 20–30 min later. Transports placenta with mother to hospital. | 1 | | |
| Places sanitary napkin between mother's legs. Massages lower abdomen in a firm circular motion. | 1 | | |
| Places mother in Trendelenburg position, provides $O_2$, monitor vital signs. | 1 | | (CPI) |
| Evaluates infant vital signs/APGAR. Provides interventions as necessary. | 1 | | (CPI) |

Must receive 14 out of 18 points.

Comments:_____

Failure of any of the CPIs is an automatic failure.

Evaluator: _____   NSP ID:_____

PASS      FAIL

# Chapter Review

## Chapter Summary

Because women have unique anatomical structures that function in reproduction, OEC Technicians can be faced with unique situations when providing care for a woman. These situations include vaginal bleeding, reproductive system infections, problems with internal reproductive organs, and of course situations related to a normal or an abnormal pregnancy. By understanding the female anatomy, the pathological processes that are unique to females, and pregnancy, OEC Technicians will have the knowledge they need to help women who have reproductive system–related medical problems.

Most women with any gynecologic or obstetrical complaint will require further evaluation by a physician at a medical facility. Whether this is done emergently or within a short time is the important determination that OEC Technicians must make and recommend to their patients. The initial care you provide could be life saving to the woman, or to the child she is carrying if she is pregnant.

## Remember...

1. Gynecologic emergencies are related to a woman's reproductive organs.
2. Always consider the possibility of pregnancy in a female of reproductive age.
3. The goals for managing OB/GYN emergencies are rapid identification of a potentially serious or life-threatening condition, immediate care, and evacuation to definitive care.
4. A pregnant woman may lose 30–35 percent of her blood volume from hemorrhage before showing signs of shock.
5. Maternal hemorrhage places the fetus at high risk for shock.
6. Treat all pregnant trauma patients for shock.
7. Prevent maternal hypotension by placing the patient on her left side.
8. Always respect a woman's privacy.

# Chapter Questions

## Multiple Choice

Choose the correct answer.

1. What do you do next if after 1 minute of resuscitation (rescue breathing) you find that a newborn's pulse has increased to 100 beats per minute? _____
   a. Gradually reduce the rate and pressure with the BVM until the newborn can breathe on its own and maintains good color.
   b. Increase the breath rate and pressure with the BVM until the newborn can breathe on its own and maintains good color.
   c. Immediately stop ventilating the newborn.
   d. Continue rescue breathing at the same rate until more advanced medical help arrives.

2. What should you do next if after 30 seconds of receiving ventilations and supplemental oxygen a newborn's pulse rate has increased from 60 to 80? _____
   a. Continue with the ventilations and check the pulse again in 30 seconds.
   b. Begin CPR.
   c. Administer blow-by oxygen.
   d. Stop ventilations and allow the newborn to breathe on its own because its pulse rate has improved.

3. Which of the following statements regarding trauma during pregnancy is false? _____
   a. Because of protection from the maternal bony pelvis, the amniotic fluid, and an increase in maternal blood volume, it takes a fairly major incident—such as a high-speed collision—to cause fetal or maternal injury or death due to trauma.
   b. Most cases of trauma during pregnancy can be handled by taking care of the ABCDs, by placing the woman on her left side (or tilting a backboard to the left), by administering oxygen, and by rapidly transporting the woman to definitive medical care.
   c. Uterine rupture may present with minimal signs or symptoms even as the fetus and the woman are slipping into shock.
   d. The fetus is less protected from shock when the woman goes into shock.

4. Other than maternal death, what is the *most common* cause of fetal death due to major or minor trauma? _____
   a. a collision that results in uterine rupture
   b. a shearing force that results in abruptio placentae
   c. a fall that results in premature labor
   d. a uterine perforation

5. Which of the following questions is *not* appropriate to ask a female of childbearing age who has been injured? _____
   a. Have you been sexually active?
   b. Could you possibly be pregnant?
   c. When was your last normal menstrual period?
   d. When is your next period expected?

6. Which of the following questions are important questions to ask an ill or injured woman who is known to be pregnant? (check all that apply)
   _____ a. When is the expected due date?
   _____ b. What is your blood type?
   _____ c. Have you had any prenatal care?
   _____ d. Do you have any unique prenatal or preexisting medical conditions such as gestational diabetes, or a history of high blood pressure or twins?
   _____ e. When did you last urinate?
   _____ f. Has your water broken? or Have your membranes ruptured?
   _____ g. Have you noted any vaginal bleeding since the injury?
   _____ h. Have you felt the baby move since the injury?
   _____ i. Do you know who the baby's father is?

## Short Answer

Name some of the dangerous consequences of a fall or collision during pregnancy.

_____

_____

_____

## Sequence

Number the following actions in the correct sequence for an imminent field delivery.

_____ **a.** Check to see if the baby's head is crowning; apply gentle pressure with your gloved hand as the head emerges to decrease risk of perineal tearing.

_____ **b.** Prepare your site by gathering the necessary supplies.

_____ **c.** Feel for the umbilical cord around the infant's neck. If it is present, lift and remove it, or clamp and cut it if you cannot remove it.

_____ **d.** Place the patient on a firm, padded surface on her back in a semi-Fowler's position with a blanket or pillow lifting her buttocks 2–4 inches.

_____ **e.** Wait for the baby's head to rotate; then suction out the baby's mouth.

_____ **f.** Suction out the baby's airway if there is a visible obstruction.

_____ **g.** Use your non-dominant hand to control the baby's head, and slide your dominant hand alongside the baby's body as it emerges.

_____ **h.** Time the woman's contractions.

_____ **i.** Use a gloved hand on either side of the baby's head to guide the baby down slightly and help deliver the baby's shoulder.

_____ **j.** Record the time of birth.

_____ **k.** Rotate the baby 180 degrees and suction out the baby's mouth and nose.

## Matching

Match each of the following terms to its description.

_____ **1.** abruptio placentae

_____ **2.** dysmenorrhea

_____ **3.** eclampsia

_____ **4.** ectopic pregnancy

_____ **5.** gestation

_____ **6.** miscarriage

_____ **7.** placenta previa

**a.** a premature separation of a normally situated but improperly implanted placenta, resulting in severe pain, a firm, contracted uterus, and bright-red vaginal bleeding

**b.** a placenta placed abnormally low over the cervix, presenting with dark-red, painless, vaginal bleeding

**c.** painful menstruation with cramps in the lower abdomen

**d.** a pregnancy occurring elsewhere than within the uterus

**e.** a syndrome characterized by maternal hypertension, edema of the face and hands, and seizures

**f.** the period during which a woman is pregnant; in humans it is about 266 days from the fertilization of the egg until birth

**g.** a term for spontaneous abortion occurring prior to 20 weeks of gestation

# Scenario

*In response to a call from the Ski Shop, you arrive to find a woman who is lying on her back in pain, crying out for help. You ask her what could be wrong and she says, "I am pregnant and think I am delivering the baby." She also tells you that this is her first pregnancy and that she needs to have a bowel movement.*

*You secure the area and direct the shop clerk to clear the area of patrons.*

1. Your first action should be to _____
   a. show the woman where the women's toilet is, so she can have a bowel movement before going into labor.
   b. lower the woman to the floor and place her in the Semi-Fowler's position.
   c. lower the woman to the floor and place her in the Trendelenburg position.
   d. lower the woman to the floor and place her in the recovery position.

*You inspect her vaginal area for crowning and time her contractions. You can see a 2-inch diameter patch of hair on the top of the baby's head. The woman's contractions are less than 2 minutes apart and last for about 30 seconds each.*

2. What stage of labor is the woman in? _____
   a. first
   b. second
   c. third
   d. fourth

3. Based on the timing of the contractions, what is your next step? _____
   a. Call for an ambulance but be prepared to deliver the baby in the shop.
   b. Call for an ambulance and deliver the patient to the hospital.
   c. Move the patient to the first-aid room for treatment.
   d. Attempt to find other family members and have them get their car for transporting the woman to the hospital.

*As the woman starts pushing, the baby's head is expelled.*

4. Which of the following are not part of the OB-GYN kit?_____
   a. a scalpel
   b. a suture kit
   c. the umbilical cord ties
   d. sterile non-latex gloves

*The baby's delivery is complete. You note the time of birth, wrap the baby in a blanket to prevent hypothermia.*

5. The order of suctioning is_____
   a. the mouth.
   b. the nose first, then the mouth.
   c. the nose, then the mouth, then the nose again.
   d. the mouth first, then the nose.

*The baby's delivery is complete. You note the time of birth, wrap the baby in a blanket to prevent hypothermia, and continue to suction the baby's airway. The baby is breathing on his own within a few seconds. An OEC Technician next measures the baby's APGAR score and then repeats the process in five minutes.*

*The baby's heart rate is 104 beats per minute, his respirations are rated based on a weak cry, his muscle tone shows some motion, he is weakly crying, and his body is pink but his extremities are blue.*

6. What is the first APGAR score? _____
   a. 8
   b. 7
   c. 6
   d. 5

*The ambulance arrives, and the new mom and her healthy newborn are transferred to a gurney and taken to the hospital. The plastic bag containing the placenta is labeled with the woman's name and the date and the time and is sent with the two patients in the ambulance.*

## Suggested Reading

The American Congress of Obstetricians and Gynecologists. 2003. *Exercise During Pregnancy.* Patient education pamphlet accessed at http://www.acog.org/publications/patient_education/bp119.cfm

Cusick, S. S., and C. D. Tibbles. 2007. "Trauma in Pregnancy." *Emergency Medicine Clinics of North America* 25(3): 861–872, xi.

Daniels, R. V., and C. McCuskey. 2003. "Abnormal Vaginal Bleeding in the Non-pregnant Patient." *Emergency Medicine Clinics of North America* 21(3): 751–772.

DeCock, M. F. 2007. "Premature Infant Delivery in the Prehospital Setting." *Journal of Emergency Medical Services* 32(2): 72–83.

EXPLORE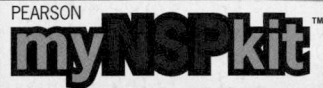

Please go to www.myNSPkit.com. Under Student Resources, you will find animations, videos, web links, and games related to this chapter—and much more. Look for information on breech presentation, ectopic pregnancy, neonatal resuscitation and more.

Register your access code from the front of your book by going to www.myNSPkit.com and selecting the appropriate links. If the in-cover access code has been redeemed, go to www.myNSPkit.com and follow links to **Buy Access.**

# Special Operations and Ambulance Operations

**35**

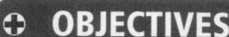

Denis M. Meade, MA, EMTP

Michael G. Millin, MD, MPH, FACEP

Rick King, NSP National Mountain Travel & Rescue Program Director, National Ski Patrol System, Inc.

Howard M. Laney, National Avalanche Program Director, National Ski Patrol System, Inc.

Frank Rossi, Pacific Northwest Division Mountain Travel and Rescue Advisor, National Ski Patrol System, Inc.

## ⊕ OBJECTIVES

**Upon completion of this chapter, the OEC Technician will be able to:**

**35-1**   Define special operations.

**35-2**   List several public safety activities that are classified as special operations.

**35-3**   Describe the basic operational tasks or objectives of various special operations groups.

**35-4**   List and describe the disaster response agencies that OEC Technicians are encouraged to join.

**35-5**   Describe HAZWOPER.

**35-6**   Identify the purpose of the International Hazard Classification System diamond placard system.

**35-7**   List and describe the three hazard control zones.

*continued*

## Chapter Overview

OEC Technicians are trained and prepared to manage a variety of medical and trauma emergencies. They also are able to identify and mitigate hazards, direct the actions of other rescuers at an emergency scene, and triage patients. Despite their superb training, OEC Technicians will occasionally encounter incidents that exceed the scope of their training and expertise. In these rare situations, OEC Technicians may need to summon rescuers with specialized skills and equipment to assist in managing the situation.

*continued*

## HISTORICAL TIMELINE

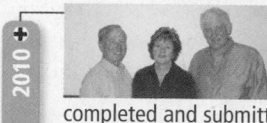

**2010**   *OEC* Fifth Edition is completed and submitted to production due to the great efforts of the NSP committee and many contributing writers.

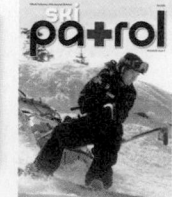

**2010**   OEC 5th Edition manuscript is introduced at the National Director's Meeting.

**35-8** Describe the purpose of and the mechanism of action for the contents of a nerve-agent antidote kit.

**35-9** Describe and demonstrate how to properly self-administer the contents of a nerve-agent antidote kit.

### ⊕ KEY TERMS

| | | |
|---|---|---|
| **CBRNE,** *p. 1109* | **high-angle rescue (HAR),** *p. 1123* | **search,** *p. 1118* |
| **cold zone,** *p. 1114* | **hot zone,** *p. 1114* | **special operations,** *p. 1101* |
| **extrication,** *p. 1105* | **low-angle rescue (LAR),** *p. 1124* | **terrorism,** *p. 1109* |
| **HAZWOPER,** *p. 1114* | **rescue,** *p. 1118* | **warm zone,** *p. 1114* |

This chapter provides an overview of the special operations situations in which OEC Technicians are most likely to become involved: natural and human-caused disasters, hazardous materials incidents, and searches. This chapter also includes a basic overview of ambulance operations. Although most OEC Technicians do not operate an ambulance, many of the principles presented apply to other equipment that OEC Technicians operate and maintain. Other topics covered in this chapter are community-based emergency response groups, rope rescues, and basic fire ground operations. The indications for and the self-administration of nerve-agent auto-injectors are also described.

The material in this chapter is intended to keep OEC Technicians safe when working on an incident involving specialized response personnel; it is not intended to either be all-encompassing or to replace specialized training. Additionally, the material presented is intended to encourage OEC Technicians to obtain additional training to better meet the needs of their respective resort areas and communities, and it is included so that rescuers can meet the requirements for achieving emergency first-responder status. Ski patrollers may find the information on avalanche rescue particularly valuable.

OEC Technicians are thoroughly trained to manage a variety of medical and trauma emergencies, to identify and mitigate hazards, to triage patients, and to direct the actions of other rescuers at the scene of an emergency. Despite this superb training, OEC Technicians occasionally encounter incidents that exceed the scope of their training and their expertise. **Special operations** is a generic term that denotes the various infrequently performed activities that require specialized training, skills, and equipment in remote and/or difficult settings. Additionally, numerous public safety activities are also classified as "special operations," including vehicle extrication, disaster management, search and rescue operations, low-angle rescues, lift evacuations, and avalanche rescues.

## Ambulance Operations

OEC Technicians frequently interact with ambulance crews (Figure 35-1■). Depending on the design of the emergency care system, OEC Technicians may even be asked to assist in a patient's care during transport to the hospital, so it is important that OEC Technicians have a basic understanding of ambulance operations and a familiarity with some of the nuances of working within such a confined environment.

OEC Technicians may encounter three basic ambulance designs:

+ A *Type I* ambulance has a truck-style chassis with a separate driver's compartment and a modular, box-style patient's compartment (Figure 35-2a■).

⊕ **35-1** Define special operations.

⊕ **35-2** List several public safety activities that are classified as special operations.

**special operations** infrequently performed activities requiring specialized training and equipment in remote and/or difficult settings.

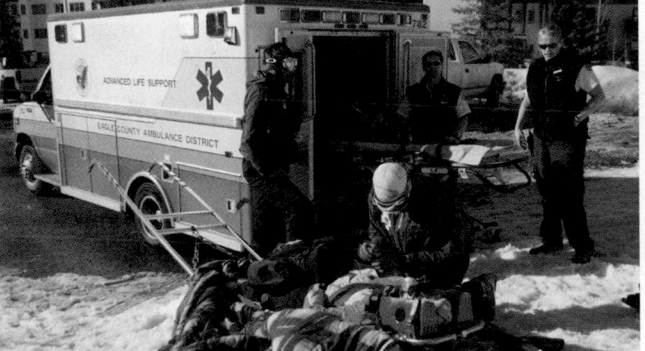

**Figure 35-1** OEC Technicians frequently interact with ambulance crews.
Copyright Scott Smith

A Type II ambulance has a van-style design that has a long wheelbase and direct access between the patient's compartment and the driver's compartment (Figure 35-2b■).

✚ A Type III ambulance has a van-style driver's compartment with direct access to an integral, modular patient's compartment (Figure 35-2c■).

Individual states, counties, or cities may impose rules and regulations regarding ambulance operations, including essential equipment requirements, minimum crew configurations and certification requirements, who may operate an ambulance, and when lights and sirens may be used. The next sections describe basic operational tasks and objectives for ambulance operations.

### Preparing for a Call

An ambulance must be maintained in a state of readiness and be fully stocked at all times (Figure 35-3■). Such readiness is made possible by regular maintenance, equipment checks, and routine cleaning. In most EMS systems, rescuers perform equipment inspections daily or at the beginning of each work period. Additionally, durable equipment (e.g., a stretcher, long spine boards) is cleaned after each use, and disposable equipment is replaced as needed to maintain minimum supply levels.

In accordance with federal recommendations, ambulances are strategically positioned within their geographic response area to reduce the response time to a request for assistance.

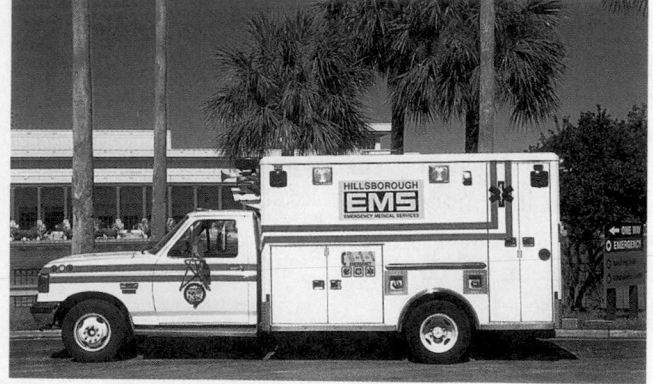

**Figure 35-2a** A Type I ambulance.

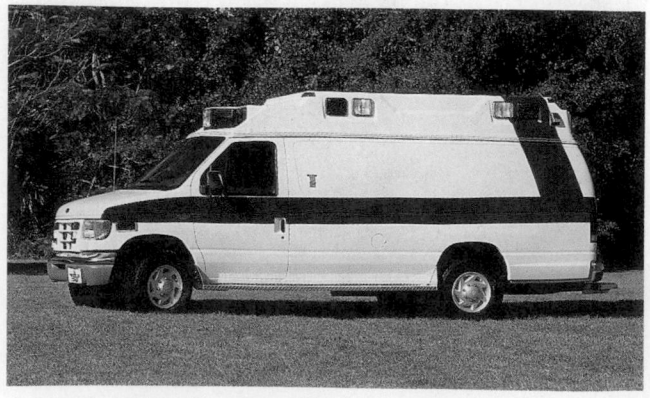

**Figure 35-2b** A Type II ambulance.

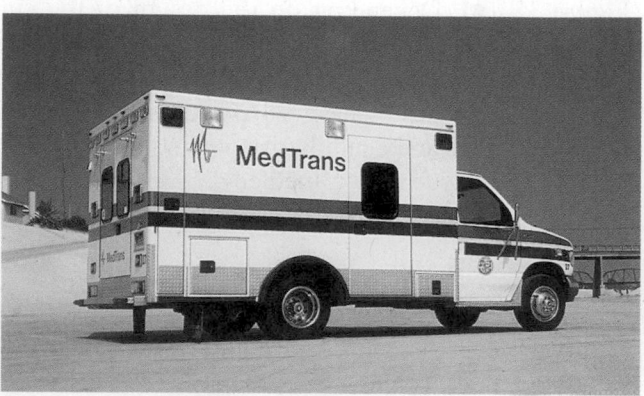

**Figure 35-2c** A Type III ambulance.

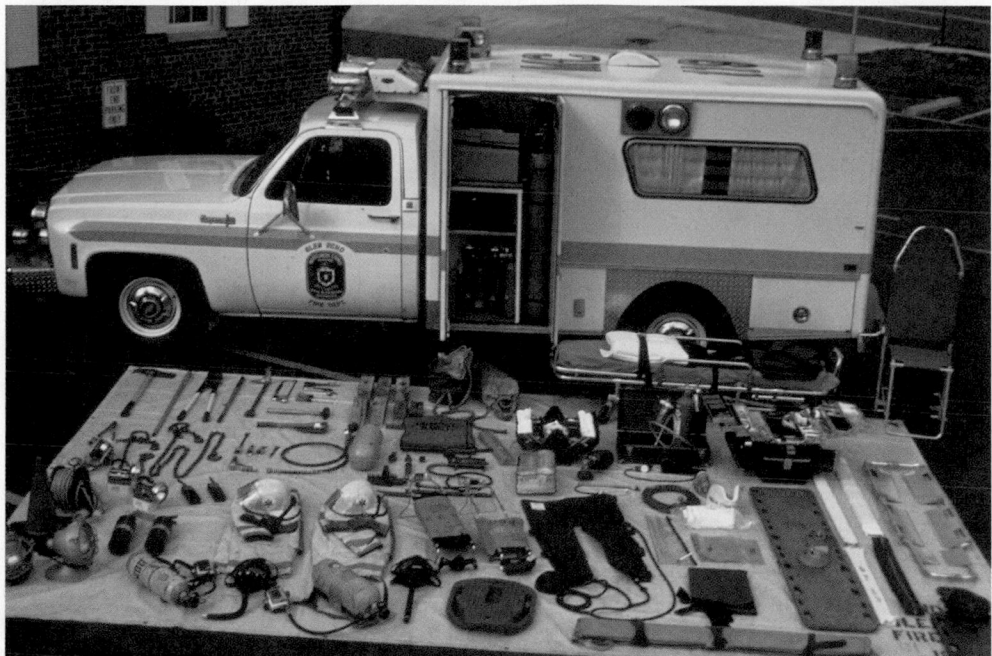

**Figure 35-3** Ambulances must be organized and properly maintained to respond quickly to a call.

## Responding to a Call

When an OEC Technician requests an ambulance to transport a patient, many things must occur if the ambulance is to arrive in a timely manner. For instance, the ambulance crew must receive accurate information regarding the location and nature of the emergency, and the crew must safely navigate to the scene despite possible dense traffic, hazardous road conditions, and/or inclement weather.

Most states and provinces have strict regulations regarding when lights and sirens may be used. As a rule, ambulance operators must obey all traffic laws, regardless of whether or not lights and siren are in use, although some exceptions may exist. The driver of an emergency vehicle must at all times observe "due regard for the safety of others," including that of the ambulance crew, the patient, passengers, other motorists, and the public at large. The following standard driving rules apply:

+ Observe all traffic laws, except as allowed by law.
+ Use the most appropriate route to and from the scene of the emergency.
+ Maintain a safe distance from other vehicles.
+ Use warning devices (e.g., lights and sirens) only as authorized by law or policy.

Intersections are the location of most ambulance accidents; the majority of collisions occur during daylight hours and in dry conditions (Figure 35-4■). When approaching an intersection, the ambulance crew must visually "clear" the intersection by ensuring that all other vehicles have come to a complete stop before the ambulance enters the intersection. Ideally, the ambulance operator should make eye contact with other drivers before proceeding through the intersection.

## Arriving at the Scene

The location in which an ambulance is parked depends on the circumstances. Whenever possible, the ambulance should be parked in a designated parking space, away from traffic. If law

**Figure 35-4** The most dangerous situation for a responding ambulance is entering an intersection during daylight hours.

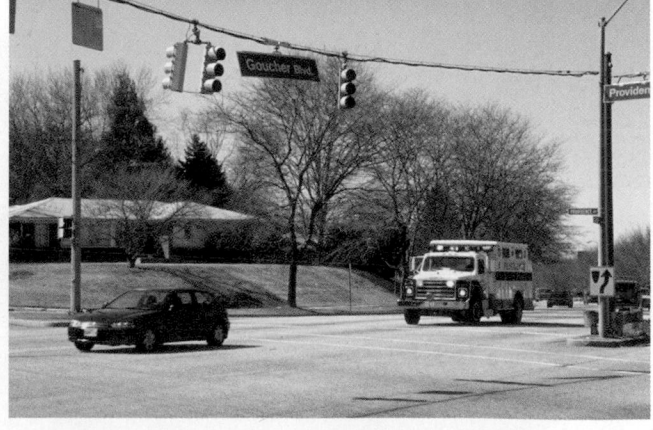

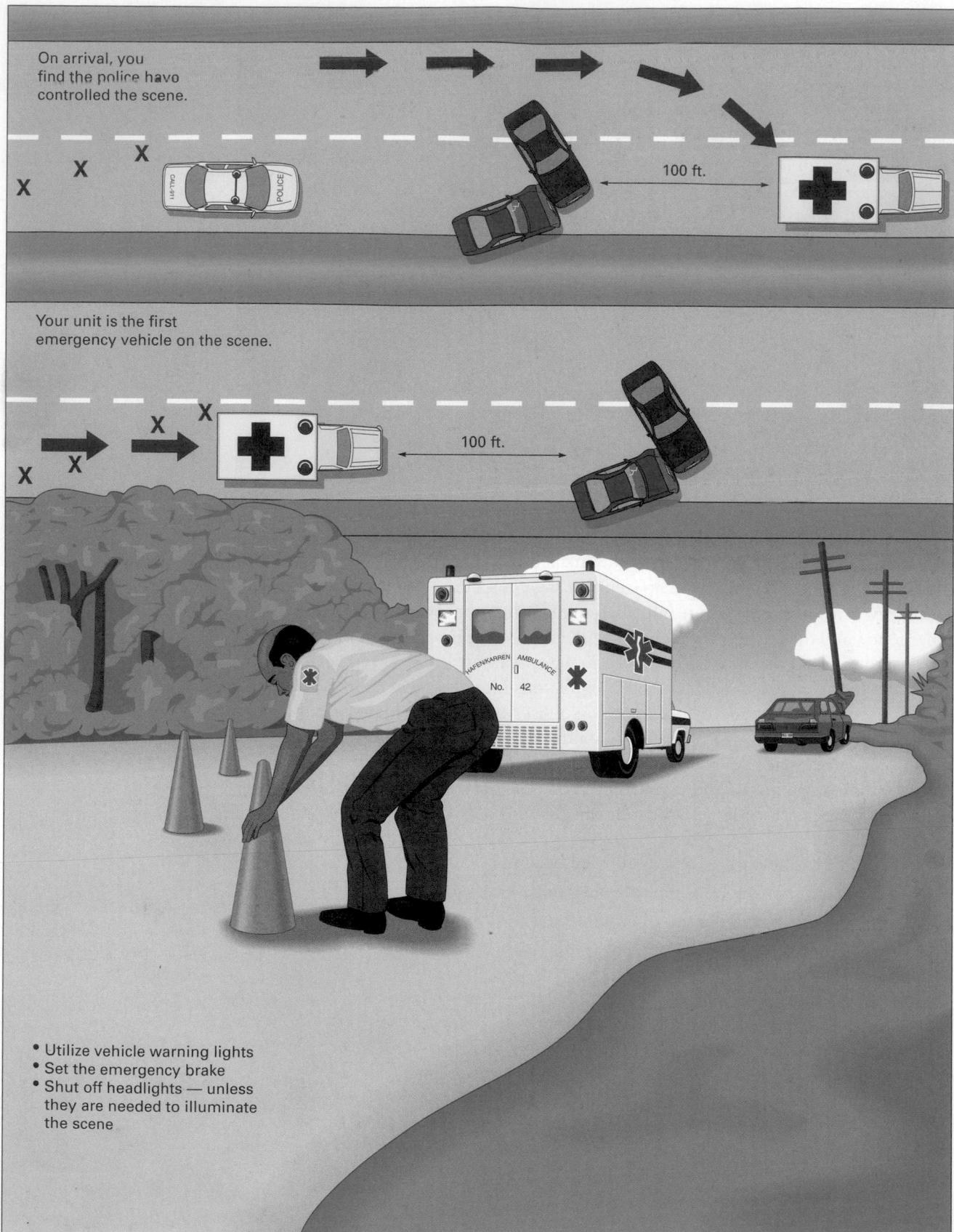

Figure 35-5 Proper parking plans for an ambulance at a collision scene.

enforcement personnel or fire equipment are at the scene, the ambulance should be parked 50–100 feet *beyond* the scene; if the scene has not yet been secured, the ambulance should be parked approximately 50–100 feet *before* the scene, using the ambulance to protect the scene, the rescuers, and bystanders (Figure 35-5■). The parking brake should be set after the vehicle is placed in "Park," and warning lights should be left on to visually alert drivers to the presence of an accident scene.

The area around the ambulance and accident scene is known as the "ambulance operation zone" and is designed to provide a safety barrier. When moving back and forth between the ambulance and the scene, walk along the side of the ambulance that is *farthest* from traffic.

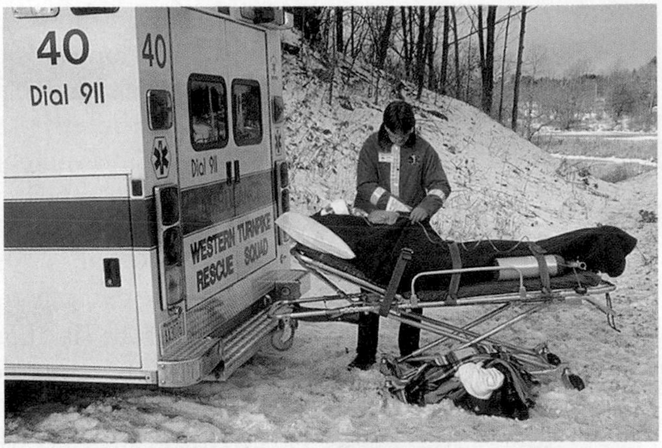

**Figure 35-6** The use of straps to secure a patient to a stretcher; straps may also be used as restraints for an agitated patient.

## Transferring Patients

Patients are generally moved to and from an ambulance on a wheeled ambulance stretcher, which typically can be raised and lowered by as few as two people. Specific ambulance stretcher operations vary, so check the manufacturer's instructions or contact the EMS agencies you work with to obtain training on the use of this device. The patient is secured to the stretcher by straps that are usually placed over the chest, the abdomen or upper thighs, and the lower legs (Figure 35-6■). For patients who are agitated, the strap buckles can be turned toward the patient to prevent unbuckling. Loading and unloading an ambulance stretcher may be performed by one or two people, typically by the ambulance operator and an assistant.

OEC Technicians may be asked to assist an ambulance crew in caring for a patient during transport to a definitive-care facility. When this occurs, OEC Technicians should be prepared to provide the full range of their OEC skills, including CPR, airway management, hemorrhage control, bandaging, and splinting. Under certain circumstances, they also may be asked to *assist* an advanced life support provider (e.g., an advanced EMT, a Paramedic), as described in Chapter 36, ALS Interface.

The patient's compartment of most ambulances generally is organized so that essential equipment is close at hand. For instance, airway equipment and oxygen are typically stored near the head of the stretcher, whereas bandaging supplies and splints are usually placed in cabinets near the middle of the stretcher.

Working in the back of a moving ambulance can be extremely dangerous and is much different than providing care on a stable, stationary surface. Accordingly, OEC Technicians asked to assist in the back of a moving ambulance must be very careful when standing or moving around because of the risk of losing their balance and becoming seriously injured. Unless absolutely necessary, remain seated at all times, either at the patient's head or side, or as instructed by the ambulance crew. While seated, use restraining devices, if available. Stand only long enough to perform the required task and then sit down again. Some ambulances are equipped with track-mounted harnesses that facilitate standing while the vehicle is in motion.

Be aware of any sharp objects (e.g., needles, edges) that may be present. Secure or stow loose objects and equipment to prevent them from becoming missiles in the event of a sharp turn or sudden braking. Keep your center of gravity low at all times. If you have any questions regarding how to operate safely in the back of a moving ambulance, consult a member of the ambulance crew.

## Extricating a Patient from a Vehicle

**Extrication** is the process of removing a trapped person (as from a vehicle that has been involved in a collision) when the removal of the person via a conventional exit (e.g.,

**extrication** the process of removing a trapped person (as from a vehicle that has been involved in a collision) when conventional means of exit are impossible or inadvisable.

a door, a window) is impossible or inadvisable. Examples in which OEC Technicians may become involved in extrication from a vehicle include an automobile crash, an overturned snowcat or groomer, or an airplane or helicopter crash.

Vehicle extrication is a time-consuming process involving several basic operational tasks and objectives, including assessment, stabilization, gaining access to the patient, and the initial care and removal of the patient.

### Assessment

Conduct a scene size-up to identify potential hazards and to form a general impression of the situation. During this step, assess the vehicle's position (e.g., upright, on its side, or upside down), stability (e.g., what is needed to keep the vehicle from inadvertently moving), and overall condition (e.g., leaking fuel, smoking, fire possible or already present). Mitigate all hazards (e.g., sharp edges, fuel or chemical leaks, undeployed airbags, or high-voltage batteries) before beginning extrication efforts. Gather basic patient information during this step (e.g., the total number of patients, priority of extrication, triage status).

To prevent injuries during extrication efforts, all rescuers must use proper personal protective equipment. Ski patrollers should keep their helmets, goggles, and gloves on at all times. Other OEC Technicians should wear, at a minimum, an approved safety helmet, impact-resistant glasses, and heavy leather work gloves.

### Stabilization

A vehicle that has been involved in a crash must be properly stabilized (Figure 35-7■). This is especially true if the vehicle is found on its side or, worse, upside down. Even a vehicle that is upright must be stabilized to prevent accidental movement during rescue operations.

Standard vehicle stabilization-related tasks include shutting down the vehicle's engine, de-energizing the electrical system by disconnecting the battery cables, engaging the parking brake, and cribbing the vehicle (placing 4-inch by 4-inch or 6-inch by 6-inch wood blocks at strategic points to stabilize the vehicle and keep it from moving). If needed, a vehicle may be further stabilized using chains or come-alongs attached to nearby trees, rocks, or rescue vehicles.

### Gaining Access to the Patient

Whenever a patient must be extricated from a vehicle, rescuers create an imaginary 10-foot radius around the vehicle known as the "working area" or "inner circle." Access into this area is generally restricted to personnel who are directly involved in the extrication process or who are providing life-saving interventions to the patient.

As a rule, experts recommend that rescuers "try before you pry"—that is, check all of the vehicle's doors before attempting a forcible entry to reach a patient. A door on the opposite side of the vehicle is often undamaged and fully functional. Using this door may save precious minutes or even hours of unnecessary extrication efforts.

Gaining access to a patient can involve moving or cutting away parts of the vehicle so that rescue personnel can make physical contact with the patient. This action also provides an exit through which the patient may be removed from the vehicle. A variety of tools may be used, ranging from simple hand tools such as a spring-loaded punch, a screwdriver, or a crowbar (Table 35-1■), to complex hydraulic tools such as cutters,

**Anatomy of a Vehicle Extrication Scene**

NOTE

*Front*

*Driver's side of vehicle*

*Passenger's side of vehicle*

*Rear of vehicle*

*Working area (inner circle; 10 feet around outside of vehicle)*

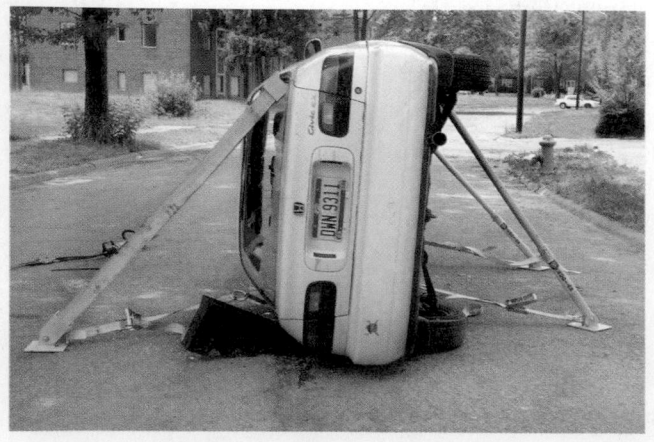

**Figure 35-7** Always stabilize a vehicle for everyone's safety before beginning rescue operations.

**Table 35-1** Simple Hand Tools

| Tool | Use(s) |
| --- | --- |
| Belt cutter | To cut seat belts, restraining straps, or other cloth materials |
| Bolt cutter | For cutting thick metal objects such as locks, Nader pins, hinges, or thick wires |
| Center punch | To break safety glass to gain access through a window |
| Chock/Step chock | To stabilize the wheels of a vehicle; may incorporate multiple "steps" for wheels of different heights |
| Come-along | To provide a mechanical advantage in pulling apart metal and gaining access to the patient compartment |
| Cribbing (a set of wood blocks) | To stabilize a vehicle or provide support to an unsteady object |
| Hack saw | To cut metal, typically small metal objects or sheet metal |
| Hammer/sledge hammer | To make sharp edges blunt; to pound parts of the vehicle to gain access to the inside |
| High-lift jack | To provide a mechanical advantage for lifting heavy or unstable objects |
| Pry bar/Crow bar | To serve as a fulcrum to open doors or to move twisted metal aside |
| Screwdriver | To remove screws or to pry open narrow spaces |
| Wedge | To mechanically hold a door open |
| Wire cutters | For cutting thin metal objects such as retaining clips or wires |

spreaders, or saws (Figure 35-8■). Additionally, chains, ratchet straps, come-alongs, airbags, and winches may be used, especially if large parts of the vehicle must be moved, lifted, or pulled away. OEC Technicians should be familiar with and be able to appropriately use a variety of simple hand tools.

If extrication is required, all windshields, rear window and side window glass in the immediate area should be carefully removed. In addition, any vehicle restraint devices such as seatbelts or harnesses should be cut away. If necessary, the vehicle's door(s) or top may be removed, a third "door" may be cut, or the dashboard may be moved.

### Initial Care and Removal of the Patient

The removal of a patient follows the general principles described in other chapters and centers on correcting threats to life and protecting the patient's spine. Care may need to be initiated while the patient is still inside the vehicle. Long spine boards, vest-type immobilization devices, and short boards are commonly used to remove a patient from a vehicle (Figure 35-9■).

**Figure 35-8** Parts of the vehicle may need to be cut away so that rescue personnel can make physical contact with a patient.

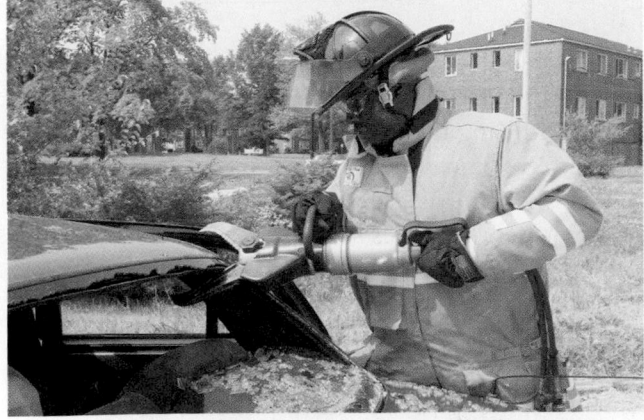

**Figure 35-9** The focuses of extricating a patient are the ABCDs and protecting the patient's spine.

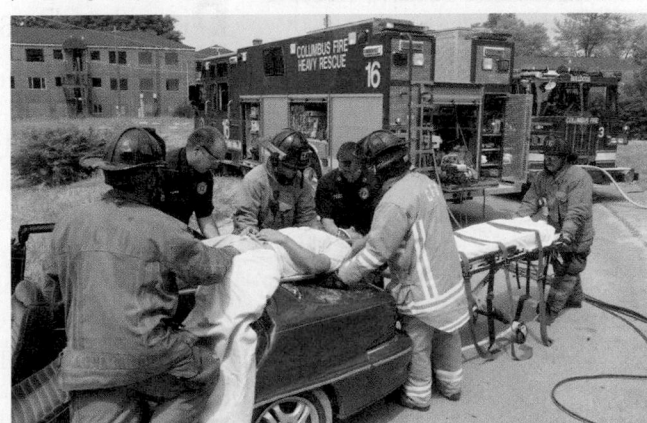

## STOP, THINK, UNDERSTAND

### Multiple Choice
Choose the correct answer.

1. The area around an ambulance and an accident scene is known as the _____
   a. ambulance operation zone.
   b. danger zone.
   c. safety zone.
   d. accident rescue zone.

2. Where should an ambulance be parked if the scene has not yet been secured? _____
   a. At least 5 feet before the scene
   b. 50–100 feet before the scene
   c. 25–50 feet beyond the scene
   d. At least 50 feet beyond the scene

3. Where should an ambulance be parked if law enforcement personnel or fire equipment are at the scene? _____
   a. 25–50 feet beyond the scene
   b. 25–50 feet before the scene

   c. 50–100 feet beyond the scene
   d. 50–100 feet before the scene

4. What are the basic operational tasks and objectives for ambulance operations? _____
   a. preparing for a call, responding to a call, and documenting a call
   b. preparing for a call and responding to a call
   c. responding to a call and documenting a call
   d. preparing for a call and documenting a call

5. A general rule in extricating a patient from a vehicle is_____
   a. "cut first."
   b. "break the glass, then cut."
   c. "pry before breaking the glass."
   d. "try before you pry."

## ✚ CASE UPDATE ✚

Arriving on scene, you find no immediate hazards, and when you look inside the car, you find two victims, both unresponsive but apparently breathing. One patient is bleeding from the mouth. You cannot open either door of the coupe. You contact dispatch and request immediate assistance, backboards, a trauma pack with oxygen, an ALS ambulance, and law enforcement personnel. You also request the fire department to come and extricate the patients from the vehicle, and you summon your patrol's low-angle rescue team.

*What should you do now?*

---

**⊕ 35-3** Describe the basic operational tasks or objectives of various special operations groups.

**⊕ 35-4** List and describe the disaster response agencies that OEC Technicians are encouraged to join.

# Disaster Response

Chapter 4, Incident Command and Triage, discussed the management of multiple-casualty incidents (MCIs), including the structure of the National Incident Management System (NIMS), the process of utilizing the Incident Command System (ICS), and methods for triaging patients into treatment priorities. Most MCIs can be managed using local resources or by enlisting the assistance of resources from the surrounding areas. However when an incident becomes so large that outside resources are needed, the situation is considered a disaster. Although rare, disasters often have serious consequences. The key to effective disaster management is preparedness.

Disasters are typically grouped into two broad categories: natural disasters and human-caused disasters. Examples of natural disasters include floods, tornados, hurricanes (Figure 35-10■), wild-land fires, droughts, and earthquakes (Figure 35-11■).

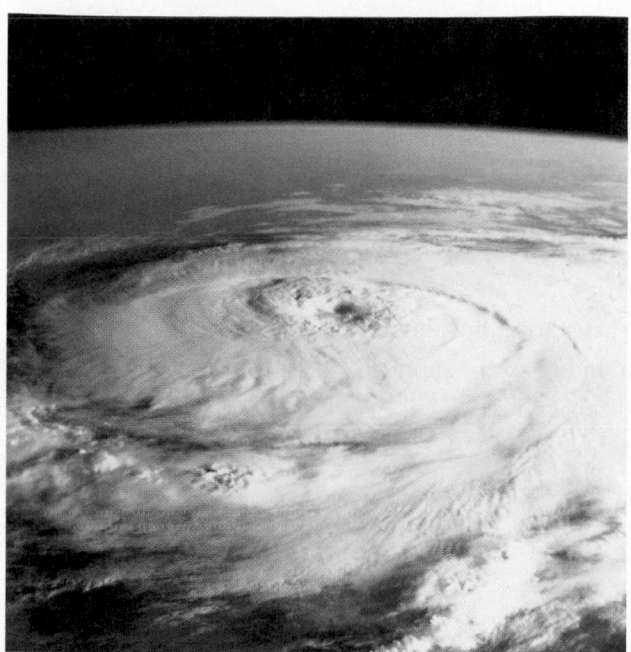

**Figure 35-10** A hurricane, as seen from space, is one kind of natural disaster.
Copyright Dorling Kindersley Media Library

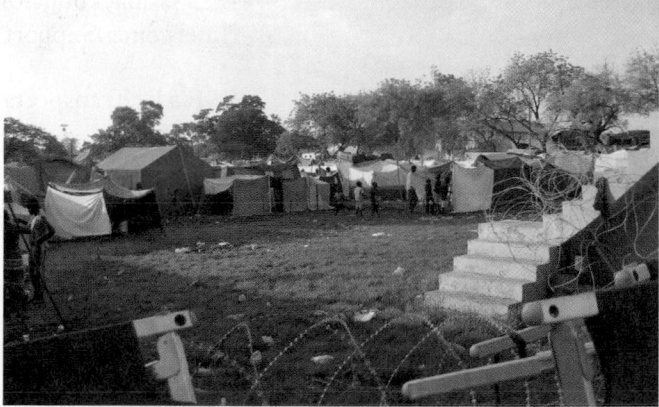

**Figure 35-11** Tent cities in Haiti after the 2010 earthquake.
Copyright Edward McNamara

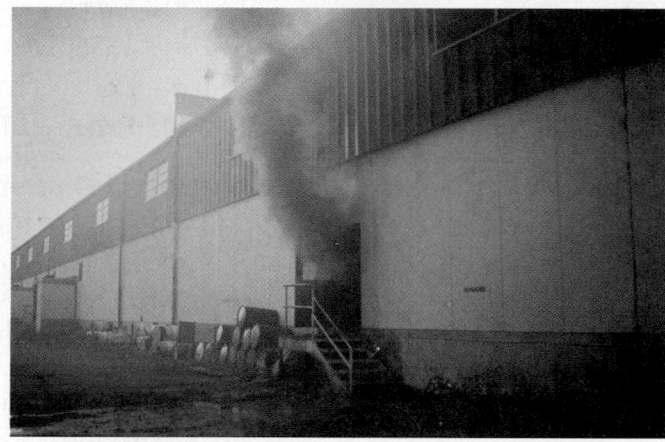

**Figure 35-12** An unintentional human-caused disaster at a warehouse.

Human-caused disasters can be subdivided into unintentional or intentional disasters. Examples of unintentional disasters include failure of an electrical power grid, an explosion at a power plant requiring mass evacuation of the local population, or a fire in a warehouse (Figure 35-12■). Intentional disasters often are due to an act of **terrorism** and are typically classified by the substance involved using the mnemonic **CBRNE**, (SEE-Burn) which represents chemical, biological, radiological, nuclear, and explosive.

Whether natural or man-made, a disaster often brings temporary chaos to a local or regional community. Fortunately, an organized system is in place in the United States to respond to disasters, whether local or national in scale. Trained individuals who are not part of this organized system often want to volunteer to help in the response to disasters, but because organized disaster teams have specific tasks and procedures that typically require specialized training, the presence of unofficial disaster responders can actually impede the overall mission. Therefore, if you wish to participate in disaster response, consider becoming a member of an established disaster response team, such as a local Civilian Emergency Response Team (CERT), a local Disaster Medical Assistance Team (DMAT), a regional Medical Resource Corps (MRC), or the national Urban Search and Rescue (USAR) group. These groups are part of the country's National Response Framework (NRF).

Developed by the Department of Homeland Security, the NRF provides guidelines for the all-hazards response to any incident within the United States, identifies the key principles to the response, and delineates the responsibilities of all entities that may participate in the response. The NRF is supported by five principles: engaged partnerships, a tiered response, scalable operational capabilities, a unified command, and readiness to act.

**terrorism** a human-caused event that is intended to inflict fear and can involve hazardous materials.

**CBRNE** a mnemonic for the common types of human-caused disasters; represents chemical, biologic, radiological, nuclear, and explosive.

The backbone of the NRF consists of the following 15 specialized groups called Emergency Support Function (ESF) annexes:

ESF #1  Transportation
ESF #2  Communications
ESF #3  Public works and engineering
ESF #4  Firefighting
ESF #5  Emergency management
ESF #6  Mass care, emergency assistance, housing, and human services
ESF #7  Logistics management and resource support
ESF #8  Public health and medical services
ESF #9  Search and rescue
ESF #10 Oil and hazardous materials response
ESF #11 Agriculture and natural resources
ESF #12 Energy
ESF #13 Public safety and security
ESF #14 Long-term community recovery
ESF #15 External affairs

## National Disaster Medical System (NDMS)

The Office of the Assistant Secretary for Preparedness and Response (ASPR) within the U.S. Department of Health and Human Services (DHHS) oversees the administration of ESF #8, public health and medical services. The mobilization and operation of ESF #8 is largely carried out by the National Disaster Medical System (NDMS). The primary purpose of NDMS is to supplement local and regional public health and medical resources in dealing with the medical effects of major disasters. NDMS has three primary components:

+ Medical response to a disaster
+ Movement of patients from a disaster site to an unaffected area
+ Definitive medical care at participating hospitals in unaffected areas

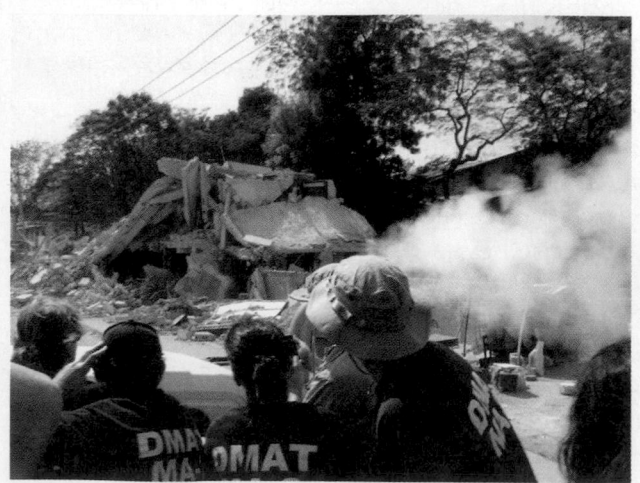

**Figure 35-13** This DMAT team is part of a federal medical response team within NDMS.
Copyright Edward McNamara

Disaster response within NDMS is carried out through the following five types of specialized response teams:

+ Disaster Medical Assistance Teams (DMAT)
+ Disaster Mortuary Operational Response Teams (DMORT)
+ National Veterinary Response Teams (NVRT)
+ National Nurse Response Teams (NNRT)
+ National Pharmacy Response Teams (NPRT)

Of the five response teams within NDMS, disaster medical assistance teams (DMATs) are responsible for the medical aspects of disaster response (Figure 35-13■). DMATs are trained to deploy to disaster sites and are equipped with sufficient supplies to be self-sustainable for 72 hours. Each team consists of physicians, nurses, paramedics, pharmacists, mental health professionals, communication specialists, logistics specialists, and administrative support personnel. To ensure continuous availability for disaster medical response, DMAT team members are employed part-time by DHHS and dedicate a portion of their professional time to disaster response.

Although a fully deployed team typically consists of 35 members, the team may also deploy in five-member strike teams. DMATs are able to set up and run a self-supporting field hospital (Figure 35-14■). They may also supplement local health-care resources by providing staff at first-aid stations and/or within hospitals.

Given their expertise in providing emergency care in outdoor settings, OEC Technicians are encouraged to join a DMAT. For more information about DMATs, go to http://www.hhs.gov/aspr/opeo/ndms/teams/dmat.html.

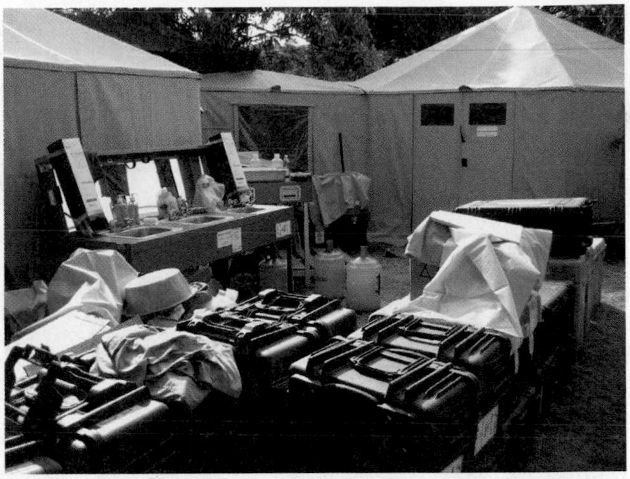

**Figure 35-14** DMATs can set up self-supporting field hospitals.
Copyright Edward McNamara

## Medical Reserve Corps (MRC)

In addition to the formalized structure of the NDMS, another asset available for the local, regional, and national disaster response is the volunteer Medical Reserve Corps (MRC). On a national level, MRCs are organized through the Office of the Surgeon General. At the unit level, MRCs are community based, composed of volunteer medical professionals who have agreed to help in the event of a disaster. Although the training and time commitment are not as intense as that for a DMAT, MRC team members are required to complete basic disaster training and maintain a minimum set of credentials. Many MRCs are given specific goals for strengthening the national public-health infrastructure. Because the OEC curriculum is accepted by MRCs, OEC Technicians are encouraged to join their local or regional MRC. For more information about MRC or to find a local unit, go to http://www.medicalreservecorps.gov.

## Community Emergency Response Team (CERT)

Each local community needs citizens trained in basic disaster response, and these needs extend well beyond medical care. Communities affected by disasters need assistance with evacuation, search and rescue, fire suppression, communications, and other forms of basic assistance. A community emergency response team (CERT) is designed specifically for this purpose. Although organized through the Federal Emergency Management Agency (FEMA), CERTs are composed of local volunteers that support local public-safety officials and provide immediate assistance to victims during a disaster. Members receive basic training in emergency response, search and rescue, and other topics specifically related to disaster management. The federal CERT program and the NSP have been working together for several years to encourage patrollers to join their local CERT teams. For more information about CERT or to find a local unit, go to http://www.citizencorps.gov/cert.

The NSP encourages ski patrollers and OEC Technicians to serve on their local MRC or CERT so they can be mobilized to provide assistance in the event of a national, regional, or local disaster. In serving in this capacity, OEC Technicians continue the legacy of volunteerism established by NSP founder Charles "Minnie" Dole.

# Hazardous Materials Response

A hazardous material (HazMat) is any substance that, because of its quantity, concentration, or physical or chemical characteristics, is capable of harming people, property, or the environment. Hazardous materials can be solids, gas, or liquids (Figure 35-15■). Control of hazardous materials in the United States is under the

**35-5** Describe HAZWOPER.

**35-6** Identify the purpose of the International Hazard Classification System diamond placard system.

**35-7** List and describe the three hazard control zones.

**35-8** Describe the purpose of and the mechanism of action for the contents of a nerve-agent antidote kit.

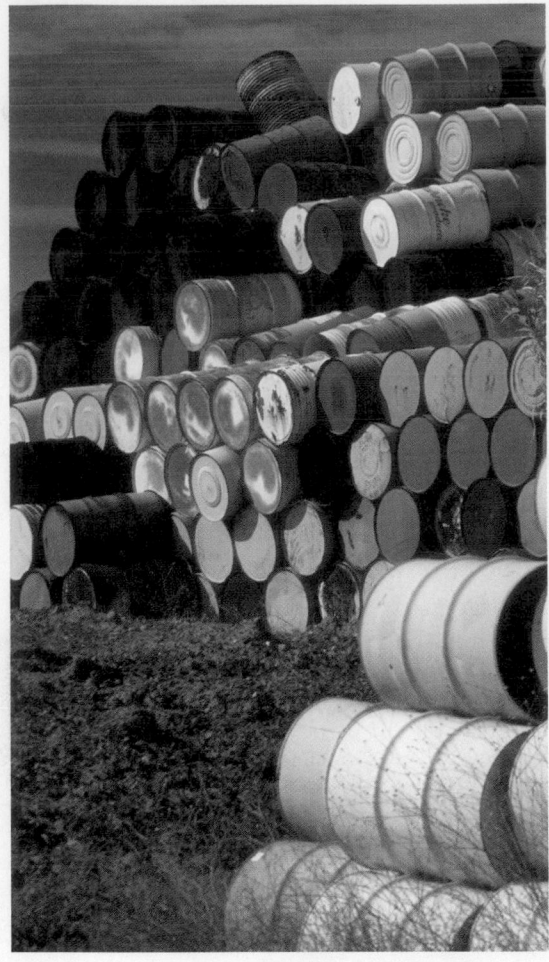

**Figure 35-15** Hazardous materials (HazMats) are substances that, because of their quantity, concentration, or physical or chemical characteristics, are capable of harming people, property, or the environment. HazMats may be housed in or transported through your community.

authority of the U.S. Department of Transportation (DOT), which uses the International Hazard Classification System to distinguish the following nine types of HazMats:

+ Explosives
+ Gases
+ Flammable/combustible liquids
+ Flammable solids
+ Oxidizers and organic peroxides
+ Poisonous materials and infectious substances
+ Radioactive substances
+ Corrosive materials
+ Miscellaneous hazardous materials

As required by the DOT and the National Fire Protection Association (NFPA), each hazardous material that is in transit must be identified by a specific placard known as the NFPA safety diamond. This diamond-shaped placard contains four smaller, color-coded diamond-shaped fields, each of which identifies the known hazards for a given material—flammability (red), health hazard (blue), chemical reactivity (yellow), and special precautions (white)—as shown in Figure 35-16■. Table 35-2■ provides an explanation of the numerals and symbols that can appear in each of the four colored fields.

HazMat incidents are managed using the incident command system (ICS). Within the ICS structure, a HazMat safety officer reports directly to an incident commander and ensures the safety of personnel responding to the incident. The HazMat ICS operations branch includes a HazMat entry team with backup personnel (Figure 35-17■), decontamination personnel, and medical sector personnel. Fortunately, the majority of HazMat incidents in the United States are unintentional.

**Figure 35-17** Placing HazMat protective equipment on a member of a response entry team.

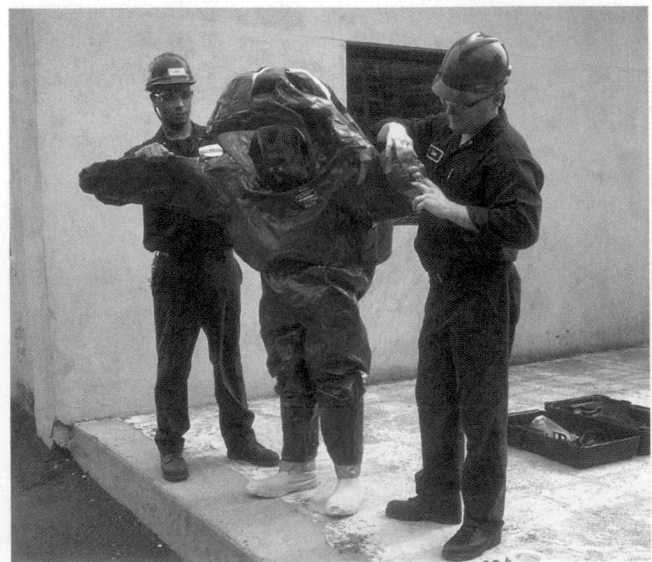

**Figure 35-16** A diamond-shaped NFPA 704 hazardous materials placard.

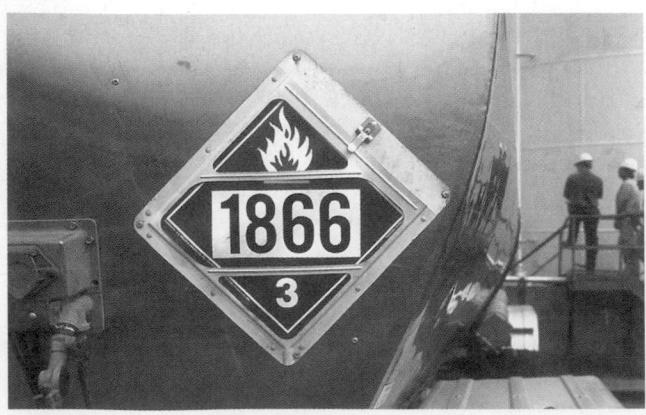

**Table 35-2** NFPA Safety Diamond

| FLAMMABILITY (RED): THE SUSCEPTIBILITY OF A MATERIAL TO BURNING | | |
|---|---|---|
| **SYMBOL** | **EXPLANATION** | **EXAMPLE** |
| 0 | Materials that will not burn | Water |
| 1 | Materials that must be pre-heated before ignition can occur | Corn oil |
| 2 | Materials that must be moderately heated or exposed to relatively high ambient temperature before ignition can occur | Diesel fuel oil |
| 3 | Liquids and solids that can be ignited under almost all ambient temperature conditions | Gasoline |
| 4 | Materials that will rapidly or completely vaporize at atmospheric pressure and normal ambient temperature, or that are readily dispersed in air and will burn readily | Propane gas |

| HEALTH HAZARD (BLUE): THE TYPE OF POSSIBLE INJURY THE MATERIAL CAN INFLICT | | |
|---|---|---|
| **SYMBOL** | **EXPLANATION** | **EXAMPLE** |
| 0 | Materials that on exposure under fire conditions would offer no hazard beyond that of ordinary combustible material | Peanut oil |
| 1 | Materials that on exposure would cause irritation but only minor residual injury | Turpentine |
| 2 | Materials that on intense or continued but not chronic exposure could cause temporary incapacitation or possible residual injury | Ammonia gas |
| 3 | Materials that on short exposure could cause serious temporary or residual injury | Chlorine gas |
| 4 | Materials that on very short exposure could cause death or major residual injury | Hydrogen cyanide |

| REACTIVITY (YELLOW): THE MATERIAL'S SUSCEPTIBILITY TO BURNING | | |
|---|---|---|
| **SYMBOL** | **EXPLANATION** | **EXAMPLE** |
| 0 | Materials that in themselves are normally stable, even under fire exposure conditions, and are not reactive with water | Liquid nitrogen |
| 1 | Materials that in themselves are normally stable, but which can become unstable at elevated temperatures and pressures | Phosphorus (red or white) |
| 2 | Materials that readily undergo violent chemical change at elevated temperatures and pressures, or that react violently with water, or that may form explosive mixtures with water | Calcium metal |
| 3 | Materials that in themselves are capable of detonation or explosive decomposition or reaction but require a strong initiating source, or that must be heated under confinement before initiation, or that react explosively with water | Fluorine gas |
| 4 | Materials that in themselves are readily capable of detonation or of explosive decomposition or reaction at normal temperatures and pressures | Trinitrotoluene (TNT) |

| SPECIAL PRECAUTIONS/PROTECTIVE GEAR NEEDED (WHITE): SPECIAL HANDLING OR OTHER IMPORTANT INFORMATION | | |
|---|---|---|

Symbols specified in National Fire Codes, section 704:

| SYMBOL | EXPLANATION | EXAMPLE |
|---|---|---|
| W̶ | Materials that show unusual reactivity with water (i.e., do not put water on them) | Magnesium metal |
| OX | Materials that possess oxidizing properties | Ammonium nitrate (fertilizer used in Oklahoma City bombing) |

Other symbols commonly used:

| | | |
|---|---|---|
| ACID | Material is an acid | |
| ALK | Material is a base (alkaline) | |
| COR | Material is corrosive | |
| ☢ | Material is radioactive | |
| | If the white field is blank, there are no special hazards or precautions | |

### NOTE

### HAZWOPER

Several levels of HAZWOPER training and certification are available: the Awareness, Operations, Technician, and Commander levels. Awareness-level personnel receive an overview of HazMat response and typically perform tasks in the outer "safe" zone. Operations-level personnel receive more specialized training and typically operate within the warm zone. Technician-level personnel are trained to function in any of the hazard zones, whereas Commander-level personnel supervise the overall management of response and clean-up efforts.

**HAZWOPER** stands for **HAZ**ardous **W**aste **OP**erations and **E**mergency **R**esponse; refers to federally mandated training for anyone who may encounter uncontrolled hazardous materials.

**Figure 35-18** The safety control zones at the site of a hazardous materials emergency.

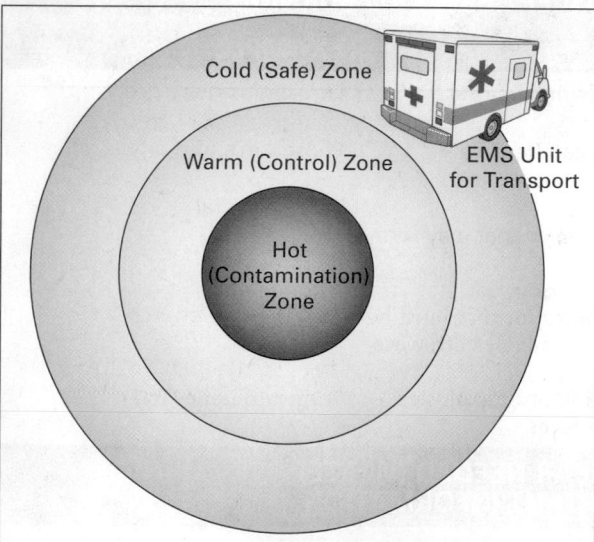

### Hot (Contamination) Zone

Contamination is actually present.
Personnel must wear appropriate protective gear.
Number of rescuers limited to those absolutely necessary.
Bystanders never allowed.

### Warm (Control) Zone

Area surrounding the contamination zone.
Vital to preventing spread of contamination.
Personnel must wear appropriate protective gear.
Lifesaving emergency care is performed.

### Cold (Safe) Zone

Normal triage, stabilization, and treatment performed.
Rescuers must shed contaminated gear before entering the cold zone.

However, there is always the potential for an intentional HazMat incident, which is considered an act of terrorism. Management of a HazMat terrorist event also utilizes the ICS structure, with the addition that all terrorist events are considered criminal acts and fall under the jurisdiction of the federal government.

The response to and decontamination of a hazardous materials site are conducted in accordance with Occupational, Health, and Safety Administration (OSHA) standards and is referred to as **HAZWOPER,** which stands for **HAZ**ardous **W**aste **OP**erations and **E**mergency **R**esponse.

The federal government mandates HAZWOPER training for any worker (paid or volunteer) who works in an environment in which uncontrolled hazardous materials may be encountered. Training and certification needs depend on the type(s) of substances to which an employee may be exposed and the worker's expected duties when responding to a HazMat-related incident. Typical training includes the types of hazardous materials present and their associated risks, recognition of hazardous materials, hazardous materials response, personal protective equipment, and containment and decontamination procedures. Training requirements generally include classroom and practical training, formal certification, and annual refresher training.

The most important step in the initial management of a HazMat incident is to prevent members of the public from contacting the hazardous material by establishing an isolation perimeter to prevent their entry. The boundary may be established by placing traffic cones at street intersections or by stringing barrier tape around buildings. Emergency responders may need to enforce the boundary with their physical presence.

Once the isolation perimeter is set, the next step is to establish three hazard-control zones, which establish the working areas of the incident (Figure 35-18■). The zone surrounding the incident, which is considered to be the most dangerous and the most contaminated, is known as the **hot zone**. Only personnel with specialized training and equipment are permitted to enter this zone. The **warm zone** surrounds the hot zone and is a transition zone in which decontamination occurs. As for the hot zone, only personnel with training in decontamination techniques should enter this zone. The outer **cold zone** is that part of the incident area that contains support personnel and equipment; it is considered safe to operate in this zone without specialized protective equipment. Located within the cold zone are the command post and the triage, treatment, and transport areas to which OEC Technicians are typically assigned to assist in the medical care of ill or injured patients. Once a patient has been removed from the hot zone and has been decontaminated in the warm zone, medical treatment can begin in the cold zone (Figure 35-19■).

At times a member of the incident response team will require treatment due to exposure to a hazardous material. One potential hazard is organophosphate poisoning. As discussed in Chapter 12, Substance Abuse and Poisoning, organophosphates cause excessive pulmonary secretions that can lead to respiratory failure. Signs and symptoms of organophosphate poisoning can be remembered

| **SLUDGE** | **DUMBELS** |
|---|---|
| **Table 35-3** The Signs and Symptoms of Organophosphate Poisoning: SLUDGE and DUMBELS | |
| S: Salivation | D: Defecation |
| L: Lacrimation (tearing) | U: Urination |
| U: Urination | M: Miosis (constriction of the pupils) |
| D: Defecation | B: Bronchorrhea (coughing mucus from the lungs) |
| G: GI irritation (vomiting) | E: Emesis (vomiting) |
| E: Eye (pupil) constriction | L: Lacrimation (tearing) |
| | S: Salivation |

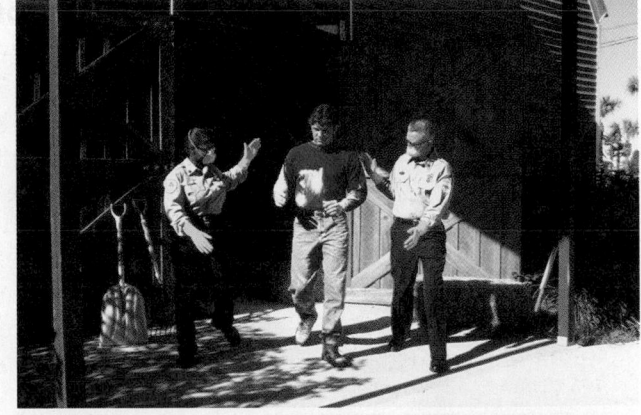

**Figure 35-19** Treatment begins after the patient has been moved from or has left the hot zone, has completed the decontamination process, and has entered the cold zone.

using the acronyms DUMBELS or SLUDGE (Table 35-3■). The treatment for organophosphate poisoning is the administration of IV atropine, often in large doses, by ALS providers. The treatment for organophosphate exposure in mass-casualty settings, in which IV access is often impractical, is self-administration of a nerve-agent antidote kit. Two common kits are the Mark I kit and the DuoDote kit.

In the event that you have been exposed to an organophosphate or a chemical nerve agent, OEC Technicians may need to self-administer a nerve-agent antidote. Administration of the antidote kit can be life saving. Each kit contains two medications: atropine and pralidoxime chloride (2-PAM Cl). The Mark I kit (Figure 35-20■) administers the medications in two auto-injectors, whereas the DuoDote kit (Figure 35-21■) administers the medications in a single auto-injector. The kits also include step-by-step directions.

**hot zone** the area closest to the center of a CBRNE incident; is the most dangerous and most contaminated area.

**warm zone** a transition area surrounding the hot zone; the zone in which decontamination occurs.

**cold zone** the area outside the warm zone, in which it is safe to operate without specialized equipment.

**Figure 35-21** The DuoDote nerve-agent antidote kit, which administers the medications in a single auto-injector.

**Figure 35-20** The Mark I nerve-agent antidote kit, which administers the medications in two auto-injectors.

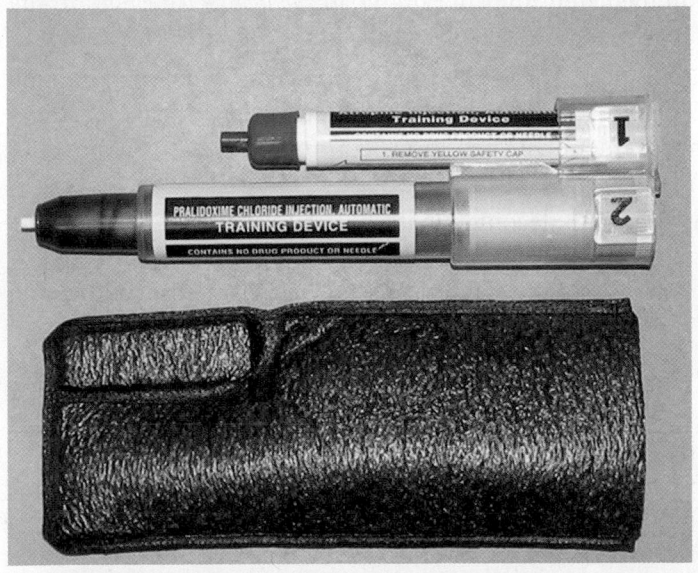

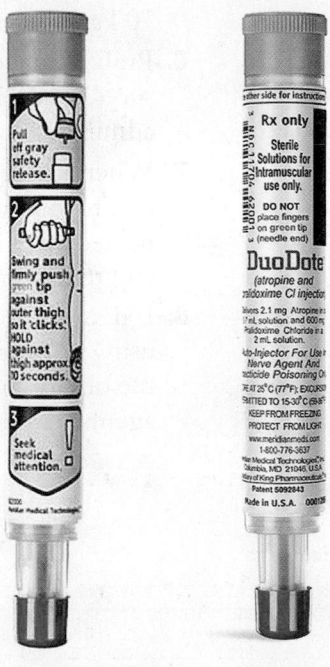

## Mechanism of Action of Nerve Agents

The nervous system controls bodily functions by secreting various chemical transmitters, which act as "instructions" to nerves, muscles, and glands. These neurological instructions are of two types: those that stimulate activity by muscles and glands, and those that signal inactivity in those structures. The presence of a nerve agent interferes with the normal instructions of chemical transmitters in a way that overstimulates the nerve endings, so muscles and certain glands overreact. The results are excessive salivation, tearing, airway secretions, respiratory distress, and depressed mental status. The initial treatment for a nerve-agent exposure consists of a two-part antidote: atropine (to dry up secretions) and 2-PAM Chloride (to reverse the action of the nerve agent).

⊕ 35-9 Describe and demonstrate how to properly self-administer the contents of a nerve-agent antidote kit.

## Recommended Dosing Schedules for Exposure to a Nerve Agent

If you have been exposed to a nerve agent and have mild symptoms, self-administer one kit containing both drugs. If excessive salivation and mental status changes become present, self-administer two atropine auto-injectors and one 2-PAM Cl injector. In assisting with a patient who has been exposed, remove secretions (using suction if necessary) and maintain the patient's airway. If severe signs and symptoms are present, the EMS providers will administer three atropine auto-injectors and three 2-PAM Cl injectors in rapid succession. Note the following information concerning the administration of nerve-agent antidote medications:

1. The medications are administered in a similar manner as used for an Epi-Pen. Follow the directions on the nerve-agent antidote kit.
2. When assisting with another patient support ventilations with a bag-valve mask, if needed.
3. Repeat dosages will be administered by EMS as needed.
4. If signs and symptoms resolve, then only continued monitoring is necessary.
5. Premeasured doses of auto-injectors should be safe in most adults. Note, however, that auto-injectors were designed for a "standard military profile"—that is, for an individual who is healthy, is approximately 18–35 years old, weighs about 70 kg (154 lbs.), and has no preexisting medical conditions.
6. Pralidoxime chloride (2-PAM Cl) is most effective, especially for severe exposures, if administered immediately after poisoning and *following* (not before) the administration of atropine.
7. When the nerve agent has been ingested, exposure may continue for some time due to slow absorption from the lower bowel, and fatal relapses have been reported after initial improvement. In such cases, continued medical monitoring and transport are mandatory.
8. If dermal exposure has occurred, decontamination is critical and should be done using standard decontamination procedures. Monitoring should be directed to the observation of the same signs and symptoms seen with all exposures to nerve agents.

## STOP, THINK, UNDERSTAND

### Multiple Choice

Choose the correct answer.

1. How many Emergency Support Functions (ESF) annexes make up the backbone of the National Response Framework (NRF)? _____

   a. 5
   b. 10
   c. 15
   d. 20

2. Which of the following is not a disaster response team? _____

   a. Disaster Emergency Response Team (DERT)
   b. Regional Medical Resource Corps (MRC)
   c. National Urban Search and Rescue (USAR)
   d. Civilian Emergency Response Team (CERT)

3. What is the purpose of the National Fire Protection Association (NFPA) diamond placard system? _____

   a. to identify the known safety hazards for gases
   b. to identify the known safety hazards for solids
   c. to identify the known safety hazards for liquids
   d. to identify the known safety hazards for a given material

4. Which of the following operations does not occur in the cold zone? _____

   a. decontamination
   b. command Post
   c. treatment
   d. triage

### List

List the three primary components of the National Disaster Medical System (NDMS).

1. _____
2. _____
3. _____

### Short Answer

1. What is the purpose of a Mark I Kit or a DuoDote Kit?

   _____

   _____

   _____

2. List the two medications found in a Mark I Kit or a DuoDote Kit, and indicate what each medication does.

   _____

   _____

   _____

   _____

# Search and Rescue

**search** a methodical process of actively gathering information about a person or group in distress or danger and then physically looking for them.

**rescue** the process of extracting a person or group from distress or danger.

A search and rescue (SAR) operation has two interrelated components: a **search**, the methodical process of actively gathering information about and then physically looking for one or more individuals in distress or imminent danger, and a **rescue**, the process of extracting such individuals from distress or danger. Efforts can quickly shift from one component to the other. For instance, upon locating a missing individual, the search portion of the mission is terminated, but if the individual is trapped and/or injured, the focus of the mission shifts to rescue operations (Figure 35-22■).

Among the many search and rescue disciplines are combat, mountain, urban, ground, air, and sea operations (Figure 35-23■). Even though the term *search and rescue* is used generically, each SAR discipline has distinctly different missions, roles, training and staffing requirements, equipment needs, and operational procedures.

Search and rescue work is dangerous. Among the countless challenges a SAR team faces are difficult terrain, inclement weather, extremes of temperature, time of day, size of the area to be searched, and the total number of people missing. Additionally, natural or human-caused hazards can further complicate a SAR team's mission. These variables, and others, must be considered whenever a SAR team organizes its plan of action because they can turn a relatively simple search into a technical evacuation that requires additional personnel, advanced training, and specialized equipment.

Ski patrollers and other OEC Technicians at many ski resorts routinely engage in the most basic type of search—that is, looking for a person who has become separated from family or friends (Figure 35-24■). Many ski areas have developed a protocol manual that specifically identifies the steps to be taken when searching for a lost person. Because of their backcountry expertise, OEC Technicians are often asked to join a SAR team or to assist a team during a mission.

Because many ski and recreational areas around the country are typically close to or adjacent to state or federal lands, SAR efforts often require assistance from multiple local emergency management and response agencies. Under these circumstances, the need for cross-jurisdictional coordination and common procedures and systems becomes critical. Accordingly, SAR teams within the United States operate under the federal NIMS structure and use the Incident Command System to manage SAR-related incidents.

**Figure 35-23** A successful conclusion to a rescue at sea.
Copyright Dorling Kindersley Media Library

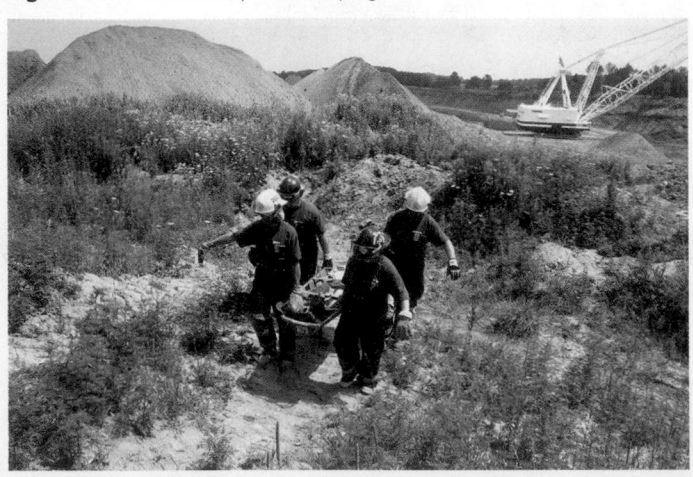

**Figure 35-22** A rescue operation in progress.

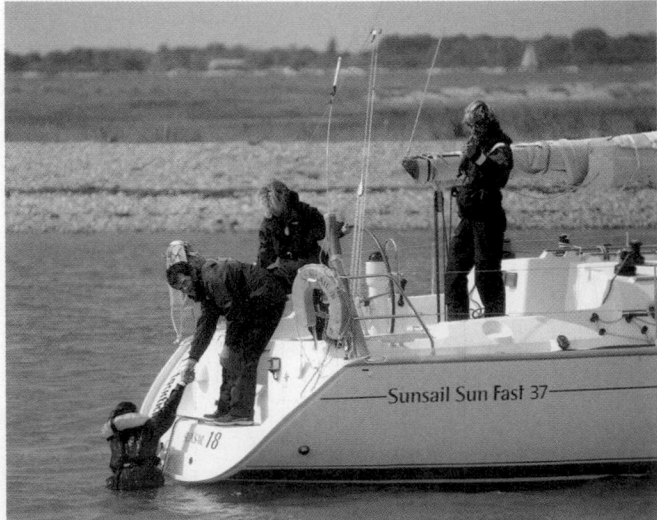

Although complex, SAR operations can be broken down to five basic tasks:

1. **Mobilization.** Once the team is informed of a mission, it assembles and responds to the site of the incident. Each team member has a specific role; team leaders are typically cross-trained in multiple roles.

2. **Intelligence Gathering.** Team members gather information about the lost person(s), typically by asking the following questions:
   - Where was the person last seen? (This helps to narrow the search area.)
   - What was the person's intended destination? (This helps to establish a search grid and identify possible travel routes the person may use.)
   - How physically fit is the person? (A person who is fit can travel farther and faster than one who is not.)
   - What is the person's mental status? (Does the person have a known mental illness? Is the person in a rational state of mind? Is the person depressed or suicidal?)
   - What equipment does the person have? (A person who is well equipped can survive longer than one who has minimal supplies.)
   - What type of terrain exists within the search area? (A person can travel faster and farther on flat ground than in mountainous terrain.)

3. **Containment.** Using the information gathered, the team establishes a containment area, an area with defined boundaries within which the party was last seen and might still be located. For ski patrollers, containment may include patrolling the boundaries of the ski area to look for tracks or signs that the missing person left the containment area.

4. **Search.** Once the search area has been defined, it is divided into a search grid consisting of smaller areas (Figure 35-25■). Based on available information, search teams are deployed to search the grid(s) in which the person is most likely located.

5. **Rescue.** A person who has been found may require medical care, evacuation, or other assistance. In the event of a fatal outcome, the body must be recovered and removed.

SAR skills are something that every patroller and OEC Technician should acquire through additional training. It is not a matter of *if* patrollers or OEC Technicians will

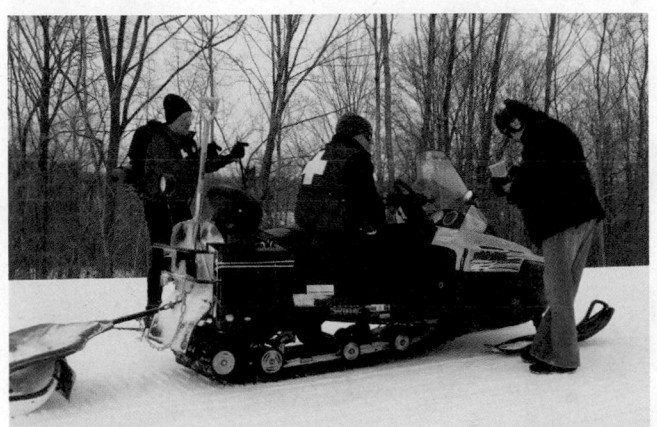

**Figure 35-24** OEC Technicians and ski patrollers working together on a search and rescue operation.
Copyright Beverly Henrickson

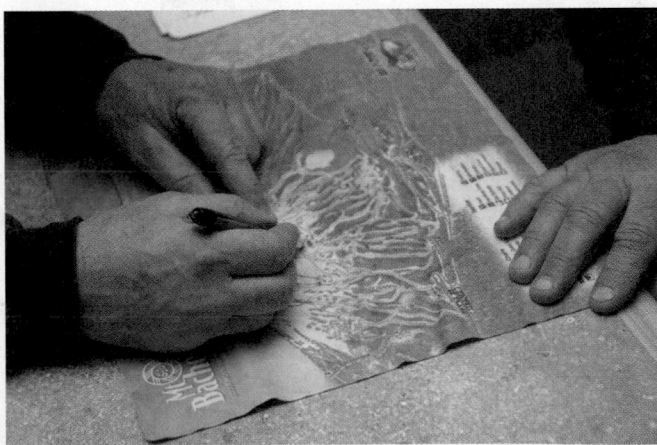

**Figure 35-25** This map might be used to set up search grids.
Copyright Studio 404

**Figure 35-26** NSP programs for Mountain Travel and Rescue and Avalanche courses teach important SAR techniques.
Copyright Studio 404

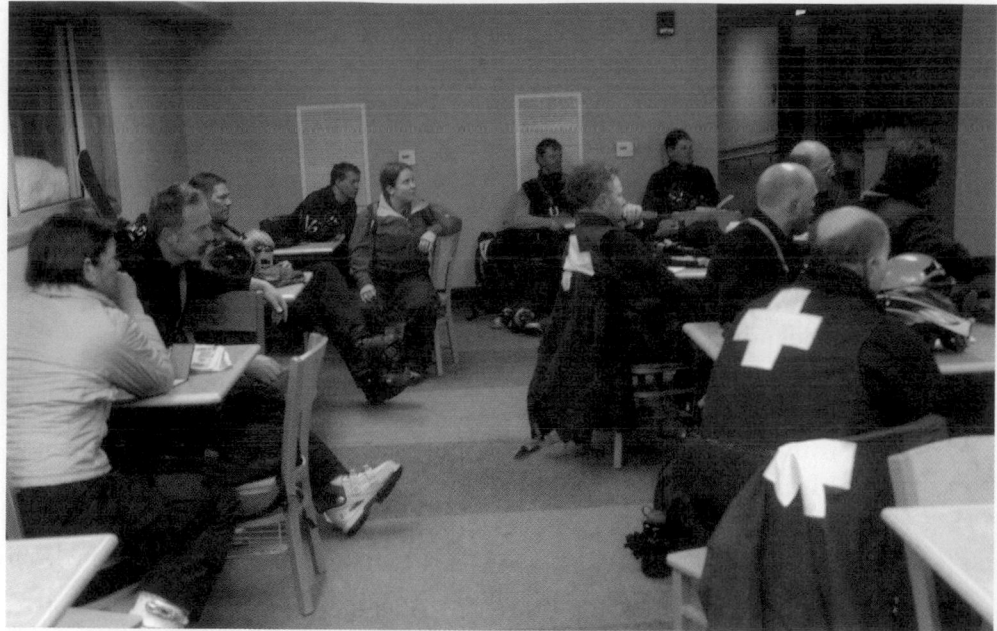

be asked to participate in a search and rescue operation, but *when* they will be asked to participate. SAR training can be acquired through NSP Mountain Travel and Rescue and Avalanche courses (Figure 35-26■) or through local SAR teams, which are usually operated by a local law-enforcement agency.

## Avalanche Rescue

Burial in an avalanche is a true medical emergency, and small avalanches can be just as deadly as large avalanches (Figure 35-27■). Although most avalanches occur primarily during winter, they have claimed lives during every month of the year and in every kind of weather. What's more, they are not confined to remote, high alpine terrain and can occur on any steep, snow-covered slope (Figure 35-28■), even rooftops.

**Figure 35-27** Even small avalanches can be dangerous!
Copyright Dave Saville—FEMA

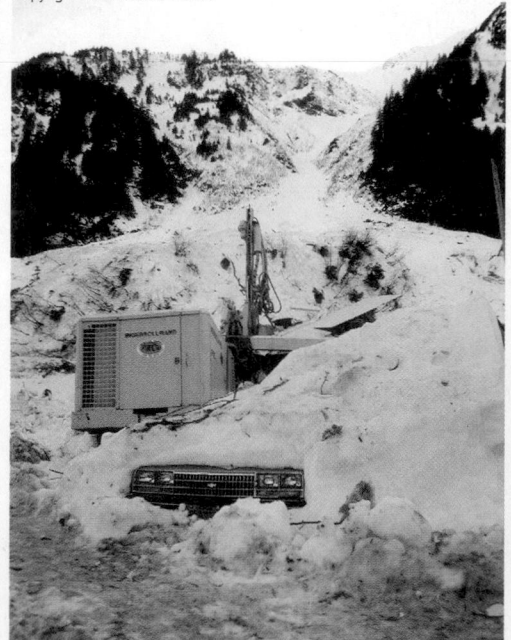

**Figure 35-28** Avalanches can occur anywhere that there is a steep, snow-covered slope.
Copyright Alex Kerney

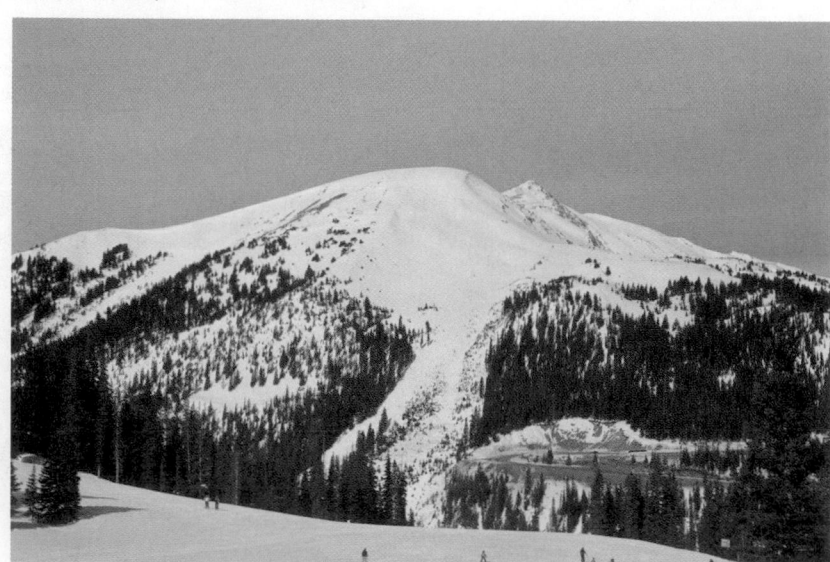

Because the chances of surviving complete burial decrease rapidly with time, dropping to 50 percent within the first 30 minutes, rescue operations must be initiated as soon as possible, preferably by a companion who was not caught in the avalanche. However, companion rescue efforts alone are not often successful without the additional resources provided by organized rescue operations. There is minimal likelihood of survival when avalanche victims are buried for more than 35 minutes with an obstructed airway and in cardiac arrest upon extrication.

Avalanche rescue operations within the United States are conducted using ICS. Operational effectiveness is greatly enhanced by using technology, including wireless communications, which enable rescuers to quickly learn of incidents, and helicopters, which enable rescuers to reach the scene within minutes. Avalanche transceivers and the RECCO system have also improved rescue efforts by dramatically reducing search time. The use of rescue dog teams has also shortened search times. Specially trained and equipped rescuers, including OEC Technicians, can provide life-saving emergency medical care in the field.

An organized avalanche rescue consists of four basic functions:

+ **The immediate search.** Get rescuers to the site as quickly as possible to find and uncover the victim(s).
+ **Medical care.** Provide emergency care for the victims.
+ **Transportation/evacuation.** Get the victims out of the field and to advanced medical care, if needed.
+ **Support (logistics).** Care for the rescuers in the field (provide food, shelter, rest, and replacements).

These functions are not sequential and may be performed simultaneously, depending on need and the availability of resources.

Although many variables affect avalanche incidents and the resulting response, most rescue operations follow a similar sequence of events.

1. *The Incident Is Reported* (Figure 35-30■).
   • If physically present, a team member interviews the reporting party and, if he is a witness, arranges for transport back to the site.
   • If the report was patched through from a 911 call, a team member gets as much detail as possible on the location and number of buried victims as well as a call-back number.
2. *The Team Is Alerted and Responds.*
   • Rescue headquarters is notified.
   • A pre-designated Incident Commander takes charge and initiates the rescue operation according to pre-established plans.
   • The immediate search team is assembled (including witnesses), equipped (including a dog team, avalanche receivers, and a RECCO detector, if available), and dispatched (Figure 35-31■).
   • A permanent Site Leader is appointed and dispatched.
   • A medical team is assembled, equipped, and dispatched.

**RECCO**

RECCO is a highly effective avalanche rescue system that enables rescuers to quickly locate an avalanche victim using harmonic radar. The system consists of two parts: a small reflector that is usually sewn into a person's clothing, and a hand-held detector that enables rescuers to locate a buried avalanche victim (Figure 35-29■).

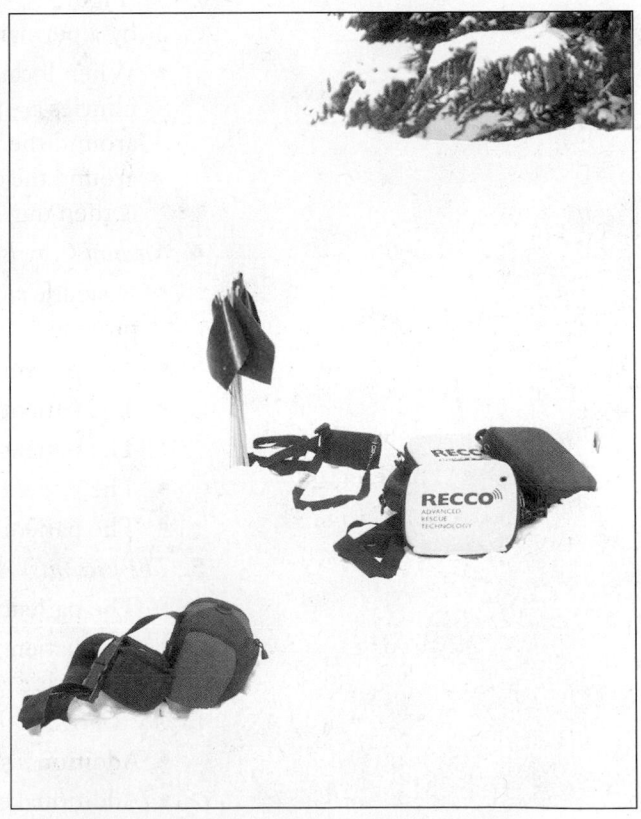

**Figure 35-29** Use of the RECCO system has dramatically reduced search times for victims of avalanches.
Copyright Studio 404

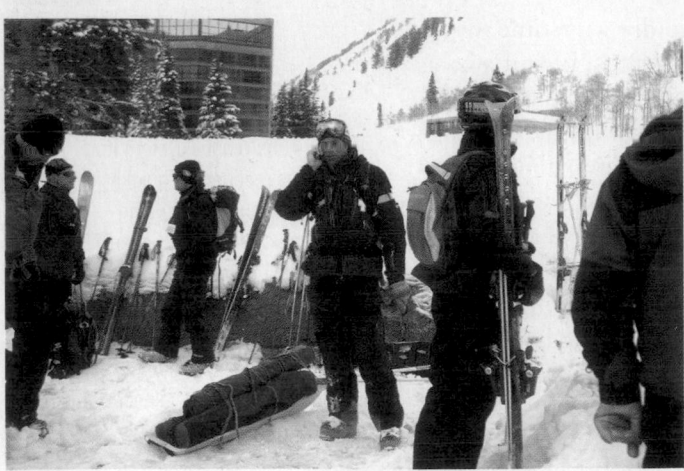

**Figure 35-30** An avalanche incident is reported.
Copyright Studio 404

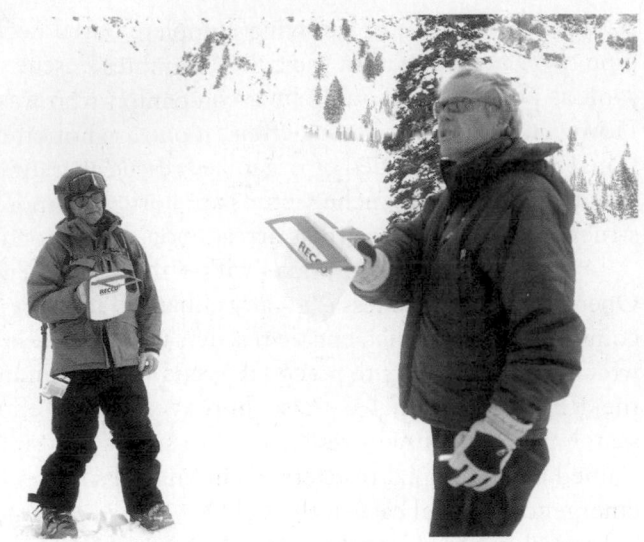

**Figure 35-31** Search team members respond by assembling themselves and specialized equipment.
Copyright Studio 404

- Logistics support for dispatched teams and incoming resources is organized.
- Additional teams are assembled and dispatched to perform a variety of functions as needed.

3. *The Victim(s) Are Located/Extricated.*
   - The Immediate Search Team Leader determines and marks a safe route to the incident site, assesses scene safety, initiates the search, and incorporates resources (personnel and equipment) into the search effort as they arrive (Figure 35-32■). As the operation grows, this team member may be replaced by a permanent Site Leader.
   - When located, the victim is dug out as quickly and safely as possible. (Spine injuries are presumed until proven otherwise.) Snow is quickly removed from around the victim's face and an airway is established, followed by excavating around the chest to enable chest-wall expansion. The rest of the victim's body is then dug completely free to allow extrication and other emergency care.

4. *Medical Care Is Provided* (Figure 35-33■).
   - Basic life support (and advanced life support, ALS, if needed and available) is provided.
   - The patient is moved to a safer location, if necessary.
   - The patient's other injuries are treated.
   - The patient is assessed and treated for hypothermia.
   - The patient is protected from further injury or cooling.
   - The patient's condition is continually monitored.

5. *The Victim(s) Are Evacuated.*
   - The patient is prepared for transport (in a litter or sled).
   - The patient is transported to an appropriate medical facility for more definitive care.

6. *The Operation Is Given Logistical Support.*
   - Additional searchers are made available.
   - Additional equipment is made available.

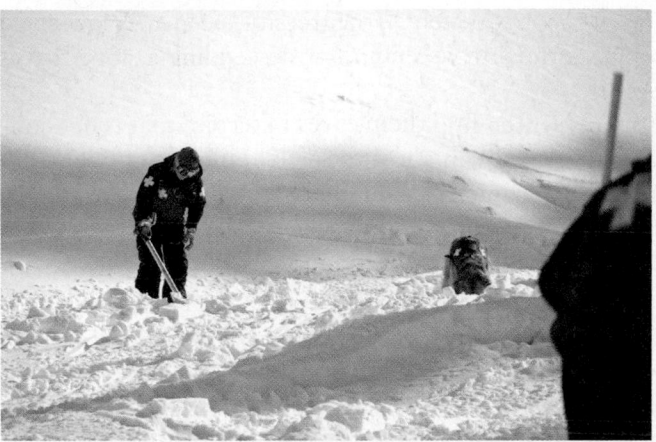

**Figure 35-32** Team members search for victims.
Copyright Alex Kerney

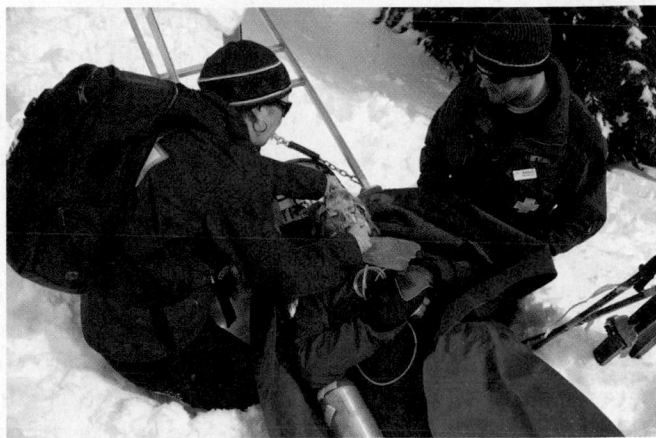

**Figure 35-33** Team members provide medical care for this extricated avalanche victim.
Copyright Tristan Roberson

- Care for rescuers (food, water, shelter, sanitation, etc.) is arranged.
- Transport of rescuers and equipment back to base is arranged.

As with any incident, rescuer safety is the top priority. The fact that an avalanche has occurred should strongly suggest a high probability for similar conditions along the route and on the slopes adjacent to the incident site. Upon arrival, the Immediate Search Team Leader, who is highly trained and experienced in managing avalanche-related incidents, assesses overall site safety. If there is a significant residual avalanche hazard at the site, the hazard must be mitigated before the team proceeds.

During prolonged operations, team leaders must ensure that rescuers are properly cared for and supported. Because rescuers who are dehydrated, cold, or exhausted could divert precious resources from the rescue effort by becoming additional casualties, all members of the avalanche rescue team must be physically fit, thoroughly trained, and properly equipped for the operation (Figure 35-34■).

Buried avalanche victims often have life-threatening conditions associated with asphyxia, trauma, and hypothermia. Cardiac problems can occur also, either immediately or subsequently as a consequence of asphyxia, traumatic shock, or hypothermia. OEC Technicians should assess and manage these injuries in the usual fashion, as described in previous chapters.

Whenever possible, a helicopter equipped with ALS providers and equipment should be dispatched and landed close to the incident site. If multiple patients are buried or injured, standard triage methods are employed in which patients with vital signs take priority over those without vital signs.

## Low-Angle Rescue

A rope rescue is any technical rescue operation involving static ropes, anchors, belaying devices, and other equipment that provides a mechanical advantage. The ski patrol recognizes two types of rope rescue: high-angle rescue and low-angle rescue. A **high-angle rescue (HAR)** is any rescue work performed by

**high-angle rescue (HAR)** any rescue work done by ascending or descending a slope steeper than approximately 45 degrees.

**Figure 35-34** Assembling the proper equipment is essential for any avalanche rescue operation.
Copyright Dave King/Dorling Kindersley Media Library

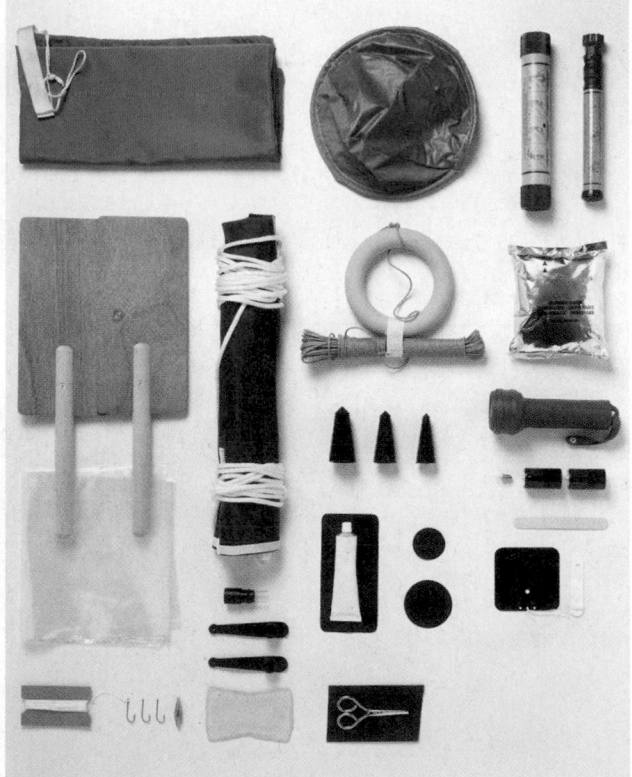

**low-angle rescue (LAR)** any rescue work done by ascending or descending a slope that is less than approximately 45 degrees.

ascending or descending a slope of approximately 45 degrees or steeper. A **low-angle rescue (LAR)** is any rescue work performed by ascending or descending a slope that is less than approximately 45 degrees.

Given that patrollers and rescuers often find themselves in terrain that is not conducive to an easy rescue or evacuation, knowing how to safely remove a patient from sloped terrain is a skill that all OEC Technicians should possess (Figure 35-35■).

Of the many sources of information regarding LAR, some are geared toward crevasse rescue for mountaineering and climbing, whereas others focus on emergency rescue for SAR teams or fire departments. The information in these LAR guidelines covers the basics: raising and lowering systems; setting up anchors, pulleys, and prusiks; and safety concerns.

One of the first decisions that rescuers must make in a low-angle rescue is whether to lower or raise the patient out of the incident zone, the area in which the patient is located (Figure 35-36■). As with all rescue operations, the safety of the rescuers and the patient is the primary concern in LAR operations, but the simplicity of the rescue system should also be considered. Generally, if it is a viable option, it is easier to lower a patient to a safe zone while letting gravity do some of the work. If the incident zone does not allow for the patient to be easily lowered to a safe zone, additional rescuers and equipment may be required to pull the patient up to a safe zone. For more information about low-angle rescue, contact the National Ski Patrol or your local search and rescue team.

Rope rescues, which fall under the Operations section, should be performed using the ICS. Ideally, you should have two teams: a technical rope team that is responsible for providing safe access to the patient and for extricating the patient and rescuers, and a second team that is responsible for providing medical care to the patient. The technical rope team and the medical team should each have a team commander.

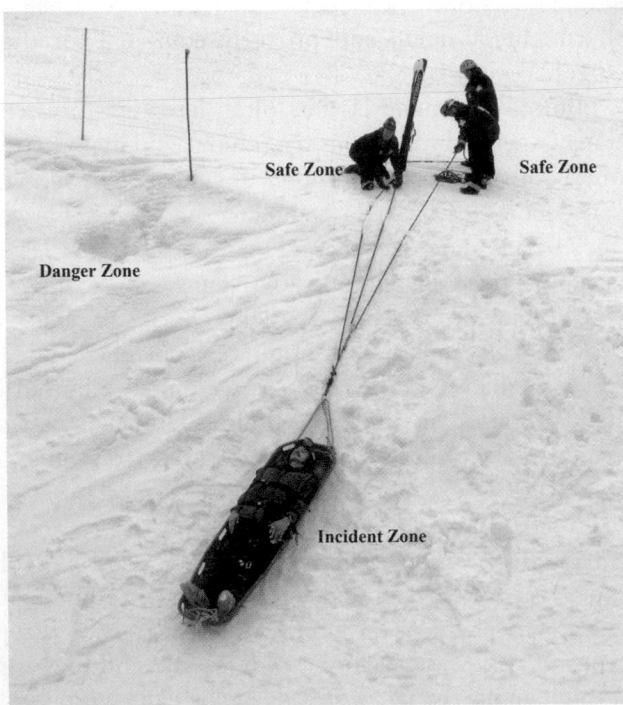

**Figure 35-36** Of the different zones of a low-angle rescue, the incident zone is where the patient is located.
Copyright Rick King

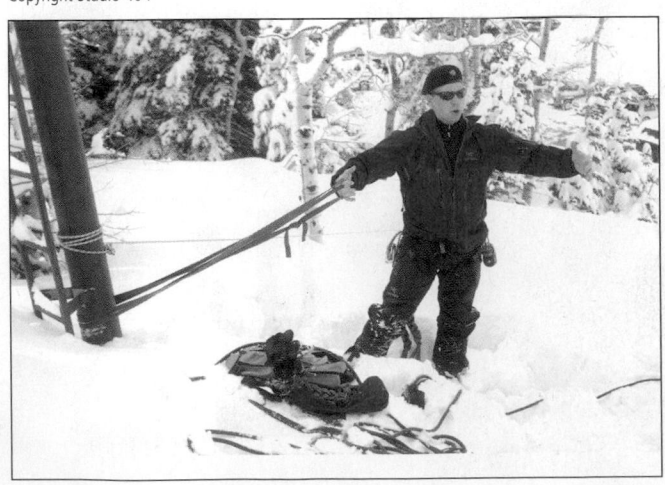

**Figure 35-35** This instructor is demonstrating low-angle rescue skills during a class.
Copyright Studio 404

Depending on the situation, it may be necessary to initiate medical treatment for a patient before a completed rope system is in place. Providing rapid medical treatment requires that members of the medical team can safely access the patient. Safe access may be accomplished by rappelling down to the patient using a separate rope, and then tying off to a tree or some other natural anchor near the patient.

## Confined Space Rescue

A confined space rescue is a type of rescue involving an enclosed area that has limited or restricted means of entry or exit. The confined space may be natural or human-made. Rock caves, ice caverns, and fissures, for instance, are natural confined spaces, whereas underground pipes, tunnels, mine shafts, wells, storage tanks, and trenches are human-made confined spaces. A confined space may also be created in the rubble following a building collapse.

Many confined space rescues may be facilitated not only by equipment, but also by a specially trained search dog. The exceptional sense of smell and trainability of dogs makes them ideally suited for finding objects or people. Search dogs can be trained to "alert" when they detect the odor of almost anything, including humans, even when that odor is part of a complex mixture of odors. Avalanche dogs are probably the most common search dogs that ski patrollers will encounter.

A well-trained avalanche dog can be a great asset in a search operation, especially if buried victims lack avalanche transceivers (Figure 35-37■). Under favorable conditions, dogs can easily search an area much faster than is possible using a probe line, and in cases involving large search areas, dogs work faster than transceiver searches. Many patrols at ski resorts in avalanche country have dogs on duty so that they can respond quickly to incidents within and near the resort's boundaries. Many alpine SAR groups also have dog teams with handlers on call so that they can be deployed into the field quickly. If an area or a rescue agency does not have a dog team on staff, its alerting and rescue plan should identify available local dog resources and the procedures for mobilizing them.

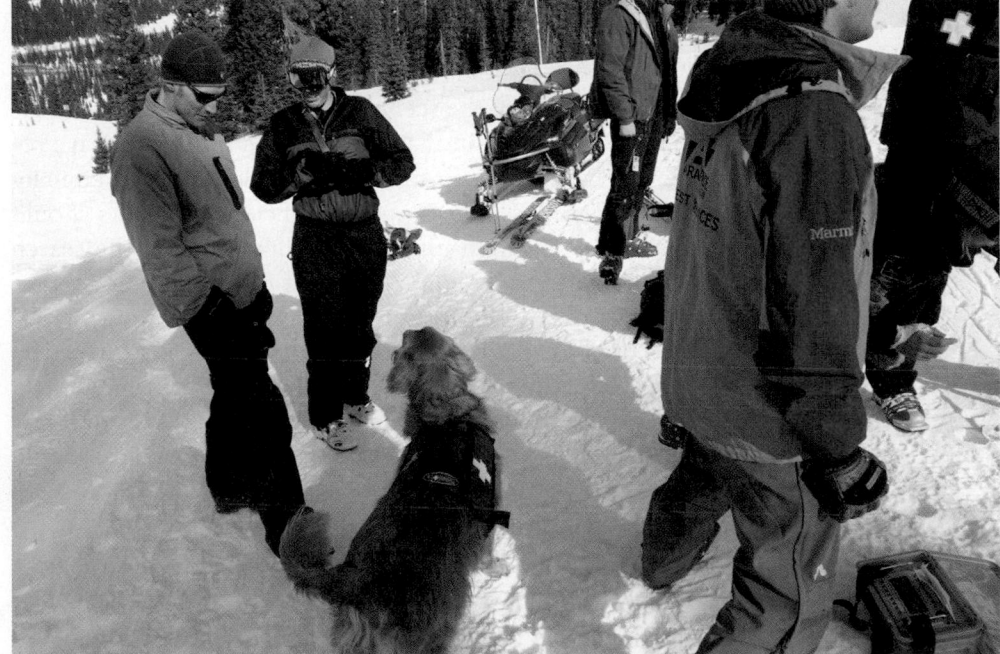

**Figure 35-37** Avalanche dogs are invaluable members of a search and rescue team.
Copyright Alex Kerney

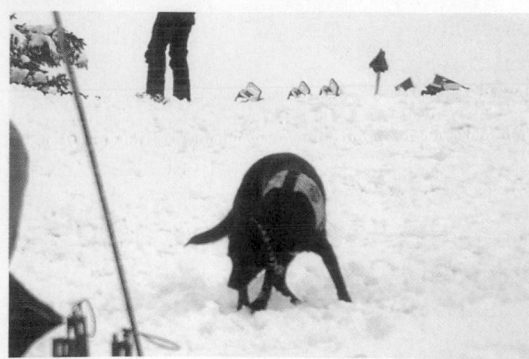

**Figure 35-38** Station a dog downwind of the search area before the search begins.
Copyright Studio 404

Several avalanche dog training organizations and certification standards are in place within the United States. Because these organizations have slightly different training methods, the ways search dogs behave in the field can vary. An initiative to establish international standards for the training and certification of avalanche rescue dogs is currently underway.

### Scent Factors

Dogs follow a cone-shaped scent trail in the air to the victim or to some other source of the scent. In order to be detected, the scent of a person buried in an avalanche must first reach the surface of the snow. The time it takes for a scent to reach the surface depends on both the depth of burial and the scent's rate of diffusion through the snow, which in turn depends on the temperature and density of the snow. In general, colder snow temperatures speed the diffusion rate, whereas greater snow density slows the diffusion rate. These rates can vary from less than 1 min/meter in dry powder snow to 15 min/meter in wet packed snow.

A scent does not always travel in a straight line up through the snow—it follows the path of least resistance. Scent may move horizontally between blocks of snow or rocks or be channeled by running water or trees to emerge a significant distance from the actual burial location. A dog will "alert" wherever this scent emerges from the snow, which is not necessarily directly over the victim. Steady winds of low to moderate velocity provide ideal conditions for dogs; strong, gusty winds make searching more difficult. Dogs are best positioned downwind of the search area before the search begins (Figure 35-38■).

### Dog Capabilities

A dog's sense of smell is so sensitive it can not only discriminate among individuals, but also between individuals and articles of their clothing, and between a live victim and a dead body. Thus in alpine avalanche rescue situations, it is advantageous for dogs to "alert" on the victim's clothing and equipment, in addition to the victim's scent, to provide clues that can reduce the size of the search area. Air temperature does not seem to affect the sensitivity of a dog's sense of smell, so dogs are a huge asset in alpine avalanche rescue operations (Figure 35-39■).

**Figure 35-39** Well trained dogs are a huge asset in an avalanche burial search effort.
Copyright Andrea Booher/FEMA

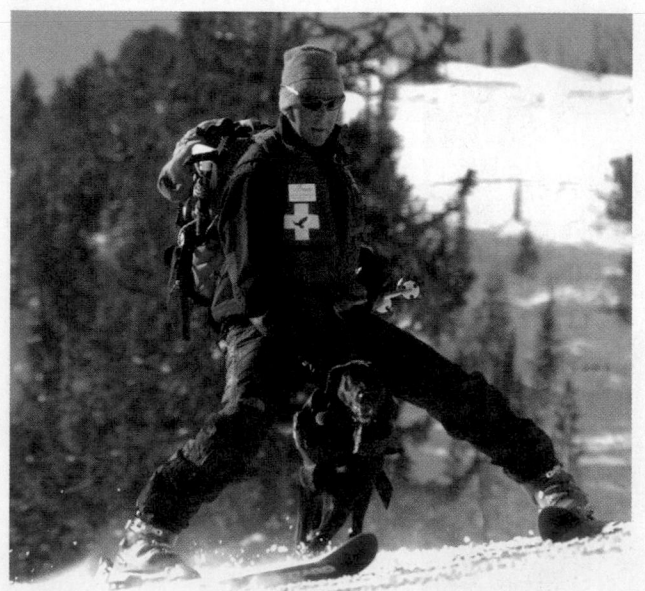

### Simplifying the Search

Because dogs detect all the scents around them, they must in effect ignore every scent but that of the buried victim to earn a reward for their search. Their task can be made easier by reducing as many competing scents as possible, and thus rescuers should keep bystanders and non-essential personnel out of the search zone (Figure 35-40■). It is more difficult for a rescue dog to detect the scent of a buried victim in an avalanche run out zone if the area contains distracting scents. For this reason, rescuers should stage equipment and food away from the area (preferably downwind); should avoid leaving any kind of litter or body wastes (including saliva or urine) in the search area; and should even avoid sitting on the snow.

### Search Dog Etiquette

Even though dog teams are trained to work around other rescuers and equipment, the only person giving commands to a dog should

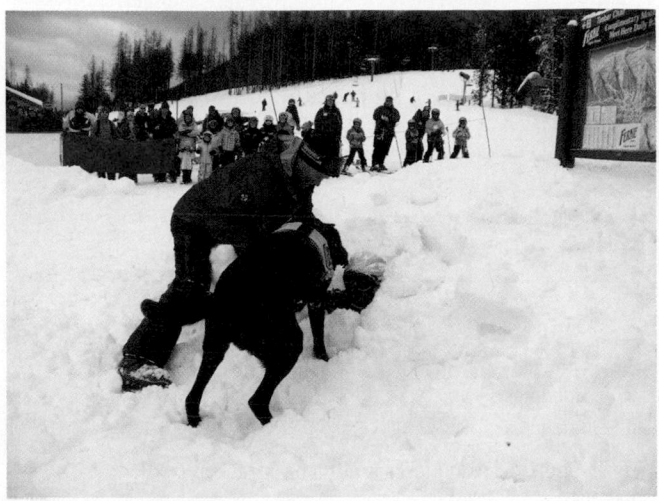

**Figure 35-40** To reduce distracting scents, rescuers should keep all nonessential items and personnel away from the immediate search area.
Copyright Fernie Alpine Resort

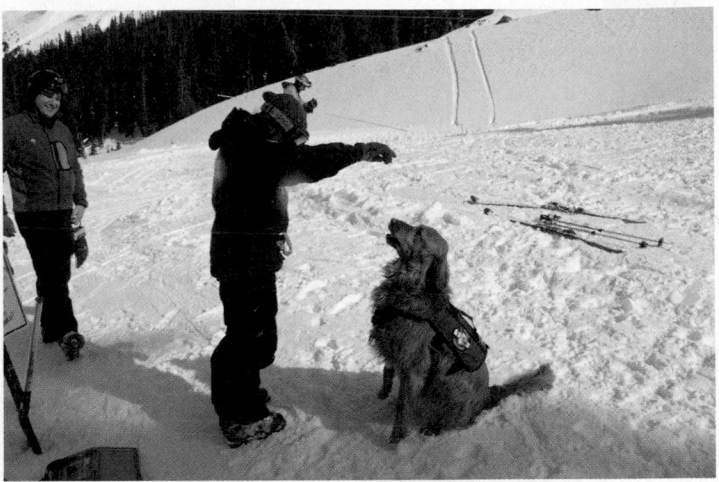

**Figure 35-41** Only the dog's handler should give commands to the dog.
Copyright Alex Kerney

be the dog's handler, who often uses hand signals to communicate with the dog (Figure 35-41■). During an avalanche rescue, obey the rule "silence is golden" to avoid distracting the dog. If the dog comes over to investigate you, it is only doing so to rule out your scent; ignore it and stay focused on your job. Never approach, touch, or feed a rescue dog without its handler's permission.

## Dog Alerts

A dog "alerts" when it locates the source of a human scent coming off the surface of the snow. It communicates this alert to the handler in different ways—sometimes by barking, sometimes by digging, sometimes by both. It is up to the handler to decide whether the dog's behavior constitutes an alert. When a dog alerts, immediately spot probe the area. Because the scent may leave the surface some distance from the actual burial site, shoveling before attaining a probe strike may waste precious time and should be avoided unless the probe pole is shorter than the depth of the debris.

It usually does not hurt for a dog to dig aggressively where it alerts, but the dog's handler should call the dog off as soon as a probe strike is made so that rescuers can dig out the victim using appropriate shoveling techniques. This course of action protects the dog and allows rescuers to safely excavate, extricate the patient, and provide emergency medical care.

**Figure 35-42** FEMA-trained dogs are used to find people that are still alive but trapped within wrecked structures.
Copyright Andrea Booher/FEMA

## Incidents Involving Structures

In situations involving multiple casualties of people trapped in buildings such as resort structures, urban search dogs certified by the Federal Emergency Management Agency (FEMA) may be superior to dogs trained specifically for alpine avalanche SAR (Figure 35-42■). FEMA-trained dogs are familiarized with scents found in buildings and are trained to alert to live humans only, rather than to dead bodies, clothing, or other items. These dogs are trained to explore cavities, and they work without wearing harnesses, which makes them less likely to be caught on wreckage debris in tight spaces.

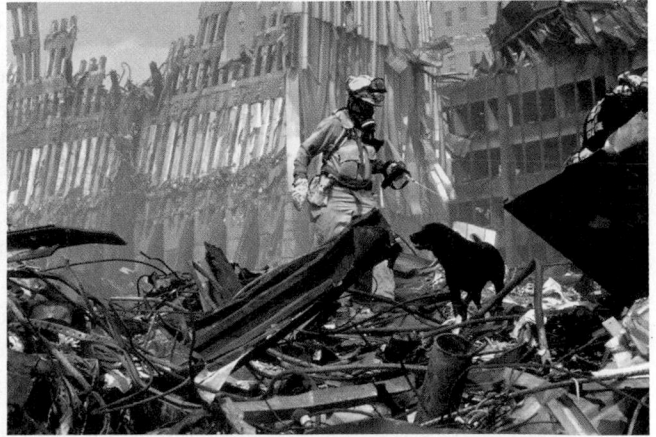

## Water Rescue

Water rescue is another type of specialized rescue operation and includes swift water rescue, flood rescue, ice rescue, and dive rescue. The basic principles of water rescue are covered in Chapter 29, Water Emergencies.

# STOP, THINK, UNDERSTAND

## Multiple Choice
Choose the correct answer.

1. What is the top priority in an avalanche rescue? _____
   a. establish the victim's airway
   b. locate the victim/victims
   c. provide support for the rescuers (logistics)
   d. assure rescuer safety

2. What degree of slope defines a low-angle rescue (as distinguished from a high-angle rescue)? _____
   a. 45 degrees
   b. 40 degrees

   c. 35 degrees
   d. 30 degrees

3. Which of the following tasks is not a basic task of a SAR operation?_____
   a. containment
   b. support
   c. intelligence gathering
   d. mobilization

## List
List six challenges a SAR team may face.

1. _____
2. _____
3. _____
4. _____
5. _____
6. _____

## Short Answer
Describe the RECCO system.

_____
_____
_____

# Fire Ground Operations

Fire-ground operations (fire operations at a structure, brush fire, hazmat incident etc.) are usually conducted in accordance with National Fire Protection Association (NFPA) standards because most fire departments adopt NFPA standards as part of their standard operating procedures. On occasion, OEC Technicians may be requested to provide medical support at the scene of a fire, most often to triage, treat, and transport patients, including injured firefighters (Figure 35-43■). OEC Technicians also may be asked to assist with firefighter rehabilitation, a process that involves monitoring the medical condition of firefighters following a work period and identifying those who are medically fit to return to duty. According to NFPA standards, firefighter rehabilitation should occur at any fire or prolonged rescue scene in which on-scene activities potentially exceed a safe level of physical or mental endurance.

Fire ground operations focus on the following key tasks, which are listed from highest priority to lowest priority:

+ Size-up: identifying building size and type of construction, and whether flames are visible
+ Accountability: identifying the locations of people within the scene
+ Rescue/life safety: helping people
+ Confinement: keeping the fire contained and from damaging other structures
+ Control: extinguishing the fire
+ Ventilation: making an opening in the structure to allow flames, smoke, and toxic vapors to exhaust
+ Property conservation

If called to a fire scene, you will likely be requested to report to one of possibly several staging areas until needed. The staging area may be located near the incident or several miles away. In the United States, fire ground operations are managed using the National Incident Management System, which is described in Chapter 4, Incident Command and Triage.

You can do several things to assist fire personnel if you arrive at the scene of a fire before they do. First, report the fire, including its exact location and the type of structure involved, using the following standard terminology:

+ Residence (including general size, such as large or small)
+ Apartments (includes multi-unit dwellings)
+ Commercial (such as warehouses, stores, or office building)
+ High rise (four floors or taller)

In addition, provide basic information about the current fire conditions using the following common terms:

+ Fire showing (flames are visible)
+ Smoke showing (smoke is visible)
+ Nothing showing (neither flames nor smoke is visible)

While you await the arrival of firefighters, attempt to gather information from witnesses or people evacuating the building. Among the questions to ask are the following:

+ Is everyone out of the building? How do you know?
+ How many people are still inside the building? How do you know?
+ Where in the building are the people located? How do you know?
+ Exactly where in the building is the fire located? How do you know?

Provide this information to the first fire officer to arrive on scene because it can save precious time and might save lives.

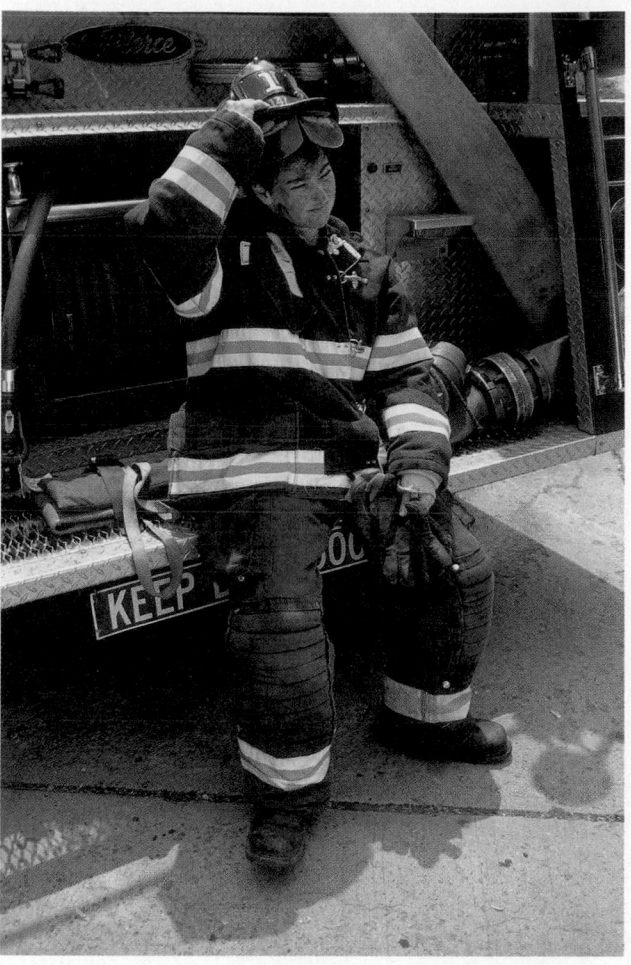

**Figure 35-43** On occasion, OEC Technicians may be asked to care for an injured firefighter.
Copyright Lynton Gardiner/Dorling Kindersley Media Library

---

### Fire Ground Anatomy

As you stand directly in front of a building, each of its sides is given a designation:

*Side A (the front of the building)*
*Side B (the left side of the building)*
*Side C (the back of the building)*
*Side D (the right side of the building)*

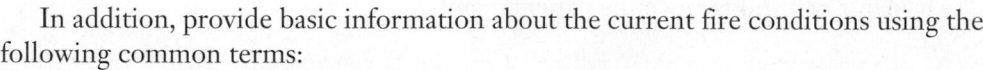

NOTE

Firefighting is strenuous, even life-threatening work. Each year, tens of thousands of firefighters are injured, and approximately 100 firefighters are killed in the line of duty. Any injured firefighters will be evacuated as quickly as possible, and as an OEC Technician, you may be asked to help care for them. Firefighters wear protective gear, including a self-contained breathing apparatus (SCBA). To effectively treat an injured firefighter, you will likely need to remove this equipment. To remove the personal protective gear and SCBA of a firefighter who has suspected spinal injuries, perform the following procedure:

1. Rescuer #1: Manually stabilize the patient's head and neck in neutral anatomic alignment.

2. Rescuers #2 and #3: Log-roll the patient onto his side.

3. Rescuer #4:
   a. Remove the regulator mounted on the face piece.
   b. Unstrap and remove the patient's helmet.
   c. Slide the flame-resistant hood back.
   d. Loosen the straps on the face shield.
   e. Remove the firefighter's face shield.
   f. Open the throat strap of the patient's turn-out coat.
   g. Loosen the shoulder and waist straps on the SCBA, and remove the SCBA.
   h. Remove the patient's uppermost arm from the sleeve of the turn-out coat.
   i. Roll the remaining portion of the jacket toward the ground.

4. Rescuers #1, #2, and #3: Log-roll the patient into a supine position on a long spine board.

5. Rescuer #4:
   a. Gently remove the patient's other arm from the turn out coat.
   b. Remove or cut the patient's suspenders.

6. Rescuer #2 and #3:
   a. Remove the patient's boots.
   b. Unfasten and remove the patient's pants.

 **CASE DISPOSITION**

After establishing yourself as the Incident Commander, you define a safe work zone by creating a perimeter. Soon, other OEC Technicians and your patrol's low-angle rescue team arrive. Rescuers quickly begin taking care of the patients. After the fire department's vehicle extrication team has removed the two patients from the wreckage, you give the patients additional care, package them, and raise them up the embankment to a safe zone. EMTs and a paramedic arrive, and they assume patient care. One patient has life-threatening injuries and is airlifted by helicopter to a trauma center. The other patient has suspected spinal injuries and is taken to a hospital by ground ambulance. Both are expected to recover from their injuries.

## Skill Guide

Date: _____

(CPI) = Critical Performance Indicator

Candidate: _____

Start time: _____

End time: _____

## Nerve Agent Administration

**Objective:** To demonstrate ability to correctly administer nerve agent antidote.

| Skill | Max Points | Skill Demo | |
|---|---|---|---|
| Determines scene is safe. | 1 | | (CPI) |
| Introduces self, obtains permission to treat/help. | 1 | | |
| Initiates Standard Precautions. | 1 | | (CPI) |
| Minimizes further exposure. | 1 | | (CPI) |
| Identifies substance. | 1 | | |
| If nerve gas is suspected, obtains nerve gas antidote kit. | 1 | | (CPI) |
| Observes patient for excessive salivation (pneumonic SLUDGE-DUMBELS). | 1 | | |
| Evaluates patient mental status. | 1 | | |
| Clears/maintains airway and manages secretions. | 1 | | (CPI) |
| If SEVERE signs/symptoms exists— Administers 3 atropine & 3 2-PAM CL injections in rapid succession. | 1 | | (CPI) |
| Maintains airway, uses BVM or suction if needed. Monitor vitals. | 1 | | (CPI) |
| Re-evaluates patient, monitor vitals. | 1 | | (CPI) |
| Arranges for rapid transport. | 1 | | (CPI) |

Must receive 11 out of 13 points.

Comments: _____

Failure of any of the CPIs is an automatic failure.

Evaluator: _____ NSP ID: _____

PASS      FAIL

# ♦ Chapter Review

## Chapter Summary

As part of their regular duties, OEC Technicians may become involved in a special operations incident. Although these situations occur infrequently, all rescuers, including OEC Technicians, should be able to identify the types of incidents to which special operations personnel may be summoned. By having a fundamental understanding of the mission and basic operational procedures of special operations groups, OEC Technicians will be better able to assist those groups and provide care to outdoor recreationalists in need of help.

HAZWOPER training is an essential part of HazMat response and is required for anyone who works in environments in which uncontrolled hazardous materials may be encountered.

OEC Technicians who are ski patrollers provide a specialized service to public safety officials and as such constitute a type of special operation group. It is for this reason that the leaders of the National Ski Patrol encourage all its members to become more involved with disaster response teams. By becoming involved, patrollers and OEC Technicians help to perpetuate Minnie Dole's dream of volunteerism and of creating a nationally recognized rescue organization.

## Remember...

1. Special operations require specialized training, skills, and equipment.
2. OEC Technicians need a basic understanding of basic special operations-related tasks and objectives so that they can safely assist EMS crews.
3. When encountering a victim trapped in a vehicle, always "try before you pry."

4. OEC Technicians are encouraged to join a CERT, MRC, DMAT, or USAR team.
5. The care for organophosphate exposure is self-administration of nerve-agent antidote medications available in a kit (Mark I or DuoDote).
6. The National Response Framework (NRF) is the organized system for disaster response in the United States.

## Chapter Questions

### Multiple Choice

Choose the correct answer.

1. Which of the following operations is not considered a special operation?_____
   a. avalanche rescue
   b. low-angle rescue
   c. vehicle extrication
   d. backboarding someone with a suspected back injury

2. Which of the following is not a basic operational task or an objective for vehicle extrication?_____
   a. assessing the scene
   b. stabilizing the patient
   c. gaining access
   d. providing initial care and removing the patient

3. Which of the following teams is not one of the specialized response teams within the National Disaster Medical System? _____
   a. National Pharmacy Response Team (NPRTS)
   b. National EMT Response Team (NERT)
   c. National Veterinary Response Team (NVRT)
   d. Disaster Mortuary Response Team (DMORT)

4. Which of the following hazard control zones is considered the most dangerous and contaminated zone? _____
   a. containment zone
   b. warm zone
   c. hot zone
   d. cold zone

5. Which of the following statements concerning ways to simplify an avalanche rescue operation involving a trained dog is false? _____
   a. Rescuers should avoid sitting in the snow.
   b. Rescuers should avoid leaving any litter or body waste in the search area.
   c. Rescuers should stage equipment (especially food) away from the area, preferably downwind.
   d. Rescuers should be stationed 100 feet downwind of the search area while the dog is working.

6. Which of the following lists places the focus of fire ground operations in the correct order? _____
   a. rescue/life safety, size-up, accountability, confinement, control, ventilation, property conservation
   b. size-up, accountability, rescue/life safety, confinement, control, ventilation, property conservation
   c. accountability, size-up, rescue/life safety, confinement, control, ventilation, property conservation
   d. control, size-up, accountability, rescue/life safety, confinement, control, ventilation, property conservation

7. What does the blue portion of the NFPA safety diamond indicate? _____
   a. flammability
   b. health hazard
   c. susceptibility to burning (chemical reactivity)
   d. special precautions/protective gear needed

8. What does the yellow portion of the NFPA safety diamond indicate? _____
   a. flammability
   b. health hazard
   c. susceptibility to burning (chemical reactivity)
   d. special precautions/protective gear needed

9. What does the white portion of the NFPA safety diamond indicate? _____
   a. flammability
   b. health hazard
   c. susceptibility to burning (chemical reactivity)
   d. special precautions/protective gear needed

10. What does the numeral 3 within the red diamond of an NFPA label indicate? _____
   a. A material that must be preheated before ignition can occur.
   b. Liquids and solids that can be ignited under almost all ambient temperature conditions.
   c. A material that would cause only minor irritation upon exposure.
   d. A material that is normally stable but can become unstable at elevated temperatures and pressures.

## Short Answer

1. Define special operations, and indicate when they should be called upon for help.

_____

_____

_____

_____

2. What does HAZWOPER stand for?

_____

_____

_____

_____

3. Who is required to take HAZWOPER training?

_____

_____

_____

_____

# Scenario

A small avalanche occurred in the backcountry of a state park, and one individual was able to free herself and call 911 on a cell phone to request help. A small party of rescuers gathers and responds while a call for additional community help is made by one of the rescuers using his radio.

The search party locates the cell phone caller and starts the interviewing process to narrow the search area.

SAR is the process of looking for and providing aid to people who are in distress or imminent danger.

1. SAR consists of what two components? _____
   a. search operations and recovery operations
   b. search operations and rapid extrication
   c. stabilization of operations and rapid removal
   d. search operations and rescue operations

Complex SAR operations are broken down into five basic tasks.

2. The first task of SAR is _____
   a. intelligence gathering.
   b. mobilization.
   c. containment.
   d. search.

3. Using the information gathered, the team establishes a_____ area with defined boundaries.
   a. search
   b. rescue
   c. containment
   d. recovery

*On operations involving an avalanche rescue, recovery time is critical.*

**4.** The chance of surviving a complete burial decreases rapidly and is_____

    **a.** 50 percent within the first 30 minutes.

    **b.** 10 percent within the first 30 minutes.

    **c.** 50 percent within 60 minutes.

    **d.** 60 percent within 60 minutes.

*When a rescue involves a chemical or a substance, check for the NFPA safety diamond on the container's packaging.*

## Suggested Reading

http://www.citizencorps.gov/cert

http://www.medicalreservecorps.gov

http://www.hhs.gov/aspr/opeo/ndms/teams/dmat.html

http://www.fema.gov/hazard/index.shtm

EXPLORE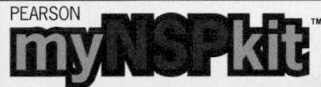

Please go to www.myNSPkit.com. Under Student Resources, you will find animations, videos, web links, and games related to this chapter—and much more. Look for information on triage simulation, hazardous materials, aeromedical evacuation, and more.

Register your access code from the front of your book by going to www.myNSPkit.com and selecting the appropriate links. If the in-cover access code has been redeemed, go to www.myNSPkit.com and follow links to **Buy Access.**

# ALS Interface

Jamie A. Goodis, MD
Paul S. Auerbach, MD, MS, FACEP, FAWM

36

## ⊕ OBJECTIVES

**Upon completion of this chapter, the OEC Technician will be able to:**

**36-1** Define advanced life support (ALS).

**36-2** List the roles and responsibilities of an ALS provider.

**36-3** Describe the roles of OEC Technicians in *assisting* an ALS provider.

**36-4** List the indications for each of the following advanced procedures:
- advanced airway management
- intravenous therapy
- cardiac monitoring (electrocardiogram: ECG or EKG)
- electrical therapy
- medication administration

**36-5** Describe how to assess proper placement of an endotracheal tube.

**36-6** Describe how to properly set up a mechanical ventilator.

**36-7** Describe how to properly set up an intravenous solution for administration.

**36-8** Describe how to properly set up a four-lead ECG.

**36-9** List common respiratory, cardiac, and analgesic medications ALS providers use.

**36-10** Describe how to properly set up a metered-dose inhaler for use.

**36-11** List the "five rights" of safe medication administration.

## ⊕ KEY TERMS

**analgesic,** *p. 1164*
**cricothyrotomy,** *p. 1149*

**electrocardiogram (ECG or EKG),** *p. 1159*

**endotracheal intubation,** *p. 1141*

## Chapter Overview

As an OEC Technician, you will often be the first health care provider to arrive at the scene of an outdoor emergency, and so a great deal of responsibility will rest on your shoulders. At this point in your OEC training, you should be able to evaluate, treat, package, and transport a seriously ill or injured patient. In addition, you are expected to be able to identify the need for additional resources at the scene, convey

*continued*

## HISTORICAL TIMELINE

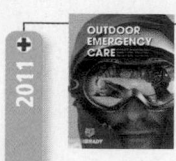

**2011** *OEC* Fifth Edition is published.

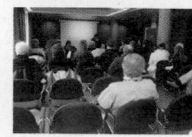

**2011** Classes begin using OEC 5th edition.

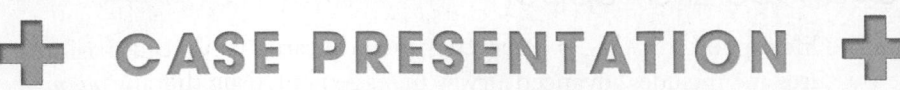

# CASE PRESENTATION

A 42-year-old man skis into a lift tower, striking both his body and his head. He is found unconscious and unresponsive to painful stimuli. He is not wearing a helmet, and he has massive facial injuries and is bleeding profusely from both the mouth and nose. His airway is obstructed with blood, broken teeth, snow, and vomit. He also has an obvious deformity of the right wrist and a large bruise on his right anterior chest.

*What should you do?*
*What does this victim need as soon as possible?*

all the information you know about the patient in a standardized manner, and facilitate the patient's smooth transition to the next level of care (Figure 36-1■). Your training has prepared you to manage a wide variety of traumatic and medical emergencies commonly encountered by OEC Technicians. At times, however, your patient's injuries or illness will be beyond the scope of your knowledge and skills. Such situations can be especially difficult and challenging because you will be working in a difficult environment with limited resources: no electricity or running water, and scant support equipment, supplies, and medications.

Patients can present with a wide range of injuries or illnesses that can vary in severity from relatively minor to life threatening, and your ability to recognize the signs and symptoms of a critical patient, initiate treatment, and swiftly transport them to a higher level of care can mean the difference between life and death. The longer it takes to initiate definitive care for critically injured or ill individuals, the higher the morbidity and mortality, and thus recognizing *when* advanced care is urgently needed is a skill that every OEC Technician must possess.

This chapter presents a basic overview of advanced life support (ALS), including indications for ALS, the roles of ALS providers, and common ALS procedures and medications. The chapter also explains the ways in which OEC Technicians may *assist* an ALS provider in treating a severely ill or injured patient, and the circumstances under which it is allowable for them to assist:

- when the resort where you are an OEC Technician permits you to do so
- when a physician has accepted responsibility for supervising your assistance and provides medical direction
- when the state or province in which you are an OEC Technician legally allows you to do so

As an OEC Technician, you are not legally permitted to perform any skills beyond those that have been presented in previous chapters. The skills and uses of medications described in the following pages are *not* part of an OEC Technician's scope of practice. Your understanding of when these procedures are indicated, combined with your ability and willingness to help an ALS provider, may help to save the life of a critically ill or injured patient. When assisting an ALS provider, always use BSI and wear personal protective equipment.

The "take-home" message for OEC Technicians: know when ALS care is needed, and promptly call for help.

**Figure 36-1** It is important that OEC Technicians help smooth the transition of patients to a higher level of care.
Copyright Scott Smith

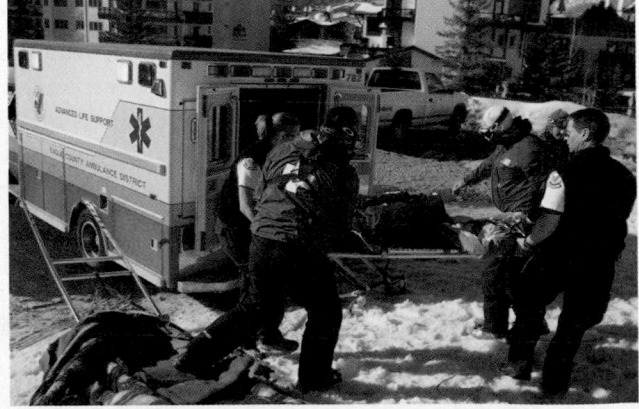

⊕ **36-1** Define advanced life support (ALS).

⊕ **36-2** List the roles and responsibilities of an ALS provider.

# Advanced Life Support

Advanced life support, or ALS, is emergency medical care that exceeds basic life support measures and includes advanced airway management, drug therapy, *manual* electrical therapy (for the heart), and other procedures. ALS is commonly required whenever basic life support (BLS) measures have proven ineffective. In cases requiring ALS there is little time to waste, and prompt initiation of advanced care could mean the difference between survival and death. Indications for ALS care include, but are not limited to, the following conditions:

+ altered level of responsiveness (GCS less than 12)
+ severe head, facial, oral, or neck injuries (including burns)
+ severe respiratory difficulties (including allergic reactions)
+ acute chest pain
+ irregular heart beat
+ cardiac/respiratory arrest
+ unresponsiveness
+ stroke/TIA
+ seizures
+ multi-system trauma
+ shock or severe blood loss
+ relief for severe pain

ALS providers—which include AEMTs, paramedics, some RNs and PAs, and physicians—bring unique knowledge and skill sets to the scene and can help stabilize a patient's condition before and during transport to a definitive-care facility. These highly skilled clinicians can provide the following components of ALS:

+ advanced airway management
+ intravenous therapy
+ cardiac monitoring
+ electrical therapy
+ administration of medications
+ invasive procedures

Initiated early, each of these therapies can potentially decrease the rates of patient morbidity and mortality.

## Transition of Care to ALS Providers

⊕ **36-3** Describe the roles of OEC Technicians in *assisting* an ALS provider.

If ALS providers are summoned to a scene, they—like you—have a legal and ethical duty to respond. Upon their arrival, the most highly trained prehospital ALS provider on scene assumes care of the patient.

If the responding ALS providers are part of your patrol or rescue unit, policies and procedures governing their activation and authority should already exist. If the ALS providers are not part of your patrol or rescue unit but instead are, for example, bystanders who identify themselves as ALS providers, then it is essential that you first check their credentials to ensure that they are in fact ALS providers. Obviously, if a paramedic arrives in an ambulance and in uniform, this formality may not be necessary.

Next, thank the Bystander ALS providers for their willingness to lend assistance. Then, remind them that once they assume medical care of a patient, they must ac-

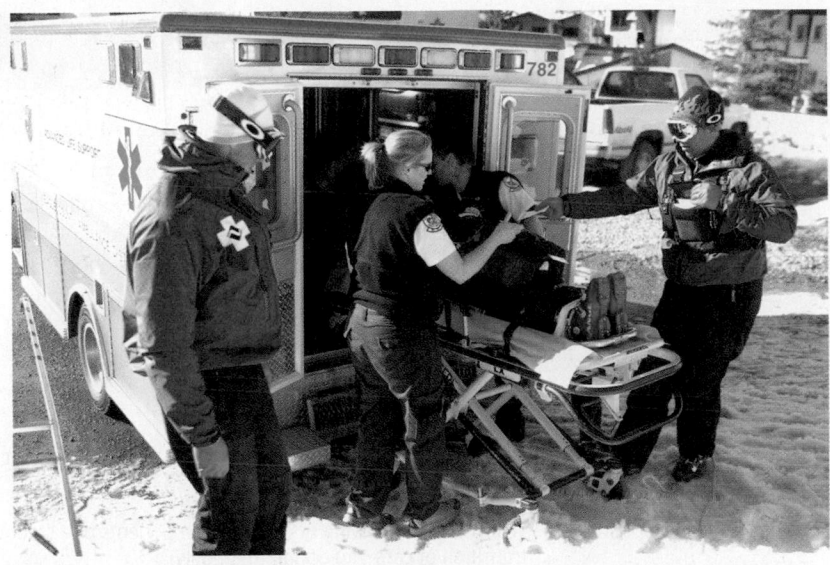

**Figure 36-2** Give ALS providers a concise and accurate hand-off report concerning the patient's condition and needs.
Copyright Scott Smith

company that patient to a definitive-care facility to ensure continuity of care. Bystander ALS providers may find performing the skills they have been taught to be difficult (if not impossible) in the field when pertinent specialized equipment is not available.

To facilitate a smooth transition of care, it is essential that you give ALS providers a brief hand-off report about the patient's current condition and immediate medical needs, and your perceived need for specific ALS interventions. ALS providers depend on you to provide an accurate and concise hand-off report that focuses on the key facts the ALS team will need to make subsequent critical care decisions (Figure 36-2■). The SOAP and CHEATED acronyms, described in Chapter 8, Medical Communications and Documentation, are excellent methods for assembling the information needed for an effective hand-off report.

Once you have finished delivering your report, be sure to ask the ALS providers if they have any questions. This allows them to obtain additional information about the incident, the scene, and the initial care provided. They, in turn, will relay this information in their hand-off report to the definitive-care facility's staff. Once the patient hand-off is complete, ask the ALS providers if they need any help, if you are permitted to do so. At this point the ALS providers may request that you assist them as they initiate advanced care.

Like OEC Technicians, ALS providers begin treatment by carefully assessing the ABCDs, and they may need your help in retrieving ALS equipment, ventilating a patient with an advanced airway, monitoring vital signs, assembling and preparing IV fluids, taping down IV catheters, attaching pressure infusers for IV fluids, assisting in securing ET tubes once in place, applying ECG electrodes, assisting patients with their own medications, assisting with the administration of nebulized medications, applying and interpreting pulse oximeters, and using electronic blood glucose determination devices. OEC Technicians may not assemble, test, or insert an advanced airway (EOA/ET), assemble drugs for administration, use ECG paddles or a manual defibrillator to cardiovert a patient. The exception is the use of an automated electronic defibrillator by OEC Technicians who have been trained in using one. Your ability to competently and expeditiously perform these skills will allow ALS providers to focus their attention on the patient, thereby ensuring the continuity of care.

# STOP, THINK, UNDERSTAND

## Multiple Choice

Choose the correct answer.

1. Which of the following statements is true? _____
   a. Only ALS providers have a duty to respond.
   b. Patient care is assumed by the most highly trained prehospital provider on scene.
   c. It is not necessary for the first OEC Technician on scene to ascertain that an incoming bystander ALS provider is actually credentialed as such.
   d. The ALS provider who assumes patient care is not responsible for accompanying the patient to a definitive-care facility.

2. Which of the following skills are within the scope of an OEC Technician's practice? (check all that apply)
   _____ a. recognizing *when* advanced care is needed
   _____ b. intubating a patient
   _____ c. administering $O_2$ to a patient
   _____ d. inserting an oropharyngeal airway
   _____ e. suctioning a patient's airway
   _____ f. administering IV fluids to combat hypovolemic shock
   _____ g. assisting with the set up of an endotracheal tube
   _____ h. defibrillating a patient with an AED

3. Which of the following skills may ALS providers offer in the field? (check all that apply)
   _____ a. advanced airway maintenance
   _____ b. IV therapy
   _____ c. electrical therapy
   _____ d. administration of medications
   _____ e. cardiac monitoring
   _____ f. pain management
   _____ g. reattachment of an amputated finger
   _____ h. minor surgery

4. Which of the following actions are components of a smooth transition of care? (check all that apply)
   _____ a. Providing incoming ALS providers a brief report.
   _____ b. Providing incoming ALS providers information about the patient's immediate medical needs.
   _____ c. Providing incoming ALS providers an accurate list of vital signs.
   _____ d. Providing incoming ALS providers SOAP/CHEATED information.
   _____ e. Providing incoming ALS providers a list of names of all OEC Technicians who cared for the patient.

## Matching

1. Match each of the following terms with its description.

   _____ 1. ALS
   _____ 2. BLS
   _____ 3. AED
   _____ 4. paramedic
   _____ 5. OEC Technician

   a. a prehospital provider who is not allowed to perform advanced skills
   b. a medical device used by ALS and BLS providers on a patient during cardiac arrest
   c. the level of care that a paramedic is allowed to perform
   d. a prehospital provider that may provide advanced skill and medication under physician direction
   e. the level of care that OEC Technicians are trained to provide

2. Indicate whether each of the following situations warrants BLS or ALS.

   _____ 1. basic life support (BLS)
   _____ 2. advanced life support (ALS)

   a. a patient with a concussion and a GCS score of 15
   b. a patient with a concussion and a GCS score of 12
   c. a patient with burns to the face, neck, and hands
   d. a patient with a rash after touching poison oak
   e. a patient with a prior history of anaphylaxis to latex who complains of respiratory distress after accidental exposure to latex gloves
   f. a 23-year-old male having a seizure (no prior history)
   g. a 16-year-old female with a dislocated shoulder who has little pain
   h. a patient with multi-system trauma
   i. a patient with a fractured humerus who is in severe pain
   j. a semi-conscious 17-year-old male with a respiratory rate of 12 following an alcohol overdose
   k. a patient suffering from an irregular pulse, with or without chest pain

# Advanced Airway Management

Preservation of the ABCDs is essential for patient survival, and the first step of airway management, of course, is to recognize the need for it. Signs of airway compromise, which are described in Chapter 9, Airway Management, include agitation, confusion, pallor, cyanosis, chest wall/sternal retractions, and very fast or very slow breathing. If the situation is not immediately obvious, an easy way to assess the need for an advanced airway is to ask yourself the following four questions:

1. Is the airway patent? (Is the airway in the mouth free of blood/teeth? Are facial trauma and/or oral swelling present?)
2. Is the patient ventilating well? (Is he breathing regularly and deeply without assistance?)
3. Is the patient oxygenating well? (Is the skin pink? Does pulse oximetry indicate normal oxygen saturation?)
4. Are conventional methods for managing the airway—suction, supplemental oxygen, a nasopharyngeal airway, an oropharyngeal airway, or a bag-valve mask—effective?

A "No" answer to any of these questions indicates a clear need for an advanced airway. There are three primary methods for achieving and maintaining a patent airway using advanced airway procedures: endotracheal intubation, other advanced airway adjuncts, and cricothyrotomy. Again, only ALS providers may perform these procedures; however OEC Technicians should recognize the need for an advanced airway and call for an ALS provider.

## Endotracheal Intubation

**Endotracheal intubation** involves inserting a breathing tube into a patient's trachea (Figure 36-3■). Once in place within the trachea, a balloon around the end of the tube is inflated, "sealing" the tube within the airway and preventing contaminants from entering. The tube is connected to the universal adapter on a bag-valve device, and ventilation is performed using a bag valve device connected to an oxygen source.

An ALS provider can perform two types of endotracheal intubation: orotracheal (or oral) intubation, which involves passing a breathing tube through the open mouth, through the vocal cords, and into the trachea; and nasotracheal (or nasal) intubation, which involves passing a breathing tube through the nose and into the trachea. Oral intubation is performed more often than is nasal intubation.

### Indications/Contraindications of Endotracheal Intubation

Endotracheal intubation is indicated whenever traditional methods for securing an airway are not effective. Nasotracheal intubation is indicated when C-spine precautions are required while establishing an airway, when a patient's airway must be immediately secured (e.g., due to airway burns, a severe asthma attack, or unresponsiveness to medication), or when injury or physiology prevents the patient's jaw from being opened sufficiently to allow orotracheal intubation.

The relative contraindication to endotracheal intubation is the presence of a gag reflex; in its presence, any intubation attempt could induce vomiting that in turn could compromise airway patency. However, there may be instances in which an endotracheal tube may be inserted into a responsive patient with an intact gag

**⊕ 36-4** List the indications for each of the following advanced procedures:

- advanced airway management
- intravenous therapy
- cardiac monitoring (electrocardiogram: ECG or EKG)
- electrical therapy
- medication administration

**endotracheal intubation** the process of placing a tube into the trachea and maintaining it to provide an airway while preventing aspiration of foreign material into the bronchi (and lungs).

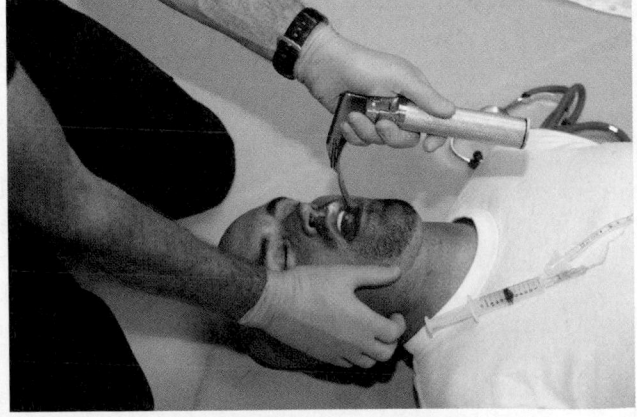

**Figure 36-3** Inserting an endotracheal tube into a patient.
Copyright Mike Halloran

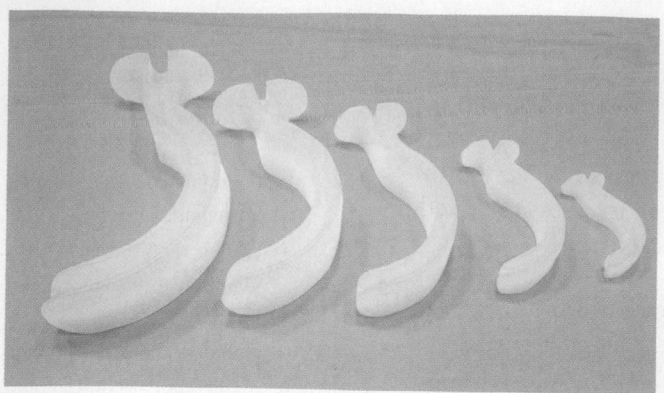

**Figure 36-4** Oral airways.
Copyright Edward McNamara

reflex to help the patient breathe more effectively. Cervical spine injury is a relative contraindication to orotracheal intubation, but this procedure can be safely performed if assisting rescuers use their hands to stabilize the patient's C-spine by maintaining in-line positioning (*not* traction).

Nasotracheal intubation is contraindicated in the presence of severe facial injuries or fractures, or in a suspected basilar skull fracture, because the procedure can worsen existing injuries or cause other complications. Nasotracheal intubation is relatively contraindicated in an apneic patient because the lack of air movement significantly increases the difficulty of the procedure.

**Equipment and Set-Up** The following equipment is needed to properly perform endotracheal intubation:

+ laryngoscope handle
+ laryngoscope blades
+ endotracheal tube
+ water-based lubricant
+ flexible stylet
+ 10–12 cc syringe
+ device or tape for securing the tube
+ suction device with rigid suction catheter
+ digital wave form or colorimetric (older type) $CO_2$ detector
+ bag valve with reservoir (a mask is not needed because the device connects directly to the endotracheal tube)
+ oxygen tank
+ tubing to connect to the oxygen supply
+ oral airway or bite block (Figure 36-4■)

Set-up is a two-step process that involves assembling the equipment and checking each item's readiness for performing its proper function. Many ALS providers organize their advanced airway equipment in a special kit, package, or roll-up bag that greatly reduces the time needed to locate the equipment and ensures that each item needed is readily available. Some items are available in multiple sizes, and such kits ensure that an adequate size assortment is on hand. Next, ALS providers assemble and check each item, beginning with the laryngoscope blade and handle.

**Figure 36-5** A laryngoscope handle (at top), three Miller blades (at left), and three MacIntosh ("Mac") blades (at right).
Copyright Edward McNamara

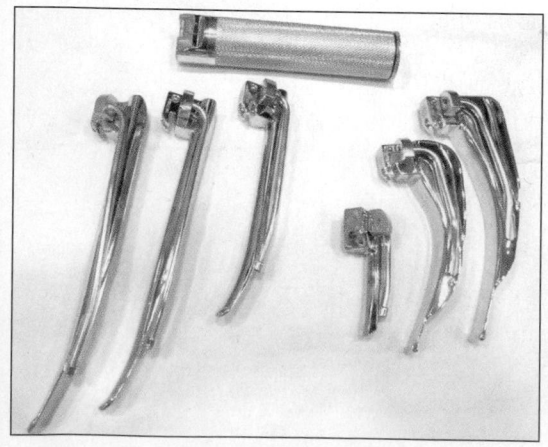

There are two basic types of laryngoscope blades: straight blades, known as Miller blades, and curved blades, known as Macintosh or "Mac" blades (Figure 36-5■). Blades come in different sizes, ranging from "0" for infants to "4" for large adults, and are available in disposable plastic or reusable stainless steel. The blade size may be indicated on the large end of the blade. The blade type and size used depend on the ALS provider's preference (Figure 36-6■ and Figure 36-7■).

Most blades include an integrated light source built into the end of the blade. The light, which may be fiberoptic or simply a small light bulb, is powered by batteries within the laryngoscope handle. When the attached blade is opened, the integrated light illuminates the airway, which facilitates the placement of the tube.

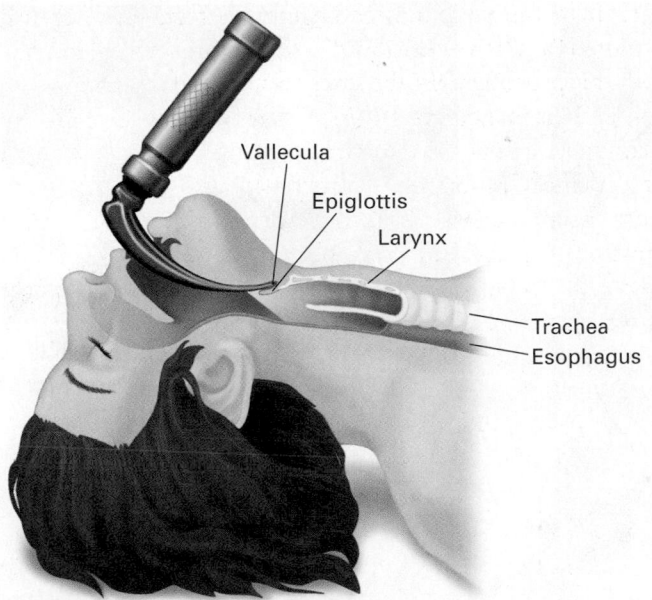

**Figure 36-6** Use of a laryngoscope with a curved or MacIntosh ("Mac") blade.

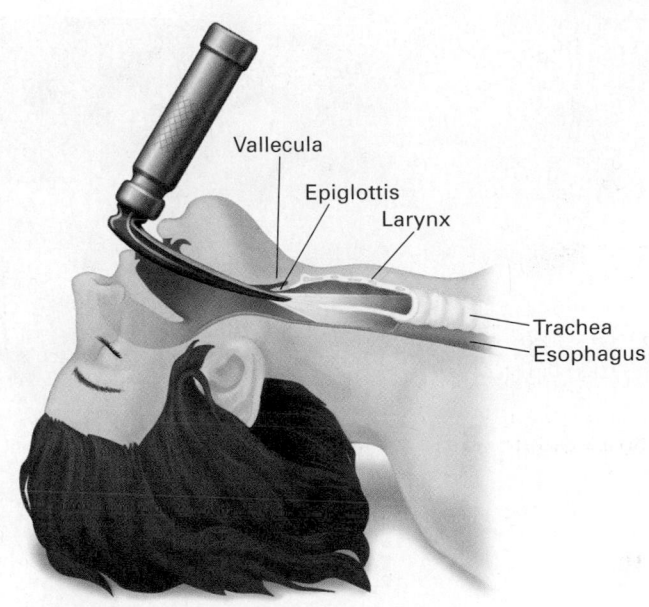

**Figure 36-7** Use of a laryngoscope with a straight or Miller blade.

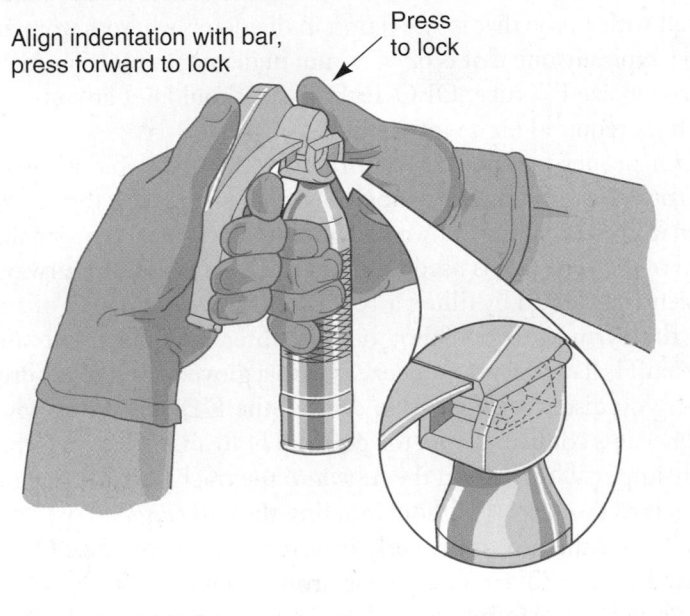

Align indentation with bar, press forward to lock

Press to lock

(a)

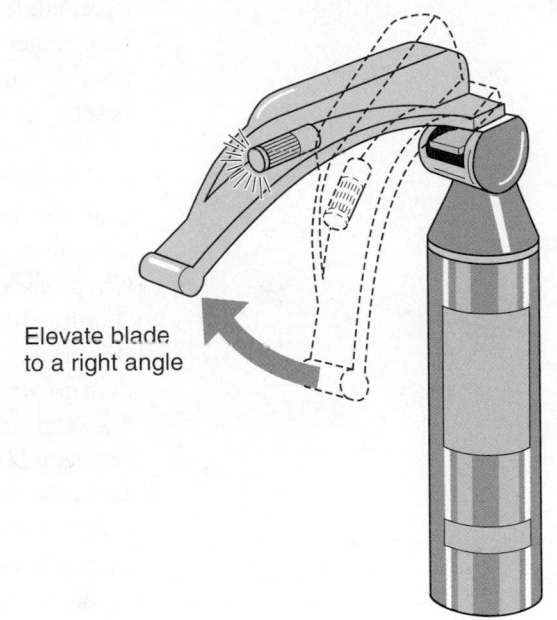

Elevate blade to a right angle

(b)

**Figure 36-8** Always check to make sure that the blade is securely attached to the handle and that the light is functional.

It is crucial to check that the blade attaches properly to the handle and that the light is functional before attempting to use the equipment. To check the handle and blade for proper functioning, attach the blade to the handle by inserting the notched end of the blade into the small bar atop the handle (Figure 36-8■). Then raise the blade until it "clicks" into position. The light should immediately come on. To turn the light off (thereby conserving the battery), fold the blade down out of the "clicked and locked" position while leaving it attached to the handle. The handle and blade are now ready for use.

Endotracheal (ET) tubes come in a variety of sizes, ranging from 3.0 mm for infants to 9.0 mm for very large adults (Figure 36-9■). A good rule of thumb for selecting a

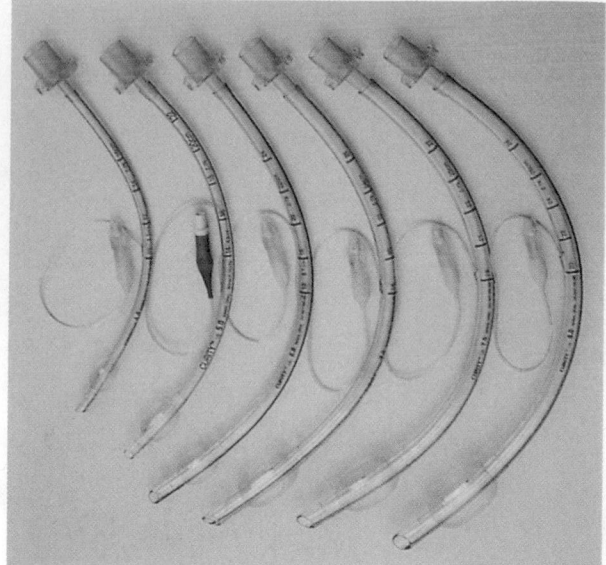

**Figure 36-9** Endotracheal tubes come in an assortment of sizes.

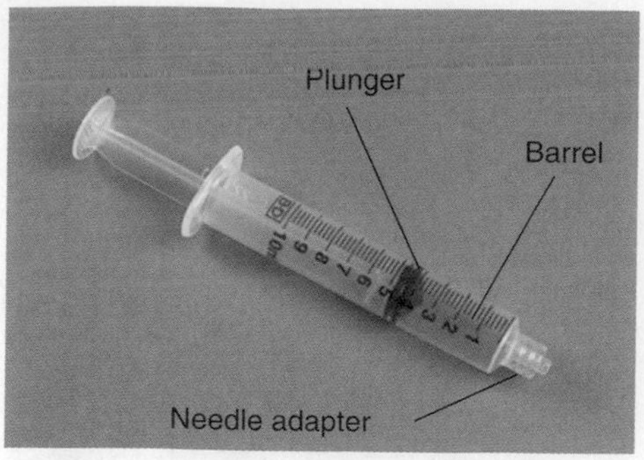

**Figure 36-10** Fill a syringe like this one with 10 cc of air to check the cuff.

tube of the appropriate size is that the ET tube should be approximately the same diameter as the patient's nostril or little finger. This works for children and adults alike. Most adult men will do well with a tube that is 7.5–8 mm in diameter, whereas women tend to need a smaller tube, typically one that is 6.5–7.5 mm in diameter. Only an ALS provider may select the proper size ET tube; OEC Technicians should not attempt to determine the size of ET tube required for an intubation.

To check an ET tube for proper functioning, first remove the tube from its protective package. Arising from midway along the tube's shaft is a small tube that ends at a small bulb and adapter. This small bulb, known as a pilot bulb, connects to a small, inflatable "cuff" at the end of the tube and is used to inflate the cuff to seal the airway. Check the integrity of the inflatable cuff by filling a 10–12 cc syringe with 10 cc of air (Figure 36-10■). Attach the syringe to the pilot bulb adapter and inject the air (Figure 36-11■). After the cuff inflates, gently squeeze it with a gloved hand to ensure that no air leaks from it. If you discover an air leak, discard the ET tube, get a new one, and repeat the test. Once it is confirmed that the cuff will hold air, deflate it. Otherwise, it is difficult (usually impossible) to insert the tube into the trachea. Add 10 cc of air to the syringe and attach it to the adapter without inflating the cuff (Figure 36-12■). It can now be inflated easily after the tube is properly inserted into the trachea. Only ALS providers are permitted to test ET equipment for proper functionality.

Most ALS providers prefer to perform orotracheal intubation using a flexible stylet. (Nasotracheal intubation does not require the use of a stylet.) The stylet, a section of flexible wire is inserted into the tube as a way of keeping it in a desired position. Most often it is bent at the end, making it resemble a hockey stick. This allows for easier insertion of the tube into the trachea. (Figure 36-13■). Many ALS providers find it helpful to lightly lubricate both the stylet and the tip of the ET tube with a water-based lubricant (a "jelly") before insertion (Figure 36-14■). When placing the stylet into the tube, ensure that it does not extend beyond the sidewall opening at the end of the tube, because it could then damage (gouge) the airway when the tube is inserted. Fold the top end of the stylet over to prevent it from inadvertently sliding farther down the tube. The ET tube is now ready for use. In general, ALS providers are responsible for the assembly and testing of their own advanced airway (ET/EOA/etc.) equipment; OEC Technicians may assist ALS providers by retrieving the equipment and gathering items specifically requested by the ALS providers.

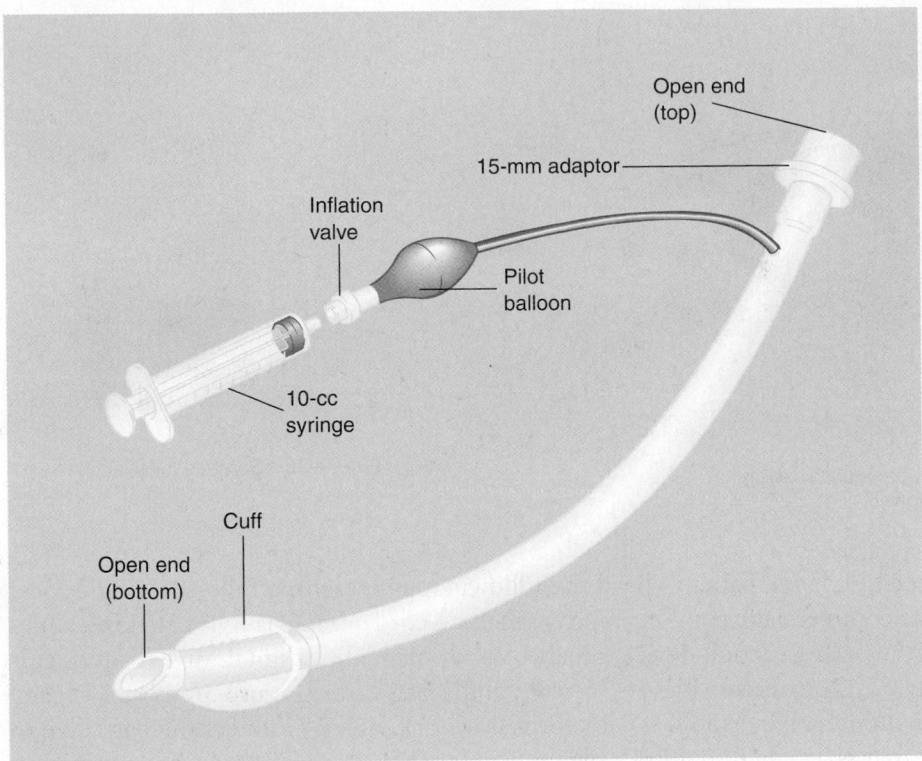

**Figure 36-11** Inject air into the pilot bulb adapter. Gently squeeze the inflated cuff with gloved fingers to check for an air leak.

**Figure 36-12** An endotracheal tube and syringe assembled for intubation.

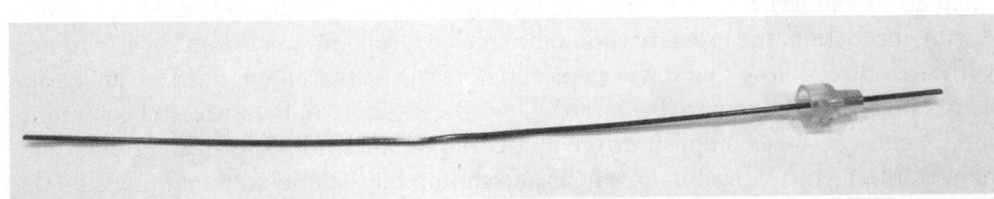

**Figure 36-13** A flexible stylet.
Copyright Edward McNamara

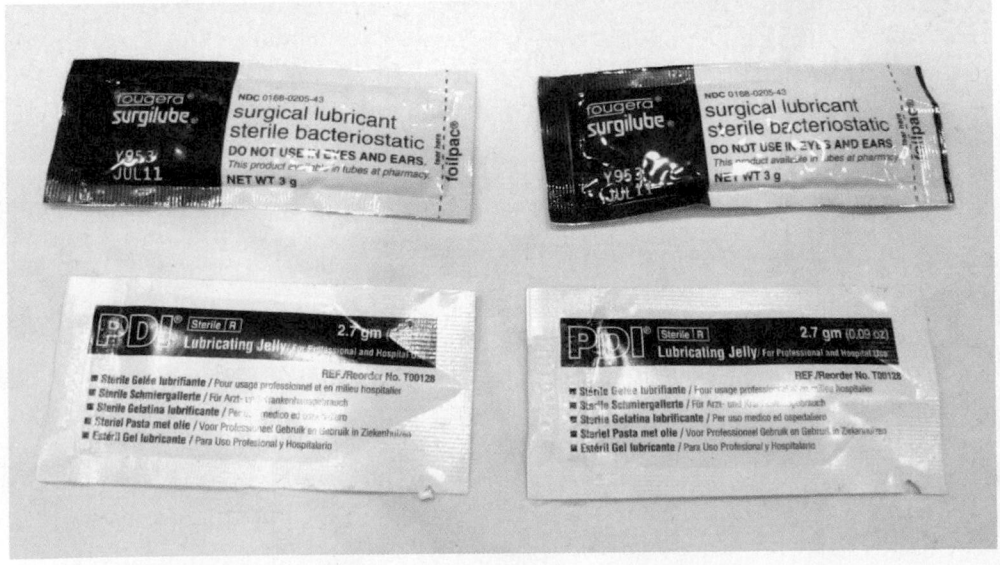

**Figure 36-14** Lubricants for use with ET tubes.
Copyright Edward McNamara

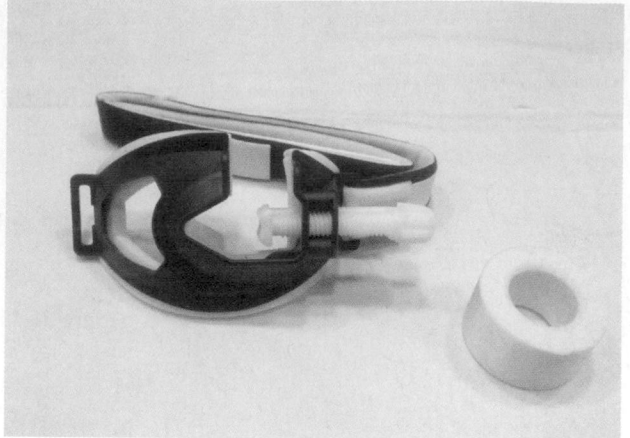

**Figure 36-15** Tube securing devices.
Copyright Edward McNamara

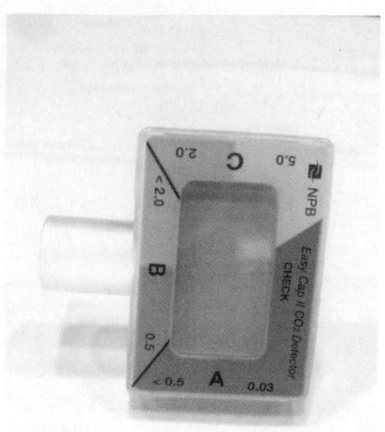

**Figure 36-16** A colorimetric $CO_2$ detector.
Copyright Edward McNamara

Place beside the patient's head the following equipment: a tube-securing device, whether commercially made or improvised (with cord or tape) (Figure 36-15■); a suction catheter and suction device (mechanical or manual); a digital wave form or colorimetric $CO_2$ detector (Figure 36-16■); and a bag valve (Figure 36-17■). In many states a digital waveform $CO_2$ detector is now mandatory. Connect the bag valve to tubing that is attached to a full oxygen cylinder (Figure 36-18■). All the equipment needed to perform endotracheal intubation is now in place and ready for use.

Before and during intubation, an ALS provider may direct you to exert external pressure on the patient's cricoid cartilage to facilitate placement of the ET tube. The routine use of cricoid pressure to prevent aspiration in cardiac arrest is not recommended by the AHA. If, however, cricoid pressure is requested by an ALS provider during intubation, the pressure should be adjusted, relaxed, or released in accordance with their direction so that it will assist and not impede placement of an advanced airway. The BURP maneuver (Backward, Upward, Rightward, Pressure) is a commonly used technique to accomplish external cricoid pressure. To perform the BURP maneuver, place your gloved index finger and thumb on the cricoid membrane and deliver *light* pressure in backward (toward the spine), upward (toward the head), and rightward (toward the patient's right side) directions (Figure 36-19■).

**Figure 36-17** A bag valve with a reservoir.
Copyright Edward McNamara

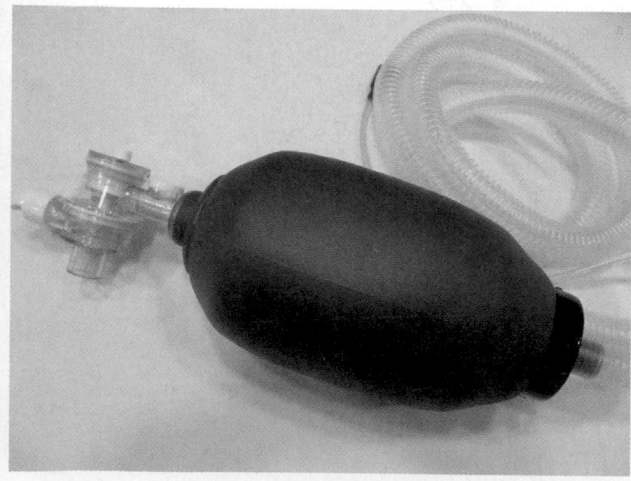

**Figure 36-18** An oxygen tank.
Copyright Edward McNamara

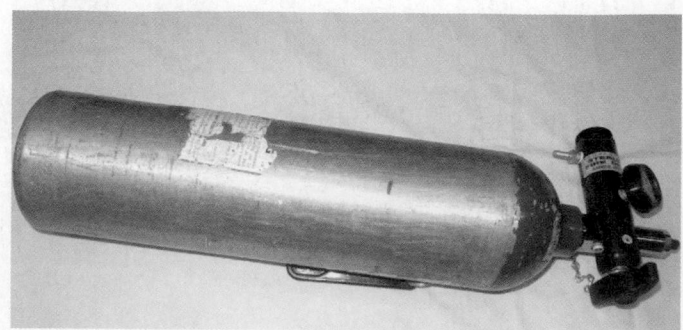

Perhaps the most important types of assistance an OEC Technician can provide to ALS providers during advanced airway interventions are assisting with excellent BVM ventilation to pre-oxygenate the patient and providing suctioning to protect the airway. Excellent BLS airway management allows an ALS provider to concentrate on performing advanced airway procedures.

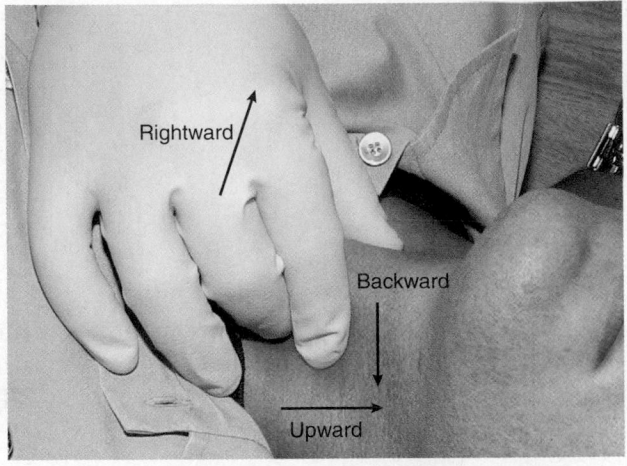

**Figure 36-19** The use of the BURP maneuver on the cricoid cartilage to facilitate endotracheal tube placement.

# STOP, THINK, UNDERSTAND

## Multiple Choice

Choose the correct answer.

1. You are caring for an asthmatic patient and find her growing agitated. Her lips are blue, her pulse rate is 28, and her pulse oximetry reading is 86. What is your next best step?

   _____

   a. Administer $O_2$, immediately call for ALS, and prepare to transport the patient.
   b. Administer $O_2$, but do not call ALS until you have a second full set of vital signs.
   c. Help the patient use her inhaler, after which no call to 911 will be needed.
   d. Place the patient in the recovery position and transport her to the nearest medical facility.

2. What are the two types of laryngoscope blades? _____
   a. Smith and Wesson
   b. Debeer and Yankauer
   c. Auerbach and Johe
   d. Miller and Macintosh

3. The diameter of a correctly sized ET tube should be approximately

   _____

   a. the diameter of the patient's pinkie finger or nostril.
   b. the width of the patient's cricoid cartilage.
   c. half the width of the patient's tongue.
   d. the distance from a corner of the patient's mouth to the earlobe on the same side.

## Short Answer

List some of the signs or symptoms of airway compromise.

_____

_____

_____

_____

_____

## Sequence

Place the following actions that an ALS provider takes during an endotracheal intubation in order from first (1) to last (8).

_____ a. Place securing device, suction device, and colometric $CO_2$ indicator near the patient's head.
_____ b. Disengage blade and turn light off, but leave blade and light source connected.
_____ c. Check integrity of pilot bulb and cuff by inflating bulb with 10–12 cc of air.
_____ d. Attach blade to handle and be sure light source works.
_____ e. Lubricate stylet and tip of ET tube with water-soluble lubricant and insert sytlet into tube.
_____ f. Choose and check the desired blade.
_____ g. Deflate pilot bulb and refill the syringe with 10 cc of air.
_____ h. Connect the BVM to the oxygen cylinder.

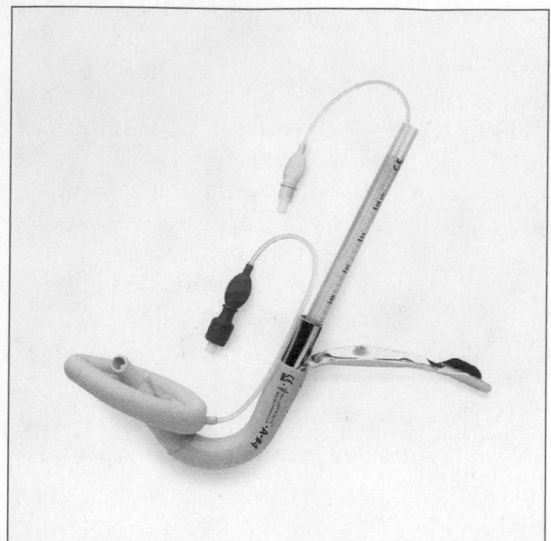

**Figure 36-20** A laryngeal mask airway (LMA).

## Other Advanced Airway Adjuncts

Increasingly, ALS providers are using a variety of other devices to obtain an advanced airway. Among the most widely used adjuncts are the King™ airway, the laryngeal mask airway™ (LMA) (Figure 36-20■) and the Combitube™ airway (Figure 36-21■). These devices are inserted blindly though the mouth into the airway. The LMA covers the opening to the trachea, whereas the King airway has an obturator that fits into the trachea. Once in place, inflation of a donut-shaped cuff seals the airway from contaminants. The patient is ventilated in the same manner as with an endotracheal tube. Both devices are growing in popularity and are available in several sizes.

The Combitube™ is a dual-lumen airway that has two inflatable cuffs. Like the King™ airway, the Combitube™ is inserted blindly. In most cases, the device enters the esophagus. Because it has two lumens, one connects with the trachea and the other connects with the esophagus. Therefore when inserted, one of the two lumens, which will make the connection with and provide air to the trachea, is used for bag-valve mask ventilation. After being correctly inserted, the proximal balloon is inflated with 80–100 cc of air, and then the distal balloon is inflated with 15 cc of air. The ALS provider then attempts to ventilate using the blue (#1) tube. If the patient's chest does not rise and lung sounds are not heard bilaterally, the ALS provider will attempt to ventilate using the clear (#2) tube and then reassesses to ensure adequate ventilations. Unlike the King™ airway and the LMA, the Combitube™ is not available in pediatric sizes and can be used only in patients over 4 feet tall.

**Figure 36-21** A Combitube™ airway.

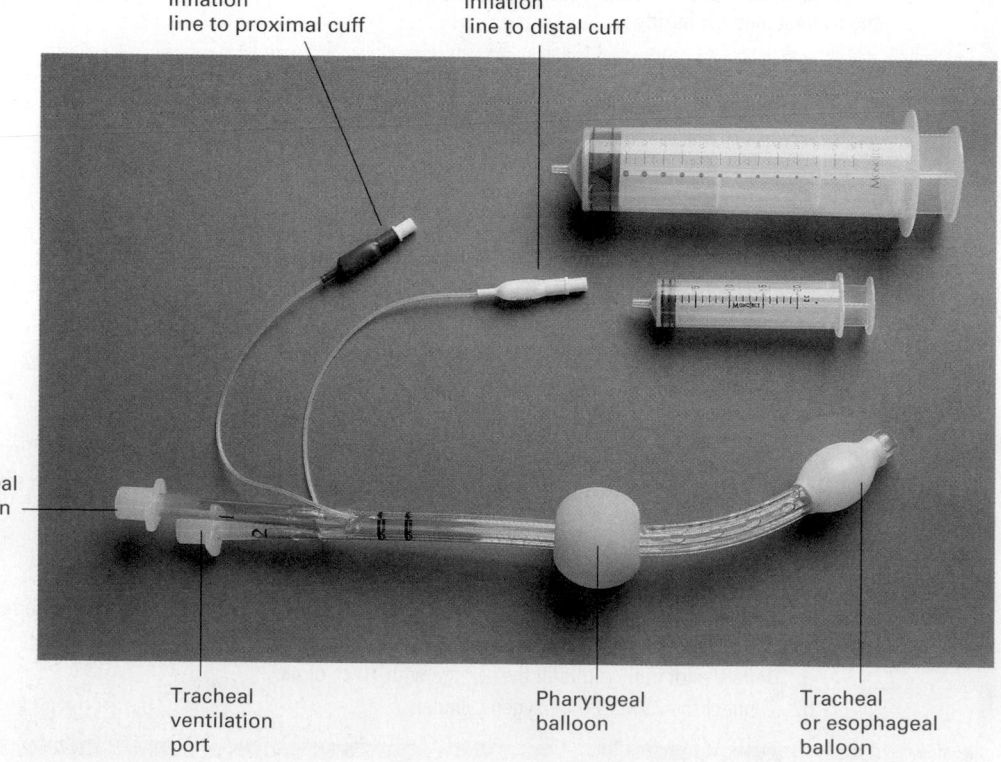

Inflation line to proximal cuff

Inflation line to distal cuff

Pharyngeal ventilation port

Tracheal ventilation port

Pharyngeal balloon

Tracheal or esophageal balloon

## Cricothyrotomy

In some cases all the usual forms of airway control, including endotracheal intubation, fail to secure a patent airway. When this occurs, ALS providers may elect to obtain an airway using a technique known as a **cricothyrotomy** (or "cric"). A cricothyrotomy can be of one of two types: surgical or non-surgical.

A surgical cricothyrotomy involves creating a small opening through both the skin of the anterior neck and the cricothyroid membrane, through which a cricothyrotomy tube, a tracheostomy tube, or a modified (cut off) endotracheal tube is placed. The distal end of the tube sits above the level at which the trachea divides into right and left mainstem bronchi, which enables inflation of both lungs. The procedure is hazardous because numerous vital anatomical structures are near the site of the incision, which is why cricothyrotomy is generally considered an airway procedure of last resort.

A non-surgical cricothyrotomy involves inserting a large-bore hypodermic needle through the cricothyroid membrane or using a special "gun" or a prefashioned cricothyrotomy kit, which inserts a small (sometimes rigid) tube through the membrane (Figure 36-22■).

**Indications/Contraindications of Cricothyrotomy**   Cricothyrotomy is indicated in adults who have experienced direct laryngeal trauma or a severe orofacial injury. Because of anatomical concerns, cricothyrotomy is generally not recommended in children younger than 12 years of age.

Cricothyotomy is *not* indicated simply because an ALS provider has not been successful in placing an endotracheal tube. In fact, numerous studies indicate that proper airway management can be performed using basic airway adjuncts, such as an OPA, when combined with timely suctioning and effective bag-valve mask ventilation.

**Equipment and Set-Up**   A cricothyrotomy is typically performed in one of three ways: using a commercially available product such as the Nutrake system, using a large-bore IV catheter, or using a scalpel. Even though both intubation and cricothyrotomy use much of the same equipment (e.g., a 6.0 ET tube, a tube-securing device, suction, oxygen, a bag-valve device, and a $CO_2$ detector), each of the three methods has some specific equipment needs.

A standard "cric kit" contains a scalpel, a tracheostomy tube, hemostats, a large-bore over-the-needle IV catheter, and a 3.0 ET tube adaptor (for connecting the catheter to the bag-valve device should a non-surgical cricothyrotomy be performed).

**cricothyrotomy**   an incision through the cricothyroid membrane for the purpose of inserting a tube to establish a "surgical airway"; is usually performed as a part of advanced airway management; is beyond the scope of practice for OEC Technicians.

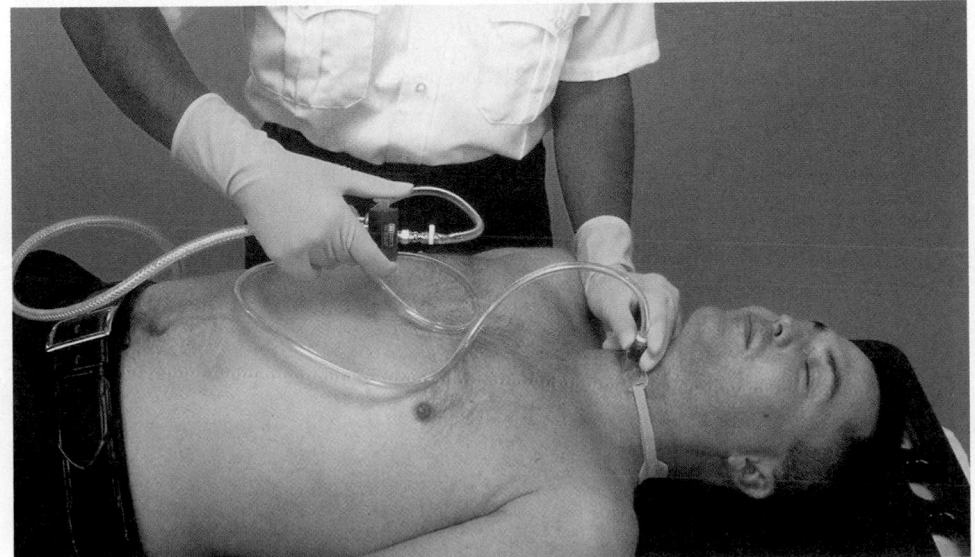

**Figure 36-22** Ventilation using a cricothyrotomy kit.

Commercial cricothyrotomy kits, such as the Nutrake system, contain a proprietary "gun" that "injects" the tube through the cricothyroid membrane. As the procedure is optimally performed under sterile conditions, all components are contained within sterile packaging.

**36-5** Describe how to assess proper placement of an endotracheal tube.

### Assessing Proper Advanced Airway Placement

Once an advanced airway has been inserted, an ALS provider will attach the tube to a bag-valve device, which in turn is connected to 100 percent oxygen. At this point the ALS provider must assess the tube for proper placement (Figure 36-23■), which is indicated by one or more of the following findings:

1. clear and equal breath sounds on auscultation
2. absence of sounds on auscultation of the stomach
3. equal bilateral chest rise with ventilation
4. fogging of the tube
5. a change in color of a colorimetric $CO_2$ detector to purple
6. pulse oximetry reading of 94 percent or higher
7. waveform capnography (an electronic device that evaluates ventilator status by monitoring carbon dioxide levels in exhaled breath)

ALS providers may also confirm proper endotracheal tube placement via direct visualization of the tube passing through the vocal cords. At the hospital, a chest X-ray is typically taken to confirm proper placement of an endotracheal or cricothyrotomy tube.

Often, ALS providers will direct you to ventilate the patient while they listen for bilateral breath sounds, which indicate that the tube is properly placed. The use of colorimetric $CO_2$ detectors is increasing. This device is attached such that the ventilator or bag-valve device operates through the ET tube; once a change in the color of the device from yellow to purple in response to the presence of $CO_2$ indicates the tube's proper placement within the trachea, the device can be removed. Waveform capnography, which provides a graph of the respirations, has replaced colorimetric $CO_2$ detectors in some states.

Once proper tube placement is confirmed, the tube is then secured in place so that it does not slip out of position (Figure 36-24■). Although specialized devices are available for this purpose, adhesive tape works just fine if these devices are not available.

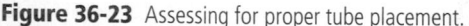

**Figure 36-23** Assessing for proper tube placement.

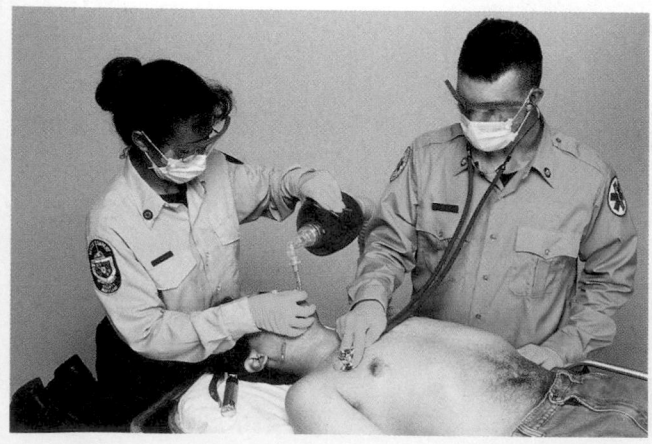

**Figure 36-24** Once proper tube placement is confirmed, secure the tube in place.

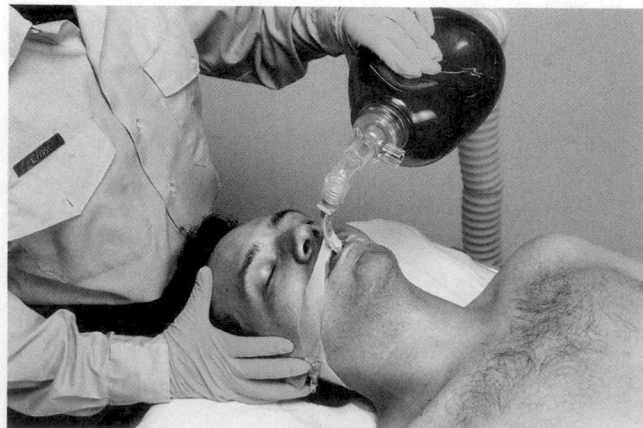

Generally, tape is placed on the patient's cheek and is wrapped around the tube once or twice before being applied to the other side of the face. This procedure may be repeated to ensure stability of the ET tube. ALS providers often place an OPA to serve as a bite block in the event the patient begins to awaken. One advantage of stable placement of the ET tube is that chest compressions during CPR need not be interrupted because the tube supplies air directly to the lungs.

## STOP, THINK, UNDERSTAND

### Multiple Choice

Choose the correct answer.

1. What does BURP stand for? _____
   a. a rude GI noise
   b. backward upward rightward pressure
   c. breathing unconscious regular pulse
   d. best upper respiratory path

2. When is a cricothyrotomy performed? _____
   a. when a patient's stomach fills with air
   b. when a patient's respiratory rate falls below 10 breaths/minute
   c. when a patient stops breathing altogether
   d. when all other forms of airway control fail

3. Which of the following statements regarding cricothyrotomy is true? _____
   a. It is a hazardous procedure and thus considered a "last resort."
   b. It is a relatively safe, quick procedure and thus is a good choice for rapidly establishing an emergency airway in the field.
   c. In some areas, medical directives allow OEC Technicians to perform this procedure.
   d. It is the procedure of choice for establishing an emergency airway in children ages 3–8 years.

4. Which of the following actions is the best course of action for an ALS provider who is unable to secure a patient's airway with an endotracheal tube? _____
   a. performing a cricothyrotomy
   b. performing a needle thoracostomy

   c. resorting to BLS airway management procedures such as an oropharyngeal airway and BVM
   d. immediately summoning or transporting the patient to another ALS provider

5. For which of the following patients is a cricothyrotomy indicated? _____
   a. a patient with direct laryngeal trauma or severe orofacial injuries
   b. a 3-year-old with a very small airway
   c. a patient that an ALS provider is unable to intubate with an endotracheal tube
   d. a cricothyrotomy is indicated for all of these patients.

6. A "cric kit" contains which of the following pieces of equipment? _____
   a. an OA, an NA, a BVM, a Yankauet tip, and a 3.0 ET tube adaptor
   b. an ET tube and a blade, a BVM and an NA, a hemostat, and a scalpel
   c. a scalpel, a trach tube hemostat, a large-bore needle/catheter, and a 3.0 ET tube adaptor
   d. a scalpel, a large-bore needle, an OA, and an NPA

### List

List the seven procedures or findings that can indicate the correct placement of an airway (ET or "cric") in a patient.

1. _____
2. _____
3. _____
4. _____
5. _____
6. _____
7. _____

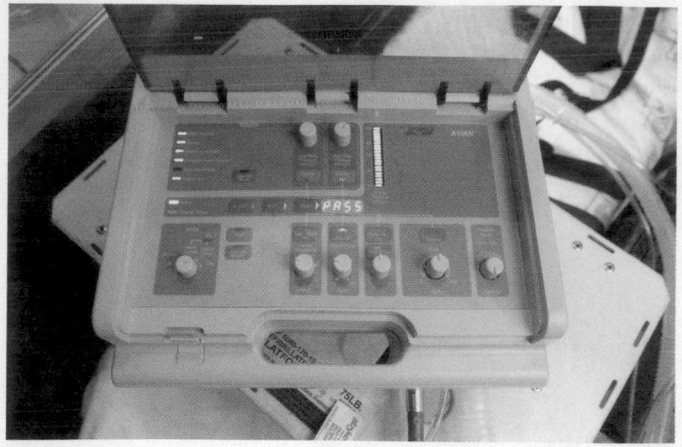

**Figure 36-25** A mechanical ventilator.

# Mechanical Ventilators

Ventilating a patient over an extended period of time is an exhausting endeavor that is even more difficult in outdoor environments or when a patient must be moved over long distances. A mechanical ventilator delivers respirations at a consistent rate and volume (Figure 36-25■). Additionally, it protects the airway while improving pulmonary gas exchange, relieving respiratory distress, assisting with lung healing, preventing exhaustion of rescuers, and reducing rescuer-caused complications such as overventilation or hyperventilation.

## Indications for Mechanical Ventilation

Mechanical ventilation is indicated for intubated patients that require prolonged transport; for patients with a primary lung injury (e.g., a severe inhalation injury or severe chest trauma); for patients with chronic obstructive pulmonary disease (COPD) or asthma whose symptoms are not relieved using conventional methods; for patients with acute respiratory acidosis; and for patients with cardiac or respiratory arrest. Ventilators are especially desirable during difficult situations because they allow ALS providers freedom to perform other procedures the patient needs.

## Equipment Set-Up

⊕ **36-6** Describe how to properly set up a mechanical ventilator.

Most ventilators are pre-programmed, so plugging them in or turning them on is the only set-up required. Typically a tube connects the ventilator to the ET tube. Once the ventilator and ET tube are connected and an ALS provider has selected the proper ventilator settings, mechanical ventilation of the patient can begin. The details of ventilator management are beyond the scope of this chapter, but in general the accepted initial settings are as follows:

- tidal volume (volume per breath)—average: 400–500 mL
- respiratory rate—average: 12–20 breaths/min
- PEEP (peak end expiratory pressure, the pressure that remains in the lungs at the end of a breath)—average: 5 mmHg
- $FiO_2$ (percent inhaled oxygen, which at sea level is 21 percent)—begin at 40–60 percent and titrate to a pulse oximetry (oxygen saturation) value greater than 94 percent

## Complications

Unfortunately, airway management does not always go smoothly, and complications may arise. Among the most common problems encountered with an intubated patient is rupture of the endotracheal tube cuff, in which case the airway is no longer adequately protected, and oxygenation and ventilation are reduced. A leak or rupture of the cuff is often detected by hearing a strange sound known as "phonation," the sound of air passing through the vocal cords, which should not be audible if the cuff is properly inflated. Because this sound may be difficult to hear in outdoor environments, ALS providers may have to rely on other signs, such as a sudden decrease in oxygen saturation level, decreased chest wall movement, or an ashen or cyanotic appearance. Another good way to determine if the cuff has ruptured is to squeeze the small pilot bulb; if it is deflated or has little or no tension, the distal cuff may be leaking or ruptured. If any of these signs are noted, an ALS provider may need to replace the tube. Again, have suction at hand at all times.

## Needle Thoracostomy

In addition to a cuff leak or failure, ongoing airway compromise may result from a variety of other factors, such as bleeding within the upper airway, an internal injury or, (infrequently) a tension pneumothorax. Even proper intubation does not guarantee that a secure airway will persist, and barotrauma (pressure-induced lung damage) can result any time an ET tube is placed and the patient is ventilated. Because a pneumothorax can grow and lead to a tension pneumothorax—especially during mechanical ventilation—whenever a tension pneumothorax is suspected, the tension must be released. An ALS provider can release this pressure by performing a needle thoracostomy.

A needle thoracostomy, also known as "venting the chest," involves placing a large-bore (typically 12 gauge or 14 gauge) over-the-needle IV catheter into either the second or third intercostal space in the mid-clavicular line, or into the fourth or fifth intercostal space in the mid-axillary line. Insertion of the needle between the ribs, through the skin and muscles, and into the pleural space alleviates the internal thoracic pressure by establishing an escape route for trapped air. Many ALS providers, disaster teams, and military personnel carry commercial "field darts" that quickly accomplish this escape of air (Figure 36-26■). Other ALS providers may perform a variation of a needle thoracostomy by inserting a chest tube.

The only indication for a needle thoracostomy is a patient who exhibits signs and symptoms associated with a tension pneumothorax.

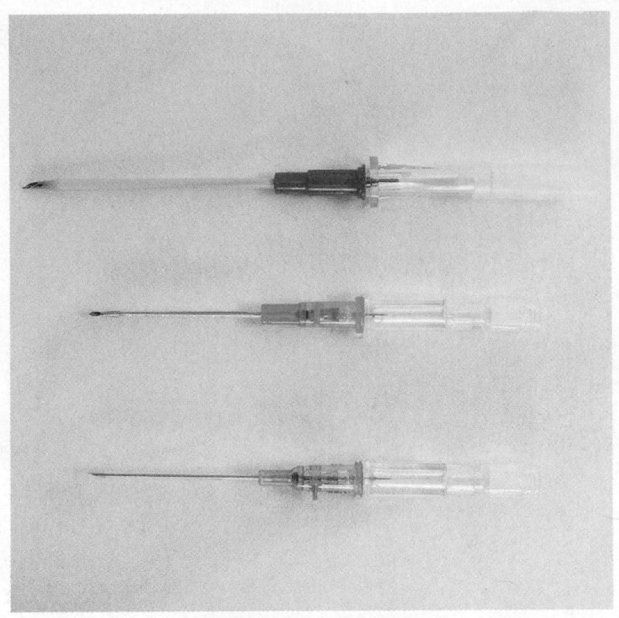

**Figure 36-26** Three "field darts" that can be used to relieve pressure caused by a tension pneumothorax.

# Metered-Dose Inhaler/Nebulizer

You may be requested to assist an ALS provider in administering an asthma patient's metered dose inhaler (MDI), a device that contains a respiratory medicine. A nebulizer is a device that is connected to an oxygen source and aerosolizes respiratory medications so that they can be inhaled. The patient breathes the medicine into their lungs, enabling it to reach the lower airway passages (e.g., bronchioles), where it exerts its effects. A variety of respiratory medications may be delivered via an MDI or a nebulizer; which medication is used depends on the severity of the patient's condition and the ALS provider's medical protocols.

⊕ **36-10**   Describe how to properly set up a metered-dose inhaler for use.

### Indications

A nebulizer treatment (Figure 36-27■) is indicated for patients with a history of asthma who are having an asthma attack, and for patients who are experiencing shortness of breath and wheezing.

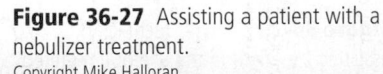

**Figure 36-27** Assisting a patient with a nebulizer treatment.
Copyright Mike Halloran

### Equipment and Set-Up

A variety of nebulizer set-ups are available (Figure 36-28■). A typical nebulizer comes prepackaged and contains six components: a mouthpiece, a two-part nebulizer bowl that converts the medication to a fine mist, a corrugated tube reservoir, a plastic "T" fitting, and oxygen connecting tubing. To set up the device:

1. Ensure that BSI precautions are observed.
2. Connect the mouthpiece to one of the two large holes on the "T" fitting.

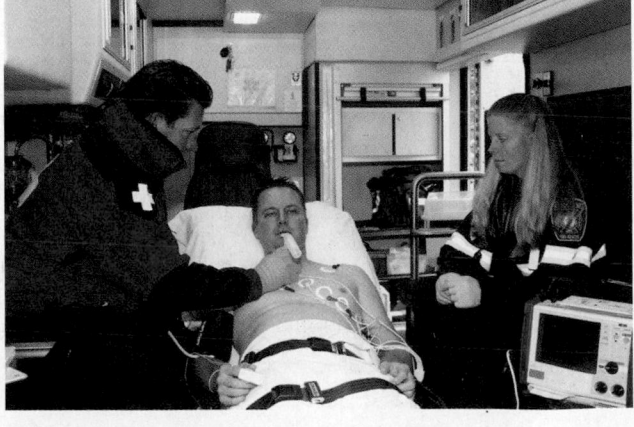

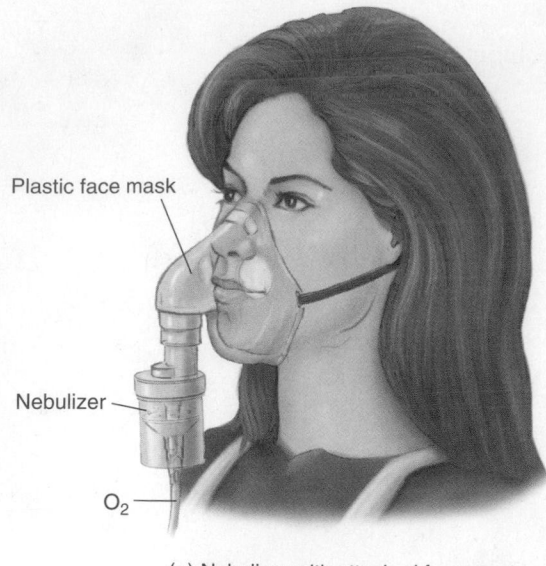

(a) Nebulizer with attached face mask

Plastic face mask

Nebulizer

$O_2$

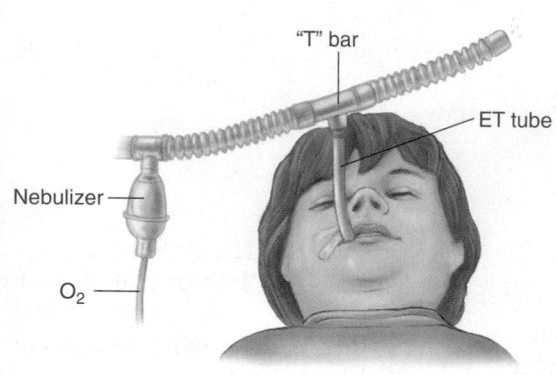

(b) Nebulizer with endotracheal tube

"T" bar

Nebulizer

ET tube

$O_2$

(c) Nebulizer with bag-valve unit

$O_2$

Reservoir

Bag-valve unit

Valve

90° elbow

ET tube

Nebulizer

**Figure 36-28** Three different nebulizer set-ups.

**Figure 36-29** An OEC Technician assisting a patient in the use of a metered dose inhaler.

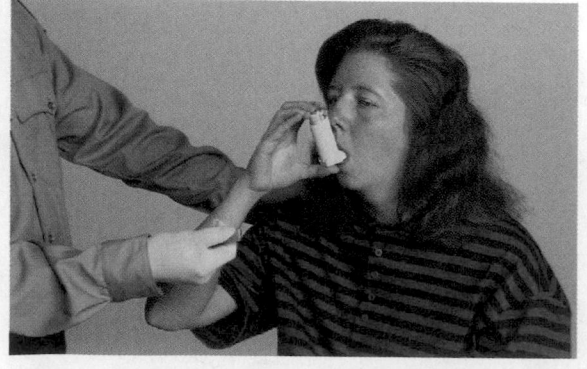

**3.** Connect the corrugated tube reservoir to the other large hole on the "T" fitting.

**4.** Attach the "T" fitting to the top of the nebulizer bowl.

**5.** Attach the oxygen tubing to the oxygen port located beneath the nebulizer bowl.

The nebulizer is now ready for an ALS provider to add the desired medication and to screw the two bowls together carefully. The oxygen flow rate is set at 6–10 LPM, at which point a fine mist should be seen exiting the end of the corrugated reservoir.

Patients typically carry their own MDI (metered dose inhaler), which usually consists of two parts: a mouthpiece and unit body, and a pressurized medication container. The pressurized medication container is inserted into the unit body, and then the MDI is ready for use, either by the patient or with assistance from an OEC Technician (Figure 36-29■).

How Can I Assist an ALS Provider?

Upon request, and in accordance with state and local protocol, OEC Technicians may perform the following tasks related to advanced airway management:

+ Perform the BURP maneuver (i.e., cricoid pressure).
+ Attach a bag-valve device to either an endotracheal tube or a cricothyrotomy device.
+ Manually ventilate an intubated patient or a cricothyrotomy patient.
+ Attach a colorimetric $CO_2$ detector to an ET tube or to a cricothyrotomy device.
+ Help secure in place an ET tube or a cricothyrotomy device.
+ Gather the mechanical ventilator, oxygen tubing, and oxygen tank.
+ Attach the mechanical ventilator to an oxygen tank.
+ Attach the mechanical ventilator to the patient.
+ Retrieve the requested equipment for performing a needle thoracostomy.
+ Retrieve requested nebulizer equipment.
+ Prepare a nebulizer for use (with the exception of adding the medication).

# STOP, THINK, UNDERSTAND

## Multiple Choice

Choose the correct answer.

1. One of the most common problems encountered with an intubated patient is_____
   a. occlusion of the ventilator tube.
   b. displacement of the airway.
   c. cricoid pressure.
   d. rupture of endotracheal cuff.

2. Phonation is best described as_____
   a. the communication system between an ALS provider and a hospital.
   b. the hissing sound a ventilator makes when it is working properly.
   c. a strange sound caused by air passing through an intubated patient's vocal cords.
   d. the sound picked up on auscultation of the lungs when an ET tube is properly placed.

3. Lung barotrauma is best defined as_____
   a. pressure-induced lung damage.
   b. damage to a barometric ventilator.
   c. chest trauma.
   d. a ruptured esophagus.

4. A needle thoracostomy relieves the pressure of a tension pneumothorax through_____
   a. a small puncture in the upper lobe of the lung.
   b. an escape route for air trapped in the bronchioles.

   c. an escape route for air trapped in the pleural space.
   d. A needle thoracostomy does not relieve a tension pneumothorax.

5. After an ET tube has been properly placed in a patient, a problem that can arise is_____
   a. a ruptured esophagus.
   b. a tension pneumothorax.
   c. a viral infection of the oropharynx.
   d. asthma.

6. MDI stands for_____
   a. metric diameter insertion.
   b. metered dose inhaler.
   c. motion detection indicator.
   d. measured diffusion inspirometer.

7. Which of the following findings could indicate that a patient's ET tube is not working correctly? (check all that apply)
   _____ a. an ashen/cyanotic appearance in the patient
   _____ b. a deflated pilot bulb
   _____ c. a pilot bulb with little or no tension
   _____ d. an increase in the patient's BP
   _____ e. an increase in the patient's respiratory rate
   _____ f. a decrease in PSAT (pulse oximetry) level

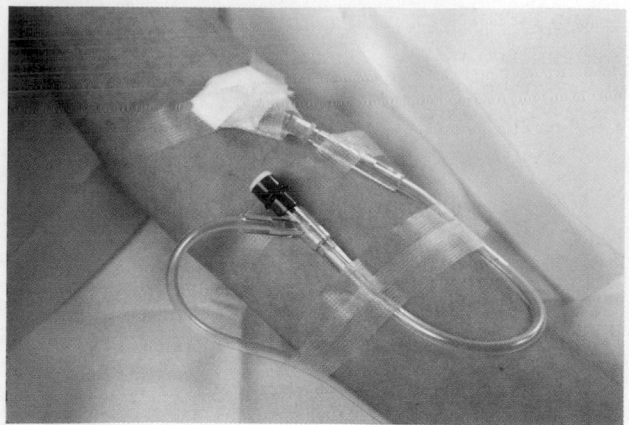

**Figure 36-30** IV therapy is a good way to rehydrate patients or give them medications.

## Intravenous (IV) Therapy

The physical demands of outdoor activities increase the body's metabolic needs. When patients suffer an illness or injury in outdoor settings, they often require rehydration or the administration of medications, which can be achieved using intravenous (IV) therapy (Figure 36-30■).

### Indications for IV Therapy

The two primary purposes for IV therapy are to replace fluids and to administer intravenous medications. Among the situations in which IV therapy is commonly initiated are diabetes, long bone fractures, joint dislocations, severe dehydration, and any conditions that require endotracheal intubation, cricothyrotomy, needle thoracostomy, rapid medication administration, or mechanical ventilation.

⊕ **36-7** Describe how to properly set up an intravenous solution for administration.

### Equipment and Set-Up

The set-up for IV therapy consists of two parts: preparing the IV solution for administration, and preparing the IV needle for insertion. Setting up an IV requires the following equipment (Figure 36-31■):

+ IV solution
+ IV tubing
+ IV needles/catheters
+ venous tourniquet
+ antiseptic swabs (alcohol, betadine)
+ 1-inch tape (cloth or plastic)
+ see-through IV site cover
+ 4-inch by 4-inch bandages
+ red "sharps" container for disposal of IV needles/catheters
+ BSI equipment such as gloves

**Figure 36-31** Equipment required to set up an IV.

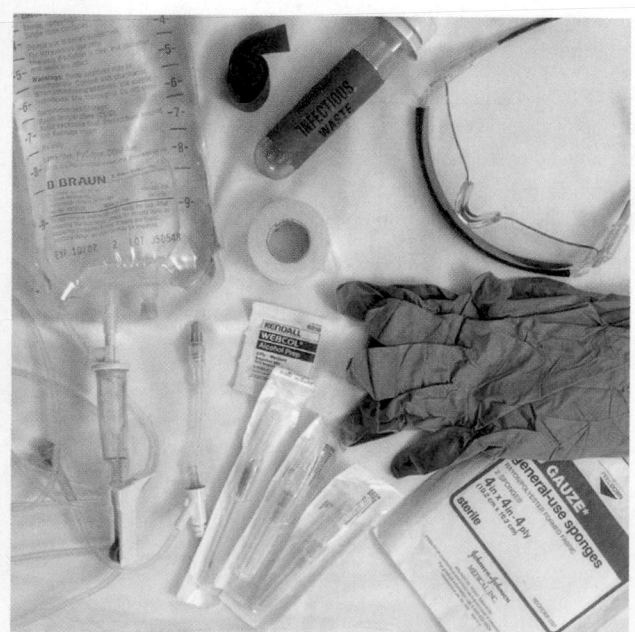

ALS providers use two main types of intravenous solutions: saline-based solutions and glucose-based solutions. Saline-based solutions contain small concentrations of sodium chloride (salt), which helps the solution remain within the bloodstream. Although saline solutions come in a variety of concentrations, ALS providers typically use 0.9% normal saline. This solution very nearly approximates the sodium chloride concentration of blood, which makes it an ideal volume expander for emergency use, especially in cases involving shock, hypovolemia, or profound dehydration. Another saline-based IV solution is lactated Ringer's solution.

Glucose-based solutions contain small amounts of sugar and also come in a variety of concentrations; ALS providers most commonly use 5% dextrose in water ($D_5W$). Glucose solutions are ideal for patients that require intravenous administration of a medication, because the solution helps to move the drug out of the bloodstream and into the tissues. IV solutions for field use are typically available in flexible, plastic containers (bags).

IV tubing serves as a means of transferring an IV solution from its container to the patient. OEC Technicians should be familiar with two types of IV tubing: macrodrop IV tubing and microdrip IV tubing. Macrodrop tubing is typically used with saline-based solutions, whereas microdrip tubing is generally used with glucose-based solutions. To differentiate the two types of tubing, either check the package label or look at the IV drip chamber; microdrip IV tubing has a small needle hanging down within the top of the chamber.

The steps in the process of preparing an IV for use are illustrated in OEC Skill 36-1. First, select the appropriate IV tubing for the solution being used and remove it from its package. Next, remove the IV solution from its protective wrapper, and remove the protective plastic covering located at the bottom of the bag to reveal the IV tubing port. Be careful not to expose either the solution or the tubing ends to contaminants. Check the condition of the bag and the solution: the bag should be free of rips, tears, or leaks; the expiration date on the bag must be today's date or some date in the future; and the solution should be clear and contain no visible particles. Next, turn the bag upside down so that you are holding it by its "neck." Close the sliding clamp lock beneath the drip chamber; otherwise, when the tubing is attached to the bag, the solution will pour out. The IV tubing has a beveled spike at one end, directly above the drip chamber. Remove the plastic cap covering the sharp spike and push the spike point down into the IV tubing port to puncture the sterile seal within the port, a process known as "spiking the (IV) bag." Return the bag to an upright position, which initiates the flow of the solution into the tubing. Next, gently squeeze the IV drip chamber until it is approximately half full. Then, slowly release the sliding lock beneath the drip chamber to allow the solution to flow through the tube and force any air out of the tubing, which prevents air bubbles from entering the patient's bloodstream. Once a tiny amount of solution begins to leak from the protective cap at the end of the IV tubing, close the sliding lock. The solution and IV tubing are now ready for use.

### Intravenous Needles

IV needles, also known as catheters, come in different sizes (Figure 36-32■). The larger the needle's inner diameter, the faster fluid can flow through it. Catheter sizes range from 24 gauge to 14 gauge. The *smaller* the gauge number, the *larger* the needle diameter. Larger-diameter needles, such as 16 gauge and 14 gauge, are typically used to infuse large amounts of volume expanders such as normal saline or lactated Ringer's. Should a blood transfusion be needed later, it should be administered through an 18-gauge or larger needle, to prevent damage to the blood cells. An 18-gauge needle is the most common size used in emergency medicine. In general, the larger the IV needle that can be placed, the better, but it is better to have a smaller IV in place than no IV at all. Immediately place used IV needles into a red, hard-sided "sharps" container to prevent accidental injury to the patient, rescuers, or bystanders. Once the IV is started and infusing, it is best to hold or hang the bag at a level above the patient's heart.

### How Can I Assist an ALS Provider?

Upon request, and in accordance with state and local protocol, OEC Technicians may perform the following tasks related to intravenous therapy:

+ Retrieve the requested IV solution.
+ Retrieve the requested IV drip set.
+ Prepare the IV solution and drip set for use.
+ Select other appropriate IV therapy equipment (e.g., antiseptic swabs, tape, tegaderm, etc.)
+ Hold the bag of IV fluids higher than the patient's heart. (Figure 36-33■)

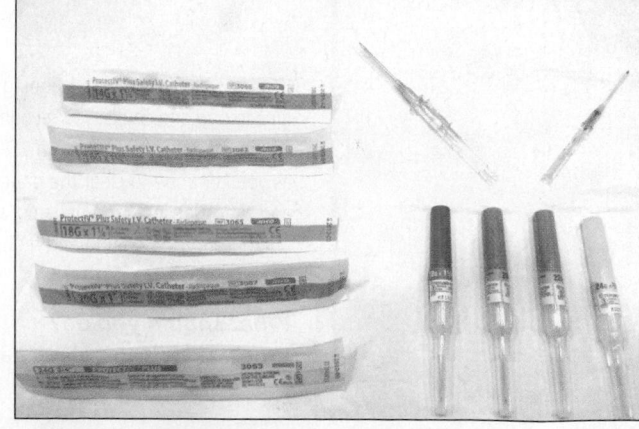

**Figure 36-32** Types of IV needles (catheters).
Copyright Edward McNamara

**Figure 36-33** A patroller assisting an
ALS provider with IV equipment.
Copyright Mike Halloran

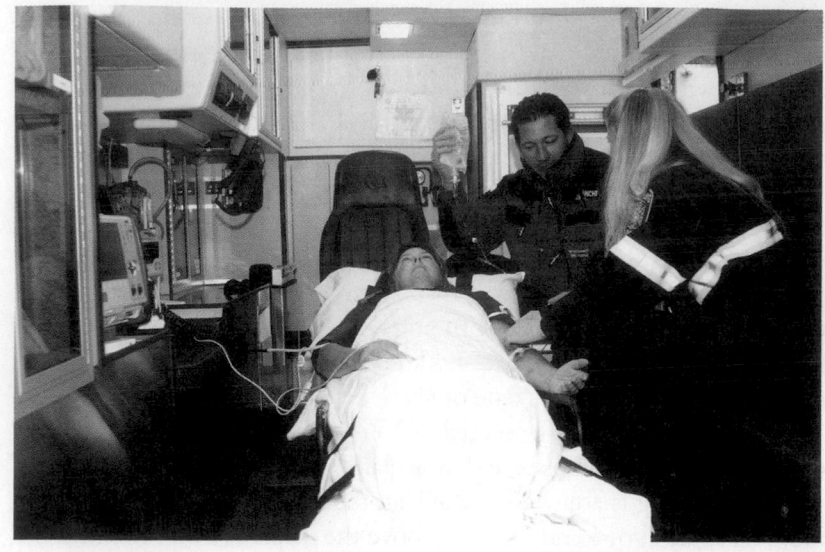

# STOP, THINK, UNDERSTAND

## Multiple Choice

Choose the correct answer.

1. The two main types of IV solutions are_____
   a. adrenalin and epinephrine-based solutions.
   b. sterile water-based solutions and ritalin-based solutions.
   c. saline-based solutions and glucose-based solutions.
   d. blood and sterile water-based solutions.

2. Saline IV solutions work as_____
   a. volume expanders.　　c. glucose stabilizers.
   b. adrenalin administrators.　d. detoxifiers.

3. Normal saline is primarily used to_____
   a. treat shock, dehydration. and hypovolemia.
   b. treat severe hypoglycemia.
   c. administer medications.
   d. detoxify poisons and reverse overdoses.

4. D$_5$W stands for_____
   a. a 5:1 ratio of drug to water.
   b. a solution of 5% dextrose in water.
   c. a solution of 5% digoxin in water.
   d. a diastolic reading after a 5-minute wait.

5. Which of the following statements about IV needles is true?
   _____
   a. A 21-gauge needle is larger than a 16-gauge needle.
   b. An 18-gauge needle is the most common size used in emergency medicine.
   c. The smaller the IV needle the better, to prevent vein damage.
   d. IV needles come in different sizes because they must be correctly matched to the size of the patient.

 # CASE UPDATE

You immediately begin suctioning the patient's airway. Despite your best efforts, bleeding persists and the victim begins to gag and choke. You recognize that the patient has a potentially life-threatening airway problem that requires advanced airway management. Other patrollers arrive, and they quickly immobilize the patient on a long spine board as you continue to clear the patient's airway. You notify ALS providers of the patient's status and immediate needs and then transport the patient down slope to awaiting ALS providers. While you ride with the patient you provide ongoing oral suctioning and high-flow oxygen by bag-valve mask. Suddenly, the bag-valve mask becomes difficult to compress.

***What should you do?***
***What do you think has happened?***

# Cardiac Monitoring and Electrical Therapy

Many medical and traumatic disorders adversely affect the performance of the heart. ALS providers can often identify potentially life-threatening cardiac abnormalities by monitoring the heart's electrical activity as shown in an **electrocardiogram (ECG or EKG)**, which is obtained by a device called an electrocardiograph. It is sometimes necessary to deliver an electrical shock to the heart, either to initiate a heartbeat (as in cardiac arrest) or to help the heart beat in a more organized way (as when a patient's heart is beating too fast). This action is known as either defibrillation or cardioversion. Thus, a cardiac monitor/defibrillator is actually two machines in one—one for monitoring heart rhythm, and one for delivering an electrical shock to the heart.

## Indications

Cardiac monitoring is indicated for patients that have any cardiac-related illness, altered mental status, syncope, or dizziness, or for any person who is found unresponsive. Electrical therapy is indicated for very specific heart rhythm disturbances that are recognized by ALS providers.

## Equipment and Set-Up

Cardiac monitoring and electrical therapy are performed using the following equipment:

+ a cardiac monitor/defibrillator
+ a monitor cable
+ electrodes
+ defibrillation/cardioversion pads

A standard cardiac monitor/defibrillator includes a small LCD screen to view a graph of the heart's electrical rhythm (an electrocardiogram) and a control panel that is used to turn the machine on and off, to select different views of the heart, and to choose different electricity settings. The monitor cable plugs into the monitor and is connected to numerous self-adherent electrodes that are attached to bare skin on the patient's chest.

Connect the leads at the end of the monitor cord to the electrodes before applying the electrodes to the patient. The leads are generally color coded white, green, black, and red and are placed as follows (Figure 36-34■):

1. The RA (right arm) electrode is white and is placed just below the right clavicle in the mid-clavicular line.
2. The RL (right leg) electrode is green and is placed on the lower abdomen just below and to the right of the umbilicus.
3. The LA (left arm) electrode is black and is placed just below the left clavicle in the mid-clavicular line.
4. The LL (left leg) electrode is red and is placed on the lower abdomen just above and left of the umbilicus.

A good way to remember the proper lead placements is "*White and green to the right, and smoke over fire,*" meaning the white electrode goes above the green electrode on the right side of the chest, whereas the black electrode is placed above the red electrode on the left side of the chest.

**electrocardiogram (ECG or EKG)** a record of the electrical activity of the heart, which provides important information concerning the functioning of the different parts of the heart.

**⊕ 36-8** Describe how to properly set up a four-lead ECG.

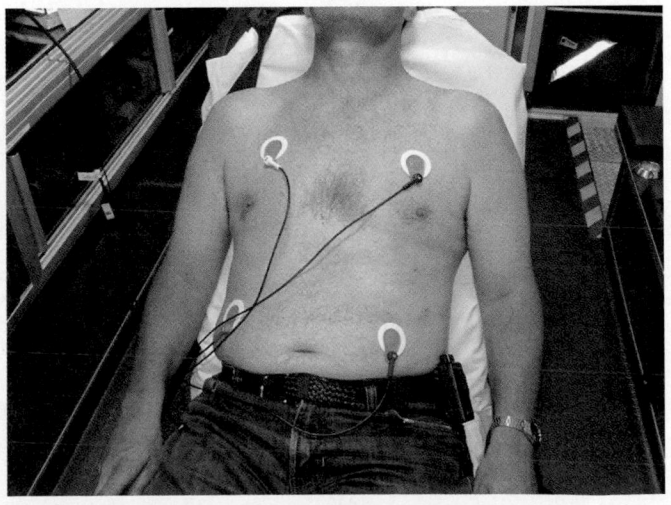

**Figure 36-34** The locations of the leads of a cardiac monitor on a male patient.
Copyright Edward McNamara

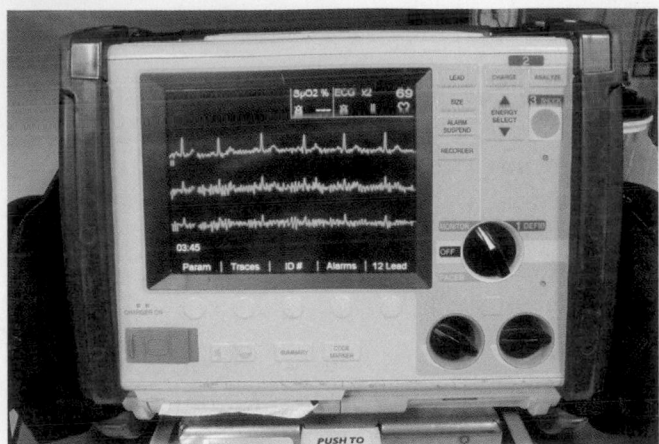

**Figure 36-35** An electrocardiograph monitor.
Copyright Edward McNamara

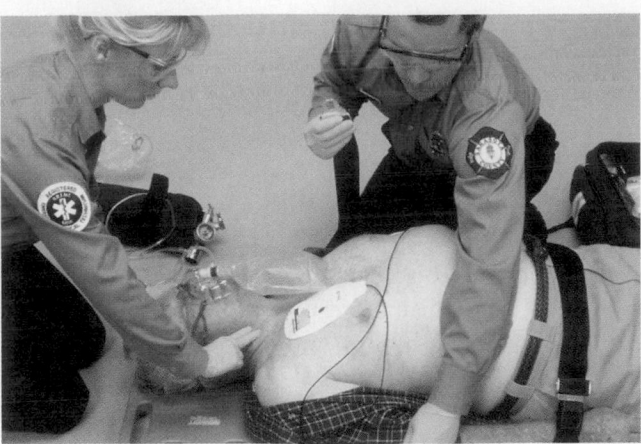

**Figure 36-36** Special defibrillation pads are used to deliver an electric shock to the heart.

Electrodes tend not to adhere well to individuals with abundant chest hair. An ALS provider may elect to clip or shave excess hair to ensure good contact with the skin. If the skin is dirty or is slick from body oil, blood, or sweat, an ALS provider may instruct you to clean or wipe the electrode site with a dry 4-inch by 4-inch dressing before applying the electrodes. Also, electrodes should not be applied over bony prominences or along skin folds, because such placement could obscure the transmission of electrical impulses. Once the leads and electrodes have been applied at their proper locations, plug the monitor cable into the monitor. The electrocardiograph monitor is now ready to be switched on (Figure 36-35■).

When ready, the ALS provider will turn the machine on and check for an ECG waveform by selecting the most appropriate lead for monitoring the patient. Most ALS providers select lead II because it generally provides the clearest image of the heart's rhythm.

## Electrical Therapy

The defibrillator portion of a cardiac monitor/defibrillator is used to deliver a specific dose of electricity to the heart. The electrical shock is delivered safely through large self-adherent pads, known as defibrillation or "defib" pads, which contain a conductive medium (to prevent contact burns) and are connected to the defibrillator by lead wires (Figure 36-36■). Depending on the equipment being used and the size/age of the patient, defibrillator pads are applied using one of two methods: the anterior method or the anterior-posterior method. As with ECG electrodes, defibrillator pads are placed directly on the patient's skin; to ensure proper contact with the skin, clip excess hair and dry the area before applying the pad. During an emergency, it may be more effective on a patient with a lot of chest hair to put on a set of defibrillator pads, pull them off (thereby removing the hair), and then apply another set of defibrillator pads.

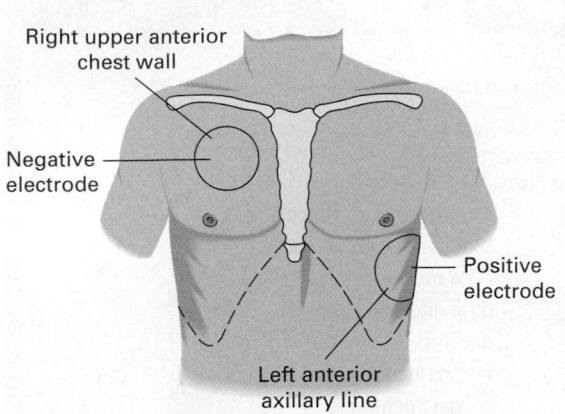

Right upper anterior
chest wall

Negative
electrode

Positive
electrode

Left anterior
axillary line

**Figure 36-37a** In the anterior method, the negative pad is placed on the upper right chest, and the positive pad is placed beneath the left nipple.

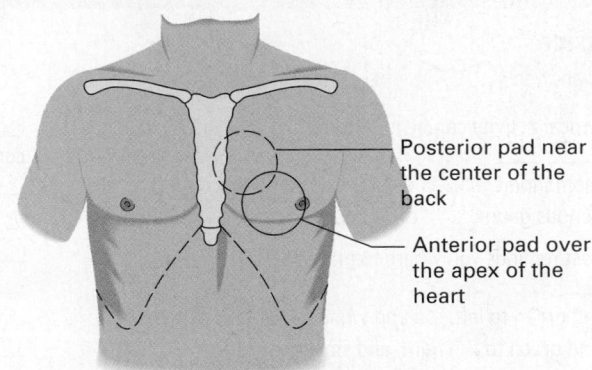

Alternative Placement
of Defibrillator Electrodes

Posterior pad near
the center of the
back

Anterior pad over
the apex of the
heart

**Figure 36-37b** In the anterior-posterior method, the positive (anterior) pad is placed on the chest in front of the heart, and the negative (posterior) pad is placed between the shoulder blades.

### Anterior Method

With this method, both pads are applied to the chest: the negative pad is placed on the upper right chest beneath the clavicle on the mid-clavicular line, whereas the positive pad is placed approximately 2–3 inches beneath the left nipple and 3–4 inches to the side along the anterior axillary line (Figure 36-37a■).

### Anterior-Posterior Method

With this method, the positive (anterior) pad is placed over the left precordium (lower part of the chest in front of the heart), whereas the negative (posterior) pad is placed on the back, between the shoulder blades (Figure 36-37b■).

Any time electrical therapy is administered, it is imperative that no one is touching the patient or any metal on the bed or stretcher, because the electrical current will traverse whatever is in direct contact with the patient. Most ALS providers are taught to announce their intention to shock the patient by loudly stating, *"I'm clear, you're clear, everybody clear,"* before administering a shock.

### How Can I Assist an ALS Provider?

Upon request, and in accordance with state and local protocol, OEC Technicians may perform the following tasks related to ECG monitoring/electrical therapy:

+ Gather the appropriate equipment to perform an ECG (e.g., electrodes, monitor cable).
+ Prepare the patient's skin for electrode placement (e.g., scrub, dry off).
+ Connect the monitor leads to the electrodes.
+ Place the electrodes on the patient.
+ Connect the monitor cable to the ECG monitor.
+ Place defibrillation pads on the patient.

# STOP, THINK, UNDERSTAND

## Multiple Choice

Choose the correct answer.

1. A heart's electrical activity can be monitored through_____
   - a. a sphygmomanometer.
   - c. electrocardiogram.
   - b. an intravenous gauge.
   - d. a heart catheter.

2. Which ditty best reminds you where to place EKG electrodes?
   _____
   - a. "Black and green to left, red and white to right."
   - b. "White and green to the right, and smoke over fire."
   - c. "Black and white go right, red and green left over."
   - d. "Black as night and white are right, then red and green go up and over."

3. Cardiac monitoring is indicated for which of the following conditions? (check all that apply)
   - _____ a. any cardiac-related illness
   - _____ b. altered mental status
   - _____ c. a broken metacarpal
   - _____ d. halitosis
   - _____ e. syncope
   - _____ f. dizziness
   - _____ g. gastroenteritis
   - _____ h. lack of consciousness and unresponsiveness
   - _____ i. crushing chest pain and shortness of breath

## Short Answer

What does it mean when you hear an ALS provider say, "I'm clear, you're clear, everybody clear"?

_____

_____

_____

_____

## Matching

Match each of the four electrodes to its correct placement. Placements may be used more than once.

- _____ 1. right arm
- _____ 2. right leg
- _____ 3. left arm
- _____ 4. left leg
- _____ 5. white
- _____ 6. green
- _____ 7. black
- _____ 8. red

- a. just below the left clavicle in the mid-clavicular line
- b. on the lower abdomen just below and to the right of the umbilicus
- c. below the right clavicle at the mid-clavicular line
- d. on the lower abdomen just above and to the left of the umbilicus

## Medication Administration

Even though medications are routinely administered by ALS personnel but not by OEC Technicians, it is good for OEC Technicians to recognize the types of medications ALS providers commonly administer (Figure 36-38■). Although ALS providers have access to a great variety of medications, most are used to treat respiratory or cardiac emergencies or to alleviate pain. Because OEC Technicians are often the first medically trained individuals on the scene, it is important that they not only recognize and begin treating common respiratory and cardiac ailments, but that they also quickly recognize when more advanced care is needed and to summon advanced providers as soon as possible.

## Respiratory Medications

Among the more common respiratory problems that may require treatment with medications are asthma, chronic obstructive pulmonary disease (COPD), and anaphylaxis. Of these, asthma is the most common respiratory ailment that OEC Technicians will likely encounter. COPD is also quite common, especially in older individuals, and may clinically resemble asthma during an acute attack. The first medication ALS providers administer to treat asthma or COPD is albuterol (Proventil®, Ventolin®), which is commonly delivered via metered dose inhaler or a nebulizer. Should the patient's respiratory distress not be resolved using albuterol therapy, ALS providers may elect to administer ipratropium (as a nebulized solution) or epinephrine (either as an IM injection or via IV push). Epinephrine is the drug of choice for the treatment of anaphylaxis when airway compromise is either present or imminent. Other medications used to treat respiratory emergencies include racemic epinephrine (Vaponephrine®), and ipratropium (Atrovent®).

## Cardiac Medications

OEC Technicians trained to use an AED should not hesitate to use it when appropriate. In nearly all instances after successful cardioversion with an AED, ALS providers also need to administer cardiac medications. This is why it is so important for OEC Technicians to summon ALS backup *early* whenever a cardiac-related situation arises. At times, ALS providers will administer electrical therapy in conjunction with cardiac medications. The primary goal when using cardiac medications is to restore or maintain adequate cerebral and coronary perfusion. Common cardiac medications that OEC Technicians may encounter when assisting an ALS provider include the following drugs (Figure 36-39■):

+ epinephrine (adrenaline)
+ atropine
+ adenosine (Adenocard®)
+ lidocaine (Xylocaine®)
+ amiodarone (Cordarone®)
+ dopamine
+ nitroglycerin

**36-9** List common respiratory, cardiac, and analgesic medications ALS providers use.

**Figure 36-38** Some of the medications ALS providers commonly administer.
Copyright Edward McNamara

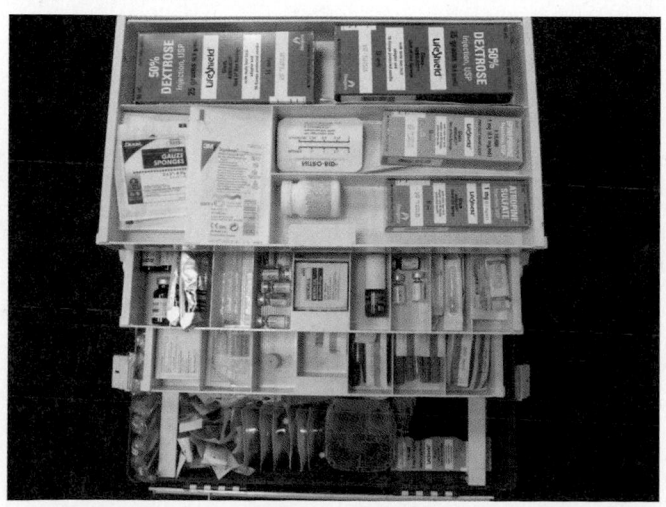

**Figure 36-39** Some common cardiac medications.
Copyright Edward McNamara

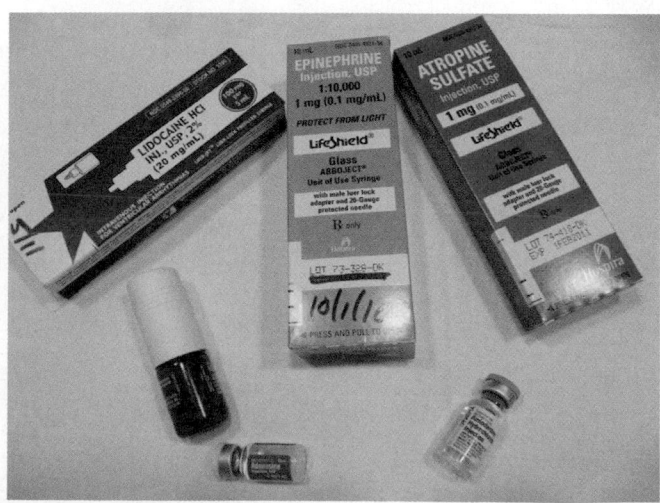

Both epinephrine and atropine are used to increase a patient's heart rate, whereas adenosine is used to slow heart rate. Both lidocaine and amiodarone are used to make the heart rhythm more regular. Dopamine is used to raise blood pressure, whereas nitroglycerin may be used to either reduce blood pressure or alleviate cardiac pain due to ischemia.

### Analgesic Medications

Because pain is a common medical complaint, OEC Technicians should be familiar with pain medications, known as **analgesics**, including their side effects and, importantly, the specific antidote in the event of an overdose. Analgesics ALS providers commonly administer include the following medications (Figure 36-40■):

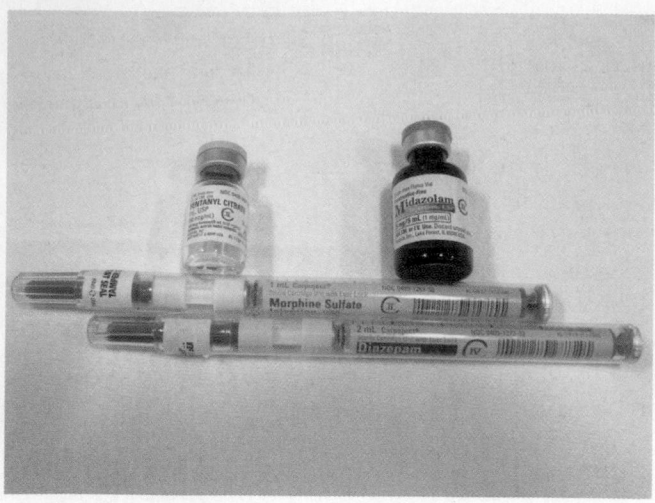

**Figure 36-40** Analgesics that ALS providers commonly administer.
Copyright Edward McNamara

**analgesic**   a drug that relieves pain.

+ morphine
+ fentanyl (Duragesic®)
+ meperidine (Demerol®)
+ hydromorphone (Dilaudid®)

Pain medication is chosen, in part, according to the source and amount of pain the patient is suffering. The primary concern (and main side effect) of any opioid analgesic is respiratory depression: as a rule, the more opioid medication given, the higher the risk for respiratory depression. Thus, it is essential that any person receiving an analgesic be carefully monitored for signs of respiratory depression, which include drowsiness, slow or shallow breathing with poor respiratory effort, and decreased oxygen saturation levels. Should any of these signs be noted, an ALS provider will likely try to reverse these adverse effects by administering the narcotic antagonist drug naloxone (Narcan®). Because naloxone has a much shorter duration of effect than most opioids, the patient may fall back into respiratory depression once the naloxone wears off and must be observed carefully in case additional naloxone must be administered to maintain the desired effect. The most commonly encountered side effect of IV narcotic pain medication is nausea, so be prepared to use suction to keep the airway open in the event of vomiting.

### Other Medications

While assisting an ALS provider, OEC Technicians may also encounter the following medications:

+ diazepam (Valium®)
+ midazolam (Versed®)
+ dextrose 50% in water ($D_{50}$)

Both diazepam and midazolam are used to reduce patient anxiety and can also be used to stop seizures, whereas dextrose 50% in water is used to rapidly elevate a hypoglycemic patient's blood sugar.

How Can I Assist an ALS Provider?

Upon request, and in accordance with state and local protocol, OEC Technicians may perform the following tasks related to the administration of medications:

+ Select the proper medication as requested.
+ Check and confirm the "five rights" of administering medication:

1. The right patient
2. The right medication
3. The right dose
4. The right route
5. The right time

⊕ **36-11** List the "five rights" of safe medication administration.

# Working and Moving as a Team

As with all aspects in medicine, the basic tenet, "*First, do no harm,*" must prevail. Thus, if at any time you see something or even suspect something that could potentially harm a patient or that doesn't appear correct, speak up! If, for example, you are the first person to notice that some IV tubing is leaking or contains a large air bubble, or that the pilot bulb of an endotracheal tube no longer seems to be holding pressure, immediately notify an ALS provider. During moving or transporting a patient, OEC Technicians must remember that ECG leads, ET tubes, IVs, and other medical equipment may be inadvertently tugged or snagged, so they must take care to ensure that all leads and tubes are secured before moving a patient to avoid dislodging crucial catheters or causing harm. The best way to do this is to work together as a team and to constantly exhibit excellent communication. Count down before moving a patient so that everyone involved knows precisely when to perform their actions.

# Ambulance Stretcher Operation

Knowing the basics of operating an ambulance stretcher will better enable you to assist ALS providers and ambulance crews. All primary ambulance stretchers are collapsible and have wheels. On some stretchers, the wheels automatically fold upon touching the back of the ambulance; on others, the top of the stretcher locks into place, and a handle must be squeezed to effect folding of the wheels. Newer stretchers may have other features, such as a collapsible IV pole, an EKG monitor stand, or an oxygen tank rack. Some stretchers can be shortened for navigation through narrow passageways. Nearly all ambulance stretchers have levers on both sides and at the foot of the stretcher that allow the stretcher to be manually raised or lowered.

OEC Technicians are encouraged to contact their local EMS agency or ambulance provider to obtain more information about how to operate their particular ambulance stretchers.

# STOP, THINK, UNDERSTAND

## Multiple Choice

Choose the correct answer.

1. What is naloxone (Narcan®), and why is it administered? _____

   a. It is an analgesic that relieves pain.
   b. It is a beta-blocker that lowers blood pressure.
   c. It is a paralytic that controls a combative patient.
   d. It is a narcotic antagonist that reverses the effect of opioid analgesics.

2. What are the "five rights"? _____

   a. The right patient, the right reason, the right level of provider, and the right medication by the right route.
   b. The patient's right to be treated with compassion, the patient's right to privacy, the patient's right to be involved in the course of treatment, the patient's right to be transported to a hospital of their choosing, the patient's right to refuse care.

   c. The right patient, the right medication, the right dose, the right route, at the right time.
   d. The right type of administration device, the right medication, the right injection site, the right expiration date, and the right vital signs after administration.

3. The most important thing to remember when assisting an ALS provider is_____

   a. "First, do no harm."
   b. "First, protect yourself."
   c. "First, protect your colleagues."
   d. "First, check the ALS provider's identification."

## Short Answer

What is the most common (and worrisome) side effect you must look for in a patient who has received morphine?

_____

_____

_____

_____

## Matching

Match each of the following medications to its action. Some actions may have more than one medication that applies.

_____  1. adenosine
_____  2. amiodarone
_____  3. atropine
_____  4. dopamine
_____  5. epinephrine
_____  6. lidocaine
_____  7. nitroglycerin

a. raises heart rate
b. lowers heart rate
c. regulates cardiac rhythm
d. raises blood pressure
e. reduces cardiac pain or lowers blood pressure

##  CASE DISPOSITION

You inform the ALS provider of the difficulty in ventilating the patient, and the provider immediately performs a needle thoracostomy. You set up an IV of normal saline while the ALS provider inserts an IV catheter. The patient is transported by ambulance to a local trauma center, where he undergoes surgery for severe maxillofacial fractures and oral trauma. Quick action by you and the other OEC Technicians to recognize the severity of the patient's injuries, and then clearing and maintaining the patient's airway, saved the patient's life.

# OEC SKILL 36-1 | Preparing a Set-up for IV Therapy

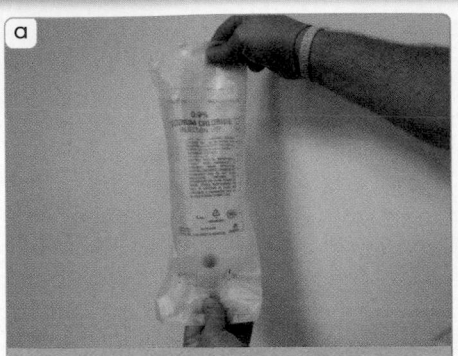

**a**

Select the appropriate bag.
Copyright Edward McNamara

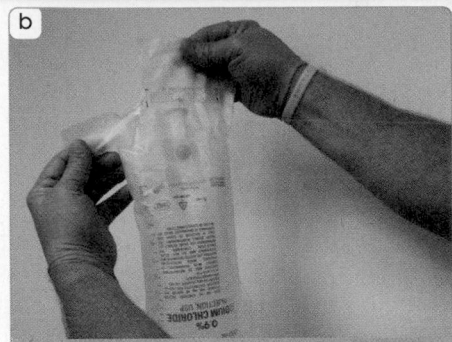

**b**

Turn the bag upside down and remove the plastic covering at the bottom of the bag.
Copyright Edward McNamara

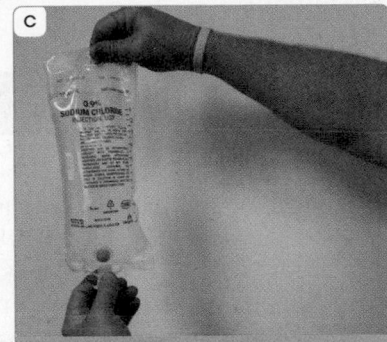

**c**

Inspect the bag for damage and proper expiration date, and inspect the solution's color and clarity.
Copyright Edward McNamara

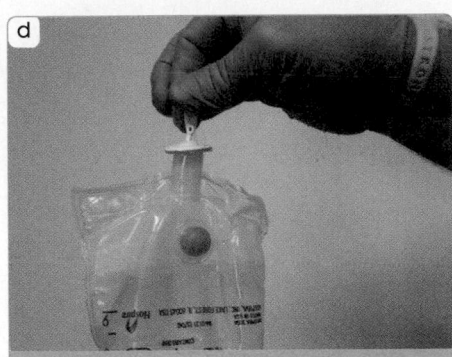

**d**

Turn the bag upside down and hold it by the "neck."
Copyright Edward McNamara

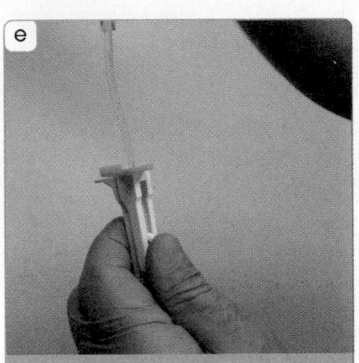

**e**

Close the sliding clamp lock beneath the drip chamber.
Copyright Edward McNamara

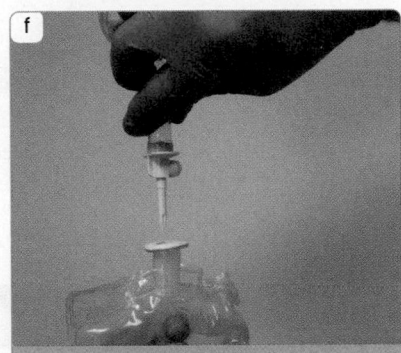

**f**

Remove the plastic cap covering the sharp spike, and then push the point into the IV tubing port, an action known as "spiking the bag."
Copyright Edward McNamara

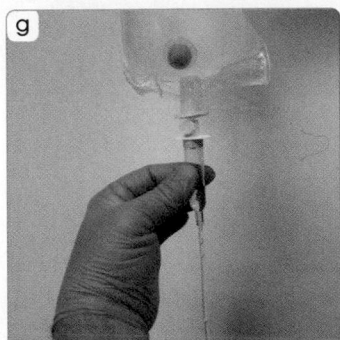

**g**

Return the bag to the upright position and gently squeeze the IV drip chamber until it is approximately half full. Then slowly release the sliding lock beneath the drip chamber to allow the solution to flow and to force any air out of the tubing.
Copyright Edward McNamara

# Chapter Review

## Chapter Summary

It is quite likely that you will encounter ALS providers numerous times during your career as an OEC Technician. At those times it is essential that you can accurately communicate the patient's needs and properly *assist* the ALS providers to ensure effective continuity of care. Doing so requires you to have a basic understanding of the roles of ALS providers, their capabilities, the procedures they may perform, the ways to set up commonly used ALS equipment, and ways to transition patients to ALS care. By taking the time to learn these skills, you are helping to ensure that your critically injured or ill patients receive the highest quality of care possible and have the greatest chances for survival.

## Remember...

1. *Early recognition of the need for ALS can save a patient's life.*
2. OEC Technicians may *not* perform ALS procedures.
3. OEC Technicians may set up ALS equipment only when requested by, and under the direct supervision of, an ALS provider in accordance with state and local protocols.
4. ALS procedures include endotracheal intubation, cricothyrotomy, needle thoracostomy, IV therapy, cardiac monitoring, electrical therapy, and administration of medications.
5. Assisting the ALS provider can improve a patient's survival.

## Chapter Questions

### Multiple Choice

Choose the correct answer.

1. Which of the following statements is false? _____
   a. Only ALS providers have a duty to respond.
   b. Patient care begins by the first person on the scene.
   c. It is necessary for the first OEC Technician on scene to ascertain that an incoming bystander ALS provider is actually credentialed as such.
   d. The ALS provider who assumes patient care is responsible for accompanying the patient to a definitive-care facility.

2. OEC Technicians may set up ALS equipment_____
   a. only when requested by, and under the direct supervision of medical direction.
   b. only when requested by, and under the direct supervision of an ALS provider in accordance with state and local protocols.
   c. only when requested by, and under the direction of the OEC Technician's supervisor.
   d. only when requested by, and under the direction of a trained EMT or AEMT.

## Short Answer

You are working on an injured patient on a ski slope when a woman skis up to you and tells you she is a physician and will be glad to take over care of this patient. What do you do?

_____

_____

_____

_____

## Matching

**1.** Match each of the following terms to its description.

_____ **1.** cricothyrotomy

_____ **2.** electrical therapy

_____ **3.** endotracheal intubation

_____ **4.** intravenous therapy

_____ **5.** nebulizer

_____ **6.** needle thoracostomy

_____ **7.** short report

**a.** a method by which an abnormal cardiac rhythm is restored

**b.** a method used to rehydrate a patient or quickly administer a medication

**c.** a simple method to open an airway when C-spine damage is suspected

**d.** a "last resort" method of airway control

**e.** a metered dose inhaler for medication to treat an asthmatic attack

**f.** a procedure used to treat a tension pneumothorax

**g.** information given to an incoming paramedic, including vital signs and a brief history

**2.** For each of the medications a through n, indicate the type of ailment it treats.

_____ **1.** cardiac disorders

_____ **2.** pain

_____ **3.** respiratory disorders

**a.** lidocaine
**b.** Proventil
**c.** albuterol
**d.** amiodarone
**e.** Ventolin
**f.** epinephrine
**g.** atropine
**h.** nitroglycerin
**i.** morphine
**j.** dopamine
**k.** fentanyl
**l.** Dilaudid
**m.** Atrovent
**n.** adenosine

## Scenario

_A call from dispatch advises you of a "person down" in the lower lodge. You arrive to find a man in his late 50s who is breathless and pulseless when you check his ABCDs. You call for the AED, O₂, more help, and ALS. You start CPR first providing compressions at a rate greater than 100 per minute and then using a pocket mask to provide rescue breathing._

_The AED arrives, the pads are applied, and a shock is delivered. The man's pulse returns but he remains breathless. You provide bag-valve ventilations with oxygen. ALS arrives with a crew of two. It will take over 20 minutes to reach the nearest medical facility. The patient is loaded into the ambulance with an OPA and AED attached. You are asked to ride along and assist the paramedic during transport._

*En route the paramedic will secure the airway with an endotracheal tube.*

1. You will assist the paramedic by_____
   a. starting an IV.
   b. inserting the ET tube through the patient's vocal cords.
   c. maintaining in-line C-spine positioning.
   d. performing nasal suctioning.

2. The correct size of endotracheal tube for a normal-sized adult male is_____
   a. 3.5 or 4.0 mm.
   b. 5.0 or 6.5 mm.
   c. 6.5 or 7.5 mm.
   d. 7.5 or 8 mm.

*Once the endotracheal tube is inserted, a securing device is attached to the patient's face to hold the tube in place.*

3. Located between the tube and the bag valve is_____
   a. an $O_2$ detector.
   b. a colormetric $CO_2$ detector.
   c. a pH detector.
   d. a nitrogen detector.

4. While attempting to insert the tube, the paramedic may request that you exert external pressure on the_____
   a. cricoid cartilage.
   b. thyroid cartilage.
   c. trachea.
   d. sternocleidomastoid muscle.

# Suggested Reading

American Heart Association. 2010. *AHA Guidelines for CPR and ECC*. Dallas: AHA.

Auerbach, P. 2007. *Wilderness Medicine*, Fifth Edition. Philadelphia: Mosby Elsevier.

Mahadevan, S., and G. Garmel. 2006. *Introduction to Clinical Emergency Medicine*. New York: Cambridge University Press.

Roberts, J. R., J. R. Hedges, and C. Custalow. 2004. *Clinical Procedures in Emergency Medicine*, Fourth Edition, Philadelphia: Saunders.

EXPLORE **PEARSON myNSPkit**™

Please go to www.myNSPkit.com. Under Student Resources, you will find animations, videos, web links, and games related to this chapter—and much more. Look for information on difficult airway management, intubation, and more.

Register your access code from the front of your book by going to www.myNSPkit.com and selecting the appropriate links. If the in-cover access code has been redeemed, go to www.myNSPkit.com and follow links to **Buy Access.**

# Appendix A
## SURVIVAL: The Rule of Threes

A large number of books pertaining to survival are on the market, from self-help for dealing with the stresses of life to the *SAS Survival Guide*. Indeed, our own *Outdoor Emergency Care, Fifth Edition*, and *Mountain Travel & Rescue* contain a huge amount of information that can contribute to the survival of OEC Technicians.

No single book or manual can cover the wide range of options one could use to survive a dangerous situation, because survival is very situational. The actions an individual needs to take to survive a plane crash, for example, are different from those needed to survive a night in the woods. Accordingly, this appendix is not intended to provide all the knowledge or tools you might need to survive a life-threatening situation; instead, it presents a set of principles you can use to prioritize the actions you must take to survive. This set of principles, set forth by the wilderness medicine/survival community, is called the **Rule of Threes**.

The Rule of Threes helps you prioritize your decisions concerning the seriousness of the conditions you face and the allocation of the resources at your disposal, the most important of which is time. Thus the Rule of Threes is a timeline of priorities:

- **3 Seconds** to decide to survive
- **3 Minutes** to get air
- **3 Hours** to get shelter
- **3 Days** to get water
- **3 Weeks** to get food

Let's consider each aspect of this crucial timeline.

## 3 Seconds

In a plane crash with fire and smoke, to take one example, you must make a quick decision about how to get out of the aircraft. The longer you wait, the less visibility you will have, and the less chance of getting to an exit before it is blocked. You may only have three seconds to decide which way to go.

Or consider this: As you are driving to your ski area on a wintry day, a car coming toward you starts to spin out of control, and if you do nothing, it will hit you. Some people will turn to avoid the crash; others will "lock up the brakes" and steer directly into danger. The first three seconds, and your ability to respond in that time frame, may determine the outcome of the incident.

One of the best texts on the psychology of survival is Laurence Gonzalez's *Deep Survival—Who Lives, Who Dies,*

*and Why*. In this book he analyzes the psychology of survival, and he looks at some of the faulty decisions people make. Among his recommendations for survival are to maintain situational awareness, anticipate problems that may arise, and have a preformed plan of action. Military squad leaders do this when they approach an area that might contain an ambush: they approach the area carefully, looking for dangers; they anticipate threats from likely directions; and before entering the area they plan responses to attack.

These same strategies can be useful for many of us. A group of backcountry skiers getting ready to cross an area that might slide should stop, assess the situation (including formulating a series of "what ifs"), and plan their responses at different danger points if the slope should slide. This way, they have "rehearsed" their actions at specific points, and they don't need to think about what their next action should be. A person who has mentally rehearsed an action is less likely to "freeze." Anticipating potential adverse situations and quickly developing "escape plans" can help in negotiating the critical first three seconds.

## 3 Minutes

Once you have decided to survive and have taken action to ensure your immediate survival, your next priority is to ensure adequate access to air. Many of us have experienced a temporary loss of air, whatever the exact circumstances, so we understand how getting air becomes our primary concern.

One of the primary settings in which ensuring access to air becomes a priority is burial beneath an avalanche. Most survival guides recommend that individuals caught in an avalanche should try to cover the nose and mouth, both to prevent snow from being forced into the airway and to provide a small pocket of air when the snow stops moving. Even a small pocket can provide some additional air, and perhaps enough air to give victims the critical minutes they need to survive until rescue.

## 3 Hours

Several stories in *Deep Survival* tell of people who venture into the outdoors for a day trip without checking local conditions or being adequately prepared. In one story, the weather is nice and warm at noon and the mountain beckons a group of hikers clad in cotton T-shirts and shorts, but three hours later a storm crests a nearby ridge and soaks the hapless hikers. In another story, a raft overturns in a cold river, dumping everybody into the water, and although they all get to shore, they are soaked, and much of their gear is floating down the river.

At this point in the stories, our hikers and rafters are not threatened with a crisis that requires an immediate decision, and they don't have to fight for air. For unprepared individuals in bad weather, the next threat is hypothermia. Under these conditions, people can quickly become incapable of clear thought and lose the ability to manipulate the tools they need to survive, so getting shelter and maintaining core body temperature is the next task for survival. In many areas, even if it is fully daylight, the sun drops quickly, and then temperatures plummet.

Constructing a reliable shelter—one that protects its occupants from moisture and insulates them from heat loss—can be a challenge in the wilderness, but it is one of the early priorities. It will likely take longer than you think, so get started right away. Don't use the remaining daylight to collect food or water while planning to set up your shelter at dusk; you need light to gather the materials for your shelter and to set it up. You can survive a night of being thirsty and hungry, but you may not survive a night of being cold and wet from the rain. Even a basic inexpensive item such as a plastic tablecloth can be stretched across some logs to form the basis of a waterproof shelter, and reduce delay in protecting your core temperature. Thinking about the "what ifs" of an outing, and then taking along some very simple items, can make this survival step much easier. You can learn about more complex forms of shelter in numerous publications or on line.

## 3 Days

After securing air and shelter, the next priority in survival is finding a source of water. An individual's water demands vary according to weather, temperature, and activity. In most environments a person can go without water for up to three days. For the average person, failure to find water within three days results in severe dehydration and renal failure. In very dry areas with high temperatures, the three-day window may actually be shorter.

If a water source is nearby, you are in luck, and you need only worry about contamination. Drinking contaminated water can make you sick and give you severe diarrhea. Still, you must weigh the relative dangers posed by drinking the water (diarrhea) versus not drinking it (dehydration and renal failure), especially if rescue is likely to occur soon. Various methods of purification are explained in numerous texts.

If your source of water is some distance from your shelter, you may decide to construct a new shelter closer to the water. As before, be sure you have enough light to complete the project. The alternative is using something that can carry/store water. Prepared individuals carry a water bottle, many of which can hold up to a liter. But something as simple as a plastic sandwich bag can be used, even though it is subject to tearing.

## 3 Weeks

It isn't pleasant, but most people can survive up to three weeks without food. In some areas at some times of year, obtaining food is easy, but for the most part, finding and securing food is a very time-consuming effort, and it should be one of your last priorities for survival. Knowing the available edible plants in the area helps, and having some simple tools, such as a knife, gives you the option of making traps and spears.

## Summary

This appendix provides a list of priorities to accomplish when your survival is at stake. Even though the *methods* you might use may vary according to conditions, the *priority* of tasks remains the same in all situations. Those interested in learning more about survival and mountain skills should consider taking one or more of the National Ski Patrol's Mountain Travel & Rescue courses, which offer material at a variety of levels from beginner to advanced.

## Selected Bibliography

Auerbach, P. (Editor). 2007. *Wilderness Medicine*, Fifth Edition. Philadelphia: Mosby Elsevier.

Craighead, F., Jr., and Craighead, J. 1984. *How to Survive on Land and Sea*. Annapolis, MD: Naval Institute Press.

Department of the Army, 1970. *Department of the Army Field Manual 21-76*. Washington, DC: Department of the Army.

Gonzalez, L. 2003. *Deep Survival—Who Lives, Who Dies, and Why*. New York: W. W. Norton and Company.

Mason, E. 1995. *Mountain Travel and Rescue*. Lakewood, CO: NSP.

May, W. G. 1973. *Mountain Search and Rescue Techniques*. Boulder, CO: Rocky Mountain Rescue Group.

Sweeney, M. S. 2008. *Complete Survival Manual*. Washington, DC: National Geographic.

Wiseman, J. 1993. *SAS Survival Guide*. New York, NY: Harper Collins Publishers.

# Appendix B
## Student OEC Skill Guide

**Candidate Name:** _____

In order to be eligible to take the OEC Practical Final Evaluation, you must master each of the skills in the following list. An OEC Instructor can sign off on this sheet after you have demonstrated a mastery of the skills, which includes obtaining a score of at least 80 percent of the points allowable and performing all of the Critical Performance Indicators (CPIs) listed on each of the skill guides. The skill guides are found in the chapter in which the skill is introduced and discussed.

Failure to master the skills or to obtain the required signatures will prevent you from being allowed to participate in the OEC Practical Final Evaluation.

| SKILL | CHAPTER | OEC INSTRUCTOR | DATE |
|---|---|---|---|
| Removing Contaminated Gloves | 3 | | |
| Bridge/BEAN Lift | 5 | | |
| Multiple Person Direct Ground Lift | 5 | | |
| Patient Assessment | 7 | | |
| Pt. Assessment—Trauma Patient | 7 | | |
| Pt. Assessment—Medical Patient | 7 | | |
| Pt. Assessment—Assessing Pupils | 7 | | |
| Pt. Assessment—Assessing Pulse | 7 | | |
| Assessing Respiration Rate | 7 | | |
| Obtaining a Blood Pressure by Auscultation | 7 | | |
| Suctioning a Patient's Airway | 9 | | |
| Inserting a Nasopharyngeal Airway (NPA) | 9 | | |
| Inserting an Oropharyngeal Airway (OPA) | 9 | | |
| Oxygen Tank Set-up and Breakdown | 9 | | |
| Shock Management | 10 | | |
| Auscultation of Breath Sounds | 13 | | |
| Assisting with a Metered-Dose Inhaler | 13 | | |
| Administration with an Auto-Injector | 14 | | |
| Controlling Bleeding | 18 | | |
| Stabilizing an Impaled Object | 18 | | |
| Figure Eight Application | 20 | | |
| Splinting an Upper Extremity Injury | 20 | | |
| Blanket Roll Splint for Shoulder | 20 | | |

*Continued on next page*

| SKILL | CHAPTER | OEC INSTRUCTOR | DATE |
|---|---|---|---|
| Posterior S/C Dislocation Reduction | 20 | | |
| Splinting a Lower Extremity Injury | 20 | | |
| Traction Splinting | 20 | | |
| Boot Removal | 20 | | |
| Manual Spine Stabilization | 21 | | |
| Sizing and Applying a Cervical Collar | 21 | | |
| Supine Patient: Log Roll onto a Long Spine Board | 21 | | |
| Short Board Immobilization | 21 | | |
| Removing a Helmet from a Lying Patient | 21 | | |
| Immobilizing a Standing Patient | 21 | | |
| Stabilizing of an Impaled Object in the Eye | 22 | | |
| Managing an Open Chest Wound | 23 | | |
| Pelvic Stabilization | 24 | | |
| Patient Restraint | 33 | | |
| Assisting with Normal Childbirth | 34 | | |
| Nerve Agent Administration | 35 | | |

# Appendix C
## Emergency Care Equipment

The equipment needs of an OEC Technician vary widely according to the activity being supported, the environment in which that activity takes place, and the unique skills required when participating with special teams. One of the main limitations in providing prehospital care in outdoor settings is that a rescuer cannot have access to unlimited supplies or personnel. When deciding what will be included in a rescue pack, each OEC Technician must decide what must be carried and what is too much to carry. The basic question that should guide the selection and preparation of the gear you take is "What injuries or illnesses do I expect to treat?" Another consideration is proximity to a higher level of care, which may be as nearby as a Patrol Room, or may be much farther away. Decreasing proximity (longer transport time) almost always requires an increase in a patroller's load.

The equipment specified in each of the following lists represents the minimum OEC Technicians need to treat the majority of injuries or illnesses they are likely to encounter in the most common outdoor activities: thus lists are provided for an alpine pack, a universal survival kit, a bike kit, a white water kit, and a Nordic kit. Working in some environments and terrains requires specialized gear; accordingly, equipment needed in areas with high avalanche risk is listed in a separate list.

### Alpine Pack (Figure ApxC-1 ■)

#### Suggested Items

- Two to four (2–4) pairs disposable non-latex medical gloves
- SAM™ splint
- Four (4) cravats
- Six (6) or more 4-inch by 4-inch gauze pads
- Two (2) 2-inch gauze wraps (or Kling)
- Hard candy (for diabetic emergencies)
- 3-inch roller bandage
- Two (2) abdominal pads
- Two (2) large trash bags (for use as a full body covering to prevent hypothermia)
- Pocket mask
- Roll of 1-inch adhesive tape
- Various sizes of adhesive bandages (e.g., Band-Aids™)

- Trauma shears (small enough to fit in the pack but strong enough to cut what you need to cut)
- A fine-tipped permanent marker (to write patient information on tape; is freeze- and smear-resistant)
- Multi-tool (Leatherman™ style, including pliers, knife, screwdriver (both flat and Phillips head) for binding anchors
- Sandwich bags (used for occlusive bandage, as a cooling pack when filled with snow or cool water, or to transport small, amputated body parts)
- Four (4) sizes of airways
- Small flashlight (with extra batteries)
- Space blanket
- Aspirin/Tylenol (for personal use)

#### Optional Items

- Stethoscope
- Forceps
- Hemostats
- Small pipe cutter
- Topical antibiotic packet
- Small tube of sun block

**Figure ApxC-1** An alpine pack.
Copyright Chuck Clements

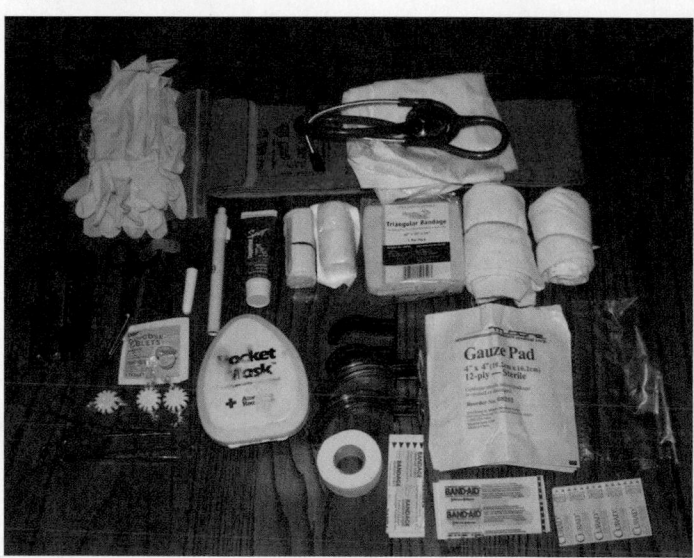

## Universal Survival Kit

A survival kit should be lightweight, small enough to throw in a bag or a car or to hook to a belt, and useful in any outdoor environment.

### Suggested Items

- One (1) 1-liter water bottle
- Multi-tool (with knife blade)
- Waterproof matches or butane lighter
- Poncho (small pouch)
- Small flashlight or head lamp (with extra batteries)
- Space blanket (keep in original package)
- 50 feet of parachute (#550) cord
- Hard candy
- Aspirin/Tylenol (for personal use)
- Whistle
- Candle (survival-specific type)
- Signal mirror
- Small compass
- Water purification tablets
- Wire saw

(Depending on the size of items, the items listed above can be stored in a 1-liter Nalgene™ bottle.)

### Optional Items

- Water filter
- Plastic table cloth (may be used as a tarp or a shelter)
- Power bars
- Cell phone and/or GPS
- Commercial fire starter
- 50 feet of #20 fishing line

## Bike Kit

Because a bike rider will likely not want to carry much weight, this list is shorter than that for an Alpine pack. Still, these items will cover most injuries (Figure ApxC-2■).

### Suggested Items

- Two to four (2–4) pairs of disposable non-latex medical gloves
- SAM™ Splint
- Two (2) cravats
- Six (6) 4-inch by 4-inch gauze pads
- Kerlix wrap (or Kling)
- Roll of 1-inch adhesive tape
- Various sizes of Band-Aids™
- Pocket mask

### Optional Items

- Cell phone and/or GPS
- Sun block

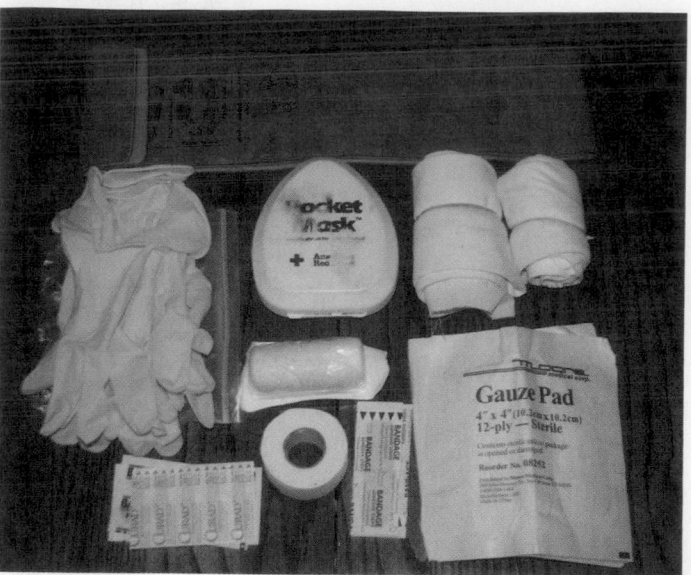

**Figure ApxC-2** A bike kit.
Copyright Chuck Clements

## White Water Kit

Items for a white water kit should be kept in a waterproof container that floats (Figure ApxC-3■).

### Suggested Items

- Two to four (2–4) disposable non-latex medical gloves
- SAM™ Splint
- Four (4) cravats
- Three (3) 2-inch gauze wraps (or Kling)
- Pocket mask
- Roll of 1-inch adhesive tape
- Various sizes of adhesive bandages (Band-Aids™)

**Figure ApxC-3** A white water kit.
Copyright Chuck Clements

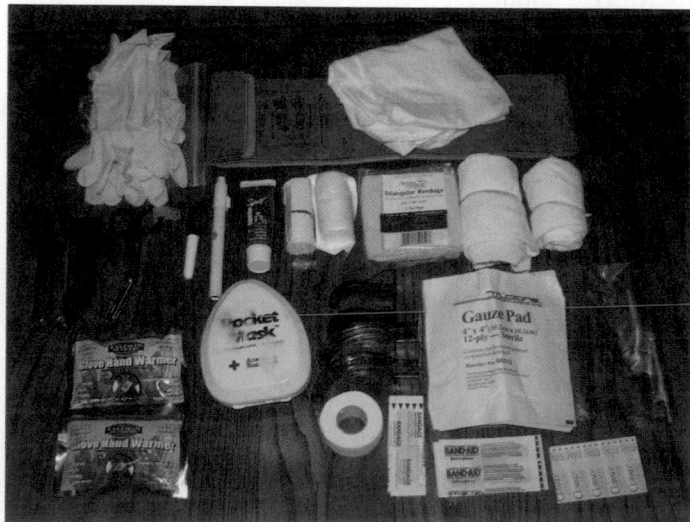

- Trauma shears
- Penlight
- Permanent marker
- Multi-tool, with knife blade
- Ziplock™ plastic bags
- Two (2) heat packs
- Sun block (with SPF of 30 or higher)
- Three or four sizes of airways

## Nordic Kit (Figure ApxC-4■)

### Suggested Items

- Two to four (2–4) disposable non-latex medical gloves
- SAM™ Splint
- Four (4) 4-inch by 4-inch gauze pads
- Four (4) cravats
- Two (2) 2-inch gauze wraps (or Kling)
- Pocket mask
- Roll of 1-inch adhesive tape
- Various sizes of adhesive bandages (Band-Aids™)
- Trauma shears
- Penlight/headlamp
- Permanent marker
- Thermometer

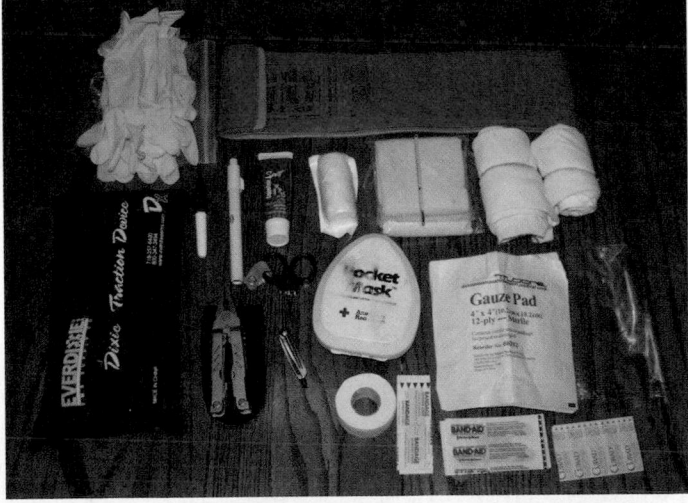

**Figure ApxC-4** A Nordic kit.
Copyright Chuck Clements

- Multi-tool, with knife blade
- Plastic bag
- Kendrick traction device (KTD) or adapter for ski poles

### Optional Items

- One (1) 1-liter water bottle
- Tube tent
- Waterproof matches or butane lighter
- Small compass
- Small poncho
- Wire saw
- Small flashlight (with extra batteries)
- Space blanket (keep in original package)
- 50 feet of parachute (#550) cord
- Whistle
- Candle (survival-specific type)

### Additional Equipment to Consider in an Avalanche Risk Area (Alpine or Nordic)

- Snow shovel
- Transceiver
- Snow probe
- Radio or cell phone

## Medications

The medications to consider for inclusion in your personal wilderness kit are listed in Table C-1■. The National Ski Patrol does not recommend dispensing or administering any medication to an injured patient.

Before you take any medicines, seek the advice of a licensed provider. Your medical advisor can provide information regarding limitations on the use of medications. Although many of these medications are available by prescription only, they can be obtained for self-use through your personal physician. Other medications are controlled medicines and can only be obtained from a licensed provider registered with the Drug Enforcement Agency.

As a rule, all medications should be kept in their original containers to avoid errors in dispensing. For many prescribed medications, it is a legal requirement that the medication remain in the original container so that the prescriber's information can be read on the container's label.

Table **C-1**

| High Altitude | | | |
|---|---|---|---|
| **Medication** | **Dose** | **When Taken** | **Indication** |
| Acetazolamide* | 250 mg | Twice a day | Mountain sickness |
| Albuterol inhaler* | | As needed | Respiratory distress |
| Ciprofloxacin* | 500 mg | Twice a day | Diarrhea/urinary infection |
| Compazine* | 10 mg | Every 6 hours | Nausea |
| Cyclopentolate opth* | 1% | 1–2 drops | Snow blindness |
| Dexamethasone* | 4 mg | Every 6 hours | Mountain sickness |
| Epi-Pen* | 0.3 mg | As needed | Severe allergic reaction |
| Nifedipine* | 30 mg | Twice a day | Pulmonary edema |
| Tylenol | 500 mg | Every 4 hours | Pain |
| **White Water** | | | |
| **Medication** | **Dose** | **When Taken** | **Indication** |
| Augmentin* | 875 mg | Twice a day | Skin/respiratory infection |
| Ciprofloxacin* | 500 mg | Twice a day | Diarrhea/urinary infection |
| Diphenhydramine | 50 mg | Every 6 hours | Allergies/itch |
| Epi-Pen* | 0.3 mg | As needed | Severe allergic reaction |
| Hydrocodone** | 5 mg | Every 6 hours | Severe pain |
| **Nordic** | | | |
| **Medication** | **Dose** | **When Taken** | **Indication** |
| Albuterol inhaler* | | As needed | Respiratory distress |
| Ciprofloxacin* | 500 mg | Twice a day | Diarrhea/urinary infection |
| Cyclopentolate opth* | 1% | 1–2 drops | Snow blindness |
| Epi-Pen* | 0.3 mg | As needed | Severe allergic reaction |
| Tylenol No. 3** | 30 mg | Every 4 hours | Pain |
| **Bike** | | | |
| **Medication** | **Dose** | **When Taken** | **Indication** |
| Albuterol inhaler* | | As needed | Respiratory distress |
| Epi-Pen* | 0.3 mg | As needed | Severe allergic reaction |
| Hydrocodone** | 5 mg | Every 6 hours | Severe pain |
| Tylenol No. 3** | 30 mg | Every 4 hours | Pain |

* Medication available only by prescription.

**Controlled medication that can be obtained only from a licensed provider registered with the Drug Enforcement Agency.

# Glossary

**A**

**abandonment** to withdraw one's support or help from, especially in spite of duty, allegiance, or responsibility.

**abdominal** pertaining to the abdomen.

**abduction** to move away from the midline of the body.

**abrasion** a rubbed or scraped area of skin.

**abruptio placentae** premature separation of a normally situated but improperly implanted placenta; it usually occurs late in pregnancy but may occur during labor.

**absence seizure** a sudden, temporary loss of mental awareness and physical activity lasting a few seconds to several minutes; also known as a petit mal seizure.

**accessory muscles of respiration** various muscles of the neck, chest, and abdomen that may become active when depth of respiration must be significantly increased.

**acclimatization** the body's physiologic process of gradual adjustment to changes in such factors as light, temperature, or altitude.

**acromioclavicular (A/C) joint** joint of the shoulder in which the acromion (top of the scapula) and the clavicle articulate.

**acute mountain sickness (AMS)** a usually mild medical condition that is caused by exposure to high altitude.

**acute myocardial infarction (AMI)** the interruption of blood supply to part of the heart, causing death of heart muscle. Also known as a heart attack.

**acute stress response** (also called *acute stress reaction*) a state of hyperarousal arising in response to a threat or a terrifying event.

**adaptive athlete** a person with a physical or intellectual disability who participates in a sport.

**adaptive equipment** modified sport gear that helps its user overcome a functional impairment.

**addendum** (plural: **addenda**) something added; an addition.

**adduction** to move toward the midline of the body.

**adjunct** a medical device that is used to assist the OEC Technician in providing patient care.

**adolescent** an individual ages 13–18 years; focus shifts from parents to peers; decision making, abstract thinking, and complex memorization skills develop.

**adrenalin(e)** (also called *epinephrine*) a hormone produced by the body; when administered as a medication, it increases heart rate, contracts blood vessels, dilates air passages, and participates in the fight-or-flight response.

**Advanced Emergency Medical Technician (AEMT)** an intermediate-level technician who has successfully completed an NHTSA-approved Advanced EMT course or its equivalent and is authorized to provide both basic and intermediate life support.

**advanced life support (ALS)** a level of EMS care for which providers are trained and authorized to insert advanced airway devices, initiate intravenous lines, and give medications.

**afterdrop** a continued drop in core temperature after removal from cold exposure.

**airway** a natural passageway that allows air to enter and exit the lungs.

**airway patency** a condition in which an airway is open and unobstructed.

**alkaline chemical** (also called a *base* or a *base chemical*) a substance capable of neutralizing an acid; has the properties of or contains an alkali; Alkaline chemicals can be very damaging: some (e.g., lye) can be harmful.

**allergen** a foreign substance (antigen) whose presence in the body stimulates an allergic reaction.

**allergic reaction** a series of signs and symptoms that occur in response to exposure to an allergen.

**allergy** an exaggerated immune response to a substance that does not normally cause a reaction.

**alpha radiation** a very heavy, slow-moving, poorly penetrating particle that is stopped by clothing or the outer layer of the skin. This type of radiation particle is a very serious contaminant when ingested or inhaled.

**altered mental status** a condition in which a person's level of awareness or responsiveness has changed.

**alternating current (AC)** electrical current that periodically flows in opposite directions.

**altitude** vertical height above sea level; elevation.

**altitude illness** encompasses all types of illness due to altitude (AMS, HAPE, and HACE).

**alveoli** tiny air sacs within the lungs; the sites at which oxygen and carbon dioxide are exchanged between inhaled air and the bloodstream.

**ambient temperature** the temperature in the immediate environment.

**Americans with Disabilities Act (ADA)** legislation passed in 1990 designed to prevent discrimination against individuals with disabilities.

**amniotic fluid** the fluid within the amniotic sac and around a fetus.

**amniotic sac** a thin, transparent membrane that holds the fetus suspended in amniotic fluid; also called "the bag of waters."

**amp (A)** a unit of current produced by 1 volt acting through the resistance of 1 ohm.

**amputation** the complete or nearly complete separation of a body part or limb.

**analgesic** a drug that relieves pain.

**anaphylaxis** a severe allergic reaction that can result in serious cardiac or respiratory compromise.

**anatomy** the study of human and animal structures, including gross anatomy (structures that can be seen with the unaided eye) and microscopic anatomy (structures visible only through a microscope).

**aneurysm** ballooning of an artery that weakens it and predisposes it to rupture.

**angina pectoris** sudden chest pain due to an inadequate supply of oxygen to the heart muscle; also called angina.

**angioedema** swelling that occurs beneath the skin or mucosa as a result of an allergic reaction.

**angulation** a sharp bend in a broken bone; a broken bone that is visibly crooked.

**anisocoria** unequal size of the pupils.

**anoxia**    a condition characterized by the lack of an oxygen supply.

**antegrade amnesia**    loss of memory of events that occurred *after* a traumatic event to the brain; an inability to recall new information.

**antibody**    a protein that is produced by the body to neutralize or destroy specific antigens.

**anticoagulant**    a medication that prevents blood from clotting; a "blood-thinner."

**antigen**    a foreign substance that when introduced into the body stimulates the production of an antibody; can be a variety of substances, including toxins, bacteria, foreign blood cells, or the cells of transplanted organs.

**antimicrobial ointment**    a semisolid, oil-based preparation that kills or inhibits the growth of bacteria (antibacterial activity) or fungi (antifungal activity).

**antivenom**    a biological material (antibodies) administered to a patient to counteract exposure to a specific kind of venom; is produced by injecting the venom into an animal and then harvesting the antibodies that the animal makes against the venom.

**anus**    the terminal opening of the digestive tract.

**aorta**    the large muscular artery that originates at the heart and serves as the main trunk of the arterial system.

**aortic aneurysm**    an abnormal dilation, bulging, or ballooning of the aorta.

**aphasia**    an inability to communicate through speech; is often an after-effect of a stroke (CVA).

**apnea**    the absence of breathing.

**apocrine gland**    a gland having a duct that opens into hair follicles in the pubic, anal, axillary, and mammary areas; these glands secretes a substance that can produce and become odorous when it comes into contact with bacteria on the skin, causing what is commonly referred to as "body odor."

**appendicular skeleton**    the periphery of the skeleton; the bones of the arms and legs.

**arachnoid mater**    the middle of the three meninges, or membranes that cover the brain and spinal cord; lies between the dura mater and the pia mater.

**arrhythmia**    abnormal heart rhythm.

**arterial gas embolism (AGE)**    a condition that occurs immediately after rapid ascent in which air bubbles enter the bloodstream from a ruptured alveolus and lodge in an artery.

**articular cartilage**    the cartilage that is affixed to the end of a bone within a joint.

**articulation**    the site at which the ends of two or more bones come together to form a joint.

**assault**    placing somebody into a position where he or she reasonably fears that battery will occur.

**assessment**    the act of determining the nature of a patient's injuries and illnesses.

**assumption of risk**    the voluntary and knowing acceptance of the potential hazards associated with an activity; a defense commonly used in cases in which injuries occur during risky recreational activities such as skiing, paragliding, and scuba diving.

**asystole**    absence of a heartbeat due to lack of cardiac electrical activity.

**ataxia**    uncoordinated muscle movements; at high altitudes, it is associated with HACE.

**atherosclerosis**    a form of arteriosclerosis in which cholesterol and lipid plaques form within the walls of arteries.

**athetoid cerebral palsy**    a form of CP that causes slow, writhing muscle contractions.

**attention deficit disorder**    a behavioral syndrome that causes short attention span, impulsive behavior, and restlessness.

**aura**    a subjective sensation that precedes a seizure.

**auscultation**    the act of listening for sounds within the body, typically using a stethoscope.

**autism spectrum disorders (ASDs)**    developmental disabilities that impair communication with others.

**autoimmune disorder**    a disease that results when the immune system attacks the body's own cells as if they were pathogens; examples are systemic lupus erythematosus, rheumatoid arthritis, and multiple sclerosis.

**auto-injector**    a spring-loaded device that pushes a hypodermic needle through the skin and injects a medication when the tip of the device is pressed firmly against the body.

**automated external defibrillator (AED)**    a medical device used to deliver an electrical shock to a patient in an effort to restore an effective heart rhythm.

**automatic implantable cardioverter defibrillator (AICD)**    an implantable defibrillator that recognizes common lethal heart rhythms and then delivers an electrical shock to the heart to restore an effective heart rhythm.

**autonomic dysreflexia (AD)**    abnormal function of the nervous system associated with spinal cord injuries; can lead to dangerously high blood pressure.

**autonomic nervous system**    the part of the peripheral nervous system that controls involuntary motor functions. This includes intestinal function, heart rate, glandular function, breathing and other involuntary functions.

**AVPU**    a mnemonic for assessing neurologic function; represents Awake or alert, responds to Verbal stimuli or Pain, Unresponsive.

**avulsion**    the tearing away of soft tissue, or a piece of soft tissue hanging as a flap.

**axial**    pertaining to the axis of a body part.

**axial loading**    a method of lifting a heavy object safely by distributing the object's weight evenly down the entire spinal column through the pelvis to the bones of the legs.

**axial skeleton**    the central core of the bony skeleton, consisting of the skull, spine, and supporting thoracic bones.

**axon**    long, slender projection of a nerve cell (neuron) that conducts electrical impulses away from the neuron's cell body.

# B

**bacteria**    primitive, ubiquitous, single-celled microorganisms, some of which are capable of causing disease in humans.

**bag-valve mask (BVM)**    a manually operated resuscitator consisting of three components: a bag reservoir, a one-way flow valve, and a face mask; used to assist patient ventilations.

**bandage**    a strip or roll of gauze or other material used for wrapping or binding a body part.

**barometric pressure**    atmospheric pressure as indicated by a barometer; the pressure exerted by the earth's atmosphere at any given point.

**barotrauma**    trauma that is caused by differences in pressure between the body and the environment.

**basal metabolism**    the minimal amount of energy needed for maintenance of life when an individual is at rest.

**base chemical** (also called a *base* or an *alkaline chemical*) a substance with a pH greater than 7, capable of neutralizing an acid; has the properties of or contains an alkali; some (e.g., lye) can be harmful.

**basic life support (BLS)** a basic level of EMS care for which providers are trained and authorized to provide basic interventions, including noninvasive airway devices, application of oxygen, CPR, and basic first aid.

**basket stretcher** a lightweight device used to transport a patient during a backcountry rescue; sometimes called a "Stokes" stretcher.

**battery** the act of touching someone without his or her consent.

**Beck's triad** the combination of falling systolic pressure, rising jugular venous pressure, and suppressed heart sounds; findings that are typical of cardiac tamponade.

**behavior** an individual's actions or reactions in response to external or internal stimuli.

**behavioral emergency** a situation in which a person acts in a way that is unacceptable or intolerable to others and oftentimes poses a danger to themselves or others.

**beta radiation** low-speed, low-energy particles that are common products of radioactive fallout and are easily stopped by 6–10 feet of air, by clothing, or by the first few millimeters of skin; this type of radiation is a serious threat if ingested (contaminated foods) or inhaled (airborne particles).

**bi-ski** a sit-ski with two skis attached to the bottom of the device.

**blanket drag** a means of moving patients by dragging them on a blanket; is used when hazards or time constraints do not permit the extra move to a device.

**blast injury** an injury caused by the detonation of explosives; the effects are compounded when the explosion takes place in a confined space.

**blister** a pocket of serous fluid between the epidermis and the dermis; can be caused by a chemical or by a physical factor such heat, frostbite, or friction.

**blood pressure (BP)** the pressure of the blood on the interior walls of the arteries.

**blood thinners** (also called *anticoagulants*) medications administered to stop thrombosis or the clotting of blood.

**blowout fracture** an injury caused by direct trauma to the eye or face that fractures the bony eye socket; can entrap the muscles that enable normal eye movement.

**blunt injury** (also called *blunt-force trauma*) an injury caused by a blow that does not penetrate the skin or other body tissues.

**body mechanics** the proper use of body movement in daily activities to prevent problems associated with posture.

**body substance isolation (BSI)** the practice of isolating all bodily substances (blood, urine, tears, feces, and so on) of patients from rescuers in order to decrease disease transmission.

**body system** a group of organs and other structures that work together to perform specific functions.

**bone crepitus** a noise or palpable feeling of crackling when fractured bone ends rub together.

**Boyle's law** the concept that at a given temperature, the volume of a gas is inversely proportional to its pressure.

**bradycardia** a slow pulse rate; a pulse rate below 60 beats per minute in an adult.

**bradypnea** a decreased respiration rate; in adults, less than 10 rpm.

**brain stem** the lower part of the brain, adjoining and structurally continuous with the spinal cord.

**breach of duty** the failure to perform a promised act or obligation of due care.

**breath sounds** the noises produced by the pulmonary structures during respiration.

**breathing** the process of inhaling air into and exhaling air out of the lungs.

**bronchi** (singular: **bronchus**) the two (left and right) large airways that branch off the trachea and enter the lungs.

**bronchodilator** an agent that causes expansion of the air passages within the lungs.

**bronchospasm** the involuntary contraction of the bronchioles.

**bucket** the seat of a sit-ski, which may have one or two skis mounted to the base of the seat.

**bullae** large blisters containing clear or bloody fluid.

**burn** a lesion of the skin caused by thermal or frictional heat, chemicals, electricity, or nuclear radiation.

## C

**callus** material at a fracture site that forms from a hematoma and later becomes bone.

**capacity** indicates the patient has normal decision-making abilities and whose judgment is not impaired.

**cardiac arrest** cessation of a functional heartbeat.

**cardiac contractility** the capacity of cardiac muscle cells for becoming shorter (contracting) in response to a suitable stimulus.

**cardiac muscle** specialized muscle of the heart that contracts regularly without stopping.

**cardiac output** the volume of blood pumped out of the heart each minute.

**cardiogenic shock** a condition whereby body tissues are oxygen deprived due to the heart's inability to adequately pump blood; may follow a large acute myocardial infarction.

**cardiopulmonary resuscitation** a procedure to revive a patient who is pulseless and not breathing.

**cardiovascular** pertaining to the circulatory system, which is composed of the heart (cardio) and the blood vessels (vascular).

**cardioversion** the restoration of a normal rhythm of the heart by electrical shock.

**carry** the act of taking or supporting the movement of a person from one location to another.

**cartilage** a tough, elastic, fibrous connective tissue found in various parts of the body, including the joints, outer ear, and end of the nose.

**cataract** clouding of the lens of the eye due to pathologic changes making the lens of the eye opaque.

**caustic substance** an agent capable of burning, corroding, dissolving, or eating away by chemical action; is destructive to tissues.

**CBRNE** a mnemonic for the common types of human-caused disasters; represents chemical, biologic, radiological, nuclear, and explosive.

**cell** the basic unit of all living tissue.

**cellular hypoxia** insufficient levels of oxygen in tissues.

**central nervous system (CNS)** the part of the nervous system that includes the brain and spinal cord.

**cerebellum** posterior part of the brain that plays an important role in the integration of sensory perception and motor control, especially for coordination.

**cerebral** pertaining to the cerebrum, the largest part of the brain.

**cerebral palsy (CP)** a brain injury before, during, or shortly following birth that results in a non-progressive, non-contagious muscular motor disorder.

**cerebrospinal fluid** serum-like fluid that functions in shock absorption for central nervous system structures; circulates through passages within the brain and within the meninges surrounding the brain and spinal cord.

**cerebrum** region on the top of the brain that integrates sensory perception and motor control and is involved in attention and the processing of language, music, and other sensory stimuli.

**chain of custody** (also called *chain of evidence*) the path that objects of evidence (such as bullets, knives, or clinical specimens) must take if they are to be legally accepted as evidence in court; includes formal documentation that establishes both the continuity of possession by every person that had custody of the evidence and the integrity of the evidence collected.

**chair carry** a method in which two rescuers form a chair with their arms to move a patient who is able to sit up without assistance.

**channel** a band of radio frequencies assigned for a particular purpose; a course or pathway through which information is transmitted; a passageway or groove that conveys fluid.

**Charles Minot "Minnie" Dole** the founder and creator of the National Ski Patrol.

**chemical burn** a burn caused by a caustic substance, such as an acid or a base.

**chief complaint** the symptom or group of symptoms about which the patient is concerned.

**chilblains** a skin condition resembling frost nip that results from prolonged exposure to cold, wet conditions.

**child abuse** any act or failure to act on the part of a parent, a caregiver, or any adult that results in serious physical or emotional harm or imminent risk of harm to a child.

**child neglect** a failure to act on the part of a parent, a caregiver, or other responsible adult to provide for the physical, emotional, educational, safety, or social needs of a child to the extent that emotional, developmental, or physical harm may occur.

**chronic obstructive pulmonary disease (COPD)** a condition in which the airways and alveoli become damaged, typically by long-term smoke exposure; its two most important forms are chronic bronchitis and chronic emphysema.

**Cincinnati Stroke Scale** a system that assesses a patient using three specific criteria on examination that may indicate that a patient is having a stroke; even one abnormal finding indicates the need for immediate transport to a hospital.

**circulatory system** a group of organs and other structures that transport blood and other nutrients throughout the body.

**cirrhosis** a chronic disease of the liver characterized by the loss of functional liver cells and their replacement by fibrous tissue; can result from alcohol abuse, nutritional deprivation, or infection (especially by hepatitis viruses).

**clinical findings** (also called *clinical signs*) observations made during the assessment of a patient.

**clinical picture** the chief features of a patient's symptoms and clinical findings.

**clonic activity** the spasmodic jerking of muscles during a seizure.

**closed chest injury** a chest injury without penetration of the chest cavity.

**closed injury** damage beneath the skin or a mucous membrane from trauma while the overlying skin remains intact.

**cognitive disability** an impairment of brain function that limits the ability to process information.

**cold zone** the area outside the warm zone, in which it is safe to operate without specialized equipment.

**coma** an abnormal loss of responsiveness during which the patient cannot be aroused by external stimuli.

**commotio cordis** sudden cardiac death due to blunt thoracic trauma without any observable thoracic or cardiac damage.

**communicable disease** a disease that can be transmitted from one person to another.

**communication** a process by which a message is transmitted from one person to another.

**comorbidity** the simultaneous presence of additional, unrelated pathologic condition(s) or diseases.

**comparative negligence** a partial legal defense that reduces the amount of damages a plaintiff can recover in a negligence-based claim based upon the degree to which the plaintiff's own negligence contributed to causing the damages; a modification of the doctrine of contributory negligence, which disallows any recovery by a plaintiff whose negligence contributed, even minimally, to causing the damages.

**compartment syndrome** a condition in which the swelling of injured muscles within their connective tissue coverings causes pressure that can damage tissue and cut off blood flow.

**competent** properly or sufficiently qualified; capable; legally qualified or fit to perform an act.

**compression dressing** an occlusive dressing that applies some pressure to a bleeding wound; it should not compromise circulation, movement, or sensation distal to the wound.

**conduction** a form of heat exchange in which heat transfers from a warmer object to a cooler object through direct contact.

**confidentiality** the nondisclosure of personal information except to an authorized person with the need to know.

**congestive heart failure** failure of the heart to efficiently pump blood to body tissues.

**consent** to give permission or approval to something proposed or requested.

**contagious disease** a disease communicable by contact with a patient suffering from it, or by contact with some secretion of or object touched by such a patient.

**contamination** soiling of an object, water, or air by foreign material such as dirt, debris, bodily fluids, or radiation.

**continuity of care** uninterrupted health care for a medical condition from the first contact between a patient and a health care provider until the point of resolution or the initiation of long-term maintenance.

**contributory negligence** the situation in which plaintiffs have, through their own negligence, contributed to causing the damages they incurred as a result of defendants' negligence.

**contusion** a bruise or soft tissue injury to a body part without a break in the skin.

**convection** direct transfer of heat through circulating air; is increased when skin is exposed to wind.

**core body temperature** the temperature in the part of the body that contains the vital organs.

**cornea** the clear but highly sensitive surface of the eye that refracts light entering into the visual system.

**coronary artery bypass grafting (CABG)** an operation that uses grafts of healthy blood vessels to bypass diseased arteries that supply the heart tissue.

**coronary artery disease (CAD)** narrowing of the coronary arteries, which supply blood and oxygen to the heart muscle.

**cortex** the hard outer layer of a bone.

**crepitus** a "crackling" feel of the skin of the chest that is detected by palpation; is caused by the presence of air trapped beneath the skin.

**cricoid cartilage** a ring-shaped structure that circles the trachea at the lower edge of the larynx; also called the cricoid ring.

**cricoid pressure** pressure applied to the cricoid cartilage to bring the vocal cords into view when a patient is being intubated.

**cricothyrotomy** an incision through the cricothyroid membrane for the purpose of inserting a tube to establish a "surgical airway"; is usually performed as a part of advanced airway management; is beyond the scope of practice for OEC Technicians.

**crisis** a state of emotional turmoil within an individual in which the balance between thoughts and emotions is lost.

**cross-contamination** the transfer of an infection or a foreign substance either directly (from one person or object to another) or indirectly (from one person or object to another via some third, intermediate source).

**crush injury** compression injury in which a great amount of force is applied to the body.

**cumulative stress response** a response of a patient to repeated physical or emotional stresses that build up over time and thus exceed the degree of stress expected by a rescuer or caregiver.

**cyanotic** marked by a bluish or gray discoloration of the skin or mucous membranes due to a lack of oxygen.

**cystitis** an inflammation of the bladder, usually caused by a bacterial infection.

# D

**Dalton's law** the concept that the pressure exerted by a mixture of nonreacting gases is equal to the sum of the partial pressures of the individual gases in the mixture.

**DCAP-BTLS** a mnemonic for assessing trauma-related injuries; represents Deformity; Contusions; Abrasions and avulsions; Punctures and penetrations; Burns, bleeding, and bruises; Tenderness; Lacerations; and Swelling.

**decerebrate posturing** abnormal extension of arms and legs, downward pointing of toes, and arching of the head; due to an injury to the brain at the level of the brainstem.

**decoding** the process by which a received message is translated and interpreted.

**decompensated shock** shock that results from the body's inability to compensate for low blood volume or inadequate tissue perfusion.

**decompression sickness (DCS)** formation of nitrogen bubbles in tissues from a too-rapid ascent.

**decontamination** the process of rendering an object, person, or area free of harmful substances such as bacteria, poison, gas, and radiation.

**decorticate posturing** abnormal flexing of the arms, clenching fists, and extending legs; due to an injury along the nerve pathway between the brain and spinal cord.

**definitive care** the level of care at which a recommended treatment can be fully brought to completion.

**dehydration** the loss of body water and electrolytes in excess to the amount needed for normal body function.

**delirium** a state of mental confusion and/or excitement characterized by disorientation with respect to time and place; may be associated with delusions and hallucinations.

**dementia** a broad impairment of intellectual function (cognition) that usually is progressive and that interferes with normal social and occupational activities.

**dendrite** a slender, typically branched projection of a nerve cell that typically receives and conducts an electrical impulse.

**density** in general, the quality of being compact or dense; specifically, the quantity of matter (mass) per unit of space (volume).

**dependent lividity** a purplish discoloration of the skin in the lowest parts of the body due to the settling of blood following death; also called livor mortis.

**depression** a clinical state marked by feelings of sadness and self-loathing.

**dermal poison** a toxin absorbed through the skin.

**dermis** the inner layer of the skin; contains hair follicles, sweat glands, nerve endings, and blood vessels.

**designer drug** a drug constructed by a chemist to produce unique and specific effects.

**diabetes mellitus** a term that refers to a complex group of syndromes having in common a disturbance in the use of glucose; a condition that is often a result of a malfunction of the beta cells of the pancreas, whose function is the production and release of insulin.

**diaphoresis** inappropriate excessive sweating.

**diffuse axonal injury** the most common and devastating types of traumatic brain injury; results when damage occurs over a more widespread area than in focal brain injury.

**dilation** the widening (increase in diameter) of a circular or tubular structure, such as the pupil of the eye or a blood vessel.

**direct current (DC)** electrical current that flows in one direction only.

**direct ground lift** a method of lifting and carrying a patient from ground level to a stretcher in which two or more rescuers kneel, place their arms beneath the patient, curl the patient to their chests, stand, and then uncurl their arms to lower the patient onto the stretcher.

**disability** any condition that impairs normal function or daily activity.

**disc (disk)** the pad of cartilage between two adjacent vertebrae.

**disease transmission** transfer of illness from an infected individual to a healthy individual.

**disinfection** the process beyond cleaning in which an agent such as alcohol or bleach (a disinfectant) is used to free something (typically an object) of microorganisms or to render them inert.

**dislocation** a separation or displacement of the bones of a joint.

**distal** farther away from the torso.

**distracting injury** any injury that directs the patient's attention away from the exam that is being performed by the rescuer.

**doctrine of abandonment** principle of withdrawing one's support or help, especially in spite of duty, allegiance, or responsibility; can result in legal consequences to the health care provider who withdraws care.

**doctrine of public reliance** when the general public has been given a reasonable expectation that an OEC Technician has the ability and duty to provide first-aid services.

**documentation** the creation of formal written or recorded information regarding a patient or incident that later may be used legally.

**dorsal** toward the back of the body or of a body part.

**dorsiflex** to move a part of the body dorsally (toward the back).

**Down syndrome (DS)** a genetic disability that causes intellectual impairment and physical anomalies.

**drag** a method of moving a patient on the ground to another location.

**draw sheet lift** (also called *draw-sheet method*) a method for lifting and moving a patient a short distance or for transferring a patient from a bed to a stretcher by grasping and pulling a loosened bed sheet or a sheet of strong fabric or plastic placed beneath the patient.

**dressing** any material (preferably sterile) used for covering and protecting a wound.

**drowning** suffocation by submersion in water.

**dry drowning** a condition in which the lungs are unable to extract oxygen from the air; may be due to persistent spasm of the larynx during immersion in liquid; also may be due to a puncture wound that reduces the diaphragm's ability to create respiratory movement, to paralysis of muscles of respiration in a cervical spine injury, or to damage to the lungs' oxygen-absorbing tissues; see also *wet drowning*.

**duty to act** a person's legal obligation to provide something to another individual.

**duty to rescue** a circumstance in which an individual can be held liable for failing to come to the rescue of another individual in peril.

**dyslexia** an impairment of information processing that makes learning new information difficult.

**dysmenorrhea** painful menstruation including cramps in the lower abdomen.

**dyspnea** difficult or labored breathing accompanied by feeling short of breath.

**dystonic cerebral palsy** a form of CP associated with extreme muscle rigidity.

# E

**ecchymosis** a bruise; discoloration of the skin associated with a closed wound; signifies bleeding within the skin.

**eccrine glands** sweat glands that function in body temperature regulation; are widely distributed but are particularly abundant on the palms the soles, and the forehead.

**eclampsia** a potentially life-threatening disorder in pregnant women that is characterized by hypertension, generalized edema, and proteinuria (protein in the urine); involves the seizures of the convulsive stage of preeclampsia-eclampsia syndrome, which are not attributable to another cerebral condition such as epilepsy.

**ectopic pregnancy** a pregnancy occurring in a site other than within the uterus.

**edema** abnormal buildup of fluid in body tissues.

**electrical current** a stream of electricity that moves along a conductor.

**electrocardiogram (ECG or EKG)** a record of the electrical activity of the heart, which provides important information concerning the functioning of the different parts of the heart.

**electrolyte** a chemical compound that separates into charged particles (ionizes) in a solution; examples are sodium chloride (NaCl) and potassium chloride (KCl).

**embolism** a blockage of a vessel by a clot or foreign material brought to the site through the bloodstream.

**embolus** a blood clot, fat, or other solid material in the venous system that breaks loose and is carried in the bloodstream, lodging in another site in the body.

**embryo** the developing infant during the period from fertilization through the eighth week of development.

**emergency care system** a network of specially trained personnel, equipment, facilities, and other resources that respond to medical emergencies. See *emergency medical services*.

**emergency medical dispatcher (EMD)** a person who has been trained to provide emergency medical advice and instructions over the telephone.

**Emergency Medical Responder (EMR)** any trained individual who is first to respond on scene at a medical emergency; renders immediate care to the patient and continues care until care is assumed by a person with higher medical training.

**emergency medical services (EMS)** a network of services, including rescue operations, prehospital emergency care, ambulance transportation, emergency department services, and public education, for treating victims of illness or injury. See *emergency care system*.

**Emergency Medical Technician (EMT)** a basic-level technician who has successfully completed an NHTSA-approved EMT course or its equivalent and is authorized to provide basic life support.

**emollients** substances that soften or soothe the skin.

**encephalitis** inflammation of the brain; can be the result of infection with the influenza, measles, rabies, or smallpox viruses.

**encoding** the process of converting the information in a message into some other form, as in a code.

**endocrine system** a group of organs and other structures that produce chemical substances that act as messages throughout the body.

**endotracheal intubation** the process of placing a tube into the trachea and maintaining it to provide an airway while preventing aspiration of foreign material into the bronchi (and lungs).

**envenomation** poisonous effects caused by bites or stings.

**epidermis** the outer layer of skin that acts as a watertight protective covering.

**epidural hematoma** a traumatic brain injury in which a buildup of blood occurs between the dura mater and the skull.

**epiglottis** a thin, leaf-shaped structure posterior to the tongue; covers the larynx when swallowing, preventing food or liquid from entering the airway.

**epiglottitis** an inflammation and swelling of the epiglottis, the small, leaf-shaped structure that covers the larynx when a person swallows and prevents food from entering the trachea.

**epinephrine** (also known as *adrenaline*) a hormone produced by the body; when administered as a medication, it increases heart rate, contracts blood vessels, dilates air passages and participates in the fight-or-flight response.

**epistaxis**   nosebleed.

**erythrocyte**   a red blood cell.

**esophageal sphincter**   a ringlike muscle that when contracted prevents the movement of food or liquid from the stomach back into the esophagus.

**esophagus**   the tube that leads from the pharynx to the stomach.

**ethical**   relating to ethics; conforming to accepted professional standards of conduct.

**ethical standards**   universally accepted guidelines for behavior and conduct.

**ethics**   the science (study) of morality or behavior that defines what is "good" or "right."

**evacuation chair**   (also called a "*stair chair*") a lightweight portable stretcher used to transport a patient in a seated position; its wheels and handles enable it to be maneuvered in tight spaces such as in stair wells.

**evaporation**   a form of heat exchange that occurs when a liquid converts to a gas.

**evisceration**   the protrusion of organs through an open abdominal wound.

**exhalation**   the act of expelling breath or air out of the lungs.

**expressed consent**   consent given when a competent injured person gives permission to provide first aid treatment and transportation.

**expressive aphasia**   the inability to express speech normally.

**exsanguination**   massive blood loss resulting in death; the process of bleeding to death.

**external auditory canal**   the passageway through the outer ear that ends at the tympanic membrane.

**extravascular**   outside of a blood vessel.

**extremity lift**   a two-person method of lifting and carrying a patient in which one rescuer slips hands under the patient's armpits and grasps the patient's wrists while another rescuer grasps the patient's knees.

**extrication**   the process of removing a trapped person (as from a vehicle that has been involved in a collision) when conventional means of exit are impossible or inadvisable.

## F

**facility**   any primary work area in or around an incident in which incident-related activities are planned, organized, directed, or conducted.

**fallopian tubes**   (also called *uterine tubes*) thin, flexible, tubular structures that extend between the uterus and the ovaries.

**fascia**   the sheet of tissue that covers the outside of muscles and various other organs.

**feces**   a waste product that contains food that cannot be digested and is expelled from the body (defecated).

**feet drag**   a method used to move a patient urgently that involves grasping the patient by the feet and dragging the person a short distance.

**femoral neck**   the portion of the femur that joins the femoral shaft to ball of the femur.

**fetus**   the developing infant during the period from the eighth week of development until birth.

**field care notes**   notes written by OEC Technicians at the scene of a patient rescue; include a time line, vital signs, witnesses' names, and other pertinent information.

**fight-or-flight response**   (also called *hyperarousal* or the *acute stress response*) the body's reaction to threats that involves a general discharge of the sympathetic nervous system and primes a person for fighting or fleeing; the first stage of a general adaptation syndrome that regulates stress responses.

**first-degree burn**   a burn that affects the epidermis only, causing reddening of the skin and mild edema but no blisters.

**flail chest**   a condition in which two or more adjacent ribs are fractured in two or more places, causing a free-floating segment of the chest wall.

**flat spinal plane**   the position of the body in which the occiput (back of the head), shoulders, buttocks, calves, and heels are all in alignment in the same flat plane.

**flutter valve**   a one-way valve, used primarily for treating a sucking chest wound or a pneumothorax, that allows air to escape out of the pleural space but prevents its entry into the chest cavity.

**fontanel**   an unfused suture between the bones of the skull of a newborn that allows expansion of the growing brain; the fontanels close at approximately 18–20 months of age.

**four tracker**   a skier with two legs (one or both of which may be a prosthetic) who also uses two outriggers.

**fourth-degree burn**   a burn that extends into muscle and bone.

**fracture**   a break in a bone's cortex.

**frostbite**   damage to tissues from freezing due to the formation of ice crystals between and within cells, rupturing the cells and leading to cell death.

**full-thickness burn**   a third-degree or fourth-degree burn.

## G

**gamma radiation**   a type of powerful and penetrating radiation associated with the fallout of a nuclear detonation or with a nuclear reactor accident; is similar to X-ray radiation.

**Gamow bag**   a portable hyperbaric chamber that is used to treat high-altitude sickness.

**gastric distention**   inflation of the stomach with air; can lead to vomiting.

**gastrointestinal system**   a group of organs and other structures that break down food and absorb nutrients into the body.

**generalized seizure**   a seizure consisting of the sudden onset of unresponsiveness, tonic contraction of muscles, loss of postural control, and a cry caused by contraction of respiratory muscles that forces an exhalation; clonic contractions of muscles occur, followed by a period of somulence.

**genitourinary disorder**   an abnormality of the organs of the reproductive and/or urinary systems.

**geriatric**   pertaining to elderly persons or to the aging process.

**gestation**   the period during which a female is pregnant; in humans it is about 266 days, from fertilization of the egg until birth.

**gestational period**   the time from the first day of a woman's last normal menstrual period before fertilization, which is about 2 weeks before fertilization, until birth.

**Glasgow Coma Scale**   a method for assessing neurologic function (i.e., level of responsiveness, movement).

**glucagon**   a hormone that stimulates the breakdown of glycogen, a storage form of glucose in the liver; is sometimes administered by injection to temporarily raise glucose levels in patients with symptomatic hypoglycemia.

**glucose** a simple sugar that is the end product of carbohydrate digestion in the body and the chief source of energy for most cells, especially neurons.

**glycogen** a stored form of glucose or carbohydrate that is made by the body; located primarily in liver or muscle.

**golden hour** the first 60 minutes following a serious traumatic event, during which prompt medical treatment may prevent death.

**Good Samaritan laws** laws that protect a person from legal liability when the person volunteers to perform an act to help someone else.

**grand mal seizure** a generalized seizure characterized by sudden onset of unconsciousness, tonic contraction of muscles, loss of postural control, and a cry (caused by contraction of respiratory muscles, forcing exhalation); clonic contractions of muscles also occur, followed by a period of unresponsiveness.

**gross negligence** in health care, reckless regard or care for a person that is clearly below the standards of accepted medical practice, either without regard for the potential consequences or with willful and wanton disregard for the rights and/or well-being of a patient.

**guarding** an involuntary action in which the abdomen becomes rigid upon examination.

**gynecologic** pertaining to gynecology.

**gynecology** the branch of medicine specializing in conditions of the female reproductive system.

# H

**handicap** any condition that impairs normal physical or intellectual function.

**hand-off report** an oral report given at the transfer of a patient from one provider to another.

**hazardous materials (HazMat)** substances that have the potential to harm people, animals, or the environment.

**HAZWOPER** stands for HAZardous Waste OPerations and Emergency Response; refers to federally mandated training for anyone who may encounter uncontrolled hazardous materials.

**head-tilt, chin-lift maneuver** a method to open a patient's airway; a process that involves tilting the patient's head backward while simultaneously lifting the patient's chin.

**Health Insurance Portability and Accountability Act (HIPAA)** a law that addresses the confidentiality of the electronic transmission of medical records; applies to medical personnel who are compensated for service.

**heart contractility** the capacity of cardiac muscle cells to shorten in response to a suitable stimulus.

**heat acclimatization** adaptation of the body over time to a hot environment.

**heat cramps** painful muscle cramps that result from dehydration and electrolyte imbalances.

**heat exhaustion** a condition characterized by fatigue, dizziness, nausea, and headache caused by dehydration and elevated core body temperature.

**heat index** a measure of the risk for heat illness; combines the effects of increasing ambient temperature and increasing humidity.

**heat stroke** a life-threatening elevation of core body temperature associated with shock and a deteriorating level of responsiveness.

**heat-related syncope** fainting secondary to pooling of the blood in the extremities due to increased core body temperature.

**hematemesis** vomiting up blood.

**hematochezia** the passage of bloody stools.

**hematoma** an extravascular collection of blood within the body's tissues or in a body cavity.

**hematuria** blood in the urine.

**hemoglobin** oxygen-carrying protein in red blood cells.

**hemopneumothorax** the abnormal presence of both blood and air in the chest cavity.

**hemoptysis** coughing up blood.

**hemorrhage** the escape of blood from the vessels; bleeding.

**hemostatic dressing** a surgical gauze/mesh impregnated with a material that stops arterial and venous bleeding in seconds.

**hemothorax** an accumulation of blood in the pleural space.

**Henry's Law** the principle that the amount of a gas dissolved at equilibrium in a given quantity of a liquid is proportional to the pressure of the gas in contact with the liquid.

**hepatitis** inflammation of the liver; may be caused by an infectious agent such as a virus, a toxin or a chemical.

**hepatitis A** (also called *infectious hepatitis*) inflammation of the liver caused by infection with hepatitis A virus, which is transmitted by ingestion of food or water contaminated by the feces of an infected person; has a shorter incubation period and generally milder symptoms than hepatitis B.

**hepatitis B** (also called *serum hepatitis*) inflammation of the liver caused by infection with hepatitis B virus, which is transmitted in several ways: via contaminated needles or sharp instruments; through contact with contaminated blood at mucous membranes, open wounds, or abraded skin; by sexual contact with an infected person; or through contaminated blood or blood derivatives in transfusions.

**herniation** protrusion of a body structure through a rupture in smooth muscle or fibrous tissue.

**herpes simplex** a sexually transmitted infection with the herpes simplex virus that typically produces clusters of small, temporary (but sometimes painful) blisters on the skin and mucous membranes, especially on the mouth, lips, face, or genitals; may recur intermittently and may affect the nervous system.

**high voltage** electricity with a voltage greater than 1,000 V (AC) or 1,500 V (DC).

**high-altitude cerebral edema (HACE)** a potentially deadly condition in which the brain swells in individuals at high altitude.

**high-altitude pulmonary edema (HAPE)** a condition in which fluid accumulates in the lungs of individuals at high altitude.

**high-angle rescue** any rescue work done by ascending or descending a slope steeper than approximately 45 degrees.

**high-Fowler position** a sitting position with the patient's body bent at the waist to 90 degrees; is typically used for patients who are experiencing severe breathing problems.

**histamine** a chemical that is released in the body as a result of an allergic reaction.

**history of present illness** a description of the circumstances surrounding the events of an incident; includes all subjective descriptions presented by the patient (or a bystander, if the patient cannot tell you).

**hives** red, itchy, usually raised blotches on the skin that often result from allergic reactions.

**homeostasis**   the body's ability to regulate its inner environment to ensure stability and to respond to changes in the outside environment.

**hormone**   a chemical substance, secreted by an endocrine gland and transported in the bloodstream, that affects the functioning of one or more target tissues.

**hot zone**   the area closest to the center of a CBRNE incident; is the most dangerous and most contaminated area.

**human crutch** (one-person assist)   a common method for helping a patient move down a slope or trail in which a lone rescuer acts as a crutch to take the weight off an injured lower extremity.

**human immunodeficiency virus (HIV)** the virus (a retrovirus) that causes AIDS.

**humidity**   the amount of water vapor in the air.

**hydration**   the process of giving water or other fluids (usually by mouth or IV) to a person to restore or maintain fluid balance.

**hyperbaric chamber**   a chamber used to treat "the bends" and other SCUBA diving injuries by returning an injured diver to the higher pressures experienced at depth; is also called a compression chamber, a diving chamber, or a recompression chamber.

**hyperextend**   to extend a joint beyond its normal range of motion.

**hyperglycemia**   an excess of glucose in the blood; when severe, may be associated with confusion or changes in mental status.

**hypersensitivity**   an exaggerated immune response to an allergen, drug, or other foreign substance.

**hypertension**   abnormally high blood pressure.

**hyperthermia**   elevated core body temperature.

**hyperventilation**   a state characterized by fast breathing (tachypnea) and deep breathing (hyperpnea).

**hyphema**   blood in the anterior chamber of the eye.

**hypnotic**   a drug that induces sleep.

**hypodermis**   the subcutaneous layer of loose connective tissue; contains a variable number of fat cells.

**hypoglycemia**   an insufficient amount of glucose in the blood; may be associated with a myriad of signs and symptoms such as tremor, diaphoresis, drowsiness,

headache, confusion, and lack of responsiveness.

**hyponatremia**   dilution of the sodium level in the blood.

**hypotension**   low blood pressure.

**hypothalamus**   a portion of the brain just below the thalamus that controls body temperature, appetite, sleep, sexual desire, and emotions; regulates the release of pituitary hormones; and regulates the parasympathetic and sympathetic nervous systems.

**hypothermia**   an abnormally low body temperature; below 95°F (35°C).

**hypoxemia**   insufficient oxygenation of the blood.

**hypoxia**   a reduction in oxygen supply to a tissue.

**hypoxic**   characterized by insufficient oxygen.

**hypoxic drive**   the respiratory control system that stimulates breathing when oxygen levels fall.

**hypoxic ventilatory response**   breathing as a result of hypoxic drive.

# I

**ictal**   of or relating to a seizure or convulsion.

**immobilization**   the process of holding an object in place, as for a fracture by a cast or internal orthopedic hardware.

**immobilized**   unable to move or fixed in position (as with a splint or cast).

**immune**   having resistance to infection of a specific pathogen or being unaffected by a given influence; exempt from (not subject to) an obligation.

**immune system**   the body's set of defense mechanisms against invasion by disease-causing organisms or foreign substances.

**immunity**   the state of being protected from a disease, especially an infectious disease.

**impairment**   any loss or limitation of physical or intellectual function.

**impaled object**   a foreign object that remains in the body in a puncture wound.

**implied consent**   a form of consent that is not expressly granted by a person, but instead is inferred from a person's actions and the facts and circumstances of a particular situation.

**improvised carries**   ways of moving a sick or injured individual using the materials available in one's environment.

**improvised litter**   a litter created using the materials available in one's environment.

**incident**   anything out of ordinary day-to-day activities that necessitates a response (e.g., emergencies, disasters, outbreaks, vaccination programs, important meetings or conferences).

**Incident Command System (ICS)**   a formal, organized method for managing an incident, regardless of its cause, size, scope, or complexity.

**Incident Commander (IC)**   the person who provides overall leadership at an incident.

**incident report forms**   forms provided by the National Ski Area Association, a ski resort, or an insurance carrier and used by OEC Technicians to document an incident; the forms include the circumstances leading to injury.

**incision**   a cut that has clean, smooth edges.

**incontinence**   the lack of voluntary control of excretory functions such as urination or defecation.

**incubation period**   the interval of time from the initial exposure to an infectious agent and the first symptoms of illness.

**index of suspicion**   when evaluating a patient who has sustained trauma, the initial impression of what could be injured and how bad the injury is, based on the mechanism of injury.

**infant**   a child ages 2–12 months.

**infarction**   formation of an area of dead tissue due to inadequate blood flow.

**influenza**   an infection caused by the influenza virus of the respiratory system characterized by chills, fever, body aches, and fatigue; commonly called "the flu."

**informed consent**   consent a person gives based upon an appreciation and understanding of the facts, implications, and possible future consequences of an action.

**ingested poison**   a toxin that enters the body through the mouth.

**inhalation**   act of drawing breath or air into the lungs.

**inhaled poison**   a toxin that is absorbed through the lungs.

**injected poison**   a toxin injected into a vein or another tissue.

**injury pattern** a combination of injuries commonly seen in a patient based on the mechanism of injury.

**insulin** a hormone produced in the pancreas that regulates blood sugar levels.

**integumentary system** a group of specialized tissues that protect the body, retain fluids, and help prevent infection; the skin.

**intellectual disability** any condition that impairs normal information processing.

**intracranial** pertaining to inside the skull.

**intracranial pressure** the pressure within the skull; can also be exerted on the brain tissue and cerebrospinal fluid.

**invasive** refers to any medical procedure in which an instrument perforates, cuts through, or penetrates into the skin or body.

**irrigate** to wash out (a body cavity or wound) with water or a medicated fluid.

**ischemia** a deficiency in blood supply (and thus a deficiency of nutrients) to a tissue; if prolonged, may result in infarction.

## J

**"jams and pretzels"** a phrase that refers to the process by which someone who is injured and an awkward position is returned to normal supine anatomical position while maintaining spinal alignment.

**jaundice** a condition, characterized by yellowing of the skin, the whites of the eyes, mucous membranes, and body fluids, that typically indicates liver failure or disease.

**jaw-thrust maneuver** a method used to open a patient's airway by displacing the jaw forward; commonly used whenever spine injury is suspected because it helps to maintain cervical spine alignment.

**joint** a site at which two or more bones meet.

**joint capsule** a sheet of fibrous connective tissue enclosing a synovial joint.

## K

**Kehr's sign** pain in an uninjured shoulder caused by the accumulation of blood beneath the diaphragm; a painful right shoulder indicates a lacerated liver, whereas a painful left shoulder indicates a lacerated spleen.

**keratin** a hard protein substance of which hair, nails, and epidermal cells are made.

**khumbu cough** a dry, persistent cough caused by inhaling excessively cold dry air that is typical at high altitude; also known as high-altitude bronchitis.

**kinematics** the branch of mechanics that studies the movement of body segments without consideration given to its mass or the forces making it move.

**kinetic energy** the energy generated by a body in motion; mathematically expressed as mass × velocity.

**kyphosis** abnormally increased dorsal curvature of the thoracic spine.

## L

**laceration** a jagged open wound.

**lachrymal glands** glands that produce tears, which irrigate the surface of the eye.

**landing zone (LZ)** an area used to land a helicopter; for fixed wing aircraft, the LZ is a temporary runway.

**laryngospasm** spasm of the vocal cords that prevents air movement through the respiratory tract.

**lateral recumbent position** a position in which a patient is lying on the left or right side.

**leukocytes** (also called *white blood cells* or *WBCs*) blood cells produced by the immune system that travel through the bloodstream to attack and kill any foreign invaders (such as bacteria or viruses) that have entered the body.

**level I trauma center** a facility that provides the highest level of surgical care to trauma patients; requires the presence of certain number of surgeons and anesthesiologists at all times; provides 24-hour-a-day in-house coverage by general surgeons and prompt availability of care in orthopedic surgery, neurosurgery, emergency medicine, radiology, internal medicine, oral and maxillofacial surgery, and critical care.

**level II trauma center** a facility that collaborates with a level I trauma center to provide patients comprehensive trauma care; it supplements the clinical expertise of a level I institution and provides all essential specialties, personnel, and equipment 24 hours a day.

**level III trauma center** a facility that provides emergency medical care to trauma patients who do not need the services of a level I or a level II trauma center.

**level IV trauma center** a facility that provides the stabilization and treatment of severely injured patients in remote areas in which no alternative care is available.

**level of responsiveness (LOR)** the degree of cognitive function and arousal of the brain; ranges from fully alert to unresponsive.

**lift** the act of raising a person from a lower position to a higher position.

**ligament** tissue that connects a bone to another bone; connective tissue that provides structure for a joint.

**litter** a flat supporting framework, such as a piece of canvas stretched between two parallel shafts, for carrying a person; a stretcher.

**livor mortis** a purplish discoloration of the skin in the lowest parts of the body due to the settling of blood following death; also called dependent lividity.

**lockjaw** closure of the jaw due to a tonic spasm of the chewing muscles; is a potential sign of tetanus, a serious acute infection of the central nervous system caused by a bacterial infection of a wound (typically a puncture wound); also called trismus.

**long spine board (LSB)** a long rectangular board, 16 inches wide by 72 inches long, on which a patient with a spinal injury is placed.

**lordosis** abnormally increased anterior curvature of the spine (usually the lumbar spine).

**low voltage** electricity with a voltage of 50–1,000 V (AC) or 120–1,500 V (DC).

**low-angle rescue** any rescue work done by ascending or descending a slope that is less than approximately 45 degrees.

**lucid period** a short period during which the condition of a patient with a traumatic brain injury temporarily improves before again deteriorating.

**lymphatic system** a group of organs and other structures that remove extra fluid from tissues, absorbs and transports fats from the circulatory system, and transports immune cells to and from the lymph nodes.

## M

**mammalian diving reflex** a reflexive response to diving in many mammals that is characterized by physiological changes that decrease oxygen consumption (including slowed heart rate and decreased blood flow to the abdominal organs and muscles) until breathing resumes.

**mandated reporter**    an individual (such as a social worker, physician, teacher, police, EMT, or counselor) who is required to report to the appropriate authorities certain types of injuries or the suspicion of specific crimes.

**mandible**    the jaw bone.

**mast cell**    a type of connective tissue cell with numerous large cytoplasmic granules containing chemicals that are released during allergic reactions.

**material safety data sheet (MSDS)**    a form that contains relevant information pertaining to a specific substance, with a focus on the hazards it poses to workers.

**maxilla**    the bone of the mid-face; the cheek bone.

**mechanical hoist**    a device for lifting people from the ground; is often affixed to military and public safety helicopters.

**mechanisim of injury (MOI)**    the kind of force that acts on the body to cause injury; the method of trauma causing an injury.

**medical director**    a physician who is responsible for ensuring and evaluating the appropriate level and quality of care throughout an emergency care system. Also referred to as a medical advisor or physician supervisor.

**medical oversight**    the process by which a physician monitors the quality of medical care rendered to patients and provides assistance and guidance to prehospital providers and emergency care systems.

**melena**    black, tarry stools.

**meninges**    the three membranes that cover the brain and spinal cord: the arachnoid mater, pia mater, and dura mater.

**meningitis**    an inflammation of the membranes covering the spinal cord and brain; may be caused by viruses or bacteria.

**meningococcal**    of or relating to the meningococcus (the bacterium *Neisseria meningitidis*), the organism that causes epidemic cerebrospinal meningitis.

**meniscus**    a specialized cartilage found in some joints; such as the knee and the acromioclavicular (A/C) joint.

**metabolic rate**    the amount of energy expended in a given period of time.

**metabolic toxin**    a toxin that interferes with the normal energy- and chemical-producing mechanisms of the body.

**metabolism**    the chemical processes occurring within a living cell or organism that are necessary for the maintenance of life.

**microorganisms**    (also called *microbes*) microscopic (too small to be seen with the unaided eye) living organisms, including bacteria, fungi, and single-celled parasites (but excluding viruses and prions).

**minor consent**    consent a parent or legal guardian gives for the treatment of a minor because legally the minor is not competent to give consent to medical treatment; the ability to provide such consent varies among states.

**miscarriage**    a common term for a spontaneous abortion; the spontaneous termination of a pregnancy before about 20 weeks of gestation, at which time the fetus is not yet sufficiently developed to survive.

**mono-ski**    a sit-ski with one ski attached to the bottom of the device.

**morbidity**    illness; the rate of illness, expressed as the number of ill individuals in a particular population in a given period of time.

**mortality**    death; the death rate, expressed as the number of deaths in a particular population in a given period of time.

**move**    the passage of a patient from one location to another.

**mucous membrane**    a thin structure that lines those body passageways that communicate with the external environment and typically contains gland cells that produce mucus.

**multi-agency coordination system (MACS)**    a process for managing an incident in which multiple agencies that have different command structures and communication capabilities are participating.

**multiple casualty incident (MCI)**    an incident involving two or more patients or an incident in which the number of patients exceeds the capability of local resources.

**multiple sclerosis (MS)**    a progressive neurologic syndrome that causes weakness, paralysis of the extremities, and visual deficits.

**multisystem trauma**    trauma in which more than one major body system is involved.

**muscular dystrophy (MD)**    a syndrome characterized by progressive muscle degeneration.

**muscular system**    a group of specialized tissues that allow movement of the body, movement within the organs of the digestive system, and the beating of the heart.

**musculosketetal system (MS)**    the combination of the bony skeleton, the voluntary muscles, and other supporting structures that gives the body form and enables movement.

**myocardial contusion**    a bruise of the heart muscle.

**myocardium**    heart muscle tissue.

# N

**N95 mask**    a NIOSH mask that filters out 95 percent of airborne particulates.

**naris**    (plural: **nares**)    a nostril, one of the two channels of the nose.

**nasal cannula (NC)**    an airway adjunct that consists of plastic tubing with two open prongs that are inserted into the patient's nostrils; provides low-flow oxygen when connected to an oxygen source.

**nasopharyngeal airway (NPA)**    a trumpet-shaped airway adjunct made from soft rubber or silicone that is inserted into the nostril to maintain a patent airway.

**National Highway Traffic Safety Administration (NHTSA)**    an agency of the Executive Branch of the U.S. Government, part of the Department of Transportation, whose mission is "Save lives, prevent injuries, reduce vehicle-related crashes."

**National Incident Management System (NIMS)**    a federally mandated "all hazards" method for responding to and managing an incident; was created as a result of Homeland Security Presidential Directive-5.

**National Medical Advisor**    a licensed physician, MD, or DO with an interest in outdoor/wilderness medicine and ski patrolling, who is appointed by the National Ski Patrol's chairman and approved by the National Ski Patrol's board of directors to serve the NSP in all matters of medical concern; chairs the National Medical Committee.

**National Medical Committee**    a group of physicians that includes one doctor from each division of the National Ski Patrol, the National OEC Program Director and other physicians selected at large, and the National Medical Advisor.

**National OEC Program Committee**    a committee composed of all Division OEC Supervisors and the National Medical

Advisor, and chaired by the National OEC Program Director; provides insight and guidance to the Board of Directors annually on matters related to the functioning of the OEC program.

**National OEC Program Director** a National Ski Patrol member who is an active specialist in the field of outdoor medicine; is appointed by the NSP chairman and confirmed by the NSP board of directors; is responsible to the board for the effective management and operation of the national OEC program. This individual also chairs the national OEC Program Committee and serves as a member of the National Education Committee and the National Medical Committee.

**National OEC Refresher Committee** committee appointed and supervised by the National OEC Program Director; is responsible for developing the annual OEC Refresher program.

**National Ski Patrol System, Inc. (NSP)** the largest winter rescue group in the world, as recognized by the United States Congress under Title 36 of the United States Code; is the premier snow sports rescue organization in the United States.

**nature of illness (NOI)** evaluation to determine the type of medical illness present.

**near-drowning** survival for at least 24 hours after being suffocated by submersion in water.

**necrosis** death of tissue.

**negligence** the failure to exercise the care that a reasonably prudent person with similar training would exercise in a similar circumstance.

**nephron** the smallest functional unit of the kidney.

**nervous system** a group of organs and other structures that regulate all body functions.

**neural ischemia** a condition in which part of the brain or spinal cord receives too little oxygenated blood; damage to these organs results after only a few minutes of anoxia.

**neurologic** pertaining to the nervous system.

**neurologic compromise** impairment of the nervous system by disease, toxicity, or injury.

**neuron** nerve cell.

**neurosis** a condition in which a person exhibits abnormal behavior but remains able to understand the normal boundaries of reality.

**neurotransmitter** a chemical substance that transmits nerve impulses across a synapse from one nerve to another nerve.

**newborn** a child in the first month of life; children in this stage are also said to be in the neonatal period.

**nitrogen narcosis** intoxication caused by high nitrogen pressure during deep SCUBA diving.

**non-invasive** refers to a medical procedure that neither penetrates the skin nor enters the body.

**nonrebreather mask (NRB)** an oxygen delivery device that has a mask, a one-way flow valve, and a reservoir bag; when connected to an oxygen tank, provides a high concentration of supplemental oxygen.

**nonurgent move** the moving of a patient when no immediate threat to life exists.

**nutrition** the body's process of utilizing food substances needed for growth and the maintenance of life.

## O

**obstetrical** pertaining to obstetrics.

**obstetrics** the branch of medicine that treats women during pregnancy, childbirth, and immediately after childbirth.

**occlusive dressing** dressing made of Vaseline® gauze, aluminum foil, or plastic wrap that prevents air and liquids from entering or exiting a wound.

**occult** hidden.

**occupational exposure** an event in which a worker comes into contact with a bodily fluid or hazardous material while on the job.

**omentum** a fatty apron-like structure (fold of peritoneum) that covers the anterior surface of the intestines within the abdominal cavity.

**oocyte** a cell from which an egg or ovum develops.

**open chest injury** a chest injury that involves penetration of the chest wall.

**open injury** an injury in which a break in the skin or a mucous membrane exposes deeper tissue to potential contamination.

**opiate** a narcotic drug that is derived from and has the same effect as opium.

**OPQRST** a mnemonic that is used in the assessment of a patient's chief complaint: represents Onset, Provocation and palliation, Quality, Radiation, Severity, and Time.

**orbit** the bony socket of the eyeball.

**organ** a structure containing similar tissues that act together to perform specific body functions.

**oropharyngeal airway (OPA)** a rigid plastic airway adjunct that is inserted into the oropharynx to maintain a patent airway.

**oropharynx** the portion of the pharynx that lies directly behind the mouth.

**orthopedic** pertaining to orthopedics, the branch of medicine concerned with the function of the musculoskeletal system.

**orthopedic stretcher** a two-piece device that is slightly concave and has an open center section; is used to transport a patient; also called a "scoop" stretcher.

**osteoporosis** a disease process that leads to a reduction in bone mass.

**ostium** a small opening.

**ostomy bag** a bag for collecting urine or feces that attaches to the body with adhesive tape.

**Outdoor Emergency Care (OEC)** a course of medical instruction developed and taught by National Ski Patrol.

**Outdoor Emergency Care (OEC) Technician** a provider who has successfully completed the NSP's OEC course and has kept his annual refresher requirement current. CPR training, including AED training, are required of this individual.

**Outdoor First Care (OFC) Provider** a person who has completed the NSP's Outdoor First Care course and is trained to render basic first aid in outdoor, nonurban environments.

**outriggers** short skis mounted on crutch-type ski poles that provide better balance for a disabled skier.

**ova** (singular: **ovum**) female sex cells or gametes produced by an ovary; an ovum that has fused with a sperm cell develops into an embryo.

**ovarian cysts** sacs that develop on the surface of an ovary and contain either fluid or a semisolid material.

**ovaries** the female gonads, located on either side of the lower abdominopelvic region, which produce ova and the hormones estrogen and progesterone.

**ovulation**   the release of an ovum from an ovary.

**oxygen saturation**   the degree to which oxygen has bound to hemoglobin.

**oxygenation**   a process in which oxygen is added to the body's tissues.

# P

**pacemaker**   a device that substitutes for the pace-making tissue of the heart; can be surgically implanted.

**pallor**   paleness or an absence of normal skin coloration.

**palm method (palm rule)**   a method for estimating the extent of a patient's burns in which the burned area is compared to the surface area of the patient's palm, which equals about 1 percent of the body's surface area.

**palmar**   on the palm side of the hand.

**palpation**   during examination, touching or feeling with the hand; a pulse, for example, may be palpated with the fingertips.

**papillary dermis**   the topmost layer of the dermis, which consists primarily of loose connective tissue and is characterized by papillae (fingerlike projections) that interdigitate with the epidermis.

**paradoxical motion**   inward movement of a flail chest segment upon inhalation.

**paralysis**   loss or impairment of motor function in a part of the body.

**paramedic**   an allied health care professional who has successfully completed an NHTSA-approved paramedic course or its equivalent and is trained to deliver both basic and advanced life support.

**paraplegic**   people who do not have use of their legs.

**parasympathetic nervous system**   that part of the involuntary nervous system that slows the heart rate, regulates digestion, and dilates the pupils, along with other functions, and is antagonistic to the sympathetic nervous system.

**paresthesia**   sensation of tingling, pricking, or numbness of a person's skin, or the feeling of "pins and needles" or a limb being "asleep."

**partial pressure**   the pressure of a single gas within a mixture of gases; the partial pressure of each gas in a mixture of gases is equal to the pressure that gas would exert if it occupied the same volume alone at the same temperature.

**partial-thickness burn**   a second-degree burn.

**patency**   the state of being patent(open or unblocked).

**pathogen**   an infectious agent that can cause disease or illness.

**pathophysiology**   the study of the functional changes of the human body associated with or resulting from disease or injury.

**patient assessment**   the procedures performed to determine a patient's condition, especially any immediately life-threatening injuries or conditions; forms the basis for decisions about emergency medical care and transport.

**patient care report**   a report that documents a patient's complaints and past medical history, plus a chronological account of the examination and treatment of the patient; is a legal document.

**patient package**   the combination of the patient, any equipment needed to care for the patient, and the device used to transport the patient.

**pediatric assessment triangle**   an assessment tool that utilizes a pediatric patient's appearance (mental status, body position, and muscle tone), work of breathing (visible movement, effort, and audible sounds), and circulation (skin color) to assess the patient's well-being.

**pelvic binder**   a device that is either purchased commercially or made from a folded sheet and is used to compress the pelvis and control bleeding in a traumatic injury.

**pelvic inflammatory disease (PID)**   an inflammatory condition of the female reproductive tract, particularly the fallopian tubes; is usually caused by sexually transmitted microorganisms.

**pelvic**   pertaining to the pelvis, the basin-shaped bony structure that supports the spine and is the point of proximal attachment for the lower extremities.

**penetrating injury**   an injury caused when an object passes through the skin or other body tissues.

**perfusion**   the delivery of oxygen and nutrient-rich blood to tissues.

**pericardial fluid**   the serous fluid contained in the pericardium (the sac surrounding the heart).

**pericardial tamponade**   the accumulation of blood or other fluid within the pericardial sac.

**pericarditis**   inflammation of the pericardium or sac surrounding the heart, causing chest pain.

**perineum**   the anatomic region between the vulva in females or the scrotum in males, and the anus.

**periosteum**   the thin outer covering of a bone.

**peripheral blood flow**   circulation to areas outside the body's core (that is, to the skin and to the extremities).

**peripheral edema**   the accumulation of fluids (swelling of tissues) in the body's periphery, usually in the lower part of the legs.

**peripheral nervous system**   the part of the nervous system outside the central nervous system.

**peristalsis**   rhythmic contractions of a tubular organ (such as the intestines) that propel the contents of the organ forward.

**peritoneal fluid**   the fluid that lubricates surfaces in the abdominal cavity to prevent friction between the peritoneal membrane and internal organs.

**peritonitis**   an inflammation (irritation) of the peritoneum, the thin tissue that lines the inner wall of the abdomen and covers most of the abdominal organs.

**PERRL**   a mnemonic for assessing the eyes (i.e., Pupils Equal, Round, Reactive to Light).

**personal protective equipment (PPE)**   items worn by medical providers, including gloves, mask, safety eyeglasses (or mask with shield), and gown, to protect them from bodily fluids.

**petit mal seizure**   a seizure consisting of a sudden, temporary loss of mental awareness and physical activity lasting a few seconds to several minutes.

**pharynx**   the passageway that extends from the nose and mouth to the larynx; consists of three parts: nasopharynx, oropharynx, and laryngopharynx.

**physical examination (physical exam)**   an evaluation of the body and its functions using inspection, palpation, and auscultation (listening).

**physiologic**   pertaining to physiology (that is, to normal, healthy body functioning), as opposed to pathology (abnormal body functioning).

**physiology** the study of how living organisms function (e.g., movement or reproduction).

**pia mater** the innermost of the three membranes (meninges) covering the brain and the spinal cord.

**pitting edema** swelling usually of the ankles that, when pressed with a finger tip, leaves a temporary indentation.

**placenta** the vascular organ, consisting of both maternal and embryonic tissues, that forms in the uterus during pregnancy and is the site of the transfer of oxygen and nutrients from mother to fetus, and removes fetal wastes.

**placenta previa** low implantation of the placenta such that it partially or completely covers the internal opening of the uterus; upon the onset of any contractions and cervical dilation, or when the cervix begins to dilate at the onset of labor, the placenta is stretched and pulled from the uterine wall, producing painless bleeding that may be life threatening to both mother and fetus.

**plantarflex** movement of the foot or toes downward, toward the sole of the foot.

**platelets** solid elements in the blood that aid in clotting.

**pleura** the thin serous membrane that envelops each lung and folds back to line the chest cavity.

**pleural fluid** the thin film of serous fluid that surrounds and lubricates the surfaces of the lungs.

**pleural space** the potential space that lies within the pleura covering the outside of the lungs and the inside of the chest wall.

**pleuritic pain** chest wall pain resulting from inflammation of the pleura (thin serous membrane) that envelops each lung.

**pneumococcal** of, derived from, or caused by the pneumococcus (the bacterium *Streptococcus pneumoniae*), the most common cause of bacterial pneumonia.

**pneumothorax** an abnormal collection of air within the pleural space.

**pocket mask** a barrier device; a folding mask with an oxygen inlet valve that is used for artificial ventilation; may be used with or without supplemental oxygen.

**poison** any substance that is injurious to health or dangerous to life.

**polydipsia** excessive thirst and fluid intake.

**polyphagia** excessive hunger.

**polypharmacy** the simultaneous use of several medications in combination.

**polyuria** excessive excretion of urine.

**popliteal fossa** posterior part of the knee.

**portable stretcher** a litter consisting of an aluminum frame and a vinyl-coated platform, with cut-outs for the rescuer's hands at each corner and along each side to facilitate carrying by multiple rescuers.

**positional asphyxia** a fatal condition in which a patient's body weight impairs the ability to breathe, resulting in suffocation.

**post-ictal** after a seizure.

**post-ictal state** the recovery period following the clonic phase of a generalized seizure, during which the patient commonly appears weak, exhausted, confused, and disoriented but progressively improves.

**power grip** a technique for gripping that places as much hand surface as possible in contact with the object being lifted, all fingers bent at the same angle, the two hands at least 10 inches apart.

**power lift** a technique that combines optimal anatomic positioning with good body mechanics to enable lifting a heavy object without becoming injured.

**pre-ictal** before a seizure.

**preeclampsia** a toxemia during pregnancy characterized by high blood pressure and edema of the hands or face; also called pregnancy-induced hypertension (PIH).

**prehospital care** any medical care rendered by trained personnel prior to arrival at a hospital.

**prehospital provider** a person who is specially trained to render medical care to a patient outside of a hospital or medical care facility.

**preschool period** the period of childhood during ages 3–6 years; a time in which a child gains fine motor skills and greater independence.

**pressure dressing** a dressing that closes bleeding blood vessels by compressing the wound.

**primary assessment** the initial assessment of an ill or injured patient that includes evaluating the airway, breathing, circulation, and disability (mental status and neurologic function).

**primary blast injury** an injury that results when the shock wave of an explosion moves from solid and liquid-filled organs (which are not subject to primary blast injury) to gas-filled organs (the lungs, gastrointestinal tract, and middle ear).

**privileged communication** a communication that cannot be disclosed without the consent of the person who made it.

**prophylactic** refers to something that protects against or prevents, especially disease; an agent that tends to ward off disease or pregnancy.

**protocols** written procedures for assessing, treating, and transporting a patient. Protocols are generally written by a team of emergency care professionals and managed by a medical director.

**pruritis** severe itching of the skin.

**pruritus** severe itching; frequently occurs in the skin during mild and moderate allergic reactions.

**psychosis** a condition in which a person exhibits abnormal behavior and has altered perceptions of reality.

**pulmonary** pertaining to the lungs.

**pulmonary blood vessels** the vessels that serve the lungs; include the pulmonary arteries, which carry deoxygenated blood from the right ventricle to the lungs, and the pulmonary veins, which carry oxygenated blood from the lungs to the left heart and then to the rest of the body.

**pulmonary contusion** a bruise of the lung tissue.

**pulmonary edema** accumulation of fluid in the lungs.

**pulmonary embolism** a condition in which a clot or other obstruction (an embolus) partially or completely blocks a pulmonary artery.

**pulse** rhythmic expansion of an artery caused by the movement of blood.

**pulse oximeter** a device that attaches to a patient's finger, toe, or earlobe and photoelectrically measures blood oxygen content as percent of oxygen saturation.

**pulse pressure** the difference between the maximum (systolic) and minimum (diastolic) blood pressures during a single heartbeat.

**pulsus paradoxus** a decrease in pulse strength (a reduction in blood pressure of more than 10 mmHg) during inhalation; results from increased intrathoracic pressure that suppresses the filling of the ventricles with blood.

**puncture** a penetrating wound resulting from a sharp, pointed object.

## Q

**quadriplegic** people who have lost function in all four extremities are called quadriplegics.

**quaternary blast injury** any blast injury that is not classified as a primary, secondary, or tertiary blast injury, including burns, crushing injuries, and respiratory injuries.

## R

**rabies** an acute, infectious, often fatal viral disease of the nervous system transmitted via the saliva by the bite of infected animals.

**radiation** a form of heat exchange in which energy is transmitted in waves (electromagnetic, ultraviolet, infrared) through space.

**rash** a temporary eruption on the skin.

**reasonable force** the minimum force needed to keep a patient from hurting themselves or others.

**receptor** a cell component with which a chemical messenger combines to alter the function of the cell.

**recurrent traumatic brain injury** a condition in which the head suffers multiple, successive injuries before a previous injury has fully healed; subsequent injuries can be much more severe due to the occurrence of previous injuries.

**referred pain** pain that originates in one part of the body but is felt in another part of the body.

**refresher** annual required continuing education training, usually given each year in the fall, that covers one-third of topics taught in the OEC curriculum.

**repetitive head injury (RHI)** a condition in which the head suffers multiple, successive injuries before a previous injury has fully healed; the most recent injury can be much more severe due to cumulative effects.

**reproductive age** the portion of the life cycle in which individuals can produce offspring—typically, years 15–50 among women, although some women can become pregnant at a younger age or at an older age.

**reproductive system** a group of organs and other structures responsible for human reproduction.

**rescue** the process of extracting a person or group from distress or danger.

**resistance blood vessel** a small artery whose wall contains muscle cells capable of contraction; as a result, such vessels can constrict and dilate to redistribute blood flow.

**resource** an individual, a single piece of equipment and its personnel complement, or a crew or team of individuals with an identified work supervisor, that can be used at an incident.

**respiration** the act of breathing in and out; also, the act of taking in of oxygen and nutrients and giving off of carbon dioxide and waste products by a cell.

**respiratory system** a group of organs and other structures that bring oxygen in the air into the body and eliminate carbon dioxide into the air through a process called breathing or respiration.

**restraint** any method, physical or mechanical, that restricts the movement of a patient.

**reticular dermis** the deepest layer of the dermis, consisting chiefly of dense fibrous tissue.

**retina** the structure at the back of the eye that has light receptor cells responsible for vision.

**retinal detachment** separation of the retina from the inside of the posterior wall of the eyeball.

**retraction** the condition in which muscles pull in between the ribs and above the sternum upon inhalation.

**retrograde amnesia** loss of memory of events that occurred before a traumatic event to the brain; an inability to recall old information.

**reverse squeeze** pain or injury to a gas-containing part of the body (for example, the sinuses) during decompression (that is, ascent) while diving.

**rigor mortis** stiffening of the body after death.

**Rothberg position** a sitting position in which the patient's upper body is raised 45 degrees and the knees are slightly bent; is used often for patients who are experiencing chest pain or a suspected heart attack.

**rule of nines** a method for estimating the surface extent of a burn, in which each of 11 defined surface areas of the body represents 9 percent of an adult's body surface, with the genital area representing the remaining 1 percent.

**ruptured aorta** development of a leak in the largest blood vessel in the body; results in massive bleeding that is usually fatal.

## S

**salinity** the degree of saltiness.

**SAMPLE** an acronym used to obtain medical history information during the assessment process; refers to Signs/symptoms, Allergies, Medications, Past medical history, Last oral intake, Events leading up to present incident.

**scald** an injury caused by a hot liquid or a hot, moist vapor.

**scenario** a simulated problem that mimics a real-life medical situation.

**scene safety** the process of assessing the site of an accident or disaster and making it safe for rescuers to enter.

**scene size-up** the first step of the assessment process, consisting of four components: scene safety, mechanism of injury, total number of patients involved, and the need for additional resources.

**schizophrenia** a psychiatric disorder in which a person cannot distinguish what is real from what is not real.

**school-aged child** a child ages 6–12 years.

**scoliosis** abnormal lateral curvature of the spine.

**"Scope of Practice"** a set of rules, regulations, and ethical considerations that define the extent, boundaries, and limitations of a prehospital provider's duties.

**search** a methodical process of actively gathering information about a person or group in distress or danger and then physically looking for them.

**sebaceous glands** glands in the skin that produce sebum, a substance that lubricates the skin's surface; also called oil glands.

**second-degree burn** a burn that affects the epidermis and the dermis and results in blisters.

**secondary assessment** the thorough, systematic physical examination that follows a primary assessment and any immediate resuscitation.

**secondary blast injury** an injury due to bomb fragments, shrapnel, and other objects propelled by an explosion; may produce visible hemorrhage or extensive but inapparent internal hemorrhage into body cavities.

**secondary drowning** the death of a drowning victim at some significant period after the immersion event.

**Section Chief** the head of a functional area within the Incident Command System.

**semi-Fowler position** a sitting position in which the patient's upper body is raised to 45 degrees; is commonly used for patients who are awake and are not suspected of having a serious injury or illness.

**sensory nerves** nerves that send signals to the brain for perception of touch, pressure, heat, cold, and pain.

**sepsis** a serious medical condition caused by the presence of pathogenic organisms or their toxins in the blood leading to a systemic inflammatory response.

**shaken baby syndrome** a condition in which an infant or toddler is picked up and violently shaken, causing a traumatic brain injury.

**sharps** a term for needles, scalpels, or any other pointed objects that could cause wounds or punctures to personnel handling them.

**shock** failure of the circulatory system to maintain adequate blood flow to tissues.

**sign** any objective finding that can be seen, heard, smelled, or measured; typically discovered during a physical exam (e.g., a bruise, the patient's blood pressure).

**simple chest wall contusion** swelling, bruising, and pain due to chest wall trauma in the absence of damage to any underlying structures.

**sit-board** a device in which a bucket used for sitting is attached to a snowboard.

**sit-ski** a device consisting of two basic components: a "bucket" or seat on which the adaptive athlete sits, and one or two skis attached to the bucket.

**skeletal muscle** type of muscle that attaches to the bony skeleton and is controlled voluntarily by the nervous system; functions to move joints to perform physical activities.

**skeletal system** a group of specialized tissues that provide support to the body, provide attachment points for muscles, protect internal organs, allow movement, store minerals, and constitute one of the sites where blood cells are made; the bones.

**ski bra** a device that attaches near the tips of each ski to hold the skis apart so the tips cannot cross.

**sleeping altitude** the altitude to which a climber descends to sleep to prevent AMS; is typically 500–1,000 feet below the highest elevation of that day's ascent.

**sliding board** a flat board, 12 inches by 36 inches, made of smooth wood or plastic, used to transfer someone to or from a wheelchair.

**sling and swathe** a soft splint used to immobilize many upper extremity injuries.

**smooth muscle** type of muscle found in organs of the body; is controlled by the autonomic nervous system; functions to push food through the intestine, contract blood vessels, and regulate other internal functions.

**snoring** an abnormal respiratory sound caused by partial obstruction of the airway.

**snow blindness** sunburn-like injury to the eye caused by excessive exposure to sunlight; can be so painful that victims cannot keep their eyes open and therefore cannot see; occurs especially at high altitudes and when sunlight reflects off of snow; also called ultraviolet keratitis or solar keratitis.

**solar keratitis** see *snow blindness*.

**span of control** the total number of individuals or resources supervised by a single person; usually 3–7 individuals or resources.

**spastic cerebral palsy** a form of CP that causes constant, involuntary muscle contractions.

**special operations** infrequently performed activities requiring specialized training and equipment in remote and/or difficult settings.

**spina bifida (SB)** a congenital malformation that results in gaps within the bony spine that expose the spinal cord to injury.

**spinal cord** tubular bundle of nervous tissue and support cells that extends from the brain downward to the sacrum within the vertebral canal; part of the central nervous system.

**spinal cord injury (SCI)** damage to the spinal cord due to trauma.

**spine** the bony structures (vertebrae) that serve as the body's backbone.

**spleen** an organ in the left upper abdominal quadrant that filters the blood and serves as a body's reservoir of blood.

**splint** a mechanical device used to prevent a part of the body from moving, protecting it from further injury.

**sprain** a stretched or torn ligament.

**squeeze** a term for a type of barotrauma in which various gas-containing areas of the body, such as the lungs or inner ear, are injured during underwater diving.

**stabilized extrication** keeping a patient's spine anatomically aligned during removal from an accident, therefore preventing any neurologic damage.

**stair chair** a portable evacuation chair that enables a patient to be transported in a seated position.

**standard of care** a level of care an OEC Technician must render based on OEC training, local medical protocols, and the requirements of a state's emergency medical system.

**standard of training** the training of National Ski Patrol OEC Technicians as set forth in the OEC course, using this text as a reference.

**Standard Precautions** the practice of protecting health care workers from exposure to bodily fluids based on the assumption that all patients are potentially infectious.

**START** a triage system commonly used by public safety personnel; an acronym for Simple Triage and Rapid Treatment.

**sterile** free from living microorganisms such as bacteria, viruses, or spores that may cause infection.

**sternocleidomastoid muscle** the powerful muscle at the sides of the neck that facilitate turning of the head.

**Stokes stretcher** (Stokes litter) a wire or plastic basket, shaped to accommodate an adult in a supine position, into which a victim is strapped for transport.

**stoma** a surgical port created in the body.

**stopping distance** the minimum distance required for a particular vehicle to stop at a given speed.

**straddle injury** an injury to the pelvis and the internal organs between the genitals and anus that results when a patient forcefully straddles a fixed object.

**strain** a stretched or torn muscle or tendon.

**stretcher** a litter.

**strike team** a group of resources of the same size or type that is managed by a strike team leader (e.g., a group of Nordic Patrollers).

**stroke volume** the volume of blood pumped out of the heart's left ventricle per contraction.

**subcutaneous emphysema** air-filled bubbles that are palpable underneath the skin; indicates an injury to an airway structure.

**subcutaneous tissue** tissue between the dermis and the fascia overlying the muscle; contains fat, nerves, and blood vessels.

**subdural hematoma** an accumulation of blood between the outer covering of the brain (dura mater) and the surface of the brain.

**subjective** arising out of an individual's perceptions of some internal state; the opposite of objective, thus a symptom is subjective because it can be identified by the patient only, whereas a sign is objective (can be detected by some outside observer).

**subluxation** an event in which a joint dislocates partially and returns to its normal anatomical position.

**submersion injuries** bodily insults caused by being immersed; examples are drowning or near-drowning and hypothermia.

**substance abuse** the intentional misuse of a substance that results in significant impairment.

**subungual hematoma** a painful extra-vascular collection of blood under a nail.

**sucking chest wound** a chest wound that penetrates the pleura or lung, allowing air to be "sucked" into the pleural space upon each inspiration.

**suctioning** a procedure that uses negative pressure to remove an object or a fluid.

**sudden cardiac arrest (SCA)** the abrupt cessation of an effective heartbeat.

**sudden infant death syndrome** the sudden, unexplained death of an infant in which a postmortem examination fails to determine the cause of death.

**suicide** the intentional taking of one's own life.

**sunburn** inflammation of the skin caused by overexposure to sunlight.

**superficial burn** a first-degree burn.

**supine** lying on the back.

**swelling** an enlargement of body tissue caused by an accumulation of excess fluid.

**symphysis pubis** the site on the anterior pelvis at which the two pubic bones are joined together.

**symptom** a subjective finding that a patient experiences and can be identified only by the patient (e.g., pain, blurred vision).

**synapse** the junction between two neurons at which an impulse is transmitted from one to the other, usually by a chemical neurotransmitter.

**syncope** a transient loss of consciousness resulting from inadequate cerebral blood flow.

**synovial fluid** the fluid, secreted by the synovial membrane, that lubricates the movement of bones in a synovial joint.

**synovium** the inner layer of the joint capsule whose cells make a viscous fluid that lubricates joints.

## T

**tachycardia** a heart rate greater than 100 beats per minute in adults.

**tachypnea** an increased respiration rate; in adults, greater than 30 rpm.

**task force** a combination of different resources with common communications that is managed by a task force leader (e.g., a sheriff's deputy, an NSP alpine patrol, and a search-and-rescue team).

**tendon** the non-contractile continuation of a muscle that gives it a mechanical advantage.

**tension** the amount of force necessary to stretch something; when used to refer to aligning a fractured long bone, the force required to straighten out the affected limb (usually 7–8 pounds).

**tension pneumothorax** the accumulation of pressurized air within the pleural space; causes the displacement of the great vessels, tracheal deviation, distention of the jugular veins, and compression of the other lung.

**tepid** lukewarm.

**terrorism** a human-caused event that is intended to inflict fear and can involve hazardous materials.

**tertiary blast injury** a blunt trauma injury (such as a bone fracture or a coup-contrecoup injury) caused when an individual experiencing an explosion becomes a missile and is thrown against other objects.

**tetanus** a serious acute infection of wounds caused by the bacterium *Clostridium tetani*, which releases a toxin that damages central nervous system structures.

**tether** a strap (or pair of straps) that is attached to an adaptive skier's waist or to a sit-ski to guide the skier and prevent excessive speed.

**thermal** pertaining to heat.

**thermoregulation** the process of maintaining normal body temperature.

**third-degree burn** a burn that destroys the epidermis and the dermis and extends into the subcutaneous tissue.

**thoracic** pertaining to the chest.

**three tracker** a skier with one leg who uses one ski and outriggers on both arms.

**thrombus** a clot in the blood.

**thymus gland** an endocrine structure in the upper chest that, as a part of the immune response, secretes a hormone (thymosin) that stimulates the development and maturation of T lymphocytes.

**tissue** a collection of cells acting together to perform a specific body function.

**toddler** a child ages 12–36 months; the stage at which a child begins to explore, climb, and speak simple words or phrases.

**tonic activity** a general stiffening of the muscles.

**tonicity** a property of solutions that relates to the concentration of solutes (such as salt) it contains, and how the water in a solution moves across a cell membrane; water in a solution crosses a cell membrane from the side that has the lower tonicity (a hypotonic solution) to the side that has the higher tonicity (a hypertonic solution); pure water is hypotonic to the solution within cells because that solution contains salts.

**tonsil tip** (also called *tonsil sucker*) a rigid plastic tube that is part of a suctioning system.

**tourniquet** an instrument that when tightened around an arm or leg temporarily arrests the flow of blood through a large artery.

**toxicological event** an event where a patient has been exposed to a harmful substance OR an incident in which the intentional or unintentional use of a substance or poison either endangers public safety and/or results in a medical emergency.

**toxin** a noxious or poisonous substance produced by an organism.

**trachea** the respiratory system structure that connects the pharynx to the bronchi; the "windpipe."

**traction** the amount of force required to straighten a limb and keep it in alignment; for a fractured femur, typically 10 percent of the patient's body weight, or approximately 15 pounds.

**traction splint** a splint used on a lower extremity to align a fracture, such as a mid-shaft fracture of the femur.

**transfer flat** a large sheet-like device, used to lift large and heavy patients, that is constructed of thick, reinforced material and has both load-bearing straps and handles sewn into the device.

**transport** to convey from one place to another.

**transport vehicles** various engine-powered vehicles (such as all-terrain vehicles or ATVs, snow machines, golf carts, automobiles, ambulances, etc.) used to transport patients.

**trauma** physical injury caused by an external force.

**trauma center** a specialized hospital providing 24-hour trauma care, including stabilization, critical care, subspecialty care, and nursing care.

**trauma surgeon** a physician who specializes in trauma care.

**traumatic asphyxia** the inability to breathe and hypoxia that results from the inability of the chest wall to expand due to external pressure or massive crushing trauma.

**traumatic brain injury** physical trauma to the brain; can be localized or diffuse.

**traumatologist** a surgeon who specializes in trauma care.

**Trendelenburg position** a position in which the patient's head is lowered 15–30 degrees (below the level of the heart) while the feet are simultaneously raised approximately 15–30 degrees; is generally used for patients who are in shock.

**triage** a process of prioritizing patients for treatment and transportation based on their clinical signs and symptoms.

**tripod position** a position in which a patient sits upright and leans forward onto outstretched arms; the head and chin are thrust forward in an attempt to keep the airway open.

**tuberculosis (TB)** an infectious bacterial disease, caused by the tubercle bacillus (*Myocobacterium tuberculosis*), that most commonly causes inflammation and calcification within the respiratory system and may infect other body organs.

**two track skiing** the use of two skis only by an adaptive skier; can include the use of adaptive equipment such as tethers and ski bras.

**two-person assist** a method in which two rescuers (on each side) assist a patient to move down a slope or trail in the same manner used in the human crutch.

# U

**ultraviolet keratitis** see *snow blindness*.

**ultraviolet radiation** waves of solar energy that are beneficial in small amounts but harmful to the skin and eyes upon overexposure.

**umbilical cord** the fetal structure containing the blood vessels that carry blood to and from the placenta.

**umbilicus** the navel.

**universal dressing** sterile, soft, highly absorbent, individually wrapped dressing that provides superior padding and protection for major wounds; usually measures 12 inches by 30 inches; also called *trauma dressing*.

**Universal Precautions** the use of equipment, including gloves, gowns, masks, and protective eyewear, to prevent the transmission of blood-borne pathogens in any bodily secretion whenever first aid or health care is provided; under Universal Precautions, rescuers *always* consider the blood and body fluids of *any* patient to be potentially infectious.

**urgent move** prompt transport of a patient whenever the patient's condition or dangerous location poses an immediate threat to life.

**urinary system** a group of organs and structures that remove wastes and toxins from the blood and excrete them in urine.

**urine** fluid waste product of humans that is produced by filtration and secretion of the kidneys.

**urticaria** hives or rashes that accompany an allergic reaction.

**uterus** the muscular abdominal female organ in which a fetus develops; the womb.

# V

**vaccination** a process for providing protection against communicable diseases by stimulating the immune system to produce antibodies against that disease; also called immunization.

**vaccine** a preparation that contains all or part of a disease agent (rendered non-infectious) and is typically administered to an individual to prevent infection with that agent.

**vagina** the birth canal.

**valgus** medial (inward) angulation of a bone or joint (toward the midline).

**varicella-zoster virus** the virus that causes chickenpox and herpes zoster.

**varus** lateral (outward) angulation of a bone or joint (away from the midline).

**vasoconstriction** the narrowing of the lumen of a blood vessel.

**vasodilation** the widening of the lumen of a blood vessel.

**ventilation** the process by which air moves into and out of the lungs, so that oxygen can be exchanged for carbon dioxide in the alveoli.

**ventral** on the front of the body.

**ventricular fibrillation** chaotic and ineffective contraction of the ventricles that leads to cardiac arrest.

**ventricular tachycardia** rapid contraction of the ventricles that can lead to ineffective blood flow to body tissues and eventually cardiac arrest.

**vertebrae** (singular: **vertebra**) the 33 bones of the spinal column.

**viruses** a group of infectious particles, smaller than cells and not generally considered living, many of which cause disease in humans.

**visceral nerves** a collection of nerves that convey impulses between a part of the central nervous system and a viscus, such as an internal organ in the chest or abdomen.

**visual impairment** a range of visual disabilities that include legal blindness, partial sightedness, and complete blindness.

**vital capacity** the maximum amount of air that can be expired following a maximum inhalation.

**vital signs** the key objective findings used to evaluate a patient's overall condition; includes pulse rate, respiratory rate, blood pressure, temperature, and level of responsiveness.

**volar** on the front of the body.

**volt (V)** a unit of electric potential or electromotive force, equal to 1 watt per ampere or 1 joule per coulomb.

# W

**warm zone** a transition area surrounding the hot zone; the zone in which decontamination occurs.

**wet drowning** a submersion injury in which the victim breathes (aspirates) water into the lungs.

**wheezing** a high-pitched respiratory sound caused by a narrowing of the tubular airways.

**white blood cells** blood cells (leukocytes) that fight infection and produce substances that fight infection.

**wind chill** the apparent temperature felt on exposed skin; is a function of the air temperature and wind speed.

**withdrawal** the physical and mental readjustment that accompanies the discontinued use of an addictive substance.

# Y

**Yankauer tip (suction catheter)** a rigid metal or plastic tube that is curved at its distal end to aid in the removal of thick secretions during oropharyngeal suctioning.

# Z

**zone of injury** the area that is close to or surrounding an injury of an extremity, such as a sprain or fracture.

# Answer Key

## Chapter 1
### STOP, THINK, UNDERSTAND *(p. 14)*
**Multiple Choice**

1. b (p. 8)
2. d (p. 27)
3. b (p. 6)
4. d (p. 15)

**Short Answer**

1. River guides, bike patrollers, law enforcement personnel, mountain guides, personnel of various government agencies. (p. 7)
2. The Tenth Mountain Division was a mountain warfare unit in World War II. The division came into being after "Minnie" Dole convinced General George C. Marshall of the value of a winter warfare unit. Thus, the NSP became the only civilian agency ever authorized to recruit for the armed forces, getting seven volunteers. In 1944 the "Tenth" performed with distinction in combat in Italy. The ski run at Vail named Riva Ridge honors the men who participated in an assault in Italy. After the war many members of the "Tenth" came home and became leaders in the ski industry. (p. 4)

### STOP, THINK, UNDERSTAND *(p. 26)*
**Multiple Choice**

1. c (p. 15)
2. d (p. 23)
3. d (p. 21)
4. b (p. 22)

**Short Answer**

1. Good Samaritan laws are designed to encourage volunteer rescuers to provide first-aid care without fear of being held liable for their actions. (p. 15)
2. *Standard of training* is the minimum level of training taught in NSP's Outdoor Emergency Care program. (p. 20) *Standard of care* includes the training set forth in the OEC text but also includes (but may not be limited to) an area's local protocols; a state's emergency medical services restrictions, laws, and procedures; and the geographic area and circumstances in which the rescuer is located. (p. 21)

**Matching**

1. c (p. 17)
2. d (p. 18)
3. b (p. 23)
4. e (p. 18)
5. a (p. 17)
6. f (p. 18)
7. g (p. 18)

### CHAPTER QUESTIONS *(p. 27)*
**Multiple Choice**

1. b (p. 19)
2. c (p. 11)
3. a (p. 8)
4. c (p. 17)
5. a (p. 22)

**Short Answer**

1. (any 10 of the following) assess safety and maintain it at a rescue scene; use proper body substance isolation techniques; assess a patient's level of responsiveness; establish and maintain an airway; assess respiration and provide adequate ventilation; provide oxygen when necessary; assess perfusion of blood to the body's tissues; control bleeding; identify and care for life-threatening problems, including shock; obtain a medical history of the patient; assess and provide specific care for different injuries; assess and provide care for medical illness; understand the assessment and treatment nuances in special populations; be able to splint or immobilize various body parts, including the spine; learn the concept of triage, and be able to help in a mass-casualty incident; be able to use rescue equipment, and pack your rescue pack appropriately; understand your role in prehospital care; be able to document care rendered in a way all medical personnel can understand; understand your ski area management's needs and interface with management; be able to identify the names of common medications and describe their basic actions (p. 10)
2. To maintain your OEC certification, you must complete an annual OEC refresher course. Each year the NSP develops a continuing education program that enables OEC technicians to "refresh" their knowledge and skills. One-third of the curriculum is presented each year. Refreshers are primarily a "hands-on" learning experience, allowing the OEC Technician to demonstrate proficiency in the skills needed to care for a patient. Upon successful completion of the refresher *each subsequent* year after completion of a full OEC course, the OEC Technician maintains the certification for another year. The refresher is developed annually by the NSP OEC Refresher Committee, and the curriculum is provided to NSP instructors. (p. 11)

**Scenario**

1. c (p. 21)
2. b (p. 15)
3. d (p. 12)
4. a (p. 17)
5. d (p. 20)
6. a (p. 17)

## Chapter 2
### STOP, THINK, UNDERSTAND *(p. 44)*
**Multiple Choice**

1. d (p. 40)
2. b (p. 42)
3. d (p. 35)
4. a (p. 40)

**Short Answer**

1. (any six of the following) integration of health services; research; legislation and regulation; system finance; human resources; medical direction; education system; public education; prevention; public access; communication system; clinical care; information systems; evaluation (pp. 35–36)
2. Continuity of care is the seamless delivery of high-quality emergency medical care as patients transition from their initial contact with a first responder through definitive treatment. (p. 41)

### CHAPTER QUESTIONS *(p. 52)*
**Multiple Choice**

1. a (p. 47)
2. b (p. 50)
3. a (p. 46)
4. d (p. 49)
5. c (p. 49)
6. c (p. 48)
7. a (p. 48)
8. b (p. 32)
9. d (p. 38)

**Matching**

1.
   1. c, f (p. 39)
   2. a, g (p. 39)
   3. e (p. 40)
   4. b, d (p. 40)
2.
   1. a, d (p. 50)
   2. c, f (p. 50)
   3. b, e (p. 50)

**Labeling**

a. IO (p. 49)
b. DO (p. 49)
c. DO (p. 49)
d. IO (p. 49)
e. DO (p. 49)

**Short Answer**

OEC Technicians are an essential part of the emergency care system and provide emergency assistance and transportation to patients not served by traditional 911 providers. (pp. 51–52)

**Scenario**

1. c (p. 40)
2. c (p. 47)
3. a (p. 48)
4. c (p. 49)

## Chapter 3
### STOP, THINK, UNDERSTAND *(p. 72)*
**Multiple Choice**

1. d (p. 61)
2. a (p. 59)
3. b (p. 62)
4. b (p. 66)
5. d (p. 70)

**Fill in the Blank**

1. arm, leg (p. 62)
2. (any four of the following) inadequate sleep, poor nutrition, physical or emotional stress, alcohol abuse, chemotherapy, diabetes, smoking, steroid use, chronic infection (p. 63)
3. Cotton (p. 66)
4. warm, cold (p. 59)

**Matching**

1. d (p. 59)
2. a (p. 60)
3. c (p. 60)
4. b (p. 60)

## STOP, THINK, UNDERSTAND *(p. 83)*

### Multiple Choice

**1.** c (p. 74)  **4.** c (p. 75)
**2.** b (p. 79)  **5.** d (p. 73)
**3.** a (p. 74)

### Fill in the Blank

direct contact, indirect contact, airborne, ingestion, vector-borne (pp. 71–73)

### Matching

**1.** d (p. 61)  **6.** d (p. 73)
**2.** e (p. 73)  **7.** a (p. 71)
**3.** a (p. 71)  **8.** b (p. 72)
**4.** e (p. 73)  **9.** b (p. 72)
**5.** c (p. 72)  **10.** c (p. 72)

## CHAPTER QUESTIONS *(p. 95)*

### Multiple Choice

**1.** d (p. 76)  **11.** d (pp. 60–61)
**2.** c (p. 59)  **12.** a. X (p. 85)
**3.** a (p. 62)  b.
**4.** d (p. 57)  c. X (p. 85)
**5.** b (p. 90)  d.
**6.** d (p. 82)  e. X (p. 85)
**7.** c (p. 94)  f. X (p. 85)
**8.** b (p. 71)  g.
**9.** a (p. 77)  h. X (p. 85)
**10.** d (p. 86)  i.

### Fill in the Blank

**1.** (any four of the following) waterproof matches, flashlight, carabiner, multipurpose tool, sunblock, whistle, radio, cell phone, signal mirrors, map, compass (pp. 67–68)
**2.** The base layer is usually tight against the skin, helping to retain heat while allowing moisture to be transferred toward the exterior, a process known as wicking. (p. 66)
**3.** The middle layer serves as the insulating layer and helps to trap warm air. (p. 66)

### Scenario

**1.** d (p. 66)  **2.** b (p. 67)

# Chapter 4

## STOP, THINK, UNDERSTAND *(p. 113)*

### Multiple Choice

**1.** c (pp. 100–101)  **3.** b (pp. 98–99)
**2.** d (p. 104)

### Fill in the Blank  See Incident Command Structure below.

## STOP, THINK, UNDERSTAND *(p. 122)*

### Multiple Choice

**1.** c (p. 120)  **3.** d (p. 120)
**2.** a (p. 114)  **4.** a (p. 114)

### Matching

**1.** c (p. 115)  **3.** a (p. 115)
**2.** b (p. 115)  **4.** d (p. 115)

## CHAPTER QUESTIONS *(p. 123)*

### Multiple Choice

**1.** b (p. 120)  **5.** b (p. 123)
**2.** d (p. 107)  **6.** a (p. 104)
**3.** a (p. 100)  **7.** d (p. 115)
**4.** d (p. 104)

### Matching

**1.** a, e, g, j (p. 116)  **3.** b, f, h (p. 117)
**2.** c, i (p. 116)  **4.** d (p. 117)

### Scenario

**1.** d (p. 104)  **5.** d (p. 116)
**2.** d (p. 104)  **6.** a (p. 117)
**3.** a (p. 120)  **7.** c (p. 116)
**4.** d (p. 116)

# Chapter 5

## STOP, THINK, UNDERSTAND *(p. 140)*

### Multiple Choice

**1.** d (p. 128)  **4.** b (p. 136)
**2.** d (p. 130)  **5.** b (pp. 136–137)
**3.** a (p. 130)  **6.** c (p. 135)

### Short Answer

**1.** How heavy is the object? What type of terrain is involved? Which carrying device will work best for the situation? (p. 129)
**2.** Does the patient have a suspected spinal injury? Does the patient need to be moved immediately? (p. 136)

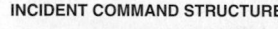

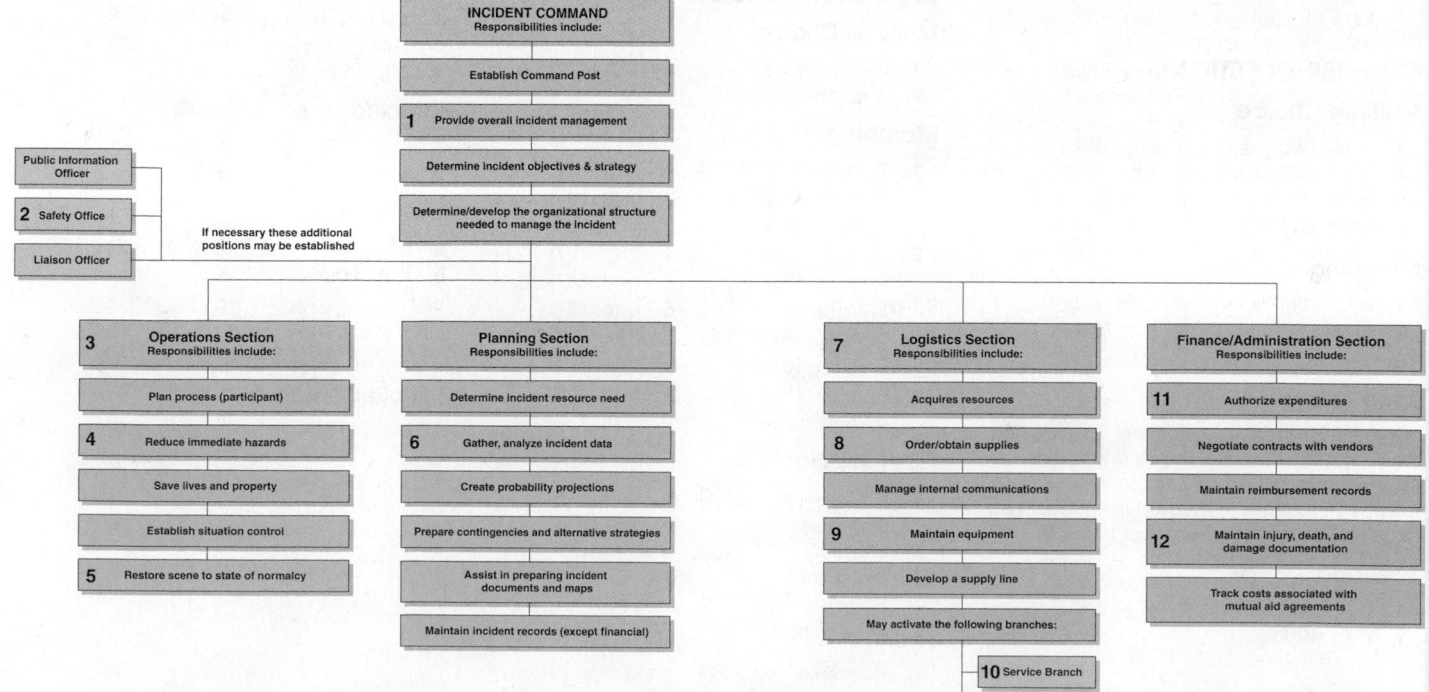

**INCIDENT COMMAND STRUCTURE**

**INCIDENT COMMAND**
Responsibilities include:

Establish Command Post

**1** Provide overall incident management

Determine incident objectives & strategy

Determine/develop the organizational structure needed to manage the incident

Public Information Officer

**2** Safety Office

Liaison Officer

If necessary these additional positions may be established

**3** **Operations Section**
Responsibilities include:

Plan process (participant)

**4** Reduce immediate hazards

Save lives and property

Establish situation control

**5** Restore scene to state of normalcy

**Planning Section**
Responsibilities include:

Determine incident resource need

**6** Gather, analyze incident data

Create probability projections

Prepare contingencies and alternative strategies

Assist in preparing incident documents and maps

Maintain incident records (except financial)

**7** **Logistics Section**
Responsibilities include:

Acquires resources

**8** Order/obtain supplies

Manage internal communications

**9** Maintain equipment

Develop a supply line

May activate the following branches:

**10** Service Branch

Support Branch

**Finance/Administration Section**
Responsibilities include:

**11** Authorize expenditures

Negotiate contracts with vendors

Maintain reimbursement records

**12** Maintain injury, death, and damage documentation

Track costs associated with mutual aid agreements

3. In axial loading, the spine is in a straight or anatomical position, with the weight evenly distributed to the vertebrae and intervertebral discs. This allows the weight to be distributed evenly down the entire spinal column through the pelvis to the bones of the legs. The shoulders must be aligned over the spine, not in front or behind the upright spine. (p. 129)

4. An urgent move is used in situations in which the patient and/or rescuer must move quickly to a safe location or when the patient's medical condition is life threatening and requires immediate transport. (p. 136)

## STOP, THINK, UNDERSTAND (p. 159)
### Multiple Choice
1. b (p. 129)    5. d (p. 142)
2. a (p. 144)    6. b (p. 143)
3. b (p. 144)    7. d (p. 143)
4. b (p. 145)

### Matching
1. e (p. 146)    4. d (p. 146)
2. c (p. 146)    5. b (p. 147)
3. a (p. 146)

### Short Answer
1. The patroller at the front handles the toboggan, drives the sled, and determines the route down the hill. (p. 150)
2. The patroller on the tail rope acts as a backup and ensures that the tail of the sled stays in the fall line. (p. 150)
3. Climbing rope, foam pad, trekking poles, skis, pack frames, oars or paddles, sleeping bag (pp. 153–154)
4. weather, altitude, outside temperature, weight, time of day, and area required to land (p. 155)

## CHAPTER QUESTIONS (p. 164)
### Multiple Choice
1. d (p. 148)    5. c (p. 131)
2. d (p. 148)    6. b (p. 136)
3. d (p. 156)    7. a (p. 137)
4. b (p. 130)

### Matching
1. e (p. 146)    4. c (p. 146)
2. a (p. 146)    5. d (p. 146)
3. b (p. 147)

### Short Answer
Approach the helicopter from the front; do not approach the helicopter unless signaled or escorted by a crew member; remain in sight of the pilot at all times; stay low; take off your hat; do not hold anything above your head. (p. 157)

### Scenario
1. a (p. 138)    3. d (p. 144)
2. c (p. 129)

# Chapter 6
## STOP, THINK, UNDERSTAND (p. 173)
### Multiple Choice
1. c (p. 167)    5. d (p. 171)
2. c (pp. 167–168)    6. b (p. 173)
3. a (p. 170)    7. c (p. 171)
4. b (p. 170)

### Matching
1. j (p. 169)    7. l (p. 170)
2. h (p. 170)    8. d (p. 170)
3. k (p. 170)    9. b (p. 169)
4. g (p. 170)    10. a (p. 170)
5. i (p. 169)    11. e (p. 170)
6. f (p. 170)    12. c (p. 169)

### Fill in the Blank
thoracic (p. 171)

## STOP, THINK, UNDERSTAND (p. 182)
### Multiple Choice
1. c (p. 174)    5. d (p. 174)
2. b (p. 174)    6. d (p. 176)
3. c (p. 174)    7. a (p. 177)
4. a (p. 174)

### Fill in the Blank
1. air is moved in and out of the lungs to exchange oxygen and carbon dioxide between body tissues and the environment. (p. 175)
2. heart, blood vessels, blood (p. 176)
3. red blood cells, white blood cells, platelets, plasma (p. 180)
4. oxygenated, away from; deoxygenated, back to (p. 180)

## STOP, THINK, UNDERSTAND (p. 189)
### Multiple Choice
1. b (p. 183)    3. b (p. 189)
2. d (p. 186)

### Matching
1. 1. a (p. 183)    4. 1. j (p. 189)
   2. c (p. 183)       2. h (p. 187)
   3. b (p. 183)       3. c (p. 187)
2. 1. b (p. 183)       4. g (p. 187)
   2. a (p. 183)       5. e (p. 187)
   3. c (p. 183)       6. a (p. 187)
3. 1. b (p. 187)       7. i (p. 187)
   2. c (p. 187)       8. f (p. 187)
   3. e (p. 187)       9. b (p. 189)
   4. a, d (p. 187)    10. d (p. 189)

### Fill in the Blank
1. brain, spinal    3. a.
   cord (p. 183)       b. X (p. 186)
2. buoyancy,           c. X (p. 186)
   protection,         d.
   chemical            e. X (p. 186)
   stability (p. 183)  f.

## STOP, THINK, UNDERSTAND (p. 202)
### Multiple Choice
1. c (p. 195)    4. d (p. 198)
2. a (p. 195)    5. c (p. 198)
3. b (p. 197)    6. b (p. 189)

### Matching
1. 1. i (p. 191)    10. b (p. 191)
   2. c (p. 191)    11. d (p. 191)
   3. e (p. 191)    12. a (p. 191)
   4. k (p. 191)  2. 1. c (p. 198)
   5. g (p. 191)     2. b (p. 198)
   6. j (p. 191)     3. d (p. 198)
   7. l (p. 191)     4. a (p. 198)
   8. f (p. 191)     5. e (p. 198)
   9. h (p. 191)

### Fill in the Blank
1. integumentary (p. 195)
2. skin (p. 195)
3. dermis (p. 195)
4. epidermis (p. 195)
5. subcutaneous (p. 195)
6. protection of the body from injury, bacteria, and other disease-producing pathogens; fluid regulation; regulation of body temperature (p. 195)
7. bones, ligaments, 206 (pp. 195, 197)
8. cranium, face (p. 197)
9. chest, ribs, sternum, thoracic spine (p. 198) skull, spinal column, thorax, pelvis, upper extremities, lower extremities (p. 197)
10. cervical: 7; thoracic: 12; lumbar: 5; sacral: 5; coccyx: 4 (p. 198)

## STOP, THINK, UNDERSTAND (p. 208)
### Multiple Choice
1. c (p. 199)    5. c (p. 206)
2. a (p. 201)    6. a (p. 206)
3. a (p. 203)    7. d (p. 206)
4. d (p. 206)

### Matching
1. c (p. 199)    3. b (p. 199)
2. a (p. 199)

### Fill in the Blank
a. X (p. 206)    d. X (p. 206)
b. X (p. 206)    e.
c.               f.

## CHAPTER QUESTIONS (p. 210)
### Multiple Choice
1. b (p. 176)    2. a (p. 197)

## Matching

**1.** 1. e (p. 171)
2. h (p. 171)
3. a (p. 181)
4. c (p. 170)
5. i (p. 171)
6. b (This is not in text; ask your instructor.)
7. f (p. 171)
8. g (p. 170)
9. d (p. 171)
**2.** 1. c (p. 171)
2. b (p. 171)
3. a (p. 171)
4. e (p. 171)
5. d (p. 171)
**3.** 1. g (p. 176)
2. h (p. 191)

3. c (p. 187)
4. i (p. 195)
5. a (p. 206)
6. j (p. 199)
7. e (p. 183)
8. f (p. 201)
9. d (p. 174)
10. k (p. 199)
11. b (p. 191)
**4.** 1. d (p. 180)
2. b (p. 181)
3. c (p. 187)
4. a (p. 181)
**5.** 1. b (pp. 201–206)
2. a (p. 183)
3. e (p. 187)
4. c (p. 197)
5. d (p. 197)

## Fill in the Blank

**1.** pelvic (p. 198)
**2.** a. X (p. 199)
b.
c. X (p. 199)

d. X (p. 199)
e. X (p. 199)
f. X (p. 199)
g.

## Scenario

**1.** b (p. 169)
**2.** b (p. 171)
**3.** b (p. 146)
**4.** a (p. 189)

# Chapter 7
## STOP, THINK, UNDERSTAND *(p. 225)*
### Multiple Choice

**1.** c (p. 215)
**2.** b (p. 217)
**3.** a (p. 218)
**4.** d (p. 218)
**5.** b (p. 220)
**6.** c (p. 220)

**7.** a (p. 220)
**8.** a (p. 222)
**9.** b (p. 222)
**10.** a (p. 223)
**11.** c (p. 224)

### Fill in the Blank

**1.** breathing through pursed lips, flaring of nostrils on inspiration, tripoding, unequal movement of chest, rising and falling of shoulder muscles with each breath (p. 220)
**2.** alert, verbal, pain, unresponsive (p. 222)

## STOP, THINK, UNDERSTAND *(p. 236)*
### Multiple Choice

**1.** d (p. 226)
**2.** a (p. 226)
**3.** all (p. 217)
**4.** a (p. 226)
**5.** d (p. 230)
**6.** b (p. 217)
**7.** c (p. 224)

**8.** c (p. 224)
**9.** a (p. 227)
**10.** all (p. 229)
**11.** e (p. 228)
**12.** c (p. 230)
**13.** a (p. 239)

## Sequence

**a.** 5 (p. 232)
**b.** 1 (p. 230)
**c.** 7 (p. 233)
**d.** 6 (p. 232)
**e.** 2 (p. 231)
**f.** 3 (p. 231)

**g.** 9 (p. 234)
**h.** 4 (p. 230)
**i.** 10 (p. 234)
**j.** 11 (p. 234)
**k.** 8 (p. 233)

## Matching

**1.** b, d, e, f, h, i (p. 227)
**2.** a, c, g, j (p. 227)

## STOP, THINK, UNDERSTAND *(p. 247)*
### Multiple Choice

**1.** a (p. 230)
**2.** c (p. 230)
**3.** c (p. 238)
**4.** d (p. 238)
**5.** d (p. 238)
**6.** all (p. 238)
**7.** d (p. 239)

**8.** d (p. 239)
**9.** a (p. 239)
**10.** a (p. 240)
**11.** b (p. 240)
**12.** c (p. 241)
**13.** c (p. 239)
**14.** a (p. 242)

### Fill in the Blank

pulse pressure (pp. 239–240)

### Matching

**1.** 1. b, d (p. 239)
2. a, c (p. 239)
**2.** 1. carotid c (p. 241)
2. femoral b (p. 241)
3. radial a (p. 241)

## CHAPTER QUESTIONS *(p. 260)*
### Multiple Choice

**1.** a. X (p. 245)
b. X (p. 245)
c. X (p. 245)
d. X (p. 245)
e. X (p. 245)
f. X (p. 245)
g. X (p. 245)
h. X (p. 245)
**2.** b (p. 246)
**3.** a (p. 215)
**4.** c (p. 215)
**5.** a (p. 235)

**6.** a (p. 238)
**7.** b (p. 240)
**8.** b (p. 240)
**9.** c (p. 242)
**10.** c (p. 242)
**11.** d (pp. 243–244)
**12.** a (p. 244)
**13.** a (p. 246)
**14.** c (p. 239)
**15.** a (p. 238)
**16.** b (p. 240)
**17.** d (p. 214)

### Matching

**1.** e (pp. 222–223)
**2.** a (pp. 228–229)
**3.** b (p. 232)

**4.** d (pp. 226–228)
**5.** c (p. 230)
**6.** f (p. 218)

### Scenario

**1.** d (p. 228)
**2.** a (p. 228)

**3.** d (p. 229)
**4.** a (p. 229)

# Chapter 8
## STOP, THINK, UNDERSTAND *(p. 281)*
### Multiple Choice

**1.** c (p. 268)
**2.** b (p. 269)
**3.** d (p. 271)

**4.** a (p. 277)
**5.** d (p. 271)

### Short Answer

**1.** to formulate an on-scene treatment plan, to assist in decisions about long-term care of the patient, to determine diagnosis and prognosis, and to reduce legal risks (p. 264)
**2.** to deliver a message in a manner that is understood by the recipient (p. 267)
**3.** oral, written, nonverbal (p. 267)
**4.** a specialized form of communication used to transmit health care–related data (p. 268)
**5.** [answers will vary] (p. 269)

## CHAPTER QUESTIONS *(p. 288)*
### Multiple Choice

**1.** d (p. 279)
**2.** a (p. 279)
**3.** c (p. 278)
**4.** c (p. 284)

**5.** c (p. 273)
**6.** a (p. 265)
**7.** d (p. 272)

### Short Answer

**1.** The patient's privacy must be protected. (p. 269)
**2.** (any four of the following) resort managers, insurers, patrol educators, medical advisors, patrol representatives (p. 269)

### Fill in the Blank

FACTUAL-OEC: Facts, Accurate, Complete, Terms, Unbiased, Avoid slang, Legible/Legal, Organized, Error free, Checked (p. 278)

SAILER: Sex of patient, Age of patient, Incident chief complaint, Location of accident, Equipment needed, Resources needed (p. 269)

CHEATED: Chief complaint, History, Examination, Assessment, Treatment, Evaluation, Disposition (p. 278)

SOAP: Subjective, Objective, Assessment, Plan (p. 277)

### Scenario

**1.** b (p. 270)
**2.** a (p. 270)
**3.** b (p. 278)

**4.** b (p. 279)
**5.** a (pp. 282–286)

# Chapter 9
## STOP, THINK, UNDERSTAND *(p. 294)*
### Multiple Choice

**1.** c (p. 292)
**2.** a (p. 293)

**3.** a, e, f (pp. 298–299)
**4.** b (p. 294)

## STOP, THINK, UNDERSTAND (p. 301)

### Multiple Choice

1. d (pp. 294–295)
2. d (p. 295)
3. a. This is correct
   b. X (pp. 298–299)
   c. X (pp. 298–299)
   d. X (pp. 298–299)
   e. This is correct
   f. This is correct
4. a. X (p. 295)
   b. X (p. 295)
   c. X (p. 295)
   d. X (p. 295)
   e. X (p. 295)
5. a. X (pp. 297–300)
   b. X (pp. 297–300)
   c. X (pp. 297–300)
6. a. X (pp. 295–300)
   b. X (pp. 295–300)
   c. X (pp. 295–300)

## STOP, THINK, UNDERSTAND (p. 303)

### Multiple Choice

1. d (p. 302)                  f. OPA (p. 302)
2. a. OPA (p. 301)             g. OPA (p. 302)
   b. OPA (p. 301)             h. NPA (p. 302)
   c. NPA (p. 301)             i. NPA (p. 301)
   d. NPA (p. 300)             j. NPA (p. 301)
   e. NPA (p. 301)             k. NPA (p. 301)

### Short Answer

The content for this answer appears after this question. When the patient begins to gag, when a more advanced airway adjunct is inserted by an ALS provider. (p. 304)

## STOP, THINK, UNDERSTAND (p. 310)

### Multiple Choice

1. a (p. 306)         9. b (p. 308)
2. c (p. 306)        10. d (p. 308)
3. d (p. 306)        11. a. X (p. 310)
4. c (p. 306)             b. X (p. 310)
5. d (p. 307)             c. X (p. 310)
6. a (p. 307)             d. X (p. 310)
7. c (p. 307)             e. X (p. 310)
8. a (p. 308)             f. X (p. 310)

## STOP, THINK, UNDERSTAND (p. 316)

### Multiple Choice

1. d (p. 315)         3. d (pp. 315–316)
2. c (p. 315)

### Fill in the Blank

1. nasal cannula, nonrebreather mask, bag-valve mask (p. 311)
2. nail polish, cold weather, shock, carbon monoxide poisoning, low red blood cell count, device malfunction (p. 315)

## CHAPTER QUESTIONS (p. 326)

### Multiple Choice

1. b (p. 307)
2. b (pp. 308–309) [(1500 − 200) × 0.16]/15 LPM = 13.9 minutes

### Fill in the Blank

1. a. jaw thrust (p. 295)
   b. head-tilt, chin-lift (p. 295)
   c. head-tilt, chin-lift (p. 295)
   d. jaw thrust (p. 295)
   e. head-tilt, chin-lift (p. 295)
   f. jaw thrust (p. 295)
2. 1. a, k (p. 298)
   2. b, c, f, (p. 311)
   3. d, g, h, j (p. 312)
   4. e, g (p. 313)
   5. i, l (p. 304)
   6. i (p. 304)
3. If encouraging the patient to use the mask fails, apply a nasal cannula. (p. 312)

### Scenario

1. c (p. 295)         3. a (p. 304)
2. c (p. 303)         4. d (p. 302)

# Chapter 10
## STOP, THINK, UNDERSTAND (p. 334)

### Multiple Choice

1. a (p. 329)         5. a (p. 332)
2. d (p. 330)         6. c (p. 332)
3. b (p. 332)         7. d (p. 332)
4. b (p. 332)         8. d (p. 333)

### Matching

1. d (p. 334)         3. c (p. 332)
2. b (p. 332)         4. a (p. 333)

### Fill in the Blank

failure of the circulatory system to maintain adequate blood flow, resulting in a state of inadequate tissue perfusion (p. 329)

## STOP, THINK, UNDERSTAND (p. 343)

### Multiple Choice

1. b (p. 338)         2. b (p. 339)

### Matching

1. 1. c (p. 335)
   2. a (p. 335)
   3. b (p. 335)
2. 1. a, i, l (p. 342)
   2. c, d, h, j and k (p. 339)
   3. b, e, g (p. 336)
   4. f (p. 339)

### Fill in the Blank

1. compensated, decompensated, irreversible (p. 335)
2. heart, blood vessels, blood (p. 331)
3. hypovolemic, cardiogenic, distributive, obstructive (p. 337)

4. a. X (p. 330)         e. X (p. 335)
   b. X (p. 335)         f.
   c.                    g. X (p. 335)
   d. X (p. 335)

## STOP, THINK, UNDERSTAND (p. 348)

### Multiple Choice

1. a (p. 340)         6. b (p. 344)
2. c (p. 341)         7. d (p. 347)
3. b (p. 345)         8. b (p. 347)
4. c (p. 345)         9. c (p. 352)
5. d (p. 344)

### Matching

1. c, d (p. 341)      4. f (p. 340)
2. a (p. 340)         5. g, b (p. 336)
3. e, h (p. 339)

## CHAPTER QUESTIONS (p. 352)

### Multiple Choice

1. a and c are both correct (p. 335)

### Matching

1. 1. a, d, e, g (p. 342)
   2. b, h (p. 342)
   3. c, f (p. 342)
2. 1. c (p. 345)
   2. a (p. 345)
   3. b (p. 345)
   4. d (p. 345)

### Fill in the Blank

1. a. X (p. 344)         e.
   b. X (p. 344)         f. X (p. 345)
   c.                    g.
   d.                    h. X (p. 345)
   e.                    i. X (p. 345)
   f.                    j. X (p. 345)
   g.                    k. X (p. 345)
2. a. X (p. 345)         l. X (p. 345)
   b. X (p. 345)         m.
   c. X (p. 345)         n. X (p. 345)
   d. X (p. 345)         o. X (p. 345)

### Scenario

1. a (p. 336)         4. c (p. 335)
2. c (p. 335)         5. d (p. 341)
3. b (p. 335)         6. a (p. 347)

# Chapter 11
## STOP, THINK, UNDERSTAND (p. 360)

### Multiple Choice

1. d (p. 356)         3. b (p. 358)
2. a (p. 358)

### Fill in the Blank

1. brain stem, cerebellum, cerebrum (p. 356)
2. insulin, glucagon (p. 358)

**Matching**

1. d (p. 356)        3. a (p. 356)
2. b (p. 356)        4. c (p. 356)

**STOP, THINK, UNDERSTAND** (p. 369)

**Multiple Choice**

1. c (p. 360)

**Fill in the Blank**

1. a. G (p. 359)
   b. G (p. 359)
   c. F (p. 359)
   d. G (p. 359)
   e. F (p. 359)
   f. F (p. 359)
   g. F (p. 359)
   h. G (p. 359)
   i. G (p. 359)
2. a. Type 1 (p. 366)
   b. Type 2 (p. 367)
   c. Type 2 (p. 367)
   d. Type 1 (p. 366)
   e. Type 2 (p. 367)
   f. Type 1 (p. 366)
   g. Type 2 (p. 367)
   h. Type 1 (p. 366)
   i. Type 1, Type 2 (p. 366)
   j. Type 2 (p. 367)
3. a. hypoglycemia (p. 367)
   b. hyperglycemia (p. 368)
   c. hypoglycemia (p. 367)
   d. hyperglycemia (p. 368)

**Matching**

1. b (p. 360)        5. g (p. 366)
2. d (p. 365)        6. c (p. 360)
3. a (p. 362)        7. f (p. 366)
4. e (p. 364)

**CHAPTER QUESTIONS** (p. 382)

**Multiple Choice**

1. d (p. 363)        4. f (p. 378)
2. c (p. 365)        5. c (p. 380)
3. d (p. 373)        6. b (p. 379)

**Fill in the Blank**

1. a. pre-ictal (p. 364)
   b. post-ictal (p. 365)
   c. ictal (p. 364)
2. hypoxia, hypoglycemia (p. 377)
3. level of consciousness assessment using the Glasgow Coma Scale, pupillary exam, motor-sensory exam, higher cortical function exam, vocal/speech exam (p. 374)
4. assessing the equality of limbs (ability to move in unison and in a directed fashion), assessing the patient's ability to sense and differentiate touch (p. 374)
5. answers will vary. Possible answer includes having the patient perform a task consisting of multiple steps (p. 375)
6. a. X (p. 375)
   b. X (p. 375)
   c. X (p. 375)

d. X (p. 375)
e. X (p. 375)
f. X (p. 375)
g. X (p. 375)
h.
i.
j. X (p. 375)
k. X (p. 375)
l. X (p. 375)
m. X (p. 375)
n.
7. a. X (p. 376)
   b.
   c. X (p. 376)
8. airway (p. 377)
9. Ensure that the patient can follow simple commands; ask the patient to hold a cup of water, determine if the patient's gag reflex is intact; ask the patient to drink a sip of water; have the patient swallow 15–20 grams of glucose. (p. 378)

**Matching**

1. 1. c, e, f (p. 371)
   2. a, b, h, i (p. 371)
   3. d, g, j, k (p. 371)
2. a. P and G (pp. 363–364)
   b. P (p. 363)
   c. P (p. 363)
   d. G (p. 364)
   e. P (p. 363)
   f. P (p. 363)
   g. G (p. 364)
   h. P (p. 363)
   i. G (p. 364)
   j. G (p. 364)
   k. G (p. 364)
   l. P (p. 363)
   m. P (p. 363)

**Scenario**

1. c (p. 363)        3. a (p. 376)
2. b (p. 373)

# Chapter 12

**STOP, THINK, UNDERSTAND** (p. 390)

**Multiple Choice**

1. d (p. 387)        4. b (p. 388)
2. b (p. 389)        5. d (p. 387)
3. a (p. 388)

**STOP, THINK, UNDERSTAND** (p. 395)

**Multiple Choice**

1. a (p. 394)        3. d (p. 390)
2. d (p. 392)

**Matching**

1. r (p. 394)        9. d (p. 391)
2. p (p. 394)       10. t (p. 392)
3. j (p. 391)       11. v (p. 394)
4. k (p. 394)       12. c (p. 391)
5. f (p. 393)       13. l (p. 391)
6. s (p. 392)       14. g (p. 394)
7. e (p. 391)       15. x (p. 392)
8. o (p. 394)       16. q (p. 394)

**STOP, THINK, UNDERSTAND** (p. 401)

**Multiple Choice**

1. c (p. 400)        4. c (p. 398)
2. b (p. 400)        5. a (p. 398)
3. d (p. 393)

**CHAPTER QUESTIONS** (p. 403)

**Multiple Choice**

1. c (p. 398)        4. b (p. 397)
2. c (p. 393)        5. a (p. 401)
3. b (p. 389)

**Short Answer**

1. Ensure scene safety and Standard Precautions; determine that a poisoning event or a substance abuse event has occurred; search the scene for evidence of a substance or poison (e.g., pill bottles, spray cans); examine the patient, looking for evidence of toxic exposure, and then manage and transport the patient (p. 396)
2. Activated charcoal absorbs and binds toxins. (p. 399)
3. 1-800-222-1222 (p. 401)
4. ingestion, inhalation, transdermal absorption, injection (p. 387)
5. manage ABCDs, apply high-flow oxygen, reduce exposure, reduce absorption, provide rapid transport to definitive care (p. 398)

**Matching**

1. d (p. 397)        6. a (p. 397)
2. j (p. 397)        7. e (p. 397)
3. b (p. 397)        8. c (p. 397)
4. i (p. 397)        9. f (p. 397)
5. g (p. 397)       10. h (p. 397)

**Scenario**

1. c (p. 397)        3. a (p. 389)
2. b (p. 391)

# Chapter 13

**STOP, THINK, UNDERSTAND** (p. 409)

**Multiple Choice**

1. a. X (p. 414)        2. c (p. 407)
   b. X (p. 413)        3. c (p. 407)
   c. X (p. 415)        4. d (p. 407)
   d. X (p. 415)
   e. (p. 414)
   f. X (p. 416)

**STOP, THINK, UNDERSTAND** (p. 413)

**Multiple Choice**

1. b (p. 408)        6. a (p. 412)
2. c (p. 408)        7. a (p. 412)
3. b (p. 408)        8. b (p. 412)
4. d (p. 410)        9. a (p. 411)
5. a (p. 410)

**Fill in the Blank**

1. Alveoli (p. 411)        2. diaphragm (p. 411)

## STOP, THINK, UNDERSTAND *(p. 417)*

### Multiple Choice

d (p. 413)

### Fill in the Blank

epiglottis (p. 413)

### Matching

**1.**
1. b (p. 414)
2. c (p. 413)
3. a (p. 413)
4. f (p. 414)
5. d (p. 415)
6. e (p. 416)

**2.**
1. b (p. 414)
2. d (p. 415)
3. e (p. 414)
4. c (p. 417)
5. a (p. 414)

## STOP, THINK, UNDERSTAND *(p. 423)*

### Multiple Choice

**1.** b (p. 418)   **3.** c (p. 421)
**2.** b (p. 418)   **4.** b (p. 422)

### Matching

**1.** a, j, o (p. 418)
**2.** d, f, k, n (p. 418)
**3.** b, l, m (p. 418)
**4.** g, i, q (p. 418)
**5.** a, e, h, m, p, q (p. 424)

### Labeling

**a.** M (p. 412)   **f.** S (p. 418)
**b.** S (p. 418)   **g.** S (p. 418)
**c.** S (p. 418)   **h.** M (p. 418)
**d.** M (p. 412)   **i.** S (p. 418)
**e.** S (p. 418)   **j.** M (p. 418)

## CHAPTER QUESTIONS *(p. 430)*

### Multiple Choice

**1.** a (p. 418)   **6.** c (p. 421)
**2.** c (p. 424)   **7.** c (p. 421)
**3.** a (p. 424)   **8.** d (p. 422)
**4.** a (p. 421)   **9.** a (p. 424)
**5.** b (p. 424)

### True or False

**a.** F (p. 424)   **e.** F (p. 424)
**b.** T (p. 424)   **f.** T (p. 424)
**c.** T (p. 424)   **g.** F (p. 424)
**d.** T (p. 424)

### Scenario

**1.** a (p. 425)   **5.** c (p. 424)
**2.** d (p. 418)   **6.** a (p. 422)
**3.** c (p. 425)   **7.** b (p. 424)
**4.** b (p. 412)

# Chapter 14

## STOP, THINK, UNDERSTAND *(p. 438)*

### Multiple Choice

**1.** b (p. 436)   **4.** d (p. 437)
**2.** c (p. 436)   **5.** b (p. 437)
**3.** a (p. 436)   **6.** d (p. 437)

### Fill in the Blank

**a.** X (p. 435)   **d.** X (p. 436)
**b.** X (p. 436)   **e.** X (p. 436)
**c.** X (p. 436)

## STOP, THINK, UNDERSTAND *(p. 445)*

### Multiple Choice

**1.** a (p. 439)   **5.** c (p. 441)
**2.** d (p. 439)   **6.** b (p. 443)
**3.** b (p. 445)   **7.** a (p. 444)
**4.** d (p. 445)

### Fill in the Blank

**a.** less than 90 mmHg (p. 445)
**b.** greater than 20 rpm (p. 445)
**c.** greater than 110 bpm (p. 445)
**d.** anxious or decreased GCS less than 14 (p. 445)
**e.** 90% (p. 445)

### Matching

**1.** a, b (p. 444)
**2.** e, j (p. 444)
**3.** c, d, f, g, h, i (p. 444)

## STOP, THINK, UNDERSTAND *(p. 449)*

### Multiple Choice

**1.** a (p. 446)   **4.** a (p. 447)
**2.** b (p. 447)   **5.** a (p. 447)
**3.** c (p. 446)

## CHAPTER QUESTIONS *(p. 454)*

### Multiple Choice

**1.** c (p. 447)   **3.** d (p. 446)
**2.** a (p. 437)

### Short Answer

Answers may vary and may include assess and correct ABCDs, open the patient's airway, apply $O_2$ with a nonrebreather mask at 15 LPM, place the patient in the shock position, remove the stinger, activate EMS, ask the patient about an EpiPen, and assist the patient as needed. (p. 447)

### Matching

**1.** h (p. 437)   **6.** e (p. 436)
**2.** b (p. 439)   **7.** g (p. 436)
**3.** i (p. 438)   **8.** a (p. 437)
**4.** j (p. 437)   **9.** d (p. 439)
**5.** c (p. 440)   **10.** f (p. 439)

### Scenario

**1.** b (p. 440)   **3.** b (p. 443)
**2.** d (p. 443)

# Chapter 15

## STOP, THINK, UNDERSTAND *(p. 471)*

### Multiple Choice

**1.** b (p. 464)   **f.** X (p. 465)
**2.** d (p. 465)   **g.** X (p. 465)
**3.** a. X (p. 465)   **h.** X (p. 465)
   b. X (p. 465)   **4.** b (p. 465)
   c. X (p. 465)   **5.** a (p. 466)
   d. X (p. 465)   **6.** d (p. 466)
   e. X (p. 465)

### Fill in the Blank

**1.** aneurysm (p. 469)
**2.** angina pectoris (p. 400)

### Matching

**1.** d (p. 466)   **7.** j (p. 469)
**2.** e (p. 467)   **8.** g (p. 469)
**3.** f (p. 468)   **9.** i (p. 469)
**4.** b (p. 468)   **10.** k (p. 468)
**5.** a (p. 468)   **11.** c (p. 468)
**6.** h (p. 469)

### True or False

**a.** F (p. 470)   **c.** T (p. 470)
**b.** F (p. 470)   **d.** F (p. 470)

## STOP, THINK, UNDERSTAND *(p. 488)*

### Multiple Choice

**1.** c (p. 466)   **4.** c (p. 472)
**2.** d (p. 486)   **5.** a (p. 472)
**3.** a (p. 486)   **6.** c (p. 475)

### Short Answer

**1.** early access (p. 476), early CPR (p. 476), early defibrillation (p. 476), early advanced care (p. 476), integrated post-cardiac arrest care (p. 476)
**2.** Give chest compressions at a rate of 100 times per minute and a depth of 1.5–2 inches, allowing for complete recoil. (p. 477)
**3.** Apply a nasal cannula at 4–6 LPM (p. 485)
**4.** Answers will vary, but should include heart attack; OPQRST, SAMPLE, assisting with any medications, administering $O_2$ with a nonrebreather mask at 15 LPM, monitoring vital signs, calling ahead to have medical attention waiting at the gate, placing the patient in position of comfort (p. 487)

### Matching

**1.** l (p. 472)   **7.** h (p. 475)
**2.** a, b, f (p. 474)   **8.** i (p. 475)
**3.** e (p. 474)   **9.** k (p. 476)
**4.** m (p. 476)   **10.** j (p. 475)
**5.** c (p. 475)   **11.** g (p. 474)
**6.** d (p. 475)

## CHAPTER QUESTIONS *(p. 491)*

### Multiple Choice

**1.** c (p. 458)   **7.** a (p. 486)
**2.** d (p. 459)   **8.** c (p. 486)
**3.** a (p. 474)   **9.** b (p. 487)
**4.** d (p. 480)   **10.** c (p. 486)
**5.** b (p. 475)   **11.** c (p. 466)
**6.** c (p. 481)   **12.** c (p. 476)

### True or False

**a.** F (p. 470)   **c.** T (p. 470)
**b.** T (p. 465)   **d.** F (p. 476)

### Scenario

**1.** d (p. 474)   **3.** c (p. 475)
**2.** a (p. 486)   **4.** b (p. 487)

# Chapter 16
## STOP, THINK, UNDERSTAND (p. 499)
### Multiple Choice
**1.** c (p. 494)  **3.** a (p. 495)
**2.** b (p. 496)  **4.** c (p. 496)

### Short Answer
**1.** a. RUQ: liver, gallbladder, portion of the colon (p. 496)
   b. LUQ: stomach, spleen, portion of the colon (p. 496)
   c. RLQ: appendix, portion of the large intestine, portion of the small intestine (p. 496)
   d. LLQ: portion of the large intestine, portion of the small intestine (p. 496)
**2.** venae cavae, aorta (p. 496)

### Matching
**1.** c (p. 496)  **5.** b (p. 496)
**2.** d (p. 496)  **6.** g (p. 496)
**3.** e (p. 496)  **7.** a (p. 496)
**4.** f (p. 496)

## STOP, THINK, UNDERSTAND (p. 507)
### Multiple Choice
**1.** a (p. 500)  **3.** b (p. 506)
**2.** b (p. 505)  **4.** d (p. 505)

### Matching
**1.** c (p. 500)  **4.** a (p. 500)
**2.** e (p. 500)  **5.** b (p. 500)
**3.** d (p. 500)

## STOP, THINK, UNDERSTAND (p. 511)
### Multiple Choice
**1.** b (p. 496)  **4.** b (p. 509)
**2.** d (p. 508)  **5.** a (p. 509)
**3.** c (p. 509)  **6.** d (p. 510)

### Short Answer
**a.** X (p. 508)  **f.** X (p. 510)
**b.** X (p. 510)  **g.**
**c.** X (p. 510)  **h.** X (p. 510)
**d.** X (p. 504)  **i.** X (p. 510)
**e.**

## CHAPTER QUESTIONS (p. 512)
### Multiple Choice
**1.** c (p. 508)  **5.** a (p. 512)
**2.** d (p. 502)  **6.** c (p. 495)
**3.** a (p. 506)  **7.** b (p. 496)
**4.** b (pp. 474, 500)

### Matching
**1.** 1. e (p. 500)   10. b (p. 502)
   2. h (p. 504)   11. g (p. 500)
   3. c (p. 503)   12. k (p. 503)
   4. f (p. 502)   13. j (p. 502)
   5. a (p. 500)   14. i (p. 500)
   6. d (p. 504)  **2.** 1. c (p. 506)
   7. l (p. 508)     2. d (p. 506)
   8. n (p. 501)     3. a (p. 506)
   9. m (p. 504)     4. b (p. 506)

### Short Answer
Hollow organs move material, whereas solid organs are highly vascular. Thus, when material leaks out of a hollow organ, peritonitis occurs, whereas damage to solid organs can cause internal bleeding and lead to hemorrhagic shock. (p. 495)

### Scenario
**1.** d (p. 504)  **4.** b (p. 502)
**2.** d (p. 499)  **5.** a (p. 510)
**3.** d (p. 500)

# Chapter 17
## STOP, THINK, UNDERSTAND (p. 529)
### Multiple Choice
**1.** b (p. 519)  **3.** d (p. 526)
**2.** a (p. 519)

### List
speed, stopping distance (p. 519)

### Matching
**1.** 1. h (p. 523)  **2.** 1. b, e (p. 527)
   2. c, d, f (p. 522)     2. b, d, e (p. 527)
   3. b, f, (p. 523)     3. c (p. 527)
   4. a, i (p. 522)     4. a (p. 528)
   5. e, g, j (p. 522)     5. a (p. 528)

## CHAPTER QUESTIONS (p. 534)
### Multiple Choice
**1.** a (p. 530)  **4.** c (p. 532)
**2.** a (p. 525)  **5.** c (p. 532)
**3.** d (p. 532)

### List
**1.** assess the mechanism of injury (MOI); determine how many patients there are; assess the need for additional resources (p. 530)
**2.** mechanism of injury (p. 521)
**3.** the forces involved; treatment rendered before your arrival (p. 531)
**4.** Onset; Provocation; Quality; Radiation/Region; Severity; Time (See Chapter 7)

### Short Answer
**1.** Answer depends on your individual patrol protocol.
**2.** Answer depends on your individual patrol protocol.

### Scenario
**1.** d (p. 525)  **3.** d (p. 531)
**2.** b (p. 522)  **4.** c (p. 520)

# Chapter 18
## STOP, THINK, UNDERSTAND (p. 541)
### Multiple Choice
**1.** c (p. 540)  **2.** d (p. 540)

### True or False
**a.** F (p. 540)  **d.** T (p. 540)
**b.** T (p. 540)  **e.** T (p. 540)
**c.** T (p. 540)

### Matching
**1.** d (p. 540)  **4.** e (p. 540)
**2.** b (p. 540)  **5.** a (p. 540)
**3.** c (p. 540)

### Short Answer
**1.** epidermis, dermis (p. 539)
**2.** Hairs become erect to trap warm air near the skin's surface; blood vessels constrict to shunt blood away from the skin. (p. 540)
**3.** Blood vessels dilate, allowing heat to radiate away from the body; sweat glands secrete sweat that evaporates, cooling the skin. (p. 540)

## STOP, THINK, UNDERSTAND (p. 544)
### Multiple Choice
**1.** c (p. 540)  **2.** d (p. 542)

### Matching
**1.** 1. V (p. 542)  **2.** 1. b (p. 543)
   2. A (p. 542)     2. a (p. 543)
   3. A (p. 542)     3. d (p. 545)
   4. V (p. 542)     4. c (p. 543)
   5. V (p. 542)     5. e (p. 543)
   6. A (p. 542)
   7. C (p. 542)

### Sequence
**a.** 3 (p. 542)  **d.** 1 (p. 542)
**b.** 4 (p. 542)  **e.** 5 (p. 542)
**c.** 6 (p. 542)  **f.** 2 (p. 542)

### List
closed injuries, open injuries, burns (p. 542)

## STOP, THINK, UNDERSTAND (p. 549)
### Multiple Choice
**1.** b (p. 545)  **3.** a (p. 548)
**2.** c (p. 547)  **4.** c (p. 549)

### Matching
**1.** e (p. 546)  **5.** f (p. 546)
**2.** a (p. 546)  **6.** c (p. 547)
**3.** g (p. 547)  **7.** h (p. 548)
**4.** b (p. 546)  **8.** d (p. 549)

### Short Answer
Both terms refer to the appearance of a wound: linear wounds are regular like incisions, whereas stellate wounds are irregular in appearance. (p. 546)

## STOP, THINK, UNDERSTAND (p. 552)
### Multiple Choice
**1.** d (p. 551)  **3.** c (p. 552)
**2.** b (p. 547)  **4.** d (p. 551)

## Short Answer

Gently wash the finger tip. Use a lighter, match, or open flame to heat the end of a paper clip (or the blunted end of a needle or pin). Touch the hot tip of the paper clip to the center of the affected nail and gently push down to allow the paper clip to burn through the nail. (The trapped blood will escape suddenly as the pressure is released, providing immediate relief from pain.) Immediately remove the paper clip to prevent it from penetrating the nail bed. Dress and bandage the wound. (p. 545)

## STOP, THINK, UNDERSTAND (p. 557)

### Multiple Choice

1. c (p. 552)
2. b (p. 553)
3. b (p. 554)
4. a (p. 554)
5. a. X (p. 554)
   b. X (p. 554)
   c. X (p. 554)
   d.
   e.
6. d (p. 555)
7. a. X (p. 555)
   b. X (p. 555)
   c. X (p. 555)
   d.
8. d (p. 555)
9. d (p. 555)

### True or False

a. T (p. 553)
b. T (p. 553)
c. F (p. 553)
d. F (p. 553)
e. T (p. 553)
f. F (p. 553)

## STOP, THINK, UNDERSTAND (p. 564)

### Multiple Choice

1. c (p. 556)
2. d (p. 556)
3. a (p. 558)
4. d (p. 558)
5. b (p. 561)
6. c (p. 542)
7. a. X (p. 560)
   b. X (p. 560)
   c. X (p. 560)
   d. X (p. 560)
   e.
8. a.
   b. X (p. 560)
   c. X (p. 561)
   d.
   e.
   f. X (pp. 552, 561)
   g. X (p. 555)
   h. X (p. 560)

## Matching

1. e (p. 559)
2. c (p. 560)
3. f (not in chapter)
4. a (p. 558)
5. b (p. 559)
6. d (p. 559)

## CHAPTER QUESTIONS (p. 576)

### Multiple Choice

1. c (p. 551)
2. a (p. 554)
3. b (p. 555)
4. a (p. 547)

### Matching

1. 1. d (p. 558)
   2. a (p. 561)
   3. e (p. 561)
   4. f (p. 558)
   5. b (p. 561)
   6. d (p. 559)
   7. c (p. 562)
   8. g (p. 553)
2. a. L, G (p. 555)
   b. L (p. 555)
   c. G (p. 555)
   d. L (p. 555)
   e. G (p. 555)
   f. L (p. 556)
   g. G (p. 555)
   h. L, G (p. 556)
   i. L, G (p. 556)

### Short Answer

Wrap the amputated part in a sterile dressing moistened with sterile saline or water; place this bundle into a zip-lock plastic bag; place this bag into a second bag containing 1 part ice to 3 parts water (1/4 cup ice to 3/4 cup water). (p. 556)

### Scenario

1. d (p. 546)
2. b (p. 561)

# Chapter 19

## STOP, THINK, UNDERSTAND (p. 587)

### Multiple Choice

1. b (p. 581)
2. a (p. 581)
3. d (p. 584)
4. a (p. 581)
5. b (p. 586)

### Fill in the Blank

1. second (p. 586)
2. first (p. 585)
3. third (p. 586)

## STOP, THINK, UNDERSTAND (p. 596)

### Multiple Choice

1. a (p. 589)
2. d (pp. 589–590)
3. b (p. 594)
4. a (p. 593)
5. d (p. 595)

### Short Answer

1. (any four of the following answers) obvious burns involving the head, face, or neck; singed hair, eyebrows, nose hairs, or facial hair; soot around the face or mouth; hoarseness/voice changes; airway swelling; darkened oral/nasal discharge (carbonaceous sputum) (p. 588)
2. the safety of OEC Technicians and other rescuers (p. 591)

## CHAPTER QUESTIONS (p. 598)

### Multiple Choice

1. d (p. 579)
2. b (p. 586)
3. c (p. 583)
4. d (p. 586)
5. c (p. 591)

### Short Answer

(any six of the following answers) burns to a child or elderly person; burns involving more than one body part; burns involving the head, neck, hands, feet, genitals, or major joints; inhalation injury/burns; difficulty breathing or hoarseness; chemical or electrical burns; partial-thickness burns with greater than 10% TBSA; any full-thickness burn; burns associated with trauma; burns with a serious underlying medical disorder; burns in a patient requiring special social, emotional, or physical needs; exposure to radioactive materials (p. 590)

**Labeling** See Rule of Nines at bottom of the page.

### Scenario

1. d (p. 581)
2. c (p. 582)
3. d (p. 586)
4. a (p. 581)
5. b (p. 589)

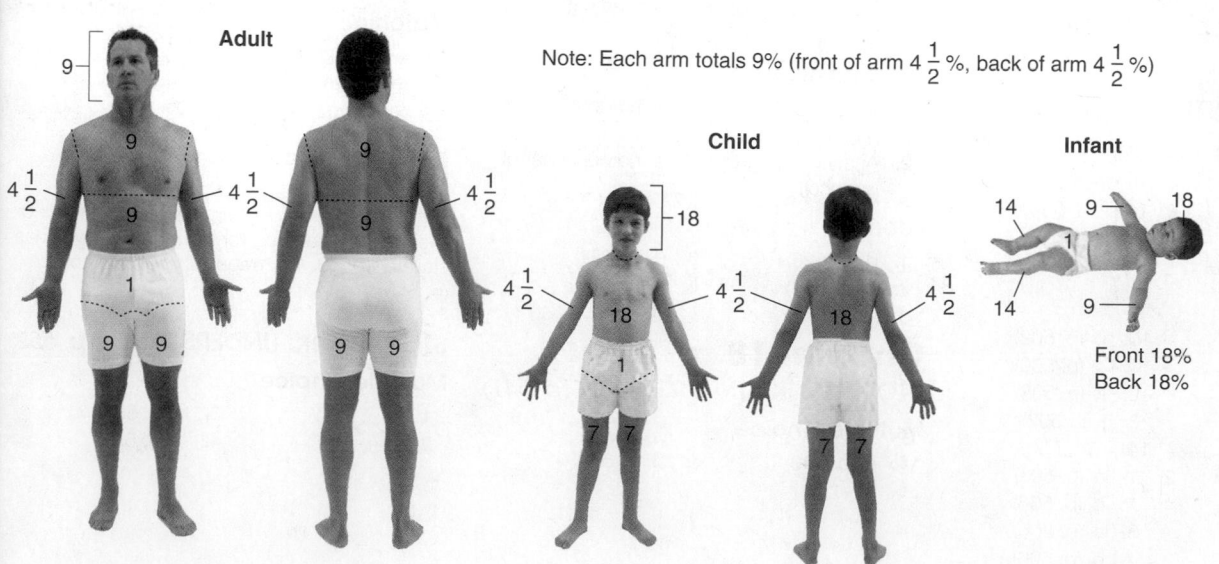

Note: Each arm totals 9% (front of arm $4\frac{1}{2}$ %, back of arm $4\frac{1}{2}$ %)

# Chapter 20
## STOP, THINK, UNDERSTAND (p. 605)
### Multiple Choice
1. d (p. 604)
2. a (p. 604)
3. b (p. 604)

### Matching
1. 1. a (p. 604)
   2. c (p. 604)
   3. b (p. 604)
2. 1. a (p. 604)
   2. b (p. 604)
   3. c (p. 604)

### List
1. protects internal organs (p. 603)
2. provides human form (p. 603)
3. produces red blood cells (p. 603)

### Short Answer
1. The axial skeleton consists of 80 bones: the skull, the vertebrae, and the thoracic cage; it is responsible for upright position of the human body. (p. 604)
2. The appendicular skeleton consists of 126 bones: the shoulders, arms, pelvis, and legs; it is responsible for manipulating objects and locomotion. (p. 604)

### Fill in the Blank
1. epiphysis, diaphysis (p. 604)
2. axial, appendicular (p. 604)

## STOP, THINK, UNDERSTAND (p. 611)
### Multiple Choice
1. a.
   b. X (p. 606)
   c.
   d. X (p. 608)
   e. X (p. 606)
   f. X (p. 606)
2. a (p. 606)
3. a (p. 607)
4. d (p. 608)
5. a. X (p. 608)
   b.
   c. X (p. 608)
   d. X (p. 608)
   e.
6. c (p. 608)
7. b (p. 609)
8. c (p. 610)
9. c (p. 610)
10. d (p. 610)
11. a (p. 610)
12. b (p. 610)

### Matching
1. 1. b (p. 607)
   2. a (p. 607)
   3. d (p. 607)
   4. c (p. 607)
   5. e (p. 607)
2. 1. b (p. 607)
   2. a (p. 607)
   3. d (p. 607)
   4. f (p. 608)
   5. c (p. 608)
   6. e (p. 607)

## STOP, THINK, UNDERSTAND (p. 616)
### Multiple Choice
1. d (p. 612)
2. a (p. 612)
3. a (p. 612)
4. b (p. 613)
5. c (p. 615)
6. c (p. 615)
7. b (p. 615)
8. d (p. 616)
9. b (p. 616)

## STOP, THINK, UNDERSTAND (p. 621)
### Multiple Choice
1. d (p. 617)
2. c (p. 619)
3. a (p. 619)
4. b (p. 619)
5. a (p. 619)
6. c (p. 619)
7. c (p. 620)
8. c (p. 619)

### Matching
1. a (p. 621)
2. b (p. 620)
3. c (p. 621)
4. d (p. 621)
5. e (p. 621)

## STOP, THINK, UNDERSTAND (p. 628)
### Multiple Choice
1. b (p. 622)
2. c (p. 623)
3. d (p. 624)
4. c (p. 624)
5. a (p. 624)
6. c (p. 625)
7. b (p. 625)
8. b (p. 625)
9. c (p. 625)
10. a (p. 625)
11. b (p. 626)
12. c (p. 626)
13. d (p. 626)
14. a (p. 626)
15. b (p. 627)
16. b (p. 627)
17. d (p. 628)
18. b (p. 628)

### Short Answer
1. "guarding" the injury site and engaging in self-stabilization by holding the forearm near to the body. (p. 622)
2. It indicates a severe MOI. (p. 625)

## STOP, THINK, UNDERSTAND (p. 637)
### Multiple Choice
1. a (p. 630)
2. a (p. 631)
3. a (p. 631)
4. c (p. 631)
5. c (p. 632)
6. c (p. 633)
7. b (p. 633)
8. c (p. 634)
9. d (p. 635)
10. b (p. 636)
11. c (p. 636)
12. b (p. 636)
13. c (p. 636)
14. c (p. 634)

### Matching
1. 1. b (p. 631)
   2. d (p. 632)
   3. e (p. 633)
   4. a (p. 634)
   5. c (p. 632)
2. 1. c (p. 635)
   2. d (p. 635)
   3. b (p. 634)
   4. a (p. 634)

### Short Answer
1. a ball and socket joint (p. 630)
2. when the knee is forced into a position of extreme "knock-knee" (p. 632)
3. common causes are sprains of the mid-foot and the great toe joint (p. 636)

## STOP, THINK, UNDERSTAND (p. 648)
### Multiple Choice
1. c (p. 639)
2. a (p. 648)
3. a (p. 648)
4. d (p. 647)
5. a (p. 646)
6. a. X (p. 644)
   b. X (p. 644)
   c. X (p. 644)
   d. X (p. 644)
   e. X (p. 644)
   f. X (p. 644)
   g.
   h.
   i.
   j.
   k.

### Short Answer
1. a. air, rigid, malleable, blanket/pillow (p. 642)
   b. traction, quick splint, rigid (pp. 643, 644)
   c. quick splint, vacuum, malleable metal (pp. 641, 643)
   d. long board (p. 641)
   e. cravats (p. 640)
   f. pelvic binder (p. 642)
   g. rigid, air, malleable metal (pp. 642, 643)
   h. airplane, blanket, roll/pillow, vacuum (pp. 641, 643)
   i. rigid (pp. 642, 646)
2. magazine: forearm, foot, or ankle (p. 645); plastic: utensil fingers (p. 646); blanket/pillow: forearm, shoulder, ankle (p. 641); ski poles: leg, knee, hip (p. 646); tree branches: hip, leg, knee, arm/elbow (p. 646); oar: hip, leg, knee (p. 646)
3. (any three of the following) check CMS before and after splinting (p. 646); manually stabilize the injury in the position found (p. 646); select the appropriate splint (p. 646); properly size the splint (p. 646); pad the splint, if needed (p. 646); position the splint (p. 646); secure the splint (p. 647)

### Fill in the Blank
1. 15 (p. 646)
2. 7 (p. 647)

## STOP, THINK, UNDERSTAND (p. 658)
### Multiple Choice
1. b (p. 650)
2. b (p. 653)
3. c (p. 652)
4. d (p. 650)
5. a. X (p. 652)
   b. X (p. 653)
   c. X (p. 652)
   d.
   e.
   f. X (p. 655)
   g.
6. a (p. 656)
7. b (p. 656)
8. b (p. 656)
9. d (p. 657)

### Short Answer
1. The cravat could be placed directly over the fracture site. (p. 652)
2. at the side of the neck, to prevent pressure on the back of the neck (p. 650)
3. to allow for CMS checks (p. 650)

## STOP, THINK, UNDERSTAND (p. 663)
### Multiple Choice
1. c (p. 659)
2. c (p. 660)
3. c (p. 660)
4. b (p. 660)
5. d (p. 660)
6. c (p. 660)
7. b (p. 661)
8. a (p. 661)
9. d (p. 663)
10. b (p. 661)
11. d (p. 662)
12. a (p. 661)
13. a (p. 663)

## Short Answer

when it is not mechanically effective due to loosening or incorrect application; when you are assisting an EMT who is required to remove a boot to assess CMS prior to transport (p. 662)

## STOP, THINK, UNDERSTAND *(p. 671)*

### Multiple Choice

| | | | |
|---|---|---|---|
| **1.** | c (p. 665) | **8.** | a (p. 668) |
| **2.** | b (p. 665) | **9.** | b (p. 669) |
| **3.** | a (p. 665) | **10.** | a (p. 669) |
| **4.** | c (p. 665) | **11.** | b (p. 670) |
| **5.** | a (p. 666) | **12.** | d (p. 671) |
| **6.** | c (p. 666) | **13.** | c (p. 671) |
| **7.** | c (p. 668) | **14.** | c (p. 670) |

### Short Answer

1. Apply manual stabilization; make one attempt to axially align the knee and the splint straight in the frontal plane with slight knee flexion. (p. 665)
2. The popliteal artery can occlude several hours after the initial injury. (p. 665)

## STOP, THINK, UNDERSTAND *(p. 675)*

### Multiple Choice

| | | | |
|---|---|---|---|
| **1.** | d (p. 673) | **3.** | b (p. 674) |
| **2.** | a (p. 673) | **4.** | c (p. 674) |

### List

**a.** head (p. 674)  **d.** calves (p. 674)
**b.** shoulders (p. 674)  **e.** heels (p. 674)
**c.** buttocks (p. 674)

## CHAPTER QUESTIONS *(p. 692)*

### Multiple Choice

| | | | |
|---|---|---|---|
| **1.** | c (p. 660) | **9.** | a. X (p. 661) |
| **2.** | d (pp. 624, 627) | | b. X (p. 661) |
| **3.** | a (p. 624) | | c. X (p. 661) |
| **4.** | d (p. 624) | | d. X (p. 661) |
| **5.** | c (p. 625) | | e. |
| **6.** | b (p. 625) | | f. X (p. 661) |
| **7.** | a (p. 636) | | g. |
| **8.** | c (p. 652) | | h. X (p. 661) |
| | | **10.** | c |

### Short Answer

1. Early and late complications can occur, including nerve damage, arterial interruption, and crooked healing or muscle damage from a loss of blood supply. (p. 626)
2. The sciatic nerve can also be injured, resulting in temporary partial or complete paralysis of the ankle and foot; additionally, the major blood vessels to the ball of the hip can be damaged. (p. 631)
3. Quickly align the injured limb and splint it anatomically; place the patient on a spine board, treat for shock with high-flow oxygen, and provide rapid transport. (p. 647)
4. Use sterile solution or clean boiled or disinfected water to wash the fracture site; use gentle axial tension to help the bone to

go back into the soft tissue and then bandage and splint the fracture site; continue to assess neurovascular status. (p. 648)
5. Use proper stabilization of the zone of injury with a figure eight bandage; allow the patient to walk out; check CMS frequently because cravats or tape may become too tight as the foot swells. (p. 670)

### Matching

| | | | |
|---|---|---|---|
| **1.** | 1. d (p. 620) | | 8. m (p. 615) |
| | 2. e (p. 621) | | 9. k (p. 612) |
| | 3. b (p. 620) | | 10. j (p. 614) |
| | 4. a (p. 621) | | 11. g (p. 613) |
| | 5. c (p. 621) | | 12. h (p. 613) |
| **2.** | 1. o (p. 615) | | 13. e (p. 613) |
| | 2. l (p. 612) | | 14. i (p. 613) |
| | 3. c (p. 615) | | 15. b (p. 615) |
| | 4. a (p. 615) | | 16. q (p. 615) |
| | 5. d (p. 615) | | 17. p (p. 615) |
| | 6. f (p. 613) | | 18. r (p. 615) |
| | 7. n (p. 613) | | |

### Scenario

| | | | |
|---|---|---|---|
| **1.** | c (p. 619) | **3.** | b (p. 659) |
| **2.** | d (p. 620) | | |

# Chapter 21
## STOP, THINK, UNDERSTAND *(p. 701)*

### Multiple Choice

| | | | |
|---|---|---|---|
| **1.** | b (p. 698) | | e. X (p. 699) |
| **2.** | c (p. 698) | | f. X (p. 699) |
| **3.** | a (p. 698) | | g. X (p. 699) |
| **4.** | a. X (p. 699) | | h. |
| | b. X (p. 699) | | i. X (p. 699) |
| | c. X (p. 699) | **5.** | a (p. 699) |
| | d. | **6.** | d (p. 700) |

### Matching

| | | | |
|---|---|---|---|
| **1.** | b (p. 700) | **4.** | d (p. 700) |
| **2.** | c (p. 700) | **5.** | e (p. 700) |
| **3.** | a (p. 700) | | |

**Labeling** See art at bottom of the page.

## STOP, THINK, UNDERSTAND *(p. 708)*

### Multiple Choice

| | | | |
|---|---|---|---|
| **1.** | b (p. 705) | **3.** | d (p. 708) |
| **2.** | c (p. 705) | | |

### Labeling

| | | | |
|---|---|---|---|
| **a.** | MO (p. 705) | **d.** | MI (p. 705) |
| **b.** | MO (p. 705) | **e.** | MI (p. 705) |
| **c.** | SC (p. 705) | **f.** | MI (p. 705) |

### Fill in the Blank

1. retrograde (p. 707)
2. anterograde (p. 707)

### List

(any three of the following) rapid deceleration, rapid acceleration, compression injury to the spinal column, penetrating or impaled object, near drowning, hypothermia or hyperthermia, electrical injury including lightning strike (p. 702)

### Matching

| | | | |
|---|---|---|---|
| **1.** | d (p. 703) | **4.** | e (p. 704) |
| **2.** | a (p. 703) | **5.** | c (pp. 704–705) |
| **3.** | b (p. 704) | | |

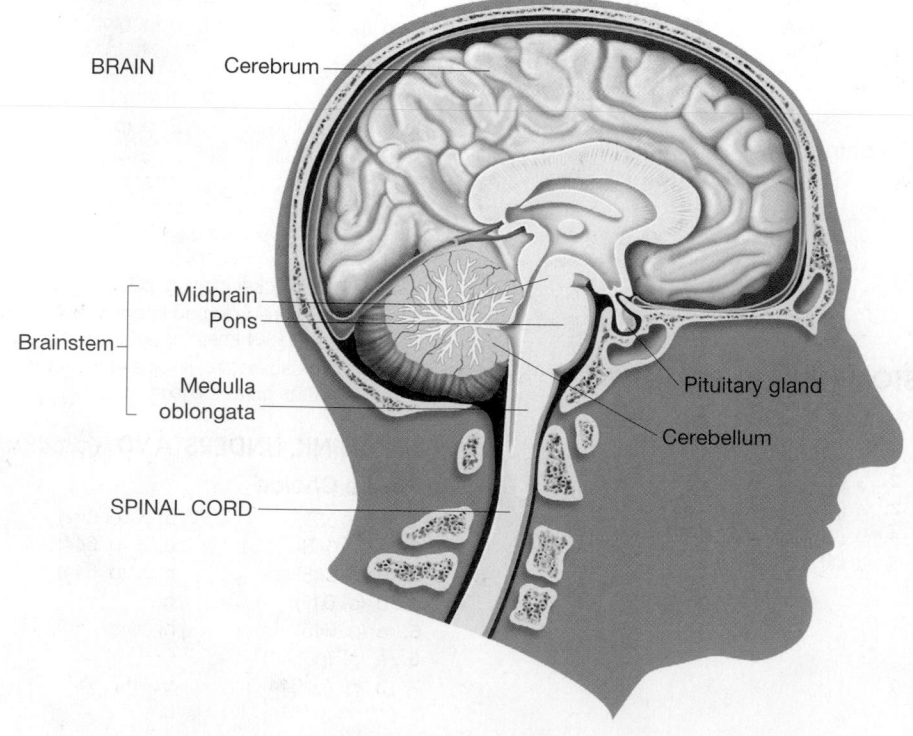

BRAIN  Cerebrum

Brainstem {
  Midbrain
  Pons
  Medulla oblongata
}

Pituitary gland

Cerebellum

SPINAL CORD

## STOP, THINK, UNDERSTAND (p. 713)

### Multiple Choice

1. a (p. 708)
2. b (p. 708)
3. a (p. 710)
4. c (p. 710)
5. d (p. 711)

### Matching

1. 1. a (p. 711)
   2. b (p. 711)
   3. c (p. 711)
   4. d (p. 712)
2. a. E (p. 709)
   b. S (p. 710)
   c. S (p. 710)
   d. B (pp. 709–710)
   e. E (p. 709)
   f. E (p. 709)
   g. S (p. 710)
   h. S (p. 710)
   i. E (p. 710)

### Short Answer

Because the cranium is an enclosed space, a hematoma within this space can compress the brain and result in serious damage. (p. 709)

## STOP, THINK, UNDERSTAND (p. 718)

### Multiple Choice

1. a (p. 714)
2. b (p. 715)
3. c (p. 705)
4. d (pp. 705, 717)
5. b (p. 718)
6. c (p. 715)

## STOP, THINK, UNDERSTAND (p. 726)

### Multiple Choice

1. a (pp. 720, 722)
2. b (pp. 721, 722)
3. a.
   b.
   c. X (p. 725)
   d. X (p. 725)
   e. X (p. 725)
   f. X (p. 725)
   g.
4. c (p. 725)

## CHAPTER QUESTIONS (p. 738)

### Multiple Choice

1. a (p. 712)
2. c (p. 712)
3. a (p. 718)
4. d (p. 707)
5. c (p. 719)
6. a.
   b. X (p. 714)
   c. X (p. 714)
   d. X (p. 714)
   e.
   f. X (p. 714)
   g. X (p. 714)
   h. X (p. 714)
   i. X (p. 714)
   j. X (p. 714)

### Matching

1. c (p. 183)
2. b (p. 699)
3. d (p. 700)
4. o (p. 699)
5. g (p. 700)
6. e (p. 700)
7. m (p. 710)
8. k (p. 183)
9. h (p. 709)
10. n (p. 183)
11. a (p. 712)
12. f (p. 700)
13. i (p. 700)
14. p (p. 183)
15. j (p. 699)
16. l (p. 710)

### Scenario

1. d (p. 714)
2. c (p. 716)
3. b (p. 724)
4. c (p. 711)

# Chapter 22

## STOP, THINK, UNDERSTAND (p. 748)

### Multiple Choice

1. a (p. 747)
2. c (p. 743)
3. b (p. 744)
4. b (p. 744)
5. d (p. 744)

### Matching

1. j (p. 746)
2. k (p. 744)
3. d (p. 744)
4. a (p. 745)
5. e (p. 745)
6. b (p. 745)
7. c (p. 745)
8. i (p. 745)
9. f (p. 746)
10. h (p. 745)
11. g (p. 745)
12. l (p. 747)

### Short Answer

1. blunt trauma, penetrating trauma, environmental exposure, chemical burns, cold weather injuries (p. 742)
2. closed head injuries and cervical spine injuries (p. 743)
3. sight, hearing, smell, and taste (p. 743)
4. large blood vessels and generous blood supply located in these areas of the body (p. 747)
5. They are only protected by thin layers of skin and muscle. (p. 747)

## STOP, THINK, UNDERSTAND (p. 752)

### Multiple Choice

1. b (p. 749)
2. c (p. 749)
3. c (p. 749)
4. c (p. 749)
5. a (p. 751)

### Matching

1. i (p. 745)
2. m (p. 744)
3. e (p. 744)
4. h (p. 749)
5. c (p. 745)
6. b (p. 749)
7. o (p. 745)
8. g (p. 751)
9. a (p. 746)
10. l (p. 743)
11. j (p. 743)
12. f (p. 744)
13. n (p. 751)
14. k (p. 747)
15. d (p. 756)

### Short Answer

1. direct trauma, drying of mucous membranes, nose picking (p. 749)
2. loud noises, pressure buildup inside the ear, fluid buildup inside the ear (p. 750)
3. They are frequently associated with severe swelling or formation of a hematoma that can compromise the airway. (p. 751)
4. The concentrated force of the injury can crush the larynx or trachea. (p. 751)

## STOP, THINK, UNDERSTAND (p. 757)

### Multiple Choice

1. b (p. 754)
2. a (p. 755)
3. c (p. 755)
4. c (p. 756)
5. d (p. 757)
6. a (p. 757)
7. c (p. 757)
8. a. X (p. 757)
   b. X (p. 757)
   c.
   d.
   e. X (p. 757)
   f.
   g. X (p. 757)

### Short Answer

1. a ruptured carotid artery or jugular vein (p. 756)
2. Airway compromise and swelling may not be immediately apparent. (p. 756)
3. direct pressure (p. 757)

## STOP, THINK, UNDERSTAND (p. 764)

### Multiple Choice

1. c (p. 759)
2. b (p. 760)
3. c (p. 759)
4. a (p. 760)

### True or False

a. T (p. 761)
b. T (p. 761)
c. F (p. 761)
d. T (p. 761)
e. F (p. 761)
f. T (p. 762)

## CHAPTER QUESTIONS (p. 767)

### Multiple Choice

1. c (p. 745)
2. b (p. 760)
3. a (p. 757)
4. d (p. 759)
5. c (p. 760)

### Short Answer

1. air embolism, cardiac arrest, pulmonary air embolism, hypoxia, aspiration of gastric contents (p. 763)
2. jaw-thrust maneuver (p. 756)
3. stroke (p. 759)

### Scenario

1. c (p. 756)
2. a (p. 761)
3. a (p. 757)

# Chapter 23

## STOP, THINK, UNDERSTAND (p. 773)

### Multiple Choice

1. b (p. 771)
2. d (p. 772)

### Fill in the Blank

1. base of the neck, costal margin (p. 772)
2. two, three (p. 772)
3. xiphoid process, lumbar vertebrae, lower ribs (p. 772)

### Labeling

1. See art at bottom of page 1210.
2. See art at bottom of page 1210.

## STOP, THINK, UNDERSTAND (p. 776)

### Multiple Choice

1. c (p. 775)
2. d (p. 776)
3. d (p. 772)
4. a.
   b.
   c. X (p. 772)
   d.
   e. X (p. 772)
   f.
   g.

## Matching

**1.** f (p. 774)   **4.** a (p. 775)
**2.** d (p. 774)   **5.** e (p. 775)
**3.** b (p. 775)   **6.** c (p. 775)

## Fill in the Blank

**1.** parietal, visceral (p. 772)
**2.** serous (p. 772)

## STOP, THINK, UNDERSTAND (p. 781)

### Multiple Choice

**1.** b (p. 777)       f. X (p. 777)
**2.** a.                g.
   b. X (p. 777)        h.
   c. X (p. 777)   **5.** d (p. 778)
   d. X (p. 777)   **6.** b (p. 778)
   e. X (p. 777)   **7.** c (p. 779)
   f. X (p. 777)   **8.** a. X (p. 778)
   g.                   b. X (p. 778)
**3.** a (p. 777)         c. X (p. 779)
**4.** a. X (p. 777)      d. X (p. 779)
   b. X (p. 777)        e.
   c. X (p. 777)        f.
   d. X (p. 778)   **9.** a (p. 781)
   e. X (p. 778)   **10.** b (p. 781)

## STOP, THINK, UNDERSTAND (p. 787)

### Multiple Choice

**1.** c (p. 783)   **4.** c (p. 785)
**2.** b (p. 784)   **5.** a (p. 785)
**3.** a (p. 786)

### Short Answer

Look for contusions, deformity, paradoxical movement of the chest, full chest expansion and symmetry, and potentially serious injuries such

as a sucking chest wound, an impaled object, or obvious flail segment. (p. 783)
**Auscultate** the lungs to ensure that breath sounds are present, clear, and equal bilaterally. (p. 783)
**Palpate** the entire chest, axillary regions, and upper back for tenderness and deformity. (p. 783)

## CHAPTER QUESTIONS (p. 789)

### Multiple Choice

**1.** c (p. 772)   **6.** c (p. 781)
**2.** b (p. 774)   **7.** a (p. 782)
**3.** a (p. 771)   **8.** a (p. 779)
**4.** b (p. 776)   **9.** c (p. 779)
**5.** c (pp. 777–778)

### Matching

**1.**  1. i (p. 780)       13. h (p. 777)
        2. p (p. 774)       14. f (p. 774)
        3. o (p. 780)       15. q (p. 779)
        4. j (p. 775)       16. r (p. 777)
        5. b (p. 778)       17. g (p. 777)
        6. l (p. 782)       18. n (p. 781)
        7. m (p. 778)   **2.**  1. e (p. 780)
        8. e (p. 774)            2. d (p. 780)
        9. c (p. 785)            3. b (p. 779)
        10. d (p. 774)           4. a (p. 777)
        11. k (p. 775)           5. c (p. 777)
        12. a (p. 772)           6. f (p. 781)

### Scenario

**1.** d (p. 783)   **3.** d (p. 784)
**2.** d (p. 775)   **4.** a (p. 786)

# Chapter 24

## STOP, THINK, UNDERSTAND (p. 796)

### Multiple Choice

**1.** b (p. 794)   **2.** c (p. 794)

### Labeling

See art at bottom of page 1211.

### Matching

**1.**  1. d (p. 795)   **2.**  1. c, d (p. 795)
        2. c (p. 795)           2. b (p. 795)
        3. b (p. 795)           3. a (p. 795)
        4. f (p. 795)
        5. a (p. 187)
        6. e (p. 191)

## STOP, THINK, UNDERSTAND (p. 803)

### Multiple Choice

**1.** b (p. 801)   **7.** a. X (p. 803)
**2.** d (p. 801)       b. X (p. 803)
**3.** a (p. 802)       c. (p. 803)
**4.** c (p. 802)       d. X (p. 803)
**5.** a (p. 802)       e. (p. 803)
**6.** b (p. 802)       f. X (p. 802)

### True or False

**a.** T (p. 798)   **d.** T (p. 798)
**b.** T (p. 798)   **e.** T (p. 798)
**c.** F (p. 798)   **f.** F (p. 798)

### List

pain, tenderness, visible external wounds, abdominal distension, abdominal rigidity, unexplained shock (p. 801)

## Label 1

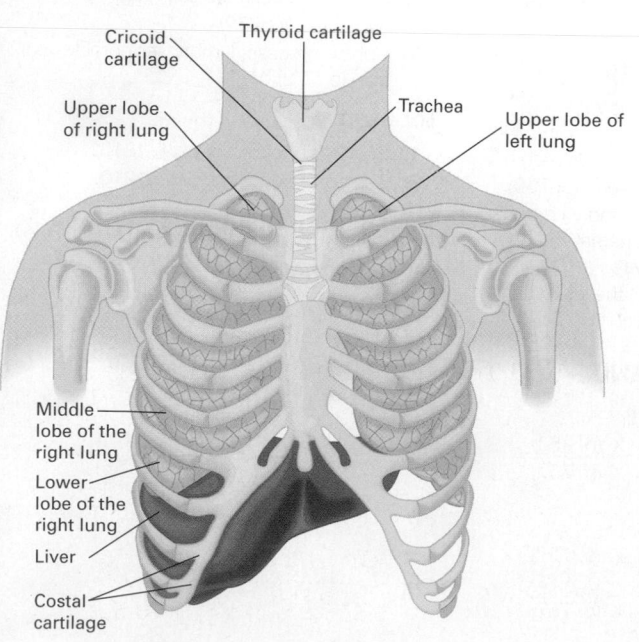

Cricoid cartilage
Thyroid cartilage
Upper lobe of right lung
Trachea
Upper lobe of left lung
Middle lobe of the right lung
Lower lobe of the right lung
Liver
Costal cartilage

## Label 2

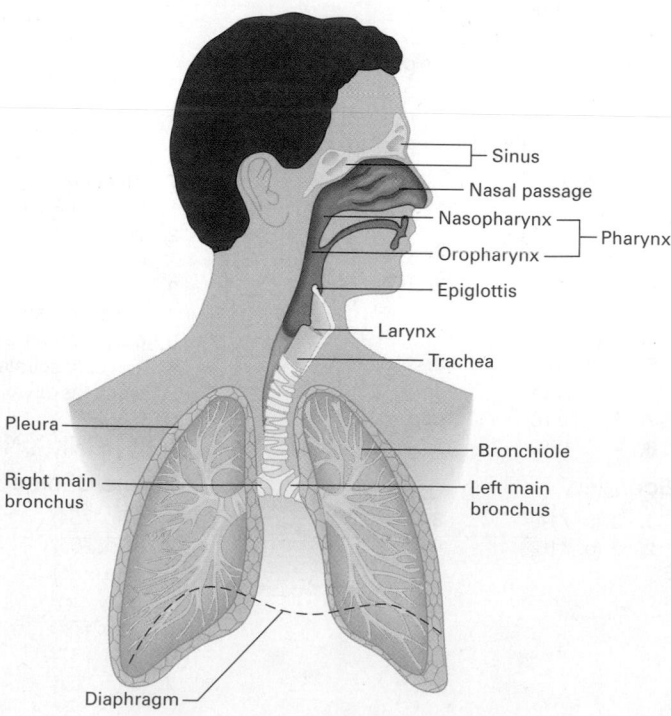

Sinus
Nasal passage
Nasopharynx
Oropharynx
Pharynx
Epiglottis
Larynx
Trachea
Pleura
Right main bronchus
Bronchiole
Left main bronchus
Diaphragm

## Matching

| | |
|---|---|
| **1.** a (p. 799) | **7.** g (p. 799) |
| **2.** c (p. 798) | **8.** h (p. 799) |
| **3.** b (p. 799) | **9.** e (p. 798) |
| **4.** d (p. 799) | **10.** f (p. 798) |
| **5.** i (p. 800) | **11.** l (p. 801) |
| **6.** j (p. 800) | **12.** k (p. 801) |

## STOP, THINK, UNDERSTAND (p. 807)

### Multiple Choice

| | |
|---|---|
| **1.** d (p. 805) | **3.** c (p. 805) |
| **2.** d (p. 805) | **4.** a (p. 806) |

## CHAPTER QUESTIONS (p. 810)

### Multiple Choice

| | |
|---|---|
| **1.** c (p. 802) | e. |
| **2.** a (p. 805) | f. X (p. 803) |
| **3.** a. X (p. 801) | g. X (p. 803) |
| b. X (p. 802) | **4.** b (p. 803) |
| c. X (p. 803) | **5.** c (p. 799) |
| d. | **6.** c (p. 805) |

### List

sheet, cravats, spine board, cervical collar, nylon cable ties, radio or cell phone (p. 806)

### Scenario

| | |
|---|---|
| **1.** d (p. 800) | **3.** b (p. 806) |
| **2.** a (p. 806) | **4.** d (p. 806) |

# Chapter 25

## STOP, THINK, UNDERSTAND (p. 823)

### Multiple Choice

| | |
|---|---|
| **1.** a (p. 815) | **3.** b (p. 818) |
| **2.** c (p. 815) | **4.** a (p. 819) |

### List

**1.** (any ten of the following) alcohol; age; freezing temperatures; high winds; high altitude; use of drugs; previous frostbite injury; overexertion; poor fitting,

inadequate, or wet clothing; dehydration; impaired circulation; poor nutrition (pp. 817–818)

**2.** (any seven of the following) know your environment; wear adequate clothing—use layering strategy; be attentive to yourself and your companions; ensure adequate nutrition and hydration; stay dry; avoid restrictive clothing and boots; change your socks; avoid alcohol, caffeine, and drugs; do not tolerate numbness in your hands or feet (pp. 821–822)

## STOP, THINK, UNDERSTAND (p. 833)

### Multiple Choice

| | |
|---|---|
| **1.** a (pp. 824–825) | **3.** a (p. 831) |
| **2.** d (p. 827) | **4.** c (p. 831) |

### List

seek shelter (p. 828); replace wet clothing (p. 828); insulate one's body from the ground (p. 828); wear a hat (p. 828); establish a vapor barrier (p. 828)

### Matching

| | |
|---|---|
| **1.** 1. b, f (p. 825) | e. yes (p. 830) |
| 2. c, d (p. 825) | f. no (p. 830) |
| 3. a, e, g (p. 826) | g. no (p. 831) |
| **2.** a. yes (p. 830) | h. yes (p. 830) |
| b. yes (p. 830) | i. no (p. 830) |
| c. yes (p. 830) | j. yes (p. 830) |
| d. no (p. 830) | |

## CHAPTER QUESTIONS (p. 835)

### Multiple Choice

| | |
|---|---|
| **1.** b (p. 815) | **4.** b (p. 831) |
| **2.** d (p. 819) | **5.** a (pp. 825, 835) |
| **3.** c (p. 828) | |

### Matching

| | |
|---|---|
| **1.** b, e (p. 816) | **3.** c (p. 817) |
| **2.** d, f (p. 817) | **4.** a (p. 817) |

### Short Answer

**1.** Passive warming relies on the retention of the patient's internal body heat; an example is shivering. Active warming involves the application of a heat source; an example is a hot water bottle. (p. 829)

**2.** prevention of heat loss (p. 828)

**3.** A hypothermic patient who is cold, rigid, and apparently lifeless may have a slow, faint heartbeat and tissue rigidity. (p. 831)

### Scenario

| | |
|---|---|
| **1.** a (p. 824) | **3.** c (p. 825) |
| **2.** d (pp. 825–826) | **4.** b (p. 830) |

# Chapter 26

## STOP, THINK, UNDERSTAND (p. 841)

### Multiple Choice

| | |
|---|---|
| **1.** c (p. 839) | c. X (p. 841) |
| **2.** b (p. 840) | d. |
| **3.** c (p. 841) | e. X (p. 841) |
| **4.** d (p. 841) | f. |
| **5.** a. | |
| b. X (p. 841) | |

## STOP, THINK, UNDERSTAND (p. 844)

### Multiple Choice

| | |
|---|---|
| **1.** b (p. 842) | **3.** b (p. 843) |
| **2.** c (p. 843) | |

### Fill in the Blank

body temperature, electrolyte balance, and body fluid balance (p. 842)

### Matching

| | |
|---|---|
| **1.** 1. b, d (p. 843) | **2.** a. 1 (p. 843) |
| 2. a, e (p. 843) | b. 4 (p. 843) |
| 3. c, f, g (p. 843) | c. 5 (p. 843) |
| 4. c (p. 843) | d. 3 (p. 843) |
| | e. 2 (p. 843) |

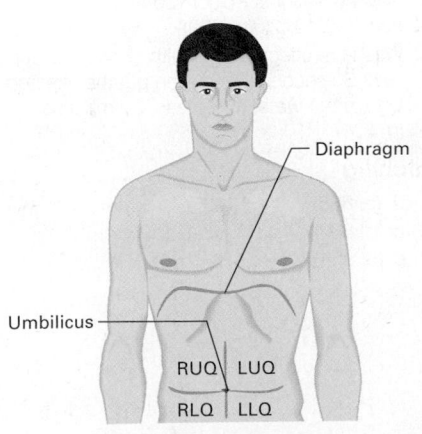

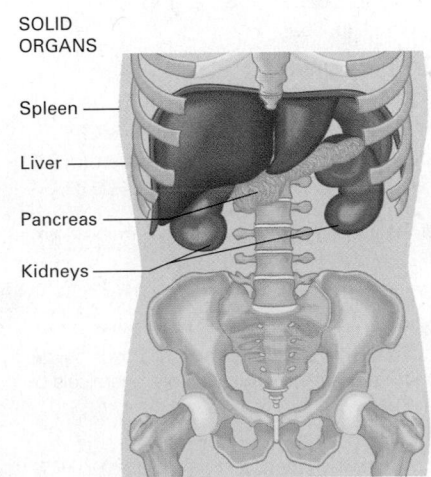

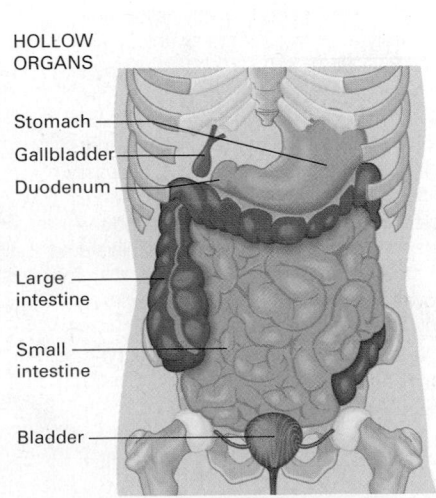

## STOP, THINK, UNDERSTAND (p. 847)
### Multiple Choice
1. d (p. 845)    4. c (p. 846)
2. b (p. 045)    5. a (p. 846)
3. a (p. 846)    6. d (p. 846)

### Short Answer
Physical sunscreens block the sunlight mechanically and are good for small areas such as the nose and lips. Chemical sunscreens rely on chemical agents to selectively absorb the harmful rays. (p. 846)

## STOP, THINK, UNDERSTAND (p. 849)
### Multiple Choice
1. b (p. 849)    d.
2. c (p. 849)    e.
3. a. (p. 848)   f. X (p. 849)
   b.            4. c (p. 851)
   c. X (p. 849)

### Fill in the Blank
1. respiratory (pp. 848–849)
2. tissue (pp. 848–849)
3. kidneys (pp. 848)
4. fern leaf or feathering (p. 848)
5. cardiac arrest (p. 848)
6. pain, paralysis, blindness, numbness, weakness, loss of hearing or speech, and unresponsiveness. (p. 848)

## STOP, THINK, UNDERSTAND (p. 855)
### Multiple Choice
1. b (pp. 852, 854)   e. X (p. 848)
2. a.                 f. X (p. 848)
   b.                 3. a (p. 853)
   c. X (p. 852)      4. c (p. 854)
   d.                 5. d (p. 854)

### Matching
1. a (p. 851)    3. d, e (pp. 852, 854)
2. b (p. 851)    4. c (p. 851)

### Short Answer
1. Remove the patient from the heat, place the patient in a supine position, elevate the patient's feet, and provide supportive oxygen. Provide cool, lightly salted or electrolyte fluids if able to swallow (pp. 852, 857)
2. Move the patient to a cool shaded environment, place the patient in a supine position, provide high-flow oxygen, and rehydrate the patient if can swallow easily. (pp. 852–853)
3. the duration of the hyperthermia and the speed with which treatment is administered (p. 853)
4. Lower the patient's body temperature by any means available. (p. 853)
5. In both cases the patient could become breathless and pulseless, resulting in the need to administer CPR. (p. 855)

## CHAPTER QUESTIONS (p. 858)
### Multiple Choice
1. d (p. 840)        5. c (p. 845)
2. c or d (p. 853)   6. c (p. 840)
3. a. X (p. 842)     7. a (p. 844)
   b. X (p. 842)     8. a.
   c. X (p. 842)        b.
   d.                   c. X (p. 849)
   e. X (p. 842)        d. X (p. 849)
   f.                   e.
   g. X (p. 842)        f. X (p. 846)
   h.                   g. X (p. 849)
   i.                   h. X (p. 849)
4. a. X (p. 845)        i.
   b.                9. b (p. 854)
   c. X (p. 845)     10. c or d (p. 854)
   d.                11. a (p. 854)
   e.
   f. X (p. 845)

### List
a fast heart rate (p. 854); a high respiratory rate (p. 854); a decreased level of consciousness (p. 854); the cessation of sweating (p. 852); shock, hypotension present (p. 854); responds rapidly to treatment (p. 854); able to treat in the field (p. 854)

### Scenario
1. c (pp. 852, 854)   3. a (p. 850)
2. d (p. 842)

# Chapter 27
## STOP, THINK, UNDERSTAND (p. 868)
### Multiple Choice
1. d (p. 862)    f. X (pp. 865–868)
2. b (p. 862)    g.
3. b (p. 862)    h. X (pp. 865–867)
4. d (p. 868)    i. X (p. 867)
5. a. X (p. 867) j. X (p. 866)
   b. X (pp. 867, 868) k. X (p. 867)
   c. X (p. 868)  l. X (pp. 865, 867)
   d.             m. X (p. 865)
   e. X (pp. 866–868)

### Matching
1. a, d (p. 862)    3 e, g (p. 862)
2. b, c, f (p. 862)

### Fill in the Blank
1. necrosis (p. 862)   4. poison (p. 862)
2. bullae (p. 864)     5. toxin (p. 862)
3. venom (p. 862)      6. jimson weed (p. 868)

### List
lily of the valley, autumn crocus, belladonna, fox glove, yew (pp. 865–867)

### Short Answer
A toxin is a poison made by a living creature, which may be a plant or an animal. A poison can come from a living creature or from chemicals or substances that do not come from living creatures. (p. 862)

## STOP, THINK, UNDERSTAND (p. 876)
### Multiple Choice
1. a (p. 874)    4. d (p. 876)
2. a (pp. 874–875) 5. c (p. 876)
3. d (p. 876)    6. b and c (p. 870)

### Fill in the Blank
amanitas (p. 870)

### List
1. 1. amanitas (p. 870)
   2. false morels (p. 871)
   3. little brown mushrooms (p. 870)
2. 1. jack-o-lantern mushrooms (p. 870)
   2. green-spored lepiota (p. 870)
3. malaria, dengue fever, yellow fever, encephalitis, West Nile virus (p. 876)

### Matching
1. b, d (p. 871)    4. c (p. 873)
2. e (p. 872)       5. g (p. 873)
3. a, f (pp. 872–873)

## STOP, THINK, UNDERSTAND (p. 882)
### Multiple Choice
1. b (p. 879)    3. d (p. 880)
2. d (p. 879)

### Matching
1. 1. d (p. 878)    2. 1. f (p. 881)
   2. b (p. 878)       2. c (p. 880)
   3. f (p. 879)       3. d (p. 880)
   4. a (p. 878)       4. e (p. 880)
   5. e (p. 878)       5. a (p. 880)
   6. c (p. 878)       6. b (p. 881)

## STOP, THINK, UNDERSTAND (p. 891)
### Multiple Choice
1. d (pp. 887–888)   7. a (p. 889)
2. b (p. 886)        8. b (p. 889)
3. c (p. 886)        9. a (p. 889)
4. a (p. 889)        10. d (p. 889)
5. a (p. 887)        11. d (p. 889)
6. c (p. 887)

### Short Answer
1. Call the National Poison Control center at 800-222-1222. (p. 890)
2. Wash the affected area with vinegar for at least 30 seconds, and then put the affected area in hot water for at least 20 minutes. (p. 889)

### Matching
1. d (p. 885)    4. a (p. 884)
2. c (p. 883)    5. f (p. 884)
3. e (p. 884)    6. b (p. 884)

## CHAPTER QUESTIONS (p. 893)

### Multiple Choice

1. c (p. 863)
2. d (p. 864)
3. c (p. 871)
4. b (p. 888)
5. a (p. 875)
6. b (p. 887)
7. c (p. 886)

8. b (pp. 887–898)
9. b (p. 889)
10. a. X (p. 889)
    b.
    c.
    d.
    e. X (p. 889)

### Short Answer

evidence of visual disturbance in the patient, spasms or seizure, unconsciousness, nausea and vomiting, cardiogenic effects, salivation, headache, dehydration, paralysis, kidney failure (pp. 868, 870)

### List

rattlesnake, copperhead, coral snake, water moccasin, massasauga (p. 878)

### Scenario

1. d (p. 865)
2. c (p. 874)
3. a (p. 875)

# Chapter 28

## STOP, THINK, UNDERSTAND (p. 908)

### Multiple Choice

1. a (p. 899)
2. d (p. 899)
3. b (p. 899)

4. a and b (p. 898)
5. c (p. 900)
6. c (p. 900)

### Matching

1. d, h (pp. 903, 904)
2. i, m, n (p. 904, 905)
3. b, g (p. 905)
4. a, f (p. 906)

5. c (p. 906)
6. j (p. 906)
7. e, k (p. 907)
8. l (p. 907)

## STOP, THINK, UNDERSTAND (p. 914)

### Multiple Choice

1. d (p. 911)
2. a (p. 909)
3. b (p. 911)

4. d (p. 912)
5. d (p. 913)
6. d (p. 912)

## CHAPTER QUESTIONS (p. 916)

### Multiple Choice

1. c (p. 899)
2. b (p. 903)
3. b (p. 902)
4. c (p. 913)

5. c (p. 913)
6. d (p. 913)
7. a (p. 905)
8. d (pp. 906, 915)

### List

1. headache, dizziness, fatigue, shortness of breath, loss of appetite, nausea, malaise, sleep disturbances, dry cough, inner chill, low urine output (p. 903)
2. 1. Make gradual ascents.
   2. Avoid rapid ascent to above 10,000 feet.
   3. Incorporate a layover of 2–3 days at an intermediate altitude (between 8,000 feet and 10,000 feet).
   4. Once above 10,000 feet, limit altitude increases to 1,000 feet per day.
   5. As you increase altitude, rest more and gain less altitude per day.
   6. Avoid heavy physical exertion for 24–48 hours at altitude.
   7. Stay hydrated.
   8. Avoid the use of alcohol and other depressant drugs. Avoid the use of tobacco.
   9. Eat a high-carbohydrate diet.
   10. If altitude illness symptoms occur, do not go higher until they resolve. (pp. 909–910)

### Scenario

1. d (p. 900)
2. b (p. 899)
3. a (pp. 903–904)
4. b (p. 911)

# Chapter 29

## STOP, THINK, UNDERSTAND (p. 924)

### Multiple Choice

1. c (p. 922)
2. d (p. 921)
3. a (p. 920)

4. b (p. 923)
5. a (p. 922)

### Fill in the Blank

1. Dry (p. 922)
2. wet (p. 922)

## STOP, THINK, UNDERSTAND (p. 932)

### Multiple Choice

1. b (p. 929)
2. d (p. 926)
3. b (p. 925)
4. c (p. 926)

5. a (p. 927)
6. b (p. 929)
7. d (p. 925)
8. c (p. 931)

### Fill in the Blank

freshwater (hypotonic), salt water (hypertonic) (p. 927)

## STOP, THINK, UNDERSTAND (p. 937)

### Multiple Choice

1. d (p. 934)
2. c (p. 934)
3. d (p. 933)
4. c (p. 934)

5. b (p. 934)
6. c (p. 934)
7. a (p. 936)

### List

1. using Standard Precautions (p. 935) or perhaps ensure personal safety and safety of others (p. 933)
2. donning a personal floatation device (p. 933)
3. wearing a helmet (p. 933)

## CHAPTER QUESTIONS (p. 938)

### Multiple Choice

1. c (p. 936)
2. d (pp. 929–931)
3. a (p. 923)
4. c (p. 923)
5. c (p. 926)

6. c (p. 922)
7. b (pp. 925–926)
8. d (p. 930)
9. b (p. 933)

### Short Answer

Reaching out to the patient with a solid object (Branch, oar, pole)
Throwing a rescue device to the patient
Rowing to a patient in a boat
Swimming to the patient (the last resort) (p. 933)

### List

1. 1. submersion injuries (p. 925)
   2. barotraumas (pp. 927–929)
   3. nitrogen narcosis (p. 929)
   4. swimmer's ear (p. 929)
   5. breath holding (p. 929)
   6. trauma (p. 930)
   7. harm by marine animals (p. 930)
   8. aggravation of existing medical conditions (p. 930)
2. 1. Something goes wrong, leading to panic (p. 922)
   2. gasping (p. 922)
   3. possible aspiration (p. 922)
   4. larynogospasm (p. 922)
   5. hypoxia (p. 922)
   6. unconsciousness (p. 922)
   7. myocardial irritability (p. 922)
   8. cardiac arrest (p. 922)
   9. relaxation of airway muscles (p. 922)
   10. aspiration of fluid (p. 922)

### Matching

1. h (p. 929)
2. i (p. 927)
3. d (p. 923)
4. j (p. 923)
5. b (p. 927)

6. c (p. 925)
7. a (p. 923)
8. f (p. 922)
9. e (p. 926)
10. g (p. 926)

### Scenario

1. b (p. 935)
2. d (p. 934)

# Chapter 30

## STOP, THINK, UNDERSTAND (p. 946)

### Multiple Choice

1. c (p. 944)
2. a. X (p. 944)
   b.
   c.
   d. X (p. 943)
   e.
   f. X (p. 943)
   g. X (p. 943)
   h.
3. d (p. 945)
4. a.
   b. X (p. 945)
   c. X (p. 945)
   d. X (p. 945)
   e. X (p. 945)
5. a (p. 945)
6. d (p. 945)
7. d (p. 945)

### Short Answer

less than. Children have a proportionally smaller blood volume than adults yet bleed at the same rate. They also have a higher heart rate and lower blood pressure. Additionally, a child's arteries are able to constrict more quickly than are an adult's arteries. This combination enables a child to compensate better *initially* to shock. (p. 945)

**STOP, THINK, UNDERSTAND** *(p. 952)*

**Multiple Choice**

1. a and b (p. 950)  3. d (p. 950)
2. h (p. 950)

**List**

1. 1. newborn (p. 947)
   2. infant (p. 947)
   3. toddler (p. 947)
   4. pre-school (p. 947)
   5. school-age (p. 948)
   6. adolescent (p. 949)
2. 1. croup (p. 950)
   2. tonsillitis (p. 950)
   3. foreign-airway obstruction (p. 950)
   4. epiglottitis (p. 951)
3. 1. bronchiolitis (p. 950)
   2. asthma (pp. 950, 951)
   3. pneumonia (pp. 950, 953)

**Short Answer**

Between birth and the age of 18, humans undergo a great variety of physical, intellectual, emotional, and social changes. It is important for OEC Technicians to understand these stages if they are to provide quality care for children. (pp. 946, 948)

**STOP, THINK, UNDERSTAND** *(p. 956)*

**Multiple Choice**

1. b (p. 954)    6. d (p. 954)
2. c (p. 954)    7. d (p. 954)
3. b (p. 953)    8. d (p. 953)
4. c (p. 954)    9. d (p. 953)
5. a (p. 954)

**Short Answer**

1. constipation or stool holding, changes in dietary or sleep patterns, and dehydration (p. 953)
2. gastroenteritis, viruses, bacteria, parasites, tainted or unfamiliar food, lack of food, and over stimulation (p. 953)
3. Children are at high risk of accidental poisoning due to their inexperience in distinguishing candy from medications or harmless plants from toxic ones. (p. 954)

**STOP, THINK, UNDERSTAND** *(p. 959)*

**Multiple Choice**

1. a (p. 957)          c.
2. d (p. 958)          d.
3. a (p. 958)
4. a (p. 958)          8. b (p. 958)
5. b (p. 958)          9. d (p. 958)
6. c (p. 958)          10. d (p. 958)
7. a. X (p. 958)       11. c (p. 958)
   b. X (p. 958)       12. c (p. 958)
                       13. d (p. 959)

**STOP, THINK, UNDERSTAND** *(p. 962)*

**Multiple Choice**

1. a. X (p. 960)       2. b and c (p. 961)
   b.                  3. a (p. 961)
   c. X (p. 960)       4. b (p. 961)
   d.                  5. a (p. 961)
   e.                  6. a (pp. 952,
   f.                     965–966)

**STOP, THINK, UNDERSTAND** *(p. 967)*

**Multiple Choice**

1. a (p. 964)          d. X (p. 964)
2. b (p. 964)          e. X (p. 965)
3. a (p. 965)          f. X (p. 965)
4. a (p. 964)          g.
5. c (p. 965)          h.
6. b (p. 965)          10. a. X (p. 963)
7. c (p. 964)              b. X (p. 963)
8. a (p. 964)              c.
9. a. X (p. 964)           d.
   b. X (p. 965)           e. X (p. 963)
   c.                      f. X (p. 963)

**Short Answer**

1. Smile; move slowly; crouch down to their eye level; speak in a calm voice; ask children what name they want to be called. (p. 966)
2. Patient sits upright in a tripod position; patient may breathe with accessory muscles; look for nasal flaring; head may bob up and down as sternocleidomastoid muscles contract; see-saw breathing may be present. (pp. 964–965)
3. Approach slowly and gently, get on their level crouching down at eye level. (p. 968)

**STOP, THINK, UNDERSTAND** *(p. 978)*

**Multiple Choice**

1. b (p. 974)          i. X (p. 969)
2. d (p. 974)          j. X (p. 969)
3. a.                  4. d (p. 971)
   b. X (p. 969)       5. a (p. 973)
   c. X (p. 969)       6. c (p. 975)
   d.                  7. c (p. 976)
   e. X (p. 969)       8. c (p. 977)
   f. X (p. 969)       9. a (p. 977)
   g. X (p. 969)       10. d (p. 974)
   h.                  11. b (p. 974)

**Fill in the Blank**

1. adolescent (p. 949)
2. child abuse (p. 960)
3. child neglect (p. 960)
4. decompensate (p. 960)
5. fontanels (p. 945)
6. nose (p. 945)

**Short Answer**

The condition of children can deteriorate quickly. (p. 975)

**CHAPTER QUESTIONS** *(p. 980)*

**Multiple Choice**

1. c (p. 954)          c. X (p. 964)
2. d (p. 956)          d.
3. a (p. 956)          e.
4. a (p. 956)          f.
5. b (p. 973)          g. X (p. 964)
6. a (p. 973)          h. X (p. 964)
7. d (p. 961)          9. b (p. 969)
8. a. X (p. 964)
   b. X (p. 964)

**Matching**

1. 1. f (p. 948)
   2. e, g, k (pp. 948, 974)
   3. a, b, d (pp. 948, 949)
   4. h, j (p. 949)
   5. c, i (p. 949)
2. 1. b (p. 951)
   2. g (p. 950)
   3. c, f (pp. 948, 950)
   4. a (p. 948)
   5. d, e (p. 951, 953)
   6. No answers are appropriate.

**List**

1. fever (p. 953)
2. hypoxia (p. 953)
3. diabetes (p. 953)
4. epilepsy (p. 953)
5. toxins (p. 953)
6. head injury (p. 953)

**Short Answer**

Status epilepticus is a seizure lasting more than 10 minutes, or a prolonged post-ictal state, or three or more seizures in a row between which the patient does not return to a normal mental status. (p. 954)

**Scenario**

1. d (pp. 943–944)    3. a (p. 954)
2. b (p. 966)         4. c (p. 954)

# Chapter 31

**STOP, THINK, UNDERSTAND** *(p. 990)*

**Multiple Choice**

1. d (p. 986)          f. X (p. 988)
2. c (p. 988)          g.
3. d (pp. 987–988)     5. c (p. 968)
4. a. X (p. 988)       6. c (p. 968)
   b. X (p. 988)       7. d (p. 969)
   c. X (p. 988)       8. c (p. 969)
   d.                  9. a (p. 969)
   e.                  10. a (pp. 989–990)

## STOP, THINK, UNDERSTAND *(p. 995)*

### Multiple Choice

1. b (p. 991)
2. a (p. 990)
3. c (p. 992)
4. b and d (p. 992)
5. a (p. 993)
6. c (p. 993)
7. b (p. 993)

### Matching

1. b (p. 994)
2. d (p. 994)
3. a (p. 994)
4. c (p. 994)

### List

1. weakness (p. 992)
2. general feeling of unease (p. 992)
3. neck pain (p. 992)
4. back pain (p. 992)
5. mild discomfort in the chest (p. 992)

## STOP, THINK, UNDERSTAND *(p. 998)*

### Multiple Choice

1. d (p. 996)
2. d (p. 996)
3. a (p. 996)
4. a (p. 996)
5. c (p. 997)
6. a. X (p. 998)
   b.
   c. X (p. 998)
   d. X (p. 998)
   e.
7. c (p. 996)

## STOP, THINK, UNDERSTAND *(p. 1004)*

### Multiple Choice

1. d (p. 1000)
2. c (p. 1002)
3. a (p. 1003)
4. b (p. 1003)
5. d (p. 993)
6. a (p. 1000)
7. d (p. 1003)
8. d (p. 1003)
9. a (p. 1003)

## CHAPTER QUESTIONS *(p. 1006)*

### Multiple Choice

1. b (pp. 000 991)
2. b (p. 996)
3. a.
   b. X (p. 1000)
   c.
   d.
   e.
   f.
   g. X (p. 1000)
   h.
4. a (p. 1003)
5. c (p. 988)

### Matching

1. 1. b (p. 989)
   2. c (p. 989)
   3. a (p. 999)
   4. d (p. 994)
2. 1. a (p. 994)
   2. c (p. 994)
3. 1. b (p. 994)
   2. d (p. 994)
3. 1. c (p. 1000)
   2. a (p. 1000)
   3. b (p. 1000)
   4. d (p. 1000)

### Scenario

1. c (p. 1002)
2. b (p. 992)
3. d (p. 1002)

# Chapter 32

## STOP, THINK, UNDERSTAND *(p. 1012)*

### Multiple Choice

1. c (p. 1011)
2. c (p. 1011)
3. c (p. 1012)

## STOP, THINK, UNDERSTAND *(p. 1014)*

### Multiple Choice

1. c (p. 1013)
2. b (p. 1013)
3. d (p. 1013)
4. a (p. 1013)
5. a (p. 1013)
6. d (p. 1013)
7. a. X (p. 1014)
   b. X (p. 1014)
   c. X (p. 1014)
   d.
   e. X (p. 1014)
   f.
   g. X (p. 1014)
   h. X (p. 1014)
   i. X (p. 1014)

### Fill in the Blank

Down syndrome, fragile X syndrome (p. 1013)

### List

(any four of the following) birth or infant asphyxia, brain trauma, lead or mercury poisoning, meningitis, Down syndrome, fragile X syndrome, fetal alcohol syndrome, syndromes that affect embryonic brain growth (p. 1013)

## STOP, THINK, UNDERSTAND *(p. 1018)*

### Multiple Choice

1. c (p. 1016)
2. d (p. 1016)
3. c (p. 1016)
4. d (p. 1016)
5. c (p. 1017)
6. b (p. 1017)

### Fill in the Blank

1. bladder catheter, urostomy, ostomy bag, ileostomy bag (p. 1016)
2. cerebral palsy (p. 1016)
3. spastic CP, athetoid, dystonic (p. 1016)

## STOP, THINK, UNDERSTAND *(p. 1027)*

### Multiple Choice

1. d (p. 1020)
2. b (No page number able to be located)
3. a.
   b. X (p. 1019)
   c. X (p. 1019)
   d.
   e.

### Fill in the Blank

1. impairment (p. 1011)
2. urostomy (p. 1016)
3. multiple sclerosis (p. 1017)
4. bi-ski (p. 1023)
5. dyslexia (p. 1012)
6. ostomy bag (p. 1016)
7. amputation (p. 1017)
8. cerebral palsy (p. 1016)
9. autonomic dysreflexia (p. 1016)
10. muscular dystrophy (p. 1017)
11. impairment (p. 1011)
12. spina bifida (p. 1017)
13. spastic (p. 1016)

### Short Answer

1. Americans with Disabilities Act; it prompted many ski resorts, for example, to begin removing physical obstacles to wheelchair access at the base area. (p. 1010)
2. Puff technology enables athletes to puff or suck on tubes using the mouth to initiate computerized motors to control, for example, a rudder and sails. (p. 1026)

## STOP, THINK, UNDERSTAND *(p. 1033)*

### Multiple Choice

1. b (p. 1028)
2. a (p. 1029)
3. c (p. 1030)
4. a (p. 1029)
5. a. X (p. 1029)
   b. X (p. 1029)
   c.
   d. X (p. 1029)
   e. X (p. 1029)
   f. X (p. 1029)
6. a. X (p. 1030)
   b. X (p. 1030)
   c. X (p. 1030)
   d. X (p. 1030)
   e. X (p. 1030)
   f. X (p. 1030)
   g. X (p. 1030)
   h.
   i. X (p. 1030)

## CHAPTER QUESTIONS *(p. 1035)*

### Multiple Choice

1. a (p. 1016)
2. d (p. 1016)
3. c (p. 1018)
4. b (p. 1031)
5. d (p. 1032)
6. d (p. 1032)
7. c (p. 1032)
8. a (p. 1032)
9. a. X (p. 1033)
   b.
   c. X (p. 1033)
   d. X (p. 1033)
   e.
   f.

### Matching

1. c (p. 1016)
2. d (p. 1017)
3. b (p. 1017)
4. a (p. 1017)

### Scenario

1. c (p. 1011)
2. c (p. 1032)
3. b (p. 1029)
4. d (p. 1029)
5. c (p. 1032)

# Chapter 33

## STOP, THINK, UNDERSTAND *(p. 1042)*

### Multiple Choice

1. c (p. 1040)
2. c (p. 1040)
3. c (p. 1040)
4. b (p. 1040)
5. a (p. 1041)

## STOP, THINK, UNDERSTAND *(p. 1046)*

### Multiple Choice

1. a (p. 1043)
2. b (p. 1043)
3. c (p. 1045)
4. a and d (p. 1045)
5. a (p. 1044)
6. c (p. 1045)
7. b (p. 1045)

### Fill in the Blank

hypoxia, hypoglycemia (pp. 993, 1042)

**Matching**

1. l (p. 1046)
2. g (p. 1045)
3. e (p. 1044)
4. k (p. 1045)
5. b (p. 1044)
6. j (p. 1044)
7. a (p. 1043)
8. f (p. 1044)
9. d (p. 1043)
10. i (p. 1045)
11. c (p. 1045)
12. h (p. 1046)

**STOP, THINK, UNDERSTAND** (p. 1049)

**Multiple Choice**

1. c (p. 1048)
2. d (p. 1049)
3. a (p. 1044)

**List**

1. 1. prolonged cardiac arrest (p. 1048)
   2. documented pulselessness and apnea for more than 30 minutes (p. 1048)
   3. livor mortis (p. 1048)
   4. rigor mortis (p. 1048)
   5. decapitation (p. 1048)
   6. obvious mortal injuries associated with cardiac arrest (p. 1048)
   7. decomposition (p. 1048)
2. 1. denial (p. 1048)
   2. anger (p. 1048)
   3. bargaining (p. 1048)
   4. depression (p. 1048)
   5. acceptance (p. 1048)

**STOP, THINK, UNDERSTAND** (p. 1057)

**Multiple Choice**

1. b (pp. 1040, 1051)
2. d (pp. 1053, 1054)
3. a (p. 1055)
4. b (p. 1055)
5. c (p. 1056)
6. c (p. 1056)
7. a. X (p. 1051)
   b. X (p. 1051)
   c. X (p. 1051)
   d.
   e. X (p. 1051)
   f.
   g.
   h.
   i.
   j. X (p. 1051)
   k.
   l. X (p. 1051)

**STOP, THINK, UNDERSTAND** (p. 1060)

**Multiple Choice**

1. a (p. 1058)
2. b (p. 1058)
3. d (p. 1059)
4. a (p. 1059)
5. c (p. 1059)
6. b (p. 1060)
7. d (pp. 1040, 1064)

**CHAPTER QUESTIONS** (p. 1060)

**Multiple Choice**

1. d (p. 1046)
2. d (p. 1053)
3. d (p. 1059)
4. b (p. 1063)

**Matching**

1. 1. a, c (p. 1043)
   2. b, d, e (p. 1043)
2. 1. a, b, d, e (pp. 1045, 1054, 1055)
   2. c, f (p. 1054)

**Scenario**

1. b (p. 1054)
2. d (p. 1045)
3. b (p. 1058)

# Chapter 34

**STOP, THINK, UNDERSTAND** (p. 1073)

**Multiple Choice**

1. b (p. 1069)
2. c (p. 1069)
3. c (p. 1071)
4. c (p. 1071)
5. a (p. 1071)

**Short Answer**

1. 28, 15, 50 (p. 1071)
2. 37 (p. 1071)

**STOP, THINK, UNDERSTAND** (p. 1076)

**Multiple Choice**

1. c (p. 1072)
2. a (p. 1072)
3. c (p. 1072)
4. a (p. 1072)
5. a (p. 1074)
6. b (p. 1075)

**Short Answer**

dizziness, diaphoresis, fainting, pallor, tachycardia, hypotension, passage of large clots (p. 1075)

**Matching**

1. 1. g (p. 1071)
   2. e (p. 1070)
   3. f (p. 1071)
   4. c (p. 1070)
   5. a (p. 1071)
   6. d (p. 1071)
   7. b (p. 1071)
2. 1. d (p. 1074)
   2. c (p. 1073)
   3. a (p. 1074)
   4. e (p. 1074)
   5. b (p. 1074)

**STOP, THINK, UNDERSTAND** (p. 1083)

**Multiple Choice**

1. b (p. 1078)
2. d (p. 1079)
3. d (p. 1079)
4. c (p. 1079)
5. c (p. 1079)
6. a. X (p. 1080)
   b. X (p. 1080)
   c.
   d. X (p. 1080)
   e. X (p. 1080)
   f. X (p. 1081)
7. a. X (p. 1079)
   b. X (p. 1079)
   c.
   d. X (p. 1079)
   e. X (p. 1079)
   f.
   g. X (p. 1080)

**Short Answer**

1. In a left lateral recumbent position; if the patient is placed on a long board supine, tilt the board slightly onto the left side (p. 1091)
2. Suctioning the nostrils before the mouth may stimulate the baby to gasp and aspirate any fluid in the nose or pharynx. (p. 1082)

3. Amniotic fluid that is not clear may be a sign of meconium in the fluid. (p. 1082)

**Matching**

1. d (p. 1078)
2. c (p. 1078)
3. a (p. 1078)
4. b (p. 1079)

**STOP, THINK, UNDERSTAND** (p. 1087)

**Multiple Choice**

1. d (p. 1085)
2. a (p. 1085)
3. d (p. 1085)
4. a (p. 1085)
5. d (p. 1085)
6. c (p. 1086)
7. b (p. 1086)
8. a (p. 1086)

**Matching**

1. a, b (pp. 1078, 1079)
2. a, c, d (p. 1078)
3. e, (p. 1078)
4. a, c, d (p. 1078)

**Short Answer**

Assess the newborn's status at 1 minute, 5 minutes, and 10 minutes after birth. Points (0, 1, or 2) are given for appearance, pulse, grimace or irritability, activity or muscle tone, and respirations. Points are added up for each time interval. The higher the number of points, the healthier the newborn. (p. 1085)

**CHAPTER QUESTIONS** (p. 1096)

**Multiple Choice**

1. a (p. 1086)
2. a (p. 1086)
3. a (p. 1088)
4. b (p. 1088)
5. a (p. 1089)
6. a. X (p. 1090)
   b.
c. X (p. 1090)
d. X (p. 1090)
e.
f. X (p. 1090)
g. X (p. 1090)
h. X (p. 1090)
i.

**Short Answer**

Ruptured uterus, abruption placenta, premature labor (p. 1088)

**Sequence**

a. 4 (pp. 1093–1094)
b. 1 (pp. 1093–1094)
c. 8 (pp. 1093–1094)
d. 2 (pp. 1093–1094)
e. 5 (pp. 1093–1094)
f. 7 (pp. 1093–1094)
g. 10 (pp. 1093–1094)
h. 3 (pp. 1093–1094)
i. 9 (pp. 1093–1094)
j. 11 (pp. 1093–1094)
k. 6 (pp. 1093–1094)

**Matching**

1. 7 (p. 1078)
2. c (p. 1073)
3. e (p. 1078)
4. d (p. 1074)
6. g (p. 1078)
5. f (p. 1071)
7. b (p. 1078)

**Scenario**

1. b (p. 1081)
2. a (p. 1079)
3. a (p. 1080)
4. b (p. 1081)
5. d (p. 1082)
6. c (p. 1085)

# Chapter 35
## STOP, THINK, UNDERSTAND *(p. 1108)*
### Multiple Choice
1. a (p. 1105)
2. b (p. 1105)
3. c (p. 1105)
4. b (p. 1102)
5. d (p. 1106)

## STOP, THINK, UNDERSTAND *(p. 1117)*
### Multiple Choice
1. c (p. 1110)
2. a (p. 1109)
3. d (p. 1112)
4. a (p. 1114)

### List
1. medical response to a disaster (p. 1110)
2. movement of patients from a disaster site to an unaffected area (p. 1110)
3. definitive medical care at participating hospitals in unaffected areas (p. 1110)

### Short Answer
1. The Mark I kit and the DuoDote kit are used to treat organophosphate exposure in mass-casualty settings, in which IV access is often impractical. (p. 1115)
2. atropine, to dry up secretions, and pralidoxime chloride (2-PAM Cl), to reverse the action of the nerve agent. (p. 1116)

## STOP, THINK, UNDERSTAND *(p. 1128)*
### Multiple Choice
1. d (p. 1121)
2. a (p. 1124)
3. b (p. 1119)

### List
1. terrain (p. 1118)
2. weather (p. 1118)
3. temperature (p. 1118)
4. time of day (p. 1118)
5. size of area to be searched (p. 1118)
6. total number of people missing (p. 1118)

### Short Answer
RECCO is a highly effective avalanche rescue system that uses harmonic radar to assist rescuers in quickly locating avalanche victims. (p. 1121)

## CHAPTER QUESTIONS *(p. 1132)*
### Multiple Choice
1. d (p. 1101)
2. b (p. 1106)
3. b (p. 1110)
4. c (p. 1114)
5. d (p. 1126)
6. b (p. 1129)
7. b (p. 1113)
8. c (p. 1113)
9. d (p. 1113)
10. b (p. 1113)

### Short Answer
1. Special operations is the generic term used to denote infrequently performed activities that require specialized training, skills, and equipment in a remote and/or austere setting. They should be called upon whenever OEC Technicians encounter incidents that exceed their scope of training and expertise. (p. 1101)
2. HAZardous Waste OPerations and Emergency Response (p. 1114)
3. Any worker, whether paid or volunteer, who works in an environment in which uncontrolled hazardous materials may be encountered is required to take HAZWOPER training. (p. 1114)

### Scenario
1. d (p. 1118)
2. b (p. 1119)
3. c (p. 1119)
4. a (p. 1121)

# Chapter 36
## STOP, THINK, UNDERSTAND *(p. 1140)*
### Multiple Choice
1. b (p. 1138)
2. a. X (p. 1137)
   b.
   c. X (p. 1137)
   d. X (p. 1137)
   e. X (p. 1137)
   f.
   g. X (p. 1137)
   h. X (p. 1137)
3. a. X (p. 1138)
   b. X (p. 1138)
   c. X (p. 1138)
   d. X (p. 1138)
   e. X (p. 1138)
   f. X (p. 1138)
   g.
   h.
4. a. X (p. 1139)
   b. X (p. 1139)
   c. X (p. 1139)
   d. X (p. 1139)
   e.

### Matching
1. 1. c (p. 1138)
   2. e (p. 1138)
   3. b (p. 1136)
   4. d (p. 1138)
   5. a (p. 1132)
2. 1. a, b, d, g, j (p. 1138)
   2. c, e, f, h, i, k (p. 1138)

## STOP, THINK, UNDERSTAND *(p. 1147)*
### Multiple Choice
1. a (p. 1141)
2. d (p. 1142)
3. a (p. 1144)

### Short Answer
Signs of airway compromise, which are described in Chapter 9 on Airway Management, include agitation, confusion, pallor, cyanosis, chest wall/sternal retractions, and very fast or very slow breathing. (p. 1141)

### Sequence
a. 5 (p. 1141)
b. 8 (p. 1141)
c. 2 (p. 1141)
d. 4 (p. 1141)
e. 7 (p. 1141)
f. 1 (p. 1141)
g. 3 (p. 1141)
h. 6 (p. 1141)

## STOP, THINK, UNDERSTAND *(p. 1151)*
### Multiple Choice
1. b (p. 1146)
2. d (p. 1149)
3. a (p. 1149)
4. c (p. 1149)
5. a (p. 1149)
6. c (p. 1149)

### List
1. clear and equal breath sounds on auscultation (p. 1150)
2. a lack of sounds on auscultation of the stomach (p. 1150)
3. equal bilateral chest rise with ventilation (p. 1150)
4. fogging of the tube (p. 1150)
5. colorimetric $CO_2$ detector with proper color change (purple) (p. 1150)
6. pulse oximetry reading (p. 1150)
7. waveform capnography (p. 1150)

## STOP, THINK, UNDERSTAND *(p. 1155)*
### Multiple Choice
1. d (p. 1152)
2. c (p. 1152)
3. a (p. 1153)
4. c (p. 1153)
5. b (p. 1153)
6. b (p. 1153)
7. a. X (p. 1152)
   b. X (p. 1152)
   c. X (p. 1152)
   d.
   e.
   f. X (p. 1152)

## STOP, THINK, UNDERSTAND *(p. 1158)*
### Multiple Choice
1. c (p. 1156)
2. a (p. 1156)
3. a (p. 1156)
4. b (p. 1156)
5. b (p. 1157)

## STOP, THINK, UNDERSTAND *(p. 1162)*
### Multiple Choice
1. c (p. 1159)
2. b (p. 1159)
3. a. X (p. 1159)
   b. X (p. 1159)
   c.
   d.
   e. X (p. 1159)
   f. X (p. 1159)
   g.
   h. X (p. 1159)
   i. X (p. 1159)

### Short Answer
The rescuer who says this is announcing the intention of providing an electrical shock to a patient. (p. 1161)

### Matching
1. c (p. 1159)
2. b (p. 1159)
3. a (p. 1159)
4. d (p. 1159)
5. a (p. 1159)
6. b (p. 1159)
7. c (p. 1159)
8. d (p. 1159)

## STOP, THINK, UNDERSTAND *(p. 1166)*
### Multiple Choice
1. d (p. 1164)
2. c (p. 1165)
3. a (p. 1165)

### Short Answer
The most worrisome side effect of morphine is respiratory depression; other side effects are headache, dizziness, and nausea. (p. 1164)

### Matching
1. b (p. 1164)
2. c (p. 1164)
3. a (p. 1164)
4. d (p. 1164)
5. a (p. 1164)
6. c (p. 1164)
7. e (p. 1164)

# CHAPTER QUESTIONS *(p. 1168)*

## Multiple Choice

**1.** a (p. 1138)  **2.** b (p. 1155)

## Short Answer

Ask the physician if she is trained in outdoor prehospital emergency care. Inform her that you are trained, and that if she starts treatment she will need to ride to the hospital with the patient. (pp. 1138– 1139)

## Matching

**1.**
1. d (p. 1149)
2. a (p. 1159)
3. c (p. 1141)
4. b (p. 1156)
5. e (p. 1153)
6. f (p. 1153)
7. g (p. 1139)

**2.**
1. a, d, f, g, h, j, n (p. 1163)
2. i, k, l (p. 1164)
3. b, c, e, f, m (p. 1163)

## Scenario

**1.** c (p. 1142)   **3.** b (p. 1146)
**2.** d (p. 1144)   **4.** a (p. 1146)

# Index

Page numbers followed by *f* indicate figures; those followed by *t* indicate tables.

## A

A (amp), defined, 583
AAA. *See* abdominal aortic aneurysm (AAA)
AAO × 4 (Awake, Alert, and Oriented to person, place, time, and situation)
  documentation tip, 715
  level of responsiveness, 222
Abandonment, defined, 17–18, 18*f*
ABCD (Airway, Breathing, Circulation, Disability) sequence
  abdominal and pelvic trauma, 801
  allergies and anaphylaxis, 443, 446–447
  altered mental status, 373, 377, 377*f*
  altitude-related emergencies, 911
  behavioral emergencies and crisis response, 1051–1052
  burned patients, 588
  cardiovascular emergencies, 472, 476
  cold-related environmental emergencies, 824
  face, eye, and neck injuries, 754
  gastrointestinal and genitourinary emergencies, 508, 510, 510*f*
  geriatric emergencies, 1001
  head and spinal injuries, 714–715
  initial care of patients and removal from a vehicle, 1107, 1107*f*
  life-threatening conditions, managing, 224–226
  lightning strikes, 852
  musculoskeletal injuries, 618, 639
  neck injuries, management of, 763
  obstetric and gynecologic emergencies, 1089, 1089*f*
  pediatric emergencies, 966
  primary assessment, 218, 218*f*
  respiratory emergencies, 418
  shock assessment, 345
  soft-tissue injuries, 551
  substance use and abuse, 396, 398
  thoracic trauma, 783
  trauma patients, 530–531, 532
  unresponsive patients, 244
  water emergency assessment, 933
Abdomen. *See also* acute abdomen
  geriatric emergencies, 993, 993*t*
  organs in, 171, 172*f*
  pain, causes of, 508*t*
  pain, with obstetrical and gynecologic emergencies
    cystitis, 1074
    dysmenorrhea, 1073–1074
    ectopic pregnancy, 1074

    ovarian cysts, 1074
    pelvic inflammatory disease, 1074
  palpation of, 509, 509*f*
  pediatric emergencies
    assessment of, 972, 972*f*, 973*f*
    injuries, 958
    pain, 953
  secondary assessment, 233, 234*f*
Abdominal and pelvic trauma
  anatomy and physiology, 794–796, 794*f*, 795*f*
  case
    disposition, 807
    presentation, 794
    update, 805
  chapter objectives, 793
  chapter overview, 793–794
  chapter review, 810–812
  common injuries
    abdominal wall contusion, 798
    diaphragm tear/rupture, 799
    evisceration, 798, 799, 800*f*
    genital injuries, 801
    hip injuries, 800, 800*f*
    impaled objects, 799, 799*f*
    intestinal tear/rupture, 799
    liver injuries, 798, 798*f*
    lower urinary tract injuries, 801
    pancreas injuries, 798–799
    pelvic fractures, 800, 800*f*
    spleen injuries, 798, 798*f*
    straddle injuries, 798, 801
    vascular injuries, 799
  Explore myNSPkit, 812
  historical timeline, 793
  key terms, 793
  patient assessment, 801–803, 802*f*, 803*f*
  patient management, 805–806
  pelvic stabilization, skill for, 808
  pelvic stabilization, skill guide for, 809, 1174
  signs and symptoms of, 801
  stop, think, understand, 796–797, 803–804, 807
  suggested reading, 812
Abdominal aortic aneurysm (AAA)
  abdominal pain, 508*t*
  cardiovascular emergency, 469
  gastrointestinal emergency, 504
  patient assessment, 475
Abdominal breathing, 418, 420
Abdominal cavity, 171, 172*f*, 495–496, 496*f*, 795
Abdominal quadrants
  described, 171, 172*f*
  organs in, 495–496, 496*f*, 795–796, 795*f*
Abdominal wall contusion, 798
Abduction
  ball and socket joints, 607
  movement, 170

Abrasions
  DCAP-BTLS assessment, 230, 230*t*
  open injuries, 545*f*, 546, 546*f*
Abruptio placentae
  defined, 1078, 1078*t*
  trauma, 1088, 1088*f*
Absence seizures
  children, 954
  defined, 364
Absorption of substances, routes for, 387–388, 388*f*
Abuse
  behavioral disorder, 1046, 1046*f*
  behavioral emergency assessment, 1056, 1056*t*
  child abuse, 960–961, 961*f*, 975, 975*t*
  elder abuse, 998
  physical abuse, 1046, 1056, 1056*t*
  sexual abuse and assault, 1046, 1056, 1056*t*, 1075–1076, 1075*f*
  verbal abuse, 1046, 1046*f*
AC (alternating current), 583
A/C joint. *See* acromioclavicular (A/C) joint
Acceleration force
  mechanism of injury, 702
  TBI, 705
Accessory muscles of respiration, 411–412, 412*f*
Accident investigation team, 286, 286*f*
"Accidental Death and Disability: The Neglected Disease of Modern Society" (National Academy of Science), 34–35
Acclimatization
  altitude, to, 902–903, 902*f*, 903*f*
  altitude illness prevention, 909, 909*f*
  defined, 902
  heat, to, 845
  personal variation, 903, 903*f*
Ace® wrap, 560
Acetaminophen
  emergency care medication, 1178*t*
  febrile seizures, 977
  infection with altered mental status, 380
  overuse and poisoning, 393
  toxicity, signs and symptoms of, 397*t*
Acetaminophen and codeine, 1178*t*
Acetaminophen and oxycodone, 392
Acetazolamide
  altitude illness prevention, 910
  emergency care medication, 1178*t*
Acetylsalicylic acid. *See* aspirin (acetylsalicylic acid)
Acidosis, 360, 361*t*, 378
Acids
  caustic substances, as contraindication to activated charcoal, 400*t*

Acids, (cont.)
  chemical burns, 582, 583f
  exposure to, 391, 391f
  toxicity, signs and symptoms of, 397t
Acquired immunodeficiency syndrome
    (AIDS). See human
    immunodeficiency virus (HIV)/
    acquired immunodeficiency
    syndrome (AIDS)
Acromioclavicular (A/C) joint
  separation of, 624–625, 624f
  upper extremity injury assessment, 623
ACS (acute coronary syndrome), 467
Activated charcoal, 399, 400f, 400t
Active warming for hypothermia,
    829–830, 829f
Acute abdomen
  causes of
    abdominal aortic aneurysm, 504
    appendicitis, 500
    bowel obstruction, 503, 503t
    cholecystitis, 502
    hepatitis, 501–502
    nephrolithiasis, 502–503
    OB/GYN-related conditions, 504
    pancreatitis, 500–501, 501f
    peptic ulcerative disease, GERD, and
        GI bleeding, 503–504, 504f
    perforated bowel, 503
    pyelonephritis, 502
  described, 499–500, 500f, 501f
  signs and symptoms, 508t
Acute coronary syndrome (ACS), 467
Acute mountain sickness (AMS)
  defined, 903, 903f
  signs and symptoms, 903–904, 903f, 904t
  treatment for, 913
Acute myocardial infarction (AMI)
  angina, distinguishing from, 474, 474f
  assessment of, 472, 473f
  cardiovascular disease, 465
  defined, 466
  described, 466–467, 467f
  geriatric emergencies, 992
  hospital care, 484–485
  silent, 474
AD (autonomic dysreflexia), 1016
ADA. See Americans with Disabilities Act
    (ADA)
Adapin. See doxepin
Adaptive athlete, defined, 1010, 1011,
    1011f. See also outdoor adaptive
    athletes
Adaptive equipment
  defined, 1018, 1019
  events for, 1019–1020
  general equipment, 1020–1022, 1020f,
    1021f, 1022f
  injury management, 1032, 1032f
  mechanism of injury, 1031, 1031f
  snow sports equipment, 1022–1025,
    1022f, 1023f, 1024f, 1025f
  warm weather sports equipment,
    1025–1026, 1026f

ADD (attention deficit disorder), 1012, 1013f
Addendums, creating, 279, 281
Adduction
  ball and socket joints, 607
  movement, 170
Adenocard®. See adenosine
Adenosine, 1163, 1164
Adenovirus, 506
Adhesive tape, allergies to, 560
Adjuncts. See also airway; airway
    management
  advanced airway adjuncts, 1148, 1148f
  airway, keeping open
    nasopharyngeal airway, 300–302, 300t,
        301f, 318, 323
    oropharyngeal airway, 300t, 302–304,
        302f, 319, 324
  defined, 300
Adolescents
  age-based assessment, 974t
  defined, 949–950, 949f
  physical, intellectual, emotional, social,
      and language development,
      948–949t
  poisoning, 954, 955f
Adrenal glands, 191, 193f, 195
Adrenalin (endocrine system), 191, 195. See
    also epinephrine
Adult-onset diabetes, 367. See also diabetes
    mellitus
Adults
  AED use, 483t
  CPR, 477–479, 477f, 478f, 482t
  vital signs, normal ranges of, 221t
Adults, older. See also geriatric emergencies
  cold injury, 818
  coup-contrecoup injury, 703
  heat illness, 842
  prescription drugs, overdose of, 392
  rib fractures, 775
  silent MI, 474
  wounds, 553
Advanced directives, 1000
Advanced Emergency Medical Technician
    (AEMT), 38, 39–40
Advanced life support (ALS)
  defined, 458
  lungs, auscultation of, 421
  musculoskeletal injuries, 639
  tension pneumothorax, 785
Advanced life support (ALS) interface
  advanced airway management
    advanced airway adjuncts, 1148, 1148f
    advanced airway placement, assessing,
        1150–1151, 1150f
    ALS providers, assisting, 1155
    cricothyrotomy, 1149–1150, 1149f
    endotracheal intubation (See
        endotracheal intubation)
    indications for, 1141
  ALS, components of, 1138
  ALS care, indications for, 1138
  ALS providers, transition of care to,
    1138–1139, 1139f

ambulance stretcher operation, 1165
cardiac monitoring and electrical therapy,
    1159–1161, 1159f, 1160f, 1161f
case
  disposition, 1166
  presentation, 1137
  update, 1158
chapter objectives, 1136
chapter overview, 1136–1137, 1137f
chapter review, 1168–1170
Explore myNSPkit, 1170
historical timeline, 1136
intravenous therapy
  ALS providers, assisting, 1157, 1158f
  equipment and set-up,
      1156–1157, 1156f
  indications for, 1156, 1156f
  intravenous needles, 1157, 1157f
  preparing a set-up for, skill for, 1167
key terms, 1136
mechanical ventilators, 1152, 1152f
medication administration, 1162–1165,
    1163f, 1164f
metered-dose inhalers and nebulizers,
    1153–1154, 1153f, 1154f
stop, think, understand, 1140, 1147,
    1151, 1155, 1158, 1162, 1166
suggested reading, 1170
working and moving as a team, 1165
AED. See automated external defibrillator
    (AED)
AEIOU-TIPS (Alcohol, acidosis, Epilepsy,
    environment, electrolytes, Insulin,
    Oxygen, overdose, Uremia,
    Trauma, tumors, Infection,
    Poisoning, psychiatric conditions,
    Seizures, stroke, syncope)
  described, 360–363, 361t, 362f, 363f
  patient assessment, 373
  patient management, 377–381, 377f, 379f
Africanized honey bees, 876
After-action reports, 51
Afterdrop, defined, 820
"Against medical advice" (A.M.A.),
    284–286, 285f
Aggrenox®. See aspirin and dipyridamole
Agitation, 1045, 1045f
AICD (automatic implantable cardioverter
    defibrillator), 484
AIDS. See human immunodeficiency virus
    (HIV)/acquired immunodeficiency
    syndrome (AIDS)
Air embolus, 752
Air splints
  ankle injuries, 669, 669f
  described, 640–641, 641f
  tourniquet, use as, 555, 555f
Air transportation
  altitude and temperature limitations, 155
  helicopter safety, 155–157, 156f,
      156t, 157f
  space and load, 155
  thoracic injuries, complicating, 782
  trauma patients, 526, 527f

types of, 154–155, 154f, 155f
weather limitations, 155
Airborne transmission of disease, 72
Airplane splint
applying, skill for, 682
described, 643, 644f
knee injuries, 665–666
Airway. *See also* ABCD (Airway, Breathing, Circulation, Disability) sequence; airway management
advanced airway management
advanced airway adjuncts, 1148, 1148f
advanced airway placement, assessing, 1150–1151, 1150f
ALS providers, assisting, 1155
cricothyrotomy, 1149–1150, 1149f
endotracheal intubation (*See* endotracheal intubation)
indications for, 1141
avalanche victims, 831
burned patients, 588
children
anatomy and physiology, 943, 944f
pediatric emergency management, 975, 975f, 976f, 977
complete obstruction, signs of, 966
defined, 291
face, eye, and neck injuries, 754, 756
facial injuries, 749, 750f
lightning strike management, 855
neck injuries, assessment of, 756
obstruction/choking emergencies, 413
plant and animal emergencies, 885
primary assessment, 218–219, 219f
Airway management
airway, clearing
finger sweep, 297–298, 297f
gravity, 297
suction, 298–300, 298f, 299f
airway, keeping open and clear
airway adjuncts, 300–304, 300t, 301f, 302f, 318–319, 323–324
barrier devices, 304–306, 304f, 305f
recovery position, 300, 300f
airway and mouth, opening
crossed-finger method, 297, 297f
head-tilt, chin-lift, 295, 296f
jaw-thrust maneuver, 295, 296f, 297
anatomy and physiology, 292–294, 293f, 294f, 295
case
disposition, 316
presentation, 293
update, 304
chapter objectives, 291–292
chapter overview, 291–292, 292f
chapter review, 326–328
Explore myNSPkit, 328
historical timeline, 291
key terms, 292
management, overview of, 294–295
oxygen therapy
bag-valve masks, 313–315, 313f, 313t, 314f, 315f

gastric distention, 315–316
indications for, 310–311
nasal cannulas, 311–312, 311f, 311t
nonrebreather masks, 312–313, 312f, 313t
oxygen containers, 306–307, 306f, 307f, 307t
oxygen cylinder set-up and breakdown, 307–308, 320–321, 325
oxygen flow duration rates, 308–309, 309t
oxygen safety, 309
pulse oximetry, 315–316f
Skill Guides
nasopharyngeal airway, inserting, 323, 1173
oropharyngeal airway, inserting, 324, 1173
oxygen cylinder, preparing for use and break down, 325, 1173
suctioning a patient's airway, 322, 1173
Skills
nasopharyngeal airway, inserting, 318
oropharyngeal airway, inserting, 319
oxygen tank set-up and breakdown, 320–321
suctioning a patient's airway, 317
stop, think, understand, 294, 301, 303, 310, 316
Airway patency, defined, 413
Alarm stage of stress reaction, 61t
Albuterol
ALS administration, 1163
common medication for respiratory conditions, 420
emergency care medication, 1178t
Alcohol intake
abdominal and pelvic trauma, 802
activated charcoal, 400t
altered mental status, 360, 361t, 377–378, 377f
behavioral emergencies, 1043, 1043f
cold injury, 817
ethanol percentages, 393
outdoor work, avoiding with, 65
overuse and poisoning, 391, 392, 393
toxicity, signs and symptoms of, 397t
Alcohol poisoning, 393
Alcohol withdrawal, 393
Allegra. *See* fexofenadine
Allergen, defined, 437
Allergic reactions
bee stings, 886, 887f
defined, 435
plants, to, 863, 863f
SAMPLE history, 227t, 228
Allergies and anaphylaxis
anatomy and physiology, 435–437, 436f, 437f
auto-injector administration, skill guide for, 453, 1173
case
disposition, 450
presentation, 436
update, 442

categories of
mild allergic reactions, 439
moderate allergic reactions, 440
severe allergic reactions, 440, 441f
causes, 438–439, 439f
chapter objectives, 434
chapter overview, 434–435, 435f
chapter review, 454–456
common medications, 443t
Explore myNSPkit, 456
historical timeline, 434
key terms, 434
patient assessment
anaphylactic shock, 445
mild allergic reaction, 444
moderate allergic reaction, 444
primary assessment and ABCDs, 443
secondary assessment, 443–445, 443f, 443t, 444f
severe allergic reaction, 444–445
patient management
epinephrine, 447–449, 448f
insect stingers, 446, 447f
severe allergic reaction, 446–449, 447f, 448f
reactions, prevention of, 440–442, 442f
Skills
auto-injector: EpiPen™, administration with, 450
auto-injector: Twinject™, administration with, 451
auto-injector: Twinject™ additional dose, administration with, 452
stop, think, understand, 438, 445–446, 449
suggested reading, 456
Allergy, defined, 434, 435
"Allergy shots," 442
Alligators
adverse effects from, 879, 879f
bites, assessment of, 887
Aloe vera ointment, 828
Alpaca injuries, 884
Alpine pack (emergency care equipment), 1175, 1175f, 1178t
Alprazolam, 391
ALS. *See* advanced life support (ALS)
Altered mental status
anatomy and physiology
brain, 356–357, 357f, 358
endocrine system, 358–359, 359f
peripheral nervous system, 357, 358f
case
disposition, 381
presentation, 357
update, 372
causes of, 359–363, 359f, 361t, 362f, 363f
chapter objectives, 355
chapter overview, 355–356, 356f
chapter review, 382–385
conditions associated with
diabetes mellitus, 365–369, 366f, 367f, 368f, 368t
epilepsy, 363

Altered mental status, *(cont.)*
   seizures, 363–365, 363*f*, 364–365*f*, 364*f*
   stroke, 370–371, 370*f*, 371*f*
defined, 356
Explore myNSPkit, 385
geriatric emergencies, 991, 991*f*
historical timeline, 355
key terms, 355–356
patient assessment
   primary assessment, 373
   secondary assessment, 373–375, 373*f*,
      374*t*, 375*f*
   stroke signs and symptoms, 375–377,
      375*f*, 376*f*
   traumatic or medical cause, 372, 372*f*
patient management, 377–381, 377*f*, 379*f*
presentations of, 359
stop, think, understand, 360, 369
suggested reading, 385
violent behavior, 381
Alternating current (AC), 583
Altitude
   aircraft operation limitations, 155
   defined, 898, 898*f*
   thoracic injuries, complicating, 782
Altitude illness, defined, 898
Altitude-related emergencies
   altitude illness, prevention of, 909–911,
      909*f*, 910*f*
   altitude physiology
      altitude, defined, 898, 898*f*
      altitude acclimatization, 902–903,
         902*f*, 903*f*
      altitude classifications, 899–902, 899*f*,
         900*f*, 901*f*
      individual response, 898–899
      rate of ascent, 898, 899*f*
   case
      disposition, 915
      presentation, 897
      update, 908
   chapter objectives, 896
   chapter overview, 896–898, 897*f*
   chapter review, 915–917
   common problems
      acute mountain sickness, 903–904,
         903*f*, 904*t*
      chilblains, 907
      concurrent medical conditions, 906
      high-altitude cerebral edema, 905, 905*f*
      high-altitude pulmonary edema,
         904–905, 905*f*
      high-altitude retinal hemorrhage, 906
      Khumbu cough, 906
      peripheral edema, 906
      radial keratotomy blindness, 906
      solar keratitis, 906–907, 906*f*
      sunburn, 907, 907*f*
   Explore myNSPkit, 918
   historical timeline, 896
   incidence of, in Rocky Mountain high-
      mountain resorts, 897, 897*f*
   key terms, 896
   patient assessment, 911–912, 911*f*

patient management, 912–914, 912*f*,
   913*f*, 914*f*
stop, think, understand, 908, 914
suggested reading, 918
Alveoli
   lower airway, 174, 176*f*
   respiratory emergencies, 411, 411*f*
A.M.A. ("against medical advice"),
   284–286, 285*f*
Amanita mushrooms, 870, 870*f*
Ambient temperature
   aircraft operation limitations, 155
   defined, 839, 840
Ambulance operations. *See also* special
      operations and ambulance
      operations
   ambulance designs, 1101–1102, 1102*f*
   arriving at the scene, 1103–1105, 1104*f*
   call, preparing for, 1102, 1103*f*
   call, responding to, 1103, 1103*f*
   extrication of patient from a vehicle,
      1105–1107, 1106*f*, 1107*f*, 1107*t*
   OEC Technicians interacting with
      ambulance crews, 1101, 1101*f*
   transferring patients, 1105, 1105*f*
American Academy of Pediatrics, 847
American Burn Association, 590, 591*f*
American College of Surgeons, 338*t*
American Red Cross (ARC)
   CPR course, 537
   *First Aid Textbook*, 8
   First-Aid training program, 56
   founding of, 34
   NSP and "Ski Safety and First Aid," 6
Americans with Disabilities Act (ADA)
   adaptive athletes, 1010
   OEC course, 12
   ski lifts, 1025
AMI. *See* acute myocardial infarction (AMI)
Aminophylline, 420
Amiodarone
   ALS administration to cardiac patients,
      1163, 1164
   cardiac medication, 487*t*
Amitriptyline
   overuse and poisoning, 391
   psychotropic agent, 1054*t*
Amnesia, 705, 707
Amniotic sac, premature rupture of,
   1088*f*, 1089
Amoxicillin and clavulanate, 1178*t*
Amp (A), defined, 583
AMPLE (Allergies, Medications, Past medical
      problems, Last meal, Events leading
      to situation) information, 275, 277*f*
Amputated parts
   care of, 547*f*, 556
   replantation of, 558
   skill for emergency care of, 569
Amputation
   adaptive athletes, 1017
   described, 556, 558
   fingers, 628
   open injuries, 545*f*, 547, 547*f*

AMS. *See* acute mountain sickness (AMS)
Analgesic
   ALS administration, 1164, 1164*f*
   defined, 1164
Anaphylactic shock
   causes of, 341*t*
   described, 337*f*, 340–341, 440
   signs and symptoms, 445
Anaphylaxis. *See also* allergies and
      anaphylaxis
   defined, 437
   process described, 440, 441*f*
Anatomical position for lifting, 129–130,
   129*f*, 130*f*
Anatomy, defined, 168
Anatomy and physiology
   body cavities, 171–173, 172*f*
   body planes and directional terms,
      168–170, 168*f*, 169*f*
   body systems
      body system, defined, 174
      cardiovascular system, 176–182, 178*f*,
         179*f*, 180*f*, 181*f*
      endocrine system, 191, 193*f*, 195
      gastrointestinal system, 187–189,
         188*f*, 189*f*
      integumentary system, 194*f*, 195, 195*f*
      lymphatic system, 206, 207*f*
      muscular system, 199–201, 200*f*, 201*f*
      nervous system, 183–187, 184*f*, 185*f*,
         186*f*, 187*f*
      reproductive system, 201, 203–206,
         204*f*, 205*f*
      respiratory system, 174–176, 175*f*,
         176*f*, 177*f*
      skeletal system, 195–199, 196*f*, 197*f*,
         198*f*, 199*f*
      urinary system, 191, 192*f*
   case
      disposition, 209
      presentation, 169
      update, 190
   chapter objectives, 167
   chapter overview, 167–168, 168*f*
   chapter review, 209–212
   Explore myNSPkit, 212
   historical timeline, 167
   homeostasis, 206, 208*f*
   key terms, 167–168
   movements, terms for, 170
   position, terms for, 169*f*, 170–171,
      170*f*, 171*f*
   stop, think, understand, 173, 182,
      189–190, 202–203, 208–209
   suggested reading, 212
Anatomy and physiology for specific
      conditions
   abdominal and pelvic trauma, 794–796,
      794*f*, 795*f*
   airway management
      lower airway, 293–294, 294*f*
      upper airway, 292–293, 293*f*
   allergies and anaphylaxis, 435–437,
      436*f*, 437*f*

altered mental status
  brain, 356–357, 357f, 358
  endocrine system, 358–359, 359f
  peripheral nervous system, 357, 358f
behavioral emergencies and crisis
    response, 1041–1042, 1041f
cardiovascular emergencies
  blood, 462, 464
  blood vessels, 460–462, 461f,
    462f, 463f
  heart, 459–460, 460f
cold-related environmental emergencies
  heat loss, mechanisms of, 816–817,
    816f, 817f
  risk factors for cold injury,
    817–818, 817f
  thermoregulation, process of, 815–816
face, eye, and neck injuries
  auditory and balance system, 744, 745f
  facial structures, 743–744, 743f
  neck anatomy, 747, 747f
  visual system, 744–746, 746f
gastrointestinal/genitourinary emergencies,
    495–496, 496f, 497f–498f
head and spinal cord injuries, 699–700,
    699f, 700f
heat-related emergencies, 839–841, 840f
immune response, 62, 62f, 63t
musculoskeletal injuries
  healing process, 610, 610f
  importance of, 602–603
  joints, 606–607, 606f, 607f
  ligaments, 607–608, 607f, 609
  movement, physiology of, 609
  muscles, 608–609, 608f, 609f
  skeleton, 603–605, 603f, 604f, 605f
  stop, think, understand, 605–606,
    611–612
  tendons, 609, 609f
obstetric and gynecologic emergencies,
    1069–1072, 1070f, 1072f
OEC Technicians learning, 8, 9f
pediatric emergencies, 943–945, 944f, 945f
plant and animal emergencies, 862, 862f
rescue basics
  "fight or flight" response, 61–62, 61t, 62f
  immune response, 62, 62f, 63t
  temperature regulation, 58–61, 58f,
    59f, 60f, 61f
respiratory emergencies
  gas exchange, 408–410, 409f
  lower airway, 410–412, 410f, 411f, 412f
  normal breathing, 412
  respiratory cycle, 410
shock
  cardiovascular system, 331–334, 331f,
    333–334f, 333f
  physiologic compensation and stages of
    shock, 335–336, 336f
skin, and burns, 580–581, 581f
soft-tissue injuries
  physiology of bleeding and clotting,
    540, 542
  skin anatomy, 539–540, 539f

substance abuse and poisoning
  body systems affected, 389–390
  physiologic actions, 387–389,
    388f, 389f
thoracic trauma, 772–773, 772f
water emergencies, 921–923, 921f,
    922f, 922t
Aneurysms. See also abdominal aortic
    aneurysm (AAA)
  aortic, 469–470, 470f, 475, 780, 780f
  brain, 470
Angel dust, 394. See also PCP
    (phencyclidine)
Angina pectoris
  described, 466, 466f
  myocardial infarction, distinguishing
    from, 474, 474f
  types of, 467t
Angioedema, defined, 440
Angioplasty, 484
Angulation, defined, 625
Animals. See also plant and animal
    emergencies
  aquatic, and water emergencies,
    930–931, 931f
  bites, management of, 889, 890, 890f
  search dogs, 1125–1127, 1125f,
    1126f, 1127f
Aniscoria, 745, 755, 755f
Ankle (traction) hitch, tying, 662, 662f
Ankles
  injury assessment, 635–636, 635f, 636f
  injury management, 668–670, 669f, 670f
Anorexia, 508t
Anoxia, defined, 415
Ant bites, 875, 876, 876f, 886–887
Antegrade amnesia
  described, 707
  post-concussive syndrome, 708
Anterior chamber of the eye, 745, 746f
Anterior (ventral) direction, 169, 169f
Anterior hip dislocation, 631, 631f
Anterior sternoclavicular (S/C)
    dislocation, 624
Antianxiety drugs, overuse of, 391
Antibody
  allergies, 436–437, 436f
  defined, 436
Anticoagulants
  coup-contrecoup injury, 704
  shock, 345
  soft-tissue injuries, 551
Antidepressants
  overuse and poisoning, 391
  toxicity, signs and symptoms of, 397t
Antigens
  allergies, 436–437, 436f
  defined, 436
Antipsychotics
  overuse and poisoning, 391
  toxicity, signs and symptoms of, 397t
Antivenom
  snake bites, 889
  spider bites, 873

Anxiety
  behavioral emergency assessment, 1055
  neurotic disorder, 1044
Aorta
  abdominal, 496, 497f
  abdominal trauma, 795
  anatomy, 179f, 180
  cardiovascular emergencies, 460, 461f
  defined, 459
Aortic aneurysm
  abdominal, 469, 475, 504, 508t
  described, 469–470, 470f
  patient assessment, 475
  thoracic trauma, 780, 780f
Aortic dissection
  described, 470, 470f, 779–780, 780f
  pain, 472
  patient assessment, 475
Aortic rupture
  described, 779–780, 780f
  fractured sternum, 776
APGAR score, 1085, 1085t
Appearance, in the pediatric assessment
    triangle, 963, 964, 964f
Appendicitis
  abdominal pain, 508t
  children, 953
  described, 500
  GI emergency, 796
Appendicular skeleton, defined,
    604, 604f
Appendix
  appendicitis, 500, 508t, 796, 953
  hollow organ, 495, 496f
  location of, 795f
Aquatic animals. See marine animals
Aqueous humor, 745
Arachnoid mater, 183, 185
ARC. See American Red Cross (ARC)
Armpits, assessment of, 783
Arrhythmia, described, 467–468
Arsenic, 400t
Arterial gas embolism (AGE), defined,
    928, 928f
Arteries. See also aorta
  anatomy of, 178f, 179f, 180, 181f
  bleeding from, 540, 542f
  cardiovascular emergencies, 460,
    461f, 462
  coronary arteries, 177, 180f
  major, of the body, 497f
  shock, 332, 333f
Arterioles, 179f, 180
Arteriosclerosis, defined, 464
Articular cartilage, 604, 605f
Articulation, defined, 633
Artificial eyes, management of, 762
Artificial joints
  elderly patients, 999, 999f
  injury to, 660
ASDs. See autism spectrum disorders (ASDs)
Asherman™ chest seal, 561, 785
Asperger's syndrome, 1013
Aspiration pneumonia, 505

Aspirin (acetylsalicylic acid)
  acute MI, 486–487, 487t
  cardiovascular emergencies, 472
  clotting process, 542
  coup-contrecoup injury, 704
  elderly patients, 994
  overuse and poisoning, 393
  toxicity, signs and symptoms of, 397t
  wounds, 553
Aspirin and dipyridamole, 345
Assault
  defined, 23–24, 24f
  sexual assault, 1075–1076, 1075f
Assessment, defined, 214. See also patient
    assessment; patient assessment for
    specific conditions
Assumption of risk, doctrine of, 18–19
Astelin. See azelastine hydrochloride
Asthma
  children, 951, 951f
  geriatric emergency management,
    1003–1004
  medications for, 1163
  respiratory emergencies, 414, 415f
Asystole, 468
Ataxia
  altitude-related emergencies, 912
  defined, 905
Atenolol
  beta-blocker use by the elderly, 994
  cardiac medication, 487t
  shock, 345
Atherosclerosis, 464–465, 464f
Athetoid cerebral palsy, 1016, 1017
Athlete's foot, 72
Ativan. See lorazepam
Atlas (C1 vertebrae), 699f, 711
Atlas-axis injuries, 711
Atmosphere, described, 922
Atorvastatin, 487t
Atria of the heart, 177, 179f
Atropine
  ALS administration to cardiac patients,
    1163, 1164
  nerve agent poisoning, 1116
  organophosphate poisoning, 1115
Atrovent®. See ipratropium
Attention deficit disorder (ADD),
    1012, 1013f
Atwater, Monty, 213
Auditory system, 744, 745f
Augmentin. See amoxicillin and clavulanate
Aura, defined, 364, 364f
Autism spectrum disorders (ASDs)
  athletes with, assessing, 1030
  defined, 1013
Autoimmune disorders, 62
Auto-injectors
  administration, skill guide for, 453, 1173
  epinephrine, 443, 885, 888–889
  EpiPen™, 447–448, 448f, 449, 450
  nerve agent and organophosphate
    poisoning, 1115, 1115f, 1116
  Twinject™, 447, 448, 448f, 449, 451, 452

Automated external defibrillator (AED)
  cardiac arrest, 482–484, 482f, 483t
  certification and recertification, 12
  defined, 465
  electrical burns, 595
  lightning strike management, 855
  moderate-to-severe hypothermia, 831
  transport of patients, 157–158
  using, skill for, 490
Automatic implantable cardioverter
    defibrillator (AICD), 484
Autonomic dysfunction (dysautonomia)
  athletes with, assessing, 1030
  cognitive disability, 1013
Autonomic dysreflexia (AD), 1016
Autonomic nervous system
  described, 187, 187f
  dysautonomia (autonomic dysfunction),
    1013, 1030
Autonomy, as ethical issue, 15
Autumn crocus, 865, 865f
Avalanche Handbook (Atwater), 213
Avalanche rescue
  equipment for, 1123, 1123f
  functions of, 1121
  hypothermia, 831–832
  overview of, 1120–1121, 1120f
  RECCO system, 1121, 1121f
  sequence of events, 1122–1123,
    1122f, 1123f
AVPU (Alert, Verbal, Pain, Unresponsive)
    scale
  altered mental status, 373
  head and spinal injury assessment, 714,
    715, 715t, 716
  musculoskeletal injuries, 618
  neurologic function, 222–223, 223t
  respiratory emergencies, 418
  soft-tissue injuries, 551
Avulsions
  DCAP-BTLS assessment, 230, 230t
  described, 556
  open injuries, 545f, 546–547, 547f
Axial drag, skill for, 728
Axial skeleton
  bones of, 699, 699f
  defined, 604, 604f
  injuries taking precedence, 638
Axis (C2 vertebrae), 699f, 711
Axons, defined, 700
Azalea, 868
Azelastine hydrochloride, 443t

## B

Back
  chest assessment, part of, 783
  secondary assessment, 233, 234f
Bacteria, and diarrhea, 506
Bacterial meningitis, 75
Bag-valve system for endotracheal tubes,
    1146, 1146f
Bag-valve mask (BVM)
  one-rescuer BVM, 314, 314f

  oxygen flow rate, 313
  oxygen therapy, 313–314, 313f
  suspected lung injury, patients
    with, 785
  two-person BVM, 314–315, 315f
  ventilation volumes, 313, 313t
Balance, and ear anatomy and physiology,
    744, 745f
Bald-faced hornets, 875f
Ball and socket joints, 607
Bandages. See also dressing and bandaging
  defined, 559
  elastic bandages, 560
  self-evacuation with ankle injuries,
    670, 670f
Bark scorpions, 874, 874f
Barotrauma
  arterial gas embolism, 928, 928f
  decompression sickness, 927–928,
    927f, 928t
  defined, 927
  squeeze and reverse squeeze, 928
Barracuda, 881, 881f, 930
Barrier devices for airway management
  described, 304, 304f
  face shield, 304–305
  pocket mask, 305–306, 305f
Barton, Clara, 34
"Baseline vitals," 238
Bases
  caustic substances, as contraindication to
    activated charcoal, 400t
  chemical burns, 582, 583f
  exposure to, 391, 391f
  toxicity, signs and symptoms of, 397t
Basic life support (BLS), 476
Basic Trauma Life Support (Campbell), 230
Basilar skull fracture, 704–705, 705f
Basket stretcher
  defined, 131
  lifting, for, 134, 134f
  patient transport, 151, 151f
Bass (fish), 881
Bats
  injuries caused by, 884, 884f
  rabies, 890
Battery, defined, 23–24, 24f
Battle's sign
  basilar skull fracture, 705, 705f
  described, 756
BEAM (body elevation and movement)
    lift, 144
BEAN (body elevation and nonmovement)
    lift, 144, 161, 162, 1173
Bear injuries, 884–885, 885f
Beck's Triad, 779
Bed linen, contaminated, 81
Bee stings
  adverse effects from, 875–876, 875f
  patient assessment, 886, 887f
  patient management, 888
Behavior
  alterations, causes of, 1044t
  defined, 1040

emergency, signs and symptoms of, 1052, 1052t, 1054–1055
violent, with altered mental status, 381
Behavioral emergencies and crisis response
anatomy and physiology, 1041–1042, 1041f
case
disposition, 1061
presentation, 1041
update, 1050
chapter objectives, 1039
chapter overview, 1039–1041, 1040f
chapter review, 1064–1066
common behavioral emergencies
behavioral conditions, 1043–1046, 1043f, 1044t, 1045f, 1046f
chemical exposures, 1043, 1043f
medical disorders, 1042, 1042f
trauma, 1043, 1043f
death and grief, 1047–1049, 1048f, 1049f
Explore myNSPkit, 1067
historical timeline, 1039
key terms, 1040
patient assessment
primary assessment, 1051–1054, 1052f, 1052t, 1053f, 1053t
scene safety, 1051, 1051f
secondary assessment, 1054–1056, 1054t, 1056t
patient management, 1056–1057, 1058–1060, 1058f, 1059f, 1060f
patient restraint, skill guide for, 1063, 1174
physical/mechanical restraint of a patient, skill for, 1062
stop, think, understand, 1042, 1046–1047, 1049–1050, 1057–1058, 1060–1061
suggested reading, 1067
Behavioral emergency, defined, 1040
Belladonna, 867
Benadryl. See diphenhydramine
"The bends," 927, 934. See also decompression sickness
Beneficence, as ethical issue, 15
Best motor response, for GCS, 716, 716f, 717f
Beta-blockers
medication use by the elderly, 994
shock, 345
Bike kit (emergency care equipment), 1176, 1176f, 1178t
Bipolar (manic-depressive) disorder
cognitive disability, 1013
psychotic disorder, 1045
Bi-ski, defined, 1023
Bison injuries, 884
Bite marks, assessment of, 885, 885f
Black widow spiders, 871, 872f
Blanket drag, 137, 137f
Blanket roll splint
described, 641
shoulder application, skill for, 678
shoulder application, skill guide for, 687, 1173
shoulder dislocation, 653

Blankets
cold-related environmental emergencies, 824, 824f
contaminated, procedures for dealing with, 81
Blast injury, categories of, 523–524, 524f
"Blast pattern triad," 524
Bleach, household, 81
Bleeding. See also hemorrhage
controlling
avalanche victims, 831
face, eye, and neck injuries, 756
lower extremity injuries, 630
neck injuries, 763, 763f
skill for, 566
skill guide for, 574, 1173
soft-tissue injuries, 551, 551f, 552
DCAP-BTLS assessment, 230, 230t
fractures, blood loss from, 615, 615t, 660
gastrointestinal, 504, 508t
physiology of, 540, 542, 542f
primary assessment, 221
Blood
cardiovascular emergencies, 462, 464
flow through heart, 177, 179f
oxygenated and oxygen-depleted, 180
plasma, 180, 181, 181f
platelets, 180, 181, 181f
red blood cells, 180–181, 181f
shock, 332–334, 333–334f
substance exposure, effects of, 390
systemic and pulmonary circulation, 177, 179f, 180
volume, during pregnancy, 1071
white blood cells, 180, 181, 181f
Blood pressure (BP)
auscultated, obtaining, procedure for, 240–241
defined, 239
explained, 181–182
normal ranges, by age, 221t
normal values by age, 971t
obtaining by auscultation, skill for, 250
obtaining by auscultation, skill guide for, 256, 1173
orthostatic blood pressure test, 242–244, 244f
palpated, obtaining, procedure for, 241, 241f
pediatric emergencies, 972, 972f
pregnancy, 1072
secondary assessment, 239–241, 240f, 241f
Blood pressure cuffs
pediatric size, 972, 972f
tourniquet, use as, 554, 554f
Blood tests for allergies, 442
Blood "thinners." See also aspirin (acetylsalicylic acid); warfarin
clotting process, 542
geriatric emergency management, 1003
medication use by the elderly, 994
Blood vessels. See also arteries; circulatory system; pulmonary circulation; veins

anatomy of, 178f, 179f, 180, 181f
cardiovascular emergencies, 460–462, 461f, 462f, 463f
coronary arteries, 177, 180f
shock, 332, 333f
systemic and pulmonary circulation, 177, 179f, 180
"Blow-by" oxygen
newborns, 1086, 1086f
pediatric emergency management, 976, 976f
Blowout fractures, 749, 750f
BLS (basic life support), 476
Blue gill fish, 881
Blunt force trauma
blunt (closed) injury, 522, 522f
common MOI, 85
eyes, 760, 760f
neck injuries, 763
Bobcat injuries, 883
Bodily distribution of substances, 389, 389f
Body cavities, 171–173, 172f, 495–496, 496f, 773, 795
Body mechanics
anatomical position for lifting, 129–130, 129f, 130f
defined, 128
human spine, 128–129, 128f
lifting, planning for, 130–131, 130f
Body substance isolation (BSI)
body fluids, list of, 77
defined, 76
disease transmission prevention, 76–77, 77f
Body surface area (BSA)
children, 944
Rule of Nines, 589–590, 590f
Body system, defined, 174
Body temperature. See also core body temperature
children, 945
cold emergencies, 819, 826–827, 826f
death, 936
heat emergencies, 839, 842, 842f, 853
normal values, by age, 221t, 971t
regulation of (See heat loss)
secondary assessment, 242, 242t
Bolin™ chest seal, 785
Bone crepitus, defined, 621
Bone marrow, 199, 199f
Bones. See skeletal system; skeleton; specific bones
Boot top fractures, 635, 635f
Boots
removal
procedure for, 670–671
skill for, 684
skill guide for, 691, 1174
tight-fitting, and cold injury, 819
Bost, Larry, 11t
Bowel obstruction
abdominal pain, 508t
causes of, 503t
described, 503

Bowman, Warren
  NSP National Medical Advisor, 494
  *Outdoor Emergency Care*, 3, 6, 7*f*, 7*t*
  positions in which patients are found, 673
  *Winter Emergency Care*, 6, 770, 793
  *Winter First Aid Manual*, 579, 861
"Boxer's" fracture, 628
Boyle's Law, 923
BP. *See* blood pressure (BP)
Brachial artery for BP measurement, 240, 240*f*
Brachial pulse
  CPR on an infant, 480
  primary assessment, 220, 221*f*
  secondary assessment, 238, 239*f*
Bradypnea, defined, 418
Brain. *See also* traumatic brain injury (TBI)
  altered mental status, 356–357, 357*f*, 358
  anatomy of, 183, 184*f*, 185, 185*f*, 186*f*
  injury, two phases of, 705
  parts of, 699–700
  trauma, and face, eye, and neck injuries, 754
Brain aneurysms, 470
Brain stem
  altered mental status, 356, 357*f*
  anatomy of, 183, 185, 185*f*, 186*f*
  defined, 700
Breasts, assessing, 203, 205*f*
Breath sounds, defined, 422
Breathing. *See also* ABCD (Airway, Breathing, Circulation, Disability) sequence
  breath, holding, under water, 929, 929*f*
  children, 943, 945
  difficulty, and head-uphill position, 149
  lightning strike management, 855
  plant and animal emergencies, 885
  primary assessment, 219–220, 220*f*, 221*t*
  rate, rhythm, and quality, 412
  stimulating, in newborns, 1085, 1085*f*
Breech delivery, 1080, 1080*f*
Brethine. *See* terbutaline
Bridge (BEAN) lift, 144, 161, 162, 1173
Brompheniramine, 443*t*
Bronchi
  lower airway, 174, 176*f*
  respiratory emergencies, 410, 410*f*
Bronchioles, 174, 176*f*
Bronchiolitis, 950
Bronchodilators, 993
Bronchospasm, 414
Brooks-Range Sled, 151
Brown recluse spiders, 872, 872*f*
Bruises, 230, 230*t*
BSA. *See* body surface area (BSA)
BSI. *See* body substance isolation (BSI)
Bucket, for a sit-ski, 1023, 1024
Bulbourethral gland, 204*f*
Bullae, defined, 864
Burn centers, transportation of patients to, 595
Burns
  anatomy and physiology, 580–581, 581*f*

burn, defined, 579–580
caring for, skill for, 597
case
  presentation, 580, 596
  update, 587
chapter objectives, 579
chapter overview, 579–580
chapter review, 598–600
children, 959
classification of
  fourth-degree burns, 585, 587*t*
  full-thickness (third-degree) burns, 585, 585*f*, 586, 586*f*, 587*t*
  partial-thickness (second-degree) burns, 585, 585*f*, 586, 586*f*, 587*t*
  superficial (first-degree) burns, 585, 585*f*, 587*t*
DCAP-BTLS assessment, 230, 230*t*
documentation of, 586
Explore myNSPkit, 600
eyes, to, 760–762, 761*f*
further care and transport, 595
historical timeline, 579
key terms, 579
lightning-caused, 848, 848*f*
outdoor hazards, 580
patient assessment
  ABCDs and primary assessment, 588, 588*f*
  scene size-up, 588
  secondary assessment, 589
  severity and extent, determining, 589–590, 590*f*, 591*f*
patient management
  ABCDs, 591–592
  bleeding, controlling, 592
  chemical burns, 593–594, 594*f*
  covering and positioning patient, 593
  dressings, 592, 592*f*
  electrical burns, 592, 594–595, 595*f*
  radiation burns, 595
  stopping the burning, 591, 591*f*, 592, 593
  thermal burns, 593, 593*f*
soft-tissue injuries, 549
stop, think, understand, 587, 596
suggested reading, 600
types of
  chemical burns, 582, 583*t*
  electrical burns, 583–584, 584*f*
  radiation burns, 584
  thermal burns, 581–582, 582*f*
BURP (Backward, Upward, Rightward, Pressure) maneuver, 1146, 1147*f*
Bush, George W., 99
Butterfly fragments in fractures, 615*t*, 635
BVM. *See* bag-valve mask (BVM)

## C

"C₃, C₄, C₅, keep the diaphragm alive," 712
CABG (coronary artery bypass grafting), 485
Cactus, 864, 864*f*

CAD (coronary artery disease), 464
Calcium, 199
Calcium-channel blockers, 994
Callus, defined, 610
Campbell, John
  *Basic Trauma Life Support*, 230
  DCAP-BTLS assessment, 230, 230*t*
Cancer, 503*t*
Canes, 1020–1021
Cannabis, 394, 886. *See also* marijuana
Capacity, defined, 284
Capillaries
  anatomy of, 178*f*, 179*f*, 180, 181*f*
  bleeding from, 540, 542*f*
  cardiovascular emergencies, 462, 462*f*
  shock, 332, 333*f*
Capillary refill test
  pediatric emergencies, 972, 972*f*
  primary assessment, 222, 222*f*
Carbon dioxide ($CO_2$)
  colorimetric $CO_2$ detectors, 1146, 1146*f*
  respiratory gas exchange, 408–410, 409*f*
Carbon monoxide (CO)
  burned patients, 589
  poisoning, 394
  poisoning, interventions for, 400
  respiratory emergencies, 416
  toxicity, signs and symptoms of, 397*t*
Cardboard splints
  described, 642–643, 643*f*
  Quick Splint, replacing, skill for, 683
Cardiac arrest
  children, 952
  CPR for adults, children, and infants, 482*t*
  CPR on a child, 479–480, 479*f*, 480*f*
  CPR on an infant, 480–481, 481*f*
  defined, 485
  early advanced care, 484
  early defibrillation, 481–484, 482*f*, 483*t*
  electrical burns, 595
  one-rescuer CPR on an adult, 477–478, 477*f*, 478*f*
  recognition of, and activation of emergency response system, 476–477, 477*f*
  two-rescuer CPR on an adult, 479
Cardiac arrhythmia, described, 467–468
Cardiac monitoring
  ALS provider, assisting, 1161
  equipment and set-up, 1159–1160, 1159*f*, 1160*f*
  indications for, 1159
  leads, placement of, 1159–1160, 1159*f*
Cardiac muscle, 199, 201*f*, 608, 609, 609*f*
Cardiac output, defined, 332
Cardiac stents, 484
Cardiac tamponade
  management of, 785
  pulsus paradoxus, 779
Cardiogenic shock
  defined, 468
  described, 337*f*, 339, 339*f*
  patient assessment, 474–475

Cardiopulmonary resuscitation (CPR)
  avalanche victims, 832
  certification and recertification, 12
  cold water submersion, 936
  cold-related environmental
    emergencies, 824
  compression technique, 477
  CPR for adults, children, and
    infants, 482t
  CPR on a child, 479–480, 479f, 480f
  CPR on an infant, 480–481, 481f
  defined, 465
  electrical burns, 595
  fractured sternum, 776
  lightning strike management, 855
  moderate-to-severe hypothermia, 831
  newborns, 477, 1086, 1086f
  one-rescuer CPR on an adult, 477–478,
    477f, 478f
  plant and animal emergencies, 887
  stopping, reasons for, 477
  transport, during, 157–159, 158f
  two-rescuer CPR on an adult, 479
Cardiovascular disease (CVD)
  common NOI, 85
  described, 464
Cardiovascular emergencies
  AED use, skill for, 490
  anatomy and physiology
    blood, 462, 464
    blood vessels, 460–462, 461f,
      462f, 463f
    heart, 459–460, 460f
  cardiovascular conditions
    angina pectoris, 466, 466f, 467t
    aortic aneurysm/aortic dissection,
      469–470, 470f
    atherosclerosis, 464–465, 464f
    cardiac arrhythmias, 467–468
    cardiogenic shock, 468
    cardiovascular diseases,
      concurrent, 470
    congestive heart failure, 465–466, 465f
    heart valve disorders, 470
    hypertension, 465
    myocardial infarction, 466–467, 467f
    pericarditis and pericardial tamponade,
      469, 469f
    pulmonary edema, 466
    sudden cardiac arrest, 468
    thromboembolism, 468–469, 469f
  case
    disposition, 489
    presentation, 459
    update, 473
  chapter objectives, 457–458
  chapter overview, 457–459, 458f
  chapter review, 491–493
  Explore myNSPkit, 493
  historical timeline, 457
  key terms, 458
  patient assessment
    angina and myocardial infarction,
      474, 474f

    aortic aneurysm/dissection, 475
    cardiogenic shock, 474–475
    congestive heart failure, 475, 475f
    hypertension, 474
    pericardial tamponade, 475
    primary assessment and ABCDs, 472
    secondary assessment, 472, 473f
    thromboembolism, 476
  patient management
    ABCDs, 476
    aspirin, 486–487
    cardiac arrest and activation of
      emergency response system,
      476–477, 477f
    common cardiac medications, 487t
    CPR for adults, children, and
      infants, 482t
    CPR on a child, 479–480, 479f, 480f
    CPR on an infant, 480–481, 481f
    early advanced care, 484
    early defibrillation, 481–484,
      482f, 483t
    hospital care of MI patients, 484–485
    nitroglycerin, 485–486, 486f
    one-rescuer CPR on an adult,
      477–478, 477f, 478f
    oxygen therapy, 485, 485f
    two-rescuer CPR on an adult, 479
  stop, think, understand, 471, 488–489
  suggested reading, 493
Cardiovascular system. See also circulatory
    system; heart; pulmonary circulation
  ALS medications, 1163–1164, 1163f
  anatomy of
    blood, 180–181, 181f
    blood vessels, 177, 178f, 179f, 180,
      180f, 181f
    heart, 176–180, 178f, 179f, 180f
  changes with aging, 987f, 988
  physiology of, 181–182
  shock, 331–334, 331f, 333f, 334f
  systemic and pulmonary circulation, 177,
    179f, 180
Cardioversion, defined, 482
Cardizem. See diltiazem
Carotid arteries
  lacerations to, 751–752
  neck anatomy and physiology, 747, 747f
Carotid pulse
  CPR on an adult, 478, 479
  CPR on an child, 479
  primary assessment, 220, 221f
  secondary assessment, 238, 238f
Carter, Jimmy, 697
Cartilage
  articular, 604, 605f
  defined, 602
  healing process, 610
  knee injuries, 633
Case reviews, 51
Castor oil plant, 866–867, 866f
Catfish, 881
Cats, injuries caused by, 883–884, 883f,
    889, 890f

Caustic agents, 400t. See also acids; bases
CBRNE (Chemical, Biological, Radiological,
    Nuclear, Explosive) disasters, 1109
CDC. See Centers for Disease Control and
    Prevention (CDC)
Cells, defined, 174
Center for Infectious Diseases (CID), 80
Centers for Disease Control and
    Prevention (CDC)
  contaminated objects, procedures for
    dealing with, 80
  TBI, incidence of, 699
  vaccination recommendations, 76
Central nervous system (CNS). See also
    brain; spinal cord
  coordinated functioning of, 698, 698f
  defined, 698
  physiology of, 186, 187f
  requirements for, 355
Cerebellum
  altered mental status, 356, 357f
  anatomy of, 183, 185, 185f, 186f
  defined, 700
Cerebral contusion
  described, 707, 708
  mortality rate, 710t
Cerebral cortex, and altered mental
    status, 358
Cerebral hematoma, types of,
    709–710, 709f
Cerebral palsy (CP), 1016–1017, 1016f
Cerebrospinal fluid (CSF)
  benefits of, 183
  defined, 700
  ear, leaking from, 755, 755f
  head and spinal injury assessment,
    717, 717f
Cerebrum
  altered mental status, 356–357,
    357f, 358
  anatomy of, 183, 185f, 186f
  defined, 700
Certification and recertification for OEC
    Technician training, 11–12, 11f, 11t
Cervical collars
  sizing and applying, 720, 720f
  sizing and applying, skill for, 727
  sizing and applying, skill guide for,
    733, 1174
Cervical spine
  axial skeleton, 699f
  face, eye, and neck injuries, 754
  fractures, 711–712, 711f
  injuries, in elderly patients, 998
  injury, assumption of, and protecting,
    224, 225
  neck injuries, assessment of, 756
  vertebrae, 196f, 198, 198f
Cervix, 1070f, 1071, 1072f
Cetirizine, 443t
"Chain of custody" for evidence, 87
Chair carry, 139, 139f
Chair lifts. See ski (chair) lifts
Charcoal, activated, 399, 400f, 400t

CHEATED (Chief complaint, History, Examination, Assessment, Treatment, Evaluation, Disposition) charting
  ALS providers, transition of care to, 1139
  described, 278
Chemical burns
  described, 582, 583f
  eyes, to, 761, 761f
  management of, 593–594, 594f
  patient assessment, 589
Chemical digestion, 187, 189, 189f
Chemical Transportation Emergency Center (CHEMTREC), 401
Chemotherapy, 63t
CHEMTREC (Chemical Transportation Emergency Center), 401, 594
Chest
  assessment of, in pediatric emergencies, 972, 973f
  secondary assessment, 232, 233f
Chest (thoracic) cavity, 171, 172f, 773
Chest injuries. See also thoracic trauma
  aortic dissection (See aortic dissection)
  aortic rupture, 776, 779–780, 780f
  children, 958, 959f
  commotio cordis, 780–781, 958
  contusions, 774, 774f
  environmental factors, 782
  flail chest, 775, 775f, 786, 786f
  fractures and dislocations, overview of, 774–775
  hemothorax, 778, 778f
  lower rib cage injury, 777
  mechanisms of injury, 774
  pericardial tamponade (See pericardial tamponade)
  pneumothorax, 416, 416f, 777–778, 778f, 782
  rib fractures, 712, 775, 785–786
  scapula fracture, 625, 712, 775
  signs and symptoms of, 784t
  sternoclavicular injury (See posterior sternoclavicular (S/C) dislocation)
  sternum fracture, 775–776
  traumatic asphyxia, 781, 781f
  traumatic death, 771
Chest pain, assessment of, 472, 473f
CHF. See congestive heart failure (CHF)
Chicken pox
  airborne transmission, 72
  common infectious disease, 74–75
  immunization for, 76t
Chief complaint
  defined, 216
  examples of, 216
  medical communications, in, 282, 282t
  medical history, 226
  patient assessment, 216–217, 217t
Chilblains, defined, 907. See also frostnip (chilblains)
Child abuse
  defined, 960–961, 961f
  signs of, 975, 975t

Child neglect, defined, 960, 961
Childbirth
  assisting with, skill for, 1092–1093
  assisting with, skill guide for, 1094–1095
  complications of, 1080–1081, 1080f
  emergency delivery, 1080, 1081–1083, 1081f, 1082f, 1083f
  stages of, 1079, 1079f
Children. See also pediatric emergencies
  AED use, 483, 483t
  assessment of, 245, 245f
  CPR, 479–480, 479f, 480f, 482t
  long spine boards, on, 720
  oral glucose, administering, 379
  respiratory emergencies, 407f
  vital signs, normal ranges of, 221t
Chlamydia, 1074
Chlorpheniramine, 443t
Chlorpromazine, 391
Chlor-Trimetron. See chlorpheniramine
Cholecystitis, 502
"Christmas tree" adapter for oxygen container regulators, 307
Chronic bronchitis, 414, 414f
Chronic obstructive pulmonary disease (COPD)
  described and incidence of, 413–414
  forms of, 414, 414f
  geriatric emergencies, 992–993, 992f
  medications for, 1163
Cialis®. See tadalafil
CID (Center for Infectious Diseases), 80
Cincinnati Prehospital Stroke Scale, 376, 376f
Ciprofloxacin, 1178t
Circulation. See also ABCD (Airway, Breathing, Circulation, Disability) sequence
  pediatric assessment triangle, 963, 964f, 965
  primary assessment, 220–222, 221f, 221t, 222f
Circulatory system. See also blood vessels; cardiovascular system
  allergic reactions, 440, 441f, 444
  defined, 174
  respiratory system, complementing, 412
CIT (Continuous Integrated Triage) method, 119
Clair, John, 919
Clarinex. See desloratadine
Claritin. See loratadine
Clark, Mark, 5
Clavicle. See also posterior sternoclavicular (S/C) dislocation
  anatomy of, 198
  injury assessment, 623–625, 623f, 624f
  injury management, 650–653, 651f
Cleaning, defined, 80
Clemastine, 443t
"Climb high and sleep low," 910
Clinical care by OEC Technicians, 36, 37–38f
Clonic activity, defined, 364, 365f

Clopidogrel
  cardiac medication, 487t
  clotting process, 542
  coup-contrecoup injury, 704
  elderly patients, 994
  shock, 345
  wounds, 553
Closed fractures
  blood loss, 615, 615t
  described, 613, 613f
Closed injury
  closed chest injury, defined, 774
  closed CNS injuries, 704, 704f
  compartment syndrome, 545
  contusions, 543, 543f
  crush injuries, 543, 543f, 545
  defined, 542
  hematomas, 543, 543f
  soft-tissue injuries, treating, skill for, 568
Closed-format patient care report, 273–274, 274f
"Clot buster" therapy, 484
"Clothesline" injuries, 751
Clothing
  contaminated, procedures for dealing with, 81
  outdoor work, preparing for, 65–67, 66f, 67f
Clotting, physiology of, 540, 542
CMS (Circulation, Movement, Sensation) evaluation
  lower extremity injury assessment, 630
  musculoskeletal injuries, 620
  traction splint application for femur fractures, 663, 663f
  upper extremity injuries, 622
CNS. See central nervous system (CNS)
CO. See carbon monoxide (CO)
$CO_2$. See carbon dioxide ($CO_2$)
Cocaine
  coronary artery vasospasm, 466
  overuse and poisoning, 392, 394
  toxicity, signs and symptoms of, 397t
Coccyx
  anatomy of, 196f, 198, 198f
  axial skeleton, 699f
Cochlear devices, 999, 1000
Cognitive disability, 1013
Cold zones, 1114, 1114f, 1115, 1115f
Cold-related emergencies
  behavioral emergencies, 1043, 1043f
  cold water submersion, 926–927, 926f, 936
Cold-related environmental emergencies
  anatomy and physiology
    heat loss, mechanisms of, 816–817, 816f, 817f
    risk factors for cold injury, 817–818, 817f
    thermoregulation, process of, 815–816
  case
    disposition, 834
    presentation, 814
    update, 823

chapter objectives, 813
chapter overview, 813–814, 814f, 815f
chapter review, 834–837
common emergencies
  afterdrop, 820
  frostnip and frostbite, 818–819, 818f, 819f
  hypothermia, 819–820, 820f
  windburn, 821
evacuation and transportation, 832
Explore myNSPkit, 837
historical timeline, 813
key terms, 813
local cold injury, stages of, 815f
patient assessment
  frostbite, 824, 824f, 825t
  hypothermia, 825–827, 825f, 825t, 826f
  overview of, 824, 824f
patient management
  frostbite, 827–828, 828f
  frostnip, 827
  hypothermia, 828–832, 829f, 831f
  other injuries/illnesses, with, 832
  windburn, 832
rescuer preparation for cold weather rescue, 821–822, 822f
stop, think, understand, 823, 833
suggested reading, 837
Colds, 72
"Cold-sores," 74
Colic, 506
Colles' fracture, 627
Collins, Henry, 742
Collisions during pregnancy, 1088, 1088f
Colon. See large intestines (colon)
Colorimetric CO₂ detectors, 1146, 1146f
Colostomies
  elderly patients, 1000
  ostomy bags, 1016
Coma, defined, 361
Combitube™ airway, 1148, 1148f
Comminuted fractures, 614f, 615f
Commonality, in emergency care systems, 42–43, 43f
Commotio cordis
  children, 958
  described, 780–781
Communicable disease, defined, 71
Communication
  aircraft, with, 156
  children, with, 968–969
  defined, 265
  elderly patients, with, 1000–1001, 1000f
  forms of, 267, 267f, 268f
  outdoor adaptive athletes, 1028–1029, 1029f
  process, components of, 267
  wilderness tips, 279
Communication systems for emergency care systems
  *EMS Agenda for the Future* (NHTSA), 36
  logistics section of incident command system, 108, 109f
  military time, 48–49, 49t

NATO phonetic alphabet, 48, 48t
radio communication, factors affecting, 47
radio etiquette, 47
radio terminology, 48, 48t
transmission pathway of radio call, 46–47, 46f, 47f
Community emergency response teams, 1111
Comparative negligence, 18
Compartment syndrome, 545
Compazine. See prochlorperazine
Compensated shock, 335
Complete fractures, 613, 614, 614f
Compression dressing, 556
Compression fractures, 615t
Compression injury, 702, 702f
Computer-generated forms, 279–281, 279f, 280f
Concurrent quality improvement, 50
Concussion
  amnesia, 705, 707
  described, 705, 707f
  post-concussive syndrome, 708
Conduction
  heat loss mechanism, 816, 816f
  temperature regulation, 59, 59f, 60f
Confidentiality, defined, 3
Confined space rescue, 1125–1127, 1125f, 1126f, 1127f
Congestive heart failure (CHF)
  described, 465–466, 465f
  geriatric emergencies, 992, 992f
  patient assessment, 475, 475f
Conical regions of the body, bandaging, 562, 563f
Conjunctiva of the eye, 744, 746f
Consent
  defined, 21
  pediatric patients, for, 964
Constipation
  children, 953
  gastrointestinal ailment, 506–507
Contact lenses, removing, 762, 762f
Contamination, defined, 73, 73f, 552
Continuing education, for emergency care systems, 51, 51f
Continuity of care, 41–42, 41f
Continuous Integrated Triage (CIT) method, 119
Contributory negligence, 18
Contusions
  abdominal wall, 798
  cerebral, 707, 708, 710t
  chest injuries, 774, 774f
  closed injury, 543, 543f
  DCAP-BTLS assessment, 230, 230t
  treatment for, 555
Convection
  heat loss mechanism, 59f, 60, 816f, 817, 817f
  heat stroke, 853
COPD. See chronic obstructive pulmonary disease (COPD)
Copperhead snakes, 878, 878f
Coral snakes, 878, 878f, 879, 879f

Cordarone®. See amiodarone
Core body temperature. See also body temperature
  heat-related emergencies, 839, 842, 842f
  lowering, with heat stroke, 853
  measuring, 825f, 826–827
Cornea of the eye, 745, 746f
Coronal (frontal) plane, 168f
Coronary arteries
  anatomy and physiology, 177, 180f
  cardiovascular emergencies, 460, 464, 464f
Coronary artery bypass grafting (CABG), 485
Coronary artery disease (CAD), 464
Cortex of bones, 604, 605f
Corticosteroids, 63t
Coumadin. See warfarin
Coup-contrecoup injury, 703–704, 703f
Coyote injuries, 882–883
CP (cerebral palsy), 1016–1017, 1016f
CPR. See cardiopulmonary resuscitation (CPR)
Crack cocaine, 392, 394
"Crackling" feel
  skin, beneath, 421
  tension pneumothorax, 778
Cranial cavity, 171, 172f
Crepitus, defined, 421
Cricoid cartilage, pressure on, during ET tube insertion, 1146, 1147f
Cricothyrotomy
  defined, 1149
  equipment and set-up, 1149–1150
  indications and contraindications, 1149
  kit for, 1149, 1149f, 1150
Crime scenes
  cordoning off, 87, 87f
  evidence, handling, 87, 88t
  management of, 87–89, 87f, 88t, 89f
  media, relations with, 88–89, 89f
  patient care taking priority over crime scene preservation, 88t
  preservation tips for, 88t
Crisis, defined, 1039, 1040
Critical incident stress management
  debriefing, 90, 90f
  teams, 1060, 1060f
Crocodile injuries, 879, 887
CroFab, 889
Crohn's disease, 503t
Crossed-finger method of opening airway, 297, 297f
Croup, 950, 950f
Crowning, defined, 1080
Crush injury
  closed injury, 543, 543f, 545
  described, 523, 523f
  open, 545f, 548, 549f
Crutches for adaptive athletes, 1021, 1022f
*Cryptosporidium* sp., 506
CSF. See cerebrospinal fluid (CSF)
Cultural diversity, 245
Cumulonimbus clouds ("thunderheads"), 848, 848f

CVD. *See* cardiovascular disease (CVD)
Cyanide, 400*t*
Cycling, by adaptive athletes, 1026, 1026*f*
Cyclopentolate ophthalmic solution, 1178*t*
Cystitis, 1074

## D

Dabigatran, 542
DAI. *See* diffuse axonal injury (DAI)
Dalton's Law, 923
DCAP-BTLS (Deformity, Contusions, Abrasions/avulsions, Punctures/ penetrations, Burns/bleeding/ bruises, Tenderness, Lacerations, Swelling) assessment
  abdominal and pelvic trauma, 802
  altered mental status, 373–374
  behavioral emergencies, 1056
  cold-related environmental emergencies, 824
  geriatric emergencies, 1002
  head and spinal injuries, 717
  musculoskeletal injuries, 619
  neck injuries, 756
  outdoor adaptive athletes, 1029
  pediatric emergencies, 972
  plant and animal emergencies, 885
  secondary assessment, 230, 230*t*
  soft-tissue injuries, 551
  substance use and abuse, 397
  thoracic trauma, 783
  trauma patients, 531
  water emergencies, 934
Deadly nightshade, 886
Death
  chest injuries, 771
  determination of, and body temperature, 936
  DNR orders, 1048
  drowning, 925, 925*f*
  moderate-to-severe hypothermia, 831, 831*f*
  obvious signs of, 1047–1048, 1048*f*
  post-injury phase of injury, 526, 527*f*
  SIDS, 957, 957*f*, 977
  suicide, 1045
  trauma in children, 957, 957*f*
Debriefing after critical incidents, 90, 90*f*
Deceleration force
  fractured sternum, 776
  mechanism of injury, 702
  TBI, 705, 707*f*
Decerebrate posturing, 224
Decompensated shock
  children, 945
  defined, 943
  described, 335
Decompression sickness
  defined, 927–928, 927*f*
  signs and symptoms, 928, 928*t*, 934
Decontamination
  bed linens, blankets, and contaminated clothing, 81

defined, 80
  disposable items, 80, 80*f*
  infectious waste, 80–81
  sharps, 82, 82*f*
  spills, 81–82, 81*f*
Decorticate posturing, 224
Deep body part, 170
*Deep Survival - Who Lives, Who Dies, and Why* (Gonzalez), 1171
Deep venous thrombosis (DVT)
  described, 468–469
  patient assessment, 476
  pulmonary embolism, 415
Deer injuries, 884, 884*f*
Deer ticks, 874–875, 874*f*
DEET (N, N-Diethyl-meta-toluamide), 876
Defibrillation. *See* electrical therapy (defibrillation)
Deformity, with musculoskeletal injuries, 619, 619*f*, 620
Dehydration, 505, 506
Delayed stress response (DSR), 90
Delayed (Yellow)(turtle) category for triage, 115*t*, 116, 116*f*
Delirium, 359
Dementia, 362
Demerol™. *See* meperidine
Dengue fever, 876
Department of Homeland Security, 1109
Dependent lividity, 1048
Depressants
  overuse and poisoning, 391
  toxicity, signs and symptoms of, 397*t*
Depressed skull fracture, 704
Depression
  behavioral emergency assessment, 1055
  neurotic disorder, 1044
Dermal poison, defined, 392
Dermis
  burns, 581, 581*f*
  defined, 539*f*, 540
  integumentary system, 195, 195*f*
  plant and animal emergencies, 862
Designer drugs (club drugs), 391
Desloratadine, 443*t*
Dexamethasone
  altitude illness prevention, 911
  emergency care medication, 1178*t*
Dextrose 50% in water (D$_{50}$), 1164
Diabetes mellitus
  altered mental status, 378–379, 379*f*
  autoimmune disorder, 62
  defined, 366
  gestational, 367
  hyperglycemia, 368–369
  hypoglycemia, 367–368, 368*f*, 368*t*
  immune system, affecting, 63*t*
  overview of, 365–366
  rare types, 367
  signs and symptoms, 366, 366*f*
  silent MI, 474
  type I, 366–367, 367*f*
  type II, 367
Dialysis shunts, 1000

Diamox. *See* acetazolamide
Diaphoresis
  defined, 472
  shock, 345
Diaphragm (muscle)
  respiration, 411, 412*f*
  tears and ruptures, 799
  thoracic trauma A & P, 772, 772*f*
Diarrhea
  children, 953
  gastrointestinal ailment, 506
  pediatric emergency management, 977
Diastolic blood pressure, 221*t*
Diazepam
  ALS administration, 1164
  overuse and poisoning, 391
Diffuse axonal injury (DAI)
  defined, 704
  described, 710
  mechanisms of injury, 710, 710*f*
  mortality rates, 710*t*
Digestion
  chemical, 187, 189, 189*f*
  mechanical, 187
Digitalis, 866
Dilaudid™. *See* hydromorphone
Diltiazem, 994
Dimetane. *See* brompheniramine
Diphenhydramine
  allergies, 443*t*
  emergency care medication, 1178*t*
  plant toxins, 888
Dipyridamole and aspirin, 345
Direct blow fractures, 635
Direct contact transmission of disease, 71
Direct current (DC), 583
Direct ground lift, 143–144, 160–161, 163, 1173
Direct medical oversight in emergency care systems, 49, 49*f*, 50
Direct pressure soft-tissue injuries, 553, 553*f*
Directional terms for the body, 169–170, 169*f*
Disability. *See also* ABCD (Airway, Breathing, Circulation, Disability) sequence
  common disabilities, among adaptive athletes
    cognitive disabilities, 1013
    combined physical and intellectual disability, 1018–1019, 1019*f*
    intellectual difficulties, 1013–1014, 1014*f*
    intellectual disabilities, 1012–1013, 1013*f*
    overview of, 1011–1012, 1011*f*
    physical disabilities, 1015–1017, 1015*f*, 1016*f*, 1017*f*
    visual and hearing impairments, 1018, 1019*f*
  defined, 1010, 1011
  impairment, comparison to, 1012
  primary assessment, 222–224, 223*t*, 224*f*
Disaster Medical Assistance Team, 1110–1111, 1110*f*, 1111*f*

Disaster response
community emergency response teams, 1111
human-caused disasters, 1109, 1109f
Medical Reserve Corps, 1111
National Disaster Medical System, 1110–1111, 1110f, 1111f
National Response Framework, 1109–1110
natural disasters, 1108, 1109f
Disease, protection from
common infectious diseases, 74–76
contamination, 73, 73f
decontamination, 80–82, 80f, 81f, 82f
disease transmission, 71–73
occupational exposure, 79–80, 79f
personal protective equipment, 77–79, 78f, 91–93, 1173
Standard Precautions and body substance isolation, 76–77, 77f
stop, think, understand, 83
vaccination recommendations, 76, 76t
Disease transmission, defined, 80
Disinfection, defined, 80
Dislocations
chest injuries, overview of, 774–775
defined, 602
described, 615–616, 615f
signs and symptoms, 621
Dispatchers (communication systems), 42, 269, 269f, 269t
Displaced fractures, 613, 614f
Displaced proximal femur fracture, 631
Disposable items, contaminated, 80, 80f
Distal direction, 169f, 170
Distracting injuries, 230
Distributive shock
anaphylactic shock, 337f, 340–341, 341t, 440
neurogenic shock, 337f, 341–342, 712
overview of, 337f, 339–340, 340f
psychogenic shock, 342
septic shock, 337f, 340, 341f
Diuretics, 994
Divers' Alert Network, 936
Diverticulitis, 503t
Do Not Resuscitate (DNR) orders, 1048
Doctrine of public reliance, 17
Documentation
emergency care systems, in, 50
preparing, 19–20, 19f
restraints, 1059
shooting or stabbing incidents, 552
Dog ticks, 875, 875f
Dogs, injuries caused by, 882–883, 883f, 889, 890f
Dogs for search and rescue
confined space rescue, 1125–1127, 1125f, 1126f, 1127f
dog alerts, 1127
scent factors for search dogs, 1126, 1126f
search, simplifying, 1126, 1127f
search capabilities, 1126, 1126f

search dog etiquette, 1126–1127, 1127f
structures, searches in, 1127, 1127f
Dole, Charles Minot "Minnie"
broken leg, 264
military unit composed of skiers, 56
National Ski Hall of Fame, induction into, 329
National Ski Patrol, founding, 3, 4–5, 5f
ski accident, 1
10th Mountain Division, recruits for, 126
Dole, Jane, 4, 5f
Dopamine, 1163, 1164
Dorsal, defined, 628
Dorsal (posterior) direction, 169, 169f
Dorsalis pedis pulse, 630f
Dorsiflex, defined, 630
Down syndrome, 1018–1019, 1019f
Doxepin, 1054t
Drag, long-axis, 136–138, 137f
Draw-sheet lift (transfer flat), 131, 145–146, 145f
Dressing and bandaging
bandaging principles, 560, 560f
dressings, types of, 558–559, 559f
hemostatic dressings, 561–562
occlusive dressings, 561
pressure dressings, 561, 561f
problem areas, 562–563, 562f, 563f, 564f
self-evacuation with ankle injuries, 670, 670f
stabilizing dressings, 561, 561f, 562f
Dressings
burned patients, 592, 592f
defined, 552
dry dressings, 828
soft-tissue injuries, 553
Drowning
autism spectrum disorders, 1013
deaths from, 925, 925f
defined, 925
dry drowning, 922
factors contributing to, 925–926, 925f
near-drowning, 702, 926–927, 926f
pathophysiology of, 921, 922f, 922t
Drugs, illicit. See also substance abuse and poisoning
abdominal and pelvic trauma, 802
behavioral emergencies, 1043, 1043f
designer drugs (club drugs), 391
Dry drowning, 922
Dry gangrene, 824
"Dry" (ischemic) stroke, 370, 370f
DSR (delayed stress response), 90
DUMBELS (Defecation, Urination, Miosis, Bronchorrhea, Emesis, Lacrimation, Salivation)
organophosphate exposure, 1115, 1115t
organophosphate or nerve agent exposure, 397t
Duodenum, 794f
DuoDote kit, 400, 1115, 1115f
Dura mater, 183, 185f
Duragesic®. See fentanyl
Duty to rescue/duty to act, 17, 18

DVT. See deep venous thrombosis (DVT)
Dyazide. See triamterene
Dysautonomia. See autonomic dysfunction (dysautonomia)
Dyslexia, 1012
Dysmenorrhea, 1073–1074
Dyspnea
common complaint, 407
defined, 410
respiratory emergencies, 418
Dystonic cerebral palsy, 1016, 1017

# E

Early (superficial) cold injury, 815f, 819, 825t. See also frostnip
Ears
anatomy and physiology, 744, 745f
injuries, 749–750, 750f, 755–756, 755f, 758–759
Ecchymosis
defined, 543
musculoskeletal injuries, 619f, 620
Eclampsia, 1078
Ecstasy, 391
Ectopic pregnancy, 1074, 1078t
Edema
congestive heart failure, 475
defined, 466
peripheral, and altitude-related problems, 906
Edson, Frank, 1, 4
Edson, Jean, 4
Education for emergency care systems, 36
87th Mountain Infantry Regiment, 5, 98
Elastic bandages, 560
Elavil. See amitriptyline
Elbows
dislocation, 626, 626f
injuries, 626, 626f
injury management, 654–656, 654f, 655f
rigid splint application, skill for, 679
Elder abuse, 998
Electrical burns and injuries
children, 959
described, 583–584, 584f
entry and exit points, 589, 595, 595f
heart conduction, 592
management of, 594–595, 595f
mechanism of injury, 703
patient assessment, 589
Electrical current, 583
Electrical therapy (defibrillation). See also automated external defibrillator (AED)
ALS provider, assisting, 1161
anterior method, 1161, 1161f
anterior-posterior method, 1161, 1161f
defibrillation, described, 1160
defibrillators, internal, 999, 1000
early, in cardiac arrest, 481–484, 482f, 483t
pads, placement of, 1160, 1160f, 1161, 1161f
Electrocardiogram (ECG or EKG), defined, 1159. See also cardiac monitoring

Electrolyte balance
  altered mental status, 361, 361t, 378
  changes with aging, 989
Elk, injuries caused by, 884
Emancipated minors, 964
Embolus, defined, 468, 469, 469f
Emergency care systems
  case
    disposition, 51
    presentation, 32
    update, 44
  chapter objectives, 31
  chapter overview, 31–33, 33f
  chapter review, 51–55
  commonality in emergency care systems, 42–43, 43f
  communications systems, 46–49, 46f, 47f, 48t, 49t
  continuing education, 51, 51f
  continuity of care, 41–42, 41f
  documentation, 50
  emergency care, history of, 33–38, 34f, 35t, 37–38f
  emergency care protocols, 50
  emergency care system, defined, 32
  emergency care systems and public health, 43–45
  emergency facilities, 40–41
  emergency personnel, levels of, 38–39f, 38–40
  Explore myNSPkit, 55
  historical timeline, 31
  key terms, 31
  medical oversight, 49–50, 49f
  quality improvement, 50–51
  research, role of, 45, 45f
  stop, think, understand, 44
  suggested reading, 55
Emergency facilities, types of, 40–41
Emergency medical dispatcher, 42. See also dispatchers (communication systems)
Emergency Medical Responders (EMRs), 20, 20f, 38–39f, 39
Emergency medical services (EMS)
  defined, 35
  essential components, 35t
  regulations for, 25
Emergency Medical Services Act of 1973, 35, 35t
Emergency Medical Technician (EMT), 38, 39
Emergency personnel, levels of, 38–39f, 38–40
Emergency situations, assessing
  mechanism of injury, 84, 85, 85f
  number of patients and need for additional resources, 85, 86f
  scene safety, 82–84, 84f
Emergency Support Function annexes, 1110
Emphysema
  pulsus paradoxus, 779
  respiratory emergencies, 414, 414f

EMS. See emergency medical services (EMS)
EMS Agenda for the Future (NHTSA), 35–36, 37–38f
EMT (Emergency Medical Technician), 38, 39
Encephalitis
  mosquitoes, 876
  vector-borne transmission of disease, 73
Endocrine system
  altered mental status, 358–359, 359f
  anatomy of, 191, 193f
  changes with aging, 990
  defined, 191
  physiology of, 191, 195
Endotracheal intubation
  defined, 1141, 1141f
  equipment and set-up
    bag valve and oxygen, 1146, 1146f
    blades, 1142, 1142f, 1143f
    CO2 detector, 1146, 1146f
    endotracheal tubes, 1143–1144, 1144f, 1145f
    handles, 1142–1143, 1142f, 1143f
    list of, 1142, 1142f
    stylets and lubricant, 1144, 1145f
  indications and contraindications for, 1141–1142
  pre-oxygenation, 1147, 1147f
  process for, 1146–1147, 1146f, 1147f
Endotracheal tubes, 1143–1144, 1144f, 1145f
Enoxaparin
  elderly patients, 994
  shock, 345
Environment. See also cold-related environmental emergencies; heat-related emergencies
  altered mental status, 360–361, 361t, 378
  capillary refill test, 222
  considerations for patient assessment, 245–246
  outdoor work, preparing for, 63, 63f
  related problems, as common NOI, 85
  thoracic injuries, complicating, 782
Epidermis
  burns, 581, 581f
  defined, 539–540, 539f
  integumentary system, 195, 195f
  plant and animal emergencies, 862
Epididymis, 204f
Epidural hematoma
  described, 709–710, 709f
  mortality rate, 710t
EpiE-Z pen™, 447
Epiglottis
  airway management, 292, 293, 293f
  anatomy of, 174, 175f, 176f
Epiglottitis, 951–952, 951f
Epilepsy, 360, 361t, 363, 378. See also seizures
Epinephrine. See also EpiPen™; Twinject™
  allergies and anaphylaxis, 443
  auto-injectors, 443, 885, 888–889

  cardiac patients, 1163, 1164
  plant and animal emergencies, 885, 888–889
  racemic, 1163
  respiratory conditions, 420
  severe allergic reactions, 447–449, 448f
EpiPen™
  administration, skill for, 450
  emergency care medication, 1178t
  severe allergic reactions, for, 447–448, 448f, 449
Epiphyses (growth plates)
  anatomy in children, 945, 945f
  bone injuries in children, 958
  epiphyseal line in bones, 604, 605f
  fractures, 615t
Epistaxis
  defined, 749
  facial injuries, 757, 757f
Equipment
  emergency care
    alpine pack, 1175, 1175f, 1178t
    bike kit, 1176, 1176f, 1178t
    medications, 1177–1178, 1178t
    Nordic kit, 1177, 1177f, 1178t
    universal survival kit, 1176
    white water kit, 1176–1177, 1176f, 1178t
  endotracheal intubation
    bag valve and oxygen, 1146, 1146f
    blades, 1142, 1142f, 1143f
    CO2 detector, 1146, 1146f
    endotracheal tubes, 1143–1144, 1144f, 1145f
    handles, 1142–1143, 1142f, 1143f
    list of, 1142, 1142f
    stylets and lubricant, 1144, 1145f
  medical, remaining with patient during transport, 150
  outdoor work, preparing for
    clothing, 65–67, 66f, 67f
    first aid kit, 65
    skin and eye protection, 69–70, 69f
    survival kit, 67–69, 67f, 68t
  tools for gaining access to patients, in a vehicle, 1106–1107, 1107t
Erectile dysfunction, 486
Errors in written communication, correcting, 279, 279f
Erythrocytes, 332–333, 333f, 334. See also red blood cells
Escherichia coli, 506
Esophagus, 187, 188f, 747
Ethical and legal issues
  abandonment, 17–18, 18f
  assault and battery, 23–24, 24f
  documentation, 19–20, 19f
  EMS system regulations, 25
  ethical issues facing OEC technicians, 15
  Good Samaritan Laws and duty to act, 15–17, 16f
  importance of, 13, 15
  Joint Statement of Understanding, 21
  judgment, 24

negligence and breach of duty, 18
patient's consent, 21–23, 22f
privacy laws, 25
refusal of care, 22, 22f, 23
risk, assumption of, 18–19
scope of training, 20, 20f
standard of training *versus* standard of care, 20–21
teamwork, 25
training, 24, 24f
Ethics, defined, 15. *See also* ethical and legal issues
Ethmoid bone, 198f
Ethylene glycol, 394, 397t
Eustachian tube obstruction, 928
Evacuation chairs, 152–153, 153f
Evaluations
emergency care systems, 36
OEC Technician training, 9, 10f
Evaporation
heat loss mechanism, 59f, 60–61, 61f, 816f, 817
heat stroke, 853
Events leading up to incident, 227t, 228
Eversion, defined, 636
Evidence
handling, at crime scenes, 87, 88t
preservation of, 19–20, 19f
Evidence-based medicine, 8
Evidence-based research, 45, 45f
Evisceration
abdominal trauma, 805
defined, 798
described, 799, 800f
Exhalation (expiration)
airway management, 294, 295
respiratory cycle, 410
Exhaustion stage of stress reaction, 61t
Expectant (Black cross) category for triage, 115t, 117–118, 118f
Expiration (exhalation). *See* exhalation (expiration)
Explosive force as MOI, 85
Expressed consent, 21–22
Expressive aphasia, 1031
Exsanguination
defined, 554
femur fractures, 660
Extension (movement), 170
Extensor posturing, 716, 716f
External auditory canal
ear injuries, 749–750
foreign body in, 759
External body part, 170
Extraocular movement
eye injuries, assessment of, 754
secondary assessment, 232, 232f
Extraocular muscles, 744
Extravascular, defined, 543
Extreme altitude, described, 900, 901f
Extremities. *See also* lower extremities; upper extremities
assessment of, in pediatric emergencies, 972, 972f

injuries in children, 958
secondary assessment, 234–235, 235f
Extremity lift, 143, 143f
Extrication
defined, 1105
patients from a vehicle, 1105–1107, 1106f, 1107f, 1107t
stabilized extrication and transfer, 673–674, 673–674f
Eyeballs, lacerations of, 760
Eyelids, lacerations of, 760
Eyes
artificial, management of, 762
assessment of, 231–232, 231f, 232f
impaled objects
described, 751, 751f
management of, 760, 760f
skill for treatment of, 765
skill guide for stabilization of, 766, 1174
injuries
assessment of, 754–755, 754f, 755f
described, 751, 751f
management of, 759–762, 759f, 760f, 761f, 762f
substance exposure
effects of, 390
reducing, 398, 399f
uninjured, synchronous movement of, 760
Eyewear, protective
contaminated spills, procedures for dealing with, 81
outdoor work, preparing for, 69–70, 69f
personal protective equipment, as, 78, 78f
sunglasses, 69, 69f, 906f, 907

**F**

FAA (U.S. Federal Aviation Administration), 155
Face
facial structures, 743–744, 743f
injuries
described, 749–750, 750f
management of, 757, 757f
pediatric emergencies, 973, 973f
trauma and environmental injuries, vulnerability to, 749, 749f
Face, eye, and neck injuries
anatomy and physiology
auditory and balance system, 744, 745f
facial structures, 743–744, 743f
neck anatomy, 747, 747f
visual system, 744–746, 746f
case
disposition, 764
presentation, 744
update, 753
chapter objectives, 742
chapter overview, 742–743
chapter review, 767–769
common injuries
exposed area, 749, 749f

eye injuries, 751, 751f
face injuries, 749–750, 750f
neck injuries, 751–752, 751f
Explore myNSPkit, 769
historical timeline, 742
impaled object in the eye, stabilizing, skill guide for, 766, 1174
impaled object in the eye, treating, skill for, 765
key terms, 742–743
patient assessment
ABCDs and primary assessment, 754
ears, 755–756, 755f
eyes, 754–755, 754f, 755f
facial injury, significant, 756
mid-face and nose, 755, 755f
mouth, 755
neck, 756, 756f
secondary assessment, 754
patient management
ear injuries, 758–759
eye injuries, 759–762, 759f, 760f, 761f, 762f
facial injuries, 757, 757f
neck injuries, 763, 763f
overview of, 756–757
stop, think, understand, 748–749, 752–753, 757–758, 764
suggested reading, 769
Face shields, 304–305
Facility, defined, 107–108, 107f
FACTUAL-OEC (Facts, Accurate, Complete, Terms, Unbiased, Avoid slang, Legible/legal) report writing, 278–279
Fallopian tubes
female reproductive system, 203, 205f
obstetric and gynecologic emergencies, 1070, 1070f
Falls
elderly patients, 996–997
mechanism of injury, 217t
pregnancy, during, 1088, 1088f
False morels, 870–871, 870f
Fang marks, 885, 885f
Fatigue, 64
"Feathering" burn pattern, 848, 848f
Febrile seizures
children, 954
pediatric emergency management, 977
Federal Emergency Management Agency (FEMA) search dogs, 1127, 1127f
Feet drag, 137–138
Females
reproductive system
anatomy of, 203, 205f
physiology of, 206
silent MI, 474
urethra, 191, 192f
Femoral neck fractures, 806
Femoral pulse
abdominal aortic aneurysm, 504
CPR on an child, 479
secondary assessment, 239, 239f

Femur
  anatomy of, 196f, 198
  distal fractures, management of, 663
  femoral neck fractures, 806
  fracture and concurrent tibia fracture, 668, 668f
  fractures, assessment of, 631–632, 632f
  fractures, bleeding from, 615t, 660
  fractures, management of, 660–663, 660f, 662f, 663f, 665
  fractures, realignment of, 663, 663f, 665
  traction splint application, skill for, 681
Fentanyl, 1164
"Ferning" burn pattern, 848, 848f
Fetal movement, 1090
Fever. See hyperthermia
"Fever blisters," 74. See also herpes simplex infections
Fexofenadine, 443t
Fibula
  anatomy of, 196f, 198
  fractures, bleeding from, 615t
  injuries, management of, 667–668
  injury assessment, 634–635, 635f
  "tib-fib" fractures, 634–635, 667–668, 683
Fidelity, as ethical issue, 15
Field care notes, 272, 272f
Fifth metatarsal fracture, 636, 636f
"Fight-or-flight" response
  autonomic nervous system, 187
  endocrine system, 191
  stress, 61–62, 61t, 62f, 1041
Figure-eight splint
  application, skill guide for, 685, 1174
  clavicle fracture, 652
  creating and applying, skill for, 677
Figure-eight pattern for bandages, 670, 670f
Finance Chief, 105t, 110
Finance/administration section of incident command system
  ICS organization, 101, 104f, 105t
  responsibilities, 109
  units of, 110
Financial foundation for emergency medical systems, 36
Finger sweep of mouth for clearing airway, 297–298, 297f
Fingers
  bandaging, 563, 564f, 573
  injuries, 628, 628f, 657–658, 657f
Fire ants, 875, 876, 876f
Fire ground operations, 1128–1130, 1129f
First aid
  American Red Cross training program, 56
  first aid kits, 65
  local protocols, 21
First Aid Textbook (ARC), 8
First-degree (superficial) burns, 585, 585f, 587t
Fish, injuries caused by, 881, 881f
Fitzpatrick Skin Phototypes System, 846t

Fixed-wing aircraft, 154–155, 154f
Flail chest
  described, 775, 775f
  management of, 786, 786f
Flank areas, examination of, 510
"Flash pulmonary edema," 475
Flat bones, 197, 604, 604f
Fleas, 876
Flexible suction catheters, 299
Flexion (movement), 170
Flexor posturing, 716, 716f
Flies, adverse effects from, 876
"Floating knee" injury
  femoral traction splint, 645
  management of, 668, 668f
Fluoxetine
  overuse and poisoning, 391
  psychotropic agent, 1054t
Fluvoxamine, 1054t
Fontanels, 945
Foot injuries
  assessment, 636, 636f
  management, 670
Force. See also specific types of force
  trauma patient assessment, 531
  types of, producing injury, 85, 521, 521f, 702, 702f
Fore and aft carry, 140, 141f
Forearm
  fracture, splinting, skill for, 680
  injuries, described, 626–627, 627f
  injuries, management of, 656
Foreign bodies. See also impaled objects
  airway obstruction
    children, 950, 977
    Heimlich maneuver, 424
  external auditory canal, 759
  eyes, in, 759, 759f
Four trackers, 1024
Fourth-degree burns, 585, 587t
Foxes
  injuries caused by, 882–883
  rabies, 890
Foxglove, 866, 866f
Fractures. See also under specific bones
  blood loss due to, 615, 615t, 660
  chest injuries, overview of, 774–775
  classification of, 613–614, 613f, 614f
  defined, 610
  facial injuries, 749, 750f
  immobilizing, 976–977
  signs and symptoms, 621, 621f
  types of, 614, 614f, 615t
  vertebral, 711–712, 711f
Freely movable joints, 606, 606f
Fresh water, near-drowning in, 927
Frontal bone, 198f
Frontal (coronal) plane, 168f
Frostbite
  assessment of, 824, 824f
  common sites for, 819
  described, 818–819, 818f, 819f
  evacuation and transportation, 832
  frostbitten tissue, how to warm, 828, 828f

frostbitten tissue, when to warm, 827
frostbitten tissue, where to warm, 827–828
hypothermia, concurrent with, 828
management of, 827–828, 828f
signs and symptoms, 825t
Frostnip (chilblains)
  chilblains, defined, 907
  described, 818, 819
  management of, 827
  signs and symptoms, 825t
  superficial cold injury, 815f, 819, 825t
Full-thickness cold injury (frostbite), 819, 825t. See also frostbite
Full-thickness (third-degree) burns, 585, 585f, 586, 586f, 587t
Fundus of the uterus, 1070f, 1071, 1072f
Funnel web spiders, 873, 873f
Furosemide
  cardiac medication, 487t
  diuretic use by the elderly, 994
  nonhemorrhagic hypovolemia, 339

# G

Gallbladder
  GI system, 187, 188f, 189
  hollow organ, 495, 496f, 794f
  location of, 795f
Gamma hydroxybutyric acid (GHB), 391
Gamma radiation, 584
Gamow bag, 913, 913f
Ganja, 394. See also marijuana
Gastric distention, 315–316
Gastritis, 508t
Gastroenteritis
  children, 953
  gastrointestinal ailment, 505
  ingestion transmission of disease, 73
Gastro-esophageal reflux disease (GERD), 503, 505
Gastrointestinal and genitourinary emergencies
  acute abdomen
    abdominal aortic aneurysm, 504
    appendicitis, 500
    bowel obstruction, 503, 503t
    cholecystitis, 502
    hepatitis, 501–502
    nephrolithiasis, 502–503
    OB/GYN-related conditions, 504
    pancreatitis, 500–501, 501f
    peptic ulcerative disease, GERD, and GI bleeding, 503–504, 504f
    perforated bowel, 503
    pyelonephritis, 502
    recognition, importance of, 499–500, 500f, 501f
  case
    disposition, 511
    presentation, 495
    update, 507
  chapter objectives, 494
  chapter overview, 494–495, 495f

chapter review, 512–515
Explore myNSPkit, 515
gastrointestinal ailments
  colic, 506
  constipation, 506–507
  diarrhea and blood stool, 506
  gastroenteritis, 505
  indigestion, 505
  nausea and vomiting, 505
  viruses, protozoa, and bacteria, 506
GI/GU anatomy and physiology, 495–496, 496f, 497–498f
historical timeline, 494
key terms, 494
patient assessment
  ABCDs, 508
  acute abdomen, signs and symptoms of, 508t
  acute abdominal pain, causes of, 508t
  physical exam, 509–510, 509f
patient management, 510, 510f
stop, think, understand, 499, 507, 511
suggested reading, 515
Gastrointestinal (GI) system
  allergic reactions, 440
  anatomy of, 187, 188f
  changes with aging, 987f, 988, 989f
  common NOI, 85
  defined, 187
  physiology of, 189, 189f
"Gateway drug," 394
GCS. See Glasgow Coma Scale (GCS)
GDM (gestational diabetes mellitus), 367
Gender, in medical communications, 282, 282t
Generalized seizures
  children, 953
  defined, 364
  phases of, 364–365, 364–365f, 364f
Geneva Basin ski patrol, 494
Genital injuries, 801, 802–803. See also gastrointestinal and genitourinary emergencies
GERD (gastro-esophageal reflux disease), 503, 505
Geriatric, defined, 987
Geriatric emergencies. See also adults, older
  advancements, considerations for
    advanced directives, 1000
    artificial joints, 999, 999f
    communicating with elderly patients, 1000–1001, 1000f
    external openings, ports, and apparatus, 1000
    implantable devices, 999–1000
  case
    disposition, 1005
    presentation, 986
    update, 996
  chapter objectives, 985
  chapter overview, 985–987, 986f
  chapter review, 1005–1008
  common illnesses and conditions
    abdominal emergencies, 993, 993t

altered mental status, 991, 991f
chronic obstructive pulmonary disease, 992–993, 993f
congestive heart failure, 992, 992f
hypertension, 991
myocardial infarction, 992
stroke, 992
syncope, 992
elder abuse, 998
Explore myNSPkit, 1008
historical timeline, 985
key terms, 985
medication use, 993–994, 993f
patient assessment, 1001–1003, 1001f, 1002t
patient management, 1003–1004, 1003f
physiologic effects of aging, 987–990, 987f, 988f, 989f
stop, think, understand, 990, 995, 998–999, 1004–1005
suggested reading, 1008
trauma considerations, 996–998, 997f
Gestation, defined, 1071
Gestational diabetes mellitus (GDM), 367
Gestational period, defined, 1071
GHB (gamma hydroxybutyric acid), 391
GI system. See gastrointestinal (GI) system
Giardia lamblia, 506
Giardia sp.
  ingestion transmission of disease, 73
  near-drowning, 927
Gingko biloba, 911
Glasgow Coma Scale (GCS)
  altered mental status, 373
  head and spinal injuries, 714, 715, 715t, 716, 716f, 717f
  musculoskeletal injuries, 618
  neurologic function, 222, 223–224, 223t
  pediatric emergencies, 971t
  respiratory emergencies, 418
Gliding joints, 607
Globe ruptures, 751, 751f
Gloves
  personal protective equipment, as, 77–78, 91–93
  putting on, 78
  removing, 78, 91–93, 1173
Glucagon
  altered mental status, 358–359, 359f
  endocrine system, 191
Glucose
  CNS requirement, 355
  defined, 356
  oral, for diabetics, 378–379, 379f
Glucose blood levels
  endocrine system, 191
  monitoring, 368, 368f
  normal values, 365
Glycogen, 359
Goals, common, in emergency care systems, 42, 43f
Golden hour, after injuries, 526, 527f
Gonorrhea
  direct contact transmission of disease, 71
  pelvic inflammatory disease, 1074

Gonzalez, Laurence, 1171
Good Samaritan laws
  Colorado Good Samaritan law, 16–17
  OEC Technicians protected by, 15–17, 16f
Gowns
  contaminated spills, procedures for dealing with, 81
  personal protective equipment, as, 79
Grass, 394. See also marijuana
Gravity method of clearing airway, 297
Gray matter of the brain, 700
Green-spored lepiota mushrooms, 870, 871, 871f
Greenstick fractures
  children, 945, 958
  described, 614f, 615t
Gregg, Walter, 434
Grief
  described, 1048, 1048f
  phases of, 1048–1049
Gross negligence, defined, 16
Ground transport of patients
  basket stretchers/litters, 151, 151f
  common methods for, 146
  evacuation (stair) chair, 152–153, 153f
  improvised litters, 153, 153f, 154f
  packaging a patient, 148–151, 148f, 149f, 150f, 151f
  toboggan or sled, 147–148, 148f
  wheeled ambulance stretcher, 151–152, 152f
Growth and development
  adolescents, 948–949t, 949–950, 949f
  infants, 947, 947f, 948–949t
  newborns, 947, 947f, 948–949t
  preschoolers, 947–948, 947f, 948–949t
  school-age children, 948–949, 948–949t, 949f
  stages of, 946–947, 948–949t
  toddlers, 947, 947f, 948–949t
Growth plates. See epiphyses (growth plates)
Guarding
  defined, 500
  musculoskeletal injuries, 619, 619f
  upper extremity injuries, 622, 623f

**H**
H. influenzae vaccination, 952
HACE. See high-altitude cerebral edema (HACE)
HAINES (High Arm In Endangered Spine) recovery position, 300, 300f
Hair
  follicles, anatomy and physiology of, 539f, 540
  integumentary system, 194f, 195, 195f
Haldol. See haloperidol
Hallucinations
  behavioral emergencies, 1044
  plants causing, 886

Hallucinogens
  overuse and poisoning, 391
  toxicity, signs and symptoms of, 397t
"Halo test" for CSF, 717, 717f
Haloperidol, 391
Hand
  bandaging, 562–563, 564f
  injuries, 628, 628t
  splinting, skill for, 680
Hand injuries, 657, 658, 659
Handicap, defined, 1010, 1011
Hand-off report, 269–271, 270f
Handwashing, 79, 79f
Hangman's fracture, 711, 711f
Hank's solution, 757
Hantavirus, 884
HAPE. See high-altitude pulmonary edema (HAPE)
HAR (high-angle rescue), 1123–1124
Hare traction splint
  "floating knee" injury, 668
  tibia fracture, 645, 645f, 668
HARH (high-altitude retinal hemorrhage), 906
Haskins, Charles, 537
Hays, George P., 167
Hazard-control zones, 1114, 1114f, 1115f
Hazardous materials (HazMat)
  dealing with, 85–87, 86f
  defined, 85
  material safety data sheets, 86–87
  warning placards, 86, 86f
Hazardous materials (HazMat) response
  hazardous materials, types of, 1111–1112, 1112f
  HazMat entry teams, 1112, 1112f
  HazMat incident management, 1114–1115, 1114f, 1115f, 1115t
  nerve agent medications, dosing schedules for, 1116
  nerve agents, mechanism of action of, 1116
  NFPA safety diamond, 1112, 1112f, 1113t
Hazardous Materials (HazMat) teams
  burned patients, 588
  chemical burns, 594
  HazMat entry teams, 1112, 1112f
  radiation burns, 595
  substance use and abuse, 396
HAZWOPER (HAZardous Waste OPerations and Emergency Response) training and certification, 1114
HCTZ. See hydrochlorothiazide (HCTZ)
Head. See also head and spinal injuries
  assessment of, in pediatric emergencies, 973, 973f
  bandaging, 562, 563f
  children, 943–944, 944f, 945
  injuries
    behavioral emergencies, 1043, 1043f
    children, 958
    head-uphill position, 149
    presentations of, 704
    sports-related, 698

  secondary assessment, 230–232, 231f, 232f
Head and spinal injuries
  anatomy and physiology, 699–700, 699f, 700f
  case
    disposition, 726
    presentation, 699
    update, 714
  chapter objectives, 697
  chapter overview, 697–699, 698f
  chapter review, 738–740
  closed and open injuries, 704, 704f
  coup-contrecoup injury, 703–704, 703f
  Explore myNSPkit, 741
  head and brain injuries (See also brain; head, injuries)
    cerebral contusion, 708
    cerebral hematoma, 709–710, 709f
    concussion, 705, 707–708, 707f
    diffuse axonal injury, 710, 710f, 710t
    intracerebral hemorrhage, 711
    recurrent traumatic brain injury, 708
    scalp injuries, 704
    skull fractures, 704–705, 705f
    traumatic brain injury, 705, 706f, 706t, 707f, 707t
  historical timeline, 697
  increased intracranial pressure, 703
  key terms, 698
  mechanisms of injury, 702–703, 702f
  patient assessment
    mini-neurologic exam, 715–716, 715t, 716f
    primary assessment, 714–715
    scene size-up, 714, 714f
    secondary assessment, 715–718, 715t, 716f, 717f
  patient management
    cervical collar sizing and application, 720, 720f
    guidelines for, 719, 719f
    helmet removal, 724–725, 724f, 725f
    long spine board, placing patient on, 720–724, 721f
  Skill Guides
    cervical collar, sizing and applying, 733, 1174
    helmet removal, 736, 1174
    manual spine stabilization, 732, 1174
    short board immobilization, 735, 1174
    standing patient, immobilizing, 737, 1174
    supine patient, log rolling onto a long spine board, 734, 1174
  Skills
    axial drag, 728
    cervical collar, sizing and applying, 727
    helmet removal, 731
    manual spine stabilization, 727
    seated patient, immobilizing, 729–730
    securing the patient onto a long spine board, 729
    standing patient, immobilizing, 730

  supine patient, log rolling onto a long spine board, 728
  spinal injuries (See also spinal injuries)
    neurogenic shock, 712
    soft-tissue injuries, 711
    vertebral fractures, 711–712, 711f
  stop, think, understand, 701, 708–709, 713, 718, 726
  suggested reading, 741
Head-tilt, chin-lift maneuver
  airway, 219, 219f
  airway, opening, 295, 296f
  pediatric emergency management, 975, 976f
Head-to-toes approach for physical exam, 969, 972
Head-uphill position
  breathing difficulties and head injuries, 149
  chest trauma management, 786
Healing process
  musculoskeletal tissues, 610, 610f
  smoking, 610
Health Insurance Portability and Accountability Act of 1996 (HIPAA), 25, 268
Health services, integration of, 35
Hearing
  auditory system, 744, 745f
  impairment, and adaptive athletes, 1018, 1019f
Heart. See also cardiovascular system
  anatomy of, 176–180, 178f, 179f, 180f
  blood flow, 177, 179f
  blood pathway through, 459, 460f
  cardiovascular emergencies, 459–460, 460f
  chambers of, 177, 179f
  coronary arteries, 177, 180f
  distant or muffled sounds, and pericardial tamponade, 475
  electrical conduction system
    described, 459–460, 460f
    electrical burns, 592, 595
  pacemaker cells, 177, 180
  shock, 331f, 332
  substance exposure, effects of, 390
  thoracic trauma A & P, 772–773, 772f
"Heart attack," 465. See also acute myocardial infarction (AMI)
Heart contractility, defined, 994
Heart rate
  acclimatization to altitude, 902
  pregnancy, 1071
Heart valves
  artificial, in elderly patients, 999
  disorders of, 470
Heat acclimatization, 845
Heat cramps
  assessment, 851
  described, 843
  management, 852
Heat exhaustion
  assessment, 851

core body temperature, 842f
described, 843
heat stroke, differentiating from, 854, 854f, 854t
management, 852–853, 853f
Heat illness
prevention measures, 845, 845f
signs and symptoms, 843, 844f
types of, described, 842–843, 842f, 844f
Heat index, defined, 840, 840f
Heat loss. *See also* thermoregulation
mechanisms of
cold-related environmental emergencies, 816–817, 816f, 817f
heat-related emergencies, 839–840f, 840
rescue basics, 59–61, 59f, 60f, 61f
prevention of, 828
skin regulation of body temperature, 540
Heat stroke
assessment, 852
core body temperature, 842f
described, 843
heat exhaustion, differentiating from, 854, 854f, 854t
management, 853–854
Heat-related emergencies
anatomy and physiology, 839–841, 840f
case
disposition, 856
presentation, 839
update, 850
chapter objectives, 838
chapter overview, 838–839, 839f
chapter review, 857–860
common emergencies
heat illness, 842–843, 842f, 844f
heat-related illness prevention, 845, 845f
lightning, 848–849, 848f
sunburn, 845–847, 846t
Explore myNSPkit, 860
historical timeline, 838
key terms, 838
patient assessment
guidelines for, 850, 851f
heat cramps, 851
heat exhaustion, 851
heat stroke, 852
heat-induced syncope, 850–851
lightning strikes, 852
sunburn, 852
patient management
guidelines for, 852, 852f
heat cramps, 852
heat exhaustion, 852–853, 853f, 854, 854f, 854t
heat stroke, 853–854, 854f, 854t
heat-induced syncope, 852
lightning strikes, 855
moving patients to cooler location, 852, 852f
sunburn, 854

stop, think, understand, 841, 844–845, 847, 849–850, 855–856
suggested reading, 860
Heat-related syncope
assessment, 850–851
described, 843
management, 852
Heimlich maneuver, 424
Helicopters (rotary-wing aircraft)
altitude and temperature limitations, 155
medical transportation, for, 34, 34f
patient transportation, for, 154–155, 154f, 155f
safety issues
ground operations, 156–157, 157f
ground-to-air communications, 156
landing zone, 155–156, 156f, 156t
space and load, 155
special transport tactics, 157
Helmets
outdoor work, preparing for, 67, 67f
removal from a lying patient, skill for, 731
removal from a lying patient, skill guide for, 736, 1174
removing from a patient, 724–725, 724f, 725f
Hematemesis
acute abdomen, 508t
defined, 504
Hematochezia
acute abdomen, 508t
defined, 504
Hematocrit, and shock, 334
Hematoma
cerebral, 709–710, 709f
closed injury, 543, 543f
Hematuria
acute abdomen, 508t
cystitis, 1074
HemCon® Bandage, 562
Hemoglobin, and shock, 333, 333f, 334
Hemopneumothorax, 778
Hemoptysis, 782, 783
Hemorrhage. *See also* bleeding
postpartum, 1078t
pregnancy, during, 1078, 1078t
soft-tissue injuries, 552
Hemorrhagic shock
classification system for, 338–339, 338t
described, 336–338, 337f, 338f
Hemorrhagic stroke, 370f, 371
Hemostatic dressings, 561–562
Hemothorax, 778, 778f
Henry's Law, 923
Hepatitis
common infectious disease, 74
described, 501–502
hepatitis A, 73, 74
hepatitis B, 71, 74
hepatitis B vaccine, 74, 76, 76t, 919
hepatitis C, 74
postexposure prophylaxis, 80
Heroin, 392

Herpes simplex infections
common infectious disease, 74
direct contact transmission of disease, 71
High altitude, described, 899–900, 900f
High-altitude cerebral edema (HACE)
described, 905, 905f
treatment for, 913, 914f
High-altitude pulmonary edema (HAPE)
described, 904–905, 905f
treatment for, 913, 913f
High-altitude retinal hemorrhage (HARH), 906
High-angle rescue (HAR), 1123–1124
High-Fowler position
defined, 171
respiratory emergencies, 424
transporting patients, 146, 146f
High-pressure injection injuries, 548–549, 549f
High-risk events, and mechanism of injury, 217t
High-velocity crashes, as mechanism of injury, 217t
High-velocity wounds, 522
Highway Safety Act of 1966, 35
Hinge joints, 607
"Hip fractures," 631. *See also* hips, fractures
HIPAA. *See* Health Insurance Portability and Accountability Act (HIPAA) of 1996
Hips
dislocations, management of, 660, 806
fractures, 631, 997, 997f
injuries, and abdominal injuries, 800, 800f
injury assessment, 630–631, 631f
Histamine, 437
History, medical. *See also* SAMPLE (Signs and Symptoms, Allergies, Medications, Pertinent past medical history, Last oral intake, Events leading to incident) history
chief complaint, 226
importance of, 226, 227f
OPQRST assessment, 227t, 228–229
past medical history, 282t, 283
pediatric emergencies, 966, 966f
SAMPLE history, 226–228, 227t
trauma with medical problem, 226
History of present illness (HPI), 282–283, 282t
HIV. *See* human immunodeficiency virus (HIV)/acquired immunodeficiency syndrome (AIDS)
Hobo spiders, 872–873
Hodgdon, David, 516
Hollow organs
abdominal and pelvic, 495–496, 496f, 794f
kinetic energy, absorption of, 519–520, 520f
Homeostasis
anatomy and physiology, 206, 208f
defined, 58, 206

Honesty, in approaching children, 968
Honeybees, 875f
Horizontal (transverse) plane, 168f
Hormones (reproductive), 201, 203
Hornets, 875–876, 875f
Horses, injuries caused by, 883f, 884
Hot zones, 1114, 1114f, 1115
HPI (history of present illness), 282–283, 282t
Human crutch, 138, 138f
Human immunodeficiency virus (HIV)/ acquired immunodeficiency syndrome (AIDS)
  common infectious disease, 75
  direct contact transmission of disease, 71
  immune system, affecting, 63t
  postexposure prophylaxis, 80
Human resources for emergency medical systems, 36
Human-caused disasters, 1109, 1109f
Humerus
  anatomy of, 196f, 198
  fractures, 625–626
  fractures, bleeding from, 615t
  fractures, management of, 653–654, 653f
  fractures, rigid splint application for, 679
Humidity, and heat-related emergencies, 839–840, 840f
HVS (hyperventilation syndrome), 414–415
Hydration
  altitude illness prevention, 909, 910f
  heat-related emergencies, 841
  outdoor work, preparing for, 70, 70f, 71t
Hydrochlorothiazide (HCTZ)
  cardiac medication, 487t
  diuretic use by the elderly, 994
Hydrocodone, 1178t
Hydrocodone and acetaminophen, 392
Hydromorphone
  ALS administration, 1164
  overuse and poisoning, 392
Hyper- (movement), 170
Hyperbaric chambers, 936
Hyperglycemia
  altered mental status, 368–369, 374, 374t
  defined, 368
Hypersensitivity, defined, 437
Hypertension
  defined, 465
  geriatric emergencies, 991
  patient assessment, 474
  pregnancy-induced, 1078
Hyperthermia
  acute abdomen, 508t
  altered mental status, 374
  defined, 242, 242t, 843
  mechanism of injury, 703
Hyperventilation
  breath holding, under water, 929, 929f
  paresthesia, 421
Hyperventilation syndrome (HVS), 414–415
Hyphema
  blunt trauma to eyes, 760, 760f
  eye injuries, 751, 751f

Hypoglycemia
  altered mental status, 367–368, 368f, 368t, 373, 374t
  blood glucose levels, monitoring, 368, 368f
  causes of, 367, 368t
  defined, 367
Hyponatremia, 841
Hypotension
  acute abdomen, 508t
  cardiovascular patients, 485
  pericardial tamponade, 475
Hypothalamus, 58, 58f, 191
Hypothermia
  assessment of, 825–827, 825f, 825t, 826f
  behavioral emergencies, 1043, 1043f
  classification of, 820, 821f
  core body temperature, 842f
  defined, 242, 242t, 819
  evacuation and transportation, 832
  extricated avalanche burial victims, 831–832
  frostbite, concurrent with, 828
  heat loss prevention, 828
  management of, 828–832, 829f, 831f
  mechanism of injury, 703
  mild hypothermia, management of, 830
  moderate-to-severe hypothermia, management of, 830–831, 831f
  predisposing factors, 819
  primary hypothermia, 819–820, 820f, 821f
  secondary hypothermia, 820
  warming methods, 829–830, 829f
  water emergencies, 936, 936f
Hypothermia wraps, 830
Hypovolemic shock
  hemorrhagic, 336–339, 337f, 338f, 338t
  nonhemorrhagic, 337f, 339, 339f
Hypoxemia, 900
Hypoxia
  altered mental status, 373
  level of responsiveness, 222
Hypoxic ventilatory response, 902, 902f

**I**

Ibuprofen, 380
ICS. See Incident Command System (ICS)
Ictal phase of seizures, 364–365, 364–365f
ID-ME triage system
  delayed category, 115t, 116, 116f
  expectant category, 115t, 117–118, 118f
  immediate category, 115–116, 115f, 115t
  minimal category, 115t, 117, 117f
IFR (instrument flight rules), 155
Ilium, 196f, 198, 199f
Imipramine, 1054t
Immediate (Red)(rabbit) category for triage, 115–116, 115f, 115t
Immersion hypothermia, 819–820, 820f
Immobilization, and bone healing, 610
Immunity (immune response)
  defined, 62, 62f

factors affecting, 63t
immune system changes with aging, 987f, 990
Impacted fractures, 614f, 615f
Impairment
  defined, 1010, 1011
  disability, comparison to, 1012
Impaled objects
  abdominal injuries, 799, 799f, 805
  defined, 547, 548f
  described, 558, 558f
  eye injuries, 751, 751f, 760, 760f
  eyes, skill for treatment of, 765
  eyes, skill guide for stabilization of, 766, 1174
  management of, 786
  mechanism of injury, 702, 702f
  neck injuries, management of, 763
  removing, 558
  stabilizing, skill for, 570
  stabilizing, skill guide for, 575, 1173
  stabilizing dressings for, 561, 561f, 562f
Implantable devices, 999–1000
Implied consent, 21, 22, 22f
Impression, in medical communications, 282t, 283
Incident, defined, 99–100
Incident command
  command staff, 104, 105t
  ICS organization, 101, 103f
  key responsibilities, 104, 104f
Incident command and triage
  case
    disposition, 122
    presentation, 99
    update, 114
  chapter objectives, 98
  chapter overview, 98, 99f
  chapter review, 123–125
  Explore myNSPkit, 125
  historical timeline, 98
  incident command system
    defined, 101
    finance/administration section, 109–110
    incident command, 104, 104f, 105t
    logistics section, 107–109, 107f, 109f
    operations section, 105–106, 105t, 106f
    organization of, 101, 102–103f
    planning section, 106–107, 107f
  incident command system and the OEC Technician, 110–112, 111f
  key terms, 98
  National Incident Management System, 98, 99–101, 100f, 101f
  stop, think, understand, 113, 122
  suggested reading, 125
  triage
    defined, 114
    ID-ME categorization, 115–118, 115f, 115t, 116f, 117f, 118f
    triage methods, 119–122, 120f, 121f
    triage tags, 118, 119f

Incident Command System (ICS)
  defined, 101
  finance/administration section, 109–110
  incident command, 104, 104f, 105t
  logistics section, 107–109, 107f, 109f
  OEC Technicians and, 110–112, 111f
  operations section, 105–106, 105t, 106f
  organization of, 101, 102–103f
  planning section, 106–107, 107f
Incident Commander (IC)
  defined, 104
  functions of, 100f
Incident report forms
  defined, 271
  information to include, 271
  NSAA incident report forms,
    272–273, 273f
Incident zone, for low-angle rescue,
    1124, 1124f
Incisions, 546, 546f
Incomplete fractures, 613–614, 614f
Independence, as ethical issue, 15
Inderal®. See propranolol
Index of suspicion
  injuries, with, 525
  soft-tissue injuries, 551, 551f
Indigestion, 505
Indirect contact transmission of disease, 72
Indirect medical oversight in emergency
    care systems, 49–50
Infants
  AED use, 483, 483t
  age-based assessment, 974t
  coup-contrecoup injury, 703
  CPR, 480–481, 481f, 482t
  defined, 947, 947f
  head trauma signs and symptoms, 710
  heat illness, 842
  physical, intellectual, emotional, social,
    and language development,
    948–949t
  sun, protecting from, 847
  vital signs, normal ranges of, 221t
Infarction, defined, 465. See also acute
    myocardial infarction (AMI)
Infection
  altered mental status, 361t, 362, 380
  chronic, affecting immune system, 63t
  lymphatic system, 206
Infectious disease
  common diseases, 74–76
  defined, 71
  Standard Precautions and body substance
    isolation, 76–77, 77f
  transmission of, 71–73
  vaccination recommendations, 76, 76t
Infectious waste, dealing with, 80–81
Inferior direction, 169, 169f
Inferior nasal concha, 198f
Inferior vena cava, 496, 498f
Influenza
  airborne transmission of disease, 72
  common infectious disease, 74
  vaccine for, 76, 76t

Information systems for emergency medical
    systems, 36
Informed consent, 21
Infusion pumps, implanted, 999, 1000
Ingested poison
  absorption, reducing with activated
    charcoal, 399, 400f, 400t
  absorption of substances, 387–388, 388f
  defined, 394
  further exposure, reducing, 398
Ingestion transmission of disease, 72–73
Inhalants
  overuse and poisoning, 391
  toxicity, signs and symptoms of, 397t
Inhalation (inspiration), 410
Inhalation injuries
  airway compromise with burns, 590
  burned patients, 582, 582f, 588, 588f
  signs and symptoms, 588
  smoke from toxic plants, 888
Inhaled poison
  absorption of substances, 388, 388f
  airway management, 294, 295
  further exposure, reducing, 398, 399f
  interventions for, 400, 400f
Inhalers. See metered-dose inhalers (MDIs)
"Inherent risk," 19
Injected, defined, 394
Injection absorption of substances, 388, 388f
Injury, phases of
  injury phase, 525–526, 525f
  post-injury phase, 526, 526f, 527f
  pre-injury phase, 525, 525f
Injury pattern, defined, 517
Injury phase of injury, 525–526, 525f
"Injury uphill" principle for transporting
    patients, 148–149
Insect bites and stings
  patient assessment, 886–887
  patient management, 888–889, 888f
  stingers, removing, 446, 447f
Inspiration (inhalation), 410
Instrument flight rules (IFR), 155
Insulin and altered mental status
  AEIOU-TIPS, 361, 361t
  defined, 358–359, 359f
  diabetes type I, 366–367, 367f
  diabetes type II, 367
  patient management, 378–379, 379f
Insulin resistance, 367
Insulin-dependent diabetes mellitus
    (IDDM), 366. See also diabetes
    mellitus
Insurance, 17
Integumentary system
  allergic reactions, 439, 440, 444
  anatomy of, 194f, 195, 195f
  changes with aging, 987f, 989–990
  defined, 195
  physiology of, 195
Intellectual difficulties, described,
    1013–1014, 1014f
Intellectual disability
  athletes with, assessing, 1029–1030

autism spectrum disorders, 1013
  defined, 1012
  learning disorders, 1012, 1012f
Intermediate altitude, described, 899
"Intermediate" outdoor medical care,
    concept of, 6
Internal body part, 170
Internal defibrillators, 999, 1000
Internal drug pumps, 999, 1000
Internet, and the NSP home page, 1009
Intestines
  large, 187, 188f, 189, 495, 496f,
    794f, 795f
  small, 187, 188f, 189, 495, 496f,
    794f, 795f
  tears and ruptures, 799
Intracerebral bleed/hemorrhage, 709f, 711
Intracranial pressure
  increased, actions of, 703
  secondary CNS injuries, 703
Intravenous (IV) therapy
  ALS providers, assisting, 1157, 1158f
  equipment and set-up, 1156–1157, 1156f
  indications for, 1156, 1156f
  intravenous needles, 1157, 1157f
  preparing a set-up for, skill for, 1167
Inversion, defined, 635
Ipratropium, 420, 1163
Iris of the eye, 745, 746f
Iron supplements
  activated charcoal, 400t
  poisoning, 394
Irregular bones, 604, 604f
Irreversible shock, 335–336
Irrigation of eyes, 761, 761f
Ischemia, defined, 466
Ischemic stroke, 370, 370f
Ischium, 196f, 198, 199f
Isopropyl (rubbing) alcohol, 393
Isoptin. See verapamil
IV therapy. See intravenous (IV) therapy

**J**

Jack-o-lantern mushrooms, 870, 871
"Jams and pretzels," 673–674, 673–674f
Jantoven. See warfarin
Jaundice
  acute abdomen, 508t
  hepatitis, 502
Jaw-thrust maneuver
  airway, 219, 219f
  airway, opening, 295, 296f, 297
Jefferson fracture, 711
Jellyfish, injuries caused by, 880, 881f,
    889, 889f
Jewelry removal, 650
Jimson weed, 868, 868f
Johe, David H., 7t
Joint capsule, 606
Joint Statement of Understanding, 21
Joints
  bandaging, 562, 562f
  defined, 602

Joints, (cont.)
  movability of, 606–607, 606f
  parts of, 606
  skeletal system, 197, 197f
  types of, 607, 607f
Judd, William R., 291
Judgment
  impairment, causes of, 284
  OEC Technicians learning to use, 24
Jugular vein
  lacerations to, 751–752
  neck anatomy and physiology, 747, 747f
Junior Ski Patrol, 264
Justice, as ethical issue, 15
Juvenile-onset diabetes, 366. See also
      diabetes mellitus

## K

Kehr's sign, 802
Kerlix™, 559
Ketamine, 391
Khumbu cough
  defined, 906
  treatment for, 913, 914f
Kidneys
  location of, 496, 496f, 795f
  solid organ, 794f
  urinary system, 191, 192f
"Killer bees," 876
Kinematics
  body's internal structures, 519–520, 520f
  defined, 517
  kinetic energy, 518–519, 519–520f
  Newton's laws of motion, 518, 518f, 519f
  stopping distance, 519, 520f
Kinetic energy
  calculation of, 518–519, 519–520f
  defined, 518
Kinetic injury, calculation of, 521
King™ airway, 1148
Kling™, 559
Knees
  dislocation, management of, 665
  dislocations, 633–634, 633f
  fractures near, 633
  injuries, management of, 665–667, 665f
  injury assessment, 632–634, 633f, 634f
  ligaments, 607–608, 607f
Knights of St. John, 33–34
Kübler-Ross, Elisabeth, 1048
Kyphosis, 989

## L

Lacerations
  DCAP-BTLS assessment, 230, 230t
  open injuries, 545f, 546, 546f
  scalp, 538f
Lachrymal glands, 746, 746f
Lacrimal apparatus, 746–747, 746f
Lacrimal bone, 198f
Lacrimal (tear) ducts, 746f, 747
Landing zone (LZ) for aircraft

  defined, 155
  selection of, 156, 156f, 156t
Langley, Roger, 4
Language, common, in emergency care
      systems, 42–43
L.A.P. (Look, Auscultate, Palpate)
  altitude-related emergencies, 911, 911f
  chest assessment, 783–784
LAR (low-angle rescue), 1123–1125, 1124f
Large intestines (colon)
  GI system, 187, 188f, 189
  hollow organ, 495, 496f, 794f
  location of, 795f
Larrey, Dominique Jean, 34, 114
Laryngeal mask airway, 1148, 1148f
Laryngopharynx, anatomy of, 175f
Laryngoscope blades, 1142, 1142f, 1143f
Laryngoscope handles, 1142–1143,
      1142f, 1143f
Laryngospasm, 922
Larynx
  neck anatomy and physiology, 747, 747f
  respiratory emergencies, 410, 410f
  upper airway, 174, 175f, 176f
Lasik surgery, 906
Lasix®. See furosemide
Last oral intake, in SAMPLE history,
      227t, 228
Late (deep) cold injury, 815f. See also
      frostbite
Lateral collateral ligament injury, 632–633
Lateral direction, 169–170, 169f
Latex allergy
  medical supplies and equipment, 439
  outdoor adaptive athletes, 1028
Latitude change and oxygen
      concentration, 902
Law enforcement officials, 1058, 1059, 1059f
Law of conservation of energy, 518
LBMs (little brown mushrooms), 870,
      871, 871f
Leap frog CPR method, 158–159
Learning disorders, 1012, 1013f
Left direction of the body, 169f, 170
Left lateral recumbent position
  airway, keeping open, 300, 300f
  alcohol intoxication, 377, 377f
  defined, 171, 171f
Left ventricular failure, 779
Left-sided CHF, 466, 475
Leg injuries, 630, 630f. See also femur; "tib-
      fib" fractures; tibia
Legal duty to act, 17
Legal issues, 552. See also ethical and legal
      issues
Legislation, for emergency medical
      systems, 35
Lens of the eye, 745, 746f
Level of responsiveness (LOR)
  decreased, as contraindication to
      activated charcoal, 399
  defined, 238, 715
  head and spinal injury assessment, 715,
      715t, 716

  primary assessment, 222
  respiratory emergencies, 418
Levitra®. See vardenafil HCl
Lice, 72
Lidocaine, 1163, 1164
Life jackets, 1026, 1026f
Life-threatening conditions
  encountered by OEC Technicians, 84
  managing, 224–226
Lift, defined, 143
"Lift Evacuation Technical Manual," 537
Lifting the patient
  BEAM lift, 144
  BEAN lift, 144, 161, 162, 1173
  direct ground lift, 143–144, 160–161,
      163, 1173
  draw-sheet lift, 145–146, 145f
  extremity lift, 143, 143f
  overview of, 141
  power grip, 142, 142f
  power lift, 142–143, 142f
Ligaments
  anatomy and physiology, 197, 197f
  defined, 602
  healing process, 610
  sprains, 612, 613
  structure and function, 607–608, 607f
  tendons, difference from, 609
Light burns to eyes, 762
Lightning injuries
  assessment, 852
  cumulonimbus clouds, 848, 848f
  lightning-caused injuries, facts about,
      848, 848f
  management, 855
  risks, reducing, 848–849
Lily of the valley, 866, 866f
Linear skull fracture, 704
Lipitor. See atorvastatin
Liquids, hot, and thermal burns, 589, 593
Lisinopril, 487t
Lithium, 400t
Litters for patient transport, 151, 153,
      153f, 154f
Little brown mushrooms (LBMs), 870,
      871, 871f
Liver
  abdominal injuries, 798, 798f
  GI system, 187, 188f, 189
  location of, 795f
  solid organ, 496, 496f, 794f
Livor mortis, 1048
Llama injuries, 884
"Load and go" situations, 784, 785
Lofstrand crutches, 1021, 1022f, 1023, 1023f
Log rolling patient onto an LSB
  skill for, 728
  skill guide for, 734, 1174
Logistics Chief, 105t, 107, 108
Logistics section of incident command
      system
  branches and units, 108–109, 109f
  facilities, 107–108, 107f
  ICS organization, 101, 104f, 105f

Long bones, 197, 604, 604f, 605f
Long spine boards (LSBs)
    children, 724
    defined, 131
    head stabilization, 720, 720f, 721f
    lifting, for, 131–132, 131t, 132f, 133f
    patient care and, 132
    placing patient on, 720–724, 721f
    securing patient to, skill for, 729
    securing patients to, 722–723
    vomiting, 724
Long-axis drags
    blanket drag, 137, 137f
    feet drag, 137–138
    shoulder drag, 137, 137f
    underarm-wrist drag, 137, 137f
    unresponsive patient, 136
Longfellow, Livingston, 31
Longitudinal traction, 644
"Look, Listen, and Feel" for breathing
    assessment, 219
Lopressor®. See metoprolol
LOR. See level of responsiveness (LOR)
Loratadine, 443t
Lorazepam, 391
Lordosis, 989
Lovenox®. See enoxaparin
Low altitude, described, 899, 899f
Low-angle rescue (LAR), 1123–1125, 1124f
Lower airway
    airway management, 293–294, 294f
    anatomy of, 174–175, 175f, 176f
    respiratory emergencies, 410–412, 410f,
        411f, 412f
Lower extremities
    anatomy of, 196f, 198
    musculoskeletal injury assessment
        ankle injuries, 635–636, 635f, 636f
        femur fractures, 631–632, 632f
        foot and toe injuries, 636, 636f
        hip and pelvis injuries, 630–631, 631f
        knee injuries, 632–634, 633f, 634f
        overview of, 630, 630f
        tibia and fibula injuries,
            634–635, 635f
    musculoskeletal injury management
        ankle injuries, 668–670, 669f, 670f
        femur and tibia fracture in the same
            leg, 668, 668f
        femur fractures, 660–663, 660f, 662f,
            663f, 665
        foot and toe injuries, 670
        hip dislocations, 660
        knee injuries, 665–667, 665f
        pelvic fractures, 659–660
        tibia and fibula injuries, 667–668
    splinting injuries, skill guides for,
        689–690, 1174
    splinting injuries, skills for, 681–683
Low-velocity wounds, 522
LSBs. See long spine boards (LSBs)
LSD (lysergic acid diethylamide)
    overuse and poisoning, 391, 394
    toxicity, signs and symptoms of, 397t

Lubricants for endotracheal tubes,
    1144, 1145f
Lucid period, described, 710
Lumbar spine
    anatomy of, 196f, 198, 198f
    axial skeleton, 699f
Lungs
    auscultation of
        respiratory emergencies, 421–422, 421f
        skill for, 426
        skill guide for, 428, 1173
    lower airway, 174, 176f
    thoracic trauma A & P, 772, 772f
Luvox. See fluvoxamine
Lyme disease
    deer ticks, 875
    vector-borne transmission of disease, 73
Lymph nodes, 206, 207f
Lymphatic system
    anatomy of, 206, 207f
    defined, 206
    physiology of, 206
Lymphatic vessels, 206, 207f
Lynx injuries, 883
LZ for aircraft. See landing zone (LZ) for
    aircraft

**M**

Macintosh laryngoscope blades, 1142,
    1142f, 1143f
Malaria
    mosquitoes, 876
    vector-borne transmission of disease, 73
Males
    erectile dysfunction, 486
    reproductive system
        anatomy of, 203, 204f
        physiology of, 203
    urethra, 191, 192f
Mammalian diving reflex, 922
Mammals, injuries caused by
    described, 882–885, 883f, 884f, 885f
    patient assessment, 887, 887f
    patient management, 889, 890, 890f
Mandated reporter, defined, 286. See also
    reporting, situations requiring
Mandible, 196f, 198f, 743, 743f
Manic-depressive disorder. See bipolar
    (manic-depressive) disorder
Manual suction device, 298, 298f
Marijuana
    overuse and poisoning, 392, 394
    plant emergencies, 886
    toxicity, signs and symptoms of, 397t
Marine animals
    injuries caused by
        described, 880–881, 880f, 881f
        patient assessment, 887
        patient management, 889, 889f
    water emergencies, 930–931, 931f
Mark I antidote kit, 400, 1115, 1115f
Marmots, 884
Marshall, George C., 5

Mary Jane, 394. See also marijuana
"Mask" reverse squeeze, 928
Masks, oxygen. See also oxygen therapy
Masks, protective
    NIOSH-approved N95, 79
    surgical, 78–79, 78f
Mass casualty incidents, 85, 86f
MASS (Move, Assess, Sort, Send) triage
    method, 119
Massasauga snakes, 878
Mastoid process, 198f
Material safety data sheets (MSDS), 86–87
Maxilla, 196f, 198f, 743, 743f
McNamara, Edward, 11t
MD (muscular dystrophy), 1017, 1017f
MDIs. See metered-dose inhalers (MDIs)
MDMA (methylenedioxy-
    methamphetamine), 391
Measles, 76
Measles, mumps, rubella (MMR)
    vaccine, 76t
Mechanical digestion, 187
Mechanical tattooing, 549
Mechanical ventilators
    complications, 1152
    described, 1152, 1152f
    equipment set-up, 1152
    indications for, 1152
Mechanism of injury (MOI)
    adaptive athletes, assessing, 0131f, 1031
    chest injuries, 774
    chief complaint, 216–217, 217t
    common MOIs, 85
    defined, 216
    demonstrable, lack of, and possibility of
        major injury, 217
    diffuse axonal injury, 710, 710f
    emergency situations, assessing, 84,
        85, 85f
    femur fractures, 632, 632f
    head and spinal injury assessment, 714
    head and spine injuries, 702–703, 702f
    knee dislocation, 634
    lower extremity injury assessment, 630
    musculoskeletal injuries, 618f, 619
    pathophysiology
        blast injury, 523–524, 524f
        blunt injury, 522, 522f
        crush injury, 523, 523f
        force producing the injury, 521, 521f
        MOI, major types of, 521
        penetrating injury, 522, 522f
        rotational injury, 522–523, 523f
    pediatric emergencies, 963
    posterior hip dislocation, 631
    thoracic trauma, 783
    trauma patient assessment, 530, 530f
Media, at crime scenes, 88–89, 89f
Medial collateral ligament sprain, 632
Medial direction, 169–170, 169f
Medial malleolus fracture, 636, 636f
Median nerve, 628, 628t
Median (sagittal) plane, 168f
Medical alert ID/tag, 1030

Medical communications and documentation
case
disposition, 287
presentation, 266
update, 282
chapter objectives, 264
chapter overview, 264–266, 265f, 266f
chapter review, 287–290
communication, forms of, 267, 267f, 268f
communication basics, 267
Explore myNSPkit, 290
historical timeline, 264
key terms, 265
medical communication, and privacy, 268
medical communications, essential content of, 282–286, 282t, 285f, 286f
oral communication, 268–271, 269f, 269t, 270f
stop, think, understand, 281
suggested reading, 290
written communication
errors, addendums, and computer-generated forms, 279–281, 279f, 280f
field care notes, 272, 272f
good report writing, characteristics of, 278–279
NSAA incident report form, 272–273, 273f
patient care reports, 273–278, 274f, 275f, 276f, 277f
types of, 271
Medical conditions
behavioral emergencies, 1042, 1042f
behavioral emergencies and crisis response, 1056
concurrent, and altitude-related problems, 906
water emergencies, aggravation with, 931
Medical direction for emergency medical systems, 36
Medical director, defined, 42
Medical Emergency Triage tag (METTAG), 118, 119f
Medical history. See history, medical
Medical oversight
emergency care systems, in, 49–50, 49f
public health in emergency care systems, 45
Medical Reserve Corps, 1111
Medications
ALS personnel, medications administered by, 1162–1165, 1163f, 1164f
ALS provider, OEC Technician assisting, 1165
altitude illness prevention, 910–911, 910f
analgesic medications, 1164, 1164f
behavioral emergencies and crisis response, 1054, 1054t
cardiac medications, 1163–1164, 1163f
elderly, use by, 993–994, 993f
emergency care equipment, 1177, 1178t

prescription and OTC drugs, 392–393
respiratory medications, 1163
SAMPLE history, 227t, 228
shock, 345
Medulla oblongata, 183, 185f, 186f
Melena, defined, 504
Meninges, anatomy of, 183, 185f
Meningitis
airborne transmission of disease, 72
children, 954
common infectious disease, 75
Meningococcal vaccine, 76t
Meniscus, defined, 633
Menstrual cycle, 206
Mental illness and cognitive disability, 1013
Mental preparedness for outdoor work, 63–64
Mental retardation, described, 1013
Mental status
altered, as common NOI, 85
GCS values by age, 971t
Meperidine
ALS administration, 1164
overuse and poisoning, 392
Metabolism
hydration needs, 70
rate of, in children, 945
substances, of, 389
temperature regulation, 59
Metal splints, 643–644, 644f
Metered-dose inhalers (MDIs)
ALS providers, assisting, 1153, 1154, 1154f
assisting with, skill for, 427
assisting with, skill guide for, 429, 1173
respiratory emergencies, 420, 420f, 424–425, 425f
Meth, 394. See also methamphetamine
Methamphetamine
coronary artery vasospasm, 466
overuse and poisoning, 392, 394
toxicity, signs and symptoms of, 397t
Methane
poisoning, 394
toxicity, signs and symptoms of, 397t
Methanol toxicity, 393
Methylenedioxymethamphetamine (MDMA), 391
Metoprolol
beta-blocker use by the elderly, 994
cardiac medication, 487t
shock, 345
METTAG (Medical Emergency Triage tag), 118, 119f
MI (myocardial infarction). See acute myocardial infarction (AMI)
Mid-axillary line on the body, 169f
Midazolam, 1164
Mid-clavicular location on the body, 169f
Middle nasal concha, 198f
Midline location on the body, 169f
Mild allergic reactions
described, 439
signs and symptoms, 444
Mild hypothermia

assessment of, 825, 825f, 825t
described, 821f
management of, 830
Military time, 48–49, 49t
Miller laryngoscope blades, 1142, 1142f, 1143f
Millin, Michael, 7t
Minimal (Green) (crossed-out ambulance) category for triage, 115t, 117, 117f
Minimal movement in joints, 607
Mini-neurologic exam, 715–716, 715t, 716f
Minor consent, defined, 21, 23
Miscarriage, 1078–1079
Mixed-format patient care report, 275, 276f
MMR (measles, mumps, rubella) vaccine, 76t
Moderate allergic reactions
described, 440
signs and symptoms, 444
Moderate hypothermia
assessment of, 825–826, 825t
described, 821f
management of, 830–831, 831f
Moderate-to-severe hypothermia, 832
MOI. See mechanism of injury (MOI)
Monkshood, 865, 865f
Mononucleosis, 71
Mono-ski, defined, 1023
"Montezuma's revenge," 506
Moose injuries, 884
Moral duty to act, 17
Moray eels
injuries caused by, 880, 880f
water emergencies, 930, 931f
Morgan, John E. P., 56, 126
Morphine
ALS administration, 1164
overuse and poisoning, 392
Mosquito bites, 876, 876f, 886–887
Motorized transport vehicles, 153, 154f
Mountain lion injuries, 883
Mountain Travel & Rescue, 1171
Mouse injuries, 884f
"Mousetrap" fall, 627
Mouth
GI system, 187, 188f, 189, 189f
injuries, assessment of, 755
Move, defined, 135
Movement, physiology of, 609
Moving, lifting, and transporting patients. See also transporting patients
body mechanics of lifting, 128–131, 128f, 129f, 130f
case
disposition, 160
presentation, 128
update, 141
chapter objectives, 126
chapter overview, 126–128, 127f
chapter review, 164–166
CPR during transport, 157–159, 158f
devices and equipment
basket ("Stokes") stretcher, 131, 134, 134f

long spine board, 131–132, 131t, 132f, 133f

orthopedic stretcher, 131, 132–133, 133f, 134f

portable stretcher, 131, 133, 134f

short spine board and vest-type lifting/immobilization devices, 131, 134–135, 135f

sitting lifting device, 131, 135, 135f

transfer flat, 131

Explore myNSPkit, 166

historical timeline, 126

key terms, 127

lifting the patient
  BEAM lift, 144
  BEAN lift, 144, 161, 162, 1173
  direct ground lift, 143–144, 160–161, 163, 1173
  draw-sheet lift (transfer flat), 145–146, 145f
  extremity lift, 143, 143f
  overview of, 141
  power grip, 142, 142f
  power lift, 142–143, 142f
  skills for, 160–163, 1173

moving a patient
  nonurgent moves, 138–140, 138f, 139f, 141f
  overview of, 135–136
  special moving situations, 141
  urgent moves, 136–138, 137f

stop, think understand, 140, 159–160

suggested reading, 166

transporting patients
  air transportation, limitations for, 155
  air transportation, means for, 154–155, 154f, 155f
  basket stretchers/litters, 151, 151f
  evacuation chairs, 152–153, 153f
  ground transport, common methods for, 146
  helicopter safety, 155–157, 156f, 156t, 157f
  improvised litters, 153, 153f, 154f
  motorized transport vehicles, 153, 154f
  packaging a patient, 148–151, 148f, 149f, 150f, 151f
  positions for, 146, 146f, 147f
  special transport tactics, 157
  toboggans and sleds, 147–148, 148f
  wheeled ambulance stretchers, 151–152, 152f

MS (multiple sclerosis), 1017

MSDS (material safety data sheets), 86–87

Mules, injuries caused by, 884

Multi-agency coordination system, 100

Multiple casualty, 114

Multiple sclerosis (MS), 1017

Multiple victims of lightning strikes, 855

Murrett, Mary, 11t

Muscles
  healing process, 610
  strains, 612–613

structure and function, 608, 608f

types of, 608–609, 609f

Muscular dystrophy (MD), 1017, 1017f

Muscular system
  anatomy of, 199, 200f, 201f
  defined, 199
  physiology of, 201

Musculoskeletal injuries
  anatomy and physiology
    healing process, 610, 610f
    importance of, 602–603
    joints, 606–607, 606f, 607f
    ligaments, 607–608, 607f, 609
    movement, physiology of, 609
    muscles, 608–609, 608f, 609f
    skeleton, 603–605, 603f, 604f, 605f
    stop, think, understand, 605–606, 611–612
    tendons, 609, 609f
  case
    disposition, 675
    presentation, 603
    update, 617
  chapter objectives, 601, 617, 639
  chapter overview, 601–602
  chapter review, 692–696
  Explore myNSPkit, 696
  historical timeline, 601
  key terms, 602
  patient assessment
    ankle injuries, 635–636, 635f, 636f
    axial skeleton injuries, 638
    clavicle and shoulder injuries, 623–625, 623f, 624f
    elbow injuries, 626, 626f
    femur fractures, 631–632, 632f
    foot and toe injuries, 636, 636f
    forearm injuries, 626–627, 627f
    hand and finger injuries, 628, 628f, 628t
    hip and pelvis injuries, 630–631, 631f
    humerus fractures, 625–626
    knee injuries, 632–634, 633f, 634f
    lower extremities, overview of, 630, 630f
    overview of, 617–620, 617f, 618f, 619f, 620f
    signs and symptoms, 620–621, 621f
    stop, think, understand, 621–622, 628–629, 637–638
    tibia and fibula injuries, 634–635, 635f
    upper extremities, overview of, 622–623, 623f
    wrist injuries, 627
  patient management
    ankle injuries, 668–670, 669f, 670f
    boot removal, 670–671
    elbow injuries, 654–656, 654f, 655f
    femur and tibia fracture in the same leg, 668, 668f
    femur fractures, 660–663, 660f, 662f, 663f, 665
    foot and toe injuries, 670
    forearm injuries, 656
    guidelines for, 639–640

hand and finger injuries, 657–658, 657f

hip dislocations, 660

humerus fractures, 653–654, 653f

knee injuries, 665–667, 665f

pelvic fractures, 659–660

shoulder, clavicle, and scapula injuries, 650–653, 651f

specific injuries, caring for, 649

splinting (See splints)

stabilized extrication and transfer, 673–674, 673–674f

stop, think, understand, 648–649, 658–659, 663–664, 671–672, 675

tibia and fibula injuries, 667–668

wrist injuries, 656–657, 657f

Skill Guides
  blanket roll splint for shoulder, 687, 1173
  boot removal, 691, 1174
  figure eight application, 685, 1174
  lower extremity injury, splinting, 689, 1174
  posterior S/C dislocation reduction, 688, 1174
  traction splinting, 690, 1173
  upper extremity injury, splinting, 686, 1174

Skills
  airplane splint, applying, 682
  blanket roll splint, applying to a shoulder, 678
  boot, removing, 684
  figure eight splint, creating and applying, 677
  forearm fracture, splinting, 680
  hand immobilization, splinting for, 680
  humerus fracture, splinting with a rigid splint, 679
  injured elbow, rigid splint fixation of, 679
  posterior sternoclavicular injury, reducing, 678
  Quick Splint, applying, 682
  Quick Splint, replacing with a cardboard splint, 683
  sling and swathe, applying, 676
  tib-fib fracture, immobilizing with two rigid splints, 683
  traction splint application to a femur, 681

suggested reading, 696

types of injuries
  dislocations, 615–616, 615f
  fractures, 613–615, 613f, 614f, 615t
  multiple musculoskeletal injuries, 616
  ruptured tendons, 613
  sprains, 612, 613
  stop, think, understand, 616
  strains, 612–613
  zone of injury, 612, 612f

Musculoskeletal system
  changes with aging, 987f, 989, 989f
  children, 945, 945f
  defined, 602

Mushrooms
  patient assessment, 886
  patient management, 888
  poisonous, 870–871, 870f, 871f
Muskellunge, 881
Myocardial contusion, defined, 774
Myocardial infarction (MI). *See* acute myocardial infarction (AMI)
Myocardium, defined, 459

# N

Nails, 194f, 195
Naloxone, 1164
Narcan®. *See* naloxone
Narcotic toxicity, signs and symptoms of, 397t
Nardil. *See* phenelzine
Nasal bone, 198f
Nasal cannula (NC)
  oxygen delivery and flow rate, 311, 311t
  oxygen therapy, 311–312, 311f
Nasopharyngeal airway (NPA)
  contraindications to, 301
  described, 300–301, 301f
  indications for, 301
  inserting, skill for, 318
  inserting, skill guide for, 323, 1173
  insertion of, 301–302
  oropharyngeal airway, comparison to, 300t
  removal of, 302
Nasopharynx, anatomy of, 174, 175f, 176f
National Academy of Science, 34–35
National Capital Poison Center Help Hotline, 401
National Disaster Medical System (NDMS)
  components of, 1110
  specialized response teams, 1110–1111, 1110f, 1111f
National Fire Protection Association (NFPA)
  fire-ground operations, standards for, 1128
  safety diamond, 1112, 1112f, 1113t
National First Aid Committee, 386
National Highway Traffic Safety Administration (NHTSA)
  defined, 35
  *EMS Agenda for the Future*, 35–36, 37–38f
National Incident Management System (NIMS)
  benefits of, 100
  components of, 100–101, 100f, 101f
  incident, defined, 99–100
  ski patrollers using, 98
National Institute for Occupational Safety and Health (NIOSH)
  back injuries, 128
  contaminated objects, procedures for dealing with, 80
  NIOSH-approved N95 masks, 79
National Medical Advisor position, defined, 6

National Medical Committee
  defined, 11
  first meeting of, 386
"National Notes," 457
National Oceanic and Atmospheric Administration (NOAA), 401
National OEC Program Committee, 11
National OEC Program Director
  defined, 12
  functions, 11
  list of directors, 11t
"National Patroller," 457
National Poison Center, 890
National Response Framework, 1109–1110
National Safety Council Distinguished Service to Safety Award, 601
National Senior Auxiliary program, 942
National Ski Areas Association (NSAA)
  incident report form, 272–273, 273f
  joint statement of understanding with NSP, 21
National Ski Association, 4
National Ski Hall of Fame, 329
National Ski Patrol European Division, 264
National Ski Patrol System, Inc. (NSP)
  code of ethics, 896
  Creed of Service and Safety, 8
  defined, 4
  establishment of, 3, 4, 5f, 31
  federal charter, 697
  first education director, 770
  Joint Statement of Understanding with the National Ski Areas Association, 21
  membership growth, 457
  OEC course, 6, 7f, 7t
  OEC Refresher Committee, 12
  Outdoor Emergency Care course, 1
  Senior Program, 838, 861
  ski patrollers, training, 7, 7f
  Student patroller classification, 896
  World War II, 4–5, 6f
National Weather Service, 849
NATO phonetic alphabet, 48, 48t
Natural disasters, 1108, 1109f
Nature of illness (NOI)
  common NOIs, 85
  defined, 216
  emergency situations, assessing, 84
Nausea
  acute abdomen, 508t
  gastrointestinal ailment, 505
  pediatric emergencies, 953, 977
NC. *See* nasal cannula (NC)
NDMS. *See* National Disaster Medical System (NDMS)
Near-drowning
  cold-water submersion, 926–927, 926f
  death from, 926
  debris and pathogens in water, 927
  defined, 926
  mechanism of injury, 702
  salinity of water, 927
  warm-water submersion, 926, 927

Nebulizers
  ALS providers, assisting, 1153
  assisting patients with, 1153f
  equipment and set-up, 1153–1154, 1154f
  indications for, 1153
Neck
  anatomy and physiology, 747, 747f
  assessment of, in pediatric emergencies, 973, 973f
  injuries
    assessment of, 756, 756f
    children, 958
    described, 751–752, 751f
    management of, 763, 763f
  secondary assessment, 232, 233f
  trauma and environmental injuries, vulnerability to, 749, 749f
Neck veins, distended, 475
Necrosis, defined, 862
Needle sticks, 79, 79f
Needle thoracostomy, 1153, 1153f
Negligence
  defined, 18
  gross negligence, 16
Nephrolithiasis, 502–503
Nephron, described, 989
Nerve agents
  antidote administration, skill guide for, 1131
  mechanism of action, 1116
  medication for, 1116
  overuse and poisoning, 392
  poisoning, interventions for, 400
  toxicity, signs and symptoms of, 397t
Nervous system. *See also* central nervous system (CNS); peripheral nervous system
  aging, changes with, 987f, 988
  anatomy of
    central nervous system, 183–186, 184f, 185f, 186f
    peripheral nervous system, 183, 184f, 186
  breathing process, 412
  defined, 183
  nerve endings in the skin, 539f, 540
  neuron, defined, 700
  physiology of, 186–187, 187f
  substance exposure, effects of, 389
Neural ischemia, 712
Neurogenic shock, 337f, 341–342, 712
Neuron, defined, 700. *See also* nerves
Neurosis, 1043, 1043f
Neurostimulators, 999
Neurotic disorders
  agitation, 1045, 1045f
  anxiety, 1044
  depression, 1044
  paranoia, 1044–1045
Neurovascular status
  lower extremity injury assessment, 630
  musculoskeletal injuries, 620
  upper extremity injury assessment, 622

Newborn period/newborns
  basic care of, 1085–1086, 1085f,
    1085t, 1086f
  CPR, 477, 481
  defined, 947, 947f
  heat illness, 842
  physical, intellectual, emotional, social,
    and language development,
    948–949t
Newton, Isaac, 518
Newton's first law of motion, 518, 518f
Newton's third law of motion, 518, 519f
NFPA. *see* National Fire Protection
    Association (NFPA)
NHTSA. *See* National Highway Traffic
    Safety Administration (NHTSA)
Nifedipine
  calcium-channel blocker use by the
    elderly, 994
  emergency care medication, 1178t
Night flight operations, 155
"Nightstick" fractures, 627
NIMS. *See* National Incident Management
    System (NIMS)
NIOSH. *See* National Institute for
    Occupational Safety and Health
    (NIOSH)
Nitrogen narcosis, 929
Nitroglycerin
  ALS administration to cardiac patients,
    1163, 1164
  angina, 467t
  cardiac medication, 472, 485–486,
    486f, 487t
  contraindications for, 485–486
  described, 472
NOAA (National Oceanic and Atmospheric
    Administration), 401
NOI. *See* nature of illness (NOI)
Nondisplaced fractures, 613
Nonhemorrhagic shock, 337f, 339, 339f
Non-immersion hypothermia, 820, 821f
Non-insulin dependent diabetes mellitus
    (NIDDM), 367. *See also* diabetes
    mellitus
Nonmaleficence, as ethical issue, 15
Nonrebreather mask (NRB), 312–313,
    312f, 313t
Nonurgent moves
  chair carry, 139, 139f
  fore and aft carry, 140, 141f
  human crutch, 138, 138f
  two-person assist, 138–139, 139f
Nonverbal communication, 267, 268f
Noradrenalin (norepinephrine), 191, 195
Nordic kit (emergency care equipment),
    1177, 1177f, 1178t
Norepinephrine (noradrenalin), 191, 195
Normal anatomical position, defined,
    169f, 170
Northern pike (fish), 881
Nortriptyline, 1054t
Nose
  injuries, and epistaxis, 749, 750f

injuries, assessment of, 755, 755f
  nasal bone, 198f
"Nose, navel, and toes" alignment for
    urgent moves, 136
Nose candy, 394. *See also* cocaine
Notes
  ABCDs, assessing, 218
  activated charcoal, contraindication
    to, 399
  acute coronary syndrome (ACS), 467
  AEDs, described, 484
  airway compromise with burns, 590
  airway obstruction, complete, 966
  artificial joints, injury to, 660
  aspirin, action of, 487
  atmosphere, described, 922
  avulsed tooth, 757
  bag-valve mask, using for patients with
    suspected lung injury, 785
  behavior and injury, 1059
  blood pressure, accurate measurement
    of, 240
  boots, tight-fitting, and cold injury, 819
  Boyle's Law, 923
  brain injury, two phases of, 705
  bubbling in carbonated beverages, 923
  burns, documentation of, 586
  burns, extensive, 595
  chemical burns, 594
  chest assessment, including upper back
    and armpits for, 783
  children on LSBs, 724
  common medications for respiratory
    conditions, 420
  contact lenses, removing, 762
  CPR technique, 477
  Dalton's Law, 923
  death and warm temperature, 936
  disability and impairment, comparison
    of, 1012
  Divers' Alert Network, 936
  documentation of AAO X 4 scale, 715
  ear drum rupture, 759
  emergency delivery, being prepared
    for, 1080
  emergency documentation, 278
  entrance and exit wounds from electrical
    burns, 595
  ethanol percentages, 393
  facial injury, significant, 756
  fire ground anatomy, 1129
  fractures, signs and symptoms of, 621
  Gamow bag, 913, 913f
  geriatric/pediatric coup-contrecoup
    injury, 703
  hallucinations, 1044
  HAZWOPER training and certification,
    1114
  head trauma in infants, 710
  Henry's Law, 923
  implantable devices, 484
  insect stingers, removing, 446, 447f
  kinetic injury, 521
  knee joint trauma, 634

National Poison Center, 890
nitroglycerin, 472
one victim and two patients, 1088
open fracture, prolonged rescue time
    for, 648
oral glucose, administering to pediatric
    patients, 379
Paralympic Games adaptive sports, 1020
partial pressure, 923
pediatric patient, general impression
    of, 965
pediatric trauma, 958
personal protective equipment for burn
    sources, 588
pole and strap injury, 628
position of function for wrist injuries,
    656, 657f
posterior sternoclavicular (S/C)
    dislocation, 624
pregnant trauma patients, first steps in
    treating, 1089
psychogenic shock, 342
pulmonary blood vessels, 462
pulse, taking, 239
pulsus paradoxus, 779
rabies, 890
RECCO system, 1121, 1121f
respirations, quality of, 240
seizures, 365
shoulder injuries, differentiating, 625
shoulder pads, removing, 275f, 725
silent MI, 474
smoking and healing, 610
square knot, tying, 650, 651f
strain *versus* sprain, 613
subungual hematoma, relieving pressure
    of, 545
systolic BP for various pulse points, 241
tendons and ligaments, difference
    between, 609
tension pneumothorax, advanced life
    support for, 785
Thomas Splint, 645, 646f
toxic alcohols, 393
toxic plants, 394
traction hitch, 662, 662f
traction *versus* tension, 646
traveler's diarrhea, preventing, 506
vehicle extrication scene, anatomy
    of, 1106
vomiting by patients on LSBs, 724
water-related rescue methods, 933, 933f
wilderness tips, 279
wounds, geriatric considerations for, 553
NPA. *See* nasopharyngeal airway (NPA)
NRB. *See* nonrebreather mask (NRB)
NRB (nonrebreather mask), 312–313,
    312f, 313t
NSAA. *See* National Ski Areas Association
    (NSAA)
NSAA incident report form, 272–273, 273f
NSP. *See* National Ski Patrol System, Inc.
    (NSP)
Nursemaid's elbow, 626

Nutrake cricothyrotomy system, 1150
Nutrition
    immune system, 62, 63t
    outdoor work, preparing for, 64, 64f, 65t

## O

Oak-N-Ivy, 888, 888f
Oblique fractures, 614f, 615t
Obstetric and gynecologic emergencies. *See also* pregnancy
    acute abdomen, 504
    anatomy and physiology, 1069–1072, 1070f, 1072f
    case
        disposition, 1092
        presentation, 1070
        update, 1089
    chapter objectives, 1068
    chapter overview, 1068–1069, 1069f
    chapter review, 1095–1098
    childbirth
        assisting with, skill for, 1092–1093
        assisting with, skill guide for, 1094–1095
        complications of, 1080–1081, 1080f
        emergency delivery, 1080, 1081–1083, 1081f, 1082f, 1083f
        stages of, 1079, 1079f
    common emergencies
        abdominal pain, causes of, 1073–1074
        cystitis, 1074
        dysmenorrhea, 1073–1074
        ectopic pregnancy, 1074
        gynecological trauma, 1075
        ovarian cysts, 1074
        pelvic inflammatory disease, 1074
        sexual assault, 1075–1076, 1075f
        vaginal bleeding, 1075
    Explore myNSPkit, 1099
    historical timeline, 1068
    key terms, 1069
    newborns, basic care of, 1085–1086, 1085f, 1085t, 1086f
    patient assessment, 1089–1090, 1089f
    patient management, 1091, 1091f
    pregnancy
        complications, 1078–1079, 1078t
        normal physiologic changes, 1077
        trauma during, 1088–1089, 1088f
    questions to ask, 1089–1090
    stop, think, understand, 1073, 1076–1077, 1083–1084, 1087
    suggested reading, 1099
Obstetric delivery kit, 1081, 1081f
Obstructive shock
    causes of, 337f, 342, 343f
    described, 342
Occipital bone, 198f
Occlusive dressings
    soft-tissue injuries, 559, 559f
    sucking chest wounds, 785, 785f
    types and purposes of, 561
    using, skill for, 571

Occult blood loss, 337
Occupational exposure
    disease, protection from, 79–80, 79f
    postexposure prophylaxis, 80
OEC. *See Outdoor Emergency Care* (OEC)
OEC Technicians
    adaptive skiers as, 1033f
    Disaster Medical Assistance Team, joining, 1111
    emergency care, giving, 3, 3f
    training for
        anatomy and physiology, 8, 9f
        evaluation and correction from instructors, 9, 10f
        knowledge and skills goals, 10
        patient assessment, 8, 9f
        scenarios, 9, 10f
Olympic Winter Games (1980), 697
*On Death and Dying* (Kübler-Ross), 1048
Onset of symptoms
    altered mental status, 373
    OPQRST assessment, 227t, 228–229
    stroke, 376
OPA. *See* oropharyngeal airway (OPA)
Open chest injury
    defined, 774
    managing, skill guide for, 788, 1174
Open CNS injuries, 704, 704f
Open crush injury, 545f, 548, 549f
Open fractures
    blood loss, 615, 615t
    described, 613, 613f
    prolonged rescue time, 648
    tibia, 635, 635f
Open injury. *See also* specific injuries
    abrasions, 545f, 546, 546f
    amputation, 545f, 547, 547f
    avulsions, 545f, 546–547, 547f
    defined, 546
    high-pressure injection, 548–549, 549f
    incisions, 546, 546f
    lacerations, 545f, 546, 546f
    management of, 555–556, 556f
    mechanical tattooing, 549
    open crush injury, 545f, 548, 549f
    overview of, 545–546
    punctures, 545f, 547, 548f
Open-format patient care report, 274–275, 275f, 277–278, 277f
Operations Chief in incident command system, 105, 105t
Operations section
    ICS organization, 101, 103f, 105t
    responsibilities and branches of, 105–106, 106f
Opiates, 392
OPQRST (Onset, Provocation and palliation, Quality, Radiation, Severity, Time) assessment
    abdominal and pelvic trauma, 802
    altitude-related emergencies, 911, 911f
    behavioral emergency assessment, 1056
    cardiovascular emergencies, 472
    face, eye, and neck injuries, 754

gastrointestinal and genitourinary emergencies, 508
    geriatric emergencies, 1002
    obstetric and gynecologic emergencies, 1089
    outdoor adaptive athletes, 1029
    pediatric emergencies, 969
    secondary assessment, 227t, 228–229
    trauma patient assessment, 531
Oral airways for endotracheal intubation, 1142, 1142f
"Oral hypoglycemia agents," 367
Oral medical communication
    dispatchers, 269, 269f
    hand-off report, 269–271, 270f
    SAILER information protocol, 269
    users of, 268, 269t
Orbit, defined, 744
Organophosphates
    exposure to, 1114–1115
    overuse and poisoning, 392
    poisoning, interventions for, 400
    poisoning, signs and symptoms of, 397t, 1115, 1115t
    treatment for, 1115, 1115f
Organs, defined, 171
Oropharyngeal airway (OPA)
    bite block, used as, 302
    described, 302, 302f
    indications for, 302
    insertion, skill for, 319
    insertion, skill guide for, 324, 1173
    insertion of, 302–303
    nasopharyngeal airway, comparison to, 300t
    removal of, 304
Oropharynx, anatomy of, 174, 175f, 176f
Orthopedic ("scoop") stretcher
    defined, 131
    lifting, for, 132–133, 133f, 134f
Orthostatic blood pressure test, 242–244, 244f
Orthostatic hypotension, causes of, 243
Os of the cervix, 1071
Osteoporosis, 989
Ostomy bag, 1016
OTC (over-the-counter) medications, 392–393
Outdoor adaptive athletes
    adaptive equipment
        defined, 1018, 1019
        events for, 1019–1020
        general equipment, 1020–1022, 1020f, 1021f, 1022f
        snow sports equipment, 1022–1025, 1022f, 1023f, 1024f, 1025f
        warm weather sports equipment, 1025–1026, 1026f
    adaptive skiers as OEC Technicians, 1033f
    case
        disposition, 1034
        presentation, 1011
        update, 1028
    chapter objectives, 1009

chapter overview, 1009–1011, 1010f
chapter review, 1035–1038
common disabilities
    cognitive disabilities, 1013
    combined physical and intellectual
        disability, 1018–1019, 1019f
    intellectual difficulties,
        1013–1014, 1014f
    intellectual disabilities,
        1012–1013, 1013f
    overview of, 1011–1012, 1011f
    physical disabilities, 1015–1017, 1015f,
        1016f, 1017f
    visual and hearing impairments,
        1018, 1019f
Explore myNSPkit, 1038
historical timeline, 1009
key terms, 1010
patient assessment
    challenges of, 1028, 1028f
    intellectual disabilities, athletes with,
        1029–1030
    physical disabilities, athletes with,
        1030–1031, 1031f
    primary and secondary assessment,
        1028–1029, 1029f
patient management
    guidelines for, 1031–1032, 1032f
    lift evacuation considerations, 1033
    stop, think, understand, 1012,
        1014–1015, 1018, 1027–1028,
        1033–1034
    suggested reading, 1038
*Outdoor Emergency Care* (OEC)
    certification and recertification
        requirements, 11–12, 11f, 11t
    course, described, 2–3, 2f
    curriculum, establishment of, 6, 7f
    fifth edition, publication of, 1100, 1136
    Fourth Edition, 1068
    National Medical Advisors, 7t
    National Program directors, 11, 11t, 12
    National Ski Patrol creating, 1
    *Outdoor Emergency Care* (Bowman), 6, 7f
    outdoor environments, working in,
        12–13, 12f, 13f
    program overview, 7–8, 7f
    second edition, publication of, 919
    survival, 1171
    third edition, publication of, 1039
    training as program focus, 8–10, 9–10f
Outdoor emergency care, introduction to
    case
        disposition, 26
        presentation, 3
        update, 14
    chapter objectives, 1–2
    chapter overview, 1–3, 2f, 3f
    chapter review, 27–29
    ethical and legal issues
        abandonment, 17–18, 18f
        assault and battery, 23–24, 24f
        documentation, 19–20, 19f
        EMS system regulations, 25

        ethical issues facing OEC technicians, 15
        Good Samaritan laws and duty to act,
            15–17, 16f
        importance of, 13, 15
        Joint Statement of Understanding, 21
        judgment, 24
        negligence and breach of duty, 18
        patient's consent, 21–23, 22f
        privacy laws, 25
        refusal of care, 22, 22f, 23
        risk, assumption of, 18–19
        scope of training, 20, 20f
        standard of training *versus* standard of
            care, 20–21
        teamwork, 25
        training, 24, 24f
    Explore myNSPkit, 30
    historical timeline, 1
    key terms, 2
    National Ski Patrol, early years, 4–6, 5f,
        6f, 7f, 7t
    OEC today
        certification and recertification
            requirements, 11–12, 11f, 11t
        outdoor environments, working in,
            12–13, 12f, 13f
        program, overview of, 7–8, 7f
        training as focus of OEC program,
            8–10, 9–10f
    Stop, Think, Understand, 14, 26
    suggested reading, 30
Outdoor Emergency Care (OEC)
    Technicians, defined, 32–33, 33f
Outdoor environment, working in, 12–13,
    12f, 13f
*Outdoor First Care*, 1009
Outdoor First Care (OFC) Providers, 32
Outdoor work, preparing for
    environmental considerations, 63, 63f
    equipment, 65–70, 66f, 67f, 68t, 69f
    hydration, 70, 70f, 71t
    mental preparedness, 63–64
    physical fitness, 64–65, 64f, 65t
    prolonged rescue response, 71, 71f
Outriggers, 1023, 1023f
Ovarian cysts, 1074
Ovaries
    endocrine system, 191, 193f
    female reproductive system, 203, 205f
    obstetric and gynecologic emergencies,
        1070, 1070f
    ovarian cysts, 1074
    solid organ, 496
Overdose, described, 361, 361t, 379
Over-the-counter (OTC) medications,
    392–393
Oxycodone
    bowel obstruction, 503t
    overuse and poisoning, 392
Oxycodone and acetaminophen, 392
OxyContin. *See* oxycodone
Oxygen
    altered mental status, 361, 361t, 379
    blood concentration

        altitude, change with, 900, 901f
        latitude, change in, 902
    respiratory gas exchange, 408–410, 409f
Oxygen saturation
    secondary assessment, 242, 243f
    shock, 333
Oxygen therapy
    altered mental status, 377
    altitude-related emergencies, 912, 912f
    avalanche victims, hypothermia in, 831
    bag-valve masks, 313–315, 313f, 313t,
        314f, 315f
    cardiovascular patients, 485, 485f
    childbirth, imminent, 1081, 1081f
    COPD, 993, 993f
    endotracheal tubes, 1146, 1146f
    face, eye, and neck injuries, 757
    gastric distention, 315–316
    GI/GU problems, 510
    indications for, 310–311
    inhaled poisons, 400, 400f
    musculoskeletal injuries, 639
    nasal cannulas, 311–312, 311f, 311t
    newborns, 1086, 1086f
    nonrebreather masks, 312–313, 312f, 313t
    obstetric and gynecologic emergency
        management, 1091
    oxygen containers, 306–307, 306f,
        307f, 307t
    oxygen cylinder set-up and breakdown,
        307–308, 320–321, 325, 1173
    oxygen cylinder size constants, 309, 309t
    oxygen flow duration rates, 308–309, 309t
    oxygen safety, 309
    pediatric emergencies, 976, 976f
    plant and animal emergencies, 887
    pregnant trauma patients, 1089
    pulse oximetry, 315–316f
    respiratory emergencies, 424
    severe allergic reactions, 446–447
    thoracic trauma, 784, 785, 786,
        786f, 786t
    trauma patients, 532, 532f
Oxygenated blood, 180
Oxygenation, defined, 246
Oxygen-depleted blood, defined, 180

**P**

Pacemaker cells of the heart, 177, 180f
Pacemakers
    described, 484
    elderly patients, 999–1000
Packaging patients for transport
    "injury uphill" principle, 148–149
    positioning for, 149–150
    steps in, 148, 148f, 149f
    transport devices, placing patient on,
        150–151, 150f, 151f
Pain
    abdominal and pelvic trauma, 802
    acute abdomen, 508t
    musculoskeletal injuries, 619, 619f
    OPQRST assessment, 227t, 228–229

Pain, (cont.)
  painful stimuli and neurologic function, 224, 224f
  parietal and visceral, 500
Palliation, 227t, 229
Palmedo, Roland, 4, 167
Pamelor. See nortriptyline
Pancreas
  abdominal injuries, 798–799
  altered mental status, 358–359, 359f
  endocrine system, 191, 193f
  GI system, 188f, 189
  location of, 795f
  pancreatitis, 500–501, 501f, 508t
  solid organ, 496, 496f, 794f
Pancreatitis
  abdominal pain, 508t
  described, 500–501, 501f
Paradoxical motion, with flail chest, 775
Paralympic Games, 1019, 1019f, 1020
Paralysis, defined, 224
Paramedics. See also advanced life support
    (ALS) interface
  cardiac arrest, 484
  defined, 38, 40
Paranoia
  behavioral emergency assessment, 1055
  neurotic disorder, 1044–1045
Paraplegic adaptive athletes, 1016
Parasympathetic nervous system, 187, 187f
Parathyroid gland, 193f
Paresthesia
  defined, 224
  hyperventilation, 421
Parietal bone, 198f
Parietal pain, defined, 500
Parietal pleura, thoracic, 772
Parnate. See tranylcypromine
Paroxetine, 1054t
Partial pressure, defined, 923
Partial seizures
  altered mental status, 363–364
  children, 953
Partial-thickness cold injury (frostbite), 819, 825t
Partial-thickness (second-degree) burns, 585, 585f, 586, 586f, 587t
Passive warming, 829, 829f
Past medical history
  medical communications, in, 282t, 283
  SAMPLE history, 227t, 228
Patella
  anatomy of, 196f, 198
  dislocations, 633, 665
  fractures, 633
Patellar ligament, rupture of, 634
Pathogens, 62, 62f
Pathologic fractures, 615t
Patient assessment. See also patient
    assessment for specific conditions
  case
    disposition, 248
    presentation, 215
    update, 237

chapter objectives, 213–214
chapter review, 213–214, 260–263
Explore myNSPkit, 263
historical timeline, 213
key terms, 214
medical patients, skill for, 251
medical patients, skill guide for, 255–256, 1173
OEC Technicians learning, 8, 9f
primary assessment
  ABCD sequence, 218, 218f
  airway, 218–219, 219f
  breathing, 219–220, 220f, 221t
  circulation, 220–222, 221f, 221t, 222f
  disability, 222–224, 223t, 224f
  life-threatening conditions, managing, 224–226
  purpose of, 217
  unresponsive adult, 217–218
reassessment, 246
scene size-up, 215–217, 215f, 217t
secondary assessment
  blood pressure, 239–241, 240f, 241f
  body temperature, 242, 242t
  level of responsiveness, 238
  medical history, 226–229, 227f, 227t
  orthostatic blood pressure test, 242–244, 244f
  oxygen saturation level, 242, 243f
  physical exam, 230–235, 231f, 232f, 233f, 234f, 235f
  physical exam, importance of, 229–230, 229f, 230f, 230t
  pulse, 238–239, 238f, 239f
  respirations, 239, 240
Skill Guides
  blood pressure, obtaining by auscultation, 117, 256
  medical patient assessment, 255–256, 1173
  patient assessment, 252–253, 1173
  pulse assessment, 257, 1173
  pupil assessment, 258, 1173
  respiration rate assessment, 259, 1173
  trauma patient assessment, 253–254, 1173
Skills
  blood pressure, obtaining by auscultation, 250
  medical patient assessment, 251
  patient assessment, 250–251
  pulse assessment, 249
  pupil assessment, 248
  respiration rate assessment, 249
  trauma patient assessment, 252
special considerations, 244–246, 245f
stop, think, understand, 236–237, 247–248
suggested reading, 263
Patient assessment for specific conditions
  abdominal and pelvic trauma, 801–803, 802f, 803f
  allergies and anaphylaxis
    anaphylactic shock, 445

    mild allergic reaction, 444
    moderate allergic reaction, 444
    primary assessment and ABCDs, 443
    secondary assessment, 443–445, 443f, 443t, 444f
    severe allergic reaction, 444–445
  altered mental status
    primary assessment, 373
    secondary assessment, 373–375, 373f, 374t, 375f
    stroke signs and symptoms, 375–377, 375f, 376f
    traumatic or medical cause, 372, 372f
  altitude-related emergencies, 911–912, 911f
  behavioral emergencies and crisis response
    primary assessment, 1051–1054, 1052f, 1052t, 1053f, 1053t
    scene safety, 1051, 1051f
    secondary assessment, 1054–1056, 1054t, 1056t
  burns
    ABCDs and primary assessment, 588, 588f
    scene size-up, 588
    secondary assessment, 589
    severity and extent, determining, 589–590, 590f, 591f
  cardiovascular emergencies
    angina and myocardial infarction, 474, 474f
    aortic aneurysm/dissection, 475
    cardiogenic shock, 474–475
    congestive heart failure, 475, 475f
    hypertension, 474
    pericardial tamponade, 475
    primary assessment and ABCDs, 472
    secondary assessment, 472, 473f
    thromboembolism, 476
  cold-related environmental emergencies
    frostbite, 824, 824f, 825t
    hypothermia, 825–827, 825f, 825t, 826f
    overview of, 824, 824f
  face, eye, and neck injuries
    ABCDs and primary assessment, 754
    ears, 755–756, 755f
    eyes, 754–755, 754f, 755f
    mid-face and nose, 755, 755f
    mouth, 755
    neck, 756, 756f
    secondary assessment, 754
  gastrointestinal and genitourinary emergencies
    ABCDs, 508
    acute abdomen, signs and symptoms of, 508t
    acute abdominal pain, causes of, 508t
    physical exam, 509–510, 509f
  geriatric emergencies, 1001–1003, 1001f, 1002t
  head and spinal injuries
    mini-neurologic exam, 715–716, 715t, 716f

primary assessment, 714–715
scene size-up, 714, 714f
secondary assessment, 715–718, 715t, 716f, 717f
heat-related emergencies
guidelines for, 850, 851f
heat cramps, 851
heat exhaustion, 851
heat stroke, 852
heat-induced syncope, 850–851
lightning strikes, 852
sunburn, 852
musculoskeletal injuries
ankle injuries, 635–636, 635f, 636f
axial skeleton injuries, 638
clavicle and shoulder injuries, 623–625, 623f, 624f
elbow injuries, 626, 626f
femur fractures, 631–632, 632f
foot and toe injuries, 636, 636f
forearm injuries, 626–627, 627f
hand and finger injuries, 628, 628f, 628t
hip and pelvis injuries, 630–631, 631f
humerus fractures, 625–626
knee injuries, 632–634, 633f, 634f
lower extremities, overview of, 630, 630f
overview of, 617–620, 617f, 618f, 619f, 620f
signs and symptoms, 620–621, 621f
stop, think, understand, 621–622, 628–629, 637–638
tibia and fibula injuries, 634–635, 635f
upper extremities, overview of, 622–623, 623f
wrist injuries, 627
obstetric and gynecologic emergencies, 1089–1090, 1089f
outdoor adaptive athletes
challenges of, 1028, 1028f
intellectual disabilities, athletes with, 1029–1030
physical disabilities, athletes with, 1030–1031, 1031f
primary and secondary assessment, 1028–1029, 1029f
pediatric emergencies
history, 966, 966f
honesty, trust, and communication, 968–969, 968f
physical exam, 969–975, 971f, 971t, 972f, 973f, 974t, 975t
primary assessment, 965–966, 966f
scene size-up, MOI, and consent, 963–965, 964f, 965f
plant and animal emergencies
bee stings, 886, 887f
guidelines for, 885, 885f
mammals, injuries caused by, 887, 887f
marine animals, injuries caused by, 887
mosquito, insect, and ant bites, 886–887
plants and mushrooms, 886
reptile bites, 887

spiders and scorpions, 886, 886f
tick bites, 886, 886f
respiratory emergencies
primary assessment and ABCDs, 418
respiratory distress, signs and symptoms of, 418–420, 419f
secondary assessment, 420–423, 420f, 421f
soft-tissue injuries, 551–552, 551f
substance use and abuse, 396–397, 396t, 397t
thoracic trauma, 783–784, 784t
trauma, principles of, 530–532, 530f, 531f
water emergencies, 933–934, 933f
Patient care and crime scene preservation, 88t
Patient care report (PCR)
AMPLE information, 275, 277f
CHEATED charting, 278
closed-format PCR, 273–274, 274f
defined, 273
documentation, importance of, 278
mixed-format PCR, 275, 276f
open-format PCR, 274–275, 275f, 277–278, 277f
SOAP charting, 277
Patient management for specific conditions
abdominal and pelvic trauma, 805–806
allergies and anaphylaxis
epinephrine, 447–449, 448f
insect stingers, 446, 447f
severe allergic reaction, 446–449, 447f, 448f
altered mental status, 377–381, 377f, 379f
altitude-related emergencies
AMS treatment, 913
concurrent medical problems, 914
descent to a lower altitude, 912, 912f
general management, 912–913, 912f
HACE treatment, 913, 914f
HAPE treatment, 913, 913f
Khumbu cough treatment, 913, 914f
behavioral emergencies and crisis response
critical incident stress, 1060, 1060f
overview of, 1056–1057
restraints, 1058–1059, 1058f, 1059f
burns
ABCDs, 591–592
bleeding, controlling, 592
chemical burns, 593–594, 594f
covering and positioning patient, 593
dressings, 592, 592f
electrical burns, 592, 594–595, 595f
radiation burns, 595
stopping the burning, 591, 591f, 592, 593
thermal burns, 593, 593f
cardiovascular emergencies
ABCDs, 476
aspirin, 486–487
cardiac arrest, and activation of emergency response system, 476–477, 477f

common cardiac medications, 487t
CPR for adults, children, and infants, 482t
CPR on a child, 479–480, 479f, 480f
CPR on an infant, 480–481, 481f
early advanced care, 484
early defibrillation, 481–484, 482f, 483t
hospital care of MI patients, 484–485
nitroglycerin, 485–486, 486f
one-rescuer CPR on an adult, 477–478, 477f, 478f
oxygen therapy, 485, 485f
two-rescuer CPR on an adult, 479
cold-related environmental emergencies
frostbite, 827–828, 828f
frostnip, 827
hypothermia, 828–832, 829f, 831f
other injuries/illnesses, with, 832
windburn, 832
face, eye, and neck injuries
ear injuries, 758–759
eye injuries, 759–762, 759f, 760f, 761f, 762f
facial injuries, 757, 757f
neck injuries, 763, 763f
overview of, 756–757
gastrointestinal and genitourinary emergencies, 510, 510f
geriatric emergencies, 1003–1004, 1003f
head and spinal injuries
cervical collar sizing and application, 720, 720f
guidelines for, 719, 719f
helmet removal, 724–725, 724f, 725f
long spine board, placing patient on, 720–724, 721f
heat-related emergencies
guidelines for, 852, 852f
heat cramps, 852
heat exhaustion, 852–853, 853f, 854, 854f, 854t
heat stroke, 853–854, 854f, 854t
heat-induced syncope, 852
lightning strikes, 855
sunburn, 854
musculoskeletal injuries
ankle injuries, 668–670, 669f, 670f
boot removal, 670–671
elbow injuries, 654–656, 654f, 655f
femur and tibia fracture in the same leg, 668, 668f
femur fractures, 660–663, 660f, 662f, 663f, 665
foot and toe injuries, 670
forearm injuries, 656
guidelines for, 639–640
hand and finger injuries, 657–658, 657f
hip dislocations, 660
humerus fractures, 653–654, 653f
knee injuries, 665–667, 665f
pelvic fractures, 659–660
shoulder, clavicle, and scapula injuries, 650–653, 651f

Patient management for specific conditions, (*cont.*)
  specific injuries, caring for, 649
  splinting (*See* splints)
  stabilized extrication and transfer, 673–674, 673–674*f*
  stop, think, understand, 648–649, 658–659, 663–664, 671–672, 675
  tibia and fibula injuries, 667–668
  wrist injuries, 656–657, 657*f*
 obstetric and gynecologic emergencies, 1091, 1091*f*
 outdoor adaptive athletes
  guidelines for, 1031–1032, 1032*f*
  lift evacuation considerations, 1033
 pediatric emergencies, 975–977, 975*f*, 976*f*, 977*f*
 plant and animal emergencies
  animal bites, care for, 889, 890, 890*f*
  biting and stinging creatures, 888–889, 888*f*
  guidelines for, 887–888
  ingested plant and mushroom toxins, 888
  large animal-related trauma, 890
  marine creatures, injuries caused by, 889, 889*f*
  plant contact toxicity, 888, 888*f*
  snake bites, 889, 889*f*
 respiratory emergencies, 424, 424*f*
 soft-tissue injuries
  amputations, 556, 558
  avulsions, 556
  contusions, 555
  direct pressure, 553, 553*f*
  dressings, 553
  impaled objects, 558, 558*f*
  open injuries, 555–556, 556*f*
  overview of, 552
  tourniquet, 553–555, 554*f*, 555*f*
 substance abuse and poisoning
  ABCDs and primary assessment, 398
  absorption, reducing, 399, 400*f*, 400*t*
  further exposure, reducing, 398, 399*f*
  help, calling for, 401
  personal safety, 398, 398*f*
  specific interventions, 400–401, 400*f*
 thoracic trauma, 784–786, 785*f*, 786*f*, 786*t*
 trauma patients, 532, 532*f*
 water emergencies, 934–936, 934*f*, 935*f*, 936*f*
Patient package, defined, 127
Patient refusal form, 379
Patients. *See also* positioning patients
 approaching, with behavioral emergencies, 1052, 1052*f*, 1053–1054, 1053*t*
 continuum of responses, with behavioral emergencies, 1052–1053, 1053*f*
 extrication from a vehicle, 1105–1107, 1106*f*, 1107*f*, 1107*t*
 gaining access to, in a vehicle, 1106–1107, 1107*f*, 1107*t*
 initial care and removal from a vehicle, 1107, 1107*f*

 number of, in assessing emergency situations, 85, 86*f*
 removing from the water, 934, 934*f*
 transferring to an ambulance, 1105, 1105*f*
Paxil. *See* paroxetine
PCP (phencyclidine)
 overuse and poisoning, 391, 392, 394
 toxicity, signs and symptoms of, 397*t*
PCR. *See* patient care report (PCR)
PCS (post-concussive syndrome), 708
PE. *See* pulmonary embolism (PE)
Peanut allergy, 439, 439*f*
Pediatric assessment triangle, 963, 964–965, 964*f*, 965*f*
Pediatric emergencies. *See also* children
 anatomy and physiology, 943–945, 944*f*, 945*f*
 case
  disposition, 979
  presentation, 944
  update, 963
 chapter objectives, 942
 chapter overview, 942–943, 943*f*
 chapter review, 980–983
 common illnesses and injuries
  abdominal pain, 953
  airway problems, 950–952, 950*f*, 951*f*
  burns and electrocutions, 959
  child abuse and neglect, 960–961, 961*f*
  meningitis, 954
  nausea, vomiting, and diarrhea, 953
  poisoning, 954, 955*f*
  respiratory failure and cardiac arrest, 952, 952*f*
  seizures, 953–954
  shock, 961–962, 962*f*
  sudden infant death syndrome, 957, 957*f*
  trauma, 957–958, 957*f*, 959*f*
 Explore myNSPkit, 984
 historical timeline, 942
 human growth and development, 946–950, 947*f*, 948–949*t*, 949*f*
 key terms, 943
 patient assessment
  history, 966, 966*f*
  honesty, trust, and communication, 968–969, 968*f*
  physical exam, 969–975, 971*f*, 971*t*, 972*f*, 973*f*, 974*t*, 975*t*
  primary assessment, 965–966, 966*f*
  scene size-up, MOI, and consent, 963–965, 964*f*, 965*f*
 patient management, 975–977, 975*f*, 976*f*, 977*f*
 stop, think, understand, 946, 952–953, 956–957, 959–960, 962, 967–968, 978–979
 suggested reading, 984
Pediatric trauma centers, 528
Pelvic binders
 described, 642, 642*f*
 pelvic fracture, management of, 806
Pelvic cavity
 described, 171, 172*f*

 organs in, protection for, 795
 vascular structures, 496
Pelvic inflammatory disease (PID), 1074
Pelvis
 anatomy of, 196*f*, 198, 199*f*
 assessment of, in pediatric emergencies, 972, 972*f*
 fractures, and abdominal injuries, 800, 800*f*
 fractures, bleeding from, 615*t*
 fractures, in elderly patients, 997
 fractures, management of, 659–660, 806
 injury assessment, 630, 630*f*, 631
 palpation of, with trauma, 802, 802*f*
 secondary assessment, 234, 235*f*
 stabilization, skill for, 808
 stabilization, skill guide for, 809, 1174
Penetrating force, as MOI, 85
Penetrating injuries
 DCAP-BTLS assessment, 230, 230*t*
 described, 522, 522*f*
 mechanism of injury, 702, 702*f*
 open pneumothorax, 777, 778*f*
 punctures, 230, 230*t*, 545*f*, 547, 548*f*
Penis, 203, 204*f*
Peptic ulcerative disease (PUD), 503–504, 504*f*
Percocet™. *See* oxycodone and acetaminophen
Perforated bowel
 abdominal pain, 508*t*
 described, 503
Perfusion
 defined, 472
 overview of, 921, 921*f*
Pericardial tamponade
 described, 469, 469*f*, 778–779, 779*f*
 obstructive shock, 337*f*, 342, 343*f*
 patient assessment, 475
 signs of, 475
Pericarditis, 469
Perineum, 1071, 1072*f*
Periosteum, 604, 605*f*
Peripheral nervous system
 altered mental status, 357, 358*f*
 anatomy of, 183, 184*f*, 186
 defined, 700
 physiology of, 186, 187*f*
Peripheral vascular disease, 63*t*
Peritonitis
 defined, 500, 798
 hollow organ, rupture of, 495–496
PERRL (Pupils are Equal, Round, and Reactive to Light), 232
Personal protective equipment (PPE)
 burned patients, 588
 chemical burns, 593–594
 defined, 77
 eye protection, 78, 78*f*
 gloves, 77–78, 91–93, 1173
 gowns, 79
 masks, 78–79, 78*f*
 soft-tissue injuries, 551
Peyote
 adverse effects, 886
 overuse and poisoning, 391

Pharynx, 292, 293f
Phencyclidine. *See* PCP (phencyclidine)
Phenelzine, 1054t
Philadelphia Cervical Collars, 720
"Phonation," 1152
Phrenic nerves, 772
Physical abuse
    behavioral emergency assessment,
        1056, 1056t
    described, 1046
Physical disabilities
    amputations, 1017
    athletes with, assessing, 1030–1031, 1031f
    cerebral palsy, 1016–1017, 1016f
    guides, using, 1015, 1015f
    intellectual disabilities, combined with,
        1018–1019, 1019f
    multiple sclerosis, 1017
    muscular dystrophy, 1017, 1017f
    sensory impairments, 1015, 1015f,
        1018, 1019f
    spina bifida, 1017
    spinal cord injuries, 1016
Physical exam
    acute abdominal or pelvic pain,
        509–510, 509f
    medical communications, in, 282t, 283
    pediatric emergencies
        age-based assessment, 974t
        child abuse, 975, 975t
        extremities, abdomen, and chest, 972,
            972f, 973f
        order for performance, 969
        reassessments, 973, 975
        spine, head, and neck, 973, 973f
        tips for, 970–971
        vital signs, 971–972, 971f, 971t, 972f
    secondary assessment
        abdomen, 233, 234f
        back, 233, 234f
        chest, 232, 233f
        extremities, 234–235, 235f
        head, 230–232, 231f, 232f
        head-to-toe assessment, importance of,
            229–230, 229f, 230f
        mnemonic for assessment, 230, 230t
        neck, 232, 233f
        pelvis, 234, 235f
Physical fitness and outdoor work, 64–65,
        64f, 65t
Physiology. *See also* anatomy and physiology
    aging process
        cardiovascular changes, 987f, 988
        gastrointestinal changes, 987f, 988, 989f
        integumentary, endocrine, and immune
            system changes, 987f, 989–990
        musculoskeletal changes, 987f, 989, 989f
        neurological changes, 987f, 988
        overview of, 987–988, 987f, 988f
        renal function and electrolyte balance
            changes, 987f, 989
        respiratory changes, 987f, 988
    defined, 168
Pia mater, 183, 185f

PID (pelvic inflammatory disease), 1074
Pika injuries, 884
Pillow splints
    ankle injuries, 669, 669f
    described, 641, 642f
Pineal gland, 191, 193f
Piranha, 881
Pit vipers, 878–879, 878f
Pitting edema, 475
Pituitary gland, 191, 193f, 195
Pivot joints, 607
Placenta, delivery of, 1082–1083, 1083f
Placenta previa, 1078, 1078t
Plague, 884
Planes of the body, 168, 168f
Planning Chief of the incident command
        system, 105t, 106
Planning section of the incident command
        system
    ICS organization, 101, 103f, 105t
    responsibilities and units of, 106–107, 107f
Plant and animal emergencies
    anatomy and physiology, 862, 862f
    animals, adverse effects from
        ants, 875, 876, 876f
        bees, wasps, and hornets, 875–876, 875f
        mammals, 882–885, 883f, 884f, 885f
        marine creatures, 880–881, 880f, 881f
        mosquitoes, fleas, and biting flies,
            876, 876f
        reptiles, 878–879, 878f, 879f
        scorpions, 874, 874f
        spiders, 871–873, 872f, 873f
        ticks, 874–875, 874f, 875f
    case
        disposition, 890
        presentation, 862
        update, 885
    chapter objectives, 861
    chapter overview, 861–862
    chapter review, 892–895
    Explore myNSPkit, 895
    historical timeline, 861
    key terms, 861
    patient assessment
        bee stings, 886, 887f
        guidelines for, 885, 885f
        mammals, injuries caused by, 887, 887f
        marine animals, injuries caused by, 887
        mosquito, insect, and ant bites, 886–887
        plants and mushrooms, 886
        reptile bites, 887
        spiders and scorpions, 886, 886f
        tick bites, 886, 886f
    patient management
        animal bites, care for, 889, 890, 890f
        biting and stinging creatures,
            888–889, 888f
        guidelines for, 887–888
        ingested plant and mushroom
            toxins, 888
        large animal-related trauma, 890
        marine creatures, injuries caused by,
            889, 889f

plant contact toxicity, 888, 888f
snake bites, 889, 889f
plants and fungi, adverse effects and
        emergencies from
    autumn crocus, 865, 865f
    belladonna, 867
    cactus, 864, 864f
    castor oil plant, 866–867, 866f
    foxglove, 866, 866f
    jimson weed, 868, 868f
    lily of the valley, 866, 866f
    monkshood, 865, 865f
    mushrooms, 870–871, 870f, 871f
    poison ivy, oak, and sumac,
        863–864, 863f
    pokeweed, 867, 867f
    rhododendron, azalea, 868, 868f
    stinging nettle, 864, 864f
    water hemlock, 867
    yew, 867, 867f
stop, think, understand, 868–869,
    876–877, 882, 891–892
suggested reading, 895
Plantarflex, defined, 630
Plants
    ingested, management for, 888
    ingestion toxicity, 865–868, 865f, 866f,
        867f, 868f
    patient assessment, 886
    poisoning, interventions for, 401
    skin toxicity, 863–864, 863f, 864f
    skin toxicity, management for,
        888, 888f
    toxic, 394
Plaque, arterial, 464–465, 464f
Plasma, 180, 181, 181f
Platelets
    bone marrow, production in, 199
    described, 180, 181, 181f
    shock, 333, 334f
Plavix®. *See* clopidogrel
Pleura
    defined, 411
    thoracic trauma A & P, 772
Pleural space, defined, 411
Pneumococcal vaccine, 76t
Pneumonia
    children, 951
    common infectious disease, 74
    respiratory emergencies, 416
Pneumothorax
    altitude complicating, 782
    causes, 777
    defined, 777
    hemopneumothorax, 778
    open pneumothorax, 777, 778f
    spontaneous, 416, 416f, 778
    tension pneumothorax (*See* tension
        pneumothorax)
Pocket mask for airway management,
    305–306, 305f
Poison ivy, 863–864, 863f, 888
Poison oak, 863–864, 863f, 888
Poison sumac, 863–864, 863f, 888

Poisoning. *See also* substance abuse and poisoning
  altered mental status, 361t, 362, 380
  children, 954, 955f
  plant and animal emergencies, 862
  poison, defined, 390
  signs and symptoms, 955f
Pokeweed, 867, 867f
Pole and strap injury, 628
Pollard, Harry, 406
Polydipsia, 366
Polypharmacy, defined, 392, 993–994
Polyuria, 366
Pons, anatomy of, 183, 185f, 186f
Popliteal fossa, 633
Portable stretcher for lifting, 131, 133, 134f
Positional asphyxia, 1059
Positioning patients
  chest trauma management, 786
  childbirth, imminent, 1081, 1081f
  obstetric and gynecologic emergency management, 1091, 1091f
  position for patient transport, 149–150
  position of comfort for GI/GU problems, 510, 510f
  pregnancy, during, 150, 1072, 1079, 1089
Positions. *See also* supine position
  head-downhill, 149
  head-uphill, 149, 786
  high-Fowler, 146, 146f, 171, 424
  left lateral recumbent, 171, 171f, 300, 300f, 377, 377f
  neutral anatomical, 673, 673f, 674, 674f
  normal anatomical, 169f, 170
  position of function for wrist injuries, 656, 657f
  positions in which patients are found, 673–674f
  prone, 149, 170, 170f
  recovery, 171, 300, 300f
  reference points for aligning patients, 674, 674f
  right lateral recumbent position, 171
  semi-Fowler, 146, 146f, 171, 171f
  terms for, 169f, 170–171, 170f, 171f
  transport, for, 150
  Trendelenburg, 146, 147f, 171, 171f
  "tripod," 220, 220f, 418, 419f, 424, 964–965
Post-concussive syndrome (PCS), 708
Posterior chamber of the eye, 745, 746f
Posterior (dorsal) direction, 169, 169f
Posterior hip dislocation, 631, 631f
Posterior sternoclavicular (S/C) dislocation
  chest injury, 776
  reducing, skill for, 678
  reducing, skill guide for, 688, 1174
  reduction of, 652–653
  signs and symptoms, 624
Posterior tibialis pulse, 630f
Postexposure prophylaxis, 80
Post-ictal phase of seizures, 365, 365f
Post-injury phase of injury, 526, 526f, 527f
Post-traumatic stress disorder (PTSD)

dealing with, 90
  signs of, 1049, 1049f
Pot, 394. *See also* marijuana
"Powderfall," 942
Power grip, 142, 142f
Power lift, 142–143, 142f
Powered suction device, 298–299, 298f
PPE. *See* personal protective equipment (PPE)
Pradaxa. *See* dabigatran
Pralidoxime chloride (2-PAM-Cl)
  nerve agent exposure, 1116
  organophosphate exposure, 1115
Prednisone, 420
Preeclampsia, 1078
Pregnancy. *See also* obstetric and gynecologic emergencies
  altitude-related problems, 906
  anatomy and physiology, 1071–1072, 1072f
  complications, 1078–1079, 1078t
  normal physiologic changes, 1077
  one victim and two patients, 1088
  positioning pregnant patients, 1072, 1079, 1089
  side position for transport, 150
  trauma during, 1088–1089, 1088f
Pregnancy-induced hypertension, 1078
Prehospital care, defined, 3
Prehospital providers, defined, 38
Pre-ictal phase of seizures, 364, 364f
Pre-injury phase of injury, 525, 525f
Pre-oxygenation of patient before suctioning airway, 299
Preschool period/preschoolers
  age-based assessment, 974t
  defined, 947–948, 947f
  physical, intellectual, emotional, social, and language development, 948–949t
Prescription drugs, 392
Pressure dressings
  defined, 553
  described, 561, 561f
Pressure sores, 132
Prevention, in emergency care systems, 36
Primary assessment
  ABCD sequence, 218, 218f
  airway, 218–219, 219f
  allergies and anaphylaxis, 443, 446
  altered mental status, 373
  behavioral emergencies and crisis response, 1051–1054, 1052f, 1052t, 1053f, 1053t
  breathing, 219–220, 220f, 221t
  cardiovascular emergencies, 472
  circulation, 220–222, 221f, 221t, 222f
  cold-related environmental emergencies, 824
  disability, 222–224, 223t, 224f
  face, eye, and neck injuries, 754
  geriatric emergencies, 1001–1002, 1002t
  head and spinal injuries, 714–715
  heat-related emergencies, 850, 851f
  life-threatening conditions, 224–226

musculoskeletal injuries, 618–619, 618f, 639
  outdoor adaptive athletes, 1028–1029, 1029f
  patient assessment, 588
  pediatric emergencies, 965–966, 966f
  plant and animal emergencies, 885
  purpose of, 217
  respiratory emergencies, 418
  shock, 345
  soft-tissue injuries, 551, 551f
  substance abuse and poisoning, 396, 398
  thoracic trauma, 783
  trauma patients, 530–531
  unresponsive adult, 217–218
Primary blast injury, 523, 524f
Primary hypothermia, 819–820, 820f, 821f
Prinivil. *See* lisinopril
Prinzmetal's angina, 467t
Privacy
  laws regarding, 25
  medical communications, 268
"Privileged communications," 268
Procardia. *See* nifedipine
Prochlorperazine, 1178t
Professional Ski Instructors Association, 985
Prolonged rescue response, 71, 71f
Prone position
  defined, 170, 170f
  packaging patients for transport, 149
Propranolol
  beta-blocker use by the elderly, 994
  shock, 345
Prospective quality improvement, 50
Prostate gland, 203, 204f
Prosthetic limbs
  adaptive athletes, 1020, 1021, 1021f
  injury management, 1032
Protocols, in emergency care systems, 50
Protozoa, 506
Proventil®. *See* albuterol
Provocation, in OPQRST assessment, 227t, 229
Proximal direction, 169f, 170
Proximal tibia compression fractures, 634, 635f
Prozac. *See* fluoxetine
Pruritus, 439
Psilocybin mushrooms, 886
Psychiatric conditions
  altered mental status, 361t, 362, 363f, 380
  neurotic disorders, 1044–1045, 1045f
  psychotic disorders, 1013, 1043–1044, 1043f, 1045, 1055–1056
Psychogenic shock, 342
Psychosis, defined, 1043–1044, 1043f
Psychotic disorders
  behavioral emergency assessment, 1055–1056
  bipolar disorder, 1013, 1045
  psychosis, 1043–1044, 1043f
  schizophrenia, 1013, 1045
PTSD. *See* post-traumatic stress disorder (PTSD)

Pubis bone, 196f, 198, 199f
Public access, in emergency medical systems, 36
Public education, in emergency medical systems, 36
Public health and emergency care systems, 43, 45
Public image of ski patrollers, 15, 15f
PUD (peptic ulcerative disease), 503–504, 504f
"Pulled muscle," 612. *See also* strains
Pulmonary circulation
    acclimatization to altitude, 902
    anatomy and physiology, 177, 179f, 180
    described, 462, 462f
Pulmonary contusion, 774, 774f
Pulmonary edema, 466
Pulmonary embolism (PE)
    described, 469, 469f
    obstructive shock, 337f, 342, 343f
    pain, 472
    patient assessment, 476
    pulsus paradoxus, 779
    respiratory emergencies, 415–416, 415f
Pulse
    assessing, skill for, 249
    assessing, skill guide for, 257, 1173
    defined, 220
    lightning strike management, 855
    lower extremity injury assessment, 630, 630f
    normal ranges, by age, 221t
    normal values by age, 971t
    pediatric emergencies, 971, 972f
    plant and animal emergencies, 885
    quality of, in secondary assessment, 239
    secondary assessment, 238–239, 238f, 239f
Pulse oximeter
    defined, 315–316f
    normal values by age, 971t
    respiratory emergencies, 422–423, 424
Pulse pressure, 182, 779
Pulseless ventricular tachycardia, 468
Pulsus paradoxus, 779
Punctures. *See also* penetrating injuries
    DCAP-BTLS assessment, 230, 230t
    open injuries, 545f, 547, 548f
Pupils
    assessing, skill for, 248
    assessing, skill guide for, 258, 1173
    eye anatomy and physiology, 745, 746f
    eye injuries, assessment of, 754, 754f
    pupillary exam
        defined, 716
        head and spinal injury assessment, 714, 715, 715t, 716
    secondary assessment, 231, 231f, 232
Pyelonephritis, 502

## Q

Quadriceps tendon rupture, 634
Quadriplegic adaptive athletes, 1016

Quality, in OPQRST assessment, 227t, 229
Quality improvement, 50–51
Quality of normal breathing, 412
Quaternary blast injury, 523–524
Quick Splint
    applying, skill for, 682
    cardboard splint, replacing with, skill for, 683
    described, 643
    distal femur fractures, 663
    "floating knee" injury, 668, 668f
    knee injuries, 665, 666
    tibia fracture, 645, 668
Quickclot® Bandage, 562

## R

Rabbits, injuries caused by, 884
Rabies
    common infectious disease, 75–76
    skunks and bats, 884
    vector-borne transmission of disease, 73
"Raccoon eyes," 705, 705f
Raccoons
    injuries caused by, 884
    rabies, 890
Racemic epinephrine, 1163
Radial head fracture, 626
Radial keratotomy blindness, 906
Radial nerve, 628, 628t
Radial pulse
    primary assessment, 220, 221f
    secondary assessment, 238
Radiation (heat loss mechanism), 59f, 60, 816f, 817
Radiation burns
    described, 584
    management of, 595
Radiation of pain, in OPQRST assessment, 227t, 229
Radio communications for emergency care systems
    military time, 48–49, 49t
    NATO phonetic alphabet, 48, 48t
    radio communication, factors affecting, 47
    radio etiquette, 47
    radio terminology, 48, 48t
    transmission pathway of radio call, 46–47, 46f, 47f
Radius
    anatomy of, 196f, 198
    fractures, 626–627, 627f
Rape, described, 1046
"Rapture of the deep," 929
Rash, defined, 864
Rate of ascent, and altitude illness, 898, 899f
Rats, injuries caused by, 884
Rattlesnakes
    adverse effects from, 878–879, 878f
    patient management, 889f
Reach, Throw, Row, Go, 933, 933f
Reasonable force, 1058
Reassessment of patients, 246

"Rebound tenderness," 509
RECCO system for avalanche victims, 1121, 1121f
Recovery position
    airway, keeping open, 300, 300f
    defined, 171
Recurrent traumatic brain injury (TBI), 708
Red blood cells
    bone marrow, production in, 199
    described, 180–181, 181f
    production, and altitude, 902
    shock, 332–333, 333f, 334
"Red" (hemorrhagic) stroke, 370f, 371
Referred pain, defined, 500, 501f
Refresher courses, 12
Refusal of care
    altered mental status in diabetics, 379
    defined, 22, 22f, 23
    documentation of, 284–286, 295f
Regulation, in emergency medical systems, 35
Regulator for oxygen containers, 307, 307f
Remedial training, in emergency care systems, 51
Renal failure, and immune system, 63t
Renal system changes with aging, 987f, 989
Reporting, situations requiring
    child abuse, 961
    elder abuse, 998
    mandated reporter, defined, 286
Reproductive age, 1073
Reproductive cycle, 1071–1072, 1072f
Reproductive system. *See also* obstetric and gynecologic emergencies
    defined, 201
    erectile dysfunction, 486
    females
        anatomy of, 203, 205f
        physiology, 206
    genital injuries, 801, 802–803
    hormones, 201, 203
    males
        anatomy of, 203, 204f
        physiology of, 203
Reptile injuries
    adverse effects from, 878–879, 878f, 879f
    patient assessment, 887
Rescue. *See also* search and rescue
    defined, 1118
    prolonged time, and open fractures, 648
Rescue basics
    anatomy and physiology
        "fight or flight" response, 61–62, 61t, 62f
        immune response, 62, 62f, 63t
        temperature regulation, 58–61, 58f, 59f, 60f, 61f
    case
        disposition, 90
        presentation, 58
        update, 73
    chapter objectives, 56
    chapter overview, 56–57, 57f
    chapter review, 94–97

Rescue basics, (cont.)
  contaminated glove removal
      skill for, 91–92
      skill guide for, 93, 1173
  crime scene management, 87–89, 87f, 88t, 89f
  disease, protection from
      common infectious diseases, 74–76
      contamination, 73, 73f
      decontamination, 80–82, 80f, 81f, 82f
      disease transmission, 71–73
      occupational exposure, 79–80, 79f
      personal protective equipment, 77–79, 78f, 91–93, 1173
      Standard Precautions and body substance isolation, 76–77, 77f
      vaccination recommendations, 76, 76t
  emergency situations, assessing
      mechanism of injury, 84, 85, 85f
      number of patients and need for additional resources, 85, 86f
      scene safety, 82–84, 84f
  Explore myNSPkit, 97
  hazardous materials, dealing with, 85–87, 86f
  historical timeline, 56
  key terms, 57
  outdoor work, preparing for
      environmental considerations, 63, 63f
      equipment, 65–70, 66f, 67f, 68t, 69f
      hydration, 70, 70f, 71t
      mental preparedness, 63–64
      physical fitness, 64–65, 64f, 65t
      prolonged rescue response, 71, 71f
  stop, think, understand, 72, 83
  stress, dealing with, 89–90, 89f, 90f
  suggested reading, 97
Research
  emergency care systems, role in, 45, 45f
  EMS Agenda for the Future (NHTSA), 35
Resistance blood vessels, 332, 333f
Resistance stage of stress reaction, 61t
Resource, defined, 100
Respiration
  acclimatization to altitude, 902, 902f
  defined, 239
  quality of, in secondary assessment, 240
  respiratory effort, pediatric, 963, 964–965, 964f, 965f
  respiratory failure in children, 952, 952f
  respiratory problems as NOI, 85
Respiratory cycle, 410
Respiratory emergencies
  anatomy and physiology
      gas exchange, 408–410, 409f
      lower airway, 410–412, 410f, 411f, 412f
      normal breathing, 412
      respiratory cycle, 410
  case
      disposition, 425
      presentation, 408
      update, 417
  chapter objectives, 406–407
  chapter overview, 406–408, 407f

  chapter review, 430–433
  common respiratory emergencies
      asthma, 414, 415f
      carbon monoxide exposure, 416
      chronic obstructive pulmonary disease, 413–414, 414f
      hyperventilation syndrome, 414–415
      obstruction/choking, 413
      overview, 412
      pneumonia, 416
      pulmonary embolism, 415–416, 415f
      spontaneous pneumothorax, 416, 416f
  Explore myNSPkit, 433
  historical timeline, 406
  inhalers, use of, 424–425, 425f
  key terms, 407
  patient assessment
      primary assessment and ABCDs, 418
      respiratory distress, signs and symptoms of, 418–420, 419f
      secondary assessment, 420–423, 420f, 421f
  patient management, 424, 424f
  Skill Guides
      lung sounds, auscultation of, 428, 1173
      metered-dose inhaler, assisting with, 429, 1173
  Skills
      lung sounds, auscultation of, 426
      metered-dose inhaler, assisting with, 427
  stop, think, understand, 409, 413, 417, 423
Respiratory rate
  assessing, skill for, 249
  assessing, skill guide for, 259, 1173
  normal ranges, by age, 221t
  normal rates by age, 412
  normal values by age, 971t
  patient assessment, 421
  pediatric emergencies, 971, 971f
  secondary assessment, 239
Respiratory system
  allergic reactions, 440, 441f, 444
  ALS medications, 1163
  anatomy of, 174–175, 175f, 176f
  changes with aging, 987f, 988
  defined, 174
  physiology of, 175–176, 177f
  pregnancy, 1071–1072
Response to treatment, in medical communications, 282t, 283
Restraints
  behavioral emergencies and crisis response, 1058–1059, 1058f, 1059f
  patient restraint, skill guide for, 1063, 1174
  physical/mechanical restraint of a patient, skill for, 1062
Retina
  anatomy and physiology, 746, 746f
  retinal detachment, 760
Retractions, intercostal, 945
Retrograde amnesia, 708

Retroperitoneal space, 496
Retrospective quality improvement in emergency care systems, 50–51
Reverse squeeze, 928
"Reverse triage," 855
Rheumatoid arthritis, 62
Rhododendron, 868, 868f
Rhythm of normal breathing, 412
Ribs
  anatomy of, 196f, 198
  fractures, 712, 775, 785–786
  lower rib cage injury, 777
  thoracic trauma, 772, 772f
RICES (Rest, Ice, Compression, Elevation, Splint) treatment for soft-tissue injuries, 555
Ricin, 867
Right direction of the body, 169f, 170
Right lateral recumbent position, 171
Right sided CHF, 465, 465f, 475
Rigid splints
  elbow application, skill for, 679
  humerus fracture application, skill for, 679
  tib-fib fracture, 667
  tib-fib fracture immobilization, skill for, 683
Rigor mortis, 1048
Risk, assumption of, 18–19
Risk managers, 271
Risk-management programs, 20
Rock, 394. See also cocaine
Rocky Mountain Spotted Fever
  tick bites, 875
  vector-borne transmission of disease, 73
Rodent injuries, 884, 884f
Rohypnol, 391
Roller gauze, 559, 642, 643f
Roosevelt, Franklin D., 56
Rope, for improvised litter, 153, 153f
Rotary-wing aircraft. See helicopters (rotary-wing aircraft)
Rotational force as MOI, 85
Rotational injury, 522–523, 523f
Rotavirus, 506
Rothberg position, 146
Royal Flying Doctors of Australia, 34
Rubbing (isopropyl) alcohol, 393
Rule of Nines for determining body surface area, 589–590, 590f
Rule of Threes for survival, 68–69, 1171–1172
Rusty, the NSP mascot, 579

## S

Sacrum
  anatomy, 196f, 198, 198f
  axial skeleton, 699f
"Saddle embolus," 416, 469
Safety issues
  ensuring, 57, 57f
  helicopters, 155–157, 156f, 156t, 157f
  oxygen therapy, 309

scene safety, 82–84, 84f

substance abuse and poisoning scene, 398, 398f

water emergencies, 933, 933f

Sager traction splints, 646

Sagittal (median) plane, 168f

SAILER (Sex, Age, Incident/chief complaint, Location, Equipment needed, Resources needed) information protocol, 269

Salivary glands, 188f, 189, 189f

*Salmonella* sp.

diarrhea, 506

ingestion transmission of disease, 73

SALT (Sort, Assess, Life saving, Triage) method, 119

Salt water, near-drowning in, 927

SAM™ (Structural, Aluminum, Malleable) splints, 644, 644f

SAMPLE (Signs and Symptoms, Allergies, Medications, Pertinent past medical history, Last oral intake, Events leading to incident) history

abdominal and pelvic trauma, 801

allergies and anaphylaxis, 443, 443f, 443t

altered mental status, 373

altitude-related emergencies, 911, 911f

behavioral emergencies and crisis response, 1054

burned patients, 589

cardiovascular emergencies, 472

cold-related environmental emergencies, 824

face, eye, and neck injuries, 754

gastrointestinal and genitourinary emergencies, 508

geriatric emergencies, 994, 1002

head and spinal injuries, 717

heat-related emergencies, 850

musculoskeletal injuries, 619

obstetric and gynecologic emergencies, 1089

outdoor adaptive athletes, 1029

pediatric emergencies, 966

plant and animal emergencies, 885

respiratory emergencies, 420

secondary assessment, 226–228, 227t

shock, 345

soft-tissue injuries, 551

trauma patients, 531

Sarin, 392

*SAS Survival Guide*, 1171

SB (spina bifida), 1017

SCA (sudden cardiac arrest), 468

Scald, defined, 581

Scalp injuries, 704

Scapula

anatomy of, 196f, 198

fractures of, 625, 712, 775

injury management, 650–652, 651f

Scenario, in OEC Technician training, 9, 10f

Scene safety, 82–84, 84f

Scene size-up

abdominal and pelvic trauma, 801

altered mental status, 372

burned patients, 588

cold-related environmental emergencies, 824

extrication of patients from a vehicle, 1106

geriatric emergencies, 1001

head and spinal injuries, 714, 714f

heat-related emergencies, 850

lightning strikes, 852

musculoskeletal injuries, 617–618, 617f, 639

patient assessment, 215–217, 215f, 217t

pediatric emergencies, 963

plant and animal emergencies, 885

safety, in behavioral emergencies, 1051, 1051f

shock, 345, 345f

soft-tissue injuries, 551, 551f

thoracic trauma, 783

trauma patients, 530, 530f

Scheinberg, Sam, 644

Schizophrenia

cognitive disability, 1013

psychotic disorder, 1045

Schobinger, Charles W., 355

School-age children

age-based assessment, 974t

defined, 948–949, 949f

physical, intellectual, emotional, social, and language development, 948–949t

SCI. *See* spinal cord injury (SCI)

Sciatic nerve, 631

Scoliosis, 989

Scoop stretcher. *See* orthopedic ("scoop") stretcher

"Scope of Practice" of prehospital provider's duties, 38, 39

Scope of training, as legal issue, 20, 20f

Scorpions

adverse effects from, 874, 874f

patient assessment, 886

patient management, 888

Sea urchin injuries, 881

Search, defined, 1118

Search and rescue

avalanche rescue, 1120–1123, 1120f, 1121f, 1122f, 1123f

basic tasks of, 1119, 1119f

confined space rescue, 1125–1127, 1125f, 1126f, 1127f

low-angle rescue, 1123–1125, 1124f

OEC Technician participation, 1119–1120, 1120f

overview of, 1118, 1118f, 1119f

water rescue, 1128

"Seat belt sign," 802, 802f

Seated patients

immobilizing, skill for, 729–730

immobilizing, skill guide for, 735, 1174

LSBs, placing on, 723

Sebaceous glands, 581, 581f

Secondary assessment

allergies and anaphylaxis, 443–445, 443f, 443t, 444f

altered mental status, 373–375, 373f, 374t, 375f

behavioral emergencies and crisis response, 1054–1056, 1054t, 1056t

blood pressure, 239–241, 240f, 241f

body temperature, 242, 242t

burned patients, 589

cardiovascular emergencies, 472, 473f

cold-related environmental emergencies, 824

face, eye, and neck injuries, 754

geriatric emergencies, 1002–1003

head and spinal injuries, 715–718, 715t, 716f, 717f

heat-related emergencies, 850

level of responsiveness, 238

medical history

chief complaint, 226

importance of, 226, 227f

OPQRST assessment, 227t, 228–229

SAMPLE history, 226–228, 227t

trauma with medical problem, 226

musculoskeletal injuries, 619–620, 619f, 620f

orthostatic blood pressure test, 242–244, 244f

outdoor adaptive athletes, 1029

oxygen saturation level, 242, 243f

pediatric emergencies

history, 966, 966f

honesty, trust, and communication, 968–969, 968f

physical exam, 969–975, 971f, 971t, 972f, 973f, 974t, 975t

physical exam, 230–235, 231f, 232f, 233f, 234f, 235f

physical exam, importance of, 229–230, 229f, 230f, 230t

plant and animal emergencies, 885, 885f

pulse, 238–239, 238f, 239f

respirations, 239, 240

respiratory emergencies, 420–423, 420f, 421f

soft-tissue injuries, 551–552, 551f

steps in, 226

substance use and abuse, 397

thoracic trauma, 783–784, 784t

trauma patients, 531

water emergencies, 934

Secondary blast injury, 523, 524f

Secondary drowning (near-drowning), 702, 926–927, 926f

Secondary hypothermia, 820

Second-degree (partial-thickness) burns, 585, 585f, 586, 586f, 587t

Section Chiefs of incident command system, 104, 105t

Sedatives

overuse of, 391

toxicity, signs and symptoms of, 397t

Seizures
  altered mental status, 361t, 362, 363, 380
  children, 953–954
  cognitive disability, 1013
  epilepsy, 360, 361t, 363, 378
  generalized seizures, 364–365,
      364–365f, 364f
  hyperventilation syndrome, 415
  other conditions, differentiating
      from, 365
  partial seizures, 363–364
  pediatric emergencies, 977, 977f
  severity of signs and symptoms, 363, 363f
  status epilepticus, 365, 954
Self-adhering roller bandage
  types of, 559
  using, skill for, 571
Self-evacuation
  ankle injuries, 670, 670f
  warming frostbitten tissue, 827
Semi-Fowler position
  defined, 171, 171f
  transporting patients, 146, 146f
Seminal vesicles, 203, 204f
Senior Program for NSP, 838
Sensory nerves, 500
Sepsis, defined, 340
Septic shock, 337f, 340, 341f
Sertraline
  overuse and poisoning, 391
  psychotropic agent, 1054t
Service animals, 1032, 1032f
Severe allergic reactions
  described, 440, 441f
  patient management, 446–449, 447f, 448f
  signs and symptoms, 444–445
Severe hypothermia
  assessment of, 825t, 826
  described, 821f
  management of, 830–831, 831f
Severity, in OPQRST assessment, 227t, 229
Sexual abuse
  behavioral emergency assessment,
      1056, 1056t
  described, 1046
Sexual assault, 1075–1076, 1075f
Shaken baby syndrome, 961
Sharks
  injuries caused by, 880f
  water emergencies, 930
Sharp instruments, 82, 82f
*Shigella* sp., 73
Shivering, 815–816
Shock
  abdominal and pelvic trauma, 795,
      803, 806
  anatomy and physiology
    cardiovascular system, 331–334, 331f,
      333–334f, 333f
    physiologic compensation and stages of
      shock, 335–336, 336f
  burned patients, 593
  case
    disposition, 349

  presentation, 330
  update, 344
  chapter objectives, 329
  chapter overview, 329–331, 330f
  chapter review, 352–354
  chest trauma, 786
  cycle of, 336f
  defined, 329–330
  Explore myNSPkit, 354
  factors affecting, 344–345
  head-downhill position, 149
  historical timeline, 329
  key terms, 329
  patient assessment, 345–346, 345f,
      346f, 347f
  patient management
    overview of, 347–348, 348f
    skill for, 350
    skill guide for, 351, 1173
  pediatric emergencies, 945, 961–962,
      962f, 977
  physiologic compensation, 335–336, 336f
  pregnancy, during, 1072, 1089
  signs and symptoms, 345–346, 346f, 347f
  soft-tissue injuries, 552
  stop, think, understand, 334, 343–344,
      348–349
  suggested reading, 354
  types of
    cardiogenic, 337f, 339, 339f, 468,
      474–475
    distributive (See distributive shock)
    hypovolemic, 336–339, 337f, 338f,
      338t, 339f
    obstructive, 337f, 342, 343f
    psychogenic, 342
  various conditions, associated with,
      330–331, 330f
"Short haul" technique for rescues, 157
Short spine boards, 131, 134–135, 135f
Shoulder drag, 137, 137f
Shoulder girdle, assessment of, 623–625,
      623f, 624f
Shoulder pads, removing, 725, 725f
"Shoulder separation," 624–625, 624f
Shoulders
  blanket roll splint application, skill guide
      for, 687, 1173
  dislocation, 624–625
  dislocation, management of, 653
  injury assessment, 623–625, 623f, 624f
  injury management, 650–653, 651f
Shriver, Eunice Kennedy, 1019
"SIC" (Size, Insert, Check) for
      oropharyngeal airways, 302–303
Side position for patient transport, 150
SIDS. *See* sudden infant death syndrome
      (SIDS)
Sign, defined, 227, 227t
Sildenafil citrate, 486
Sinus squeeze, 928
Sit-board, defined, 1023
Sit-ski, for adaptive athletes, 1023–1024,
      1023f, 1024f

Sitting lifting devices, 131, 135, 135f
SKED device, 151, 151f
Skeletal muscle, 199, 201f, 608, 609, 609f
Skeletal system. *See also* musculoskeletal
      injuries
  anatomy of
    joints and ligaments, 197, 197f
    lower extremities, 196f, 198
    pelvis, 196f, 198, 199f
    skull, 196f, 197–198, 198f
    spinal column, 196f, 198, 198f
    thorax, 196f, 198, 198f
    upper extremities, 196f, 198
  children, 945, 945f
  defined, 195
  functions of, 195, 196f
  healing process, 610, 610f
  physiology of, 199, 199f
Skeleton
  axial and appendicular, 604, 604f
  bones, parts of, 604, 605f
  bones, types of, 604, 604f, 605f
  major bones of, 603, 603f
Ski bra, 1024
Ski (chair) lifts
  adaptive athletes, 1023–1024, 1024f
  adaptive skiers, 1025, 1025f
  evacuation considerations, 1033
*Ski Patrol Magazine*, 813
*Ski Patroller's Manual* (NSP), 56, 264
"Ski Safety and First Aid" (Thompson), 6
Skier's thumb, 628, 628f
Skill Guides
  auto-injector, assisting with
      administration of, 453, 1173
  blanket roll splint for shoulder, 687, 1173
  bleeding, controlling, 574, 1173
  blood pressure, obtaining by auscultation,
      256, 1173
  boot removal, 691, 1174
  bridge/Bean lift, 162, 1173
  cervical collar, sizing and applying,
      733, 1174
  childbirth, assisting with, 1094–1095, 1174
  contaminated gloves, removing, 93, 1173
  figure eight application, 685, 1174
  helmet removal, 736, 1174
  impaled object, stabilizing, 575, 1173
  impaled objects in the eye, stabilization
      of, 766, 1174
  lower extremity injury, splinting, 689, 1174
  lungs, auscultation of (breath sounds),
      428, 1173
  manual spine stabilization, 732, 1174
  medical patient assessment, 255–256, 1173
  metered-dose inhalers, assisting with,
      429, 1173
  multiple person direct ground lift,
      163, 1173
  nasopharyngeal airway, inserting,
      323, 1173
  nerve agent antidote administration,
      1131, 1174
  open chest wound, managing, 788, 1174

oropharyngeal airway, inserting, 324, 1173
oxygen cylinder, preparing for use, and break down, 325, 1173
patient assessment, 252–253, 1173
patient restraint, 1063, 1174
pelvic stabilization, 809, 1174
posterior S/C dislocation reduction, 688, 1174
pulse, assessing, 257, 1173
pupils, assessing, 258, 1173
respiration rate, assessing, 259, 1173
shock management, 351, 1173
short board immobilization, 735, 1174
standing patient, immobilizing, 737, 1174
student inventory, 1173–1174
suctioning a patient's airway, 322, 1173
supine patient, log rolling onto a long spine board, 734, 1174
traction splinting, 690, 1173
trauma patient assessment, 253–254, 1173
upper extremity injury, splinting, 686, 1174
Skills
    AED use, 490
    airplane splint, applying, 682
    amputated part, emergency care for, 569
    auto-injector: EpiPen™, administration with, 450
    auto-injector: Twinject™, administration with, 451
    auto-injector: Twinject™ additional dose, administration with, 452
    axial drag, 728
    blanket roll splint, applying to a shoulder, 678
    bleeding, controlling, 566
    blood pressure, obtaining by auscultation, 250
    boot, removing, 684
    bridge/Bean lift, 161
    burns, caring for, 597
    cervical collar, sizing and applying, 727
    childbirth, assisting with, 1092–1093
    closed soft-tissue injuries, treating, 568
    contaminated gloves, removing, 91–93
    figure eight splint, creating and applying, 677
    finger, bandaging, 573
    forearm fracture, splinting, 680
    hand immobilization, splinting for, 680
    helmet removal, 731
    humerus fracture, splinting with a rigid splint, 679
    impaled object, stabilizing, 570
    impaled object in the eye, treatment of, 765
    injured elbow, rigid splint fixation of, 679
    IV therapy set-up, preparing, 1167
    lung sounds, auscultation of, 426
    manual spine stabilization, 727
    medical patient assessment, 251
    metered-dose inhalers, assisting with, 427
    multiple person direct ground lift, 160–161
    nasopharyngeal airway, inserting, 318
    occlusive dressing, using, 571

oropharyngeal airway, inserting, 319
oxygen tank set-up and breakdown, 320–321
patient assessment, 250–251
pelvic stabilization, 808
physical/mechanical restraint of a patient, 1062
posterior sternoclavicular injury, reducing, 678
pulse, assessing, 249
pupils, assessing, 248
Quick Splint, applying, 682
Quick Splint, replacing with a cardboard splint, 683
respiration rate, assessing, 249
seated patient, immobilizing, 729–730
securing the patient onto a long spine board, 729
self-adhering roller bandage, using, 571
shock management, 350
sling and swathe, applying, 676
standing patient, immobilizing, 730
suctioning a patient's airway, 317
supine patient, log rolling onto a long spine board, 728
tib-fib fracture, immobilizing with two rigid splints, 683
tourniquet, applying, 567
traction splint application, 681
trauma patient assessment, 252
triangular bandage bandana wrap, using, 572
Skin. *See also* integumentary system
    anatomy, 539–540, 539*f*
    anatomy and physiology, 194*f*, 195, 195*f*
    burns, 580–581, 581*f*
    color, and respiratory emergencies, 420
    color and temperature, and assessment of circulation, 221–222, 221*f*, 222*f*
    functions of, 538, 540, 580–581
    outdoor work, protection for, 69
    plant and animal emergencies, 862, 862*f*
    plants toxic to, 863–864, 863*f*, 864*f*
Skin tests
    allergies, 442, 442*f*
    tuberculosis, 76
Skull
    anatomy of, 196*f*, 197–198, 198*f*
    axial skeleton, 699, 699*f*
    fractures, 704–705, 705*f*
Skunks
    injuries caused by, 883
    rabies, 890
Sledge (sled) hockey, 1025, 1025*f*
Sleds
    CPR on, 158
    ground transport of patients, 147–148
    patient transport, 151
Sleep
    altitude for, 903, 910
    outdoor work, preparing for, 64
Sleeping altitude
    altitude illness prevention, 910
    defined, 903

"SLIC" (Size, Lubricate, Insert, Check) for NPA, 301–302
Sliding board, defined, 1022, 1022*f*
Slightly movable joints, 606*f*, 607
Sling, application of, 650–652, 651*f*
Sling and swathe
    application of, 650
    applying, skill for, 676
    described, 640, 641*f*
    sternoclavicular (S/C) dislocation, 652
SLUDGE (Salivation, Lacrimation, Urination, Defecation, GI irritation, Eye [pupillary] constriction)
    organophosphate or nerve agent exposure, 397*t*
    organophosphate poisoning, 1115, 1115*t*
Small intestines
    GI system, 187, 188*f*, 189
    hollow organ, 495, 496*f*, 794*f*
    location of, 795*f*
SMART tagging system, 119, 120*f*
"Smith's" fracture, 627
Smoking, and the healing process, 610
Smooth muscle, 199, 201*f*, 608, 609, 609*f*
Snake bites
    patient assessment, 887
    patient management, 889, 889*f*
Snow, 394. *See also* cocaine
"Snow blindness"
    eye injuries, 751, 906–907, 906*f*
    eye protection, 69, 69*f*, 906*f*, 907
Snow sports equipment for adaptive athletes, 1022–1025, 1022*f*, 1023*f*, 1024*f*, 1025*f*
Snow-bikes for adaptive athletes, 1025
Snowblower injuries, 628
Snowboarders
    NSP, joining, 985
    talus fracture, 636
Snow-sliders for adaptive athletes, 1025
"Snuff box" area for wrist injuries, 627
SOAP (subjective, Objective, Assessment, Plan) charting, 277, 1139
Soft-tissue injuries
    anatomy and physiology
        physiology of bleeding and clotting, 540, 542
        skin anatomy, 539–540, 539*f*
        soft tissues, anatomy of, 538*f*
    case
        disposition, 565
        presentation, 539
        update, 550
    chapter objectives, 537
    chapter overview, 537–538, 538*f*
    chapter review, 576–577
    dressing and bandaging
        bandaging principles, 560, 560*f*
        dressings, types of, 558–559, 559*f*
        hemostatic dressings, 561–562
        occlusive dressings, 561
        pressure dressings, 561, 561*f*
        problem areas, 562–563, 562*f*, 563*f*, 564*f*
        stabilizing dressings, 561, 561*f*, 562*f*

Soft-tissue injuries, (cont.)
  Explore myNSPkit, 578
  historical timeline, 537
  key terms, 537–538
  neck and back, 711
  patient assessment, 551–552, 551f
  patient management
    amputations, 556, 558
    avulsions, 556
    contusions, 555
    direct pressure, 553, 553f
    dressings, 553
    impaled objects, 558, 558f
    open injuries, 555–556, 556f
    overview of, 552
    tourniquet, 553–555, 554f, 555f
  Skill Guides
    bleeding, controlling, 574, 1173
    impaled object, stabilizing, 575, 1173
  Skills
    amputated part, emergency care
      for, 569
    bleeding, controlling, 566
    closed soft-tissue injuries, treating, 568
    finger, bandaging, 573
    impaled object, stabilizing, 570
    occlusive dressing, using, 571
    self-adhering roller bandage,
      using, 571
    tourniquet, applying, 567
    triangular bandage bandana wrap,
      using, 572
  stop, think, understand, 541, 544,
    549–550, 552, 557, 564–565
  suggested reading, 578
  types of
    burns, 549
    closed injuries, 542–543, 543f, 545
    open injuries, 545–549, 545f, 546f,
      547f, 548f, 549f
Solar keratitis ("snow blindness"), 69, 69f,
  751, 906–907, 906f
Solid organs
  abdominal and pelvic, 496, 496f, 794f
  kinetic energy, absorption of,
    519–520, 520f
Soman poisoning, 392
Span of control, of the NIMS, 100
Spastic cerebral palsy (CP), 1016, 1017
Speaking ability
  breathing, assessing, 220
  choking, determining, 424, 424f
  stroke, 375, 375f
Special insertion and extraction (SPIE) lines
  for rescues, 157
Special Olympics, founding of, 1019
Special operations, defined, 1101
Special operations and ambulance
  operations
  ambulance operations
    ambulance designs, 1101–1102, 1102f
    arriving at the scene, 1103–1105, 1104f
    call, preparing for, 1102, 1103f
    call, responding to, 1103, 1103f

extrication of patient from a vehicle,
    1105–1107, 1106f, 1107f, 1107t
  OEC Technicians interacting with
    ambulance crews, 1101, 1101f
  transferring patients, 1105, 1105f
  case
    disposition, 1130
    presentation, 1102
    update, 1108
  chapter objectives, 1100–1101
  chapter overview, 1100–1101
  chapter review, 1132–1135
  disaster response
    community emergency response
      teams, 1111
    human-caused disasters, 1109, 1109f
    Medical Reserve Corps, 1111
    National Disaster Medical System,
      1110–1111, 1110f, 1111f
    National Response Framework,
      1109–1110
    natural disasters, 1108, 1109f
  Explore myNSPkit, 1135
  fire ground operations, 1128–1130, 1129f
  hazardous materials response
    hazardous materials, types of,
      1111–1112, 1112f
    HazMat entry teams, 1112, 1112f
    HazMat incident management,
      1114–1115, 1114f, 1115f, 1115t
    nerve agent medications, dosing
      schedules for, 1116
    nerve agents, mechanism of action
      of, 1116
    NFPA safety diamond, 1112,
      1112f, 1113t
  historical timeline, 1100
  key terms, 1101
  nerve agent administration, skill guide
    for, 1131
  search and rescue
    avalanche rescue, 1120–1123, 1120f,
      1121f, 1122f, 1123f
    basic tasks of, 1119, 1119f
    confined space rescue, 1125–1127,
      1125f, 1126f, 1127f
    low-angle rescue, 1123–1125, 1124f
    OEC Technician participation,
      1119–1120, 1120f
    overview of, 1118, 1118f, 1119f
    water rescue, 1128
  stop, think, understand, 1108, 1117, 1128
  suggested reading, 1135
Speech. See speaking ability
Speed, 394. See also methamphetamine
Sphenoid bone, 198f
Spider bites
  adverse effects from, 871–873, 872f, 873f
  patient assessment, 886, 886f
  patient management, 888
SPIE (special insertion and extraction) lines
  for rescues, 157
Spills, contaminated, dealing with, 81–82, 81f
Spina bifida (SB), 1017

Spinal cavity, defined, 171, 172f
Spinal cord
  anatomy of, 183, 184f, 185–186
  divisions of, 700, 700f
Spinal cord injury (SCI)
  adaptive athletes, 1016
  incidence, causes, and costs of, 699
Spinal injuries. See also head and spinal
    injuries
  neurogenic shock, 712
  shock management, 347–348, 348f
  soft-tissue injuries, 711
  vertebral fractures, 711–712, 711f
Spinal protection
  altered mental status, 377
  electrical burn management, 595
  geriatric emergency management,
    1003, 1003f
  head and spinal injuries, 719, 719f
  head and spinal injury assessment,
    714–715
  initial care of patients and removal from a
    vehicle, 1107, 1107f
  lightning strike management, 855
  manual, skill for, 727
  manual, skill guide for, 732, 1174
  pediatric emergency management,
    975–976, 976f
  taking, importance of, 712
  thoracic trauma management, 784, 785
  trauma patient assessment, 530, 530f
  trauma patient management, 532
  water emergencies, 934, 935f
  water emergency assessment, 933
Spine
  alignment, during urgent moves, 136
  anatomy of, 196f, 198, 198f
  assessment of, in pediatric emergencies,
    973, 973f
  bones of, 197, 699, 699f
  lifting, 128–129, 128f
Spiny aquatic animal injuries, 881, 881f
Spiral fractures
  described, 614f, 615t
  tibia and fibula, 635
Spleen
  abdominal injuries, 798, 798f
  location of, 795f
  lymphatic system, 206, 207f
  solid organ, 496, 496f, 794f
Splints
  commercial, types of, 640, 641f
  defined, 602
  improvised splints, 645–646, 646f
  rigid or semi-rigid
    airplane splint, 643, 644f
    cardboard, wood, or metal splints,
      642–643, 643f
    malleable metal splints, 643–644, 644f
    Quick Splint, 643, 645
  soft splints
    air splints, 640–641, 641f
    blanket roll/pillow splints, 641, 642f
    pelvic binders, 642, 642f

sling and swathe splints, 640, 641f
vacuum splints, 641, 642f
splinting, principles of, 646–648, 647f
splinting, reasons for, 640
traction splints, 644–645, 645f, 646f
Sports
equipment removal, 724–725, 724f, 725f, 731, 736, 1174
head injuries, 698
snow sports equipment for adaptive athletes, 1022–1025, 1022f, 1023f, 1024f, 1025f
warm weather sports equipment for adaptive athletes, 1025–1026, 1026f
Sprains
defined, 602
described, 612, 613
signs and symptoms, 620–621
Square knot
bandaging, 560
tying, instructions for, 650, 651f
Squeeze, defined, 928
Squirrel injuries, 884
Stabilization of vehicles for extrication of patients, 1106, 1106f
Stabilized extrication and transfer
musculoskeletal injuries, 673–674, 673–674f
stabilized extrication, defined, 674
Stabilizing impaled objects. See also impaled objects
Stable angina, 467t
Stafford Act, 109
Stair chair, 152–153, 153f
Standard of care
defined, 21
versus standard of training, 20–21
Standard of training
defined, 21
versus standard of care, 20–21
Standard Precautions
burned patients, 588
contaminated objects, procedures for dealing with, 81
defined, 76
disease transmission prevention, 76–77, 77f
face, eye, and neck injuries, management of, 756
musculoskeletal injuries, 639
plant and animal emergencies, 887
trauma patient assessment, 530
Standing patients
immobilizing, skill for, 730
immobilizing, skill guide for, 737, 1174
LSBs, placing on, 723–724
Staphylococcus sp., 506
START (Simple Triage and Rapid Treatment) method
factors for assessment, 120–121, 121f
SMART tagging system, 119, 120f
"30-2-Can Do," 120–121
widespread use of, 119–120
Status asthmaticus, 414
Status epilepticus

children, 954
described, 365
Sternoclavicular (S/C) injuries. See posterior sternoclavicular (S/C) dislocation
Sternocleidomastoid muscles, 747
Sternum
anatomy of, 196f, 198
fracture of, 775–776
thoracic trauma A & P, 772, 772f
Stifneck cervical collars, 720f
Stimulants
overuse and poisoning, 392
toxicity, signs and symptoms of, 397t
Stinging nettle, 864, 864f
Stingray injuries, 880, 880f
Stoma
athletes with, assessing, 1031
ostomy bag, 1016
Stomach
GI system, 187, 188f, 189
hollow organ, 495, 496f, 794f
location of, 795f
"Stop, Drop, and Roll," 593
Stopping distance, 519, 520f
Straddle injuries, 798, 801
Strains
defined, 602
described, 612–613
signs and symptoms, 621
Stress
body's reactions to, 61–62, 61t, 62f
dealing with, 89–90, 89f, 90f
defined, 1041, 1041f
physical and mental, for OEC Technicians, 12–13, 13f
warning signs of, 89–90, 89f
Stretchers
operation of, 1165
wheeled ambulance stretchers, 151–152, 152f
Strike team, defined, 105
Stroke
altered mental status, 361t, 362, 363, 380–381
defined, 370
geriatric emergencies, 992
hemorrhagic, 370f, 371
ischemic, 370, 370f
signs and symptoms, 370f, 371f, 375–377, 375f, 376f
transient ischemic attack, 371
Stroke volume, defined, 332
Stylets for endotracheal tubes, 1144, 1145f
Subcutaneous emphysema
causes of, 421
neck injuries, assessment of, 756
tension pneumothorax, 778
Subcutaneous tissue
anatomy, 539f, 540
defined, 538
integumentary system, 195, 195f
plant and animal emergencies, 862

Subdural hematoma
described, 709f, 710
mortality rate, 710t
Subluxation, defined, 616
Submersion injuries
drowning, 925–926, 925f
near-drowning/secondary drowning, 926–927, 926f
overview of, 924–925
Substance abuse. See also drugs, illicit
common NOI, 85
defined, 390
outdoor work, preparing for, 65
Substance abuse and poisoning
accidental or intentional, determining, 386–387, 387f
anatomy and physiology
body systems affected, 389–390
physiologic actions, 387–389, 388f, 389f
case
disposition, 402
presentation, 388
update, 396
chapter objectives, 386
chapter overview, 386–387, 387f
chapter review, 402–404
commonly abused substances and poison-related emergencies, 390–394, 391f, 394f
Explore myNSPkit, 405
historical timeline, 386
key terms, 387
patient assessment, 396–397, 396t, 397t
patient management
ABCDs and primary assessment, 398
absorption, reducing, 399, 400f, 400t
further exposure, reducing, 398, 399f
help, calling for, 401
personal safety, 398, 398f
specific interventions, 400–401, 400f
stop, think, understand, 390, 395, 401
substance abuse, defined, 390
suggested reading, 405
Subungual hematoma
defined, 543
treating, 545
Sucking chest wounds
defined, 777
management of, 785, 785f
occlusive dressings, 561
Suctioning
defined, 298
devices for, 298–299, 298f
patient's airway, skill for, 317
patient's airway, skill guide for, 322, 1173
principles of, 299–300, 299f
rigid and flexible catheters for, 299
Sudden cardiac arrest (SCA), 468
Sudden infant death syndrome (SIDS)
defined, 957, 957f
pediatric emergency management, 977
Sugar tong splints
described, 644
forearm injuries, 656

Suicide
  incidence of, 1045
  methods of, 1045–1046
Sunburn
  assessment, 852
  described, 845–846
  high altitude, 907, 907f
  management, 854
  prevention of, 846–847
  sensitivity by skin types, 846, 846t
Sunfish injuries, 881
Sunglasses
  snow blindness, 69, 69f
  wraparound, 906f, 907
Sunscreen, 846–847
Superficial body part, 170
Superficial (first-degree) burns, 585, 585f, 587t
Superficial (early) cold injury, 815f, 819, 825t. See also frostnip
Superior direction, 169, 169f
Supine hypotensive syndrome, 1079
Supine position
  defined, 170, 170f
  LSBs, placing patients on, 721–723
  packaging patients for transport, 149
  severe allergic reactions, 447, 447f
  transporting patients, 146, 147f, 149
Supracondylar fracture of the elbow, 626
Surgical masks, 78–79, 78f
Survival kits, 67–69, 67f, 68t. See also equipment
Survival psychology and priorities in, 1171–1172
Suture joints, 607, 607f
Sweat glands
  anatomy and physiology, 539f, 540
  burns, 581, 581f
Sweating, and heat-related emergencies, 839, 840f, 841
Swelling
  DCAP-BTLS assessment, 230, 230t
  knee joint trauma, 634
  musculoskeletal injuries, 619–620, 619f
Swimmer's ear, 929, 929f
Swordfish injuries, 881
Sympathetic nervous system, 187, 187f
Symphysis pubis, 801
Symptom, defined, 227, 227t
Syncope
  altered mental status, 361t, 362, 363, 381
  geriatric emergencies, 992
Synovium, defined, 606
Syringes for endotracheal tube cuffs, 1144, 1144f, 1145f
Systemic circulation, 177, 179f, 180
Systolic blood pressure, 221t

T
Tabun, 392
Tachycardia
  acute abdomen, 508t
  compensated shock, 335

Tachypnea
  compensated shock, 335
  defined, 418
Tadalafil, 486
Talus fracture, 636
Task force, defined, 105
Tavist. See clemastine
Taylor, Edward
  NSP National Director, 213
  Ski Patrol Manual, 264
TB. See tuberculosis (TB)
TBI. See traumatic brain injury (TBI)
Teamwork
  ALS personnel, working with, 1165
  OEC Technicians as part of, 13, 13f, 25
Tecnu, 888, 888f
Teeth
  avulsed, management of, 757
  injuries, 750
Teller Lift collapse, 118
Temporal bone, 198f
Tenderness
  DCAP-BTLS assessment, 230, 230t
  musculoskeletal injuries, 619, 619f
Tendons
  defined, 602
  described, 609, 609f
  healing process, 610
  ligaments, difference from, 609
  ruptured, 613, 621
Tenormin®. See atenolol
Tension
  "floating knee" injury, 668
  force for splinting, 645, 646
  splinting, principles of, 647, 647f
  tendon healing, 610
Tension pneumothorax
  advanced life support, 785
  described, 777, 778f
  hallmark signs of, 777–778
  management of, 784–785
  obstructive shock, 337f, 342, 343f
10th Mountain Division, 5, 6f, 126, 167
"Tenting up" of skin over fractured clavicle, 624, 624f
Terbutaline, 420
Terrorism, defined, 1109
Tertiary blast injury, 523, 524f
Testes
  endocrine system, 191, 193f
  male reproductive system, 203, 204f
Tetanus, 75
Tetanus, diphtheria, and pertussis vaccine (Tdap), 76t
Tetanus and diphtheria vaccine (Td), 76t
Tetanus immunization
  animal bites, 889
  burned patients, 589
Tethers for adaptive athletes, 1023, 1023f
Thermal burns
  described, 581–582, 582f
  eyes, to, 761
  management, 593, 593f
  patient assessment, 589

Thermoregulation. See also heat loss
  burns, extensive, 595
  defined, 815
  heat-related emergencies, 839, 840
  process of, 815–816
Third-degree (full-thickness) burns, 585, 585f, 586, 586f, 587t
"30-2-Can Do" rule for START triage method, 120–121
"30/30" rule for lightning strikes, 849
Thomas, Hugh Owen, 646
Thomas Splint
  described, 645, 646f
  development of, 34
  "floating knee" injury, 668
Thompson, L. M., 6
Thoracic (chest) cavity
  described, 171, 172f
  thoracic trauma A & P, 773
Thoracic spine
  axial skeleton, 699f
  described, 196f, 198, 198f
  fractures of, 712
  thoracic trauma A & P, 772
Thoracic trauma. See also chest injuries
  anatomy and physiology, 772–773, 772f
  case
    disposition, 787
    presentation, 771
    update, 782
  chapter objectives, 770
  chapter overview, 770–771
  chapter review, 789–792
  chest injuries
    aortic rupture and dissection, 779–780, 780f
    commotio cordis, 780–781
    contusions, 774, 774f
    environmental factors, 782
    flail chest, 775, 775f
    fractures and dislocations, overview of, 774–775
    hemothorax, 778, 778f
    lower rib cage injury, 777
    mechanisms of injury, 774
    pericardial tamponade, 778–779, 779f
    pneumothorax, 777–778, 778f
    rib fractures, 775
    scapula fracture, 775
    sternoclavicular injury, 776
    sternum fracture, 775–776
    traumatic asphyxia, 781, 781f
  Explore myNSPkit, 792
  historical timeline, 770
  key terms, 770
  open chest wound, skill guide for, 788, 1174
  patient assessment, 783–784, 784t
  patient management, 784–786, 785f, 786f, 786t
  stop, think, understand, 773, 776, 781–782, 787
  suggested reading, 792
Thoracolumbar junction, 712

Thorax, anatomy of, 196*f*, 198, 198*f*
Thorazine. *See* chlorpromazine
"Threatened abortion," 1078, 1078*t*
Three trackers, defined, 1024, 1024*f*
"Thresholds of injury," 520
Thromboembolism
    described, 468–469, 469*f*
    patient assessment, 476
Thrombolytic therapy, 484
Thrombus, defined, 468
"Thunderheads" (cumulonimbus clouds), 848, 848*f*
Thymus gland
    endocrine system, 193*f*
    lymphatic system, 206, 207*f*
Thyroid cartilage of the larynx, 747, 747*f*
Thyroid gland
    endocrine system, 191, 193*f*
    neck anatomy and physiology, 747, 747*f*
TIAs. *See* transient ischemic attacks (TIAs)
"Tib-fib" fractures
    described, 634–635
    rigid splint immobilization, skill for, 683
    splints for, 667–668
Tibia
    anatomy of, 196*f*, 198
    fracture and concurrent femur fracture, 668, 668*f*
    fractures, bleeding from, 615*t*
    injuries, management of, 667–668
    injury assessment, 634–635, 635*f*
    "tib-fib" fractures, 634–635, 667–668, 683
Ticks
    adverse effects from, 874–875, 874*f*, 875*f*
    bites, assessment of, 886, 886*f*
    removal of, 886, 886*f*
Tiered approach to emergency personnel deployment, 39
Time, in OPQRST assessment, 227*t*, 229
Tissues, defined, 174
Tobaggans
    ground transport of patients, 147–148, 148*f*
    handling skills for patient transport, 150–151, 150*f*
Toddlers
    age-based assessment, 974*t*
    defined, 947, 947*f*
    physical, intellectual, emotional, social, and language development, 948–949*t*
Toes
    injuries, management of, 670
    injury assessment, 636
Toes-to-head approach for physical exam, 969
Tofranil. *See* imipramine
Tongue lacerations, 757
Tonic activity, defined, 364, 365*f*
Tonicity, defined, 927
"Tonsil tip" suction catheter, 299
Tonsillitis, 950
Tonsils, 206, 207*f*

Tools for gaining access to patients, in a vehicle, 1106–1107, 1107*t*
Toprol. *See* metoprolol
Tourniquets
    applying, skill for, 567
    defined, 552
    soft-tissue injuries, 553–555, 554*f*, 555*f*
Toxicological events
    general approach to, 396, 396*t*
    Hazardous Materials (HazMat) teams, 396
Toxin
    defined, 390
    plant and animal emergencies, 862
Trachea
    anatomy of, 174, 175*f*, 176*f*
    neck anatomy and physiology, 747, 747*f*
Traction hitch, tying, 662, 662*f*
Traction splints
    defined, 644
    femoral traction splints, 644–645, 645*f*, 646*f*, 647
    femur application, skill for, 681
    femur fractures, 660–663, 660*f*, 662*f*, 663*f*
    skill guide for, 690, 1173
    splinting, principles of, 647
    tension *versus*, 646
Training of OEC Technicians, legal risks of, 24, 24*f*
Tranquilizers, 391
Transdermal route for substances
    absorption, 388, 388*f*
    further exposure, reducing, 398, 399*f*
Transfer flat (draw sheet lift), 131, 145–146, 145*f*
Transient ischemic attacks (TIAs)
    altered mental status, 371
    geriatric emergencies, 992
Transport equipment, list of, 131*t*
Transportation group, in incident command system, 112
Transporting patients. *See also* moving, lifting, and transporting patients; packaging patients for transport
    air transportation
        altitude and temperature limitations, 155
        helicopter safety, 155–157, 156*f*, 156*t*, 157*f*
        space and load, 155
        types of, 154–155, 154*f*, 155*f*
        weather limitations, 155
    burned patients, 595
    ground transport
        basket stretchers/litters, 151, 151*f*
        common methods for, 146
        evacuation (stair) chair, 152–153, 153*f*
        improvised litters, 153, 153*f*, 154*f*
        packaging a patient, 148–151, 148*f*, 149*f*, 150*f*, 151*f*
        toboggan or sled, 147–148, 148*f*
        wheeled ambulance stretcher, 151–152, 152*f*

head and spinal injuries, 719, 719*f*
motorized transport vehicles, 153, 154*f*
musculoskeletal injuries, 620
obstetric and gynecologic emergency management, 1091, 1091*f*
patient with cold-related emergencies, 832
positions for, 146, 146*f*
severe allergic reactions, 449
special transport tactics, 157
trauma patient assessment, 531–532, 531*f*
trauma patient management, 532, 532*f*
Transverse fractures, 614*f*, 615*t*
Transverse (horizontal) plane, 168*f*
Tranylcypromine, 1054*t*
Trauma
    altered mental status, 361–362, 361*t*, 362*f*, 379
    behavioral emergencies, 1043, 1043*f*
    children, 957–958, 957*f*, 958*f*, 977, 977*f*
    DCAP-BTLS assessment, 230, 230*t*
    defined, 517
    elderly patients
        cervical spine injury, 998
        falls, 996–997
        hip and pelvic fractures, 997, 997*f*
        traumatic brain injury, 997, 997*f*
    gynecologic, 1075
    medical problem with, 226
    pregnancy, during, 1088–1089, 1088*f*
    restraints on patients, 1059
    water emergencies, 924, 924*f*, 930, 930*f*
Trauma, principles of
    case
        disposition, 533
        presentation, 517
        update, 530
    chapter objectives, 516
    chapter overview, 516–517
    chapter review, 533–536
    Explore myNSPkit, 536
    historical timeline, 516
    injury, phases of, 525–526, 525*f*, 526*f*, 527*f*
    key terms, 516
    kinematics, 517–520, 517*f*, 518*f*, 519*f*, 520*f*
    pathophysiology and mechanisms of injury
        blast injury, 523–524, 524*f*
        blunt injury, 522, 522*f*
        crush injury, 523, 523*f*
        force producing the injury, 521, 521*f*
        penetrating injury, 522, 522*f*
        rotational injury, 522–523, 523*f*
    patient assessment, 530–532, 530*f*, 531*f*
    patient management, 532, 532*f*
    stop, think, understand, 529
    suggested reading, 536
    trauma systems, 526–528, 527*f*, 528*f*, 528*t*
Trauma centers
    defined, 526
    levels of, 527–528, 528*f*, 528*t*
Trauma (universal) dressing, 558, 559*f*
Trauma surgeon, defined, 527, 528*f*

Trauma systems
    evacuation of patients to trauma centers, 526–527, 527f
    pediatric trauma, 528
    trauma centers, levels of, 527–528, 528f, 528t
    trauma surgeons, 527, 528f
Traumatic asphyxia
    described, 781, 781f
    management of, 784–785
Traumatic brain injury (TBI)
    children, 944
    cognitive disability, 1013
    costs of, 699
    defined, 698
    demographics of, 705, 706t
    described, 705, 706f
    elderly patients, 997, 997f
    long-term or lifelong deficits from, 699
    mechanisms of action, 705, 707f
    recurrent, 708
    signs and symptoms, 707t
"Traveler's diarrhea," 506
Treatment
    medical communications, in, 282t, 283
    rendered previously, in trauma patient assessment, 531
Treatment group for incident command system, 112
Trendelenburg position
    defined, 171, 171f
    transporting patients, 146, 147f
Triage
    defined, 114
    ID-ME categorization
        delayed category, 115t, 116, 116f
        expectant category, 115t, 117–118, 118f
        immediate category, 115–116, 115f, 115t
        minimal category, 115t, 117, 117f
    ongoing process, as, 121–122, 121f
    triage methods, 119–122, 120f, 121f
    triage tags, 118, 119f
Triage group in incident command system, 111–112, 111f
Triamterene, 994
Triangular bandages, 572
"Triple A" (Awareness, Avoidance, Action) approach to preventing allergic reactions, 441
"Tripod" position
    breathing, assessing, 220, 220f
    children assuming, 964–965
    respiratory emergencies, 418, 419f, 424
Trust, importance of, with children, 968, 968f
"Try before you pry" rule for extrication, 1106
Tuberculosis (TB)
    airborne transmission of disease, 72
    common infectious disease, 75
    NIOSH-approved N95 masks, 79
    test for, recommendations for, 76
Tularemia, 884

Tumors, and altered mental status, 361t, 362, 379
Twinject™
    additional dose administration, skill for, 452
    administration, skill for, 451
    severe allergic reactions, for, 447, 448, 448f, 449
Twisting force as MOI, 85
2-PAM-Cl. See pralidoxime chloride (2-PAM-Cl)
Two-person assist, 138–139, 139f
Two-track skiing, 1024
Tylenol. See acetaminophen
Tylenol No. 3. See acetaminophen and codeine
Tympanic membrane, rupture of, 750, 759

## U

Ulna
    anatomy of, 196f, 198
    fractures, 626–627, 627f
Ulnar nerve, 628, 628f
Ultraviolet keratitis, 69
Ultraviolet radiation, and eye protection, 69, 69f
Umbilical cord
    cutting, 1082, 1082f
    prolapse, 1080, 1080f
Underarm-wrist drag, 137, 137f
United Ski Association, 4
Universal dressing, defined, 558, 559f
Universal survival kit (emergency care equipment), 1176
"Universal" time, 48–49, 49t
Unresponsive patients
    airway occlusion, 295, 295f
    assessment of, 244–245
    finger sweep of mouth, 297–298, 297f
    primary assessment, 217–218
Unstable angina, 467t
Upper airway
    airway management, 292–293, 293f
    anatomy of, 174, 175f, 176f
Upper extremities
    anatomy of, 196f, 198
    musculoskeletal injury assessment
        clavicle and shoulder injuries, 623–625, 623f, 624f
        elbow injuries, 626, 626f
        forearm injuries, 626–627, 627f
        hand and finger injuries, 628, 628f, 628t
        humerus fractures, 625–626
        overview of, 622–623, 623f
        wrist injuries, 627
    musculoskeletal injury management
        elbow injuries, 654–656, 654f, 655f
        forearm injuries, 656
        hand and finger injuries, 657–658, 657f
        humerus fractures, 653–654, 653f
        shoulder, clavicle, and scapula injuries, 650–653, 651f

        wrist injuries, 656–657, 657f
    musculoskeletal injury management, skill guide for, 686, 1174
Upper respiratory infections, 74
Uremia, 361, 361t, 379
Ureters
    anatomy and physiology, 191, 192f
    hollow organ, 495, 496f
    location of, 795f
    retroperitoneal location, 496, 496f
Urethra
    female, 191, 192f
    male, 191, 192f
Urgent evacuation and transport
    indications for, 136
    long-axis drags, types of, 136–138, 137f
    plant and animal emergencies, 887
    principles for, 136
Urinary bladder, 191, 192f, 495, 496f
Urinary system. See also gastrointestinal and genitourinary emergencies
    anatomy of, 191, 192f, 495, 496f
    cystitis, 1074
    defined, 191
    lower urinary tract, injuries of, 801
    physiology of, 191
Urticaria, 439
Urushiol oil, 864
U.S. Congress, and NSP federal charter, 4, 5f
U.S. Department of Transportation Emergency Medical Technician (EMT) National Standard Curriculum, 7
U.S. Federal Aviation Administration (FAA), 155
Uterine atony, 1078t
Uterus
    female reproductive system, 203, 205f
    obstetric and gynecologic emergencies, 1070f, 1071, 1072f
    uterine rupture
        trauma during pregnancy, 1088–1089
        vaginal bleeding, 1078t

## V

Vaccinations, recommendations for, 76, 76t
Vacuum splints
    described, 641, 642f
    tib-fib fracture, 667–668
Vagina
    female reproductive system, 203, 205f
    obstetric and gynecologic emergencies, 1070f, 1071, 1072f
    vaginal bleeding, 1075
Valgus position, defined, 632
Valium®. See diazepam
Vaponephrine®. See racemic epinephrine
Vardenafil HCl, 486
Varicella zoster vaccine, 76t
Varicella zoster virus, 74
Varus position, 632

Vas deferens, 204f
Vaseline® gauze, 561, 785
Vector-borne transmission of disease, 73
Veins
    anatomy of, 178f, 179f, 180, 181f
    bleeding from, 540, 542f
    cardiovascular emergencies, 462, 463f
    major, of the body, 498f
    shock, 332, 333f
Venom, defined, 862
Ventilation. See also mechanical ventilators
    avalanche victims, 831
    defined, 407
    overview of, 921, 921f
Ventolin®. See albuterol
Ventral (anterior) direction, 169, 169f
Ventricles of the heart, 177, 179f
Ventricular fibrillation (VF)
    defibrillation, early, 481
    defined, 468
Ventricular tachycardia (VT)
    defibrillation, early, 481
    defined, 468
Venules, 179f, 180
Verapamil, 994
Verbal abuse, 1046, 1046f
Verbal communication, 267, 267f. See also
    oral medical communication
Versed®. See midazolam
Very high altitude, described, 900, 901f
Vestibular system, 744, 745f
Vest-style immobilization devices
    lifting, for, 131, 134–135, 135f
    pediatric emergency management,
        976, 976f
VF. See ventricular fibrillation (VF)
VFR (visual flight rules), 155
Viagra®. See sildenafil citrate
Vicodin™. See hydrocodone and
    acetaminophen
Violence
    altered mental status, 381
    behavioral disorder, 1046
Viral meningitis, 75
Viruses, 506
Visceral nerves, 500
Visceral pain, 500
Visceral pleura, thoracic, 772
Visual flight rules (VFR), 155
Visual impairment
    adaptive athletes, 1018
    defined, 1015, 1015f
    double vision, with blowout
        fractures, 749
    skiing, 1025, 1025f
Visual system, 744–747, 746f
Vital capacity, defined, 988
Vital signs
    "baseline vitals," 238
    cardiovascular emergencies, 472
    defined, 238
    geriatric emergencies, 1002, 1003
    GI/GU problems, 510

head and spinal injury assessment,
    717, 718
normal ranges, by age, 221t
obstetric and gynecologic emergencies,
    1089, 1089f
pediatric emergencies, 971–972, 971f,
    971t, 972f
respiratory emergencies, 421
secondary assessment
    baseline vitals, 238
    blood pressure, 239–241, 240f, 241f
    body temperature, 242, 242t
    level of responsiveness, 238
    orthostatic blood pressure test, 242,
        244, 244f
    oxygen saturation level, 242, 243f
    pulse, 238–239, 238f, 239f
    respirations, 239, 240
thoracic trauma assessment, 784
trauma patient assessment, 531, 531f
Vitreous humor, 745
Volar surface of the forearm, 656
Volt (V), defined, 583
Voluntary nervous system, 187
Vomiting
    acute abdomen, 508t
    children, 953
    gastrointestinal ailment, 505
    LSBs, patients on, 720
    pediatric emergency management, 977
    side position for transport, 150
VT. See ventricular tachycardia (VT)
Vulva
    female reproductive system, 203, 205f
    obstetric and gynecologic
        emergencies, 1071
VX (nerve agent), 392

W

Walleye injuries, 881
Warfarin
    cardiac medication, 487t
    clotting process, 542
    coup-contrecoup injury, 704
    elderly, use by, 994
    shock, 345
    wounds, 553
Warm weather sports equipment for adaptive
    athletes, 1025–1026, 1026f
Warm zones, 1114, 1114f, 1115
Warming measures
    altitude-related emergencies, 912, 912f
    hypothermia, 829–830, 829f
Warm-water submersion, 926, 927
Wasps, adverse effects from, 875–876, 875f
Water
    hydration needs, 70
    purification methods, 70, 70f, 71t
    salinity, and near-drowning, 927
Water emergencies
    anatomy and physiology, 921–923, 921f,
        922f, 922t

case
    disposition, 937
    presentation, 920
    update, 932
chapter objectives, 919
chapter overview, 919–920, 920f
chapter review, 938–941
common emergencies
    aquatic animals, injuries by,
        930–931, 931f
    barotrauma, 927–928, 927f, 928f, 928t
    breath holding, 929, 929f
    existing conditions, aggravating, 931
    nitrogen narcosis, 929
    submersion injuries, 924–927,
        925f, 926f
    swimmer's ear, 929, 929f
    trauma, 924, 924f, 930, 930f
Explore myNSPkit, 941
historical timeline, 919
key terms, 919
patient assessment, 933–934, 933f
patient management, 934–936, 934f,
    935f, 936f
preventing, 931, 931f
specialized rescue operation, 1128
stop, think, understand, 924, 932, 937
suggested reading, 941
Water hemlock, 867
Water moccasins, 878, 878f
Weapons, and behavioral emergencies,
    1051, 1051f
Weather
    air transport, 155
    protecting patient from, during
        transport, 150
Weed, 394. See also marijuana
Wendel, Franz, 1019
Wesson, George, 126
West Nile virus
    mosquitoes, 876
    vector-borne transmission of
        disease, 73
Wet drowning, described, 922
"Wet" (hemorrhagic) stroke, 370f, 371
Wheelchairs for adaptive athletes, 1020,
    1020f, 1021–1022, 1022f
Wheezing
    allergic reactions, 440
    defined, 418
    respiratory emergencies, 422
White blood cells
    anatomy and physiology, 180, 181, 181f
    bone marrow, production in, 199
    shock, 333, 333f
White matter of the brain, 700
"White" (ischemic) stroke, 370, 370f
White water kit (emergency care
    equipment), 1176–1177,
    1176f, 1178t
White-faced hornets, 875f
Williams, Donald, 601
Wind chill, 817, 817f

Windburn
   described, 821
   management of, 832
*Winter Emergency Care* (Bowman)
   adoption by NSP, 793
   field trials, 770
   publication of, 6
*Winter First Aid Manual* (Bowman)
   instructor manual for, 861
   second edition, publication of, 579
Withdrawal, defined, 390
Wolf injuries, 882–883
Wolf spiders, 873, 873*f*
Wood splints, 643
Wood ticks, 875
World War I emergency medical services,
      34, 34*f*
World War II
   ambulance airplanes, 34
   National Ski Patrol, 4–5, 6*f*
Wound care for open injuries, 555, 556*f*

Wrist injuries, 627, 656–657, 657*f*
Written communication
   addendums, creating, 279, 281
   computer-generated forms, 279–281,
      279*f*, 280*f*
   described, 267
   errors, correcting, 279, 279*f*
   field care notes, 272, 272*f*
   good report writing, characteristics of,
      278–279
   NSAA incident report form,
      272–273, 273*f*
   patient care reports, 273–278, 274*f*, 275*f*,
      276*f*, 277*f*
   types of, 271
Written refusal of care, defined, 23

X

Xanax. *See* alprazolam
Xylocaine®. *See* lidocaine

Y

Yankauer suction catheter, 299
Yellow fever, 876
Yellow hornets, 875*f*
Yellow jackets, 875*f*
Yew, 867, 867*f*

Z

Zesteril. *See* lisinopril
Zoloft. *See* sertraline
Zone of injury, defined, 612, 612*f*
Zyrtec. *See* cetirizine